CW00551292

TEXTBOOK OF PATHOLOGY

To deeds alone hast thou a right and
never at all to its fruits;
let not the fruits of deeds be thy motive;
neither let there be in thee
any attachment to non-performance.

The Bhagvadgita (Chapter II, verse 47)

To my wife Praveen,
for her profound love and constant support;
and our daughters: Tanya and Sugandha,
for endurance during their encroached time.

TEXTBOOK OF PATHOLOGY

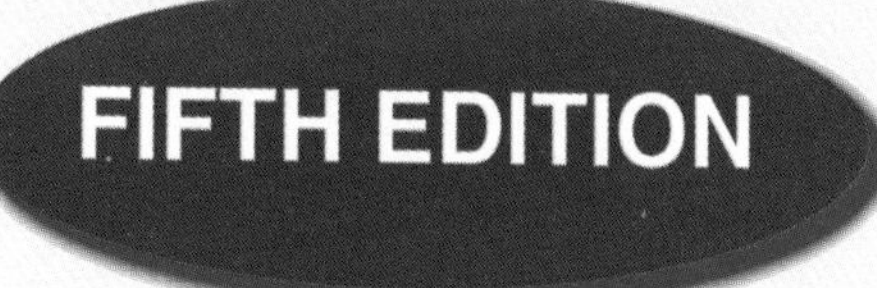

Harsh Mohan
MD, MNAMS, FICPath, FUICC
Professor & Head
Department of Pathology
Government Medical College
Sector-32 A, Chandigarh-160030
INDIA
&
Editor-in-Chief
The Indian Journal of Pathology & Microbiology
E mail: drharshmohan@yahoo.com

JAYPEE BROTHERS
MEDICAL PUBLISHERS (P) LTD
New Delhi

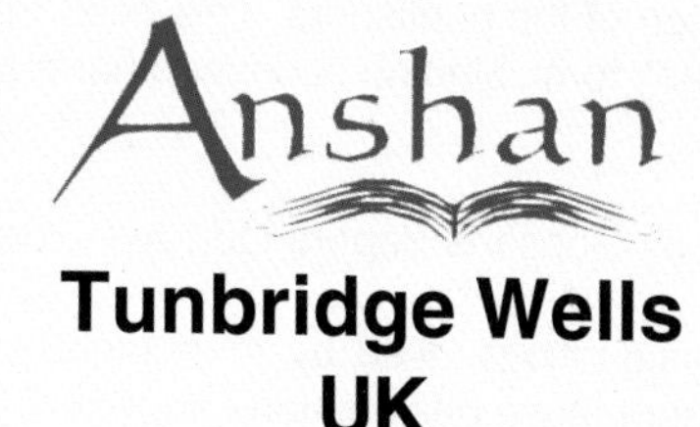

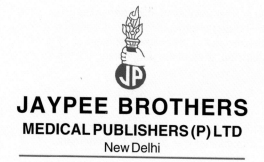

Tunbridge Wells
UK

First published in the UK by

Anshan Ltd
in 2005
6 Newlands Road
Tunbridge Wells
Kent TN4 9AT, UK

Tel/Fax: +44 (0)1892 557767
E-mail: info@anshan.co.uk
www.anshan.co.uk

Copyright © 2005 by (author)

The right of (author) to be identified as the author of this work has been asserted in accordance with the Copyright, Designs and Patents act 1988.

ISBN 1 904798 195

British Library Cataloguing in Publication Data
A catalogue record for this book is available from the British Library

All rights reserved. No part of this publication may be reproduced, stored in a retrieval system, or transmitted in any form or by any means, electronic, mechanical, photocopying, recording and/or otherwise without the prior written permission of the publishers. This book may not be lent, resold, hired out or otherwise disposed of by way of trade in any form, binding or cover other than that in which it is published, without the prior consent of the publishers.

Printed in India by Gopsons Papers Ltd., A-14, Sector 60, Noida

Many of the designations used by manufacturers and sellers to distinguish their products are claimed as trademarks. Where those designations appear in this book and where the publisher was aware of a trademark claim, the designations have been printed in initial capital letters.

Foreword

Ivan Damjanov, MD, PhD

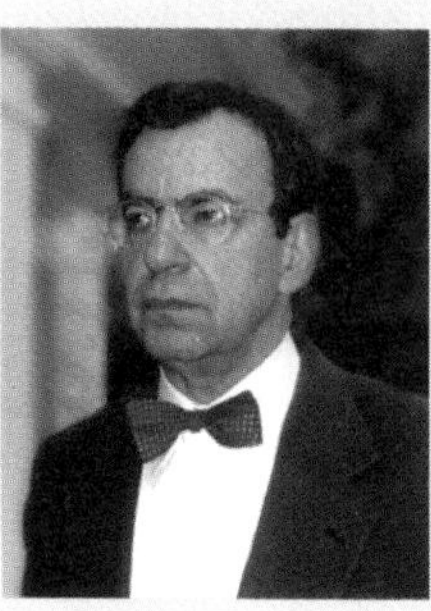

As the Book Review Editor of the journal Modern Pathology, the official journal of the United States-Canadian Academy of Pathology I am used to receiving medical books. These books are sent to my office from publishers, with a standard request for a potential review in the Journal. Nevertheless a recent package from New Delhi caught me by surprise.

As you already might have guessed, the parcel contained a copy of the 5th Edition of the *Textbook of Pathology* written by Professor Harsh Mohan, together with the Second Edition of the pocket size companion ***Pathology Quick Review and MCQs.*** Included was also a friendly letter from Mr JP Vij, the Publisher. I acknowledged the receipt of the books by email, and also congratulated the Publisher on a job well done. A brief electronic exchange between Kansas City and New Delhi ensued, whereupon Mr Vij asked me to write a foreword for the Reprint of 5th Edition of the Textbook. I accepted the invitation with pleasure.

Even though there were no specific instructions attached to the request, I assumed that I should address my notes primarily to Indian undergraduate and graduate students of Pathology. Furthermore, I decided to write the Foreword in the form of answers to the questions that I would have had if I were a medical student entering the field of Pathology. Since I do not know much about the teaching of Pathology in India, and do not personally know any Indian medical students I hope that these hypothetical questions and answers of mine will be of interest to the readers of this Textbook.

Question 1: *Is this a good book?*
Answer: Yes. This is a modern Textbook written by an expert who knows his pathology; an experienced teacher who knows what is important and what is not, and who has obviously taught pathology for many years; a well informed academician who is *au courant* with modern trends in medical education, and knows how to present pathology as a preparatory step for future clinical education of medical students.

Question 2: *How does the book compare with the leading textbooks of pathology in the USA, Great Britain and Germany?*
Answer: Very favorably. This Indian Textbook covers more or less the same topics as the equivalent Textbooks currently used in the Western Hemisphere. Like the Western textbooks it covers the traditional fields of General and Systemic Pathology: one-third of the book is devoted to General Pathology, whereas the remaining two-thirds cover Systemic Pathology.

The emphasis is on classical anatomic pathology. In that respect the Indian textbook resembles more the European than the American textbooks, which have become more clinically-oriented. In my opinion this approach gives excellent results, but only if the students have enough time to devote to Pathology. In most US medical schools this is not the case any more, and thus pathology is not taught as extensively as before. Histopathology has been deleted from most curricula, and most American medical students do not know to use efficiently the microscope, which is unfortunate. I hope that the Indian curriculum still allows students enough time for pathology, which in my opinion is the best preparation for the clinics.

Question 3: *Is the material presented in a "student-friendly" manner?*
Answer: The material is presented in a systematic manner in the best tradition of classical British textbooks, a tradition that can be traced to the classical writers of ancient Greece and Rome. This time tested teaching will be most appreciated by students who are methodical and do not take shortcuts in their effort to acquire encyclopedic knowledge of pathology. On the other hand, even if your learning method is based on "cherry-picking" i.e., you concentrate only on the most important facts in each chapter, the structure of the text will allow you to do it quite easily as well. There are no ideal books that would satisfy everybody in every respect, but there is no doubt that Professor Mohan's book is close to ideal for a classical pathology course and I predict that it will be popular with many students.

Question 4: *What are the most salient features of this textbook?*
Answer: ***Clear writing.*** As we all know clear writing reflects clear thinking, and clear thinking in my opinion, is an absolute prerequisite for good teaching. Judging from the book at hand, Professor Mohan (whom I do not know personally) is not only a clear thinker, but he must be also an exceptionally talented teacher.

Clear and visually pleasing presentation. The exposition is logical and well structured. Each chapter is subdivided into smaller entities, which are further divided into paragraphs, ideally suited for easy reading. Color coded headings and the added emphasis in form of words printed in bold or capital letters are additional attractions that facilitate learning.

Exceptionally good illustrations, flow-charts and tables. Unique to this Textbook are the numerous hand-drawn color illustrations, including many renditions of histopathologic slides. These drawings are simple, but to the point and well annotated. Students will most likely understand them much easier than the relatively impersonal original microphotographs of the same histopathologic lesions. Flow-charts are most efficiently used to explicate the pathogenesis of various lesions or the pathophysiology of disease processes. The tables are good for classifications and comparative listings of closely related diseases and their pathologic features.

***Companion pocket book* ("baby-book of pathology").** I always recommend to my students to buy a major textbook and a smaller review book containing a digest of the most important concepts; or a book of questions and answers, so that the student could test his/her knowledge of pathology and the understanding of the material in the main textbook. I was pleased to see that Professor Mohan shares my teaching philosophy and has taken upon himself to prepare for his students a shorter version of main text. This pocket book is also garnered with review questions.

The medical students are thus getting a bargain— two books for the price of one. At the same time they have a unique opportunity to see, from the example set by their teacher, on how the same material can be approached from two points of view, and presented in two formats. The old adage, that you have never learned anything unless you have seen it at least from two sides is clearly illustrated here. For the students of medicine the message is clear: if you understand the material presented in both the shorter and the longer version you can be assured that you know your Pathology inside out; and you are ready for the final examination and clinical training.

Question 5: *Do I have to know all that is in this book for my final examination?*

Answer: No!! This is the most common question my students ask me and I hope that you believe me when I say that you do not have to know it all. First of all, neither I nor Professor Mohan know it all. Second, few of us have photographic memory and infinite storage space in our brains and thus even theoretically, very few of us could learn this book by heart. I can assure you that the book was not written for those geniuses, but for the average persons like most of us. Third, your goal should not be to memorize all the facts listed in the textbook, but rather to understand the main concepts. Since the concepts cannot be fully understood or taught without specific examples, by necessity you will have to learn "some nitty-gritty details". The more details you know, the deeper your understanding of the basic concepts will be. Memorizing the details without the understanding of concepts that hold them together is not something that I would recommend. The beauty of it all is that you can decide for yourself how deep to dig in, when to stop, what to keep and memorize, and what to eliminate. And remember, deciding on what to eliminate is almost as important as choosing what to retain. As the educational gurus teach us, that is the gist of what they call active learning. And to repeat again, this Textbook is ideally suited for that approach.

At the end, let me repeat how excited I was perusing this excellent book. I hope that you will be similarly excited and I hope that it will inspire in you enthusiasm for Pathology.

Remember also the words of the great clinician William Osler, one of the founders of modern medicine in late 19th and early 20th Century, who said that our clinical practice will be only as good as our understanding of Pathology.

I hope that I have answered most of the questions that you might have had while opening this book. If you have any additional questions that I did not anticipate, please feel free to send me an email at idamjano@kumc.edu. Good luck!

Ivan Damjanov, MD, PhD
Professor of Pathology
The University of Kansas School of Medicine
Kansas City, Kansas, USA

Dr Damjanov is Professor of Pathology at the University of Kansas School of Medicine, Kansas City, Kansas, USA. He earned his Medical degree from the University of Zagreb, Croatia in 1964, and a PhD degree in Experimental Pathology from the same University in 1970. He received his Pathology training in Cleveland, New York and Philadelphia. Thereafter he served as Professor of Pathology at the University of Connecticut, Farmington, Connecticut, Hahnemann University and Thomas Jefferson University,Philadelphia, Pennsylvania. For the last ten years he has been on the Faculty of the University of Kansas School of Medicine dividing his time between teaching, practice of surgical pathology and medical publishing. He is the author of more than 300 biomedical articles, and has written or edited more than 20 medical books.

Preface

It is indeed an honour to present the fifth revised edition of *Textbook of Pathology* on successful completion of twelve years of steady progress by the textbook. The wide acceptance and popularity of previous editions of the book have encouraged us to bring about a major metamorphosis in fifth edition. In the redesigned and updated edition, the textbook has now matured into an international edition with introduction of full colour printing, which not only makes it more appealing to the eye but, more significantly, allows the user to understand and learn the illustrations, schematic representations, figures and the text clearly and more readily.

In recent times, there has been vast accumulation of knowledge on our understanding of the mechanisms of diseases, especially on genetics and molecular pathology, so much so that the word 'idiopathic' in pathogenesis of most diseases in literature is slowly disappearing. Modern-time student cannot be deprived of the fruits of these contemporary concepts on disease phenomena. However, keeping the requirement of a beginner of pathology in mind, and true to the well-accepted earlier style of the book, these aspects have been covered in the present edition by an easy-to-understand and quick recall approach.

Some of the *Key Features* of the Fifth Edition are as follows:

Updated Contents: There is emphasis on clarity and accuracy of the subject in the thoroughly revised and updated material with recent useful information inserted in different topics, including the current concepts in molecular pathology and genetics in pathogenesis of various diseases. In order to accommodate recent advances, some subjects have, in fact, been totally rewritten; e.g. Amyloidosis, Carcinogenesis, Lymphomas, Diabetes Mellitus, just to name a few.

Organisation of the Book: The book is divided into 2 sections—General Pathology (Chapter 1 to 10) and Systemic Pathology (Chapter 11 to 29), preceded by Colour Atlas (having 144 labeled photomicrographs) while at the end are appended Normal Values, References for Further Reading, and Index. Some of the chapters have been rearranged in the present edition to make the learning linked to relevant topics; e.g. chapter on Techniques in Pathology brought next to Introduction to Pathology; chapter on Diagnostic Cytopathology integrated into study of Systemic Pathology to highlight its significance, etc.

Figures, Atlas, Tables: All the illustrations in the Fifth Edition have been redrawn which are now in full colour. In doing so, weaknesses noticed in them in previous edition have been removed while their quality and clarity of features have been enhanced, making understanding clearer. This has been achieved by a meticulous blend of modern computer technology and free-hand labeled line-drawings which can be easily understood and reproduced by the beginner in pathology. Besides, there is addition of about 100 new figures (now total about 900) and 50 new tables (now total about 250) to enrich the student with a lot of material in a short space. Colour Atlas in the initial pages of the book has also undergone revision in content as well as presentation by having labeled photomicrographs.

User-friendliness: Rational use of various levels of headings, subheadings and italicized words has been done in order to help the user to undertake an in-depth study of the subject quickly with simultaneous self-assessment, and to enable the student later to revise it quickly, thus making the book truly user-friendly.

Pathology Quick Review and MCQs: With the revised edition of textbook comes its new baby-book with additional set of MCQs. This small book has been found profoundly useful by the students just before practical examination to face *viva voce* when they need to revise huge course content in a short time, or by those preparing to take postgraduate entrance examinations.

In essence, the revised edition is a comprehensive text of pathology meant primarily for students of pathology but the practicing clinicians and students of other branches of medicine, dentistry, pharmacy, alternate system of medicine, and paramedical courses would also find it useful.

ACKNOWLEDGEMENTS

The revision work was indeed a mammoth task to accomplish and would not have been possible without active cooperation from colleagues and sustained encouragement from well-wishers in general, and my departmental staff in particular. The profusely illustrated present format of the book in colour as envisioned by me has been made possible by the most valuable and selfless assistance rendered by my colleague, Dr Amanjit, MD, DNB, Senior Lecturer, Department of Pathology, who literally worked as 'artwork director' in preparing innumerable colour illustrations with Mr Satish Kaushik, BFA, Senior Artist, both of whom worked tirelessly for endless hours for months, much to the sacrifice of their personal comfort and time of their families. Dr Amanjit has also revised chapter on Diagnostic Cytopathology and has shown remarkable perseverance, immense enthusiasm and dedication in achieving perfection in the entire task and I find it hard to put my thanks in words. I also thank Dr Prashant Jain for his unfailing help in compilation of Colour Atlas. Here, I also recall and gratefully acknowledge again the help by Dr Sanjay Sangwan (now pursuing his residency in Philadelphia, US) in preparation of the original Black and White illustrations for the first edition of the textbook with me, which have now outlived their utility and hence replaced. As always, I remain indebted to those from whom I had the opportunity to learn pathology; in particular to Prof K Joshi, MD, PhD, PGIMER, Chandigarh, Prof TS Jaswal, MD, and Prof Uma Singh, MD, PGIMS, Rohtak.

During the completion of work, the Department of Medical Education and Research, Chandigarh Administration, has been extending constant strategic support and encouragement, which is gratefully acknowledged.

I must confess that I have been highly demanding on quality and accuracy from all staff members of the M/s Jaypee Brothers Medical Publishers (P) Ltd., sometimes rather impatiently, but all of them have been quite accommodating. In particular, I would like to thank profusely Mr Manoj Pahuja, Computer Art Designer, for being conscientious and patient worker, Ms Y Kapoor, Senior Desktop Operator, in acceding to all my requests for amendments smilingly and ungrudgingly till the very last minute, and Mr PS Ghuman, Senior Production Manager, for sincere efforts by him and his team in doing a thorough job in proof-reading and in styling the book. All through the project, Mr Tarun Duneja, General Manager (Publishing), M/s Jaypee Brothers Medical Publishers (P) Ltd., has been highly cooperative and is an example of a leader who leads his team from the front.

Lastly, present edition has been the brainchild of Mr JP Vij, Chairman and Managing Director of M/s Jaypee Brothers Medical Publishers (P) Ltd., and he has been highly supportive and imaginative in this project, much above the business interests. Full credit goes to Mr Nitin Goel, Gopsons, Noida, for the admirably fine quality of printing.

Finally, the users of previous editions are gratefully acknowledged for having brought this textbook at this pedestal. In the past, I have gained profitably by suggestions from colleagues and students and I urge them to continue to give their valuable suggestions and point out errors, if any, so that I may improve the future edition.

Harsh Mohan, MD, MNAMS, FICPath, FUICC
Professor & Head
Department of Pathology

Government Medical College
Sector-32 A, Chandigarh-160030
INDIA
E mail: drharshmohan@yahoo.com

ADDENDUM

I must thank profusely the early users of 5th Edition of my Textbook, who have afforded me an opportunity so soon after its initial release, to bring out the Reprint of this edition, and in the process I have been able to carry out small printing corrections. In addition, I express my hearty appreciation and gratitude to Prof. Ivan Damjanov, MD, PhD, who has been very kind to accede to our request to write its Foreword.

Contents

Index to Colour Plates

Based on

Chapter 3: Cell Injury and Cellular Adaptations

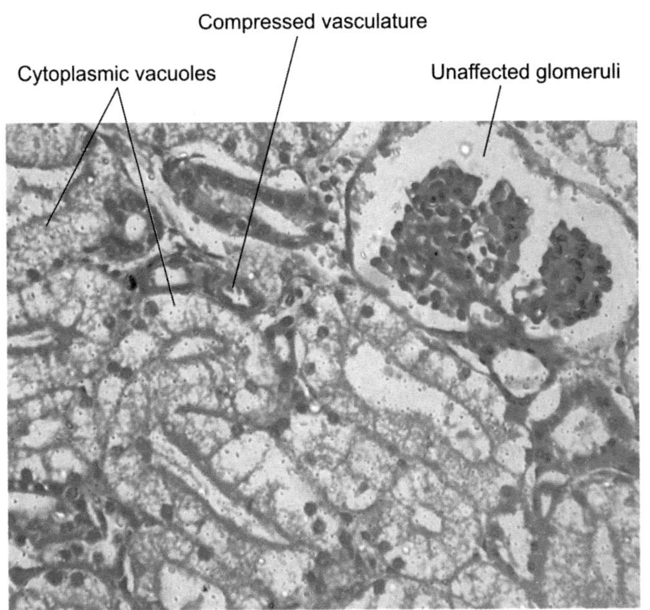

CL 1. Vacuolar nephropathy
(H & E, × 200). Details on p 41.

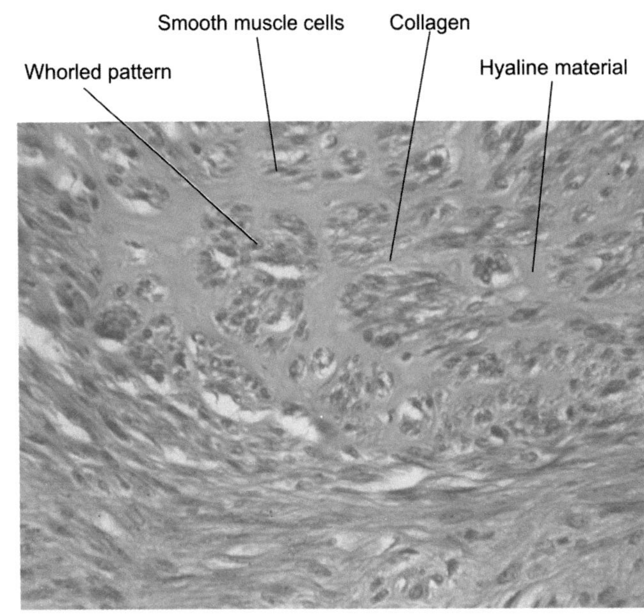

CL 2. Hyaline change in leiomyoma
(H & E, × 200). Details on p 42, 762.

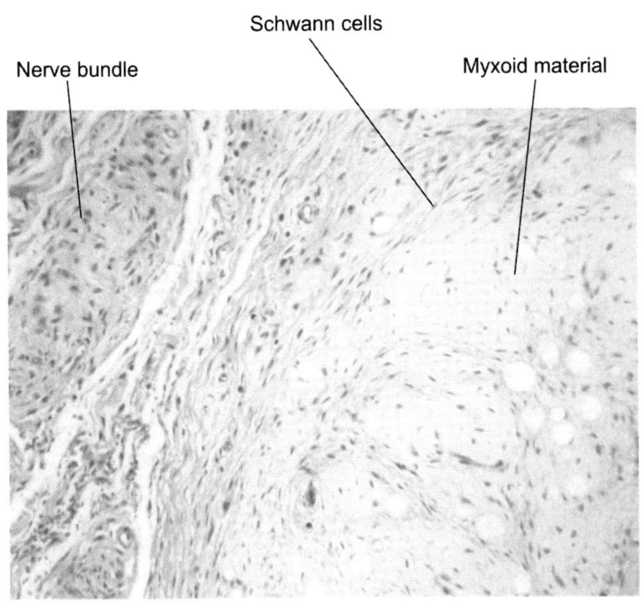

CL 3. Myxoid change in neurofibroma
(H & E, × 200). Details on p 42, 919.

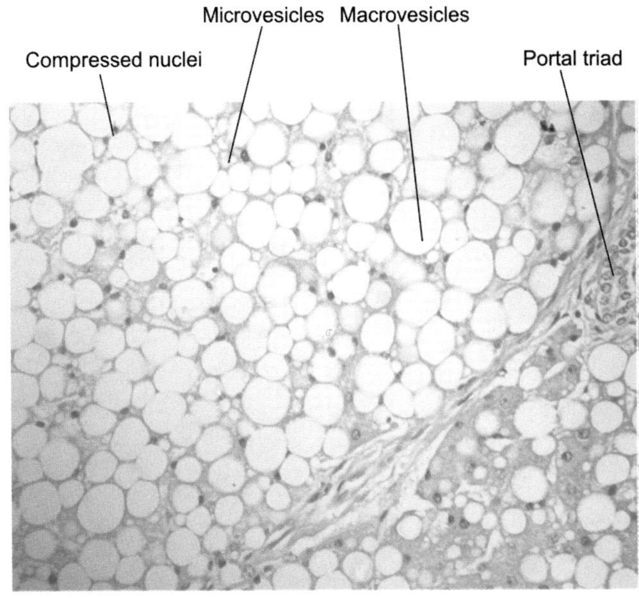

CL 4. Fatty change liver
(H & E, × 100). Details on p 44, 642.

Based on

Chapter 3: Cell Injury and Cellular Adaptations

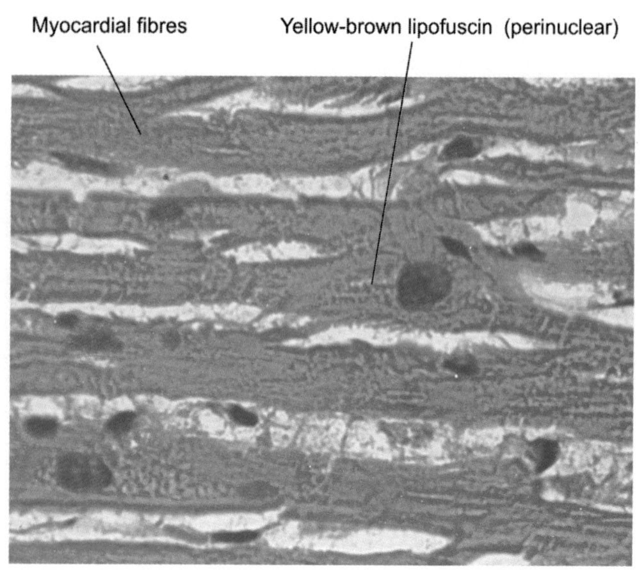

CL 5. Brown atrophy heart
(H & E, × 400). Details on p 49.

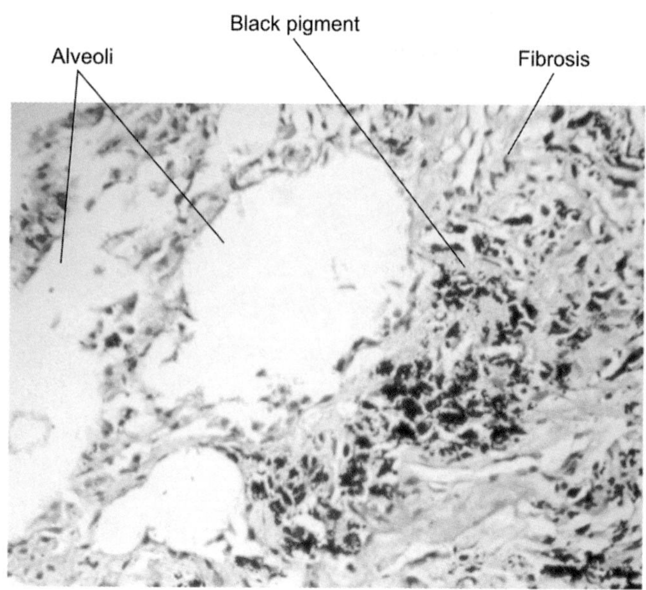

CL 6. Anthracotic pigment lung
(H & E, 100). Details on p 49, 496.

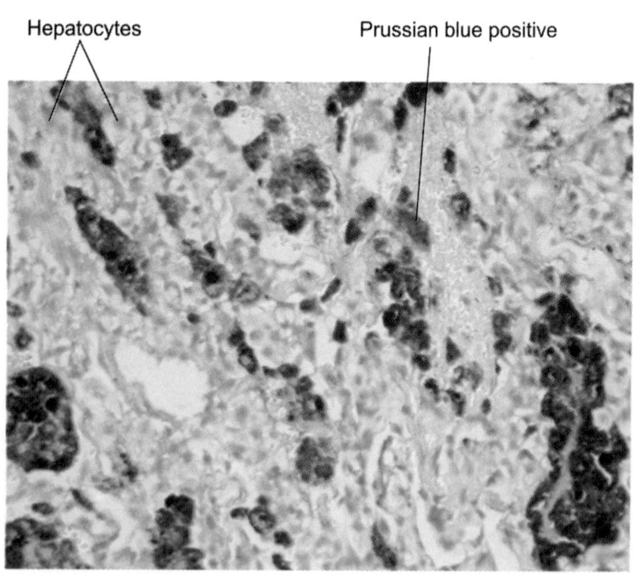

CL 7. Haemosiderin pigment in liver
(Prussian blue, × 200). Details on p 47, 647.

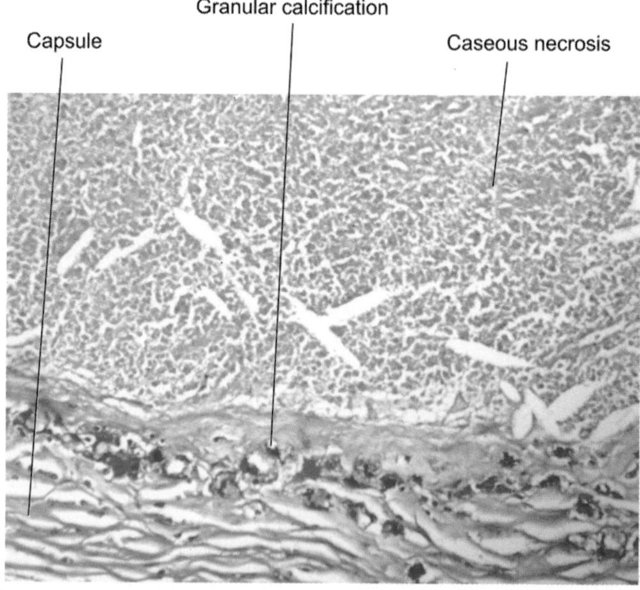

CL 8. Dystrophic calcification in tuberculous lymph node
(H & E, × 200). Details on p 56, 161.

Based on

Chapter 3: Cell Injury and Cellular Adaptations

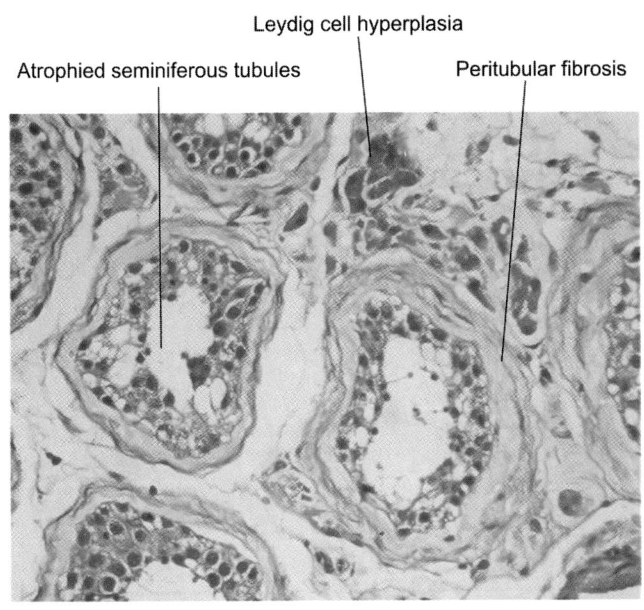

CL 9. Testicular atrophy
(H & E, × 200). Details on p 59, 728.

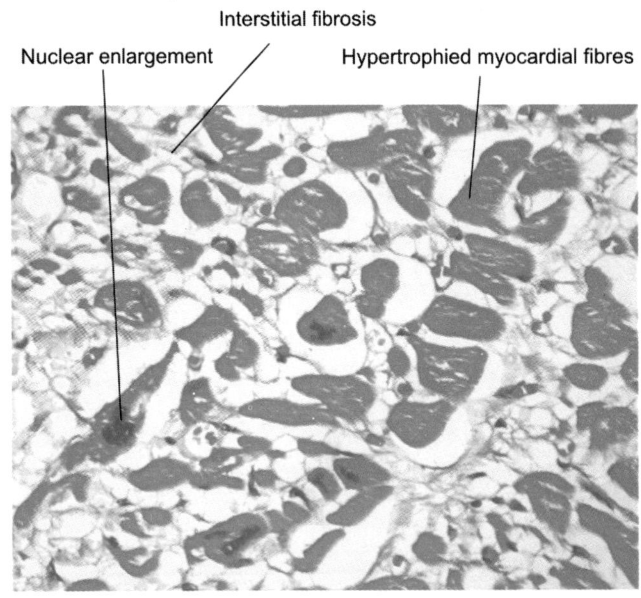

CL 10. Myocardial hypertrophy
(H & E, × 200). Details on p 60, 310.

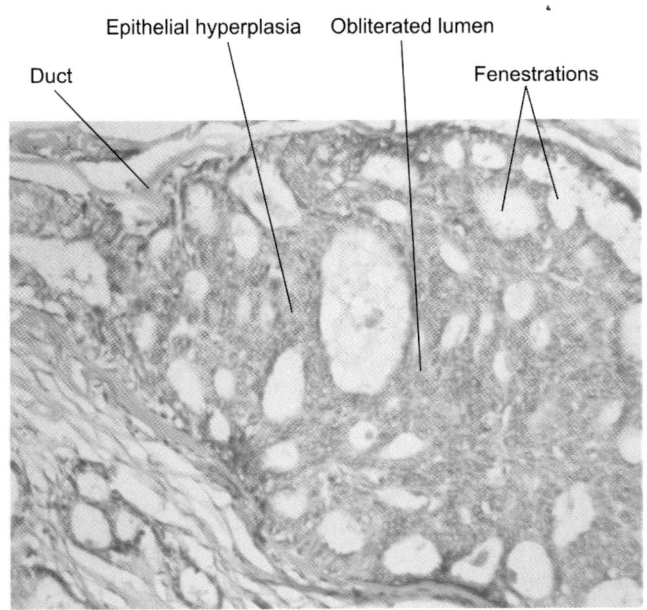

CL 11. Intraductal epithelial hyperplasia breast
(H & E, × 100). Details on p 60, 783.

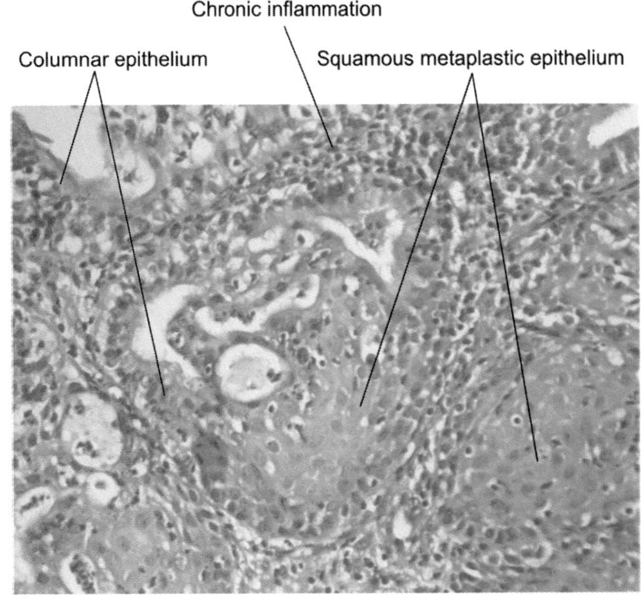

CL 12. Squamous metaplasia cervix
(H & E, × 200). Details on p 61, 752, 927.

Based on

Chapters 3, 4: Cell Injury and Cellular Adaptations; Immunopathology Including Amyloidosis

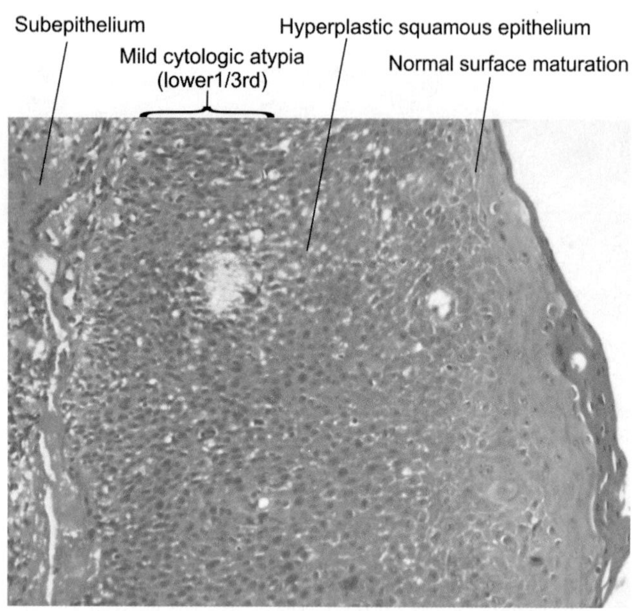

CL 13. Low-grade squamous intraepithelial lesion (L-SIL)
(H & E, × 200). Details on p 62, 754, 927.

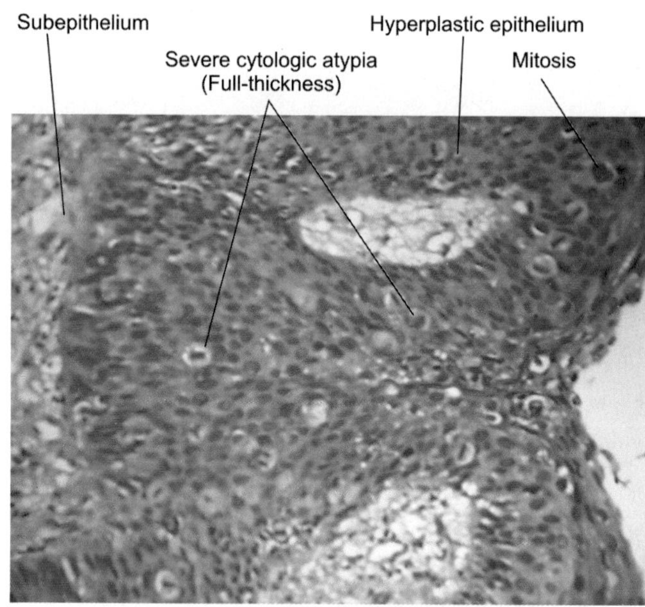

CL 14. High-grade squamous intraepithelial lesion (H-SIL)
(H & E, × 200). Details on p 62, 753, 927.

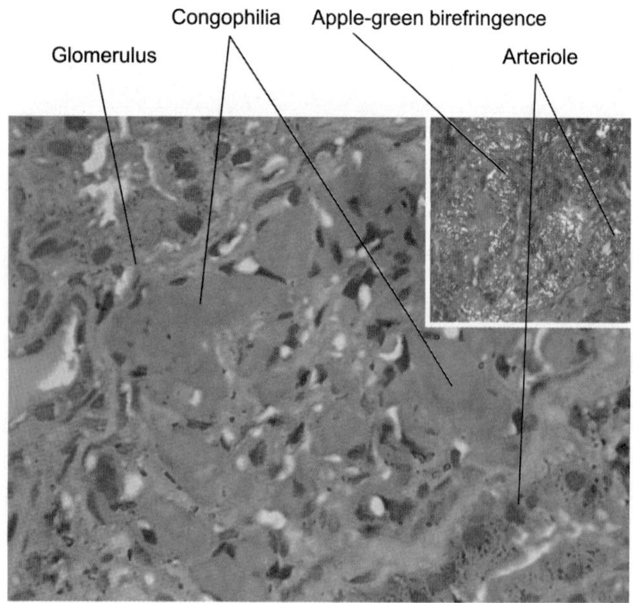

CL 15. Amyloidosis kidney
(Congo red, × 200; inbox under polarising light). Details on p 90.

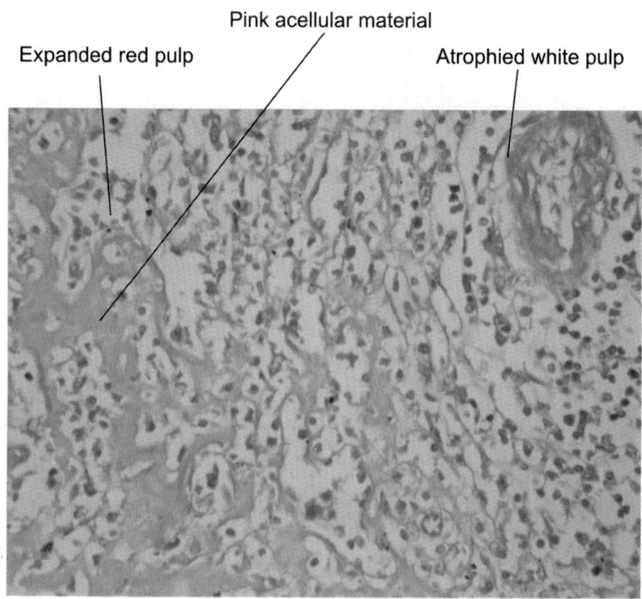

CL 16. Amyloidosis spleen
(H & E, × 200). Details on p 91.

Based on

Chapter 5: Haemodynamic Disorders

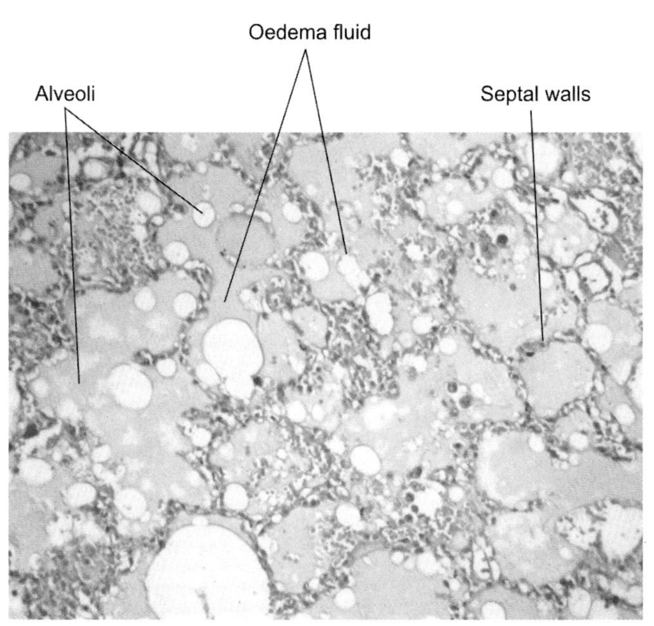

CL 17. Pulmonary oedema
(H & E, × 100). Details on p 102.

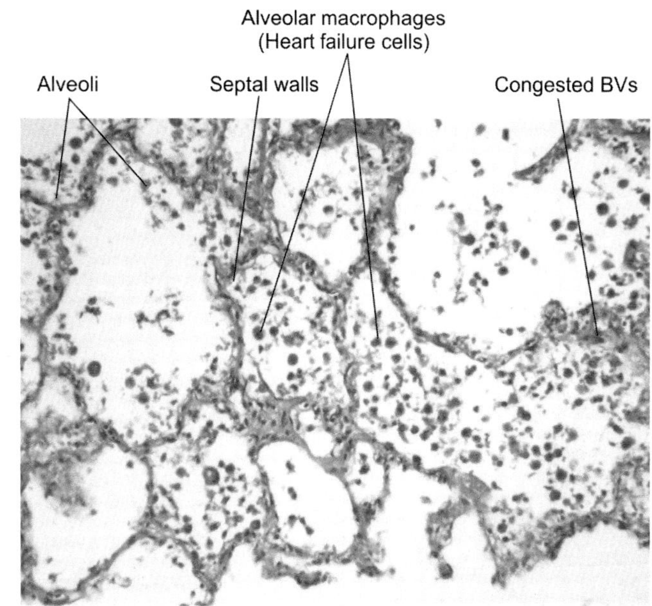

CL 18. CVC lung
(H & E, × 100). Details on p 107.

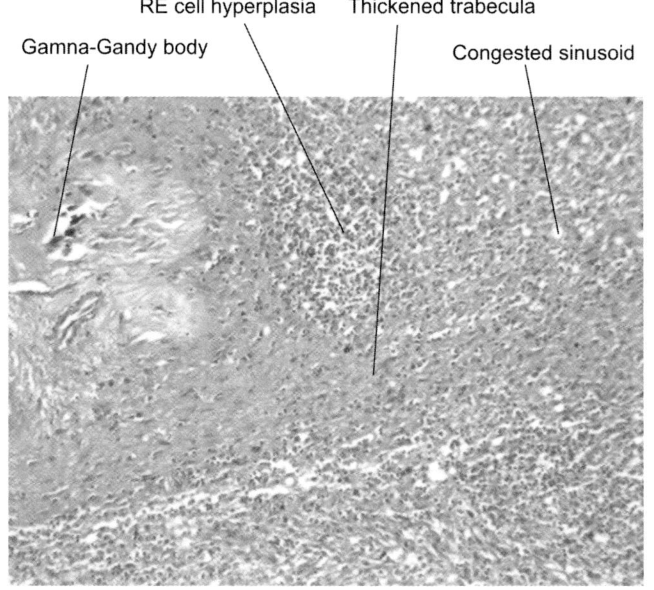

CL 19. CVC spleen
(H & E, × 100). Details on p 108, 465.

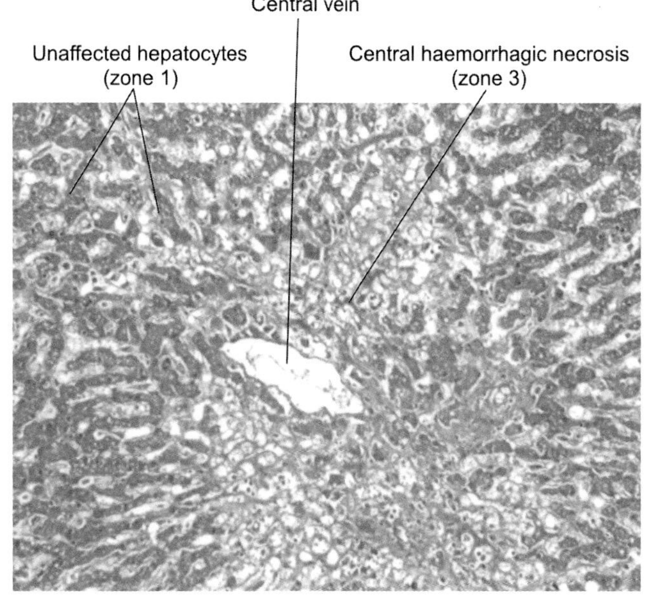

CL 20. CVC liver
(H & E, × 100). Details on p 107, 649.

Based on
Chapter 5: Haemodynamic Disorders

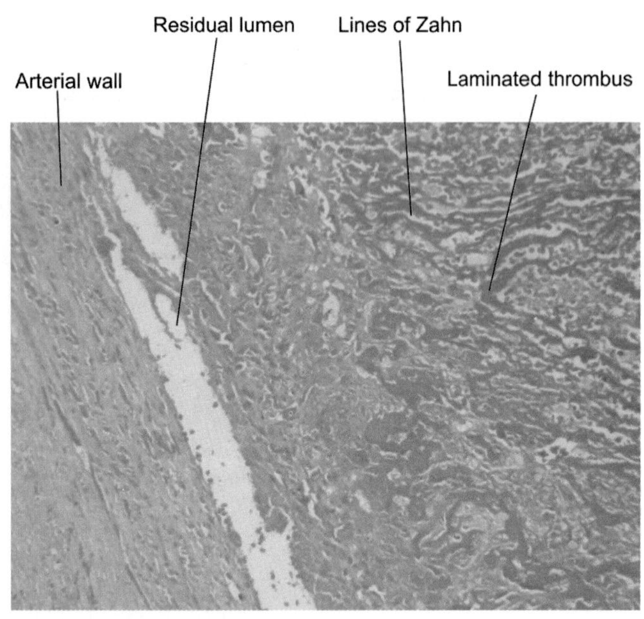

CL 21. Thrombus artery
(H & E, × 40). Details on p 118.

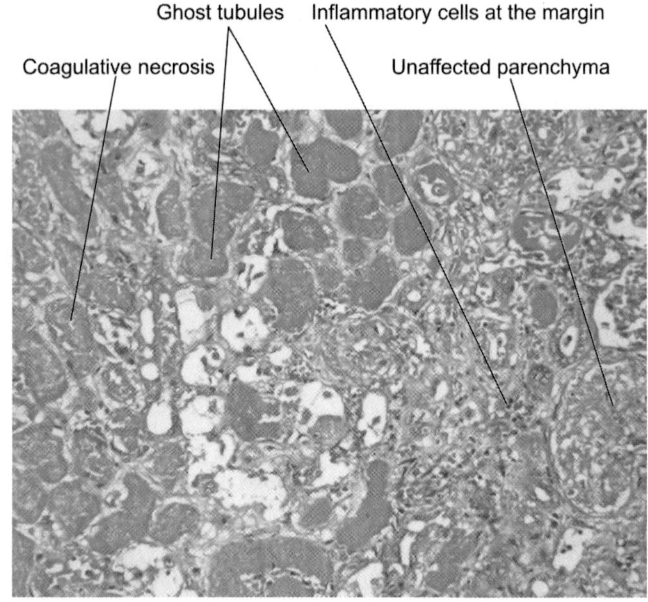

CL 22. Pale infarct kidney
(H & E, × 100). Details on p 130.

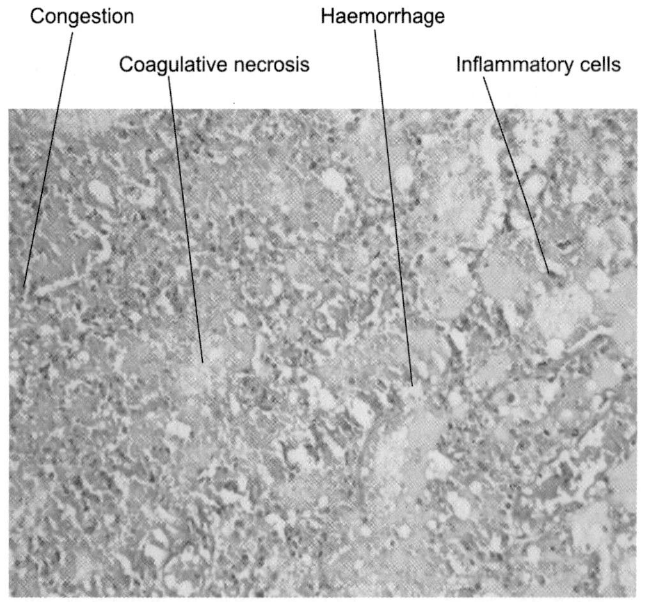

CL 23. Haemorrhagic infarct lung
(H & E, × 100). Details on p 130.

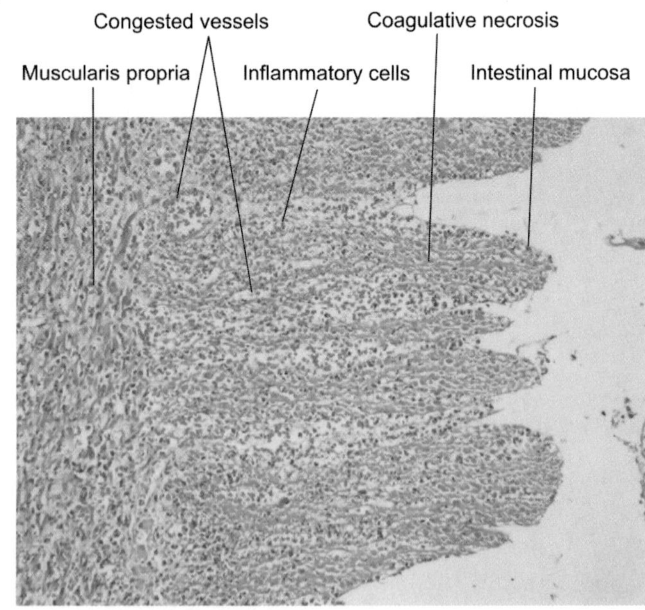

CL 24. Gangrene small bowel
(H & E, × 40). Details on p 55.

Based on

Chapter 6: Inflammation and Healing

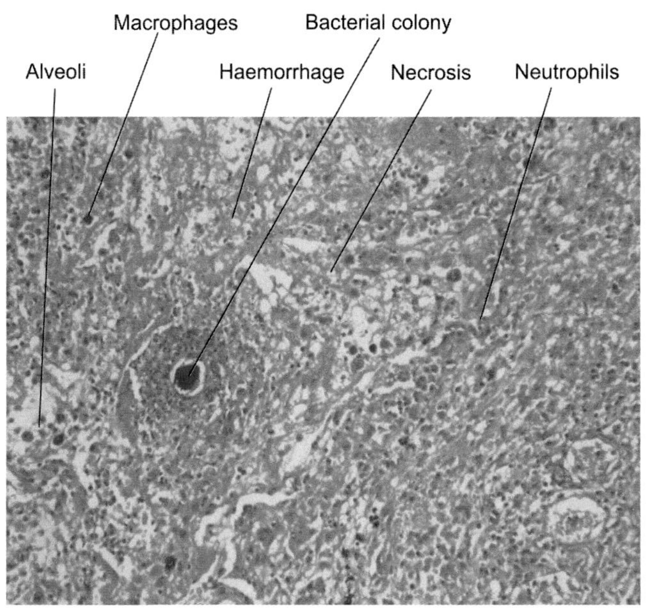

CL 25. Abscess lung
(H & E, × 100). Details on p 150, 483.

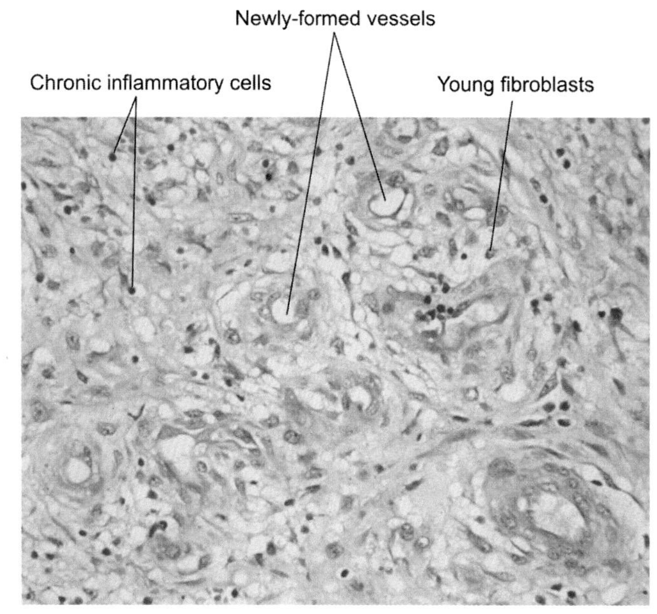

CL 26. Chronic inflammatory granulation tissue
(H & E, × 200). Details on p 153.

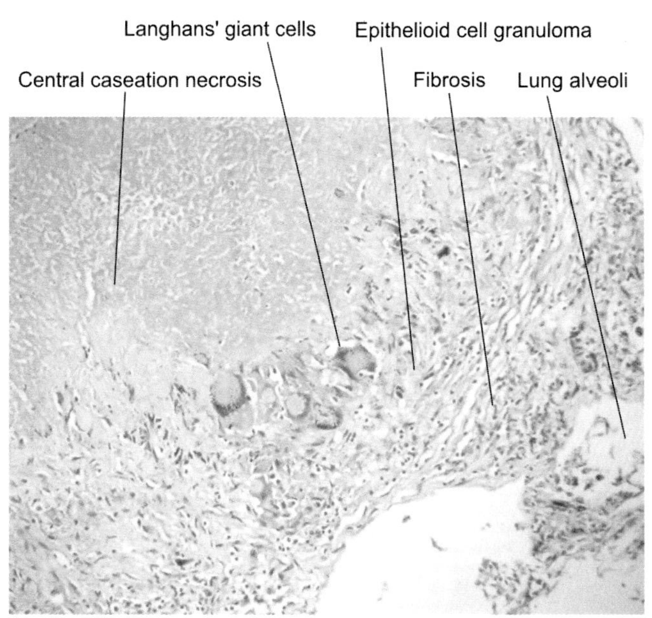

CL 27. Tuberculosis lung
(H & E, × 100). Details on p 159.

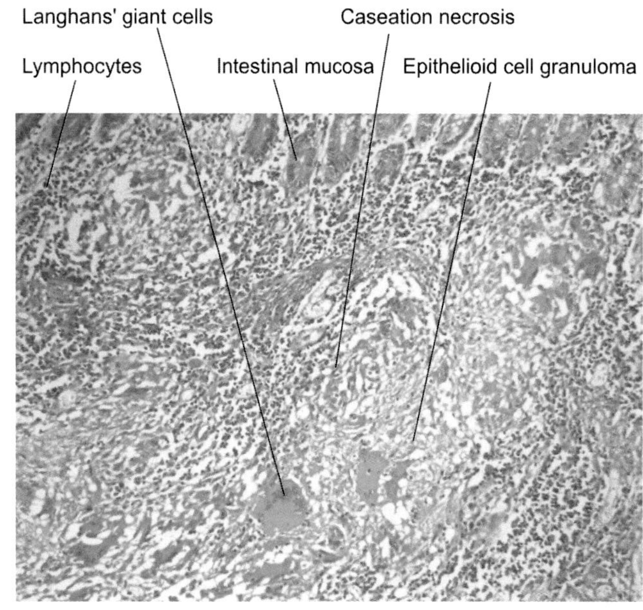

CL 28. Tuberculosis intestine
(H & E, × 100). Details on p 162, 585.

Based on

Chapter 6: Inflammation and Healing

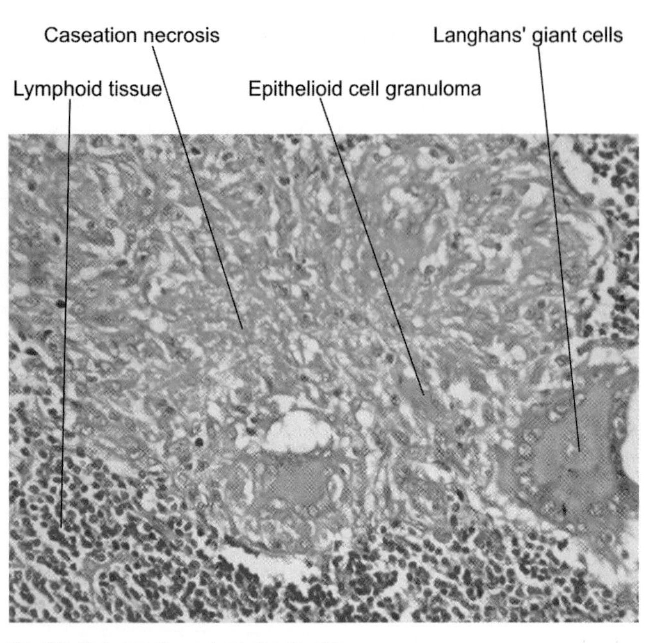

CL 29. Tuberculous lymphadenitis
(H & E, × 200). Details on p 159.

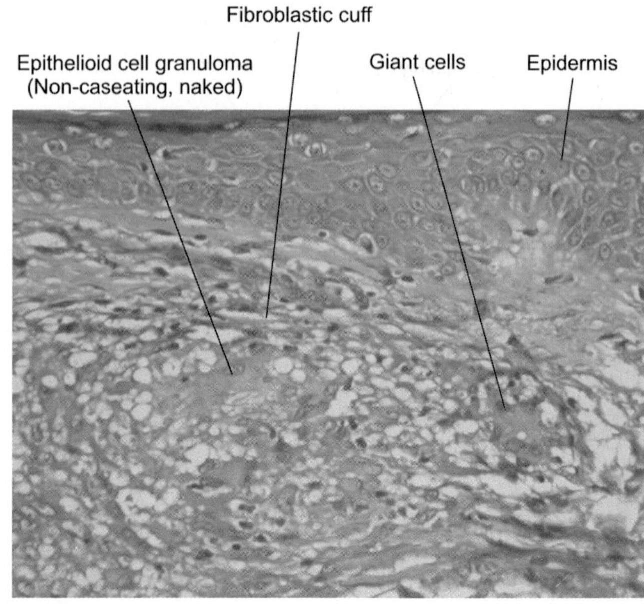

CL 30. Sarcoidosis skin
(H & E, × 200). Details on p 170.

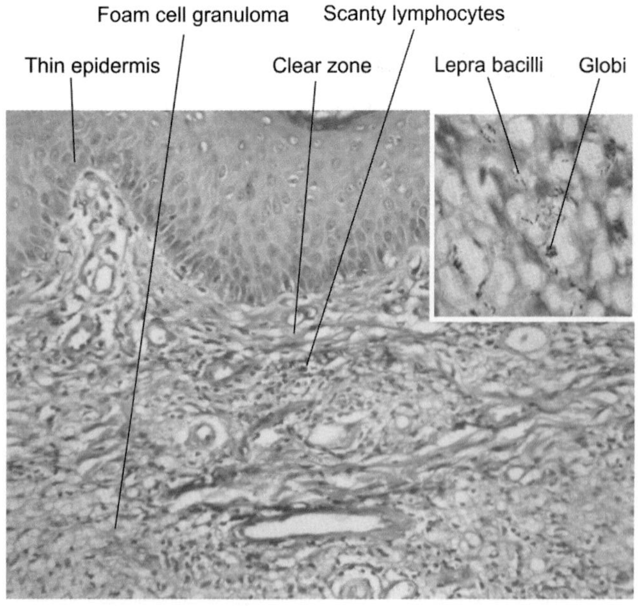

CL 31. Lepromatous leprosy (LL)
(H & E, × 100; inbox Fite Faraco, × 1000 oil). Details on p 165.

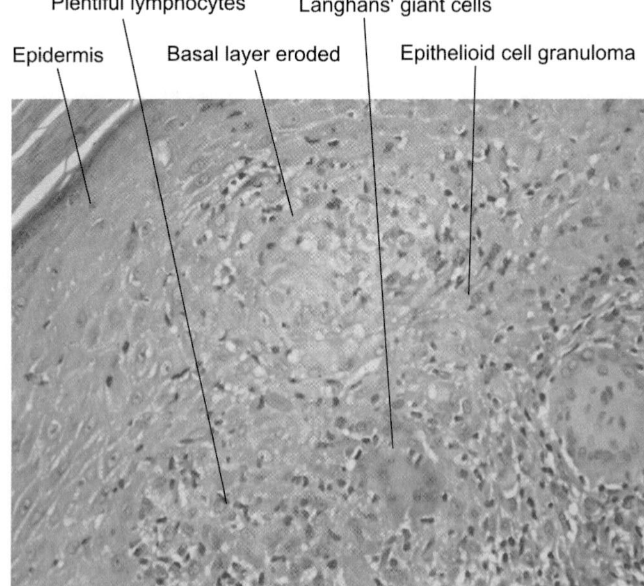

CL 32. Tuberculoid leprosy (TT)
(H & E, × 100). Details on p 165.

Based on

Chapter 7: Infectious and Parasitic Diseases

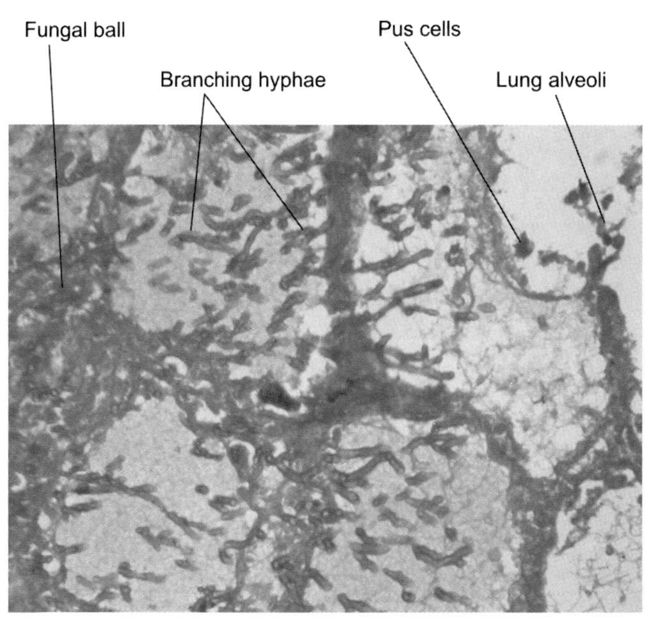

CL 33. Aspergillosis lung
(H & E, × 200). Details on p 188, 484.

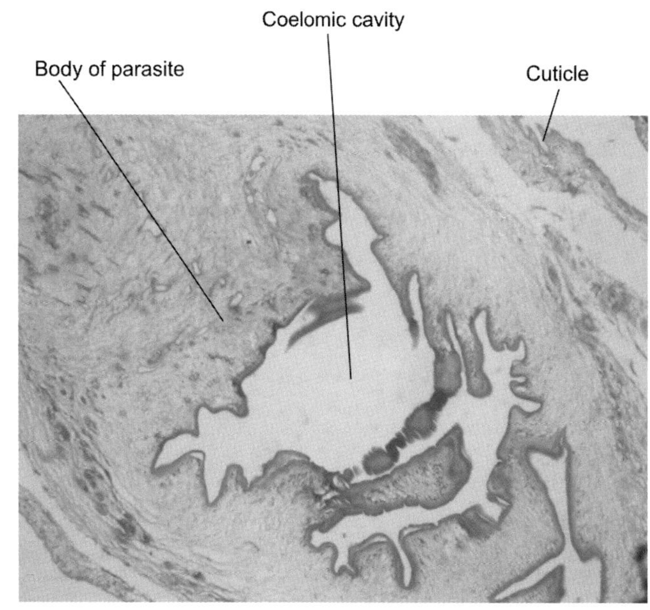

CL 34. Cysticercosis muscle
(H & E, × 40). Details on p 195.

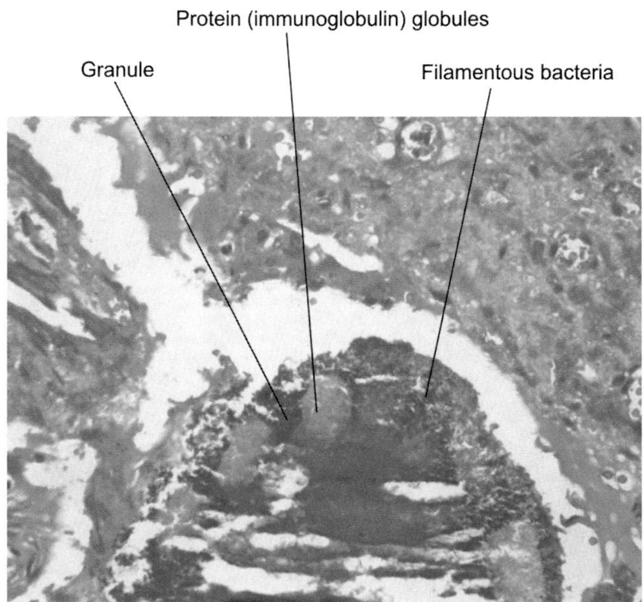

CL 35. Actinomycosis
(H & E, × 200) Details on p 169.

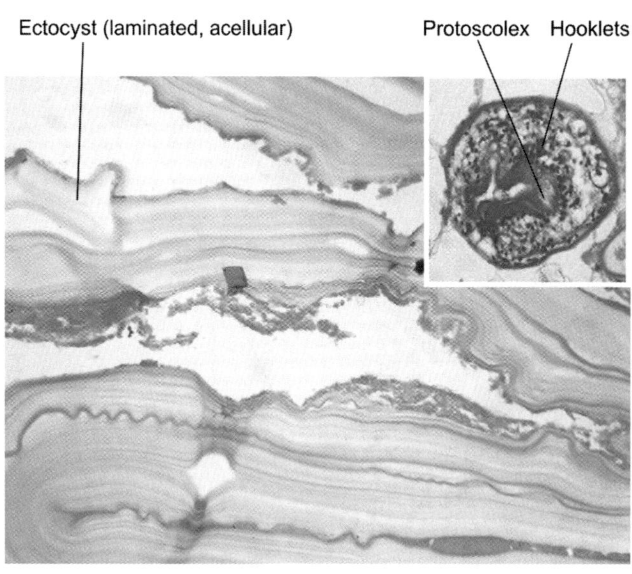

CL 36. Hydatid cyst
(H & E, × 100; inbox shows a scolex). Details on p 193, 636.

Based on

Chapters 8, 24: Neoplasia; The Skin

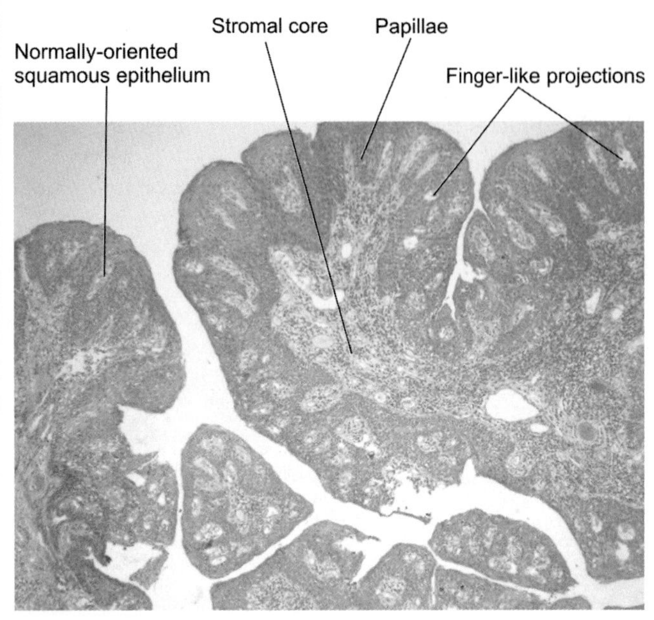

CL 37. Squamous cell papilloma
(H & E, x 40). Details on p 199, 804.

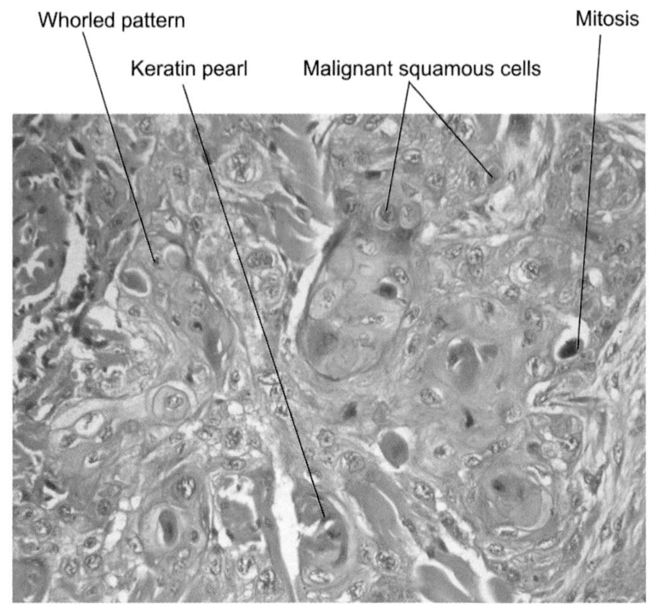

CL 38. Squamous cell carcinoma skin
(H & E, x 200). Details on p 199, 740, 806.

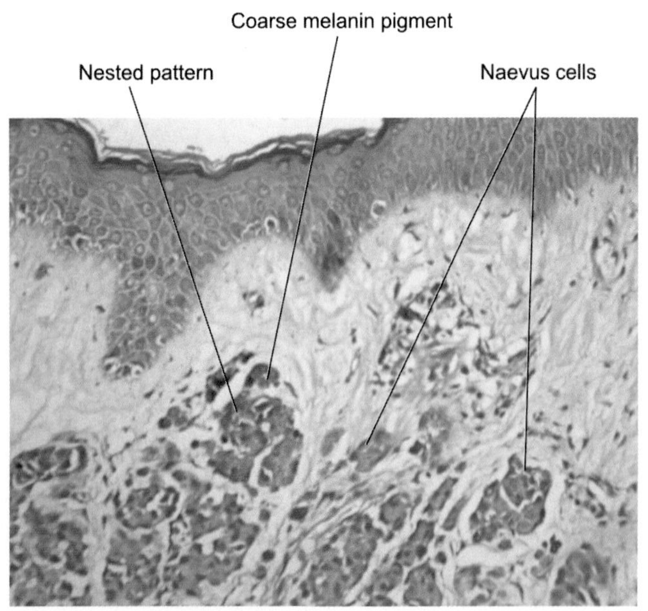

CL 39. Intradermal naevus
(H & E, x 100). Details on p 199, 810.

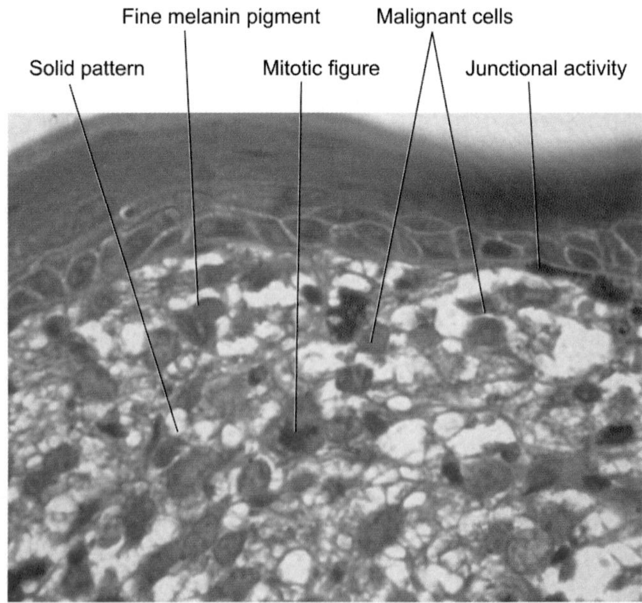

CL 40. Malignant melanoma
(H & E, x 400). Details on p 199, 522, 811.

Based on

Chapters 8, 27: Neoplasia; Soft Tissue Tumours

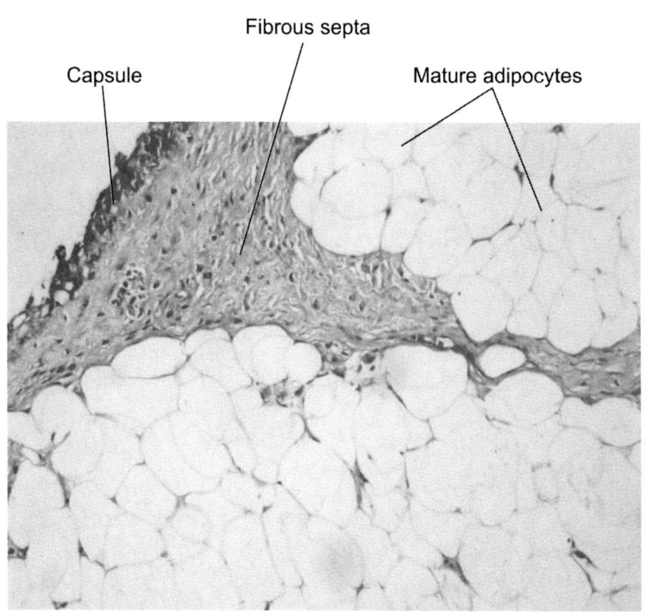

CL 41. Lipoma
(H & E, × 100). Details on p 199, 890.

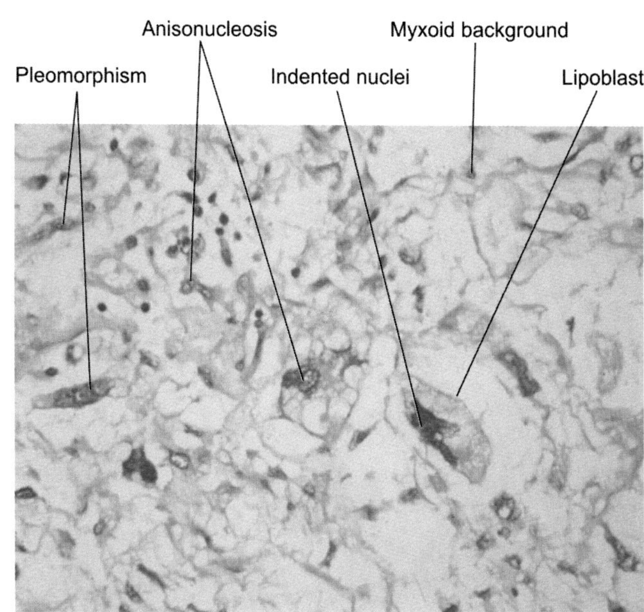

CL 42. Liposarcoma
(H & E, × 400). Details on p 199, 890.

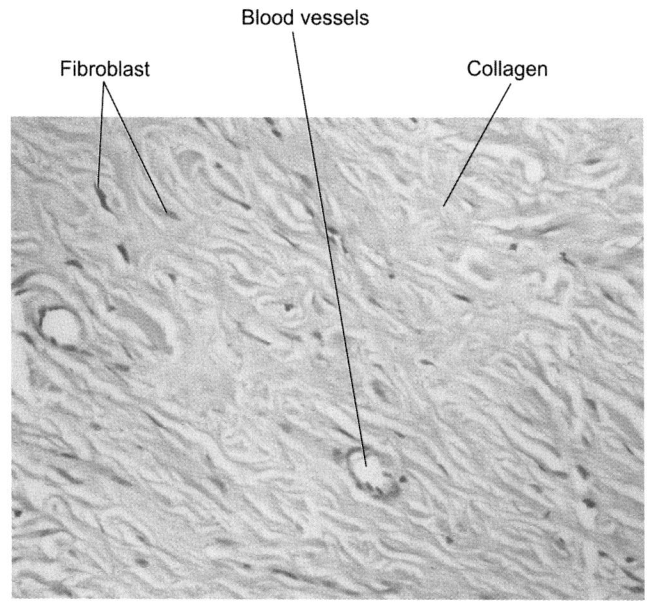

CL 43. Fibroma
(H & E, × 100). Details on p 199, 887.

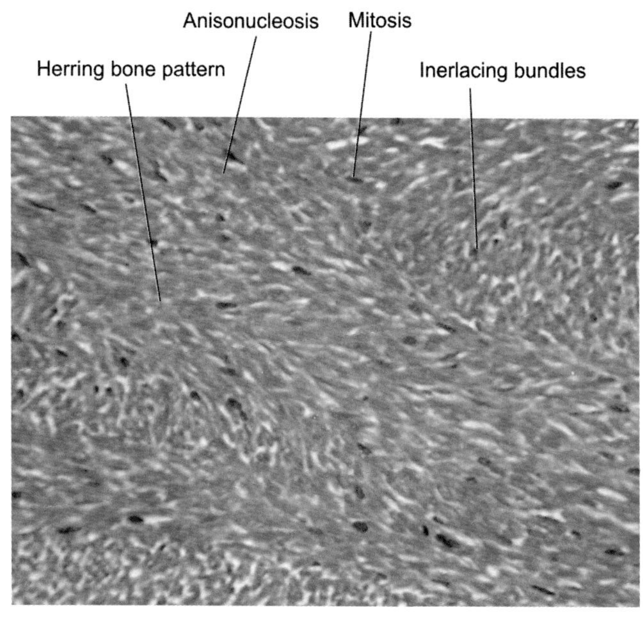

CL 44. Fibrosarcoma
(H & E, × 200). Details on p 199, 888.

Based on

Chapter 8: Neoplasia

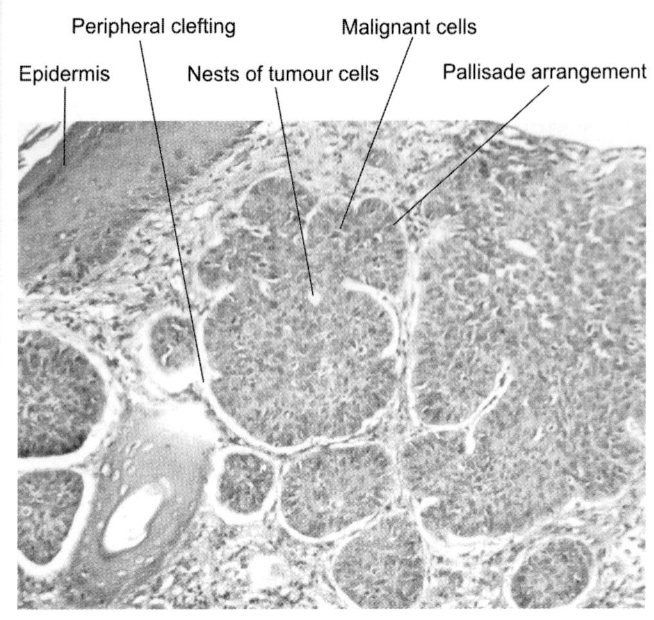

CL 45. Basal cell carcinoma skin
(H & E, x 100). Details on p 199, 807.

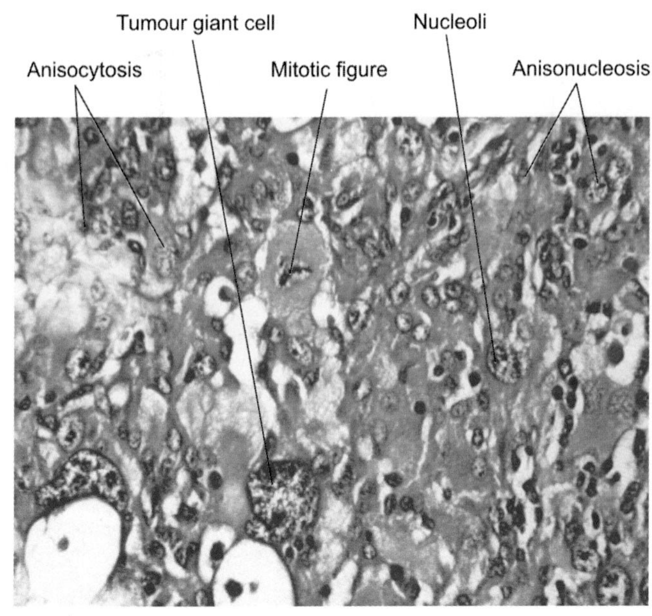

CL 46. Characteristics of malignant cells
(H & E, x 400). Details on p 202.

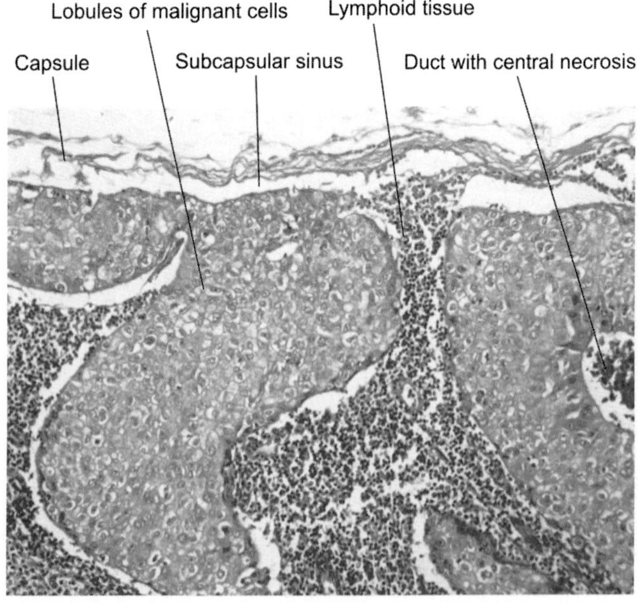

CL 47. Metastatic carcinoma lymph node
(H & E, x 200). Details on p 205, 458.

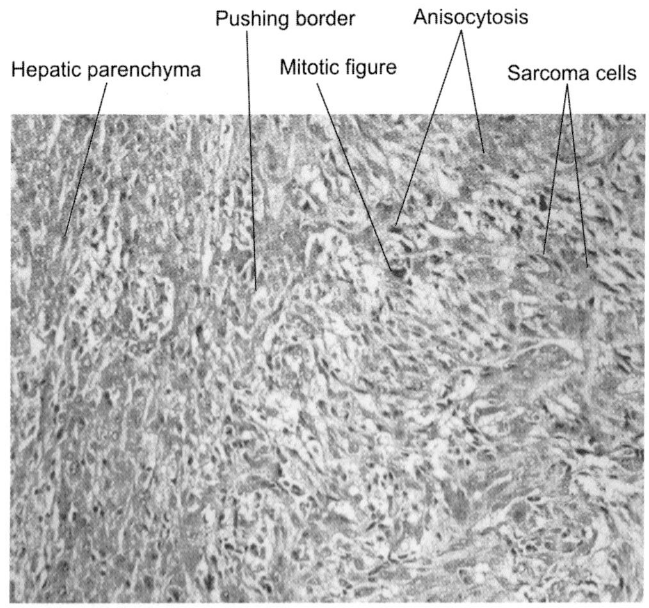

CL 48. Metastatic sarcoma liver
(H & E, x 200). Details on p 206, 657.

Based on

Chapter 11: The Blood Vessels and Lymphatics

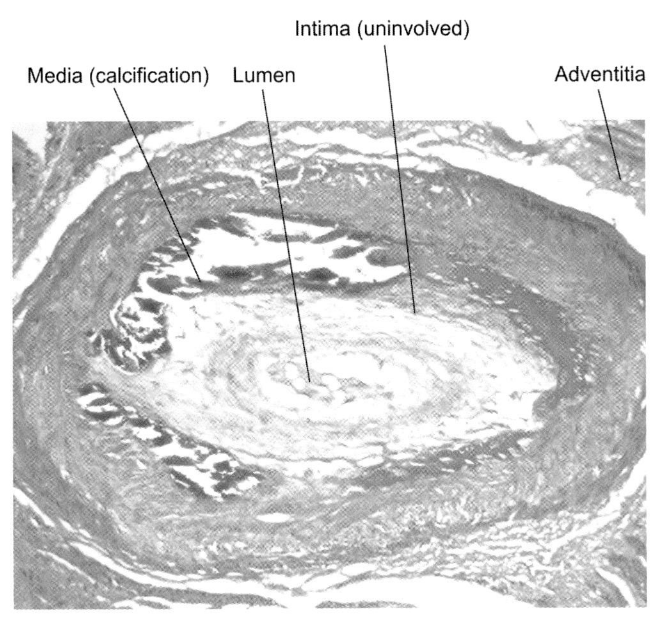

CL 49. Mönckeberg's arteriosclerosis
(H & E, × 100). Details on p 57, 279.

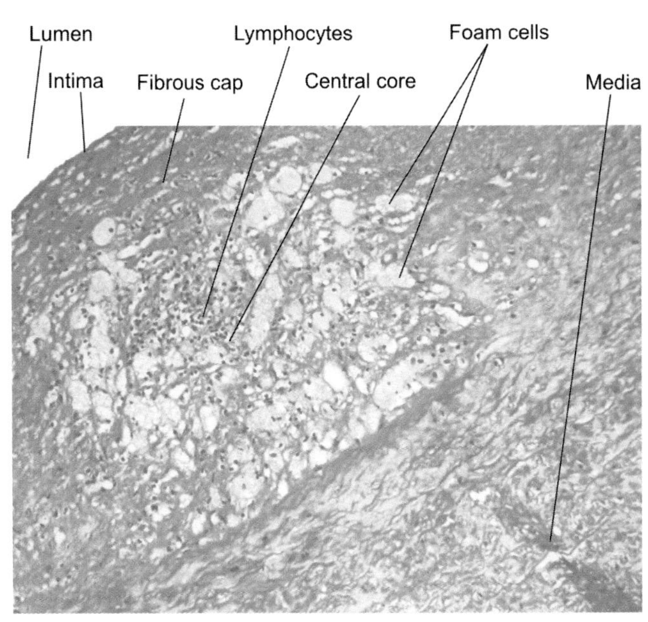

CL 50. Atheromatous plaque aorta
(H & E, × 100). Details on p 286.

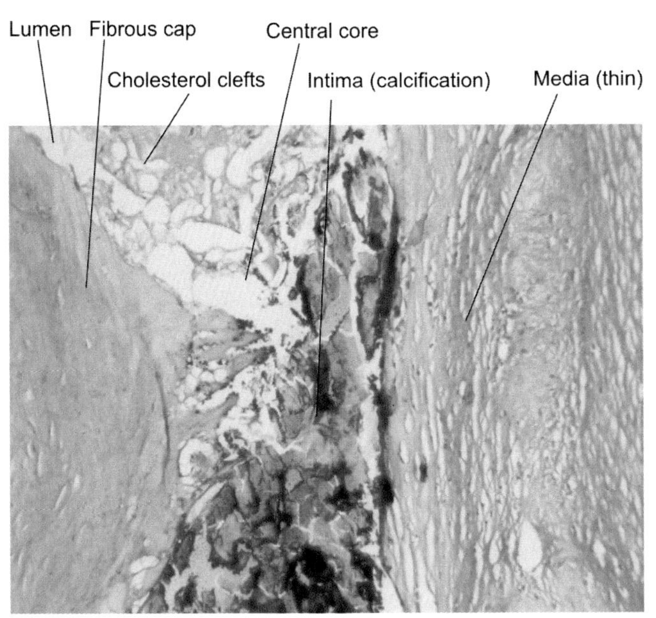

CL 51. Complicated plaque lesion coronary artery
(H & E, × 40). Details on p 286, 317.

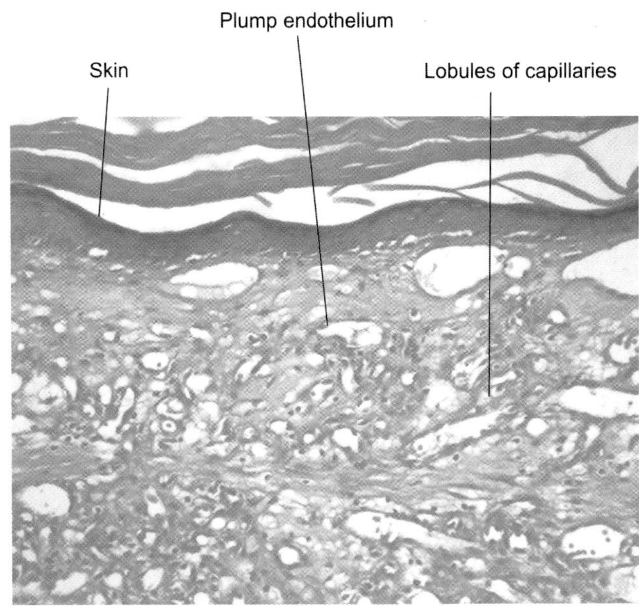

CL 52. Capillary haemangioma skin
(H & E, × 100). Details on p 300.

Based on

Chapter 11: The Blood Vessels and Lymphatics

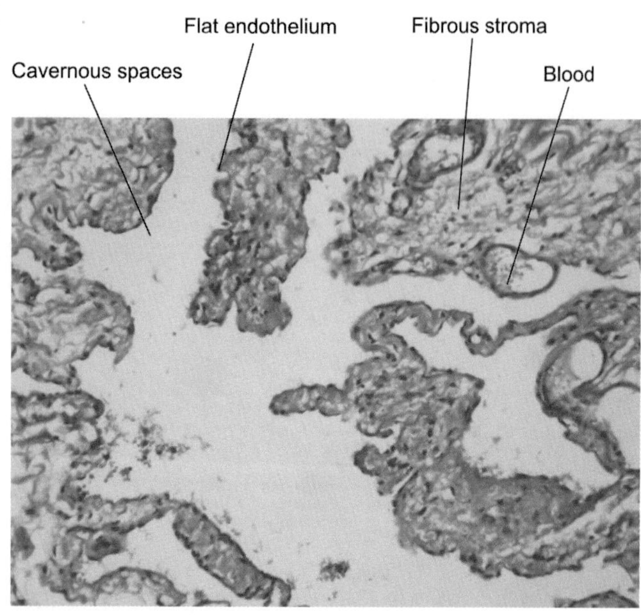

CL 53. Cavernous haemangioma
(H & E, × 100). Details on p. 301, 654.

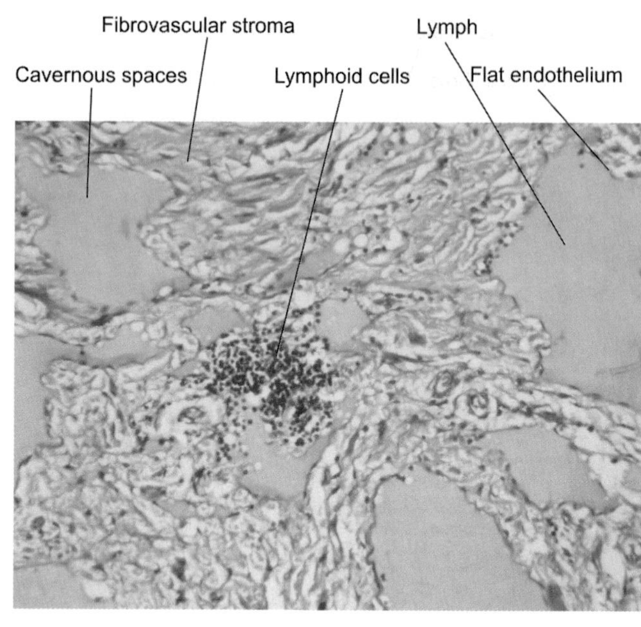

CL 54. Lymphangioma tongue
(H & E, × 100). Details on p 301.

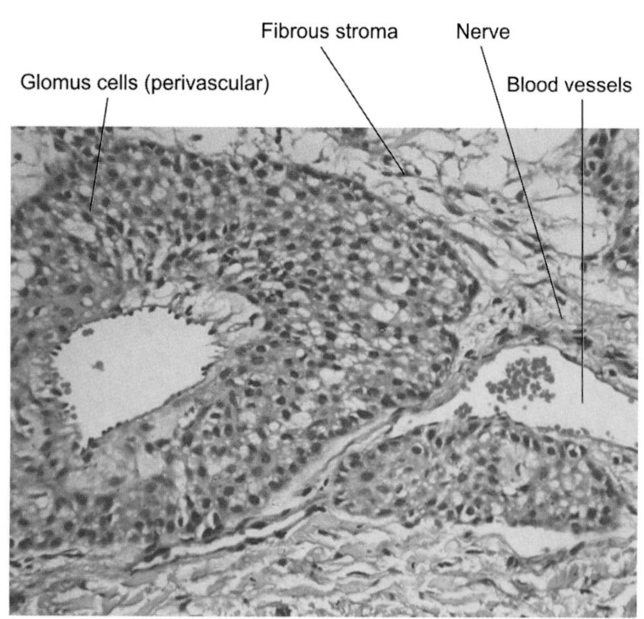

CL 55. Glomus tumour
(H & E, × 200). Details on p 302.

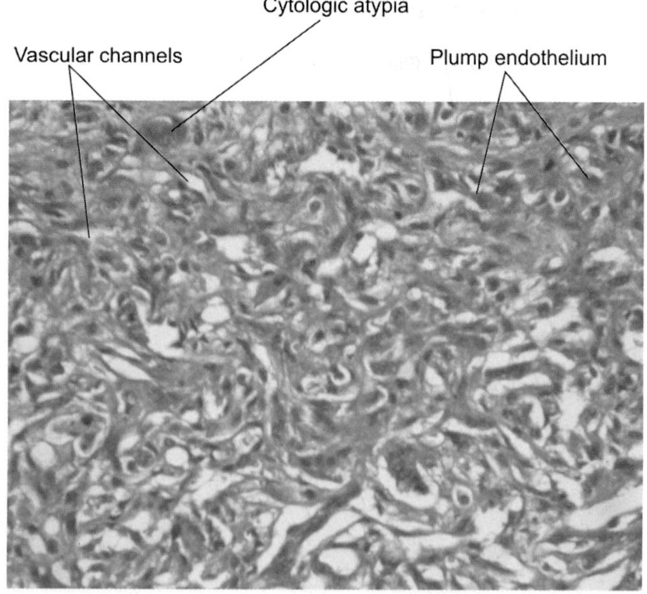

CL 56. Angiosarcoma
(H & E, x 200). Details on p 303.

Based on

Chapter 12: The Heart

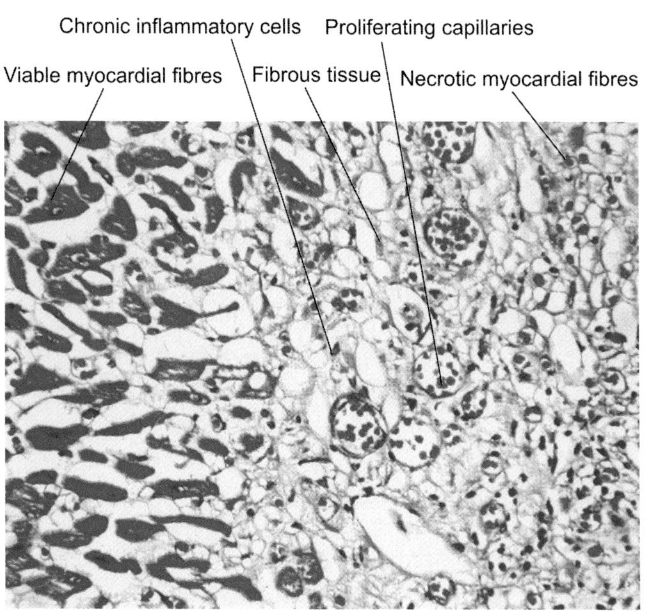

CL 57. Myocardial infarct (3-weeks old)
(H & E, × 200). Details on p 320.

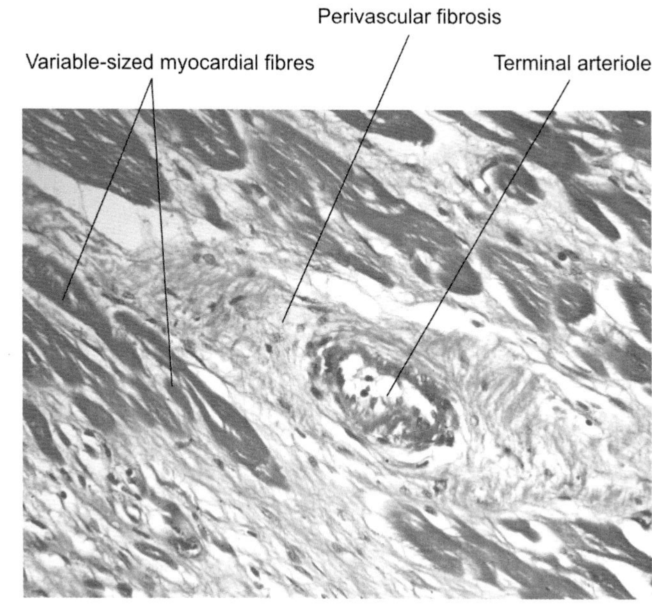

CL 58. Chronic ischaemic heart disease
(H & E, × 200). Details on p 326.

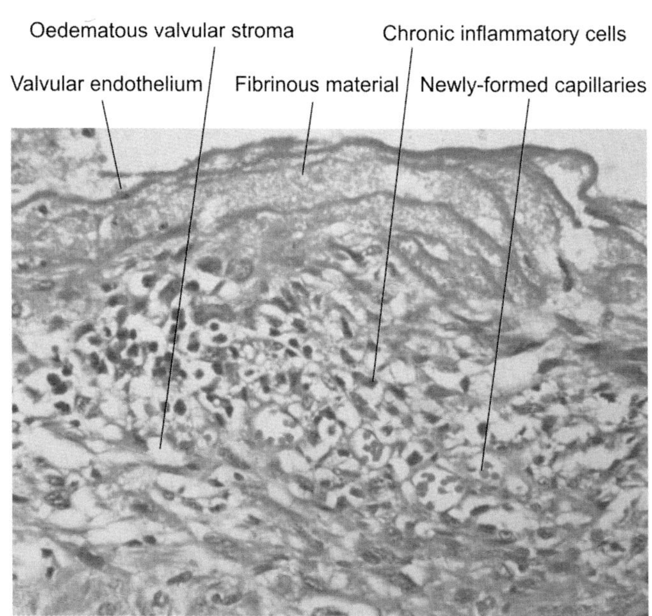

CL 59. Infective endocarditis
(H & E, × 200). Details on p 338.

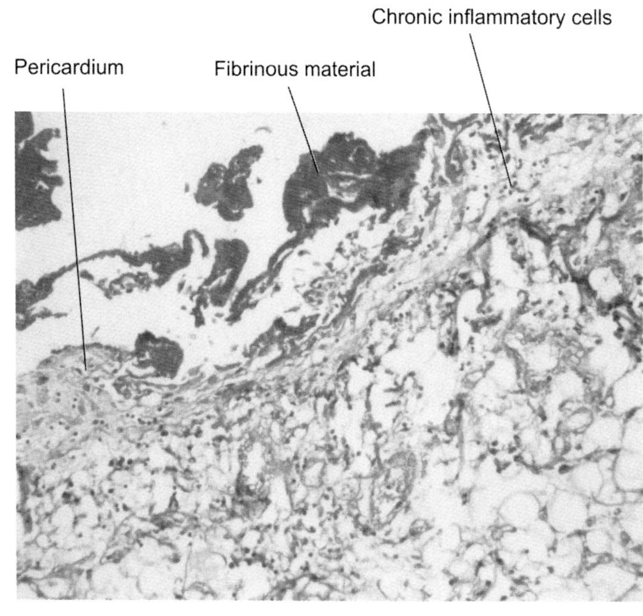

CL 60. Serofibrinous pericarditis
(H & E, × 100). Details on p 351.

Based on

Chapter 13: The Haematopoietic System

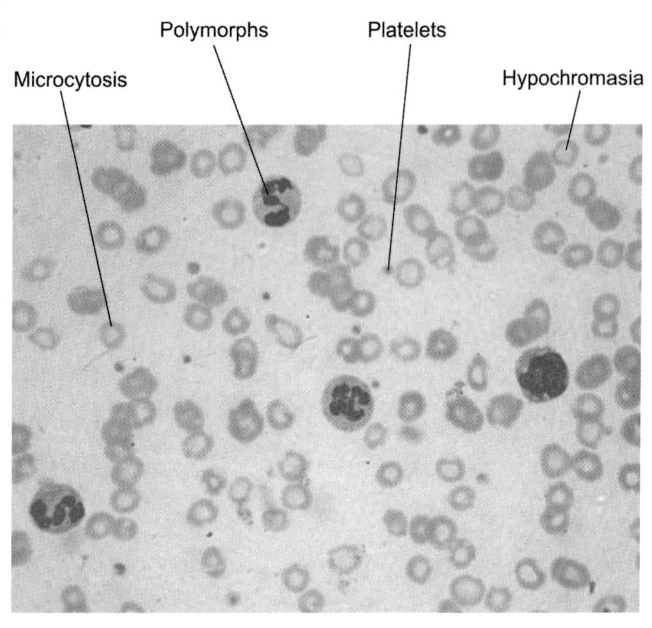

CL 61. PBF in microcytic hypochromic anaemia
(Leishman's, × 400). Details on p 372.

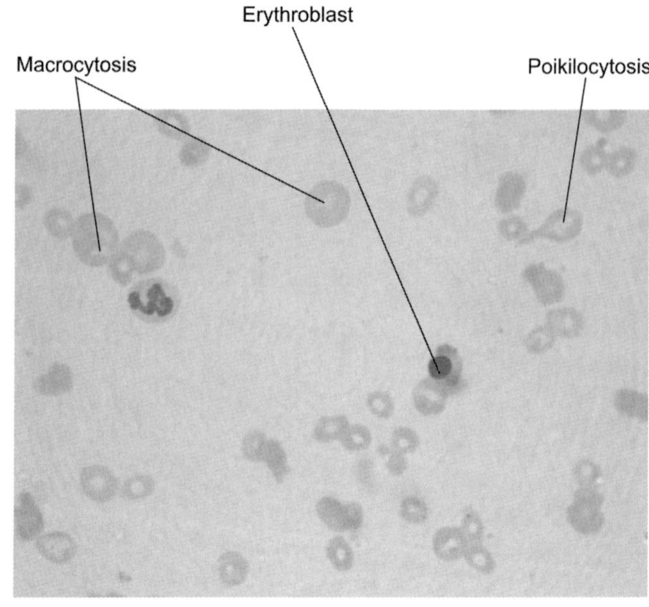

CL 62. PBF in macrocytic anaemia
(Leishman's, × 400). Details on p 381.

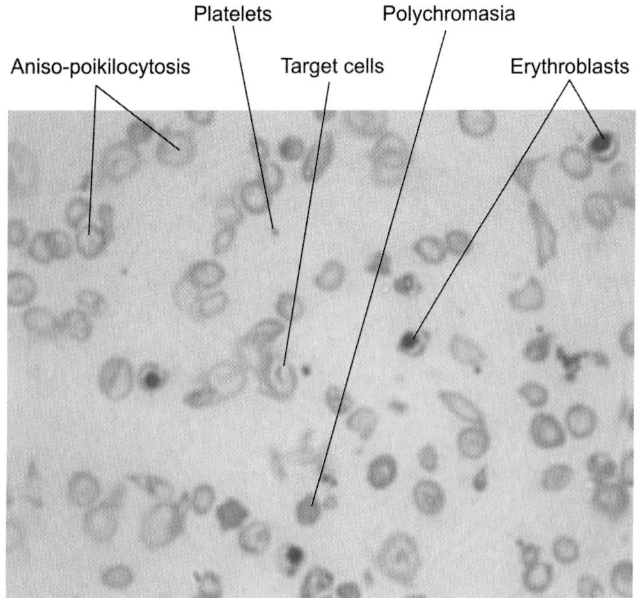

CL 63. PBF in haemolytic anaemia (Thalassaemia)
(Leishman's, × 400). Details on p 400.

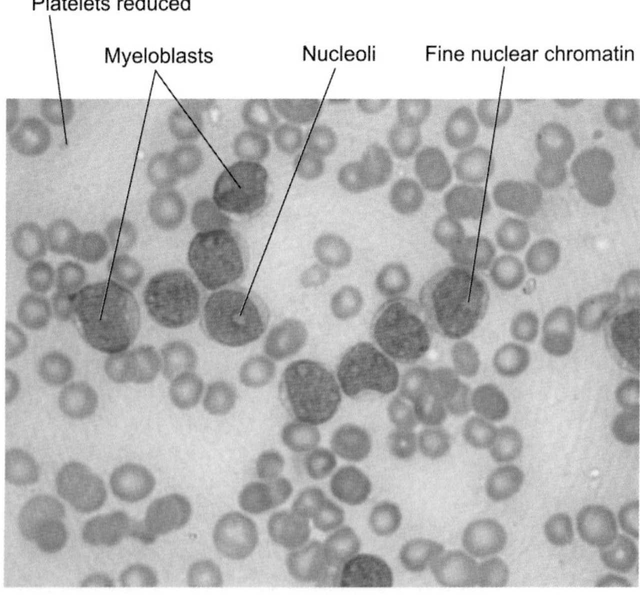

CL 64. PBF in acute myeloblastic leukaemia
(Leishman's, × 400). Details on p 417.

Based on

Chapter 13: The Haematopoietic System

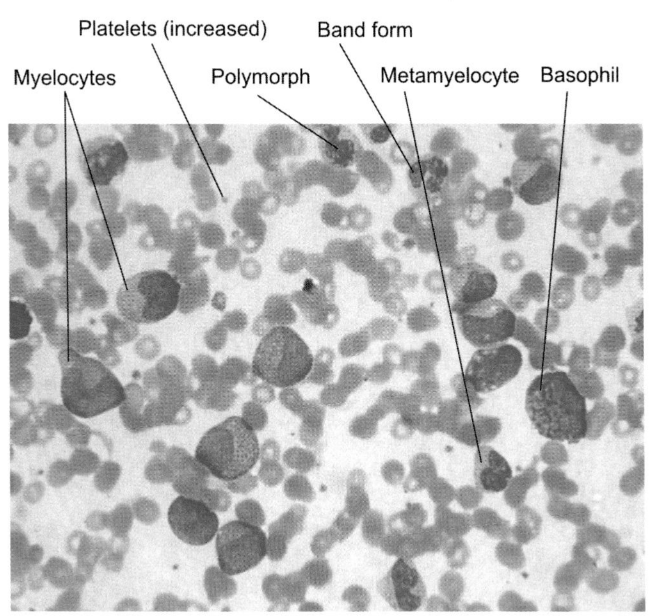

CL 65. PBF in chronic myeloid leukaemia
(Leishman's, × 400). Details on p 421.

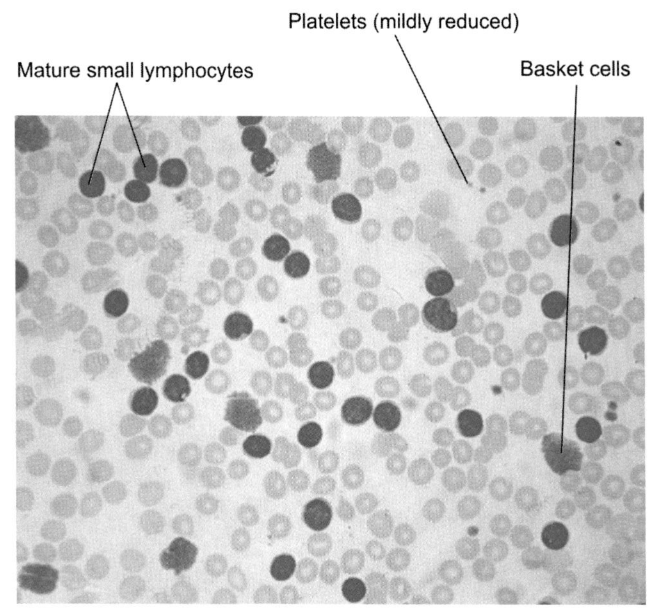

CL 66. PBF in chronic lymphocytic leukaemia
(Leishman's, × 400). Details on p 422.

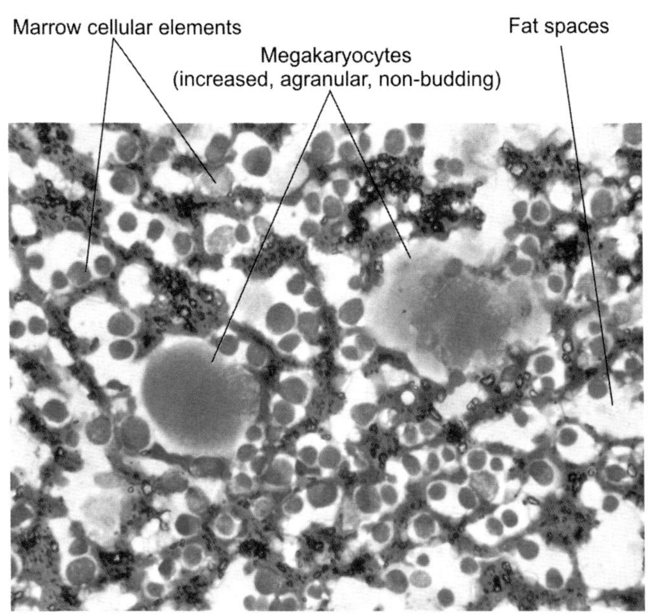

CL 67. Bone marrow aspirate in ITP
(Leishman's, × 200). Details on p 432.

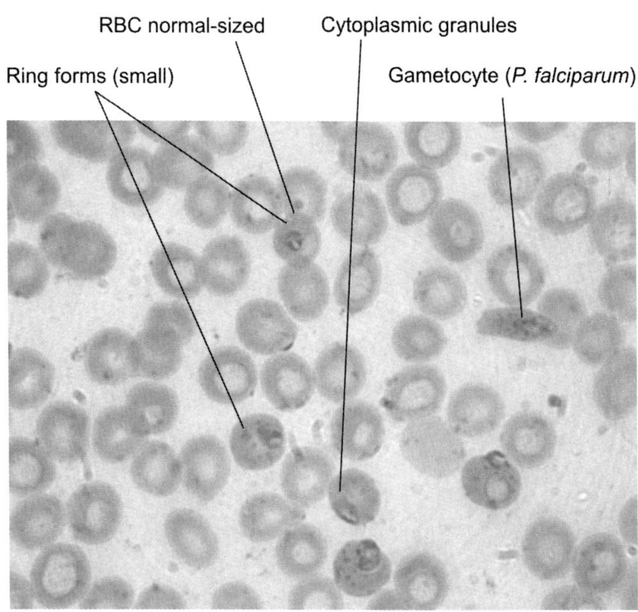

CL 68. Malarial parasite in PBF (*P. falciparum*)
(Leishman's, × 1000 oil). Details on p 194, 390.

Based on

Chapter 14: The Lymphoid System

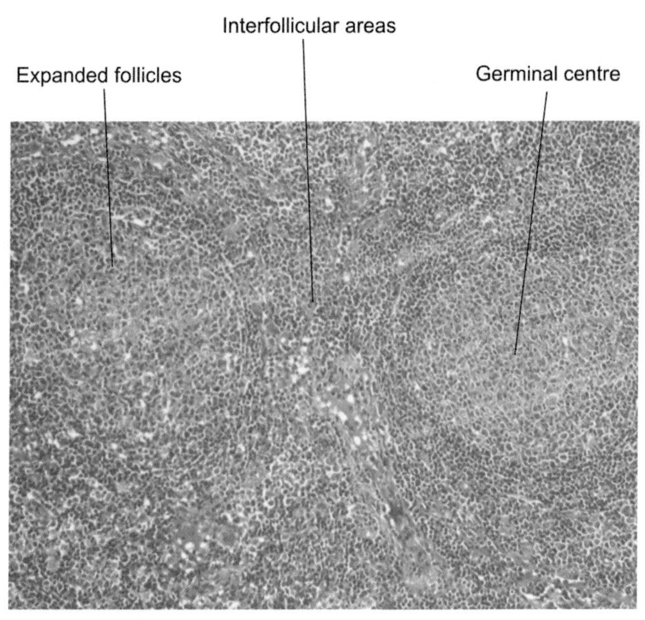

CL 69. Chronic reactive lymphadenitis
(H & E × 100). Details on p 444.

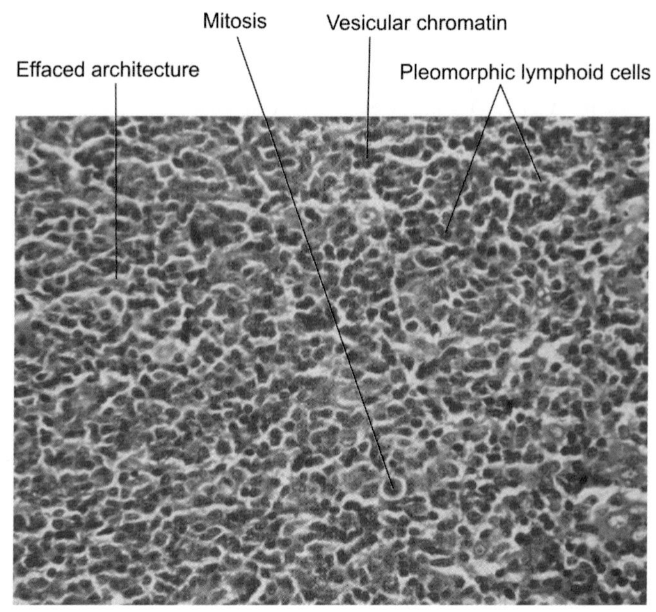

CL 70. Non-Hodgkin's lymphoma, diffuse large cell type
(H & E, × 400). Details on p 455.

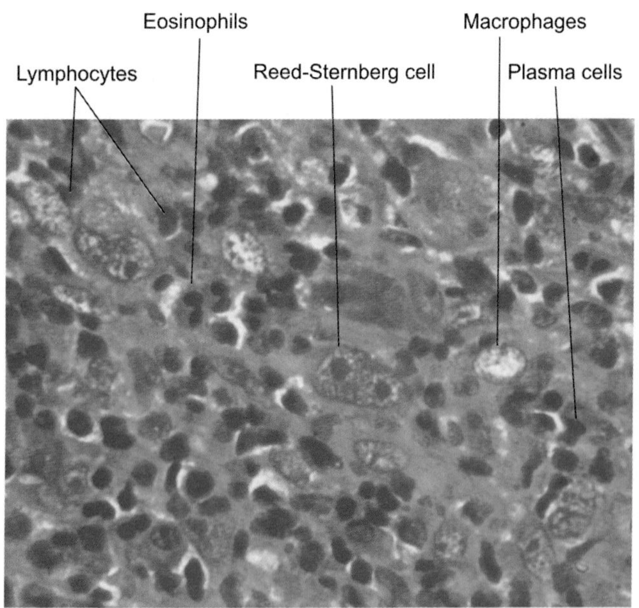

CL 71. Hodgkin's disease, mixed cellularity
(H & E × 400). Details on p 448.

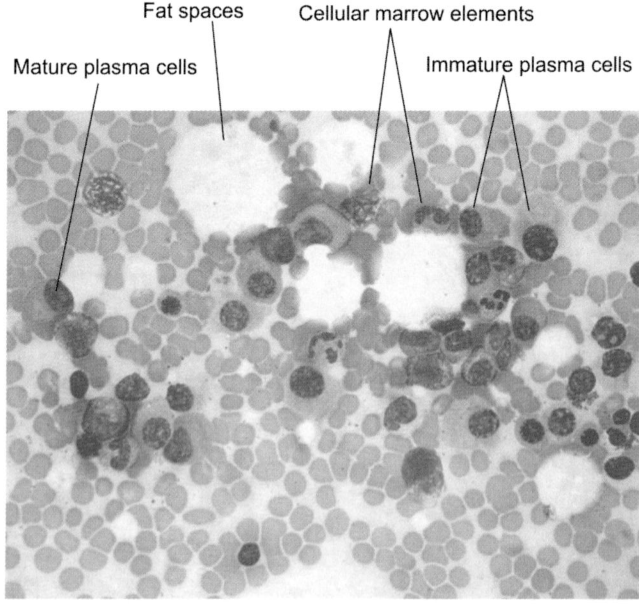

CL 72. Bone marrow aspirate in myeloma
(Leishman's, × 200). Details on p 460.

Based on

Chapter 15: The Respiratory System

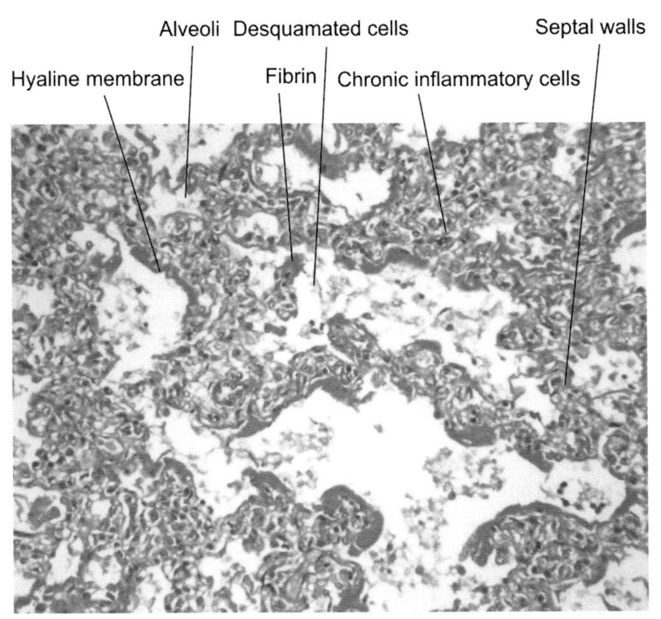

CL 73. Hyaline membrane disease
(H & E, × 200). Details on p 471.

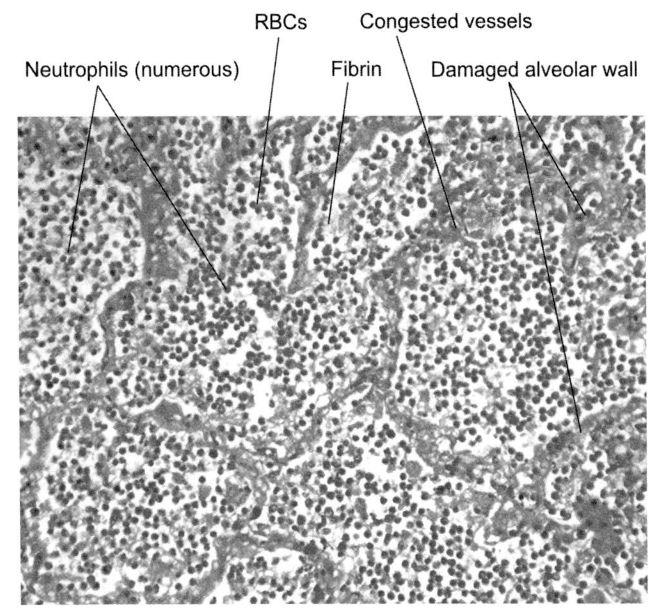

CL 74. Lobar pneumonia, red hepatisation
(H & E, × 100). Details on p 477.

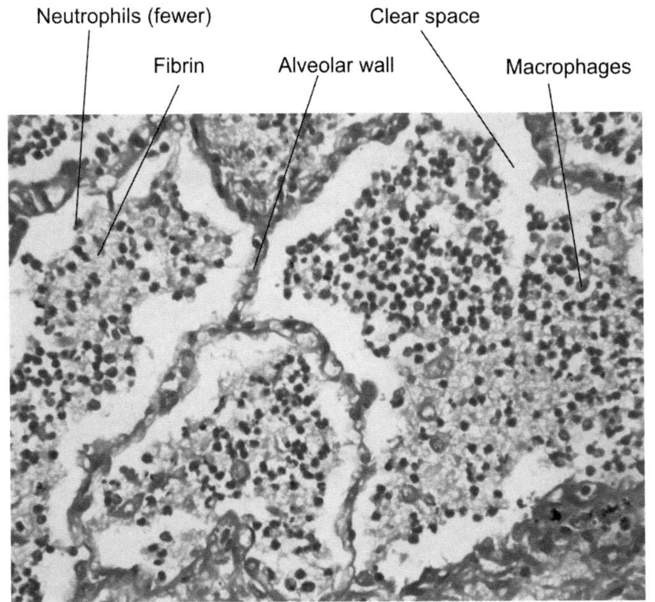

CL 75. Lobar pneumonia, grey hepatisation
(H & E, × 200). Details on p 477.

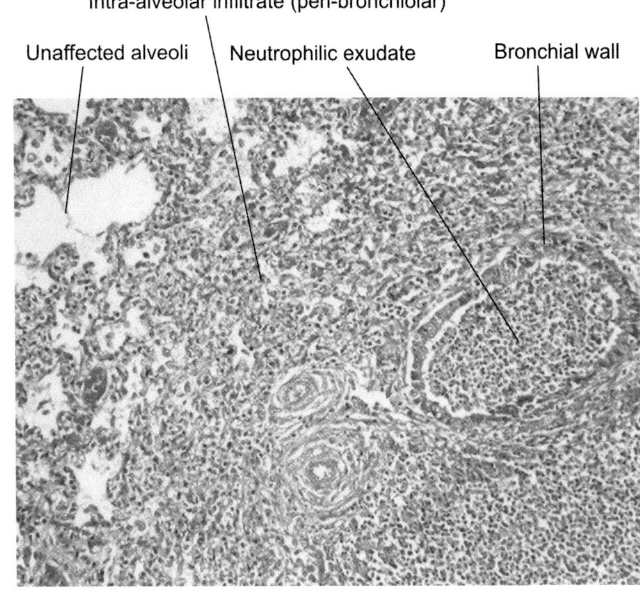

CL 76. Bronchopneumonia
(H & E, × 100). Details on p 479.

Based on

Chapter 15: The Respiratory System

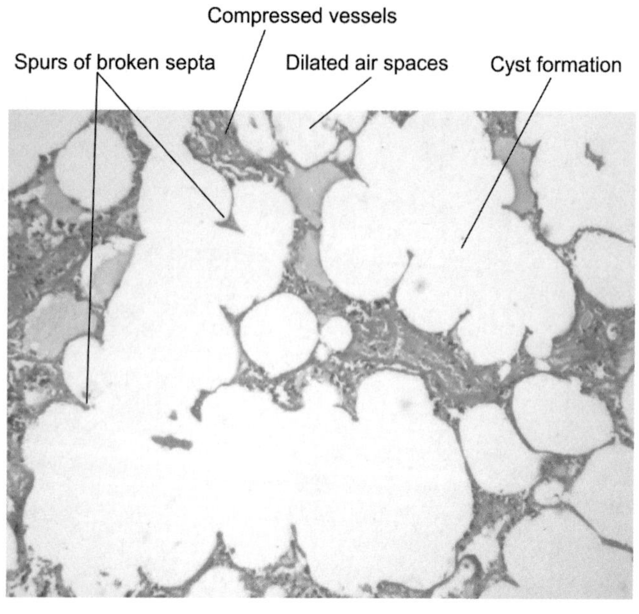

CL 77. Emphysema
(H & E, × 40). Details on p 488.

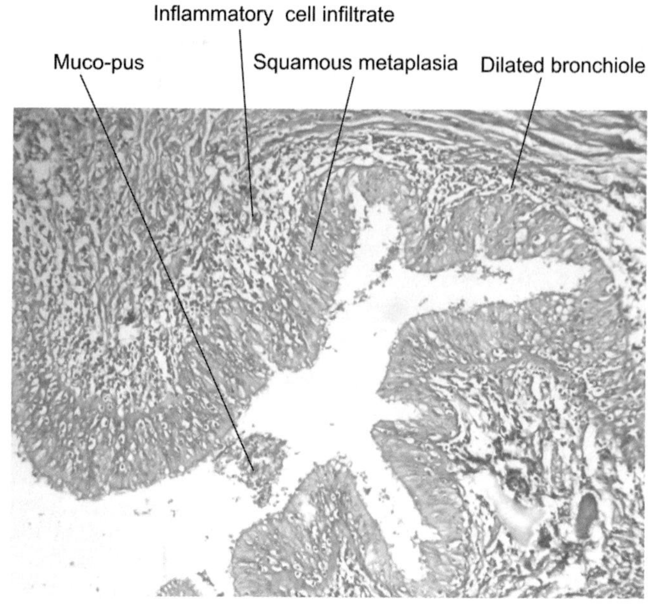

CL 78. Bronchiectasis
(H & E, × 100). Details on p 493.

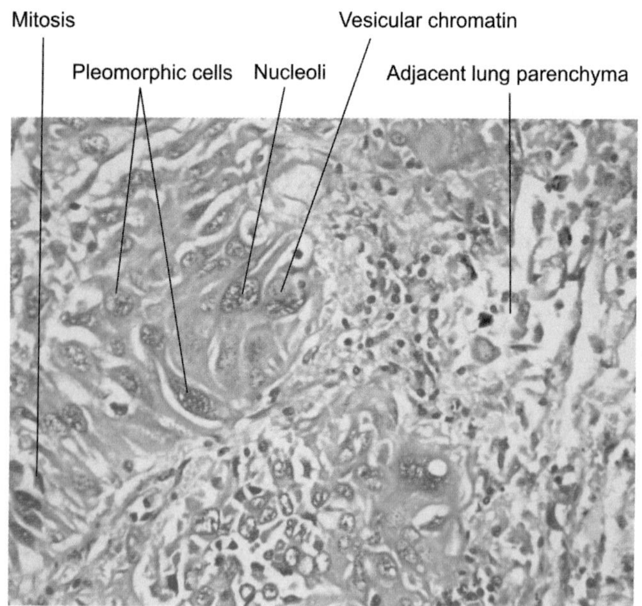

CL 79. Squamous cell carcinoma lung
(H & E, × 200). Details on p 509.

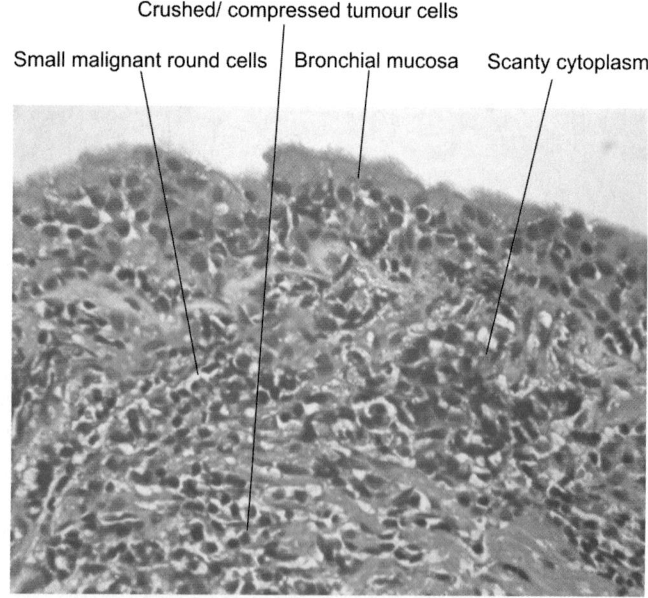

CL 80. Small cell carcinoma lung
(H & E, × 200). Details on p 510.

Based on

Chapter 16: The Eye, ENT and Neck

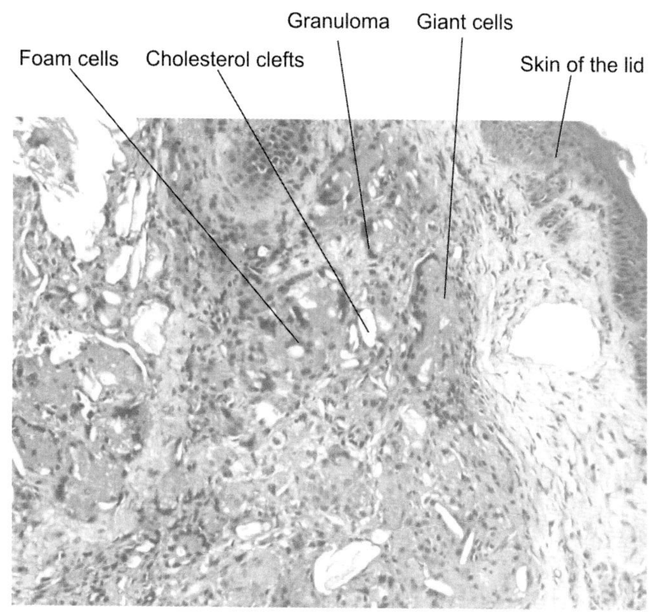

CL 81. Chalazion
(H & E, × 40). Details on p 518.

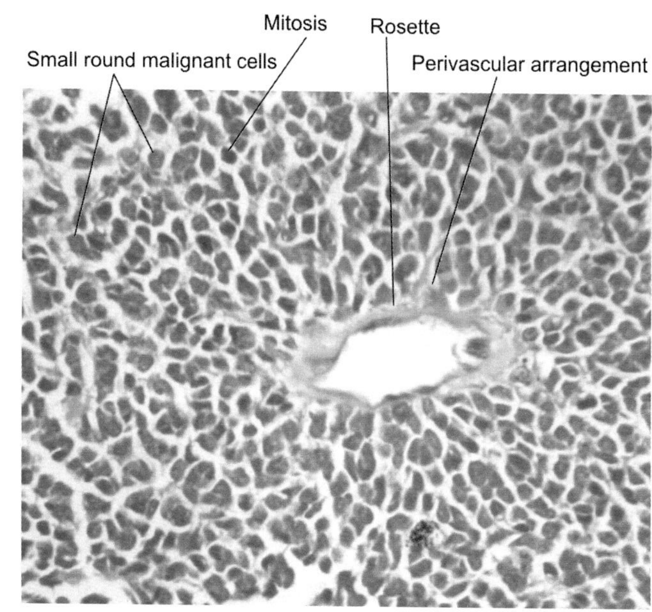

CL 82. Retinoblastoma
(H & E, × 100). Details on p 523.

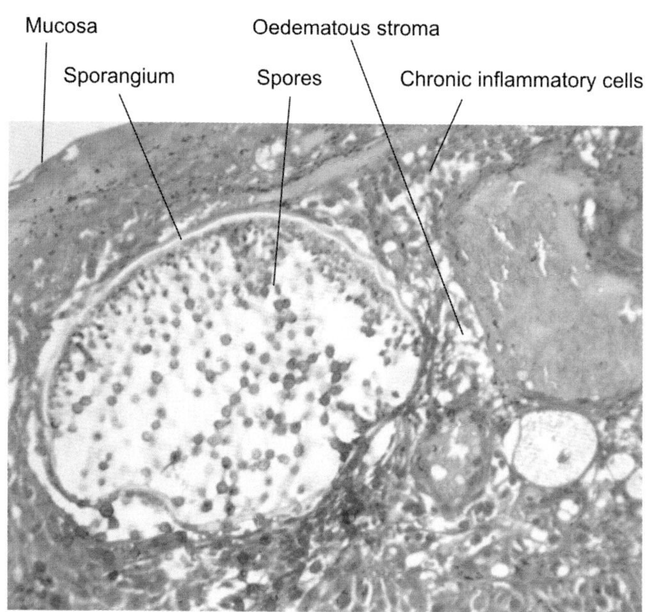

CL 83. Rhinosporidiosis nose
(H & E, × 100). Details on p 188, 527.

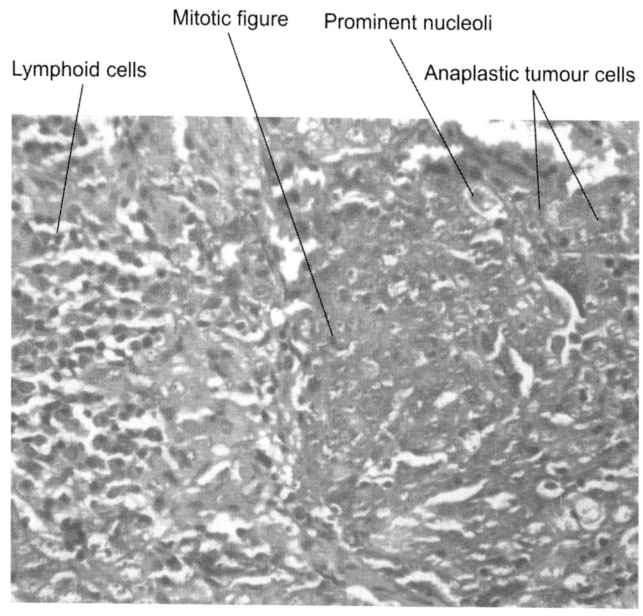

CL 84. Nasopharyngeal carcinoma
(H & E, × 200). Details on p 529.

Based on

Chapter 17: The Oral Cavity and Salivary Glands

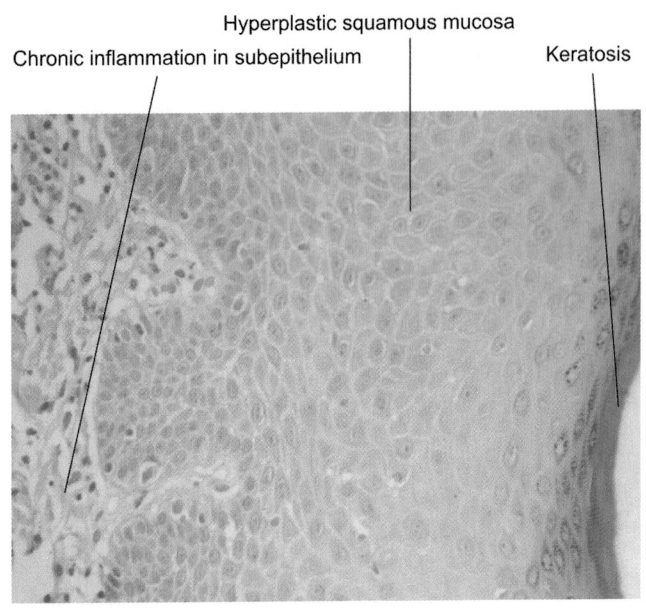

CL 85. Leukoplakia oral cavity
(H & E, × 100). Details on p 537.

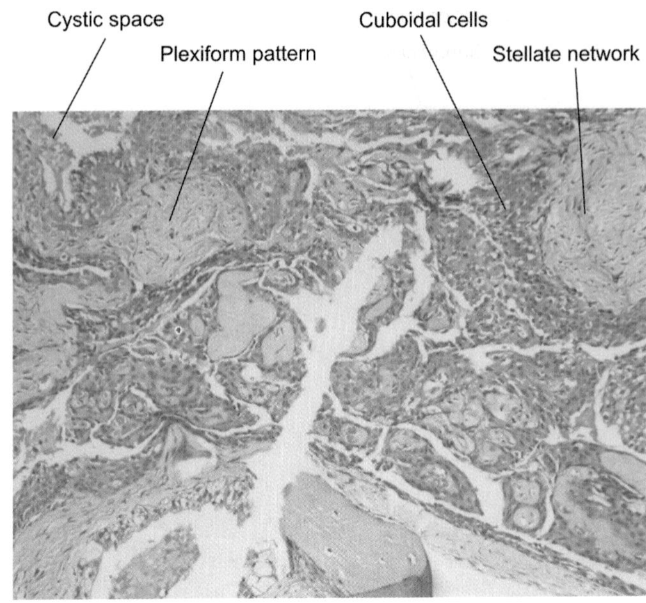

CL 86. Ameloblastoma
(H & E, × 100). Details on p 542.

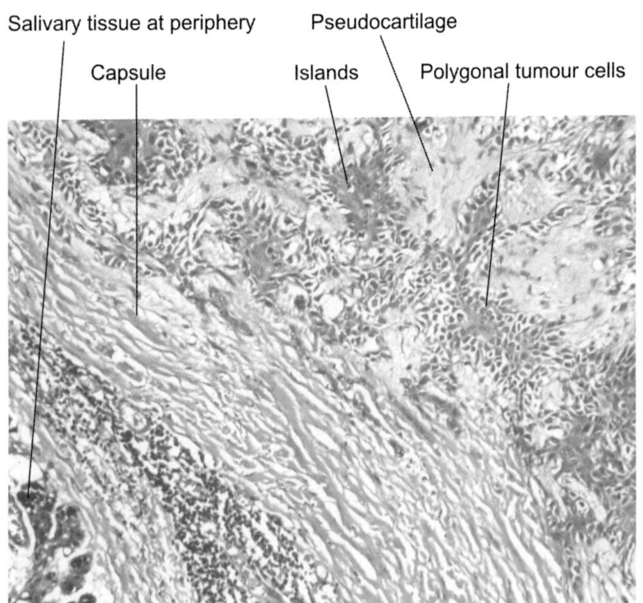

CL 87. Pleomorphic adenoma (mixed salivary tumour)
(H & E, × 100). Details on p 546.

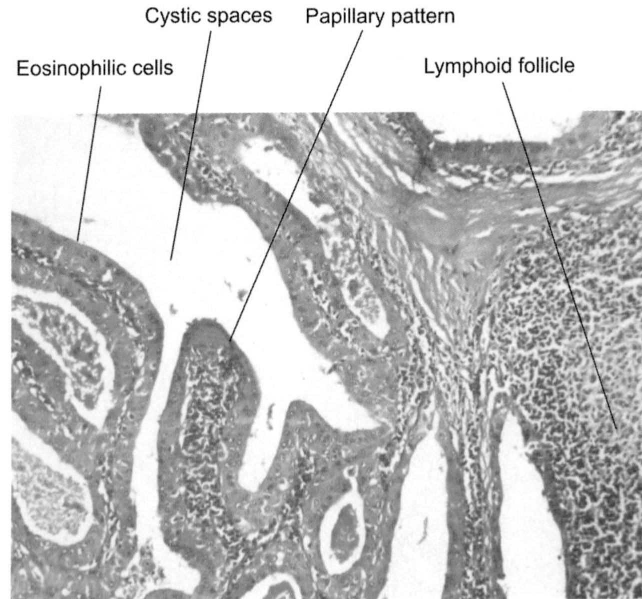

CL 88. Warthin's tumour
(H & E, × 100). Details on p 547.

Based on

Chapter 18: The Gastrointestinal Tract

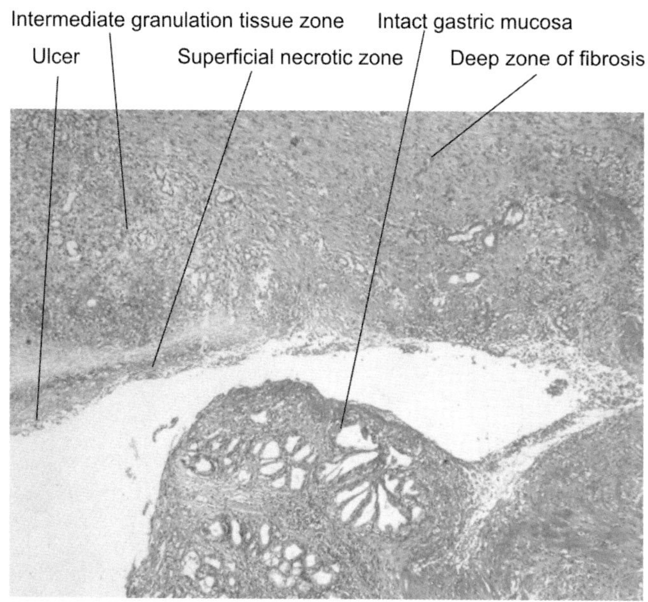

CL 89. Peptic ulcer
(H & E, × 100). Details on p 567.

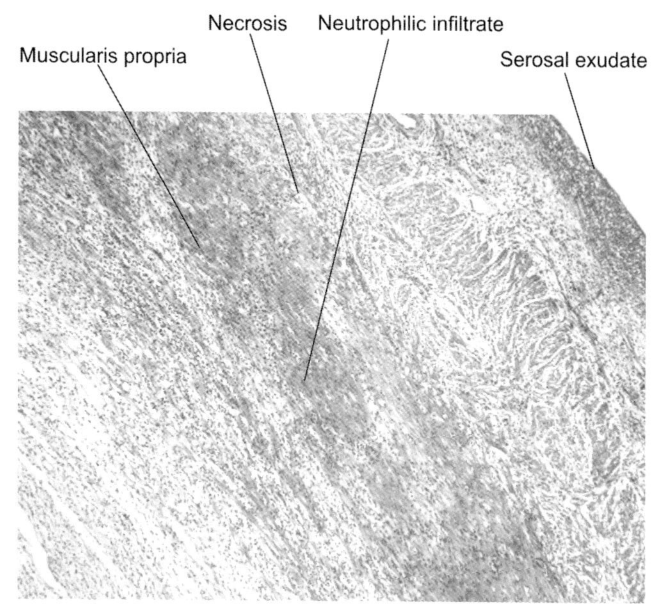

CL 90. Acute appendicitis
(H & E, × 100). Details on p 593.

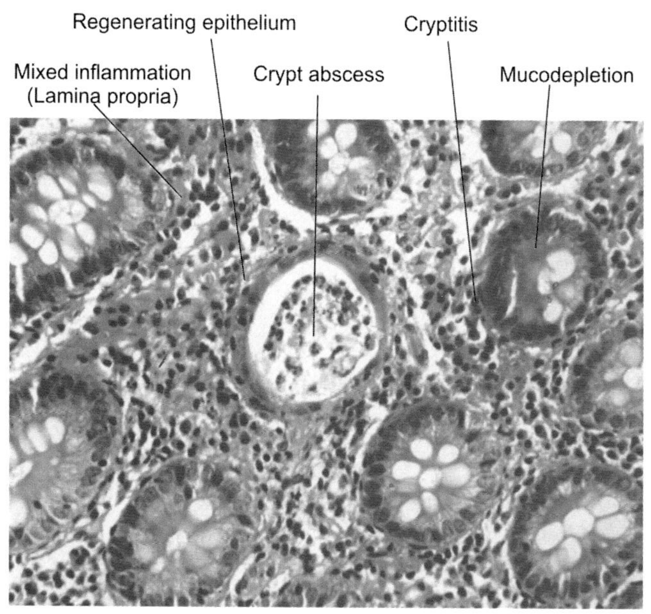

CL 91. Ulcerative colitis
(H & E, × 200). Details on p 583.

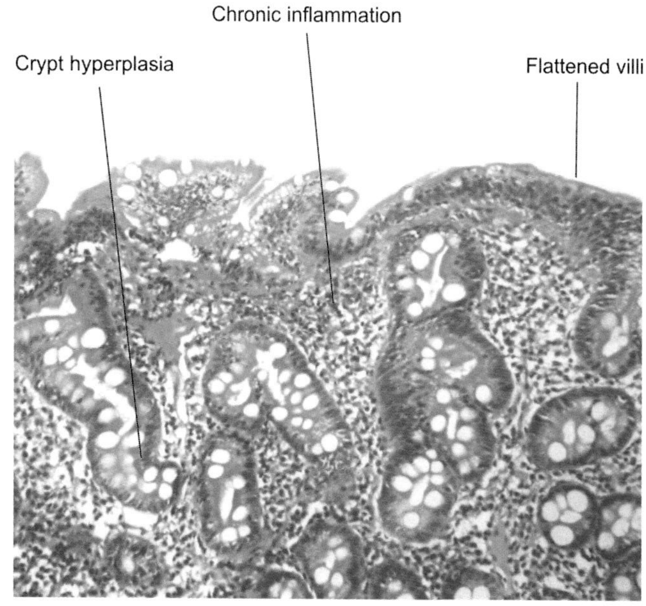

CL 92. Subtotal villous atrophy
(H & E × 100). Details on p 590.

Based on

Chapter 18: The Gastrointestinal Tract

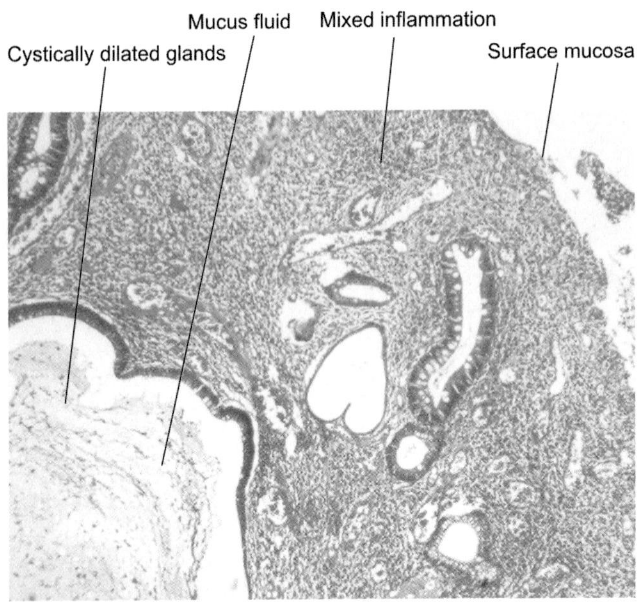

CL 93. Juvenile polyp
(H & E, × 40). Details on p 598.

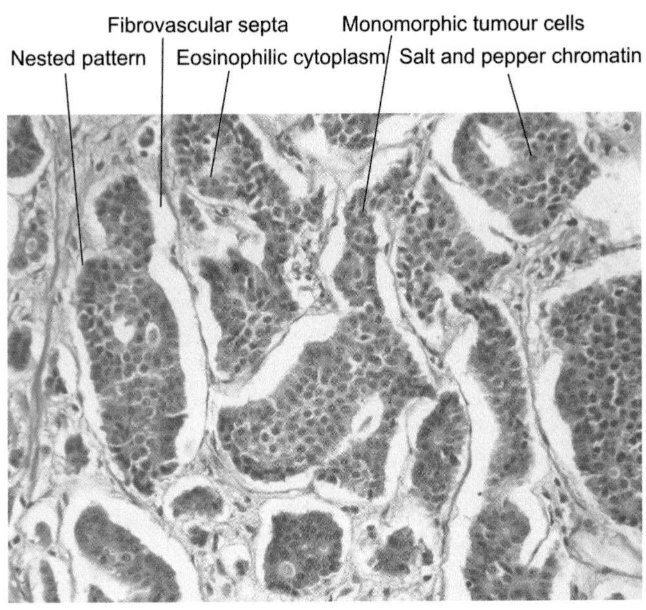

CL 94. Carcinoid tumour small intestine
(H & E, × 200). Details on p 592.

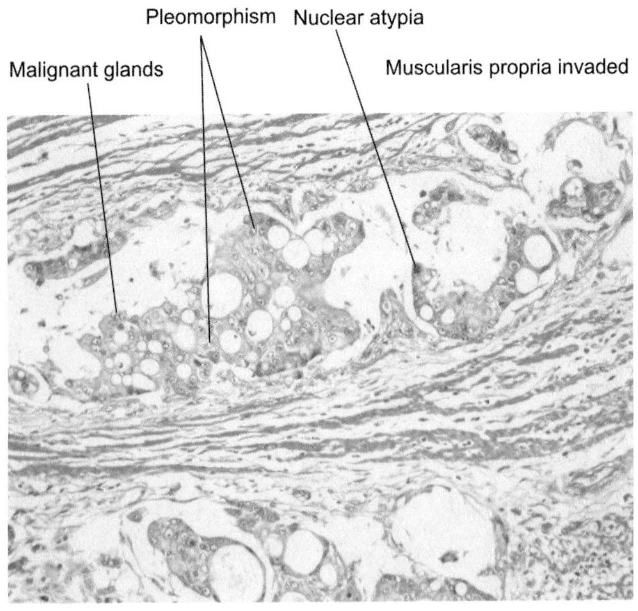

CL 95. Adenocarcinoma alimentary tract
(H & E, × 100). Details on p 573, 604.

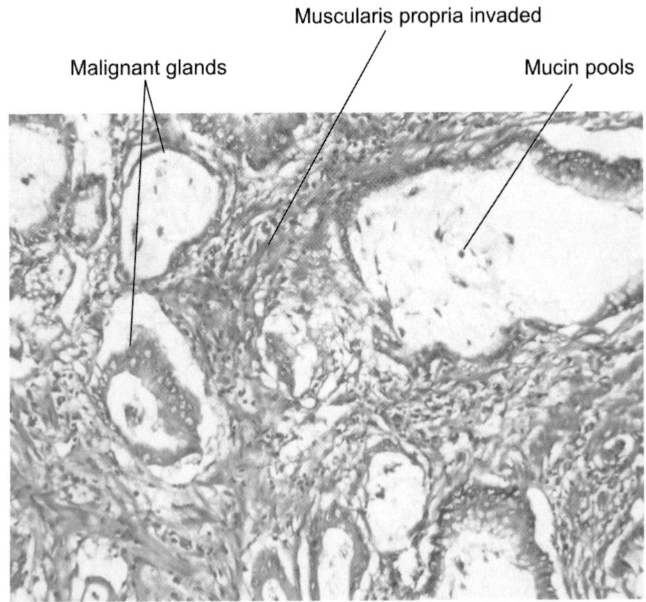

CL 96. Mucin-secreting adenocarcinoma alimentary tract
(H & E, × 100). Details on p 573, 604.

Based on

Chapter 19: The Liver, Biliary Tract and Exocrine Pancreas

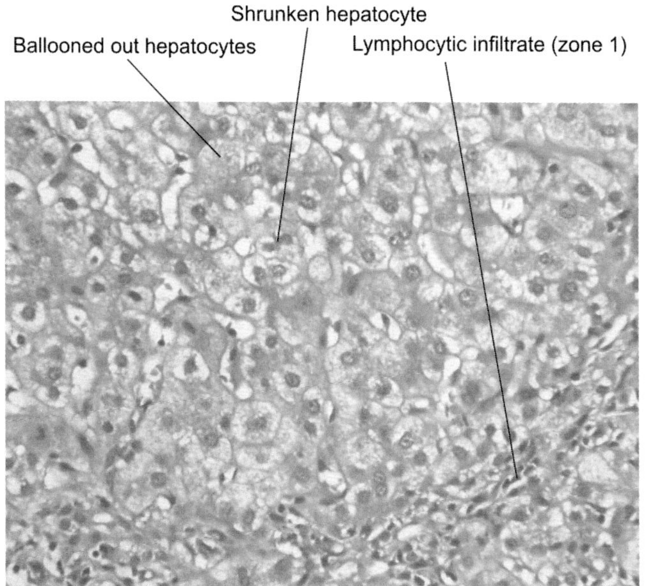

CL 97. Acute viral hepatitis
(H & E, × 200). Details on p 631.

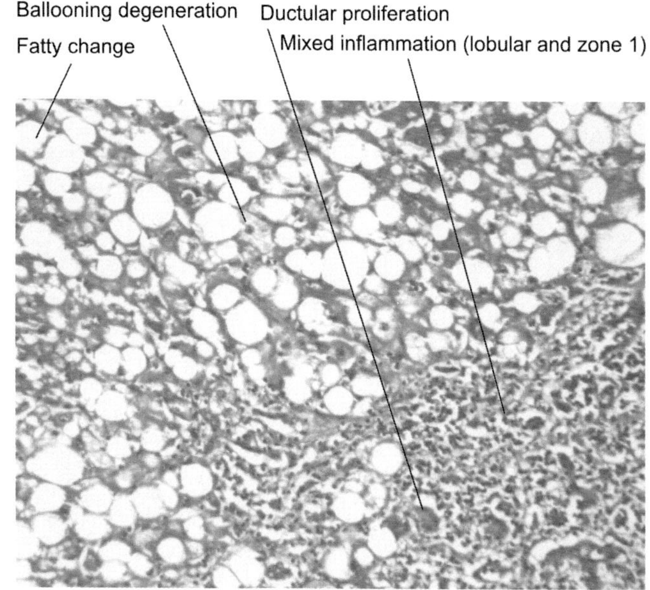

CL 98. Alcoholic hepatitis
(H & E, × 100). Details on p 642.

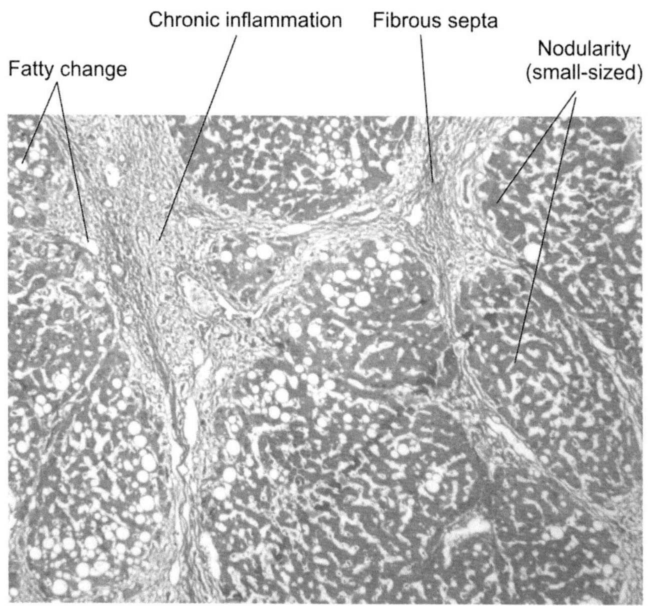

CL 99. Alcoholic (micronodular) cirrhosis
(H & E, × 40). Details on p 643.

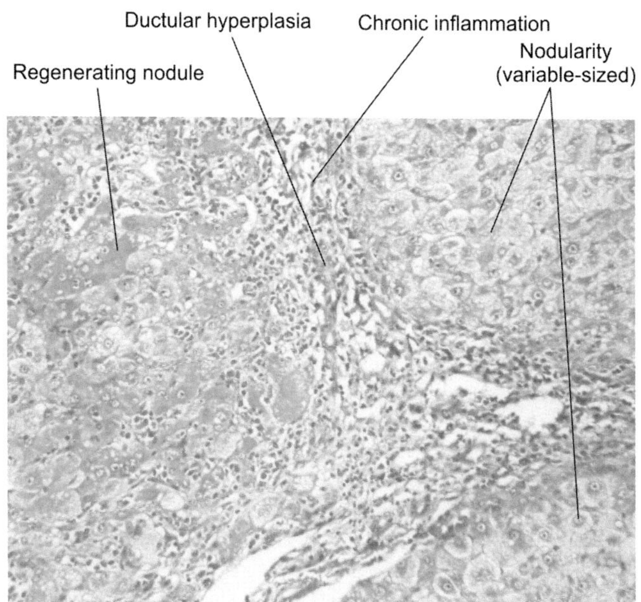

CL 100. Post-necrotic (macronodular) cirrhosis
(H & E, × 100). Details on p 644.

Based on

Chapter 19: The Liver, Biliary Tract and Exocrine Pancreas

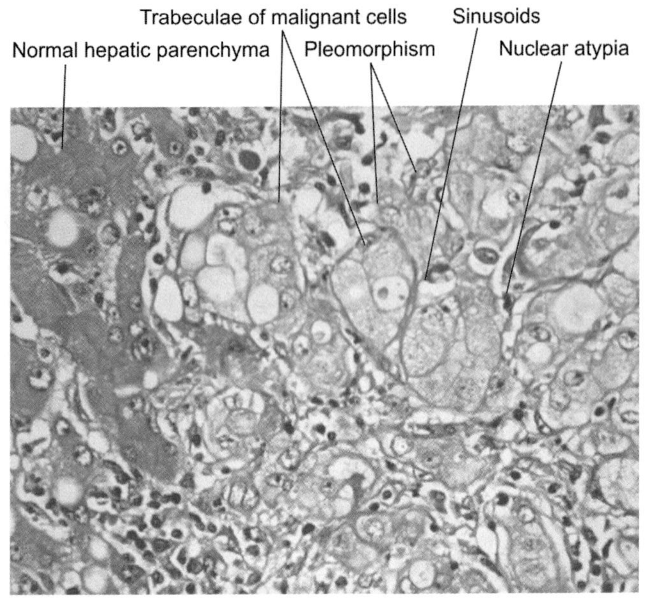

CL 101. Hepatocellular carcinoma
(H & E, × 100). Details on p 655.

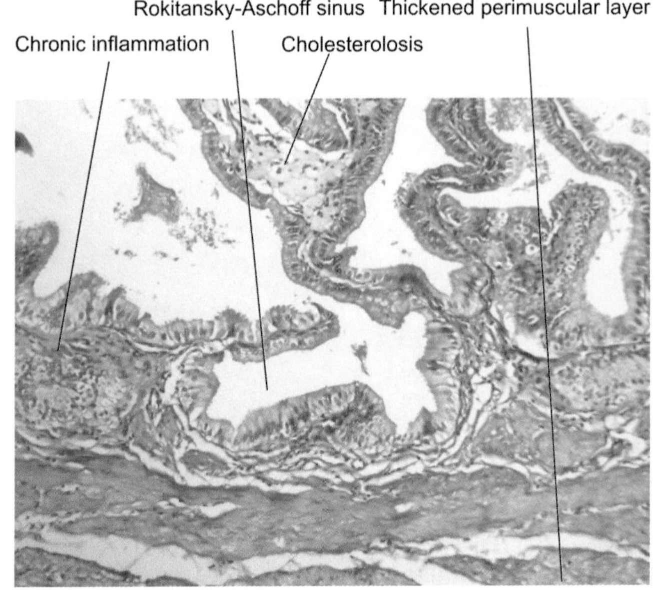

CL 102. Chronic cholecystitis with cholesterolosis
(H & E, × 100). Details on p 662.

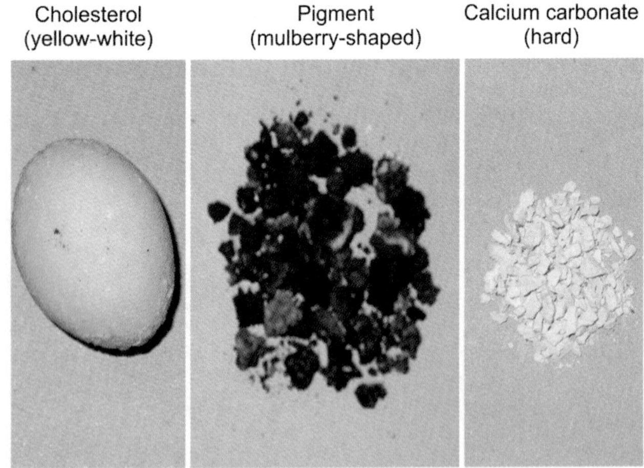

CL 103. Gallstones, pure types
Details on p 660.

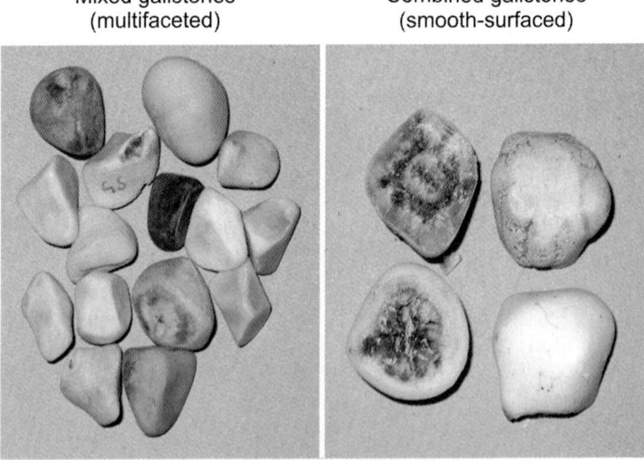

CL 104. Gallstones, mixed and combined types
Details on p 660.

Based on
Chapter 20: The Kidney and Lower Urinary Tract

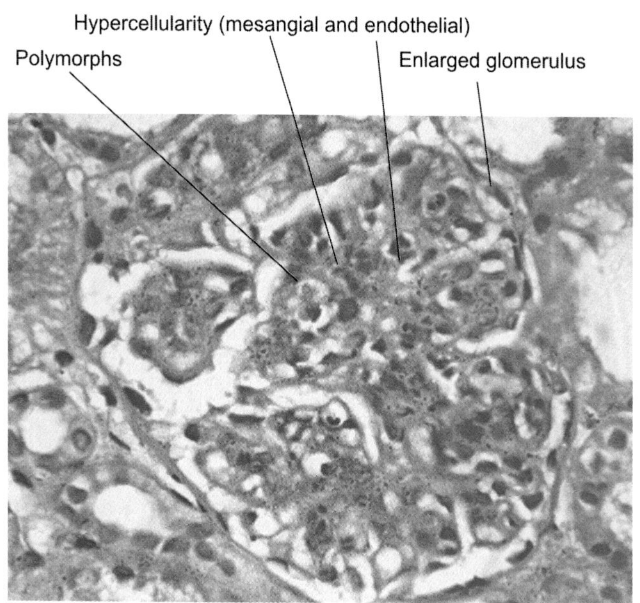

CL 105. Acute glomerulonephritis
(H & E, × 400). Details on p 690.

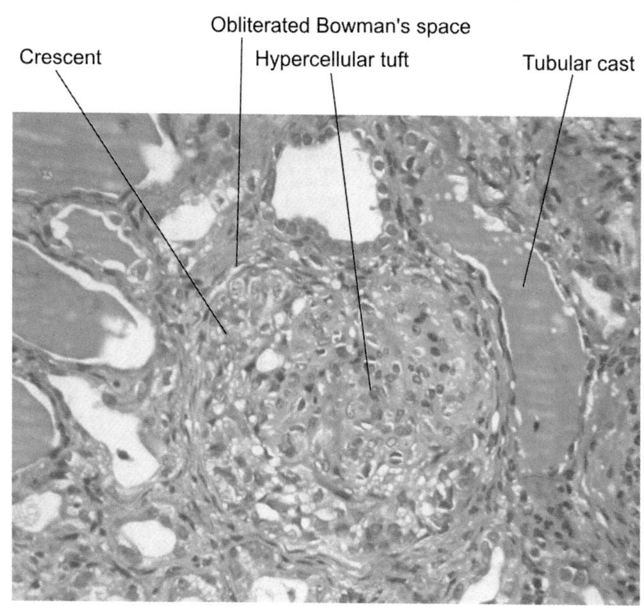

CL 106. Rapidly progressive glomerulonephritis
(H & E, × 200). Details on p 691.

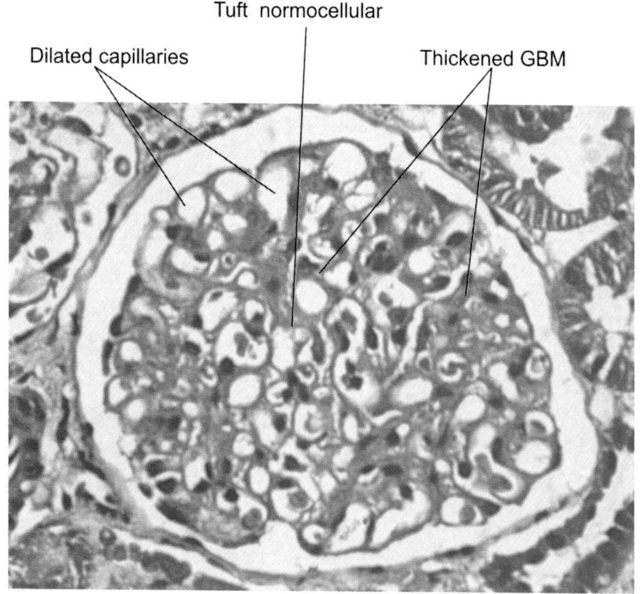

CL 107. Membranous glomerulonephritis
(H & E, × 400). Details on p 694.

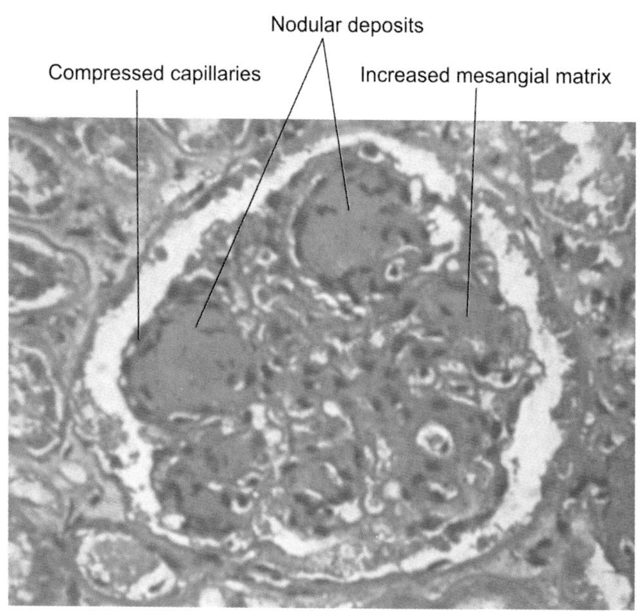

CL 108. Diabetic glomerulosclerosis: nodular (KW) lesions
(H & E, × 400). Details on p 701.

Based on

Chapter 20: The Kidney and Lower Urinary Tract

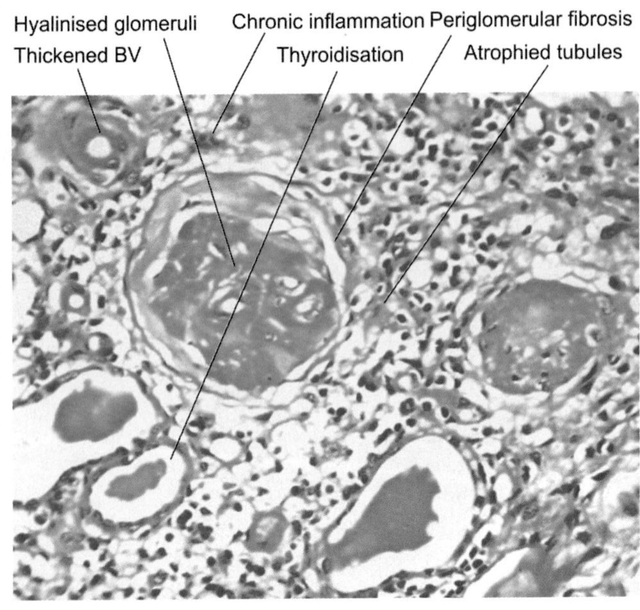

CL 109. Chronic pyelonephritis
(H & E, × 200). Details on p 707.

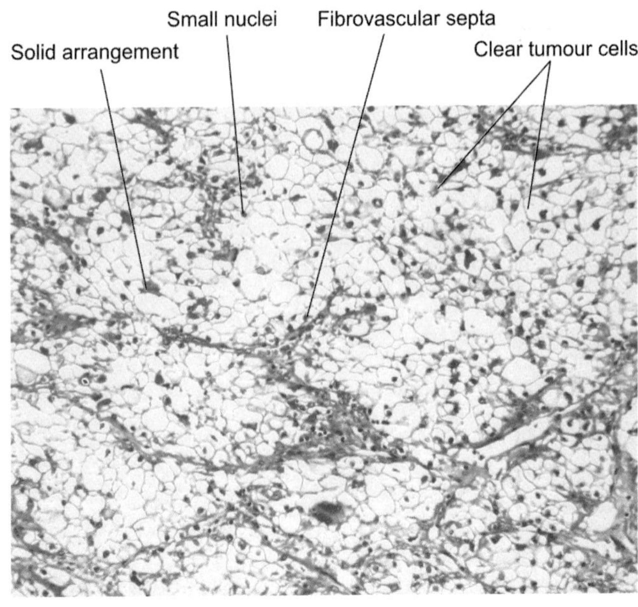

CL 110. Adenocarcinoma kidney
(H & E, × 100). Details on p 720.

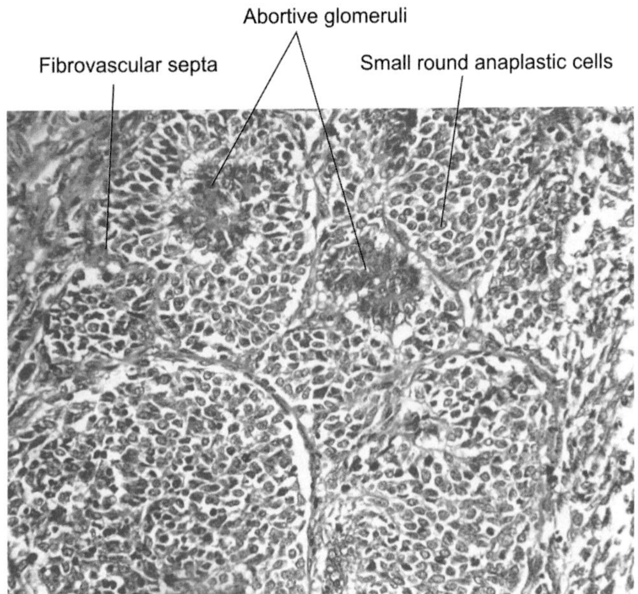

CL 111. Wilms' tumour
(H & E, × 200). Details on p 721.

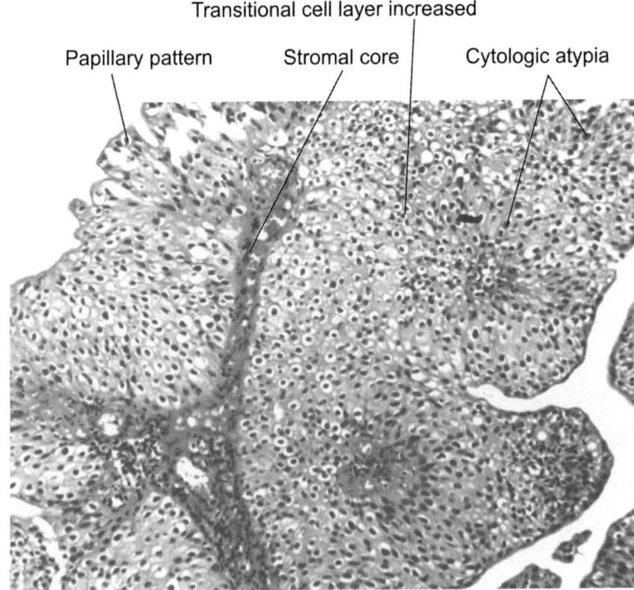

CL 112. Transitional cell carcinoma urinary bladder
(H & E, × 100). Details on p 725.

Based on

Chapter 21: The Male Reproductive System and Prostate

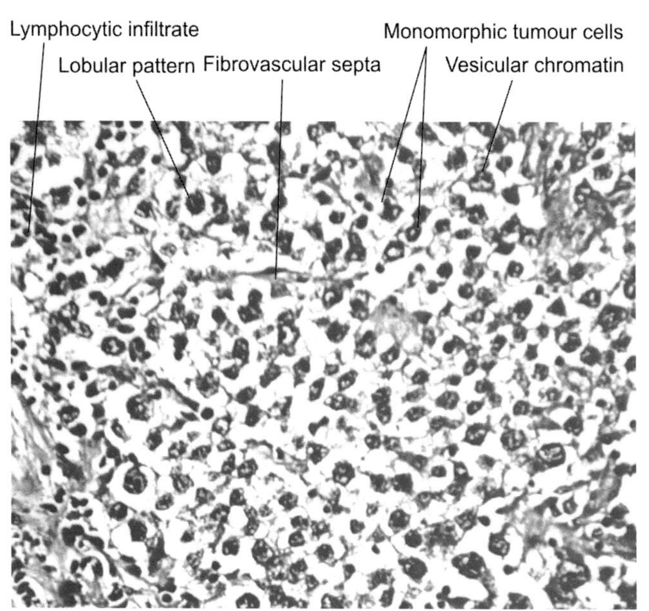

CL 113. Seminoma testis
(H & E, × 200). Details on p 735.

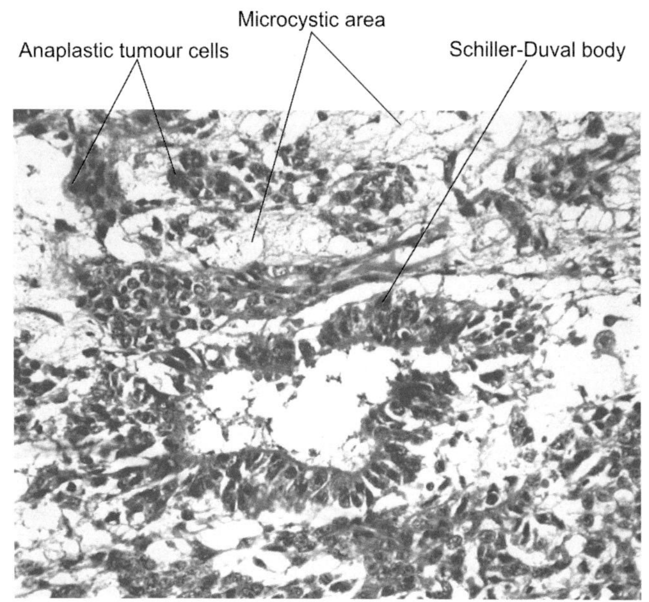

CL 114. Yolk sac tumour testis
(H & E, × 200). Details on p 736.

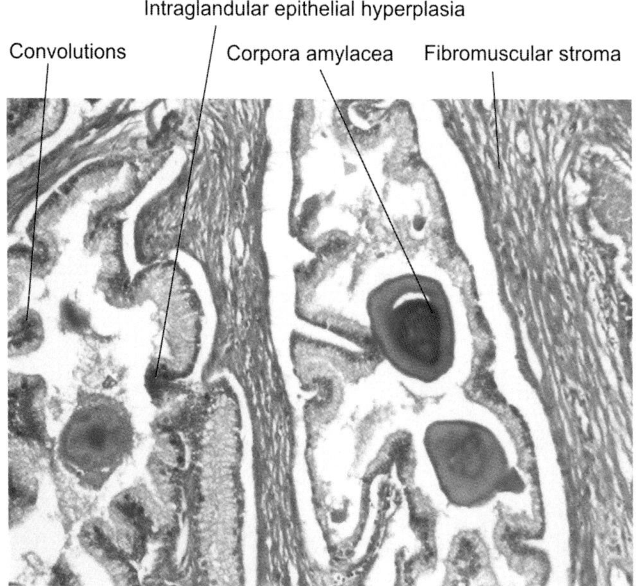

CL 115. Nodular hyperplasia prostate
(H & E, × 100). Details on p 743.

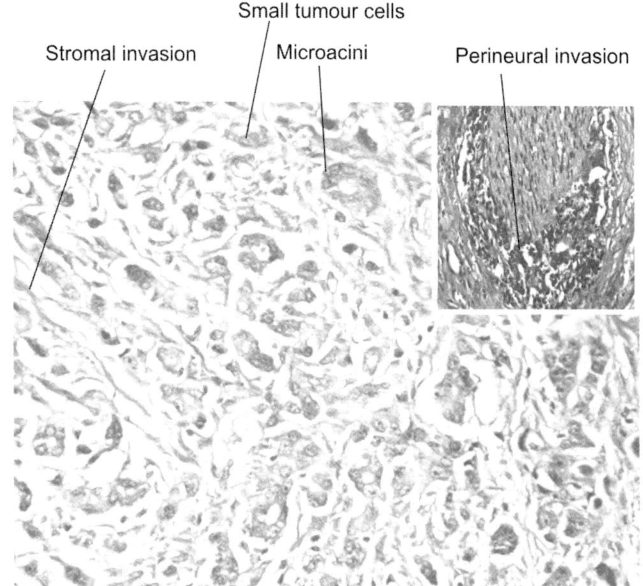

CL 116. Adenocarcinoma prostate
(H & E, × 100; inbox shows perineural invasion). Details on p 744.

Based on

Chapter 22: The Female Genital Tract

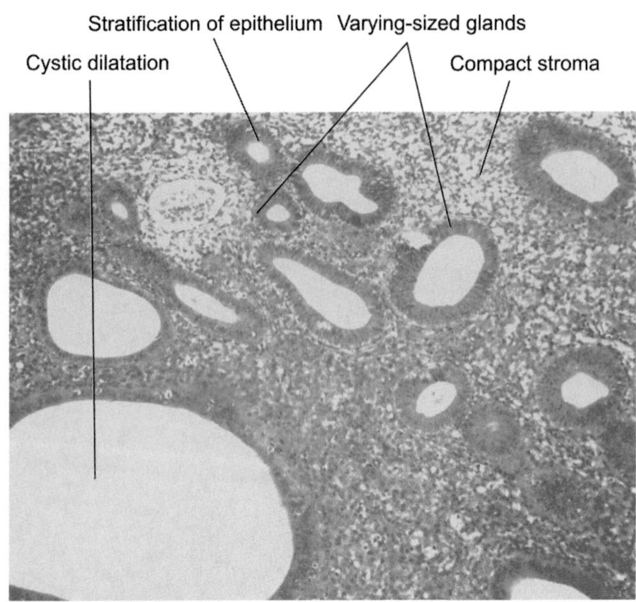

CL 117. Simple hyperplasia endometrium
(H & E, x 100). Details on p 759.

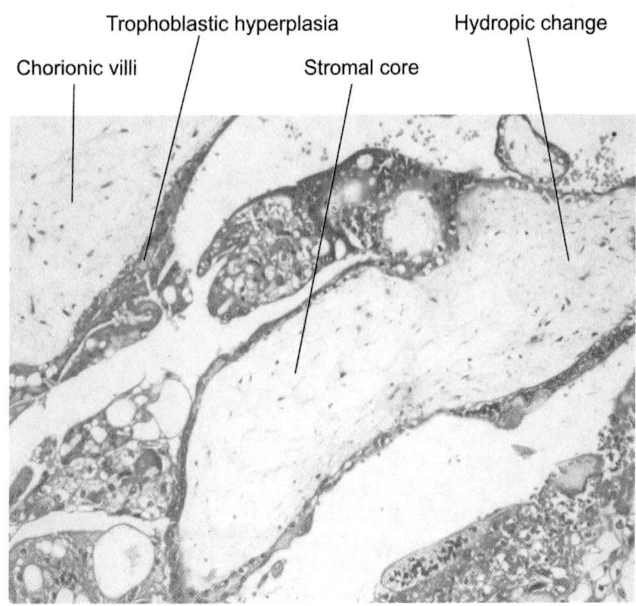

CL 118. Hydatidiform mole
(H & E, x 100). Details on p 777.

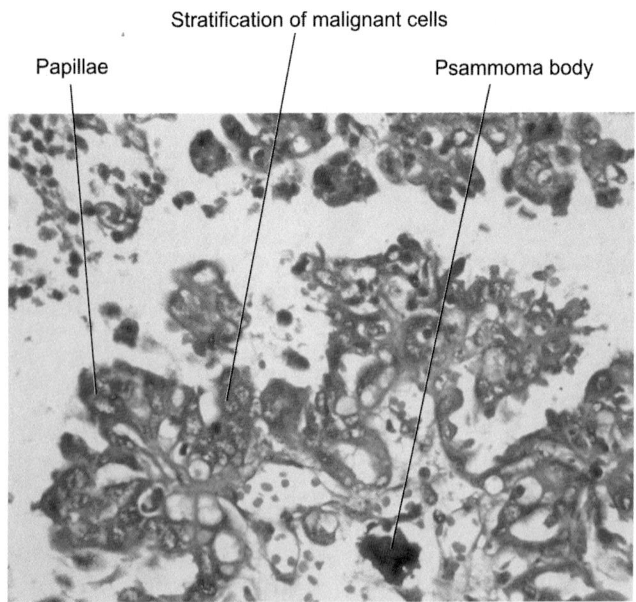

CL 119. Serous cystadenocarcinoma ovary
(H & E, x 200). Details on p 769.

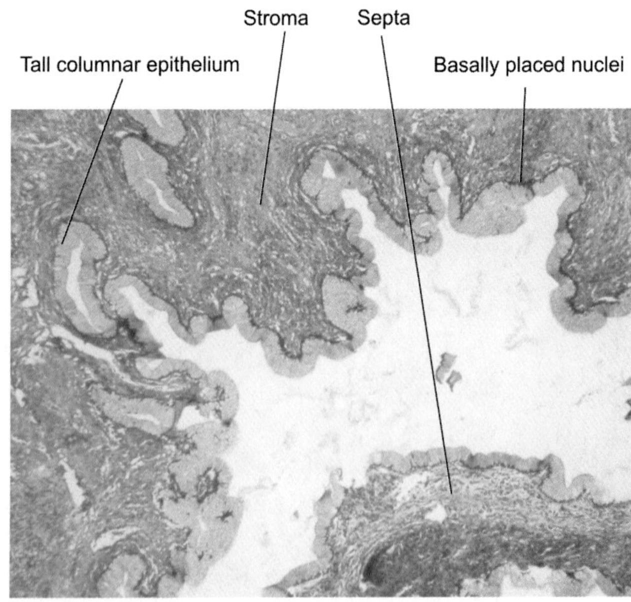

CL 120. Mucinous cystadenoma ovary
(H & E, x 100). Details on p 769.

Based on

Chapters 22, 23: The Female Genital Tract; The Breast

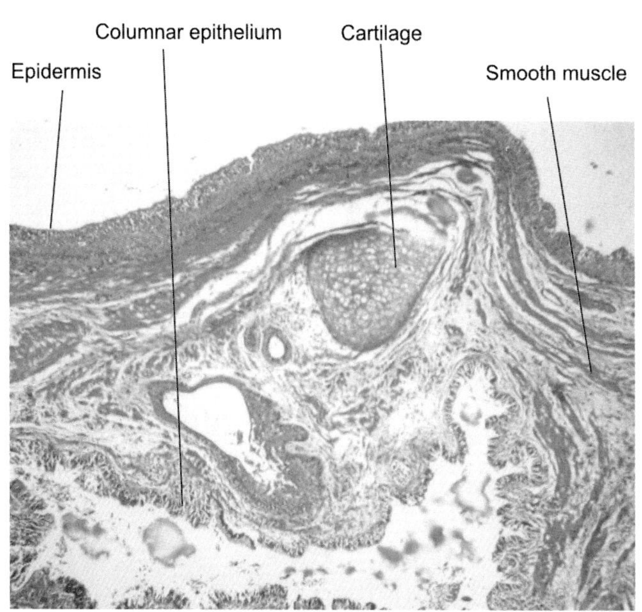

CL 121. Benign cystic teratoma ovary
(H & E, x 100). Details on p 772.

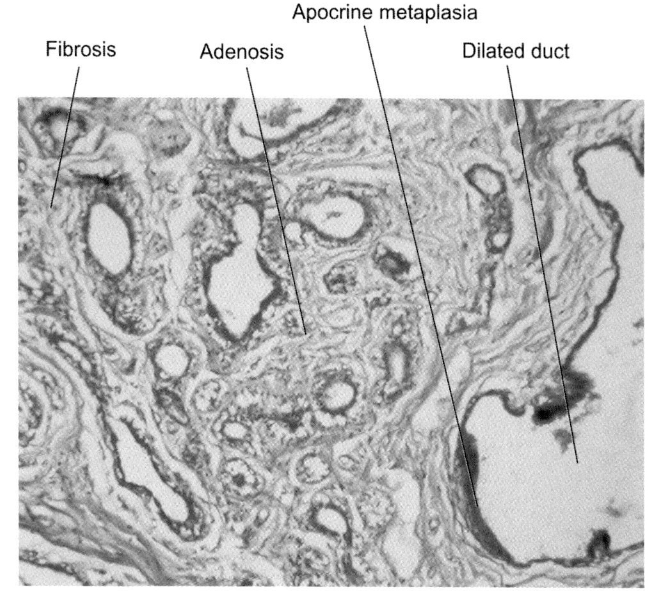

CL 122. Fibrocystic change breast
(H & E, x 100). Details on p 782.

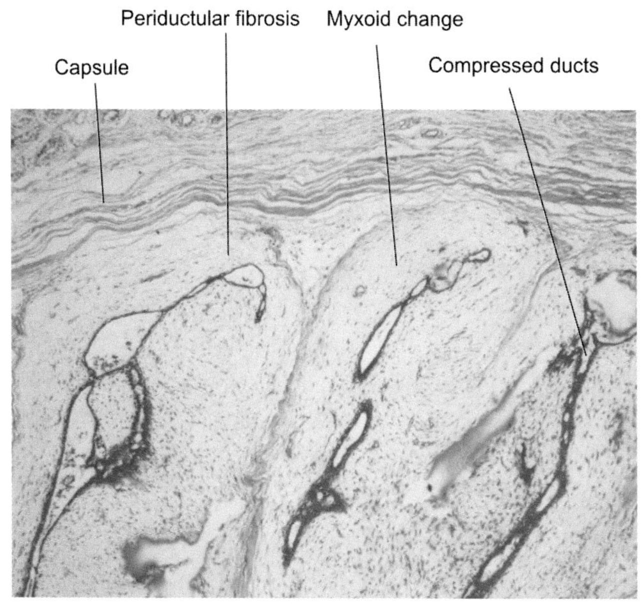

CL 123. Fibroadenoma breast
(H & E, x 100). Details on p 784.

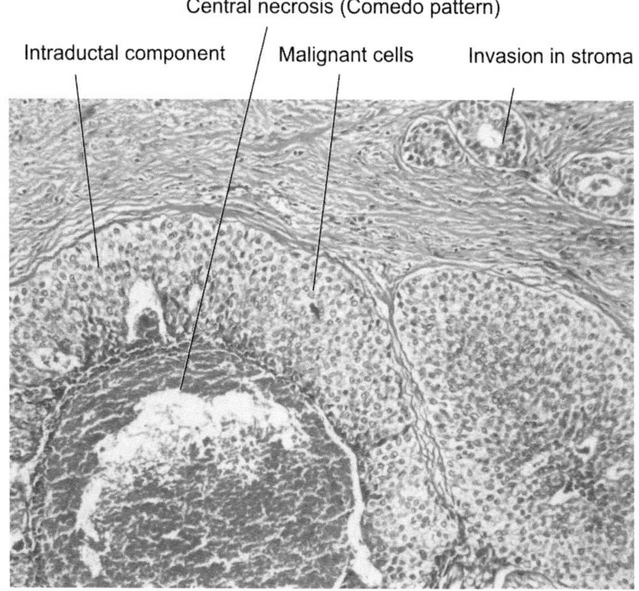

CL 124. Infiltrating duct carcinoma breast, NOS
(H & E, x 200). Details on p 788.

Based on

Chapter 25: The Endocrine System

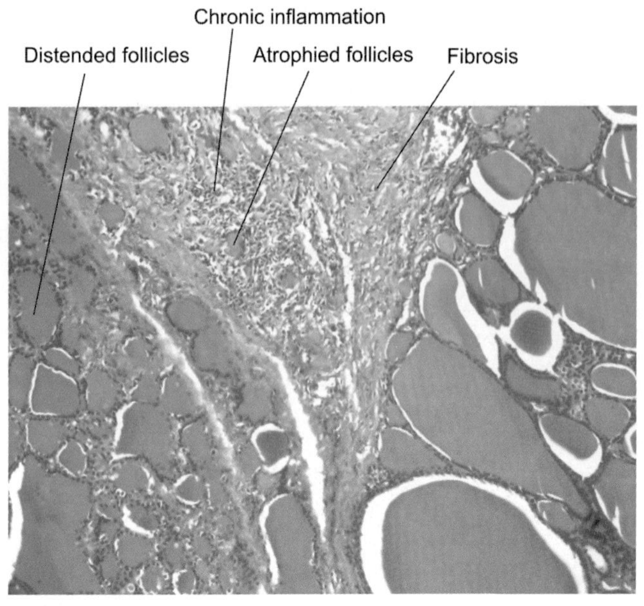

CL 125. Nodular goitre
(H & E, × 100). Details on p 833.

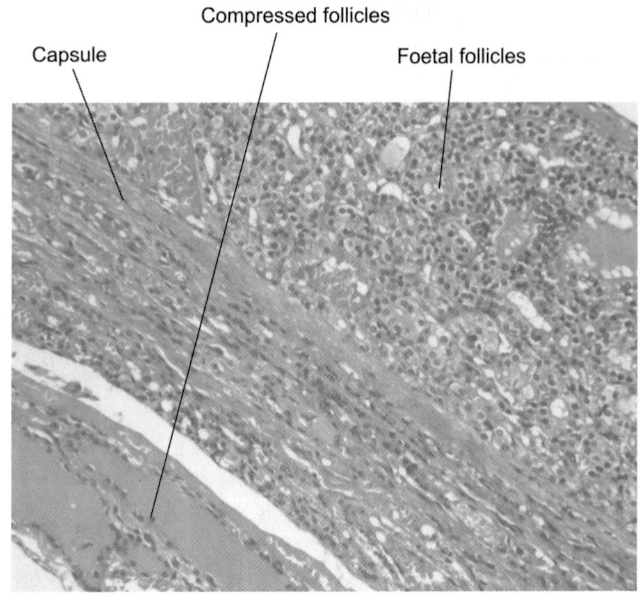

CL 126. Follicular adenoma thyroid
(H & E, × 100). Details on p 834.

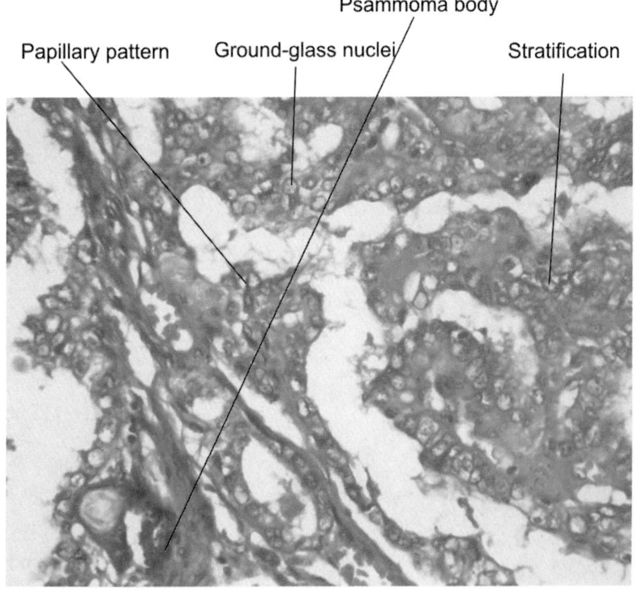

CL 127. Papillary carcinoma thyroid
(H & E, × 200). Details on p 836.

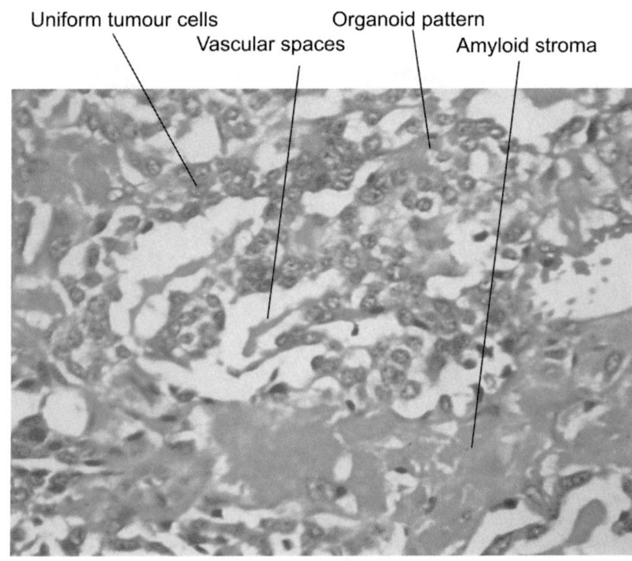

CL 128. Medullary carcinoma thyroid
(H & E, × 200). Details on p 838.

Based on

Chapter 26: The Musculoskeletal System

Chronic inflammatory cells
Acute inflammatory cells
Necrotic bone

CL 129. Chronic osteomyelitis
(H & E, × 200). Details on p 857.

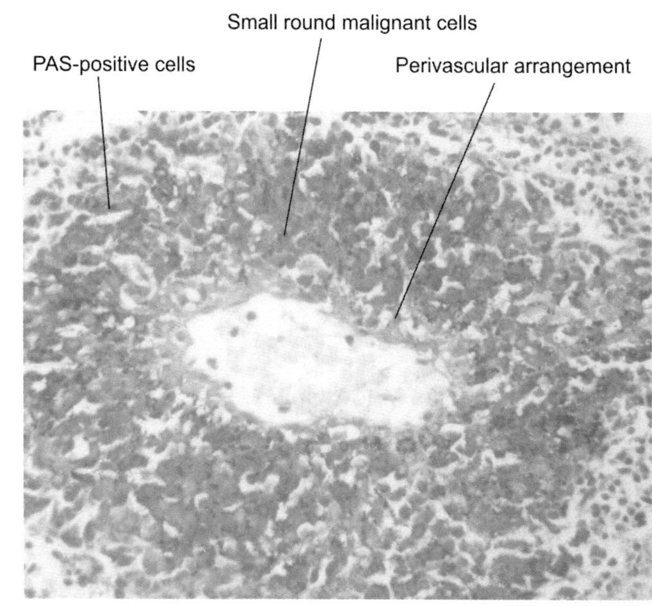

CL 130. Ewing's sarcoma
(PAS, × 400). Details on p 873.

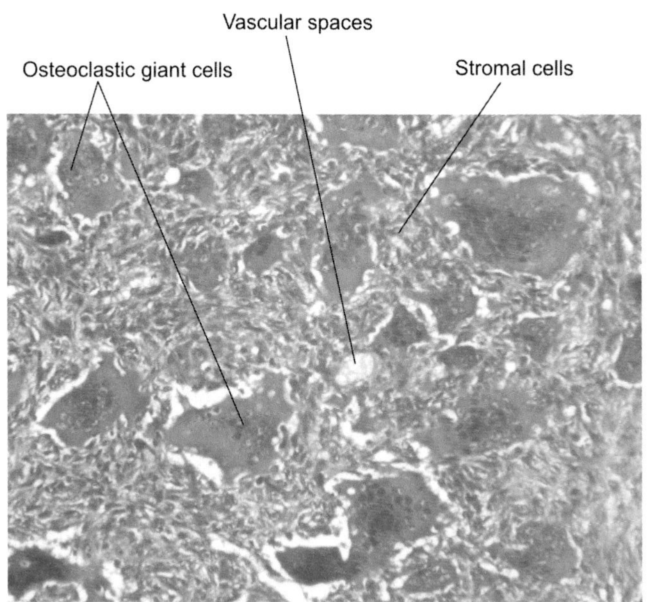

CL 131. Osteoclastoma
(H & E, × 100). Details on p 871.

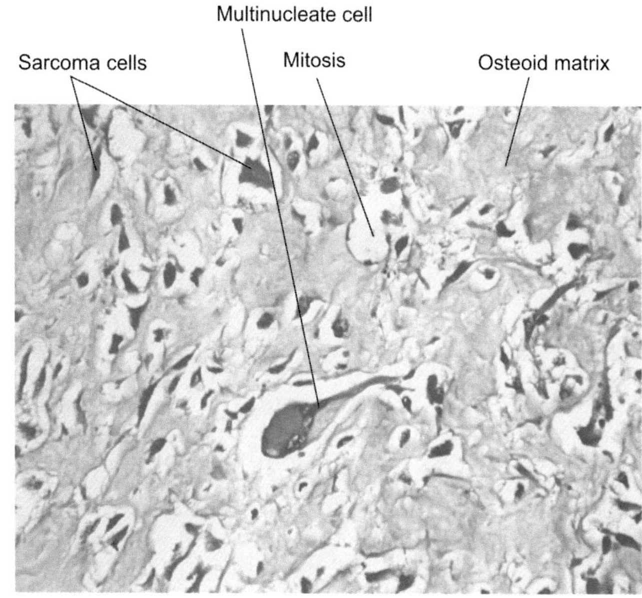

CL 132. Osteosarcoma
(H & E, × 400). Details on p 867.

Based on

Chapters 26, 28: The Musculoskeletal System; The Nervous System

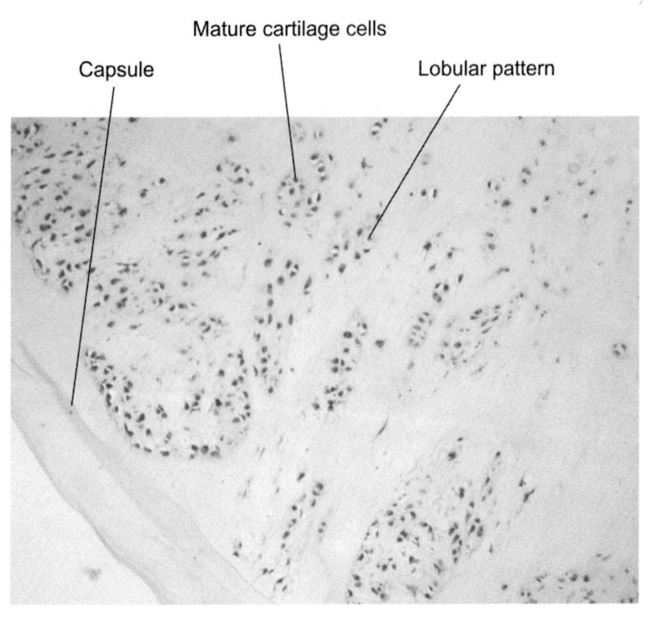

CL 133. Enchondroma
(H & E, × 100). Details on p 869.

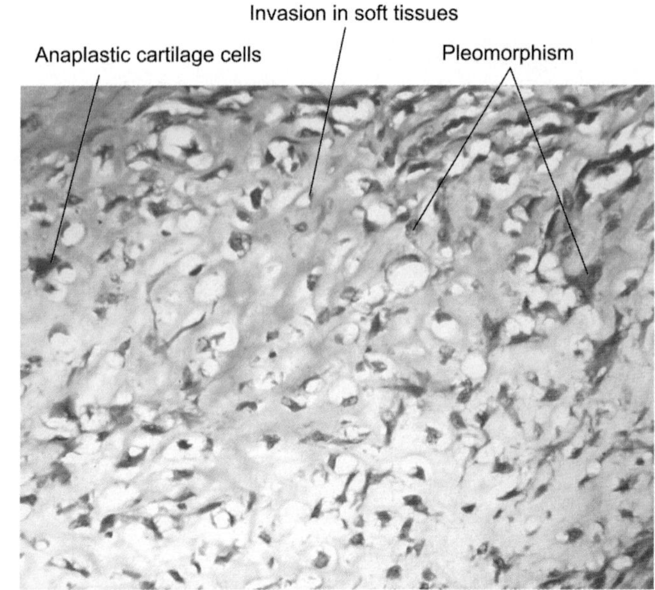

CL 134. Chondrosarcoma
(H & E, × 200). Details on p 871.

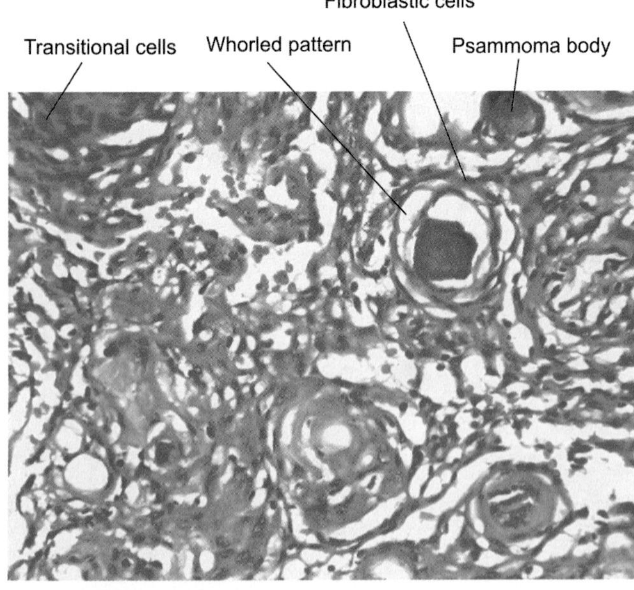

CL 135. Meningioma
(H & E, × 100). Details on p 916.

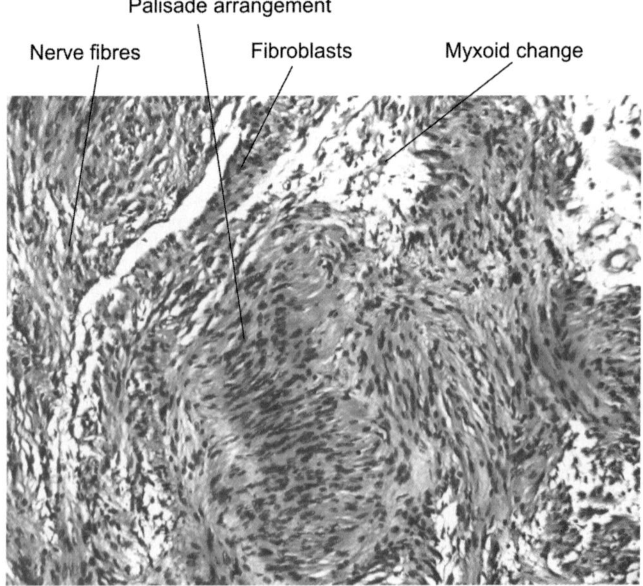

CL 136. Neurilemmoma
(H & E, × 100). Details on p 919.

Based on

Chapter 29: Diagnostic Cytopathology

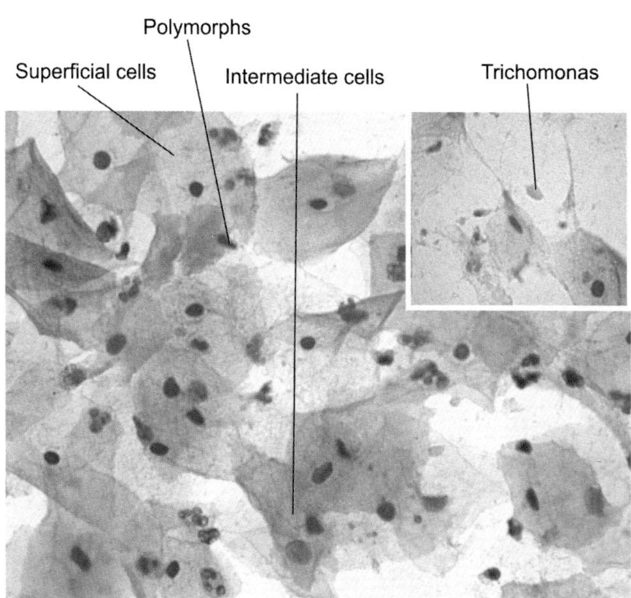

CL 137. Pap smear, inflammatory
(Pap, × 400; inbox shows Trichomonas). Details on p 924.

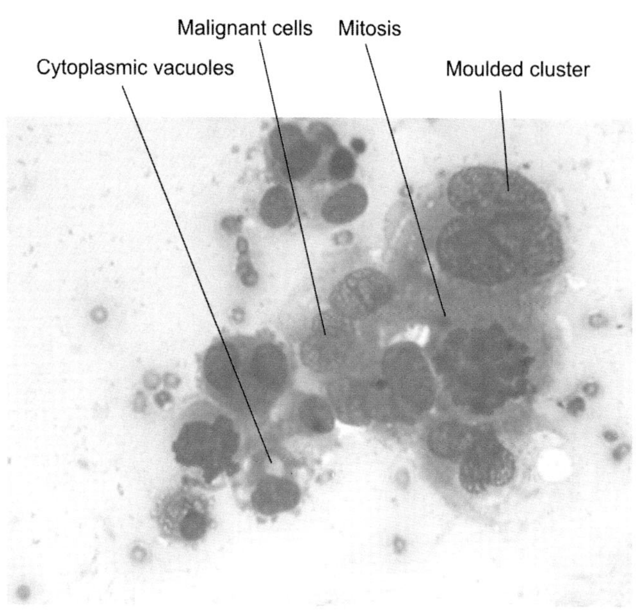

CL 138. Adenocarcinoma in ascitic fluid
(MGG, × 400). Details on p 929.

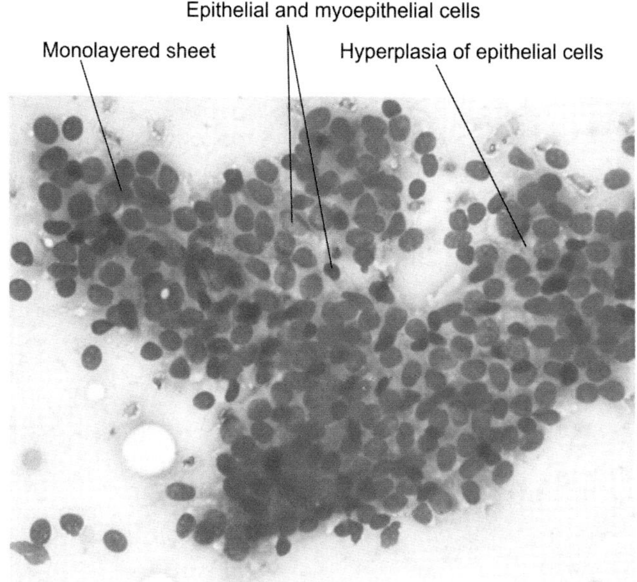

CL 139. FNA breast, fibroadenoma
(H & E, × 200). Details on p 934.

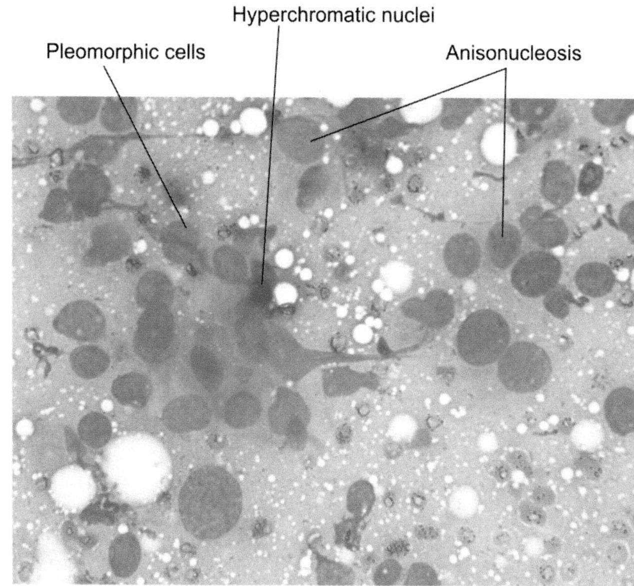

CL 140. FNA breast, infiltrating duct carcinoma
(MGG, × 400). Details on p 934.

Based on
Chapter 29: Diagnostic Cytopathology

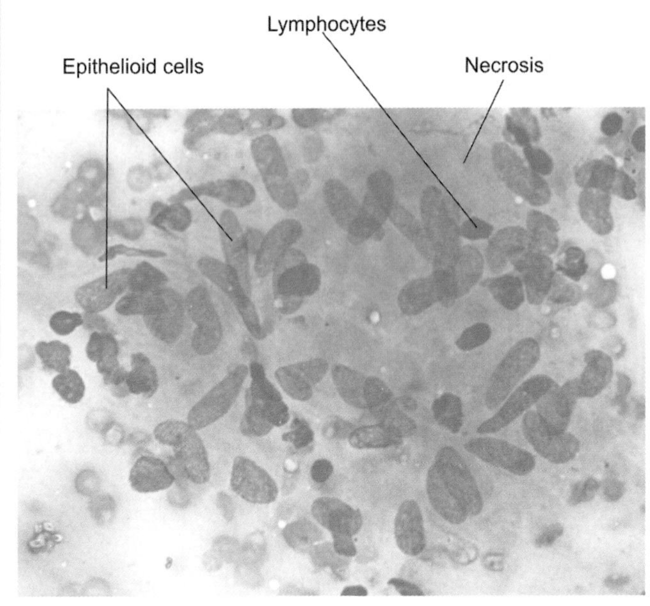

CL 141. FNA lymph node, tuberculosis
(MGG, × 400). Details on p 934.

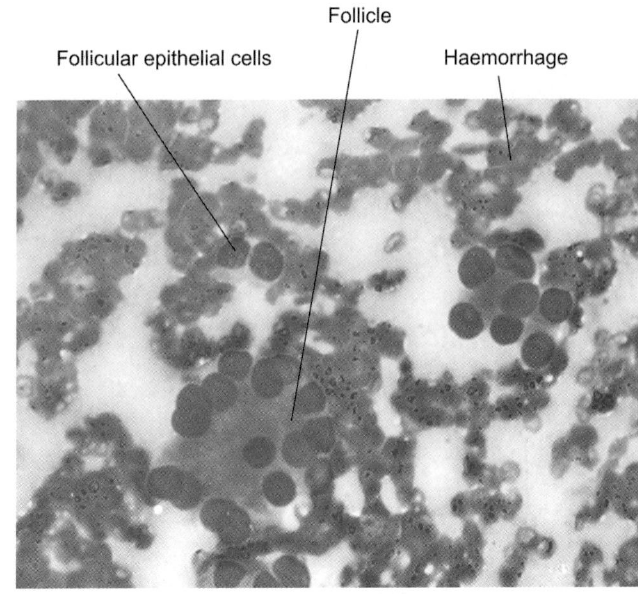

CL 142. FNA thyroid, follicular neoplasm
(MGG, × 400). Details on p 934.

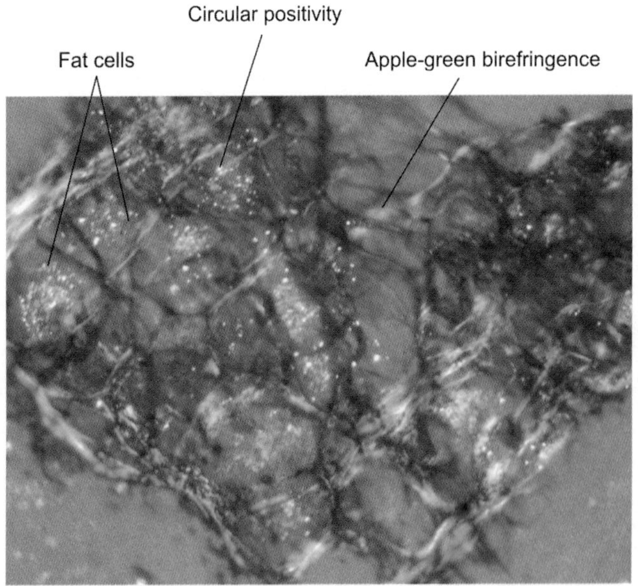

CL 143. Amyloidosis: abdominal fat aspirate
(Congo red under polaring light × 400). Details on p 938.

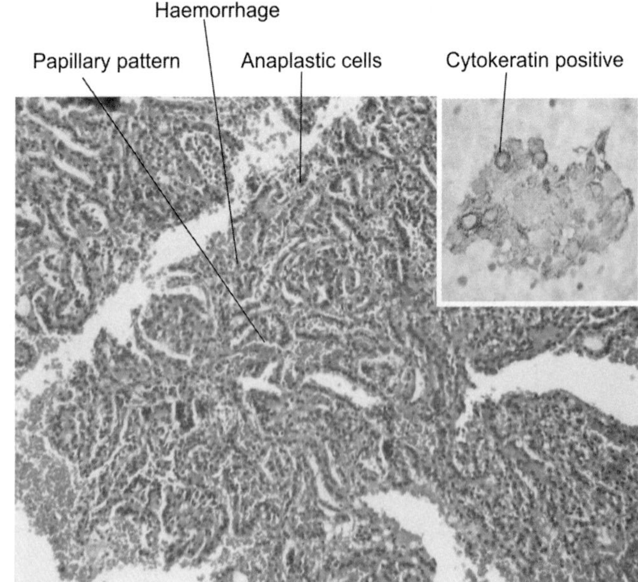

CL 144. Section of cell block: renal cell carcinoma
(H & E, × 100; inbox shows positive cytokeratin). Details on p 937.

SECTION I

GENERAL PATHOLOGY

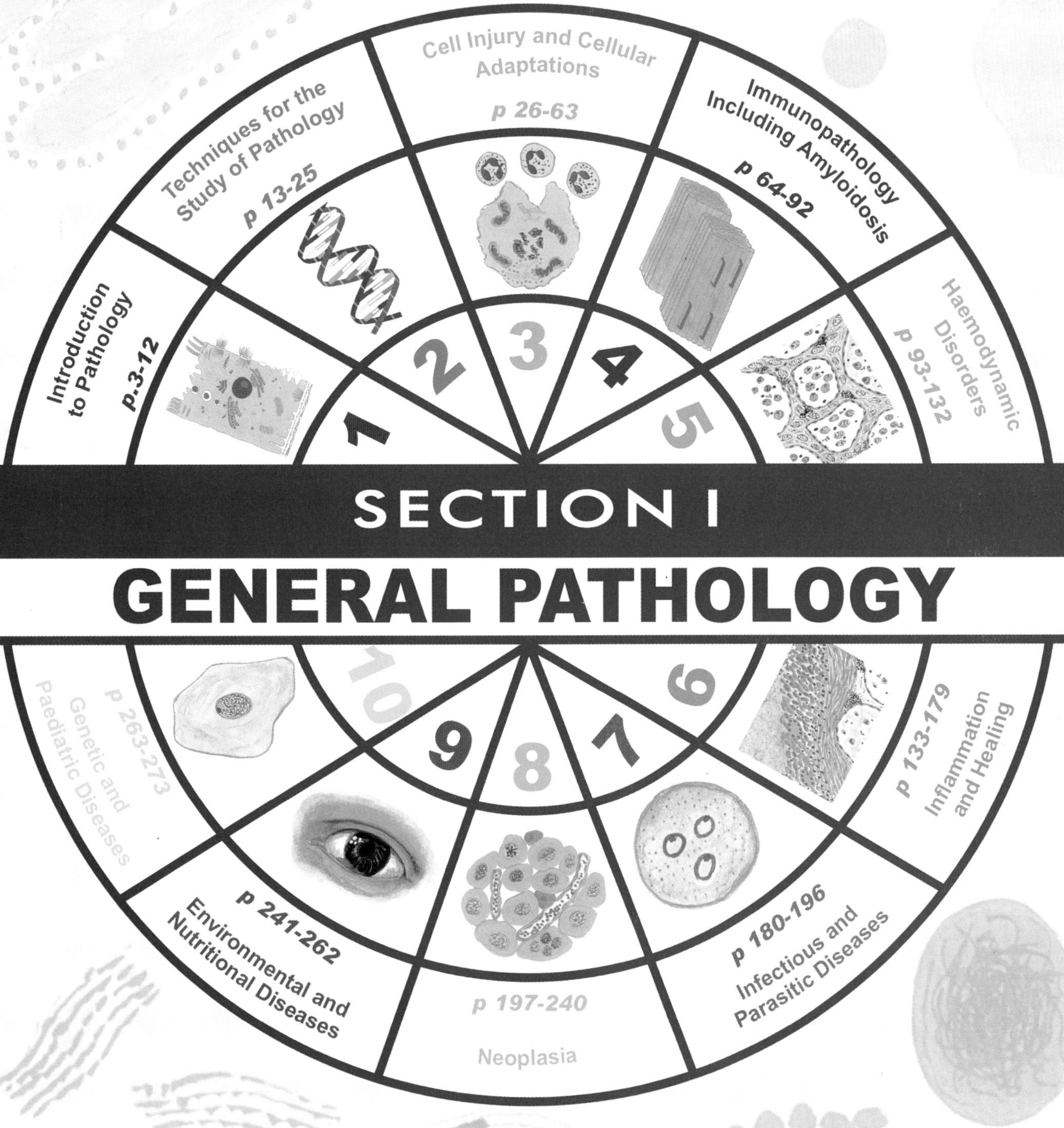

Introduction to Pathology

1

DEFINITION OF PATHOLOGY

The word *'Pathology'* is derived from two Greek words—*pathos* meaning suffering, and *logos* meaning study. Pathology is, thus, scientific study of structure and function of the body in disease; it deals with causes, effects, mechanisms and nature of disease. The knowledge and understanding of pathology is essential for all would-be doctors as well as general practitioners and specialists since unless they know the causes and mechanisms of disease and understand the language spoken by the pathologist in the form of laboratory reports, they would not be able to institute appropriate treatment or suggest preventive measures to the patient. For the medical student, the discipline of pathology forms a vital bridge between initial learning phase of preclinical sciences and the final phase of clinical subjects.

As we shall see in the pages that follow, pathology has evolved over the years as a distinct discipline from other branches—anatomy, medicine and surgery, in that sequence. After having emerged as a laboratory phase of medicine (and surgery), pathology is now not confined to laboratories alone, particularly in fields such as aspiration cytology and haematology which involve cytopathologist and haematologist in laboratory as well as in clinical phase of patientcare.

HEALTH AND DISEASE

Since pathology is the study of disease, then what is *disease*? In simple language, disease is opposite of health i.e. what is not healthy is disease. But the terms health and disease are difficult to define. *Health* is a condition when the individual is in complete accord with the surroundings, while *disease* is loss of ease to the body (dis-ease). However, it must be borne in mind that there is a wide range of 'normality' in health e.g. in height, weight, blood and tissue chemical composition etc. The confusion is further compounded by changes in health at cellular level since the cells display wide range of activities within the broad area of health similar to what is seen in diseased cells. In short, health and disease are not absolute but are considered as relative states.

A term commonly confused with disease is *illness*. While disease suggests an entity with a cause, illness is the reaction of the individual to disease in the form of symptoms (complaints of the patient) and physical signs (elicited by the clinician). Not to be ignored are the individual differences in reaction to disease. Though disease and illness are not separable, the study of diseases is done in pathology while the learning of illnesses will be done in wards and clinics.

In addition to disease and illness, there are *syndromes* (meaning running together) characterised by combination of symptoms caused by altered physiologic processes.

TERMINOLOGY IN PATHOLOGY

It is important for a beginner in pathology to be familiar with the language used in pathology:

- *Patient* is the person affected by disease.
- *Lesions* are the characteristic changes in tissues and cells produced by disease in an individual or experimental animal.
- *Pathologic changes* or *morphology* consist of examination of diseased tissues.

■ The pathologic changes can be recognised with the naked eye *(gross or macroscopic changes)* or studied by *microscopic examination* of tissues.
■ The causal factors responsible for the lesions are included in *etiology* of disease ('why' of disease).
■ The mechanism by which the lesions are produced is termed *pathogenesis* of disease ('how' of disease).
■ The functional implications of the lesion felt by the patient are *symptoms* and those discovered by the clinician are the *physical signs.*
■ The clinical significance of the morphologic and functional changes together with results of other investigations help to arrive at an answer to what is wrong *(diagnosis),* what is going to happen *(prognosis),* what can be done about it *(treatment),* and finally what should be done to avoid complications and spread *(prevention)* ('what' of disease).

EVOLUTION OF PATHOLOGY

The concept of disease is as old as life itself. Since the beginning of mankind, there has been desire as well as need to know more about the causes and mechanisms of disease. The answers to these questions have evolved over the centuries—from supernatural beliefs to the present state of our knowledge of modern pathology. However, pathology is not separable from other multiple disciplines of medicine and owes its development to interaction and interdependence on advances in diverse neighbouring branches of science and strides made in medical technology.

The brief review of fascinating history of pathology and its many magnificent personalities with their outstanding contribution in the opening pages of the book is meant to pay our obeisance to those great personalities who have laid glorious foundations of our speciality. Life and works of those whose names are cited below (which is far from complete) are linked to some disease or process—the aim being to stimulate the inquisitive beginner in pathology as to how this colourful speciality emerged.

FROM RELIGIOUS BELIEFSTO RATIONAL APPROACH (ANTIQUITYTO AD 1500)

The earliest concepts of disease were the religious beliefs that affliction or disease was the outcome of 'curse' or 'evil eye of spirits.' To ward them off, priests through prayers and sacrifices used to invoke supernatural powers to please the gods. The link between medicine and religion became so firmly established throughout the world that Greeks had *Aesculapius* as the god of healing, just as orthodox Indians pray to *Mata Sheetla* as goddess of healing for cure of smallpox.

The period of ancient religious beliefs was followed by the philosophical and rational approach to disease by the methods of observations. This happened at the time when great Greek philosophers—*Socrates, Plato* and *Aristotle,* introduced philosophical concepts to all natural phenomena.

But the real practice of medicine began with *Hippocrates* (460–377 BC), the great Greek clinical genius of all times and regarded as 'the father of medicine' (Fig. 1.1). He first stressed study of patient's symptoms and described methods of diagnosis. According to him, disturbances in equilibrium of the body resulted in an illness. He recorded his observations on cases in writing which remained the mainstay of medicine for nearly two thousand years. The most famous work of Hippocrates was his aphorisms based on his vast experience, many of which have turned into medical proverbs e.g.

'Those naturally very fat are more liable to sudden death than the thin.'

'In acute diseases, coldness of extremities is bad' etc.

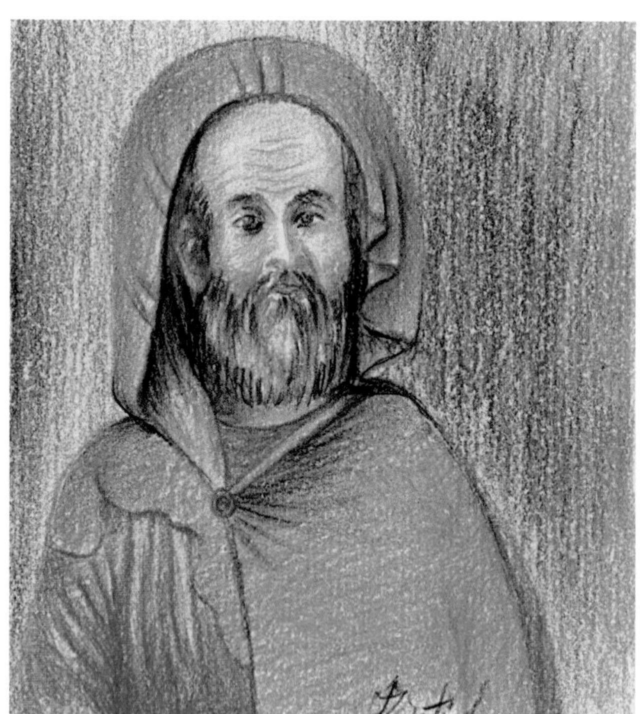

FIGURE 1.1

Hippocrates (460-377 BC). The great Greek clinical genius and regarded as 'the father of medicine'. He introduced ethical aspects to medicine.

Hippocrates introduced ethical concepts in the practice of medicine and is revered by the medical profession by taking *'Hippocratic Oath'* at the time of entry into practice of medicine.

Hippocratic teaching was further propagated in Rome by Roman physicians, notably by *Cornelius Celsus* (53 BC-7 AD) who first described four cardinal signs of inflammation—rubor (redness), tumor (swelling), calor (heat), and dolor (pain).

The hypothesis of disequilibrium of elements constituting the body *(Dhatus)* similar to Hippocratic doctrine finds mention in ancient Indian medicine books—*Charaka Samhita*, a finest document of the rational age by *Charaka* on medicine, and *Sushruta Samhita,* similar book of surgical sciences by *Sushruta,* both of which were compiled about AD 200. This concept of disease was hypothesised on fault caused by action of air *(vayu),* bile *(pitta)* and phlegm *(kapha).*

Around the same time, *Cladius Galen* (130–200 AD) in Rome postulated humoral theory, later called Galenic theory. This theory suggested that the illness resulted from imbalance between *four humors* (or body fluids): blood, lymph, black bile (believed to be from the spleen), and biliary secretion from the liver. Galen regarded himself as a disciple of Hippocrates but unlike the simplicity of his mentor who could say 'I do not know', Galen considered himself infallible and dictator in medicine and had an answer to every problem and every phenomena. Galen wrote about 80 books on diverse fields of medicine which were read by the students of the art of the healing for centuries.

The end of Medieval period was marked by backward steps in medicine. There were widespread and devastating epidemics which reversed the process of rational thinking again to supernatural concepts and divine punishment for 'sins.' The dominant belief during this period was that life was due to influence of vital substance under the control of soul *(theory of vitalism).* Dissection of human body was strictly forbidden as that would mean hurting the 'soul.'

ERA OF GROSS PATHOLOGY (AD 1500 TO 1800)

The backwardness of Medieval period was followed by the Renaissance period i.e. revival of leaning. The Renaissance began from Italy in late 15th century and spread to whole of Europe. During this period, there was quest for advances in art and science. Since there was freedom of thought, there was emphasis on philosophical and rationalistic attitudes again.

The beginning of the development of human anatomy took place during this period with the art works of famous Italian painter *Leonardo da Vinci* (1452–1519). Dissection of human body was started by *Vesalius* (1514–1564) and his pupils, *Gabriel Fallopius* (1523–1562) who described human oviducts (Fallopian tubes) and *Fabricius* who discovered lymphoid tissue around the intestine of birds (bursa of Fabricius).

von Leeuwenhoek (1632–1723), draper by profession, during his spare time invented the first ever microscope by grinding the lenses himself. He also introduced histological staining in 1714 using saffron to examine muscle fibres.

Marcello Malpighi (1624–1694) used microscope extensively and observed the presence of capillaries and described the malpighian layer of the skin, and lymphoid tissue in the spleen (malpighian corpuscles). Malpighi is known as 'the father of histology.'

The credit for beginning of the study of morbid anatomy (pathologic anatomy), however, goes to Italian anatomist-pathologist, *Giovanni B. Morgagni* (1682–1771). Morgagni was an excellent teacher in anatomy, a prolific writer as well as a practicing clinician. He published his life time experiences based on 700 postmortems and clinical findings at the age of 79 and laid the foundations of clinicopathologic methodology in the study of disease. Thus, with Morgagni, pathology had made its beginning on the autopsy table and the concept of clinicopathologic correlation (CPC) had been introduced, establishing a coherent sequence of cause, lesions, symptoms, and outcome of disease.

Sir Percival Pott (1714–1788), famous surgeon in England, identified the first ever occupational cancer in the chimney sweeps in 1775 and discovered chimney soot as the first carcinogenic agent.

John Hunter (1728–1793) was a student of Sir Percival Pott and rose to become greatest surgeon-anatomist of all times and he, together with his elder brother *William Hunter* (1718–1788) who was a reputed anatomist-obstetrician, started the first ever museum of pathologic anatomy. John Hunter made a collection of more than 13,000 surgical specimens from his flourishing practice, arranged them into separate organ systems, made comparison of specimens from animals and plants with humans, and included many clinical pathology specimens as well, and thus developed the first museum of comparative anatomy and pathology in the world which later became the Hunterian Museum in England (Fig. 1.2). Hunter also described syphilitic chancre (Hunterian chancre) and adductor canal (Hunterian canal).

Amongst of many pupils John Hunter was *Edward Jenner* (1749–1823). In fact, Jenner's work on inoculation in smallpox can be traced back to the earlier experiment

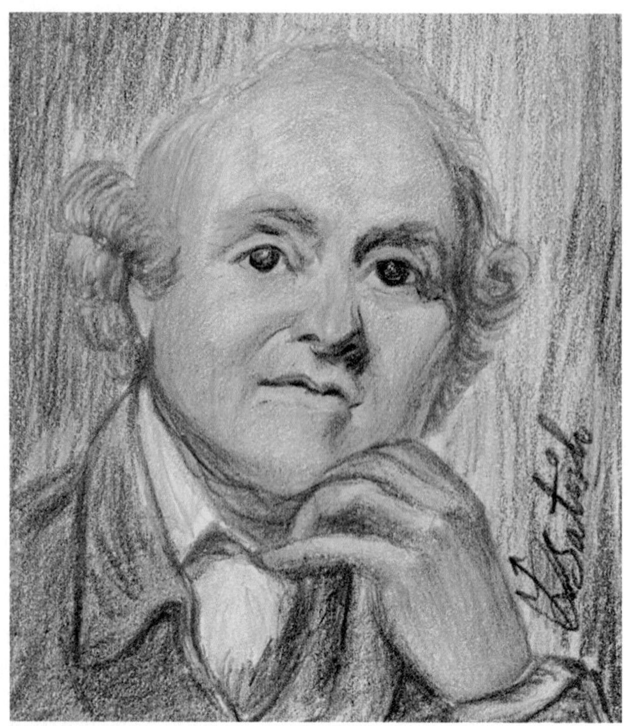

FIGURE 1.2

John Hunter (1728-1793). Scottish surgeon, regarded as the greatest surgeon-anatomist of all times and father of museum in pathology. He established first ever unique collection of pathological specimens that later resulted in the Hunterian Museum of the Royal College of Surgeons, London.

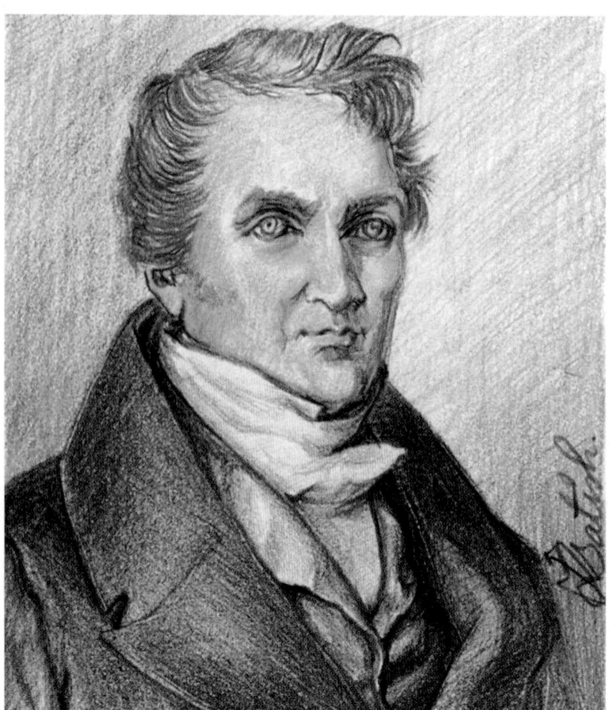

FIGURE 1.3

RTH Laennec (1781-1826). French physician, who invented stethoscope, contributed to the understanding of diseases of chest (emphysema, bronchiectasis, tuberculosis), and micronodular (Laennec's) cirrhosis associated with heavy intake of alcohol.

done by John Hunter on himself by self-inoculation of a venereal lesion from a prostitute on his own glans by a lancet which resulted in delay of his marriage for three years for getting cured.

Towards the end of 18th century, *Xavier Bichat* (1771–1802) in France described that organs were composed of tissue and divided the study of morbid anatomy into General Pathology and Systemic Pathology. Another prominent English pathologist was *Matthew Baillie* (1760–1823), nephew of Hunter brothers, who published first-ever systematic textbook of morbid anatomy in 1793.

R.T.H. Laennec (1781–1826), French physician, dominated the early part of 19th century by his numerous discoveries. He described several lung diseases (tubercles, caseous lesions, miliary lesions, pleural effusion, bronchiectasis), chronic sclerotic liver disease (later called Laennec's cirrhosis) and invented stethoscope (Fig. 1.3).

Morbid anatomy attained its zenith with appearance of *Carl F. von Rokitansky* (1804–1878), self-taught German pathologist who performed nearly 30,000 autopsies himself. He described acute yellow atrophy of the liver, wrote an outstanding monograph on diseases of arteries and congenital heart defects. He later wrote a book on pathologic anatomy which attracted a lot of criticism from his arch rival and contemporary, Rudolf Virchow, because of his own numerous theories in it. Unlike most other surgeons of that time, Rokitansky never practiced surgery and introduced the concept that pathologists confine themselves to making diagnosis which became the accepted role of pathologist later.

The era of gross pathology had three more illustrious and brilliant physician-pathologists in England who were colleagues at Guy's Hospital in London:

- *Richard Bright* (1789–1858) who described non-suppurative nephritis, later termed glomerulonephritis or Bright's disease;
- *Thomas Addison* (1793–1860) who gave an account of chronic adrenocortical insufficiency termed Addison's disease; and
- *Thomas Hodgkin* (1798–1866), who observed the complex of chronic enlargement of lymph nodes, often with enlargement of the liver and spleen, later called Hodgkin's disease.

ERA OFTECHNOLOGY DEVELOPMENT AND CELLULAR PATHOLOGY (AD 1800TO 1950s)

Upto middle of the 19th century, correlation of clinical manifestations of disease with pathological findings at autopsy became the major method of study of disease. Sophistication in surgery led to advancement in pathology. The anatomist-surgeons of earlier centuries got replaced largely with surgeon-pathologists in the 19th century.

Pathology started developing as a diagnostic discipline in later half of the 19th century with the evolution of cellular pathology which was closely linked to technology advancements in machinery manufacture for cutting thin sections of tissue, improvement in microscope, and development of chemical industry and dyes for staining.

The discovery of existence of disease-causing micro-organisms was made by French chemist *Louis Pasteur* (1822–1895). Subsequently, *G.H.A. Hansen* (1841–1912) identified Hansen's bacillus as causative agent for leprosy (Hansen's disease) in 1873. While the study of infectious diseases was being made, the concept of immune tolerance and allergy emerged which formed the basis of immunisation initiated by Edward Jenner.

Developments in chemical industry helped in switch over from earlier dyes of plant and animal orgin to synthetic dyes; aniline violet being the first such synthetic dye prepared by *Perkin* in 1856. This led to emergence of a viable dye industry for histological and bacteriological purposes. The impetus for the flourishing and successful dye industry came from the works of numerous pioneers as under:

- *Paul Ehrlich* (1854–1915), German physician, conferred Nobel Prize for his work in immunology, described Ehrlich's test for urobilinogen using Ehrlich's aldehyde reagent, staining techniques of cells and bacteria, and laid the foundations of haematology (Fig. 1.4).
- *Christian Gram* (1853–1938), Danish physician, who developed bacteriologic staining by crystal violet;
- *D.L. Romanowsky* (1861–1921), Russian physician, who developed stain for peripheral blood film using eosin and methylene blue derivatives;
- *Robert Koch* (1843–1910), German bacteriologist who, besides Koch's postulate and Koch's phenomena, developed techniques of fixation and staining for identification of bacteria, discovered tubercle bacilli in 1882 and cholera vibrio organism in 1883;
- *May-Grunwald* in 1902 and *Giemsa* in 1914 developed blood stains and applied them for classification of blood cells and bone marrow cells;

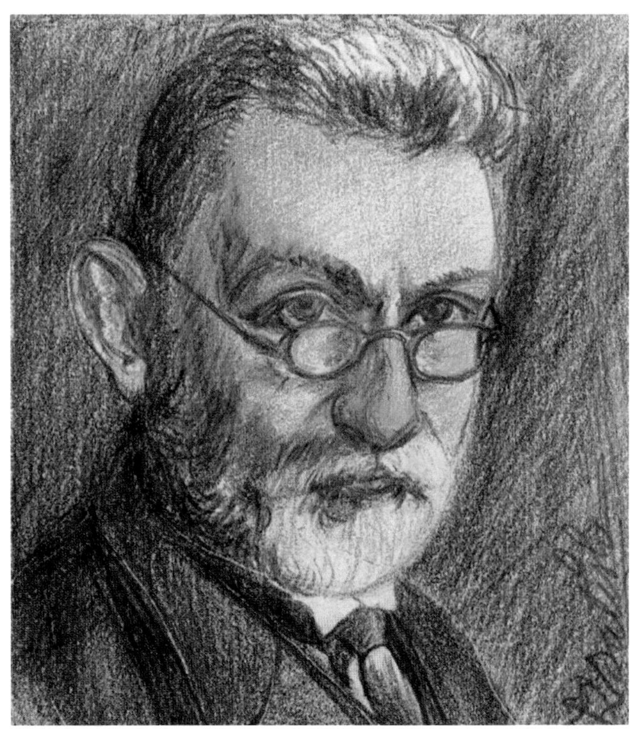

FIGURE 1.4

Paul Ehrlich (1854-1915). German physician, conferred Nobel Prize for his work in immunology, described Ehrlich's test for urobilinogen, staining techniques of cells and bacteria, and laid the foundations of haematology.

- *Sir William Leishman* (1865–1926) who described Leishman's stain for blood films in 1914 and observed Leishman-Donovan bodies (LD bodies) in leishmaniasis; and
- *Robert Feulgen* (1884–1955) who described Feulgen reaction for DNA staining and laid the foundations of cytochemistry and histochemistry.

Simultaneous technological advances in machinery manufacture led to development and upgradation of microtomes for obtaining thin sections of organs and tissues for staining by dyes for enhancing detailed study of sections.

Though the presence of cells in thin sections of non-living object cork had been first demonstrated by *Robert Hooke* in 1667, it was revived as a unit of living matter in the 19th century by *F.T. Schwann* (1810–1882), the first neurohistologist, and *Claude Bernarde* (1813–1878), pioneer in pathophysiology.

Rudolf Virchow (1821–1905) in Germany is credited with the beginning of histopathology as a method of investigation by examination of diseased tissues at cellular level. Virchow gave two major hypotheses:

- All cells come from other cells.
- Disease is an alteration of normal structure and function of these cells.

Virchow is aptly known as the 'father of cellular pathology' (Fig. 1.5). Thus, sound foundation of diagnostic pathology had been laid which was followed and promoted by numerous brilliant successive workers. Virchow also described etiology of embolism (Virchow's triad—slowing of blood stream, changes in the vessel wall, changes in the blood itself), metastatic spread of tumours (Virchow's lymph node), and diseases of blood (especially leukaemias).

Until the end of the 19th century, the study of morbid anatomy had remained largely autopsy-based and thus had remained a retrospective science. Soon, knowledge and skill gained by giving accurate diagnosis on postmortem findings was applied to surgical biopsy and thus emerged the discipline of surgical pathology.

The concept of frozen section examination when the patient was still on the operation table had been introduced by Virchow's student, *Julius Cohnheim* (1839–1884). In fact, during the initial period of development of surgical pathology around the turn of the 19th century, frozen section was considered more acceptable by the surgeons. Then there was the period when morphologic examination of cells by touch imprint smears was favoured for diagnostic purposes than actual tissue sections. Subsequently, further advances in surgical pathology were made possible by improved machinery and development of dyes and stains.

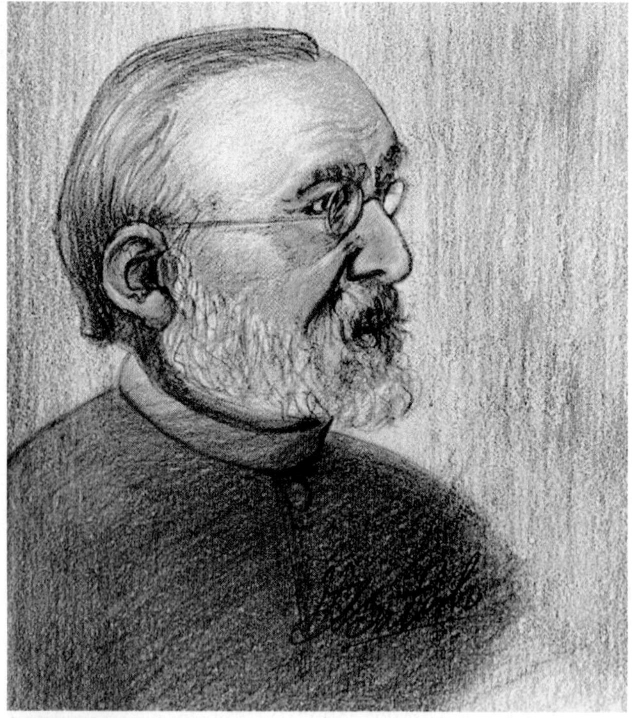

FIGURE 1.5

Rudolf Virchow (1821-1905). German pathologist regarded as 'the father of cellular pathology'.

The concept of surgeon-pathologist started in the 19th century continued as late as the middle of the 20th century in surgical departments. Assigning surgical pathology work to some faculty member in the department of surgery was common practice; that is why some of the notable pathologists of the first half of 20th century had background of clinical training e.g. *James Ewing* (1866–1943), *Pierre Masson* (1880–1958), *A.P. Stout* (1885–1967) and *Lauren Ackerman* (1905–1993).

Other landmarks in further evolution of modern pathology in this era are as follows:

- *Karl Landsteiner* (1863–1943) described the existence of human blood groups in 1901 and was awarded Nobel Prize in 1930.
- *Ruska* and *Lorries* in 1933 developed electron microscope which aided the pathologist to view ultrastructure of cell and its organelles.
- The development of exfoliative cytology for early detection of cervical cancer began with *George N. Papanicolaou* (1883–1962), a Greek-born American pathologist, in 1930s who is known as 'father of exfoliative cytology' (Fig. 1.6).

Another pioneering teacher in pathology in the 20th century was *William Boyd* (1885–1979), psychiatrist-turned pathologist whose textbooks—'Pathology for Surgeons' (first edition 1925) and 'Textbook of Pathology' (first edition 1932), dominated and inspired the students of pathology all over the world due to his flowery language and lucid style for about 50 years till 1970s. *M.M. Wintrobe* (1901–1986), a pupil of Boyd who discovered haematocrit technique, regarded him as a very stimulating teacher with keen interest in the development of museum.

MODERN PATHOLOGY (1950s TO DAWN OF 21ST CENTURY)

The strides made in the latter half of 20th century until the beginning of 21st century have made it possible to study diseases at molecular level, and provide an evidence-based and objective diagnosis and therapy. The major impact of advances in molecular biology are in the field of diagnosis and treatment of genetic disorders, immunology and in cancer. Some of the revolutionary discoveries during this time are as under:

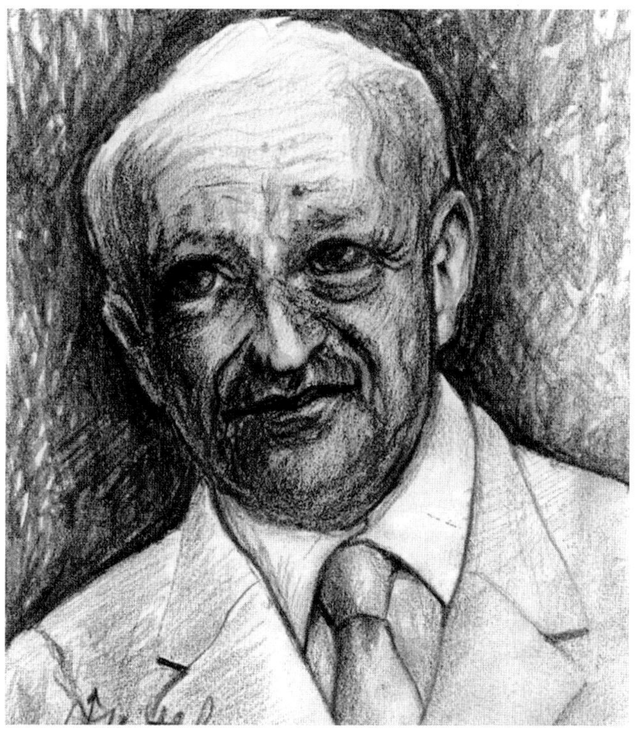

FIGURE 1.6

George N. Papanicolaou (1883-1962). American pathologist, who developed Pap test for diagnosis of cancer of uterine cervix and regarded as 'father of exfoliative cytology.'

■ Description of the structure of DNA of the cell by *Watson* and *Crick* in 1953.

■ Identification of chromosomes and their correct number in humans (46) by *Tijo* and *Levan* in 1956.

■ Identification of Philadelphia chromosome t(9;22) in chronic myeloid leukaemia by *Nowell* and *Hagerford* in 1960 as the first chromosomal abnormality in any cancer.

■ *In Situ Hybridization* introduced in 1969 in which a labeled probe is employed to detect and localize specific RNA or DNA sequences *'in situ'* (i.e. in the original place).

■ *Recombinant DNA technique* developed in 1972 using restriction enzymes to cut and paste bits of DNA.

■ In 1983, Kary Mullis introduced *polymerase chain reaction* (PCR) i.e. "xeroxing" DNA fragments which revolutionised the diagnostic molecular genetics.

■ The flexibility and dynamism of DNA invented by *Barbara McClintock* for which she was awarded Nobel Prize in 1983.

■ In 1997, *Ian Wilmut*, a Scottish scientist and his colleagues at Roslin Institute in Edinburgh, successfully used a technique of somatic cell nuclear transfer to create the clone of a sheep; the cloned sheep was named Dolly. This has set in the era of *mammalian cloning*.

■ In June 2000, discovery of chemicals of the approximately 80,000 genes that make up the human body, their structure and position on chromosomes (i.e. *mapping of the human genome*) has been successfully carried out. The functions of most of the genes that comprise human genome have also been identified. All this has opened new ways in treating and researching an endless list of diseases that are currently incurable.

■ Recent report in April 2004 suggests that Prof Wilmut's group, which first cloned the sheep Dolly, has applied to the regulatory authorities for *therapeutic cloning of human embryos* for use in treating motor neuron disease, and the embryo will be destroyed after therapeutic use. Apparently, at present time this has raised serious ethical issues and reservations. For the students, it should be known that this stage of molecular biology has been reached due to availability of *human stem cell research* in which embryonic stem cells obtained from *in vitro* fertilisation will be used for cell therapy e.g. introducing insulin-producing cells into the pancreas in a patient of insulin-dependent diabetes mellitus, or using embryonic stem cells cultured in the laboratory in lieu of a whole organ transplant. It seems that time is not far when organs for transplant may be 'harvested' from the embryo.

These inventions have set in an era of human molecular biology which is no longer confined to research laboratories but is ready for application as a modern diagnostic and therapeutic tool. Modern day human molecular biology is closely linked to information technology; the best recent example is the availability of molecular profiling by *cDNA microarrays* in which by a small silicon chip, expression of thousands of genes can be simultaneously measured.

Table 1.1 summarises the entire chronology in the evolution of the speciality of pathology.

SUBDIVISIONS OF PATHOLOGY

After a retrospective into the historical aspects of pathology, and before plunging into the study of pathology in the chapters that follow, we first introduce ourselves with the branches of human pathology.

Depending upon the species studied, there are various disciplines of pathology such as human pathology, animal pathology, plant pathology, veterinary pathology, poultry pathology etc. *Comparative pathology*

TABLE 1.1: Chronology in Evolution of Pathology.

	NAME AND COUNTRY	PERIOD	MAJOR CONTRIBUTIONS
FROM RELIGIOUS BELIEFS TO RATIONAL APPROACH (ANTIQUITY TO AD 1500)			
01.	Hippocrates (Greece)	460–377 BC	• Permanently dissociated medicine from religious mysticism • Started study of patient's symptoms as method of diagnosis • Stressed moralistic attitude for practice of medicine ('Hippocratic oath')
02.	Cornelius Celsus (Rome)	53 BC–7 AD	• Described 4 cardinal signs of inflammation (redness, heat, swelling, pain)
03.	Charaka and Sushruta (India)	200 AD	• Disequilibrium of *Dhatus* (elements constituting the body) as the cause of disease
04.	Claudius Galen (Rome)	130–200 AD	• Postulated humoral theory i.e. disease results from imbalance of four body fluids
ERA OF GROSS PATHOLOGY (AD 1500 TO 1800)			
05.	Marcello Malpighi (Balogna)	1624–1694	• Father of histology • Described malpighian layer of skin, malpighian corpuscles in spleen and presence of capillaries
06.	von Leeuwenhoek (Holland)	1632–1723	• Invented the first microscope • Introduced histological staining in 1714 • First described spermatozoa, red blood cells and giardia
07.	Giovanni B Morgagni (Italy)	1682–1771	• Introduced clinicopathologic correlation (CPC) in the study of disease
08.	Sir Percival Pott (England)	1714–1788	• Identified first occupational cancer (chimney soot) as carcinogenic agent
09.	John Hunter (Scotland)	1728–1793	• Introduced pathology museum in the study of disease
10.	Edward Jenner (France)	1749–1823	• Introduced inoculation for smallpox
11.	Xavier Bichat (France)	1771–1802	• Divided study of pathology into General Pathology and Systemic Pathology
12.	Matthew Baille (England)	1760–1823	• Authored first ever systematic textbook of morbid anatomy
13.	R.T.H. Laennec (France)	1781–1826	• Described several lung diseases such as various tuberculous lesions of lungs, bronchiectasis • Described cirrhosis of liver (later called Laennec's cirrhosis) • Invented stethoscope
14.	Carl F. von Rokitansky (Germany)	1804–1878	• Conducted 30,000 autopsies • Described acute yellow atrophy of the liver • Monograph on diseases of arteries and congenital heart defects
15.	Richard Bright (England)	1789–1858	• Described non-suppurative nephritis (glomerulonephritis)
16.	Thomas Addison (England)	1793–1860	• Described chronic adrenocortical insufficiency (Addison's disease)
17.	Thomas Hodgkin (England)	1798–1866	• Described complex of lymphoreticular involvement called Hodgkin's disease
ERA OF TECHNOLOGY DEVELOPMENT AND CELLULAR PATHOLOGY (AD 1800 TO 1950s)			
18.	Rudolf Virchow (Germany)	1821–1905	• Father of cellular pathology • Introduced histopathology as a diagnostic branch by his cellular theory • Described etiology of embolism (Virchow's triad—slowing of blood stream, changes in the vessel wall, changes in the blood itself), metastatic spread of tumours (Virchow's lymph node), diseases of blood (especially leukaemias)
19.	Julius Cohnheim (Germany)	1839–1884	• Introduced frozen section
20.	Louis Pasteur (France)	1822–1895	• Discovery of disease-causing micro-organisms
21.	G.H.A.Hansen (Germany)	1841–1912	• Identified first ever disease-causating organism, leprosy (Hansen's) bacillus
22.	Paul Ehrlich (Germany)	1854–1915	• Ehrlich's test for urobilinogen; developed stains for cells and bacteria, laid foundations of immunology and haematology
23.	Christian Gram (Denmark)	1853–1938	• Developed bacterial stain
24.	D.L.Romanowsky (Russia)	1861–1921	• Developed stain for blood film employing eosin and methylene blue derivatives
25.	Robert Koch (Germany)	1843–1910	• Koch's postulate, discovered tubercle and cholera bacilli

Contd...

TABLE 1.1 Contd...

	NAME AND COUNTRY	PERIOD	MAJOR CONTRIBUTIONS
26.	Sir William Leishman (England)	1865–1926	• Leishman stain for blood film, LD bodies in leishmaniasis
27.	Robert Feulgen (Germany)	1884–1955	• DNA staining • Founder of cytochemistry and histochemistry
28.	Karl Landsteiner (USA)	1863–1943	• Described human blood groups in 1901
29.	Ruska and Lorries	1933*	• First developed electron microscope
30.	George N. Papanicolaou (USA)	1883–1962	• Father of exfoliative cytology • Developed Pap smear for detection of cervical cancer in 1930s
31.	William Boyd (Canada)	1995–1979	• Author of widely read textbooks: Textbook of Pathology and Pathology for Surgeons for over 50 years
MODERN PATHOLOGY (1950s TO DAWN OF 21ST CENTURY)			
32.	Watson and Crick	1953*	• Described the structure of DNA
33.	Tijo and Levan	1956*	• Identification of chromosomes and their correct number of humans (46)
34.	Nowell and Hagerford	1960*	• Philadelphia chromosome in CML i.e. t(9;22)
35.	Gall & Pardue, Buongiorno-Nardelli & Amaldi, and John et al	1969*	• *In Situ* Hybridization
36.	Paul Berg	1972*	• Recombinant DNA technique
37.	Kary Mullis	1983*	• Introduced polymerase chain reaction (PCR)
38.	Barbara McClintock	1983*	• Discovered flexibility and dynamism of DNA
39.	Ian Wilmut (Scotland)	1997*	• Cloned sheep named Dolly; set in the era of *mammalian cloning*
40.	NIH, US & Wellcome Trust	2000*	• Mapping of the human genome consisting of the approximately 80,000 genes
41.	Ian Wilmut	2004*	• Therapeutic cloning of human embryos for use in treating motor neuron disease; era of human stem cell research

*Indicates the year of their discovery

deals with the study of diseases in animals in comparison with those found in man.

Human pathology is the largest branch of pathology. It is conventionally divided into *General Pathology* dealing with general principles of disease, and *Systemic Pathology* that includes study of diseases pertaining to the specific organs and body systems. With the advancement of diagnostic tools, the broad principles of which are outlined in the next chapter, the speciality of pathology has come to include the following subspecialities:

A. HISTOPATHOLOGY. Histopathology, used synonymously with anatomic pathology, pathologic anatomy, or morbid anatomy, is the classic method of study and still the most useful one which has stood the test of time. The study includes structural changes observed by naked eye examination referred to as gross or macroscopic changes, and the changes detected by light and electron microscopy supported by numerous special staining methods including histochemical and immunological techniques to arrive at the most accurate diagnosis. Modern time anatomic pathology includes super-specialities such as cardiac pathology, pulmonary pathology, neuropathology, renal pathology, gynaecologic pathology, dermatopathology, gastrointestinal pathology, oral pathology, and so on. Anatomic pathology includes the following 3 main subdivisions:

1. *Surgical pathology* deals with the study of tissues removed from the living body. It forms the bulk of tissue material for the pathologist and includes study of tissue by paraffin embedding techniques and by frozen section for rapid diagnosis.

2. *Forensic pathology and autopsy work* includes the study of organs and tissues removed at postmortem. In this, the pathologist attempts to reconstruct the course of events how they happened in the patient and culminated in his death. The postmortem anatomic diagnosis is helpful to the clinician to enhance his knowledge about the disease and his judgement. The significance of a careful postmortem examination can be summed up in the old saying 'the dead teach the living'.

3. *Cytopathology,* though a branch of anatomic pathology, has developed as a distinct subspeciality in recent times. It includes study of cells shed off from the lesions (exfoliative cytology) and fine-needle aspiration cytology (FNAC) of superficial and deep-seated lesions for diagnosis (Chapter 29).

B. HAEMATOLOGY. Haematology deals with the diseases of blood. It includes laboratory haematology and clinical haematology; the latter covers the management of patient as well.

C. CHEMICAL PATHOLOGY. Analysis of biochemical constituents of blood, urine, semen, CSF etc is included in this branch of pathology.

D. IMMUNOLOGY. Detection of abnormalities in the immune system of the body comprises immunology and immunopathology.

E. EXPERIMENTAL PATHOLOGY. This is defined as production of disease in the experimental animal and its study. However, all the findings of experimental work in animals may not be applicable to man due to species differences.

F. GEOGRAPHIC PATHOLOGY. The study of differences in distribution of frequency and type of diseases in populations in different parts of the world forms geographic pathology.

G. MEDICAL GENETICS. This is the branch of human genetics that deals with the relationship between heredity and disease. There have been important developments in the field of medical genetics e.g. in blood groups, inborn errors of metabolism, chromosomal aberrations in congenital malformations and neoplasms etc.

H. MOLECULAR PATHOLOGY. The detection and diagnosis of abnormalities at the level of DNA of the cell is included in molecular pathology. Recent advancements in molecular biologic techniques have resulted in availability of these methods not only for research purposes but also as a tool in diagnostic pathology.

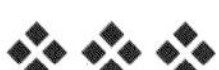

Techniques for the Study of Pathology

2

For learning contemporary pathology effectively, it is essential that the student is familiar with the various laboratory methods, techniques and tools employed for the study of pathology. This chapter is devoted to the basic aspects of various such methods as are available—ranging from the basic microscopy to the most recent methods, in a modern pathology laboratory.

AUTOPSY PATHOLOGY

Professor William Boyd in his unimitable style wrote 'Pathology had its beginning on the autopsy table'. The significance of study of autopsy in pathology is summed up in Latin inscription in an autopsy room reproduced in English as "The place where death delights to serve the living'. As stated in the previous chapter, G.B. Morgagni in Italy (1682-1771) and T.H.A. Laennec (1781-1826) in France started collecting the case records of hospital cases and began correlation of clinical features with the lesions observed at autopsy and thus marked the beginning of clinicopathologic correlation (CPC). CPC continues to be the most important form of clinical teaching activity in medical institutions worldwide.

There is still no substitute for a careful postmortem examination which enlightens the clinician about the pathogenesis of disease, reveals hazardous effects of therapy administered, and settles the discrepancies finally between antemortem and postmortem diagnosis.

Traditionally, there are two methods for carrying out autopsy, either of which may be followed:

1. Block extraction of abdominal and thoracic organs.
2. *In situ* organ-by-organ dissection.

In conditions where multiple organs are expected to be involved, complete autopsy should be performed. But if a particular organ-specific disease is suspected, a mini-autopsy or limited autopsy may be sufficient.

The study of autopsy throws new light on the knowledge and skills of both physician as well as pathologist. The main **purposes** of autopsy are as under:

1. *Quality assurance of patientcare* by:
   i) confirming the cause of death;
   ii) establishing the final diagnosis; and
   iii) study of therapeutic response to treatment.
2. *Education of the entire team* involved in patientcare by:
   i) making autopsy diagnosis of conditions which are often missed clinically e.g. pneumonia, pulmonary embolism, acute pancreatitis, carcinoma prostate;
   ii) discovery of newer diseases made at autopsy e.g. Reye's syndrome, Legionnaire's disease, SARS;
   iii) study of demography and epidemiology of diseases; and
   iv) affords education to students and staff of pathology.

Declining autopsy rate throughout world in the recent times is owing to the following reasons:

1. Higher diagnostic confidence has been made possible by advances in imaging techniques e.g. CT, MRI etc.
2. Physician's fear of legal liability on being wrong.

Continued support for advocating autopsy by caring physicians as well as by discernible pathologists in tertiary-care hospitals is essential for improved patient-care and progress in medical science.

SURGICAL PATHOLOGY

HISTORICAL PERSPECTIVE

The term surgical pathology is currently applied synonymously with histopathology, morbid anatomy, anatomic pathology and cellular pathology. Surgical pathology is the classic and time-tested method of tissue diagnosis made on gross and microscopic study of tissues.

As discussed already, surgical pathology made its beginning from pathologic study of tissues made available at autopsy. Surgeons of old times relied solely on operative/gross findings and, thereafter, discarded the excised tissues, without affording an opportunity to the pathologist to make microscopic diagnosis. However, with technology development and advances made in the dye industry in the initial years of this century, the speciality of diagnostic surgical pathology by biopsy developed.

In the beginning, this task was assigned to a surgeon faculty member in the surgery departments and appropriately called 'surgical pathologist'. Currently, the field of surgical pathology has expanded so much that several subspecialities have developed e.g. nephropathology, neuropathology, haematopathology, dermatopathology, gynaecologic pathology cytopathology, paediatric pathology, and so on.

SCOPE AND LIMITATIONS OF SURGICAL PATHOLOGY

Surgical pathology services in any large hospital depend largely on inputs from surgeons and physicians familiar with the scope and limitations inherent in the speciality. Thus it is vital that clinician and pathologist communicate freely—formally as well as informally, through request forms, verbally, and at different fora such as tissue committees and interdepartmental conferences.

SURGICAL PATHOLOGY PROTOCOL

1. REQUEST FORMS. The first and foremost task of the clinician requesting tissue diagnosis is to send a completed request form that accompanies the surgical pathology specimen. It must contain the entire relevant information about the case and the disease (history, physical and operative findings, results of other relevant biochemical/haematological/radiological investigations, and clinical and differential diagnosis).

2. TISSUE ACCESSION. Tissue received in the surgical pathology laboratory must have proper identification of the specimen matching with that on the accompanied request form. For routine tissue processing by paraffin-embedding technique, the tissue must be either in appropriate fixative solution (most commonly 10% formol-saline or 10% buffered formalin) or received fresh-unfixed. For frozen section, the tissue is always transported fresh-unfixed. The frozen section is employed for rapid diagnosis and for demonstration of certain constituents which are normally lost in processing in alcohol or xylene e.g. fat, enzymes etc. Microwave fixation may also be used in the laboratory for rapid fixation of routine surgical specimens.

3. GROSS ROOM. Gross examination of the specimen received in the laboratory is the next most important step. Proper gross dissection, description and selection of tissue sample is a crucial part of the pathologic examination of tissue submitted. Complacency at this step cannot be remedied at a later stage and might require taking the tissue pieces afresh if the specimen is large enough and delay the report, or if the tissue biopsy is small the entire surgical procedure may have to be done again. In recent times, gross description can be recorded by a speech-recognition system without the aid of an assistant to do it.

Calcified tissues and bone are subjected to decalcification to remove the mineral and soften the tissue by treatment with decalcifying agents such as acids and chelating agents (most often aqueous nitric acid).

It is mandatory that all the gross-room personnel follow strict precautions in handling the tissues infected with tuberculosis, hepatitis, HIV and other viruses.

4. HISTOPATHOLOGY LABORATORY. Tissue cassettes alongwith unique number given in the gross room to the tissue sample is carried throughout laboratory procedures. Majority of histopathology departments use automated tissue processors (Fig. 2.1, A) having 12 separate stages completing the cycle in about 18 hours by overnight schedule as under:

- 10% formalin for fixation;
- ascending grades of alcohol (70%, 95% through 100%) for dehydration for about 5 hours in 6-7 jars,
- xylene/toluene/chloroform for clearing for 3 hours in two jars; and
- paraffin impregnation for 6 hours in two thermostat-fitted waxbaths.

In order to avoid contamination of the laboratory with vapour of formalin and alcohols, vacuum tissue processors having closed system are also available.

Embedding of tissue is done in molten wax, blocks of which are prepared using L (Leuckhart's) mould. Now-a-days, plastic moulds in different colours for

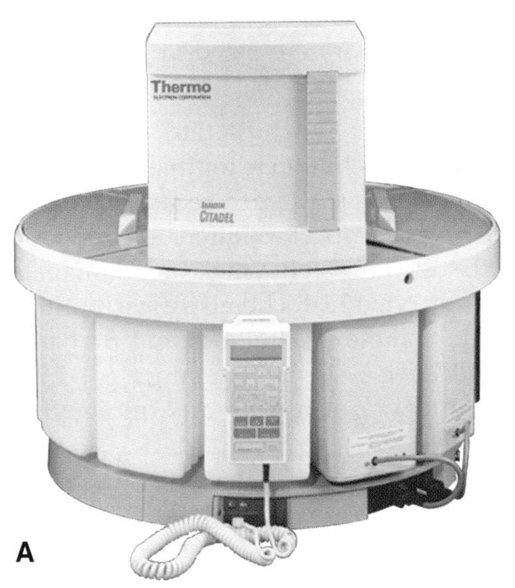

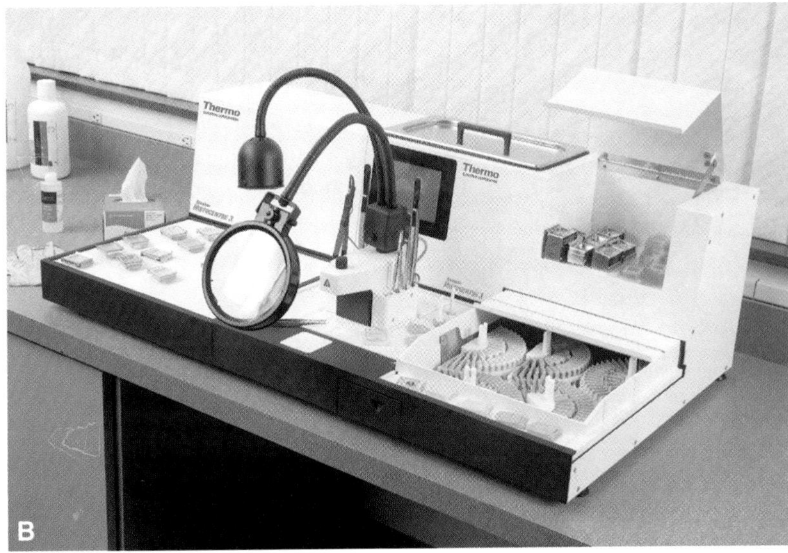

FIGURE 2.1

Automatic tissue processor (A) and tissue embedding centre (B) (both Thermo Shandon, UK). Courtesy: Towa Optics (India) Pvt. Ltd., New Delhi.

blocking are also available and the entire process can be temperature-controlled for which tissue embedding centres are available (Fig. 2.1,B). The blocks are then trimmed followed by sectioning by microtomy, most often by rotary microtome, employing fixed knife or disposable blades (Fig. 2.2).

Cryostat or frozen section eliminates all the steps of tissue processing and paraffin-embedding. Instead the tissue is frozen to ice at about –25°C which acts as embedding medium and then sectioned (Fig. 2.3). Sections are then ready for staining. It is a quick diagnostic procedure for tissues before proceeding to a major radical surgery. This is also used for demonstration of some special substances in the cells and tissues e.g. fat, enzymes. This procedure can be carried out in operation theatre complex near the operating table.

Paraffin-embedded sections are routinely stained with haematoxylin and eosin (H & E). Frozen section is stained with rapid H & E or toluidine blue routinely. Special stains are employed for either of the two methods according to need. The sections are mounted and submitted for microscopic study.

5. SURGICAL PATHOLOGY REPORT. The final and the most important task of pathology laboratory is issuance of a prompt, accurate, brief, and prognostically significant report. The ideal report must contain five aspects:

i) History (as available to the pathologist including patient's identity).

ii) Precise gross description.

iii) Brief microscopic findings.

iv) Morphologic diagnosis which must include the organ for indexing purposes using SNOMED (*S*cientific *No*menclature in *Med*icine) codes.

v) Additional comments in some cases.

6. QUALITY CONTROL. An internal quality control by mutual discussion in controversial cases and

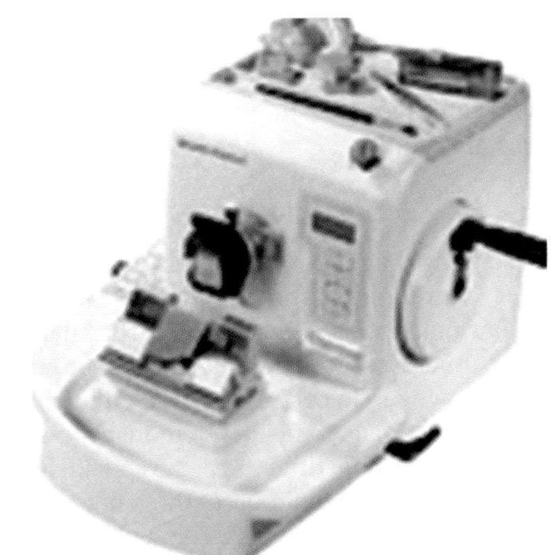

FIGURE 2.2

Rotary microtome (Thermo Shandon, UK). Courtesy: Towa Optics (India) Pvt. Ltd., New Delhi.

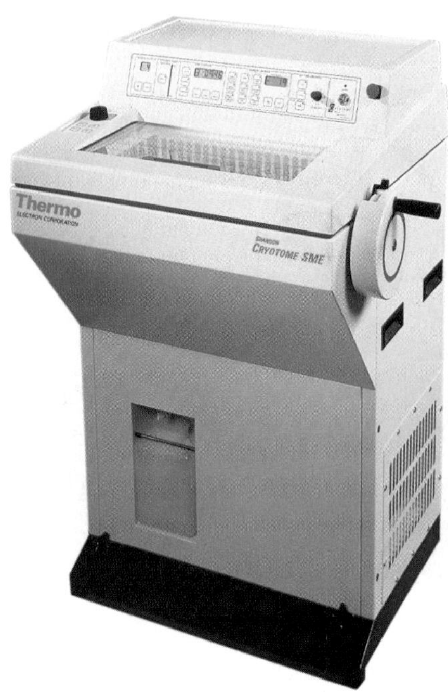

FIGURE 2.3

Cryostat (Model Cryotome, Thermo Shandon, UK). Courtesy: Towa Optics (India) Pvt. Ltd., New Delhi.

self-check on the quality of sections are important for accuracy and efficacy of the procedure.

7. **HISTOPATHOLOGIST AND THE LAW.** Problem of allegations of negligence and malpractice in laboratory medicine too have come to the forefront now just as with other clinical disciplines. In equivocal biopsies, it is desirable to have more opinions from other histopathologists. Besides, the duties of sensitive reporting work should never be delegated unless the superior is confident that the delegatee has sufficient experience and ability.

SPECIAL STAINS

In H & E staining, haematoxylin stains nuclei and eosin is used as counterstain for cytoplasm and various extracellular material. H & E staining is routinely used to diagnose microscopically vast majority of surgical specimens. However, in certain 'special' circumstances when the pathologist wants to demonstrate certain specific substances/constituents of the cells/tissues to confirm etiologic, histogenic or pathogenetic components, special stains are employed. The staining depends upon either physical, chemical or differential solubility of the stain with the tissues. The principles of some of the staining procedures are well known while those of others are unknown.

Some of the commonly used special stains in a surgical pathology laboratory are listed in Table 2.1.

ENZYME HISTOCHEMISTRY

Enzyme histochemical techniques for tissue section require special preparations of fresh tissues and can not be applied to paraffin-embedded sections or formalin-fixed tissues since enzymes are damaged rapidly. Currently, enzyme histochemistry has limited applications due to complex techniques and preparations required and have been largely superseded by immunohistochemical procedures and molecular pathology techniques.

Some of the commonly used enzyme histochemical stains are given in Table 2.2.

BASIC MICROSCOPY

Microscope is the basic tool of the pathologist just as is the stethoscope for the physician and scalpel for the surgeon. It is an instrument which produces greatly enlarged images of minute objects. The usual type of microscope used in clinical laboratories is called *light microscope.*

In general, there are two types of light microscopes:

Simple microscope. This is a simple hand magnifying lens. The magnification power of hand lens is from 2x to 200x.

Compound microscope. This has a battery of lenses which are fitted in a complex instrument. One type of lens remains near the object (objective lens) and another type of lens near the observer's eye (eye piece lens). The eye piece and objective lenses have different magnification. The compound microscope can be *monocular* having single eye piece or *binocular* which has two eye pieces (Fig. 2.4). *Multi-headed microscopes* are used as an aid to teaching and for demonstration purposes.

VARIANTS OF LIGHT MICROSCOPY. Besides the light microscopes, other modifications for special purposes in the clinical laboratories are as under:

Dark ground illumination (DGI). This method is used for examination of unstained living micro-organisms e.g. *Treponema pallidum.* The micro-organisms are illuminated by an oblique ray of light which does not pass through the micro-organism. The condenser is blackened in the centre and light passes through its periphery illuminating the living micro-organism on a glass slide.

TABLE 2.1: Common Special Stains in Surgical Pathology (in Alphabetic Order of Constituents).

STAIN	COMPONENT/TISSUE	DYES	INTERPRETATION
A. AMYLOID			
1. *Congo red with polarising light*	Amyloid	Congo red	Green-birefringence: amyloid
2. *Toluidine blue*	Amyloid	Toluidine blue	Orthochromatic blue: amyloid
B. CARBOHYDRATES			
3. *Periodic acid-Schiff (PAS)*	Carbohydrates, (particularly glycogen), all mucins	Periodic acid, Schiff reagent (basic fuchsin)	Glycogen and other carbohydrates: magenta Nuclei: blue
4. *Mucicarmine/Best's carmine*	Acidic mucin	Carmine	Mucin: red Nuclei: blue
5. *Alcian blue (AB)*	Acidic mucin	Alcian blue (at pH 2.5)	Acid mucin: blue Nuclei: red
6. *Combined AB-PAS*	Neutral mucin	Alcian blue	Acid mucin: blue Neutral mucin: magenta Nuclei: pale blue .
C. CONNECTIVE TISSUES			
7. *Van Gieson's*	Extracellular collagen	Picric acid, acid fuchsin, celestin blue-haemalum	Nuclei: blue/black Collagen: red Other tissues: yellow
8. *Masson's trichrome*	Extracellular collagen	Acid fuchsin, phosphomolybdic acid, methyl blue, celestin blue-haemalum	Nuclei: blue/black Cytoplasm, muscle, red cells: red Collagen: blue
9. *Phosphotungstic acid-haematoxylin (PTAH)*	Muscle and glial filaments	Haematoxylin, phosphotungstic acid, permanganate, oxalic acid	Muscle striations, neuroglial fibres, fibrin: dark blue Nuclei: blue Cytoplasm: pale pink
10. *Verhoeffs elastic*	Elastic fibres	Haematoxylin, Ferric chloride, iodine, potassium iodide	Elastic fibres: black Other tissues: counter-stained
11. *Gordon and Sweet's*	Reticular fibres	Silver nitrate	Reticular fibres: black Nuclei: black or counterstained
D. LIPIDS			
12. *Oil red O*	Fats (unfixed cryostat)	Oil red O	Mineral oils: red Unsaturated fats, Phospholipids: pink
13. *Sudan Black B*	Fats (unfixed cryostat)	Sudan black B	Unsaturated fats: blue black
14. *Osmium tetroxide*	Fats (unfixed cryostat)	Osmium tetroxide	Unsaturated lipids: brown black Saturated lipids: unstained
E. MICRO-ORGANISMS			
15. *Gram's*	Bacteria (cocci, bacilli)	Crystal violet, Lugol's iodine, neutral red	Gram-positive, keratin, fibrin: blue Gram-negative: red
16. *Ziehl-Neelsen's (Acid-fast)*	Tubercle bacilli	Carbol fuchsin, methylene blue (differentiate in acid-alcohol)	Tubercle bacilli, hair shaft, actinomyces: red Background: pale blue

Contd...

TABLE 2.1 Contd...

STAIN	COMPONENT/TISSUE	DYES	INTERPRETATION
17. *Fite-Wade*	Leprosy bacilli	Carbol fuchsin, methylene blue (decolorise in 10% sulfuric acid)	Lepra bacilli: red Background: blue
18. *Grocott's silver methanamine*	Fungi	Sodium tetraborate, silver nitrate, methanamine	Fungi, *Pneumocystis:* black Red cells: yellow Background: pale green
19. *Giemsa*	Parasites	Giemsa powder	Protozoa: dark blue Nuclei: blue
20. *Shikata's orcein*	Hepatitis B surface antigen (HBsAg)	Acid permanganate, orcein, tetrazine	HBsAg positive: brown to black Background: yellow
F. NEURAL TISSUES			
21. *Luxol fast blue*	Myelin	Luxol fast blue, cresyl violet	Myelin: blue/green Cells: violet/pink
22. *Bielschowsky's silver*	Axons	Silver nitrate	Axon and neurofibrils: black
G. PIGMENTS AND MINERALS			
23. *Perl's Prussian blue*	Haemosiderin, iron	Pot. ferrocyanide	Ferric iron: blue Nuclei: red
24. *Masson-Fontana*	Melanin, argentaffin cells	Silver nitrate	Melanin, argentaffin, chromaffin, lipofuscin: black Nuclei: red
25. *Alizarin red S*	Calcium	Alizarin red S	Calcium deposits: orange red
26. *von Kossa*	Mineralised bone	Silver nitrate, safranin O	Mineralised bone: black Osteoid: red
27. *Rubeanic acid*	Copper	Rubeanic acid	Copper: greenish-black Nuclei: pale red
28. *Pigment extraction*	Removal of formalin pigment and malarial pigment	Alcoholic picric acid	Formalin pigment/malarial pigment: removed
29. *Grimelius'*	Argyrophil cells	Silver nitrate	Argyrophil granules: brown-black
H. PROTEINS AND NUCLEIC ACIDS			
30. *Feulgen reaction*	DNA	Pot. metabisulphite	DNA: red purple Cytoplasm: green
31. *Methyl green-pyronin*	DNA, RNA	Methyl green, pyronin-Y	DNA: green-blue RNA: red

Polarising microscope. This method is used for demonstration of birefringence e.g. amyloid, foreign body, hair etc. The light is made plane polarised. After passing through a disc, the rays of light vibrate in a single plane at right angle to each other. Two discs made up of prism are placed in the path of light, one below the object known as polariser and another placed in the body tube which is known as analyser. The lower disc is rotated to make the light plane polarised.

Fluorescent microscope and electron microscope are discussed separately below.

IMMUNOFLUORESCENCE

Immunofluorescence technique is employed to localise antigenic molecules on the cells by microscopic examination. This is done by using specific antibody against the antigenic molecule forming antigen-antibody complex at the specific antigenic site which is made

TABLE 2.2: Common Enzyme Histochemical Stains.

	STAIN	COMPONENT/TISSUE	DYES	INTERPRETATION
1.	Alkaline phosphatase	Cell membranes (cryostat)	Sod.β-glycerophosphate (final pH 9.0)	Alk.phosph. activity: brown/black Nuclei: green
2.	Acid phosphatase	Lysosomes (cryostat)	Sod. β-glycerophosphate (final pH 5.0)	Acid phosph. activity: black Nuclei: green or red
3.	Acetyl cholinesterase (ACE)	Nerve fibres in Hirschsprung's disease (cryostat)	Acetylcholine iodide	Nerve fibres positive for ACE: red brown
4.	Nonspecific esterases	Esterase, lipase, cholinesterase (cryostat)	α-naphthyl acetate	Esterase: reddish brown Nuclei: green
5.	Tyrosinase-DOPA reaction	Melanin (cryostat)	L-tyrosine, DL-DOPA	DOPA oxidase: brown Nuclei: blue
6.	Dehydrogenase	Endogenous dehydrogenase (cryostat)	Tetrazolium soln (NBT)	Positive: purple formazan deposits Nuclei: green
7.	ATPase	Myopathies (cryostat)	ATP	Type I fibres: dark Type 2 fibres: pale

visible by employing a fluorochrome which has the property to absorb radiation in the form of ultraviolet light so as to be within the visible spectrum of light in microscopic examination.

The immunofluorescent method has the following essential components:

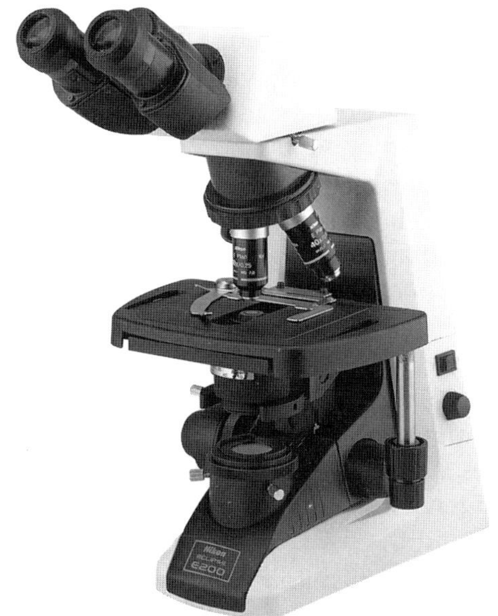

FIGURE 2.4

Binocular light microscope (Model E 400, Nikon, Japan). Courtesy: Towa Optics (India) Pvt. Ltd., New Delhi.

FLUORESCENCE MICROSCOPE. Fluorescence microscopy is based on the principle that the exciting radiation from ultraviolet light of shorter wavelength (360 nm) or blue light (wavelength 400 nm) causes fluorescence of certain substances and thereafter re-emits light of a longer wavelength.

- Some substances fluoresce naturally; this is termed *primary fluorescence* or *autofluorescence* though UV light is required for visualising them better e.g. vitamin A, porphyrin, chlorophyll.
- *Secondary fluorescence* is more common by employed and is production of fluorescence on addition of dyes or chemicals called fluorochromes.

Source of light. Mercury vapour and xenon gas lamps are used as source of light for fluorescence microscopy.

Filters. A variety of filters are used between the source of light and objective: *first,* heat absorbing filter; *second,* red-light stop filter; and *third* exciter filter to allow the passage of light of only the desired wavelength. On passing through the specimen, light of both exciting and fluorescence wavelength collects. Exciter light is removed by another filter called *barrier filter* between the objective and the observer to protect the observer's eyes so that only fluorescent light reaches the eyes of observer.

Condenser. Dark-ground condenser is used in fluorescence microscope so that no direct light falls into the objective and instead gives dark contrast background to the fluorescence.

TECHNIQUES. There are two types of fluorescence techniques both of which are performed on cryostat sections of fresh unfixed tissue: direct and indirect.

■ In *direct technique,* first introduced by Coons (1941) who did the original work on immunofluorescence, antibody against antigen is directly conjugated with the fluorochrome and then examined under fluorescence microscope.

■ In *indirect technique,* also called sandwich technique, there is interaction between tissue antigen and specific antibody, followed by a step of washing and then addition of fluorochrome for completion of reaction. Indirect immunofluorescence technique is applied to detect autoantibodies in patient's serum.

APPLICATIONS. Immunofluorescence methods are applied for the following purposes:

1. *Detection of autoantibodies in the serum* e.g. smooth muscle antibodies (SMA), antinuclear antibodies (ANA), antimitochondrial antibody (AMA), thyroid microsomal antibody etc.
2. *In renal diseases* for detection of deposits of immunoglobulins, complement and fibrin in various types of glomerular diseases by frozen section as discussed in Chapter 20.
3. *In skin diseases* to detect deposits of immunoglobulin by frozen section, particularly at the dermo-epidermal junction and in upper dermis e.g. in various bullous dermatosis (Chapter 24).
4. For study of *mononuclear cell surface markers* using monoclonal antibodies.
5. For specific diagnosis of *infective disorders* e.g. viral hepatitis.

IMMUNOHISTOCHEMISTRY

Immunohistochemistry is the application of immunologic techniques to the cellular pathology. The technique is used to detect the status and localisation of particular antigen in the cells by use of specific antibodies which then helps in determining cell lineage specifically, or is used to confirm a specific infection.

In the last decade, significant advances have been made in techniques for immunohistochemistry so much so that routinely processed paraffin-embedded tissue blocks can be used for the purpose, thus making profound impact on diagnostic surgical pathology. Earlier, diagnostic surgical pathology used to be considered a subjective science with inter-observer variation, particularly in borderline lesions and lesions of undetermined origin, but use of immunohistochemical techniques has added *objectivity, specificity* and *reproducibility* to the surgical pathologist's diagnosis.

Overview of Immunohistochemistry

■ The evolution of immunohistochemistry can be traced to *immunofluorescence methods* in which antibodies labelled with fluorescent compound could localise the specific antigen in the cryostat section.

■ The need for fluorescent microscope was obviated by subsequent development of *horseradish peroxidase enzymatic labelling technique* with some colorogenic system instead of fluorochrome so that the frozen section with labelled antibody could be visualised by light microscopy. *Chromogens* commonly used in immunohistochemical reaction are diaminobenzidine tetrahydrochloride (DAB) and aminoethyl carbazole (AEC), both of which produce stable dark brown reaction end-product.

■ Subsequently, immunoperoxidase technique employing labelled antibody method to *formalin-fixed paraffin sections* was developed which is now widely used.

■ Currently, the two most commonly used procedures are:

i) *Peroxidase-antiperoxidase (PAP) method* in which PAP reagent is pre-formed stable immune-complex which is linked to the primary antibody by a bridging antibody.

ii) *Avidin-biotin conjugate (ABC) immunoenzymatic technique* in which biotinylated secondary antibody serves to link the primary antibody to a large preformed complex of avidin, biotin and peroxidase.

■ The selection of antibody/antibodies for performing immunohistochemical staining is done after making differential diagnosis on H & E sections. Generally, *a panel of antibodies* is preferable over a single test to avoid errors.

■ Antibodies for immunohistochemistry are produced by polyclonal and *monoclonal (hybridoma) techniques;* the latter is largely used to produce specific high-affinity antibodies. At present, vast number of antibodies against cell antigens for immunohistochemical stains are available and the list is increasing at a steady rate.

■ Immunohistochemical stains should always be done with appropriate *positive controls* i.e. tissue which is known to express particular antigen acts as a control. 'Sausage' tissue block technique combines the staining of multiple tissues in a single slide with a single staining procedure and is quite economical.

■ For interpretation of results of immunohistochemical stains, it is important to remember that *different antigens are localised at different sites in cells* and accordingly positive staining is seen and interpreted at those sites e.g. membranous staining for leucocyte common antigen (LCA); nuclear staining for progesterone receptors etc.

■ Immunohistochemical stains *cannot be applied* to distinguish between neoplastic and non-neoplastic lesions, or between benign and malignant tumours. These distinctions have to be done by traditional methods in surgical pathology.

Applications of Immunohistochemistry

At present, immunohistochemical stains are used for the following purposes, in order of utility:

1. Tumours of uncertain histogenesis. Immunohistochemical methods have brought about a revolution in approach to diagnosis of tumours of uncertain origin, primary as well as metastatic from an unknown primary tumour. A panel of antibodies is chosen to resolve such diagnostic problem cases; the selection of antibodies being made is based on clinical history, morphologic features, and results of other relevant investigations. Immunohistochemical stains for *intermediate filaments* (keratin, vimentin, desmin, neurofilaments and glial fibillary acidic proteins) expressed by the tumour cells are of immense value besides others listed in Table 2.3.

2. Prognostic markers in cancer. The second important application of immunohistochemical stains is to predict the prognosis of tumours by identification of enzymes, tumour-specific antigens, oncogenes, tumour suppressor genes and tumour cell proliferation markers. Analysis of tumours by these methods is a significant improvement over the conventional prognostic considerations by clinical staging and histologic grading.

3. Prediction of response to therapy. Immunohistochemical methods are widely used to predict therapeutic response in two important tumours—carcinoma of breast and prostate. Both these tumours are under the growth regulation of hormones—oestrogen and androgen, respectively. The specific receptors for these growth regulating hormones are located on respective tumour cells. Tumours expressing high level of receptor positivity would respond favourably to removal of the endogenous source of such hormones (oophorectomy in oestrogen-positive breast cancer and orchiectomy in androgen-positive prostatic carcinoma), or hormonal therapy is administered to lower their levels: oestrogen therapy in prostatic cancer and androgen therapy in breast cancer. The results of oestrogen-receptors and progesterone-receptors in breast cancer have significant prognostic correlation, though the results of androgen-receptor studies in prostatic cancer have limited prognostic value.

TABLE 2.3: Common Immunohistochemical Stains for Tumours of Uncertain Origin.

TUMOUR	IMMUNOSTAIN
1. *Epithelial tumours (Carcinomas)*	i) Pankeratin ii) Epithelial membrane antigen (EMA) iii) Carcinoembryonic antigen (CEA) iv) Neuron-specific enolase (NSE)
2. *Mesenchymal tumours (Sarcomas)*	i) Vimentin (general mesenchymal) ii) Desmin (for general myogenic) iii) Muscle specific actin (for general myogenic) iv) Myoglobin (for skeletal myogenic) v) α-1-anti-chymotrypsin (for malignant fibrous histiocytoma) vi) Factor VIII (for vascular tumours)
3. *Special groups*	
a) Melanoma	i) Vimentin ii) S-100 iii) HMB-45 (most specific)
b) Lymphoma	i) Leucocyte common antigen (LCA/CD45) ii) Pan-B iii) Pan-T iv) RS cell marker (for Hodgkin's)
c) Neural and neuroendocrine tumours	i) Neurofilaments (NF) ii) NSE iii) GFAP (for glial tumours) iv) Chromogranin (for neuroendocrine) v) Synaptophysin

4. Infections. More recently, immunohistochemical methods are being applied to confirm infectious agent in tissues by use of specific antibodies against microbial DNA or RNA e.g. in CMV, HPV, *Pneumocystis carinii* etc.

ELECTRON MICROSCOPY

Electron microscope (EM) first developed in 1930s in Germany has undergone modifications so as to add extensive new knowledge to our understanding the structure and function of normal and diseased cells at the level of cell organelles. However, more recently, widespread use of diagnostic immunohistochemistry in surgical pathology has restricted the application of EM to the following areas of diagnostic pathology:

1. In renal pathology in conjunction with light microscopy and immunofluorescence (Chapter 20).
2. Ultrastructure of tumours of uncertain histogenesis.
3. Subcellular study of macrophages in storage diseases.
4. For research purposes.

TYPES OF EM

There are two main types of EM:

1. Transmission electron microscope (TEM). TEM is the tool of choice for pathologist for study of ultrastructure of cell at organelle level. In TEM, a beam of electrons passes through ultrathin section of tissue. The magnification obtained by TEM is 2,000 to 10,000 times.

2. Scanning electron microscope (SEM). SEM scans the cell surface architecture and provides three-dimensional image. For example, for viewing the podocytes in renal glomerulus.

Technical Aspects

Following are some of the relevant salient technical considerations pertaining to EM:

1. Fixation. Whenever it is planned to undertake EM examination of tissue, small thin piece of tissue not more than 1 mm thick should be fixed in 2-4% buffered glutaraldehyde or mixture of formalin and glutaraldehyde. Following fixation, the tissue is post-fixed in buffered solution of osmium tetroxide to enhance the contrast.

2. Embedding. Tissue is plastic-embedded with resin on grid.

3. Semithin sections. First, semithin sections are cut at a thickness of 1 μm and stained with methylene blue or toluidine blue. Sometimes, paraffin blocks can also be cut for EM study but generally are not quite satisfactory due to numerous artefacts. Semithin sections guide in making the differential diagnosis and in selecting the area to be viewed in ultrathin sections.

4. Ultrathin sections. For ultrastructural examination, ultrathin sections are cut by use of diamond knife. In order to increase electron density, thin sections may be stained by immersing the grid in solution of lead citrate and urinyl acetate.

CYTOGENETICS

Applied aspects of cytogenetics have been discussed in Chapter 10. Here, we shall concentrate on brief technical considerations only.

Human somatic cells are diploid and contain 46 chromosomes: 22 pairs of autosomes and one pair of sex chromosomes (XX in the case of female and XY in the males). Gametes (sperm and ova) contain 23 chromosomes and are called *haploid cells.* All ova contain 23X while sperms contain 23X or 23Y chromosomes. Thus the sex of the off spring is determined by paternal chromosomal contribution i.e. if the ovum is fertilised by X-bearing sperm, female zygote results, while an ovum fertilised by Y-bearing sperm forms male zygote.

Karyotyping

Karyotype is defined as the sequence of chromosomal alignment on the basis of size, centromeric location and banding pattern. The structure of chromosome is described in Chapter 3.

Determination of karyotype of an individual is an important tool in cytogenetic analysis. Broad outlines of karyotyping are as under:

1. Cell selection. Cells capable of growth and division are selected for cytogenetic analysis. These include: cells from amniotic fluid, chorionic villus sampling (CVS), peripheral blood lymphocytes, bone marrow, lymph node, solid tumours etc.

2. Cell culture. The sample so obtained is cultured in mitogen media. A *mitogen* is a substance which induces mitosis in the cells e.g. PPD, phytohaemagglutinin (PHA), pokeweed mitogen (PWM), phorbol ester (TPA) etc. The dividing cells are then arrested in metaphase by the addition of colchicine or colcemid, both of which are inhibitory to microtubule formation. Subsequently, the cells are lysed by adding hypotonic solution.

The metaphase cells are then fixed in methanol-glacial acetic acid mixture.

3. Staining/banding. When stained, the chromosomes have the property of forming alternating dark and light bands. For this purpose, the fixed metaphase preparation is stained by one of the following banding techniques:

a) *Giemsa banding* or *G-banding,* the most commonly used.

b) *Quinacrine banding* or *Q-banding* used to demonstrate bands along chromosomes.

c) *Constitutive banding* or *C-banding* is used to demonstrate constitutive heterochromatin.

d) *Reverse staining Giemsa banding* or *R-banding* gives pattern opposite to those obtained by G-banding.

4. Microscopic analysis. Chromosomes are then photographed by examining the preparation under the microscope. From the photograph, chromosomes are cut and then arranged according to their size, centromeric location and banding patterns. The pairs of chromosomes are identified by the arm length of chromosomes. The centromere divides the chromosome into a short upper arm called *p arm* (p for *petit* in French meaning 'short') and a long lower arm called *q arm* (letter q next to p).

Applications

The field of cytogenetics has widespread applications in diagnostic pathology (Chapter 10). In brief, karyotyping is employed for the following purposes:

i) *Chromosomal numerical abnormalities* e.g. Down's syndrome (trisomy 21 involving autosome 21), Klinefelter's syndrome (trisomy 46), Turner's syndrome (monosomy 45, XO), spontaneous abortions.

ii) *Chromosome structural abnormalities* include translocations {e.g. Philadelphia chromosome t (9;22), cri-du-chat (5p) syndrome, repeated spontaneous miscarriages}, deletions, insertions, isochromosome, and ring chromosome formation.

iii) *Cancer* is characterised by multiple and complex chromosomal abnormalities which include increase or decrease in the number as well as structural alterations in a way that chromosomal material is deleted, duplicated or rearranged.

MOLECULAR PATHOLOGY

During the last quarter of the century, rapid strides have been made in the field of molecular biology. As a result, molecular techniques which were earlier employed for research purposes only have now been made available for diagnostic purposes. These techniques detect abnormalities at the level of DNA or RNA of the cell.

Broadly speaking, all the DNA/RNA-based molecular techniques employ hybridisation technique based on recombinant technology. Specific region of DNA or RNA is detected by labelling it with a probe (*Probe* is a chain of nucleotides consisting of certain number of known base pairs). Probes are of different sizes and sources as under:

1. *Genomic probes* is derived from a region of DNA of cells.
2. *cDNA probe* is derived from RNA by reverse transcription.
3. *Oligonucleotide probe* is a synthetic probe contrary to genomic DNA and cDNA probe both of which are derived from cellular material.
4. *Riboprobe* is prepared by *in vitro* transcription system.

Molecular Methods

Following is a brief account of various molecular techniques available as diagnostic tool in surgical pathology:

1. *IN SITU* HYBRIDISATION. *In situ* hybridisation (ISH) is a molecular hybridisation technique which allows localisation of nucleic acid sequence directly in *the intact cell* (i.e. *in situ)* without DNA extraction unlike other hybridisation-based methods described below. ISH involves specific hybridisation of a single strand of a labelled nucleic acid probe to a single strand of complementary target DNA or RNA in the tissue. The end-product of hybridisation is visualised by radioactive-labelled probe (^{32}P, ^{125}I), or non-radioactive-labelled probe (e.g. biotin, digoxigenin).

Applications. ISH is used for the following:

i) In *viral infections* e.g. HPV, EBV, HIV, CMV, HCV etc.

ii) In *human tumours* for detection of gene expression and oncogenes.

iii) In *chromosomal disorders,* particularly by use of fluorescent *in situ* hybridisation (FISH).

2. FILTER HYBRIDISATION. In this method, target DNA or RNA is extracted from the tissue, which may either be fresh, frozen and unfixed tissue, or formalin-fixed paraffin-embedded tissue. Extracted target DNA or RNA is then immobilised on nitrocellulose filter or nylon. Hybridisation of the target DNA is then done with labelled probe. DNA analysis by filter hybridisation includes various methods as under:

i) *Slot and dot blots* in which the DNA sample is directly bound to the filter without fractionation of nucleic acid size.

ii) *Southern blot* which is similar to dot-blot but differs in performing prior DNA-size fractionation by gel electrophoresis (E.M. Southern is the name of scientist who described Southern blot technique).

iii) *Northern blot* is similar to Southern blot but involves size fractionation of RNA (Northern is, however, opposite direction of southern and not someone's name).

iv) *Western blot* is analogous to the previous two methods but is employed for protein fractionation and in this method antibodies are used as probes.

Applications. In view of high degree of specificity and sensitivity of the molecular hybridisation techniques, these techniques have widespread applications in diagnostic pathology:

i) *In neoplasia,* haematologic as well as non-haematologic.

ii) *In infectious diseases* for actual diagnosis of causative agent, epidemiologic studies and identification of newer infectious agents.

iii) *In inherited genetic diseases* for carrier testing, prenatal diagnosis and direct diagnosis of the genetic disease.

iv) *In identity determination* for tissue transplantation, forensic pathology, and parentage testing.

3. POLYMERASE CHAIN REACTION. Polymerase chain reaction (PCR) is a revolutionary technique for molecular genetic purpose with widespread applications in diagnostics and research. The technique is based on the *principle* that a single strand of DNA has limitless capacity to duplicate itself to form millions of copies. In PCR, a single strand of DNA generates another by DNA polymerase using a short complementary DNA fragment; this is done using a *primer* which acts as an initiating template.

A *cycle of PCR* consists of three steps:

i) *Heat denaturation* of DNA (at 94°C for 60-90 seconds).

ii) *Annealing* of the primers to their complementary sequences (at 55°C for 30-120 seconds).

iii) *Extension* of the annealed primers with DNA polymerase (at 72°C for 60-180 seconds).

Repeated cycling can be done in automated thermal cycler and yields large accumulation of the target sequence since each newly generated product, in turn, acts as template in the next cycle.

Applications. PCR analysis has the same applications as for filter hybridisation techniques and has many advantages over them in being more rapid, can be automated by thermal cyclers and a need for low level of starting DNA/RNA. However, PCR suffers from the risk of contamination; thus extreme caution is required in the laboratory during PCR technique.

FLOW CYTOMETRY

Flow cytometry is a more recent tool in the study of properties of cells suspended in a single moving stream. Flow cytometry, thus, overcomes the problem of subjectivity involved in microscopic examination of cells and tissues in histopathology and cytopathology.

Flow cytometer has a laser-light source for fluorescence, cell transportation system in a single stream, monochromatic filters, lenses, mirrors and a computer for data analysis. Flow cytometer acts like a cell sorter to physically sort out cells from liquid suspension flowing in a single-file. Since single-cell suspensions are required for flow cytometry, its applications are limited to flow assays e.g. leucocytes, erythrocytes and their precursors; body fluids, and sometimes solid tissues made into cell suspensions.

Applications. Currently, flow cytometric analysis finds uses in clinical practice in the following ways:

1. *Immunophenotyping* by detailed antigenic analysis of various haematopoietic neoplasias e.g. acute and chronic leukaemias, lymphomas (Hodgkin's and non-Hodgkin's), and plasmacytic neoplasms.
2. *Diagnosis and prognostication of immunodeficiency* e.g. in AIDS by CD4 + T lymphocyte counts. Patients with CD4 + T cell counts below 500/μl require antiviral treatment.
3. To *diagnose the cause of allograft rejection* in renal transplantation in end-stage renal disease by CD3 + T cell counts. Patients with CD3 + T cells below 100-200/μl have lower risk of graft rejection.
4. *Diagnosis of autoantibodies* in ITP, and autoimmune neutropenia.
5. *Measurement of nucleic acid content* e.g. counting reticulocytes which contain RNA.
6. *DNA ploidy* studies in various types of cancers.

OTHER METHODS FOR CELL PROLIFERATION ANALYSIS

Besides flow cytometry, the degree of proliferation of cells in tumours can be determined by various other methods. These include the following:

1. Mitotic count. This is the oldest but still widely used method in routine diagnostic pathology work. The number of cells in mitosis are counted per high power field e.g. in categorising various types of smooth muscle tumours.

2. Radioautography. In this method, the proliferating cells are labelled *in vitro* with thymidine and then the tissue processed for paraffin-embedding. Thymidine-labelled cells (corresponding to S-phase) are then counted per 2000 tumour cell nuclei and expressed as thymidine-labelling index. The method is employed as prognostic marker in breast carcinoma.

3. Microspectrophotometric analysis. The section is stained with Feulgen reaction which imparts staining to DNA content of the cell and then DNA content is measured by microspectrophotometer. The method is tedious and has limited use.

4. Immunohistochemistry. The nuclear antigen specific for cell growth and division is stained by immunohistochemical method and then positive cells are counted under the microscope or by an image analyser. Such proliferation markers include Ki-67, Ki-S1, and cyclins.

5. Nucleolar organiser region (NOR). Nucleolus contains ribosomal components which are formed at chromosomal regions containing DNA called NORs. NORs have affinity for silver. This property is made use in staining the section with silver (Ag NOR technique). NORs appear as black intranuclear dots while the background is stained yellow-brown.

COMPUTERS IN PATHOLOGY LABORATORY

A busy pathology laboratory has a lot of data to be communicated to the clinicians. Pathologist too requires access to patient's data prior to reporting of results on specimens received. It is, therefore, imperative that a modern pathology laboratory has laboratory information system (LIS) which should be ideally connected to hospital information system (HIS).

Besides, the laboratory staff and doctors should have adequate computer literacy on these systems.

LIS includes: computer system, speech recognition system and image analysis system.

COMPUTER SYSTEMS. There are two main purposes of having computers in the laboratory:

- for the *billing* of patients' investigations; and
- for *reporting* of results of tests in numeric, narrative and graphic format.

Applications. Application of computers in the pathology laboratory has several advantages as under:

1. The laboratory as well as the hospital staff have access to information pertaining to the patient which helps in *improving patientcare.*
2. The *turn-around time* (i.e. time between specimen collection and reporting of results) of any test is shortened.
3. It *improves productivity* of laboratory staff at all levels who can be utilised for other jobs.
4. *Coding and indexing* of results and data of different tests is possible on computer system.
5. For *research purposes* and getting accredition so as to get grants for research, computerised data of results are mandatory.

SPEECH RECOGNITION SYSTEM. Computer systems are now available which can recognise and transform spoken words of gross and microscopic description of reports through dictaphone into text without the use of secretarial staff.

IMAGE ANALYSERS. Image analyser is a form of computer that can capture image formed by microscopic viewing of slide and transform it into digital image which can be used for various purposes e.g.

1. *Morphometric studies* of cells as regards their features.
2. *Quantitative nuclear DNA ploidy* measurement.
3. *Evaluation of immunohistochemical staining quantitatively.*
4. *Storage and retrieval of laboratory data to* save time and space occupied by the records.

The concept of *'tele-pathology'* (similar to *'tele-radiology'* for filmless radiology departments) instantaneously moves information on pathology work and also pass relevant literature on-line from one place to another far off place through internet information superhighway.

cDNA MICROARRAYS ANALYSIS. This is the latest application of silicon chip technology for simultaneous analysis of large volume of data pertaining to human genes for molecular profiling of tumours. The method eliminates use of DNA probes and instead fluorescent labelling of cDNA is used. High resolution laser scanners are used for detecting fluorescent signals while level of gene expression by different samples is measured by application of bioinformatics.

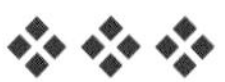

Cell Injury and Cellular Adaptations 3

Human body, unlike unicellular amoeba, is quite complex and is made of 70,000 billion cells which comprise different tissues and organs, each of which is assigned predetermined specific function. In health, these cells remain in accord with each other. However, most forms of diseases begin with cell injury and consequent loss of cellular function. *Cell injury is defined as a variety of stresses a cell encounters as a result of changes in its internal and external environment.* All cells of the body have inbuilt mechanism to deal with changes in environment to an extent. The cellular response to stress varies and depends upon the following variables:

i) The type of cell and tissue involved.
ii) On extent and type of cell injury.

Cellular responses to injury may be as follows (Fig. 3.1):

1. When there is increased functional demand, the cell may adapt to the changes which are expressed morphologically and then revert back to normal after the stress is removed *(cellular adaptations, see* Fig. 3.22).
2. When the stress is mild to moderate, the injured cell may recover *(reversible cell injury)*, while when the injury is persistent the cell may die *(irreversible cell injury)*.
3. The residual effects of reversible cell injury may persist in the cell as evidence of cell injury at subcellular level *(subcellular changes)*, or metabolites may accumulate within the cell *(intracellular accumulations)*.

In order to learn the fundamentals of disease processes, therefore, it is essential to have an understanding of the causes and mechanisms of cell injury and cellular adaptations. But before that, a brief review of structure of a normal mammalian cell and its functions is outlined below.

THE NORMAL CELL

Different types of cells of the body possess features which distinguish one type from another. However, most mammalian cells have an overall common structure and function.

CELL STRUCTURE

Under normal conditions, cells are dynamic structures existing in fluid environment. A cell is enclosed by cell membrane that extends internally to enclose nucleus and various subcellular organelles suspended in cytosol (Fig. 3.2).

I. Cell Membrane

Electron microscopy has shown that cell membrane or plasma membrane has a trilaminar structure having a total thickness of about 7.5 nm and is known as *unit membrane*. The three layers consist of two electron-dense

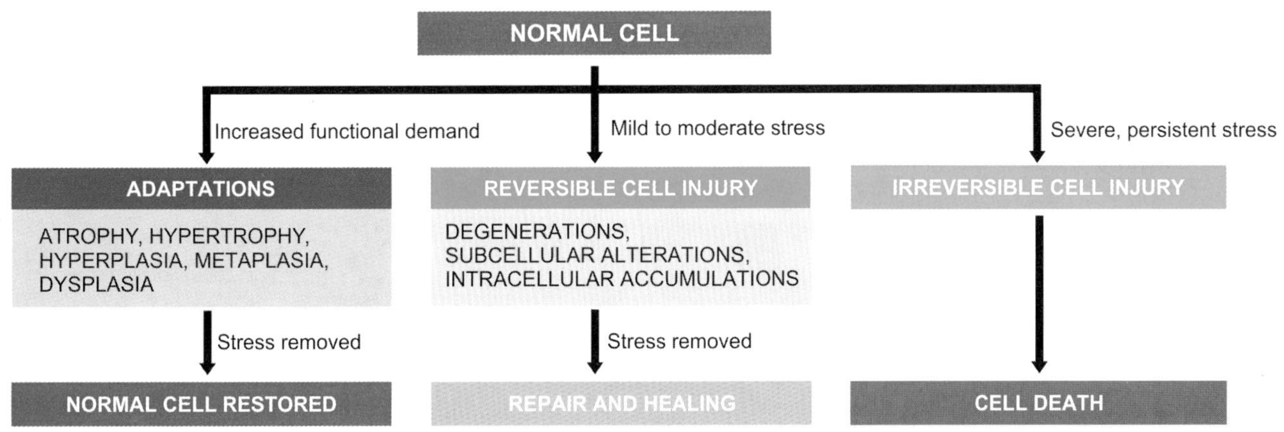

FIGURE 3.1

Cellular responses to cell injury.

layers separated by an electronlucent layer. Biochemically, the cell membrane is composed of complex mixture of phospholipids, glycolipids, cholesterol, proteins and carbohydrates. These layers are in a gel-like arrangement and are in a constant state of flux. The outer surface of some types of cells shows a coat of mucopolysaccharide forming a fuzzy layer called *glycocalyx*. Proteins and glycoproteins of the cell membrane may act as antigens (e.g. blood group antigens), or may form receptors (e.g. for viruses, bacterial products, hormones, immunoglobulins and many enzymes). The cell receptors are probably related to the microtubules and microfilaments of the underlying cytoplasm. The microtubules connect one receptor with the next. The microfilaments are contractile structures so that the receptor may move within the cell membrane. Bundle of microfilaments along with cytoplasm and protein of cell membrane may form projections on the surface of the cell called *microvilli*. Microvilli are especially numerous on the surface of absorptive and secretory cells (e.g. small intestinal mucosa) increasing their surface area.

In brief, the cell membrane performs the following important functions:

i) Selective permeability that includes diffusion, membrane pump ('sodium pump') and pinocytosis ('cell drinking').

ii) Membrane antigens (e.g. blood group antigens, transplantation antigen).

iii) Cell receptors for cell-cell recognition and communication.

II. Nucleus

The nucleus consists of an outer nuclear membrane enclosing nuclear chromatin and nucleoli.

1. NUCLEAR MEMBRANE. The nuclear membrane is the outer envelop consisting of 2 layers of the unit membrane which are separated by a 40-70 nm wide space. The outer layer of the nuclear membrane is studded with ribosomes and is continuous with endoplasmic reticulum. The two layers of nuclear membrane at places are fused together forming circular nuclear pores which are about 50 nm in diameter.

2. NUCLEAR CHROMATIN. The main substance of the nucleus is comprised by the nuclear chromatin which is in the form of shorter pieces of thread-like structures called *chromosomes* of which there are 23 pairs (46 chromosomes) together measuring about a metre in length in a human diploid cell. Of these, there are 22 pairs (44 chromosomes) of *autosomes* and one pair of *sex chromosomes*, either XX (female) or XY (male). Each chromosome is composed of two chromatids connected at the centromere to form 'X' configuration having variation in location of the centromere. Depending upon the length of chromosomes and centromeric location, 46 chromosomes are categorised into 7 groups from A to G according to *Denver classification* (adopted at a meeting in Denver, USA).

Chromosomes are composed of 3 components, each with distinctive function. These are: deoxyribonucleic acid (DNA) comprising about 20%, ribonucleic acid (RNA) about 10%, and the remaining 70% consists of

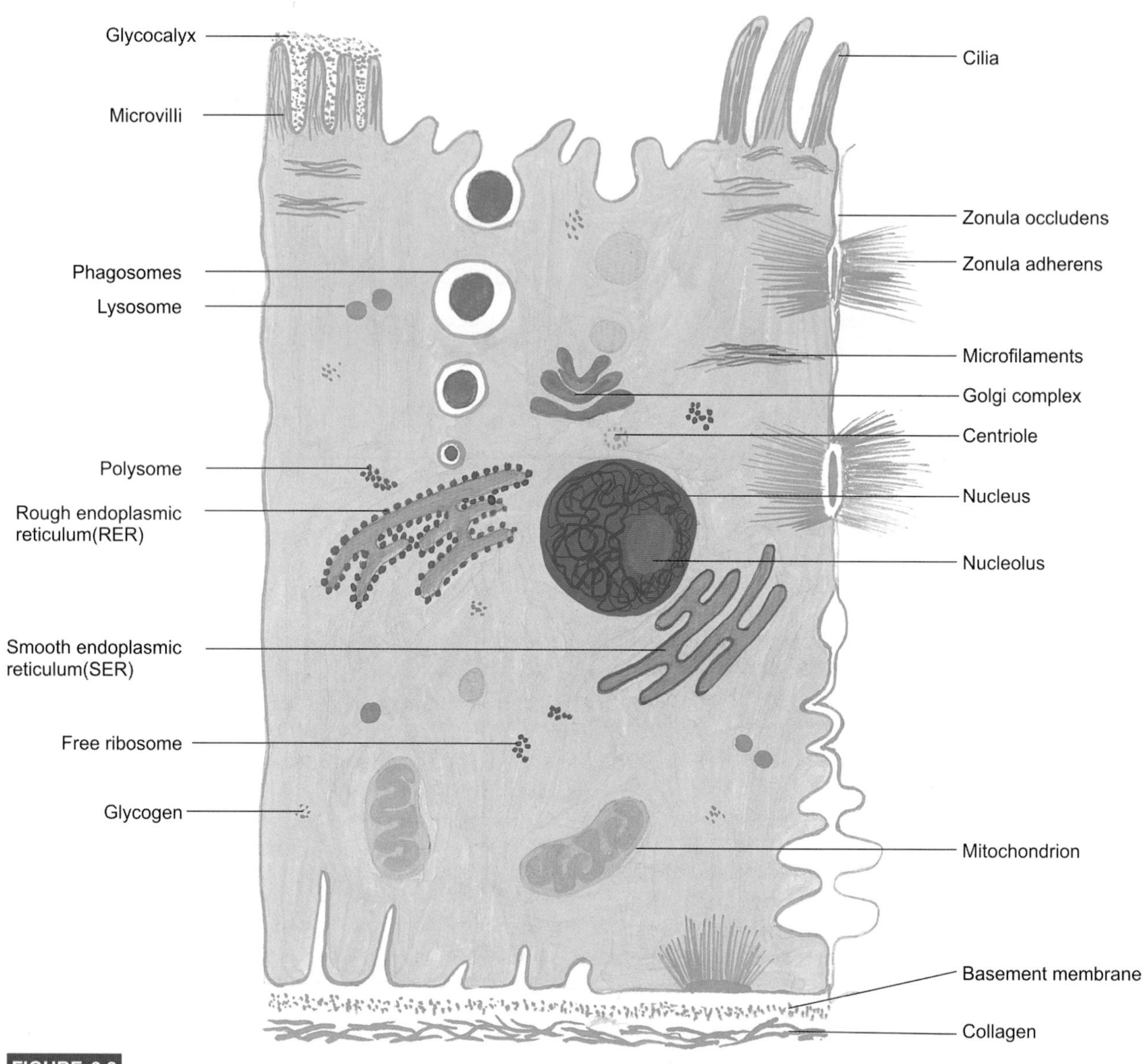

FIGURE 3.2

Schematic diagram of the structure of an epithelial cell.

nuclear proteins that include a number of basic proteins (histones), neutral proteins, and acid proteins. DNA of the cell is largely contained in the nucleus. The only other place in the cell that contains small amount of DNA is mitochondria. Nuclear DNA along with histone nuclear proteins form bead-like structures called nucleosomes which are studded along the coils of DNA. Nuclear DNA carries the genetic information that is passed via RNA into the cytoplasm for manufacture of proteins of similar composition. During cell division, one half of DNA molecule acts as a template for the manufacture of the other half by the enzyme, DNA polymerase, so that the genetic characteristics are transmitted to the next progeny of cells *(replication)*.

The **DNA molecule** as proposed by Watson and Crick in 1953 consists of two complementary polypeptide chains forming a double helical strand which is wound spirally around an axis composed of pentose sugar-phosphoric acid chains. The molecule is spirally twisted in a ladder-like pattern the steps of which are composed of *4 nucleotide bases: two purines* (adenine and guanine i.e. A and G) and *two pyrimidines* (cytosine and thymine i.e. C and T); however, A pairs specifically with T while G pairs with C (Fig. 3.3). The sequence of these nucleotide base pairs in the chain, of which there are thousands, determines the information contained in the DNA molecule or constitutes the genetic code.

In the interphase nucleus (i.e. between mitosis), part of the chromatin that remains relatively inert metabolically and appears deeply basophilic due to condensation of chromosomes is called *heterochromatin,* while the part of chromatin that is lightly stained or vesicular due to dispersed chromatin is called *euchromatin*. For example, in lymphocytes there is predominance of heterochromatin while the nucleus of a hepatocyte is mostly euchromatin.

3. NUCLEOLUS. The nucleus may contain one or more rounded bodies called nucleoli. Nucleolus is the site of synthesis of ribosomal RNA. Nucleolus is composed of granules and fibrils representing newly synthesised ribosomal RNA.

III. Cytosol and Organelles

The cytosol or the cytoplasm is the gel-like ground substance in which the organelles (meaning *little organs*) of the cells are suspended. These organelles are the site of major enzymatic activities of the cell which are possibly mediated by enzymes in the cytosol. The major organelles are the cytoskeleton, mitochondria, ribosomes, endoplasmic reticulum, Golgi apparatus or complex, lysosomes, and microbodies or peroxisomes.

1. CYTOSKELETON. Microfilaments, intermediate filaments, and microtubules are responsible for maintaining cellular form and movement and are collectively referred to as cytoskeleton.

i) Microfilaments are long filamentous structures having a diameter of 6-8 nm. They are composed of contractile proteins, actin and myosin, and diverse materials like parts of microtubules and ribonucleoprotein fibres. Bundles of microfilaments are especially prominent close to the plasma membrane and form *terminal web*. Extension of these bundles of microfilaments alongwith part of plasma membrane on the surface of the cell form *microvilli* which increase the absorptive surface of the cells.

ii) Intermediate filaments are filamentous structures, 10 nm in diameter, and are cytoplasmic constituent of a number of cell types. They are composed of proteins. There are 5 principal types of intermediate filaments:

a) *Cytokeratin* (found in epithelial cells).

b) *Desmin* (found in skeletal, smooth and cardiac muscle).

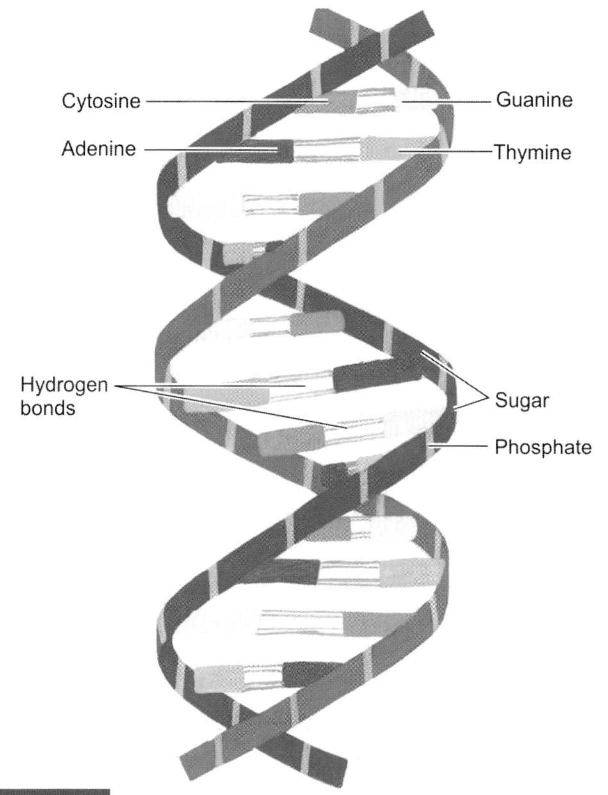

FIGURE 3.3

Diagrammatic structure of portion of DNA molecule.

c) *Vimentin* (found in cells of mesenchymal origin).

d) *Glial fibrillary acidic protein* (present in astrocytes and ependymal cells).

e) *Neurofilaments* (seen in neurons of central and peripheral nervous system).

Their main function is to mechanically integrate the cell organelles within the cytoplasm.

iii) Microtubules are long hollow tubular structures about 25 nm in diameter. They are composed of protein, tubulin. *Cilia* and *flagella* which project from the surface of cell are composed of microtubules enclosed by plasma membrane and are active in locomotion of the cells. *Basal bodies* present at the base of each cilium or flagellum and *centriole* located at the mitotic spindle of cells are the two other morphologically similar structures composed of microtubules.

2. MITOCHONDRIA. Mitochondria are oval structures and are more numerous in metabolically active cells. They are enveloped by two layers of membrane—the outer smooth and the inner folded into incompete septa or sheaf-like ridges called *cristae*. Chemically and structurally, membranes of mitochondria are similar to cell membrane. The inner membrane, in addition, contains lollipop-shaped globular structures projecting into the matrix present between the layers of membrane. The matrix of the mitochondria contains enzymes required in the Krebs' cycle by which the products of carbohydrate, fat and protein metabolism are oxidised to produce energy which is stored in the form of ATP in the lollipop-like globular structures. Mitochondria are not static structures but undergo changes in their configuration during energised state by alteration in matrix and intercristal space; the outer membrane is, however, less elastic. Aside from their role in metabolism, mitochondria possess DNA and ribosomes but no histones, and may have a role in synthesising membrane-bound proteins of mitochondria.

3. RIBOSOMES. Ribosomes are spherical particles which contain 80-85% of the cell's RNA. They may be present in the cytosol as 'free' unattached form, or in 'bound' form when they are attached to membrane of endoplasmic reticulum. They may lie as 'monomeric units' or as 'polyribosomes' when many monomeric ribosomes are attached to a linear molecule of messenger RNA. Ribosomes are the protein-synthesising units.

4. ENDOPLASMIC RETICULUM. Endoplasmic reticulum is composed of vesicles and intercommunicating canals whose main function is the manufacture of protein. It is composed of unit membrane which is continuous with both nuclear membrane and the Golgi apparatus, and possibly with the cell membrane. Morphologically, there are 2 forms of endoplasmic reticulum: rough or granular, and smooth or agranular.

i) *Rough endoplasmic reticulum (RER)* is so-called because its outer surface is rough or granular due to attached ribosomes on it. RER is especially well developed in cells active in protein synthesis e.g. Russell bodies of plasma cells, Nissl granules of nerve cells.

ii) *Smooth endoplasmic reticulum (SER)* is devoid of ribosomes on its surface. SER and RER are generally continuous with each other. SER contains many enzymes which metabolise drugs, steroids, cholesterol, and carbohydrates and partake in muscle contraction.

5. GOLGI APPARATUS OR COMPLEX. The Golgi apparatus or complex is generally located close to the nucleus. Morphologically, it appears as vesicles, sacs or lamellae composed of unit membrane and is continuous with the endoplasmic reticulum. The Golgi apparatus is particularly well developed in exocrine glandular cells. Its main functions are synthesis of carbohydrates and complex proteins and packaging of proteins synthesised in the RER into vesicles. Some of these vesicles may contain lysosomal enzymes and specific granules such as in neutrophils and in beta cells of the pancreatic islets.

6. LYSOSOMES. Lysosomes are rounded to oval membrane-bound organelles containing powerful lysosomal digestive (hydrolytic) enzymes. There are 3 forms of lysosomes:

i) *Primary lysosomes or storage vacuoles* are formed from the various hydrolytic enzymes synthesised by the RER and packaged in the Golgi apparatus.

ii) *Secondary lysosomes or autophagic vacuoles* are formed by fusion of primary lysosomes with the parts of damaged or worn-out cell components.

iii) *Residual bodies* are indigestible materials in the lysosomes e.g. lipofuscin.

7. CENTRIOLE OR CENTROSOME. These are seen as two small structures composed of electron-dense fibrils. They perform the function of formation of cilia and flagellae and form the spindle of fibrillary protein during mitosis.

IV. Intercellular Junctions

Plasma membranes of epithelial and endothelial cells, though closely apposed, are separated from each other by 20 nm wide space. These cells communicate across this space through intercellular junctions or junctional complexes visible under electron microscope and are of 4 types (Fig. 3.4):

1. Occluding junctions (Zonula occludens). These are tight junctions situated just below the luminal margin of adjacent cells. As a result, the regions of occluding zones are impermeable to macromolecules. The examples of occluding zones are seen in renal tubular epithelial cells, intestinal epithelium, and vascular endothelium in the brain constituting blood-brain barrier.

2. Adhering junctions (Zonula adherens). These are located just below the occluding zones between the adjacent cells and are permeable to tracer particles. These zones are in contact with actin microfilaments, e.g. in small cell carcinoma of the lung.

3. Desmosomes (Macula densa). These are tiny adhesion plates present focally between the adjacent epithelial cells, especially numerous in the epidermis. Bundles of intermediate filaments (termed tonofilaments in the case of epidermis) project from the intercellular desmosomes and radiate into the cytoplasm. Hemidesmosomes are a variant of desmosomes, occurring at the basal region of epithelial cells between plasma membrane and the basement membrane.

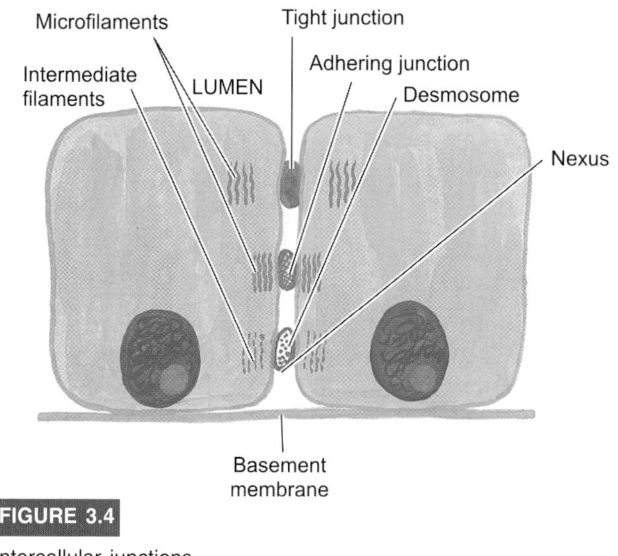

FIGURE 3.4

Intercellular junctions.

4. Gap junctions (Nexus). Gap junctions or nexus are the regions on the lateral surfaces of epithelial cells where the gap between the adjoining plasma membranes is reduced from 20 nm to about 2 nm in width. Pits or holes are present in the regions of gap junctions so that these regions are permeable to small tracer particles.

MOLECULAR INTERACTIONS BETWEEN CELLS

All cells in the body, including those in circulation, constantly exchange information with each other. This process is accomplished in the cells by chemical agents, also called as molecular agents or factors. Following categories are common to most cells in the body:

1. Cell adhesion molecules (CAMs)
2. Cytokines
3. Membrane receptors

1. Cell Adhesion Molecules (CAMs)

These are chemicals which mediate the interaction between cells (cell-cell interaction) as well as between cells and extracellular matrix (cell-ECM interaction).The *ECM* is the ground substance or matrix of connective tissue which provides environment to the cells and consists of 3 components:

i) fibrillar structural proteins (collagen, elastin);

ii) adhesion proteins (fibronectin, laminin, fibrillin, osteonectin, tenacin); and

iii) molecules of proteoglycans and glycosaminoglycans (heparan sulphate, chondroitin sulphate, dermatan sulphate, keratan sulphate, hyaluronic acid).

CAMs participate in fertilisation, embryogenesis, tissue repair, haemostasis, cell death by apoptosis and in inflammation. CAMs may be detected on the surface of cells as well as free in circulation. There are 5 groups of CAMs:

i) Integrins: They have alpha (or CD11*) and beta (CD18) subunits and have a role in cell-ECM interactions and in leucocyte-endothelial cell interaction.

ii) Cadherins: These are calcium-dependent adhesion molecules which bind adjacent cells together and prevent invasion of ECM by cancer cells. Various types of cadherins include: E-cadherin (epithelial cell), N-cadherin (nerve cell), M-cadherin (muscle cell), P-cadherin (placenta).

iii) Selectins: Also called as lectins, these CAMs contain lectins or lectin-like protein molecules which bind to glycoproteins and glycolipids on the cell surface. Their major role is in movement of leucocytes and platelets and develop contact with endothelial cells. Selectins are of 3 types: *P-selectin* (from platelets, also called CD62), *E-selectin* (from endothelial cells, also named ECAM), and *L-selectin* (from leucocytes, also called LCAM).

iv) Immunoglobulin superfamily: This group consists of a variety of immunoglobulin molecules present on most cells of the body. These partake in cell-to-cell contact through various other CAMs and cytokines. They have a major role in recognition and binding of immunocompetent cells. This group includes ICAM-1,2 (intercellular adhesion molecule, also called CD54), VCAM (vascular cell adhesion molecule, also named CD106), NCAM (neural cell adhesion molecule).

v) CD44: The last group of adhesion molecules is a break away from immunoglobulin superfamily. CD44 molecule binds to hyaluronic acid and is expressed on leucocytes. It is involved in leucocyte-leucocyte-endothelial interactions as well as in cell-ECM interactions.

2. Cytokines

These are soluble proteins secreted by haemopoietic and non-haemopoietic cells in response to various stimuli. Their main role is in activation of immune system. Presently, about 50 cytokines have been identified which are grouped in 6 categories:

i) interferons (IFN),

ii) interleukins (IL),

iii) tumour necrosis factor (TNF, cachectin),

*CD number (for Cluster of Differentiation) is the nomenclature given to the clone of cells which carry these molecules on their cell surface or in their cytoplasm.

iv) transforming growth factor (TGF),
v) colony stimulating factor (CSF), and
vi) growth factors.

The examples of growth factors are platelet-derived growth factor (PDGF), epidermal growth factor (EGF), fibroblast growth factor (FGF), endothelial-derived growth factor (EDGF), transforming growth factor (TGF).

All these cytokines have further subtypes as alpha, beta, or are identified by numbers. Cytokines involved in leucocyte-endothelial cell interaction are called *chemokines* while growth factors and other cytokines are named *crinopectins*.

3. Cell Membrane Receptors

Cell receptors are molecules consisting of proteins, glycoproteins or lipoproteins and may be located on the outer cell membrane, inside the cell, or may be trans-membranous. These receptor molecules are synthesised by the cell itself depending upon their requirement, and thus there may be upregulation or downregulation of number of receptors. There are 3 main types of receptors:

i) Enzyme-linked receptors: These receptors are involved in control of cell growth e.g. tyrosine kinase associated receptors take part in activation of synthesis and secretion of various hormones.

ii) Ion channels: The activated receptor for ion exchange such as for sodium, potassium and calcium and certain pepetide hormones determines inward or outward movement of these molecules.

iii) G-protein receptors. These are trans-membranous receptors and activate phosphorylating enzymes for metabolic and synthetic functions of cells. The activation of adenosine monophosphate-phosphatase cycle (c-AMP) by the G-proteins (guanosine nucleotide binding regulatory proteins) is the most important signal system, also known as 'second messenger' activation. The activated second messenger (cyclic-AMP) then regulates other intracellular activities.

CELL CYCLE

Multiplication of the somatic (mitosis) and germ (meiosis) cells is the most complex of all cell functions. Mitosis is controlled by genes which encode for release of specific proteins molecules that promote or inhibit the process of mitosis at different steps. Mitosis promoting protein molecules are *cyclins A, B and E.* These cyclins activate *cyclin-dependent kinases (CDKs)* which act in conjunction with cyclins. After the mitosis is complete, cyclins and CDKs are degraded and the residues of used molecules are taken up by cytoplasmic caretaker proteins, *ubiquitin,* to the peroxisome for further degradation.

Period between the mitosis is called *interphase*. The *cell cycle* is the phase between two consecutive divisions (Fig. 3.5). There are 4 sequential phases in the cell cycle: G_1 (gap 1) phase, S (synthesis) phase, G_2 (gap 2) phase, and M (mitotic) phase.

G_1 (Pre-mitotic gap) phase is the stage when messenger RNAs for the proteins and the proteins themselves required for DNA synthesis (e.g. DNA polymerase) are synthesised. The process is under control of cyclin E and CDKs.

S phase involves replication of nuclear DNA. Cyclin A and CDKs control it.

G_2 (Pre-mitotic gap) phase is the short gap phase in which correctness of DNA synthesised is assessed. This stage is promoted by cyclin B and CDKs.

M phase is the stage in which process of mitosis to form two daughter cells is completed. This occurs in 4 sequential stages: *prophase, metaphase, anaphase,* and *telophase* (i.e. PMAT).

- *Prophase.* Each chromosome divides into 2 chromatids which are held together by centromere. The centriole divides and the two daughter centrioles move towards opposite poles of the nucleus and the nuclear membrane disintegrates.
- *Metaphase.* The microtubules become arranged between the two centrioles forming spindle, while the chromosomes line up at the equatorial plate of the spindle.
- *Anaphase.* The centromeres divide and each set of separated chromosomes moves towards the opposite poles of the spindle. Cell membrane also begins to divide.
- *Telophase.* There is formation of nuclear membrane around each set of chromosomes and reconstitution of the nucleus. The cytoplasm of the two daughter cells completely separates.

G_0 phase. The daughter cells may continue to remain in the cell cycle and divide further, or may go out of the cell cycle into resting phase, called G_0 phase.

Stimulation of mitosis can be studied in a number of ways as under:

- *Compensatory stimulation* of mitosis by removal of part of an organ.
- *Reparative stimulation* of mitosis occurs when a tissue is injured.

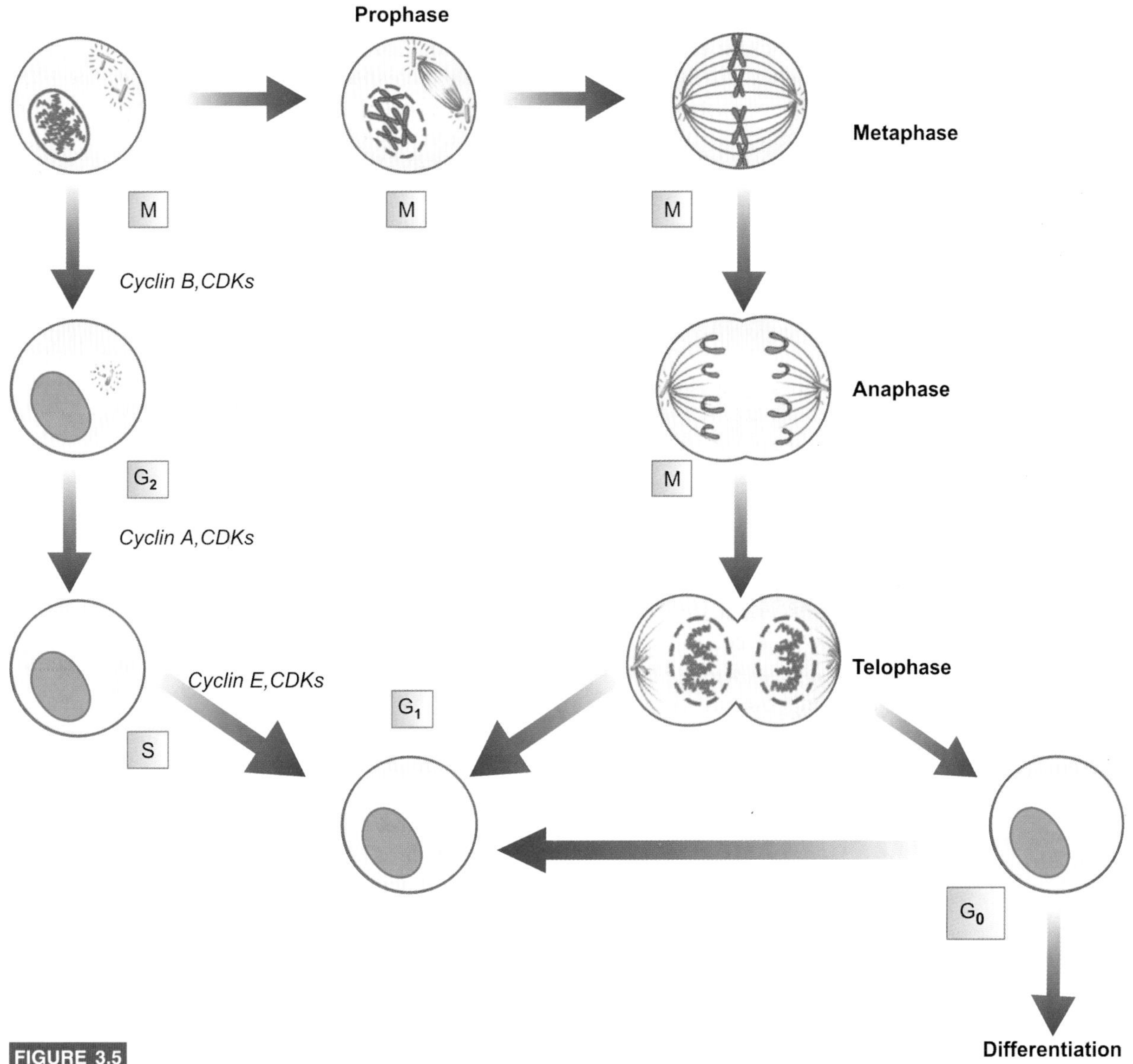

FIGURE 3.5

The cell cycle in mitosis. Premitotic phases are the G_1, S and G_2 phase while M (mitotic) phase is accomplished in 4 sequential stages: prophase, metaphase, anaphase, and telophase. On completion of cell division, two daughter cells are formed which may continue to remain in the cell cycle or go out of it in resting phase, the G_0 phase. (CDK = *cyclin dependent kinase*).

■ *Target organ stimulation* of mitosis occurs under the influence of specific hormones which have mitogenic effect on cells of the target organ.

ETIOLOGY OF CELL INJURY

The causes of cell injury, reversible or irreversible, may be broadly classified into two large groups:

A. Genetic causes
B. Acquired causes

The genetic causes of various diseases are discussed in Chapter 10. The acquired causes of disease comprise vast majority of common diseases afflicting mankind. Based on underlying agent, the acquired causes of cell injury can be further categorised as under:

1. Hypoxia and ischaemia
2. Physical agents
3. Chemical agents and drugs
4. Microbial agents
5. Immunologic agents
6. Nutritional derangements
7. Psychological factors.

In a given situation, more than one of the above etiologic factors may be involved.

1. HYPOXIA AND ISCHAEMIA. Cells of different tissues essentially require oxygen to generate energy and perform metabolic functions. Deficiency of oxygen or hypoxia results in failure to carry out these activities by the cells. Hypoxia is the most common cause of cell injury. The causes of hypoxia are as under:

- The most common mechanism of hypoxic cell injury is by reduced supply of blood to cells i.e. ischaemia.
- However, oxygen deprivation of tissues may result from other causes as well e.g. in anaemia, carbon monoxide poisoning, cardiorespiratory insufficiency, and increased demand of tissues.

2. PHYSICAL AGENTS. Physical agents in causation of disease are:

- mechanical trauma (e.g. road accidents);
- thermal trauma (e.g. by heat and cold);
- electricity;
- radiation (e.g. ultraviolet and ionising); and
- rapid changes in atmospheric pressure.

3. CHEMICALS AND DRUGS. An ever increasing list of chemical agents and drugs may cause cell injury. Important examples include:

- chemical poisons such as cyanide, arsenic, mercury;
- strong acids and alkalis;
- environmental pollutants;
- insecticides and pesticides;
- oxygen at high concentrations;
- hypertonic glucose and salt;
- social agents such as alcohol and narcotic drugs; and
- therapeutic administration of drugs.

4. MICROBIAL AGENTS. Injuries by microbes include infections caused by bacteria, rickettsiae, viruses, fungi, protozoa, metazoa, and other parasites.

Diseases caused by biologic agents are discussed in Chapter 7.

5. IMMUNOLOGIC AGENTS. Immunity is a 'double-edged sword'—it protects the host against various injurious agents but it may also turn lethal and cause cell injury e.g.

- hypersensitivity reactions;
- anaphylactic reactions; and
- autoimmune diseases.

Immunologic diseases are discussed in Chapter 4.

6. NUTRITIONAL DERANGEMENTS. A deficiency or an excess of nutrients may result in nutritional imbalances.

- Nutritional deficiency diseases may be due to overall deficiency of nutrients (e.g. starvation), of protein calorie (e.g. marasmus, kwashiorkor), of minerals (e.g. anaemia), or of trace elements.
- Nutritional excess is a problem of affluent societies resulting in obesity, atherosclerosis, heart disease and hypertension.

Nutritional diseases are discussed in Chapter 9.

7. PSYCHOLOGIC FACTORS. There are no specific biochemical or morphologic changes in common acquired mental diseases due to mental stress, strain, anxiety, overwork and frustration e.g. depression, schizophrenia. However, problems of drug addiction, alcoholism, and smoking result in various organic diseases such as liver damage, chronic bronchitis, lung cancer, peptic ulcer, hypertension, ischaemic heart disease etc.

PATHOGENESIS OF CELL INJURY

The underlying alterations in biochemical systems of cells for reversible and irreversible cell injury by various agents listed above is complex and varied. However, in general, the following principles apply in pathogenesis of most forms of cell injury by various agents:

1. Type, duration and severity of injurious agent: The extent of cellular injury depends upon type, duration and severity of the stimulus e.g. small dose of chemical toxin or short duration of ischaemia cause reversible cell injury while large dose of the same chemical agent or persistent ischaemia cause cell death.

2. Type, status and adaptability of target cell: The type of cell as regards its susceptibility to injury, its nutritional and metabolic status, and adaptation of the cell to hostile environment determine the extent of cell injury e.g. skeletal muscle can withstand hypoxic injury for long time while cardiac muscle suffers irreversible cell injury after 30-60 minutes of persistent ischaemia.

3. Underlying intracellular phenomena: Irrespective of other factors, two essential biochemical phenomena underlie all forms of cell injury to distinguish between reversible and irreversible cell injury:

i) Inability to reverse mitochondrial dysfunction by reperfusion or reoxygenation.

ii) Disturbance in membrane function in general, and in plasma membrane in particular.

4. Morphologic consequences: All forms of biochemical changes underlying cell injury are expressed in terms of morphologic changes. The ultrastructural changes become apparent earlier than the light microscopic alterations. The morphologic changes of reversible cell injury (e.g. hydropic swelling) appear earlier than morphologic alterations in cell death (e.g. in myocardial infarction).

The interruption of blood supply (ischaemia) and impaired oxygen supply to the tissues (hypoxia) are most common form of cell injury in human beings. Pathogenesis of hypoxic and ischaemic cell injury is, therefore, discussed in detail below followed by brief discussion on pathogenesis of chemical and physical (ionising radiation) agents. Immunologic tissue injury (Chapter 4) and nutritional factors (Chapter 9) are discussed in respective chapters.

Pathogenesis of Ischaemic and Hypoxic Injury

Ischaemia and hypoxia are common causes of cell injury. The underlying intracellular processes and mechanisms involved in reversible and irreversible cell injury by hypoxia and ischaemia are as under:

REVERSIBLE CELL INJURY. If the ischaemia or hypoxia is of short duration, the effects are reversible on rapid restoration of circulation e.g. in coronary artery occlusion, myocardial contractility, metabolism and ultrastructure are reversed if the circulation is quickly restored. The sequential changes in reversible cell injury are as under (Fig. 3.6):

1. Decreased generation of cellular ATP. ATP is essentially required for a variety of cellular functions such as membrane transport, protein synthesis, lipid synthesis and phospholipid metabolism. ATP in human cell is derived from 2 sources—*firstly,* by aerobic respiration or oxidative phosphorylation (which requires oxygen) in the mitochondria, and *secondly,* by anaerobic glycolytic pathway (in which ATP is generated from glucose/glycogen in the absence of oxygen). Ischaemia and hypoxia both limit the supply of oxygen to the cells, thus causing decreased ATP generation from ADP. But in *ischaemia,* aerobic respiration as well as glucose availability are both compromised resulting in more severe effects of cell injury. On the other hand, in *hypoxia* anaerobic glycolytic energy production continues and thus cell injury is less severe. Secondly, highly specialised cells such as myocardium, proximal tubular cells of the kidney, and neurons of the CNS are dependent on aerobic respiration for ATP generation and thus these tissues suffer from ill-effects of ischaemia more severely and rapidly.

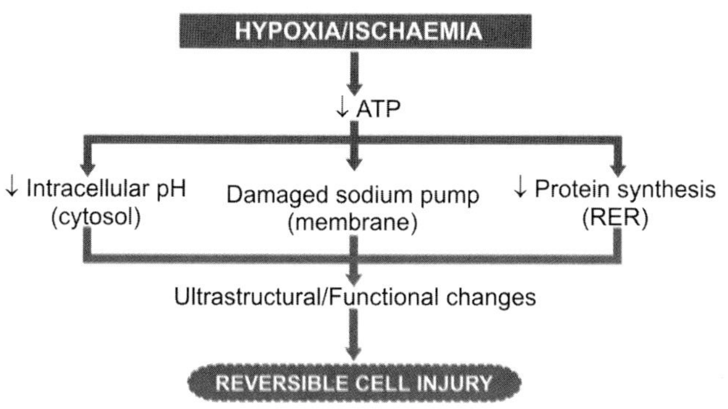

FIGURE 3.6

Sequence of events in the pathogenesis of reversible cell injury caused by hypoxia/ischaemia.

2. Reduced intracellular pH. Due to low oxygen supply to the cell, aerobic respiration by mitochondria fails first. This is followed by switch to anaerobic glycolytic pathway for the energy (i.e. ATP) requirement. This results in rapid depletion of glycogen and accumulation of lactic acid lowering the intracellular pH. Early fall in intracellular pH (i.e. intracellular acidosis) results in clumping of nuclear chromatin.

3. Damage to plasma membrane sodium pump. Normally, the energy (ATP)-dependent sodium pump ($Na^+ - K^+$ ATPase) operating at the plasma membrane allows active transport of sodium out of the cell and diffusion of potassium into the cell. Lowered ATP in the cell and consequent increased ATPase activity interfere with this membrane-regulated process. This results in intracellular accumulation of sodium and diffusion of potassium out of cell. The accumulation of sodium in the cell leads to increase in intracellular water to maintain iso-osmotic conditions (hydropic swelling, discussed later in the chapter).

4. Reduced protein synthesis. As a result of continued hypoxia, ribosomes are detached from granular endoplasmic reticulum and polysomes are degraded to monosomes, thus causing reduced protein synthesis.

5. Functional consequences. Reversible cell injury may result in functional disturbances e.g. myocardial contractility ceases within 60 seconds of coronary occlusion but can be reversed if circulation is restored.

6. Ultrastructural changes. Reversible injury to the cell causes the following ultrastructural changes (Fig. 3.7,A):

i) *Endoplasmic reticulum:* Distension of cisternae by fluid and detachment of membrane-bound polyribosomes from the surface of RER.

ii) *Mitochondria:* Mitochondrial swelling and phospholipid-rich amorphous densities.

iii) *Plasma membrane:* Loss of microvilli and focal projections of the cytoplasm ('blebs').

iv) *Myelin figures:* These are structures lying in the cytoplasm or present outside the cell. They are derived

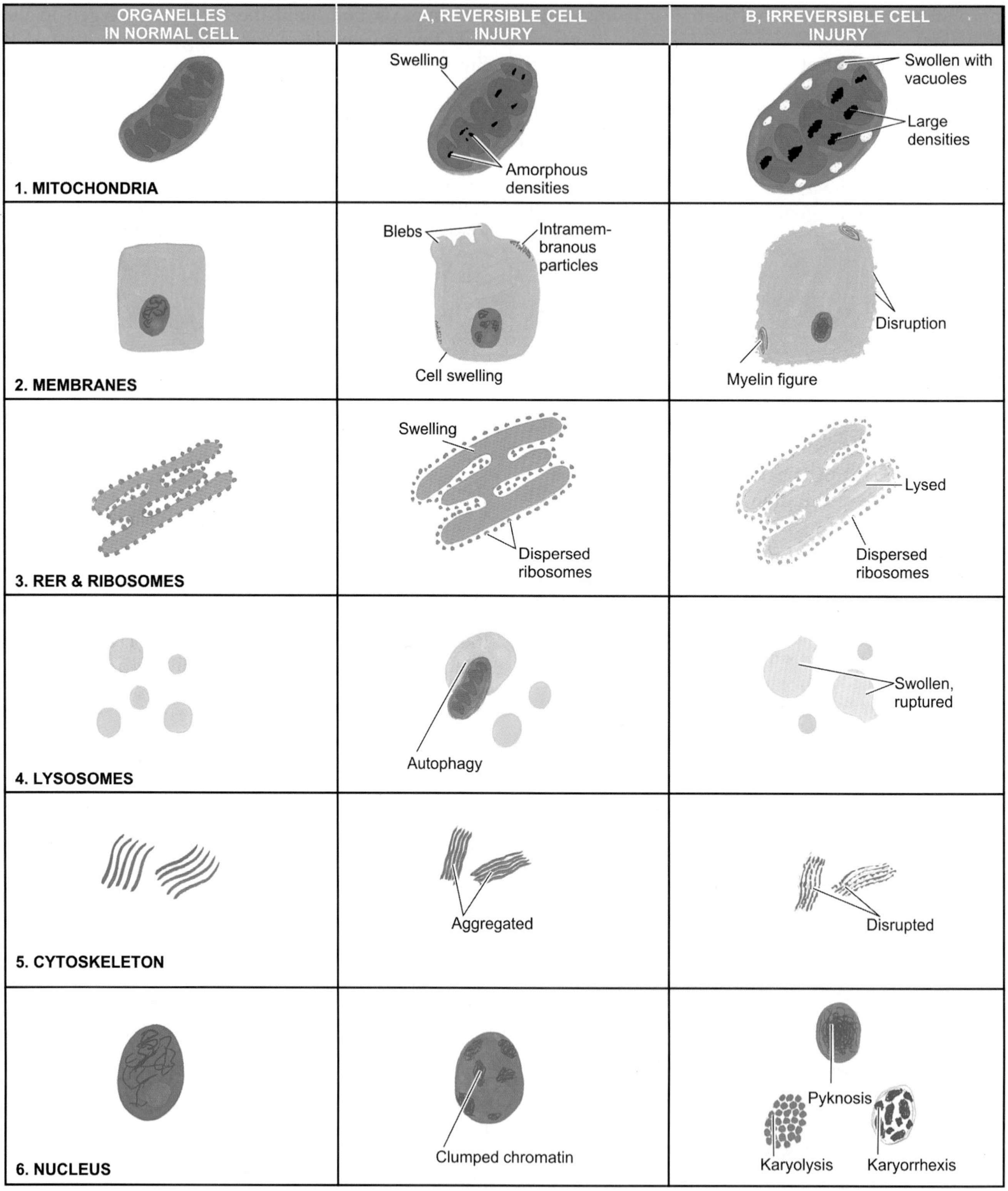

ORGANELLES IN NORMAL CELL	A, REVERSIBLE CELL INJURY	B, IRREVERSIBLE CELL INJURY
1. MITOCHONDRIA	Swelling; Amorphous densities	Swollen with vacuoles; Large densities
2. MEMBRANES	Blebs; Intramembranous particles; Cell swelling	Disruption; Myelin figure
3. RER & RIBOSOMES	Swelling; Dispersed ribosomes	Lysed; Dispersed ribosomes
4. LYSOSOMES	Autophagy	Swollen, ruptured
5. CYTOSKELETON	Aggregated	Disrupted
6. NUCLEUS	Clumped chromatin	Pyknosis; Karyolysis; Karyorrhexis

FIGURE 3.7

Ultrastructural changes during cell injury due to hypoxia-ischaemia.

from membranes (plasma or organellar) enclosing water and dissociated lipoproteins between the lamellae of injured membranes.

v) *Nucleolus:* There is segregation of granular and fibrillar components of nucleolus and reduced synthesis of ribosomal RNA.

Upto this point, withdrawal of acute stress that resulted in reversible cell injury can restore the cell to normal state.

IRREVERSIBLE CELL INJURY. Persistence of ischaemia or hypoxia results in irreversible changes in structure and function of the cell (cell death). The stage at which this *point of no return* is reached from reversible cell injury is unclear but the sequence of events is a continuation of reversibly injured cell. Two essential phenomena always distinguish irreversible from reversible cell injury (Fig. 3.7,B):

- Inability of the cell to reverse *mitochondrial dysfunction* on reperfusion or reoxygenation; and
- *Disturbance in cell membrane function* in general, and in plasma membrane in particular.

In addition, there is continued depletion of proteins, leakage of lysosomal enzymes into the cytoplasm, reduced intracellular pH and further reduction in ATP.

1. Mitochondrial dysfunction. As a result of continued hypoxia, a large cytosolic influx of Ca^{++} ions occurs, especially after reperfusion of irreversibly injured cell, which is taken up by mitochondria and is the cause of mitochondrial dysfunction. Morphologically, mitochondrial changes seen are vacuoles in the mitochondria and deposits of amorphous calcium salts in the mitochondrial matrix.

2. Membrane damage. Defect in membrane function in general, and plasma membrane in particular, is the most important event in irreversible cell injury in ischaemia. The mechanisms underlying membrane damage are as under (Fig. 3.8):

i) *Accelerated degradation of membrane phospholipid.* Oxygen deprivation causes shift of calcium from mitochondria and endoplasmic reticulum into the cytosol. Increased level of calcium in the cytosol activates endogenous phospholipases from ischaemic tissue which degrade membrane phospholipids progressively which are the main constituent of the lipid bilayer membrane. An alternate hypothesis is decreased replacement-synthesis of membrane phospholipids due to reduced ATP.

ii) *Cytoskeletal damage.* The normal intermediate filaments of the cytoskeleton which are anchored to the cell membrane are damaged due to degradation by activated intracellular proteases or by physical effect of cell swelling producing irreversible cell membrane injury.

iii) *Toxic oxygen radicals.* Another important mechanism of irreversible cell injury is free-radical induced (described below). Reactive oxygen-derived species—superoxide (O'_2), hydrogen peroxide (H_2O_2) and hydroxyl radicals ($\dot{O}H^-$), are increased in ischaemia. These oxygen radicals are produced during reperfusion by incoming polymorphs. Free radical injury is operative not only in hypoxia but also in radiation injury, chemical injury, microbial killing, aging, atherosclerosis, carcinogenesis.

iv) *Break down products of lipid.* The lipid break down products and catabolic products which accumulate in the injured cell cause further damage to various cell membranes.

v) *Reperfusion damage.* Normally, the concentration of calcium ions in extracellular fluid is 10^{-3} M while that in the cytosol is much low 10^{-7} M (M for millimole). Upon reperfusion of irreversibly injured cell, calcium homeostasis is disturbed and there is large cytosolic influx of calcium ions. An increased cytosolic calcium concentration may activate membrane phospholipases leading to phospholipid degradation, or calcium-dependent proteases may get activated to bring about membrane damage.

3. Hydrolytic enzymes. Damage to lysosomal membranes is followed by liberation of *hydrolytic enzymes* (RNAase, DNAase, proteases, glycosidases, phosphatases, and cathepsin) which on activation cause enzymatic digestion of cellular components and induce the nuclear changes (pyknosis, karyolysis and karyorrhexis) and hence cell death. The dead cell is eventually replaced by masses of phospholipids called *myelin figures* which are either phagocytosed by macrophages or there may be formation of calcium soaps.

4. Serum estimation of liberated intracellular enzymes. Liberated enzymes just mentioned leak across the abnormally permeable cell membrane into the serum, the estimation of which may be used as clinical parameters of cell death. For example, in myocardial infarction, estimation of elevated serum glutamic oxaloacetic transaminase (SGOT), lactic dehydrogenase (LDH), isoenzyme of creatine kinase (CK-MB), and more recently cardiac troponins (cTn) are useful guides for death of heart muscle.

Ischaemia-Reperfusion Injury

Depending upon the duration of ischaemia/hypoxia, restoration of blood flow may result in the following 3 different consequences:

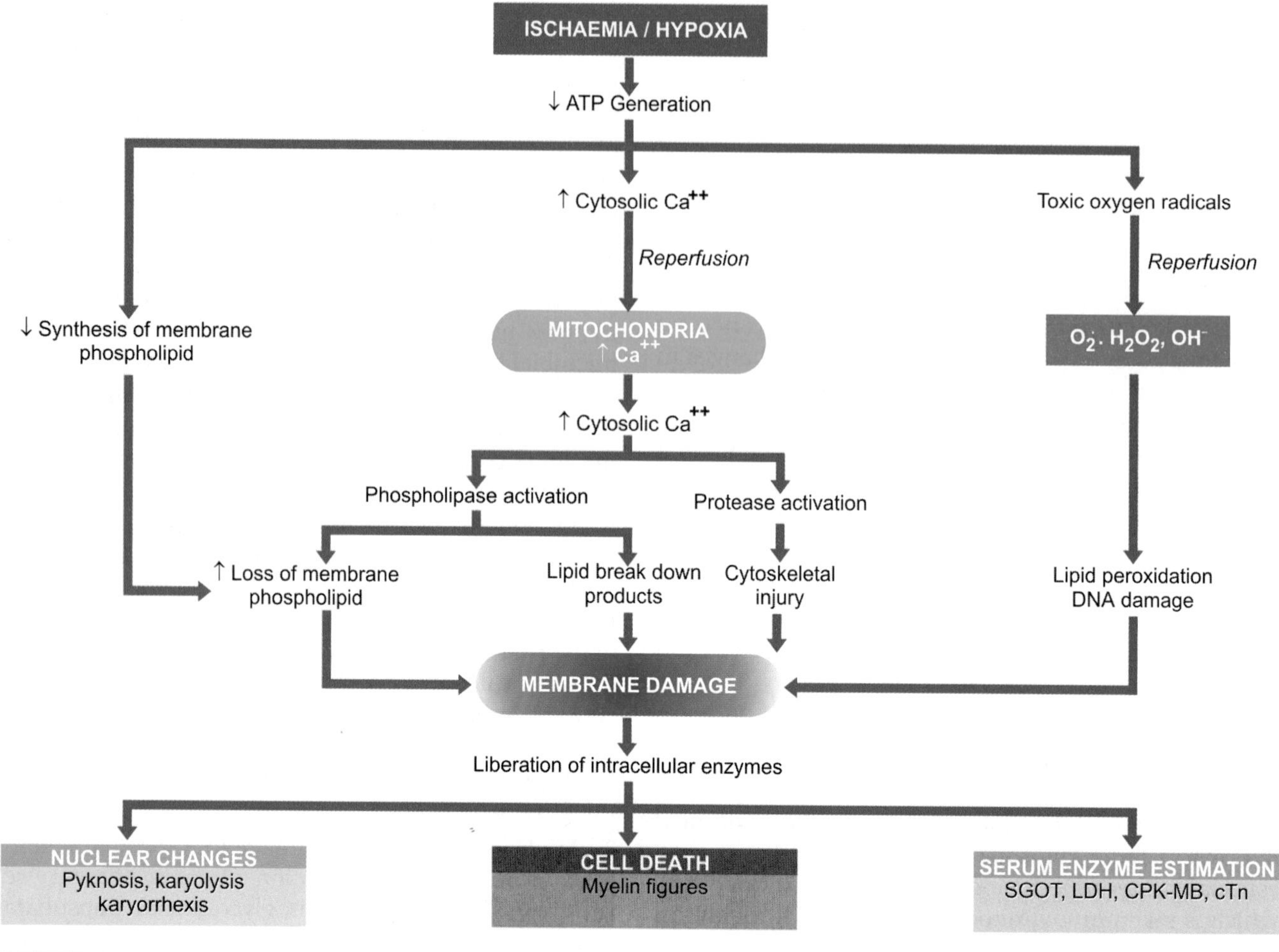

FIGURE 3.8

Possible sequence of events in the pathogenesis of irreversible cell injury with ischaemia.

1. *When the period of ischaemia is of short duration,* reperfusion with resupply of oxygen restores the structural and functional state of the injured cell i.e. reversible cell injury.

2. *When ischaemia is for longer duration,* then rather than restoration of structure and function of the cell, reperfusion paradoxically deteriorates the already injured cell. This is termed ischaemia-reperfusion injury. The main proposed mechanism in ischaemia-reperfusion injury is that upon reoxygenation there is increased generation of oxygen free radicals or activated oxygen species (superoxide, H_2O_2, hydroxyl radicals) from incoming inflammatory cells. Alternatively, during reperfusion activated oxygen species may be generated by adhesion and activation of circulating neutrophils. Besides, ischaemia also damages the cellular antioxidant defense mechanism favouring further accumulation of oxygen free radicals.

3. *Longer period of ischaemia* may also produce irreversible cell injury *during ischaemia itself* without any role of reperfusion. Cell death in such cases is not attributed to formation of activated oxygen species. But instead on reperfusion there is marked intracellular excess of sodium and calcium ions due to cell membrane damage.

Free Radical-Mediated Cell Injury

Although oxygen is the lifeline of all cells and tissues, its molecular forms as oxygen free radicals (or reactive oxygen intermediates) can be most devastating for the cells. Free radical-mediated cell injury plays an important role in the following situations:

i) In ischaemic reperfusion injury (as mentioned above in mechanism of membrane damage in hypoxia).
ii) In ionising radiation by causing radiolysis of water
iii) In chemical toxicity
iv) Hyperoxia (toxicity due to oxygen therapy)
v) Cellular aging
vi) Killing of exogenous biologic agents
vii) Inflammatory damage
viii) Destruction of tumour cells
ix) Chemical carcinogenesis
x) Atherosclerosis.

Generation of oxygen free radicals begins within mitochondrial inner membrane when cytochrome oxidase catalyses the four electron reduction of oxygen (O_2) to water (H_2O). Intermediate between reaction of O_2 to H_2O, three partially reduced species of oxygen are generated depending upon the number of electrons transferred. These are:

- Superoxide oxygen (O'_2): one electron
- Hydrogen peroxide (H_2O_2): two electrons
- Hydroxyl radical (OH^-): three electrons.

A few other oxygen radicals which may be generated in reactions other than those during O_2 to H_2O are: hypochlorous acid (HOCl), peroxynitrate ion (ONOO), nitric oxide (NO) generated by various body cells (endothelial cells, neurons, macrophages etc), and release of superoxide free radical in Fenton reaction (see below).

FREE RADICAL GENERATION. The three partially reduced intermediate species between O_2 to H_2O are derived from enzymatic and non-enzymatic reaction as under (Fig. 3.9):

1. *Superoxide (O'_2):* Superoxide anion O'_2 may be generated by direct auto-oxidation of O_2 during mitochondrial electron transport reaction. Alternatively, O^-_2 is produced enzymatically by xanthine oxidase and cytochrome P_{450} in the mitochondria or cytosol. O^-_2 so formed is catabolised to produce H_2O_2 by superoxide dismutase (SOD).

2. *Hydrogen peroxide (H_2O_2):* H_2O_2 is reduced to water enzymatically by catalase (in the peroxisomes) and glutathione peroxidase GSH (both in the cytosol and mitochondria).

3. *Hydroxyl radical (OH^-):* OH^- radical is formed by 2 ways in biologic processes: by radiolysis of water and by reaction of H_2O_2 with ferrous (Fe^{++}) ions; the latter process is termed as Fenton reaction.

FREE RADICAL REACTIONS. The hydroxyl radical is the most reactive species. It may produce membrane damage by the following mechanisms (Fig. 3.10):

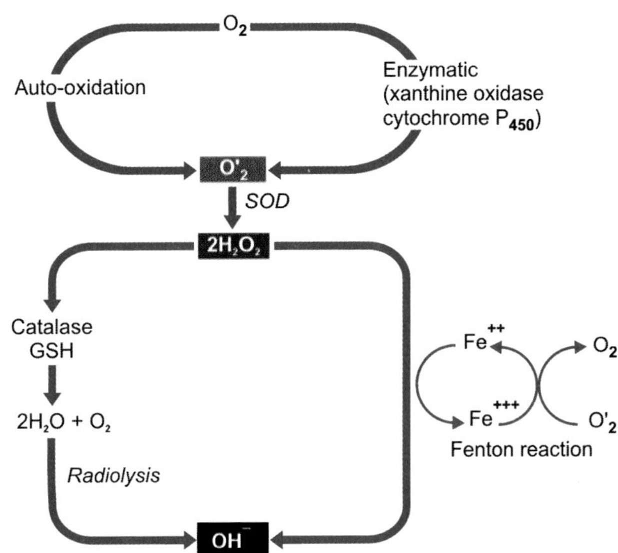

FIGURE 3.9
Mechanisms of generation of free radicals by free radicals. (SOD = *superoxide dismutase;* GSH = *glutathione peroxidase*).

i) *Lipid peroxidation.* Polyunsaturated fatty acids (PUFA) of membrane are attacked repeatedly and severely by oxygen-derived free radicals to yield highly destructive PUFA radicals—lipid hydroperoxy radicals and lipid hypoperoxides. This reaction is termed lipid peroxidation. The lipid peroxides are decomposed by transition metals such as iron. Lipid peroxidation is propagated to other sites causing widespread membrane damage and destruction of organelles.

ii) *Oxidation of proteins.* Oxygen-derived free radicals cause cell injury by oxidation of protein macromolecules of the cells, cross linking of labile amino acids as well

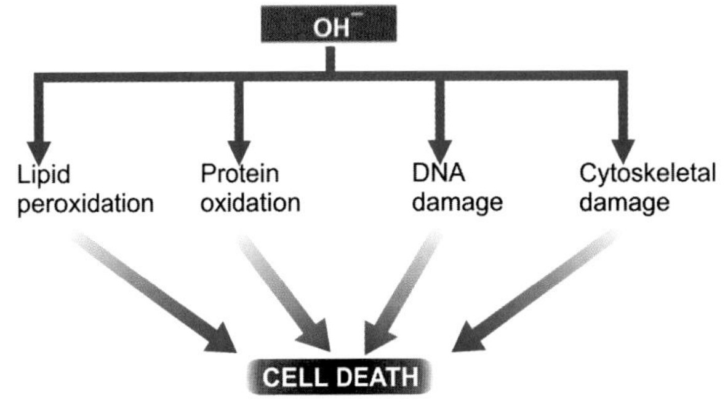

FIGURE 3.10
Mechanism of cell death by hydroxyl radical, the most reactive oxygen species.

as by fragmentation of polypeptides directly. The end-result is degradation of cytosolic neutral proteases and cell destruction.

iii) *DNA damage.* Free radicals cause breaks in the single strands of the nuclear and mitochondrial DNA. This results in cell injury; it may also cause malignant transformation of cells.

iv) *Cytoskeletal damage.* Reactive oxygen species are also known to interact with cytoskeletal elements and interfere in mitochondrial aerobic phosphorylation and thus cause ATP depletion.

ANTI-OXIDANTS. Anti-oxidants are endogenous or exogenous substances which inactivate the free radicals. These substances include:

- Vitamins E, A and C (ascorbic acid)
- Sulfhydryl-containing compounds e.g. cysteine and glutathione.
- Serum proteins e.g. ceruloplasmin and transferrin.

Free radicals are formed in physiologic as well as pathologic processes. However, oxygen radicals are basically unstable and are destroyed spontaneously. The rate of spontaneous destruction is determined by catalytic action of certain enzymes such as superoxide dismutase (SOD), catalase and glutathione peroxidase. The net effect of free radical injury in physiologic and disease states, therefore, depends upon the rate of free radical formation and rate of their elimination.

Pathogenesis of Chemical Injury

Chemicals induce cell injury by one of the following two mechanisms:

DIRECT CYTOTOXIC EFFECTS. Some chemicals combine with components of the cell and produce direct cytotoxicity without requiring metabolic activation. The cytotoxic damage is usually greatest to cells which are involved in the metabolism of such chemicals e.g. in mercuric chloride poisoning, the greatest damage occurs to cells of the alimentary tract and kidney. Cyanide kills the cell by poisoning mitochondrial cytochrome oxidase thus blocking oxidative phosphorylation.

Examples of directly cytotoxic chemicals include chemotherapeutic agents used in treatment of cancer, toxic heavy metals such as mercury, lead and iron.

CONVERSION TO REACTIVE TOXIC METABOLITES. This mechanism involves metabolic activation to yield ultimate toxin that interacts with the target cells. The target cells in this group of chemicals may not be the same cell that metabolised the toxin. Example of cell injury by conversion of reactive metabolites is toxic liver necrosis caused by carbon tetrachloride (CCl_4), acetaminophen (commonly used analgesic and antipyretic) and bromobenzene. Cell injury by CCl_4 is classic example of an industrial toxin (used in dry-cleaning industry) that produces cell injury by products produced from the body's drug-metabolising P_{450} enzyme system. The underlying mechanisms include free radical injury, and direct toxic effect on cell membrane and nucleus.

Pathogenesis of Physical Injury

Injuries caused by mechanical force are of medicolegal significance. But they may lead to a state of shock. Injuries by changes in atmospheric pressure (e.g. decompression sickness) are detailed in Chapter 5. Radiation injury to human by accidental or therapeutic exposure is of importance in treatment of persons with malignant tumours as well as may have carcinogenic influences (Chapter 8).

Killing of cells by *ionising radiation* is the result of direct formation of hydroxyl radicals from radiolysis of water (Fig. 3.11). These hydroxyl radicals damage the cell membrane as well as may interact with DNA of the target cell. In proliferating cells, there is inhibition of DNA replication and eventual cell death by apoptosis

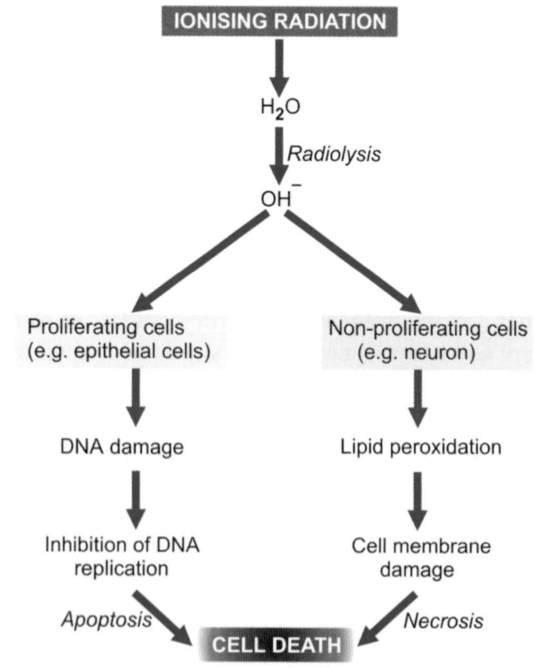

FIGURE 3.11

Mechanisms of cell injury by ionising radiation.

(e.g. epithelial cells). In non-proliferating cells there is no effect of inhibition of DNA synthesis and in these cells there is cell membrane damage followed by cell death by necrosis (e.g. neurons).

MORPHOLOGY OF CELL INJURY

After having discussed the molecular and biochemical mechanisms of various forms of cell injury, we now turn to light microscopic morphologic changes of reversible and irreversible cell injury.

Depending upon the severity of cell injury, degree of damage and residual effects on cells and tissues are variable. In general, morphologic changes in various forms of cell injury can be classified as shown in Table 3.1 and are discussed below.

MORPHOLOGY OF REVERSIBLE CELL INJURY

In conventional description of morphologic changes, the term degeneration has been used to denote morphology of reversible cell injury. However, now it is realised that this term does not provide any information on the nature of underlying changes and thus currently more acceptable terms of *retrogressive changes* or simply reversible cell injury are applied to non-lethal cell injury.

Following morphologic forms of reversible cell injury are included under this heading:
1. Cellular swelling (hydropic change, or vacuolar degeneration)
2. Fatty change
3. Hyaline change
4. Mucoid change

Cellular Swelling

This is the commonest and earliest form of cell injury from almost all causes. Other synonyms of cellular swelling used in the past are *cloudy swelling* (for gross appearance of the affected organ), *hydropic change* (accumulation of water within the cell), and *vacuolar degeneration* (due to cytoplasmic vacuolation).

TABLE 3.1: Classification of Morphologic Forms of Cell Injury.

MECHANISM OF CELL INJURY	NOMENCLATURE
1. *Reversible cell injury*	Retrogressive changes (older term: degenerations)
2. *Irreversible cell injury*	Cell death—necrosis
3. *Programmed cell death*	Apoptosis
4. *Residual effects of cell injury*	Subcellular alterations
5. *Deranged cell metabolism*	Intracellular accumulation of lipid, protein, carbohydrate
6. *After-effects of necrosis*	Gangrene, pathologic calcification

The common causes of cellular swelling include: bacterial toxins, chemicals, poisons, burns, high fever, intravenous administration of hypertonic glucose or saline etc.

Cloudy swelling results from impaired regulation of cellular volume, especially for sodium. This regulation is operative at 3 levels: at the plasma membrane itself, at the sodium pump on the plasma membrane, and at the supply of ATP. Injurious agent may interfere with these regulatory mechanisms and result in accumulation of sodium in the cell which, in turn, leads to inflow of water to maintain iso-osmotic conditions and hence cellular swelling occurs.

Grossly, the affected organ such as kidney, liver or heart muscle is enlarged due to swelling. The cut surface bulges outwards and is slightly opaque.

Microscopically, it is characterised by the following features (Fig. 3.12) (COLOUR PLATE I: CL 1):

1. The cells are swollen and the microvasculature compressed. The cellular swelling is due to increased influx of sodium and extracellular water into the cell and escape of potassium.
2. Small clear vacuoles are seen in the cells and hence the term vacuolar degeneration. These vacuoles represent distended cisternae of the endoplasmic reticulum.

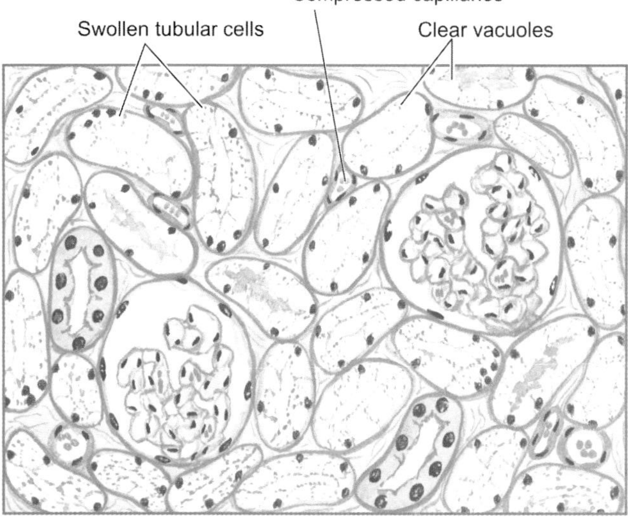

FIGURE 3.12

Hydropic change kidney. The tubular epithelial cells are distended with cytoplasmic vacuoles while the interstitial vasculature is compressed.

Ultrastructural changes in hydropic swelling include the following:

i) Dilatation of endoplasmic reticulum.
ii) Detachment of polysomes from the surface of RER.
iii) Mitochondrial swelling.
iv) Blebs on the plasma membrane.
v) Loss of fibrillarity of nucleolus.

It may be mentioned here the hydropic swelling is entirely reversible if the injurious agent is removed.

Hyaline Change

The word 'hyaline' means glassy (*hyalos* = glass). Hyaline is a descriptive histologic term for glassy, homogeneous, eosinophilic appearance of material in haematoxylin and eosin-stained sections and does not refer to any specific substance. Hyaline change is associated with heterogeneous pathologic conditions and may be intracellular or extracellular.

INTRACELLULAR HYALINE. Intracellular hyaline is mainly seen in epithelial cells. For example:

1. *Hyaline droplets* in the proximal tubular epithelial cells in cases of excessive reabsorption of plasma proteins.
2. *Hyaline degeneration* of voluntary muscle, also called Zenker's degeneration, occurs in rectus abdominalis muscle in typhoid fever. The muscle loses its fibrillar staining and becomes glassy and hyaline.
3. *Mallory's hyaline* represents aggregates of intermediate filaments in the hepatocytes in alcoholic liver cell injury.
4. Nuclear or cytoplasmic *hyaline inclusions* seen in some viral infections.
5. *Russell's bodies* representing excessive immunoglobulins in the rough endoplasmic reticulum of the plasma cells.

EXTRACELLULAR HYALINE. Extracellular hyaline is seen in connective tissues. A few examples of extracellular hyaline change are:

1. Hyaline degeneration in *leiomyomas* of the uterus (**COLOUR PLATE I: CL 2**).
2. Hyalinised *old scar* of fibrocollagenous tissues.
3. *Hyaline arteriolosclerosis* is renal vessels in hypertension and diabetes mellitus.
4. Hyalinised glomeruli in *chronic glomerulonephritis*.
5. *Corpora amylacea* are rounded masses of concentric hyaline laminae seen in the prostate in the elderly, in the brain and in the spinal cord in old age, and in old infarcts of the lung.

Though fibrin and amyloid have hyaline appearance, they have distinctive features and staining reactions and can be distinguished from non-specific hyaline material.

Mucoid Change

Mucus secreted by mucous glands is a combination of proteins complexed with mucopolysaccharides. *Mucin*, a glycoprotein, is its chief constituent. Mucin is normally produced by epithelial cells of mucous membranes and mucous glands, as well as by some connective tissues like in the umbilical cord. Epithelial mucin stains positively with periodic acid-Schiff (PAS), while connective tissue mucin is PAS negative but is stained positively with colloidal iron. Both are, however, stained by alcian blue.

EPITHELIAL MUCIN. Some examples of functional excess of epithelial mucin are:

1. Catarrhal inflammation of mucous membrane (e.g. of respiratory tract, alimentary tract, uterus).
2. Obstruction of duct leading to mucocele in the oral cavity and gall bladder.
3. Cystic fibrosis of the pancreas.
4. Mucin-secreting tumours (e.g. of ovary, stomach, large bowel etc).

CONNECTIVE TISSUE MUCIN. A few examples of disturbances of connective tissue mucin are:

1. Mucoid or myxoid degeneration in some tumours e.g. myxomas, neurofibromas (**COLOUR PLATE I: CL 3**), soft tissue sarcomas etc.
2. Dissecting aneurysm of aorta due to Erdheim's medial degeneration and Marfan's syndrome.
3. Myxomatous change in the dermis in myxoedema.
4. Myxoid change in the synovium in ganglion on the wrist.

SUBCELLULAR ALTERATIONS IN CELL INJURY

Certain morphologically distinct alterations at subcellular level are noticeable in both acute and chronic forms of cell injury. These occur at the level of cytoskeleton, lysosomes, endoplasmic reticulum and mitochondria:

1. CYTOSKELETAL CHANGES. Components of cytoskeleton may show the following morphologic abnormalities:

i) Defective microtubules:

- In Chédiak-Higashi syndrome characterised by poor phagocytic activity of neutrophils.

- Poor sperm motility causing sterility.
- Immotile cilia syndrome (Kartagener's syndrome) characterised by immotile cilia of respiratory tract and consequent chronic infection due to defective clearance of inhaled bacteria.
- Defects in leucocyte function of phagocytes such as migration and chemotaxis.

ii) Defective microfilaments:

- In myopathies
- Muscular dystrophies

iii) Accumulation of intermediate filaments: Various classes of intermediate filaments (cytokeratin, desmin, vimentin, glial fibrillary acidic protein, and neurofilament) may accumulate in the cytosol. For example:

- Mallory's body or alcoholic hyaline as intracytoplasmic eosinophilic inclusion seen in alcoholic liver disease which is collection of cytokeratin intermediate filaments.
- Neurofibrillary tangles, neurities and senile plaques in Alzheimer's disease are composed of neurofilaments and paired helical filaments.

2. LYSOSOMAL CHANGES. Lysosomes contain powerful hydrolytic enzymes. Heterophagy and autophagy are the two ways by which lysosomes show morphologic changes of phagocytic function.

i) Heterophagy. Phagocytosis (cell eating) and pinocytosis (cell drinking) are the two forms by which material from outside is taken up by the lysosomes of cells such as polymorphs and macrophages to form *phagolysosomes.* This is termed heterophagy. Microbial agents and foreign particulate material are eliminated by this mechanism.

ii) Autophagy. This is the process by which worn out intracellular organelles and other cytoplasmic material form autophagic vacuole that fuses with lysosome to form *autophagolysosome*.

iii) Indigestible material. Some indigestible exogenous particles such as carbon or endogenous substances such as lipofuscin may persist in the lysosomes of the cells for a long time as residual bodies.

iv) Storage diseases. As discussed in Chapter 10, a group of lysosomal storage diseases due to hereditary deficiency of enzymes may result in abnormal collection of metabolites in the lysosomes of cells.

3. S.E.R. HYPERTROPHY. Hypertrophy of smooth endoplasmic reticulum of liver cells as an adaptive change may occur in response to prolonged use of barbiturates.

4. MITOCHONDRIAL CHANGES. Mitochondrial injury plays an important role in cell injury. Morphologic changes of cell injury in mitochondria may be seen in the following conditions:

i) *Megamitochondria.* Megamitochondria consisting of unusually big mitochondria are seen in alcoholic liver disease and nutritional deficiency conditions.

ii) Alterations in the *number of mitochondria* may occur. Their number increases in hypertrophy and decreases in atrophy.

iii) *Oncocytoma* in the salivary glands, thyroid and kidneys consists of tumour cells having very large mitochondria.

iv) *Myopathies* having defect in mitochondria have abnormal cristae.

5. HEAT SHOCK PROTEINS AND UBIQUITIN. Heat shock proteins (HSP), more appropriately called *stress proteins*, are a variety of intracellular carrier proteins present in most cells for physiologic function. However, in response to stresses of various types (e.g. toxins, drugs, poisons, ischaemia), their level goes up both inside the cell as well as leak out into the plasma, and hence the name stress proteins. They perform the role of *chaperones* (house-keeping) i.e. they direct and guide metabolic molecules to the sites of metabolic activity e.g. protein folding, disaggregation of protein-protein complexes and transport of proteins into various intracellular organelles (*protein kinesis*).

In experimental studies HSPs have been shown to limit tissue necrosis in ischaemic reperfusion injury in myocardial infarcts. In addition, they have also been shown to have a central role in protein aggregation in amyloidosis.

Another related stress protein, *ubiquitin* (so named due to its ubiquitous or universal presence in the cells of the body), has been found to be involved in activation of genes for protein synthesis in neurodegenerative diseases such as in Alzheimer's disease, Creutzfeldt-Jakob disease, Parkinson's disease.

INTRACELLULAR ACCUMULATIONS

Intracellular accumulation of substances in abnormal amounts can occur within the cytoplasm (especially lysosomes) or nucleus of the cell. This phenomenon was previously referred to as *infiltration*, implying thereby that something unusual has infiltrated the cell from outside which is not always the case. Intracellular accumulation of the substance in mild degree causes reversible cell injury while more severe damage results in irreversible cell injury.

Such abnormal intracellular accumulations can be divided into 3 groups:

i) *Accumulation of constituents of normal cell metabolism produced in excess* e.g. accumulations of lipids (fatty change, cholesterol deposits), proteins and carbohydrates. In addition, deposits of amyloid and urate are discussed later.

ii) *Accumulation of abnormal substances* produced as a result of abnormal metabolism due to lack of some enzymes e.g. storage diseases or inborn errors of metabolism. These are discussed in Chapter 10.

iii) *Accumulation of pigments* e.g. endogenous pigments under special circumstances, and exogenous pigments due to lack of enzymatic mechanisms to degrade the substances or transport them to other sites.

These pathologic states are discussed below.

FATTY CHANGE (STEATOSIS)

Fatty change, steatosis or fatty metamorphosis is the intracellular accumulation of neutral fat within parenchymal cells. It includes the older, now abandoned, terms of *fatty degeneration* and *fatty infiltration* because fatty change neither necessarily involves degeneration nor infiltration. The deposit is in the cytosol and represents an absolute increase in the intracellular lipids. It is especially common in the liver but may occur in other non-fatty tissues like the heart, skeletal muscle, kidneys (lipoid nephrosis or minimum change disease) and other organs.

Fatty Liver

Liver is the commonest site for accumulation of fat because it plays central role in fat metabolism. Depending upon the cause and amount of accumulation, fatty change may be mild and reversible, or severe producing irreversible cell injury and cell death.

ETIOLOGY. The commonest causes of fatty liver include the following:

i) excess alcohol consumption (most common);
ii) starvation;
iii) malnutrition;
iv) obesity;
v) diabetes mellitus;
vi) chronic illnesses (e.g. tuberculosis);
vii) late pregnancy;
viii) hypoxia (e.g. anaemia, cardiac failure);
ix) hepatotoxins (e.g. carbon tetrachloride, chloroform, ether, aflatoxins and other poisons);
x) certain drugs (e.g. administration of oestrogen, steroids, tetracycline etc); and
xi) Reye's syndrome.

PATHOGENESIS. Pathogenesis of fatty liver depends upon the stage at which the individual etiologic agent acts in the normal fat transport and metabolism (Fig. 3.13).

Lipids as free acids enter the liver cell from either of the following 2 sources:

- *From diet* as chylomicrons (containing triglycerides and phospholipids) and as free fatty acids; and
- *From adipose tissue* as free fatty acids.

Normally, a small part of fatty acids is synthesised from acetate in the liver cells. Most of fatty acid is esterified to triglycerides by the action of α-glycerophosphate and only a small part is changed into cholesterol, phospholipids and ketone bodies. Intracellular triglycerides require 'lipid acceptor protein' to form lipoprotein, the form in which lipids are normally excreted from the liver cells.

In fatty liver, intracellular accumulation of triglycerides can occur due to defect at one or more of the following *6 steps* in the normal fat metabolism:

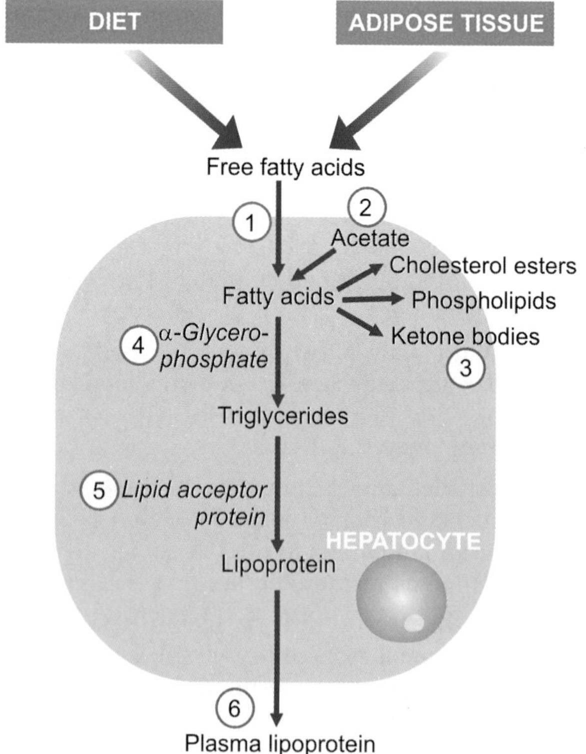

FIGURE 3.13

Lipid metabolism in the pathogenesis of fatty liver. Defects in any of the six numbered steps (corresponding to the description in the text) can produce fatty liver by different etiologic agents.

1. Increased entry of free fatty acids into the liver.
2. Increased synthesis of fatty acids by the liver.
3. Decreased conversion of fatty acids into ketone bodies resulting in increased esterification of fatty acids to triglycerides.
4. Increased α-glycerophosphate causing increased esterification of fatty acids to triglycerides.
5. Decreased synthesis of 'lipid acceptor protein' resulting in decreased formation of lipoprotein from triglycerides.
6. Block in the excretion of lipoprotein from the liver into plasma.

In most cases of fatty liver, one of the above mechanisms is operating. But in the case of liver cell injury by chronic alcoholism, many factors are implicated which includes:

- increased lipolysis;
- increased free fatty acid synthesis;
- decreased triglyceride utilisation;
- decreased fatty acid oxidation to ketone bodies; and
- block in lipoprotein excretion.

Even a severe form of liver cell dysfunction may be reversible; e.g an alcoholic who has not developed progressive fibrosis in the form of cirrhosis, the enlarged fatty liver may return to normal if the person becomes teetotaller.

PATHOLOGIC CHANGES. Grossly, the fatty liver is enlarged with a tense, glistening capsule and rounded margins. The cut surface bulges slightly and is pale-yellow to yellow and is greasy to touch.

Microscopically, there are numerous lipid vacuoles in the cytoplasm of hepatocytes.

i) The vacuoles are initially small and are present around the nucleus *(microvesicular)*.

ii) But with progression of the process, the vacuoles become larger pushing the nucleus to the periphery of the cells *(macrovesicular)* (COLOUR PLATE I: CL 4).

iii) At times, the hepatocytes laden with large lipid vacuoles may rupture and lipid vacuoles coalesce to form fatty cysts (Fig. 3.14).

iv) Infrequently, *lipogranulomas* may appear consisting of collections of lymphocytes, macrophages, and some multinucleated giant cells.

v) Fat in the tissue can be demonstrated by frozen section followed by *fat stains* such as Sudan dyes (Sudan III, IV, Sudan black), oil red O and osmic acid.

CHOLESTEROL. Intracellular deposits of cholesterol and its esters in macrophages may occur when there is

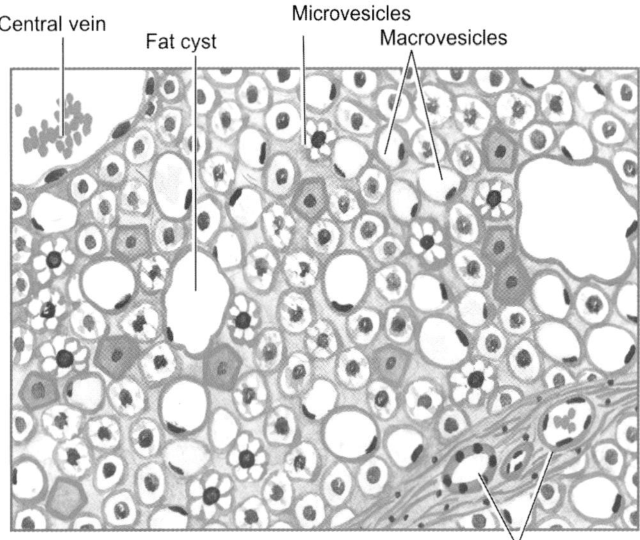

FIGURE 3.14

Fatty liver. Many of the hepatocytes are distended with fat vacuoles pushing the nuclei to the periphery, while others show multiple small vacuoles in the cytoplasm.

hypercholesterolaemia. This turns macrophages into foam cells. The examples are:

1. *Fibrofatty plaques* of atherosclerosis (Chapter 11).
2. Clusters of foam cells in tumour-like masses called *xanthomas* and *xanthelasma*.

Stromal Fatty Infiltration

This form of lipid accumulation is quite different from fatty change just described. Stromal fatty infiltration is the deposition of mature adipose cells in the stromal connective tissue in contrast to intracellular deposition of fat in the parenchymal cells in fatty change. The condition occurs most often in patients with obesity. The two commonly affected organs are the heart and the pancreas. Thus, heart can be the site for intramyocardial fatty change as well as epicardial (stromal) fatty infiltration. The presence of mature adipose cells in the stroma generally does not produce any dysfunction. In the case of heart, stromal fatty infiltration is associated with increased adipose tissue in the epicardium.

INTRACELLULAR ACCUMULATION OF PROTEINS

Pathologic accumulation of proteins in the cytoplasm of cells may occur in the following conditions.

1. In *proteinuria*, there is excessive renal tubular reabsorption of proteins by the proximal tubular epithe-

lial cells which show pink hyaline droplets in their cytoplasm. The change is reversible so that with control of proteinuria the protein droplets disappear.

2. The cytoplasm of actively functioning plasma cells shows pink hyaline inclusions called *Russell's bodies* representing synthesised immunoglobulins.

3. In *α_1-antitrypsin deficiency*, the cytoplasm of hepatocytes shows eosinophilic globular deposits of a mutant protein.

4. *Mallory's body* or alcoholic hyaline in the hepatocytes is intracellular accumulation of intermediate filaments of cytokeratin and appear as amorphous pink masses.

INTRACELLULAR ACCUMULATION OF GLYCOGEN

Conditions associated with excessive accumulation of intracellular glycogen are as under:

1. In *diabetes mellitus*, there is intracellular accumulation of glycogen in different tissues because normal cellular uptake of glucose is impaired. Glycogen deposits in diabetes mellitus are seen in epithelium of distal portion of proximal convoluted tubule and descending loop of Henle, in the hepatocytes, in beta cells of pancreatic islets, and in cardiac muscle cells. Deposits of glycogen produce clear vacuoles in the cytoplasm of the affected cells. Best's carmine and periodic acid-Schiff (PAS) staining may be employed to confirm the presence of glycogen in the cells.

2. In *glycogen storage diseases or glycogenosis*, there is defective metabolism of glycogen due to genetic disorders. These conditions along with other similar genetic disorders are discussed in Chapter 10.

PIGMENTS

Pigments are coloured substances present in most living beings including humans. There are 2 broad categories of pigments: endogenous and exogenous.

A. ENDOGENOUS PIGMENTS

Endogenous pigments are either normal constituents of cells or accumulate under special circumstances e.g. melanin, ochronosis, haemoprotein-derived pigments, and lipofuscin.

Melanin

Melanin is the brown-black, non-haemoglobin-derived pigment normally present in the hair, skin, choroid of the eye, meninges and adrenal medulla. It is synthesised in the melanocytes and dendritic cells, both of which are present in the basal cells of the epidermis and is stored in the form of cytoplasmic granules in the phagocytic cells called the melanophores, present in the underlying dermis. Melanocytes possess the enzyme tyrosinase necessary for synthesis of melanin from tyrosine. However, sometimes tyrosinase is present but is not active and hence no melanin pigment is visible. In such cases, the presence of tyrosinase can be detected by incubation of tissue section in the solution of dihydroxy phenyl alanine (DOPA). If the enzyme is present, dark pigment is identified in pigment cells. This test is called as *DOPA reaction* and is particularly useful in differentiating amelanotic melanoma from other anaplastic tumours.

Various disorders of melanin pigmentation cause generalised and localised hyperpigmentation and hypopigmentation:

i) Generalised hyperpigmentation:

a) In *Addison's disease*, there is generalised hyperpigmentation of the skin, especially in areas exposed to light, and of buccal mucosa.

b) *Chloasma* observed during pregnancy is the hyperpigmentation on the skin of face, nipples, and genitalia and occurs under the influence of oestrogen. A similar appearance may be observed in women taking oral contraceptives.

c) In *chronic arsenical poisoning*, there is characteristic rain-drop pigmentation of the skin.

ii) Focal hyperpigmentation:

a) *Cäfe-au-lait spots* are pigmented patches seen in neurofibromatosis and Albright's syndrome.

b) *Peutz-Jeghers syndrome* is characterised by focal perioral pigmentation.

c) *Melanosis coli* is pigmentation of the mucosa of the colon.

d) *Melanotic tumours*, both benign such as pigmented naevi, and malignant such as melanoma, are associated with increased melanogenesis.

e) *Lentigo* is a pre-malignant condition in which there is focal hyperpigmentation on the skin of hands, face, neck, and arms.

f) *Dermatopathic lymphadenitis* is an example of deposition of melanin pigment in macrophages of the lymph nodes draining skin lesions.

iii) Generalised hypopigmentation: *Albinism* is an extreme degree of generalised hypopigmentation in which tyrosinase activity of the melanocytes is genetically defective and no melanin is formed. Albinos have blond hair, poor vision and severe photophobia. They are highly sensitive to sunlight. Chronic sun exposure may lead to precancerous lesions and squamous and basal cell cancers of the skin in such individuals.

iv) Localised hypopigmentation:

a) *Leucoderma* is a form of partial albinism and is an inherited disorder.

b) *Vitiligo* is local hypopigmentation of the skin and is more common. It may have familial tendency.

c) *Acquired focal hypopigmentation* can result from various causes such as leprosy, healing of wounds, DLE, radiation dermatitis etc.

Ochronosis

Ochronosis is an autosomal recessive disorder in which there is deficiency of an oxidase enzyme required for break down of homogentisic acid which then accumulates in the tissues and is excreted in the urine. The pigment is melanin-like and is deposited both intracellularly and intercellularly. Most commonly affected tissues are the cartilages, capsules of joints, ligaments and tendons. In almost all the cases, alkaptonuria is present in which homogentisic acid is excreted by the kidneys. The urine of these patients, if allowed to stand for some hours in air, turns black due to oxidation of homogentisic acid.

Haemoprotein-derived Pigments

Haemoproteins are the most important endogenous pigments derived from haemoglobin, cytochromes and their break down products. For an understanding of disorders of haemoproteins, it is essential to have knowledge of normal iron metabolism and its transport which is described in Chapter 13. In disordered iron metabolism and transport, haemoprotein-derived pigments accumulate in the body. These pigments are haemosiderin, acid haematin (haemozoin), bilirubin, and porphyrins.

1. HAEMOSIDERIN. Iron is stored in the tissues in 2 forms:

- *Ferritin,* which is iron complexed to apoferritin and can be identified by electron microscopy.
- *Haemosiderin,* which is formed by aggregates of ferritin and is identifiable by light microscopy as golden-yellow to brown, granular pigment, especially within the mononuclear phagocytes of the bone marrow, spleen and liver where break down of senescent red cells takes place. Haemosiderin is ferric iron that can be demonstrated by Prussian blue reaction. In this reaction, colourless potassium ferrocyanide reacts with ferric ions of haemosiderin to form deep blue *ferric-ferrocyanide* (COLOUR PLATE II: CL 7).

Excessive storage of haemosiderin occurs in situations when there is increased break down of red cells, or systemic overload of iron due to primary (idiopathic, hereditary) haemochromatosis, and secondary (acquired) causes such as in thalassaemia, sideroblastic anaemia, alcoholic cirrhosis, multiple blood transfusions etc.

Accordingly, the effects of haemosiderin excess are as under (Fig. 3.15):

a) Localised haemosiderosis. This develops whenever there is haemorrhage into the tissues. With lysis of red cells, haemoglobin is liberated which is taken up by macrophages where it is degraded and stored as haemosiderin. For example:

- The changing colours of a bruise or a *black eye* are caused by the pigments like biliverdin and bilirubin which are formed during transformation of haemoglobin into haemosiderin.
- Another example of local haemosiderosis is *brown induration* in the lungs as a result of small haemorrhages as occur in mitral stenosis and left ventricular failure. Microscopy reveals the presence of 'heart failure cells' which are haemosiderin-laden alveolar macrophages.

b) Generalised (Systemic or Diffuse) haemosiderosis. Systemic overload with iron may result in generalised haemosiderosis. There can be two types of patterns:

- *Parenchymatous deposition of haemosiderin* occurs in the parenchymal cells of the liver, pancreas, kidney, and heart.
- *Reticuloendothelial deposition* occurs in the liver, spleen, and bone marrow.

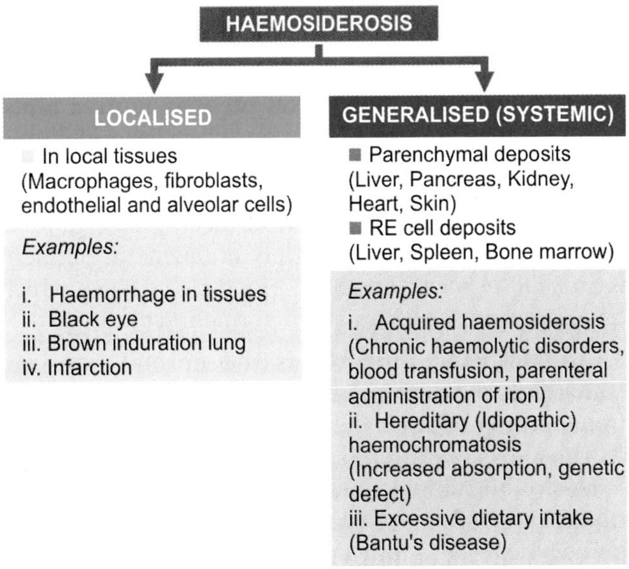

HAEMOSIDEROSIS
LOCALISED
In local tissues
(Macrophages, fibroblasts, endothelial and alveolar cells)
Examples:
i. Haemorrhage in tissues
ii. Black eye
iii. Brown induration lung
iv. Infarction
GENERALISED (SYSTEMIC)
Parenchymal deposits
(Liver, Pancreas, Kidney, Heart, Skin)
RE cell deposits
(Liver, Spleen, Bone marrow)
Examples:
i. Acquired haemosiderosis
(Chronic haemolytic disorders, blood transfusion, parenteral administration of iron)
ii. Hereditary (Idiopathic) haemochromatosis
(Increased absorption, genetic defect)
iii. Excessive dietary intake
(Bantu's disease)

FIGURE 3.15

Effects of haemosiderosis.

Generalised or systemic overload of iron may occur due to following causes:

*i) **Increased erythropoietic activity:*** In various forms of chronic haemolytic anaemia, there is excessive break down of haemoglobin and hence iron overload. The problem is further compounded by treating the condition with blood transfusions (transfusional haemosiderosis) or by parenteral iron therapy. The deposits of iron in these cases, termed as *acquired haemosiderosis,* are initially in reticuloendothelial tissues but may secondarily affect other organs.

*ii) **Excessive intestinal absorption of iron:*** A form of haemosiderosis in which there is excessive intestinal absorption of iron even when the intake is normal, is known as *idiopathic or hereditary haemochromatosis.* It is an autosomal dominant disease associated with much more deposits of iron than cases of acquired haemosiderosis. It is characterised by *triad* of pigmentary liver cirrhosis, pancreatic damage resulting in diabetes mellitus, and skin pigmentation. On the basis of the last two features the disease has come to be termed as *'bronze diabetes'*.

*iii) **Excessive intake of dietary iron:*** A common example of excessive intake of iron is *Bantu's disease* in black tribals of South Africa who conventionally brew their alcohol in cast iron pots that serves as a rich source of additional dietary iron. The excess of iron gets deposited in various organs including liver causing cirrhosis.

2. ACID HAEMATIN (HAEMOZOIN). Acid haematin or haemozoin is a haemoprotein-derived brown-black pigment containing haem iron in ferric form in acidic medium. But it differs from haemosiderin because it can not be stained by Prussian blue (Perl's) reaction, probably because of formation of complex with a protein so that it is unable to react in the stain. Haematin pigment is seen most commonly in chronic malaria and in mismatched blood transfusions. Besides, the *malarial pigment* can also be deposited in macrophages and in the hepatocytes. Another variety of haematin pigment is *formalin pigment* formed in blood-rich tissues which have been preserved in acidic formalin solution.

3. BILIRUBIN. Bilirubin is the normal non-iron containing pigment present in the bile. It is derived from porphyrin ring of the haem moiety of haemoglobin. Normal level of bilirubin in blood is less than 1 mg/dl. Excess of bilirubin causes an important clinical condition called jaundice. Normal bilirubin metabolism and pathogenesis of jaundice are described in Chapter 19. Briefly, jaundice appears in one of the following 3 ways:

a) *Prehepatic or haemolytic,* when there is excessive destruction of red cells.

b) *Posthepatic or obstructive,* which results from obstruction to the outflow of conjugated bilirubin.

c) *Hepatocellular* that results from failure of hepatocytes to conjugate bilirubin and inability of bilirubin to pass from the liver to intestine.

Excessive accumulation of bilirubin pigment can be seen in different tissues and fluids of the body, especially in the hepatocytes, Kupffer cells and bile sinusoids. Skin and sclerae become distinctly yellow. In infants, rise in unconjugated bilirubin may produce toxic brain injury called *kernicterus.*

4. PORPHYRINS. Porphyrins are tetrapyrrols which exist in 3 forms in nature combined with different metals:

i) *haem* contains iron;
ii) *chlorophyll* contains magnesium; and
iii) *cobalamin* contains cobalt.

Porphyria results from genetic deficiency of one of the enzymes required for the synthesis of haem so that there is excessive production of porphyrins. Often, the genetic deficiency is precipitated by intake of some drugs. Porphyrias are broadly of 2 types: erythropoietic and hepatic.

(a) Erythropoietic porphyrias. These have defective synthesis of haem in the erythrocytes. These may be further of 2 subtypes:

- *Congenital type,* in which the urine is red due to the presence of uroporphyrin I and coproporphyrin 1. The skin of these infants is highly photosensitive. Bones and skin show red brown discoloration.
- *Erythropoietic protoporphyria,* in which there is excess of protoporphyrin but no excess of porphyrin in the urine.

(b) Hepatic porphyrias. These are more common and have a defect in synthesis of haem in the liver. Its further subtypes include the following:

- *Acute intermittent porphyria* is characterised by acute episodes of 3 patterns: abdominal, neurological, and psychotic. These patients do not have photosensitivity. There is excessive delta aminolaevulinic acid and porphobilinogen in the urine.
- *Variegate porphyria* is common in the whites of South Africa. Photosensitivity occurs and there are acute attacks of colicky abdominal pain and neurological manifestations.
- *Hereditary coproporphyria* is quite rare.
- *Porphyria cutanea tarda* is the most common of all porphyrias. Porphyrins collect in the liver and small quantity is excreted in the urine. Skin lesions are similar

to those in variegate porphyria. Most of the patients have associated haemosiderosis with cirrhosis which may eventually develop into hepatocellular carcinoma.

Lipofuscin (Wear and Tear Pigment)

Lipofuscin or lipochrome is yellowish-brown intracellular lipid pigment (*lipo* = fat, *fuscus* = brown). The pigment is often found in atrophied cells of old age and hence the name 'wear and tear pigment'. It is seen in the myocardial fibres, hepatocytes, Leydig cells of the testes and in neurons in senile dementia. However, the pigment may, at times, accumulate rapidly in different cells in wasting diseases unrelated to aging.

By ***light microscopy,*** the pigment is coarse golden brown granular and often accumulates in the central part of the cells around the nuclei. In the heart muscle, the change is associated with wasting of the muscle and is commonly referred to as `brown atrophy' (Fig. 3.16) (COLOUR PLATE II: CL 5). The pigment can be stained by fat stains but differs from other lipids in being fluorescent and acid-fast.

By electron microscopy, lipofuscin appears as intra-lysosomal electron-dense granules in perinuclear location. These granules are composed of lipid-protein complexes. Lipofuscin represents the collection of indigestible material in the lysosomes after intracellular lipid peroxidation and is therefore an example of residual bodies. Unlike in normal cells, in aging or debilitating diseases the phospholipid end products of membranes damage mediated by oxygen free radicals fail to get eliminated and hence are deposited as lipofuscin pigment.

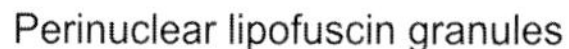

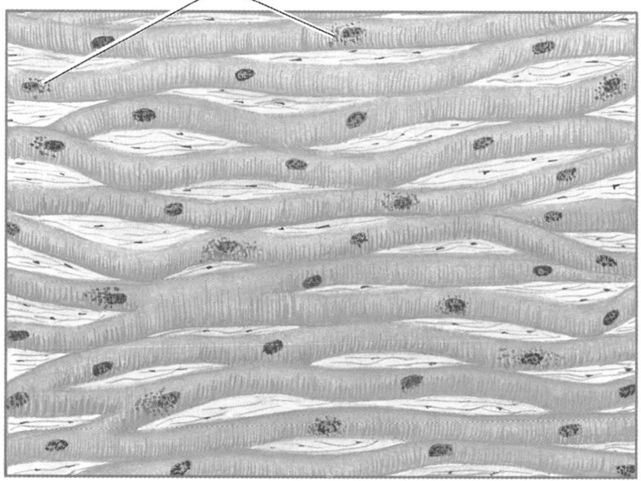

FIGURE 3.16

Brown atrophy of the heart. The lipofuscin pigment granules are seen in the cytoplasm of the myocardial fibres, especially at the poles of nuclei.

B. EXOGENOUS PIGMENTS

Exogenous pigments are those which are introduced into the body from outside such as by inhalation, ingestion or inoculation.

Inhaled Pigments

The lungs of most individuals, especially of those living in urban areas due to atmospheric pollutants and of smokers, show a large number of inhaled pigmented materials. The most commonly inhaled substances are carbon or coal dust; others are silica or stone dust, iron or iron oxide, asbestos and various other organic substances. These substances may produce occupational lung diseases called pneumoconiosis (Chapter 15). The pigment particles after inhalation are taken up by alveolar macrophages. Some of the pigment-laden macrophages are coughed out via bronchi, while some settle in the interstitial tissue of the lung and in the respiratory bronchioles and pass into lymphatics to be deposited in the hilar lymph nodes. *Anthracosis* (i.e. deposition of cabon particles) is seen in almost every adult lung and generally provokes no reaction of tissue injury (COLOUR PLATE II: CL 6). However, extensive deposition of particulate material over many years in coal-miners' pneumoconiosis, silicosis, asbestosis etc. provoke low grade inflammation, fibrosis and impaired respiratory function.

Ingested Pigments

Chronic ingestion of certain metals may produce pigmentation. The examples are as under:

i) *Argyria* is chronic ingestion of silver compounds and results in brownish pigmentation in the skin, bowel, and kidney.

ii) *Chronic lead poisoning* may produce the characteristic blue lines on teeth at the gumline.

iii) *Melanosis coli* results from prolonged ingestion of certain cathartics.

iv) *Carotenaemia* is yellowish-red coloration of the skin caused by excessive ingestion of carrots which contain carotene.

Injected Pigments (Tattooing)

Pigments like India ink, cinnabar and carbon are introduced into the dermis in the process of tattooing where the pigment is taken up by macrophages and lies permanently in the connective tissue. The examples of injected pigments are prolonged use of ointments containing mercury, dirt left accidentally in a wound, and tattooing by pricking the skin with dyes.

MORPHOLOGY OF IRREVERSIBLE CELL INJURY (CELL DEATH)

Cell death is a state of irreversible injury. It may occur in the living body as a local or focal change (i.e. autolysis, necrosis and apoptosis) and the changes that follow it (i.e. gangrene and pathologic calcification), or result in end of the life (somatic death). These pathologic processes involved in cell death are described below.

AUTOLYSIS

Autolysis *('self-digestion')* is disintegration of the cell by its own hydrolytic enzymes liberated from lysosomes. Autolysis can occur in the living body when it is surrounded by inflammatory reaction *(vital reaction)*, or may occur as postmortem change in which there is complete absence of surrounding inflammatory response. Autolysis is *rapid* in some tissues rich in hydrolytic enzymes such as in the pancreas, and gastric mucosa; *intermediate* in tissues like the heart, liver and kidney; and *slow* in fibrous tissue. Morphologically, autolysis is identified by homogeneous and eosinophilic cytoplasm with loss of cellular details and remains of cell as debris.

NECROSIS

Necrosis is defined as focal death along with degradation of tissue by hydrolytic enzymes liberated by cells. It is invariably accompanied by inflammatory reaction.

Necrosis can be caused by various agents such as hypoxia, chemical and physical agents, microbial agents and immunological injury. Two essential changes bring about irreversible cell injury in necrosis—cell digestion by lytic enzymes and denaturation of proteins. These processes are morphologically identified by characteristic cytoplasmic and nuclear changes in necrotic cell (Fig. 3.17,A). The cytoplasm appears homogeneous and intensely eosinophilic. Occasionally, it may show vacuolation or dystrophic calcification. The nuclear changes include condensation of nuclear chromatin *(pyknosis)* which may either undergo dissolution *(karyolysis)* or fragmentation into many granular clumps *(karyorrhexis)* (see Fig. 3.7).

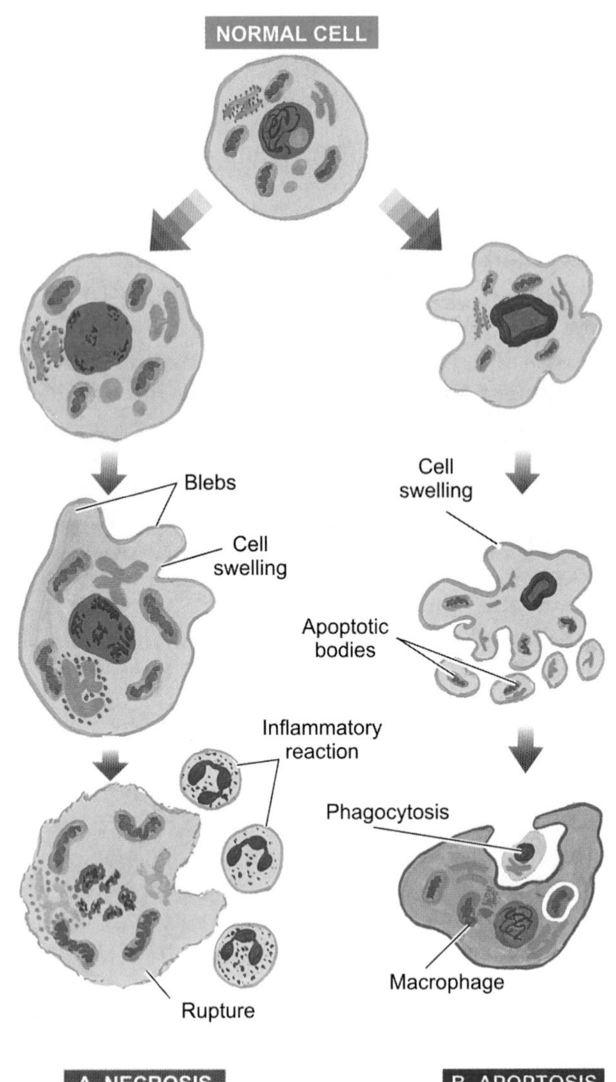

FIGURE 3.17

Necrosis and apoptosis. A, Cell necrosis is identified by homogeneous, eosinophilic cytoplasm and nuclear changes of pyknosis, karyolysis, and karyorrhexis. B, Apoptosis consists of condensation of nuclear chromatin and fragmentation of the cell into membrane-bound apoptotic bodies which are engulfed by macrophages.

Types of Necrosis

Morphologically, 5 distinct types of necrosis are identified: coagulative, liquefaction (colliquative), caseous, fat, and fibrinoid necrosis.

1. COAGULATIVE NECROSIS. This is the most common type of necrosis caused by irreversible focal injury, mostly from sudden cessation of blood flow (ischaemia), and less often from bacterial and chemical agents. The organs commonly affected are the heart, kidney, and spleen.

Grossly, foci of coagulative necrosis in the early stage are pale, firm, and slightly swollen. With progression, they become more yellowish, softer, and shrunken. ***Microscopically***, the hallmark of coagulative necrosis is the conversion of normal cells into their 'tombstones' i.e. outlines of the cells are retained so that the cell type can still be recognised but their cytoplasmic and nuclear details are lost. The necrosed cells are swollen and appear more eosinophilic than the normal, along with nuclear changes described above. This pattern of microscopic change results from 2 processes: denaturation of proteins and enzymatic digestion of the cell. But cell digestion and liquefaction fail to occur (*c.f.* liquefaction necrosis). Eventually, the necrosed focus is infiltrated by inflammatory cells and the dead cells are phagocytosed leaving granular debris and fragments of cells (Fig. 3.18,A).

2. LIQUEFACTION (COLLIQUATIVE) NECROSIS. Liquefaction or colliquative necrosis occurs commonly due to ischaemic injury and bacterial or fungal infections. It occurs due to degradation of tissue by the action of powerful hydrolytic enzymes. The common examples are infarct brain and abscess cavity.

Grossly, the affected area is soft with liquefied centre containing necrotic debris. Later, a cyst wall is formed.

Microscopically, the cystic space contains necrotic cell debris and macrophages filled with phagocytosed material. The cyst wall is formed by proliferating capillaries, inflammatory cells, and gliosis (proliferating glial cells) in the case of brain and proliferating fibroblasts in the case of abscess cavity (Fig. 3.18,B).

3. CASEOUS NECROSIS. Caseous necrosis is found in the centre of foci of tuberculous infections. It combines features of both coagulative and liquefactive necrosis.

Grossly, foci of caseous necrosis, as the name implies, resemble dry cheese and are soft, granular and yellowish. This appearance is partly attributed to the histotoxic effects of lipopolysaccharides present in the capsule of the tubercle bacilli, *Mycobacterium tuberculosis*.

Microscopically, the necrosed foci are structureless, eosinophilic, and contain granular debris (Fig. 3.18,C). The surrounding tissue shows characteristic granulo-

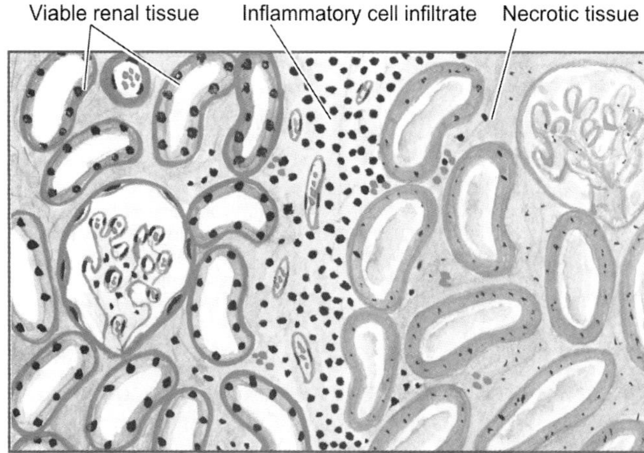

A, COAGULATIVE NECROSIS (KIDNEY)

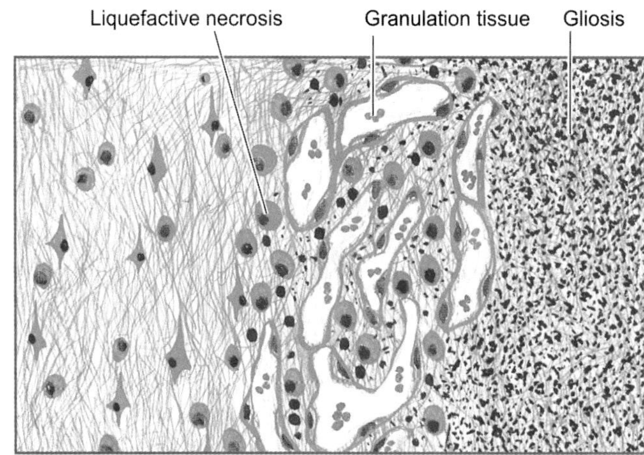

B, LIQUEFACTIVE NECROSIS (BRAIN)

Viable lymphoid tissue
Granulomatous inflammation
Caseous necrosis

C, CASEOUS NECROSIS (LYMPH NODE)

FIGURE 3.18

Principal types of necrosis. (For details, consult the text).

matous inflammatory reaction consisting of epithelioid cells with interspersed giant cells of Langhans' or foreign body type and peripheral mantle of lymphocytes **(COLOUR PLATE VIII: CL 29).**

4. FAT NECROSIS. Fat necrosis is a special form of cell death occurring at two anatomically different locations but morphologically similar lesions. These are: following *acute pancreatic necrosis,* and *traumatic fat necrosis* commonly in breasts.

In the case of pancreas, there is liberation of pancreatic lipases from injured or inflamed tissue that results in necrosis of the pancreas as well as of the fat depots throughout the peritoneal cavity, and sometimes, even affecting the extra-abdominal adipose tissue.

Fat necrosis in either of the two instances results in hydrolysis of neutral fat present in adipose cells into glycerol and free fatty acids. The damaged adipose cells assume cloudy appearance when only free fatty acids remain behind, after glycerol leaks out. The leaked out free fatty acids, on the other hand, complex with calcium to form calcium soaps (saponification) discussed later under dystrophic calcification.

Grossly, fat necrosis appears as yellowish-white and firm deposits. Formation of calcium soaps imparts the necrosed foci firmer and chalky white appearance.

Microscopically, the necrosed fat cells have cloudy appearance and are surrounded by an inflammatory reaction. Formation of calcium soaps is identified in the tissue sections as amorphous, granular and basophilic material.

5. FIBRINOID NECROSIS. Fibrinoid necrosis or fibrinoid degeneration is characterised by deposition of fibrin-like material which has the staining properties of fibrin. It is encountered in various examples of immunologic tissue injury (e.g. in immune complex vasculitis, autoimmune diseases, Arthus reaction etc), arterioles in hypertension, peptic ulcer etc.

Microscopically, fibrinoid necrosis is identified by brightly eosinophilic, hyaline-like deposition in the vessel wall or on the luminal surface of a peptic ulcer. Local haemorrhages may occur due to rupture of these blood vessels.

APOPTOSIS

Apoptosis is a form of 'coordinated and internally programmed cell death' which is of significance in a variety of physiologic and pathologic conditions (*apoptosis* is a Greek word meaning 'falling off' or 'dropping off'). The term was first coined in 1972 as distinct from necrosis.

PATHOLOGIC CHANGES. The characteristic morphologic changes in apoptosis as seen in histologic and electron microscopic examination are as under (Fig. 3.17,B):

1. Involvement of *single cells or small clusters of cells* in the background of viable cells. The apoptotic cells are round to oval shrunken masses of intensely eosinophilic cytoplasm containing condensed or fragmented nuclear chromatin. Characteristically, unlike necrosis, inflammatory response around apoptosis is absent.
2. *Shrinkage of cell* with dense cytoplasm and almost-normal organelles.
3. Convolutions of the cell membrane with formation of membrane-bound near-spherical bodies called *apoptotic bodies* containing compacted organelles.
4. *Chromatin condensation* around the periphery of nucleus.
5. Characteristically, there is *no acute inflammatory reaction.*
6. *Phagocytosis* of apoptotic bodies by macrophages takes place at varying speed. There may be swift phagocytosis, or loosely floating apoptotic cells after losing contact, with each other and basement membrane as single cells, or may result in major cell loss in the tissue without significant change in the overall tissue structure.

BIOCHEMICAL CHANGES. Biochemical processes underlying the morphologic changes are as under:

1. Proteolysis of cytoskeletal proteins.
2. Protein-protein cross linking.
3. Fragmentation of nuclear chromatin by activation of nuclease.
4. Appearance of phosphatidylserine on the outer surface of cell membrane.
5. In some forms of apoptosis, appearance of an adhesive glycoprotein thrombospondin on the outer surface of apoptotic bodies.
6. Appearance of phosphatidylserine and thrombospondin on the outer surface of apoptotic cell facilitates early recognition by macrophages for phagocytosis prior to appearance of inflammatory cells.

IDENTIFYING APOPTOTIC CELLS. Identifying and counting of apoptotic cells is possible by following methods:

1. Staining of chromatin condensation (by haematoxylin, Feulgen, or acridine orange).
2. Flow cytometry to visualise rapid cell shrinkage.
3. DNA changes detected by *in situ* techniques or by gel electrophoresis.
4. Annexin V as marker for apoptotic cell membrane having phosphatidylserine on the cell exterior.

MOLECULAR MECHANISMS OF APOPTOSIS. Several physiologic and pathologic processes activate apoptosis in a variety of ways. However, in general the following events sum up the sequence involved in apoptosis:

1. Initiators of apoptosis. Stimuli for signalling programmed cell death act either at the cell membrane or intracellularly. These include:
i) Absence of stimuli required for normal cell survival (e.g. absence of certain hormones, growth factors, cytokines).
ii) Activators of programmed cell death (e.g. receptors for TNF).
iii) Intracellular stimuli include heat, radiation, hypoxia etc.

2. Regulators of apoptosis. After a cell has been initiated into apoptosis by above-mentioned signals, next comes the phase in which certain proteins convert death signals to the final programmed cell death and thus determine the outcome. These regulator proteins include the following:

i) *BCL-2. BCL*-2 protein is a human counterpart of *CED-9* (cell *d*eath) gene found in programmed cell death of nematode worm *C. elegans. BCL-2* is located in the outer mitochondrial membrane and may regulate the apoptotic process by binding to some other related proteins e.g to *BAX* and *BAD* for promoting apoptosis, and *BCL-XL* for inhibiting apoptosis. Another important *BCL-2* binding protein in the cytosol is the pro-*a*poptotic *p*rotease *a*ctivating *f*actor *(apaf-1)* which is a mammalian counterpart of gene *CED-4* of nematode. The net effect on the mitochondrial membrane is thus based on the pro-apoptotic and anti-apoptotic members of *BCL-2* protein family.

ii) *Other apoptotic regulator proteins.* Besides *BCL-2,* other important regulator proteins of apoptosis are TP53 *(p53)* protein, *caspases, BAX* and certain viruses (adenovirus, papillomavirus, hepatitis B virus).

3. Programmed cell death. The final outcome of apoptotic regulators in the programmed cell death involves the following pathways:

i) *FAS receptor activation.* Cell surface receptor *FAS* (CD 95) is present on cytotoxic (CD 8+) T cells. On coming in contact with the target cell, the *FAS* receptor is activated. This leads to activation of caspases and subsequent proteolysis.

ii) *Ceramide generation.* Due to hydrolysis of phospholipid sphingomyelin of the plasma membrane, ceramide is generated. Ceramide is implicated in further mitochondrial injury.

iii) *DNA damage.* Damage to DNA produced by various agents such as ionising radiation, chemotherapeutic agents, activated oxygen species lead to apoptosis. DNA damage affects nuclear protein TP53 *(p53)* which induces the synthesis of cell death promoting protein *BAX.*

4. Phagocytosis. The dead apoptotic cells and their fragments possess cell surface receptors which facilitate their identification by adjacent phagocytes. The phagocytosis is unaccompanied by any other inflammatory cells.

The mechanism of apoptosis is schematically represented in Fig. 3.19.

APOPTOSIS IN BIOLOGIC PROCESSES. Apoptosis is responsible for mediating cell death in a wide variety of physiologic and pathologic processes as under:

Physiologic Processes:
1. Organised cell destruction in sculpting of tissues during *development of embryo.*

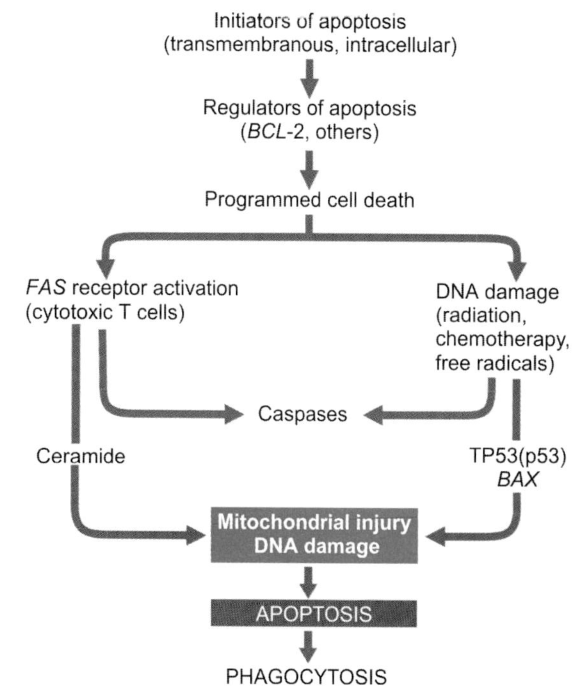

FIGURE 3.19
Mechanism of apoptosis.

2. Physiologic involution of cells in *hormone-dependent tissues* e.g. endometrial shedding, regression of lactating breast after withdrawal of breast feeding.

3. Normal cell destruction followed by *replacement proliferation* such as in intestinal epithelium.

4. *Involution of the thymus* in early age.

Pathologic Processes:

1. Cell death in tumours exposed to *chemotherapeutic agents.*

2. *Cell death by cytotoxic T cells* in immune mechanisms such as in graft-versus-host disease and rejection reactions.

3. *Cell death in viral infections* e.g. formation of Councilman bodies in viral hepatitis.

4. *Pathologic atrophy* of organs and tissues on withdrawal of stimuli e.g. prostatic atrophy after orchiectomy, atrophy of kidney or salivary gland on obstruction of ureter or ducts, respectively.

5. Progressive *depletion of CD4+T cells* in the pathogenesis of AIDS.

6. Cell death in response to *injurious agents* involved in causation of necrosis e.g. radiation, hypoxia and mild thermal injury.

7. In *degenerative diseases of CNS* e.g. in Alzheimer's disease, Parkinson's disease, and chronic infective dementias.

The contrasting features of apoptosis and necrosis are illustrated in Fig. 3.17 and summarised in Table 3.2.

GANGRENE

Gangrene is a form of necrosis of tissue with superadded putrefaction. The type of necrosis is usually coagulative due to ischaemia (e.g. in gangrene of the bowel, gangrene of limb). On the other hand, *gangrenous or necrotising inflammation* is characterised by primarily inflammation provoked by virulent bacteria resulting in massive tissue necrosis. Thus, the end-result of necrotising inflammation and gangrene is the same but the way the two are produced, is different. The examples of necrotising inflammation are: gangrene lung, gangrenous appendicitis, and noma (cancrum oris).

There are 3 main forms of gangrene—dry, wet and gas gangrene. In either type of gangrene, coagulative necrosis undergoes liquefaction by the action of putrefactive bacteria.

Dry Gangrene

This form of gangrene begins in the distal part of a limb due to ischaemia. The typical example is the dry gangrene in the toes and feet of an old patient due to arteriosclerosis. Other causes of dry gangrene foot include thromboangiitis obliterans (Buerger's disease), Raynaud's disease, trauma, ergot poisoning. It is usually initiated in one of the toes which is farthest from the blood supply, containing so little blood that even the invading bacteria find it hard to grow in the necrosed tissue. The gangrene spreads slowly upwards until it reaches a point where the blood supply is adequate to keep the tissue viable. A *line of separation* is formed at this point between the gangrenous part and the viable part.

PATHOLOGIC CHANGES. ***Macroscopically,*** the affected part is dry, shrunken and dark black, resembling the foot of a mummy. It is black due to liberation of haemoglobin from haemolysed red blood cells which is acted upon by hydrogen disulfide (H_2S)

TABLE 3.2: Contrasting Features of Apoptosis and Necrosis.

FEATURE	APOPTOSIS	NECROSIS
1. *Definition*	Programmed and coordinated cell death	Cell death along with degradation of tissue by hydrolytic enzymes
2. *Causative agents*	Physiologic and pathologic processes	Hypoxia, toxins
3. *Morphology*	i) No Inflammatory reaction ii) Death of single cells iii) Cell shrinkage iv) Cytoplasmic blebs on membrane v) Apoptotic bodies vi) Chromatin condensation vii) Phagocytosis of apoptotic bodies by macrophages	i) Inflammatory reaction always present ii) Death of many adjacent cells. iii) Cell swelling initially iv) Membrane disruption v) Damaged organelles vi) Nuclear disruption vii) Phagocytosis of cell debris by macrophages
4. *Molecular changes*	i) Lysosomes and other organelles intact ii) Genetic activation by proto-oncogenes and oncosuppressor genes, and cytotoxic T cell-mediated target cell killing	i) Lysosomal breakdown with liberation of hydrolytic enzymes ii) Cell death by ATP depletion, membrane damage, free radical injury

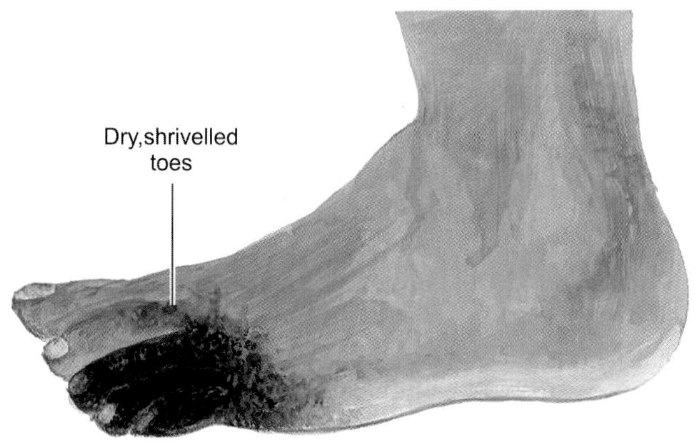

FIGURE 3.20

Dry gangrene of foot. The gangrenous area is dry, shrunken and dark and is separated from the viable tissue by clear line of separation.

produced by bacteria resulting in formation of black iron sulfide. The line of separation usually brings about complete separation with eventual falling off of the gangrenous tissue if it is not removed surgically (Fig. 3.20).

Histologically, there is necrosis with smudging of the tissue. The line of separation consists of inflammatory granulation tissue.

Wet Gangrene

This occurs in naturally moist tissues and organs such as the mouth, bowel, lung, cervix, vulva etc. Diabetic foot is another example of wet gangrene due to high sugar content in the necrosed tissue which favours growth of bacteria. *Bed sores* occurring in a bed-ridden patient due to pressure on sites like the sacrum, buttocks and heels are the other important clinical conditions included in wet gangrene. Wet gangrene usually develops rapidly due to blockage of venous and less commonly arterial blood flow from thrombosis or embolism. The affected part is stuffed with blood which favours the rapid growth of putrefactive bacteria. The toxic products formed by bacteria are absorbed causing systemic manifestations of septicaemia, and finally death. The spreading wet gangrene lacks clear-cut line of demarcation and may spread to peritoneal cavity causing peritonitis.

PATHOLOGIC CHANGES. ***Macroscopically,*** the affected part is soft, swollen, putrid, rotten and dark. The classic example is gangrene of bowel, commonly due to strangulated hernia, volvulus or intussusception. The part is stained dark due to the same mechanism as in dry gangrene (Fig. 3.21,A).

Histologically, there is coagulative necrosis with stuffing of affected part with blood. There is ulceration of the mucosa and intense inflammatory infiltration. Lumen of the bowel contains mucus and blood. The line of demarcation between gangrenous segment and viable bowel is generally not clear-cut (Fig. 3.21,B) (COLOUR PLATE VI: CL 24).

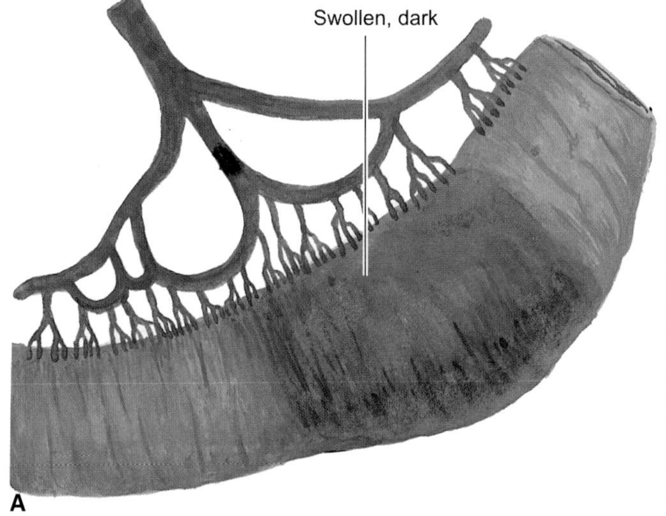

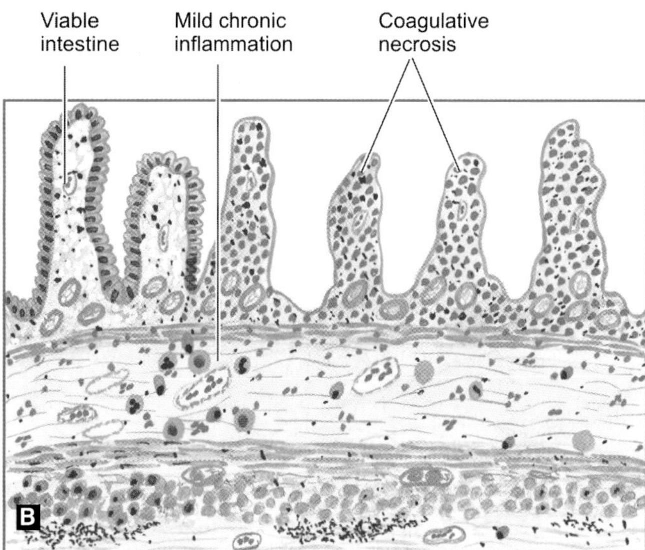

FIGURE 3.21

A, Wet gangrene of small bowel. The affected part is soft, swollen and dark. Line of demarcation between gangrenous segment and the viable bowel is not clear-cut. B, Microscopy shows coagulative necrosis of the affected bowel wall stuffed with blood while the junction with normal intestine shows an inflammatory infiltrate.

TABLE 3.3: Contrasting Features of Dry and Wet Gangrene.

	FEATURE	DRY GANGRENE	WET GANGRENE
1.	*Site*	Commonly limbs	More common in bowel
2.	*Mechanisms*	Arterial occlusion	More commonly venous obstruction, less often arterial occlusion
3.	*Macroscopy*	Organ dry, shrunken and black	Part moist, soft, swollen, rotten and dark
4.	*Putrefaction*	Limited due to very little blood supply	Marked due to stuffing of organ with blood
5.	*Line of demarcation*	Present at the junction between healthy and gangrenous part	No clear line of demarcation
6.	*Bacteria*	Bacteria fail to survive	Numerous present
7.	*Prognosis*	Generally better due to little septicaemia	Generally poor due to profound toxaemia

Contrasting features of two main forms of gangrene are summarised in Table 3.3.

Gas Gangrene

Gas gangrene is a special form of wet gangrene caused by gas-forming clostridia (gram-positive anaerobic bacteria) which gain entry into the tissues through open contaminated wounds, especially in the muscles, or as a complication of operation on colon which normally contains clostridia. Clostridia produce various toxins which produce necrosis and oedema locally and are also absorbed producing profound systemic manifestations.

PATHOLOGIC CHANGES. ***Grossly,*** the affected area is swollen, oedematous, painful and crepitant due to accumulation of gas bubbles within the tissues. Subsequently, the affected tissue becomes dark black and foul smelling.

Microscopically, the muscle fibres undergo coagulative necrosis with liquefaction. Large number of gram-positive bacilli can be identified. At the periphery, a zone of leucocytic infiltration, oedema and congestion are found. Capillary and venous thrombi are common.

PATHOLOGIC CALCIFICATION

Deposition of calcium salts in tissues other than osteoid or enamel is called pathologic or heterotopic calcification. Two distinct types of pathologic calcification are recognised:

- *Dystrophic calcification*, which is characterised by deposition of calcium salts in dead or degenerated tissues with normal calcium metabolism and normal serum calcium levels.
- *Metastatic calcification*, on the other hand, occurs in apparently normal tissues and is associated with deranged calcium metabolism and hypercalcaemia.

Etiology and pathogenesis of the two are different but morphologically the deposits in both resemble normal minerals of the bone.

Histologically, in routine H and E stained sections, calcium salts appear as deeply basophilic, irregular and granular clumps. The deposits may be intracellular, extracellular, or at both locations. Occasionally, heterotopic bone formation (ossification) may occur. Calcium deposits can be confirmed by special stains like silver impregnation method of *von-Kossa* producing black colour, and *alizarin red S* that produces red staining. Pathologic calcification is often accompanied by diffuse or granular deposits of iron giving positive Prussian blue reaction.

Etiopathogenesis

The two types of pathologic calcification result from distinctly different etiologies and mechanisms.

DYSTROPHIC CALCIFICATION. As apparent from definition, dystrophic calcification may occur due to 2 types of causes:

- Calcification in dead tissue
- Calcification of degenerated tissue.

Calcification in dead tissue

1. *Caseous necrosis* in tuberculosis is the most common site for dystrophic calcification. Living bacilli may be present even in calcified tuberculous lesions, lymph nodes, lungs, etc (COLOUR PLATE V: CL 18).
2. *Liquefaction necrosis* in chronic abscesses may get calcified.

Chapter Three

3. *Fat necrosis* following acute pancreatitis or traumatic fat necrosis in the breast results in deposition of calcium soaps.
4. *Infarcts* may sometimes undergo dystrophic calcification.
5. *Thrombi,* especially in the veins, may produce phleboliths.
6. *Haematomas* in the vicinity of bones may undergo dystrophic calcification.
7. *Dead parasites* like in hydatid cyst, Schistosoma eggs, and cysticercosis are some of the examples showing dystrophic calcification.
8. Calcification in *breast cancer* detected by mammography.
9. *Congenital toxoplasmosis* involving the central nervous system visualised by calcification in the infant brain.

Calcification in degenerated tissues

1. *Dense old scars* may undergo hyaline degeneration and subsequent calcification.
2. *Atheromas* in the aorta and coronaries frequently undergo calcification (COLOUR PLATE XIII: CL 52).
3. *Mönckeberg's sclerosis* shows calcification in the tunica media of muscular arteries in elderly people (Chapter 11) (COLOUR PLATE XIII: CL 49).
4. *Stroma of tumours* such as uterine fibroids, breast cancer, thyroid adenoma, goitre etc show calcification. Some tumours show characteristic spherules of calcification called *psammoma bodies* or calcospherites such as in meningioma, papillary serous cystadenocarcinoma of the ovary and papillary carcinoma of the thyroid.
5. *Cysts* which have been present for a long time may show calcification of their walls e.g. epidermal and pilar cysts.
6. *Calcinosis cutis* is a condition of unknown cause in which there are irregular nodular deposits of calcium salts in the skin and subcutaneous tissue.
7. *Senile degenerative changes* may be accompanied by dystrophic calcification such as in costal cartilages, tracheal or bronchial cartilages, and pineal gland in the brain etc.

The **pathogenesis** of dystrophic calcification is not quite clear. A few factors like local alteration of pH in the necrotic tissue and release of enzymes (e.g. alkaline phosphatase) from necrotic or degenerated tissue have been implicated which favour deposition of calcium salts. The process of dystrophic calcification has been likened to the formation of normal hydroxyapatite in the bone involving 2 phases: initiation and propagation.

■ *Initiation* is the phase in which calcium and phosphates begin to accumulate intracellularly in the mitochondria, or extracellularly in membrane-bound vesicles.

■ *Propagation* is the phase in which minerals deposited in the initiation phase are propagated to form mineral crystals.

METASTATIC CALCIFICATION. Since metastatic calcification occurs in normal tissues due to hypercalcaemia, its causes would include one of the following two conditions:

■ Excessive mobilisation of calcium from the bone.
■ Excessive absorption of calcium from the gut.

Excessive mobilisation of calcium from the bone. These causes are more common and include the following:

1. *Hyperparathyroidism* which may be primary such as due to parathyroid adenoma, or secondary such as from parathyroid hyperplasia, chronic renal failure etc.
2. *Bony destructive lesions* such as multiple myeloma, metastatic carcinoma.
3. *Prolonged immobilisation* of a patient results in disuse atrophy of the bones and hypercalcaemia.

Excessive absorption of calcium from the gut. Less often, excess calcium may be absorbed from the gut causing hypercalcaemia and metastatic calcification. These causes are as under:

1. *Hypervitaminosis D* results in increased calcium absorption.
2. *Milk-alkali syndrome* caused by excessive oral intake of calcium in the form of milk and administration of calcium carbonate in the treatment of peptic ulcer.
3. *Hypercalcaemia of infancy* is another condition in which metastatic calcification may occur.

Metastatic calcification may occur in any normal tissue of the body but affects the following organs more commonly:

■ *Kidneys,* especially at the basement membrane of tubular epithelium and in the tubular lumina causing nephrocalcinosis.
■ *Lungs,* especially in the alveolar walls.
■ *Stomach,* on the acid-secreting fundal glands.
■ *Blood vessels,* especially on the internal elastic lamina.
■ *Cornea* is another site affected by metastatic calcification.

The **pathogenesis** of metastatic calcification at the above mentioned sites is based on the hypothesis that these sites have relatively high (alkaline) pH which favours the precipitation of the calcium.

The distinguishing features between the two types of pathologic calcification are summarised in Table 3.4.

TABLE 3.4: Differences between Dystrophic and Metastatic Calcification.

	FEATURE	DYSTROPHIC CALCIFICATION	METASTATIC CALCIFICATION
1.	*Definition*	Deposits of calcium salts in dead and degenerated tissues	Deposits of calcium salts in normal tissues
2.	*Calcium metabolism*	Normal	Deranged
3.	*Serum calcium level*	Normal	Hypercalcaemia
4.	*Causes*	Necrosis (caseous, liquefactive, fat), infarcts, thrombi, haematomas, dead parasites, old scars, atheromas, Mönckeberg's sclerosis, certain tumours, cysts, calcinosis cutis	Hyperparathyroidism (due to adenoma, hyperplasia, CRF), bony destructive lesions (e.g. myeloma, metastatic carcinoma), prolonged immobilisation, hypervitaminosis D, milk-alkali syndrome, hypercalcaemia of infancy
5.	*Pathogenesis*	Akin to formation of normal hydroxyapatite involving phases of initiation and propagation	Favoured by relatively high pH (alkaline) at certain sites e.g. in lungs, stomach, blood vessels and cornea

CELLULAR ADAPTATIONS

For the sake of survival on exposure to stress, the cells make adjustments with the changes in their environment (i.e. adapt) to the physiologic needs *(physiologic adaptation)* and to non-lethal pathologic injury *(pathologic adaptation)*. Broadly speaking, such physiologic and pathologic adaptations occur by following processes (Fig. 3.22):

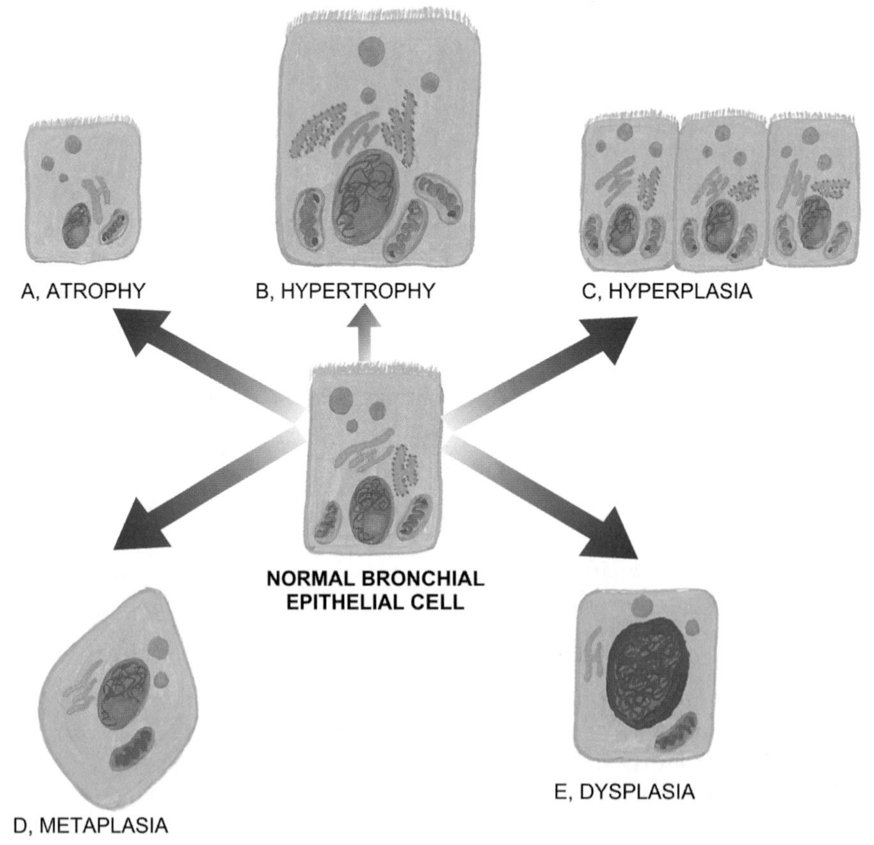

FIGURE 3.22

Adaptive disorders of growth.

- Decreasing or increasing their size i.e. *atrophy* and *hypertrophy* respectively, or by increasing their number i.e. *hyperplasia*.
- By changing the pathway of phenotypic differentiation of cells i.e. *metaplasia* and *dysplasia*.

In general, the adaptive responses are reversible on withdrawal of stimulus. However, if the irritant stimulus persists for long time, the cell may not be able to survive and may either die or progress further e.g. cell death in sustained atrophy, progression of dysplasia into carcinoma *in situ*. Thus, the concept of evolution 'survival of the fittest' holds true for adaptation as *'survival of the adaptable'*.

Various mechanisms which may be involved in adaptive cellular responses include:

- Altered cell surface receptor binding.
- Alterations in signal for protein synthesis.
- Synthesis of new proteins by the target cell such as heat-shock proteins (HSPs).

Common forms of cellular adaptive responses along with examples of physiologic and pathologic adaptations are briefly discussed below.

ATROPHY

Reduction of the number and size of parenchymal cells of an organ or its parts which was once normal is called atrophy (c.f. *hypoplasia* which is the term used for developmentally small size, and *aplasia* for extreme failure of development so that only rudimentary tissue is present).

CAUSES. Atrophy may occur from physiologic or pathologic causes.

A. Physiologic atrophy. Atrophy is a normal process of aging in some tissues which could be due to loss of endocrine stimulation or arteriosclerosis. For example:
i) Atrophy of lymphoid tissue in lymph nodes, appendix and thymus.
ii) Atrophy of gonads after menopause.
iii) Atrophy of brain.

B. Pathologic atrophy. The causes are as under:

1. *Starvation atrophy.* In starvation, there is first depletion of carbohydrate and fat stores followed by protein catabolism. There is general weakness, emaciation and anaemia referred to as cachexia seen in cancer and severely-ill patients.

2. *Ischaemic atrophy.* Gradual diminution of blood supply due to atherosclerosis may result in shrinkage of the affected organ e.g.
i) Small atrophic kidney in atherosclerosis of renal artery.
ii) Atrophy of brain in cerebral atherosclerosis.

3. *Disuse atrophy.* Prolonged diminished functional activity is associated with disuse atrophy of the organ e.g.
i) Wasting of muscles of limb immobilised in cast.
ii) Atrophy of .the pancreas in obstruction of pancreatic duct.

4. *Neuropathic atrophy.* Interruption in nerve supply leads to wasting of muscles e.g.
i) Poliomyelitis
ii) Motor neuron disease
iii) Nerve section.

5. *Endocrine atrophy.* Loss of endocrine regulatory mechanism results in reduced metabolic activity of tissues and hence atrophy e.g.
i) Hypopituitarism may lead to atrophy of thyroid, adrenal and gonads.
ii) Hypothyroidism may cause atrophy of the skin and its adnexal structures.

6. *Pressure atrophy.* Prolonged pressure from benign tumours or cyst or aneurysm may cause compression and atrophy of the tissues e.g.
i) Erosion of spine by tumour in nerve root.
ii) Erosion of skull by meningioma arising from pia-arachnoid.
iii) Erosion of sternum by aneurysm of arch of aorta.

7. *Idiopathic atrophy.* There are some examples of atrophy where no obvious cause is present e.g.
i) Myopathies.
ii) Testicular atrophy.

PATHOLOGIC CHANGES. Irrespective of the underlying cause for atrophy, the pathologic changes are similar. The organ is small, often shrunken. The cells become smaller in size but are not dead cells (Fig. 3.22, A). Shrinkage in cell size is due to reduction in cell organelles, chiefly mitochondria, myofilaments and endoplasmic reticulum. There is often increase in the number of autophagic vacuoles containing cell debris. These autophagic vacuoles may persist to form 'residual bodies' in the cell cytoplasm e.g. lipofuscin pigment granules in brown atrophy (page 49) **(COLOUR PLATE III: CL 9).**

HYPERTROPHY

Hypertrophy is an increase in the size of parenchymal cells resulting in enlargement of the organ or tissue, without any change in the number of cells.

CAUSES. Hypertrophy may be physiologic or pathologic. In both cases, it is caused either by increased functional demand or by hormonal stimulation. Hypertrophy without accompanying hyperplasia affects mainly muscles. In non-dividing cells too, only hypertrophy occurs.

A. Physiologic hypertrophy. Enlarged size of the uterus in pregnancy is an excellent example of physiologic hypertrophy as well as hyperplasia.

B. Pathologic hypertrophy. Examples of certain diseases associated with hypertrophy are as under:

1. *Hypertrophy of cardiac muscle* may occur in a number of cardiovascular diseases. A few examples producing left ventricular hypertrophy are:
i) Systemic hypertension
ii) Aortic valve disease (stenosis and insufficiency)
iii) Mitral insufficiency

2. *Hypertrophy of smooth muscle e.g.*
i) Cardiac achalasia (in oesophagus)
ii) Pyloric stenosis (in stomach)
iii) Intestinal strictures
iv) Muscular arteries in hypertension.

3. *Hypertrophy of skeletal muscle* e.g. hypertrophied muscles in athletes and manual labourers.

4. *Compensatory hypertrophy* may occur in an organ when the contralateral organ is removed e.g.
i) Following nephrectomy on one side in a young patient, there is compensatory hypertrophy as well as hyperplasia of the nephrons of the other kidney.
ii) Adrenal hyperplasia following removal of one adrenal gland.

Chapter Three

PATHOLOGIC CHANGES. The affected organ is enlarged and heavy. For example a hypertrophied heart of a patient with systemic hypertension may weigh 700-800 g as compared to average normal adult weight of 350 g. There is enlargement of muscle fibres as well as of nuclei (Fig. 3.22,B) (COLOUR PLATE III: CL 10). At ultrastructural level, there is increased synthesis of DNA and RNA, increased protein synthesis and increased number of organelles like mitochondria, endoplasmic reticulum and myofibrils.

HYPERPLASIA

Hyperplasia is an increase in the number of parenchymal cells resulting in enlargement of the organ or tissue. Quite often, both hyperplasia and hypertrophy occur together. Hyperplasia occurs due to increased recruitment of cells from G_0 (resting) phase of the cell cycle to undergo mitosis, when stimulated. All body cells do not possess hyperplastic growth potential (Chapter 6). Labile cells (e.g. epithelial cells of the skin and mucous membranes, cells of the bone marrow and lymph nodes) and stable cells (e.g. parenchymal cells of the liver, pancreas, kidney, adrenal, and thyroid) can undergo hyperplasia, while permanent cells (e.g. neurons, cardiac and skeletal muscle) have little or no capacity for regenerative hyperplastic growth. Neoplasia differs from hyperplasia in having hyperplastic growth with loss of growth-regulatory mechanism due to change in genetic composition of the cell. Hyperplasia, on the other hand, persists so long as stimulus is present.

CAUSES. As with other non-neoplastic disorders of growth, hyperplasia has also been divided into physiologic and pathologic.

A. Physiologic hyperplasia. The two most common types are as follows:

1. *Hormonal hyperplasia* i.e. hyperplasia occurring under the influence of hormonal stimulation e.g.
i) Hyperplasia of female breast at puberty, during pregnancy and lactation.
ii) Hyperplasia of pregnant uterus.
iii) Proliferative activity of normal endometrium after a normal menstrual cycle.
iv) Prostatic hyperplasia in old age.

2. *Compensatory hyperplasia* i.e. hyperplasia occurring following removal of part of an organ or a contralateral organ in paired organ e.g.
i) Regeneration of the liver following partial hepatectomy
ii) Regeneration of epidermis after skin abrasion
iii) Following nephrectomy on one side, there is hyperplasia of nephrons of the other kidney.

B. Pathologic hyperplasia. Most examples of pathologic hyperplasia are due to excessive stimulation of hormones or growth factors e.g.
i) Endometrial hyperplasia following oestrogen excess.
ii) In wound healing, there is formation of granulation tissue due to proliferation of fibroblasts and endothelial cells.
iii) Formation of skin warts from hyperplasia of epidermis due to human papilloma virus.
iv) Pseudocarcinomatous hyperplasia of the skin.
v) Intraductal epithelial hyperplasia in the breast in fibrocystic breast disease (COLOUR PLATE III: CL 11).

PATHOLOGIC CHANGES. There is enlargement of the affected organ or tissue and increase in the number of cells (Fig. 3.22,C). This is due to increased rate of DNA synthesis and hence increased mitoses of the cells.

METAPLASIA

Metaplasia (*meta* = transformation, *plasia* = growth) is defined as a reversible change of one type of epithelial or mesenchymal adult cells to another type of adult epithelial or mesenchymal cells, usually in response to abnormal stimuli, and often *reverts back to normal on removal of stimulus* (Fig. 3.22,D). However, if the stimulus persists for a long time, epithelial metaplasia may transform into cancer.

Metaplasia is broadly divided into 2 types: epithelial and mesenchymal.

A. EPITHELIAL METAPLASIA. This is the more common type. The metaplastic change may be patchy or diffuse and usually results in replacement by stronger but less well-specialised epithelium. However, the metaplastic epithelium being less well-specialised such as squamous type, results in deprivation of protective mucus secretion and hence more prone to infection. Some common types of epithelial metaplasia are as under:

1. Squamous metaplasia. Various types of epithelium are capable of undergoing squamous metaplastic change due to chronic irritation that may be mechanical, chemical or infective in origin. Some common examples of squamous metaplasia are seen at following sites:

i) In *bronchus* (normally lined by pseudostratified columnar ciliated epithelium) in chronic smokers.

ii) In *uterine endocervix* (normally lined by simple columnar epithelium) in prolapse of the uterus and in old age (Fig. 3.23, A and B) (COLOUR PLATE III: CL 12).

iii) In *gallbladder* (normally lined by simple columnar epithelium) in chronic cholecystitis with cholelithiasis.

iv) In *prostate* (ducts normally lined by simple columnar epithelium) in chronic prostatitis and oestrogen therapy.

v) In *renal pelvis* and *urinary bladder* (normally lined by transitional epithelium) in chronic infection and stones.

vi) In *vitamin A deficiency*, apart from xerophthalmia, there is squamous metaplasia in the nose, bronchi, urinary tract, lacrimal and salivary glands.

2. Columnar metaplasia. There are some conditions in which there is transformation to columnar epithelium. For example:

i) Intestinal metaplasia in healed chronic gastric ulcer.

ii) Conversion of pseudostratified columnar epithelium in chronic bronchitis and bronchiectasis to columnar type.

iii) In cervical erosion (congenital and adult type), there is variable area of endocervical glandular mucosa everted into the vagina.

B. MESENCHYMAL METAPLASIA. Less often, there is transformation of one adult type of mesenchymal tissue to another. The examples are as under:

1. Osseous metaplasia. Osseous metaplasia is formation of bone in fibrous tissue, cartilage and myxoid tissue. Examples of osseous metaplasia are as under:

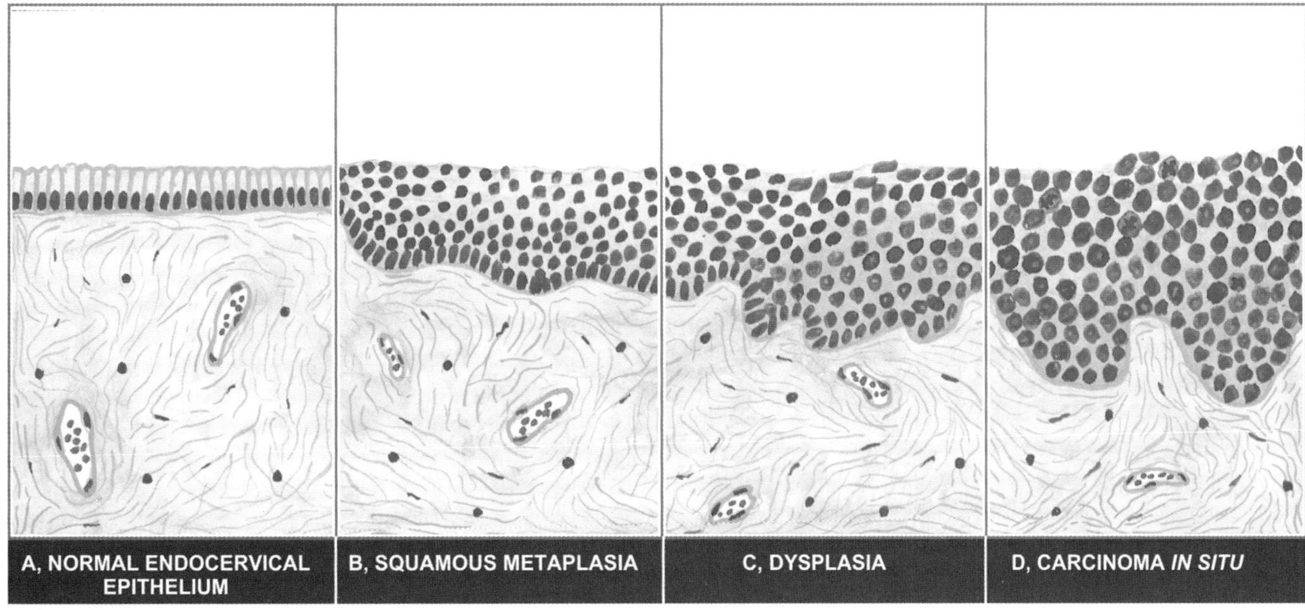

FIGURE 3.23

Schematic diagram showing sequential changes in uterine cervix from normal epithelium to development of carcinoma *in situ*. A, Normal mucus-secreting endocervical epithelium. B, Squamous metaplasia. C, Dysplastic change. D, Carcinoma *in situ*.

i) In arterial wall in old age (Mönckeberg's medial calcific sclerosis)
ii) In soft tissues in myositis ossificans
iii) In cartilage of larynx and bronchi in elderly people
iv) In scar of chronic inflammation of prolonged duration
v) In the fibrous stroma of tumour.

2. Cartilaginous metaplasia. In healing of fractures, cartilaginous metaplasia may occur where there is undue mobility.

DYSPLASIA

Dysplasia means 'disordered cellular development', often accompanied with metaplasia and hyperplasia; it is therefore also referred to as *atypical hyperplasia*. Dysplasia occurs most often in epithelial cells. Epithelial dysplasia is characterised by cellular proliferation and cytologic changes. These changes include:

1. Increased number of layers of epithelial cells
2. Disorderly arrangement of cells from basal layer to the surface layer
3. Loss of basal polarity i.e. nuclei lying away from basement membrane
4. Cellular and nuclear pleomorphism
5. Increased nucleocytoplasmic ratio
6. Nuclear hyperchromatism
7. Increased mitotic activity.

The two most common examples of dysplastic changes are the *uterine cervix* (Fig. 3.23, C) and *respiratory tract*.

Dysplastic changes often occur due to chronic irritation or prolonged inflammation. On removal of the inciting stimulus, the changes may disappear. In a proportion of cases, however, dysplasia progresses into carcinoma *in situ* (cancer confined to layers superficial to basement membrane) (Fig. 3.23, D) or invasive cancer (COLOUR PLATE IV: CL 13,14). This concept is further discussed in details in Chapters 8, 15, and 22.

The differences between dysplasia and metaplasia are contrasted in Table 3.5.

CELLULAR AGING

Old age is a concept of longevity in human beings. The consequences of aging appear after reproductive age. However, aging is distinct from mortality and disease although aged individuals are more vulnerable to disease.

The average age of death of primitive man was barely 20-25 years compared to life-expectancy now which is approaching 80 years, survival being longer in women than men (3:2). About a century ago, the main causes of death were accidents and infections. But now with greater safety and sanitation, the mortality in the middle years has sufficiently declined. However, the maximum human lifespan has remained stable at about 110 years. Higher life expectancy in women is not due to difference in the response of somatic cells of the two sexes but higher mortality rate in men is attributed to violent causes and greater susceptibility to cardiovascular disease, cancer, cirrhosis and respiratory diseases, for which cigarette smoking and alcohol consumption are important contributory factors.

In general, the life expectancy of an individual depends upon the following factors:

1. *Intrinsic genetic process* i.e the genes controlling response to endogenous and exogenous factors initiating apoptosis in senility
2. *Environmental factors* e.g. consumption and inhalation of harmful substances, diet, role of antioxidants etc.

TABLE 3.5: Differences between Metaplasia and Dysplasia.

FEATURE	METAPLASIA	DYSPLASIA
i) Definition	Change of one type of epithelial or mesenchymal cell to another type of adult epithelial or mesenchymal cell	Disordered cellular development, may be accompanied with hyperplasia or metaplasia
ii) Types	Epithelial (squamous, columnar) and mesenchymal (osseous, cartilaginous)	Epithelial only
iii) Tissues affected	Most commonly affects bronchial mucosa, uterine endocervix; others mesenchymal tissues (cartilage, arteries)	Uterine cervix, bronchial mucosa
iv) Cellular changes	Mature cellular development	Disordered cellular development (pleomorphism, nuclear hyperchromasia, mitosis, loss of polarity)
v) Natural history	Reversible on withdrawal of stimulus	May regress on removal of inciting stimulus, or may progress to higher grades of dysplasia or carcinoma *in situ*

3. *Lifestyle of the individual* such as diseases due to alcoholism (e.g.cirrhosis, hepatocellular carcinoma), smoking (e.g. bronchogenic carcinoma and other respiratory diseases), drug addiction.
4. *Age-related diseases* e.g. atherosclerosis and ischaemic heart disease, diabetes mellitus, hypertension, osteoporosis, Alzheimer's disease, Parkinson's disease etc.

CELLULAR BASIS

With age, structural and functional changes occur in different organs and systems of the human body. Although no definitive biologic basis of aging is established, most acceptable theory is the functional decline of non-dividing cells such as neurons and myocytes. The following hypotheses based on investigations explain the cellular basis of aging:

1. Experimental cellular senescence. By *in vitro* studies of tissue culture, it has been observed that cultured human fibroblasts replicate for upto 50 population doublings and then the culture dies out. It means that *in vitro* there is reduced functional capacity to proliferate with age. Studies have shown that there is either loss of chromosome 1 or deletion of its long arm (1q). Alternatively it has been observed that with every cell division there is progressive shortening of *telomere* present at the tips of chromosomes which in normal cell is repaired by the presence of RNA enzyme, *telomerase*. However, due to aging, due to inadequate presence of telomerase enzyme, lost telomere is not repaired resulting in interference in viability of cell.

2. Genetic control in invertebrates. Clock *(clk)* genes responsible for controlling the rate and time of aging have been identified in lower invertebrates e.g. *clk-1* gene mutation in the metazoa, *Caenorhabditis elegans*, results in prolonging the lifespan of the worm and slowing of some metabolic functions.

3. Diseases of accelerated aging. Aging is under genetic control in human beings supported by the observation of high concordance in lifespan of identical twins. A heritable condition associated with signs of accelerated aging process is termed *progeria* and is characterised by baldness, cataracts, and coronary artery disease. Another example is Werner syndrome, a rare autosomal recessive disease, characterised by similar features of premature aging, atherosclerosis and risk for development of various cancers.

4. Oxidative stress hypothesis. Currently, it is believed that aging is partly caused by progressive and reversible molecular oxidative damage due to persistent oxidative stress on the human cells. In normal cells, very small amount (3%) of total oxygen consumption by the cell is converted into reactive oxygen species. The rate of generation of reactive oxygen species is directly correlated with metabolic rate of the organisms.With aging, there is low metabolic rate with generation of toxic oxygen radicals which fail to get eliminated causing their accumulation and cell damage. The underlying mechanism appears to be oxidative damage to mitochondria. The role of antioxidant in retarding the oxidant damage has been reported in some studies.

ORGAN CHANGES IN AGING

Although all organs start showing deterioration with aging, following organs show evident morphologic and functional changes:

1. *Cardiovascular system:* Atherosclerosis, arteriosclerosis with calcification, Mönckeberg's medial calcification, brown atrophy of heart, loss of elastic tissue from aorta and major arterial trunks causing their dilatation.
2. *Nervous system:* Atrophy of gyri and sulci, Alzheimer's disease, Parkinson's disease.
3. *Musculoskeletal system*: Degenerative bone diseases, frequent fractures due to loss of bone density, age related muscular degeneration.
4. *Eyes:* Deterioration of vision due to cataract and vascular changes in retina.
5. *Hearing:* Disability in hearing due to senility is related to otosclerosis.
6. *Immune system:* reduced IgG response to antigens, frequent and severe infections.
7. *Skin:* Laxity of skin due to loss of elastic tissue.
8. *Cancers:* As discussed later in Chapter 8, 80% of cancers occur in the age range of 50 and 80 years.

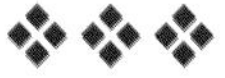

Immunopathology Including Amyloidosis

4

Immunity and immunopathology are proverbial two edges of 'double-edged sword'.

Before discussing of immunopathology which is the study of derangements in the immune system, it is important to know the structure and function of the normal immune system (immunophysiology) and to get familiarised with a few terms and definitions commonly used in any description of immunology.

- An **antigen (Ag)** is defined as a substance, usually protein in nature, which when introduced into the tissues stimulates antibody production.
- **Hapten** is a non-protein substance which has no antigenic properties, but on combining with a protein can form a new antigen capable of forming antibodies.
- An **antibody (Ab)** is a protein substance produced as a result of antigenic stimulation. Circulating antibodies are immunoglobulins (Igs) of which there are 5 classes: IgG, IgA, IgM, IgE and IgD.
- Alternatively, an antigen may induce **specifically sensitised cells** having the capacity to recognise, react and neutralise the injurious agent or organisms.
- The antigen may combine with antibody to form **antigen-antibody complex**. The reaction of Ag with Ab *in vitro* may be *primary* or *secondary phenomena*; the secondary reaction induces a number of processes. *In vivo*, the Ag-Ab reaction may cause tissue damage (Fig. 4.1).

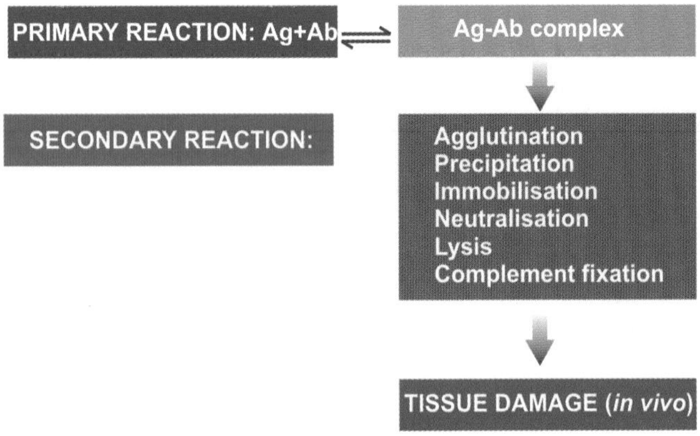

PRIMARY REACTION: Ag+Ab ⇌ Ag-Ab complex

SECONDARY REACTION: Agglutination, Precipitation, Immobilisation, Neutralisation, Lysis, Complement fixation

↓

TISSUE DAMAGE (*in vivo*)

FIGURE 4.1

Antigen-antibody reactions. Primary and secondary reactions occur *in vitro* while tissue damage results from *in vivo* Ag-Ab reaction.

COMPONENTS OF IMMUNE SYSTEM

Broadly speaking, immunity or body defense mechanism is divided into 2 types, each with humoral and cellular components:

I. Nonspecific or innate immunity is considered as the first line of defense without antigenic specificity. Its major components are:

a) *Humoral:* comprised by complement.

b) *Cellular:* consists of neutrophils, macrophages, and natural killer (NK) cells.

II. Specific or adaptive immunity is characterised by antigenic specificity. Its main components are:

a. *Humoral:* consisting of antibodies formed by B cells.

b. *Cellular:* mediated by T cells.

The various components of both types of immunity are interdependent and interlinked for their functions.

The components of innate immunity like the complement, neutrophils and macrophages are described in Chapter 6. The other components of the immune system are considered below:

Lymphocytes

Morphologically, lymphocytes appear as a homogeneous group but functionally two major lymphocyte populations are identified—T and B lymphocytes. B cells differentiate into plasma cells which form specific antibodies. T cells proliferate on coming in contact with appropriate antigen after which the non-specific accessory cells (PMNs and macrophages) play a critical role in completion of immunopathologic reaction.

B and T cells cannot be distinguished by light or electron microscopy but can be differentiated by immunologic methods (Table 4.1). B cells express specific antibodies as immunoglobulins. T cells, on the other hand, have surface molecules expressed at different stages of their development which are characterised by monoclonal antibodies according to the *cluster of differentiation* (CD).

Hybridoma Monoclonal Antibodies

Hybridoma technique is the *in vitro* method of obtaining monoclonal antibodies against any antigen by mixing (hybridising) B cells of required clone of antibodies with myeloma cells as source for continued secretion of immunoglobulin to immortalise the cell lineage. Currently, hybridoma monoclonal antibodies are produced commercially against all possible antigens such as DNA, RNA, intermediate filaments, molecular cellular proteins etc. The use of hybridoma monoclonal antibodies has helped in recognising subpopulations of T and B cells. This has been found particularly helpful in identification of benign and malignant lesions of B cell series. Antibodies labelled specifically to kappa (κ) and lambda (λ) light chains, both of which are normally present on B cells, can be used to determine whether the lesion is:

- *polyclonal*, if arising from stimulation of several clones containing κ as well as λ light chains e.g. in non-neoplastic or reactive proliferations; or

TABLE 4.1: Differences between T and B Lymphocytes.

FEATURE	T CELLS	B CELLS
1. ***Origin***	Bone marrow → Thymus	Bone marrow → Bursa (in fowl); mucosa-associated lymphoid tissue (MALT)
2. ***Life span***	Small T cells: months to years T cell blasts: several days	Small B cells: less than 1 month B cell blasts : several days
3. ***Location***		
(i) *Lymph nodes*	Perifollicular (paracortical)	Germinal centres, medullary cords
(ii) *Spleen*	Periarteriolar	Germinal centres, red pulp
(iii) *Peyer's patches*	Perifollicular	Central follicles
4. ***Presence in***		
(i) *Blood*	80%	20%
(ii) *Bone marrow*	Rarely present	Numerous
(iii) *Lymph nodes*	85%	15%
(iv) *Spleen*	65%	35%
(v) *Thymus*	90%	10%
5. ***Surface markers***		
(i) *Ag receptors*	Present	Absent
(ii) *Surface Ig*	Absent	Present
(iii) *Fc receptor*	Absent	Present
(iv) *Complement receptor*	Absent	Present
(v) *Rosettes*	E-rosettes (sheep erythrocytes)	EAC-rosettes (mouse erythrocytes)
(vi) *CD markers*	TH CD4, 3, 7, 2 TS CD8, 3, 7, 2	CD19, 21, 23
6. ***Functions***	(i) CMI via cytotoxic T cells positive for CD3 and CD4 (ii) Delayed hypersensitivity via CD4+ T cells (iii) Immunoregulation of other T cells, B cells and stem cells via T helper (CD4+) or T suppressor (CD8+) cells	(i) Role in humoral immunity by synthesis of specific antibodies (Igs) (ii) Precursors of plasma cells

■ *monoclonal,* if arising from stimulation of only one clone and thus one light chain type only e.g. in malignant tumours.

Effector Lymphocyte Subpopulations

Different subpopulations of sensitised lymphocytes ($T_{DTH,}$ CD4+ T cells, or helper T cells; $T_{CTL,}$ CD8+ T cells, or cytotoxic lymphocytes) and unsensitised cells (NK or natural killer cells) can mediate the specific immune responses (Table 4.2).

Macrophage

The role of macrophages in inflammation consisting of circulating monocytes and tissue macrophages has been described in Chapter 6. The macrophage subpopulations like the dendritic cells found in the lymphoid tissue and Langerhans' cells seen in the epidermis, are characterised by the presence of dendritic cytoplasmic processes and are active in the immune system.

The functions of macrophage subpopulations in the immune system are as follows:

i) They *recognise the antigen* for presenting to immunocompetent T or B cells.

ii) The *phagocytic function* of macrophage is performed due to location of surface receptor for Fc fragment of IgG and C_3 complement.

iii) Macrophages produce *interleukin*-1 which has a role in differentiation stage of T and B lymphocytes.

iv) Macrophages are capable of *lysing tumour cells* by secretion of toxic metabolites.

v) They act as powerful effector cells in some forms of *cell-mediated immunity* e.g. in delayed hypersensitivity reactions.

vi) They act as *mediators of inflammation* in release of prostaglandins, activation of coagulation factors and in secretion of acute phase reactant proteins by the liver.

Immune Effector Mechanism

The immune defense reactions by body against infective agent are mediated through different effector mechanisms as summarised in Table 4.3.

HUMAN LEUCOCYTE ANTIGEN (HLA) SYSTEM

Though not a component of immune system, HLA system is described here as it is considered important in the regulation of the immune system. HLA stands for Human Leucocyte Antigens because these antigens were first discovered on leucocytes. The major importance of human histocompatibility antigens of HLA system lies in matching donor and recipient for organ transplant.

Out of the various genes for histocompatibility antigens, most of the transplantation antigens are located on a portion of *chromosome 6* of all nucleated cells of the body and platelets. This is called *major histocompatibility complex (MHC) or HLA complex*. These genes occupy four regions or loci—A, B, C and D, on the short (p) arm of chromosome 6 and exhibit marked variation in allelic genes at each locus. Therefore, the product of HLA antigens is highly polymorphic. The letter w in

TABLE 4.2: Effector Lymphocyte Subpopulations.

SUBPOPULATION	FUNCTIONS
1. *T_{DTH} (CD4+, helper T) cells*	60% peripheral T cells Release lymphokines Activate macrophages Mediate delayed hypersensitivity reactions
2. *T_{CTL} (CD8+, cytotoxic suppressor T) cells*	30% peripheral T cells Specific cell-mediated cytotoxicity
3. *NK (CD11, 45, 46, 57) cells*	React without previous sensitisation React and lyse the target cells e.g. tumour cells, virus-infected cells and some normal cells
4. *K (Fc Ig receptor) cells*	Antibody-dependent cell-mediated cytotoxicity e.g. autoimmune thyroiditis
5. *TIL (activated NK) cells*	Lysis of cells more effective than NK cells

CD= Cluster of differentiation; CTL= cytotoxic T lymphocytes; NK= natural killer; K= killer; TIL= tumour infiltrating lymphocytes; Fc Ig= crystalisable fragment of immunoglobulin.

TABLE 4.3: Immune Effector Mechanisms.

INFECTIVE AGENT	IMMUNE DEFENSE MECHANISM	ORIGIN
1. *Bacteria*	Circulating antibodies (neutralising, cytotoxic, atopic or anaphylactic, immune-complex type)	Humoral
2. *Viruses*	Cellular (delayed hypersensitivity) Antibodies	Sensitised T cells Humoral
3. *Mycobacteria*	Granulomatous (delayed) Antibodies	Sensitised T cells Ab against poorly degradable Ag
4. *Protozoa*	Cellular (delayed) Antibodies	Sensitised T cells Humoral
5. *Worms*	Anaphylactic Granulomatous (delayed)	Humoral Sensitised T cells
6. *Fungi*	Granulomatous (delayed)	Sensitised T cells

some of the genes (e.g. D_{w3}, C_{w4}, B_{w15} etc) refers to the numbers allocated to them at international workshops.

Depending upon the characteristics of MHC, they have been divided into 3 classes (Fig. 4.2):

- **Class I MHC antigens** have loci as HLA-A, HLA-B and HLA-C. CD8 lymphocytes carry receptors for class I MHC and are used to identify the cells having them.
- **Class II MHC antigens** have single locus as HLA-D. These antigens have further 3 loci, DR, DQ and DP.

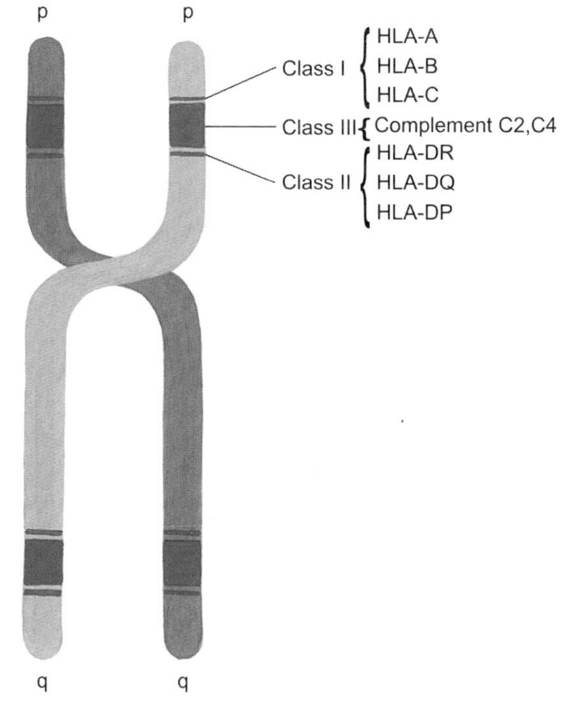

FIGURE 4.2

HLA system and loci on chromosome 6.

Class II MHC is identified by B cells and CD4 or T helper cells.

- **Class III MHC antigens** are some components of the complement system (C2 and C4) coded on HLA complex but are not associated with HLA expression and are not used in antigen identification.

In view of high polymorphism of class I and class II genes, they have a number of alleles on loci numbered serially like HLA-A 1, HLA-A 2, HLA-A 3 etc.

ROLE OF HLA COMPLEX. The HLA complex is significant in a number of ways:

1. Organ transplantation. Historically, the major importance of HLA system is in matching donor and recipient for tissue transplantation. The recipient's immune system can recognise the histocompatibility antigens on the donor organ and accordingly accept it or reject it. Both humoral as well as cell-mediated immune responses are involved in case of genetically non-identical transplants.

2. Regulation of the immune system. Class I and II histocompatibility antigens play a role in regulating both cellular and humoral immunity:

- *Class I Ags* regulate the function of cytotoxic T cells (CD8+ subpopulation) e.g. in virus infections.
- *Class II Ags* regulate the function of helper T cells (CD4+ subpopulation).

3. Association of diseases with HLA. An increasing number of diseases has been found to have association with some specific histocompatibility antigens. These disorders include the following:

i) *Inflammatory* such as ankylosing spondylitis.

ii) *Autoimmune disorders* such as rheumatoid arthritis, insulin-dependent diabetes mellitus.

iii) *Inherited disorders of metabolism* like idiopathic haemochromatosis.

The exact mechanism of such associations between the disease and HLA type is not clearly understood.

DISEASES OF IMMUNITY

The word *immunity* is synonymous with *resistance* meaning protection from particular diseases or injuries, whereas the term *hypersensitivity* is interchangeable with *allergy* meaning a state of exaggerated or altered immune response to a given agent. The diseases of the immune system are broadly classified into the following 4 groups:

I. Immunodeficiency disorders characterised by deficient cellular and/or humoral immune functions. This group is comprised by a list of *primary and secondary immunodeficiency diseases* including the dreaded *acquired immunodeficiency syndrome (AIDS).*

II. Hypersensitivity reactions characterised by hyperfunction of the immune system and cover the various mechanisms of *immunologic tissue injury.*

III. Autoimmune diseases occur when the immune system fails to recognise 'self' from 'non-self'. A growing number of *autoimmune and collagen diseases* are included in this group.

IV. Possible immune disorders in which the immunologic mechanisms are suspected in their etiopathogenesis. Classical example of this group is *amyloidosis* discussed later in this chapter.

In addition to the above groups of immunologic disorders, an account of *transplantation rejection* is appended at the end of discussion below.

IMMUNODEFICIENCY DISEASES

Failure or deficiency of immune system, which normally plays a protective role against infections, manifests by occurrence of repeated infections in an individual having immunodeficiency diseases.

Traditionally, immunodeficiency diseases are classified into 2 types:

A. *Primary immunodeficiencies* are usually the result of genetic or developmental abnormality of the immune system.

B. *Secondary immunodeficiencies* arise from acquired suppression of the immune system.

Since the first description of primary immunodeficiency by Bruton in 1952, an increasing number of primary and secondary immunodeficiency syndromes are being added to the list, the latest addition being the acquired immunodeficiency syndrome (AIDS) in 1981.

A list of most immunodeficiency diseases with the possible defect in the immune system is given in Table 4.4, while an account of AIDS is given below.

ACQUIRED IMMUNODEFICIENCY SYNDROME (AIDS)

Since the initial recognition of AIDS in the United States in 1981, tremendous advances have taken place in the understanding of this dreaded disease in the last decade as regards its epidemiology, etiology, immunology, pathogenesis, clinical features and morphologic changes in various tissues and organs of the body. But efforts at finding its definite treatment and a vaccine have not yielded success so far, and thus the prognosis remains grim. Hence the global attention is presently focussed on preventive measures.

EPIDEMIOLOGY. Although AIDS was first described in the US, the disease has now attained pandemic proportions involving all continents. Presently, developing countries comprise majority of cases and Africa alone constitutes 50% of all positive cases globally. According to a rough estimate, 1 in every 100 sexually active adults worldwide is infected with HIV. Half of all serologically positive cases are in women while children comprise 5% of all cases. According to the WHO data, the last decade has shown an alarming rise in incidence of AIDS cases in South-East Asia including Thailand, Indonesia and Indian sub-continent. However, giving exact figures of cases is pointless since the numbers are increasing by millions and all such data will be outdated with every passing year. In India, epicentre of the epidemic lies in the states of Maharashtra and Tamil Nadu which together comprise about 50% of all HIV positive cases (mostly contracted sexually), while North-East state of Manipur accounts for 8% of all cases (mostly among intravenous drug abusers).

ETIOLOGIC AGENT. AIDS is caused by a retrovirus called human immunodeficiency virus (HIV) which is a type of human T cell leukaemia-lymphoma virus (HTLV).

HIV resembles other HTLVs in shape and size and both have *tropism for CD4 molecules* present on subpopulation of T cells which are the particular targets of attack by HIV. However, *HIV differs from HTLV in being cytolytic for T cells causing immunodeficiency (cytopathic virus) while HTLV may transform the target cells into T cell leukaemia (transforming virus)* (Chapter 8). Two forms of HIV have been described, HIV1 being the etiologic agent for AIDS in the US and Central Africa, while HIV2 causes a similar disease in West Africa and parts of India.

HIV-I virion or virus particle is spherical in shape and 100-140 nm in size (Fig. 4.3):

TABLE 4.4: Immunodeficiency Diseases.

DISEASE	DEFECT
A. PRIMARY IMMUNODEFICIENCY DISEASES	
1. Severe combined immunodeficiency diseases (Combined deficiency of T cells, B cells and lgs):	
(i) Reticular dysgenesis	Failure to develop primitive marrow reticular cells
(ii) Thymic alymphoplasia	No lymphoid stem cells
(iii) Agammaglobulinaemia (Swiss type)	No lymphoid stem cells
(iv) Wiscott-Aldrich syndrome	Cell membrane defect of haematopoietic stem cells; associated features are thrombocytopenia and eczema
(v) Ataxia telangiectasia	Defective T cell maturation
2. T cell defect:	
DiGeorge's syndrome (thymic hypoplasia)	Epithelial component of thymus fails to develop
3. B cell defects (antibody deficiency diseases):	
(i) Bruton's X-linked agammaglobulinaemia	Defective differentiation from pre-B to B cells
(ii) Autosomal recessive agammaglobulinaemia	Defective differentiation from pre-B to B cells
(iii) IgA deficiency	Defective maturation of IgA synthesising B cells
(iv) Selective deficiency of other lg types	Defective differentiation from B cells to specific Ig-synthesising plasma cells
(v) Immune deficiency with thymoma	Defective pre-B cell maturation
4. Common variable immunodeficiencies (characterised by decreased lgs and serum antibodies and variable CMI):	
(i) With predominant B cell defect	Defective differentiation of pre-B to mature B cells
(ii) With predominant T cell defect	
(a) Deficient T helper cells	Defective differentiation of thymocytes to T helper cells
(b) Presence of activated T suppressor cells	T cell disorder of unknown origin
(iii) With autoantibodies to B and T cells	Unknown differentiation defect
B. SECONDARY IMMUNODEFICIENCY DISEASES	
1. Infections	AIDS (HIV virus); other viral, bacterial and protozoal infections
2. Cancer	Chemotherapy by antimetabolites; irradiation
3. Lymphoid neoplasms (lymphomas, lymphoid leukaemias)	Deficient T and B cell functions
4. Malnutrition	Protein deficiency
5. Sarcoidosis	Impaired T cell function
6. Autoimmune diseases	Administration of high dose of steroids toxic to lymphocytes
7. Transplant cases	Immunosuppressive therapy

- It contains a *core* having *core proteins*, chiefly p24 and p18, two strands of genomic RNA and the enzyme, reverse transcriptase.
- The core is covered by a *double layer of lipid membrane* derived from the outer membrane of the infected host cell during budding process of virus. The membrane is studded with *2 viral glycoproteins, gp120 and gp41,* in the positions shown.

Besides various other genes, **three important genes** which code for the respective components of virion are: *gag* for core proteins, *pol* for reverse transcriptase, and *env* for the envelope proteins. These genes and viral components act as markers for the laboratory diagnosis of HIV infection. Besides, there is *tat* gene (transactivator) for viral functions such as amplification of viral genes, viral budding and replication.

ROUTES OF TRANSMISSION. Transmission of HIV infection occurs by one of following three routes:

1. Sexual contact. Sexual contact in the main mode of spread and constitutes 75% of all cases of HIV transmission. Most cases of AIDS in the industrialised world like in the US occur in *homosexual* or *bisexual males* while *heterosexual promiscuity* seems to be the dominant mode of HIV infection in Africa and Asia. Other sexually transmitted diseases (STDs) may act as cofactors for spread of HIV, in particular gonorrhoea and chlamydia. Transmission from male-to-male and male-to-female is more potent route than that from female-to-male.

2. Parenteral transmission. This mode of transmission is the next largest group (25%) and occurs in 3 groups of high risk populations:

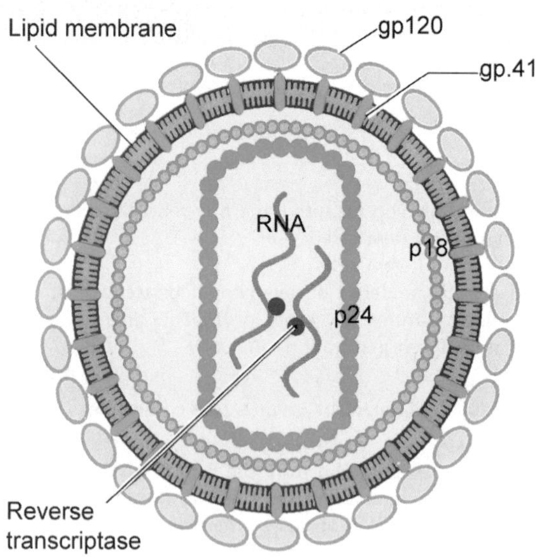

FIGURE 4.3

Schematic representation of HIV virion or virus particle. The particle has core containing proteins, p24 and p18, two strands of viral RNA, and enzyme reverse transcriptase. Bilayer lipid membrane is studded with 2 viral glycoproteins, gp120 and gp41, in the positions shown.

i) *Intravenous drug abusers* by sharing needles, syringes etc comprise a large group in the US.

ii) *Haemophiliacs* who have received large amounts of factor VIII concentrates from pooled blood components from multiple donors.

iii) *Recipients of blood and blood products* who have received multiple transfusions of whole blood or components like platelets and plasma.

3. Perinatal transmission. HIV infection occurs from infected mother to the newborn during pregnancy *transplacentally*, or in immediate post-partum period *through contamination* with maternal blood, infected amniotic fluid or breast milk.

In about 6% of cases, the risk factor cannot be determined.

Besides blood, *HIV has been isolated from a number of body fluids and tissues* such as: semen, vaginal secretions, cervical secretions, breast milk, CSF, synovial, pleural, peritoneal, pericardial and amniotic fluid.

In order to allay the fear in the public regarding spread of HIV infection, *AIDS cannot be transmitted by* casual non-sexual contact like shaking hands, hugging, sharing household facilities like beds, toilets, utensils etc.

HIV contaminated waste products can be *sterilised and disinfected by* most of the chemical germicides used in laboratories at a much lower concentration. These are: sodium hypochlorite (liquid chlorine bleach), formaldehyde (5%), ethanol (70%), glutaraldehyde (2%), β-propionolactone. HIV is also heat-sensitive and can be inactivated at 56°C for 30 min.

PATHOGENESIS. The pathogenesis of HIV infection is largely related to the *depletion of CD4+ T cells (helper T cells) resulting in profound immunosuppression.*

The sequence of events shown in Fig. 4.4 is outlined below:

1. Selective tropism and internalisation. HIV on entering the body via any route described above has *selective tropism for CD4+* cells and certain population of monocytes and macrophages. In this way, envelope glycoprotein gp120 of the virion binds to CD molecule and the virus particle is internalised into CD4+ cell.

2. Uncoating and proviral DNA integration. The virus is then uncoated and its genomic RNA is transcribed to proviral DNA by enzyme reverse transcriptase. The proviral DNA so formed may initially remain *unintegrated* in the affected cell and later gets *integrated* into the T cell genome.

3. Budding and syncytia formation. On activation, the infected CD4+ T cells bear budding viral particles due to multiplication which further attract more number of CD4+ T cells resulting in syncytia formation.

4. Cytopathic effects. In an inactive T cell, the infection may remain in *latent phase* for a long time, accounting for the long incubation period. An antigenically-activated and infected T cell develops into *cytopathic phase*. How cytopathic effects on T cells are produced is not quite clear. However, there is evidence to suggest that these effects occur due to interaction of CD4 molecule of T cell with gp120 of HIV viral envelope. The cytopathic effects on T cells are two fold: *firstly*, there is quantitative depletion of CD4+ T cells due to direct cytolysis; and *secondly*, there is qualitative defect in the form of inability of these T cells to respond to antigens.

The CD4 molecule-gp120 interaction also leads to *infection with other viruses* like CMV, hepatitis, herpes simplex etc.

5. Effects on monocytes and macrophages. Besides the cytopathic effects on CD4+ T cells, CD4 molecule-bearing subpopulations of monocytes and macrophages (e.g., dendritic cells, microglial cells) are also attacked by HIV but without causing cytopathic effects on these cells. These HIV-infected cells, thus, may act as a reservoir of HIV infection as well as may be the source of infection to other organs like the nervous system.

6. HIV infection of nervous system. Out of non-lymphoid organ involvement, HIV infection of nervous

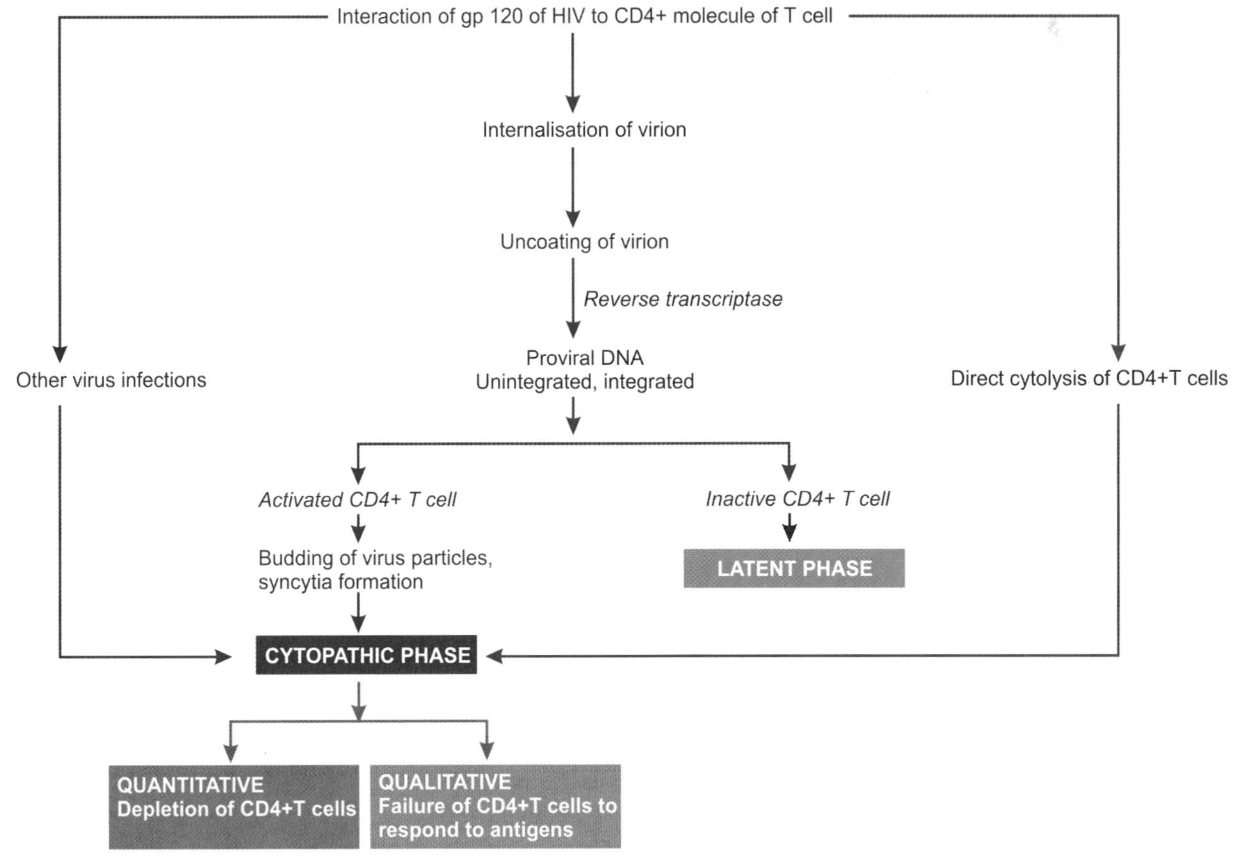

FIGURE 4.4

Sequence of events in the pathogenesis of HIV infection.

system is the most serious and can occur as a result of the following:

i) Infection carried to the microglia of the nervous system by *HIV infected CD4+ monocyte-macrophage subpopulation or endothelial cells.*

ii) *Direct infection* of astrocytes and oligodendrocytes.

iii) Neurons are not invaded by HIV but are affected due to gp120 and by release of *cytokines* by macrophages.

75-90% of AIDS patients may demonstrate some form of neurological involvement at autopsy. Various syndromes which may appear as neurological manifestations and sometimes presenting features of AIDS include the following (Chapter 28):

- acute aseptic meningitis;
- subacute encephalitis;
- vacuolar myelopathy; and
- peripheral neuropathy.

7. B cell dysfunctions. Besides affecting CD4+ cells, gpl20 of HIV envelope also produces derangements of B cell functions resulting in decreased immunoglobulin production, hypergammaglobulinaemia, polyclonal activation, circulating immune complexes.

A summary of major abnormalities in the immune system in AIDS is given in Table 4.5.

NATURAL HISTORY. As per the WHO, AIDS is defined as the existence of at least two major signs associated with at least one minor sign, in the absence of known secondary causes of immunosuppression.

- *Major signs* include:

i) weight loss of > 10% of body weight;

ii) chronic diarrhoea of > 1 month's duration; and

iii) prolonged fever (intermittent or continuous) for > 1 month.

- *Minor signs* are:

i) recurrent oropharyngeal candidiasis;

ii) persistent generalised lymphadenopathy;

iii) persistent cough for > one month;

iv) generalised pruritic dermatitis;

v) recurrent herpes zoster; and

vi) progressive disseminated herpes simplex infection.

TABLE 4.5: Major Abnormalities in Immune System in AIDS.

1. **T CELL ABNORMALITIES**
   - (i) Lymphopenia with depletion of CD4+ T cells; reversal of CD4 to CD8 cell ratio
   - (ii) Susceptibility to opportunistic infections
   - (iii) Susceptibility to neoplasms
   - (iv) Decreased delayed type hypersensitivity
   - (v) Decreased proliferative response to mitogens and soluble antigens
   - (vi) Decreased specific cytotoxicity
   - (vii) Decreased production of interleukin 2
2. **B CELL ABNORMALITIES**
   - (i) Decreased Ig production
   - (ii) Polyclonal activation
   - (iii) Hypergammaglobulinaemia
   - (iv) Circulating immune complexes
3. **ABNORMALITIES OF MONOCYTE-MACROPHAGE CELL LINE**
   - (i) Decreased chemotaxis
   - (ii) Decreased cytotoxicity
4. **NK CELL ABNORMALITIES**

   Decreased cytotoxicity

The following 3 phases are recognised (Table 4.6):

1. Acute HIV syndrome (3-12 weeks). Entry of HIV into the body of an immunocompetent host is heralded by the following sequence of events:

i) High levels of plasma *viraemia* due to replication of the virus.

ii) Virus-specific immune response as seen by *seroconversion* after 3-6 weeks of initial exposure to HIV.

iii) Initially, sudden marked reduction in *CD4+ T cells* (helper T cells) followed by return to normal levels.

iv) Rise in *CD8+ T cells* (HIV-specific cytotoxic T cells).

v) Appearance of self-limited non-specific *acute viral illness* (flu-like or infectious mononucleosis-like) in 50-70% of adults within 3-6 weeks of initial infection (CDC group 1). Manifestations include: sore throat, fever, myalgia, skin rash, and sometimes aseptic meningitis. These symptoms resolve spontaneously in 2-3 weeks.

2. Middle chronic phase (10-12 years). The initial acute seroconversion illness is followed by a phase of competition between HIV and the host immune response as under:

i) *Viraemia* due to viral replication in the lymphoid tissue continues which is initially not as high but with passage of time viral load increases due to crumbling host defenses.

ii) Chronic stage depending upon host immune system may continue as long as *10 years*.

iii) *CD 4+ T cells* continue to proliferate but net result is moderate fall in CD4+ T cell counts.

iv) Cytotoxic CD8+ T cell count remains high.

v) Clinically, it is a stage of *latency*. The patient may be asymptomatic (CDC group II), or may develop mild constitutional symptoms and persistent generalised lymphadenopathy (CDC group III).

3. Final crisis phase. This phase is characterised by profound immunosuppression and onset of full-blown AIDS and has the following features:

i) Marked increase in *viraemia*.

ii) The time period between HIV infection developing into chronic phase followed by full-blown AIDS may last *7-10 years and culminates in death.*

iii) *CD 4+ T cells* are markedly reduced (below 200 per μl).

iv) *Clinically*, the features of the final phase are categorised into following 5 subgroups (CDC group IV) (Fig. 4.5):

Subgroup A: *Constitutional disease* characterised by fever of more than one month duration, weight loss of more than 10% of body weight, and chronic diarrhoea lasting more than one month.

TABLE 4.6: Natural History of HIV Infection.

PHASE	EARLY, ACUTE	MIDDLE, CHRONIC	FINAL, CRISIS
Period after infection	3-6 weeks	10 to 12 years	Any period up to death
CDC category	Group I: Acute HIV syndrome	Group II: Asymptomatic infection Group III: PGL	Group IV: 5 Subgroups: A:Constitutional symptoms B: Neurologic disease C:Secondary infection D:Secondary neoplasms E: Other conditions
Plasma viraemia	High	Moderate	High
CD4 counts	Suddenly reduced	Moderate loss	Severely reduced (< 200/μl)

(CDC = Centres for Disease Control, Atlanta, USA; PGL = Persistent generalised lymphadenopathy).

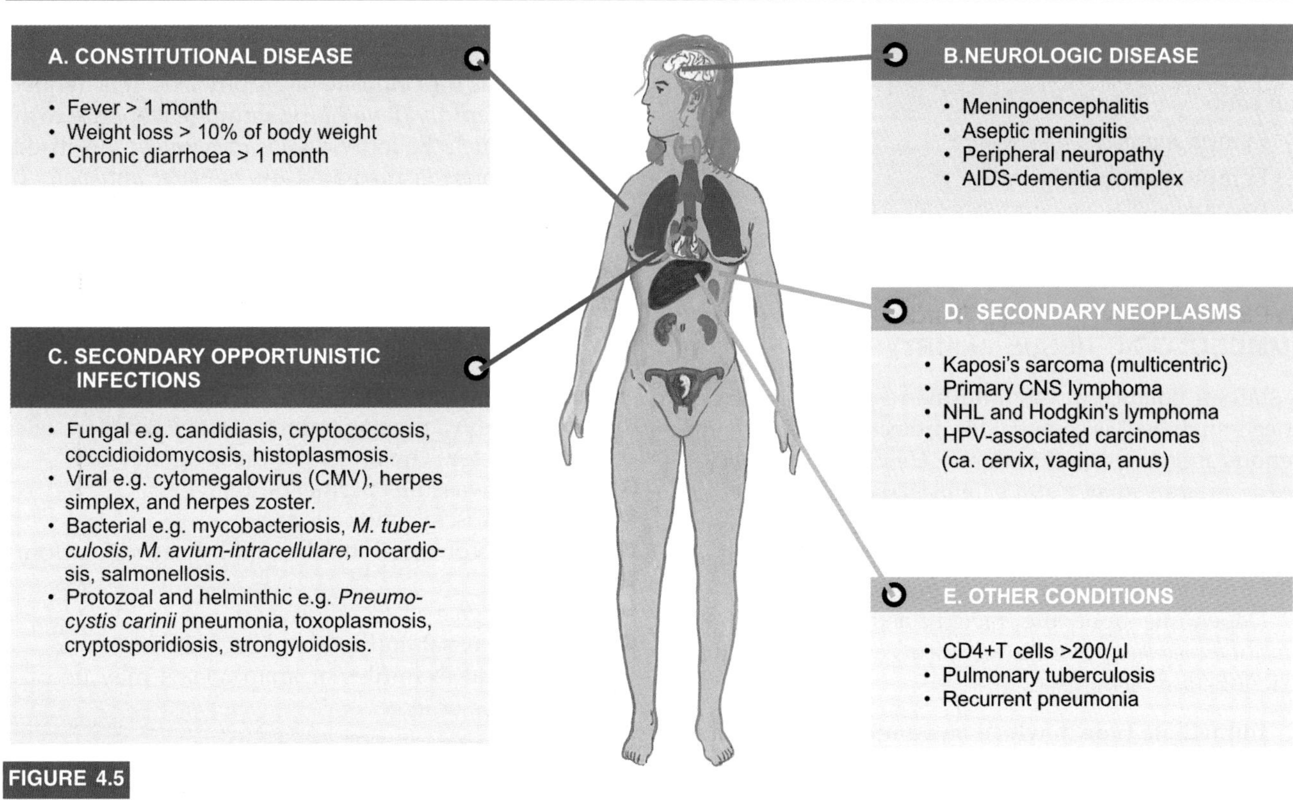

A. CONSTITUTIONAL DISEASE
• Fever > 1 month
• Weight loss > 10% of body weight
• Chronic diarrhoea > 1 month
B.NEUROLOGIC DISEASE
• Meningoencephalitis
• Aseptic meningitis
• Peripheral neuropathy
• AIDS-dementia complex
C. SECONDARY OPPORTUNISTIC INFECTIONS
• Fungal e.g. candidiasis, cryptococcosis, coccidioidomycosis, histoplasmosis.
• Viral e.g. cytomegalovirus (CMV), herpes simplex, and herpes zoster.
• Bacterial e.g. mycobacteriosis, M. tuberculosis, M. avium-intracellulare, nocardiosis, salmonellosis.
• Protozoal and helminthic e.g. Pneumocystis carinii pneumonia, toxoplasmosis, cryptosporidiosis, strongyloidosis.
D. SECONDARY NEOPLASMS
• Kaposi's sarcoma (multicentric)
• Primary CNS lymphoma
• NHL and Hodgkin's lymphoma
• HPV-associated carcinomas (ca. cervix, vagina, anus)
E. OTHER CONDITIONS
• CD4+T cells >200/μl
• Pulmonary tuberculosis
• Recurrent pneumonia

FIGURE 4.5

Major clinical manifestations of full-blown AIDS.

Subgroup B: *Neurologic disease* present in majority of cases and include viral meningoencephalitis, aseptic meningitis, peripheral neuropathy, AIDS-dementia complex.

Subgroup C: *Secondary opportunistic infections* such as fungal, viral, bacterial and parasitic.

Subgroup D: *Secondary neoplasms* such as Kaposi's sarcoma (Chapter 8), Non-Hodgkin's lymphoma (Burkitt's, immunoblastic), Hodgkin's lymphoma, primary CNS lymphoma.

Subgroup E: This recent subgroup includes < 200 CD 4+ T lymphocytes/μl, pulmonary tuberculosis and recurrent pneumonia.

The average survival after the onset of full-blown AIDS is 18-24 months.

PATHOLOGIC CHANGES. The morphological changes in AIDS are non-specific and variable depending upon the stage of the disease. In general, the autopsy findings include the following (Fig. 4.5):

1. *Lymphoid tissues* (lymph nodes, spleen, thymus and bone marrow) show predominant changes *viz.:*

- *In early stage*, there is B cell hyperplasia in the form of nonspecific follicular hyperplasia and plasmacytosis in the medulla of the lymph nodes.
- *The full blown AIDS* is characterised by universal lymphoid cell depletion, which, due to immunosuppression, may reveal evidence of opportunistic infections. Malignant lymphomas and other T cell neoplasms may occur.

2. Widespread opportunistic infections.
3. AIDS-associated cancers e.g. HPV-associated cancers such as carcinoma of uterine cervix, vagina, anus.
4. Neurological manifestations includes AIDS-associated dementia.
5. AIDS associated nephropathy characterised by focal segmental glomerulosclerosis.

LABORATORY DIAGNOSIS OF AIDS. The investigations of a suspected case of AIDS include *initial testing for antibodies against HIV by ELISA and confirmation by Western blot or immunofluorescence test.*

The various laboratory tests currently used in research and clinical laboratories are categorised into 2 groups:

1. Specific tests:

i) Serologic tests by ELISA, Western blot and immunofluorescence test

ii) Antigen detection tests using envelope and core proteins of HIV by recombinant DNA techniques

iii) Virus isolation and culture in neoplastic T cell line

iv) Polymerase chain reaction (PCR).

2. **Indirect tests:**

i) CD4 and CD8 cell counts; reversal of CD4 to CD8 cell ratio

ii) Lymphopenia

iii) Lymph node biopsy

iv) Platelet count revealing thrombocytopenia

v) Increased β-2 microglobulin levels.

HYPERSENSITIVITY REACTIONS (IMMUNOLOGIC TISSUE INJURY)

A state of balance in the immune responses (humoral or cell-mediated) is essential for protection against endogenous and exogenous antigens. *Hypersensitivity is defined as a state of exaggerated immune response to an antigen.* The lesions of hypersensitivity (immunologic tissue injury) are produced due to interaction between antigen and product of the immune response.

Depending upon the *rapidity* and *duration* of the immune response, two distinct forms of hypersensitivity reactions are recognised:

1. **Immediate type** in which on administration of antigen, the reaction occurs immediately (within seconds to minutes). Immune response in this type is mediated largely by *humoral antibodies*. Immediate type of hypersensitivity is further of 3 types—*type I, II and III.*

2. **Delayed type** in which the reaction is slower in onset and develops within 24-48 hours and the effect is prolonged. It is mainly mediated by *cellular response. Type IV reaction* is the delayed hypersensitivity reaction.

The mechanisms and examples of immunologic tissue injury by the 4 types of hypersensitivity reactions are summarised in Table 4.7.

Type I: Anaphylactic, Atopic Reaction

Anaphylaxis is the opposite of prophylaxis. It is defined as a state of rapidly developing immune response to an antigen to which the individual is previously sensitised.

The response is mediated by *humoral antibodies of IgE type or reagin antibodies.* IgE antibodies sensitise basophils of peripheral blood or mast cells of tissues leading to release of pharmacologically-active substances called *anaphylactic mediators*. These substances are histamine, serotonin, vasoactive intestinal peptide (VIP), chemotactic factors of anaphylaxis for neutrophils and eosinophils, leukotrienes B_4 and D_4, prostaglandins (thromboxane A_2, prostaglandin D_2 and E_2) and platelet activating factor. The effects of these agents are:

- increased vascular permeability;
- smooth muscle contraction;
- early vasoconstriction followed by vasodilatation;
- shock;
- increased gastric secretion; and
- increased nasal and lacrimal secretions.

The clinical examples of anaphylaxis may be of 2 types: *systemic or local.*

1. Examples of **systemic anaphylaxis** are:

i) administration of antisera e.g. anti-tetanus serum (ATS);

ii) administration of drugs e.g. penicillin; and

iii) sting by wasp or bee.

The clinical features of systemic anaphylaxis include itching, erythema, contraction of respiratory bronchioles, diarrhoea, pulmonary oedema, pulmonary haemorrhage, shock and death.

2. Examples of **local anaphylaxis** are:

i) hay fever (seasonal allergic rhinitis) due to pollen sensitisation of conjunctiva and nasal passages;

TABLE 4.7: Mechanisms of Immunologic Tissue Injury.

TYPE	MECHANISM	EXAMPLES
Type I (Anaphylactic, atopic)	Humoral Abs of IgE type → basophils/mast cells sensitised → release of anaphylactic mediators	i. Systemic anaphylaxis (administration of antisera and drugs, stings) ii. Local anaphylaxis (hay fever, bronchial asthma, food allergy, cutaneous, angioedema)
Type II (Cytotoxic)	i. Cytotoxic auto- and iso-antibodies to blood cells ii. Cytotoxic Abs to tissue components iii. Ab-dependent cell-mediated cytotoxicity (ADCC)	i. Autoimmune haemolytic anaemia, transfusion reactions, erythroblastosis foetalis, ITP, leucopenia, drug-induced ii. Myasthenia gravis, male sterility iii. Tumour cells, parasites
Type III (Immune-complex)	i. Local (Arthus reaction) Ag-Ab complexes ii. Systemic (circulating) Ag-Ab complexes or serum sickness	i. Injection of ATS, farmer's lung ii. Glomerulonephritis, collagen diseases, Goodpasture's syndrome, arthritis, uveitis, skin diseases
Type IV (Cell-mediated)	i. Classical delayed hypersensitivity mediated by CD4 + T cells ii. T cell mediated cytotoxicity by CD8+ T cells	i. Tuberculin reaction, tuberculosis, tuberculoid leprosy, typhoid, contact dermatitis ii. Virus-infected cells, tumour cells, transplant rejection

Chapter Four

ii) bronchial asthma due to allergy to inhaled allergens like house dust;

iii) food allergy to ingested allergens like fish, cow's milk etc;

iv) cutaneous anaphylaxis due to contact of antigen with skin characterised by urticaria, wheal and flare; and

v) angioedema, an autosomal dominant inherited disorder characterised by laryngeal oedema, oedema of eyelids, lips, tongue and trunk.

Local anaphylaxis is common, affecting about 10% of population. About 50% of these conditions are familial with genetic predisposition and therefore also called *atopic reactions*.

Type II: Cytotoxic Reaction

Cytotoxic reactions are defined as those reactions which cause injury to the cell by combining humoral antibodies with cell surface antigens; blood cells being affected more commonly.

Three types of mechanisms are involved in mediating cytotoxic reactions:

1. Cytotoxic antibodies to blood cells. This mechanism involves direct cytolysis of blood cells (red blood cells, leucocytes and platelets) by combining the cell surface antigen with lgG or lgM class antibodies. In the process, complement system is activated resulting in injury to the cell membrane. The cell surface is made susceptible to phagocytosis due to coating or opsonisation from serum factors or opsonins.

Examples of cytotoxicity by this mechanism are as under:

i) *Autoimmune haemolytic anaemia* in which the red cell injury is brought about by autoantibodies reacting with antigens present on red cell surface. Antiglobulin test (direct Coombs' test) is employed to detect the antibody on red cell surface (Chapter 13).

ii) *Transfusion reactions* due to incompatible or mismatched blood transfusion.

iii) Haemolytic disease of the newborn (*erythroblastosis foetalis*) in which the foetal red cells are destroyed by maternal isoantibodies crossing the placenta.

iv) *Idiopathic thrombocytopenic purpura* (ITP) is the destruction of platelets by autoantibodies reacting with surface components of normal plaletets.

v) *Leucopenia with agranulocytosis* may be caused by autoantibodies to leucocytes causing their destruction.

vi) *Drug-induced cytotoxic antibodies* are formed in response to administration of certain drugs like penicillin, methyl dopa, rifampicin etc. The drugs or their metabolites act as haptens binding to the surface of blood cells to which the antibodies combine, bringing about destruction of cells.

2. Cytotoxic antibodies to tissue components. Cellular injury may be brought about by autoantibodies reacting with some components of tissue cells in certain diseases.

Examples are as under:

i) In *Graves' disease* (primary hyperthyroidism), thyroid autoantibody is formed which reacts with the TSH receptor to cause hyperfunction and proliferation.

ii) In *myasthenia gravis*, antibody to acetylcholine receptors of skeletal muscle is formed which blocks the neuromuscular transmission at the motor end-plate, resulting in muscle weakness.

iii) In *male sterility*, antisperm antibody is formed which reacts with spermatozoa and causes impaired motility as well as cellular injury.

More recently, however, Graves' disease has been categorised separately under *type V hypersensitivity reaction (stimulatory type)*. TSH receptor on thyroid cell membrane reacts with long-acting thyroid stimulating (LATS) autoantibody which, in turn, brings about chemical overactivity (stimulatory type) of thyroid gland (i.e. hyperthyroidism).

3. Antibody-dependent cell-mediated cytotoxicity (ADCC). Cytotoxicity by this mechanism is mediated by leucocytes like monocytes, neutrophils, eosinophils and NK cells. The antibodies involved are mostly IgG class. The cellular injury occurs by lysis of antibody-coated target cells through Fc receptors on leucocytes.

The *examples* of target cells killed by this mechanism are tumour cells, parasites etc.

Type III: Immune Complex Reaction

Type III reactions result from formation of immune complexes by direct antigen-antibody (Ag-Ab) combination as a result of which the complement system gets activated causing cell injury.

Two types of antigens can cause immune complex-mediated tissue injury:

1. *Exogenous antigens* such as infectious agents (bacteria, viruses, fungi, parasites); certain drugs and chemicals.

2. *Endogenous antigens* such as blood components (immunoglobulins, tumour antigens) and antigens in cells and tissues (nuclear antigens in SLE).

Depending upon the distribution and location of antigens, type III reactions are of 2 types:

1. Local: Arthus reaction. It is a localised inflammatory reaction, usually an immune complex vasculitis of skin, in an individual with circulating antibody. Large immune complexes are formed due to excess of antibodies which precipitate locally in the vessel wall causing fibrinoid necrosis.

Examples of local immune complex disease are:

i) injection of antitetanus serum; and

ii) farmer's lung in which there is allergic alveolitis in response to bacterial antigen from mouldy hay.

2. Systemic: Circulating immune complex disease or serum sickness. The steps involved in cell injury by circulating immune complexes are as follows:

i) After the antigen is introduced into the circulation, it initiates formation of antibodies which react with antigen to form circulating Ag-Ab complexes.

ii) These complexes are then deposited at different tissue sites containing basement membrane exposed to circulating blood e.g. basement membrane of renal glomeruli, lungs, choroid plexus of brain, uveal tract of eye, synovial membrane of joints.

iii) Following deposition of Ag-Ab complexes in the tissues, there is acute inflammatory reaction and activation of the complement system with elaboration of biologically-active compounds such as chemotactic factors, vasoactive amines and anaphylatoxins. The immune complexes are phagocytosed by leucocytes drawn at the site by chemotactic factors.

Examples of circulating immune complex diseases are as under:

i) Various forms of glomerulonephritis e.g. acute glomerulonephritis, membranous glomerulonephritis, glomerulonephritis in SLE (lupus nephritis).

ii) Collagen diseases e.g. SLE, polyarteritis nodosa, scleroderma, rheumatoid arthritis, Sjögren's syndrome, dermatomyositis.

iii) Goodpasture's syndrome caused by an antibody, common to pulmonary as well as renal basement membrane, and produces glomerulonephritis associated with pulmonary haemorrhage.

iv) Arthritis occurring transiently during infections.

v) Uveitis.

vi) Skin diseases.

Type IV: Cell-Mediated Reaction

This type of hypersensitivity is mediated by specifically-sensitised T lymphocytes produced in the cell-mediated immune response.

Cell-mediated reactions are of 2 main types:

1. Classical delayed hypersensitivity. This is mediated by specifically sensitised CD4+ T cell subpopulation on contact with antigen. These cells possess surface receptors which bind to the antigen, resulting in cell injury characterised by slowly developing inflammatory response and hence the name delayed hypersensitivity.

The classical *example* of delayed hypersensitivity is the tuberculin reaction. On intradermal injection of tuberculoprotein (PPD), an unsensitised individual develops no response (tuberculin negative). On the other hand, a person who has developed cell-mediated immunity to tuberculoprotein as a result of BCG immunisation or has been exposed to tuberculous infection develops typical delayed inflammatory reaction, reaching its peak in 48 hours (tuberculin positive), after which it subsides slowly. *Microscopically,* mononuclear inflammatory cells in and around small blood vessels and oedema are seen.

Other examples of delayed hypersensitivity response are tuberculosis, tuberculoid leprosy, typhoid fever, and contact dermatitis due to allergic response to a number of chemicals and allergens.

2. T cell-mediated cytotoxicity. CD8+ subpopulation of T lymphocytes are the cytotoxic T cells (T_{CTL}) and are generated in response to antigens like virus-infected cells, tumour cells and incompatible transplanted tissue or cells.

AUTOIMMUNE DISEASES

Autoimmunity is a state in which the body's immune system fails to distinguish between 'self' and 'non-self' and reacts by formation of autoantibodies against one's own tissue antigens. In other words, there is loss of tolerance to one's own tissues; *autoimmunity is the opposite of immune tolerance.*

Immune tolerance is a normal phenomenon present since foetal life and is defined as the ability of an individual to recognise self tissue and antigens. Normally, the immune system of the body is able to distinguish self from non-self antigens by the following mechanisms:

1. *Clonal elimination.* According to this theory, during embryonic development, T cells maturing in the thymus acquire the ability to distinguish self from non-self. These T cells are then eliminated by apoptosis for the tolerant individual.

2. *Concept of clonal anergy.* According to this mechanism, T lymphocytes which have acquired the ability to distinguish self from non-self are not eliminated but instead become non-responsive and inactive.

3. *Suppressor T cells.* According to this mechanism, the tolerance is achieved by a population of specific suppressor T cells which do not allow the antigen-responsive cells to proliferate and differentiate.

PATHOGENESIS OF AUTOIMMUNITY

The mechanisms by which the immune tolerance of the body is broken causes autoimmunity. These mechanisms may be immunological, genetic, and microbial, all of which may be interacting.

1. Immunological factors. Failure of immunological mechanisms of tolerance initiates autoimmunity. These mechanisms are as follows:

i) *Polyclonal activation of B cells.* B cells may be directly activated by stimuli such as infection with micro-organisms and their products leading to bypassing of T cell tolerance.

ii) *Generation of self-reacting B cell clones* may also lead to bypassing of T cell tolerance.

iii) *Decreased T suppressor and increased T helper cell activity.* Loss of T suppressor cell and increase in T helper cell activities may lead to high levels of auto-antibody production by B cells contributing to auto-immunity.

iv) *Fluctuation of anti-idiotype network control* may cause failure of mechanisms of immune tolerance.

v) *Sequestered antigen released from tissues.* 'Self-antigen' which is completely sequestered may act as 'foreign-antigen' if introduced into the circulation later. For example, in trauma to the testis, there is formation of anti-sperm antibodies against spermatozoa; similar is the formation of autoantibodies against lens crystallin.

2. Genetic factors. There is evidence in support of genetic factors in the pathogenesis of autoimmunity as under:

i) There is increased expression of *Class II HLA antigens* on tissues involved in autoimmunity.

ii) There is increased *familial incidence* of some of the autoimmune disorders.

3. Microbial factors. Infection with microorganisms, particularly viruses (e.g. EBV infection), and less often bacteria (e.g. streptococci, *Klebsiella*) and mycoplasma, has been implicated in the pathogenesis of autoimmune diseases. However, a definite evidence in support is lacking.

TYPES AND EXAMPLES OF AUTOIMMUNE DISEASES

Depending upon the type of autoantibody formation, the autoimmune diseases are broadly classified into 2 groups:

1. Organ specific diseases. In these, the autoantibodies formed react specifically against an organ or target tissue component and cause its chronic inflammatory destruction. The tissues affected are endocrine glands (thyroid, pancreatic islets of Langerhans, adrenal cortex), alimentary tract, blood cells and various other tissues and organs.

2. Non-organ specific diseases. These are diseases in which a number of autoantibodies are formed which react with antigens in many tissues and thus cause systemic lesions. The examples of this group are various systemic collagen diseases.

However, a few autoimmune diseases overlap between these two main categories.

Based on these 2 main groups, a comprehensive list of autoimmune (or collagen) diseases is presented in Table 4.8. Some of the systemic autoimmune diseases *(marked with astrix)* are discussed in this chapter while others from both the groups are described later in the relevant chapters.

Systemic Lupus Erythematosus (SLE)

SLE is the classical example of systemic autoimmune or collagen diseases. The disease derives its name *'lupus'* from the Latin word meaning 'wolf' since initially this disease was believed to affect skin only and eat away skin like a wolf. However, now 2 forms of lupus erythematosus are described:

1. Systemic or disseminated form is characterised by acute and chronic inflammatory lesions widely scattered in the body and there is presence of various nuclear and cytoplasmic autoantibodies in the plasma.

2. Discoid form is characterised by chronic and localised skin lesions involving the bridge of nose and adjacent cheeks without any systemic manifestations. Rarely, discoid form may develop into disseminated form.

ETIOLOGY. The exact etiology of SLE is not known. However, autoantibodies against nuclear and cytoplasmic components of the cells are demonstrable in plasma by immunofluorescence tests in almost all cases of SLE. Some of the important *antinuclear antibodies (ANAs)* or antinuclear factors *(ANFs)* against different nuclear antigens are as under:

i) *Antinuclear antibodies* (*ANA*) are the antibodies against common nuclear antigen that includes DNA as well as RNA.

ii) *Antibodies to double-stranded (anti-dsDNA) or single-stranded DNA* (*anti-ssDNA*) is the most specific, present in half the cases of SLE.

iii) *Anti-Smith antigen antibodies* (*anti-SmAg*), in which antibodies appear against Smith antigen which is part of ribonucleoproteins.

TABLE 4.8: Autoimmune Diseases.

NON-ORGAN SPECIFIC (SYSTEMIC)	ORGAN SPECIFIC (LOCALISED)
1. Systemic lupus erythematosus*	1. ENDOCRINE GLANDS
2. Rheumatoid arthritis	(i) Hashimoto's (autoimmune) thyroiditis
3. Scleroderma (Progressive systemic sclerosis)*	(ii) Graves' disease
4. Polymyositis-dermatomyositis*	(iii) Insulin-dependent diabetes mellitus
5. Polyarteritis nodosa (PAN)	(iv) Idiopathic Addison's disease
6. Sjögren's syndrome*	2. ALIMENTARY TRACT
7. Reiter's syndrome*	(i) Autoimmune atrophic gastritis in pernicious anaemia
8. Mixed connective tissue disease*	(ii) Ulcerative colitis
	(iii) Crohn's disease
	3. BLOOD CELLS
	(i) Autoimmune haemolytic anaemia
	(ii) Autoimmune thrombocytopenia
	4. OTHERS
	(i) Myasthenia gravis
	(ii) Autoimmune orchitis
	(iii) Autoimmune encephalomyelitis
	(iv) Goodpasture's syndrome
	(v) Primary biliary cirrhosis
	(vi) Lupoid hepatitis
	(vii) Membranous glomerulonephritis
	(viii) Autoimmune skin diseases

**Diseases discussed in this chapter.*

iv) Anti-ribonucleoproteins (anti-RNP) are not specific for SLE but are seen more often in Sjögren's syndrome.

v) Anti-histone antibodies, seen particularly in cases of drug-induced SLE.

vi) Anti-nucleolar antibodies to nucleolar antigens.

vii) Antiphospholipid antibodies or lupus anticoagulant are quite specific for SLE and are responsible for thrombotic complications in cases of SLE.

The source of these autoantibodies as well as hypergammaglobulinaemia in SLE is the **polyclonal activation of B cells** brought about by following derangements:

1. *Immunologic factors.* These include:

i) an inherited defect in B cells;
ii) stimulation of B cells by micro-organisms;
iii) T helper cell hyperactivity; and
iv) T suppressor cell defect.

2. *Genetic factors.* Genetic predisposition to develop autoantibodies to nuclear and cytoplasmic antigens in SLE is due to the immunoregulatory function of class II HLA genes implicated in the pathogenesis of SLE.

3. *Other factors.* Various other factors express the genetic susceptibility of an individual to develop clinical disease. These factors are:

i) certain drugs e.g. penicillamine D;
ii) certain viral infections e.g. EBV infection; and
iii) certain hormones e.g. oestrogen.

PATHOGENESIS. The autoantibodies formed by any of the mechanisms explained above are the mediators of tissue injury in SLE. Two types of immunologic tissue injury can occur in SLE:

1. *Type II hypersensitivity* is characterised by formation of autoantibodies against blood cells (red blood cells, platelets, leucocytes) and results in haematologic derangement in SLE.

2. *Type III hypersensitivity* is characterised by antigen-antibody complex (commonly DNA-anti-DNA antibody; sometimes lg-anti-lg antibody complex) which is deposited at sites such as renal glomeruli, walls of small blood vessels etc.

LE CELL PHENOMENON. This was the first diagnostic laboratory test described for SLE. The test is based on the principle that ANAs cannot penetrate the intact cells and thus cell nuclei should be exposed to bind them with the ANAs. The binding of exposed nucleus with ANAs results in homogeneous mass of nuclear chromatin material which is called *LE body or haematoxylin body.*

LE cell is a phagocytic leucocyte, commonly polymorphonuclear neutrophil, and sometimes a monocyte, which engulfs the homogeneous nuclear material of the injured cell. For demonstration of LE cell phenomenon *in vitro,* the blood sample is traumatised to expose the nuclei of blood leucocytes to ANAs. This results in binding of denatured and damaged nucleus with ANAs.

The ANA-coated denatured nucleus is chemotactic for phagocytic cells.

- If this mass is engulfed by a neutrophil, displacing the nucleus of neutrophil to the rim of the cell, it is called *LE cell* (Fig. 4.6,A).
- If the mass, more often an intact lymphocyte, is phagocytosed by a monocyte, it is called *Tart cell* (Fig. 4.6,B).

LE cell test is positive in 70% cases of SLE while newer and more sensitive immunofluorescence tests for autoantibodies are positive in almost 100% cases of SLE. A few other conditions may also show positive LE test e.g. rheumatoid arthritis, lupoid hepatitis, penicillin sensitivity etc.

PATHOLOGIC CHANGES. The manifestations of SLE are widespread in different visceral organs as well as show erythematous cutaneous eruptions. The principal lesions are renal, vascular, cutaneous and cardiac; other organs and tissues involved are serosal linings (pleuritis, pericarditis); joints (synovitis); spleen (vasculitis); liver (portal triaditis); lungs (interstitial pneumonitis, fibrosing alveolitis), CNS (vasculitis) and in blood (autoimmune haemolytic anaemia, thrombocytopaenia).

Histologically, the characteristic lesion in SLE is *fibrinoid necrosis* which may be seen in the connective tissue, beneath the endothelium in small blood vessels, under the mesothelial lining of pleura and pericardium, under the endothelium in endocardium, or under the synovial lining cells of joints.

Table 4.9 summarises the morphology of lesions in different organs and tissues in SLE.

CLINICAL FEATURES. SLE, like most other autoimmune diseases, is more common in women in their 2nd to 3rd decades of life. As obvious from Table 4.9, SLE is a multisystem disease and thus a wide variety of clinical features may be present. A typical full-fledged case of SLE has the following characteristics:

- butterfly-like erythematous rash on skin of face;
- fever;
- painful joints;
- chest pain (due to pleuritis and pericarditis);
- renal involvement (proteinuria, haematuria, casts);
- haematologic derangements (haemolytic anaemia, thrombocytopenia, leucopenia); and
- neurologic disorders (seizures, psychosis).

The disease usually runs a long course of flare-ups and remissions; renal failure is the most frequent cause of death.

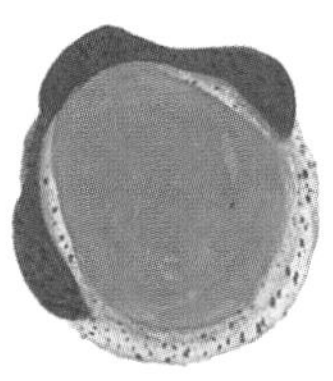
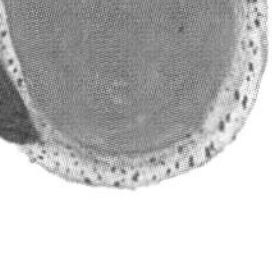
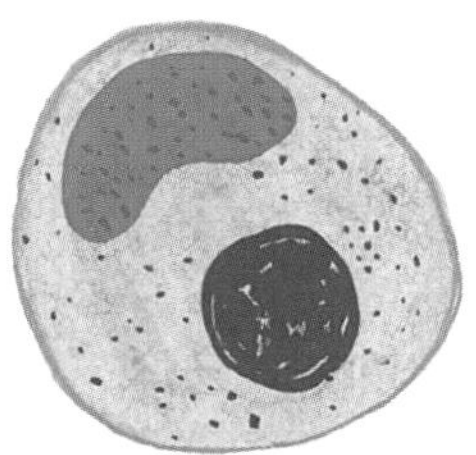

FIGURE 4.6

LE cell phenomenon. A. *Typical LE cell.* The rounded mass of amorphous nuclear material (LE body) has displaced the lobes of neutrophil to the rim of the cell. B. *Tart cell.* A lymphocyte with intact nuclear structure phagocytosed by monocyte, the nucleus of which is compressed.

Scleroderma (Progressive Systemic Sclerosis)

Just like SLE, scleroderma was initially described as a skin disease characterised by progressive fibrosis. But now, 2 main types are recognised:

1. *Diffuse scleroderma* in which the skin shows widespread involvement and may progress to involve visceral structures.
2. *CREST syndrome* of progressive systemic sclerosis characterised by Calcinosis (C), Raynaud's phenomenon (R), Esophageal hypomotility (E), Sclerodactyly (S) and Telangiectasia (T).

ETIOPATHOGENESIS. The etiology of this disease is not known. However, antinuclear antibodies are detected in majority of cases of systemic sclerosis. Immunologic mechanisms have been implicated in the pathogenesis of lesions in systemic sclerosis which finally cause activation of fibroblasts. The *immune mechanisms* leading to stimulation of fibroblasts may act in the following ways:

1. *Elaboration of cytokines* such as by fibroblast growth factor and chemotactic factors by activated T cells and macrophages.
2. *Endothelial cell injury* due to cytotoxic damage to endothelium from autoantibodies or antigen-antibody complexes. This results in aggregation and activation of platelets which increases vascular permeability and stimulates fibroblastic proliferation.

PATHOLOGIC CHANGES. Disseminated visceral involvement as well as cutaneous lesions are seen in systemic sclerosis.

1. Skin changes. Skin is involved diffusely, beginning distally from fingers and extending

TABLE 4.9: Morphology of Major Lesions in SLE.

ORGANS (MAIN LESION)	MORPHOLOGIC FEATURES
1. *Renal lesions (Lupus nephritis)*	EM-shows large deposits in mesangium, subepithelial or subendothelial. IM-shows granular deposits of immune complex (IgG and C3) on capillaries, mesangium and tubular basement membranes. Six patterns: i. Minimal disease : LM shows no change ii. Mesangial GN : LM shows increase in matrix; mesangial hypercellularity. iii. Focal proliferative GN : LM shows focal (parts of 50% glomeruli) endothelial and mesangial cell proliferation; infiltration with neutrophils. iv. Diffuse proliferative GN : LM shows all glomeruli affected; proliferation of endothelial, mesangial and epithelial cells; epithelial crescents. v. Membranous lupus GN : LM shows diffuse basement membrane thickening; features of nephrotic syndrome. vi. Sclerosing nephropathy : LM shows hyalinisation of whole of glomeruli.
2. *Small blood vessels (Acute necrotising vasculitis)*	Affects all tissues; commonly skin and muscles involved; LM shows fibrinoid deposits in the vessel wall; perivascular infiltrate of mononuclear cells.
3. *Cutaneous lesions (Erythematous eruptions)*	Butterfly area on nose and cheek; LM shows liquefactive degeneration of basal layer of epidermis; oedema at dermoepidermal junction; acute necrotising vasculitis in dermis; IM shows immune complex deposits (IgG and C3) at dermo-epidermal junction.
4. *Cardiac lesions (Libman-Sacks endocarditis)*	Vegetations on mitral and tricuspid valves, may extend to mural endocardium, chordae tendineae; LM of vegetations shows fibrinoid material, necrotic debris, inflammatory cells, haematoxylin bodies may be present; connective tissue of endocardium and myocardium may show focal inflammation and necrotising vasculitis.

(EM = electron microscopy, LM = light microscopy; IM = immunofluorescence microscopy; GN = glomerulonephritis).

proximally to arms, shoulders, neck and face. In advanced stage, the fingers become claw-like and face mask-like.

Microscopically, changes are progressive from early to late stage.

- *Early stage* shows oedema and degeneration of collagen. The small-sized blood vessels are occluded and there is perivascular infiltrate of mononuclear cells.
- *Late stage* reveals thin and flat epidermis. Dermis is largely replaced by compact collagen and there is hyaline thickening of walls of dermal blood vessels. In advanced cases subcutaneous calcification may occur.

2. Kidney changes. Involvement of kidneys is seen in majority of cases of systemic sclerosis. The lesions are prominent in the walls of interlobular arteries which develop changes resembling malignant hypertension. There is thickening of tunica intima due to concentric proliferation of intimal cells and fibrinoid necrosis of vessel wall.

3. Smooth muscle of GIT. Muscularis of the alimentary tract, particularly oesophagus, is progressively atrophied and replaced by fibrous tissue.

4. Skeletal muscle. The interstitium of skeletal muscle shows progressive fibrosis and degeneration of muscle fibres with associated inflammatory changes.

5. Cardiac muscle. Involvement of interstitium of the heart may result in heart failure.

6. Lungs. Diffuse fibrosis may lead to contraction of the lung substance. There may be epithelium-lined honey-combed cysts of bronchioles.

7. Small arteries. The lesions in small arteries show endarteritis due to intimal proliferation and may be the cause for Raynaud's phenomenon.

CLINICAL FEATURES. Systemic sclerosis is more common in middle-aged women. The clinical manifestations include:

- claw-like flexion deformity of hands;
- Raynaud's phenomenon;

- oesophageal fibrosis causing dysphagia and hypomotility;
- malabsorption syndrome;
- respiratory distress;
- malignant hypertension;
- pulmonary hypertension; and
- biliary cirrhosis.

Polymyositis-Dermatomyositis

As the name suggests, this disease is a combination of symmetric muscle weakness and skin rash.

ETIOPATHOGENESIS. The exact cause of the disease is unknown. However, antinuclear antibodies are detected in 25% of cases. Thus, an *immunologic hypothesis* has been proposed. The affected muscles are infiltrated by sensitised T lymphocytes of both T helper and T suppressor type which are considered to bring about inflammatory destruction of muscle. *Viral etiology* due to infection with coxsackie B virus has also been suggested.

PATHOLOGIC CHANGES. The skeletal muscles usually affected are of pelvis, shoulders, neck, chest and diaphragm.

Histologically, vacuolisation and fragmentation of muscle fibres and numerous inflammatory cells are present. In late stage, muscle fibres are replaced by fat and fibrous tissue.

CLINICAL FEATURES. It is a multi-system disease characterised by:

- muscle weakness, mainly proximal;
- skin rash, typically with heliotropic erythema and periorbital oedema;
- dysphagia due to involvement of pharyngeal muscles;
- respiratory dysfunction; and
- association with deep-seated malignancies.

Sjögren's Syndrome

Sjögren's syndrome is characterised by the *triad* of dry eyes *(keratoconjunctivitis sicca)*, dry mouth *(xerostomia)*, and *rheumatoid arthritis*. The combination of the former two symptoms is called *sicca syndrome*.

ETIOPATHOGENESIS. Immune mechanisms have been implicated in the etiopathogenesis of lesions in Sjögren's syndrome. Antinuclear antibodies are found in about 90% of cases; test for rheumatoid factor is positive in 25% of cases. The lesions in lacrimal and salivary glands are mediated by T lymphocytes, B cells and plasma cells.

PATHOLOGIC CHANGES. *In early stage,* the lacrimal and salivary glands show periductal infiltration by lymphocytes and plasma cells, which at times may form lymphoid follicles (pseudolymphoma). *In late stage,* glandular parenchyma is replaced by fat and fibrous tissue. The ducts are also fibrosed and hyalinised.

CLINICAL FEATURES. The disease is common in women in 4th to 6th decades of life. It is clinically characterised by:

- Symptoms *referable to eyes* such as blurred vision, burning and itching.
- Symptoms *referable to xerostomia* such as fissured oral mucosa, dryness, and difficulty in swallowing.
- Symptoms due to *glandular involvement* such as enlarged and inflamed lacrimal gland (Mikulicz's syndrome is involvement of parotid alongwith lacrimal gland).
- Symptoms due to *systemic involvement* referable to lungs, CNS and skin.

Reiter's Syndrome

This syndrome is characterised by *triad of arthritis, conjunctivitis* and *urethritis.* There may be mucocutaneous lesions on palms, soles, oral mucosa and genitalia. Antinuclear antibodies and RA factor are usually negative.

Mixed ConnectiveTissue Disease

This designation is applied to a syndrome having features of 3 collagen diseases—SLE, progressive systemic sclerosis, and dermatomyositis. High titers of antinuclear antibodies are detected. The clinical features are varied and consist of manifestations of diseases included. However, renal involvement is generally not seen and prognosis is good due to response to corticosteroid therapy.

TRANSPLANT REJECTION

According to the genetic relationship between donor and recipient, transplantation of tissues is classified into 4 groups:

1. *Autografts* are grafts in which the donor and recipient is the same individual.
2. *Isografts* are grafts between the donor and recipient of the same genotype.
3. *Allografts* are those in which the donor is of the same species but of a different genotype.
4. *Xenografts* are those in which the donor is of a different species from that of the recipient.

All types of grafts have been performed in human beings but xenografts have been found to be rejected

Chapter Four

invariably due to genetic disparity. Presently, surgical skills exist for skin grafts and for organ transplants such as kidney, heart, lungs, liver, pancreas, cornea and bone marrow. But most commonly practised are skin grafting, kidney and bone marrow transplantation. For any successful tissue transplant without immunological rejection, matched major histocompatibility locus antigens (HLA) between the donor and recipient are of paramount importance (see page 66). The greater the genetic disparity between donor and recipient in HLA system, the stronger and more rapid will be the rejection reaction.

Besides the rejection reaction, a peculiar problem occurring especially in bone marrow transplantation is graft-versus-host reaction (GVH). In humans, GVH reaction results when immunocompetent cells are transplanted to an immunodeficient recipient e.g. when severe combined immunodeficiency is treated by bone marrow transplantation. The clinical features of GVH reaction include: fever, weight loss, anaemia, dermatitis, diarrhoea, intestinal malabsorption, pneumonia and hepatosplenomegaly. The intensity of GVH reaction depends upon the extent of genetic disparity between the donor and recipient.

Mechanisms of Graft Rejection

Except for autografts and isografts, an immune response against allografts is inevitable. The development of immunosuppressive drugs has made the survival of allografts in recipients possible. Rejection of allografts involves both cell-mediated and humoral immunity.

1. CELL-MEDIATED IMMUNE REACTIONS. These are mainly responsible for graft rejection and are mediated by T cells. The lymphocytes of the recipient on coming in contact with HLA antigens of the donor are sensitised in case of incompatibility. The sensitised T cells in the form of cytotoxic T cells (T_{CTL}) as well as by hypersensitivity reactions initiated by helper T cells attack the graft and destroy it.

2. HUMORAL IMMUNE REACTIONS. Currently, in addition to the cell-mediated immune reactions, a role for humoral antibodies in certain rejection reactions has been suggested. These include: *preformed circulating antibodies* due to pre-sensitisation of the recipient before transplantation e.g. by blood transfusions and previous pregnancies, or in *non-sensitised individuals* by complement dependent cytotoxicity, antibody-dependent cell-mediated cytotoxicity (ADCC) and antigen-antibody complexes.

Types of Rejection Reactions

Based on the underlying mechanism and time period, rejection reactions are classified into 3 types: hyperacute, acute and chronic.

1. HYPERACUTE REJECTION. Hyperacute rejection appears within minutes to hours of placing the transplant and destroys it. It is mediated by preformed humoral antibody against donor-antigen.

Grossly, hyperacute rejection is recognised by the surgeon soon after the vascular anastomosis of the graft is performed to the recipient's vessels. The organ becomes swollen, oedematous, haemorrhagic, purple and cyanotic rather than gaining pink colour.

Histologically, the characteristics of Arthus reaction are present. There are numerous neutrophils around dilated and obstructed capillaries which are blocked by fibrin and platelet thrombi. Small segments of blood vessel wall may become necrotic and there is necrosis of much of the transplanted organ. Small haemorrhages are common.

Cross-matching of the donor's lymphocytes with those of the recipient before transplantation has diminished the frequency of hyperacute rejection.

2. ACUTE REJECTION. This usually becomes evident within a few days to a few months of transplantation. Acute graft rejection may be mediated by cellular or humoral mechanisms.

Acute cellular rejection is more common and is characterised by extensive infiltration in the interstitium of the transplant by lymphocytes (mainly T cells), a few plasma cells, monocytes and a few polymorphs. There is damage to the blood vessels and there are foci of necrosis in the transplanted tissue. Acute humoral rejection appears due to poor response to immunosuppressive therapy. It is characterised by acute rejection vasculitis and foci of necrosis in small vessels. The mononuclear cell infiltrate is less marked as compared to acute cellular rejection and consists mostly of B lymphocytes.

3. CHRONIC REJECTION. Chronic rejection may follow repeated attacks of acute rejection or may develop slowly over a period of months to a year or so. The underlying mechanisms of chronic rejection may be immunologic or ischaemic. Patients with chronic rejection of renal transplant show progressive deterioration in renal function as seen by rising serum creatinine levels.

PATHOLOGIC CHANGES. In chronic rejection of transplanted kidney, the changes are intimal fibrosis, interstitial fibrosis and tubular atrophy. Renal allografts may develop glomerulonephritis by transmission from the host, or rarely may be *de novo* glomerulonephritis.

AMYLOIDOSIS

Amyloidosis is the term used for a group of diseases characterised by extracellular deposition of fibrillar proteinaceous substance called amyloid having common morphological appearance, staining properties and physical structure but with variable protein (or biochemical) composition.

First described by Rokitansky in 1842, the substance was subsequently named by Virchow as 'amyloid' under the mistaken belief that the material was starch-like (*amylon* = starch). This property was demonstrable *grossly* on the cut surface of an organ containing amyloid which stained brown with iodine and turned violet on addition of dilute sulfuric acid. By *light microscopy* with H&E staining, amyloid appears as extracellular, homogeneous, structureless and eosinophilic hyaline material, which is *positive with Congo red* staining and shows apple-green birefringence on *polarising microscopy.*

The nomenclature of different forms of amyloid is done by putting the alphabet A for amyloid, followed by the suffix derived from the name of specific protein constituting amyloid of that type e.g. AL (A for amyloid, L for light chain-derived), AA, ATTR etc.

PHYSICAL AND CHEMICAL NATURE OF AMYLOID

Ultrastructural examination and chemical analysis reveal the complex nature of amyloid. *It emerges that on the basis of morphology and physical characteristics all forms of amyloid are similar in appearance, but they are chemically heterogeneous.* Based on these analysis, amyloid is composed of 2 main types of complex proteins (Fig. 4.7):

I. *Fibril proteins* comprise about 95% of amyloid.

II. *Non-fibrillar components* which include *P-component* predominanly and there are several different proteins which together constitute the remaining 5% of amyloid.

I. Fibril Proteins

By electron microscopy, it bacame apparent that major component of all forms of amyloid (about 95%) consists

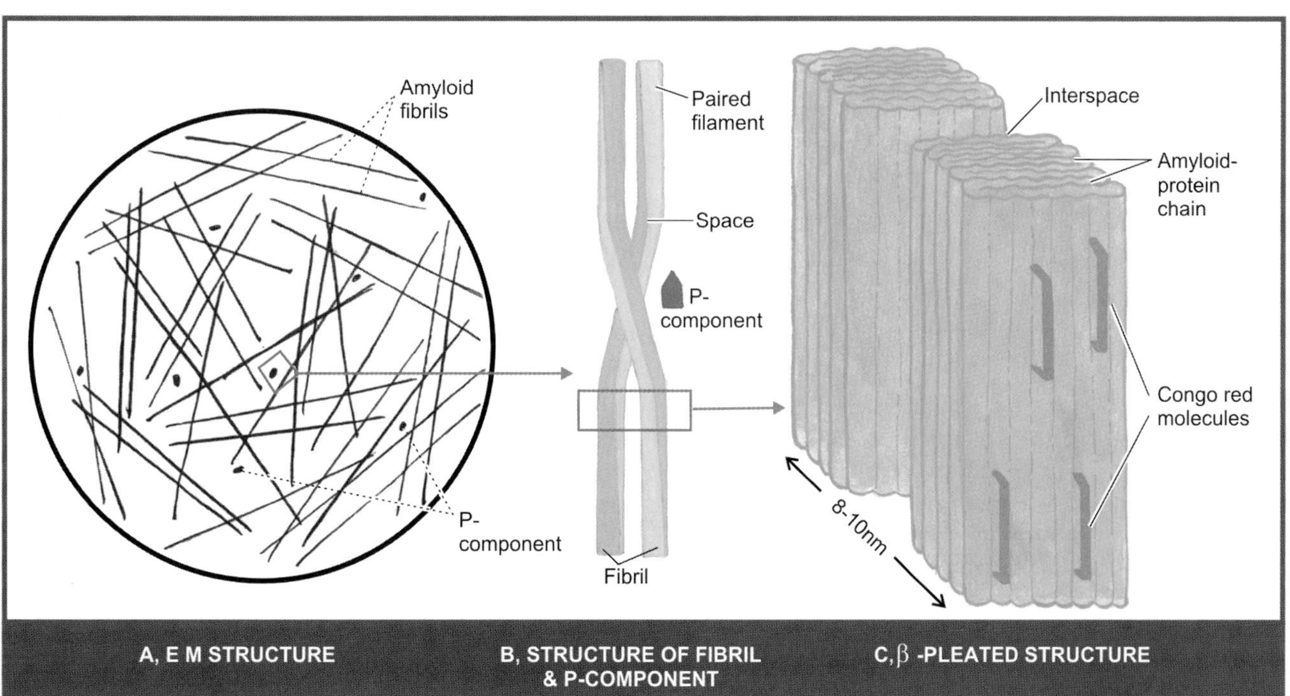

FIGURE 4.7

Diagrammatic representation of the ultrastructure of amyloid. A, Electron microscopy shows major part consisting of amyloid fibrils (95%) randomly oriented, while the minor part is essentially P-component (5%) B, Each fibril is further composed of double helix of two pleated sheets in the form of *twin filaments* separated by a clear space. P-component has a pentagonal or doughnut profile. C, X-ray crystallography and infra-red spectroscopy shows fibrils having *cross-β-pleated* sheet configuration which produces periodicity that gives the characteristic staining properties of amyloid with Congo red and birefringence under polarising microscopy.

of meshwork of fibril proteins. The *fibrils* are delicate, randomly dispersed, non-branching, each measuring 7.5-10 nm in diameter and having indefinite length. Each fibril is further composed of double helix of two pleated sheets in the form of *twin filaments* separated by a clear space. By X-ray crystallography and infra-red spectroscopy, the fibrils are shown to have *cross-β-pleated* sheet configuration which produces 1000 A° periodicity that gives the characteristic staining properties of amyloid with Congo red and birefringence under polarising microscopy. Based on these features amyloid is also referred to as *β-fibrillosis*.

Chemical analysis of fibril proteins of amyloid revealed heterogeneous nature of amyloid. Chemically two major forms of amyloid fibril proteins were first identified in 1970s while currently 20 biochemically different proteins are known to form amyloid fibrils in humans in different clinicopathologic settings. Thus these can be categorised as under:

i) AL (amyloid light chain) protein;
ii) AA (amyloid associated) protein;
iii) Other proteins.

AL PROTEIN. AL amyloid fibril protein is derived from immunoglobulin light chain, which in most cases includes amino-terminal segment of the immunoglobulin light chain and part of C region. AL fibril protein is more frequently derived from the lambda (λ) light chain than kappa (κ), the former being twice more common. However, in any given case, there is amino acid sequence homology. AL type of fibril protein is produced by immunoglobulin-secreting cells and is therefore seen in association with plasma cell dyscrasias and is seen in primary systemic amyloidosis.

AA PROTEIN. AA fibril protein is composed of protein with molecular weight of 8.5-kD which is derived from larger precursor protein in the serum called SAA (serum amyloid-associated protein) with a molecular weight of 12.5-kD. Unlike AL amyloid, the deposits of AA amyloid do not have sequence homology. In the plasma, SAA circulates in association with HDL_3 (high-density lipoprotein). SAA is an acute phase reactant protein synthesised in the liver, its level being high in chronic inflammatory and traumatic conditions. SAA fibril protein is found in secondary amyloidosis which includes the largest group of diseases associated with amyloidosis.

OTHER PROTEINS. Apart from the two major forms of amyloid fibril proteins, a few other forms of proteins are found in different clinical states:

1. **Transthyretin (TTR)** is a serum protein synthesised in the liver and *trans*ports *thy*roxine and *retin*ol normally (trans-thy-retin). It was earlier called AFp (amyloid familial prealbumin) since it precedes albumin (pre-albumin) on serum electrophoresis but is not related to serum albumin. Single amino acid substitution mutations in the structure of TTR results in variant form of protein which is responsible for amyloidosis i.e. ATTR. About 60 such mutations have been described. ATTR is the most common form of heredofamilial amyloidosis e.g. in familial amyloid polyneuropathies. However, the deposits of ATTR in the elderly primarily involving the heart (senile cardiac amyloidosis) consists of normal TTR without any mutation. Another interesting aspect in ATTR is that despite being inherited, the disease appears in middle age or elderly.

2. **Aβ_2-microglobulin (Aβ_2M)** is amyloid seen in cases of long-term haemodialysis (8-10 years). As the name suggests, β_2M is a small protein which is a normal component of major histocompatibility complex (MHC) and has β-pleated sheet structure. β_2M is not effectively filtered during haemodialysis and thus there is high serum concentration of β_2M protein in these patients. Although the deposit due Aβ_2M may be systemic in distribution, it has predilection for bones and joints.

3. **β-amyloid protein (Aβ)** is distinct from Aβ_2M and is seen in cerebral plaques as well as cerebral blood vessels in Alzheimer's disease. Aβ is derived from amyloid beta precursor protein (AβPP) which is a transmembrane glycoprotein. The normal function of AβPP is probably cell-to-matrix signalling.

4. **Immunoglobulin heavy chain amyloid (AH)** derived from truncated heavy chain of immunoglobulin is an uncommon form of systemic amyloidosis.

5. **Amyloid from hormone precursor proteins** such as pro-calcitonin, islet amyloid polypeptide, pro-insulin, prolactin, atrial nitouretic factor, and lactoferrin has also been reported in amyloid.

6. **Amyloid of prion protein (APrP)** is derived from precursor prion protein which is a plasma membrane glycoprotein. Prion proteins are proteinaceous infectious particles lacking in RNA or DNA. Amyloid in prionosis occurs due to abnormally folded isoform of the PrP.

7. **Miscellaneous heredofamilial forms of amyloid** include a variety of amyloid proteins reported recently. These include amyloid derived from: apolipoprotein I (AApoAI), gelsolin (Agel), lysozyme (ALys), fibrinogen α-chain (AFib), and cystatin C (ACys) etc.

II. Non-fibrillar Components

Non-fibrillar components comprise about 5% of the amyloid material. These include the following:
1. *Amyloid P (AP)-component* synthesised in the liver and is present in all types of amyloid. It is derived from circulating serum amyloid P-component, a glycoprotein resembling the normal serum α_1-glycoprotein and is PAS-positive. It is structurally related to C-reactive protein, an acute phase reactant, but is not similar to it. By electron microscopy, it has a pentagonal profile (P-component) or doughnut-shape with an external diameter of 9 nm and internal diameter of 4 nm.
2. *Apolipoprotein-E (apoE)*: It is a regulator of lipoprotein metabolism and is found in all types of amyloid. One allele apoE4 increases the risk of Alzheimer precursor protein (APP) deposition in Alzheimer's disease but not in all other types of amyloid deposits.
3. *Sulfated glycosaminoglycans(GAGs)*: These are constituents of matrix proteins; particulary associated is heparan sulfate in all types of tissue amyloid.
4. *α-1 anti-chymotrypsin:* It is only seen in cases of AA deposits but negative in primary amyloidosis.
5. *Protein X:* This protein has been shown to be present in cases of prionoses.
6. *Other components*: Besides above, components of complement, proteases, and membrane constituents may be seen.

PATHOGENESIS OF AMYLOIDOSIS

The earliest observation that amyloidosis developed in experimental animals who were injected repeatedly with antigen to raise antisera for human use led to the concept that amyloidogenesis was the result of immunologic mechanisms. AL variety of amyloid protein was thus first to be isolated. It is now appreciated that amyloidosis or fibrillogenesis is multifactorial and that different mechanisms are involved in different types of amyloid.

In general amyloidogenesis *in vivo* occurs in the following sequence (Fig. 4.8):
1. *Pool of amyloidogenic precursor protein* is present in circulation in different clinical settings and in response to stimuli e.g. increased hepatic synthesis of AA or ATTR, increased synthesis of AL etc.
2. *A nidus for fibrillogenesis*, meaning thereby an alteration in microenvironment to stimulate deposition of amyloid protein. This alteration involves changes and interaction between basement membrane proteins and amyloidogenic protein.
3. *Partial degradation or proteolysis* occurs prior to deposition of fibrillar protein which may occur in macrophages or reticuloendothelial cells e.g. in AL, AA, TTR, AGel, ACys, Alzheimer's disease, AApoAI.
4. *Exceptions to this generalisation* are seen in ATTR (heredofamilial type in which there are amino acid mutations in most cases), Aβ2M (in which there are elevated levels of normal β2M protein which remain unfiltered during haemodialysis) and prionosis (in which β-pleated sheet is formed *de novo*).
5. The role of *non-fibrillar components* such as AP, apoE and GAGs in amyloidosis is unclear; probably they facilitate in aggregation of proteins and protein folding leading to fibril formation, substrate adhesion and protection from degradation.

Deposition of AL and AA amyloid is schematically shown in Fig. 4.8 and is briefly outlined below.

Deposition of AL Amyloid

1. The stimulus for production of AL amyloid is some disorder of *immunoglobulin synthesis* e.g. multiple myeloma, B cell lymphoma, other plasma cell dyscrasias.
2. Excessive immunoglobulin production is in the form of *monoclonal gammopathy* i.e. there is production of either intact immunoglobulin, or λ light chain, or κ light chain, or rarely heavy chains. This takes place by monoclonal proliferation of plasma cells, B lymphocytes, or their precursors.
3. *Partial degradation* in the form of limited proteolysis of larger protein molecules occurs in macrophages which are anatomically closely associated with AL amyloid.
4. *Non-fibrillar components* like AP and GAGs play some role in folding and aggregation of fibril proteins.

Deposition of AA Amyloid

1. AA amyloid is directly related to *SAA levels.* SAA is a high density lipoprotein the levels of which are elevated in long-standing tissue destruction accompanied by chronic inflammation.
2. SAA is synthesised by the liver in response to *cytokines*, notably interleukin 1 and 6, from activated macrophages. However, SAA levels in isolation do not always lead to AA amyloid.
3. As in AL amyloid, *partial degradation* in the form of limited proteolysis takes place in reticuloendothelial cells.
4. In AA amyloid, a significant role is played by another glycoprotein, *amyloid enhancing factor (AEF)*. The exact composition of AEF is not known. It is elaborated in chronic inflammation, cancer and familial Mediterranean fever. On the basis of experimental induction of AA amyloid, AEF has been shown to accelerate AA amyloid deposition. Possibly, AEF acts as a nidus for deposition of fibrils in AA amyloid.

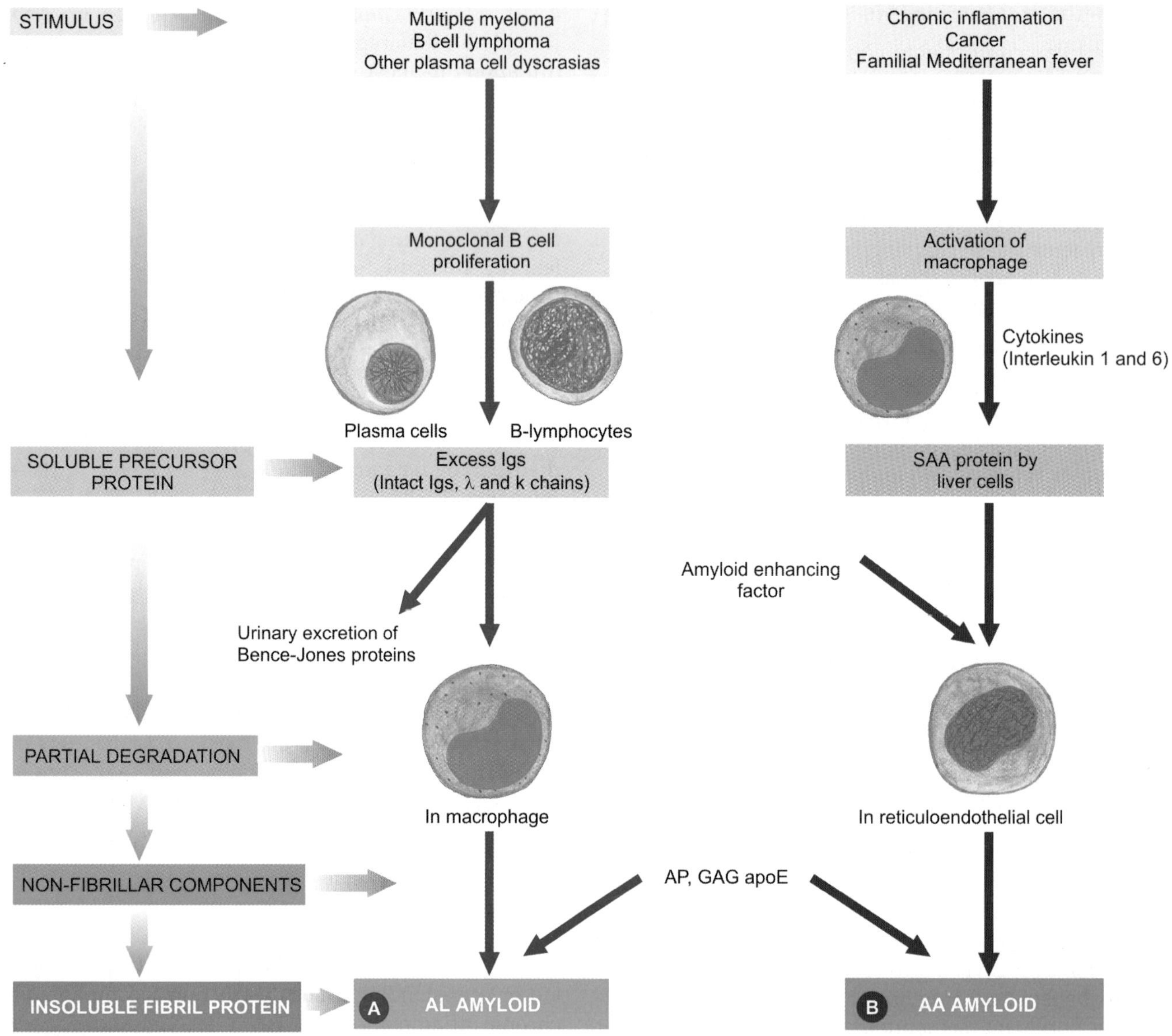

FIGURE 4.8

Pathogenesis of two main forms of amyloid deposition (AL = Amyloid light chain; AA = Amyloid-associated protein; GAG = glycosaminoglycan; AP = Amyloid P component). The sequence on left shows general schematic representation common to both major forms of amyloidogenesis.

5. As in AL amyloid, there is a role of *AP component* and *glycosaminoglycans* in the fibril protein aggregation and to protect it from disaggregation again.

CLASSIFICATION OF AMYLOIDOSIS

Amyloidosis has been classified in a number of ways in the past. These include:

- Classification of amyloidosis into *primary (mesenchymal)* and *secondary (parenchymal)* types;
- On histological basis into *pericollagenous* corresponding in distribution to primary, and *perireticulin* corresponding to secondary amyloidosis; and
- On clinical location of amyloidosis into *pattern I* (involving tongue, heart, bowel, skeletal and smooth muscle, skin and nerves), *pattern II* (principally involving liver, spleen, kidney and adrenals) and *mixed* (involving sites of both pattern I and II).

However, with availability of biochemical composition of various forms of amyloid, a biochemical-based *clinicopathologic classification* is widely acceptable (Table 4.10). According to this classification, amyloidosis can be divided into 2 major categories, each found in distinct clinical settings:

A. Systemic (generalised) amyloidosis:
1. Primary (AL)
2. Secondary/reactive/ inflammatory (AA)
3. Haemodialysis-associated ($A\beta_2M$)
4. Heredofamilial (ATTR, AA, Others)

B. Localised amyloidosis:
1. Senile cardiac (ATTR)
2. Senile cerebral (Aβ, APrP)
3. Endocrine (Hormone precursors)
4. Tumour-forming (AL)

A. SYSTEMIC AMYLOIDOSIS

1. Primary Systemic (AL) Amyloidosis

Primary amyloidosis consisting of AL fibril proteins is systemic or generalised in distribution. About 30% cases of AL amyloid have some form of plasma cell dyscrasias, most commonly multiple myeloma (in about 10% cases), and less often other monoclonal gammopathies such as Waldenström's macroglobulinaemia, heavy chain disease, solitary plasmacytoma and nodular malignant lymphoma (B cell lymphoma). The neoplastic plasma cells usually are a single clone and, therefore, produce the same type of immunoglobulin light chain or part of light chain. Almost all cases of multiple myeloma have either λ or κ light chains (Bence Jones proteins) in the serum and are excreted in the urine. However, in contrast to normal or myeloma light chains, AL is twice more frequently derived from λ light chains.

The remaining 70% cases of AL amyloid do not have evident B-cell proliferative disorder or any other associated diseases and are thus cases of true 'primary' (idiopathic) amyloidosis. However, by more sensitive methods, some plasma cell dyscrasias are detectable in virtually all patients with AL. Majority of these cases too have a single type of abnormal immunoglobulin in their serum (monoclonal) and that these patients have some degree of plasmacytosis in the bone marrow, suggesting the origin of AL amyloid from precursor plasma cells.

AL amyloid is most prevalent type of systemic amyloidosis in the USA. Primary amyloidosis is often severe in the heart, kidney, bowel, skin, peripheral nerves, respiratory tract, skeletal muscle, and other organs.

Recently, it has been possible to reproduce AL amyloid in mice by repeated injections of human

TABLE 4.10: Classification of Amyloidosis.

CATEGORY	ASSOCIATED DISEASE	BIOCHEM.TYPE	ORGANS COMMONLY INVOLVED
A. SYSTEMIC (GENERALISED) AMYLOIDOSIS			
1. ***Primary***	Plasma cell dyscrasias	AL type	Heart, bowel, skin, nerves, kidney
2. ***Secondary (Reactive)***	Chronic inflammation, cancers	AA type	Liver, spleen, kidneys, adrenals
3. ***Haemodialysis associated***	Chronic renal failure	$A\beta_2M$	Synovium, joints, tendon sheaths
4. ***Heredofamilial***			
i. *Hereditary polyneuropathies*	—	ATTR	Peripheral and autonomic nerves, heart
ii. *Familial Mediterranean fever*	—	AA type	Liver, spleen, kidneys, adrenals
iii. *Rare hereditary forms*	---	AApoAI, AGel, ALys, AFib, ACys	Systemic amyloidosis
B. LOCALISED AMYLOIDOSIS			
1. ***Senile cardiac***	Senility	ATTR	Heart
2. ***Senile cerebral***	Alzheimer's, transmissible encephalopathy	Aβ, APrP	Cerebral vessels, plaques, neurofibrillary tangles
3. ***Endocrine***	Medullary carcinoma Diabetes type II	Procalcitonin Proinsulin	Thyroid Islets of Langerhans
4. ***Tumour-forming***	Lungs, larynx, skin, urinary bladder, tongue, eye	AL	Respective anatomic location

AL= Amyloid light chain; AA= Amyloid-associated protein; $A\beta_2M$= Amyloid β_2-microglobulin; ATTR= Amyloid transthyretin; APrP=Amyloid of prion proteins, Aβ= β-amyloid protein).

amyloidogenic light chains. Treatment of AL amyloid is targetted at reducing the underlying clonal expansion of plasma cells.

2. Secondary/Reactive (AA) Systemic Amyloidosis

The second form of systemic or generalised amyloidosis is reactive or inflammatory or secondary in which the fibril proteins contain AA amyloid. Secondary or reactive amyloidosis occurs typically as a complication of chronic infectious (e.g. tuberculosis, bronchiectasis, chronic osteomyelitis, chronic pyelonephritis, leprosy, chronic skin infections), non-infectious chronic inflammatory conditions associated with tissue destruction (e.g. autoimmune disorders such as rheumatoid arthritis, inflammatory bowel disease), some tumours (e.g. renal cell carcinoma, Hodgkin's disease) and in familial Mediterranean fever, an inherited disorder (discussed below).

Secondary amyloidosis is typically distributed in solid abdominal viscera like the kidney, liver, spleen and adrenals. Secondary reactive amyloidosis is seen less frequently in developed countries due to containment of infections before they become chronic but this is the most common type of amyloidosis worldwide, particularly in underdeveloped and developing countries of the world.

AA amyloid occurs spontaneously in some birds and animals; it can also be experimentally induced in animals. Control of inflammation is the mainstay of treatment.

The contrasting features of the two main forms of systemic amyloidosis are given in Table 4.11.

3. Haemodialysis-Associated ($A\beta_2M$) Amyloidosis

Patients on long-term dialysis for more than 10 years for chronic renal failure may develop systemic amyloidosis derived from β_2-microglobulin which is normal component of MHC. The amyloid deposits are preferentially found in the vessel walls at the synovium, joints, tendon sheaths and subchondral bones. However, systemic distribution has also been observed in these cases showing bulky visceral deposits of amyloid.

4. Heredofamilial Amyloidosis

A few rare examples of genetically-determined amyloidosis having familial occurrence and seen in certain geographic regions have been described. These are as under:

i) Hereditary polyneuropathic (ATTR) amyloidosis. This is an autosomal dominant disorder in which amyloid is deposited in the peripheral and autonomic nerves resulting in muscular weakness, pain and paraesthesia, or may have cardiomyopathy. This type of amyloid is derived from transthyretin (ATTR) with single amino acid substitution in the structure of TTR; about 60 types of such mutations have been described. Though hereditary, the condition appears well past middle life.

ii) Familial Mediterranean fever (AA). This is an autosomal recessive disease and is seen in people of Mediterranean region (e.g. Sephardic jews, Armenians, Arabs and Turks). The condition is characterised by periodic attacks of fever and polyserositis i.e.

TABLE 4.11: Contrasting Features of Primary and Secondary Amyloidosis.

FEATURE	PRIMARY AMYLOID	SECONDARY AMYLOID
1. *Biochemical composition*	AL (Light chain proteins); lambda chains more common than kappa; sequence homology of chains	AA (Amyloid associated proteins); derived from larger precursor protein SAA; No sequence homology of polypeptide chain
2. *Associated diseases*	Plasma cell dyscrasias e.g. multiple myeloma, B cell lymphomas, others	Chronic inflammation e.g. infections (TB, leprosy, osteomyelitis, brochiectasis), autoimmune diseases (rheumatoid arthritis, IBD), cancers (RCC, Hodgkin's disease), FMF
3. *Pathogenesis*	Stimulus → Monoclonal B cell proliferation → Excess of Igs and light chains → Partial degradation → Insoluble AL fibril	Stimulus → Chronic inflammation → Activation of macrophages → Cytokines (IL1,6) → Partial degradation → AEF → Insoluble AA fibril
4. *Incidence*	Most common in US and other developed countries	Most common worldwide (particularly third world countries)
5. *Organ distribution*	Kidney, heart, bowel, nerves	Kidney, liver, spleen, adrenals
6. *Stains to distinguish*	Congophilia persists after permanganate treatment of section; specific immunostains anti-λ, anti-κ	Congophilia disappears after permanganate treatment of section; specific immunostain anti-AA

inflammatory involvement of the pleura, peritoneum, and synovium causing pain in the chest, abdomen and joints respectively. Amyloidosis occurring in these cases is AA type, suggesting relationship to secondary amyloidosis due to chronic inflammation. The distribution of this form of heredofamilial amyloidosis is similar to that of secondary amyloidosis.

iii) Rare hereditary forms. Heredofamilial mutations of several normal proteins have been reported e.g. apolipoprotein I (AApoAI), gelsolin (Agel), lysozyme (ALys), fibrinogen α-chain (AFib), and cystatin C (ACys) etc. These types may also result systemic amyloidosis.

B. LOCALISED AMYLOIDOSIS

1. Senile cardiac amyloidosis (ATTR). Senile cardiac amyloidosis is seen in 50% of people above the age of 70 years. The deposits are seen in the heart and aorta. The type of amyloid in these cases is ATTR but without any change in the protein structure of TTR.

2. Senile cerebral amyloidosis (Aβ, APrP). Senile cerebral amyloidosis is heterogeneous group of amyloid deposition of varying etiologies that includes sporadic, familial, hereditary and infectious. Some of the important diseases associated with cerebral amyloidosis and the corresponding amyloid proteins are:Alzheimer's disease (Aβ), Down's syndrome (Aβ) and transmissible spongiform encephalopathies (APrP) such as in Creutzfeldt-Jakob disease, fatal familial insomnia, mad cow disease, kuru.

In Alzheimer's disease, deposit of amyloid is seen as Congophilic angiopathy (amyloid material in the walls of cerebral blood vessels), neurofibrillary tangles and in senile plaques.

3. Endocrine amyloidosis (Hormone precursors). Some endocrine tumours are associated with microscopic deposits of amyloid e.g. in medullary carcinoma of the thyroid (procalcitonin), islet cell tumour of the pancreas (islet amyloid polypeptide), type 2 diabetes mellitus and insulinoma (pro-insulin), pituitary amyloid (prolactin), isolated atrial amyloid deposits (atrial nitouretic factor), and familial corneal amyloidosis (lactoferrin).

4. Localised tumour forming amyloid (AL). Sometimes, isolated tumour like formation of amyloid deposits are seen e.g. in lungs, larynx, skin, urinary bladder, tongue, eye, isolated atrial amyloid. In most of these cases, the amyloid type is AL.

STAINING CHARACTERISTICS OF AMYLOID

1. STAIN ON GROSS. The oldest method since the time of Virchow for demonstrating amyloid on cut surface of a gross specimen, or on the frozen/paraffin section is iodine stain. Lugol's iodine imparts *purple* colour to the amyloid-containing area which on addition of dilute sulfuric acid turns blue. This starch-like property of amyloid is due to AP component, a glycoprotein, present in all forms of amyloid.

Various stains and techniques employed to distinguish and confirm amyloid deposits in sections are as given in Table 4.12.

2. H & E. Amyloid by light microscopy with haematoxylin and eosin staining appears as extracellular, homogeneous, structureless and eosinophilic hyaline material, especially in relation to blood vessels. However, if the deposits are small, they are difficult to detect by routine H and E stains. Besides, a few other hyaline deposits may also take pink colour (page 42).

3. METACHROMATIC STAINS (ROSANILINE DYES). Amyloid has the property of metachromasia i.e. the dye reacts with amyloid and undergoes a colour change. Metachromatic stains employed are rosaniline dyes such as methyl violet and crystal violet which impart *rose-pink* colouration to amyloid deposits. However, small amounts of amyloid are missed, mucins also have metachromasia and that aqueous mountants are required for seeing the preparation. Therefore, this method has low sensitivity and lacks specificity.

4. CONGO RED AND POLARISED LIGHT. All types of amyloid have affinity for Congo red stain; therefore this method is used for confirmation of amyloid of all types. The stain may be used on both gross specimens and microscopic sections; amyloid of all types stains *red colour*. If the stained section is viewed in polarised light, the amyloid characteristically shows *apple-green birefringence* due to cross-β-pleated sheet configuration of amyloid fibrils. The stain can also be used to distinguish between AL and AA amyloid (primary and

TABLE 4.12: Staining Characteristics of Amyloid.

STAIN	APPEARANCE
1. *H & E*	Pink, hyaline, homogeneous
2. *Methyl violet/Crystal violet*	Metachromasia: rose-pink
3. *Congo red*	Light microscopy: pink red
	Polarising light: red-green birefringence
4. *Thioflavin-T/Thioflavin-S*	Ultraviolet light: fluorescence
5. *Immunohistochemistry (antibody against fibril protein)*	Immunoreactivity: Positive
6. *Non-specific stains:*	
i) Standard toluidine blue	Orthochromatic blue, polarising ME dark red
ii) Alcian blue	Blue-green

secondary amyloid respectively). After prior treatment with permanganate or trypsin on the section, Congo red stain is repeated—in the case of primary amyloid (AL amyloid), the Congo red positivity (congophilia) persists,* while it turns negative for Congo red in secondary amyloid (AA amyloid). Congo red dye can also be used as an *in vivo* test (described below).

5. FLUORESCENT STAINS. Fluorescent stain thioflavin-T binds to amyloid and fluoresce *yellow* under ultraviolet light, i.e. amyloid emits secondary fluorescence. Thioflavin-S is less specific.

6. IMMUNOHISTOCHEMISTRY. More recently, type of amyloid can be classified by immunohistochemical stains. Various antibody stains against the specific antigenic protein types of amyloid are commercially available. However, more useful ones are *anti-AP* for confirmation of presence of amyloid of all types, and *anti-AA*, and *anti-lambda (λ)* and *anti- kappa (κ)* antibody stains for fibril protein of specific types by positive immunoreactivity.

7. NON-SPECIFIC STAINS. A few stains have been described for amyloid at different times but they lack specificity. These are as under:

i) Standard toluidine blue: This method gives *orthochromatic blue* colour to amyloid which under polarising microscopy produces *dark red* birefringence. However, there are false positive as well as false negative results; hence not recommended.

ii) Alcian blue: It imparts *blue-green* colour to amyloid positive areas and is used for mucopolysaccharide content in amyloid but uptake of dye is poor and variable.

iii) Periodic acid Schiff (PAS): It is used for demonstration of carbohydrate content of amyloid but shows variable positivity and is not specific.

DIAGNOSIS OF AMYLOIDOSIS

Amyloidosis may be detected as an unsuspected morphologic finding in a case, or the changes may be severe so as to produce symptoms and may even cause death. The diagnosis of amyloid disease can be made from the following investigations:

1. BIOPSY EXAMINATION. Histologic examination of biopsy material is the commonest and confirmatory method for diagnosis in a suspected case of amyloidosis. Biopsy of an obviously *affected organ* is likely to offer the best results e.g. *kidney biopsy* in a case on dialysis, sural nerve biopsy in familial polyneuropathy. In systemic amyloidosis, renal biopsy provides the best detection rate, but *rectal biopsy* also has a good pick up rate. However, *gingiva* and *skin biopsy* have poor result. More recently, fine needle aspiration of abdominal *subcutaneous fat* followed by Congo red staining and polarising microscopic examination for confirmation has become an acceptable simple and useful technique with excellent result.

2. IN VIVO CONGO RED TEST. A known quantity of Congo red dye may be injected intravenously in living patient. If amyloidosis is present, the dye gets bound to amyloid deposits and its levels in blood rapidly decline. The test is, however, not popular due to the risk of anaphylaxis to the injected dye.

3. OTHER TESTS. A few other tests which are not diagnostic but are supportive of amyloid disease are protein electrophoresis, immunoelectrophoresis of urine and serum, and bone marrow aspiration.

PATHOLOGIC CHANGES IN AMYLOIDOSIS OF ORGANS

Although amyloidosis of different organs shows variation in morphologic pattern, some features are applicable in general to most of the involved organs.

Macroscopically, the affected organ is usually enlarged, pale and rubbery. Cut surface shows firm, waxy and translucent parenchyma which takes positive staining with the iodine test.

Microscopically, the deposits of amyloid are found in the extracellular locations, initially in the walls of small blood vessels producing microscopic changes and effects, while later the deposits are in large amounts causing macroscopic changes and effects of pressure atrophy.

Based on these general features of amyloidosis, the salient pathologic findings of major organ involvements are described below.

Amyloidosis of Kidneys

Amyloidosis of the kidneys is most common and most serious because of ill-effects on renal function. The deposits in the kidneys are found in most cases of secondary amyloidosis and in about one-third cases of primary amyloidosis. Amyloidosis of the kidney accounts for about 20% of deaths from amyloidosis. Even small quantities of amyloid deposits in the glomeruli can cause proteinuria and nephrotic syndrome.

*Easy way to remember: Three *ps* i.e. *p*ersistence of congophilia in *p*rimary amyloid after *p*ermanganate treatment.

Grossly, the kidneys may be normal-sized, enlarged or terminally contracted due to ischaemic effect of narrowing of vascular lumina. Cut surface is pale, waxy and translucent.

Microscopically, amyloid deposition occurs primarily in the glomeruli, though it may involve peritubular interstitial tissue and the walls of arterioles as well (Fig. 4.9):

- *In the glomeruli*, the deposits initially appear on the basement membrane of the glomerular capillaries, but later extend to produce luminal narrowing and distortion of the glomerular capillary tuft. This results in abnormal increase in permeability of the glomerular capillaries to macromolecules with consequent proteinuria and nephrotic syndrome.
- *In the tubules*, the amyloid deposits likewise begin close to the tubular epithelial basement membrane. Subsequently, the deposits may extend further outwards into the intertubular connective tissue, and inwards to produce degenerative changes in the tubular epithelial cells and amyloid casts in the tubular lumina.
- The *vascular involvement* affects chiefly the walls of small arterioles and venules, producing narrowing of their lumina and consequent ischaemic effects (COLOUR PLATE IV: CL 15)

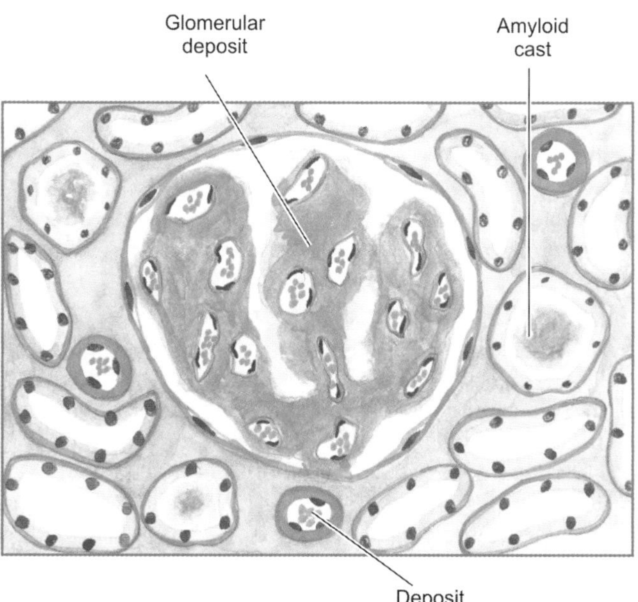

FIGURE 4.9

Amyloidosis of kidney. The amyloid deposits are seen mainly in the glomerular capillary tuft. The deposits are also present in peritubular connective tissue producing atrophic tubules and amyloid casts in the tubular lumina, and in the arterial wall producing luminal narrowing.

Amyloidosis of Spleen

Amyloid deposition in the spleen, for some unknown reasons, may have one of the following two patterns (Fig. 4.10):

1. **'SAGO SPLEEN'.** The splenomegaly is not marked and cut surface shows characteristic translucent pale and waxy nodules resembling sago grains and hence the name.

   Microscopically, the amyloid deposits begin in the walls of the arterioles of the white pulp and may subsequently replace the follicles.

2. **'LARDACEOUS SPLEEN'.** There is generally moderate to marked splenomegaly (weight up to 1 kg). Cut surface of the spleen shows map-like areas of amyloid (lardaceous-lard-like; *lard* means fat of pigs).

   Microscopically, the deposits involve the walls of splenic sinuses and the small arteries and in the connective tissue of the red pulp (COLOUR PLATE IV: CL 16).

Amyloidosis of Liver

In about half the cases of systemic amyloidosis, liver involvement by amyloidosis is seen.

Grossly, the liver is often enlarged, pale, waxy and firm.

Histologically, the features are as under (Fig. 4.11):

- The amyloid initially appears in the space of Disse (the space between the hepatocytes and sinusoidal endothelial cells).
- Later, as it increases, it compresses the cords of hepatocytes so that eventually the liver cells are shrunken and atrophic and replaced by amyloid. However, hepatic function remains normal even at an advanced stage of the disease.
- To a lesser extent, portal tracts and Kupffer cells are involved in amyloidosis.

Amyloidosis of Heart

Heart is involved in systemic amyloidosis quite commonly, more so in the primary than in secondary systemic amyloidosis. It may also be involved in localised form of amyloidosis in very old patients. Amyloidosis of the heart may produce arrhythmias due to deposition in the conduction system.

Grossly, the heart is often normal in size. However, at times it may be enlarged and show tiny nodular deposits of amyloid underneath the endocardium, subendocardially and between the myocardial fibres. Later, there may be a pressure atrophy of the

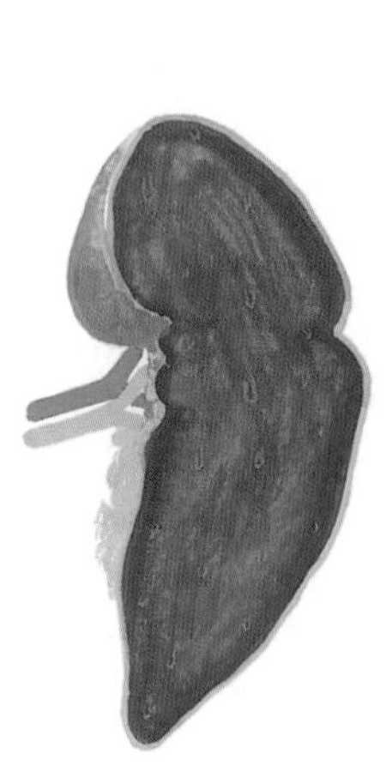

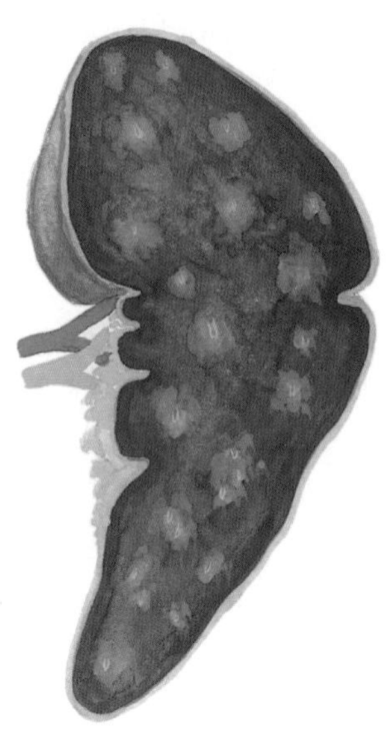

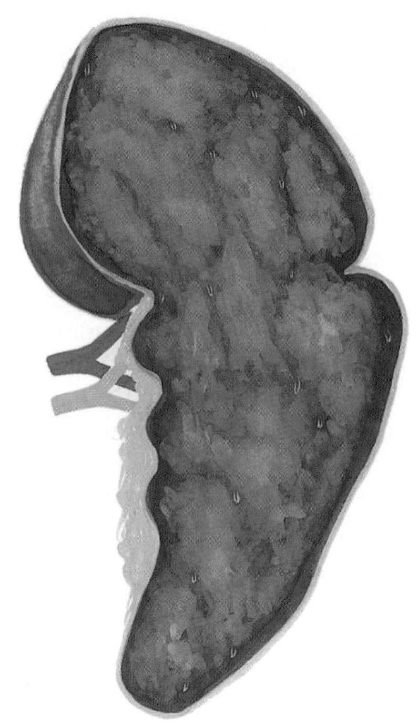

FIGURE 4.10

Macroscopic patterns of amyloidosis of the spleen.

myocardial fibres and impaired ventricular function which may produce restrictive cardiomyopathy.

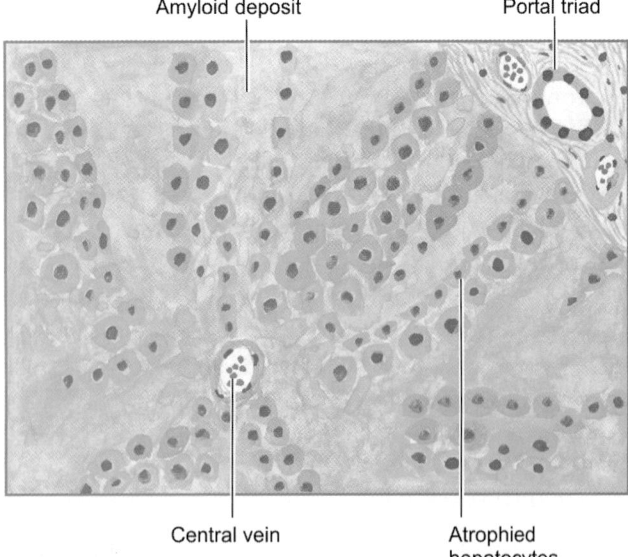

FIGURE 4.11

Amyloidosis of the liver. The deposition is extensive in the space of Disse causing compression and pressure atrophy of hepatocytes.

Amyloidosis of Alimentary Tract

Involvement of the gastrointestinal tract by amyloidosis may occur at any level from the oral cavity to the anus. Rectal and gingival biopsies are the common sites for diagnosis of systemic amyloidosis. The deposits are initially located around the small blood vessels but later may involve adjacent layers of the bowel wall. Tongue may be the site for tumour-forming amyloid, producing macroglossia.

Other Organs

Uncommonly, the deposits of amyloid may occur in various other tissues such as pituitary, thyroid, adrenals, skin, lymph nodes, respiratory tract and peripheral and autonomic nerves.

Thus, amyloidosis may be an incidental finding at autopsy or in symptomatic cases diagnosis can be made from the methods given above, biopsy examination being the most important method. The prognosis of patients with generalised amyloidosis is generally poor; between the two forms of generalised amyloidosis, however, secondary reactive amyloidosis has somewhat better outcome due to controllable underlying condition. Renal failure and cardiac arrhythmias are the most common causes of death in systemic amyloidosis.

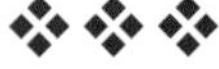

Haemodynamic Disorders

5

INTERNAL ENVIRONMENT

Many workers have pointed out that life on earth probably arose in the sea, and that the body water which is the environment of the cells, is similar to the ancient ocean from where life began. Although it appears quite tempting to draw comparison between environment of the cell and the ancient oceans but it would be rather an oversimplification in considering the cellular environment to be wholly fluid ignoring the presence of cells, fibres and ground substance.

Claude Bernarde (1949) first coined the term *internal environment or milieu interieur* for the state in the body in which the interstitial fluid that bathes the cells and the plasma, together maintain the normal morphology and function of the cells and tissues of the body. The mechanism by which the constancy of the internal environment is maintained and ensured is called the *homeostasis.* For this purpose, living membranes with varying permeabilities such as vascular endothelium and the cell wall play important role in exchange of fluids, electrolytes, nutrients and metabolites across the compartments of body fluids.

The normal composition of internal environment consists of the following components (Fig. 5.1):

1. WATER. Water is the principal and essential constituent of the body. The total body water in a normal adult male comprises 50-70% (average 60%) of the body weight and about 10% less in a normal adult female (average 50%). Thus, the body of a normal man weighing 65 kg contains approximately 40 litres of water. The total body water (assuming average of 60%) is distributed into 2 main compartments of body fluids separated from each other by membranes freely permeable to water. These are as under (Fig. 5.2):

i) Intracellular fluid compartment. This comprises about 33% of the body weight, the bulk of which is contained in the muscles.

ii) Extracellular fluid compartment. This constitutes the remaining 27% of body weight containing water. Included in this are the following 4 subdivisions of extracellular fluid (ECF):

a) Interstitial fluid including lymph fluid constitutes the major proportion of ECF (12% of body weight).

b) Intravascular fluid or blood plasma comprises about 5% of the body weight. Thus plasma content is about 3 litres of fluid out of 5 litres of total blood volume.

c) Mesenchymal tissues such as dense connective tissue, cartilage and bone contain body water that comprises about 9% of the body weight.

d) Transcellular fluid constitutes 1% of body weight. This is the fluid contained in the secretions of secretory cells of the body e.g. skin, salivary glands, mucous membranes of alimentary and respiratory tracts, pancreas, liver and biliary tract, kidneys, gonads, thyroid, lacrimal gland and CSF.

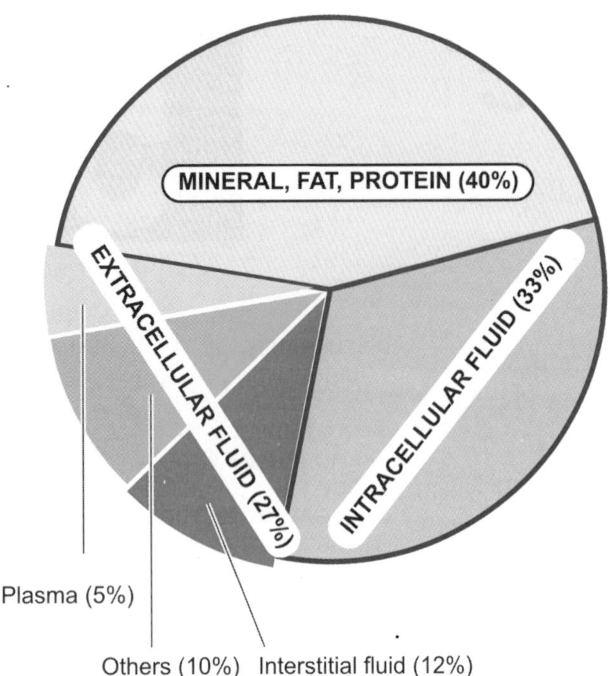

FIGURE 5.1

Body fluid compartments.

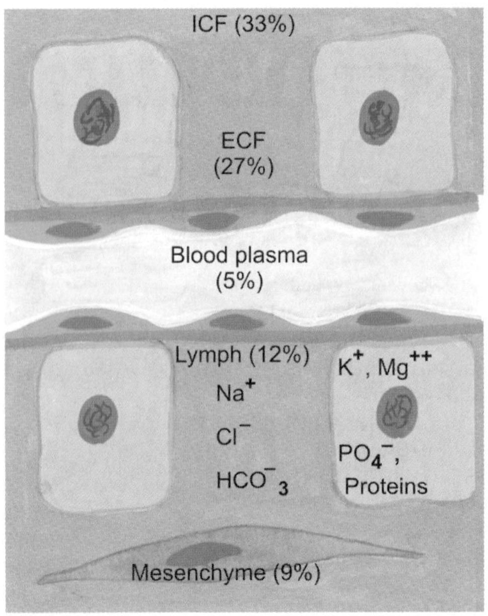

FIGURE 5.2

Body fluid compartments. (ICF = intracellular fluid compartment; ECF = extracellular fluid compartment).

2. **ELECTROLYTES.** The concentration of cations (positively charged) and anions (negatively charged) is different in intracellular and extracellular fluids:

■ *In the intracellular fluid,* the main cations are potassium and magnesium and the main anions are phosphates and proteins. It has low concentration of sodium and chloride.

■ *In the extracellular fluid,* the predominant cation is sodium and the principal anions are chloride and bicarbonate. Besides these, a small proportion of non-diffusible proteins and some diffusible nutrients and metabolites such as glucose and urea are present in the ECF.

The essential difference between the two main subdivisions of ECF is the higher protein content in the plasma than in the interstitial fluid which plays an important role in maintaining fluid balance.

The **major functions** of electrolytes are as follows:

i) Electrolytes are the main solutes in the body fluids for maintenance of acid-base equilibrium.

ii) Electrolytes maintain the proper osmolality and volume of body fluids (*Osmolality* is the solute concentration per kg water compared from *osmolarity* which is the solute concentration per litre solution).

iii) The concentration of certain electrolytes determines their specific physiologic functions e.g. the effect of calcium ions on neuromuscular excitability. The concentration of the major electrolytes is expressed in milli-equivalent (mEq) per litre so as to compare the values directly with each other. In order to convert mg per dl into mEq per litre the following formula is used:

$$\text{mEq/L} = \frac{\text{mg/dl}}{\text{Eq weight of element}} \times 10$$

NORMAL WATER AND ELECTROLYTE BALANCE (GIBBS-DONNAN EQUILIBRIUM)

Normally, a state of balance exists between the amount of water absorbed into the body and that which is eliminated from the body. The water as well as electrolytes are distributed nearly constantly in different body fluid compartments.

1. Water is normally *absorbed* into the body from the bowel or is introduced parenterally; average intake being 2800 ml per day.

2. Water is *eliminated* from the body via:

■ kidneys in the urine (average 1500 ml per day):

■ via the skin as insensible loss in perspiration or as sweat (average 800 ml per day), though there is wide variation in loss via sweat depending upon weather, temperature, fever and exercise;

■ via the lungs in exhaled air (average 400 ml per day); and

- minor losses via the faeces (average 100 ml per day) and lacrimal, nasal, oral, sexual and mammary (milk) secretions.

The cell wall as well as capillary endothelium are entirely permeable to water but they differ in their permeability to electrolytes. Capillary wall is completely permeable to electrolytes while the cell membrane is somewhat impermeable. As mentioned earlier, concentration of potassium and phosphate are high in the intracellular fluid whereas concentration of sodium and chloride are high in the ECF. The osmotic equilibrium between the two major body fluid compartments is maintained by the passage of water from or into the intracellular compartment. The 2 main subdivisions of ECF—blood plasma and interstitial fluid, are separated from each other by capillary wall which is freely permeable to water but does not allow free passage of macromolecules of plasma proteins resulting in higher protein content in the plasma.

ACID-BASE BALANCE

Besides changes in the volume of fluids in the compartments, changes in ionic equilibrium affecting the acid-base balance of fluids occur. In terms of body fluids,

- an *acid* is a molecule or ion which is capable of giving off a hydrogen ion (H^+ ion donor); and
- a base is a molecule or ion which is capable of taking up hydrogen ion (H^+ ion acceptor).

A number of acids such as carbonic, phosphoric, sulfuric, lactic, hydrochloric and ketoacids are formed during normal metabolic activity. However, carbonic acid is produced in largest amount as it is the end-product of aerobic tissue activity. In spite of these acids, the pH of the blood is kept constant at 7.4 $\pm$ 0.05 in health.

The pH of blood and acid-base balance are regulated in the body by the following factors:

1. BUFFER SYSTEM. Buffers are substances which have weak acids and strong bases and limit the change in H^+ ion concentration to the normal range. They are the first line of defense for maintaining acid-base balance and do so by taking up H^+ ions when the pH rises. The most important buffer which regulates the pH of blood is *bicarbonate-carbonic acid system* followed by *intracellular buffering action of haemoglobin* and *carbonic anhydrase* in the red cells.

2. PULMONARY MECHANISM. During respiration, CO_2 is removed by the lungs depending upon the partial pressure of CO_2 in the arterial blood. With ingestion of high quantity of acid-forming salts, ventilation is increased as seen in acidosis in diabetic ketosis and uraemia.

3. RENAL MECHANISM. The other route by which H^+ ions can be excreted from the body is in the urine. Here H^+ ions secreted by the renal tubular cells are buffered in the glomerular filtrate by:

- *combining with phosphates* to form phosphoric acid;
- *combining with ammonia* to form ammonium ions; and
- *combining with filtered bicarbonate ions* to form carbonic acid.

However, carbonic acid formed is dissociated to form CO_2 which diffuses back into the blood to reform bicarbonate ions.

PRESSURE GRADIENTS AND FLUID EXCHANGES

Aside from water and electrolytes or crystalloids, both of which are freely interchanged between the interstitial fluid and plasma, the ECF contains colloids like proteins which minimally cross the capillary wall. These substances exert pressures responsible for exchange between the interstitial fluid and plasma.

Normal Fluid Pressures (Fig. 5.3,A)

1. OSMOTIC PRESSURE. This is the pressure exerted by the chemical constituents of the body fluids. Accordingly, osmotic pressure may be of the following types:

- **Crystalloid osmotic pressure** exerted by electrolytes present in the ECF and comprises the major portion of the total osmotic pressure.
- **Colloid osmotic pressure or oncotic pressure** exerted by proteins present in the ECF and constitutes a small part of the total osmotic pressure but is more significant physiologically. Since the protein content of the plasma is higher than that of interstitial fluid, oncotic pressure of plasma is higher (average 25 mmHg) than that of interstitial fluid (average 8 mmHg).
- **Effective oncotic pressure** is the difference between the higher oncotic pressure of plasma and the lower oncotic pressure of interstitial fluid and is *the force that tends to draw fluid into the vessels.*

2. HYDROSTATIC PRESSURE. This is the capillary blood pressure.

There is considerable *pressure gradient* at the two ends of capillary loop—being higher at the arteriolar end (average 32 mmHg) than at the venular end (average 12 mmHg).

- **Tissue tension** is the hydrostatic pressure of interstitial fluid and is lower than the hydrostatic

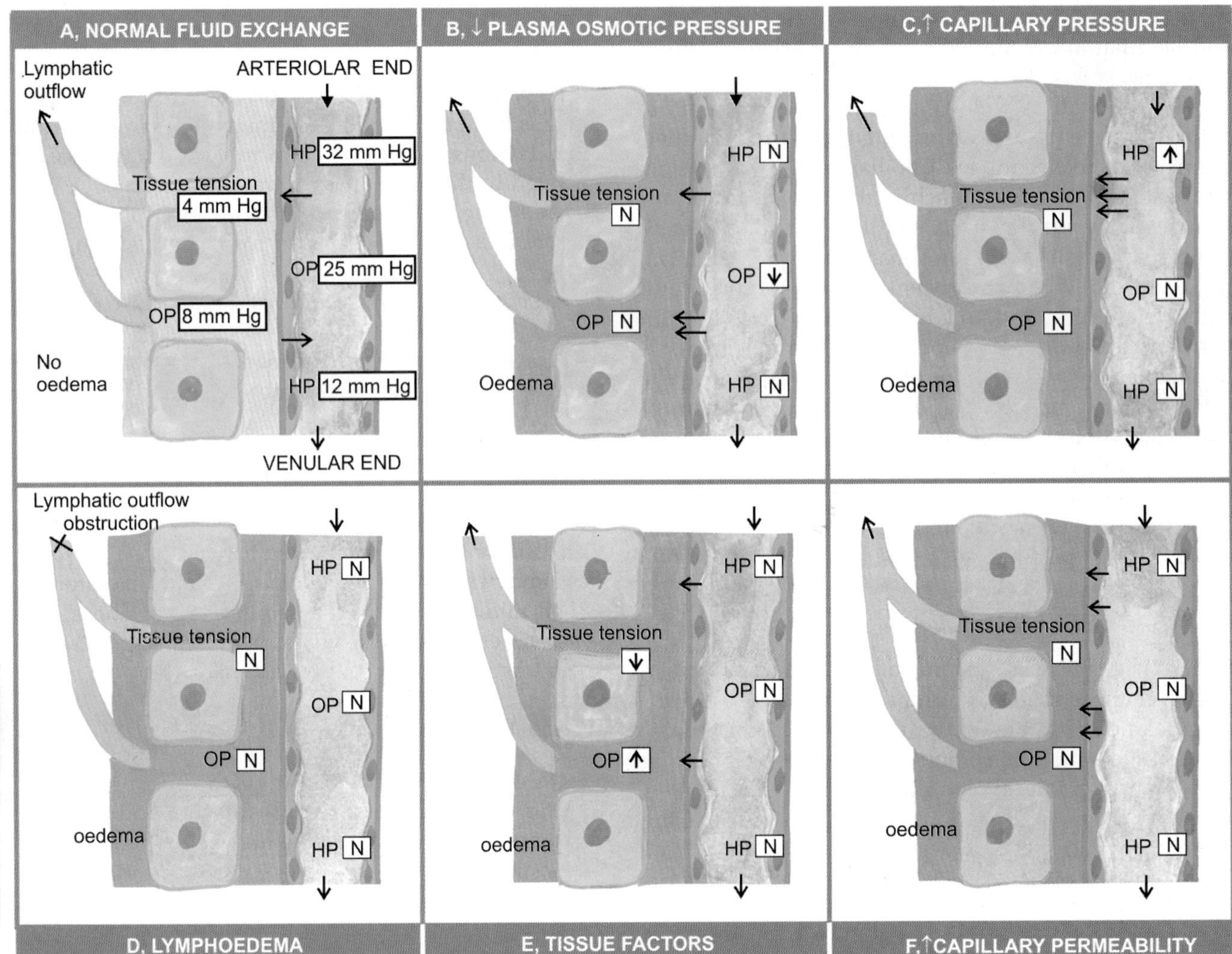

FIGURE 5.3

Diagrammatic representation of pathogenesis of oedema (OP = oncotic pressure; HP = hydrostatic pressure). A, Normal pressure gradients and fluid exchanges between plasma, interstitial space and lymphatics. B, Mechanism of oedema by decreased plasma oncotic pressure and hypoproteinaemia. C, Mechanism of oedema by increased hydrostatic pressure in the capillary. D, Mechanism of lymphoedema. E, Mechanism by tissue factors (increased oncotic pressure of interstitial fluid and lowered tissue tension). F, Mechanism of oedema by increased capillary permeability.

pressure in the capillary at either end (average 4 mmHg).

- **Effective hydrostatic pressure** is the difference between the higher hydrostatic pressure in the capillary and the lower tissue tension; it is *the force that drives fluid through the capillary wall into the interstitial space.*

Normal Fluid Exchanges

Normally, the fluid exchanges between the body compartments take place as under (Fig. 5.3,A):

- *At the arteriolar end of the capillary,* the balance between the hydrostatic pressure (32 mmHg) and plasma oncotic pressure (25 mmHg) is the hydrostatic pressure of 7 mmHg which is the outward-driving force so that a small quantity of fluid and solutes leave the vessel to enter the interstitial space.
- *At the venular end of the capillary,* the balance between the hydrostatic pressure (12 mmHg) and plasma oncotic pressure (25 mmHg) is the oncotic pressure of 13 mmHg which is the inward-driving force so that the fluid and solutes re-enter the plasma.
- *The tissue fluid* left after exchanges across the capillary wall escapes into the lymphatics from where it is finally drained into venous circulation.
- *Tissue factors* i.e. oncotic pressure of interstitial fluid and tissue tension, are normally small and insignificant

forces opposing the plasma hydrostatic pressure and capillary hydrostatic pressure, respectively.

DISTURBANCES OF BODY FLUIDS AND ELECTROLYTES

The common derangements of body fluid are as follows:
1. Oedema;
2. Overhydration; and
3. Dehydration or pure water deficiency.

These are discussed below.

OEDEMA

DEFINITION ANDTYPES

The Greek word *oidema* means swelling. *Oedema may be defined as abnormal and excessive accumulation of fluid in the interstitial tissue spaces and serous cavities.* The presence of abnormal collection of fluid within the cell is sometimes called intracellular oedema but should more appropriately be called hydropic degeneration (page 41). The accumulation of fluid in the body cavities is correspondingly known as ascites (in the peritoneal cavity), hydrothorax or pleural effusion (in the pleural cavity), and hydropericardium or pericardial effusion (in the pericardial cavity). The oedema may be of 2 main types (Fig. 5.4):

1. *Localised* in the organ or limb; and
2. *Generalised (anasarca or dropsy)* when it is systemic in distribution, particularly noticeable in the subcutaneous tissues.

Besides, there are a few special forms of oedema.

The oedema fluid lies free in the interstitial space between the cells and can be displaced from one place to another. In the case of oedema in the subcutaneous tissues, momentary pressure of finger produces a depression known as *pitting oedema*. The other variety is *non-pitting* or *solid oedema* in which no pitting is produced on pressure e.g. in myxoedema, elephantiasis. Oedema fluid may be:

- *transudate* which is more often the case, such as in oedema of cardiac and renal disease; or
- *exudate* such as in inflammatory oedema.

The differences between transudate and exudate are tabulated in Table 5.1.

PATHOGENESIS OF OEDEMA

Oedema is caused by mechanisms that interfere with normal fluid balance of plasma, interstitial fluid and lymph flow. The following six mechanisms may be operating singly or in combination to produce oedema:

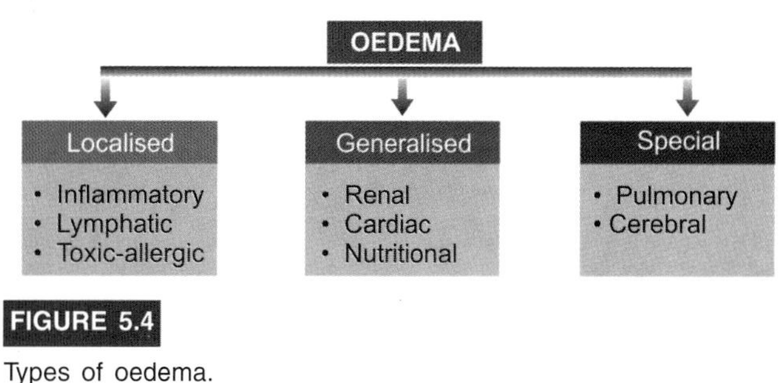

FIGURE 5.4

Types of oedema.

1. Decreased plasma oncotic pressure
2. Increased capillary hydrostatic pressure
3. Lymphatic obstruction
4. Tissue factors (increased oncotic pressure of interstitial fluid, and decreased tissue tension)
5. Increased capillary permeability
6. Sodium and water retention.

These mechanisms are discussed below and illustrated in Fig. 5.3:

1. DECREASED PLASMA ONCOTIC PRESSURE. The plasma oncotic pressure exerted by the total amount of plasma proteins tends to draw fluid into the vessels normally. A fall in the total plasma protein level (hypoproteinaemia of less than 5 g/dl), results in lowering of plasma oncotic pressure in a way that it can no longer counteract the effect of hydrostatic pressure of blood. This results in increased outward movement of fluid from the capillary wall and decreased inward movement of fluid from the interstitial space causing oedema (Fig. 5.3,B). Hypoproteinaemia usually produces generalised oedema (anasarca). Out of the various plasma proteins, albumin has four times higher plasma oncotic pressure than globulin so that it is hypoalbuminaemia (albumin below 2.5 g/dl) that results in oedema more often.

The **examples** of oedema by this mechanism are seen in the following conditions:

i) *Oedema of renal disease* e.g. in nephrotic syndrome, acute glomerulonephritis.

ii) *Ascites* of liver disease e.g. in cirrhosis.

iii) *Oedema due to other causes* of hypoproteinaemia e.g. in protein-losing enteropathy.

2. INCREASED CAPILLARY HYDROSTATIC PRESSURE. The hydrostatic pressure of the capillary is the force that normally tends to drive fluid through the capillary wall into the interstitial space by counteracting the force of plasma oncotic pressure. A rise in the hydrostatic pressure at the venular end of the capillary which is normally low (average 12 mmHg) to a level more than the plasma oncotic pressure results in

TABLE 5.1: Differences between Transudate and Exudate.

FEATURE	TRANSUDATE	EXUDATE
1. *Definition*	Filtrate of blood plasma without changes in endothelial permeability	Oedema of inflamed tissue associated with increased vascular permeability
2. *Character*	Non-inflammatory oedema	Inflammatory oedema
3. *Protein content*	Low (less than 1 g/dl); mainly albumin, low fibrinogen; hence no tendency to coagulate	High (2.5-3.5 g/dl), readily coagulates due to high content of fibrinogen and other coagulation factors
4. *Glucose content*	Same as in plasma	Low (less than 60 mg/dl)
5. *Specific gravity*	Low (less than 1.015)	High (more than 1.018)
6. *pH*	> 7.3	< 7.3
7. *LDH*	Low	High
8. *Effusion LDH/ Serum LDH ratio*	< 0.6	> 0.6
9. *Cells*	Few cells, mainly mesothelial cells and cellular debris	Many cells, inflammatory as well as parenchymal
10. *Examples*	Oedema in congestive cardiac failure	Purulent exudate such as pus

Chapter Five

minimal or no reabsorption of fluid at the venular end, consequently leading to oedema (Fig. 5.3,C).

The **examples** of oedema by this mechanism are seen in the following disorders:

i) *Oedema of cardiac disease* e.g. in congestive cardiac failure, constrictive pericarditis.

ii) *Ascites of liver disease* e.g. in cirrhosis of liver.

iii) *Passive congestion* e.g. in mechanical obstruction due to thrombosis of veins of the lower legs, varicosities, pressure by pregnant uterus, tumours etc.

iv) *Postural oedema* e.g. transient oedema of feet and ankles due to increased venous pressure seen in individuals who remain standing erect for longtime such as traffic constables.

3. LYMPHATIC OBSTRUCTION. Normally the interstitial fluid in the tissue spaces escapes by way of lymphatics so that obstruction to outflow of these channels causes localised oedema, known as lymphoedema (Fig. 5.3,D).

The **examples** of lymphoedema include the following:

i) *Removal of axillary lymph nodes* in radical mastectomy for carcinoma of the breast produces lymphoedema of the affected arm.

ii) *Pressure from outside* on the main abdominal or thoracic duct such as due to tumours, effusions in serous cavities etc may produce lymphoedema. At times, the main lymphatic channel may rupture and discharge chyle into the pleural cavity (chylothorax) or into peritoneal cavity (chylous ascites).

iii) *Inflammation of the lymphatics* as seen in filariasis (infection with *Wuchereria bancrofti*) results in chronic lymphoedema of scrotum and legs known as elephantiasis.

iv) *Occlusion of lymphatic channels* by malignant cells may result in lymphoedema.

v) *Milroy's disease or hereditary lymphoedema* is due to abnormal development of lymphatic channels. It is seen in families and the oedema is mainly confined to one or both the lower limbs (Chapter 11).

4. TISSUE FACTORS. The forces acting in the interstitial space—oncotic pressure of the interstitial space and tissue tension, are normally quite small and insignificant to counteract the effects of plasma oncotic pressure and capillary hydrostatic pressure respectively. However, in some situations, the tissue factors in combination with other mechanisms play a role in causation of oedema (Fig. 5.3,E). These are as under:

i) *Elevation of oncotic pressure of interstitial fluid* as occurs due to increased vascular permeability and inadequate removal of proteins by lymphatics.

ii) Lowered tissue tension as seen in *loose subcutaneous tissues* of eyelids and external genitalia.

5. INCREASED CAPILLARY PERMEABILITY. As described previously, an intact capillary endothelium is a semipermeable membrane which permits the free flow of water and crystalloids but allows minimal passage of plasma proteins normally. However, when the capillary endothelium is injured by various 'capillary poisons' such as toxins and their products, histamine, anoxia, venoms, certain drugs and chemicals, the capillary permeability to plasma proteins is enhanced due to development of gaps between the endothelial cells. This, in turn, causes reduced plasma oncotic pressure and elevated oncotic pressure of interstitial fluid which consequently produces oedema (Fig. 5.3,F).

The **examples** of oedema by this mechanism are seen in the following conditions:

i) *Generalised oedema* due to increased vascular permeability may occur in systemic infections, poisonings, certain drugs and chemicals, anaphylactic reactions and anoxia.

ii) *Localised oedema* such as:

- *Inflammatory oedema* as seen in infections, allergic reactions, insect-bite, irritant drugs and chemicals. It is generally exudate in nature.
- *Angioneurotic oedema* is an acute attack of localised oedema occurring on the skin of face and trunk and may involve lips, larynx, pharynx and lungs. It is possibly neurogenic or allergic in origin.

6. SODIUM AND WATER RETENTION. Before describing the mechanism of oedema by sodium and water retention, it is essential to recollect the normal regulatory mechanism of sodium and water balance.

Normally, about 80% of sodium is reabsorbed by the proximal convoluted tubule under the influence of intrinsic renal mechanism or extra-renal mechanism:

- **Intrinsic renal mechanism** is activated in response to sudden reduction in the effective arterial blood volume (hypovolaemia) as occurs in severe haemorrhage. Hypovolaemia stimulates the arterial baroreceptors present in the carotid sinus and aortic arch which, in turn, send the sympathetic outflow via the vasomotor centre in the brain. As a result of this, renal ischaemia occurs which causes reduction in the glomerular filtration rate, decreased excretion of sodium in the urine and consequent retention of sodium.

- **Extra-renal mechanism** involves the secretion of aldosterone, a sodium retaining hormone, by the *renin-angiotensin-aldosterone system*. Renin is an enzyme secreted by the granular cells in the juxta-glomerular apparatus. Its release is stimulated in response to low concentration of sodium in the tubules. Its main action is stimulation of the angiotensinogen which is α_2-globulin or renin substrate present in the plasma. On stimulation, angiotensin I, a decapeptide, is formed in the plasma which is subsequently converted into angiotensin II, an octapeptide, in the lungs and kidneys. Angiotensin II stimulates the adrenal cortex to secrete aldosterone hormone. Aldosterone increases sodium reabsorption in the renal tubules and sometimes causes a rise in the blood pressure.

- **ADH mechanism**. Retention of sodium leads to retention of water secondarily under the influence of anti-diuretic hormone (ADH) or vasopressin. This hormone is secreted by the cells of the supraoptic and paraventricular nuclei in the hypothalamus and is stored in the neurohypophysis (posterior pituitary). The release of hormone is stimulated by increased concentration of sodium in the plasma and hypovolaemia. Large amounts of ADH produce highly concentrated urine.

Excessive retention of sodium and water and their decreased renal excretion occur in response to hypovolaemia and lowered concentration of sodium in the renal tubules via stimulation of intrinsic renal and extra-renal mechanisms as well as via release of ADH (Fig. 5.5).

The **examples** of oedema by these mechanims are as under:

i) *Oedema of cardiac disease* e.g. in congestive cardiac failure.
ii) *Ascites* of liver disease e.g. in cirrhosis of liver.
iii) *Oedema of renal disease* e.g. in nephrotic syndrome, glomerulonephritis.

PATHOGENESIS AND MORPHOLOGY OF IMPORTANT TYPES OF OEDEMA

As observed from the pathogenesis of oedema just described, more than one mechanism may be involved in many examples of localised and generalised oedema. Some of the important examples are described below.

Renal Oedema

Generalised oedema occurs in certain diseases of renal origin such as in nephrotic syndrome, some types of glomerulonephritis, and in renal failure due to acute tubular injury.

1. Oedema in nephrotic syndrome. Since there is persistent and heavy proteinuria (albuminuria) in nephrotic syndrome, there is hypoalbuminaemia causing decreased plasma oncotic pressure resulting in severe generalised oedema *(nephrotic oedema)*. The hypoalbuminaemia causes fall in the plasma volume activating renin-angiotensin-aldosterone mechanism which results in retention of sodium and water, thus setting in a vicious cycle which persists till the albuminuria continues. Similar type of mechanism operates in the pathogenesis of oedema in protein-losing enteropathy, further confirming the role of protein loss in the causation of oedema.

The *nephrotic oedema* is classically more severe and marked and is present in the subcutaneous tissues as well as in the visceral organs. The affected organ is enlarged and heavy with tense capsule.

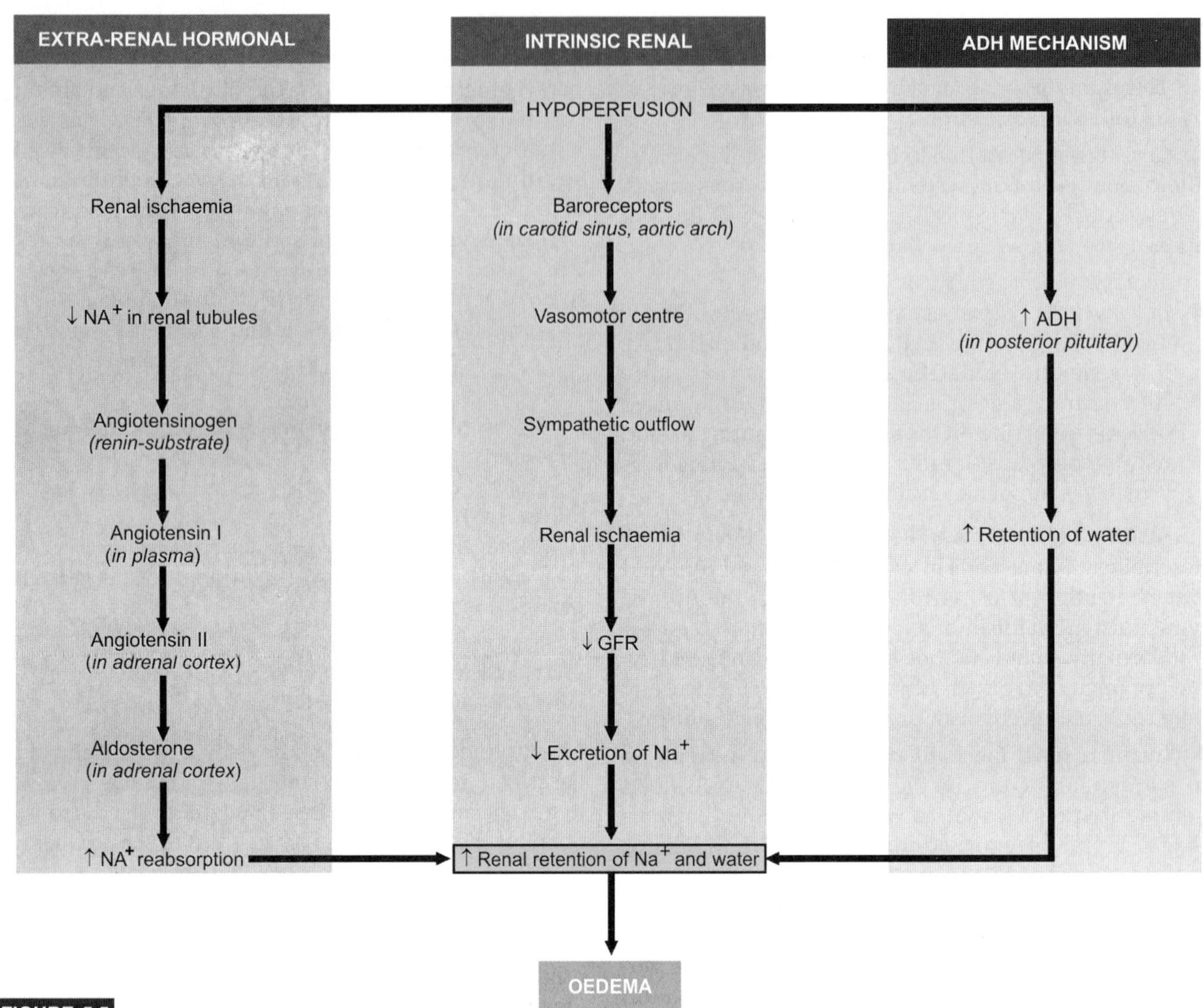

FIGURE 5.5

Mechanisms involved in oedema by sodium and water retention. On *left* and *middle* are the sequence of events in extra-renal hormonal and intrinsic-renal mechanisms respectively for sodium and water retention, whereas on *right* is shown the ADH mechanism for water retention.

Microscopically, the oedema fluid separates the connective tissue fibres of subcutaneous tissues. Depending upon the protein content, the oedema fluid may appear homogeneous, pale, eosinophilic, or may be deeply eosinophilic and granular.

2. Oedema in glomerulonephritis. Oedema occurs in conditions with diffuse glomerular disease such as in acute diffuse glomerulonephritis and rapidly progressive glomerulonephritis *(nephritic oedema).* In contrast to nephrotic oedema, nephritic oedema is not due to hypoproteinaemia but is due to excessive reabsorption of sodium and water in the renal tubules via renin-angiotensin-aldosterone mechanism. The protein content of oedema fluid in glomerulonephritis is quite low (less than 0.5 g/dl).

The *nephritic oedema* is usually mild as compared to nephrotic oedema and begins in the loose tissues such as on the face around eyes, ankles and genitalia. Oedema in these conditions is usually not affected by gravity (unlike cardiac oedema).

The salient differences between the nephrotic and nephritic oedema are outlined in Table 5.2.

3. Oedema in acute tubular injury. Acute tubular injury following shock or toxic chemicals results in gross oedema of the body. The damaged tubules lose their capacity for selective reabsorption and concentration of the glomerular filtrate resulting in increased reabsorp-

TABLE 5.2: Differences between Nephrotic and Nephritic Oedema.

FEATURE	NEPHROTIC OEDEMA	NEPHRITIC OEDEMA
1. *Cause*	Nephrotic syndrome	Glomerulonephritis (acute, rapidly progressive)
2. *Proteinuria*	Heavy	Moderate
3. *Mechanism*	↓ Plasma oncotic pressure, Na^+ and water retention	Na^+ and water retention
4. *Degree of oedema*	Severe, generalised	Mild
5. *Distribution*	Subcutaneous tissues as well as visceral organs	Loose tissues mainly (face, eyes, ankles, genitalia)

tion and oliguria. Besides, there is excessive retention of water and electrolytes and rise in blood urea.

Cardiac Oedema

Generalised oedema develops in right-sided and congestive cardiac failure. Pathogenesis of cardiac oedema is explained on the basis of the following hypotheses (Fig. 5.6):

1. Reduced cardiac output causes hypovolaemia which stimulates intrinsic-renal and extra-renal hormonal (renin-angiotensin-aldosterone) mechanisms as well as ADH secretion resulting in sodium and water retention and consequent oedema.

2. Due to heart failure, there is elevated central venous pressure which is transmitted backward to the venous end of the capillaries, raising the capillary hydrostatic pressure and consequent transudation; this is known as *back pressure hypothesis*.

3. Chronic hypoxia may injure the capillary wall causing increased capillary permeability and result in oedema; this is called *forward pressure hypothesis*. However, this theory lacks support since the oedema by this mechanism is exudate whereas the cardiac oedema is typically transudate.

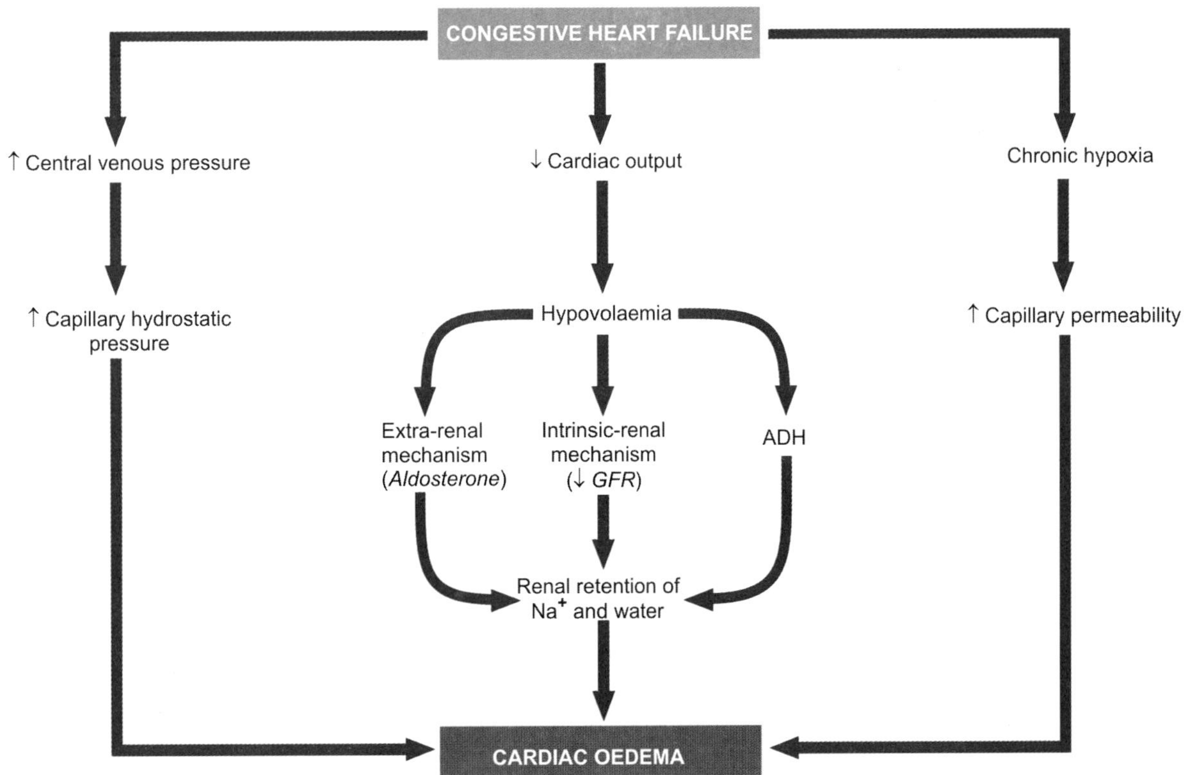

FIGURE 5.6

Mechanisms involved in the pathogenesis of cardiac oedema.

In left heart failure, the changes are, however, different. There is venous congestion, particularly in the lungs, so that pulmonary oedema develops rather than generalised oedema (described below).

Cardiac oedema is influenced by gravity and is thus characteristically *dependent oedema* i.e. in an ambulatory patient it is on the lower extremities, while in a bedridden patient oedema appears on the sacral and genital areas. The accumulation of fluid may also occur in serous cavities.

Pulmonary Oedema

Acute pulmonary oedema is the most important form of local oedema as it causes serious functional impairment but has special features. It differs from oedema elsewhere in that the fluid accumulation is not only in the tissue space but also in the pulmonary alveoli.

ETIOPATHOGENESIS. The hydrostatic pressure in the pulmonary capillaries is much lower (average 10 mmHg). Normally the plasma oncotic pressure is adequate to prevent the escape of fluid into the interstitial space and hence lungs are normally free of oedema. Pulmonary oedema can result from either the elevation of pulmonary hydrostatic pressure or the increased capillary permeability (Fig. 5.7).

1. Elevation in pulmonary hydrostatic pressure (Haemodynamic oedema). In heart failure, there is increase in the pressure in pulmonary veins which is transmitted to pulmonary capillaries. This results in imbalance between pulmonary hydrostatic pressure and the plasma oncotic pressure so that excessive fluid moves out of pulmonary capillaries into the interstitium of the lungs. Simultaneously, the endothelium of the pulmonary capillaries develops fenestrations permitting passage of plasma proteins and fluid into the interstitium. The interstitial fluid so collected is cleared by the lymphatics present around the bronchioles, small muscular arteries and veins. As the capacity of the lymphatics to drain the fluid is exceeded (about tenfold increase in fluid), the excess fluid starts accumulating in the interstitium *(interstitial oedema)* i.e. in the loose tissues around bronchioles, arteries and in the lobular septa. Next follows the thickening of the alveolar walls because of the interstitial oedema. Upto this stage, no significant impairment of gaseous exchange occurs. However, prolonged elevation of hydrostatic pressure and due to high pressure of interstitial oedema, the alveolar lining cells break and the alveolar air spaces are flooded with fluid *(alveolar oedema)* driving the air out of alveolus, thus seriously hampering the lung function.

Examples of pulmonary oedema by this mechanism are seen in left heart failure, mitral stenosis, pulmonary vein obstruction, thyrotoxicosis, cardiac surgery, nephrotic syndrome and obstruction to the lymphatic outflow by tumour or inflammation.

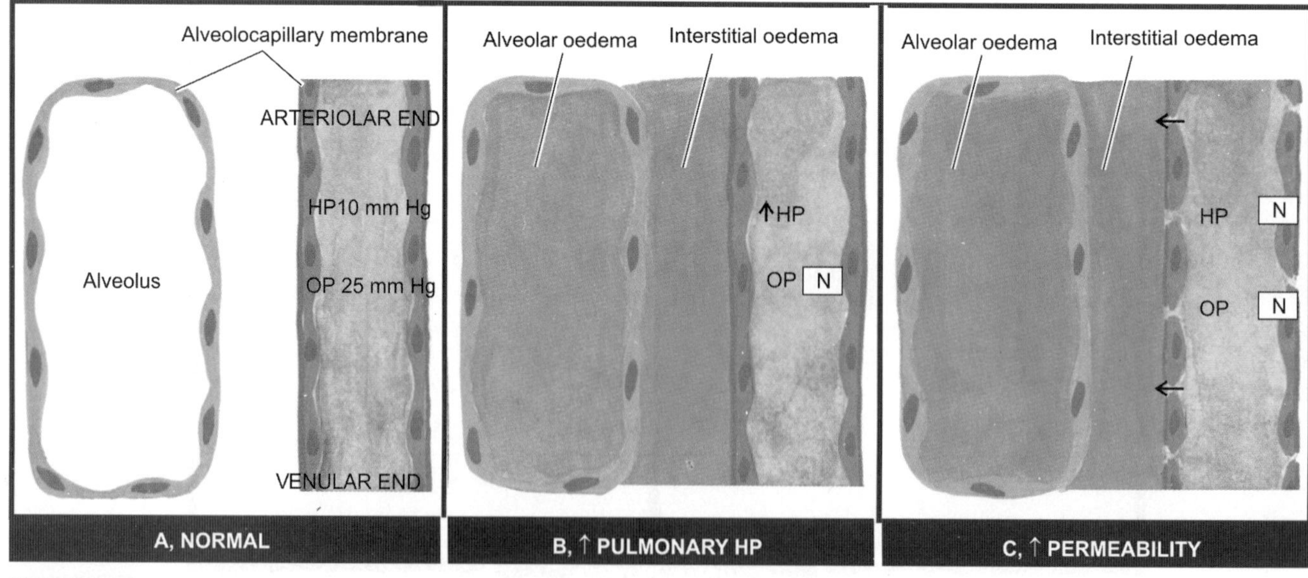

FIGURE 5.7

Mechanisms involved in the pathogenesis of pulmonary oedema. A, Normal fluid exchange at the alveolocapillary membrane (capillary endothelium and alveolar epithelium). B, Pulmonary oedema via elevated pulmonary hydrostatic pressure. C, Pulmonary oedema via increased vascular permeability.

2. Increased vascular permeability (Irritant oedema). The vascular endothelium as well as the alveolar epithelial cells (alveolo-capillary membrane) may be damaged causing increased vascular permeability so that excessive fluid and plasma proteins leak out, initially into the interstitium and subsequently into the alveoli.

This mechanism explains pulmonary oedema in *examples* such as in fulminant pulmonary and extrapulmonary infections, inhalation of toxic substances, aspiration, shock, radiation injury, hypersensitivity to drugs or antisera, uraemia and adult respiratory distress syndrome (ARDS).

3. Acute high altitude oedema. Individuals climbing to high altitude suddenly without halts and without waiting for acclimatisation to set in, suffer from serious circulatory and respiratory ill-effects. Commonly, the deleterious effects begin to appear after an altitude of 2500 metres is reached. These changes include: appearance of oedema fluid in the lungs, congestion and widespread minute haemorrhages. These changes can cause death within a few days. The underlying mechanism appears to be anoxic damage to the pulmonary vessels. However, if acclimatisation to high altitude is allowed to take place, the individual develops polycythaemia, raised pulmonary arterial pressure, increased pulmonary ventilation and a rise in heart rate and increased cardiac output.

PATHOLOGIC CHANGES. Irrespective of the underlying mechanism in the pathogenesis of pulmonary oedema, the fluid accumulates more in the basal regions of lungs. The thickened interlobular septa along with their dilated lymphatics may be seen in chest X-ray as linear lines perpendicular to the pleura and are known as *Kerley's lines.*

Grossly, the lungs in pulmonary oedema are heavy, moist and subcrepitant. Cut surface exudes frothy fluid (mixture of air and fluid).

Microscopically, the alveolar capillaries are congested. Initially the excess fluid collects in the interstitial lung spaces (interstitial oedema) but later the fluid fills the alveolar spaces (alveolar oedema). The interstitium as well as the alveolar spaces thus contain an eosinophilic, granular and pink proteinaceous material, often admixed with some RBCs and macrophages (Fig. 5.8) (COLOUR PLATE V: CL 17). This may be seen as brightly eosinophilic pink lines along the alveolar margin called *hyaline membrane.* Long-standing pulmonary oedema is prone to get infected by bacteria producing hypostatic pneumonia which may be fatal.

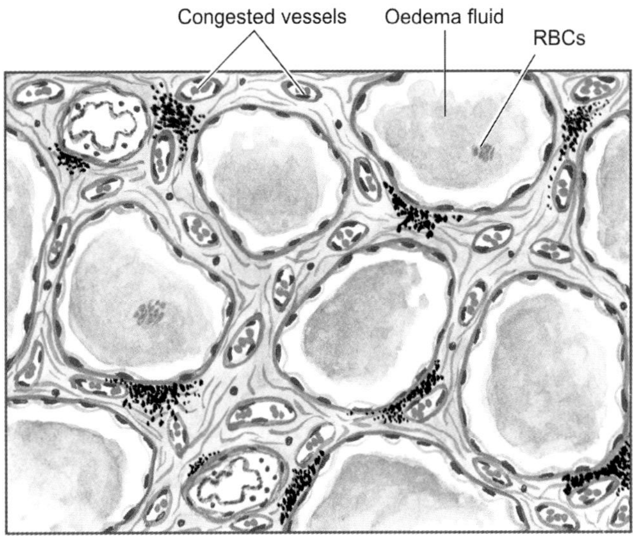

FIGURE 5.8

Pulmonary oedema. The alveolar capillaries are congested. The alveolar spaces as well as interstitium contain eosinophilic, granular, homogeneous and pink proteinaceous oedema fluid alongwith some RBCs and inflammatory cells.

In chronically elevated venous pressure, known as chronic passive congestion of lung or *brown induration,* the lungs are firm and heavy. The sectioned surface is rusty brown in colour.

Microscopically, the alveolar septa are widened and the alveolar spaces contain numerous haemosiderin-laden macrophages (heart failure cells) and, in late stage, may show variable amount of fibrosis.

Cerebral Oedema

Cerebral oedema or swelling of brain is the most threatening example of oedema. The mechanism of fluid exchange in the brain differs from elsewhere in the body since there are no draining lymphatics in the brain but instead, the function of fluid-electrolyte exchange is performed by the blood-brain barrier located at the endothelial cells of the capillaries.

Cerebral oedema can be of 3 types:

1. VASOGENIC OEDEMA. This is the most common type and corresponds to oedema elsewhere resulting from increased filtration pressure or increased capillary permeability. Vasogenic oedema is prominent around cerebral contusions, infarcts, brain abscess and some tumours.

Grossly, the white matter is swollen, soft, with flattened gyri and narrowed sulci. Sectioned surface is soft and gelatinous.

Microscopically, there is separation of tissue elements by the oedema fluid and swelling of astrocytes. The perivascular (Virchow-Robin) space is widened and clear halos are seen around the small blood vessels.

2. CYTOTOXIC OEDEMA. In this type, the blood-brain barrier is intact and the fluid accumulation is intracellular. The underlying mechanism is disturbance in the cellular osmoregulation as occurs in some metabolic derangements, acute hypoxia and with some toxic chemicals.

Microscopically, the cells are swollen and vacuolated. In some situations, both vasogenic as well as cytotoxic cerebral oedema results e.g. in purulent meningitis.

3. INTERSTITIAL OEDEMA. This type of cerebral oedema occurs when the excessive fluid crosses the ependymal lining of the ventricles and accumulates in the periventricular white matter. This mechanism is responsible for oedema in non-communicating hydrocephalus.

OVERHYDRATION

Overhydration is a state of pure water excess or water intoxication.

PATHOGENESIS. A normal healthy individual can consume large volumes of water and respond via water diuresis without producing any deleterious effects. This is because the normal individual has the capacity to excrete large volumes of dilute urine when excess of water is given without electrolytes. However, in certain conditions, the kidneys have a restricted ability to dilute the urine when large amounts of pure water are given. This results in expansion of extracellular fluid compartment with reduced osmolality and intracellular oedema. An early diuretic phase is followed by oliguria or even anuria due to damaged renal tubular epithelial cells.

CAUSES. Overhydration is encountered in the following conditions:

1. Acute and chronic renal disease
2. Severe congestive heart failure
3. Addison's disease
4. Cirrhosis of the liver
5. Tumours producing ADH e.g. bronchogenic carcinoma
6. Early postoperative period when patient is on infusion of glucose solution but is incapable of diluting the urine due to liberation of vasopressin (ADH) by the stress of surgery.

CLINICAL AND BIOCHEMICAL EFFECTS. These are as under:

- *Disordered cerebral function e.g.* nausea, vomiting, headache, confusion and in severe cases convulsions, coma, and even death.
- *Plasma changes* include reduced plasma electrolytes with decreased osmolality, lowered plasma proteins and reduced PCV.

DEHYDRATION

Dehydration or pure water deficiency is a state of deprivation of water without corresponding loss of electrolytes.

PATHOGENESIS. Decrease of body water initially affects intravascular compartment so that the blood volume is reduced. This is followed by withdrawing of fluid from the interstitial compartment with consequent hyperosmolality. This leads to shifting of intracellular water to the extracellular compartment which results in cellular dehydration as well as depletion of potassium ions from the cells. Release of ADH secretion in response to hypovolaemia results in reduced renal excretion of water. Sodium excretion is initially normal but later the renin-angiotensin-aldosterone mechanism is stimulated so that sodium is retained and its excretion decreases. Thus, this type of dehydration is characterised by water and potassium loss.

CAUSES. Pure water deficiency is less common than salt depletion but can occur in the following conditions:

1. Deficient water intake e.g. in dysphagia, obstructive lesion in oesophagus, starvation, intense weakness, coma.
2. Excessive loss of water e.g. in diabetes insipidus, hyperparathyroidism, pyrexia, hyperapnoea.

CLINICAL AND BIOCHEMICAL EFFECTS. These changes are as follows:

- *Clinical effects* are intense thirst, mental confusion, fever, oliguria.
- *Plasma changes.* In early stage, the levels of sodium, plasma proteins and PCV are unaltered but in late stage, there is rise in blood urea, serum sodium and PCV.

DISTURBANCES OF ELECTROLYTES

Changes in the concentration of sodium, potassium, chloride, bicarbonate, water and blood pH are briefly discussed below.

COMBINED SODIUM ANDWATER DEFICIENCY

Combined sodium and water deficiency is more common than deficiency of either component separately.

It is commonly called salt depletion because both sodium and chloride are lost equally.

PATHOGENESIS. Combined loss of water and sodium leads to fall in the volume of intravascular fluid first, and then reduction in extracellular fluid. Initially, there is no fall in the sodium level. But later, in response to ADH secretion, water is retained and sodium level falls. Thus, this type of dehydration is characterised by severe water and sodium loss.

CAUSES. Loss of sodium and water can occur in the following conditions:

1. Gastrointestinal disorders e.g. severe vomitings, diarrhoea.
2. Excess loss via the sweat.
3. Excess loss via urine e.g. in patients of heart failure on diuretics, Addison's disease, advanced diabetes mellitus.
4. Excess loss via blood and plasma e.g. in severe haemorrhage, extensive burns.

CLINICAL AND BIOCHEMICAL EFFECTS. These are:

- *Clinical effects* are signs and symptoms of dehydration such as sunken eyeballs, wrinkled skin, dry tongue, muscle cramps, oliguria.
- *Plasma changes.* There is reduced level of plasma sodium, and raised levels of plasma proteins, PCV and blood urea.

ABNORMALITIES OF THE pH OF BLOOD

The pH may be defined as the negative logarithm of the H^+ ion concentration of a solution. In health, the pH of blood is kept constant at 7.4 ± 0.05. In the body, pure water dissociates into very minute amounts of equal number of hydrogen ions and hydroxyl ions (10^{-7} each):

$$H_2O \rightleftharpoons H^+ + OH^-$$

An increased concentration of H^+ ions shifts the pH lower (acidosis) whereas a decreased concentration of H^+ ions shifts the pH higher (alkalosis).

The pH of the blood is normally maintained according to Henderson-Hasselbalch equation:

$$pH = pK + \log \frac{\text{conjugate base } (HCO'_3)}{\text{conjugate acid } (Pco_2)}$$

where pK is the dissociation constant of the carbonic acid which is 6.1, the concentration of the base (HCO'_3) is 24 mmol/litre, and the concentration of the acid (carbonic acid) in solution at partial pressure of CO_2 (Pco_2) of 40 mmHg (the normal alveolar tension) is 1.2 mmol/litre.

$$\text{Thus, pH of blood} = 6.1 + \log \frac{24}{1.2}$$

$$= 6.1 + \log 20$$
$$= 6.1 + 1.3$$
$$= 7.4$$

Therefore, the pH of blood depends upon 2 principal factors:

- the *concentration of bicarbonate;* and
- the *partial pressure of CO_2* that determines the concentration of carbonic acid.

Accordingly, the disorders of the pH of the blood can be of 2 types:

1. *alterations in the blood bicarbonate* levels (metabolic acidosis and alkalosis); and
2. *alteration in Pco_2* which depends upon the ventilatory function of the lungs (respiratory acidosis and alkalosis).

Metabolic Acidosis

A fall in the blood pH due to metabolic component is brought about by fall of bicarbonate level and excess of H^+ ions in the blood. This occurs in the following situations:

- Production of large amounts of lactic acid (lactic acidosis) e.g. in vigorous exercise, shock.
- Uncontrolled diabetes mellitus (diabetic ketoacidosis).
- Starvation.
- Chronic renal failure.
- Therapeutic administration of ammonium chloride or acetazolamide (diamox).

High blood levels of H^+ ions in metabolic acidosis stimulate the respiratory centre so that the breathing is deep and rapid *(air hunger or Kussmaul's respiration).* There is fall in the plasma bicarbonate levels.

Metabolic Alkalosis

A rise in the blood pH due to rise in the bicarbonate levels of plasma and loss of H^+ ions is called metabolic alkalosis. This is seen in the following conditions:

- Severe and prolonged vomitings.
- Administration of alkaline salts like sodium bicarbonate.
- Hypokalaemia such as in Cushing's syndrome, increased secretion of aldosterone.

Clinically, metabolic alkalosis is characterised by depression of respiration, depressed renal function with uraemia and increased bicarbonate excretion in the urine. The blood level of bicarbonate is elevated.

Respiratory Acidosis

A fall in the blood pH occurring due to raised Pco_2 consequent to underventilation of lungs (CO_2 retention) causes respiratory acidosis. This can occur in the following circumstances:

- Air obstruction as occurs in chronic bronchitis, emphysema, asthma.
- Restricted thoracic movement e.g. in pleural effusion, ascites, pregnancy, kyphoscoliosis.
- Impaired neuromuscular function e.g. in poliomyelitis, polyneuritis.

Clinically, there is peripheral vasodilatation and raised intracranial pressure. If there is severe CO_2 retention, patients may develop confusion, drowsiness and coma. The arterial Pco_2 level is raised.

Respiratory Alkalosis

A rise in the blood pH occurring due to lowered Pco_2 consequent to hyperventilation of the lungs (excess removal of CO_2) is called respiratory alkalosis. This is encountered in the following conditions:

- Hysterical overbreathing
- Working at high temperature
- At high altitude
- Meningitis, encephalitis
- Salicylate intoxication

Clinically, the patients with respiratory alkalosis are characterised by peripheral vasoconstriction and consequent pallor, lightheadedness and tetany. The arterial Pco_2 is lowered.

HAEMODYNAMIC DISTURBANCES

There are three main basic requirements for normal circulatory function: normal anatomic features, normal physiologic controls, and normal biochemical composition of the blood. These are essential to maintain normal blood flow and perfusion of tissues.

Derangements of blood flow or haemodynamic disturbances are considered under 2 broad headings:

I. *Disturbances in the volume of the circulating blood.* These include: hyperaemia and congestion, haemorrhage and shock.

II. *Circulatory disturbances of obstructive nature.* These are: thrombosis, embolism, ischaemia and infarction.

I. DISTURBANCES IN THE VOLUME OF CIRCULATING BLOOD

HYPERAEMIA AND CONGESTION

Hyperaemia and congestion are the terms used for increased volume of blood within dilated vessels of an organ or tissue; the increased volume from arterial and arteriolar dilatation being referred to as *hyperaemia or active hyperaemia*, whereas the impaired venous drainage is called *venous congestion or passive hyperaemia*. If the condition develops rapidly it is called *acute*, while more prolonged and gradual response is known as *chronic*.

Active Hyperaemia

The dilatation of arteries, arterioles and capillaries is effected either through sympathetic neurogenic mechanism or via the release of vasoactive substances. The affected tissue or organ is pink or red in appearance (erythema).

The *examples* of active hyperaemia are seen in the following conditions:

- Inflammation e.g. congested vessels in the walls of alveoli in pneumonia.
- Blushing i.e. flushing of the skin of face in response to emotions.
- Menopausal flush.
- Muscular exercise.
- High grade fever.

Passive Hyperaemia (Venous Congestion)

The dilatation of veins and capillaries due to impaired venous drainage results in passive hyperaemia or venous congestion, commonly referred to as *congestion*. Congestion may be acute or chronic, the latter being more common and called *chronic venous congestion* (CVC). The affected tissue or organ is bluish in colour due to accumulation of venous blood (cyanosis). Obstruction to the venous outflow may be local or systemic. Accordingly, venous congestion is of 2 types:

- *Local venous congestion* results from obstruction to the venous outflow from an organ or part of the body e.g. portal venous obstruction in cirrhosis of the liver, outside pressure on the vessel wall as occurs in tight bandage, plasters, tumours, pregnancy, hernia etc, or intraluminal occlusion by thrombosis.
- *Systemic (General) venous congestion* is engorgement of systemic veins e.g. in left-sided and right-sided heart failure and diseases of the lungs which interfere with pulmonary blood flow like pulmonary fibrosis, emphysema etc. Usually the fluid accumulates upstream to the specific chamber of the heart which is initially affected (Chapter 12). For example, in *left-sided heart failure* (such as due to mechanical overload in aortic stenosis, or due to weakened left ventricular wall as in myo-cardial infarction) pulmonary congestion results, whereas in *right-sided heart failure* (such as due to pulmonary stenosis or pulmonary hypertension) syste-

mic venous congestion results. Fig. 5.9 illustrates the mechanisms involved in passive or venous congestion of different organs.

MORPHOLOGY OF CVC OF ORGANS

Morphologic changes seen in CVC of the lungs, liver, spleen and kidney are discussed below.

CVC Lung

Chronic venous congestion of lung occurs in left heart failure, especially in rheumatic mitral stenosis so that there is consequent rise in pulmonary venous pressure.

Grossly, the lungs are heavy and firm in consistency. The sectioned surface is dark brown in colour referred to as *brown induration* of the lungs.

Histologically, the alveolar septa are widened due to the presence of interstitial oedema as well as due to dilated and congested capillaries. The septa are mildly thickened due to slight increase in fibrous connective tissue. Rupture of dilated and congested capillaries may result in minute intra-alveolar haemorrhages. The breakdown of erythrocytes liberates haemosiderin pigment which is taken up by alveolar macrophages, so called *heart failure cells,* present in the alveolar lumina. The brown induration of the cut surface of the lungs is due to the pigmentation and fibrosis (Fig. 5.10) (COLOUR PLATE V: CL 18).

CVC Liver

Chronic venous congestion of the liver occurs in right heart failure and sometimes due to occlusion of inferior vena cava and hepatic vein.

Grossly, the liver is enlarged and tender and the capsule is tense. Cut surface shows characteristic *nutmeg* liver due to red and yellow mottled appearance, corresponding to congested centre of lobules and fatty peripheral zone respectively (Fig. 5.11).

Microscopically, the changes of congestion are more marked in the centrilobular zone due to severe

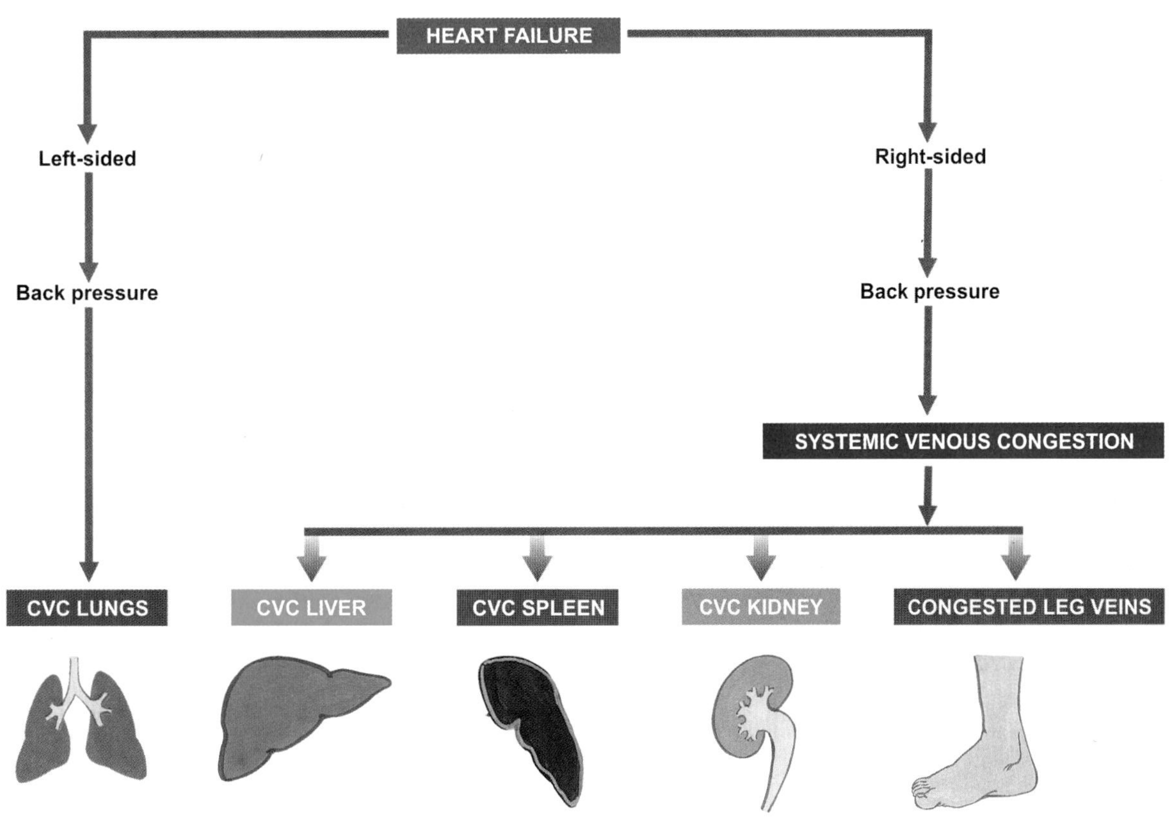

FIGURE 5.9

Schematic representation of mechanisms involved in chronic venous congestion (CVC) of different organs.

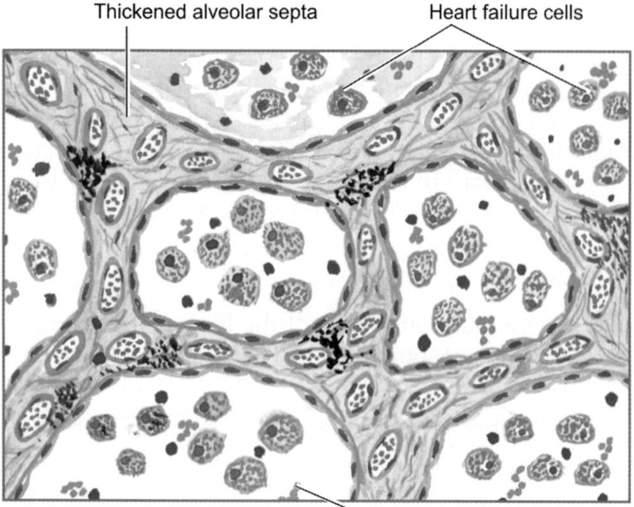

FIGURE 5.10

Histological appearance of CVC lung. The alveolar walls are widened and thickened due to congestion, oedema and mild fibrosis and the alveolar lumina contain heart failure cells.

hypoxia than in the peripheral zone. The central veins as well as the adjacent sinusoids are distended and filled with blood. The centrilobular hepatocytes undergo degenerative changes, and eventually *centrilobular haemorrhagic necrosis* may be seen. Long-standing cases may show fine centrilobular fibrosis and regeneration of hepatocytes, resulting in cardiac cirrhosis (Chapter 19). The peripheral zone of the lobule is less severely affected by chronic hypoxia and shows some *fatty change* in the hepatocytes (Fig. 5.12) (COLOUR PLATE V: CL 20).

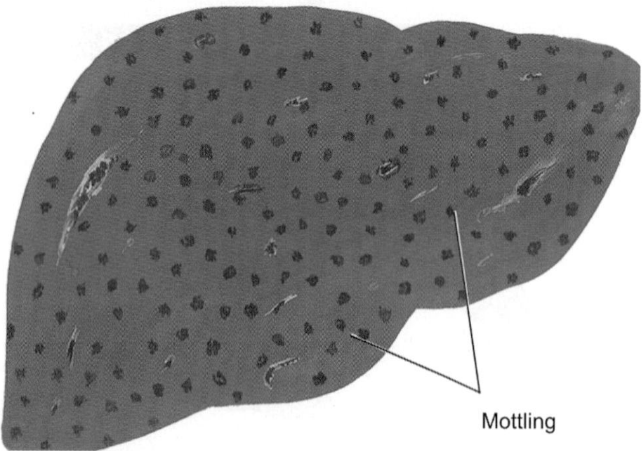

FIGURE 5.11

Nutmeg liver. The cut surface shows mottled appearance—alternate pattern of dark congestion and pale fatty change.

CVC Spleen

Chronic venous congestion of the spleen occurs in right heart failure and in portal hypertension from cirrhosis of liver.

Grossly, the spleen in early stage is slightly to moderately enlarged (upto 250 g as compared to normal 150 g), while in long-standing cases there is progressive enlargement and may weigh upto 500 to 1000 g. The organ is deeply congested, tense and cyanotic. Sectioned surface is gray tan.

Microscopically, the red pulp shows congestion and marked sinusoidal dilatation with areas of recent and old haemorrhages. These haemorrhages may get organised and form Gamna-Gandy bodies or siderofibrotic nodules which are deposits of haemosiderin pigment and calcium salts on fibrous connective tissue and elastic fibres. The reticulin-network as well as fibrous trabeculae are thickened (Fig. 5.13). In the late stage, there is hyperplasia of macrophages and fibroblasts resulting in increase in fibrous tissue of the capsule and hyperplasia of red pulp all of which account for firmness of the spleen (COLOUR PLATE V: CL 19). This advanced stage seen more commonly in hepatic cirrhosis is called *congestive splenomegaly* and is the commonest cause of hypersplenism (Chapter 14).

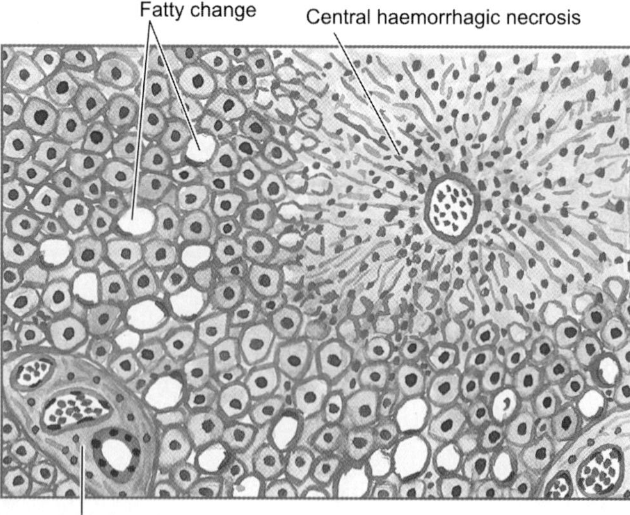

FIGURE 5.12

CVC liver. The centrilobular zone shows marked degeneration and necrosis of hepatocytes accompanied by haemorrhage while the peripheral zone shows mild fatty change of liver cells.

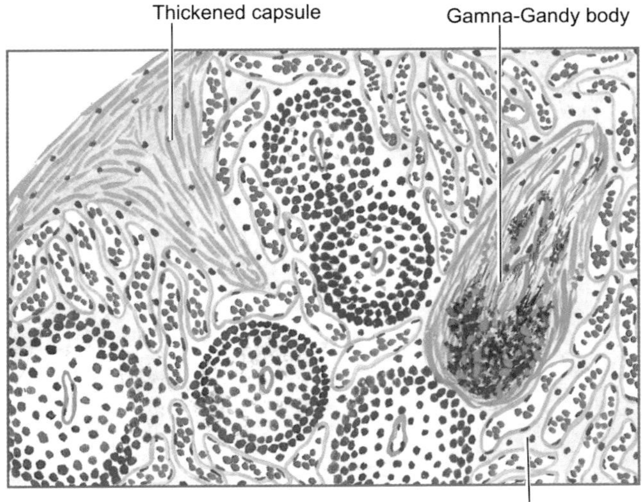

FIGURE 5.13

Histological appearance of CVC spleen. The sinuses are dilated and congested. There is increased fibrosis in the red pulp, capsule and the trabeculae. Two Gamna-Gandy bodies are also seen.

CVC Kidney

Grossly, the kidneys are slightly enlarged and the medulla is congested.

Microscopically, the changes are rather mild. The tubules may show degenerative changes like cloudy swelling and fatty change. The glomeruli may show mesangial proliferation.

HAEMORRHAGE

Haemorrhage is the escape of blood from a blood vessel. The bleeding may occur *externally, or internally* into the serous cavities (e.g. haemothorax, haemoperitoneum, haemopericardium) or into a hollow viscus. Extravasation of blood into the tissues with resultant swelling is known as *haematoma*. Large extravasations of blood into the skin and mucous membranes are called *ecchymoses*. *Purpuras* are small areas of haemorrhages (upto 1 cm) into the skin and mucous membrane, whereas *petechiae* are minute pinhead-sized haemorrhages. Microscopic escape of erythrocytes into loose tissues may occur following marked congestion and is known as *diapedesis*.

CAUSES OF HAEMORRHAGE. The blood loss may be large and sudden *(acute)*, or small repeated bleeds may occur over a period of time *(chronic)*. The various causes of haemorrhage are listed below:

1. *Trauma* to the vessel wall e.g. penetrating wound in the heart or great vessels, during labour etc.
2. *Spontaneous haemorrhage* e.g. rupture of an aneurysm, septicaemia, bleeding diathesis (such as purpura), acute leukaemias, pernicious anaemia, scurvy.
3. *Inflammatory lesions of the vessel wall* e.g. bleeding from chronic peptic ulcer, typhoid ulcers, blood vessels traversing a tuberculous cavity in the lung, syphilitic involvement of the aorta, polyarteritis nodosa.
4. *Neoplastic invasion* e.g. haemorrhage following vascular invasion in carcinoma of the tongue.
5. *Vascular diseases* e.g. atherosclerosis.
6. *Elevated pressure within the vessels* e.g. cerebral and retinal haemorrhage in systemic hypertension, severe haemorrhage from varicose veins due to high pressure in the veins of legs or oesophagus.

EFFECTS OF HAEMORRHAGE. The effects of blood loss depend upon 3 main factors:

- the amount of blood loss;
- the speed of blood loss; and
- the site of the haemorrhage.

The loss upto 20% of blood volume suddenly or slowly generally has little clinical effects because of compensatory mechanisms. A sudden loss of 33% of blood volume may cause death, while loss of upto 50% of blood volume over a period of 24 hours may not be necessarily fatal. However, chronic blood loss generally produces an iron deficiency anaemia, whereas acute haemorrhage may lead to serious immediate consequences such as hypovolaemic shock.

SHOCK

Definition and Types

Shock is defined as a clinical state of cardiovascular collapse characterised by:

- an acute reduction of effective circulating blood volume; and
- an inadequate perfusion of cells and tissues.

The end result is hypotension and cellular hypoxia and, if uncompensated, may lead to impaired cellular metabolism and death. Shock may be of 2 main types: primary (initial) and secondary (true) shock.

PRIMARY OR INITIAL SHOCK. It is transient and usually a benign vasovagal attack resulting from sudden reduction of venous return to the heart caused by neurogenic vasodilatation and consequent peripheral pooling of blood. It can occur immediately following trauma, severe pain or emotional overreaction such as due to fear, sorrow or surprise. Clinically, the patient generally develops unconsciousness, weakness, sinking sensation, pale and clammy limbs, weak and rapid pulse, and low blood pressure. The attack usually lasts for a few seconds or minutes.

SECONDARY OR TRUE SHOCK. This is the form of shock which occurs due to haemodynamic derangements with hypoperfusion of the cells. This type of shock is the true shock which is commonly referred to as 'shock' if not specified and is the type described below.

Etiology and Classification

Many types of injuries and diseases can cause shock. These causes are broadly grouped under 3 major headings, and accordingly shock is classified into 3 main etiologic forms: hypovolaemic, cardiogenic, and septic.

1. HYPOVOLAEMIC SHOCK. Reduction in blood volume induces hypovolaemic shock. The causes of hypovolaemia include the following:

i) *Severe haemorrhage* (external or internal) e.g. in trauma, surgery.

ii) *Fluid loss* e.g. in severe burns, crush injury to a limb, persistent vomitings and severe diarrhoea causing dehydration.

2. SEPTIC SHOCK. Severe bacterial infections or septicaemia induce septic shock. The predominant causes are as under:

i) Gram-negative septicaemia (endotoxic shock) e.g. infection with *E. coli, Proteus, Klebsiella, Pseudomonas* and bacteroides. Endotoxins of gram-negative bacilli have been implicated as the most important mediator of septic shock.

ii) Gram-positive septicaemia (exotoxic shock) is less common e.g. infection with streptococci, pneumococci.

As shown schematically in Fig. 5.14, lysis of gram-negative bacteria releases endotoxin, a lipopolysaccharide (LPS), into circulation where it binds to lipopolysaccharide-binding protein (LBP). The complex of LPS-LBP binds to CD14 molecule on the surface of the monocyte/macrophage which in turn is stimulated to elaborate tumour necrosis factor-α (TNF-α). TNF-α induces septic shock by endothelial cell injury by many mechanisms which include:

a) Direct cytotoxicity

b) Promotes the adherence of polymorphs to endothelium

c) Stimulates the release of interleukin-1 (IL-1)

d) Promotes the release of procoagulant tissue factor that causes thrombosis and local ischaemia.

3. CARDIOGENIC SHOCK. Acute circulatory failure with sudden fall in cardiac output from acute diseases of the heart without actual reduction of blood volume (normovolaemia) results in cardiogenic shock. The causes include the following:

i) Deficient emptying e.g.

- Myocardial infarction
- Rupture of the heart
- Cardiac arrhythmias

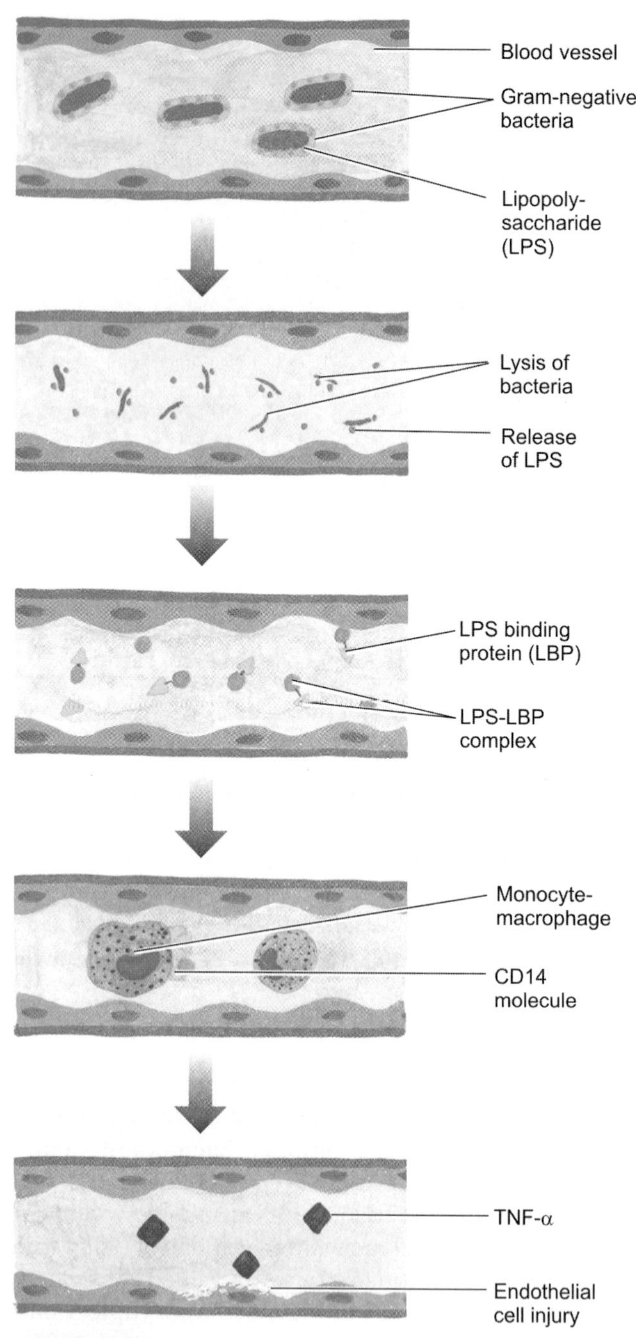

FIGURE 5.14

Pathogenesis of endotoxic shock.

ii) Deficient filling e.g.

- Cardiac tamponade from haemopericardium

iii) Obstruction to the outflow e.g.

- Pulmonary embolism
- Ball valve thrombus.

Besides the three major forms of shock described above, *neurogenic shock* (following anaesthesia or spinal cord injury) and *anaphylactic shock* are two other types of shock resulting from peripheral vasodilation with pooling of blood.

Pathogenesis

There are 2 basic features in the pathogenesis of shock:

- reduced effective circulating blood volume; and
- reduced supply of oxygen to the cells and tissues with resultant anoxia.

1. REDUCED EFFECTIVE CIRCULATING VOLUME. It may result by either of the following mechanisms:

i) by actual loss of blood volume as occurs in hypovolaemic shock; or

ii) by decreased cardiac output without actual loss of blood (normovolaemia) as occurs in cardiogenic shock and septic shock.

2. TISSUE ANOXIA. Following reduction in the effective circulating blood volume from either of the above two mechanisms and from any of the etiologic agents, there is decreased venous return to the heart resulting in decreased cardiac output. This consequently causes reduced supply of oxygen to the organs and tissues and hence tissue anoxia, and shock ensues.

In contrast to hypovolaemic and cardiogenic shock, patients in septic shock have hyperdynamic circulation due to peripheral vasodilatation and pooling of blood, as well as there is increased vascular permeability. This results in reduction of effective circulating blood volume, lowered cardiac output, reduced blood flow (hypotension) and inadequate perfusion of cells and tissues. Disseminated intravascular coagulation (DIC) is prone to develop in septic shock due to endothelial cell injury by toxins.

The sequence of events in the pathogenesis of shock is summarised in Fig. 5.15.

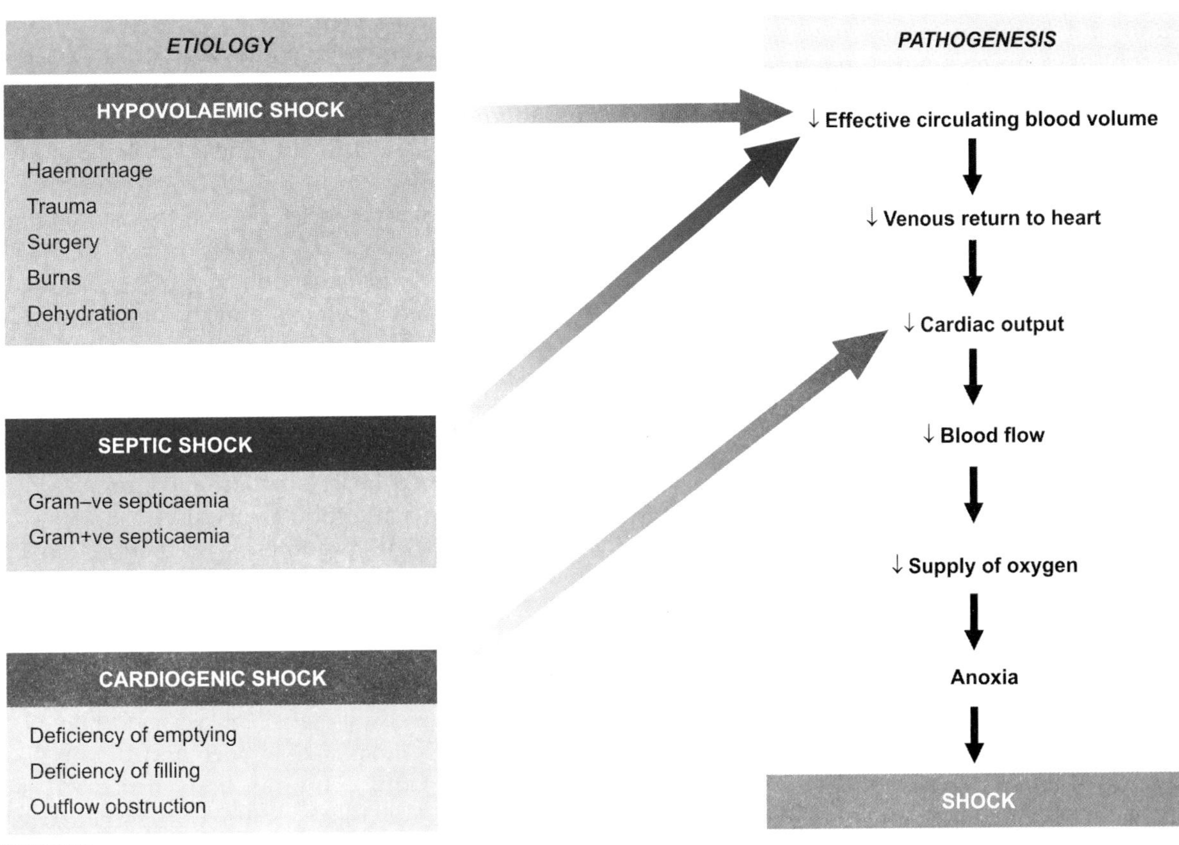

FIGURE 5.15

Etiology *(left)* and pathogenesis *(right)* of shock.

Stages of Shock

Deterioration of the circulation in shock is a progressive phenomenon and can be divided arbitrarily into 3 stages:

1. Non-progressive (initial, compensated reversible) shock.
2. Progressive decompensated shock.
3. Decompensated (irreversible) shock.

1. NON-PROGRESSIVE (INITIAL, COMPENSATED REVERSIBLE) SHOCK. In the early stage of shock, an attempt is made to maintain adequate cerebral and coronary blood supply by redistribution of blood so that the vital organs (brain and heart) are adequately perfused and oxygenated. This is achieved by activation of various neurohormonal mechanisms causing *widespread vasoconstriction* and by *fluid conservation by the kidney*. If the condition that caused the shock is adequately treated, the compensatory mechanism may be able to bring about recovery and re-establish the normal circulation; this is called compensated or reversible shock. These compensatory mechanisms are as under:

i) Widespread vasoconstriction. In response to reduced blood flow (hypotension) and tissue anoxia, the neural and humoral factors (e.g. baroreceptors, chemoreceptors, catecholamines, renin, and VEM or vasoexcitor material from hypoxic kidney) are activated. All these bring about vasoconstriction, particularly in the vessels of the skin and abdominal viscera. Widespread vasoconstriction is a protective mechanism as it causes increased peripheral resistance, increased heart rate (tachycardia) and increased blood pressure. However, in septic shock, there is initial vasodilatation followed by vasoconstriction. Besides, in severe septic shock there is elevated level of thromboxane A_2 which is a potent vasoconstrictor and may augment the cardiac output alongwith other sympathetic mechanisms. Clinically cutaneous vasoconstriction is responsible for cool and pale skin in initial stage of shock.

ii) Fluid conservation by the kidney. In order to compensate the actual loss of blood volume in hypovolaemic shock, the following factors may assist in restoring the blood volume and improve venous return to the heart:

- Release of aldosterone from hypoxic kidney.
- Release of ADH due to decreased effective circulating blood volume.
- Reduced glomerular filtration rate (GFR) due to arteriolar constriction.
- Shifting of tissue fluids into the plasma due to lowered capillary hydrostatic pressure (hypotension).

iii) Vascular autoregulation. In response to hypoxia and acidosis, regional blood flow to the heart and brain is preserved by vasodilatation of the coronary and cerebral circulation.

2. PROGRESSIVE DECOMPENSATED SHOCK. This is a stage when the patient suffers from some other stress or risk factors (e.g. pre-existing cardiovascular and lung disease) besides persistence of the shock so that there is progressive deterioration. The effects of progressive decompensated shock due to tissue hypoperfusion are as under:

a) Pulmonary hypoperfusion with resultant tachypnoea and adult respiratory distress syndrome.

b) Tissue anoxia causing anaerobic glycolysis results in metabolic lactic acidosis. Lactic acidosis lowers the tissue pH which in turn makes the vasomotor response ineffective. This results in vasodilation and peripheral pooling of blood.

Clinically at this stage the patient develops confusion and worsening of renal function.

3. DECOMPENSATED (IRREVERSIBLE) SHOCK. When the shock is so severe that in spite of compensatory mechanisms and despite therapy and control of etiologic agent which caused the shock, no recovery takes place, it is called decompensated or irreversible shock. Its effects due to widespread cell injury include the following:

a) Progressive fall in the blood pressure due to deterioration in cardiac output attributed to release of myocardial depressant factor (MDF).

b) Severe metabolic acidosis due to anaerobic glycolysis.

c) Respiratory distress due to pulmonary oedema, tachypnoea and adult respiratory distress syndrome (ARDS).

d) Ischaemic cell death of brain, heart and kidneys due to reduced blood supply to these organs.

Clinically, at this stage the patient has features of coma, worsened heart function and progressive renal failure due to acute tubular necrosis.

A number of hypotheses or factors have been described in irreversibility of shock, with tissue anoxia occupying the central role (Fig. 5.16). These are as under:

i) Persistence of widespread vasoconstriction. Although widespread vasoconstriction is a compensatory mechanism, its persistence for prolonged duration can cause anoxia of tissues and organs like the liver, spleen, kidney and intestine. Particularly significant is the postcapillary venular constriction contributing to tissue anoxia.

ii) Vasodilatation and increased vascular permeability. Anoxia damages the capillary and venular wall so that

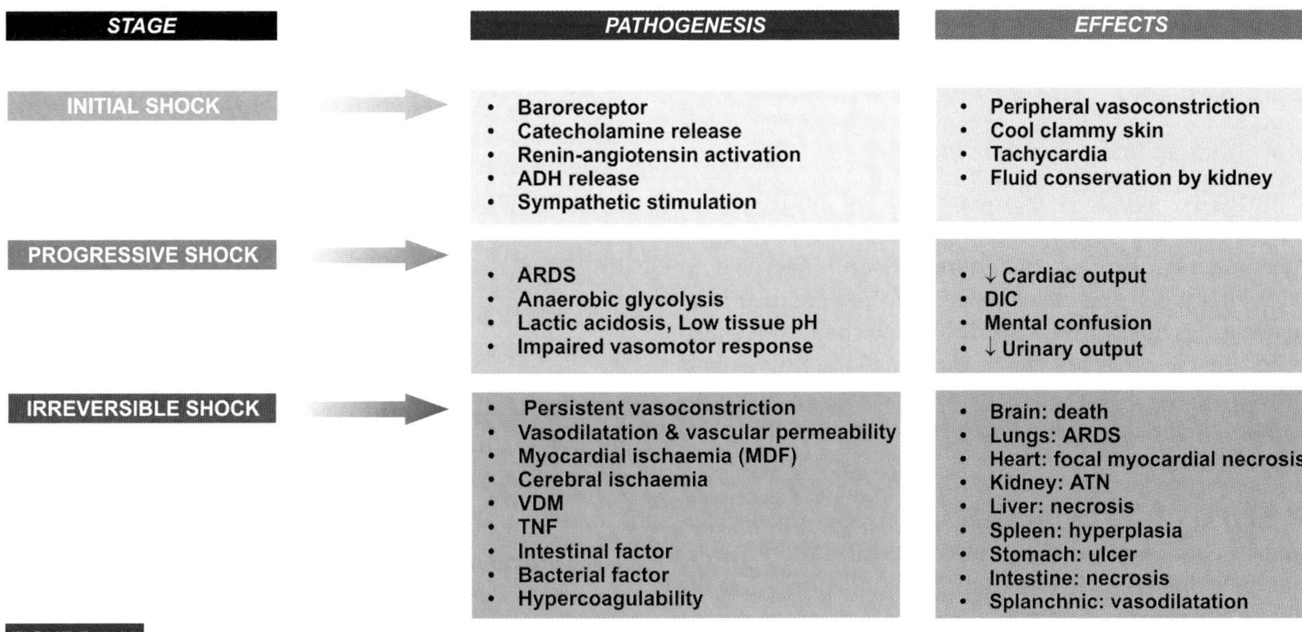

FIGURE 5.16

Mechanisms and effects of three stages of shock.

there is vasodilatation and increased vascular permeability. Vasodilatation results in peripheral pooling of blood while increased vascular permeability causes escape of fluid from circulation into the interstitial tissues, both of which further deteriorate the effective circulating blood volume.

iii) Myocardial ischaemia. Persistently reduced blood flow to myocardium causes coronary insufficiency and myocardial ischaemia due to release of myocardial depressant factor (MDF). This results in depression of cardiac function, reduced cardiac output and decreased blood flow.

iv) Cerebral ischaemia. Cerebral ischaemia resulting from persistent reduction of blood flow causes depression of the vasomotor centre. This results in vasodilatation and peripheral pooling of blood, thus reducing the venous return to the heart and consequent lowered cardiac output.

v) Vasodepressor material (VDM). VDM is a substance produced by the spleen and skeletal muscle and is normally inactivated in the liver. In severe hypoxia of the liver as occurs in irreversible shock, the mechanism of inactivation of VDM in liver is damaged so that its blood levels rise. VDM causes peripheral vasodilatation (reverse of VEM) and thus diverts blood from the systemic circulation, resulting in deterioration of the circulation.

vi) Tumour necrosis factor (TNF). In septic shock, monocyte-macrophage cell system gets activated by bacterial products causing release of substances like prostaglandins, leukotrienes, platelet activating factor and interleukins-1, 6 and 18. These substances have been implicated in producing irreversibility of endotoxic shock.

vii) Intestinal factor. Due to prolonged vasoconstriction, haemorrhagic necrosis of the intestinal tract occurs. This results in loss of blood and plasma into the intestine from haemorrhagic lesions, causing further reduction in effective circulating blood volume.

viii) Bacterial factor. Prolonged anoxic injury to the reticuloendothelial organs like the liver and spleen impairs the normal anti-bacterial defense mechanism of these organs. This results in release of undetoxified endotoxins derived from intestinal bacteria into the circulation, which cause further vasoconstriction and its harmful effects.

ix) Hypercoagulability of blood. Excessive accumulation of lactic acid in the blood in prolonged shock enhances the release of catecholamines (e.g. epinephrine) into the circulation. The effects of catecholamines include the release of clot promoting factor, release of thromboplastin and release of platelet aggregator, ADP. Excess lactic acid in the blood can also cause endothelial injury and thus initiate thrombosis. In this way, hypercoagulability of blood with consequent microthrombi impair the blood flow and may even cause tissue necrosis.

Morphologic Complications in Shock

Eventually, shock is characterised by multisystem failure. The morphologic changes in shock are due to hypoxia resulting in degeneration and necrosis in various organs. The major organs affected are the brain, heart, lungs and kidneys. Morphologic changes are also noted in the adrenals, gastrointestinal tract, liver and other organs. The predominant morphologic complications of shock are shown in Fig. 5.16 and described below.

1. HYPOXIC ENCEPHALOPATHY. Cerebral ischaemia in compensated shock may produce altered state of consciousness. However, if the blood pressure falls below 50 mmHg as occurs in systemic hypotension in prolonged shock and cardiac arrest, brain suffers from serious ischaemic damage with loss of cortical functions, coma, and a vegetative state.

Grossly, the area supplied by the most distal branches of the cerebral arteries suffers from severe ischaemic necrosis which is usually the border zone between the anterior and middle cerebral arteries (Chapter 28).
Microscopically, the changes are noticeable if ischaemia is prolonged for 12 to 24 hours. Neurons, particularly Purkinje cells, are more prone to develop the effects of ischaemia. The cytoplasm of the affected neurons is intensely eosinophilic and the nucleus is small pyknotic. Dead and dying nerve cells are replaced by gliosis.

2. HEART IN SHOCK. Heart is more vulnerable to the effects of hypoxia than any other organ. Heart is affected in cardiogenic as well as in other forms of shock. There are 2 types of morphologic changes in heart in all types of shock:

i) *Haemorrhages and necrosis.* There may be small or large ischaemic areas or infarcts, particularly located in the subepicardial and subendocardial region.

ii) *Zonal lesions.* These are opaque transverse contraction bands in the myocytes near the intercalated disc.

3. SHOCK LUNG. Lungs due to dual blood supply are generally not affected by hypovolaemic shock but in septic shock the morphologic changes in lungs are quite prominent termed 'shock lung'.

Grossly, the lungs are heavy and wet.
Microscopically, changes of adult respiratory distress syndrome (ARDS) are seen (Chapter 15). Briefly, the changes include congestion, interstitial and alveolar oedema, interstitial lymphocytic infiltrate, alveolar hyaline membranes, thickening and fibrosis of alveolar septa, and fibrin and platelet thrombi in the pulmonary microvasculature.

4. SHOCK KIDNEY. One of the important complications of shock is irreversible renal injury, first noted in persons who sustained crush injuries in building collapses in air raids in World War II. The renal ischaemia following systemic hypotension is considered responsible for renal changes in shock. The end-result is generally anuria and death.

Grossly, the kidneys are soft and swollen. Sectioned surface shows blurred architectural markings.
Microscopically, the tubular lesions are seen at all levels of nephron and are referred to as acute tubular necrosis (ATN) which can occur following other causes besides shock (Chapter 20). If extensive muscle injury or intravascular haemolysis are also associated, peculiar brown tubular casts are seen.

5. ADRENALS IN SHOCK. The adrenals show stress response in shock. This includes release of aldosterone in response to hypoxic kidney, release of glucocorticoids from adrenal cortex and catecholamines like adrenaline from adrenal medulla. In severe shock, adrenal haemorrhages may occur.

6. HAEMORRHAGIC GASTROENTEROPATHY. The hypoperfusion of the alimentary tract in conditions such as shock and cardiac failure may result in mucosal and mural infarction called haemorrhagic gastroenteropathy (Chapter 18). This type of non-occlusive ischaemic injury of bowel must be distinguished from full-fledged infarction in which case the deeper layers of gut (muscularis and serosa) are also damaged. In shock due to burns, acute stress ulcers of the stomach or duodenum may occur and are known as Curling's ulcers.

Grossly, the lesions are multifocal and widely distributed throughout the bowel. The lesions are superficial ulcers, reddish purple in colour. The adjoining bowel mucosa is oedematous and haemorrhagic.
Microscopically, the involved areas show dilated and congested vessels and haemorrhagic necrosis of the mucosa and sometimes submucosa. Secondary infection may supervene and condition may progress into pseudomembranous enterocolitis.

7. LIVER IN SHOCK. Due to effects of hypoxia on liver, VDM is released from the liver which causes vasodilatation. Besides, focal necrosis may be seen, fatty change may occur and the liver function may be impaired.

8. OTHER ORGANS. Other organs such as lymph nodes, spleen and pancreas may also show foci of necrosis in shock. In addition, the patients who survive acute phase of shock succumb to overwhelming infection due to altered immune status and host defense mechanism.

Clinical Features

The classical features of decompensated shock are characterised by *depression of 4 vital processes:*

- Very low blood pressure
- Subnormal temperature
- Feeble and irregular pulse
- Shallow and sighing respiration

In addition, the patients in shock have pale face, sunken eyes, weakness, cold and clammy skin. Renal dysfunction in shock is clinically characterised by a phase of oliguria due to ATN and a later phase of diuresis due to regeneration of tubular epithelium. Haemoconcentration is present in early oliguric phase while marked electrolyte imbalance occurs in diuretic phase. With progression of the condition, the patient may develop stupor, coma and death.

II. CIRCULATORY DISTURBANCES OF OBSTRUCTIVE NATURE

THROMBOSIS

Definition and Effects

Thrombosis is the process of formation of solid mass in circulation from the constituents of flowing blood; the mass itself is called a *thrombus*. A *blood clot* is the mass of coagulated blood formed *in vitro* e.g. in a test tube. *Haematoma* is the extravascular accumulation of blood clot e.g. into the tissues. *Haemostatic plugs* are the blood clots formed in healthy individuals at the site of bleeding e.g. in injury to the blood vessel. In other words, haemostatic plug at the cut end of a blood vessel may be considered the simplest form of thrombosis. Haemostatic plugs are useful as they stop the escape of blood and plasma, whereas thrombi developing in the unruptured cardiovascular system may be life-threatening by causing one of the following harmful effects:

1. Ischaemic injury. Thrombi may decrease or stop the blood supply to part of an organ or tissue and cause ischaemia which may subsequently result in infarction.

2. Thromboembolism. The thrombus or its part may get dislodged and be carried along in the bloodstream as embolus to lodge in a distant vessel.

Pathophysiology

Since the protective haemostatic plug formed as a result of normal haemostasis is an example of thrombosis, it is essential to describe *thrombogenesis* in relation to the normal haemostatic mechanism.

Human beings possess inbuilt system by which the blood remains in fluid state normally and guards against the hazards of thrombosis and haemorrhage. However, injury to the blood vessel initiates haemostatic repair mechanism or thrombogenesis. Virchow described three primary events which predispose to thrombus formation *(Virchow's triad):* endothelial injury, alteration in flow of blood, and hypercoagulability of blood. These events are discussed below:

1. ROLE OF BLOOD VESSEL WALL. The integrity of blood vessel wall is important for maintaining normal blood flow. An intact endothelium has the following functions:

i) It *protects* the flowing blood from the thrombogenic influence of subendothelium.

ii) It elaborates a few *anti-thrombotic* factors (thrombosis inhibitory factors) e.g.

a) Heparin-like substance which accelerates the action of antithrombin III and inactivates some other clotting factors.

b) Thrombomodulin which converts thrombin into activator of protein C, an anticoagulant.

c) Inhibitors of platelet aggregation such as ADPase, PGI_2 or prostacyclin.

d) Tissue plasminogen activator which accelerates the fibrinolytic activity.

iii) It can release a few *prothrombotic factors* which have procoagulant properties (thrombosis favouring factors) e.g.

a) Thromboplastin or tissue factor released from endothelial cells.

b) von Willebrand factor that causes adherence of platelets to the subendothelium.

c) Platelet activating factor which is activator and aggregator of platelets.

d) Inhibitor of plasminogen activator that suppresses fibrinolysis.

Vascular injury exposes the subendothelial connective tissue (e.g. collagen, elastin, fibronectin, laminin and glycosaminoglycans) which are thrombogenic and thus plays important role in initiating haemostasis as well as thrombosis. Injury to vessel wall also causes vasoconstriction of small blood vessels briefly so as to reduce the blood loss. Endothelial injury is of major significance in the formation of arterial thrombi and thrombi of the heart, especially of the left ventricle. A number of factors and conditions may cause vascular injury and predispose to the formation of thrombi. These are as under:

i) Endocardial injury in myocardial infarction, myocarditis, cardiac surgery, prosthetic valves.
ii) Ulcerated plaques in advanced atherosclerosis.
iii) Haemodynamic stress in hypertension.
iv) Arterial diseases.
v) Diabetes mellitus.
vi) Endogenous chemical agents such as hypercholesterolaemia, endotoxins.
vii) Exogenous chemical agents such as cigarette smoke.

2. ROLE OF PLATELETS. Following endothelial cell injury, platelets come to play a central role in normal haemostasis as well as in thrombosis. The sequence of events is as under:

i) Platelet adhesion. The platelets in circulation recognise the site of endothelial injury and adhere to exposed subendothelial collagen *(primary aggregation)*, von Willebrand's factor is required for such adhesion between platelets and collagen. Normal non-activated platelets have open canalicular system with cytoplasmic organelles (granules, mitochondria, endoplasmic reticulum) dispersed throughout the cytoplasm (Fig. 5.17,A). During the early adhesion process, there is dilatation of canalicular system with formation of pseudopods and the cytoplasmic organelles shift to the centre of the cell (Fig. 5.17,B).

ii) Platelet release reaction. The activated platelets then undergo release reaction by which the platelet granules are released to the exterior (Fig. 5.17,C). Two main types of platelet granules are released:

a) *Alpha granules* containing fibrinogen, fibronectin, platelet-derived growth factor, platelet factor 4 (an antiheparin) and cationic proteins.

b) *Dense bodies* containing ADP (adenosine diphosphate), ionic calcium, 5-HT (serotonin), histamine and epinephrine.

As a sequel to platelet activation and release reaction, the phospholipid complex-platelet factor 3 gets activated which plays important role in the intrinsic pathway of coagulation.

iii) Platelet aggregation. Following release of ADP, a potent platelet aggregating agent, aggregation of additional platelets takes place *(secondary aggregation)*. This results in formation of temporary haemostatic plug. However, stable haemostatic plug is formed by the action of fibrin, thrombin and thromboxane A_2.

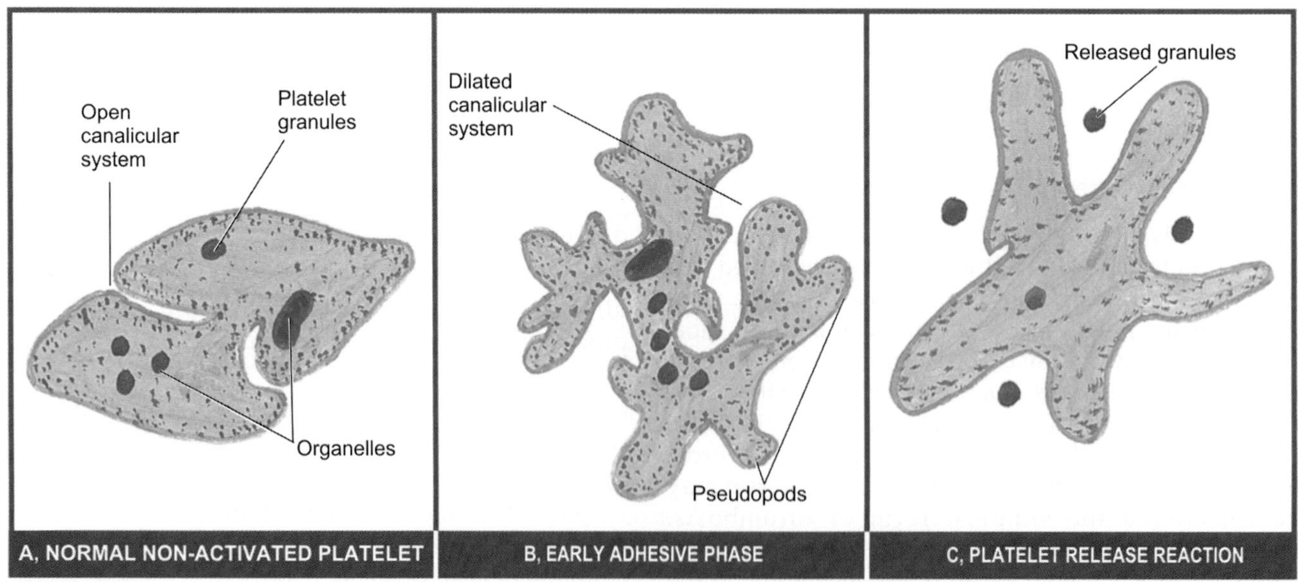

FIGURE 5.17

Activation of platelets during haemostatic plug formation and thrombogenesis. A, Normal non-activated platelet, having open canalicular system and the cytoplasmic organelles dispersed in the cell. B, Early adhesion phase, showing dilatation of the canalicular system with formation of pseudopods and the organelles present in the centre of the cell. C, Platelet release reaction, showing release of granules to the exterior.

3. ROLE OF COAGULATION SYSTEM. Coagulation mechanism is the conversion of the plasma fibrinogen into solid mass of fibrin. The coagulation system is involved in both haemostatic process and thrombus formation. Fig. 5.18 shows the schematic representation of the cascade of intrinsic (blood) pathway, the extrinsic (tissue) pathway, and the common pathway leading to formation of fibrin polymers.

i) In the intrinsic pathway, contact with abnormal surface leads to activation of factor XII and the sequential interactions of factors XI, IX, VIII and finally factor X, alongwith calcium ions (factor IV) and platelet factor 3.

ii) In the extrinsic pathway, tissue damage results in the release of tissue factor or thromboplastin. Tissue factor on interaction with factor VII activates factor X.

iii) The common pathway begins where both intrinsic and extrinsic pathways converge to activate factor X which forms a complex with factor Va and platelet factor 3, in the presence of calcium ions. This complex activates prothrombin (factor II) to thrombin (factor IIa) which, in turn, converts fibrinogen to fibrin. Initial monomeric fibrin is polymerised to form insoluble fibrin by activation of factor XIII.

iv) Regulation of coagulation system. The blood is kept in fluid state normally and coagulation system kept in check by controlling mechanisms. These are as under:

a) *Protease inhibitors.* These act on coagulation factors so as to oppose the formation of thrombin e.g. antithrombin III, protein C, C_1 inactivator, α1-antitrypsin, α2-macroglobulin.

b) *Fibrinolytic system.* Plasmin, a potent fibrinolytic enzyme, is formed by the action of plasminogen activator on plasminogen present in the normal plasma (Fig. 5.19). Two types of plasminogen activators (PA) are identified:

- *Tissue-type PA* derived from endothelial cells and leucocytes.
- *Urokinase-like PA* present in the plasma.

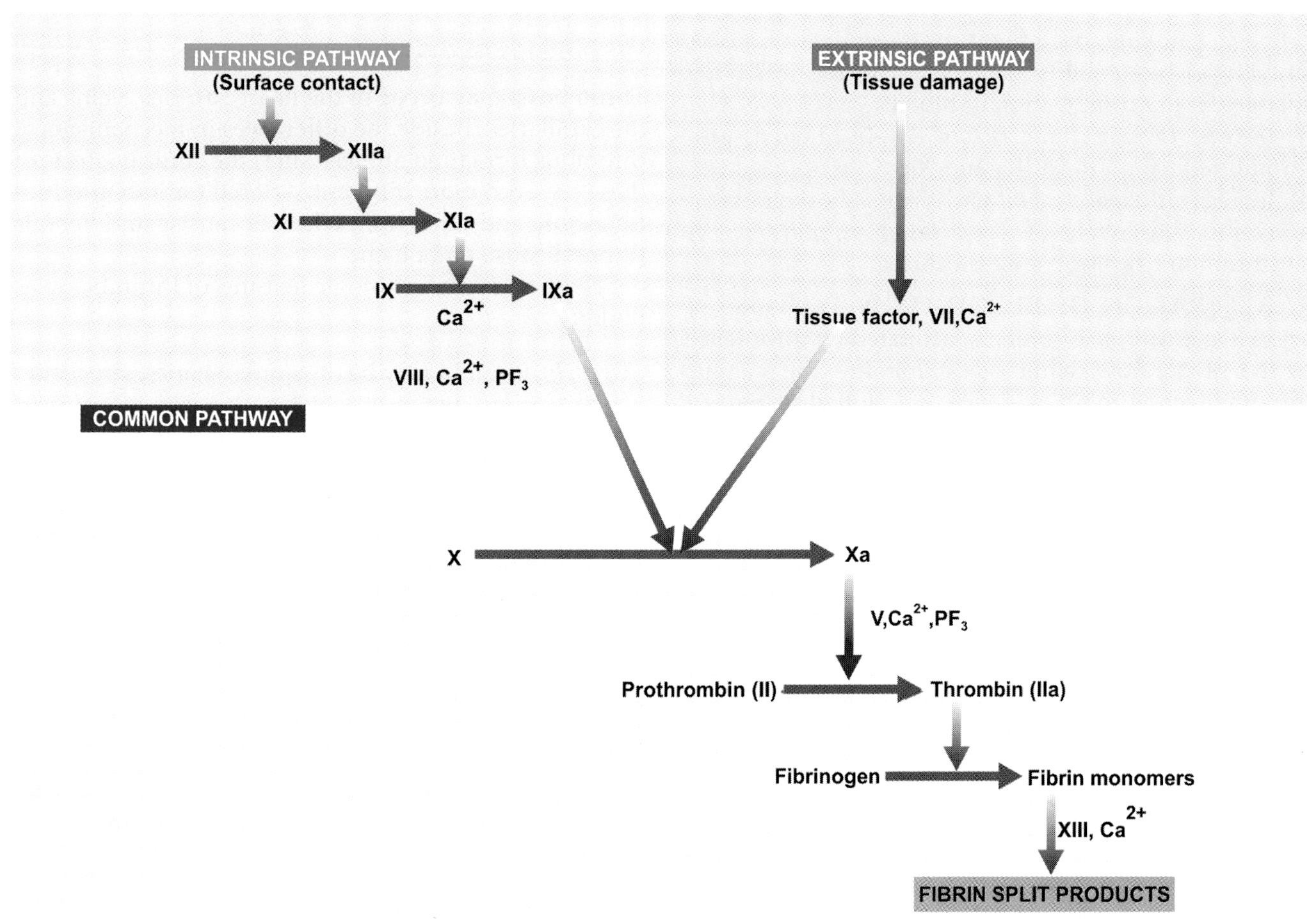

FIGURE 5.18

Schematic representation of pathways of coagulation mechanism.

Chapter Five

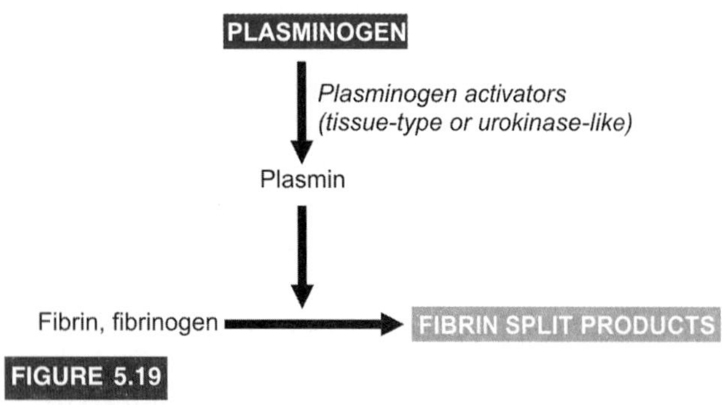

FIGURE 5.19

The fibrinolytic system.

Plasmin so formed acts on fibrin to destroy the clot and produces fibrin split products (FSP).

4. HYPERCOAGULABILITY OF BLOOD. The occurrence of thrombosis in some conditions such as in nephrotic syndrome, advanced cancers, extensive trauma, burns and during puerperium is explained on the basis of hypercoagulability of blood. The effect of hypercoagulability on thrombosis is favoured by advancing age, smoking, use of oral contraceptives and obesity. Hypercoagulability may occur by the following changes in the composition of blood:

i) *Increase in coagulation factors* e.g. fibrinogen, prothrombin, factor VIIa, VIIIa and Xa.

ii) Increase in *platelet count* and their adhesiveness.

iii) Decreased levels of *coagulation inhibitors* e.g. antithrombin III, fibrin split products.

5. ALTERATION OF BLOOD FLOW. Formation of arterial and cardiac thrombi is facilitated by turbulence in the blood flow, while stasis initiates the venous thrombi even without evidence of endothelial injury.

i) *Normally,* there is axial flow of blood in which the most rapidly-moving central stream consists of leucocytes and red cells. The platelets are present in the slow-moving laminar stream adjacent to the central stream while the peripheral stream consists of most slow-moving cell-free plasma close to endothelial layer (Fig. 5.20,A).

ii) *In turbulence and stasis,* the normal axial flow of blood is disturbed so that the platelets come into contact with the endothelium (Fig. 5.20,B).

Besides, the inhibitors of coagulation fail to reach the site of thrombus resulting in enlargement of thrombus size. Turbulence may actually injure the endothelium resulting in deposition of platelets and fibrin.

The sequence of events in thrombogenesis is illustrated in Fig. 5.21.

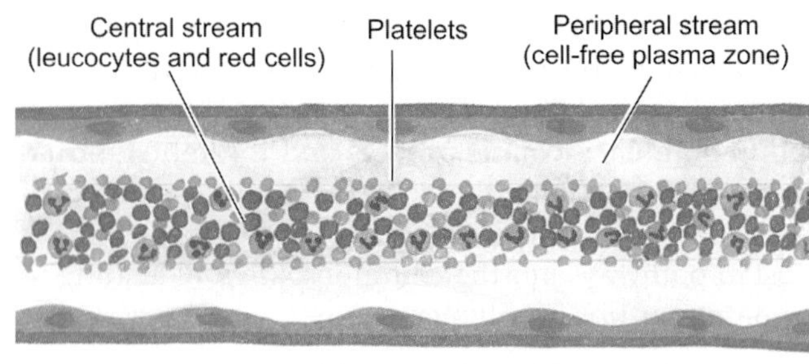

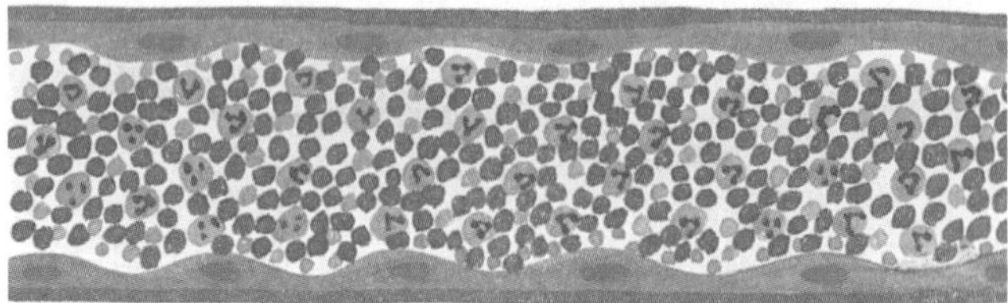

FIGURE 5.20

Alteration in flow of blood.

Morphology of Various Types

Thrombosis may occur in the heart, arteries, veins and the capillaries. Beside the differences in mechanisms of thrombus formation at these sites, the clinical effects of these are even more different. Arterial thrombi produce ischaemia and infarction, whereas cardiac and venous thrombi cause embolism.

The general morphologic features of thrombi are as under:

Grossly, thrombi may be of various shapes, sizes and composition depending upon the site of origin. Arterial thrombi tend to be white and mural while the venous thrombi are red and occlusive. Mixed or laminated thrombi are also common and consist of alternate white and red layers called lines of Zahn. Red thrombi are soft, red and gelatinous whereas white thrombi are firm and pale.

Microscopically, the composition of thrombus is determined by the rate of flow of blood i.e. whether it is formed in the rapid arterial and cardiac circulation, or in the slow moving flow in veins. The lines of Zahn are formed by alternate layers of light-staining aggregated platelets admixed with fibrin meshwork and dark-staining layer of red cells. Red (venous) thrombi have more abundant red cells, leucocytes and platelets entrapped in fibrin meshwork (COLOUR PLATE VI: CL 21). Thus, red thrombi closely resemble blood clots *in vitro* (Fig. 5.22).

Chapter Five

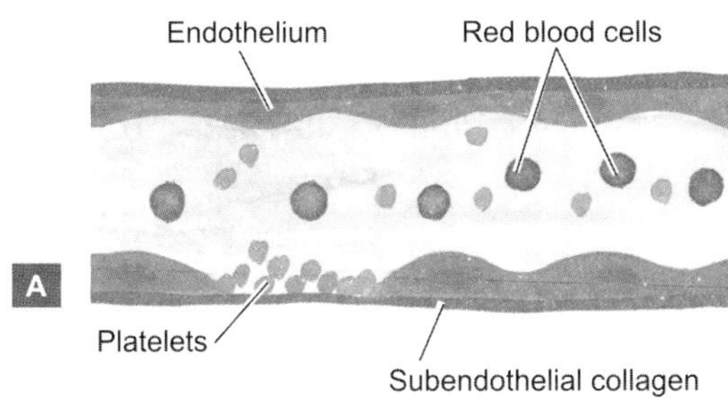

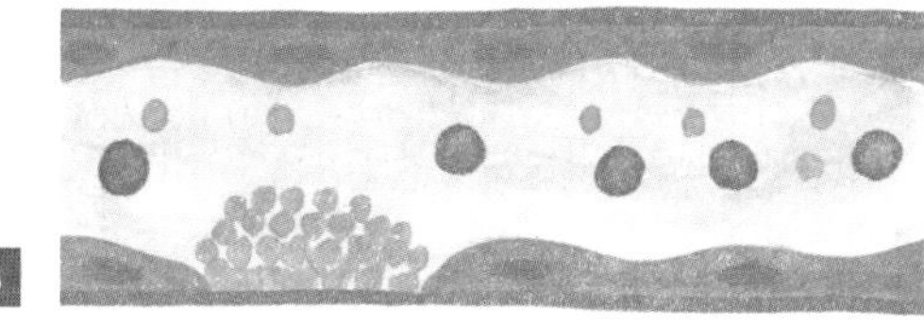

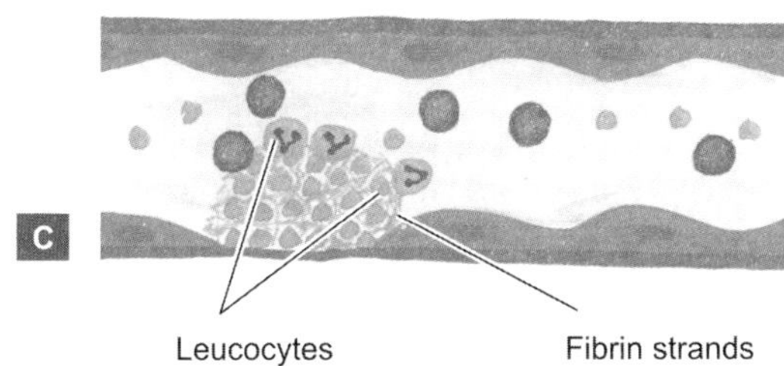

FIGURE 5.21

Sequence of events in thrombogenesis. A, Endothelial injury exposes subendothelium, initiating adherence of platelets and activation of coagulation system. B, Following platelet release reaction, ADP is released which causes further aggregation of platelets. C, Activated coagulation system forms fibrin strands in which are entangled some leucocytes and red cells.

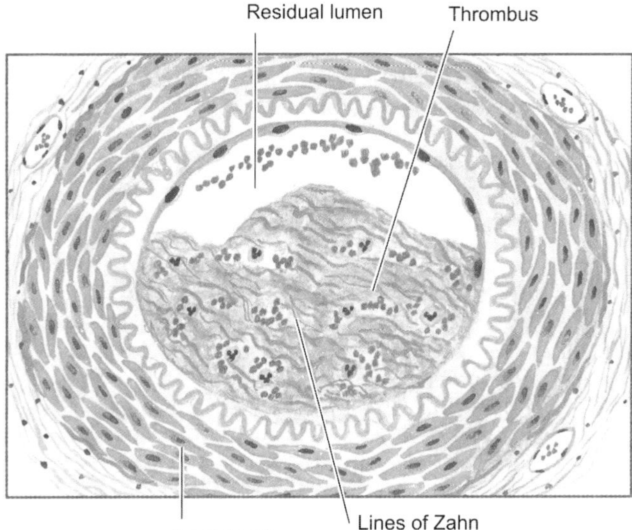

FIGURE 5.22

Thrombus in an artery. The thrombus is adherent to the arterial wall and is seen occluding most of the lumen. It shows lines of Zahn composed of granular-looking platelets and fibrin meshwork with entangled red cells and leucocytes.

Red thrombi (antemortem) have to be distinguished from postmortem clots (Table 5.3).

CARDIAC THROMBI. Thrombi may form in any of the chambers of heart and on the valve cusps. They are more common in the atrial appendages, especially of the right atrium, and on mitral and aortic valves called vegetations which may be seen in infective endocarditis and non-bacterial thrombotic endocarditis (Chapter 12). Cardiac thrombi are mural (non-occlusive) as are the mural thrombi encountered in the aorta in atherosclerosis and in aneurysmal dilatations. Rarely, large round thrombus may form and obstruct the mitral valve and is called *ball-valve thrombus*. *Agonal thrombi* are formed shortly before death and may occur in either or both the ventricles. They are composed mainly of fibrin.

ARTERIAL AND VENOUS THROMBI. The examples of major forms of vascular thrombi are as under:

Arterial thrombi:

i) Aorta: aneurysms, arteritis.
ii) Coronary arteries: atherosclerosis.
iii) Mesenteric artery: atherosclerosis, arteritis.
iv) Arteries of limbs: atherosclerosis, diabetes mellitus, Buerger's disease, Raynaud's disease.
v) Renal artery: atherosclerosis, arteritis.
vi) Cerebral artery: atherosclerosis, vasculitis.

TABLE 5.3: Distinguishing Features of Antemortem Thrombi and Postmortem Clots.

	FEATURE	ANTEMORTEM THROMBI	POSTMORTEM CLOTS
1.	*Gross*	Dry, granular, firm and friable	Gelatinous, soft and rubbery
2.	*Relation to vessel wall*	Adherent to the vessel wall	Weakly attached to the vessel wall
3.	*Shape*	May or may not fit their vascular contours	Take the shape of vessel or its bifurcation
4.	*Microscopy*	The surface contains apparent lines of Zahn	The surface is *'chicken fat'* yellow covering the underlying red *'currant jelly'*

Venous thrombi:

i) Veins of lower limbs: deep veins of legs, varicose veins.
ii) Popliteal, femoral and iliac veins: postoperative stage, postpartum.
iii) Pulmonary veins: CHF, pulmonary hypertension.
iv) Hepatic and portal vein: portal hypertension.
v) Superior vena cava: infections in head and neck.
vi) Inferior vena cava: extension of thrombus from hepatic vein.
vii) Mesenteric veins: volvulus, intestinal obstruction.
viii) Renal vein: renal amyloidosis.

Distinguishing features between thrombi formed in rapidly-flowing arterial circulation and slow-moving venous blood are given in Table 5.4.

CAPILLARY THROMBI. Minute thrombi composed mainly of packed red cells are formed in the capillaries in acute inflammatory lesions, vasculitis and in disseminated intravascular coagulation (DIC).

Fate of Thrombus

The possible fate of thrombi is as under (Fig. 5.23):

1. RESOLUTION. Thrombus activates the fibrinolytic system with consequent release of plasmin which may dissolve the thrombus completely resulting in resolution. Usually, lysis is complete in small venous thrombi while large thrombi may not be dissolved. Fibrinolytic activity can be accentuated by administration of thrombolytic substances (e.g. urokinase, streptokinase), especially in the early stage when fibrin is in monomeric form.

2. ORGANISATION. If the thrombus is not removed, it starts getting organised. Phagocytic cells (neutrophils and macrophages) appear and begin to phagocytose fibrin and cell debris. The proteolytic enzymes liberated by leucocytes and endothelial cells start digesting coagulum. Capillaries grow into the thrombus from the site of its attachment and fibroblasts start invading the thrombus. Thus, fibrovascular granulation tissue is formed which subsequently becomes dense and less vascular and is covered over by endothelial cells. The thrombus in this way is excluded from the vascular lumen and becomes part of vessel wall. The new vascular channels in it may be able to re-establish the blood flow, called recanalisation. The fibrosed thrombus may undergo hyalinisation and calcification e.g. phleboliths in the pelvic veins.

3. PROPAGATION. The thrombus may enlarge in size due to more and more deposition from the constituents of flowing blood. In this way, it may ultimately cause obstruction of some important vessel.

4. THROMBOEMBOLISM. The thrombi in early stage and infected thrombi are quite friable and may get detached from the vessel wall. These are released in part or completely in bloodstream as emboli which produce ill-effects at the site of their lodgement (page 122).

Factors Predisposing to Thrombosis

A number of primary (genetic) and secondary (acquired) factors favour thrombosis.

Primary (Genetic) factors:
i) Deficiency of antithrombin
ii) Deficiency of protein C or S
iii) Defects in fibrinolysis
iv) Mutation in factor V

Secondary (acquired) factors:
a) Risk factors:
i) Advanced age
ii) Prolonged bed-rest
iii) Immobilisation
iv) Use of oral contraceptives
v) Cigarette smoking
vi) Tissue damage e.g. trauma, fractures, burns

TABLE 5.4: Distinguishing Features of Arterial and Venous Thrombi.

FEATURE	ARTERIAL THROMBI	VENOUS THROMBI
1. *Blood flow*	Formed in rapidly-flowing blood of arteries and heart	Formed in slow-moving blood in veins
2. *Sites*	Common in aorta, coronary, cerebral, iliac, femoral, renal and mesenteric arteries	Common in superficial varicose veins, deep leg veins, popliteal, femoral and iliac veins
3. *Thrombogenesis*	Formed following endothelial cell injury e.g. in atherosclerosis	Formed following venous stasis e.g. in abdominal operations, child-birth
4. *Development*	Usually mural, not occluding the lumen completely, may propagate	Usually occlusive, take the cast of the vessel in which formed, may propagate in both directions
5. *Macroscopy*	Grey-white, friable with lines of Zahn on surface	Red-blue with fibrin strands and lines of Zahn
6. *Microscopy*	Distinct lines of Zahn composed of platelets, fibrin with entangled red and white blood cells	Lines of Zahn with more abundant red cells
7. *Effects*	Ischaemia leading to infarcts e.g. in the heart, brain etc	Thromboembolism, oedema, skin ulcers, poor wound healing

Chapter Five

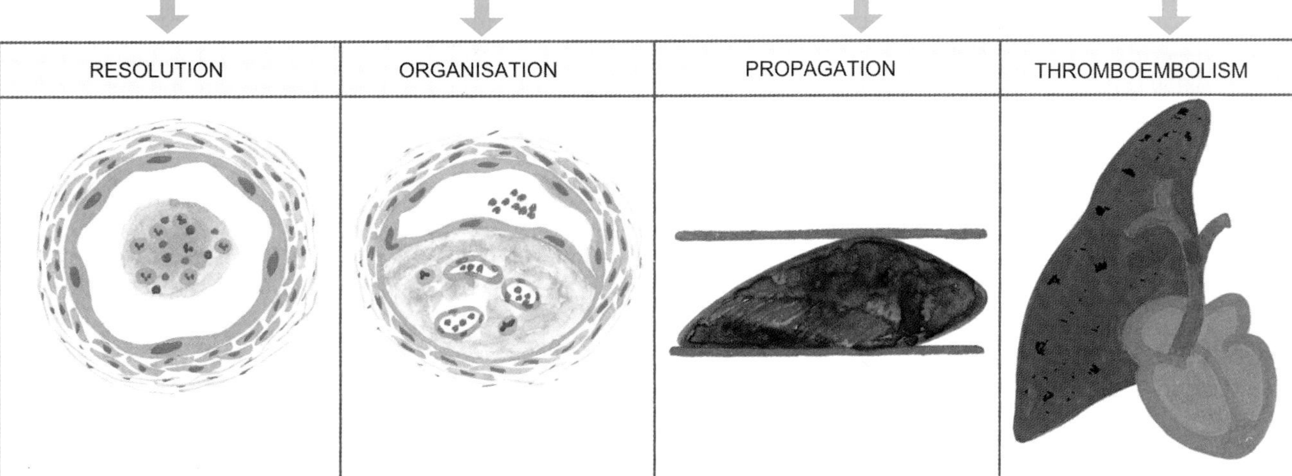

FIGURE 5.23

Fate of thrombus.

b) Clinical conditions predisposing to thrombosis:

i) Heart diseases e.g. myocardial infarction, CHF, rheumatic mitral stenosis, cardiomyopathy.
ii) Atherosclerosis
iii) Aneurysms of the aorta and other vessels
iv) Varicosities of leg veins
v) Nephrotic syndrome
vi) Disseminated cancers
vii) Late pregnancy and puerperium.

Clinical Effects of Thrombosis

These depend upon the site of thrombi, rapidity of formation, and nature of thrombi.

1. Cardiac thrombi. Large thrombi in the heart may cause sudden death by mechanical obstruction of blood flow or through thromboembolism to vital organs.

2. Arterial thrombi. These cause ischaemic necrosis of the deprived part (infarct) which may lead to gangrene. Sudden death may occur following thrombosis of coronary artery.

3. Venous thrombi (Phlebothrombosis). These may cause various effects such as:

i) Thromboembolism
ii) Oedema of area drained
iii) Poor wound healing
iv) Skin ulcer
v) Painful thrombosed veins (thrombophlebitis)
vi) Painful white leg (phlegmasia alba dolens) due to ileofemoral venous thrombosis in postpartum cases
vii) Thrombophlebitis migrans in cancer.

4. Capillary thrombi. Microthrombi in microcirculation may give rise to disseminated intravascular coagulation (DIC).

EMBOLISM

Definition and Types

Embolism is the process of partial or complete obstruction of some part of the cardiovascular system by any mass carried in the circulation; the transported intravascular mass detached from its site of origin is called an *embolus*. Most usual forms of emboli (90%) are thromboemboli i.e. originating from thrombi or their parts detached from the vessel wall.

Emboli may be of various types:

A. Depending upon the matter in the emboli, they can be:

i) Solid e.g. detached thrombi (thromboemboli), atheromatous material, tumour cell clumps, tissue fragments, parasites, bacterial clumps, foreign bodies.
ii) Liquid e.g. fat globules, amniotic fluid, bone marrow.
iii) Gaseous e.g. air, other gases.

B. Depending upon whether infected or not, they are called:

i) Bland, when sterile.
ii) Septic, when infected.

C. Depending upon the source of the emboli, they are classified as:

i) Cardiac emboli from left side of heart e.g. emboli originating from atrium and atrial appendages, infarct in the left ventricle, vegetations of endocarditis.

ii) Arterial emboli e.g. in systemic arteries in the brain, spleen, kidney, intestine.

iii) Venous emboli e.g. in pulmonary arteries.

iv) Lymphatic emboli can also occur.

D. Depending upon the flow of blood, two special types of emboli are mentioned:

i) Paradoxical embolus. An embolus which is carried from the venous side of circulation to the arterial side or vice versa is called paradoxical or crossed embolus e.g. through arteriovenous communication such as in patent foramen ovale, septal defect of the heart, and arteriovenous shunts in the lungs.

ii) Retrograde embolus. An embolus which travels against the flow of blood is called retrograde embolus e.g. metastatic deposits in the spine from carcinoma prostate. The spread occurs by retrograde embolism through intraspinal veins which carry tumour emboli from large thoracic and abdominal veins due to increased pressure in body cavities e.g. during coughing or straining.

Some of the important types of embolism are tabulated in Table 5.5 and described below:

Thromboembolism

A detached thrombus or part of thrombus constitutes the most common type of embolism. These may arise in the arterial or venous circulation (Fig. 5.24):

Arterial (systemic) thromboembolism. Arterial emboli may be derived from the following sources:

A. *Causes within the heart* (80-85%): These are mural thrombi in the left atrium or left ventricle, vegetations on the mitral or aortic valves, prosthetic heart valves and cardiomyopathy.

B. *Causes within the arteries:* These include emboli developing in relation to atherosclerotic plaques, aortic aneurysms, pulmonary veins and paradoxical arterial emboli from the systemic venous circulation.

The *effects* of arterial emboli depend upon their size, site of lodgement, and adequacy of collateral circulation. If the vascular occlusion occurs, the following ill-effects may result:

i) Infarction of the organ or its affected part e.g. ischaemic necrosis in the lower limbs (70-75%), spleen, kidneys, brain, intestine.

ii) Gangrene following infarction in the lower limbs if the collateral circulation is inadequate.

iii) Arteritis and mycotic aneurysm formation from bacterial endocarditis.

iv) Myocardial infarction may occur following coronary embolism.

v) Sudden death may result from coronary embolism or embolism in the middle cerebral artery.

Venous thromboembolism. Venous emboli may arise from the following sources:

i) Thrombi in the veins of the lower legs are the most common cause of venous emboli.

ii) Thrombi in the pelvic veins.

iii) Thrombi in the veins of the upper limbs.

iv) Thrombosis in cavernous sinus of the brain.

v) Thrombi in the right side of heart.

The most significant *effect* of venous embolism is obstruction of pulmonary arterial circulation leading to pulmonary embolism described below.

TABLE 5.5: Important Types of Embolism.

TYPE	COMMON ORIGIN
1. *Pulmonary embolism*	Veins of lower legs
2. *Systemic embolism*	Left ventricle (arterial)
3. *Fat embolism*	Trauma to bones/soft tissues
4. *Air embolism*	Venous: head & neck operations, obstetrical trauma Arterial: cardiothoracic surgery, angiography
5. *Decompression sickness*	Descent: divers Ascent: unpressurised flight
6. *Amniotic fluid embolism*	Components of amniotic fluid
7. *Atheroembolism*	Atheromatous plaques
8. *Tumour embolism*	Tumour fragments

Pulmonary Thromboembolism

DEFINITION. Pulmonary embolism is the most common and fatal form of venous thromboembolism in which there is occlusion of pulmonary arterial tree by thromboemboli. Pulmonary thrombosis as such is uncommon and may occur in pulmonary atherosclerosis and pulmonary hypertension. Differentiation of pulmonary thrombosis from pulmonary thromboembolism is tabulated in Table 5.6.

ETIOLOGY. Pulmonary emboli are more common in hospitalised or bed-ridden patients, though they can occur in ambulatory patients as well. The causes are as follows:

i) Thrombi originating from large veins of lower legs (such as popliteal, femoral and iliac) are the cause in 95% of pulmonary emboli.

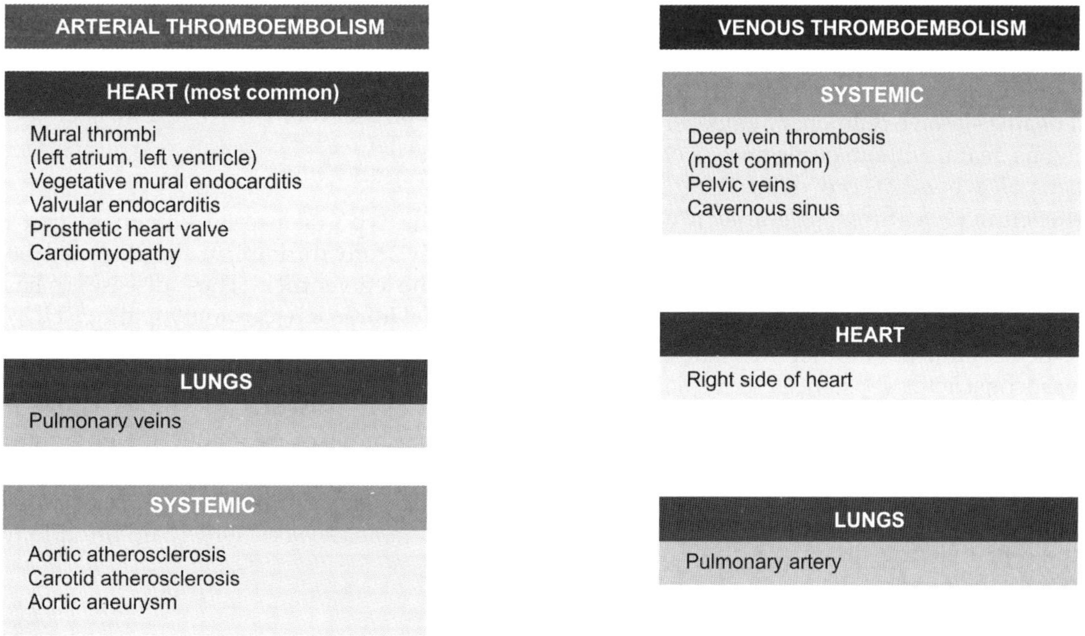

ARTERIAL THROMBOEMBOLISM

HEART (most common)

Mural thrombi
(left atrium, left ventricle)
Vegetative mural endocarditis
Valvular endocarditis
Prosthetic heart valve
Cardiomyopathy

LUNGS

Pulmonary veins

SYSTEMIC

Aortic atherosclerosis
Carotid atherosclerosis
Aortic aneurysm

VENOUS THROMBOEMBOLISM

SYSTEMIC

Deep vein thrombosis
(most common)
Pelvic veins
Cavernous sinus

HEART

Right side of heart

LUNGS

Pulmonary artery

FIGURE 5.24

Sources of arterial and venous emboli.

ii) Less common sources include thrombi in varicosities of superficial veins of the legs, and pelvic veins such as peri-prostatic, periovarian, uterine and broad ligament veins.

PATHOGENESIS. Detachment of thrombi from any of the above-mentioned sites produces a thrombo-embolus that flows through venous drainage into the larger veins draining into right side of the heart.

- If the thrombus is large, it is impacted at the bifurcation of the main pulmonary artery *(saddle embolus)*, or may be found in the right ventricle or its outflow tract.
- More commonly, there are *multiple emboli*, or a large embolus may be fragmented into many smaller emboli which are then impacted in a number of vessels, particularly affecting the lower lobes of lungs.
- Rarely, *paradoxical embolism* may occur by passage of an embolus from right heart into the left heart through atrial or ventricular septal defect. In this way, pulmonary emboli may reach systemic circulation.

CONSEQUENCES OF PULMONARY EMBOLISM. Pulmonary embolism occurs more commonly as a complication in patients of acute or chronic debilitating diseases who are immobilised for a long duration. Women in their reproductive period are at higher risk such as in late pregnancy, following delivery and with use of contraceptive pills. The effects of pulmonary embolism depend mainly on the size of the occluded

TABLE 5.6: Contrasting Features of Pulmonary Thrombosis and Pulmonary Thromboembolism.

	FEATURE	PUL. THROMBOSIS	PUL. THROMBOEMBOLISM
1.	*Pathogenesis*	Locally formed	Travelled from distance
2.	*Location*	In small arteries and branches	In major arteries and branches
3.	*Attachment to vessel wall*	Firmly adherent	Loosely attached or lying free
4.	*Gross appearance*	Head pale, tail red	No distinction in head and tail; smooth surface dry dull surface
5.	*Microscopy*	Platelets and fibrin in layers, Lines of Zahn seen	Mixed with blood clot, lines of Zahn rare

vessel, the number of emboli, and on the cardiovascular status of the patient. The following consequences can result (Fig. 5.25):

i) Sudden death. Massive pulmonary embolism results in instantaneous death, without occurrence of chest pain or dyspnoea. However, if the death is somewhat delayed, the clinical features resemble myocardial infarction i.e. severe chest pain, dyspnoea and shock.

ii) Acute cor pulmonale. Numerous small emboli may obstruct most of the pulmonary circulation resulting in acute right heart failure. Another mechanism is by release of vasoconstrictor substances from platelets or by reflex vasoconstriction of pulmonary vessels.

iii) Pulmonary infarction. Obstruction of relatively small-sized pulmonary arterial branches may result in pulmonary infarction (page 130). The clinical features include chest pain due to fibrinous pleuritis, haemoptysis and dyspnoea due to reduced functioning pulmonary parenchyma.

iv) Pulmonary haemorrhage. Obstruction of terminal branches (endarteries) leads to central pulmonary haemorrhage. The clinical features are haemoptysis, dyspnoea, and less commonly, chest pain due to central location of pulmonary haemorrhage. Sometimes, there may be concomitant pulmonary infarction.

v) Resolution. Vast majority of small pulmonary emboli (60-80%) are resolved by fibrinolytic activity. These patients are clinically silent owing to bronchial circulation so that lung parenchyma is adequately perfused.

vi) Pulmonary hypertension, chronic cor pulmonale and pulmonary arteriosclerosis. These are the sequelae of multiple small thromboemboli undergoing healing rather than resolution.

Systemic Embolism

This is the type of arterial embolism that originates commonly from thrombi in the diseased heart, especially in the left ventricle. These diseases of heart include myocardial infraction, cardiomyopathy, RHD, congenital heart disease, infective endocarditis, and prosthetic cardiac valves. These arterial emboli invariably cause infarction at the sites of lodgement which include, in descending order of frequency, lower extremity, brain, and internal visceral organs (spleen, kidneys, intestines). *Thus, the effects and sites of arterial emboli are in striking contrast to venous emboli* which are often lodged in the lungs.

Fat Embolism

Obstruction of arterioles and capillaries by fat globules constitutes fat embolism. If the obstruction in the circulation is by fragments of adipose tissue, it is called fat-tissue embolism.

ETIOLOGY. Following are the important causes of fat embolism:

i) Traumatic causes:

■ *Trauma to bones* is the most common cause of fat embolism e.g. in fractures of long bones leading to

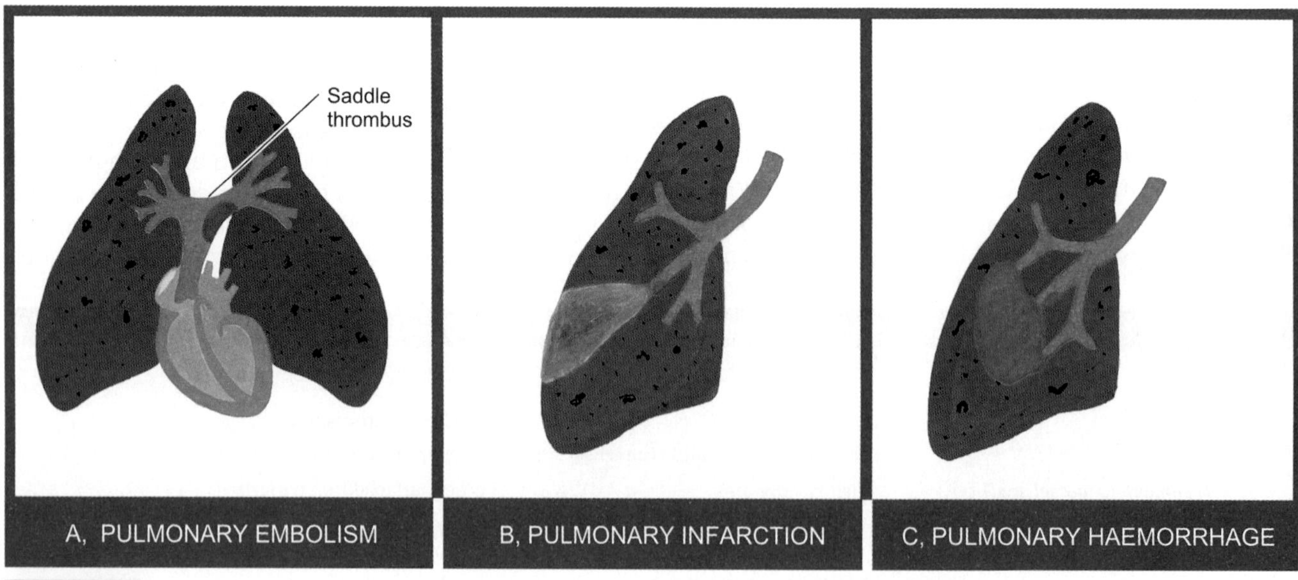

FIGURE 5.25

Three main consequences of pulmonary embolism. A, Saddle embolus, causing sudden death. B, Pulmonary infarction, commonly peripheral. C, Pulmonary haemorrhage, usually central.

passage of fatty marrow in circulation, concussions of bones, after orthopaedic surgical procedures etc.

- *Trauma to soft tissue* e.g. laceration of adipose tissue and in puerperium due to injury to pelvic fatty tissue.

ii) Non-traumatic causes:

- Extensive burns
- Diabetes mellitus
- Fatty liver
- Pancreatitis
- Sickle cell anaemia
- Decompression sickness
- Inflammation of bones and soft tissues
- Extrinsic fat or oils introduced into the body.

PATHOGENESIS. The following mechanisms are proposed to explain the pathogenesis of fat embolism. These may be acting singly or in combination.

i) Mechanical theory. Mobilisation of fluid fat may occur following trauma to the bone or soft tissues. The fat globules released from the injured area may enter venous circulation and finally most of the fat is arrested in the small vessels in the lungs. Some of the fat globules may further pass through into the systemic circulation to lodge in other organs.

ii) Emulsion instability theory. This theory explains the pathogenesis of fat embolism in non-traumatic cases. According to this theory, fat emboli are formed by aggregation of plasma lipids (chylomicrons and fatty acids) due to disturbance in natural emulsification of fat.

iii) Intravascular coagulation theory. In stress, release of some factor activates disseminated intravascular coagulation (DIC) and aggregation of fat emboli.

iv) Toxic injury theory. According to this theory, the small blood vessels of lungs are chemically injured by high plasma levels of free fatty acid, resulting in increased vascular permeability and consequent pulmonary oedema.

CONSEQUENCES OF FAT EMBOLISM. The effects of fat embolism depend upon the size and quantity of fat globules, and whether or not the emboli pass through the lungs into the systemic circulation.

i) Pulmonary fat embolism. In patients dying after fractures of bones, presence of numerous fat emboli in the capillaries of the lung is a frequent autopsy finding because the small fat globules are not likely to appreciably obstruct the vast pulmonary vascular bed. However, widespread obstruction of pulmonary circulation due to extensive pulmonary embolism can occur and result in sudden death.

Microscopically, the lungs show hyperaemia, oedema, petechial haemorrhages and changes of adult respiratory distress syndrome (ARDS). Pulmonary infarction is usually not a feature of fat embolism because of the small size of globules. In routine stains, the fat globules in the pulmonary arteries, capillaries and alveolar spaces appear as vacuoles. Frozen section is essential for confirmation of globules by fat stains such as Sudan dyes (Sudan black, Sudan III and IV), oil red O and osmic acid.

ii) Systemic fat embolism. Some of the fat globules may pass through the pulmonary circulation such as via patent foramen ovale, arteriovenous shunts in the lungs and vertebral venous plexuses, and get lodged in the capillaries of organs like the brain, kidney, skin etc.

- **Brain.** The pathologic findings in the brain are petechial haemorrhages on the leptomeninges and minute haemorrhages in the parenchyma.
Microscopically, microinfarct of brain, oedema and haemorrhages are seen. The CNS manifestations include delirium, convulsions, stupor, coma and sudden death.
- **Kidney.** Renal fat embolism present in the glomerular capillaries, may cause decreased glomerular filtration. Other effects include tubular damage and renal insufficiency.
- **Other organs.** Besides the brain and kidneys, other findings in systemic fat embolism are petechiae in the skin, conjunctivae, serosal surfaces, fat globules in the urine and sputum.

Gas Embolism

Air, nitrogen and other gases can produce bubbles within the circulation and obstruct the blood vessels causing damage to tissue. Two main forms of gas embolism—air embolism and decompression sickness are described below.

Air Embolism

Air embolism occurs when air is introduced into venous or arterial circulation.

VENOUS AIR EMBOLISM. Air may be sucked into systemic veins under the following circumstances:

i) Operations on head and neck, and trauma. The accidental opening of a major vein of the neck like jugular, or neck wounds involving the major neck veins, may allow air to be drawn into venous circulation.

ii) Obstetrical operations and trauma. During childbirth by normal vaginal delivery, caesarean section, abortions and other procedures, fatal air embolism may result from the entrance of air into the opened-up uterine venous sinuses and endometrial veins.

iii) Intravenous infusion of blood and fluid. Air embolism may occur during intravenous blood or fluid infusions if only positive pressure is employed.

iv) Angiography. During angiographic procedures, air may be entrapped into a large vein causing air embolism.

The **effects** of venous air embolism depend upon the following factors:

i) Amount of air introduced into the circulation. The volume of air necessary to cause death is variable but usually 100-150 ml of air entry is considered fatal.

ii) Rapidity of entry of a smaller volume of air is important determinant of a fatal outcome.

iii) Position of the patient during or soon after entry of air is another factor. The air bubbles may ascend into the superior vena cava if the position of head is higher than the trunk (e.g. in upright position) and reach the brain.

iv) General condition of the patient e.g. in severely ill patients, as little as 40 ml of air may have serious results.

The mechanism of death is by entrapment of air emboli in the pulmonary arterial trunk in the right heart. If bubbles of air in the form of froth pass further out into pulmonary arterioles, they cause widespread vascular occlusions. If death from pulmonary air embolism is suspected, the heart and pulmonary artery should be opened *in situ* under water so that escaping froth or foam formed by mixture of air and blood can be detected.

ARTERIAL AIR EMBOLISM. Entry of air into pulmonary vein or its tributaries may occur in the following conditions:

i) Cardiothoracic surgery and trauma. Arterial air embolism may occur following thoracic operations, thoracocentesis, rupture of the lung, penetrating wounds of the lung, artificial pneumothorax etc.

ii) Paradoxical air embolism. This may occur due to passage of venous air emboli to the arterial side of circulation through a patent foramen ovale or via pulmonary arteriovenous shunts.

iii) Arteriography. During arteriographic procedures, air embolism may occur.

The **effects** of arterial air embolism are in the form of certain characteristic features:

i) Marble skin due to blockage of cutaneous vessels.

ii) Air bubbles in the retinal vessels seen ophthalmoscopically.

iii) Pallor of the tongue due to occlusion of a branch of lingual artery.

iv) Coronary or cerebral arterial air embolism may cause sudden death by much smaller amounts of air than in the venous air embolism.

Decompression Sickness

This is a specialised form of gas embolism known by various names such as caisson's disease, divers' palsy or aeroembolism.

PATHOGENESIS. Decompression sickness is produced when the individual decompresses suddenly, either from high atmospheric pressure to normal level, or from normal pressure to low atmospheric pressure.

- In divers, workers in caissons (diving-bells), offshore drilling and tunnels, who *descend* to high atmospheric pressure, increased amount of atmospheric gases (mainly nitrogen; others are O_2, CO_2) are dissolved in blood and tissue fluids. When such an individual ascends too rapidly i.e. comes to normal level suddenly from high atmospheric pressure, the gases come out of the solution as minute bubbles, particularly in fatty tissues which have affinity for nitrogen. These bubbles may coalesce together to form large emboli.
- In aeroembolism, seen in those who *ascend* to high altitudes or air flight in unpressurised cabins, the individuals are exposed to sudden decompression from low atmospheric pressure to normal levels. This results in similar effects as in divers and workers in caissons.

EFFECTS. The effects of decompression sickness depend upon the following:

- Depth or altitude reached
- Duration of exposure to altered pressure
- Rate of ascent or descent
- General condition of the individual

The pathologic changes are more pronounced in sudden decompression from high pressure to normal levels than in those who decompress from low pressure to normal levels. The changes are more serious in obese persons as nitrogen gas is more soluble in fat than in body fluids.

Clinical effects of decompression sickness are of 2 types—acute and chronic.

- **Acute form** occurs due to acute obstruction of small blood vessels in the vicinity of joints and skeletal muscles. The condition is clinically characterised by the following:

i) 'The bends', as the patient doubles up in bed due to acute pain in joints, ligaments and tendons.

ii) 'The chokes' occur due to accumulation of bubbles in the lungs, resulting in acute respiratory distress.

iii) Cerebral effects may manifest in the form of vertigo, coma, and sometimes death.

■ **Chronic form** is due to foci of ischaemic necrosis throughout body, especially the skeletal system. Ischaemic necrosis may be due to embolism *per se*, but other factors such as platelet activation, intravascular coagulation and hypoxia might contribute. The features of chronic form are as under:

i) Avascular necrosis of bones e.g. head of femur, tibia, humerus.

ii) Neurological symptoms may occur due to ischaemic necrosis in the central nervous system. These include paraesthesias and paraplegia.

iii) Lung involvement in the form of haemorrhage, oedema, emphysema and atelactasis may be seen. These result in dyspnoea, nonproductive cough and chest pain.

iv) Skin manifestations include itching, patchy erythema, cyanosis and oedema.

v) Other organs like parenchymal cells of the liver and pancreas may show lipid vacuoles.

Amniotic Fluid Embolism

This is the most serious, unpredictable and unpreventible cause of maternal mortality. During labour and in the immediate postpartum period, the contents of amniotic fluid may enter the uterine veins and reach right side of the heart resulting in fatal complications. The amniotic fluid components which may be found in uterine veins, pulmonary artery and vessels of other organs are: epithelial squames, vernix caseosa, lanugo hair, bile from meconium, and mucus. The mechanism by which these amniotic fluid contents enter the maternal circulation is not clear. Possibly, they gain entry either through tears in the myometrium and endocervix, or the amniotic fluid is forced into uterine sinusoids by vigorous uterine contractions.

PATHOLOGIC CHANGES. Notable changes are seen in the lungs such as haemorrhages, congestion, oedema and changes of ARDS, and dilatation of right side of the heart.

These changes are associated with identifiable amniotic fluid contents within the pulmonary microcirculation.

The *clinical syndrome* is characterised by the following features:

- Sudden respiratory distress and dyspnoea
- Deep cyanosis
- Cardiovascular shock
- Convulsions
- Coma
- Unexpected death

The *cause of death* may not be obvious but can occur as a result of the following mechanisms:

i) Mechanical blockage of the pulmonary circulation in extensive embolism.

ii) Anaphylactoid reaction to amniotic fluid components.

iii) Disseminated intravascular coagulation (DIC) due to liberation of thromboplastin by amniotic fluid.

iv) Haemorrhagic manifestations due to thrombocytopenia and afibrinogenaemia.

Atheroembolism

Atheromatous plaques, especially from aorta, may get eroded to form atherosclerotic emboli which are then lodged in medium-sized and small arteries. These emboli consist of cholesterol crystals, hyaline debris and calcified material, and may evoke foreign body reaction at the site of lodgement.

PATHOLOGIC CHANGES and their effects in atheroembolism are as under:

i) Ischaemia, atrophy and necrosis of tissue distal to the occluded vessel.

ii) Infarcts in the organs affected such as the kidneys, spleen, brain and heart.

iii) Gangrene in the lower limbs.

iv) Hypertension, if widespread renal vascular lesions are present.

Tumour Embolism

Malignant tumour cells invade the local blood vessels and may form tumour emboli to be lodged elsewhere, producing metastatic tumour deposits. Notable examples are clear cell carcinoma of kidney, carcinoma of the lung, malignant melanoma etc (Chapter 8).

Miscellaneous Emboli

Various other endogenous and exogenous substances may act as emboli. These are:

i) Fragments of tissue
ii) Placental fragments
iii) Red cell aggregates (sludging)
iv) Bacteria
v) Parasites
vi) Barium emboli following enema
vii) Foreign bodies e.g. needles, talc, sutures, bullets, catheters etc.

ISCHAEMIA

DEFINITION. Ischaemia is defined as deficient blood supply to part of a tissue. The cessation of blood supply may be complete (complete ischaemia) or partial (partial ischaemia). The harmful effects of ischaemia may result from 3 ways:

1. Hypoxia due to deprivation of oxygen to tissues.
2. Inadequate supply of nutrients to the tissue such as glucose and amino acids.
3. Inadequate clearance of metabolites resulting in accumulation of metabolic waste-products in the affected tissue.

ETIOLOGY. A number of causes may produce ischaemia. These are as under:

1. Causes in the heart. Inadequate cardiac output resulting from heart block, ventricular arrest and fibrillation may cause hypoxic injury to brain.

- If the arrest continues for 15 seconds, consciousness is lost.
- If the condition lasts for more than 4 minutes, irreversible ischaemic damage to brain occurs.
- If it is prolonged for more than 8 minutes, death is inevitable.

2. Causes in the arteries. The commonest and most important causes of ischaemia are due to obstruction in arterial blood supply. These are:

i) Luminal occlusion such as due to:

- Thrombosis
- Embolism

ii) Causes in the arterial wall such as:

- Vasospasm (e.g. in Raynaud's disease)
- Hypothermia, ergotism
- Arteriosclerosis
- Polyarteritis nodosa
- Thromboangiitis obliterans (Buerger's disease)
- Severed vessel wall

iii) Outside pressure on an artery such as:

- Ligature
- Tourniquet
- Tight plaster, bandages
- Torsion.

3. Causes in the veins. Blockage of venous drainage may lead to engorgement and obstruction to arterial blood supply resulting in ischaemia. The examples include the following:

i) Luminal occlusion such as in:

- Thrombosis of mesenteric veins
- Cavernous sinus thrombosis

ii) Causes in the vessel wall such as in:

- Varicose veins of the legs

iii) Outside pressure on a vein as in:

- Strangulated hernia
- Intussusception
- Volvulus

4. Causes in the microcirculation. Ischaemia may result from occlusion of arterioles, capillaries and venules. The causes are as under:

i) Luminal occlusion such as:

- By red cells e.g. in sickle cell anaemia, red cells parasitised by malaria, acquired haemolytic anaemia, sludging of the blood.
- By white cells e.g. in chronic myeloid leukaemia
- By fibrin e.g. defibrination syndrome
- By precipitated cryoglobulins
- By fat embolism
- In decompression sickness.

ii) Causes in the microvasculature wall such as:

- Vasculitis e.g. in polyarteritis nodosa, Henoch-Schönlein purpura, Arthus reaction, septicaemia.
- Frost-bite injuring the wall of small blood vessels.

iii) Outside pressure on microvasculature as in:

- Bedsores.

FACTORS DETERMINING THE SEVERITY OF ISCHAEMIC INJURY. The extent of damage produced by ischaemia due to occlusion of arterial or venous blood vessels depends upon a number of factors. These are as under:

1. Anatomic pattern. The extent of injury by ischaemia depends upon the anatomic pattern of arterial blood supply of the organ or tissue affected. There are 4 different patterns of arterial blood supply:

i) Single arterial supply without anastomosis. Some organs receive blood supply from arteries which do not have significant anastomosis and are thus functional end-arteries. Occlusion of such vessels invariably results in ischaemic necrosis. The examples are:

- Central artery of the retina
- Interlobular arteries of the kidneys.

ii) Single arterial supply with rich anastomosis. Arterial supply to some organs has rich interarterial anastomoses so that blockage of one vessel can re-establish blood supply bypassing the blocked arterial branch, and hence the infarction is less common in such circumstances. For example:

- Superior mesenteric artery supplying blood to the small intestine.
- Inferior mesenteric artery supplying blood to distal colon.
- Arterial supply to the stomach by 3 separate vessels derived from coeliac axis.

■ Interarterial anastomoses in the 3 main trunks of the coronary arterial system.

iii) Parallel arterial supply. Blood supply to some organs and tissues is such that the vitality of the tissue is maintained by alternative blood supply in case of occlusion of one. The examples are:

■ Blood supply to brain in the region of circle of Willis.
■ Arterial supply to forearm by radial and ulnar arteries.

iv) Double blood supply. The effect of occlusion of one set of vessels is modified if an organ has dual blood supply. For example:

■ Lungs are perfused by bronchial circulation as well as by pulmonary arterial branches.
■ Liver is supplied by both portal circulation and hepatic arterial flow.

However, collateral circulation is of little value if the vessels are severely affected with spasm, atheroma or any other condition.

2. General and cardiovascular status. The general status of an individual as regards cardiovascular function is an important determinant to assess the effect of ischaemia. Some of the factors which render the tissues more vulnerable to the effects of ischaemia are:

i) Anaemias (sickle cell anaemia, in particular)
ii) Lowered oxygenation of blood (hypoxaemia)
iii) Senility with marked coronary atherosclerosis
iv) Cardiac failure
v) Blood loss
vi) Shock.

3. Type of tissue affected. The vulnerability of tissue of the body to the effect of ischaemia is variable. The mesenchymal tissues are quite resistant to the effect of ischaemia as compared to parenchymal cells of the organs. The following tissues are more vulnerable to ischaemia:

i) Brain (cerebral cortical neurons, in particular).
ii) Heart (myocardial cells).
iii) Kidney (especially epithelial cells of proximal convoluted tubules).

4. Rapidity of development. Sudden vascular obstruction results in more severe effects of ischaemia than if it is gradual since there is less time for collaterals to develop.

5. Degree of vascular occlusion. Complete vascular obstruction results in more severe ischaemic injury than the partial occlusion.

EFFECTS. The effects of ischaemia are variable and range from 'no change' to 'sudden death'.

1. No effects on the tissues, if the collateral channels develop adequately so that the effect of ischaemia fails to occur.

2. Functional disturbances. These result when collateral channels are able to supply blood during normal activity but the supply is not adequate to withstand the effect of exertion. The examples are angina pectoris and intermittent claudication.

3. Cellular changes. Partial ischaemia may produce cellular changes such as cloudy swelling, fatty change, atrophy and replacement fibrosis. Infarction results when the deprivation of blood supply is complete so as to cause necrosis of tissue affected.

4. Sudden death. The cause of sudden death from ischaemia is usually myocardial and cerebral infarction.

INFARCTION

DEFINITION. Infarction is the process of tissue necrosis resulting from some form of circulatory insufficiency; the localised area of necrosis so developed is called an *infarct*.

ETIOLOGY. All the causes of ischaemia discussed above can cause infarction. There are a few other note-worthy features in infarcts:

■ Most commonly, infarcts are caused by interrupted arterial blood supply, called *ischaemic necrosis*.
■ Less commonly, venous obstruction can produce infarcts termed *stagnant hypoxia*.
■ Generally, *sudden, complete, and continuous occlusion* by thrombosis or embolism produces infarcts.
■ Infarcts may be produced by *nonocclusive circulatory insufficiency* as well e.g. incomplete atherosclerotic narrowing of coronary arteries may produce myocardial infarction due to acute coronary insufficiency.

TYPES OF INFARCTS. Infarcts are classified depending upon different features:

1. According to their colour, infarcts may be:

■ *Pale or anaemic,* due to arterial occlusion and are seen in compact organs e.g. in the kidneys, heart, spleen.
■ *Red or haemorrhagic,* seen in soft loose tissues and are caused either by pulmonary arterial obstruction (e.g. in the lungs) or by arterial or venous occlusion (e.g. in the intestines).

2. According to their age, infarcts are classified as:

■ *Recent or fresh*
■ *Old or healed*

3. According to presence or absence of infection, they may be:

■ *Bland,* when free of bacterial contamination
■ *Septic,* when infected.

PATHOGENESIS. The process of infarction takes place as follows:

i) *Localised hyperaemia* due to local anoxaemia occurs immediately after obstruction of the blood supply.

ii) Within a few hours, the affected part becomes swollen due to *oedema and haemorrhage*. The amount of haemorrhage is variable, being more marked in the lungs and spleen, and less extensive in the kidneys and heart.

iii) *Cellular changes* such as cloudy swelling and degeneration appear early, while death of the cells or necrosis occurs in 12-48 hours.

iv) There is progressive *autolysis* of the necrotic tissue and haemolysis of the red cells.

v) *An acute inflammatory reaction and hyperaemia* appear at the same time in the surrounding tissues in response to products of autolysis.

vi) *Blood pigments*, haematoidin and haemosiderin, liberated by haemolysis are deposited in the infarct. At this stage, most infarcts become pale due to loss of red cells.

vii) Following this, there is progressive *ingrowth of granulation tissue* from the margin of the infarct so that eventually the infarct is replaced by a fibrous scar. Dystrophic calcification may occur sometimes. However, in the case of infarct brain, there is liquefactive necrosis which heals by gliosis.

PATHOLOGIC CHANGES. Some general morphological features of infarcts are described below, followed by pathologic changes in infarcts of different organs.

Grossly, infarcts of solid organs are usually wedge-shaped, the apex pointing towards the occluded artery and the wide base on the surface of the organ. Infarcts due to arterial occlusion are generally pale while those due to venous obstruction are haemorrhagic. Most infarcts become pale later as the red cells are lysed but pulmonary infarcts never become pale due to extensive amount of blood. Cerebral infarcts are poorly defined with central softening (encephalomalacia). Recent infarcts are generally slightly elevated over the surface while the old infarcts are shrunken and depressed under the surface of the organ.

Microscopically, the pathognomonic cytologic change in all infarcts is coagulative necrosis of the affected area of tissue or organ. In cerebral infarcts, however, there is characteristic liquefactive necrosis. Some amount of haemorrhage is generally present in any infarct. At the periphery of an infarct, inflammatory reaction is noted. Initially, neutrophils predominate but subsequently macrophages and fibroblasts appear. Eventually, the necrotic area is replaced by fibrous scar tissue, which at times may show dystrophic calcification. In cerebral infarcts, the liquefactive necrosis is followed by gliosis i.e. replacement by microglial cells distended by fatty material (gitter cells).

Infarcts of Different Organs

Table 5.7 summarises the gross appearance and the usual outcome of the common types of infarction. Fig. 5.26 shows the organs most commonly affected by infarction.

A few representative examples ot infarction of some organs (lungs, kidney, liver and spleen) are discussed below. Myocardial infarction (Chapter 12), cerebral infarction (Chapter 28) and infarction of small intestines (Chapter 18) are covered in detail later in respective chapters of Systemic Pathology.

INFARCT LUNG. Embolism of the pulmonary arteries may produce pulmonary infarction, though not always. This is because lungs receive blood supply from bronchial arteries as well, and thus occlusion of pulmonary artery ordinarily does not produce infarcts. However, it may occur in patients who have inadequate circulation such as in chronic lung diseases and congestive heart failure.

Grossly, the pulmonary infarcts are classically wedge-shaped with base on the pleura, haemorrhagic, variable in size, and most often in the lower lobes. Fibrinous pleuritis usually covers the area of infarct. Cut surface is dark purple and may show the blocked vessel near the apex of the infarcted area. Old organised and healed pulmonary infarcts appear as retracted fibrous scars.

Microscopically, the characteristic histologic feature is coagulative necrosis of the alveolar walls. Initially, there is infiltration by neutrophils and intense alveolar capillary congestion, but later their place is taken by haemosiderin, phagocytes and granulation tissue (COLOUR PLATE VI: CL 23).

INFARCT KIDNEY. Renal infarction is common, found in upto 5% of autopsies. Majority of them are caused by thromboemboli, most commonly originating from the heart such as in mural thrombi in the left atrium, myocardial infarction, vegetative endocarditis and aortic aneurysm. Less commonly, renal infarcts may occur due to advanced renal artery atherosclerosis, arteritis and sickle cell anaemia.

TABLE 5.7: Infarcts of Most Commonly Affected Organs.

	LOCATION	GROSS APPEARANCE	OUTCOME
1.	*Myocardial infarction*	Pale	Frequently lethal
2.	*Pulmonary infarction*	Haemorrhagic	Less commonly fatal
3.	*Cerebral infarction*	Haemorrhagic or pale	Fatal if massive
4.	*Intestinal infarction*	Haemorrhagic	Frequently lethal
5.	*Renal infarction*	Pale	Not lethal unless massive and bilateral
6.	*Infarct spleen*	Pale	Not lethal
7.	*Infarct liver*	Pale	Not lethal
8.	*Infarcts lower extremity*	Pale	Not lethal

Grossly, renal infarcts are often multiple and may be bilateral. Characteristically, they are pale or anaemic and wedge-shaped with base resting under the capsule and apex pointing towards the medulla. Generally, a narrow rim of preserved renal tissue under the capsule is spared because it draws its blood supply from the capsular vessels. Cut surface of renal infarct in the first 2 to 3 days is red and congested but by 4th day the centre becomes pale yellow. At the end of one week, the infarct is typically anaemic and depressed below the surface of the kidney (Fig. 5.27).

Microscopically, the affected area shows characteristic coagulative necrosis of renal parenchyma i.e. there are ghosts of renal tubules and glomeruli without intact nuclei and cytoplasmic content. The margin of the infarct shows inflammatory reaction—initially acute but later macrophages and fibrous tissue predominate (Fig. 5.28) (COLOUR PLATE VI: CL 22).

INFARCT SPLEEN. Spleen is one of the common sites for infarction. Splenic infarction results from occlusion of the splenic artery or its branches. Occlusion is caused most commonly by thromboemboli arising in the heart (e.g. in mural thrombi in the left atrium, vegetative endocarditis, myocardial infarction), and less frequently by obstruction of microcirculation (e.g. in myeloproliferative diseases, sickle cell anaemia, arteritis, Hodgkin's disease, bacterial infections).

Grossly, splenic infarcts are often multiple. They are characteristically pale or anaemic and wedge-shaped with their base at the periphery and apex pointing towards hilum.

Microscopically, the features are similar to those found in anaemic infarcts in kidney. Coagulative necrosis and inflammatory reaction are seen. Later, the necrotic tissue is replaced by shrunken fibrous scar.

INFARCT LIVER. Just as in lungs, infarcts in the liver are uncommon due to dual blood supply—from portal vein and from hepatic artery. Obstruction of the portal vein is usually secondary to other diseases such as hepatic cirrhosis, intravenous invasion of primary carcinoma of the liver, carcinoma of the pancreas and pylephlebitis. Occlusion of portal vein or its branches generally does not produce ischaemic infarction but

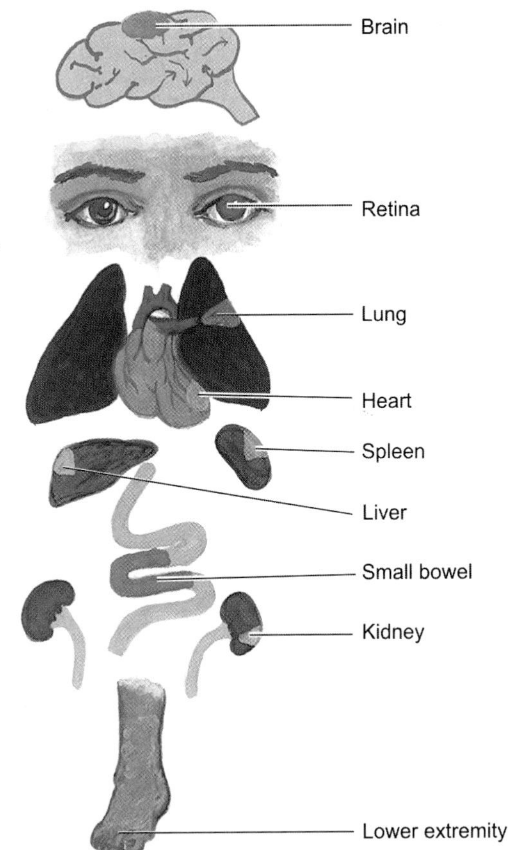

FIGURE 5.26
Common locations of systemic infarcts following arterial embolism.

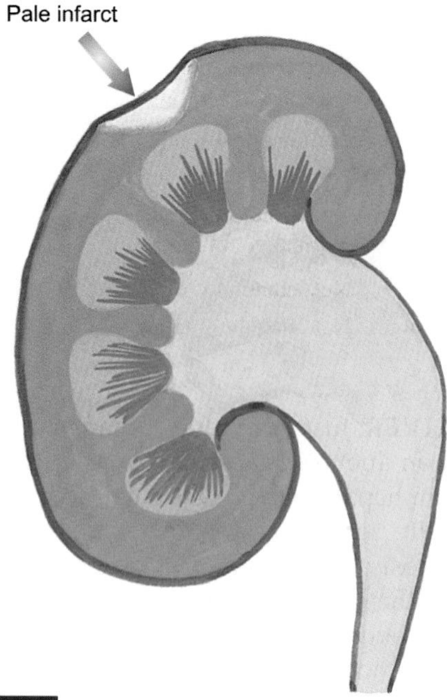

FIGURE 5.27

Infarct kidney, gross appearance. The wedge-shaped infarct is slightly depressed on the surface. The apex lies internally and wide base is on the surface. The central area is pale while the margin is haemorrhagic.

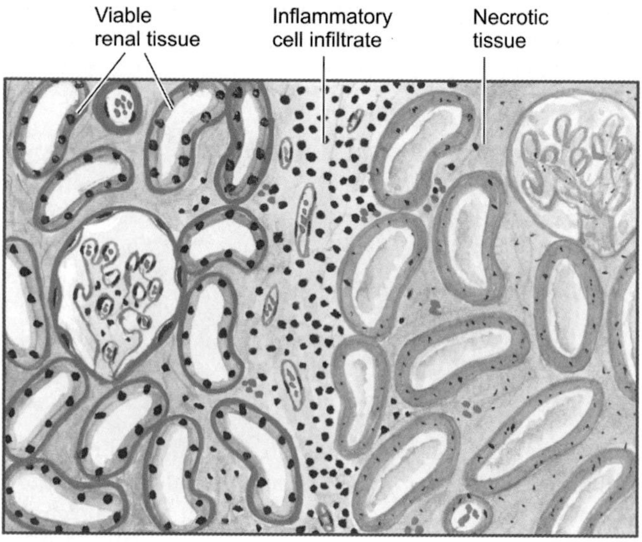

FIGURE 5.28

Microscopic appearance of renal infarct. Renal tubules and glomeruli show typical coagulative necrosis i.e. intact outlines of necrosed cells. There is dense acute inflammatory infiltrate at the periphery of the infarct.

instead reduced blood supply to hepatic parenchyma causes non-ischaemic infarct called *infarct of Zahn*. Obstruction of the hepatic artery or its branches, on the other hand, caused by arteritis, arteriosclerosis, bland or septic emboli, results in ischaemic infarcts of the liver.

Grossly, ischaemic infarcts of the liver are usually anaemic but sometimes may be haemorrhagic due to stuffing of the site by blood from the portal vein. Infarcts of Zahn (non-ischaemic infarcts) produce sharply defined red-blue area in liver parenchyma. ***Microscopically,*** ischaemic infarcts show characteristics of pale or anaemic infarcts as in kidney or spleen. Infarcts of Zahn occurring due to reduced portal blood flow result in atrophy of hepatocytes and dilatation of sinusoids.

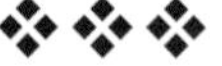

Inflammation and Healing

6

INFLAMMATION

INTRODUCTION

DEFINITION AND CAUSES. Inflammation is defined as the local response of living mammalian tissues to injury due to any agent. It is a body defense reaction in order to eliminate or limit the spread of injurious agent as well as to remove the consequent necrosed cells and tissues.

The agents causing inflammation may be as under:

1. *Physical agents* like heat, cold, radiation, mechanical trauma.
2. *Chemical agents* like organic and inorganic poisons.
3. *Infective agents* like bacteria, viruses and their toxins.
4. *Immunological agents* like cell-mediated and antigen-antibody reactions.

Thus, *inflammation is distinct from infection*—the former being a protective response by the body while the latter is invasion into the body by harmful microbes and their resultant ill-effects by toxins. Inflammation involves 2 basic processes with some overlapping, viz. early *inflammatory response* and later followed by *healing*. Though both these processes generally have protective role against injurious agents, inflammation and healing may cause considerable harm to the body as well e.g. anaphylaxis to bites by insects or reptiles, drugs, toxins, atherosclerosis, chronic rheumatoid arthritis, fibrous bands and adhesions in intestinal obstruction.

SIGNS OF INFLAMMATION. The Roman writer Celsus in 1st century A.D. named the famous 4 *cardinal signs of inflammation* as:

- *rubor* (redness);
- *tumor* (swelling);
- *calor* (heat); and
- *dolor* (pain).

To these, fifth sign *functio laesa* (loss of function) was later added by Virchow. The word inflammation means burning. This nomenclature had its origin in old times but now we know that burning is only one of the signs of inflammation.

TYPES OF INFLAMMATION. Depending upon the defense capacity of the host and duration of response, inflammation can be classified as acute and chronic.

I. *Acute inflammation* is of short duration and represents the early body reaction and is usually followed by repair.

The main features of acute inflammation are:

1. accumulation of fluid and plasma at the affected site;
2. intravascular activation of platelets; and
3. polymorphonuclear neutrophils as inflammatory cells.

II. *Chronic inflammation* is of longer duration and occurs either after the causative agent of acute inflammation persists for a long time, or the stimulus is such that it induces chronic inflammation from the beginning.

The characteristic feature of chronic inflammation is presence of chronic inflammatory cells such as lymphocytes, plasma cells and macrophages.

ACUTE INFLAMMATION

The changes in acute inflammation can be conveniently described under the following 2 headings:

I. Vascular events.
II. Cellular events.

I. VASCULAR EVENTS

Alteration in the microvasculature (arterioles, capillaries and venules) is the earliest response to tissue injury. These alterations include: haemodynamic changes and changes in vascular permeability.

Haemodynamic Changes

The earliest features of inflammatory response result from changes in the vascular flow and calibre of small blood vessels in the injured tissue. The sequence of these changes is as under:

1. Irrespective of the type of injury, immediate vascular response is of **transient vasoconstriction** of arterioles. With mild form of injury, the blood flow may be re-established in 3-5 seconds while with more severe injury the vasoconstriction may last for about 5 minutes.

2. Next follows **persistent progressive vasodilatation** which involves mainly the arterioles, but to a lesser extent, affects other components of the microcirculation like venules and capillaries. This change is obvious within half an hour of injury. Vasodilatation results in increased blood volume in microvascular bed of the area, which is responsible for redness and warmth at the site of acute inflammation.

3. Progressive vasodilatation, in turn, may elevate the **local hydrostatic pressure** resulting in transudation of fluid into the extracellular space. This is responsible for swelling at the local site of acute inflammation.

4. **Slowing or stasis** of microcirculation occurs next. Slowing is attributed to increased permeability of microvasculature that results in increased concentration of red cells, and thus, raised blood viscosity.

5. Stasis or slowing is followed by **leucocytic margination** or peripheral orientation of leucocytes (mainly neutrophils) along the vascular endothelium. The leucocytes stick to the vascular endothelium briefly, and then move and migrate through the gaps between the endothelial cells into the extravascular space. This process is known as *emigration* (discussed later in detail).

The features of haemodynamic changes in inflammation are best demonstrated by the **Lewis experiment.** Lewis induced the changes in the skin of inner aspect of forearm by firm stroking with a blunt point. The reaction so elicited is known as *triple response* or *red line response* consisting of the following (Fig. 6.1):

i) *Red line* appears within a few seconds following stroking and results from local vasodilatation of capillaries and venules.

ii) *Flare* is the bright reddish appearance or flush surrounding the red line and results from vasodilatation of the adjacent arterioles.

iii) *Wheal* is the swelling or oedema of the surrounding skin occurring due to transudation of fluid into the extravascular space.

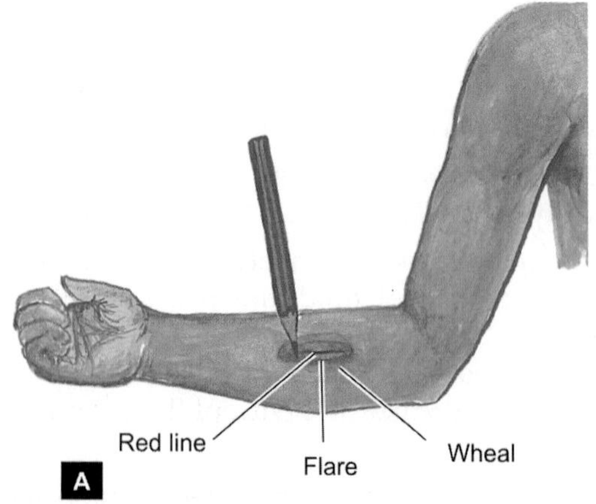

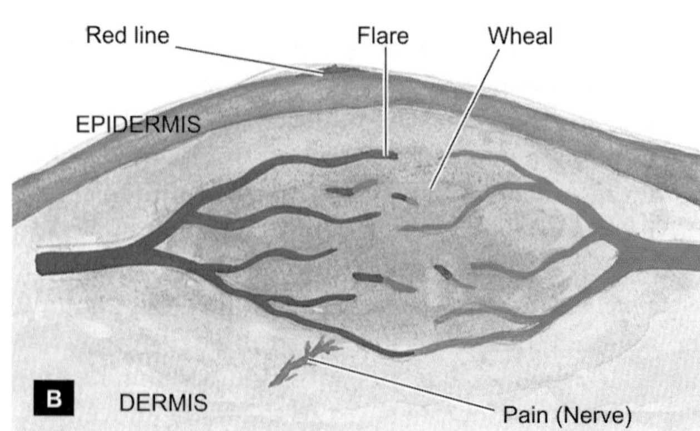

FIGURE 6.1

A, 'Triple response' elicited by firm stroking of skin of forearm with a pencil. B, Diagrammatic view of microscopic features of triple response of the skin.

These features, thus, elicit the classical signs of inflammation—redness, heat, swelling and pain.

Altered Vascular Permeability

PATHOGENESIS. In and around the inflamed tissue, there is accumulation of oedema fluid in the interstitial compartment which comes from blood plasma by its escape through the endothelial wall of peripheral vascular bed. In the initial stage, the escape of fluid is due to vasodilatation and consequent elevation in hydrostatic pressure. This is transudate in nature. But subsequently, the characteristic inflammatory oedema, exudate, appears by increased vascular permeability of microcirculation. The differences between transudate and exudate, are already summarised in Table 4.1 (*see* page 98).

The appearance of inflammatory oedema due to increased vascular permeability of microvascular bed is explained on the basis of **Starling's hypothesis**. In normal circumstances, the fluid balance is maintained by two opposing sets of forces:

i) Forces that cause **outward movement** of fluid from microcirculation are *intravascular hydrostatic pressure* and *osmotic pressure of interstitial fluid*.

ii) Forces that cause **inward movement** of interstitial fluid into circulation are *intravascular osmotic pressure* and *hydrostatic pressure of interstitial fluid*.

Whatever little fluid is left in the interstitial compartment is drained away by lymphatics and, thus, no oedema results normally (Fig. 6.2,A). However, in inflamed tissues, the endothelial lining of microvasculature becomes more leaky. Consequently, intravascular osmotic pressure decreases and osmotic pressure of the interstitial fluid increases resulting in excessive outward flow of fluid into the interstitial compartment which is exudative inflammatory oedema (Fig. 6.2,B).

MECHANISMS OF INCREASED VASCULAR PERMEABILITY. In acute inflammation, normally non-permeable endothelial layer of microvasculature becomes leaky. This is explained by one or more of the following mechanisms which are diagrammatically illustrated in Fig. 6.3.

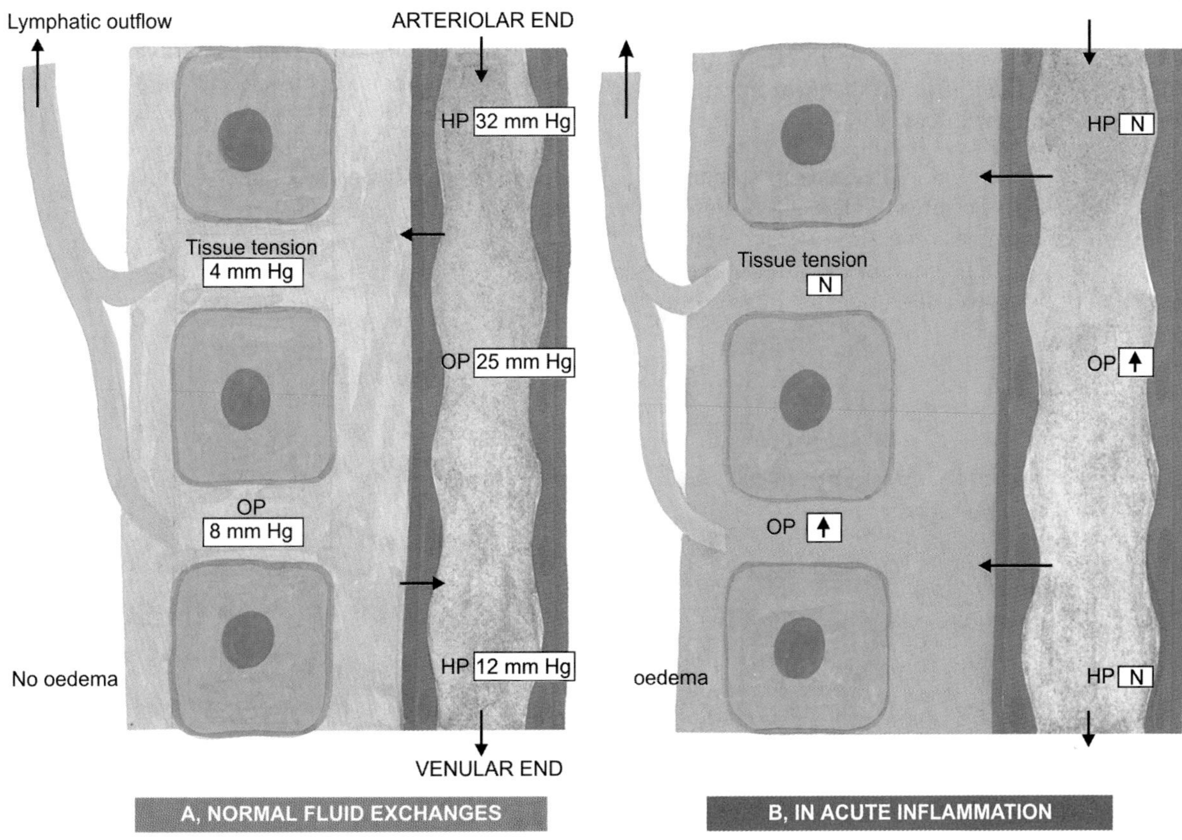

FIGURE 6.2

Fluid interchange between blood and extracellular fluid (ECF). (HP = hydrostatic pressure, OP = osmotic pressure).

TABLE 6.1: Mechanisms of Increased Vascular Permeability.

MECHANISM	MICROVASCULATURE	RESPONSE TYPE	PATHOGENESIS	EXAMPLES
1. *Endothelial cell contraction*	Venules	Immediate transient (15-30 min)	Histamine, bradykinin, others	Mild thermal injury
2. *Endothelial cell retraction*	Venules	Somewhat delayed (4-6 hrs) prolonged (24 hrs or more)	IL-1, TNF	*In vitro* only
3. *Direct endothelial cell injury*	Arterioles, venules, capillaries	Immediate prolonged (hrs to days), or delayed (2-12 hrs) prolonged (hrs to days)	Cell necrosis and detachment	Moderate to severe burns, severe bacterial infection, radiation injury
4. *Leucocyte-mediated endothelial injury*	Venules, capillaries	Delayed, prolonged	Leucocyte activation	Pulmonary venules and capillaries
5. *Neovascularisation*	All levels	Any type	Angiogenesis, VEGF	Healing, tumours

i) Contraction of endothelial cells. This is the most common mechanism of increased leakiness that affects venules exclusively while capillaries and arterioles remain unaffected. The endothelial cells develop temporary gaps between them due to their contraction resulting in vascular leakiness. It is mediated by the release of histamine, bradykinin and other chemical mediators. The response begins immediately after injury, is usually reversible, and is for short duration (15-30 minutes).

Example of such *immediate transient leakage* is mild thermal injury of skin of forearm.

ii) Retraction of endothelial cells. In this mechanism, there is structural re-organisation of the cytoskeleton of endothelial cells that causes reversible retraction at the intercellular junctions. This change too affects venules and is mediated by cytokines such as interleukin-1 (IL-1) and tumour necrosis factor (TNF). The onset of response takes 4-6 hours after injury and lasts for 2-4 hours or more *(somewhat delayed and prolonged leakage)*.

The example of this type of response exists *in vitro* experimental work only.

iii) Direct injury to endothelial cells. Direct injury to the endothelium causes cell necrosis and appearance of physical gaps at the sites of detached endothelial cells. Process of thrombosis is initiated at the site of damaged endothelial cells. The change affects all levels of microvasculature (venules, capillaries and arterioles). The increased permeability may either appear immediately after injury and last for several hours or days *(immediate sustained leakage)*, or may occur after a delay of 2-12 hours and last for hours or days *(delayed prolonged leakage)*.

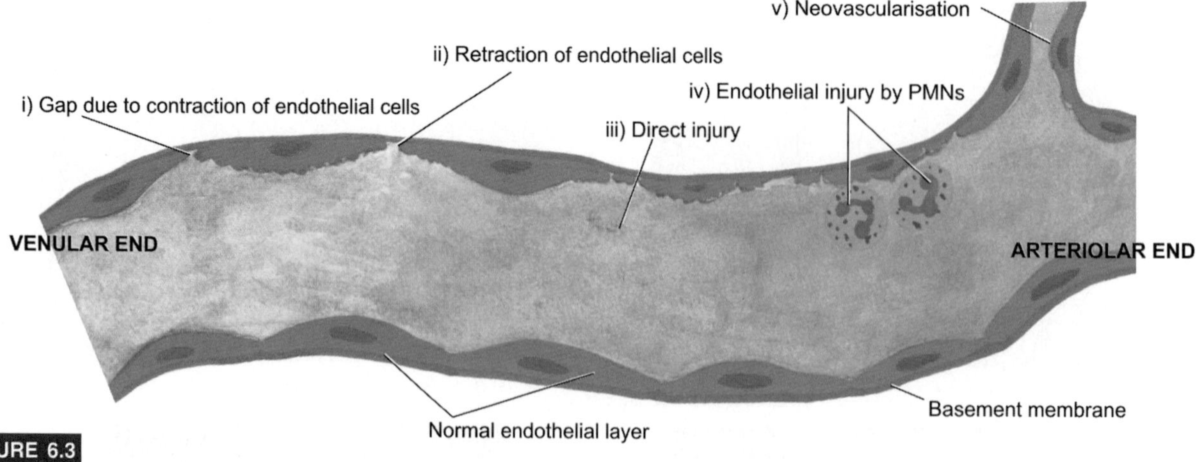

FIGURE 6.3

Schematic illustration of pathogenesis of increased vascular permeability in acute inflammation. The serial numbers in the figure correspond to 6 numbers in the text.

The examples of immediate sustained leakage are severe bacterial infections while delayed prolonged leakage may occur following moderate thermal injury and radiation injury.

iv) Endothelial injury mediated by leucocytes. Adherence of leucocytes to the endothelium at the site of inflammation may result in activation of leucocytes. The activated leucocytes release proteolytic enzymes and toxic oxygen species which may cause endothelial injury and increased vascular leakiness. This form of increased vascular leakiness affects mostly venules and is a *late response*.

The examples are seen in sites where leucocytes adhere to the vascular endothelium e.g. in pulmonary venules and capillaries.

v) Neovascularisation. In addition, the newly formed capillaries under the influence of vascular endothelial growth factor (VEGF) during the process of repair and in tumours are excessively leaky.

These mechanisms are summarised in Table 6.1.

II. CELLULAR EVENTS

The cellular phase of inflammation consists of 2 processes:

1. exudation of leucocytes; and
2. phagocytosis.

Exudation of Leucocytes

The escape of leucocytes from the lumen of microvasculature to the interstitial tissue is the most important feature of inflammatory response. In acute inflammation, polymorphonuclear neutrophils (PMNs) comprise the first line of body defense, followed later by monocytes and macrophages.

The changes leading to migration of leucocytes are as follows:

1. CHANGES IN THE FORMED ELEMENTS OF BLOOD. In the early stage of inflammation, the rate of flow of blood is increased due to vasodilatation. But subsequently, there is slowing or stasis of bloodstream. With stasis, changes in the normal axial flow of blood in the microcirculation take place. The normal axial flow consists of central stream of cells comprised by leucocytes and RBCs and peripheral cell-free layer of plasma close to vessel wall (Fig. 6.4,A). Due to slowing and stasis, the central stream of cells widens and peripheral plasma zone becomes narrower because of loss of plasma by exudation. This phenomenon is known as *margination*. As a result of this redistribution, the neutrophils of the central column come close to the vessel wall; this is known as *pavementing* (Fig. 6.4,B).

2. ROLLING AND ADHESION. Peripherally marginated and pavemented neutrophils slowly roll over the endothelial cells lining the vessel wall *(rolling phase)* (Fig. 6.4,C). This is followed by the transient bond between the leucocytes and endothelial cells becoming firmer *(adhesion phase)*. The following adhesion molecules bring about rolling and adhesion phases:

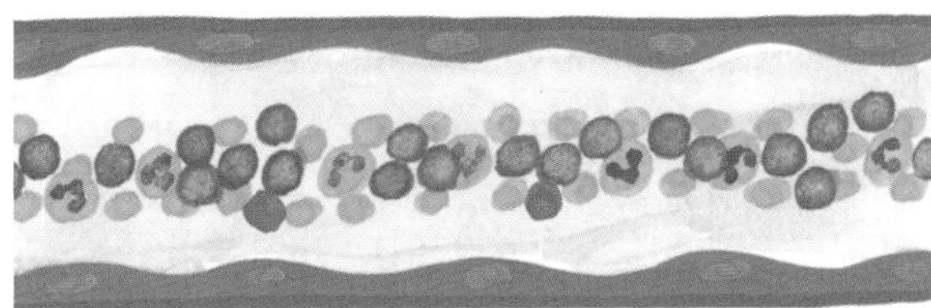
A, NORMAL AXIAL FLOW

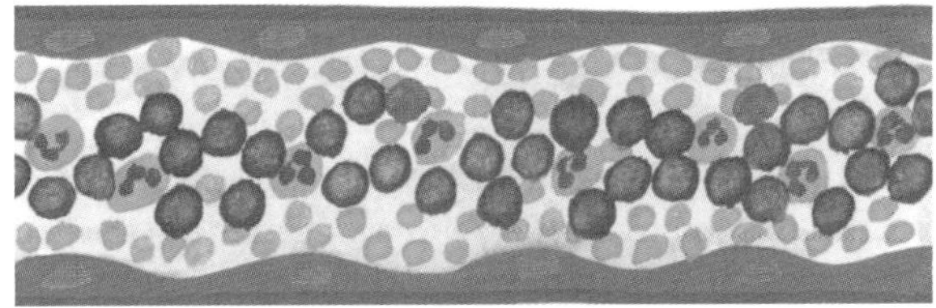
B, MARGINATION AND PAVEMENTING

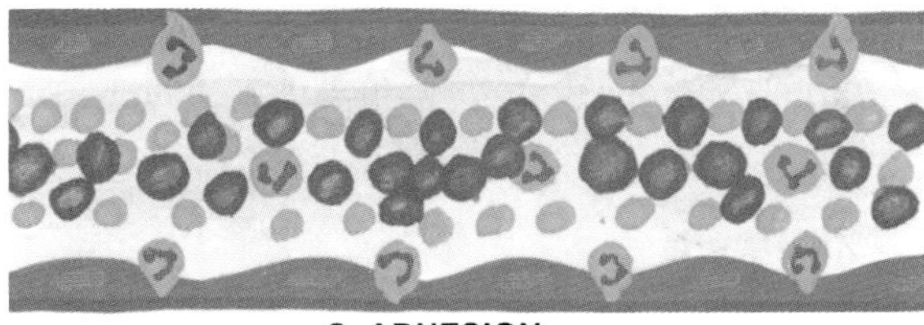
C, ADHESION

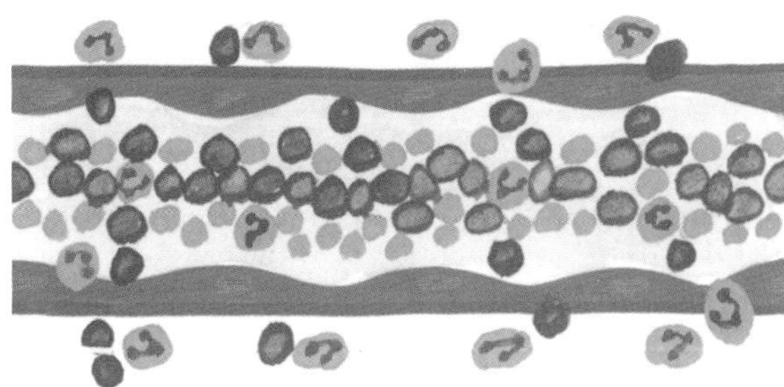
D, EMIGRATION AND DIAPEDESIS

FIGURE 6.4 Sequence of changes in the exudation of leucocytes. A, Normal axial flow of blood with central column of cells and peripheral zone of cell-free plasma. B, Margination and pavementing of neutrophils with narrow plasmatic zone. C, Adhesion of neutrophils to endothelial cells with pseudopods in the intercellular junctions. D, Emigration of neutrophils and diapedesis with damaged basement membrane.

i) **Selectins** mediate rolling of PMNs over endothelial surface. These consist of *P-selectin* (preformed and stored in endothelial cells and platelets), *E-selectin* (synthesised by cytokine-activated endothelial cells) and *L-selectin* (expressed on the surface of lymphocytes and neutrophils).

ii) **Integrins** on the endothelial cell surface are activated during the process of loose and transient adhesions between endothelial cells and leucocytes. At the same time the receptors for integrins on the neutrophils are also stimulated. This process brings about firm adhesion between leucocyte and endothelium.

iii) **Immunoglobulin superfamily adhesion molecule** such as intercellular adhesion molecule (ICAM-1, 2) help in localising leucocytes to the site of tissue injury and thus help in transmigration of PMNs.

3. EMIGRATION. After sticking of neutrophils to endothelium, the former move along the endothelial surface till a suitable site between the endothelial cells is found where the neutrophils throw out cytoplasmic pseudopods. Subsequently, the neutrophils lodged between the endothelial cells and basement membrane cross the basement membrane by damaging it locally with secreted collagenases and escape out into the extravascular space; this is known as *emigration* (Fig. 6.4,D). The damaged basement membrane is repaired almost immediately. As already mentioned, neutrophils are the dominant cells in acute inflammatory exudate in the first 24 hours, and monocyte-macrophages appear in the next 24-48 hours. However, neutrophils are short-lived (24-48 hours) while monocyte-macrophages survive much longer.

Simultaneous to emigration of leucocytes, escape of red cells through gaps between the endothelial cells, *diapedesis*, takes place. It is a passive phenomenon—RBCs being forced out either by raised hydrostatic pressure or may escape through the endothelial defects left after emigration of leucocytes. Diapedesis gives haemorrhagic appearance to the inflammatory exudate.

4. CHEMOTAXIS. The chemotactic factor-mediated transmigration of leucocytes after crossing several barriers (endothelium, basement membrane, perivascular myofibroblasts and matrix) to reach the interstitial tissues is called chemotaxis. The concept of chemotaxis is well illustrated by *Boyden's chamber experiment*. In this, a millipore filter (3 μm pore size) separates the suspension of leucocytes from the test solution in tissue culture chamber. If the test solution contains chemotactic agent, the leucocytes migrate through the pores of filter towards the chemotactic agent (Fig. 6.5).

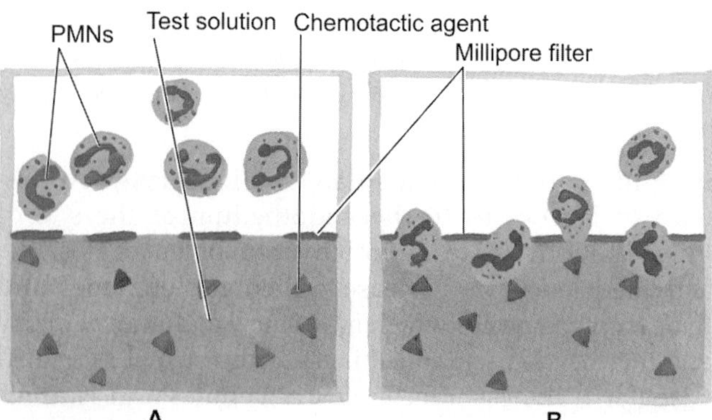

FIGURE 6.5

The Boyden's chamber with millipore filter, shown by dotted line. A, Suspension of leucocytes above is separated from test solution below. B, Lower half of chamber shows migration of neutrophils towards chemotactic agent.

The agents acting as potent chemotactic substances for different leucocytes called *chemokines* are as follows:

i) Leukotriene B_4 (LT-B_4)

ii) Platelet factor 4 (PF_4)

iii) Components of complement system (C_3, C_5 in particular)

iv) Cytokines (Interleukins IL-1, IL-5, IL-6)

v) Soluble bacterial products (such as formylated peptides)

vi) Monocyte chemoattractant protein (MCP-1)

vii) Chemotactic factor for CD_4+T cells

viii) Eotaxin chemotactic for eosinophils.

There are specific receptors for each of the chemoattractants listed above. In addition, chemotactic agents also induce leucocyte activation that includes: the production of arachidonic acid metabolites, degranulation and secretion of lysosomal enzymes, generation of oxygen metabolites, increased intracellular calcium, and increase in leucocyte surface adhesion molecules.

Phagocytosis

Phagocytosis is defined as the process of engulfment of solid particulate material by the cells (cell-eating). The cells performing this function are called *phagocytes*. There are 2 main types of phagocytic cells:

i) Polymorphonuclear neutrophils (PMNs) which appear early in acute inflammatory response, also called as *microphages*.

ii) Circulating monocytes and fixed tissue mononuclear phagocytes called as *macrophages*.

The process of phagocytosis is similar for both polymorphs and macrophages and involves the following 4 steps:

1. Recognition and attachment stage (opsonisation)
2. Engulfment stage
3. Secretion (degranulation) stage
4. Digestion or degradation stage.

1. RECOGNITION AND ATTACHMENT STAGE. The phagocytic cells are recognised and attracted to bacteria by chemotatic factors released by bacterial products as well as by tissue proteins. In order to establish a bond between bacteria and the cell membrane of phagocytic cell, the micro-organisms get coated with *opsonins* which are naturally-occurring factors in the serum. The main opsonins present in the serum and their corresponding receptors on the surface of phagocytic cells (PMNs or macrophages) are as under (Fig. 6.6,A):

i) *IgG opsonin* is the Fc fragment of immunoglobulin G; it is the naturally occurring antibody in the serum that coats the bacteria while the PMNs possess receptors for the same.

ii) C_{3b} *opsonin* is the fragment of complement; it is generated by activation of complement pathway. It is strongly chemotactic for attracting PMNs to bacteria.

iii) *Lectins* are carbohydrate-binding proteins in the plasma which bind to bacterial cell wall.

2. ENGULFMENT STAGE. The opsonised particle bound to the surface of phagocyte is ready to be engulfed. This is accomplished by formation of cytoplasmic pseudopods around the particle due to activation of actin filaments beneathe cell wall, enveloping it in a phagocytic vacuole (Fig. 6.6,B). Eventually, the plasma membrane enclosing the phagocytic vacuole breaks from the cell surface so that membrane lined phagocytic vacuole lies free in the cell cytoplasm (Fig. 6.6,C). The lysosomes of the cell fuse with the phagocytic vacuole and form phagolysosome or phagosome (Fig. 6.6,D).

3. DEGRANULATION STAGE. During this process, the preformed granule-stored products of PMNs are discharged or secreted into the phagosome and the extracellular environment. In particular, the specific or secondary granules of PMNs are discharged (e.g. lysosomes) while the azurophilic granules are fused with phagosomes. Besides the discharge of preformed granules, mononuclear phagocytes synthesise and secrete certain enzymes (e.g. interleukin 2 and 6,TNF), arachidonic acid metabolites (e.g. prostaglandins, leukotrienes, platelet activating factor) and oxygen metabolites (e.g. superoxide oxygen, hydrogen peroxide, hypochlorous acid).

4. KILLING OR DEGRADATION STAGE. Next comes the stage of killing and digestion of micro-organism completing the role of phagocytes as scavanger cells. The micro-organisms after being killed by antibacterial substances are degraded by hydrolytic enzymes. However, this mechanism fails to kill and degrade some bacteria like tubercle bacilli.

The antimicrobial agents act by either of the following mechanisms:

i) Oxygen-dependent bactericidal mechanism;
ii) Oxygen-independent bactericidal mechanism; and
iii) Nitric oxide mechanism.

i) Oxygen-dependent bactericidal mechanism. An important mechanism of microbicidal killing is by the

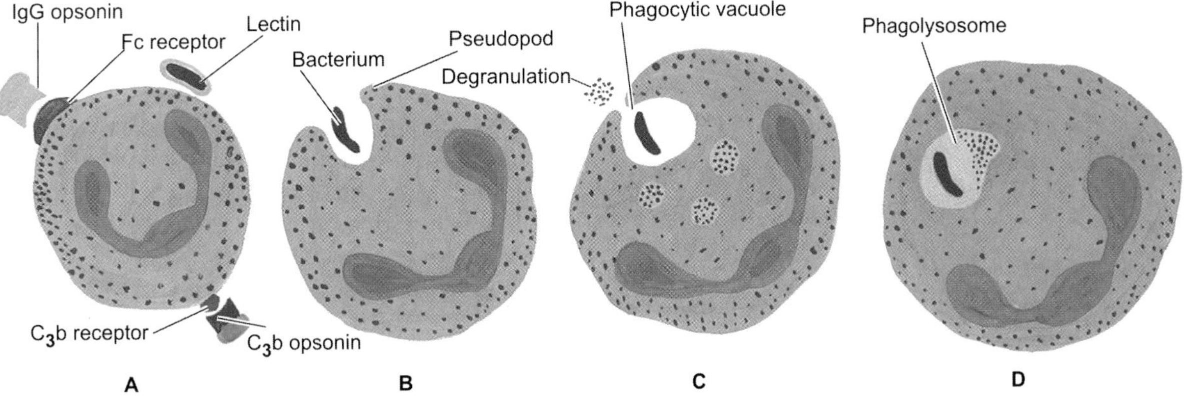

FIGURE 6.6

Stages in phagocytosis of a foreign particle. A, Opsonisation of the particle. B, Pseudopod engulfing the opsonised particle. C, Incorporation within the cell (phagocytic vacuole) and degranulation. D, Phagolysosome formation after fusion of lysosome of the cell.

production of reactive oxygen metabolites (O'_2 H_2O_2, OH′, HOCl, HOI, HOBr).

A phase of increased oxygen consumption ('respiratory burst') by activated phagocytic leucocytes requires the essential presence of NADPH oxidase.

NADPH-oxidase present in the cell membrane of phagosome reduces oxygen to superoxide ion (O'_2):

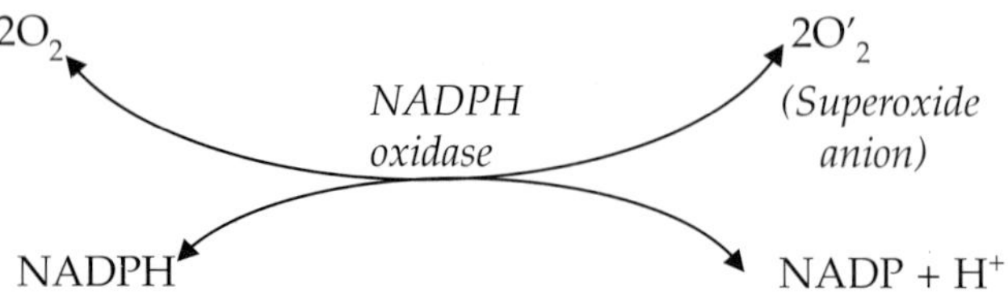

Superoxide is subsequently converted into H_2O_2 which has bactericidal properties:

$$2O'_2 + 2H^+ \longrightarrow H_2O_2 \text{ (Hydrogen peroxide)}$$

This type of bactericidal activity is carried out either via enzyme myeloperoxidase (MPO) present in the granules of neutrophils and monocytes, or independent of enzyme MPO, as under:

a) *MPO-dependent killing (H_2O_2-MPO-halide system).* In this mechanism, the enzyme MPO acts on H_2O_2 in the presence of halides (chloride, iodide or bromide) to form hypohalous acid (HOCl, HOI, HOBr) which is more potent antibacterial agent than H_2O_2:

$$H_2O_2 \xrightarrow[Cl', Br', I']{MPO} HOCl + H_2O \text{ (Hypochlorous acid)}$$

b) *MPO-independent killing.* Mature macrophages lack the enzyme MPO and they carry out bactericidal activity by producing OH^- ions and superoxide singlet oxygen (O′) from H_2O_2 in the presence of O'_2 (Haber-Weiss reaction) or in the presence of Fe^{++} (Fenton reaction):

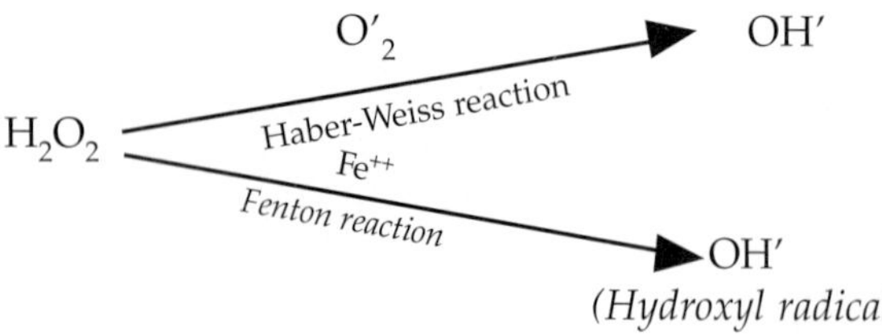

Reactive oxygen metabolites are particularly useful in eliminating microbial organisms that grow within phagocytes e.g. *M. tuberculosis, Histoplasma capsulatum.*

ii) Oxygen-independent bactericidal mechanism. Some agents released from the granules of phagocytic cells do not require oxygen for bactericidal activity. These include lysosomal hydrolases, permeability increasing factors, defensins and cationic proteins.

iii) Nitric oxide mechanism. In addition to oxygen-dependent and oxygen-independent mechanisms, recently role of nitric oxide (NO) in inflammatory reaction has been emphasised. NO is produced by endothelial cells as well as by activated macrophages. In experimental animals, NO has been shown to have fungicidal and anti-parasitic action but its role in bactericidal activity in human beings is yet not clear.

CHEMICAL MEDIATORS OF INFLAMMATION

Also called as permeability factors or endogenous mediators of increased vascular permeability, these are a large and increasing number of endogenous compounds which can enhance vascular permeability. However, currently many chemical mediators have been identified which partake in other processes of acute inflammation as well e.g. vasodilatation, chemotaxis, fever, pain and cause tissue damage.

The substances acting as chemical mediators of inflammation may be released *from the cells, the plasma, or damaged tissue* itself. They are broadly classified into 2 groups:

i) mediators released by cells; and
ii) mediators originating from plasma.

Table 6.2 presents a list of chemical mediators of acute inflammation.

Chemical mediators involved in causing increased vascular permeability and consequent oedema of tissues are shown in Fig. 6.7.

I. Cell-derived Mediators

1. VASOACTIVE AMINES. Two important pharmacologically active amines that have role in the early inflammatory response (first one hour) are histamine and 5-hydroxytryptamine (5-HT) or serotonin.

i) Histamine. It is stored in the granules of mast cells, basophils and platelets. Histamine is released from these cells by various agents as under:

a) Stimuli or substances inducing acute inflammation e.g. heat, cold, irradiation, trauma, irritant chemicals, immunologic reactions etc.
b) Anaphylatoxins like fragments of complement C_{3a}, and C_{5a}, which increase vascular permeability and cause oedema in tissues.
c) Histamine-releasing factors from neutrophils, monocytes and platelets.
d) Neuropeptides such as substance P.
e) Interleukins.

TABLE 6.2: Chemical Mediators of Acute Inflammation.

I. **CELL-DERIVED MEDIATORS**
1. Vasoactive amines (Histamine, 5-hydroxytryptamine)
2. Arachidonic acid metabolites (Eicosanoids)
   i. Metabolites via cyclo-oxygenase pathway (prostaglandins, thromboxane A_2, prostacyclin)
   ii. Metabolites via lipo-oxygenase pathway (5-HETE, leukotrienes)
3. Lysosomal components
4. Platelet activating factor
5. Cytokines (IL-1, TNF-α, TNF-β, IF-γ, chemokines)
6. Nitric oxide and oxygen metabolites

II. **PLASMA-DERIVED MEDIATORS (PLASMA PROTEASES)**
These are products of:
1. The kinin system
2. The clotting system
3. The fibrinolytic system
4. The complement system

The main *actions* of histamine are: vasodilatation, increased vascular (venular) permeability, itching and pain. Stimulation of mast cells and basophils also releases products of arachidonic acid metabolism including the release of *slow-reacting substances of anaphylaxis (SRS-As)*. The SRS-As consist of various leukotrienes (LTC_4, LTD_4 and LTE_4).

ii) 5-Hydroxytryptamine (5-HT or serotonin). It is present in tissues like chromaffin cells of GIT, spleen, nervous tissue, mast cells and platelets. The actions of 5-HT are similar to histamine but it is a less potent mediator of increased vascular permeability and vasodilatation than histamine. It may be mentioned here that carcinoid tumour is a serotonin-secreting tumour (Chapter 18).

2. ARACHIDONIC ACID METABOLITES (EICOSANOIDS). Arachidonic acid is a fatty acid, eicosatetraenoic acid, and its 2 main sources are:
- from diet directly; and
- conversion of essential fatty acid, linoleic acid to arachidonic acid.

Arachidonic acid must be first activated by stimuli or other mediators like C_{5a} so as to form arachidonic acid metabolites by one of the following 2 pathways: via cyclo-oxygenase pathway and via lipo-oxygenase pathway.

i) Metabolites via cyclo-oxygenase pathway (prostaglandins, thromboxane A_2, prostacyclin). The name 'prostaglandin' was first given to a substance found in human seminal fluid but now the same substance has been isolated from a number of other body tissues. Prostaglandins and related compounds are also called *autocoids*.

Cyclo-oxygenase is a fatty acid enzyme which acts on activated arachidonic acid to form prostaglandin endoperoxide (PGG_2). PGG_2 is enzymatically transformed into PGH_2 with generation of free radical of oxygen. PGH_2 is further acted upon by enzymes and

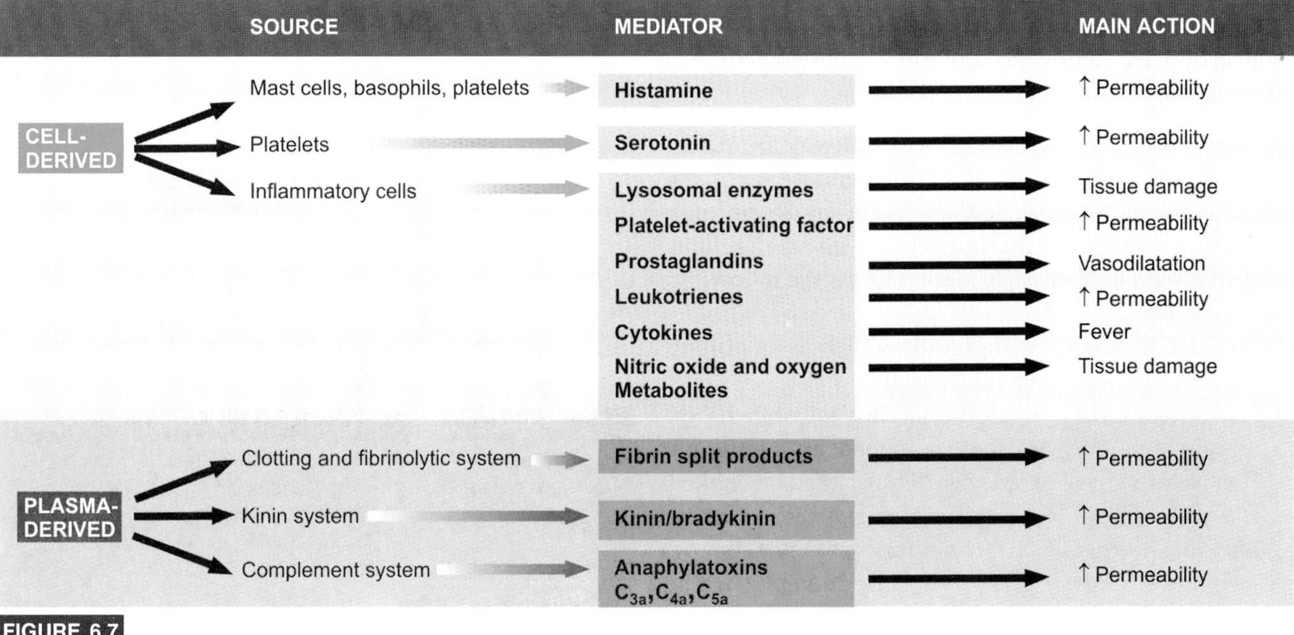

FIGURE 6.7
Chemical mediators of inflammation.

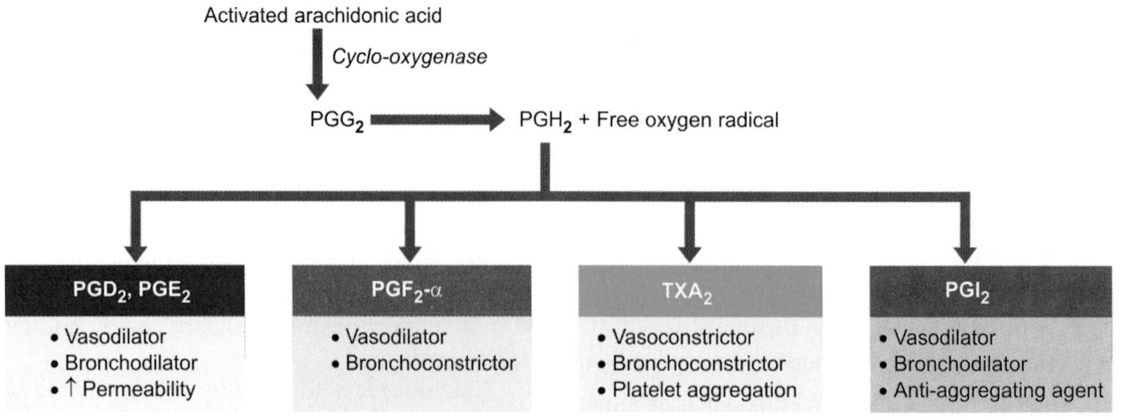

FIGURE 6.8

Arachidonic acid metabolites via cyclo-oxygenase pathway.

results in formation of the following 3 metabolites (Fig. 6.8):

a) *Prostaglandins (PGD_2, PGE_2 and PGF_2-α).* PGD_2 and PGE_2 act on blood vessels to cause increased venular permeability, vasodilatation and bronchodilatation and inhibit inflammatory cell function. PGF_2-α induces vasodilatation and bronchoconstriction.

b) *Thromboxane A_2 (TXA_2).* It is a vasoconstrictor and broncho-constrictor and enhances inflammatory cell function by causing platelet aggregation.

c) *Prostacyclin (PGI_2).* PGI_2 induces vasodilatation, bronchodilatation and inhibits inflammatory cell function by acting as anti-aggregating agent for platelets.

ii) Metabolites via lipo-oxygenase pathway (5-HETE, leukotrienes). The enzyme, lipo-oxygenase, acts on activated arachidonic acid to form hydroperoxy compound, 5-HPETE (hydroperoxy eico-satetraenoic acid) which on further peroxidation forms the following 2 metabolites (Fig. 6.9):

a) *5-HETE* (hydroxy compound) which is a potent chemotactic agent for neutrophils.

b) *Leukotrienes* (LT) or slow-reacting substances of anaphylaxis (SRS-As) are so named as they were first isolated from leucocytes. Firstly, unstable leukotriene A_4 (LTA_4) is formed which is acted upon by enzymes to form LTB_4 (chemotactic for phagocytic cells and stimulates phagocytic cell adherence) while LTC_4, LTD_4 and LTE_4 have common actions by causing smooth muscle contraction and thereby induce vasoconstriction, bronchoconstriction and increased vascular permeability.

3. LYSOSOMAL COMPONENTS. The inflammatory cells—neutrophils and monocytes, contain lysosomal granules which on release elaborate a variety of mediators of inflammation. These are as under:

i) Granules of neutrophils. These are of two types: specific or secondary, and azurophil or primary. The specific granules contain lactoferrin, lysozyme, alkaline phosphatase and collagenase while the large azurophil granules have myeloperoxidase, acid hydrolases and

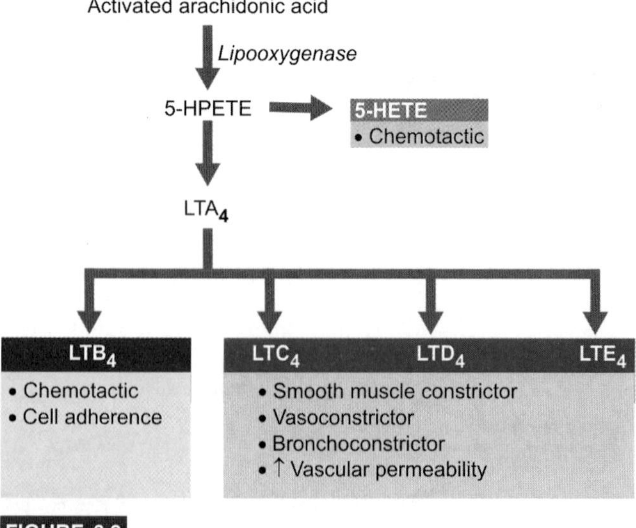

FIGURE 6.9

Arachidonic acid metabolites via lipooxygenase pathway.

neutral proteases such as elastase, collagenase and proteinase.

Acid proteases act within the cell to cause destruction of bacteria in phagolysosome while neutral proteases attack on the extracellular constituents such as basement membrane, collagen, elastin, cartilage etc.

However, degradation of extracellular components like collagen, basement membrane, fibrin and cartilage by proteases results in harmful tissue destruction which is kept in check by antiproteases like α_1-antitrypsin and α_2-macroglobulin.

ii) Granules of monocytes and tissue macrophages. These cells on degranulation also release mediators of inflammation like acid proteases, collagenase, elastase and plasminogen activator. However, they are more active in chronic inflammation than acting as mediators of acute inflammation.

4. PLATELET ACTIVATING FACTOR (PAF). It is released from IgE-sensitised basophils or mast cells, other leucocytes, endothelium and platelets. Apart from its action on platelet aggregation and release reaction, the actions of PAF as mediator of inflammation are:

- increased vascular permeability;
- vasodilatation in low concentration and vasoconstriction otherwise;
- bronchoconstriction;
- adhesion of leucocytes to endothelium; and
- chemotaxis.

5. CYTOKINES. Cytokines are polypeptide substances produced by activated lymphocytes *(lymphokines)* and activated monocytes *(monokines)*. These agents may act on 'self' cells producing them or on other cells. Currently, main cytokines acting as mediators of inflammation are: interleukin-1 (IL-1), tumour necrosis factor (TNF)-α and β, interferon (IF)-γ, and chemokines (IL-8, PF-4).

IL-1 and TNF-α are formed by activated macrophages while TNF-β and IF-γ are produced by activated T cells. The chemokines include interleukin 8 (released from activated macrophages) and platelet factor-4 from activated platelets, both of which are potent chemoattractant for inflammatory cells and hence their name.

The actions of various cytokines as mediator of inflammation are as under:

i) IL-1 and TNF-α, TNF-β induce endothelial effects in the form of increased leucocyte adherence, thrombogenicity, elaboration of other cytokines, fibroblastic proliferation and acute phase reactions.

ii) IF-γ causes activation of macrophages and neutrophils and is associated with synthesis of nitric acid synthase.

iii) Chemokines are a family of chemoattractants for inflammatory cells and include:

- IL-8 chemotactic for neutrophils;
- platelet factor-4 chemotactic for neutrophils, monocytes and eosinophils;
- MCP-1 chemotactic for monocytes; and
- eotaxin chemotactic for eosinophils.

6. NITRIC OXIDE AND OXYGEN METABOLITES. Nitric oxide (NO) was originally described as vascular relaxation factor produced by endothelial cells. It has recently been included as a mediator of inflammatory responses since activated macrophages also produce NO during the oxidation of arginine by the action of enzyme, NO synthase.

NO plays the following role in inflammation:

- Vasodilatation
- Anti-platelet activating agent
- Possibly microbicidal action.

Oxygen-derived metabolites are released from activated neutrophils and macrophages and include superoxide oxygen (O'_2), H_2O_2, OH′ and toxic NO products. These oxygen-derived free radicals have the following action in inflammation:

- Endothelial cell damage and thereby increased vascular permeability.
- Activation of protease and inactivation of antiprotease causing tissue matrix damage.
- Damage to other cells.

The actions of free radicals are counteracted by antioxidants present in tissues and serum which play a protective role (page 38).

II. Plasma-derived Mediators (Plasma Proteases)

These include the various products derived from activation and interaction of 4 interlinked systems: kinin, clotting, fibrinolytic and complement. Each of these systems has its inhibitors and accelerators in plasma with negative and positive feedback machanisms respectively.

Hageman factor (factor XII) of clotting system plays a key role in interactions of the four systems. Activation of factor XII *in vivo* by contact with basement membrane and bacterial endotoxins, and *in vitro* with glass or kaolin, leads to activation of clotting, fibrinolytic and kinin systems. In inflammation, activation of factor XII is brought about by contact of the factor leaking through the endothelial gaps. The end-products of the activated clotting, fibrinolytic and kinin systems activate the complement system that generate permeability factors. These permeability factors, in turn, further activate clotting system.

The inter-relationship between 4 systems is summarised in Fig. 6.10.

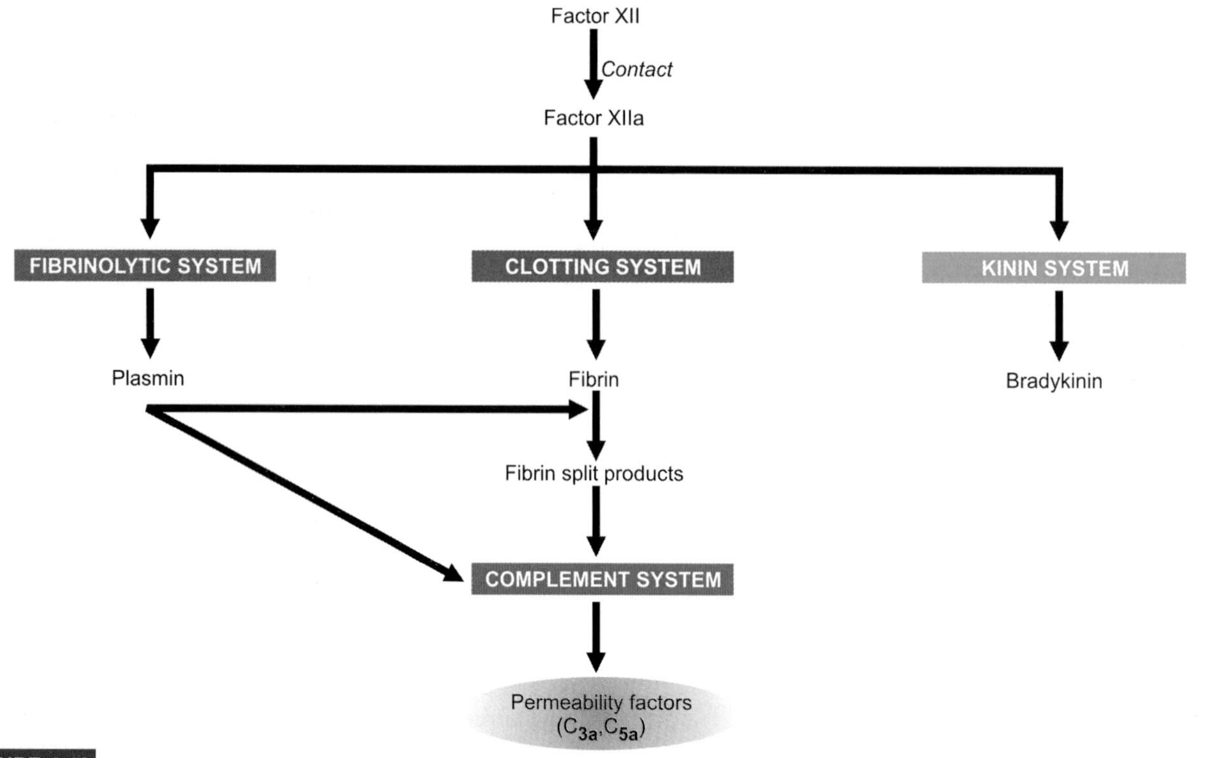

FIGURE 6.10

Inter-relationship between clotting, fibrinolytic, kinin and complement systems.

1. THE KININ SYSTEM. This system on activation by factor XIIa generates bradykinin, so named because of the slow contraction of smooth muscle it induces. First, kallikrein is formed from plasma prekallikrein by the action of prekallikrein activator which is a fragment of factor XIIa. Kallikrein then acts on high molecular weight kininogen to form bradykinin (Fig. 6.11).

Bradykinin acts in the early stage of inflammation and its effects include:

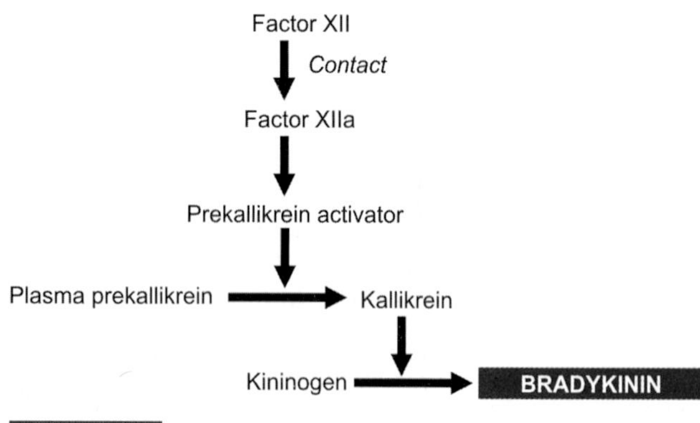

FIGURE 6.11

Pathway of the kinin system.

- smooth muscle contraction;
- vasodilatation;
- increased vascular permeability; and
- pain.

2. THE CLOTTING SYSTEM. Factor XIIa initiates the cascade of the clotting system resulting in formation of fibrinogen which is acted upon by thrombin to form fibrin and fibrinopeptides (Fig. 6.12).

The actions of fibrinopeptides in inflammation are:

- increased vascular permeability;
- chemotaxis for leucocyte; and
- anticoagulant activity.

3. THE FIBRINOLYTIC SYSTEM. This system is activated by plasminogen activator, the sources of which include kallikrein of the kinin system, endothelial cells and leucocytes. Plasminogen activator acts on plasminogen present as component of plasma proteins to form plasmin. Further breakdown of fibrin by plasmin forms fibrinopeptides or fibrin split products (Fig. 6.13).

The actions of plasmin in inflammation are:

- activation of factor XII to form prekallikrein activator that stimulates the kinin system to generate bradykinin;
- splits off complement C_3 to form C_{3a} which is a permeability factor; and

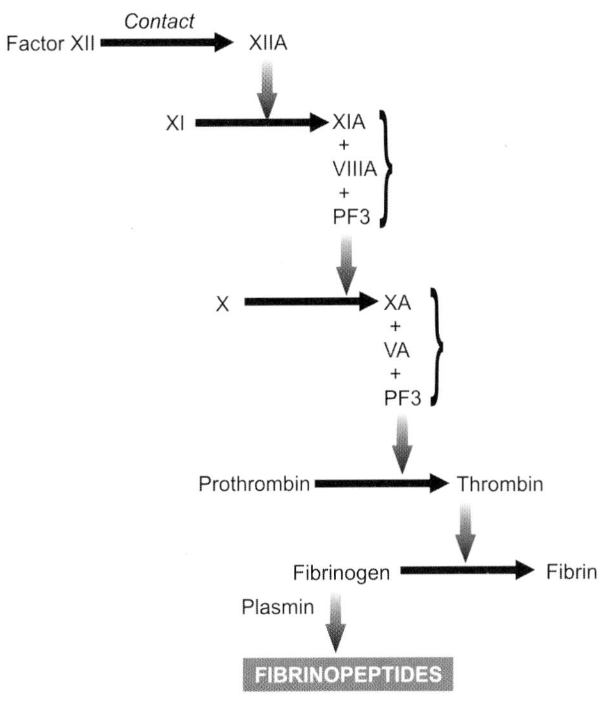

FIGURE 6.12

Pathway of the clotting system.

■ degrades fibrin to form fibrin split products which increase vascular permeability and are chemotactic to leucocytes.

4. THE COMPLEMENT SYSTEM. The activation of complement system can occur either:

i) by *classic pathway* through antigen-antibody complexes; or

ii) by *alternate pathway* via non-immunologic agents such as bacterial toxins, cobra venoms and IgA.

Complement system on activation by either of these two pathways yields anaphylatoxins C_{3a}, C_{4a} and C_{5a}, and membrane attack complex (MAC). The relative potencies of anaphylatoxins are in the descending sequence of C_{3a}, C_{5a} and C_{4a}.

The actions of *anaphylatoxins* in inflammation are:

■ release of histamine from mast cells and basophils;
■ increased vascular permeability causing oedema in tissues;
■ C_{3b} augments phagocytosis; and
■ C_{5a} is chemotactic for leucocytes.

The action of MAC is to cause pores in the cell membrane of the invading microorganisms.

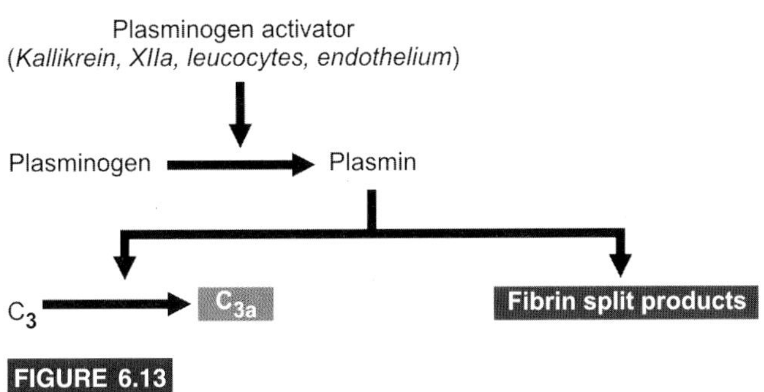

FIGURE 6.13

The activation of fibrinolytic system.

REGULATION OF INFLAMMATION

The onset of inflammatory responses outlined above may have potentially damaging influence on the host tissues as evident in hypersensitivity conditions. Such self-damaging effects are kept in check by the host mechanisms so as to resolve inflammation. These include the following mechanisms:

i) Acute phase reactants. A variety of acute phase reactant (APR) proteins are released in plasma in response to tissue trauma and infection. These include the following:

i) *Certain cellular protection factors* (α_1-antitrypsin, α_1-chymotrypsin,α_2-antiplasmin, plasminogen activator inhibitor);

ii) *Some coagulation proteins* (fibrinogen, plasminogen, von Willebrand factor, factor VIII);

iii) *Transport proteins* (ceruloplasmin, haptoglobin);

iv) *Immune agents* (serum amyloid A and P component, C-reactive protein); and

v) *Stress proteins* (heat shock proteins—HSP, ubiquitin).

The APR are synthesised mainly in the liver and to some extent in macrophages. APR combined with systemic features of fever and leucocytosis is termed *'acute phase response'*. Deficient synthesis of APR leads to severe form of disease in chronic and repeated inflammatory responses.

ii) Corticosteroids. The endogenous glucocorticoids act as anti-inflammatory agents. Their levels are raised in infection and trauma by self-regulating mechanism.

iii) Free cytokine receptors. The presence of free receptors for cytokines in the serum correlates directly with disease activity.

iv) Suppressor T cells. A prohibition of suppressor T cells is seen which inhibits the function of T and B cells.

v) Anti-inflammatory chemical mediators. As already described, PGE_2 and prostacyclin have both pro-inflammatory as well as anti-inflammatory actions.

THE INFLAMMATORY CELLS

The cells participating in acute and chronic inflammation are circulating leucocytes, plasma cells and tissue macrophages. The structure, function and production of these cells are dealt with in detail in Chapter 13. Here, it is pertinent to describe the role of these cells in inflammation. Summary of their morphology, characteristics and functions is given in Table 6.3.

1. Polymorphonuclear Neutrophils (PMN)

Commonly called as neutrophils or polymorphs, these cells alongwith basophils and eosinophils are known as granulocytes due to the presence of granules in the cytoplasm. These granules contain many substances like proteases, myeloperoxidase, lysozyme, esterase, aryl sulfatase, acid and alkaline phosphatase, and cationic proteins. The diameter of neutrophils ranges from 10 to 15 μm and are actively motile (Table 6.3,A). These cells comprise 40-75% of circulating leucocytes and their number is increased in blood (neutrophilia) and tissues in acute bacterial infections. These cells arise in the bone marrow from stem cells (Chapter 13).

The functions of neutrophils in inflammation are as follows:

i) **Initial phagocytosis** of micro-organisms as they form the first line of body defense in bacterial infection. The steps involved are adhesion of neutrophils to vascular endothelium, emigration through the vessel wall, chemotaxis, engulfment, degranulation, killing and degradation of the foreign material.

ii) **Engulfment** of antigen-antibody complexes and non-microbial material.

iii) **Harmful effect** of neutrophils is destruction of the basement membranes of glomeruli and small blood vessels.

2. Eosinophils

These are larger than neutrophils but are fewer in number, comprising 1 to 6% of total blood leucocytes (Table 6.3,E). Eosinophils share many structural and functional similarities with neutrophils like their production in the bone marrow, locomotion, phagocytosis, lobed nucleus and presence of granules in the cytoplasm containing a variety of enzymes, of which major basic protein and eosinophil cationic protein are the most important which have bactericidal and toxic action against helminthic parasites. However, granules of eosinophils are richer in myeloperoxidase than neutrophils and lack lysozyme. High level of steroid hormones leads to fall in number of eosinophils and even disappearance from blood.

The absolute number of eosinophils is increased in the following conditions and, thus, they partake in inflammatory responses associated with these conditions:

i) allergic conditions;
ii) parasitic infestations;
iii) skin diseases; and
iv) certain malignant lymphomas.

3. Basophils (Mast Cells)

The basophils comprise about 1% of circulating leucocytes and are morphologically and pharmacologically similar to mast cells of tissue. These cells contain coarse basophilic granules in the cytoplasm and a polymorphonuclear nucleus (Table 6.3,F). These granules are laden with heparin and histamine. Basophils and mast cells have receptors for IgE and degranulate when crosslinked with antigen.

The role of these cells in inflammation are:

i) in immediate and delayed type of hypersensitivity reactions; and
ii) release of histamine by IgE-sensitised basophils.

4. Lymphocytes

Next to neutrophils, these cells are most numerous of the circulating leucocytes (20-45%). Apart from blood, lymphocytes are present in large numbers in spleen, thymus, lymph nodes and mucosa-associated lymphoid tissue (MALT). They have scanty cytoplasm and consist almost entirely of nucleus (Table 6.3,C).

Besides their role in antibody formation (B lymphocytes) and in cell-mediated immunity (T lymphocytes), these cells participate in the following types of inflammatory responses:

i) *In tissues*, they are dominant cells in chronic inflammation and late stage of acute inflammation.

ii) *In blood*, their number is increased (lymphocytosis) in chronic infections like tuberculosis.

5. Plasma Cells

These cells are larger than lymphocytes with more abundant cytoplasm and an eccentric nucleus which has cart-wheel pattern of chromatin (Table 6.3,D). Plasma cells are normally not seen in peripheral blood. They develop from lymphocytes and are rich in RNA and γ-globulin in their cytoplasm. There is an interrelationship between plasmacytosis and hyperglobulinaemia. These cells are most active in antibody synthesis.

Their number is increased in the following conditions:

i) prolonged infection with immunological responses e.g. in syphilis, rheumatoid arthritis, tuberculosis;

TABLE 6.3: Morphology and Functions of Inflammatory Cells.

MORPHOLOGY	FEATURES	MEDIATORS
A, POLYMORPH	i. Initial phagocytosis of bacteria and foreign body ii. Acute inflammatory cell	i. Primary granules (MPO, lysozyme, cationic proteins, acid hydrolases, elastase) ii. Secondary granules (lysozyme, alk. phosph, collagenase, lactoferrin) iii. Tertiary granules (gelatinase, cathepsin) iv. Reactive oxygen metabolites
B, MONOCYTE/MACROPHAGE	i. Bacterial phagocytosis ii. Chronic inflammatory cell iii. Regulates lymphocyte response	i. Acid and neutral hydrolases (lysosomal) ii. Cationic protein iii. Phospholipase iv. Prostaglandins, leukotrienes v. IL-1
C, LYMPHOCYTE	i. Humoral and cell-mediated immune responses ii. Chronic inflammatory cell iii. Regulates macrophage response	i. B cells: antibody production ii. T cells: delayed hypersensitivity, cytotoxicity
D, PLASMA CELL	i. Derived from B cells ii. Chronic inflammatory cell	i. Antibody synthesis ii. Antibody secretion
E, EOSINOPHIL	i. Allergic states ii. Parasitic infestations iii. Chronic inflammatory cell	i. Reactive oxygen metabolites ii. Lysosomal (major basic protein, cationic protein, eosinophil peroxidase, neurotoxin) iii. PGE_2 synthesis
F, BASOPHIL/MAST CELL	i. Receptor for IgE molecules ii. Electron-dense granules	i. Histamine ii. Leukotrienes iii. Platelet activating factor

ii) hypersensitivity states; and
iii) multiple myeloma.

6. Mononuclear-Phagocyte System (Reticuloendothelial System)

This cell system includes cells derived from 2 sources with common morphology, function and origin (Table 6.3,B). These are as under:

Blood monocytes. These comprise 4-8% of circulating leucocytes.

Tissue macrophages. These include the following cells in different tissues:

i) Macrophages in inflammation.
ii) Histiocytes, macrophages present in connective tissues.
iii) Kupffer cells, macrophages of liver cells.
iv) Alveolar macrophages (type II pneumocytes) in lungs.
v) Macrophages/histiocytes of the bone marrow.
vi) Tingible body cells of germinal centres of lymph nodes.

vii) Littoral cells of splenic sinusoids.
viii) Osteoclasts in the bones.
ix) Microglial cells of the brain.
x) Langerhans' cells/dendritic histiocytes of the skin.
xi) Hoffbauer cells of the placenta.
xii) Mesangial cells of glomerulus.

The mononuclear phagocytes are the scavenger cells of the body as well as participate in immune system of the body. Their functions in inflammation are given below while their role in the immune system are described on page 66.

Role of macrophages in inflammation. The functions of mononuclear-phagocyte cells are as under:

i) *Phagocytosis* (cell eating) and *pinocytosis* (cell drinking).

ii) *Macrophages on activation* by lymphokines released by T lymphocytes or by non-immunologic stimuli elaborate a variety of biologically active substances as under:

a) Proteases like collagenase and elastase which degrade collagen and elastic tissue.
b) Plasminogen activator which activates the fibrinolytic system.
c) Products of complement.
d) Some coagulation factors (factor V and thromboplastin) which convert fibrinogen to fibrin.
e) Chemotactic agents for other leucocytes.
f) Metabolites of arachidonic acid.
g) Growth promoting factors for fibroblasts, blood vessels and granulocytes.
h) Cytokines like interleukin-1 and tumour necrosis factor.
i) Oxygen-derived free radicals.

7. Giant Cells

A few examples of multinucleate giant cells exist in normal tissues (e.g. osteoclasts in the bones, trophoblasts in placenta, megakaryocytes in the bone marrow). However, in chronic inflammation when the macrophages fail to deal with particles to be removed, they fuse together and form multinucleated giant cells. Besides, morphologically distinct giant cells appear in some tumours also. Some of the common types of giant cells are described below:

A. Giant cells in inflammation:

i) Foreign body giant cells. These contain numerous nuclei (up to 100) which are uniform in size and shape and resemble the nuclei of macrophages. These nuclei are scattered throughout the cytoplasm (Fig. 6.14,A). These are seen in chronic infective granulomas, leprosy and tuberculosis.

ii) Langhans' giant cells. These are seen in tuberculosis and sarcoidosis. Their nuclei are like the nuclei of macrophages and epithelioid cells. These nuclei are arranged either around the periphery in the form of horseshoe or ring or are clustered at the two poles of the giant cell (Fig. 6.14,B).

iii) Touton giant cells. These multinucleated cells have vacuolated cytoplasm due to lipid content e.g. in xanthoma (Fig. 6.14,C).

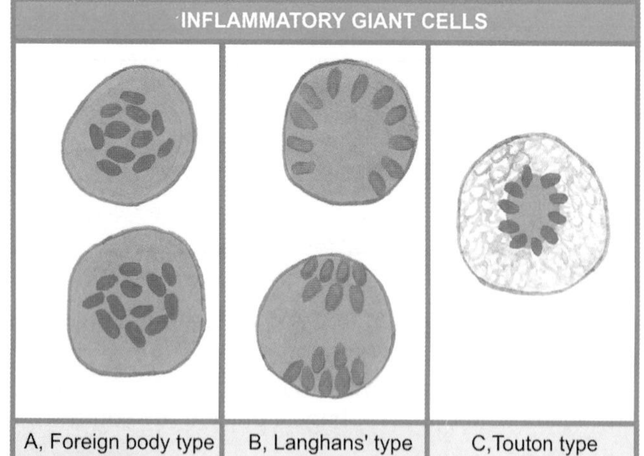

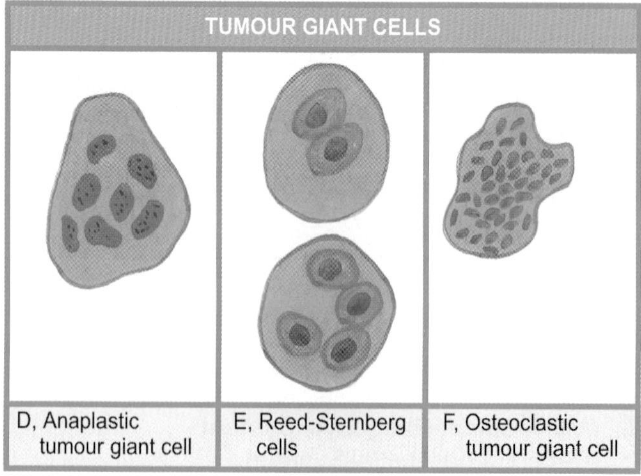

FIGURE 6.14

Giant cells of various types. A, Foreign body giant cell with uniform nuclei dispersed throughout the cytoplasm. B, Langhans' giant cells with uniform nuclei arranged peripherally or clustered at the two poles. C, Touton giant cell with circular pattern of nuclei and vacuolated cytoplasm. D, Anaplastic tumour giant cell with nuclei of variable size and shape. E, Reed-Sternberg cell. F, Osteoclastic tumour giant cell.

iv) Aschoff giant cells. These multinucleate giant cells are derived from cardiac histiocytes and are seen in rheumatic nodule (Chapter 12).

B. Giant cells in tumours:

i) Anaplastic cancer giant cells. These are larger, have numerous nuclei which are hyperchromatic and vary in size and shape (Fig. 6.14,D). These giant cells are not derived from macrophages but are formed from dividing nuclei of the neoplastic cells e.g. carcinoma of liver, various soft tissue sarcomas etc.

ii) Reed-Sternberg cells. These are also malignant tumour giant cells which are generally binucleate and are seen in various histologic types of Hodgkin's lymphomas (Fig. 6.14,E).

iii) Giant cell tumour of bone. This tumour of the bones has uniform distribution of osteoclastic giant cells spread in the stroma (Fig. 6.14,F).

FACTORS DETERMINING VARIATION IN INFLAMMATORY RESPONSE

Although acute inflammation is typically characterised by vascular and cellular events with emigration of neutrophilic leucocytes, not all examples of acute inflammation show infiltration by neutrophils. On the other hand, some chronic inflammatory conditions are characterised by neutrophilic infiltration. For example, *typhoid fever* is an example of acute inflammatory process but the cellular response in it is lymphocytic; *osteomyelitis* is an example of chronic inflammation but the cellular response in this condition is mainly neutrophilic.

The morphologic variation in inflammation depends upon a number of factors and processes. These are discussed below:

1. Factors Involving the Organisms

i) Type of injury and infection. For example, skin reacts to herpes simplex infection by formation of vesicle and to streptococcal infection by formation of boil; lung reacts to pneumococci by occurrence of lobar pneumonia while to tubercle bacilli it reacts by granulomatous inflammation.

ii) Virulence. Many species and strains of organisms may have varying virulence e.g. the three strains of *C. diphtheriae (gravis, intermedius and mitis)* produce the same diphtherial exotoxin but in different amount.

iii) Dose. The concentration of organism in small doses produces usually local lesions while larger dose results in more severe spreading infections.

iv) Portal of entry. Some organisms are infective only if administered by particular route e.g. *Vibrio cholerae* is not pathogenic if injected subcutaneously but causes cholera if swallowed.

v) Product of organisms. Some organisms produce enzymes that help in spread of infections e.g. hyaluronidase by *Clostridium welchii*, streptokinase by streptococci, staphylokinase and coagulase by staphylococci.

2. Factors Involving the Host

i) General health of host. For example, starvation, haemorrhagic shock, chronic debilitating diseases like diabetes mellitus, alcoholism etc render the host more susceptible to infections.

ii) Immune state of host. Immunodeficiency helps in spread of infections rapidly e.g. in AIDS.

iii) Leukopenia. Patients with low WBC count with neutropenia or agranulocytosis develop spreading infection.

iv) Site or type of tissue involved. For example, the lung has loose texture as compared to bone and, thus, both tissues react differently to acute inflammation.

v) Local host factors. For instance, ischaemia, presence of foreign bodies and chemicals cause necrosis and are thus harmful.

3. Type of Exudation

The appearance of escaped plasma determines the morphologic type of inflammation as under:

i) Serous, when the fluid exudate resembles serum or is watery e.g. pleural effusion in tuberculosis, blister formation in burns.

ii) Fibrinous, when the fibrin content of the fluid exudate is high e.g. in pneumococcal and rheumatic pericarditis.

iii) Purulent or suppurative exudate is formation of creamy pus as seen in infection with pyogenic bacteria e.g. abscess, acute appendicitis.

iv) Haemorrhagic, when there is vascular damage e.g. acute haemorrhagic pneumonia in influenza.

v) Catarrhal, when the surface inflammation of epithelium produces increased secretion of mucous e.g. common cold.

4. Cellular Proliferation

Variable cellular proliferation is seen in different types of inflammations.

i) There is no significant cellular proliferation in **acute bacterial infections** except in typhoid fever in which there is intestinal lymphoid hyperplasia.

ii) Viral infections have the ability to stimulate cellular proliferation e.g. epidermal cell proliferation in herpes simplex, chickenpox and smallpox.

iii)In rapidly progressive glomerulonephritis, there is proliferation of glomerular capsular epithelial cells resulting in formation of 'crescents'.

iv) In chronic inflammation, cellular proliferation of macrophages, fibroblasts and endothelial cells occurs.

5. Necrosis

The extent and type of necrosis in inflammation is variable.

i) In **gas gangrene**, there is extensive necrosis with discoloured and foul smelling tissues.

ii) In **acute appendicitis,** there is necrosis as a result of vascular obstruction.

iii) In **chronic inflammation** such as tuberculosis, there is characteristic caseous necrosis.

MORPHOLOGY OF ACUTE INFLAMMATION

Inflammation of an organ is usually named by adding the suffix-*itis* to its Latin name e.g. appendicitis, hepatitis, cholecystitis, meningitis etc. A few morphologic varieties of acute inflammation are described below:

1. PSEUDOMEMBRANOUS INFLAMMATION. It is inflammatory response of mucous surface (oral, respiratory, bowel) to toxins of diphtheria or irritant gases. As a result of denudation of epithelium, plasma exudes on the surface where it coagulates, and together with necrosed epithelium, forms false membrane that gives this type of inflammation its name.

2. ULCER. Ulcers are local defects on the surface of an organ produced by inflammation. Common sites for ulcerations are the stomach, duodenum, intestinal ulcers in typhoid fever, intestinal tuberculosis, bacillary and amoebic dysentery, ulcers of legs due to varicose veins etc. In the acute stage, there is infiltration by polymorphs with vasodilatation while long-standing ulcers develop infiltration by lymphocytes, plasma cells and macrophages with associated fibroblastic proliferation and scarring.

3. SUPPURATION (ABSCESS FORMATION). When acute bacterial infection is accompanied by intense neutrophilic infiltrate in the inflamed tissue, it results in tissue necrosis. A cavity is formed which is called an abscess and contains purulent exudate or pus and the process of abscess formation is known as suppuration. The bacteria which cause suppuration are called pyogenic.

Microscopically, pus is creamy or opaque in appearance and is composed of numerous dead as well as living neutrophils, some red cells, fragments of tissue debris and fibrin. In old pus, macrophages and cholesterol crystals are also present (Fig. 6.15) **(COLOUR PLATE VII: CL 25).**

An abscess may be discharged to the surface due to increased pressure inside or may require drainage by the surgeon. Due to tissue destruction, resolution does not occur but instead healing by fibrous scarring takes place.

Some of the common examples of abscess formation are as under:

i) *Boil or furruncle* which is an acute inflammation via hair follicles in the dermal tissues.

ii) *Carbuncle* is seen in untreated diabetics and occurs as a loculated abscess in the dermis and soft tissues of the neck.

4. CELLULITIS. It is a diffuse inflammation of soft tissues resulting from spreading effects of substances like hyaluronidase released by some bacteria.

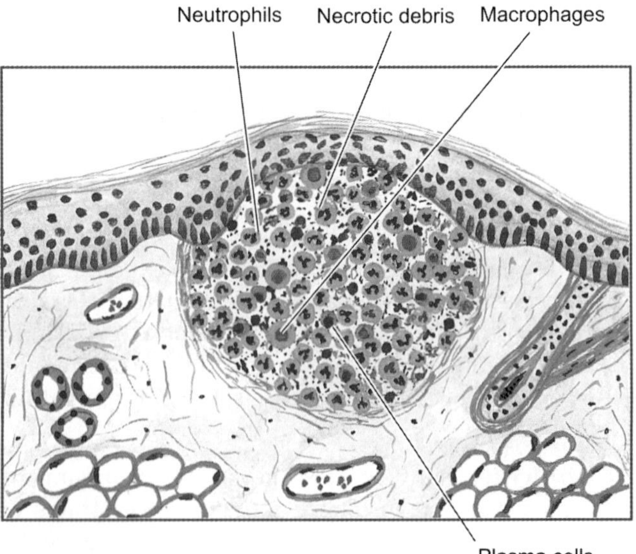

FIGURE 6.15

An abscess in the skin. It contains pus composed of necrotic tissue, debris, fibrin, RBCs and dead and living neutrophils. Some macrophages are seen at the periphery.

5. BACTERIAL INFECTION OF THE BLOOD. This includes the following 3 conditions:

i) Bacteraemia is defined as presence of small number of bacteria in the blood which do not multiply significantly. They are commonly not detected by direct microscopy. Blood culture is done for their detection e.g. infection with *Salmonella typhi, Escherichia coli, Streptococcus viridans.*

ii) Septicaemia means presence of rapidly multiplying, highly pathogenic bacteria in the blood e.g. pyogenic cocci, bacilli of plague etc. Septicaemia is generally accompanied by systemic effects like toxaemia, multiple small haemorrhages, neutrophilic leucocytosis and disseminated intravascular coagulation (DIC).

iii) Pyaemia is the dissemination of small septic thrombi in the blood which cause their effects at the site where they are lodged. This can result in pyaemic abscesses or septic infarcts.

a) *Pyaemic abscesses* are multiple small abscesses in various organs such as in cerebral cortex, myocardium, lungs and renal cortex, resulting from very small emboli fragmented from septic thrombus. Microscopy of pyaemic abscess shows a central zone of necrosis containing numerous bacteria, surrounded by a zone of suppuration and an outer zone of acute inflammatory cells (Fig. 6.16,A).

b) *Septic infarcts* result from lodgement of larger fragments of septic thrombi in the arteries with relatively larger foci of necrosis, suppuration and acute inflammation e.g. septic infarcts of the lungs, liver, brain, and kidneys from septic thrombi of leg veins or from acute bacterial endocarditis (Fig. 6.16,B).

SYSTEMIC EFFECTS OF ACUTE INFLAMMATION

The account of acute inflammation given up to now above is based on local tissue responses. However, acute

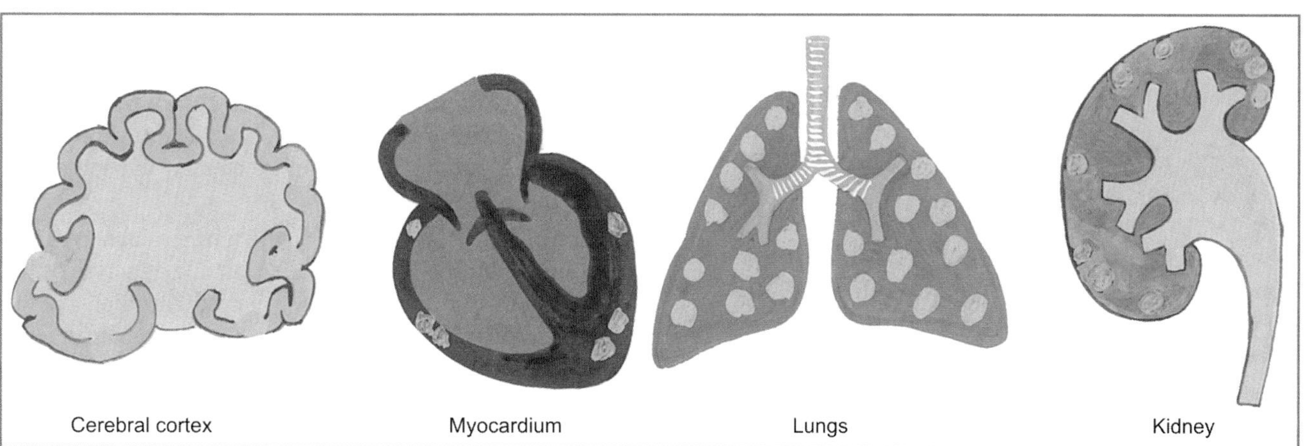

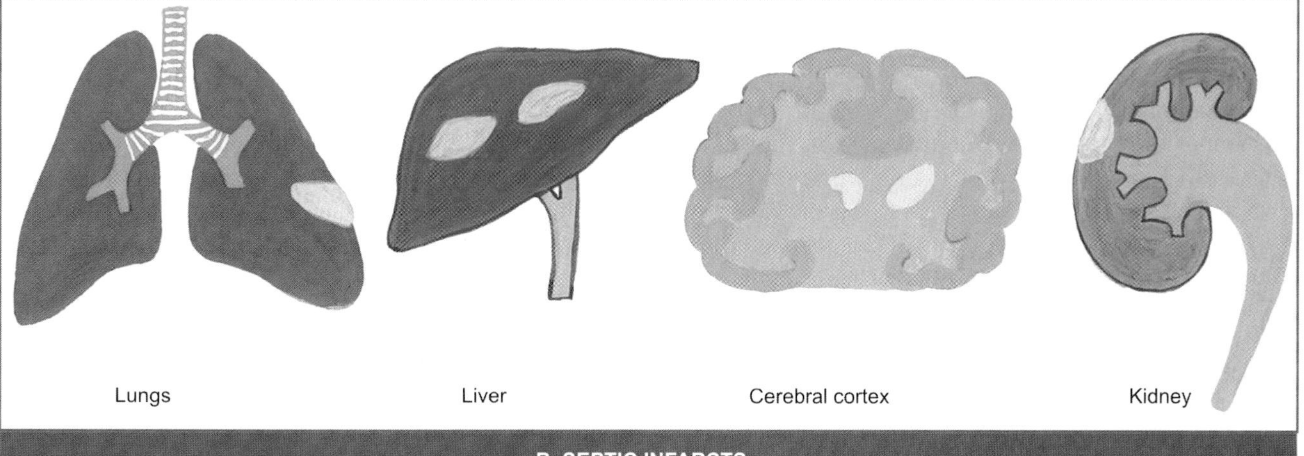

FIGURE 6.16

Sequelae of pyaemia.

inflammation is associated with systemic effects as well. These include fever, leucocytosis and lymphangitis-lymphadenitis.

1. **Fever** occurs due to bacteraemia. It is thought to be mediated through release of factors like prostaglandins, interleukin-1 and tumour necrosis factor in response to infection.

2. **Leucocytosis** commonly accompanies the acute inflammatory reactions, usually in the range of 15,000-20,000/μl. When the counts are higher than this with 'shift to left' of myeloid cells, the blood picture is described as leukaemoid reaction. Usually, in bacterial infections there is neutrophilia; in viral infections lymphocytosis; and in parasitic infestations, eosinophilia. Typhoid fever, an example of acute inflammation, however, induces leucopenia with relative lymphocytosis.

3. **Lymphangitis-lymphadenitis** is one of the important manifestations of localised inflammatory injury. The lymphatics and lymph nodes that drain the inflamed tissue show reactive inflammatory changes in the form of lymphangitis and lymphadenitis. This response represents either a nonspecific reaction to mediators released from inflamed tissue or is an immunologic response to a foreign antigen. The affected lymph nodes may show hyperplasia of lymphoid follicles (follicular hyperplasia) and proliferation of mononuclear phagocytic cells in the sinuses of lymph node (sinus histiocytosis) (Chapter 14).

4. **Shock** may occur in severe cases. Massive release of cytokine TNF-α, a mediator of inflammation, in response to severe tissue injury or infection results in profuse systemic vasodilatation, increased vascular permeability and intravascular volume loss. The net effect of these changes is hypotension and shock. Systemic activation of coagulation pathway may occur leading to microthrombi throughout the body and result in disseminated intravascular coagulation (DIC) , bleeding and death.

FATE OF ACUTE INFLAMMATION

The acute inflammatory process can culminate in one of the following 4 outcomes:

1. Resolution
2. Healing by scarring
3. Progression to suppuration
4. Progression to chronic inflammation.

1. **Resolution.** It means complete return to normal tissue following acute inflammation. This occurs when tissue changes are slight and the cellular changes are reversible e.g. resolution in lobar pneumonia.

2. **Healing by scarring.** This takes place when the tissue destruction in acute inflammation is extensive so that there is no tissue regeneration but actually there is healing by fibrosis.

3. **Suppuration.** When the pyogenic bacteria causing acute inflammation result in severe tissue necrosis, the process progresses to suppuration. Initially, there is intense neutrophilic infiltration. Subsequently, mixture of neutrophils, bacteria, fragments of necrotic tissue, cell debris and fibrin comprise pus which is contained in a cavity to form an abscess. The abscess, if not drained, may get organised by dense fibrous tissue, and in time, get calcified.

4. **Chronic inflammation.** The acute inflammation may progress to chronic inflammation in which the processes of inflammation and healing proceed side by side.

CHRONIC INFLAMMATION

DEFINITION AND CAUSES. Chronic inflammation is defined as prolonged process in which tissue destruction and inflammation occur at the same time.

Chronic inflammation can be caused by one of the following 3 ways:

1. **Chronic inflammation following acute inflammation.** When the tissue destruction is extensive, or the bacteria survive and persist in small numbers at the site of acute inflammation e.g. in osteomyelitis, pneumonia terminating in lung abscess.

2. **Recurrent attacks of acute inflammation.** When repeated bouts of acute inflammation culminate in chronicity of the process e.g. in recurrent urinary tract infection leading to chronic pyelonephritis, repeated acute infection of gallbladder leading to chronic cholecystitis.

3. **Chronic inflammation starting *de novo*.** When the infection with organisms of low pathogenicity is chronic from the beginning e.g. infection with *Mycobacterium tuberculosis*.

GENERAL FEATURES OF CHRONIC INFLAMMATION

Though there may be differences in chronic inflammatory response depending upon the tissue involved and causative organisms, there are some basic similarities amongst various types of chronic inflammation. Following general features characterise any chronic inflammation:

1. **MONONUCLEAR CELL INFILTRATION.** Chronic inflammatory lesions are infiltrated by mononuclear

inflammatory cells like phagocytes and lymphoid cells. Phagocytes are represented by circulating monocytes, tissue macrophages, epithelioid cells and sometimes, multinucleated giant cells. The macrophages comprise the most important cells in chronic inflammation. These may appear at the site of chronic inflammation from:

i) chemotactic factors and adhesion molecules for continued infiltration of macrophages;
ii) local proliferation of macrophages; and
iii) longer survival of macrophages at the site of inflammation.

The blood monocytes on reaching the extravascular space transform into tissue macrophages. Besides the role of macrophages in phagocytosis, they may get activated in response to stimuli such as cytokines (lymphokines) and bacterial endotoxins. On activation, macrophages release several biologically active substances e.g. acid and neutral proteases, oxygen-derived reactive metabolites and cytokines. These products bring about tissue destruction, neovascularisation and fibrosis.

Other chronic inflammatory cells include lymphocytes, plasma cells, eosinophils and mast cells. In chronic inflammation, lymphocytes and macrophages influence each other and release mediators of inflammation.

2. TISSUE DESTRUCTION OR NECROSIS. Tissue destruction and necrosis are central feature of most forms of chronic inflammatory lesions. This is brought about by activated macrophages which release of a variety of biologically active substances e.g. protease, elastase, collagenase, lipase, reactive oxygen radicals, cytokines (IL-1, IL-8, TNF), nitric oxide, angiogenesis growth factor etc.

3. PROLIFERATIVE CHANGES. As a result of necrosis, proliferation of small blood vessels and fibroblasts is stimulated resulting in formation of inflammatory granulation tissue. Eventually, healing by fibrosis and collagen laying takes place.

SYSTEMIC EFFECTS OF CHRONIC INFLAMMATION

Chronic inflammation is associated with following systemic features:

1. Fever. Invariably there is mild fever, often with loss of weight and weakness.

2. Anaemia. As discussed in Chapter 13, chronic inflammation is acompanied by anaemia of varying degree.

3. Leucocytosis. As in acute inflammation, chronic inflammation also has leucocytosis but generally there is relative lymphocytosis in these cases.

4. ESR. ESR is elevated in all cases of chronic inflammation.

5. Amyloidosis. Long-term cases of chronic suppurative inflammation may develop secondary systemic (AA) amyloidosis.

TYPES OF CHRONIC INFLAMMATION

Conventionally, chronic inflammation is subdivided into 2 types:

1. Non-specific, when the irritant substance produces a non-specific chronic inflammatory reaction with formation of granulation tissue and healing by fibrosis e.g. chronic osteomyelitis, chronic ulcer.

2. Specific, when the injurious agent causes a characteristic histologic tissue response e.g. tuberculosis, leprosy, syphilis.

However, for a more descriptive classification, histological features are used for classifying chronic inflammation into 2 corresponding types:

1. Chronic non-specific inflammation. It is characterised by non-specific inflammatory cell infiltration e.g. chronic osteomyelitis, lung abscess. A variant of this type of chronic inflammatory response is chronic suppurative inflammation in which infiltration by polymorphs and abscess formation are additional features e.g. actinomycosis.

2. Chronic granulomatous inflammation. It is characterised by formation of granulomas e.g. tuberculosis, leprosy, syphilis, actinomycosis, sarcoidosis etc.

GRANULOMATOUS INFLAMMATION

Granuloma is defined as a circumscribed, tiny lesion, about 1 mm in diameter, composed predominantly of collection of modified macrophages called epithelioid cells, and rimmed at the periphery by lymphoid cells. The word *'granuloma'* is derived from *granule* meaning circumscribed granule-like lesion, and *-oma* which is a suffix commonly used for true tumours but here indicates inflammatory mass or collection of macrophages.

Epithelioid cells, so called because of their epithelial cell-like appearance, are modified macrophages/ histiocytes which are somewhat elongated, having pale-staining abundant cytoplasm, vesicular and lightly-staining slipper-shaped nucleus, while the cell membrane of adjacent epithelioid cells is closely apposed due to hazy cell outline. Epithelioid cells are weakly phagocytic.

Besides the presence of epithelioid cells and lymphoid cells, granulomas may have giant cells, necrosis and fibrosis:

1. The giant cells are formed by fusion of adjacent epithelioid cells and may have 20 or more nuclei. These nuclei may be arranged at the periphery like horse-shoe or ring or clustered at the two poles (Langhans' giant cells), or they may be present centrally (foreign body giant cells). The former are commonly seen in tuberculosis while the latter are common in foreign body tissue reactions. Like epithelioid cells these giant cells are weakly phagocytic but produce secretory products which help in removing the invading agents.

2. Necrosis may be a feature of some granulomatous conditions e.g. central caseation necrosis of tuberculosis, so called because of cheese-like appearance and consistency of necrosis.

3. Fibrosis is due to proliferation of fibroblasts at the periphery of granuloma.

The following two factors favour the formation of granulomas:

i) *Presence of poorly digestible irritant* which may be organisms like *Mycobacterium tuberculosis,* particles of talc, etc.

ii) *Presence of cell-mediated immunity* to the irritant, implying thereby the role of hypersensitivity in granulomatous inflammation.

The mechanism of evolution of granuloma is graphically depicted in Fig. 6.17.

The classical example of granulomatous inflammation is the tissue response to tubercle bacilli which is called as *tubercle* seen in tuberculosis (described below). A fully-developed tubercle is about 1 mm in diameter with central area of caseation necrosis, surrounded by epithelioid cells and one to several multinucleated giant cells (commonly Langhans' type), surrounded at the periphery by lymphocytes and bounded by fibroblasts and fibrous tissue.

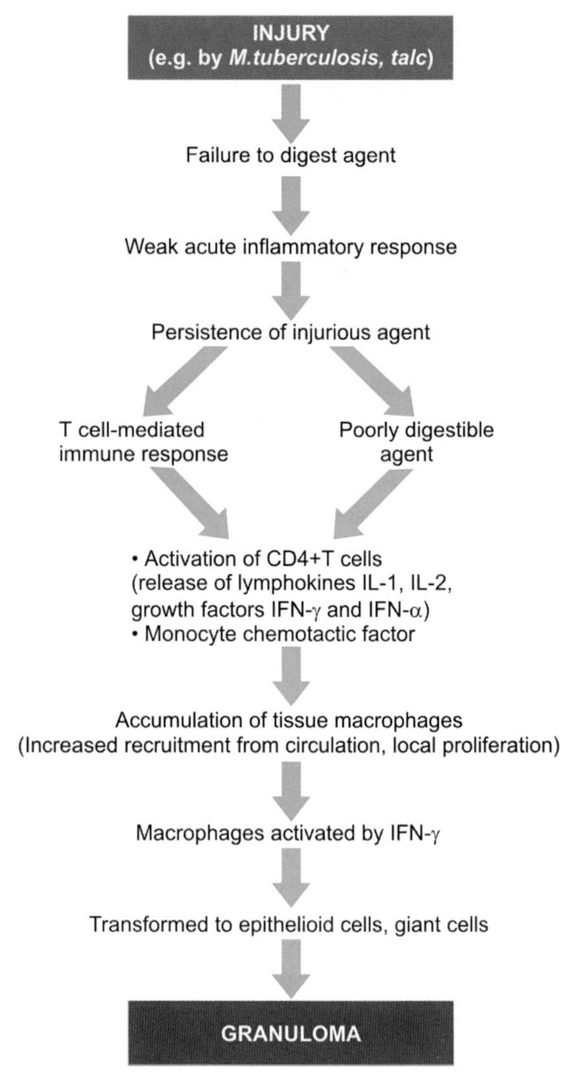

FIGURE 6.17

Mechanism of evolution of a granuloma (IL=interleukin; IFN= interferon).

EXAMPLES OF GRANULOMATOUS INFLAMMATION

Granulomatous inflammation is typical of reaction to poorly digestible agents elicited by tuberculosis, leprosy, fungal infections, schistosomiasis, foreign particles etc. A comprehensive list of important examples of granulomatous conditions, their etiologic agents and salient features is given in Table 6.4. The principal examples (marked with asterix in the table) are discussed below while a few others appear in relevant Chapters later.

TUBERCULOSIS

Tissue response in tuberculosis represents classical example of chronic granulomatous inflammation in humans.

CAUSATIVE ORGANISM. Tubercle bacillus or Koch's bacillus (named after discovery of the organism by Robert Koch in 1882) called *Mycobacterium tuberculosis* causes tuberculosis in the lungs and other tissues of the human body. The *organism is a strict aerobe and thrives best in tissues with high oxygen tension like in the apex of the lung.*

The organism has 5 distinct pathogenic strains: *hominis, bovis, avium, murine, and cold-blooded vertebrate strain.* A sixth non-pathogenic strain, *M. smegmatis*, is found in the smegma and as contaminant in the urine of both men and women. Out of these, the first two strains (*hominis* and *bovis*) are definitely infective to human

TABLE 6.4: Principal Granulomatous Conditions.

	CONDITIONS	ETIOLOGIC AGENT	SPECIAL CHARACTERISTICS
I.	**BACTERIAL**		
1.	***Tuberculosis****	*Mycobacterium tuberculosis*	Tuberculous granulomas with central caseation necrosis; acid-fast bacilli.
2.	***Leprosy****	*Mycobacterium leprae*	Foamy histiocytes with acid-fast bacilli (lepromatous); epithelioid cell granulomas (tuberculoid).
3.	***Syphilis****	*Treponema pallidum*	Gummas composed of histiocytes; plasma cell infiltration; central necrosis.
4.	***Granuloma inguinale (Donovanosis)***	*C. donovani (Donovan body)*	Anal and genital lesions; macrophages and neutrophils show Donovan bodies.
5.	***Brucellosis (Mediterranean fever)***	*Brucella abortus*	Dairy infection to humans; enlarged reticuloendothelial organs (lymph nodes, spleen, bone marrow); non-specific granulomas.
6.	***Cat scratch disease***	Coccobacillus	Lymphadenitis; reticuloendothelial hyperplasia; granulomas with central necrosis and neutrophils.
7.	***Tularaemia (Rabbit fever)***	*Francisella (Pasteurella) tularensis*	Necrosis and suppuration (acute); tubercles hard or with minute central necrosis (chronic).
8.	***Glanders***	*Actinobacillus mallei*	Infection from horses and mules; subcutaneous lesions and lymphadenitis; infective granulomas.
II.	**FUNGAL**		
1.	***Actinomycosis**** *(bacterial)*	*Actinomycetes israelii*	Cervicofacial, abdominal and thoracic lesions; granulomas and abscesses with draining sinuses; sulphur granules.
2.	***Blastomycosis***	*Blastomyces dermatitidis*	Cutaneous, systemic and lung lesions; suppuration; ulceration and granulomas.
3.	***Cryptococcosis***	*Cryptococcus neoformans*	Meninges, lungs and systemic distribution; organism yeast-like with clear capsule.
4.	***Coccidiodomycosis***	*Coccidioides immitis*	Meninges, lungs and systemic distribution; granulomas and abscesses; organism cyst containing endospores.
III.	**PARASITIC**		
	Schistosomiasis (Bilharziasis)	*Schistosoma mansoni, haematobium, japonicum*	Eggs and granulomas in gut, liver, lung; schistosome pigment; eosinophils in blood and tissue.
IV.	**MISCELLANEOUS**		
1.	***Sarcoidosis****	Unknown	Non-caseating granulomas (hard tubercles); asteroid and Schaumann bodies in giant cells.
2.	***Crohn's disease (Regional enteritis)***	Unknown ? Bacteria, ?? Viruses	Transmural chronic inflammatory infiltrates; non-caseating sarcoid-like granulomas.
3.	***Silicosis***	Silica dust	Lung lesions, fibrocollagenous nodules.
4.	***Berylliosis***	Metallic beryllium	Sarcoid-like granulomas in lungs; fibrosis; inclusions in giant cells (asteroids, Schaumann bodies, crystals).
5.	***Foreign body granulomas***	Talc, suture, oils, wood splinter etc.	Non-caseating granulomas with foreign body giant cells; demonstration of foreign body.

*Diseases discussed in this chapter.

beings while infection with avium strain *(M. avium-intracellulare)* is common in patients with AIDS.

M. tuberculosis hominis is a slender rod-like bacillus, 4 μm in length, and can be demonstrated by the following methods:

1. *Acid fast (Ziehl-Neelsen) staining.* The acid fastness of the tubercle bacilli is due to waxy content in the cell wall of the organism making it impermeable to the usual stains. It takes up stain by heated carbol fuchsin and resists decolourisation by acids and alcohols (acid fast and alcohol fast) and can be decolourised by 20% sulphuric acid.
2. *Fluorescent dye methods.*
3. *Culture* of the organism in Lowenstein-Jensen (L.J.) medium for 6 weeks.
4. *Guinea pig inoculation* method by subcutaneous injection of the organisms.

ATYPICAL MYCOBACTERIA. Occasionally, human tuberculosis may be caused by atypical mycobacteria which are non-pathogenic to guinea pigs and resistant to usual anti-tubercular drugs.

There are 4 groups of atypical mycobacteria:

Group I: Photochromogens. These organisms produce yellow pigment in the culture grown in light.

Group II: Scotochromogens. Pigment is produced, whether the growth is in light or in dark.

Group III: Non-chromogens. No pigment is produced by the bacilli and the organism is closely related to avium bacillus.

Group IV: Rapid growers. These organisms grow fast in the culture but are less pathogenic than others.

The infection by atypical mycobacteria is acquired directly from the environment, unlike person-to-person transmission of classical tuberculosis and the disease produced is known as *atypical mycobacteriosis.* The lesions produced may be granulomas, nodular collection of foamy cells, or acute inflammation.

Five patterns of the disease are recognised:

i) Pulmonary disease produced by *M. kansasii* or *M. avium-intracellulare.*

ii) Lymphadenitis caused by *M. avium-intracellulare* or *M. scrofulaceum.*

iii) Ulcerated skin lesion produced by *M. ulcerans* or *M. marinum.*

iv) Abscess caused by *M.fortuitum or M. chelonei.*

v) Bacteraemias by *M. avium-intracellulare* as seen in immunosuppressed patients of AIDS.

INCIDENCE. In spite of great advances in chemotherapy and immunology, tuberculosis still continues to be worldwide in distribution, more common in poorer countries of Africa, Latin America and Asia. Other factors contributing to higher incidence of tuberculosis are malnutrition, inadequate medical care, poverty, crowding, chronic debilitating conditions like uncontrolled diabetes, alcoholism and immunocompromised states like AIDS. However, the exact incidence of disease cannot be determined as all patients infected with *M. tuberculosis* may not develop the clinical disease and many remain reactive to tuberculin without developing symptomatic disease.

MODE OF TRANSMISSION. Human beings acquire infection with tubercle bacilli by one of the following routes:

1. *Inhalation* of organisms present in fresh cough droplets or in dried sputum from an open case of pulmonary tuberculosis.
2. *Ingestion* of the organisms leads to development of tonsillar or intestinal tuberculosis. This mode of infection of human tubercle bacilli is from self-swallowing of infected sputum of an open case of pulmonary tuberculosis, or ingestion of bovine tubercle bacilli from milk of diseased cows.
3. *Inoculation* of the organisms into the skin may rarely occur from infected postmortem tissue.
4. *Transplacental route* results in development of congenital tuberculosis in foetus from infected mother and is a rare mode of transmission.

SPREAD OF TUBERCULOSIS. The disease spreads in the body by various routes:

1. Local spread. This takes place by macrophages carrying the bacilli into the surrounding tissues.

2. Lymphatic spread. Tuberculosis is primarily an infection of lymphoid tissues. The bacilli may pass into lymphoid follicles of pharynx, bronchi, intestines or regional lymph nodes resulting in regional tuberculous lymphadenitis which is typical of childhood infections. Primary complex is primary focus with lymphangitis and lymphadenitis.

3. Haematogenous spread. This occurs either as a result of tuberculous bacillaemia because of the drainage of lymphatics into the venous system or due to caseous material escaping through ulcerated wall of a vein. This produces millet seed-sized lesions in different organs of the body like lungs, liver, kidneys, bones and other tissues and is known as miliary tuberculosis.

4. By the natural passages. Infection may spread from:

i) lung lesions into pleura (tuberculous pleurisy);

ii) transbronchial spread into the adjacent lung segments;

iii) tuberculous salpingitis into peritoneal cavity (tuberculous peritonitis);

iv) infected sputum into larynx (tuberculous laryngitis);

v) swallowing of infected sputum (ileocaecal tuberculosis); and

vi) renal lesions into ureter and down to trigone of bladder.

HYPERSENSITIVITY AND IMMUNITY IN TUBERCULOSIS. Hypersensitivity or allergy, and immunity or resistance, play a major role in the development of lesions in tuberculosis. Tubercle bacilli as such do not produce any toxins. Tissue changes seen in tuberculosis are not the result of any exotoxin or endotoxin but are instead the result of host response to the organism which is in the form of development of cell-mediated hypersensitivity (or type IV hypersensitivity) and immunity. Both these host responses develop as a consequence of several lipids present in the microorganism which include the following:

1. **mycosides** such as 'cord factor' which are essential for growth and virulence of the organism in the animals; and

2. **glycolipids** present in the mycobacterial cell wall like *'Wax-D'* which acts as an adjuvant acting along with tuberculoprotein.

It has been known since the time of Robert Koch that the tissue reaction to tubercle bacilli is different in healthy animal not previously infected (primary infection) from an animal who is previously infected (secondary infection).

1. **In the primary infection,** intradermal injection of tubercle bacilli into the skin of a healthy guinea pig evokes no visible reaction for 10-14 days. After this period, a nodule develops at the inoculation site which subsequently ulcerates and heals poorly as the guinea pig, unlike human beings, does not possess any natural resistance. The regional lymph nodes also develop tubercles. This process is a manifestation of delayed type of hypersensitivity and is comparable to primary tuberculosis in children although healing invariably occurs in children.

2. **In the secondary infection,** the sequence of changes is different. The tubercle bacilli are injected into the skin of the guinea pig who has been infected with tuberculosis 4-6 weeks earlier. In 1-2 days, the site of inoculation is indurated and dark, attaining a diameter of about 1 cm. The skin lesion ulcerates which heals quickly and the regional lymph nodes are not affected. This is called *Koch's phenomenon* and is indicative of hypersensitivity and immunity in the host.

Similar type of changes can be produced if injection of live tubercle bacilli is replaced with old tuberculin (OT).

Hypersensitivity and immunity are closely related and are initiated through T lymphocytes sensitised against specific antigens in tuberculin. As a result of this sensitisation, lymphokines are released from T cells which induce increased microbicidal activity of the macrophages.

Tuberculin (Mantoux) skin test. This test is done by intradermal injection of 0.1 ml of tuberculoprotein, purified protein derivative (PPD). Delayed type of hypersensitivity develops in individuals who are having or have been previously infected with tuberculous infection which is identified as an indurated area of more than 15 mm in 72 hours. However, patients having disseminated tuberculosis may show negative test due to release of large amount of tuberculoproteins from the endogenous lesions masking the hypersensitivity test. A positive test is indicative of cell-mediated hypersensitivity to tubercular antigens but does not distinguish between infection and disease. The test may be false positive in atypical mycobacterial infection and false negative in sarcoidosis, some viral infections, Hodgkin's disease and fulminant tuberculosis.

Immunisation against tuberculosis. Protective immunisation against tuberculosis is induced by injection of attenuated strains of bovine type of tubercle bacilli, *Bacilli Calmette Guerin* (BCG). Cell-mediated immunity with consequent delayed hypersensitivity reaction develops with healing of the lesion, but the cell-mediated immunity persists, rendering the host tuberculin-positive and hence immune.

EVOLUTION OF TUBERCLE. The sequence of events which take place when tubercle bacilli are introduced into the tissue are as under (Fig. 6.18):

1. When the tubercle bacilli are injected intravenously into the guinea pig, the bacilli are lodged in pulmonary capillaries where an *initial response of neutrophils* is evoked which are rapidly destroyed by the organisms.

2. After about 12 hours, there is *progressive infiltration by macrophages.* This is due to coating of tubercle bacilli with serum complement factors C_{2a} and C_{3b} which act as opsonins and attract the macrophages. Macrophages dominate the picture throughout the remaining life of the lesions. If the tubercle bacilli are, however, inhaled into the lung alveoli, macrophages predominate the picture from the beginning.

3. The macrophages start *phagocytosing* the tubercle bacilli and either kill the bacteria or die away

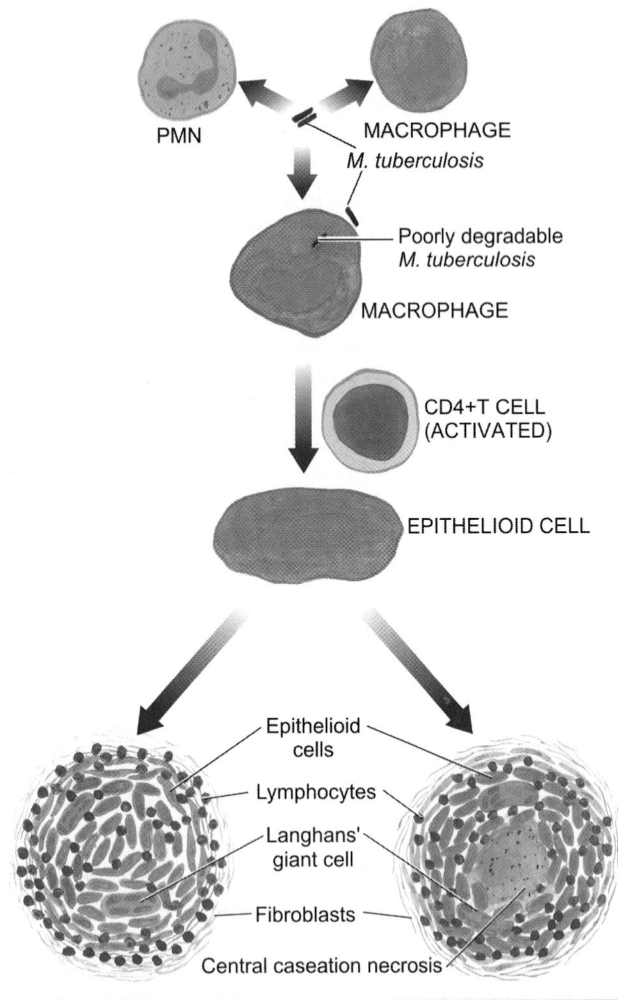

FIGURE 6.18

Schematic evolution of tubercle. In fully formed granuloma, the centre is composed of granular caseation necrosis, surrounded by epithelioid cells and Langhans' giant cells and peripheral rim of lymphocytes bounded by fibroblasts.

themselves. In the latter case, they further proliferate locally as well as there is increased recruitment of macrophages from blood monocytes.

4. As a part of body's immune response, T and B cells are activated. Activated CD4+T cells develop the cell-mediated *delayed type hypersensitivity reaction,* while B cells result in formation of antibodies which play no role in body's defence against tubercle bacilli.

5. In 2-3 days, the macrophages undergo structural changes as a result of immune mechanisms—the cytoplasm becomes pale and eosinophilic and their nuclei become elongated and vesicular. These modified macrophages resemble epithelial cells and are called *epithelioid cells.*

6. The epithelioid cells in time aggregate into tight clusters or *granulomas.* Release of cytokines in response to sensitised CD4+T cells and some constituents of mycobacterial cell wall play a role in formation of granuloma.

7. Some of the macrophages form *multinucleated giant cells* by fusion of adjacent cells. The giant cells may be Langhans' type having peripherally arranged nuclei in the form of horseshoe or ring, or clustered at the two poles of the giant cell; or they may be foreign body type having centrally-placed nuclei.

8. Around the mass of epithelioid cells and giant cells is a zone of lymphocytes, plasma cells and fibroblasts. The lesion at this stage is called *hard tubercle* due to absence of central necrosis.

9. Within 10-14 days, the centre of the cellular mass begins to undergo caseation necrosis, characterised by cheesy appearance and high lipid content. This stage is called *soft tubercle* which is the hallmark of tuberculous lesions. The development of caseation necrosis is possibly due to interaction of mycobacteria with activated T cells (CD4+ helper T cells via IF-γ and CD8+ suppressor T cells directly) as well as by direct toxicity of mycobacteria on macrophages. *Microscopically,* caseation necrosis is structureless, eosinophilic and granular material with nuclear debris.

10. The soft tubercle which is a fully-developed granuloma with caseous centre does not favour rapid proliferation of tubercle bacilli. *Acid-fast bacilli* are difficult to find in these lesions and may be demonstrated at the margins of recent necrotic foci and in the walls of the cavities.

The **fate of a granuloma** is variable:

i) The caseous material may undergo liquefaction and extend into surrounding soft tissues, discharging the contents on the surface. This is called *cold abscess* although there are no pus cells in it.

ii) In tuberculosis of tissues like bones, joints, lymph nodes and epididymis, sinuses are formed and the *sinus tracts* are lined by tuberculous granulation tissue.

iii) The adjacent granulomas may *coalesce* together enlarging the lesion which is surrounded by progressive fibrosis.

iv) In the granuloma enclosed by fibrous tissue, calcium salts may get deposited in the caseous material *(dystrophic calcification)* and sometimes the lesion may even get ossified over the years **(COLOUR PLATE II: CL 8).**

TYPES OFTUBERCULOSIS

Lung is the main organ affected in tuberculosis. Depending upon the type of tissue response and age, the infection with tubercle bacilli is of 2 main types:
A. Primary tuberculosis; and
B. Secondary tuberculosis.

A. Primary Tuberculosis

The infection of an individual who has not been previously infected or immunised is called *primary tuberculosis* or *Ghon's complex* or *childhood tuberculosis*.

Primary complex or Ghon's complex is the lesion produced at the portal of entry with foci in the draining lymphatic vessels and lymph nodes. The most commonly involved tissues for primary complex are lungs and hilar lymph nodes. The other tissues which may show primary complex are tonsils and cervical lymph nodes, and in the case of ingested bacilli the lesions may be found in small intestine and mesenteric lymph nodes.

The incidence of disseminated form of progressive primary tuberculosis is particularly high in immunocompromised host e.g. in patients of AIDS.

Primary complex or Ghon's complex in lungs consists of 3 components (Fig. 6.19):

1. Pulmonary component. Lesion in the lung is the primary focus or Ghon's focus. It is 1-2 cm solitary area of tuberculous pneumonia located peripherally under a patch of pleurisy, in any part of the lung but more often in subpleural focus in the upper part of lower lobe.

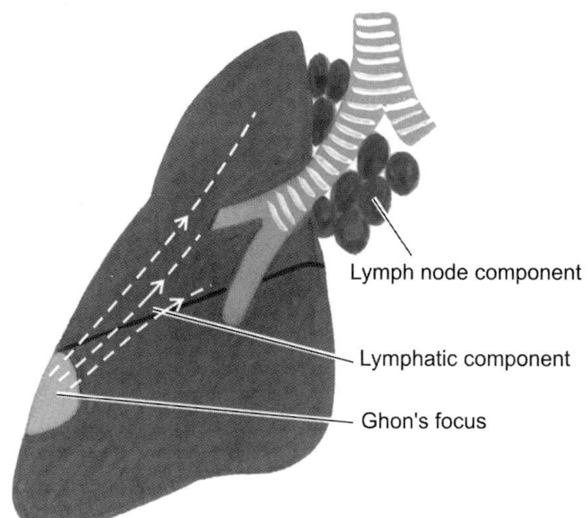

FIGURE 6.19

The primary complex composed of 3 components: Ghon's focus, draining lymphatics, and hilar lymph nodes.

Microscopically, the lung lesion consists of tuberculous granulomas with caseation necrosis.

2. Lymphatic vessel component. The lymphatics draining the lung lesion contain phagocytes containing bacilli and may develop beaded, miliary tubercles along the path of hilar lymph nodes.

3. Lymph node component. This consists of enlarged hilar and tracheo-bronchial lymph nodes in the area drained. The affected lymph nodes are matted and show caseation necrosis.

Microscopically, the lesions are characterised by extensive caseation, tuberculous granulomas and fibrosis. Nodal lesions are potential source of re-infection later (COLOUR PLATE VIII: CL 29).

In the case of primary tuberculosis of alimentary tract due to ingestion of tubercle bacilli, a small primary focus is seen in the intestine with enlarged mesenteric lymph nodes producing *tabes mesenterica*. The enlarged and caseous mesenteric lymph nodes may rupture into peritoneal cavity and cause tuberculous peritonitis.

FATE OF PRIMARY TUBERCULOSIS. Primary complex may have one of the following sequelae (Fig. 6.20):

1. The lesions of primary tuberculosis of lung commonly do not progress but instead heal by *fibrosis*, and in time undergo *calcification* and even *ossification*.

2. In some cases, the primary focus in the lung continues to grow and the caseous material is disseminated through bronchi to the other parts of the same lung or the opposite lung. This is called *progressive primary tuberculosis*.

3. At times, bacilli may enter the circulation through erosion in a blood vessel and spread to various tissues and organs. This is called *primary miliary tuberculosis* and the lesions are seen in organs like liver, spleen, kidney, brain and bone marrow.

4. In certain circumstances like in lowered resistance and increased hypersensitivity of the host, the healed lesions of primary tuberculosis may get reactivated. The bacilli lying dormant in acellular caseous material are activated and cause *progressive secondary tuberculosis*. It affects children more commonly but adults may also develop this kind of progression.

B. Secondary Tuberculosis

The infection of an individual who has been previously infected or sensitised is called *secondary*, or *post-primary* or *reinfection*, or *chronic tuberculosis*.

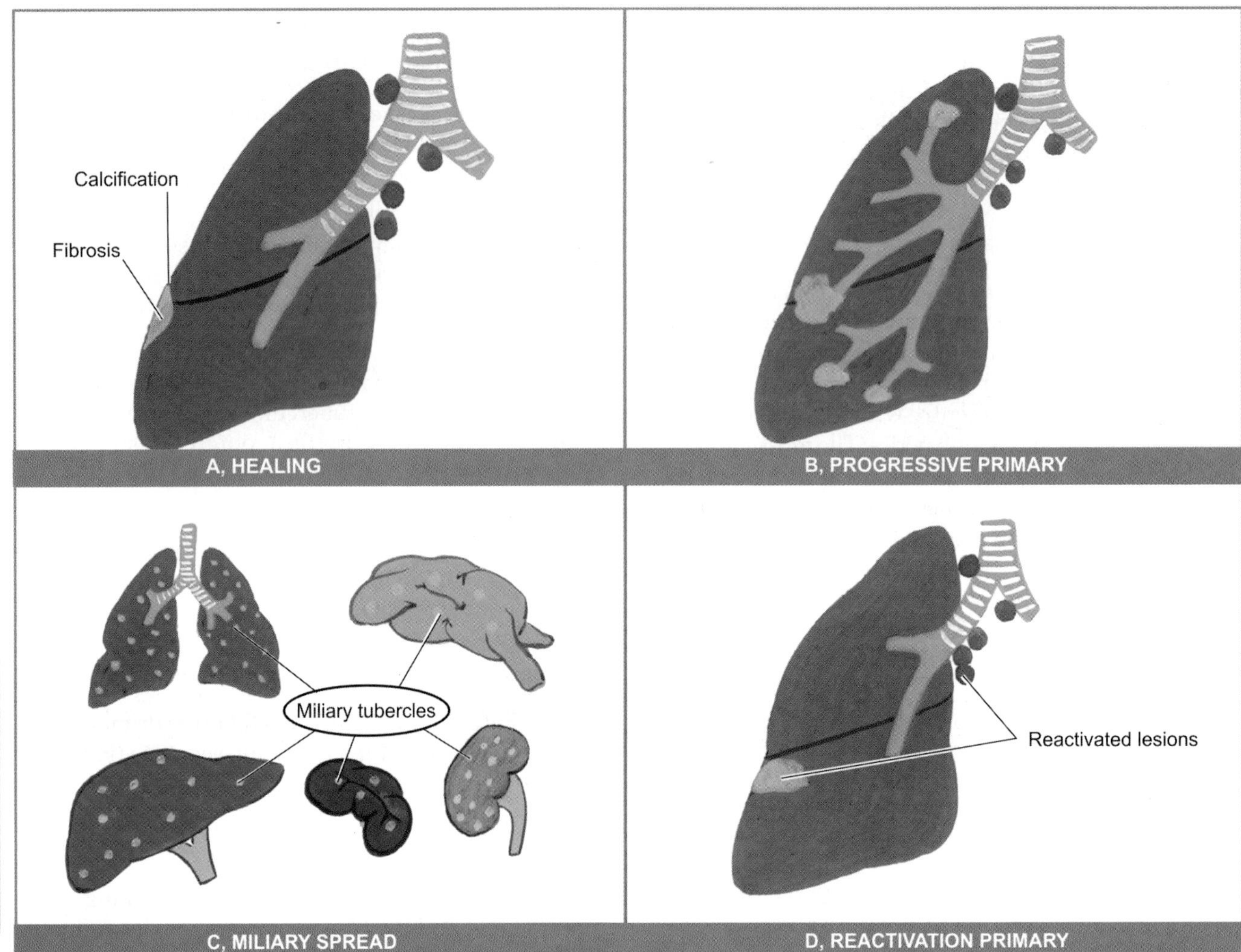

FIGURE 6.20

Sequelae of primary complex. A, Healing by fibrosis and calcification. B, Progressive primary tuberculosis spreading to the other areas of the same lung or opposite lung. C, Miliary spread to lungs, liver, spleen, kidneys and brain. D, Progressive secondary pulmonary tuberculosis from reactivation of dormant primary complex.

The infection may be acquired from (Fig. 6.21):

- *endogenous source* such as reactivation of dormant primary complex; or
- *exogenous source* such as fresh dose of reinfection by the tubercle bacilli.

Secondary tuberculosis occurs most commonly in lungs in the region of apex. Other sites and tissues which can be involved are tonsils, pharynx, larynx, small intestine and skin. Secondary tuberculosis of other organs and tissues is described in relevant chapters later while that of lungs is discussed here.

Secondary Pulmonary Tuberculosis

The lesions in secondary pulmonary tuberculosis usually begin as 1-2 cm apical area of consolidation of the lung, which may in time develop a small area of central caseation necrosis and peripheral fibrosis. It occurs by haematogenous spread of infection from primary complex to the apex of the affected lung where the oxygen tension is high and favourable for growth of aerobic tubercle bacilli. *Microscopically,* the appearance is typical of tuberculous granulomas with caseation necrosis.

Patients with HIV infection previously exposed to tuberculous infection have particularly high incidence of reactivation of primary tuberculosis and the pattern of lesions in such cases is similar to that of primary tuberculosis i.e. with involvement of hilar lymph nodes rather than cavitary and apical lesions in the lung. In addition, opportunistic infection with *M. avium-intracellulare* can occur in cases of AIDS.

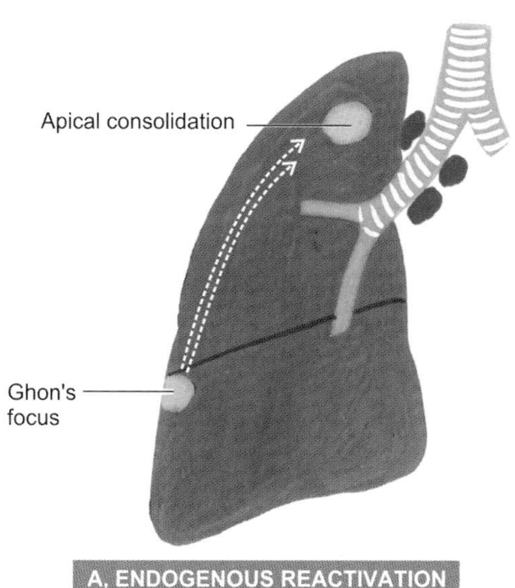

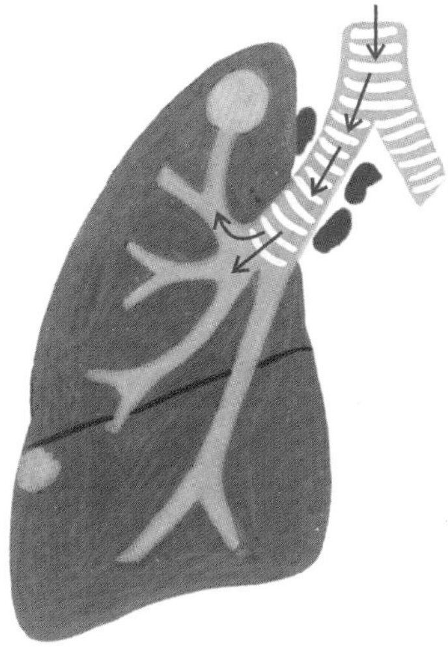

FIGURE 6.21

Progressive secondary tuberculosis. A, Endogenous infection from reactivation of dormant primary complex. B, Exogenous infection from fresh dose of tubercle bacilli.

FATE OF SECONDARY PULMONARY TUBERCULOSIS. The subapical lesions in lungs can have the following courses:

1. The lesions may *heal* with fibrous scarring and calcification.

2. The lesions may *coalesce* together to form larger area of tuberculous pneumonia and produce progressive secondary pulmonary tuberculosis with the following pulmonary and extrapulmonary involvements:

i) Fibrocaseous tuberculosis
ii) Tuberculous caseous pneumonia
iii) Miliary tuberculosis.

I. FIBROCASEOUS TUBERCULOSIS. The original area of tuberculous pneumonia undergoes massive central caseation necrosis which may:

- either break into a bronchus from a cavity *(cavitary or open fibrocaseous tuberculosis)*; or
- remain, as a soft caseous lesion without drainage into a bronchus or bronchiole to produce a non-cavitary lesion *(chronic fibrocaseous tuberculosis)*.

The cavity provides favourable environment for proliferation of tubercle bacilli due to high oxygen tension. The cavity may communicate with bronchial tree and becomes the source of spread of infection *('open tuberculosis')*. The open case of secondary tuberculosis may implant tuberculous lesion on the mucosal lining of air passages producing *endobronchial and endotracheal tuberculosis*. Ingestion of sputum containing tubercle bacilli from endogenous pulmonary lesions may produce *laryngeal and intestinal tuberculosis*.

Grossly, tuberculous cavity is spherical with thick fibrous wall, lined by yellowish, caseous, necrotic material and the lumen is traversed by thrombosed blood vessels. Around the wall of cavity are seen foci of consolidation. The overlying pleura may also be thickened (Fig. 6.22,A)

Microscopically, the wall of cavity shows eosinophilic, granular, caseous material which may show foci of dystrophic calcification. Widespread coalesced tuberculous granulomas composed of epithelioid cells, Langhans' giant cells and peripheral mantle of lymphocytes and having central caseation necrosis are seen. The outer wall of cavity shows fibrosis (Fig. 6.22,B) **(COLOUR PLATE VII: CL 27).**

Complications of cavitary secondary tuberculosis are:

a) aneurysms of patent arteries crossing the cavity producing haemoptysis;
b) extension to pleura producing bronchopleural fistula;
c) tuberculous empyema from deposition of caseous material on the pleural surface; and
d) thickened pleura from adhesions of parietal pleura.

II. TUBERCULOUS CASEOUS PNEUMONIA. The caseous material from a case of secondary tuberculosis in an individual with high degree of hypersensitivity

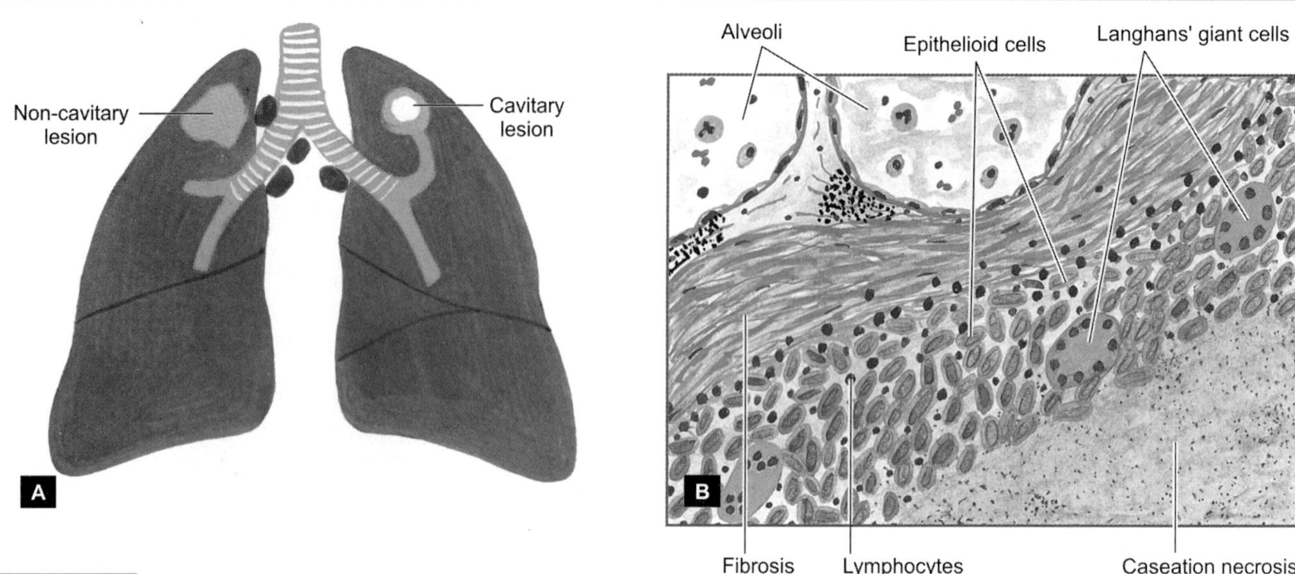

FIGURE 6.22

Fibrocaseous tuberculosis. A, Non-cavitary (chronic) fibrocaseous tuberculosis (left) and cavitary/open fibrocaseous tuberculosis (right). B, Microscopic appearance of lesions of secondary fibrocaseous tuberculosis of the lung showing wall of the cavity.

may spread to rest of the lung producing caseous pneumonia (Fig. 6.23,A).

Microscopically, the lesions show exudative reaction with oedema, fibrin, polymorphs and monocytes but numerous tubercle bacilli can be demonstrated in the exudates (Fig. 6.23,B).

III. MILIARY TUBERCULOSIS. This is lympho-haematogenous spread of tuberculous infection from primary focus or later stages of tuberculosis. The spread may occur to systemic organs or isolated organ. The spread is either by entry of infection into pulmonary vein producing disseminated or isolated organ lesion in different extra-pulmonary sites (e.g. liver, spleen, kidney, brain and bone marrow) or into pulmonary artery restricting the development of miliary lesions within the lung (Fig. 6.24,A). The miliary lesions are millet seed-sized (1 mm diameter), yellowish, firm areas without grossly visible caseation necrosis.

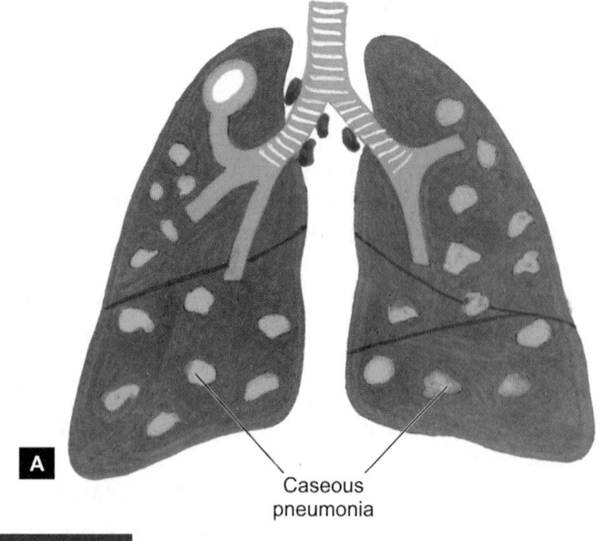

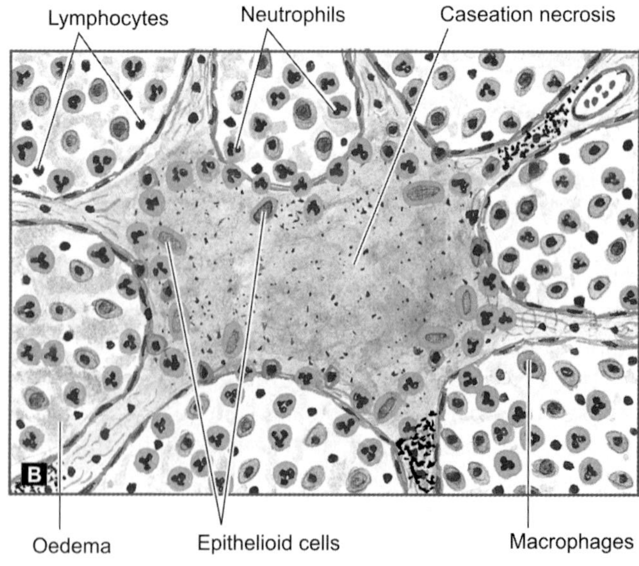

FIGURE 6.23

A, Bilateral tuberculous caseous pneumonia. B, Tuberculous caseous pneumonia showing exudative reaction. In AFB staining, these cases have numerous acid-fast bacilli (not shown here).

Microscopically, the lesions show the structure of tubercles with minute areas of caseation necrosis (Fig. 6.24,B) **(COLOUR PLATE VII: CL 28).**

Clinical Features of Tuberculosis

The clinical manifestations in tuberculosis may be variable depending upon the location, extent and type of lesions. However, in secondary pulmonary tuberculosis which is the common type, the usual clinical features are as under:

1. Referable to lungs—such as productive cough, may be with haemoptysis, pleural effusion, dyspnoea, orthopnoea etc. Chest X-ray may show typical apical changes like pleural effusion, nodularity, and miliary or diffuse infiltrates in the lung parenchyma.

2. Systemic features—such as fever, night sweats, fatigue, loss of weight and appetite. Long-standing and untreated cases of tuberculosis may develop systemic secondary amyloidosis.

Causes of death in pulmonary tuberculosis are usually pulmonary insufficiency, pulmonary haemorrhage, sepsis due to disseminated miliary tuberculosis, cor pulmonale or secondary amyloidosis.

LEPROSY

Leprosy or Hansen's disease (after discovery of the causative organism by Hansen in 1874) is a chronic infectious disease affecting mainly the cooler parts of the body such as the skin, mouth, respiratory tract, eyes, peripheral nerves, superficial lymph nodes and testis. Though the earliest and main involvement in leprosy is of the skin and nerves but in bacteraemia from endothelial colonisation or by bacilli filtered from blood by reticuloendothelial system, other organs such as the liver, spleen, bone marrow and regional lymph nodes are also involved. Advanced cases may develop secondary amyloidosis and renal disease, both of which are of immunologic origin.

Causative Organism

The disease is caused by *Mycobacterium leprae* which closely resembles *Mycobacterium tuberculosis* but is less acid-fast. The organisms in tissues appear as compact rounded masses *(globi)* or are arranged in parallel fashion like *cigarettes-in-pack.*

M. leprae can be demonstrated in tissue sections, in split skin smears by splitting the skin, scrapings from cut edges of dermis, and in nasal smears by the following techniques:

1. *Acid-fast (Ziehl-Neelsen) staining.* The staining procedure is similar as for demonstration of *M. tuberculosis* but can be decolourised by lower concentration (5%) of sulphuric acid (less acid-fast).
2. *Fite-Faraco staining* procedure is a modification of Z.N. procedure and is considered better for more adequate staining of tissue sections.
3. *Gomori methenamine silver (GMS)* staining can also be employed.

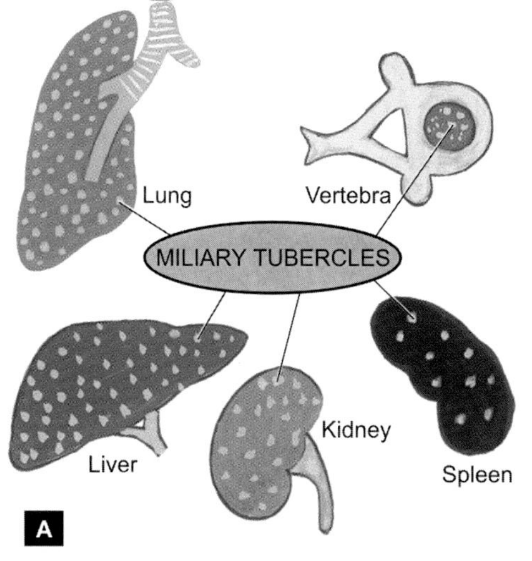

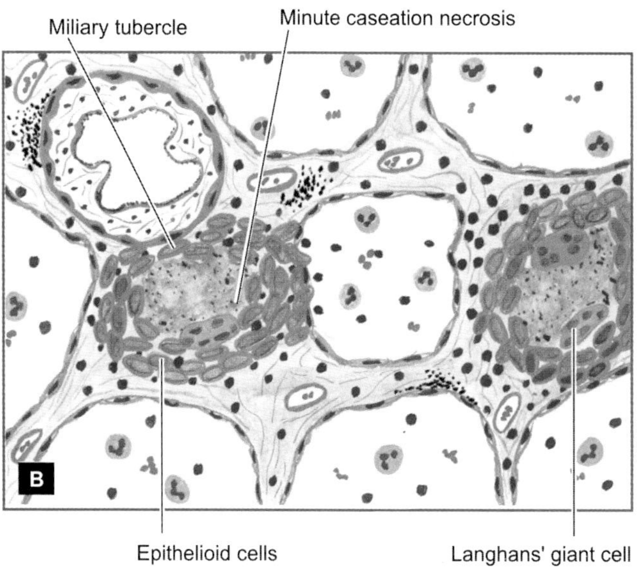

FIGURE 6.24

A, Acute miliary tuberculosis affecting different organs (lung, liver, spleen, kidney and vertebra. B, Miliary tubercles in lung having minute central caseation necrosis.

The slit smear technique gives a reasonable quantitative measure of *M. leprae* when stained with Ziehl-Neelsen method and examined under 100x oil objective for determining the density of bacteria in the lesion *(bacterial index, BI)*. B.I. is scored from 1+ to 6+ (range from 1 to 10 bacilli per 100 fields to > 1000 per field) as *multibacillary* leprosy while B.I. 0+ is termed *paucibacillary*.

Nine-banded armadillo, a rodent, acts as an experimental animal model as it develops leprosy which is histopathologically and immunologically similar to human leprosy.

Incidence

The disease is endemic in areas with hot and moist climates and in poor tropical countries. According to the WHO, five countries—India, Brazil, Indonesia, Myanmar (Burma) and Nigeria, together constitute vast majority of leprosy cases, of which India accounts for about one-third of all registered leprosy cases globally. In India, the disease is seen more commonly in regions like Tamil Nadu, Bihar, Pondicherry, Andhra Pradesh, Orissa, West Bengal and Assam. Very few cases are now seen in Europe and the United States.

Mode of Transmission

Leprosy is a slow communicable disease and the incubation period between first exposure and appearance of signs of disease varies from 2 to 20 years (average about 3 years). The infectivity may be from the following sources:

1. *Direct contact* with untreated leprosy patients who shed numerous bacilli from damaged skin, nasal secretions, mucous membrane of mouth and hair follicles.
2. *Materno-foetal transmission* across the placenta.
3. Transmission from *milk* of leprosy patient to infant.

Classification

Leprosy is broadly classified into 2 main types:

- Lepromatous type representing *low resistance*; and
- Tuberculoid type representing *high resistance*.

Salient differences between the two main forms of leprosy are summarised in Table 6.5.

Since both these types of leprosy represent two opposite poles of host immune response, these are also called *polar forms* of leprosy. Cases not falling into either of the two poles are classified as *borderline* and *indeterminate types*.

Currently, leprosy is classified into 7 groups *(modified Ridley and Jopling's classification)*. These are:

TT—Tuberculoid Polar *(High resistance)*
BT—Borderline Tuberculoid
TI—Tuberculoid Indefinite
BB—Mid Borderline
LI—Lepromatous Indefinite
BL—Borderline Lepromatous
LL—Lepromatous Polar *(Low resistance)*

In addition, not included in Ridley-Jopling's classification are cases of indeterminate leprosy, pure neural leprosy and histoid leprosy resembling a nodule of dermatofibroma and positive for lepra bacilli.

Reactions in Leprosy

There may be two types of lepra reactions: type I (borderline reactions), and type II (erythema nodosum leprosum).

TABLE 6.5: Differences between Lepromatous and Tuberculoid Leprosy.

FEATURE	LEPROMATOUS LEPROSY	TUBERCULOID LEPROSY
1. *Skin lesions*	Symmetrical, multiple, hypopigmented, erythematous, maculopapular or nodular (leonine facies).	Asymmetrical, single or a few lesions, hypopigmented and erythematous macular.
2. *Nerve involvement*	Present but sensory disturbance is less severe.	Present with distinct sensory disturbance.
3. *Histopathology*	Collection of foamy macrophages or lepra cells in the dermis separated from epidermis by a 'clear zone'.	Hard tubercle similar to granulomatous lesion, eroding the basal layer of epidermis; no clear zone.
4. *Bacteriology*	Lepra cells highly positive for lepra bacilli seen as 'globi' or 'cigarettes-in-pack' appearance.	Lepra bacilli few, seen in destroyed nerves as granular or beaded forms.
5. *Immunity*	Suppressed (low resistance).	Good immune response (high resistance).
6. *Lepromin test*	Negative.	Positive.

TYPE I: BORDERLINE REACTIONS. The polar forms of leprosy do not undergo any change in clinical and histopathological picture. The borderline groups are unstable and may move across the spectrum in either direction with upgrading or downgrading of patient's immune state. Accordingly, there may be two types of borderline reaction:

1. **Upgrading reaction** is characterised by increased cell-mediated immunity and occurs in patients of borderline lepromatous (BL) type on treatment who upgrade or shift towards tuberculoid type.

Histologically, the upgrading reaction shows an increase of lymphocytes, oedema of the lesions and reduced B.I.

2. **Downgrading reaction** is characterised by lowering of cellular immunity and is seen in borderline tuberculoid (BT) type who downgrade or shift towards lepromatous type.

Histologically, the lesions show dispersal and spread of the granulomas and increased presence of lepra bacilli.

TYPE II: ERYTHEMA NODOSUM LEPROSUM (ENL). ENL occurs in lepromatous patients after treatment. It is characterised by tender cutaneous nodules, fever, iridocyclitis, synovitis and lymph node involvement.

Histologically, the lesions in ENL show infiltration by neutrophils and prominence of vasculitis. Secondary amyloidosis may follow repeated attacks of ENL in leprosy.

Clinical Features

The two main forms of leprosy show distinctive clinical features:

1. Lepromatous Leprosy:

i) The skin lesions in LL are generally symmetrical, multiple, slightly hypopigmented and erythematous macules, papules, nodules or diffuse infiltrates. The nodular lesions may coalesce to give *leonine facies* appearance.

ii) The lesions are hypoaesthetic or anaesthetic but the sensory disturbance is not as distinct as in TT.

2. Tuberculoid leprosy:

i) The skin lesions in TT occur as either single or as a few asymmetrical lesions which are hypopigmented and erythematous macules.

ii) There is a distinct sensory impairment.

Histopathology of Leprosy

Usually, skin biopsy from the margin of lesions is submitted for diagnosis and for classification of leprosy. The histopathologic diagnosis of multibacillary leprosy like LL and BL offers no problem while the indeterminate leprosy and tuberculoid lesions are paucibacillary and their diagnosis is made together with clinical evidence.

In general, for histopathologic evaluation in all suspected cases of leprosy the following broad *guidelines* should be followed:

- cell type of granuloma;
- nerve involvement; and
- bacterial load.

The main features in various groups are given below.

1. Lepromatous leprosy:

The following features characterise lepromatous polar leprosy (Fig. 6.25,A):

i) In the dermis, there is proliferation of macrophages with foamy change, particularly around the blood vessels, nerves and dermal appendages. The foamy macrophages are called *'lepra cells' or Virchow cells.*

ii) The lepra cells are heavily laden with acid-fast bacilli demonstrated with AFB staining. The AFB may be seen as compact globular masses *(globi)* or arranged in parallel fashion like *'cigarettes-in-pack'* (COLOUR PLATE VIII: CL 31).

iii) The dermal infiltrate of lepra cells characteristically does not encroach upon the basal layer of epidermis and is separated from epidermis by a subepidermal uninvolved *clear zone.*

iv) The *epidermis* overlying the lesions is thinned out, flat and may even ulcerate (COLOUR PLATE VIII: CL 31).

2. Tuberculoid leprosy:

The polar tuberculoid form presents the following histological features (Fig. 6.25,B):

i) The dermal lesions show granulomas resembling *hard tubercles* composed of epithelioid cells, Langhans' giant cells and peripheral mantle of lymphocytes.

ii) Lesions of tuberculoid leprosy have predilection for *dermal nerves* which may be destroyed and infiltrated by epithelioid cells and lymphocytes.

iii) The granulomatous infiltrate erodes the basal layer of epidermis i.e. there is *no clear zone* (COLOUR PLATE VIII: CL 32).

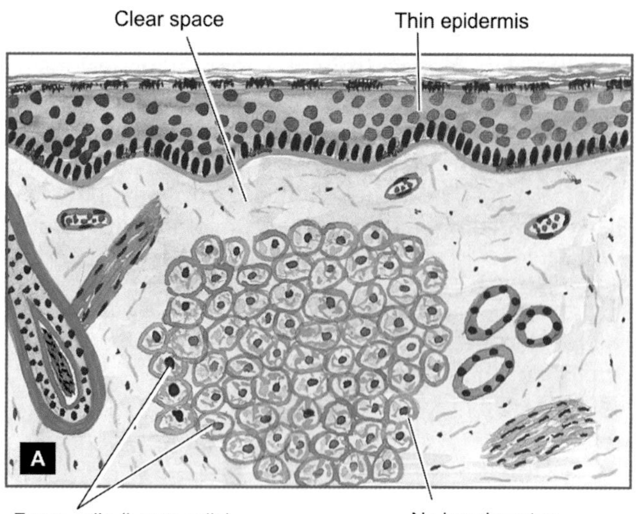

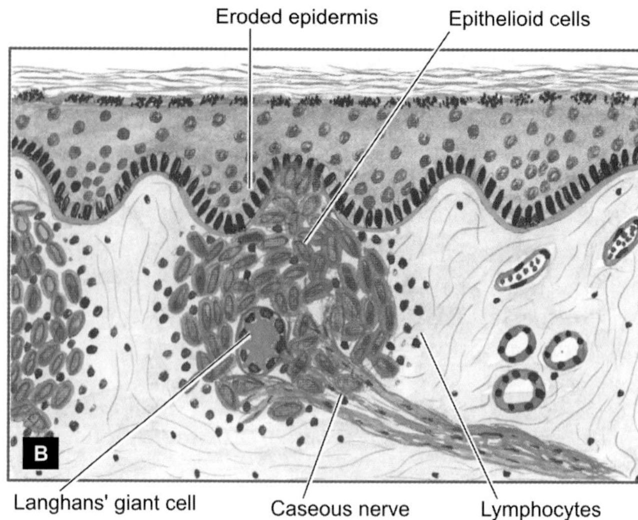

FIGURE 6.25

Polar forms of leprosy.

A, *Lepromatous leprosy (LL)*. Proliferation of lepra cells around blood vessels and dermal adnexal structures with subepidermal clear zone. These cells show 'Globi' and 'cigarettes-in-pack' appearance of bacilli in AFB staining (not shown here).

B, *Tuberculoid leprosy (TT)*. Granulomatous lesion in the vicinity of dermal nerve without clear subepidermal zone. The granuloma would show scanty and granular forms of bacilli in a destroyed nerve in AFB staining (not shown here).

iv) The *lepra bacilli* are few and seen in destroyed nerves.

3. Borderline leprosy:
The histopathologic features of the three forms of borderline leprosy are as under:

i) *Borderline tuberculoid (BT)* form shows epithelioid cells and plentiful lymphocytes. There is a narrow clear subepidermal zone. Lepra bacilli are scanty and found in nerves.

ii) *Borderline lepromatous (BL)* form shows predominance of histiocytes, a few epithelioid cells and some irregularly dispersed lymphocytes. Numerous lepra bacilli are seen.

iii) *Mid-borderline (BB)* form shows sheets of epithelioid cells with no giant cells. Some lymphocytes are seen in the peri-neurium. Lepra bacilli are present, mostly in nerves.

4. Indeterminate leprosy:
The histopathologic features are non-specific so that the diagnosis of non-specific chronic dermatitis may be made. However, a few features help in suspecting leprosy as under:

i) Lymphocytic or mononuclear cell infiltrate, focalised particularly around skin adnexal structures like hair follicles and sweat glands or around blood vessels.

ii) Nerve involvement, if present, is strongly supportive of diagnosis.

iii) Confirmation of diagnosis is made by finding of lepra bacilli.

Immunology of Leprosy

Lepromin test is not a diagnostic test but is used for classifying leprosy on the basis of immune response. Intradermal injection of lepromin, an antigenic extract of *M. leprae*, reveals delayed hypersensitivity reaction in patients of tuberculoid leprosy.

- An early positive reaction appearing as an indurated area in 24-48 hours is called *Fernandez reaction*.
- A delayed granulomatous lesion appearing after 3-4 weeks is called *Mitsuda reaction*.

Patients of lepromatous leprosy are negative by the lepromin test.

The test indicates that cell-mediated immunity is greatly suppressed in LL while patients of TT show good immune response. Delayed type of hypersensitivity is conferred by T helper cells. The granulomas of TT have sufficient T helper cells and fewer T suppressor cells at the periphery while the cellular infiltrates of LL lack T helper cells.

Though the patients of LL have humoral components like high levels of immunoglobulins (IgG, IgA, IgM) and antibodies to mycobacterial antigens but these antibodies do not have any protective role.

Anti-leprosy vaccines are now being developed and undergoing human trials but since the incubation period of leprosy is quite long, the efficacy of such vaccines will be known after a number of years.

SYPHILIS

Syphilis is a venereal (sexually-transmitted) disease caused by spirochaetes, *Treponema pallidum*. Other treponemal diseases are yaws, pinta and bejel. The word 'syphilis' is derived from the name of the mythological handsome boy, Syphilus, who was cursed by Apollo with the disease.

Causative Organism

T. pallidum is a coiled spiral filament 10 μm long that moves actively in fresh preparations. The organism cannot be stained by the usual methods and can be demonstrated in the exudates and tissues by:

1. *dark ground illumination (DGI)* in fresh preparation;
2. *fluorescent antibody technique*; and
3. *silver impregnation techniques.*

The organism has not been cultivated in any culture media but experimental infection can be produced in rabbits and chimpanzees. The organism is rapidly destroyed by cold, heat, and antiseptics.

Immunology

T. pallidum does not produce any endotoxin or exotoxin. The pathogenesis of the lesions appears to be due to host immune response.

Treponemal infection is associated with two important antibodies which are immunoglobulins. These are as under:

1. The Wassermann antibodies. Wassermann described a complement fixing antibody against antigen of human syphilitic tissue. This antigen is used in the Standard Test for Syphilis (STS) as follows:

i) Wassermann complement fixing test; and
ii) Venereal Disease Research Laboratory (VDRL) test.

2. Treponemal antibodies. Treponemal antibodies are produced which react with treponemal protein. The tests employed for detecting these antibodies are:

i) Reiter protein complement fixation (RPCF) test;
ii) Treponema pallidum immobilisation (TPI) test;
iii) Fluorescent treponemal antibody (FTA) test; and
iv) Treponemal passive haemagglutination (TPHA) test.

Mode of Transmission

Syphilitic infection can be transmitted by the following routes:

1. *Sexual intercourse* resulting in lesions on glans penis, vulva, vagina and cervix.
2. *Intimate person-to-person contact* with lesions on lips, tongue or fingers.
3. *Transfusion* of infected blood.
4. *Materno-foetal transmission* in congenital syphilis if the mother is infected.

Stages of Acquired Syphilis

Acquired syphilis is divided into 3 stages depending upon the period after which the lesions appear and the type of lesions. These are: primary, secondary and tertiary syphilis.

1. PRIMARY SYPHILIS. Typical lesion of primary syphilis is *chancre* which appears on genitals or at extra-genital sites in 2-4 *weeks* after exposure to infection (Fig. 6.26,A). Initially, the lesion is a painless papule which ulcerates in the centre so that the fully-deve-loped chancre is an indurated lesion with central ulceration accompanied by regional lymphadenitis. The chancre heals without scarring, even in the absence of treatment.

Histologically, the chancre is characterised by:

i) Dense infiltrate of lymphocytes, plasma cells and a few macrophages.
ii) Perivascular aggregation of mononuclear cells, particularly plasma cells (periarteritis and endarteritis).

Antibody tests are positive in 1-3 weeks after the appearance of chancre. Spirochaetes can be demonstrated in the exudates by DGI.

2. SECONDARY SYPHILIS. Inadequately treated patients of primary syphilis develop *mucocutaneous lesions* and painless lymphadenopathy in *2-3 months* after the exposure (Fig. 6.26,B). Mucocutaneous lesions may be in the form of the mucous patches on mouth, pharynx and vagina; and generalised skin eruptions and condyloma lata in anogenital region.

Antibody tests are always positive at this stage. Secondary syphilis is *highly infective stage* and spirochaetes can be easily demonstrated in the mucocutaneous lesions.

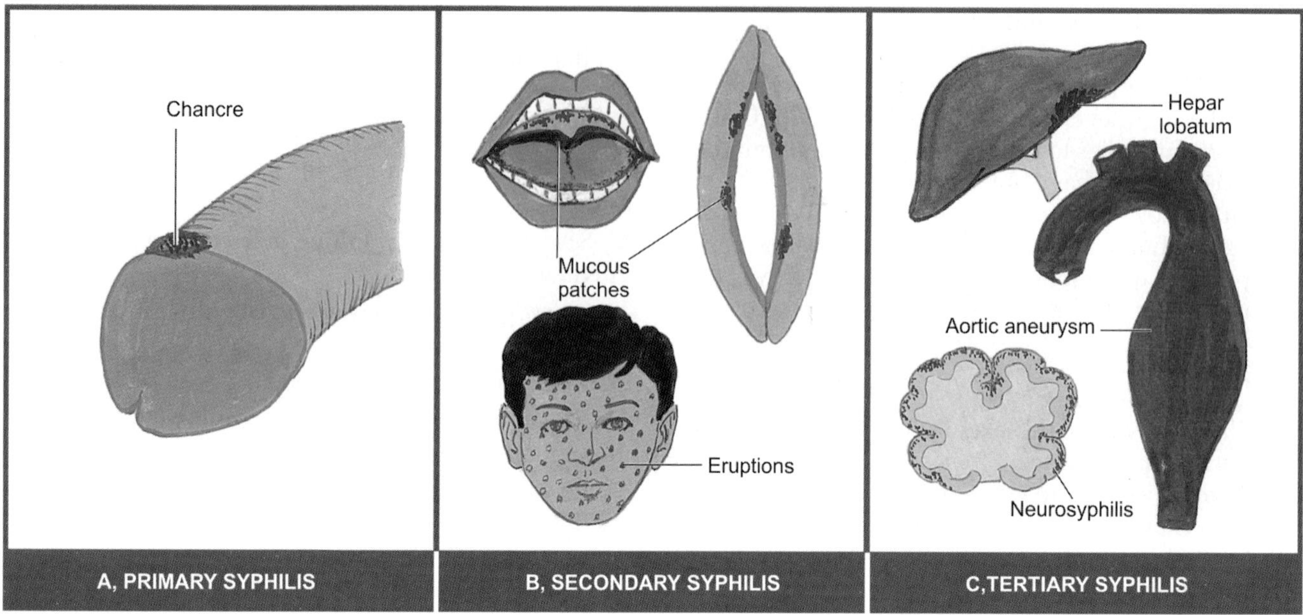

FIGURE 6.26

Organ involvement in various stages of acquired syphilis.

A, *Primary syphilis*: Primary lesion is 'chancre' on glans penis. B, *Secondary syphilis:* Mucocutaneous lesions—mucous patches on oral and vaginal mucosa and generalised skin eruptions. C, *Tertiary syphilis:* Localised lesion as gumma of liver with scarring (hepar lobatum); diffuse lesions (right) in aorta (aneurysm, narrowing of mouths of coronary ostia and incompetence of aortic valve ring) and nervous system.

3. TERTIARY SYPHILIS. After a latent period of appearance of secondary lesions and about *2-3 years* following first exposure, tertiary lesions of syphilis appear. Lesions of tertiary syphilis are much less infective than the other two stages and spirochaetes can be demonstrated with great difficulty. These lesions are of 2 main types (Fig. 6.26,C):

i) Syphilitic gumma. It is a solitary, localised, rubbery lesion with central necrosis, seen in organs like liver, testis, bone and brain. In liver, the gumma is associated with scarring of hepatic parenchyma *(hepar lobatum).*

Histologically, the structure of gumma shows (Fig. 6.27):

a) central coagulative necrosis resembling caseation but is less destructive so that outlines of necrosed cells can still be faintly seen; and

b) surrounding zone of palisaded macrophages with lymphocytes, plasma cells, giant cells and fibroblasts.

ii) Diffuse lesions of tertiary syphilis. The lesions appear following widespread dissemination of spirochaetes in the body. The diffuse lesions are predominantly seen in cardiovascular and nervous systems which are described in detail later in the relevant chapters. Briefly, these lesions are as under:

a) *Cardiovascular syphilis* mainly involves thoracic aorta. The wall of aorta is weakened and dilated due to syphilitic aortitis and results in aortic aneurysm, incompetence of aortic valve and narrowing of mouths of coronary ostia (Chapter 12).

b) *Neurosyphilis* may manifest as:

- meningovascular syphilis affecting chiefly the meninges;
- tabes dorsalis affecting the spinal cord; and
- general paresis affecting the brain.

CONGENITAL SYPHILIS. Congenital syphilis may develop in a foetus of more than 16 weeks gestation who is exposed to maternal spirochaetaemia. There can be 3 possibilities:

1. The child born dead. The child is premature, with macerated skin, enlarged spleen and liver, and with syphilitic epiphysitis.

2. The child born alive (Infantile form). The child may show mucocutaneous lesions of acquired secondary syphilis and bony lesions like epiphysitis and

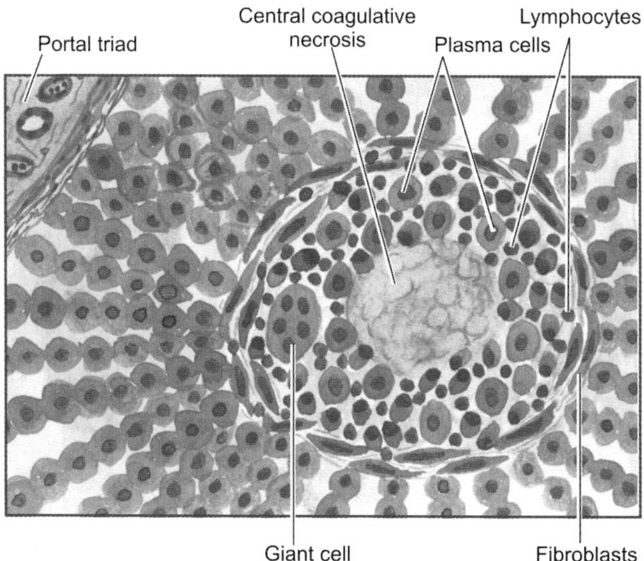

FIGURE 6.27

Typical microscopic appearance in the case of syphilitic gumma of the liver. Central coagulative necrosis is surrounded by palisades of macrophages and plasma cells marginated peripherally by fibroblasts.

periostitis. The bridge of nose may fall due to ulceration and destruction giving the characteristic 'saddle nose' appearance of congenital syphilis.

3. **The late type.** The lesions appear after some years. The characteristic 'Hutchinson's teeth' seen in this type are small, widely spaced, peg-shaped permanent teeth. Tertiary lesions like gummas and neurosyphilis may also be seen.

Histologically, mononuclear cell infiltration is seen in most internal organs in congenital syphilis. Many spirochaetes can be demonstrated in involved tissues.

ACTINOMYCOSIS

Actinomycosis is a chronic suppurative disease caused by anaerobic bacteria, *Actinomycetes israelii.* The disease is conventionally included in mycology though the causative organism is filamentous bacteria and not true fungus. The disease is worldwide in distribution. The organisms are commensals in the oral cavity, alimentary tract and vagina. The infection is always endogeneous in origin and not person-to-person. The organisms invade, proliferate and disseminate in favourable conditions like break in mucocutaneous continuity, some underlying disease etc.

PATHOLOGIC CHANGES. Depending upon the anatomic location of lesions, actinomycosis is of 4 types: cervicofacial, thoracic, abdominal, and pelvic (Fig. 6.28,A).

1. **Cervicofacial actinomycosis.** This is the commonest form (60%) and has the best prognosis. The infection enters from tonsils, carious teeth, periodontal disease or trauma following tooth extraction. Initially, a firm swelling develops in the lower jaw ('lumpy jaw'). In time, the mass breaks down and abscesses and sinuses are formed. The discharging pus contains typical tiny yellow sulphur granules. The infection may extend into adjoining soft tissues as well as may destroy the bone.

2. **Thoracic actinomycosis.** The infection in the lungs is due to aspiration of the organism from oral cavity or extension of infection from abdominal or hepatic lesions. Initially, the disease resembles pneumonia but subsequently the infection spreads to the whole of lung, pleura, ribs and vertebrae.

3. **Abdominal actinomycosis.** This type is common in appendix, caecum and liver. The abdominal infection results from swallowing of organisms from oral cavity or extension from thoracic cavity.

4. **Pelvic actinomycosis.** Infection in the pelvis occurs as a complication of intrauterine contraceptive devices (IUCD's).

Microscopically, irrespective of the location of actinomycosis, the following features are seen (Fig. 6.28,B) **(COLOUR PLATE IX: CL 35):**

i) The inflammatory reaction is a granuloma with central suppuration. There is formation of abscesses in the centre of lesions and at the periphery are seen chronic inflammatory cells, giant cells and fibroblasts.

ii) The centre of each abscess contains the bacterial colony, 'sulphur granule', characterised by radiating filaments (hence previously known as *ray fungus*) with hyaline, eosinophilic, club-like ends representative of secreted immunoglobulins.

iii) Bacterial stains reveal the organisms as gram-positive filaments, nonacid-fast, which stain positively with Gomori's methenamine silver (GMS) staining.

SARCOIDOSIS (BOECK'S SARCOID)

Sarcoidosis is a systemic disease of unknown etiology. It is worldwide in distribution and affects adults from 20-40 years of age. The disease is characterised by the presence of non-caseating epithelioid cell granulomas ('sarcoid granuloma') in the affected tissues and organs, notably lymph nodes and lungs. Other sites are the skin, spleen, uvea of the eyes, salivary glands, liver and

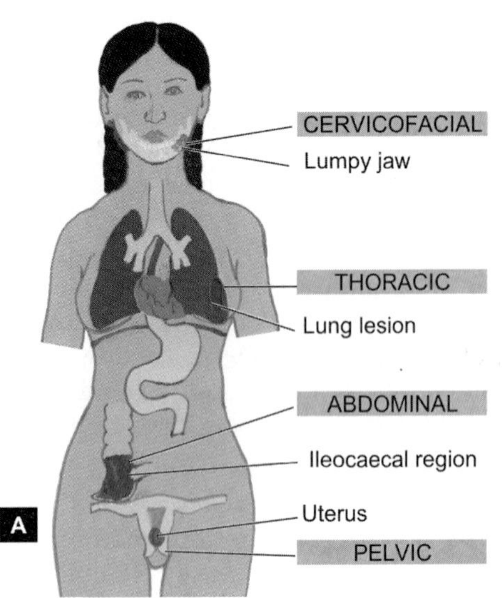

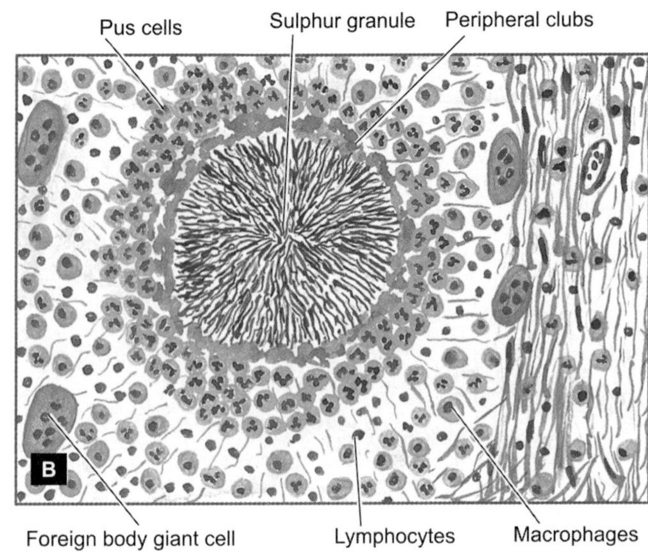

FIGURE 6.28

Morphology of actinomycosis. A, Sites and routes of infection. B, Microscopic appearance of abscess and sulphur granule.

bones of hands and feet. The histologic diagnosis is generally made by exclusion.

ETIOLOGY AND PATHOGENESIS. The cause of sarcoidosis remains unknown. Since the disease is characterised by granulomatous tissue reaction, possibility of cell-mediated immune mechanisms has been suggested. The following observations point towards a possible immune origin of sarcoidosis:

1. Just as in tuberculosis, sarcoidosis is characterised by distinctive granulomatous response against *poorly degradable antigen*, but quite unlike tuberculosis, the antigen in sarcoidosis has eluded workers so far. PCR studies on affected pulmonary tissue have given equivocal result as regards presence of mycobacterial antigen.
2. That there are immunologic abnormalities in sarcoidosis is substantiated by *high levels of CD4+T cells* lavaged from lung lesions.There is also elevation in levels of IL-2 receptors in serum and in lavaged fluid from lungs.
3. There is presence of *activated alveolar macrophages* which elaborate cytokines that initiate the formation of non-caseating granulomas.

PATHOLOGIC CHANGES. The lesions in sarcoidosis are generalised and may affect various organs and tissues at sometime in the course of disease, but brunt of the disease is borne by the lungs and lymph nodes (Fig. 6.29,A):

Microscopically, the following features are present (Fig. 6.29,B) **(COLOUR PLATE VIII: CL 30):**

1. The diagnostic feature in sarcoidosis of any organ or tissue is the *non-caseating sarcoid granuloma,* composed of epithelioid cells, Langhans' and foreign body giant cells and surrounded peripherally by fibroblasts.
2. Typically, granulomas of sarcoidosis are *'naked'* i.e. either devoid of peripheral rim of lymphocytes or there is paucity of lymphocytes.
3. In late stage, the granuloma is either *enclosed by hyalinised fibrous tissue* or is replaced by hyalinised fibrous mass.
4. The giant cells in sarcoid granulomas contain certain *cytoplasmic inclusions* like:
   - i) *Asteroid bodies* which are eosinophilic and stellate-shaped structures.
   - ii) *Schaumann's bodies or conchoid (conch like) bodies* which are concentric laminations of calcium and of iron salts, complexed with proteins.
   - iii) *Birefringent cytoplasmic crystals* which are colourless.

Similar types of inclusions are also observed in chronic berylliosis (Chapter 15).

KVIEM'S TEST. It is a useful intradermal diagnostic test. The antigen prepared from involved lymph node or spleen is injected intradermally. In a positive test, nodular lesion appears in 3-6 weeks at the inoculation

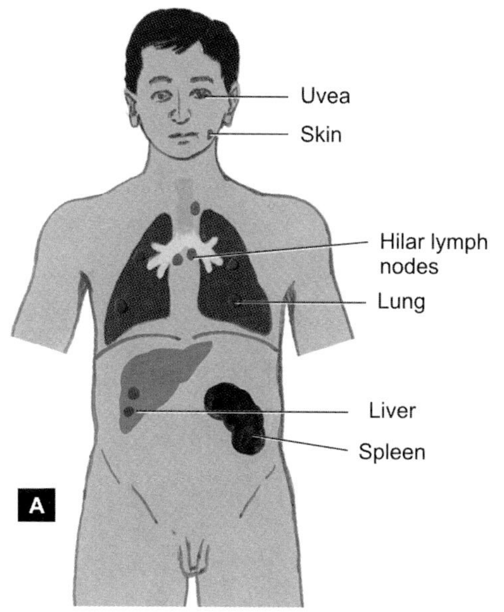

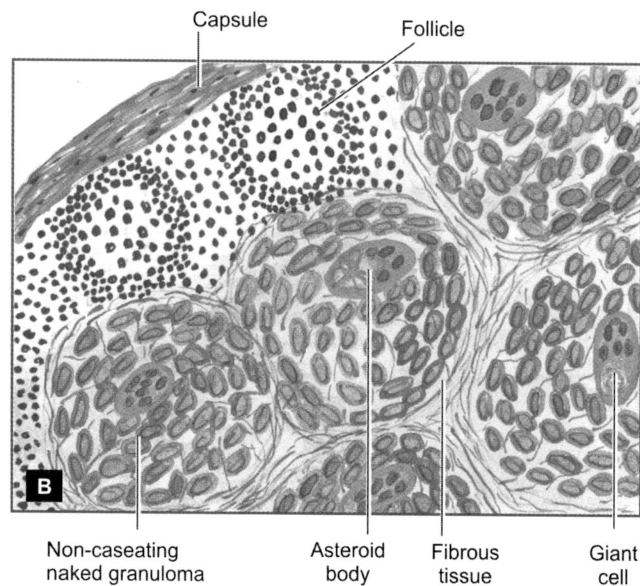

FIGURE 6.29

Morphology of sarcoidosis. A, The lesions are predominantly seen in lymph nodes and throughout lung parenchyma. B, Microscopic appearance of characteristic non-caseating sarcoid granulomas in lymph node.

site which on microscopic examination shows presence of non-caseating granulomas.

HEALING

Injury to tissue may result in cell death and tissue destruction. *Healing* on the other hand is the body response to injury in an attempt to restore normal structure and function. The process of healing involves 2 distinct processes:

- *Regeneration* when healing takes place by proliferation of parenchymal cells and usually results in complete restoration of the original tissues.
- *Repair* when the healing takes place by proliferation of connective tissue elements resulting in fibrosis and scarring.

At times, both the processes take place simultaneously.

REGENERATION

Some parenchymal cells are short-lived while others have a longer lifespan. In order to maintain proper structure of tissues, these cells are under the constant regulatory control of their cell cycle. These include growth factors such as: epidermal growth factor, fibroblast growth factor, platelet-derived growth factor, endothelial growth factor, transforming growth factor-β. *Cell cycle* (page 32) is defined as the period between two successive cell divisions and is divided into 4 unequal phases (Fig. 6.30):

- *M (mitosis) phase:* Phase of mitosis.
- *G_1 (gap 1) phase:* The daughter cell enters G_1 phase after mitosis.
- *S (synthesis) phase:* During this phase, the synthesis of nuclear DNA takes place.
- *G_2 (gap 2) phase:* After completion of nuclear DNA duplication, the cell enters G_2 phase.
- *G_0 (gap 0) phase:* This is the quiescent or resting phase of the cell after an M phase.

Not all cells of the body divide at the same pace. Some mature cells do not divide at all while others complete a cell cycle every 16-24 hours. The main difference between slowly-dividing and rapidly-dividing cells is the duration of G_1 phase.

Depending upon their capacity to divide, the cells of the body can be divided into 3 groups: labile cells, stable cells, and permanent cells.

1. **Labile cells.** These cells continue to multiply throughout life under normal physiologic conditions. These include: surface epithelial cells of epidermis, alimentary tract, respiratory tract, urinary tract, vagina, cervix, uterine endometrium, haematopoietic cells of bone marrow and cells of lymph nodes and spleen.
2. **Stable cells.** These cells decrease or lose their ability to proliferate after adolescence but retain the capacity

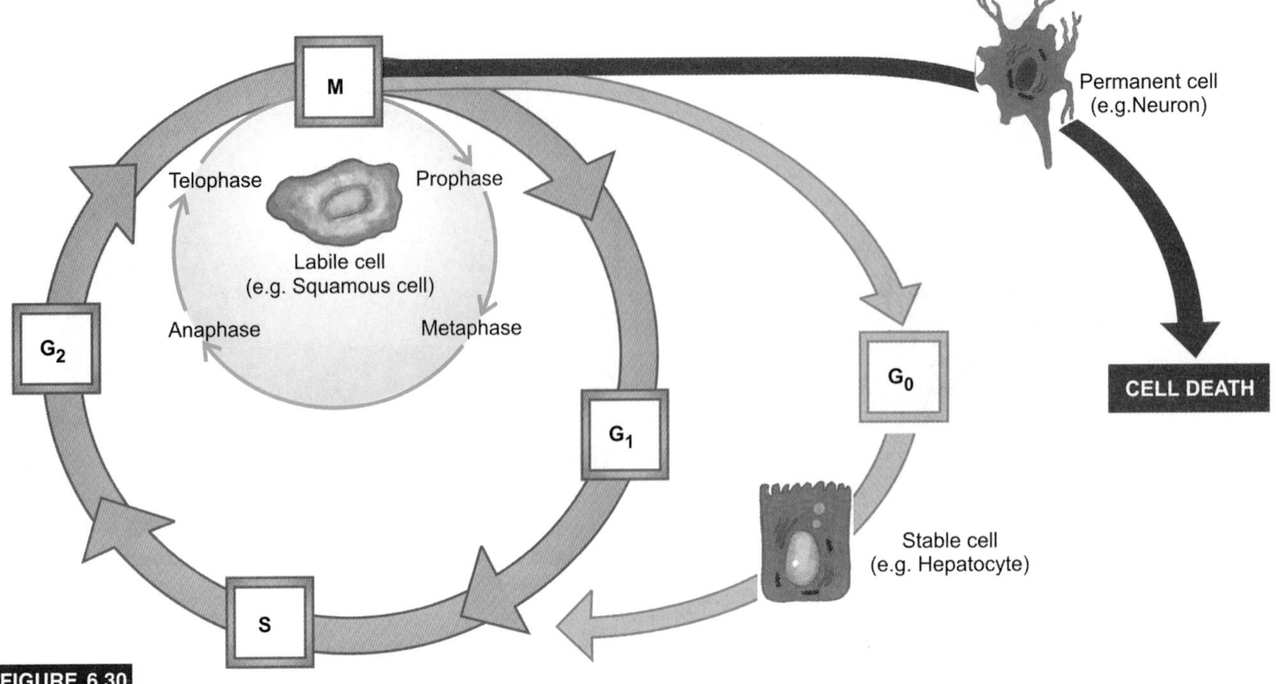

FIGURE 6.30

Parenchymal cells in relation to cell cycle (G_0–Resting phase; G_1, G_2–Gaps; S–Synthesis phase; M–Mitosis phase). The inner circle *shown with green line* represents cell cycle for labile cells; circle *shown with yellow-orange line* represents cell cycle for stable cells; and the circle *shown with red line* represents cell cycle for permanent cells. Compare them with traffic signals—green stands for *'go'* applies here to dividing labile cells; yellow-orange signal for *'ready to go'* applies here to stable cells which can be stimulated to enter cell cycle; and red signal for *'stop'* here means non-dividing permanent cells.

to multiply in response to stimuli throughout adult life. These include: parenchymal cells of organs like liver, pancreas, kidneys, adrenal and thyroid; mesenchymal cells like smooth muscle cells, fibroblasts, vascular endothelium, bone and cartilage cells.

3. **Permanent cells.** These cells lose their ability to proliferate around the time of birth. These include: neurons of nervous system, skeletal muscle and cardiac muscle cells.

RELATIONSHIP OF PARENCHYMAL CELLS WITH CELL CYCLE. If the three types of parenchymal cells described above are correlated with the phase of cell cycle (Fig. 6.30), the following inferences can be derived:

1. Labile cells which are continuously dividing cells remain in the cell cycle from one mitosis to the next.

2. Stable cells are in the resting phase (G_0) but can be stimulated to enter the cell cycle.

3. Permanent cells are non-dividing cells which have left the cell cycle and die after injury.

Regeneration of any type of parenchymal cells involves the following 2 processes:

i) Proliferation of original cells from the margin of injury with migration so as to cover the gap.

ii) Proliferation of migrated cells with subsequent differentiation and maturation so as to reconstitute the original tissue.

REPAIR

Repair is the replacement of injured tissue by fibrous tissue. Two processes are involved in repair:

1. Granulation tissue formation; and
2. Contraction of wounds.

Repair response takes place by participation of mesenchymal cells (consisting of connective tissue stem cells, fibrocytes and histiocytes), endothelial cells, macrophages, platelets, and the parenchymal cells of the injured organ.

Granulation Tissue Formation

The term granulation tissue derives its name from slightly granular and pink appearance of the tissue. Each granule corresponds histologically to proliferation of new small blood vessels which are slightly lifted on the surface by thin covering of fibroblasts and young collagen.

The following 3 phases are observed in the formation of granulation tissue (Fig. 6.31):

1. PHASE OF INFLAMMATION. Following trauma, blood clots at the site of injury. There is acute inflammatory response with exudation of plasma, neutrophils and some monocytes within 24 hours.

2. PHASE OF CLEARANCE. Combination of proteolytic enzymes liberated from neutrophils, autolytic enzymes from dead tissues cells, and phagocytic activity of macrophages clear off the necrotic tissue, debris and red blood cells.

3. PHASE OF INGROWTH OF GRANULATION TISSUE. This phase consists of 2 main processes: angiogenesis or neovascularisation, and fibrogenesis (COLOUR PLATE VII: CL 26).

i) Angiogenesis (neovascularisation). Formation of new blood vessels at the site of injury takes place by proliferation of endothelial cells from the margins of severed blood vessels. Initially, the proliferated endothelial cells are solid buds but within a few hours develop a lumen and start carrying blood. The newly formed blood vessels are more leaky, accounting for the oedematous appearance of new granulation tissue. Soon, these blood vessels differentiate into muscular arterioles, thin-walled venules and true capillaries.

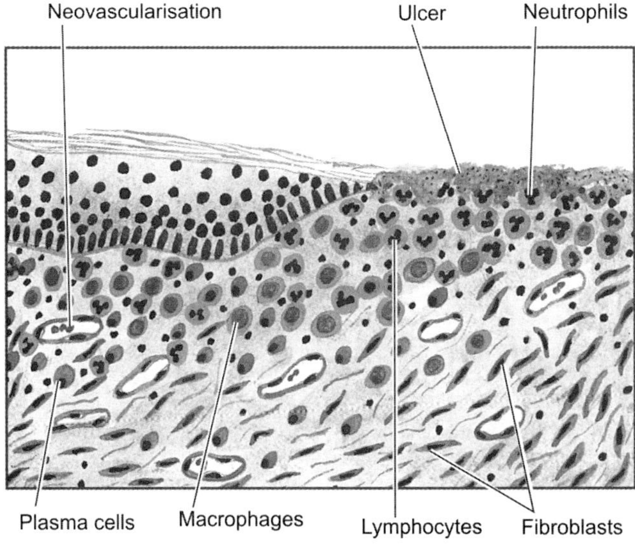

FIGURE 6.31

Active granulation tissue has inflammatory cell infiltrate, newly formed blood vessels and young fibrous tissue in loose matrix.

The process of angiogenesis is stimulated with proteolytic destruction of basement membrane and takes place under the influence of the following factors:

a) Angiogenesis takes place under the influence of vascular endothelial growth factor (VEGF) elaborated by mesenchymal cells but its receptors are present in endothelial cells only.

b) Platelet-derived growth factor (PDGF), transforming growth factor-β (TGF-β), basic fibroblast growth factor (bFGF), other cytokines and surface integrins are the factors which are associated with cellular proliferation.

ii) Fibrogenesis. The newly formed blood vessels are present in an amorphous ground substance or matrix. The new fibroblasts originate from fibrocytes as well as by mitotic division of fibroblasts. Some of these fibroblasts have combination of morphologic and functional characteristics of smooth muscle cells (*myofibroblasts*). Collagen fibrils begin to appear by about 6th day. As maturation proceeds, more and more of collagen is formed while the number of active fibroblasts and new blood vessels decreases. This results in formation of inactive looking scar known as *cicatrisation*.

Contraction of Wounds

The wound starts contracting after 2-3 days and the process is completed by the 14th day. During this period, the wound is reduced by approximately 80% of its original size. Contracted wound results in rapid healing since lesser surface area of the injured tissue has to be replaced.

In order to explain the mechanism of wound contraction, a number of factors have been proposed. These are as under:

1. *Dehydration* as a result of removal of fluid by drying of wound was first suggested but without being substantiated.

2. *Contraction of collagen* was thought to be responsible for contraction but wound contraction proceeds at a stage when the collagen content of granulation tissue is very small.

3. Discovery of *myofibroblasts* appearing in active granulation tissue has resolved the controversy surrounding the mechanism of wound contraction. These cells have features intermediate between those of fibroblasts and smooth muscle cells. Their migration into the wound area and their active contraction decreases the size of the defect. The evidences in support of this concept are both morphological as well as functional characteristics of modified fibroblasts or myofibroblasts as under:

i) Fibrils present in the cytoplasm of these cells resemble those seen in smooth muscle cells.

ii) These cells contain actin-myosin similar to that found in non-striated muscle cells.

iii) The nuclei of these cells have infoldings of nuclear membrane like in smooth muscle cells.

iv) These cells have basement membrane and desmosomes which are not seen in ordinary fibroblasts.

v) The cytoplasm of these modified cells demonstrates immunofluorescent labelling with anti-smooth muscle antibodies.

vi) The drug response of granulation tissue is similar to that of smooth muscle.

WOUND HEALING

Healing of skin wounds provides a classical example of combination of regeneration and repair described above. This can be accomplished in one of the following two ways:

- Healing by first intention *(primary union)*; and
- healing by second intention *(secondary union)*.

Healing by First Intention (Primary Union)

This is defined as healing of a wound which has the following characteristics:

i) clean and uninfected;
ii) surgically incised;
iii) without much loss of cells and tissue; and
iv) edges of wound are approximated by surgical sutures.

The sequence of events in primary union is illustrated in Fig. 6.32 and described below:

1. Initial haemorrhage. Immediately after injury, the space between the approximated surfaces of incised wound is filled with blood which then clots and seals the wound against dehydration and infection.

2. Acute inflammatory response. This occurs within 24 hours with appearance of polymorphs from the margins of incision. By 3rd day, polymorphs are replaced by macrophages.

3. Epithelial changes. The basal cells of epidermis from both the cut margins start proliferating and migrating towards incisional space in the form of epithelial spurs. A well-approximated wound is covered by a layer of epithelium in 48 hours. The migrated epidermal cells separate the underlying viable dermis from the overlying necrotic material and clot, forming *scab* which is cast off. The basal cells from the margins continue to divide. By 5th day, a multilayered new epidermis is formed which is differentiated into superficial and deeper layers.

4. Organisation. By 3rd day, fibroblasts also invade the wound area. By 5th day, new collagen fibrils start forming which dominate till healing is completed. In 4 weeks, the scar tissue with scanty cellular and vascular

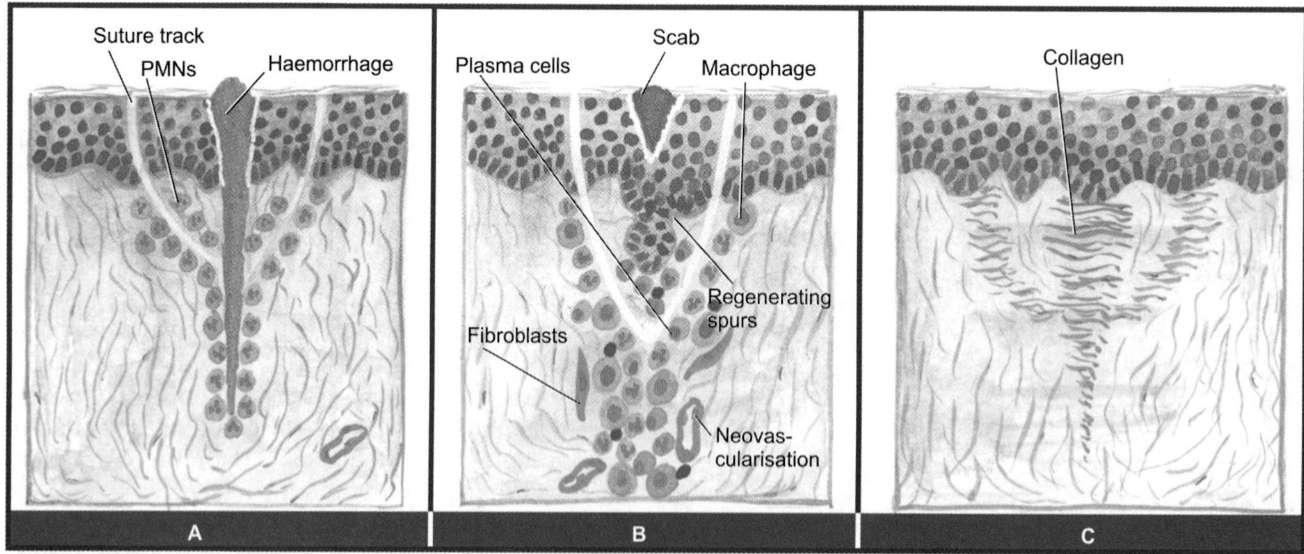

FIGURE 6.32

Primary union of skin wounds. A, The incised wound as well as suture track on either side are filled with blood clot and there is inflammatory response from the margins. B, Spurs of epidermal cells migrate along the incised margin on either side as well as around the suture track. Formation of granulation tissue also begins from below. C, Removal of suture at around 7th day results in scar tissue at the sites of incision and suture track.

elements, a few inflammatory cells and epithelialised surface is formed.

5. Suture tracks. Each suture track is a separate wound and incites the same phenomena as in healing of the primary wound i.e. filling the space with haemorrhage, some inflammatory cell reaction, epithelial cell proliferation along the suture track from both margins, fibroblastic proliferation and formation of young collagen. When sutures are removed around 7th day, much of epithelialised suture track is avulsed and the remaining epithelial tissue in the track is absorbed. However, sometimes the suture track gets infected *(stitch abscess)*, or the epithelial cells may persist in the track *(implantation or epidermal cysts)*.

Thus, the scar formed in a sutured wound is neat due to close apposition of the margins of wound; the use of adhesive tapes avoids removal of stitches and its complications.

Healing by Second Intention (Secondary Union)

This is defined as healing of a wound having the following characteristics:

i) open with a large tissue defect, at times infected;
ii) having extensive loss of cells and tissues; and
iii) the wound is not approximated by surgical sutures but is left open.

The basic events in secondary union are similar to primary union but differ in having a larger tissue defect which has to be bridged. Hence healing takes place from the base upwards as well as from the margins inwards. The healing by second intention is slow and results in a large, at times ugly, scar as compared to rapid healing and neat scar of primary union.

The sequence of events in secondary union is illustrated in Fig. 6.33 and described below:

1. Initial haemorrhage. As a result of injury, the wound space is filled with blood and fibrin clot which dries.

2. Inflammatory phase. There is an initial acute inflammatory response followed by appearance of macrophages which clear off the debris as in primary union.

3. Epithelial changes. As in primary healing, the epidermal cells from both the margins of wound proliferate and migrate into the wound in the form of epithelial spurs till they meet in the middle and re-epithelialise the gap completely. However, the proliferating epithelial cells do not cover the surface fully until granulation tissue from base has started filling the wound space. In this way, pre-existing viable connective tissue is separated from necrotic material and clot on the surface, forming *scab* which is cast off. In time, the regenerated epidermis becomes stratified and keratinised.

4. Granulation tissue. The main bulk of secondary healing is by granulations. Granulation tissue is formed by proliferation of fibroblasts and neovascularisation from the adjoining viable elements. The newly-formed granulation tissue is deep red, granular and very fragile. With time, the scar on maturation becomes pale and

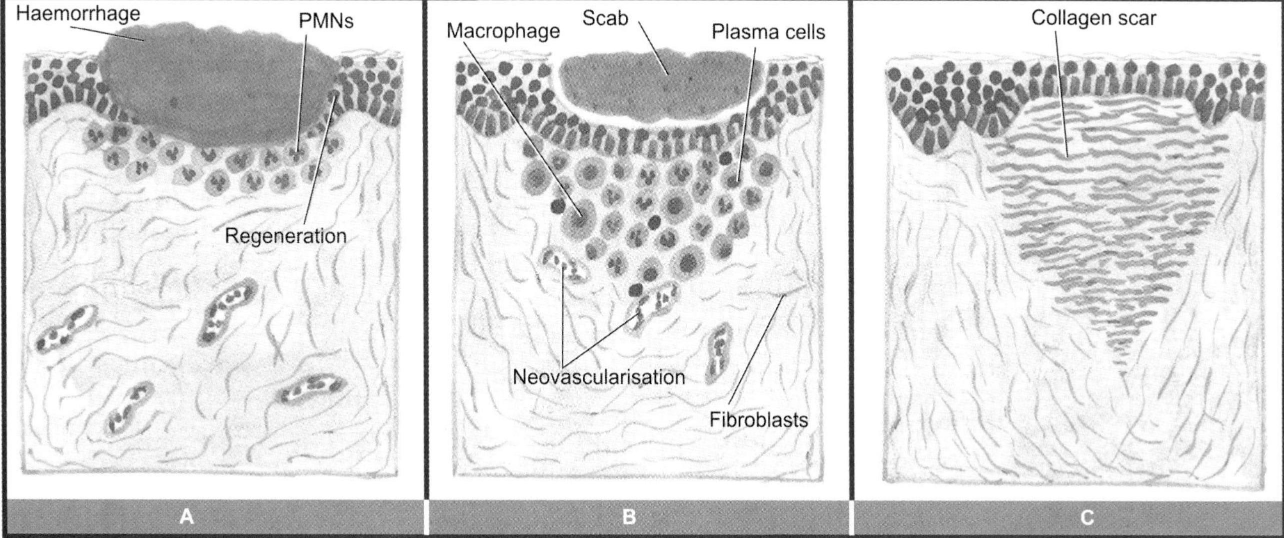

FIGURE 6.33

Secondary union of skin wounds. A, The open wound is filled with blood clot and there is inflammatory response at the junction of viable tissue. B, Epithelial spurs from the margins of wound meet in the middle to cover the gap and separate the underlying viable tissue from necrotic tissue at the surface forming scab. C, After contraction of the wound, a scar smaller than the original wound is left.

white due to increase in collagen and decrease in vascularity. The specialised structures of skin like hair follicles and sweat glands are not replaced unless their viable residues remain which may regenerate.

5. Wound contraction. Contraction of wound is an important feature of secondary healing, not seen in primary healing. Due to the action of myofibroblasts present in granulation tissue, the wound contracts to one-third to one-fourth of its original size. Wound contraction occurs at a time when active granulation tissue is being formed.

6. Presence of infection. Bacterial contamination of an open wound delays the process of healing due to release of bacterial toxins that provoke necrosis, suppuration and thrombosis. Surgical removal of dead and necrosed tissue, *debridement,* helps in preventing the bacterial infection of open wounds.

Complications of Wound Healing

During the course of healing, following complications may occur:

1. *Infection* of wound due to entry of bacteria delays the healing.
2. *Implantation (epidermal) cyst* formation may occur due to persistence of epithelial cells in the wound after healing.
3. *Pigmentation.* Healed wounds may at times have rust-like colour due to staining with haemosiderin. Some coloured particulate material left in the wound may persist and impart colour to the healed wound.
4. *Deficient scar formation.* This may occur due to inadequate formation of granulation tissue.
5. *Incisional hernia.* A weak scar, especially after a laparotomy, may be the site of bursting open of a wound (wound dehiscence) or an incisional hernia.
6. *Hypertrophied scars and keloid formation.* At times the scar formed is excessive, ugly and painful. Excessive formation of collagen in healing may result in keloid *(claw-like)* formation, seen more commonly in Blacks. Hypertrophied scars differ from keloid in that they are confined to the borders of the initial wound while keloids have tumour-like projection of connective tissue.
7. *Excessive contraction.* An exaggeration of wound contraction may result in formation of contractures or cicatrisation e.g. Dupuytren's (palmar) contracture, plantar contracture and Peyronie's disease (contraction of the cavernous tissues of penis)
8. *Neoplasia.* Rarely, scar may be the site for development of carcinoma later e.g. squamous cell carcinoma in Marjolin's ulcer i.e. a scar following burns on the skin.

Extracellular Matrix--Wound Strength

The wound is strengthened by proliferation of fibroblasts and myofibroblasts which get structural support from the extracellular matrix (ECM). In addition to providing structural support, ECM can direct cell migration, attachment, differentiation and organisation.

ECM has five main components: collagen, adhesive glycoproteins, basement membrane, elastic fibres, and proteoglycans.

1. COLLAGEN. The collagens are a family of proteins which provide structural support to the multicellular organism. It is the main component of tissues such as fibrous tissue, bone, cartilage, valves of heart, cornea, basement membrane etc.

Collagen is synthesised and secreted by a complex biochemical mechanism on ribosomes. The collagen synthesis is stimulated by various growth factors and is degraded by collagenase. Regulation of collagen synthesis and degradation take place by various local and systemic factors so that the collagen content of normal organs remains constant. On the other hand, defective regulation of collagen synthesis leads to hypertrophied scar, fibrosis, and organ dysfunction.

Depending upon the biochemical composition, 18 types of collagen have been identified called collagen *type I to XVIII*, many of which are unique for specific tissues. Type I, III and V are *true fibrillar collagen* which form the main portion of the connective tissue during healing of wounds in scars. Other types of collagen are *non-fibrillar* and amorphous material seen as component of the basement membranes.

Morphologically, the smallest units of collagen are *collagen fibrils*, which align together in parallel bundles to form *collagen fibres*, and then *collagen bundles.*

2. ADHESIVE GLYCOPROTEINS. Various adhesive glycoproteins acting as glue for the ECM and the cells consist of fibronectin, tenascin (cytotactin) and thrombospondin.

i) Fibronectin (*nectere* = to bind) is the best characterised glycoprotein in ECM and has binding properties to other cells and ECM. It is of two types—plasma and tissue fibronectin.

- *Plasma fibronectin* is synthesised by the liver cells and is trapped in basement membrane such as in filtration through the renal glomerulus.
- *Tissue fibronectin* is formed by fibroblasts, endothelial cells and other mesenchymal cells. It is responsible for the primitive matrix such as in the foetus, and in wound healing.

ii) Tenascin or cytotactin is the glycoprotein associated with fibroblasts and appears in wound about 48 hours after injury. It disappears from mature scar tissue.

iii) Thrombospondin is mainly synthesised by granules of platelets. It functions as adhesive protein for keratinocytes and platelets but is inhibitory to attachment of fibroblasts and endothelial cells.

3. BASEMENT MEMBRANE. Basement membranes are periodic acid-Schiff (PAS)-positive amorphous structures that lie underneath epithelia of different organs and endothelial cells. They consist of collagen type IV and laminin.

4. ELASTIC FIBRES. While the tensile strength in tissue comes from collagen, the ability to recoil is provided by elastic fibres. Elastic fibres consist of 2 components—elastin glycoprotein and elastic microfibril. Elastases degrade the elastic tissue e.g. in inflammation, emphysema etc.

5. PROTEOGLYCANS. These are a group of molecules having 2 components—an essential carbohydrate polymer (called polysaccharide or glycosaminoglycan), and a protein bound to it, and hence the name proteoglycan. Various proteoglycans are distributed in different tissues as under:

i) *Chondroitin sulphate*—abundant in cartilage, dermis
ii) *Heparan sulphate*—in basement membranes
iii) *Dermatan sulphate*—in dermis
iv) *Keratan sulphate*—in cartilage
v) *Hyaluronic acid*—in cartilage, dermis.

In wound healing, the deposition of proteoglycans precedes collagen laying.

The strength of wound also depends upon factors like the site of injury, depth of incision and area of wound. After removal of stitches on around 7th day, the wound strength is approximately 10% which reaches 80% in about 3 months.

Factors Influencing Healing

Two types of factors influence the wound healing: those acting locally, and those acting in general.

A. LOCAL FACTORS. These include the following factors:

1. *Infection* is the most important factor acting locally which delays the process of healing.
2. *Poor blood supply* to wound slows healing e.g. injuries to face heal quickly due to rich blood supply while injury to leg with varicose ulcers having poor blood supply heals slowly.
3. *Foreign bodies* including sutures interfere with healing and cause intense inflammatory reaction and infection.
4. *Movement* delays wound healing.
5. Exposure to *ionising radiation* delays granulation tissue formation.
6. Exposure to *ultraviolet light* facilitates healing.
7. *Type, size and location* of injury determines whether healing takes place by resolution or organisation.

B. SYSTEMIC FACTORS. These are as under:

1. *Age.* Wound healing is rapid in young and somewhat slow in aged and debilitated people due to poor blood supply to the injured area in the latter.
2. *Nutrition.* Deficiency of constituents like protein, vitamin C (scurvy) and zinc delays the wound healing.
3. *Systemic infection* delays wound healing.
4. *Administration of glucocorticoids* has anti-inflammatory effect.
5. *Uncontrolled diabetics* are more prone to develop infections and hence delay in healing.
6. *Haematologic abnormalities* like defect of neutrophil functions (chemotaxis and phagocytosis), and neutropenia and bleeding disorders slow the process of wound healing.

HEALING IN SPECIALISED TISSUES

Healing of skin wound provides an example of general process of healing by regeneration and repair. However, in certain specialised tissues, either regeneration or repair may predominate. Some of these examples are described below.

Fracture Healing

Healing of fracture by callus formation depends upon some clinical considerations whether the fracture is:

- *traumatic* (in previously normal bone), or *pathological* (in previously diseased bone);
- *complete or incomplete* like green-stick fracture; and
- *simple* (closed), *comminuted* (splintering of bone), or *compound* (communicating to skin surface).

However, basic events in healing of any type of fracture are similar and resemble healing of skin wound to some extent.

- **Primary union of fractures** occurs in a few special situations when the ends of fracture are approximated as is done by application of compression clamps. In these cases, bony union takes place with formation of medullary callus without periosteal callus formation. The patient can be made ambulatory early but there is more extensive bone necrosis and slow healing.
- **Secondary union** is the more common process of fracture healing. Though it is a continuous process, secondary bone union is described under the following 3 headings:

i) Procallus formation
ii) Osseous callus formation
iii) Remodelling

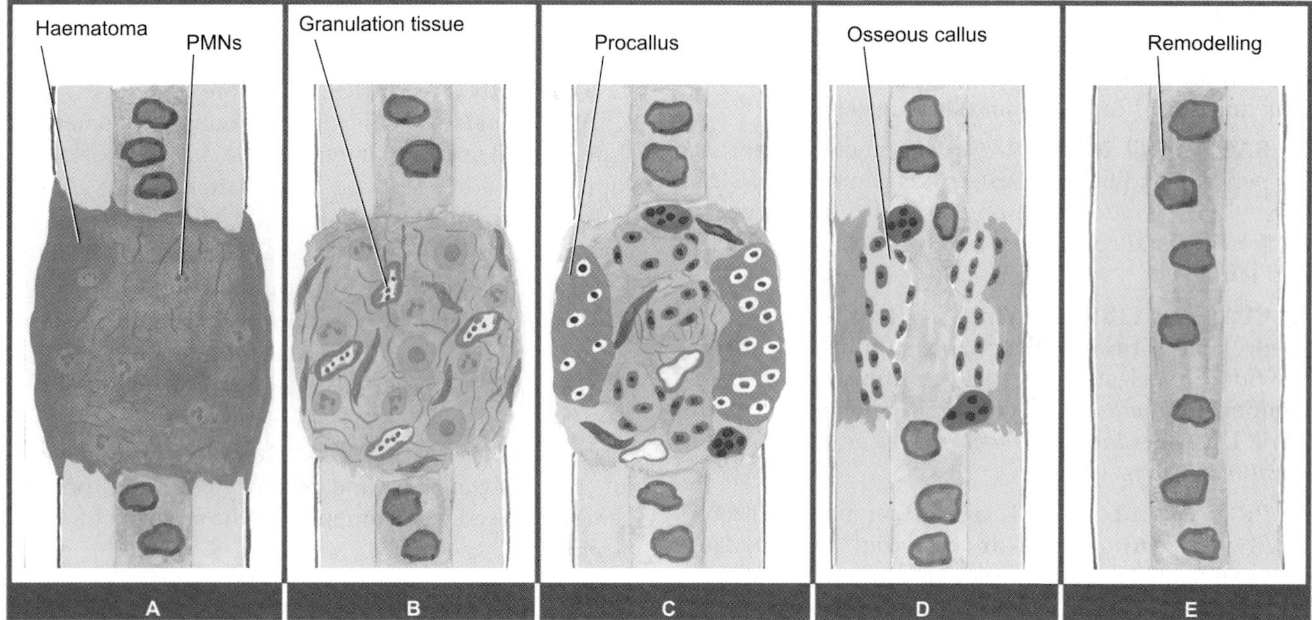

FIGURE 6.34

Fracture healing. A, Haematoma formation and local inflammatory response at the fracture site. B, Ingrowth of granulation tissue with formation of soft tissue callus. C, Formation of procallus composed of woven bone and cartilage with its characteristic fusiform appearance and having 3 arbitrary components—external, intermediate and internal callus. D, Formation of osseous callus composed of lamellar bone following clearance of woven bone and cartilage. E, Remodelled bone ends; the external callus cleared away. Intermediate callus converted into lamellar bone and internal callus developing bone marrow cavity.

These processes are illustrated in Fig. 6.34 and described below:

I. PROCALLUS FORMATION. Steps involved in the formation of procallus are as follows:

1. Haematoma forms due to bleeding from torn blood vessels, filling the area surrounding the fracture (Fig. 6.34,A). Loose meshwork is formed by blood and fibrin clot which acts as framework for subsequent granulation tissue formation.

2. Local inflammatory response occurs at the site of injury with exudation of fibrin, polymorphs and macrophages. The macrophages clear away the fibrin, red blood cells, inflammatory exudate and debris. Fragments of necrosed bone are scavenged by macrophages and osteoclasts.

3. Ingrowth of granulation tissue begins with neovascularisation and proliferation of mesenchymal cells from periosteum and endosteum. A soft tissue callus is thus formed which joins the ends of fractured bone without much strength (Fig. 6.34,B).

4. Callus composed of woven bone and cartilage starts within the first few days. The cells of inner layer of the periosteum have osteogenic potential and lay down collagen as well as osteoid matrix in the granulation tissue. The osteoid undergoes calcification and is called *woven bone callus.* A much wider zone over the cortex on either side of fractured ends is covered by the woven bone callus and united to bridge the gap between the ends, giving spindle-shaped or fusiform appearance to the union. In poorly immobilised fractures (e.g. fracture ribs), the subperiosteal osteoblasts may form cartilage at the fracture site. At times, callus is composed of woven bone as well as cartilage, temporarily immobilising the bone ends.

This stage is called provisional callus or procallus formation and is arbitrarily divided into *external, intermediate* and *internal procallus* (Fig. 6.34,C).

II. OSSEOUS CALLUS FORMATION. The procallus acts as scaffolding on which osseous callus composed of lamellar bone is formed. The woven bone is cleared away by incoming osteoclasts and the calcified cartilage disintegrates. In their place, newly-formed blood vessels and osteoblasts invade, laying down osteoid which is calcified and lamellar bone is formed by developing Haversian system concentrically around the blood vessels (Fig. 6.34,D).

III. REMODELLING. During the formation of lamellar bone, osteoblastic laying and osteoclastic removal are taking place remodelling the united bone ends, which after sometime, is indistinguishable from normal bone. The external callus is cleared away, compact bone (cortex) is formed in place of intermediate callus and the bone marrow cavity develops in internal callus (Fig. 6.34,E).

COMPLICATIONS OF FRACTURE HEALING. These are as under:

1. **Fibrous union** may result instead of osseous union if the immobilisation of fractured bone is not done. Occasionally, a false joint may develop at the fracture site (pseudo-arthrosis).
2. **Non-union** may result if some soft tissue is interposed between the fractured ends.
3. **Delayed union** may occur from causes of delayed wound healing in general such as infection, inadequate blood supply, poor nutrition, movement and old age.

Healing of Nervous Tissue

CENTRAL NERVOUS SYSTEM. The nerve cells of brain, spinal cord and ganglia once destroyed are not replaced. Axons of CNS also do not show any significant regeneration. The damaged neuroglial cells, however, may show proliferation of astrocytes called gliosis.

PERIPHERAL NERVOUS SYSTEM. In contrast to the cells of CNS, the peripheral nerves show regeneration, mainly from proliferation of Schwann cells and fibrils from distal end. The process is discussed in Chapter 28. Briefly, it consists of the following:

- Myelin sheath and axon of the intact distal nerve undergo Wallerian degeneration up to the next node of Ranvier towards the proximal end.
- The degenerated debris are cleared away by macrophages.
- Regeneration in the form of sprouting of fibrils takes place from the viable end of axon. These fibrils grow along the track of degenerated nerve so that in about 6-7 weeks, the peripheral stump consists of tube filled with elongated Schwann cells.
- One of the fibrils from the proximal stump enters the old neural tube and develops into new functional axon.

Healing of Muscle

All three types of muscle fibres have limited capacity to regenerate.

SKELETAL MUSCLE. The regeneration of striated muscle is similar to peripheral nerves. On injury, the cut ends of muscle fibres retract but are held together by stromal connective tissue. The injured site is filled with fibrinous material, polymorphs and macrophages. After clearance of damaged fibres by macrophages, one of the following two types of regeneration of muscle fibres can occur:

- If the muscle sheath is intact, sarcolemmal tubes containing histiocytes appear along the endomysial tube which, in about 3 months time, restores properly oriented muscle fibres e.g. in Zenker's degeneration of muscle in typhoid fever.
- If the muscle sheath is damaged, it forms a disorganised multinucleate mass and scar composed of fibrovascular tissue e.g. in Volkmann's ischaemic contracture.

SMOOTH MUSCLE. Non-striated muscle has limited regenerative capacity e.g. appearance of smooth muscle in the arterioles in granulation tissue. However, in large destructive lesions, the smooth muscle is replaced by permanent scar tissue.

CARDIAC MUSCLE. Destruction of heart muscle is replaced by fibrous tissue. However, in situations where the endomysium of individual cardiac fibre is intact (e.g. in diphtheria and coxsackie virus infections), regeneration of cardiac fibres may occur in young patients.

Healing of Mucosal Surfaces

The cells of mucosal surfaces have very good regeneration and are normally being lost and replaced continuously e.g. mucosa of alimentary tract, respiratory tract, urinary tract, uterine endometrium etc. This occurs by proliferation from margins, migration, multilayering and differentiation of epithelial cells in the same way as in the epidermal cells in healing of skin wounds.

Healing of Solid Epithelial Organs

Following gross tissue damage to organs like kidney, liver and thyroid, the replacement is by fibrous scar e.g. in chronic pyelonephritis and cirrhosis of liver. However, in parenchymal cell damage with intact basement membrane or intact supporting stromal tissue, regeneration may occur. For example:

- *In tubular necrosis* of kidney with intact basement membrane, proliferation and slow migration of tubular epithelial cells may occur to form renal tubules.
- *In viral hepatitis* if part of the liver lobule is damaged with intact stromal network, proliferation of hepatocytes may result in restoration of liver lobule.

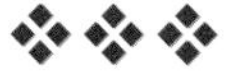

Infectious and Parasitic Diseases

7

INTRODUCTION

Microorganisms, namely bacteria, viruses, fungi and parasites, are present everywhere—in the soil, water, atmosphere and on the body surfaces, and are responsible for a large number of infectious diseases in human beings. Some microorganisms are distributed throughout the world while others are limited to certain geographic regions only. In general, tropical and underdeveloped countries are specially affected by infectious diseases than the developed countries. Certain *infectious diseases* are not so common in the developed world now but they continue to be major health problems in the under-developed countries e.g. tuberculosis, leprosy, typhoid fever, cholera, measles, pertussis, malaria, amoebiasis, pneumonia etc. *Vaccines* have been successful in controlling or eliminating some diseases e.g. smallpox, poliomyelitis, measles, pertussis etc. Insecticides have helped in controlling malaria to an extent. However, infections still rank very high *as a cause of death* in the world. Reasons for this trend are not difficult to seek:

- development of newer and antibiotic-resistant strains of microorganisms;
- administration of immunosuppressive therapy to patients with malignant tumours and transplanted organs making them susceptible to opportunistic infections;
- increasing number of patients reporting to hospital for different illnesses but instead many developing hospital-acquired infections, and
- lastly and more recently is the discovery in 1981 of previously unknown deadly disease i.e. acquired immunodeficiency syndrome (AIDS) caused by human immunodeficiency virus (HIV).

While talking of infective diseases, let us not forget the fact that many microorganisms may actually benefit mankind. Following is the range of *host-organism inter-relationship*, which may vary quite widely:

1. *Symbiosis* i.e. cooperative association between two dissimilar organisms beneficial to both.
2. *Commensalism* i.e. two dissimilar organisms living together benefitting one without harming the other.
3. *True parasitism* i.e. two dissimilar organisms living together benefitting the parasite but harming the host.
4. *Saprophytism* i.e. organisms living on dead tissues.

Besides the microorganisms, more recently a modified host protein present in the mammalian CNS has been identified called *prion protein*. Prions are transmissible agents just as infectious particles but lack nucleic acid. These agents are implicated in the etiology of spongiform encephalopathy, (including kuru), bovine spongiform encephalopathy (or mad cow disease) and Creutzfeldt-Jakob disease (associated with corneal transplantation). (Dr. Prusiner who discovered prion protein was awarded Nobel Prize in medicine in 1997).

Infectious diseases are the consequence of inter-relationship between disease-producing properties of microorganisms and host-defense capability against the invading organisms. Briefly, factors determining this host-microorganism relationship are given below:

Factors Relating to Infectious Agents

These are as under:

i) Mode of entry. Microorganisms causing infectious disease may gain entry into the body by various routes e.g.

- through ingestion (external route);
- inoculation (parenteral method);
- inhalation (respiration);
- perinatally (vertical transmission);
- by direct contact (contagious infection); and
- by contaminated water, food, soil, environment or from an animal host (zoonotic infections).

ii) Spread of infection. Microorganisms after entering the body may spread further through the phagocytic cells, blood vessels and lymphatics.

iii) Production of toxins. Bacteria liberate toxins which have effects on cell metabolism. *Endotoxins* are liberated on lysis of the bacterial cell while *exotoxins* are secreted by bacteria and have effects at distant sites too.

iv) Virulence of organisms. Many species and strains of organisms may have varying virulence e.g. the three strains of *C. diphtheriae (gravis, intermedius and mitis)* produce the same diphtherial exotoxin but in different amounts.

v) Product of organisms. Some organisms produce enzymes that help in spread of infections e.g. hyaluronidase by *Cl. welchii*, streptokinase by streptococci, staphylokinase and coagulase by staphylococci.

Factors Relating to Host

Microorganisms invade human body when defenses are not adequate. These factors include the following:

i) Physical barrier. A break in the continuity of the skin and mucous membranes allows the microorganisms to enter the body.

ii) Chemical barrier. Mucus secretions of the oral cavity and the alimentary tract and gastric acidity prevent bacterial colonisation.

iii) Effective drainage. The natural passages of the hollow organs like respiratory, gastrointestinal, urinary and genital system provide a way to drain the excretions effectively. Similarly, ducts of various glands are the conduits of drainage of secretions. Obstruction in any of these passages promotes infection.

iv) Immune defense mechanisms. These include the phagocytic leucocytes of blood (polymorphs and monocytes), phagocytes of tissues (mononuclear-phagocyte system) and the immune system as discussed in Chapter 4.

Some of the common diseases produced by pathogenic microorganisms are discussed below. Each group of microorganisms discussed here is accompanied by a list of diseases produced by them in a table. These lists of diseases are in no way complete but include only important and common examples. No attempts will be made to give details of organisms as that would mean repeating what is given in the textbooks of Microbiology. Instead, salient clinico-pathologic aspects of these diseases are highlighted.

Methods of Identification

The organisms causing infections and parasitic diseases may be identified by routine H & E stained sections in many instances. However, confirmation in most cases requires either application of special staining techniques or by molecular biologic methods (Table 7.1). In addition, culture of lesional tissue should be carried out for species identification and drug sensitivity. Generally, the organism is looked for at the advancing edge of the lesion rather than in the necrotic centre.

DISEASES CAUSED BY BACTERIA, SPIROCHAETES AND MYCOBACTERIA

In order to gain an upper hand in human host, bacteria must resist early engulfment by neutrophils. They

TABLE 7.1: Methods of Identification of Microorganisms.

1. *Bacteria*
   i. Gram stain: Most bacteria
   ii. Acid fast stain: Mycobacteria, Nocardia
   iii. Giemsa: Campylobacteria
2. *Fungi*
   i. Silver stain: Most fungi
   ii. Periodic acid-Schiff (PAS): Most fungi
   iii. Mucicarmine: Cryptococci
3. *Parasites*
   i. Giemsa: Malaria, Leishmania
   ii. Periodic acid-Schiff: Amoebae
   iii. Silver stain: Pneumocystis
4. *All classes including viruses*
   i. Culture
   ii. *In situ* hybridisation
   iii. DNA analysis
   iv. Polymerase chain reaction (PCR)

survive and damage the host in a variety of ways such as by generation of toxins (e.g. gas-forming anaerobes), by forming a slippery capsule that resists attachment to macrophages (e.g. pneumococci), by inhibition of fusion of phagocytic vacuoles with lysosomes (e.g. tubercle bacilli) etc.

Table 7.2 provides an abbreviated classification of bacterial diseases and their etiologic agents. A few common and important examples amongst these are discussed below.

PLAGUE

Plague is caused by *Yersinia (Pasteurella) pestis* which is a small gram-negative coccobacillus that grows rapidly on most culture media. Direct identification of the organism in tissues is possible by fluorescence antisera methods.

Plague has been a great killer since 14th century and is known to have wiped out populations of cities. However, the modern Europe is plague free, probably due to widespread use of arsenic as rat poison. Currently, the world over, Vietnam and Tanzania have most cases of plague. However, an outbreak in Surat in the state of Gujarat in Western part of India in 1994 alarmed the world once again that we are not totally free of this dreaded 'black death'.

Plague is a zoonotic disease and spreads by rodents, primarily by rats, both wild and domestic; others being squirrels and rabbits.

Infection to humans occurs by rat-flea or by inhalation. After the organisms enter the blood stream, they reach the draining lymph nodes where, rather than being phagocytosed by phagocytic cells, they proliferate rapidly giving rise to tender lymphadenopathy. This occurs within 24-48 hours of infection and is accompa-

TABLE 7.2: Diseases Caused by Bacteria, Spirochaetes and Mycobacteria.

DISEASE	ETIOLOGIC AGENT
1. *Typhoid (enteric) fever (Chapter 18)*	*Salmonella typhi*
2. *Plague**	*Yersinia pestis*
3. *Anthrax**	*Bacillus anthracis*
4. *Whooping cough* (pertussis)*	*Bordetella pertussis*
5. *Chancroid*	*Haemophilus ducreyi*
6. *Granuloma inguinale**	*Calymmatobacterium donovani*
7. *Gonorrhoea*	*Neisseria gonorrhoeae*
8. *Cholera*	*Vibrio cholerae*
9. *Shigellosis*	*S. dysenteriae, S. flexneri, S. boydii, S. sonnei*
10. *Brucellosis*	*B. melitensis, B. abortus, B. suis, B. canis*
11. *Diphtheria*	*Corynebacterium diphtheriae*
12. *Lobar pneumonia (Chapter 15)*	*Streptococcus pneumoniae, Staphylococcus aureus, Haemophilus influenzae, Klebsiella pneumoniae*
13. *Bronchopneumonia (Chapter 15)*	*Staphylococci, Streptococci, K. pneumoniae, H. influenzae*
14. *Bacterial meningitis (Chapter 28)*	*Escherichia coli, H.influenzae, Neisseria meningitidis, Streptococcus pneumoniae*
15. *Bacterial endocarditis (Chapter 12)*	*Staphylococcus aureus, Streptococcus viridans*
16. *Other staphylococcal infections**	*S. aureus, S. epidermidis, S. saprophyticus*
17. *Streptococcal infections**	*S. pyogenes, S. faecalis, S. pneumoniae. S. viridans*
18. *E. coli infections (Chapter 20) (Urinary tract infection)*	*Escherichia coli*
19. *Clostridial diseases**	
i) *Gas gangrene*	*C. perfringens*
ii) *Tetanus*	*C. tetani*
iii) *Botulism*	*C. botulinum*
iv) *Clostridial food poisoning*	*C. perfringens*
v) *Necrotising enterocolitis*	*C. perfringens*
20. *Tuberculosis (page 154)*	*Mycobacterium tuberculosis*
21. *Leprosy (page 163)*	*Mycobacterium leprae*
22. *Syphilis (page 167)*	*Treponema pallidum*
23. *Actinomycosis (page 169)*	*Actinomyces israelii*
24. *Nocardiosis*	*Nocardia asteroides*

*Diseases discussed in this chapter.

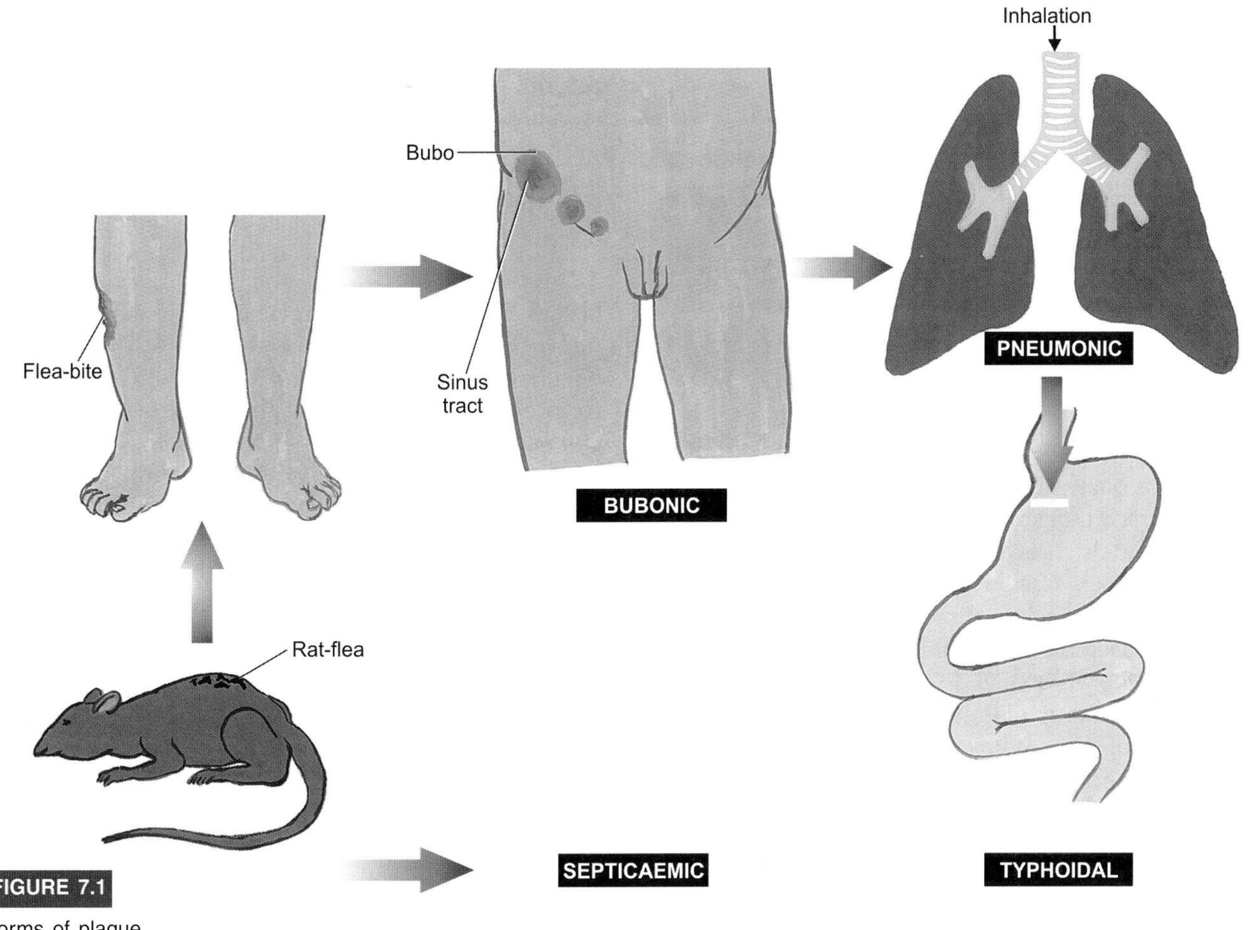

FIGURE 7.1

Forms of plague.

nied by chills, fever, myalgia, nausea, vomiting and marked prostration. If untreated, death occurs from disseminated intravascular coagulation (DIC) within 1 to 2 days with development of widespread petechiae and ecchymoses leading to gangrene and hence the name *black death.* In other cases, death results from multi-organ failure due to profound toxaemia. The patient and his fluids are highly infectious and can be transmitted by arthropods as well as person-to-person contact, giving rise to secondary cases.

Virulence of the organism *Y. pestis* is attributed to the elaboration of plague toxins: pesticin and lipopolysaccharide endotoxin.

PATHOLOGIC CHANGES. Following forms of plague are recognised (Fig. 7.1):

1. Bubonic plague, the most common
2. Pneumonic plague
3. Typhoidal plague
4. Septicaemic plague

BUBONIC PLAGUE. This form is characterised by rapid appearance of tender, fluctuant and enlarged regional lymph nodes, several centimeters in diameter, and may have discharging sinuses on the skin. ***Microscopically,*** the features are as under:

- Effaced architecture of lymph nodes due to necrosis in and around the affected nodes.
- Multiple necrotising granulomas.
- Characteristic mononuclear inflammatory response.
- Masses of proliferating bacilli in sinusoids of lymph nodes.
- Cellulitis in the vicinity.

PNEUMONIC PLAGUE. This is the most dreaded form of plague that occurs by inhalation of bacilli from air-borne particles of carcasses of animals or from affected patient's cough. It is characterised by occurrence of bronchopneumonia, with the following conspicuous microscopic features:

- Necrosis of alveolar walls.
- Intense hyperaemia and haemorrhages.
- Numerous bacilli in the alveolar lumina.
- Characteristic mononuclear inflammatory response with very scanty neutrophils.

TYPHOIDAL PLAGUE. This form of plague is unassociated with regional lymphadenopathy. The lesions in typhoidal plague are as follows:

- Necrotic foci in visceral lymphoid tissue.
- Necrotic areas in parenchymal visceral organs.
- G.I. manifestations with diarrhoea and pain abdomen.

SEPTICAEMIC PLAGUE. This is a form of progressive, fulminant bacterial infection associated with profound septicaemia in the absence of afarent regional lymphadenitis.

ANTHRAX

Anthrax is a bacterial disease of antiquity caused by *Bacillus anthracis* that spreads from animals to man. The disease is widely prevalent in cattle and sheep but human infection is rare. However, much of knowledge on human anthrax has been gained owing to fear of use of these bacteria for military purpose or for "bio-terrorism" (other microbial diseases in this list include: botulism, pneumonic plague, smallpox). Recently, the human form of disease has attracted a lot of attention of the media and the civilized world due to its use in the form of anthrax-laced letters sent by possible terrorist groups as a retaliatory biological weapon against the US interest subsequent to punitive attacks by the US on Afghanistan as an aftermath of September 11, 2001 terrorist attacks in the US. In India, anthrax in animals is endemic in South due to large unprotected and uncontrolled population of live-stock population. But anthrax is also prevalent in human beings in India; in Pondicherry alone 35 cases have been reported.

ETIOPATHOGENESIS. The causative organism, *Bacillus anthracis,* is a gram-positive, aerobic bacillus, 4.5 μm long. It is a spore-forming bacillus and the spores so formed outside the body are quite resistant. The disease occurs as an exogenous infection by contact with soil or animal products contaminated with spores.

Depending upon the portal of entry, three types of human anthrax is known to occur:

i) **Cutaneous form** by direct contact with skin and is most common.

ii) **Pulmonary form** by inhalation, also called as "wool-sorters' disease" and is most fatal.

iii) **Gastrointestinal form** by ingestion and is rare.

The mechanism of infection includes spread of bacilli from the portal of entry to the regional lymph nodes through lymphatics where the bacteria proliferate. There is delayed accumulation of polymorphs and macrophages. Macrophages also play a role in expression of bacterial toxicity; bacterial toxin is quite lethal to macrophages.

PATHOLOGIC CHANGES. The characteristic lesions of anthrax are haemorrhage, oedema and necrosis at the portal of entry.

1. **Cutaneous anthrax** is the most common and occurs in two forms: one type is characterized by necrotic lesion due to vascular thrombosis, haemorrhage and acellular necrosis, while the other form begins as a pimple at the point of entry of *B. anthracis* into the abraded exposed skin, more often in the region of hands and the head and neck. The initial lesion develops into a vesicle or blister containing clear serous or blood-stained fluid swarming with anthrax bacilli which can be identified readily by smear examination. The bursting of the blister is followed by extensive oedema and black tissue necrosis resulting in formation of severe 'malignant pustule'. Regional lymph nodes are invariably involved alongwith profound septicaemia.

2. **Pulmonary anthrax (wool-sorters' disease)** occurring from inhalation of spores of *B. anthracis* in infectious aerosols results in rapid development of malignant pustule in the bronchus. This is followed by development of primary extensive necrotising pneumonia and haemorrhagic mediastinitis which is invariably fatal.

3. **Intestinal anthrax** is rare in human beings and is quite similar to that seen in cattle. Septicaemia and death often results in this type too. The lesions consist of mucosal oedema, small necrotic ulcers, massive fluid loss and haemorrhagic mesenteric lymphadenitis.

Besides, anthrax septicaemia results in spread of infection to all other organs.

LABORATORY DIAGNOSIS. Anthrax can be diagnosed by a few simple techniques:

Smear examination: Gram stained smear shows rod-shaped, spore-forming, gram-positive bacilli. Endospores are detectable by presence of unstained defects or holes within the cell.

Culture: Anthrax bacteria grow on sheep blood agar as flat colonies with an irregular margin (medusa head).

Anthrax contaminated work surfaces, materials and equipment must be decontaminated with 5% hypochlorite or 5% phenol.

Chapter Seven

WHOOPING COUGH (PERTUSSIS)

Whooping cough is a highly communicable acute bacterial disease of childhood caused by *Bordetella pertussis*. The use of DPT vaccination has reduced the prevalence of whooping cough in different populations.

The causative organism, *B. pertussis*, has strong tropism for the brush border of the bronchial epithelium. The organisms proliferate here and stimulate the bronchial epithelium to produce abundant tenacious mucus. Within 7-10 days after exposure, catarrhal stage begins which is the most infectious stage. There is low grade fever, rhinorrhoea, conjunctivitis and excess tear production. Paroxysms of cough occur with characteristic 'whoop'. The condition is self-limiting but may cause death due to asphyxia in infants. *B. pertussis* produces a heat-labile toxin, a heat-stable endotoxin, and a lymphocytosis-producing factor called histamine-sensitising factor.

Microscopically, the lesions in the respiratory tract consist of necrotic bronchial epithelium covered by thick mucopurulent exudate. In severe cases, there is mucosal erosion and hyperaemia. The peripheral blood shows marked lymphocytosis upto 90% and enlargement of lymphoid follicles in the bronchial mucosa and peribronchial lymph nodes.

GRANULOMA INGUINALE

Granuloma inguinale is a sexually-transmitted disease affecting the genitalia and inguinal and perianal regions caused by *Calymmatobacterium donovani*. The disease is common in tropical and subtropical countries such as New Guinea, Australia and India. The organism inhabits the intestinal tract. The infection is transmitted through vaginal or anal intercourse and by autoinoculation. The incubation period varies from 2 to 4 weeks. Initially, the lesion is in the form of a papule, a subcutaneous nodule or an ulcer. Within a few weeks, it develops into a raised, soft, painless, reddish ulcer with exuberant granulation tissue. Depending upon whether the individual is heterosexual or homosexual, the lesions are located on the penis, scrotum, genitocrural folds and inguinal folds, or in the perianal and anal area respectively. Regional lymphadenopathy generally does not occur.

Microscopically, the margin of the ulcer shows epithelial hyperplasia. The ulcer bed shows neutrophilic abscesses. The dermis and subcutaneous tissues are infiltrated by numerous histiocytes containing many bacteria called *Donovan bodies,* and lymphocytes, plasma cells and neutrophils. These organisms are best demonstrated by silver impregnation techniques.

STAPHYLOCOCCAL INFECTIONS

Staphylococci are gram-positive cocci which are present everywhere—in the skin, umbilicus, nasal vestibule, stool etc. Three species are pathogenic to human beings: *Staph. aureus, Staph. epidermidis and Staph. saprophyticus.* Most staphylococcal infections are caused by *Staph. aureus.* Staphylococcal infections are among the commonest antibiotic-resistant hospital-acquired infection in surgical wounds.

A wide variety of suppurative diseases are caused by *Staph. aureus* which includes the following (Fig. 7.2):

1. Infections of skin. Staphylococcal infections of skin are quite common. The infection begins from lodgement of cocci in the hair root due to poor hygiene and results in obstruction of sweat or sebaceous gland duct. This is

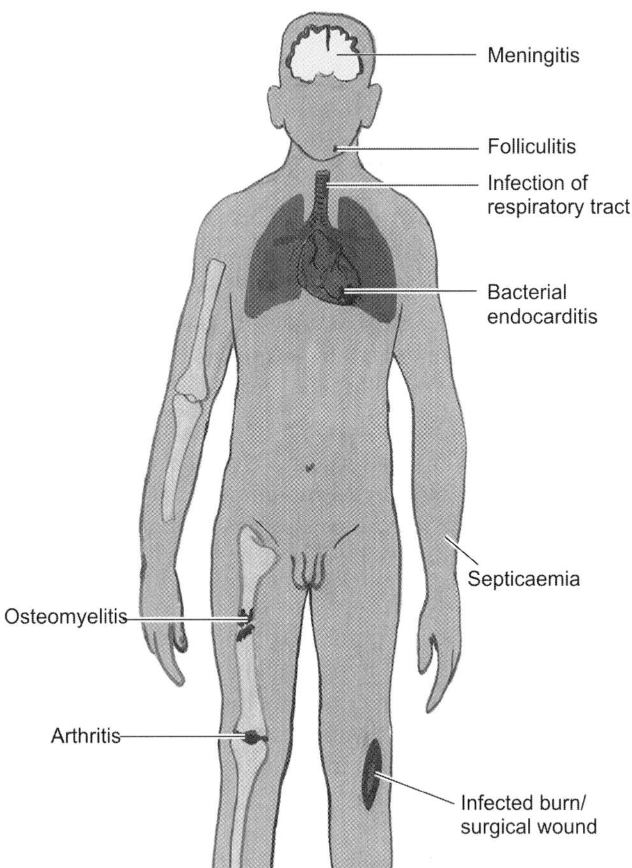

FIGURE 7.2

Suppurative diseases caused by *Staphylococcus aureus.*

termed *folliculitis.* Involvement of adjacent follicles results in larger lesions called *furuncle.* Further spread of infection horizontally under the skin and subcutaneous tissue causes *carbuncle* or *cellulitis. Styes* are staphylococcal infection of the sebaceous glands of Zeis, the glands of Moll and eyelash follicles. *Impetigo* is yet another staphylococcal skin infection common in school children in which there are multiple pustular lesions on face forming honey-yellow crusts. *Breast abscess* may occur following delivery when staphylococci are transmitted from infant having neonatal sepsis or due to stasis of milk.

2. **Infections of burns and surgical wounds.** These are quite common due to contamination from the patient's own nasal secretions or from hospital staff. Elderly, malnourished, obese and neonates have increased susceptibility.

3. **Infections of the upper and lower respiratory tract.** Small children under 2 years of age get staphylococcal infections of the respiratory tract commonly. These include pharyngitis, bronchopneumonia, staphylococcal pneumonia and its complications.

4. **Bacterial arthritis.** Septic arthritis in the elderly is caused by *Staph. aureus.*

5. **Infection of bone (Osteomyelitis).** Young boys having history of trauma or infection may develop acute staphylococcal osteomyelitis (Chapter 26).

6. **Bacterial endocarditis.** Acute and subacute bacterial endocarditis are complications of infection with *Staph. aureus* and *Staph. epidermidis* (Chapter 12).

7. **Bacterial meningitis.** Surgical procedures on central nervous system may lead to staphylococcal meningitis (Chapter 28).

8. **Septicaemia.** Staphylococcal septicaemia may occur in patients with lowered resistance or in patients having underlying staphylococcal infections. Patients present with features of bacteraemia such as shaking chills and fever (Chapter 6).

9. **Toxic shock syndrome.** Toxic shock syndrome is a serious complication of staphylococcal infection characterised by fever, hypotension and exfoliative skin rash. The condition affects young menstruating women who use tampons of some brands which when kept inside the vagina cause absorption of staphylococcal toxins from the vagina.

STREPTOCOCCAL INFECTIONS

Streptococci are also gram-positive cocci but unlike staphylococci, they are more known for their non-suppurative autoimmune complications than suppurative inflammatory responses. Streptococcal infections occur throughout the world but their problems are greater in underprivileged populations where antibiotics are not instituted readily.

The following groups and subtypes of streptococci have been identified and implicated in different streptococcal diseases (Fig. 7.3):

1. *Group A or Streptococcus pyogenes,* also called β-haemolytic streptococci, are involved in causing upper respiratory tract infection and cutaneous infections (erysipelas). In addition, beta haemolytic streptococci are involved in autoimmune reactions in the form of rheumatic heart disease (RHD).

2. *Group B or Streptococcus agalactiae* produces infections in the newborn and is involved in non-suppurative post-streptococcal complications such as RHD and acute glomerulonephritis.

3. *Group C and G streptococci* are responsible for respiratory infections.

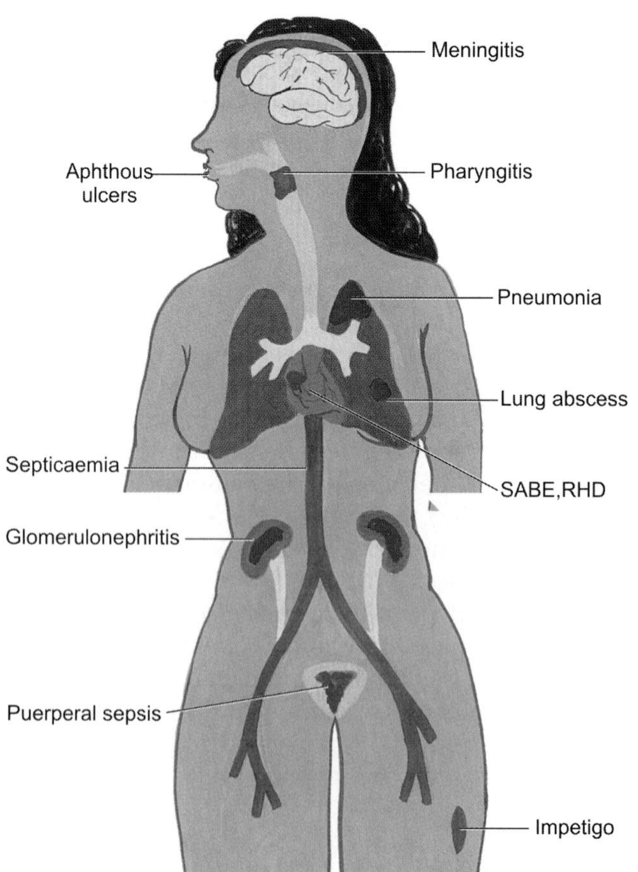

FIGURE 7.3

Diseases caused by streptococci.

4. *Group D or Streptococcus faecalis,* also called enterococci are important in causation of urinary tract infection, bacterial endocarditis, septicaemia etc.

5. *Untypable α-haemolytic streptococci* such as *Streptococcus viridans* constitute the normal flora of the mouth and may cause bacterial endocarditis.

6. *Pneumococci or Streptococcus pneumoniae* are etiologic agents for bacterial pneumonias, meningitis and septicaemia.

CLOSTRIDIAL DISEASES

Clostridia are gram-positive spore-forming anaerobic microorganisms found in the gastrointestinal tract of herbivorous animals and man. These organisms may undergo vegetative division under anaerobic conditions, and sporulation under aerobic conditions. These spores are passed in faeces and can survive in unfavourable conditions. On degeneration of these microorganisms, the plasmids are liberated which produce many toxins responsible for the following clostridial diseases depending upon the species (Fig. 7.4):

1. Gas gangrene by *C. perfringens*
2. Tetanus by *C. tetani*
3. Botulism by *C. botulinum*
4. Clostridial food poisoning by *C. perfringens*
5. Necrotising enterocolitis by *C. perfringens.*

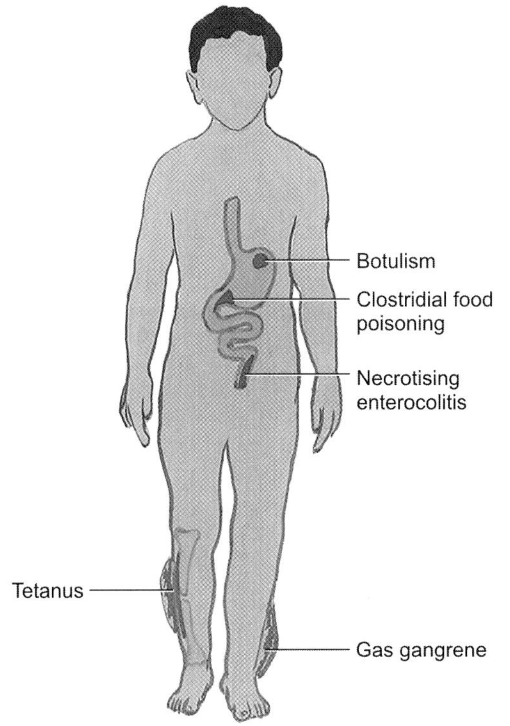

FIGURE 7.4

Diseases caused by clostridia.

GAS GANGRENE. Gas gangrene is a rapidly progressive and fatal illness in which there is myonecrosis of previously healthy skeletal muscle due to elaboration of myotoxins by some species of clostridia. In majority of cases (80-90%), the source of myotoxins is *C. perfringens* Type A; others are *C. novyi* and *C. septicum.* Generally, traumatic wounds and surgical procedures are followed by contamination with clostridia and become the site of myonecrosis (Fig. 7.4). The incubation period is 2 to 4 days. The most common myotoxin produced by *C. perfringens* Type A is the alpha toxin which is a lecithinase. The prevention of gas gangrene lies in debridement of damaged tissue in which the clostridia thrive. The lesion has serosanguineous discharge with odour and contains gas bubbles. There is very scanty inflammatory reaction at the site of gas gangrene.

TETANUS. Tetanus or 'lock jaw' is a severe acute neurologic syndrome caused by tetanus toxin, tetanospasmin, which is a neurotoxic exotoxin elaborated by *C. tetani.* The spores of the microorganism present in the soil enter the body through a penetrating wound. In underdeveloped countries, tetanus in neonates is seen due to application of soil or dung on the umbilical stump. The degenerated microorganisms liberate the tetanus neurotoxin which causes neuronal stimulation and spasm of muscles (Fig. 7.4). The incubation period of the disease is 1-3 weeks. The earliest manifestation is lock-jaw or trismus. Rigidity of muscles of the back causes backward arching or opisthotonos. Death occurs due to spasm of respiratory and laryngeal muscles.

BOTULISM. Botulism is characterised by symmetric paralysis of cranial nerves, limbs and trunk. The condition occurs following ingestion of food contaminated with neurotoxins of *C. botulinum* and less often by contamination of a penetrating wound. The spores of *C. botulinum* are capable of surviving in unfavourable conditions and contaminate vegetables and other foods, especially if improperly stored or canned. The symptoms of botulism begin to appear within 12 to 36 hours of ingestion of food containing the neurotoxins (type A to type G). The toxins resist gastric digestion and are absorbed from the upper portion of small intestine and enter the blood. On reaching the cholinergic nerve endings, the toxin binds to membrane receptors and inhibits release of acetylcholine resulting in paralysis and respiratory failure (Fig. 7.4).

CLOSTRIDIAL FOOD POISONING. Clostridial food poisoning is caused by enterotoxin elaborated by *C. perfringens.* Out of five serotypes of *C. perfringens,* type A and C produce alpha-enterotoxin that causes food poisoning (Fig. 7.4). These serotypes of organism are omnipresent in the environment and thus clostridial poisoning occurs throughout the world. Food poisoning from *C. perfringens* is mostly from ingestion of meat and its products which have been allowed to dry resulting in dehydration and anaerobic conditions suitable for growth of *C. perfringens*. The contaminated meat contains vegetative form of the organism and no preformed enterotoxin (unlike botulism where preformed neurotoxin of *C. botulinum* is ingested). On ingestion of the contaminated meat, alpha-enterotoxin is produced in the intestine. Symptoms of the food poisoning appear within 12 hours of ingestion of contaminated meat and recovery occurs within 2 days.

NECROTISING ENTEROCOLITIS. Necrotising enterocolitis or 'pig bel' is caused by beta-enterotoxin produced by *C. perfringens* Type C. The condition occurs especially in undernourished children who suddenly indulge in overeating such as was first reported participation in pig feasts by poor children in New Guinea and hence the name 'pig bel'. Adults do not develop the condition due to good antibody response.

Ingestion of contaminated pork by malnourished children who normally take protein-deficient vegetarian diet causes elaboration of beta-enterotoxin. The symptoms appear within 48 hours after ingestion of contaminated meat. These include: severe abdominal pain, distension, vomiting and passage of bloody stools. Milder form of disease runs a course similar to other forms of gastroenteritis while fulminant 'pig bel' may result in death of the child.

Grossly, the disease affects small intestine segmentally. The affected segment of bowel shows green, necrotic pseudomembrane covering the necrotic mucosa and there is associated peritonitis. Advanced cases may show perforation of the bowel wall.
Microscopically, there is transmural infiltration by acute inflammatory cell infiltrate with changes of mucosal infarction, oedema and haemorrhage (Chapter 18). The pseudomembrane consists of necrotic epithelium with entangled bacilli.

DISEASES CAUSED BY FUNGI

Of the large number of known fungi, only a few are infective to human beings. Many of the human fungal infections are opportunistic i.e. they occur in conditions with impaired host immune mechanisms. Such conditions include defective neutrophil function, administration of corticosteroids, immunosuppressive therapy and immunodeficiency states (congenital and acquired). A list of common fungal infections of human beings is given in Table 7.3. A few important representative examples are discussed below.

MYCETOMA

Mycetoma is a chronic suppurative infection involving a limb, shoulder or other tissues and is characterised by draining sinuses. The material discharged from the sinuses is in the form of grains consisting of colonies of fungi or bacteria. Mycetomas are of 2 main types:

- *Mycetomas* caused by actinomyces (higher bacteria) comprising about 60% of cases (page 169); and
- *Eumycetomas* caused by true fungi comprising the remaining 40% of the cases.

Most common fungi causative for eumycetoma are *Madurella mycetomatis* or *Madurella grisea*, both causing black granules from discharging sinuses. Eumycetomas are particularly common in Northern and tropical Africa, Southern Asia and tropical America. The organisms are inoculated directly from soil into bare feet, from carrying of contaminated sacks on the shoulders, and into the hands from infected vegetation.

PATHOLOGIC CHANGES. After several months of infection, the affected site, most commonly foot, is swollen and hence the name 'madura foot'. The lesions extend deeply into the subcutaneous tissues, along the fascia and eventually invade the bones. They drain through sinus tracts which discharge purulent material and grains. The surrounding tissue shows granulomatous reaction.

CANDIDIASIS

Candidiasis is an opportunistic fungal infection caused most commonly by *Candida albicans* and occasionally

TABLE 7.3: Diseases Caused by Fungi.

DISEASE	ETIOLOGIC AGENT
1. *Mycetoma**	*Madurella mycetomatis*
2. *Aspergillosis (Chapter 15)*	*Aspergillus fumigatus, A. flavus, A. niger*
3. *Blastomycosis*	*Blastomyces dermatitidis*
4. *Candidiasis**	*Candida albicans*
5. *Coccidioidomycosis*	*Coccidioides immitis*
6. *Cryptococcosis*	*Cryptococcus neoformans*
7. *Histoplasmosis*	*Histoplasma capsulatum*
8. *Rhinosporidiosis (Chapter 16)*	*Rhinosporidium seeberi*
9. *Superficial mycosis**	*Microsporum, Trichophyton, Epidermophyton*

*Conditions discussed in this chapter.

Chapter Seven

by *Candida tropicalis.* In human beings, Candida species are present as normal flora of the skin and mucocutaneous areas, intestines and vagina. The organism becomes pathogenic when the balance between the host and the organism is disturbed. Various predisposing factors are: impaired immunity, prolonged use of oral contraceptives, long-term antibiotic therapy, corticosteroid therapy, diabetes mellitus, obesity, pregnancy etc.

PATHOLOGIC CHANGES. Candida produces superficial infections of the skin and mucous membranes, or may invade deeper tissues as described under:

1. **Oral thrush.** This is the commonest form of mucocutaneous candidiasis seen especially in early life. Full-fledged lesions consist of creamy white pseudomembrane composed of fungi covering the tongue, soft palate, and buccal mucosa. In severe cases, ulceration may be seen.
2. **Candidal vaginitis.** Vaginal candidiasis or monilial vaginitis is characterised clinically by thick, yellow, curdy discharge. The lesions form pseudomembrane of fungi on the vaginal mucosa. They are quite pruritic and may extend to involve the vulva (vulvovaginitis) and the perineum.
3. **Cutaneous candidiasis.** Candidal involvement of nail folds producing change in the shape of nail plate (paronychia) and colonisation in the intertriginous areas of the skin, axilla, groin, infra-and intermammary, intergluteal folds and interdigital spaces are some of the common forms of cutaneous lesions caused by *Candida albicans.*
4. **Systemic candidiasis.** Invasive candidiasis is rare and is usually a terminal event of an underlying disorder associated with impaired immune system. The organisms gain entry into the body through an ulcerative lesion on the skin and mucosa or may be introduced by iatrogenic means such as via intravenous infusion, peritoneal dialysis or urinary catheterisation. The lesions of systemic candidiasis are most commonly encountered in kidneys as ascending pyelonephritis and in heart as candidal endocarditis.

SUPERFICIAL MYCOSIS

Dermatophytes are the most important example of cutaneous mycosis caused by *Microsporum, Trichophyton* and *Epidermophyton.* These superficial fungi are spread by direct contact or by fomites and infect tissues such as the skin, hair and nails. Examples of diseases pertaining to these tissues are as under:

- *Tinea capitis* characterised by patchy alopecia affecting the scalp and eyebrows.
- *Tinea barbae* is acute folliculitis of the beard.
- *Tinea corporis* is dermatitis with formation of erythematous papules.

The diagnosis of dermatophytosis is made by light microscopic examination of skin scrapings after addition of sodium or potassium hydroxide solution. Other methods include fungal culture and demonstration of fungus in tissue sections.

DISEASES CAUSED BYVIRUSES

Viral diseases are the most common cause of human illness. However, many of the viral infections remain asymptomatic while others produce viral disease. Another peculiar feature of viral infection is that a single etiologic agent may produce different diseases in the same host depending upon host immune response and age at infection e.g. varicella-zoster virus is causative for chickenpox as well as herpes zoster. Viruses are essentially intracellular parasites. Depending upon their nucleic acid genomic composition, they may be single-stranded or double-stranded, RNA or DNA viruses. A list of common viruses and diseases caused by them is given in Table 7.4. Oncogenic viruses and their role in neoplasms are discussed in Chapter 8. A few common and important viral diseases are described below.

VIRAL HAEMORRHAGIC FEVERS

Viral haemorrhagic fevers are a group of acute viral infections which have common features of causing haemorrhages, shock and sometimes death. Viruses causing haemorrhagic fevers were earlier called *ar*thropod-*bo*rne *(or arbo)* viruses since their transmission was considered to be from arthropods to humans. However, now it is known that all such viruses are not transmitted by arthropod vectors alone and hence now such haemorrhagic fevers are classified according to the routes of transmission and other epidemiologic features into 4 groups:

- Mosquito-borne (e.g. yellow fever, dengue fever, Rift Valley fever)
- Tick-borne (e.g. Crimean haemorrhagic fever, Kyasanur Forest disease)
- Zoonotic (e.g. Korean haemorrhagic fever, Lassa fever)
- Marburg virus disease and Ebola virus disease by unknown route.

Of these, mosquito-borne viral haemorrhagic fevers in which *Aedes aegypti* mosquitoes are vectors are the

TABLE 7.4: Diseases Caused by Viruses.

DISEASE	ETIOLOGIC AGENT
1. *Viral haemorrhagic fevers**	Arthropod-borne (arbo) viruses
2. *Severe acute respiratory syndrome (SARS, Bird flu)**	Influenza virus type A
3. *Viral encephalitis*	Arthropod-borne (arbo) viruses
4. *Rabies**	Rabies virus (arboviruses)
5. *Poliomyelitis*	Poliovirus
6. *Smallpox (Variola)*	Variola virus
7. *Chickenpox (varicella)**	Varicella-zoster virus
8. *Herpes simplex and herpes genitalis**	Herpes simplex virus (HSV-I) and (HSV-II)
9. *Herpes zoster**	Varicella-zoster virus
10. *Lymphogranuloma venereum**	*Chlamydia trachomatis*
11. *Cat-scratch disease**	*Bartonella henselae*
12. *Viral hepatitis (Chapter 19)*	Hepatotropic viruses
13. *Cytomegalovirus inclusion disease*	Cytomegalovirus (CMV)
14. *Infectious mononucleosis (Chapter 13)*	Epstein-Barr virus (EBV)
15. *Measles (Rubeola)*	Measles virus
16. *German measles (Rubella)*	Rubella virus
17. *Mumps (Chapter 17)*	Mumps virus
18. *Viral respiratory infections*	Adenovirus, echovirus, rhinovirus, coxsackie virus, influenza A,B and C etc.
19. *Viral gastroenteritis*	Rotaviruses, Norwalk-like viruses

*Diseases discussed in this chapter.

most common problem the world over, especially in underdeveloped countries. Two important examples of Aedes mosquito-borne viral haemorrhagic fevers are yellow fever and dengue fever, which are discussed below.

Yellow Fever

Yellow fever is the oldest known viral haemorrhagic fever restricted to some regions of Africa and South America. Monkeys carry the virus without suffering from illness and the virus is transmitted from them to humans by *Aedes aegypti* as vector.

Yellow fever is characterised by the following clinical features: Sudden onset of high fever, chills, myalgia, headache, jaundice, hepatic failure, renal failure, bleeding disorders and hypotension.

PATHOLOGIC CHANGES. Major pathologic changes are seen in the liver and kidneys.

Liver. The characteristic changes include:

i) midzonal necrosis;
ii) Councilman bodies; and
iii) microvesicular fat.

Kidneys. The kidneys show the following changes:

i) coagulative necrosis of proximal tubules;
ii) accumulation of fat in the tubular epithelium; and
iii) haemorrhages.

Patients tend to recover without sequelae and death rate is less than 5%, death resulting from hepatic or renal failure, and petechial haemorrhages in the brain.

Dengue Haemorrhagic Fever (DHF)

The word dengue is derived from African word *'denga'* meaning fever with haemorrhages. Dengue is caused by virus transmitted by bites of mosquito *Aedes aegypti;* the transmission being highest during and after rainy season when mosquitos are numerous. DHF was first described in 1953 when it struck Philippines. An outbreak of DHF occurred in Delhi and neighbouring cities in 1996 claiming several lives. In 1997 too, some cases of DHF have been reported in post-monsoon period in Delhi.

Dengue occurs in two forms:

1. *Dengue fever or break-bone fever* in an uncomplicated way is a self-limited febrile illness affecting muscles and joints with severe back pain due to myalgia (and hence the name 'break-bone' fever).
2. *Dengue haemorrhagic fever (DHF),* on the other hand, is a severe and potentially fatal form of acute febrile

illness characterised by cutaneous and intestinal haemorrhages due to thrombocytopenia, haemoconcentration, hypovolaemic shock and neurologic disturbances. DHF is most common in children under 15 years of age.

Dengue virus infects blood monocytes, lymphocytes and endothelial cells. This initiates complement activation and consumptive coagulopathy including thrombocytopenia. The entire process takes place rapidly and may evolve over a period of a few hours. If patient is treated appropriately at this stage, there is rapid and dramatic recovery. But in untreated cases, *dengue shock syndrome* develops and death occurs.

PATHOLOGIC CHANGES. The predominant *organ changes in DHF* are due to:
i) focal haemorrhages and congestion;
ii) increased vascular permeability resulting in oedema in different organs;
iii) coagulopathy with thrombocytopenia; and
iv) haemoconcentration.

The main derangement in **laboratory investigations in DHF** are:
i) Leucopenia with relative lymphocytosis, sometimes with atypical lymphocytes
ii) Thrombocytopenia
iii) Elevated haematocrit due to haemoconcentration
iv) X-ray chest showing bilateral pleural effusion
v) Deranged liver function tests (elevated transaminases, hypoalbuminaemia and reversed A:G ratio)
vi) Prolonged coagulation tests (prothrombin time, activated partial thromboplastin time and thrombin time)

Diagnosis of DHF is confirmed by:
- serologic testing for detection of antibodies;
- detection of virus by immunofluorescence method and monoclonal antibodies; and
- rapid methods such as reverse transcriptase-PCR and fluorogenic-ELISA.

At autopsy, the predominant organ changes observed are as follows:
i) *Brain:* intracranial haemorrhages, cerebral oedema, dengue encephalitis.
ii) *Liver:* enlarged; necrosis of hepatocytes and Kupffer cells, Reye's syndrome in children.
iii) *Kidneys:* petechial haemorrhages and features of renal failure.
iv) *Muscles and joints:* perivascular mononuclear cell infiltrate.

SEVERE ACUTE RESPIRATORY SYNDROME (SARS)

Severe acute respiratory syndrome (SARS) is the human form of bird flu or avian influenza having similar symptomatology. Recently, since the beginning of the year 2004, there have been outbreaks in poultry birds resulting in slaughtering of millions of infected chickens. There have been confirmed reports of spread of infection to human beings during this period in South-East Asia (particularly in Hong Kong, Vietnam, Thailand, South Korea, Japan, Indonesia, Taiwan and China) and its rapidly downhill and fatal clinical course; this has sent alarm bells all over world for quarantine.

ETIOPATHOGENESIS. Bird flu is caused by influenza viruses type A and primarily infects the birds, pigs and horses. Though it is not fatal for wild birds, it can kill poultry birds and people. Humans acquire infection through contaminated nasal, respiratory and faecal material from infected birds. An individual who has human flu and also gets infected with bird flu, then the hybrid virus so produced is highly contagious and causes lethal disease. The subtype of the virus in the current outbreak is H5N1. No person-to-person transmission has been reported. Humans do not have immune protection against avian viruses.

CLINICOPATHOLOGICAL FEATURES. Typically, the disease begins with influenza-like features such as fever, cough, sore throat, muscle aches and eye infection. Soon, the patient develops viral pneumonia and acute respiratory distress (hence the term SARS), and terminally kidney failure.

There is apprehension of an epidemic of SARS if the avian virus mutates and gains the ability to cause person-to-person infection. Since currently vaccine is yet being developed, the available measures are directed at prevention of infection and isolation of infected case.

VARICELLA ZOSTER VIRUS INFECTION

Varicella zoster virus is a member of herpes virus family and causes chickenpox (varicella) in non-immune individuals and herpes zoster (shingles) in those who had chickenpox in the past.

Varicella or chickenpox is an acute vesicular exanthem occurring in non-immune persons, especially children. The condition begins as an infection of the nasopharynx. On entering the blood stream, viraemia is accompanied by onset of fever, malaise and anorexia. Maculopapular skin rash, usually on upper trunk and face, develops in a day or two. This is followed by formation of vesicles which rupture and heal with formation of scabs. A few cases may develop complications which include pneumonia, hepatitis, encephalitis, carditis, orchitis, arthritis, and haemorrhages.

Herpes zoster or shingles is a recurrent, painful, vesicular eruption caused by reactivation of dormant varicella zoster virus in an individual who had chickenpox in the earlier years. The condition is infectious and spreads to children. The virus during the latent period resides in the dorsal root spinal ganglia or in the cranial nerve ganglia. On reactivation, the virus spreads from the ganglia to the sensory nerves and to peripheral nerves. Unlike chickenpox, the vesicles in shingles are seen in one or more of the sensory dermatomes and along the peripheral nerves. The lesions are particularly painful as compared with painless eruptions in chickenpox.

HERPES SIMPLEXVIRUS INFECTION

Two of the herpes simplex viruses (HSV)—type 1 and 2, cause 'fever blisters' and herpes genitalis respectively.

HSV-1 causes vesicular lesions on the skin, lips and mucous membranes. The infection spreads by close contact. The condition is particularly severe in immunodeficient patients and neonates while milder attacks of infection cause fever blisters on lips, oral mucosa and skin. Severe cases may develop complications such as meningoencephalitis and keratoconjunctivitis. Various stimuli such as fever, stress and respiratory infection reactivate latent virus lying in the ganglia and result in recurrent attacks of blisters.

HSV-2 causes herpes genitalis characterised by vesicular and necrotising lesions on the cervix, vagina and vulva. Like HSV-1 infection, lesions caused by HSV-2 are also recurrent and develop in non-immune individuals. Latency of HSV-2 infection is similar to HSV-1 and the organisms are reactivated by stimuli such as menstruation and sexual intercourse. The role of HSV-2 in female genital cancer has been surpassed by HPV infection (Chapter 22).

LYMPHOGRANULOMA VENEREUM

Lymphogranuloma venereum (LGV) is a sexually-transmitted disease caused by *Chlamydia trachomatis* and is characterised by mucocutaneous lesions and regional lymphadenopathy. Though described here under viral infections, chlamydia are no more considered as filterable viruses as was previously thought but are instead intracellular gram-negative bacteria. LGV is worldwide in distribution but its prevalence rate is high in tropics and subtropics in Africa, South-East Asia and India.

The condition begins as a painless, herpes-like lesion on the cervix, vagina, or penis. The organisms are carried via lymphatics to regional lymph nodes. The involved lymph nodes are tender, fluctuant and may ulcerate and drain pus.

Microscopically, the lymph nodes have characteristic stellate-shaped abscesses surrounded by a zone of epithelioid cells (granuloma). Healing stage of the acute lesion takes place by fibrosis and permanent destruction of lymphoid structure.

CAT-SCRATCH DISEASE

Another condition related to LGV, cat-scratch disease, is caused by *Bartonella henselae,* an organism linked to rickettsiae but unlike rickettsiae this organism can be grown in culture. The condition occurs more commonly in children (under 18 years of age). There is regional nodal enlargement which appears about 2 weeks after cat-scratch, and sometimes after thorn injury. The lymphadenopathy is self-limited and regresses in 2-4 months.

Microscopically the changes in lymph node are characteristics:

i) Initially, there is formation of non-caseating sarcoid-like granulomas.
ii) Subsequently, there are neutrophilic abscesses surrounded by pallisaded histiocytes and fibroblasts, an appearance simulating LGV discussed above.
iii) The organism is extracellular and can be identified by silver stains.

RABIES

Rabies is a fatal form of encephalitis in humans caused by rabies virus. The virus is transmitted into the human body by a bite by infected carnivores e.g. dog, wolf, fox and bats. The virus spreads from the contaminated saliva of these animals. The organism enters a peripheral nerve and then travels to the spinal cord and brain. A latent period of 10 days to 3 months may elapse between the bite and onset of symptoms. Since the virus localises at the brainstem, it produces classical symptoms of difficulty in swallowing and painful spasm of the throat termed hydrophobia. Other clinical features such as irritability, seizure and delirium point towards viral encephalopathy. Death occurs within a period of a few weeks.

Microscopic examination shows characteristic Negri bodies which are intracytoplasmic, deeply eosinophilic inclusions present in neurons of the brainstem.

DISEASES CAUSED BY PARASITES

Diseases caused by parasites (protozoa and helminths) are quite common and comprise a very large group of infestations and infections in human beings. Parasites may cause disease due to their presence in the lumen of the intestine, due to infiltration into the blood stream, or due to their presence inside the cells. A short list of parasitic diseases is given in Table 7.5. These diseases form a distinct subject of study called Parasitology; only a few conditions are briefly considered below.

AMOEBIASIS

Amoebiasis is caused by *Entamoeba histolytica,* named for its lytic action on tissues. It is the most important intestinal infection of man. The condition is particularly more common in tropical and subtropical areas with poor sanitation.

The parasite occurs in 2 forms: a *trophozoite form* which is active adult form seen in the tissues and diarrhoeal stools, and a *cystic form* seen in formed stools but not in the tissues. The trophozoite form can be stained positively with PAS procedure in tissue sections while amoebic cysts having four nuclei can be identified in stools. The cysts are the infective stage of the parasite and are found in contaminated water or food. The trophozoites are formed from the cyst stage in the intestine and colonise in the caecum and large bowel. The trophozoites as well as cysts are passed in stools but the trophozoites fail to survive outside or are destroyed by gastric secretions.

PATHOLOGIC CHANGES. The lesions of amoebiasis include amoebic colitis, amoeboma, amoebic liver abscess and spread to other sites (Fig. 7.5).

■ **Amoebic colitis,** the most common type of amoebic infection begins as a small area of necrosis of mucosa which may ulcerate. These ulcerative lesions may enlarge, develop undermining of margins of the ulcer due to lytic action of the trophozoite and have necrotic bed. Such chronic amoebic ulcers are described as flask-shaped ulcers due to their shape. The margin of the ulcer shows inflammatory response consisting of admixture of polymorphonuclear as well as mononuclear cells.

■ **Amoeboma** is the inflammatory thickening of the wall of large bowel resembling carcinoma of the colon. *Microscopically,* the lesion consists of inflammatory granulation tissue, fibrosis and clusters of trophozoites at the margin of necrotic with viable tissue.

TABLE 7.5: Diseases Caused by Parasites.

DISEASE	ETIOLOGIC AGENT
A. PROTOZOAL DISEASES	
1. *Chagas' disease (Trypanosomiasis)*	*Trypanosoma cruzi*
2. *Leishmaniasis (Kala-azar)*	*L. tropica, L. braziliensis, L. donovani*
3. *Malaria**	*Plasmodium vivax, P. falciparum, P. ovale, P. malariae*
4. *Toxoplasmosis*	*Toxoplasma gondii*
5. *Pneumocystosis*	*Pneumocystis carinii*
6. *Amoebiasis**	*Entamoeba histolytica*
7. *Giardiasis*	*Giardia lamblia*
B. HELMINTHIC DISEASES	
1. *Ascariasis*	*Ascaris lumbricoides*
2. *Enterobiasis (oxyuriasis)*	*Enterobius vermicularis*
3. *Hookworm disease*	*Ancylostoma duodenale*
4. *Trichinosis*	*Trichinella spiralis*
5. *Filariasis**	*Wuchereria bancrofti*
6. *Visceral larva migrans*	*Toxocara canis*
7. *Cutaneous larva migrans*	*Strongyloides stercoralis*
8. *Schistosomiasis (Bilharziasis)*	*Schistosoma haematobium*
9. *Clonorchiasis*	*Clonorchis sinensis*
10. *Fascioliasis*	*Fasciola hepatica*
11. *Echinococcosis (Hydatid disease) (Chapter 19)*	*Echinococcus granulosus*
12. *Cysticercosis**	*Taenia solium*

*Diseases discussed in this chapter

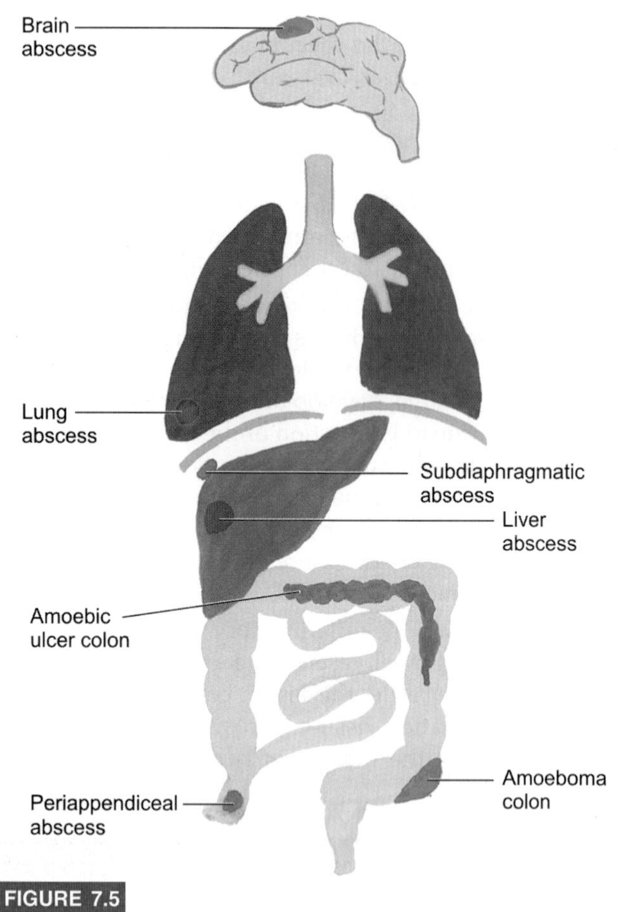

FIGURE 7.5
Complications of amoebiasis.

■ **Amoebic liver abscess** may be formed by invasion of the radicle of the portal vein by trophozoites. Amoebic liver abscess may be single or multiple (Chapter 18). The amoebic abscess contains yellowish-grey amorphous liquid material in which trophozoites are identified at the junction of the viable and necrotic tissue.

■ **Other sites** where spread of amoebic infection may occur are peritonitis by perforation of amoebic ulcer of colon, extension to the lungs and pleura by rupture of amoebic liver abscess, haematogenous spread to cause amoebic carditis and cerebral lesions, cutaneous amoebiasis via spread of rectal amoebiasis or from anal intercourse.

MALARIA

Malaria is a protozoal disease caused by any one or combination of four species of plasmodia: *Plasmodium vivax, Plasmodium falciparum, Plasmodium ovale* and *Plasmodium malariae.* While *Plasmodium falciparum* causes malignant malaria, the other three species produce benign form of illness. These parasites are transmitted by bite of female *Anopheles* mosquito. The disease is endemic in several parts of the world, especially in tropical Africa, parts of South and Central America, India and South-East Asia.

The life cycle of plasmodia is complex and is diagrammatically depicted in Fig. 7.6,A. *P. falciparum* differs from other forms of plasmodial species in 4 respects:

i) It does not have exo-erythrocytic stage.

ii) Erythrocytes of any age are parasitised while other plasmodia parasitise juvenile red cells.

iii) One red cell may contain more than one parasite.

iv) The parasitised red cells are sticky causing obstruction of small blood vessels by thrombi, a feature which is responsible for extraordinary virulence of *P. falciparum.*

The main clinical features of malaria are cyclic peaks of high fever accompanied by chills, anaemia and splenomegaly.

PATHOLOGIC CHANGES. Parasitisation and destruction of erythrocytes are responsible for major pathologic changes as under (Fig. 7.6,B):

1. Malarial pigment liberated by destroyed red cells accumulates in the phagocytic cells of the reticuloendothelial system resulting in enlargement of the spleen and liver *(hepatosplenomegaly).*
2. In falciparum malaria, there is massive absorption of haemoglobin by the renal tubules producing *blackwater fever (haemoglobinuric nephrosis).*
3. At autopsy, *cerebral malaria* is characterised by congestion and petechiae on the white matter.
4. Parasitised erythrocytes in falciparum malaria are sticky and get attached to endothelial cells resulting in obstruction of capillaries of deep organs such as of the brain leading to hypoxia and death. If the patient lives, *microhaemorrhages* and *microinfarcts* may be seen in the brain.

The diagnosis of malaria is made by demonstration of malarial parasite in thin or thick blood films or sometimes in histologic sections (COLOUR PLATE XVII: CL 68).

FILARIASIS

Wuchereria bancrofti and *Brugia malayi* are responsible for causing Bancroftian and Malayan filariasis in different geographic regions. The lymphatic vessels inhabit the adult worm, especially in the lymph nodes, testis and epididymis. Microfilariae seen in the

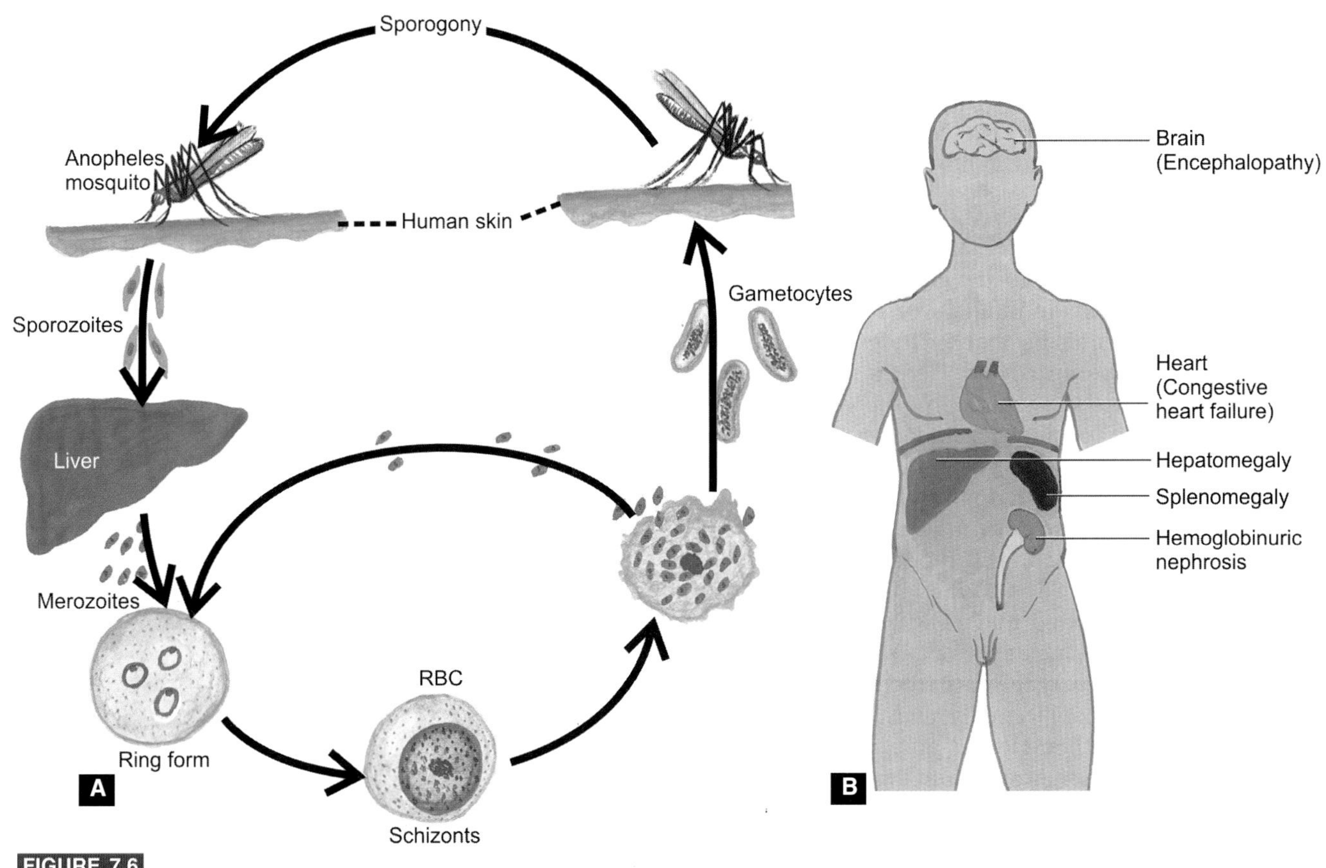

FIGURE 7.6

Life cycle of malaria (A) and major pathological changes in organs (B)

circulation are produced by the female worm. Majority of infected patients remain asymptomatic. Symptomatic cases may have two forms of disease—an acute form and a chronic form.

- *Acute form* of filariasis presents with fever, lymph-angitis, lymphadenitis, epididymo-orchitis, urticaria, eosinophilia and microfilariaemia.
- *Chronic form* of filariasis is characterised by lymph-adenopathy, lymphoedema, hydrocele and elephantiasis.

The most significant histologic changes are due to the presence of adult worms in the lymphatic vessels causing lymphatic obstruction and lymphoedema. The regional lymph nodes are enlarged and their sinuses are distended with lymph. The tissues surrounding the blocked lymphatics are infiltrated by chronic inflammatory cell infiltrate consisting of lymphocytes, histiocytes, plasma cells and eosinophils. Chronicity of the process causes enormous thickening and induration of the skin of legs and scrotum resembling the hide of an elephant and hence the name *elephantiasis*. *Chylous ascites* and *chyluria* may occur due to rupture of the abdominal lymphatics.

CYSTICERCOSIS

Cysticercosis is infection by the larval stage of *Taenia solium*, the pork tapeworm. The adult tape-worm resides in the human intestines. The eggs are passed in human faeces which are ingested by pigs or they infect vegetables. These eggs then develop into larval stages in the host, spread by blood to any site in the body and form cystic larvae termed *cysticercus cellulosae*. Human beings may acquire infection by the larval stage by eating undercooked pork ('measly pork'), by ingesting uncooked contaminated vegetables, and sometimes, by autoinfection.

PATHOLOGIC CHANGES. The cysticercus may be single or there may be multiple cysticerci in the different tissues of the body. The cysts may occur virtually anywhere in body and accordingly produce symptoms; most common sites are the brain, skeletal muscle and skin. The cysticercus consists of a round to oval white cyst, about 1 cm in diameter, contains milky fluid and invaginated scolex with birefringent hooklets. The cysticercus may remain viable for a long time and incite no inflammation. But when the embryo dies, it produces granulomatous reaction with eosinophils. Later, the lesion may become scarred and calcified (COLOUR PLATE IX: CL 34).

TORCH COMPLEX

TORCH complex refers to development of common complex of symptoms in infants due to infection with different microorganisms that include: *T*oxoplasma, *R*ubella, *C*ytomegalovirus, and *H*erpes simplex virus. The infection may be acquired by the foetus during intrauterine life, or perinatally and damage the foetus or infant. Since the symptoms produced by TORCH group of organisms are indistinguishable from each other, it is a common practice in a suspected pregnant mother or infant to test for all the four main TORCH agents.

It has been estimated that TORCH complex infections have an overall incidence of 1-5% of all live born children. All the microorganisms in the TORCH complex are transmitted transplacentally and, therefore, infect the foetus from mother. Herpes and cytomegalovirus infections are common intrapartum infections acquired venereally. An infectious mononucleosis-like disease is present in about 10% of mothers whose infants have *Toxoplasma* infection. Genital herpes infection is present in 20% of mothers whose newborn babies suffer from herpes infection. Rubella infection during acute stage in the first 10 weeks of pregnancy is more harmful to the foetus than at later stage of gestation. Symptoms of cytomegalovirus infection are present in less than 1% of mothers who display antibodies to it.

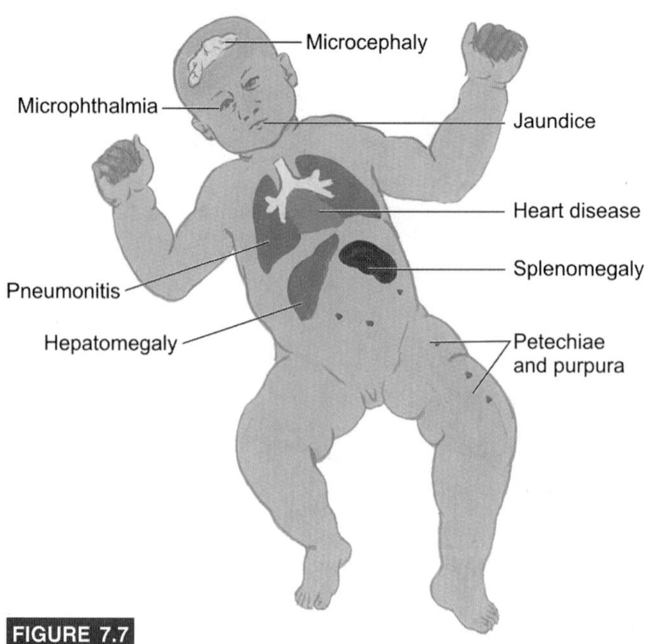

FIGURE 7.7

Lesions produced by TORCH complex infection in foetus *in utero.*

The classic features of syndrome produced by TORCH complex are seen in congenital rubella. The features include: ocular defects, cardiac defects, CNS manifestations, sensorineural deafness, thrombocytopenia and hepatosplenomegaly (Fig. 7.7).

The foetal damage caused by TORCH complex infection is irreparable and, therefore, prevention is the best mode of therapy.

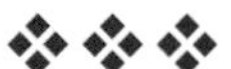

Neoplasia

8

NOMENCLATURE AND CLASSIFICATION

INTRODUCTION. The term 'neoplasia' means new growth; the new growth produced is called 'neoplasm' or 'tumour'. However, all 'new growths' are not neoplasms since examples of new growth of tissues and cells also exist in the processes of embryogenesis, regeneration and repair, hyperplasia and hormonal stimulation. The proliferation and maturation of cells in normal adults is controlled as a result of which some cells proliferate throughout life (labile cells), some have limited proliferation (stable cells), while others do not replicate (permanent cells). On the other hand, neoplastic cells lose control and regulation of replication and form an abnormal mass of tissue.

Therefore, satisfactory definition of a neoplasm or tumour is *'a mass of tissue formed as a result of abnormal, excessive, uncoordinated, autonomous and purposeless proliferation of cells'*. The branch of science dealing with the study of neoplasms or tumours is called oncology (*oncos*=tumour, *logos*=study). Neoplasms may be 'benign' when they are slow-growing and localised without causing much difficulty to the host, or 'malignant' when they proliferate rapidly, spread throughout the body and may eventually cause death of the host. The common term used for all malignant tumours is cancer. Hippocrates (460-377 BC) coined the term *karkinos* for cancer of the breast. The word 'cancer' means crab, thus reflecting the true character of cancer since 'it sticks to the part stubbornly like a crab'.

All tumours, benign as well as malignant, have 2 basic components:

- *'Parenchyma'* comprised by proliferating tumour cells; parenchyma determines the nature and evolution of the tumour.
- *'Supportive stroma'* composed of fibrous connective tissue and blood vessels; it provides the framework on which the parenchymal tumour cells grow.

The tumours derive their nomenclature on the basis of the parenchymal component comprising them. The suffix *'-oma'* is added to denote benign tumours. Malignant tumours of epithelial origin are called *carcinomas,* while malignant mesenchymal tumours are named *sarcomas* (*sarcos* = fleshy). However, some cancers are composed of highly undifferentiated cells and are referred to as *undifferentiated malignant tumours.*

Although, this broad generalisation regarding nomenclature of tumours usually holds true in majority of instances, some examples contrary to this concept are: *melanoma* for carcinoma of the melanocytes, *hepatoma* for carcinoma of the hepatocytes, *lymphoma* for malignant tumour of the lymphoid tissue, and *seminoma* for malignant tumour of the testis. *Leukaemia* is the term used for cancer of blood forming cells.

SPECIAL CATEGORIES OF TUMOURS. Following categories of tumours are examples which defy the generalisation in nomenclature given above:

1. Mixed tumours. When two types of tumours are combined in the same tumour, it is called a mixed tumour. For example:

i) *Adenosquamous carcinoma* is the combination of adenocarcinoma and squamous cell carcinoma in the endometrium.

ii) *Adenoacanthoma* is the mixture of adenocarcinoma and benign squamous elements in the endometrium.

iii) *Carcinosarcoma* is the rare combination of malignant tumour of the epithelium (carcinoma) and of mesenchymal tissue (sarcoma) such as in thyroid.

iv) *Collision tumour* is the term used for morphologically two different cancers in the same organ which do not mix with each other.

v) *Mixed tumour of the salivary gland* (or pleomorphic adenoma) is the term used for benign tumour having combination of both epithelial and mesenchymal tissue elements.

2. Teratomas. These tumours are made up of a mixture of various tissue types arising from totipotent cells derived from the three germ cell layers—ectoderm, mesoderm and endoderm. Most common sites for teratomas are ovaries and testis (*gonadal teratomas*). But they occur at *extra-gonadal sites* as well, mainly in the midline of the body such as in the head and neck region, mediastinum, retroperitoneum, sacrococcygeal region etc. Teratomas may be *benign or mature* (most of the ovarian teratomas) or *malignant or immature* (most of the testicular teratomas).

3. Blastomas. Blastomas or embryomas are a group of malignant tumours which arise from embryonal or partially differentiated cells which would normally form blastema of the organs and tissue during embryogenesis. These tumours occur more frequently in infants and children (under 5 years of age) and include some examples of tumours in this age group: neuroblastoma, nephroblastoma (Wilms' tumour), hepatoblastoma, retinoblastoma, medulloblastoma, pulmonary blastoma.

4. Hamartoma. Hamartoma is benign tumour which is made of mature but disorganised cells of tissues indigenous to the particular organ e.g. hamartoma of the lung consists of mature cartilage, mature smooth muscle and epithelium. Thus, all mature differentiated tissue elements which comprise the bronchus are present in it but are jumbled up as a mass.

5. Choristoma. Choristoma is the name given to the ectopic islands of normal tissue. Thus, choristoma is heterotopia but is not a true tumour, though it sounds like one.

CLASSIFICATION. The currently used classification of tumours is based on the histogenesis (i.e. cell of origin) and on the anticipated behaviour (Table 8.1). However, it must be mentioned here that the classification described here is only a summary. Detailed classifications of benign and malignant tumours pertaining to different tissues and body systems alongwith morphologic features of specific tumours appear in the specific chapters of Systemic Pathology later.

CHARACTERISTICS OF TUMOURS

Majority of neoplasms can be categorised clinically and morphologically into benign and malignant on the basis of certain characteristics listed below. However, there are exceptions. A small proportion of tumours have some features suggesting innocent growth while other features point towards a more ominous behaviour. Therefore, it must be borne in mind before describing characteristics of neoplasm that there is a wide variation in the degree of deviation from the normal in all the tumours.

The characteristics of tumours are described under the following headings:

I. Rate of growth
II. Clinical and gross features
III. Microscopic features
IV. Local invasion (Direct spread)
V. Metastasis (Distant spread)

Based on these characteristics, contrasting features of benign and malignant tumours are summarised in Table 8.2 and illustrated in Fig. 8.1.

I. RATE OF GROWTH

The tumour cells generally proliferate more rapidly than the normal cells. In general, benign tumours grow slowly and malignant tumours rapidly. However, there are exceptions to this generalisation. The rate at which the tumour enlarges depends upon 2 main factors:

1. Rate of division and destruction of tumour cells
2. Degree of differentiation of the tumour.

1. Rate of division and destruction of tumour cells. In general, malignant tumour cells have increased mitotic rate and slower death rate i.e. the cancer cells do not follow normal controls in cell cycle and are immortal. If the rate of cell division is high, it is likely that tumour cells in the centre of the tumour do not receive adequate nourishment and undergo ischaemic necrosis. While dead tumour cells appear as 'apoptotic figures' (Chapter 3), the dividing cells of tumours are seen as normal and abnormal 'mitotic figures' (discussed later).

TABLE 8.1: Classification of Tumours.

TISSUE OF ORIGIN	BENIGN	MALIGNANT
I. TUMOURS OF ONE PARENCHYMAL CELL TYPE		
A. Epithelial Tumours		
1. *Squamous epithelium*	Squamous cell papilloma	Squamous cell (Epidermoid) carcinoma
2. *Transitional epithelium*	Transitional cell papilloma	Transitional cell carcinoma
3. *Glandular epithelium*	Adenoma	Adenocarcinoma
4. *Basal cell layer skin*	—	Basal cell carcinoma
5. *Neuroectoderm*	Naevus	Melanoma (melanocarcinoma)
6. *Hepatocytes*	Liver cell adenoma	Hepatoma (hepatocellular carcinoma)
7. *Placenta (Chorionic epithelium)*	Hydatidiform mole	Choriocarcinoma
B. Non-epithelial (Mesenchymal) tumours		
1. *Adipose tissue*	Lipoma	Liposarcoma
2. *Adult fibrous tissue*	Fibroma	Fibrosarcoma
3. *Embryonic fibrous tissue*	Myxoma	Myxosarcoma
4. *Cartilage*	Chondroma	Chondrosarcoma
5. *Bone*	Osteoma	Osteosarcoma
6. *Synovium*	Benign synovioma	Synovial sarcoma
7. *Smooth muscle*	Leiomyoma	Leiomyosarcoma
8. *Skeletal muscle*	Rhabdomyoma	Rhabdomyosarcoma
9. *Mesothelium*	—	Mesothelioma
10. *Blood vessels*	Haemangioma	Angiosarcoma
11. *Lymph vessels*	Lymphangioma	Lymphangiosarcoma
12. *Glomus*	Glomus tumour	—
13. *Meninges*	Meningioma	Invasive meningioma
14. *Haematopoietic cells*	—	Leukaemias
15. *Lymphoid tissue*	Pseudolymphoma	Malignant lymphomas
16. *Nerve sheath*	Neurilemmoma, Neurofibroma	Neurogenic sarcoma
17. *Nerve cells*	Ganglioneuroma	Neuroblastoma
II. MIXED TUMOURS		
Salivary glands	Pleomorphic adenoma (mixed salivary tumour)	Malignant mixed salivary tumour
III. TUMOURS OF MORE THAN ONE GERM CELL LAYER		
Totipotent cells in gonads or in embryonal rests	Mature teratoma	Immature teratoma

2. Degree of differentiation. Secondly, the rate of growth of malignant tumour is directly proportionate to the degree of differentiation. Poorly differentiated tumours show aggressive growth pattern as compared to better differentiated tumours. Some tumours, after a period of slow growth, may suddenly show spurt in their growth due to development of an aggressive clone of malignant cells. On the other hand, some tumours may cease to grow after sometime. Rarely, a malignant tumour may disappear spontaneously from the primary site, possibly due to necrosis caused by good host immune attack, only to reappear as secondaries elsewhere in the body e.g. choriocarcinoma, malignant melanoma.

The regulation of tumour growth is under the control of growth factors secreted by the tumour cells. Out of various growth factors, important ones modulating tumour biology are listed below and discussed later:

i) Epidermal growth factor (EGF)
ii) Fibroblast growth factor (FGF)
iii) Platelet-derived growth factor (PDGF)
iv) Colony stimulating factor (CSF)
v) Transforming growth factors-β (TGF-β)
vi) Interleukins (IL).

TABLE 8.2: Contrasting Features of Benign and Malignant Tumours.

FEATURES	BENIGN	MALIGNANT
I. CLINICAL AND GROSS FEATURES		
1. ***Boundaries***	Encapsulated or well-circumscribed	Poorly-circumscribed and irregular
2. ***Surrounding tissue***	Often compressed	Usually invaded
3. ***Size***	Usually small	Often larger
4. ***Secondary changes***	Occur less often	Occur more often
II. MICROSCOPIC FEATURES		
1. ***Pattern***	Usually resembles the tissue of origin closely	Often poor resemblance to tissue of origin
2. ***Basal polarity***	Retained	Often lost
3. ***Pleomorphism***	Usually not present	Often present
4. ***Nucleo-cytoplasmic ratio***	Normal	Increased
5. ***Anisonucleosis***	Absent	Generally present
6. ***Hyperchromatism***	Absent	Often present
7. ***Mitoses***	May be present but are always typical mitoses	Mitotic figures increased and are generally atypical and abnormal
8. ***Tumour giant cells***	May be present but without nuclear atypia	Present with nuclear atypia
9. ***Chromosomal abnormalities***	Infrequent	Invariably present
10. ***Function***	Usually well maintained	May be retained, lost or become abnormal
III. GROWTH RATE	Usually slow	Usually rapid
IV. LOCAL INVASION	Often compresses the surrounding tissues without invading or infiltrating them	Usually infiltrates and invades the adjacent tissues
V. METASTASIS	Absent	Frequently present
VI. PROGNOSIS	Local complications	Death by local and metastatic complications

Chapter Eight

II. CLINICAL AND GROSS FEATURES

Clinically, benign tumours are generally slow growing, and depending upon the location, may remain asymptomatic (e.g. subcutaneous lipoma), or may produce serious symptoms (e.g. meningioma in the nervous system). On the other hand, malignant tumours grow rapidly, may ulcerate on the surface, invade locally into deeper tissues, may spread to distant sites (metastasis), and also produce systemic features such as weight loss, anorexia and anemia. In fact, two of the cardinal clinical features of malignant tumours are: *invasiveness and metastasis.*

The gross appearance of benign and malignant tumours may be quite variable and the features may not be diagnostic on the basis of gross appearance alone. However, certain distinctive features characterise almost all tumours—they have a different colour, texture and consistency as compared to the surrounding tissue of origin. Gross terms such as papillary, fungating, infiltrating, haemorrhagic, ulcerative and cystic are used to describe the macroscopic appearance of the tumours.

- *Benign tumours* are generally spherical or ovoid in shape. They are encapsulated or well-circumscribed, freely movable, more often firm and uniform, unless secondary changes like haemorrhage or infarction supervene (Fig. 8.1,A, E).
- *Malignant tumours,* on the other hand, are usually irregular in shape, poorly-circumscribed and extend into the adjacent tissues. Secondary changes like haemorrhage, infarction and ulceration are seen more often. Sarcomas typically have fish-flesh like consistency while carcinomas are generally firm (Fig. 8.1,C, G).

III. MICROSCOPIC FEATURES

For recognising and classifying the tumours, the microscopic characteristics of tumour cells are of greatest importance. These features which are appreciated in histologic sections are as under:

1. microscopic pattern;
2. cytomorphology of neoplastic cells (differentiation and anaplasia);
3. tumour angiogenesis and stroma; and
4. inflammatory reaction.

BENIGN | MALIGNANT

EPITHELIAL

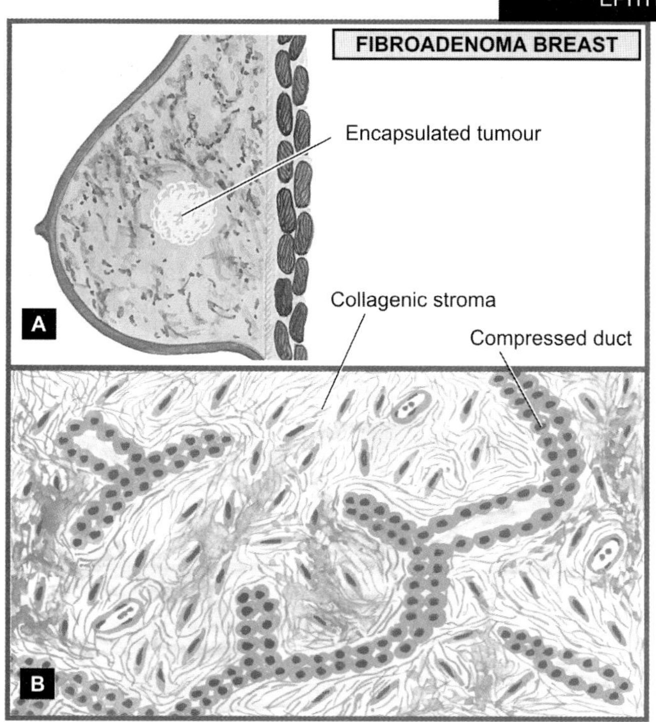

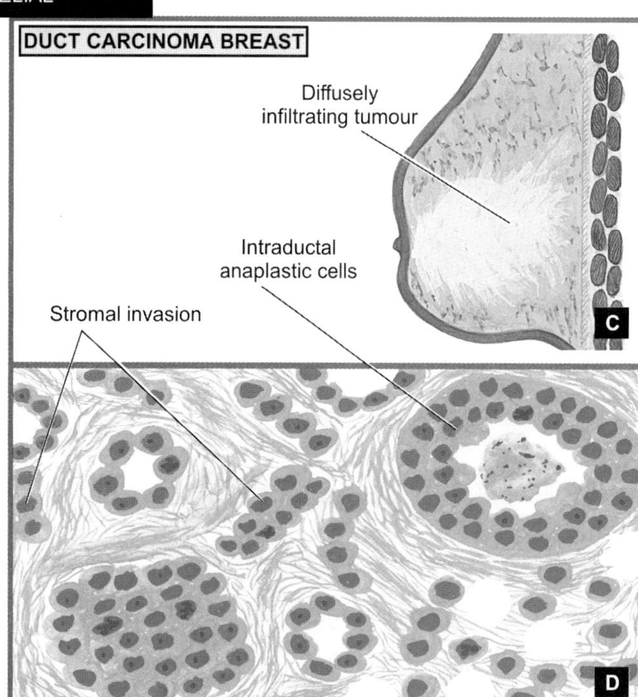

MESENCHYMAL

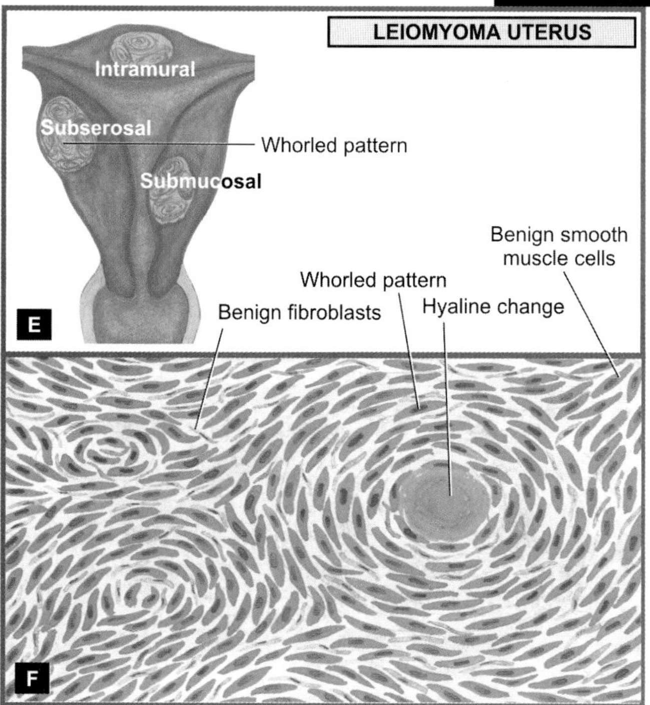

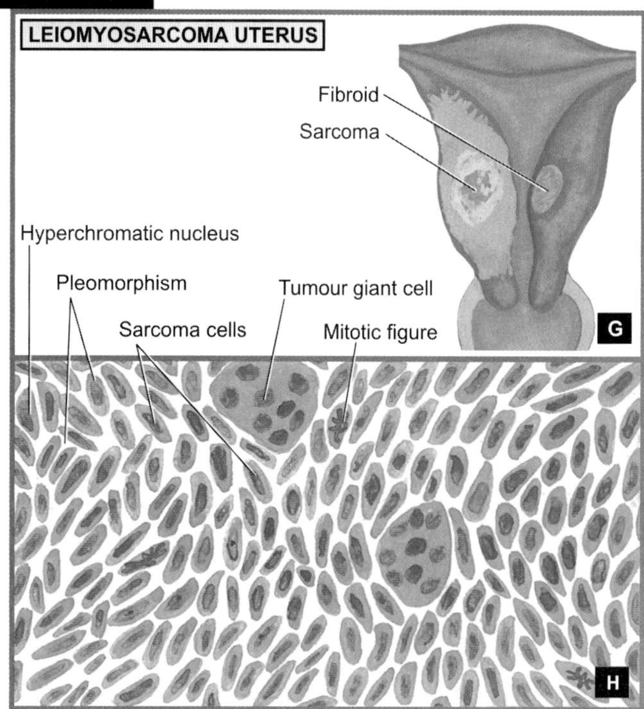

FIGURE 8.1

Gross and microscopic features of prototypes of benign *(left)* and malignant *(right)* tumours.

1. Microscopic Pattern

The tumour cells may be arranged in a variety of patterns in different tumours as under:

- The *epithelial tumours* generally consist of acini, sheets, columns or cords of epithelial tumour cells that may be arranged in solid or papillary pattern (Fig. 8.1,B, D).
- The *mesenchymal tumours* have mesenchymal tumour cells arranged as interlacing bundles, fasicles or whorls, lying separated from each other usually by the intercellular matrix substance such as hyaline material in leiomyoma (Fig. 8.1,E), cartilaginous matrix in chondroma, osteoid in osteosarcoma, reticulin network in soft tissue sarcomas etc (Fig. 8.1,H).
- Certain tumours have *mixed patterns* e.g. teratoma arising from totipotent cells, pleomorphic adenoma of salivary gland (mixed salivary tumour), fibroadenoma of the breast, carcinosarcoma of the uterus and various other combinations of tumour types.
- *Haematopoietic tumours* such as leukaemias and lymphomas often have none or little stromal support.
- Generally, most benign tumours and low grade malignant tumours *reduplicate* the normal structure of origin more closely so that there is little difficulty in identifying and classifying such tumours (Fig. 8.1,B, F). However, anaplastic tumours differ greatly from the arrangement in normal tissue of origin of the tumour and may occasionally pose problems in classifying the tumour.

Chapter Eight

2. Cytomorphology of Neoplastic Cells (Differentiation and Anaplasia)

The neoplastic cell is characterised by morphologic and functional alterations, the most significant of which are *'differentiation' and 'anaplasia'*.

- **Differentiation** is defined as the extent of morphological and functional resemblance of parenchymal tumour cells to corresponding normal cells. If the deviation of neoplastic cell in structure and function is minimal as compared to normal cell, the tumour is described as *'well-differentiated'* such as most benign and low-grade malignant tumours. *'Poorly differentiated'*, *'undifferentiated'* or *'dedifferentiated'* are synonymous terms for poor structural and functional resemblance to corresponding normal cell.
- **Anaplasia** is lack of differentiation and is a characteristic feature of most malignant tumours. Depending upon the degree of differentiation, the extent of anaplasia is also variable i.e. poorly differentiated malignant tumours have high degree of anaplasia.

As a result of anaplasia, noticeable morphological and functional alterations in the neoplastic cells are observed. These are considered below and are diagrammatically illustrated in Fig. 8.2 (COLOUR PLATE XII: CL 46):

i) Loss of polarity. Normally, the nuclei of epithelial cells are oriented along the basement membrane which is termed as basal polarity. This property is based on cell adhesion molecules, particularly selectins. Early in malignancy, tumour cells lose their basal polarity so that the nuclei tend to lie away from the basement membrane.

ii) Pleomorphism. The term pleomorphism means variation in size and shape of the tumour cells. The extent of cellular pleomorphism generally correlates with the degree of anaplasia. Tumour cells are often bigger than normal but in some tumours they can be of normal size or smaller than normal.

iii) N:C ratio. Generally, the nuclei of malignant tumour cells show more conspicuous changes. Nuclei are enlarged disproportionate to the cell size so that the nucleocytoplasmic ratio is increased from normal 1:5 to 1:1.

iv) Anisonucleosis. Just like cellular pleomorphism, the nuclei too, show variation in size and shape in malignant tumour cells.

v) Hyperchromatism. Characteristically, the nuclear chromatin of malignant cell is increased and coarsely clumped. This is due to increase in the amount of nucleoprotein resulting in dark-staining nuclei, referred to as hyperchromatism. Nuclear shape may vary, nuclear membrane may be irregular and nuclear chromatin is clumped along the nuclear membrane.

vi) Nucleolar changes. Malignant cells frequently have a prominent nucleolus or nucleoli in the nucleus reflecting increased nucleoprotein synthesis. This may be demonstrated as Nucleolar Organiser Region (NOR) by silver (Ag) staining called AgNOR material.

vii) Mitotic figures. The parenchymal cells of poorly-differentiated tumours often show large number of mitoses as compared with benign tumours and well-differentiated malignant tumours. As stated above, these appear as either normal or abnormal mitotic figures.

- *Normal mitotic figures* may be seen in some non-neoplastic proliferating cells (e.g. haematopoietic cells of the bone marrow, intestinal epithelium, hepatocytes etc), in certain benign tumours and some low grade malignant tumours; in sections they are seen as a dark

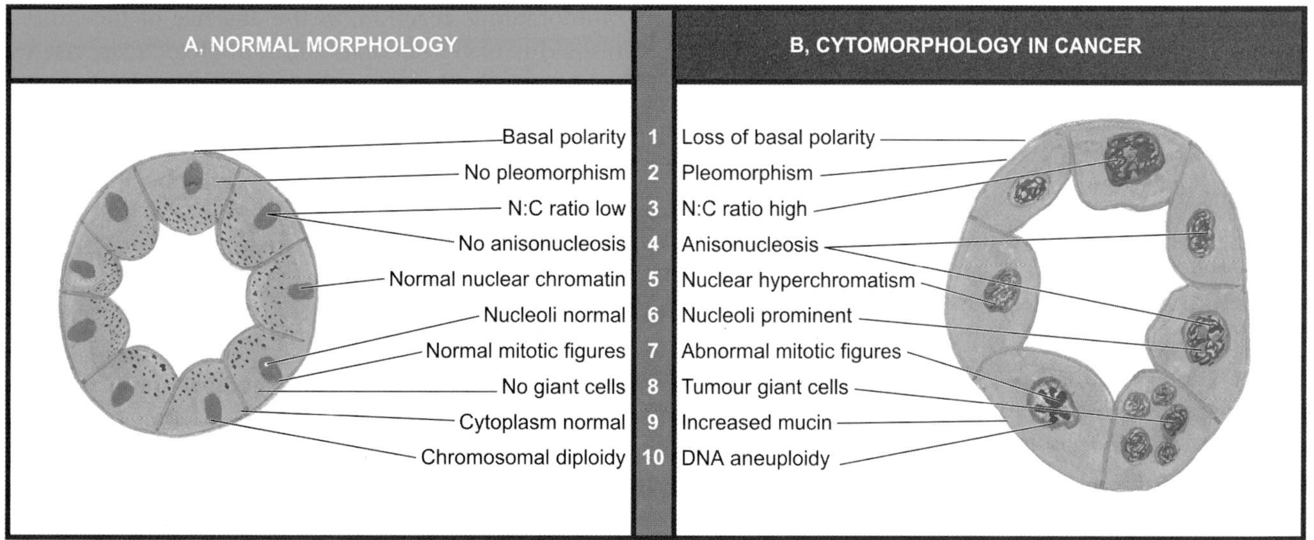

FIGURE 8.2

Diagrammatic representation of cytomorphologic features of neoplastic cells. Characteristics of cancer (B) in a gland are contrasted with the appearance of a normal mucous gland (A).

band of dividing chromatin at two poles of the nuclear spindle.

■ *Abnormal or atypical mitotic figures* are more important in malignant tumours and are identified as tripolar, quadripolar and multipolar spindles in malignant tumour cells.

viii) Tumour giant cells. Multinucleate tumour giant cells or giant cells containing a single large and bizarre nucleus, possessing nuclear characters of the adjacent tumour cells, are another important feature of anaplasia in malignant tumours.

ix) Functional (Cytoplasmic) changes. Structural anaplasia in tumours is accompanied with functional anaplasia as appreciated from the cytoplasmic constituents of the tumour cells. The functional abnormality in neoplasms may be quantitative, qualitative, or both.

■ Generally, benign tumours and better-differentiated malignant tumours continue to function well qualitatively, though there may be *quantitative* abnormality in the product e.g. large or small amount of collagen produced by benign tumours of fibrous tissue, keratin formation in well-differentiated squamous cell carcinoma. In more anaplastic tumours, there is usually quantitative fall in the product made by the tumour cells e.g. absence of keratin in anaplastic squamous cell carcinoma.

■ There may be both *qualitative and quantitative* abnormality of the cellular function in some anaplastic tumours e.g. multiple myeloma producing abnormal immunoglobulin in large quantities.

■ Endocrine tumours may cause excessive hormone production leading to characteristic clinical syndromes. Besides the production of hormones by endocrine tumours, hormones or hormone-like substances may be produced by certain tumours quite unrelated to the endocrine glands. This property of tumours is called *ectopic hormone production* e.g. oat cell carcinoma of the lung can secrete ACTH and ADH; less often it may produce gonadotropin, thyrotropin, parathormone, calcitonin and growth hormone. Ectopic erythropoietin may be produced by carcinoma of kidneys, hepatocellular carcinoma and cerebellar haemangioblastoma.

x) Chromosomal abnormalities. All tumour cells have abnormal genetic composition and on division they transmit the genetic abnormality to their progeny. The chromosomal abnormalities are more marked in more malignant tumours which include deviations in both morphology and number of chromosomes. Most malignant tumours show *DNA aneuploidy*, often in the form of an increase in the number of chromosomes, reflected morphologically by the increase in the size of nuclei.

One of the most important examples of a consistent chromosomal abnormality in human malignancy is the presence of Philadelphia chromosome (named after the city in which it was first described) in 95% cases of chronic myeloid leukaemia. In this, part of the long arm of chromosome 9 is translocated to part of the long arm of chromosome 22 (t 9; 22). Other examples of neoplasms showing chromosomal abnormalities are Burkitt's lymphoma, acute lymphoid leukaemia, multiple myeloma, retinoblastoma, oat cell carcinoma, Wilms' tumour etc.

3. Tumour Angiogenesis and Stroma

The connective tissue alongwith its vascular network forms the supportive framework on which the parenchymal tumour cells grow and receive nourishment. In addition to variable amount of connective tissue and vascularity, the stroma may have nerves and metaplastic bone or cartilage but no lymphatics.

TUMOUR ANGIOGENESIS. In order to provide nourishment to growing tumour, new blood vessels are formed from pre-existing ones (angiogenesis). How this takes place is discussed later under molecular pathogenesis of cancer. However, related morphologic features are as under:

i) Microvascular density. The new capillaries add to the vascular density of the tumour which has been used as a marker to assess the rate of growth of tumours and hence grade the tumours. This is done by counting microvascular density in the section of the tumour.

ii) Central necrosis. However, if the tumour outgrows its blood supply as occurs in rapidly growing tumours or tumour angiogenesis fails, its core undergoes ischaemic necrosis.

TUMOUR STROMA. The collagenous tissue in the stroma may be scanty or excessive. In the former case, the tumour is soft and fleshy (e.g. in sarcomas, lymphomas), while in the latter case the tumour is hard and gritty (e.g. infiltrating duct carcinoma breast). Growth of fibrous tissue in tumour is stimulated by basic fibroblast growth factor (bFGF) elaborated by tumour cells.

- If the epithelial tumour is almost entirely composed of parenchymal cells, it is called *medullary* e.g. medullary carcinoma of the breast, medullary carcinoma of the thyroid.
- If there is excessive connective tissue stroma in the epithelial tumour, it is referred to as *desmoplasia* and the tumour is hard or *scirrhous* e.g. infiltrating duct carcinoma breast, linitis plastica of the stomach.

4. Inflammatory Reaction

At times, prominent inflammatory reaction is present in and around the tumours. It could be the result of ulceration in the cancer when there is secondary infection. The inflammatory reaction in such instances may be acute or chronic. However, some tumours show chronic inflammatory reaction, chiefly of lymphocytes, plasma cells and macrophages, and in some instances granulomatous reaction, in the absence of ulceration. This is due to cell-mediated immunologic response by the host in an attempt to destroy the tumour. In some cases, such an immune response improves the prognosis.

The *examples* of such reaction are: seminoma testis, malignant melanoma of the skin, lymphoepithelioma of the throat, medullary carcinoma of the breast, choriocarcinoma, Warthin's tumour of salivary glands etc.

IV. LOCAL INVASION (DIRECT SPREAD)

BENIGN TUMOURS. Most benign tumours form encapsulated or circumscribed masses that *expand and push aside* the surrounding normal tissues without actually invading, infiltrating or metastasising.

MALIGNANT TUMOURS. Malignant tumours also enlarge by expansion and some well-differentiated tumours may be partially encapsulated as well e.g. follicular carcinoma thyroid. But characteristically, they are distinguished from benign tumours by *invasion, infiltration and destruction* of the surrounding tissue, besides distant metastasis (described below). In general, tumours invade via the route of least resistance, though eventually most cancers recognise no anatomic boundaries. Often, cancers extend through tissue spaces, permeate lymphatics, blood vessels, perineural spaces and may penetrate a bone by growing through nutrient foramina. More commonly, the tumours invade thin-walled capillaries and veins than thick-walled arteries. Dense compact collagen, elastic tissue and cartilage are some of the tissues which are sufficiently resistant to invasion by tumours.

Mechanism of invasion of malignant tumours is discussed together with that of metastasis below.

V. METASTASIS (DISTANT SPREAD)

Metastasis (*meta* = transformation, *stasis* = residence) is defined as spread of tumour by invasion in such a way that discontinuous secondary tumour mass/masses are formed at the site of lodgement. *Metastasis and invasiveness are the two most important features to distinguish malignant from benign tumours.* Benign tumours do not metastasise while all the malignant tumours with a few exceptions like gliomas of the central nervous system and basal cell carcinoma of the skin, can metastasise. Generally, larger, more aggressive and rapidly-growing tumours are more likely to metastasise but there are numerous exceptions. About one third of malignant tumours at presentation have evident metastatic deposits while another 20% have occult metastasis.

Routes of Metastasis

Cancers may spread to distant sites by following pathways:

1. Lymphatic spread
2. Haematogenous spread
3. Other routes (Transcoelomic spread along epithelium-lined surfaces, spread via cerebrospinal fluid, implantation).

1. LYMPHATIC SPREAD. *In general, carcinomas metastasise by lymphatic route while sarcomas favour haematogenous route.* However, sarcomas may also spread by lymphatic pathway. The involvement of lymph nodes by malignant cells may be of two forms:

i) Lymphatic permeation. The walls of lymphatics are readily invaded by cancer cells and may form a continuous growth in the lymphatic channels called lymphatic permeation.

ii) Lymphatic emboli. Alternatively, the malignant cells may detach to form tumour emboli so as to be carried along the lymph to the next draining lymph node. The tumour emboli enter the lymph node at its convex surface and are lodged in the subcapsular sinus where they start growing (Fig. 8.3,C) (COLOUR PLATE XII: CL 47). Later, of course, the whole lymph node may be replaced and enlarged by the metastatic tumour.

■ Generally, regional lymph nodes draining the tumour are invariably involved producing *regional nodal metastasis* e.g. from carcinoma breast to axillary lymph nodes, from carcinoma thyroid to lateral cervical lymph nodes, bronchogenic carcinoma to hilar and para-tracheal lymph nodes etc (Fig. 8.3,A, B).

■ However, all regional nodal enlargements are not due to nodal metastasis because necrotic products of tumour and antigens may also incite regional lymphadenitis of *sinus histiocytosis.*

■ Sometimes lymphatic metastases do not develop first in the lymph node nearest to the tumour because of venous-lymphatic anastomoses or due to obliteration of lymphatics by inflammation or radiation, so called *skip metastasis.*

■ Other times, due to obstruction of the lymphatics by tumour cells, the lymph flow is disturbed and tumour cells spread against the flow of lymph causing *retrograde metastases* at unusual sites e.g. metastasis of carcinoma prostate to the supraclavicular lymph nodes, metastatic deposits from bronchogenic carcinoma to the axillary lymph nodes.

■ *Virchow's lymph node* is nodal metastasis preferentially to supraclavicular lymph node from cancers of abdominal organs e.g. cancer stomach, colon, and gall bladder.

It is believed that lymph nodes in the vicinity of tumour perform multiple roles—as initial barrier filter, and in destruction of tumour cells, while later provide fertile soil for growth of tumour cells.

Mechanism of lymphatic route of metastasis is discussed later under biology of invasion and metastasis.

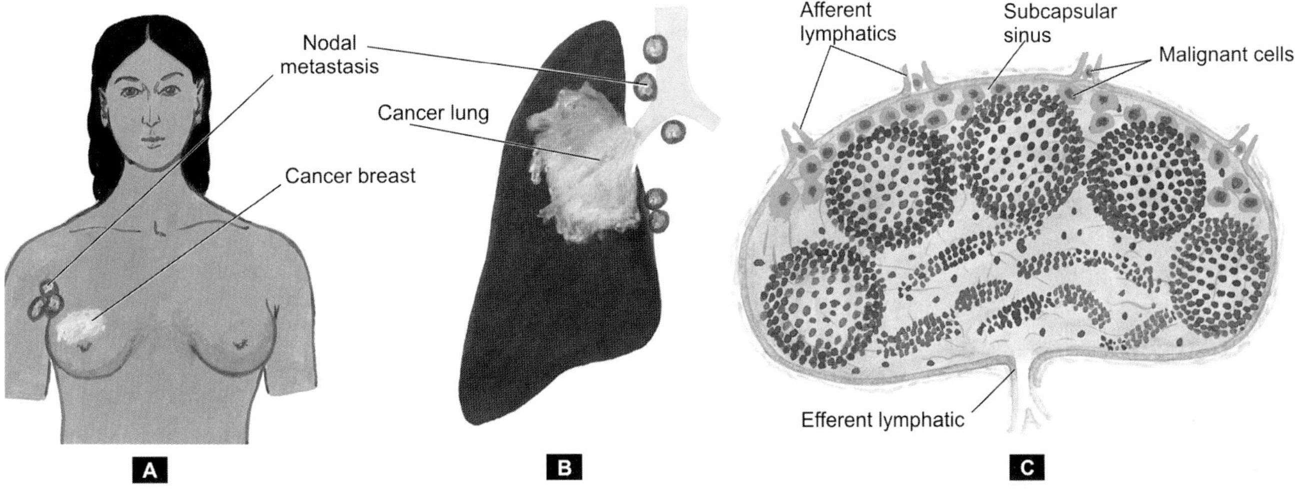

FIGURE 8.3

Regional nodal metastasis. A, Axillary nodes involved by carcinoma breast. B, Hilar and para-tracheal lymph nodes involved by bronchogenic carcinoma. C, Lymphatic spread begins by lodgement of tumour cells in subcapsular sinus via afferent lymphatics entering at the convex surface of the lymph node.

2. HAEMATOGENOUS SPREAD. *Blood-borne metastasis is the common route for sarcomas but certain carcinomas also frequently metastasise by this mode,* especially those of the lung, breast, thyroid, kidney, liver, prostate and ovary. The common sites for blood-borne metastasis are: the liver, lungs, brain, bones, kidney and adrenals, all of which provide 'good soil' for the growth of 'good seeds' (*seed-soil theory*). However, a few organs such as spleen, heart, skeletal muscle do not allow tumour metastasis to grow. Spleen is unfavourable site due to open sinusoidal pattern which does not permit tumour cells to stay there long enough to produce metastasis. In general, only a proportion of cancer cells are capable of clonal proliferation in the proper environment; others die without establishing a metastasis.

- *Systemic veins* drain blood into vena cavae from limbs, head and neck and pelvis. Therefore, cancers of these sites more often metastasise to the lungs (COLOUR PLATE XII: CL 48).
- *Portal veins* drain blood from the bowel, spleen and pancreas into the liver. Thus, tumours of these organs frequently have secondaries in the liver.
- *Arterial spread* of tumours is less likely because they are thick-walled and contain elastic tissue which is resistant to invasion. Nevertheless, arterial spread may occur when tumour cells pass through pulmonary capillary bed or through pulmonary arterial branches which have thin walls. Cancer of the lung may metastasise by pulmonary arterial route to kidneys, adrenals, bones, brain etc.
- *Retrograde spread* by blood route may occur at unusual sites due to retrograde spread after venous obstruction, just as with lymphatic metastases. Important examples are vertebral metastases in cancers of the thyroid and prostate.

Macroscopically, blood-borne metastases in an organ appear as multiple, rounded nodules of varying size, scattered throughout the organ (Fig. 8.4). Sometimes, the metastasis may grow bigger than the primary tumour. At times, metastatic deposits may come to attention first without an evident primary tumour. In such cases search for primary tumour may be rewarding, but rarely the primary tumour may remain undetected or occult. Metastatic deposits just like primary tumour may cause further dissemination via lymphatics and blood vessels.

Microscopically, the secondary deposits generally reproduce the structure of primary tumour. However, the same primary tumour on metastasis at diferent sites may show varying grades of differentiation, apparently due to the influence of local environment surrounding the tumour for its growth.

3. SPREAD ALONG BODY CAVITIES AND NATURAL PASSAGES. Uncommonly, some cancers may spread by *seeding* at other surfaces. These routes of distant spread are as under:

i) Transcoelomic spread. Certain cancers invade through the serosal wall of the coelomic cavity so that tumour fragments or clusters of tumour cells break off to be carried in the coelomic fluid and are implanted elsewhere in the body cavity. Peritoneal cavity is involved most often, but occasionally pleural and pericardial cavities are also affected. Examples of transcoelomic spread are:

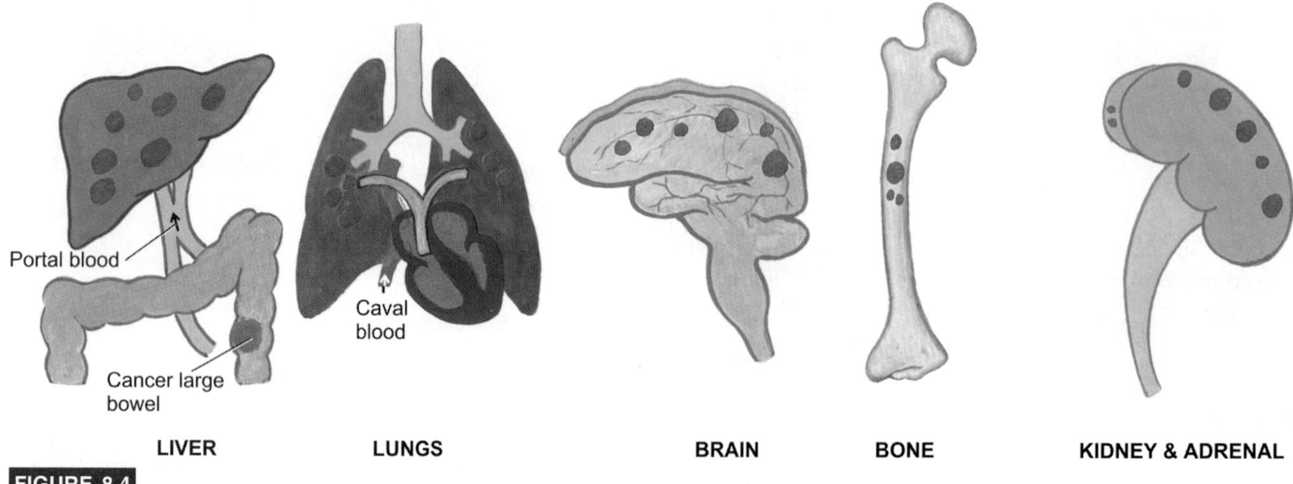

FIGURE 8.4

Gross appearance of haematogenous metastases at common sites.

a) carcinoma of the stomach seeding to both ovaries (Krukenberg tumour);

b) carcinoma of the ovary spreading to the entire peritoneal cavity without infiltrating the underlying organs;

c) pseudomyxoma peritonei is the gelatinous coating of the peritoneum from mucin-secreting carcinoma of the ovary or apppendix; and

d) carcinoma of the bronchus and breast seeding to the pleura and pericardium.

ii) Spread along epithelium-lined surfaces. It is unusual for a malignant tumour to spread along the epithelium-lined surfaces because intact epithelium and mucus coat are quite resistant to penetration by tumour cells. However, exceptionally a malignant tumour may spread through:

a) the fallopian tube from the endometrium to the ovaries or *vice-versa;*

b) through the bronchus into alveoli; and

c) through the ureters from the kidneys into lower urinary tract.

iii) Spread via cerebrospinal fluid. Malignant tumour of the ependyma and leptomeninges may spread by release of tumour fragments and tumour cells into the CSF and produce metastases at other sites in the central nervous system.

iv) Implantation. Rarely, a tumour may spread by implantation by surgeon's scalpel, needles, sutures, or may be implanted by direct contact such as transfer of cancer of the lower lip to the apposing upper lip.

MECHANISM AND BIOLOGY OF INVASION AND METASTASIS

The process of local invasion and distant spread (by lymphatic and haematogenous routes) discussed above involves passage through barriers before gaining access to the vascular lumen. This includes making the passage by the cancer cells by dissolution of extracellular matrix (ECM) at three levels— at the basement membrane of tumour itself, at the level of interstitial connective tissue, and at the basement membrane of microvasculature. The following steps are involved at the cell molecular level which are schematically illustrated in Fig. 8.5.

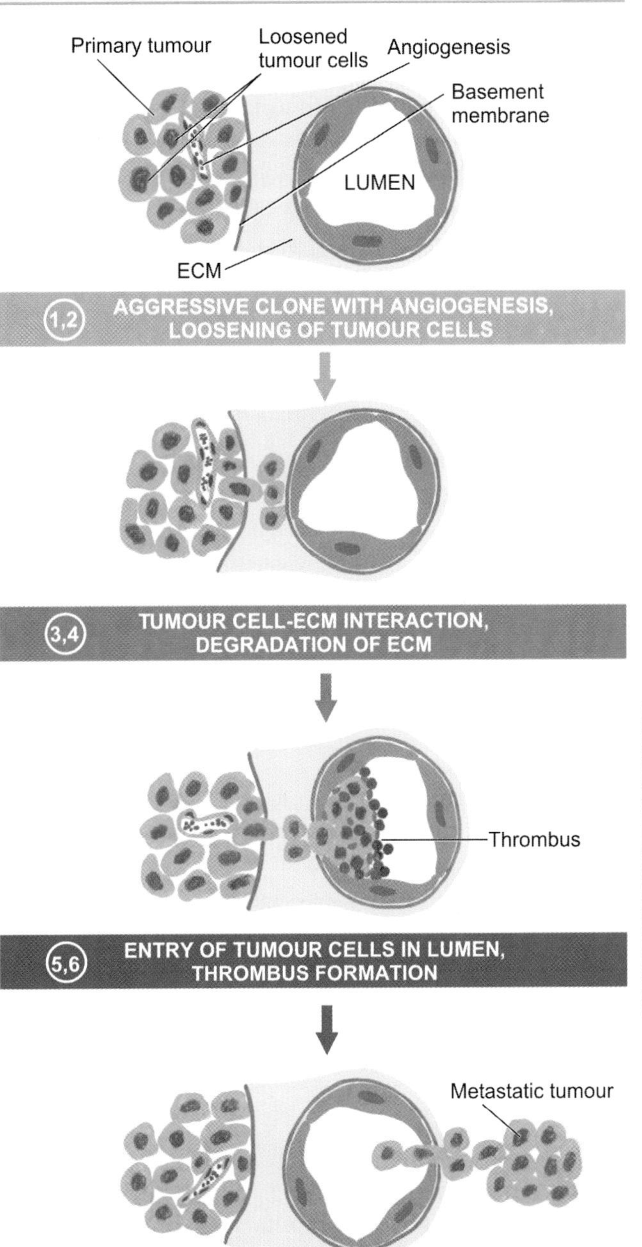

FIGURE 8.5

Mechanism and biology of local invasion and metastasis. The serial numbers in the figure correspond to their description in the text.

1. Aggressive clonal proliferation and angiogenesis. The first step in the spread of cancer cells is the development of rapidly proliferating clone of cancer cells. This is explained on the basis of *tumour heterogeneity*, i.e. in the population of monoclonal tumour cells, a subpopulation or clone of tumour cells has the right biologic characteristics to complete the steps involved in the development of metastasis. Tumour angiogenesis plays a very significant role in metastasis since the new vessels formed as part of growing tumour are more vulnerable to invasion because these evolving vessels are directly in contact with cancer cells.

2. Tumour cell loosening. Normal cells remain glued to each other due to presence of cell adhesion molecules (CAMs), E (epithelial)-cadherin. In epithelial cancers there is either loss or inactivation of E-cadherin and also other CAMs of immunoglobulin superfamily, all of which results in loosening of cancer cells.

3. Tumour cell-ECM interaction. Loosened cancer cells now are attached to ECM proteins, mainly *laminin* and *fibronectin*. This attachment is facilitated due to profoundness of receptors on the cancer cells for both these proteins. There is also loss of *integrins*, the transmembrane receptors, further favouring invasion.

4. Degradation of ECM. Tumour cells overexpress *proteases* and matrix-degrading enzymes, *metalloproteinases* that includes collagenases and gelatinase, while the inhibitors of metalloproteinases are decreased. Another protease, cathepsin D, is also increased in certain cancers. These enzymes bring about dissolution of ECM—firstly basement membrane of tumour itself, then make way for tumour cells through the interstitial matrix, and finally dissolve the basement membrane of the vessel wall.

5. Entry of tumour cells into capillary lumen. The tumour cells after degrading the basement membrane are ready to migrate into lumen of capillaries or venules for which the following mechanisms play a role:

i) *Autocrine motility factor (AMF)* is a cytokine derived from tumour cells and stimulates receptor-mediated motility of tumour cells.

ii) *Cleavage products of matrix components* which are formed following degradation of ECM have properties of tumour cell chemotaxis, growth promotion and angiogenesis in the cancer.

After the malignant cells have migrated through the breached basement membrane, these cells enter the lumen of lymphatic and capillary channels.

6. Thrombus formation. The tumour cells protruding in the lumen of the capillary are now covered with constituents of the circulating blood and form the thrombus. Thrombus provides nourishment to the tumour cells and also protects them from the immune attack by the circulating host cells. In fact, normally a large number of tumour cells are released into ciculation but they are attacked by the host immune cells. Actually a very small proportion of malignant cells (less than 0.1%) in the blood stream survive to develop into metastasis.

7. Extravasation of tumour cells. Tumour cells in the circulation (capillaries, venules, lymphatics) may mechanically block these vascular channels and attach to vascular endothelium. In this way, the sequence similar to local invasion is repeated and the basement membrane in exposed.

8. Survival and growth of metastatic deposit. The extravasated malignant cells on lodgement in the right environment grow further under the influence of growth factors produced by host tissues, tumour cells and by cleavage products of matrix components. These growth factors in particular include: PDGF, FGF, TGF-β and VEGF. The metastatic deposits grow further if the host immune defense mechanism fails to eliminate it. Metastatic deposits may further metastasise to the same organ or to other sites by forming emboli.

PROGNOSTIC MARKERS

Metastasis is a common event in malignant tumours which greatly reduces the survival of patient. In the biology of tumour, metastasis is a form of unusual cell differentiation in which the tumour cells form disorderly masses at ectopic sites and start growing there. This random phenomenon takes place in a stepwise manner involving only a subpopulation of tumour cells selectively. The process is governed by *inappropriate expression of genes which normally partake in physiologic processes* i.e. it is a genetically programmed phenomenon.

Recent evidence has shown that in metastatic tumours, survival of host is correlated with some clinical and molecular features of tumours which act as *prognostic markers*. These are as under:

i) Clinical prognostic markers: Size, grade, vascular invasion and nodal involvement by the tumour.

ii) Molecular prognostic markers: Molecular markers indicative of poor prognosis in certain specific tumours are:

a) expression of an oncogene by tumour cells *(C-met)*;
b) CD 44 molecule;
c) oestrogen receptors;
d) epidermal growth factor receptor;
e) angiogenesis factors and degree of neovascularisation; and
f) expression of *m*etastasis *a*ssociated *g*ene or *n*ucleic *a*cid (MAGNA) in the DNA fragment in metastasising tumour.

GRADING AND STAGING OF CANCER

'Grading' and 'staging' are the two systems to determine the prognosis and choice of treatment after a malignant tumour is detected. *Grading is defined as the macroscopic and microscopic degree of differentiation of the tumour, while staging means extent of spread of the tumour within the patient.*

Grading

Cancers may be graded grossly and microscopically. Gross features like exophytic or fungating appearance are indicative of less malignant growth than diffusely infiltrating tumours. However, grading is largely based on 2 important histologic features: *the degree of anaplasia, and the rate of growth.* Based on these features, cancers are categorised from grade I as the most differentiated, to grade III or IV as the most undifferentiated or anaplastic. Many systems of grading have been proposed but the one described by *Broders* for dividing squamous cell carcinoma into 4 grades depending upon the degree of differentiation is followed for other malignant tumours as well. *Broders' grading* is as under:

Grade I: Well-differentiated (less than 25% anaplastic cells).

Grade II: Moderately-differentiated (25-50% anaplastic cells).

Grade III: Moderately-differentiated (50-75% anaplastic cells).

Grade IV: Poorly-differentiated or anaplastic (more than 75% anaplastic cells).

However, grading of tumours has several shortcomings. It is subjective and the degree of differentiation may vary from one area of tumour to the other. Therefore, it is common practice with pathologists to grade cancers in descriptive terms (e.g. well-differentiated, undifferentiated, keratinising, non-keratinising etc) rather than giving the tumours grade numbers.

Staging

The extent of spread of cancers can be assessed by 3 ways—by clinical examination, by investigations, and by pathologic examination of the tissue removed. Two important staging systems currently followed are: TNM staging and AJC staging.

TNM staging. (T for primary *t*umour, N for regional *n*odal involvement, and M for distant *m*etastases) was developed by the UICC (Union Internationale Contre Cancer, Geneva). For each of the 3 components namely T, N and M, numbers are added to indicate the extent of involvement, as under:

T_0 *to* T_4: *In situ* lesion to largest and most extensive primary tumour.

N_0 *to* N_3: No nodal involvement to widespread lymph node involvement.

M_0 *to* M_2: No metastasis to disseminated haematogenous metastases.

AJC staging. (American Joint Committee staging) divides all cancers into stage 0 to IV, and takes into account all the 3 components of the preceding system (primary tumour, nodal involvement and distant metastases) in each stage.

TNM and AJC staging systems can be applied for staging most malignant tumours.

EPIDEMIOLOGY AND PREDISPOSITIONTO NEOPLASIA

CANCER INCIDENCE

The overall incidence of cancer in a population or country is known by registration of all cancer cases (cancer registry) and by rate of death from cancer. Worldwide, it is estimated that about 20% of all deaths are cancer-related. There have been changing patterns in incidence of cancers in both the sexes and in different geographic locations as outlined below. Table 8.3 shows worldwide incidence (in decending order) of different forms of cancer in men, women, and children. As evident from the Table, some types of cancers are commoner in India while others are more common in the Western populations since etiologic factors are different.

EPIDEMIOLOGIC FACTORS

A lot of clinical and experimental research and epidemiological studies have been carried out in the field of oncology so as to know the possible causes of cancer and mechanisms involved in transformation of a normal cell into a neoplastic cell. It is widely known that no single factor is responsible for development of tumours. The role of some factors in production of neoplasia is established while that of others is epidemiological and many others are still unknown.

Besides the etiologic role of some agents discussed later, the pattern and incidence of cancer depends upon the following:

A) A large number of *predisposing epidemiologic factors or cofactors* which include a number of endogenous host factors and exogenous environmental factors.

B) *Chronic non-neoplastic (pre-malignant) conditions.*

C) *Role of hormones in cancer.*

A. Predisposing Factors

1. FAMILIAL AND GENETIC FACTORS. It has long been suspected that familial predisposition and heredity play a role in the development of cancers. In general, the risk of developing cancer in relatives of a known cancer patient is almost three times higher as compared

TABLE 8.3: Most Common Malignant Tumours (*In Descending Order*).

	MEN	WOMEN	CHILDREN
1.	Lung (oral cavity in India)	Breast (cervix in India)	Acute leukaemias
2.	Prostate	Lung	CNS tumours
3.	Colon-rectum	Colon-rectum	Lymphomas
4.	Leukaemia-lymphoma	Leukaemia-lymphoma	Neuroblastoma
5.	Liver	Ovary	Bone sarcomas

to control subjects. The overall estimates suggest that genetic cancers comprise not greater than 5% of all cancers. Some of the common examples are as under:

i) Retinoblastoma. About 40% of retinoblastomas are familial and show an autosomal dominant inheritance. Carriers of such genetic composition have 10,000 times higher risk of developing retinoblastoma which is often bilateral. Such patients are predisposed to develop another primary malignant tumour, notably osteogenic sarcoma. Retinoblastoma susceptibility gene, *RB gene,* located on chromosome 13 was the first cancer-predisposing gene identified.

ii) Familial polyposis coli. This condition has autosomal dominant inheritance. The polypoid adenomas may be seen at birth or in early age. By the age of 50 years, almost 100% cases of familial polyposis coli develop cancer of the colon.

iii) Multiple endocrine neoplasia (MEN). A combination of adenomas of pituitary, parathyroid and pancreatic islets (MEN-I) or syndrome of medullary carcinoma thyroid, pheochromocytoma and parathyroid tumour (MEN-II) are encountered in families.

iv) Neurofibromatosis or von Recklinghausen's disease. This condition is characterised by multiple neurofibromas and pigmented skin spots (*cafe au lait spots*). These patients have family history consistent with autosomal dominant inheritance in 50% of patients.

v) Cancer of the breast. Female relatives of breast cancer patients have 2 to 3 times higher risk of developing breast cancer.

vi) DNA-chromosomal instability syndromes. These are a group of pre-neoplastic conditions having defect in DNA repair mechanism. A classical example is xeroderma pigmentosum, an autosomal recessive disorder, characterised by extreme sensitivity to ultraviolet radiation. The patients may develop various types of skin cancers such as basal cell carcinoma, squamous cell carcinoma and malignant melanoma.

2. RACIAL AND GEOGRAPHIC FACTORS. Differences in racial incidence of some cancers may be partly attributed to the role of genetic composition but are largely due to influence of the environment and geographic differences affecting the whole population such as climate, soil, water, diet, habits, customs etc. Some of the examples of racial and geographic variations in various cancers are as under:

i) White Europeans and Americans develop most commonly malignancies of the lung, breast, and colon. Liver cancer is uncommon in these races. Breast cancer is uncommon in Japanese women but is more common in American women.

ii) Black Africans, on the other hand, have more commonly cancers of the skin, penis, cervix and liver.

iii) Japanese have five times higher incidence of carcinoma of the stomach than the Americans.

iv) South-East Asians, especially of Chinese origin have more commonly nasopharyngeal cancer.

v) Indians of both sexes have higher incidence of carcinoma of the oral cavity and upper aerodigestive tract, while in females carcinoma of uterine cervix and of breast run parallel in incidence. Cancer of the liver in India is more due to viral hepatitis (HBV and HCV) and subsequent cirrhosis than due to alcoholism.

3. ENVIRONMENTAL AND CULTURAL FACTORS. Surprising as it may seem, we are surrounded by an environment of carcinogens which we eat, drink, inhale and touch. Some of the examples are given below:

i) Cigarette smoking is the single most important environmental factor implicated in the etiology of cancer of the oral cavity, pharynx, larynx, oesophagus, lungs, pancreas and urinary bladder.

ii) Alcohol abuse predisposes to the development of cancer of oropharynx, larynx, oesophagus and liver.

iii) Alcohol and tobacco together further accentuate the risk of developing cancer of the upper aerodigestive tract.

iv) Cancer of the cervix is linked to a number of factors such as age at first coitus, frequency of coitus, multiplicity of partners, parity etc. Sexual partners of circumcised males have lower incidence of cervical cancer than the partners of uncircumcised males.

v) **Penile cancer** is rare in the Jews and Muslims as they are customarily circumcised. Carcinogenic component of smegma appears to play a role in the etiology of penile cancer.

vi) **Betel nut cancer** of the cheek and tongue is quite common in some parts of India due to habitual practice of keeping the bolus of *paan* in a particular place in mouth for a long time.

vii) A large number of **industrial and environmental substances** are carcinogenic and are occupational hazard for some populations. These include exposure to substances like arsenic, asbestos, benzene, vinyl chloride, naphthylamine etc.

viii) **Certain constituents of diet** have also been implicated in the causation of cancer. Overweight individuals, deficiency of vitamin A and people consuming diet rich in animal fats and low in fibre content are more at risk of developing certain cancers such as colonic cancer. Diet rich in vitamin E, on the other hand, possibly has some protective influence by its antioxidant action.

4. AGE. Generally, cancers occur in older individuals past 5th decade of life, though there are variations in age incidence in different forms of cancers. It is not clear whether higher incidence of cancer in advanced age is due to alteration in the cells of the host, longer exposure to the effect of carcinogen, or decreased ability of the host immune response. Some tumours have two peaks of incidence e.g. acute leukaemias occur in children and in older age group. The biologic behaviour of tumours in children does not always correlate with histologic features. Besides acute leukaemias, *other tumours in infancy and childhood* are: neuroblastoma, nephroblastoma (Wilms' tumour), retinoblastoma, hepatoblastoma, rhabdomyosarcoma, Ewing's sarcoma, teratoma and CNS tumours.

5. SEX. Apart from the malignant tumours of organs peculiar to each sex, most tumours are generally more common in men than in women except cancer of the breast, gall bladder, thyroid and hypopharynx. Although there are geographic and racial variations, *cancer of the breast* is the commonest cancer in *women* throughout the world while *lung cancer* is the commonest cancer in *men*. The differences in incidence of certain cancers in the two sexes may be related to the presence of specific sex hormones.

B. Chronic Non-neoplastic (Pre-malignant) Conditions

Premalignant lesions are a group of conditions which predispose to the subsequent development of cancer. Such conditions are important to recognise so as to prevent the subsequent occurrence of an invasive cancer. Many of these conditions are characterised by morphologic changes in the cells such as increased nuclear-cytoplasmic ratio, pleomorphism of cells and nuclei, increased mitotic activity, poor differentiation, and sometimes accompanied by chronic inflammatory cells.

Some examples of premalignant lesions are given below:

1. Carcinoma *in situ* (intraepithelial neoplasia). When the cytological features of malignancy are present but the malignant cells are confined to epithelium without invasion across the basement membrane, it is called as carcinoma *in situ* or intraepithelial neoplasia (CIN). The common sites are:

i) Uterine cervix at the junction of ecto and endocervix
ii) Bowen's disease of the skin
iii) Actinic or solar keratosis
iv) Oral leukoplakia
v) Intralobular and intraductal carcinoma of the breast.

The area involved in carcinoma *in situ* may be single and small, or multifocal. As regards the behaviour of CIN, it may regress and return to normal or may develop into invasive cancer. In some instances such as in cervical cancer, there is a sequential transformation from squamous metaplasia, to epithelial dysplasia, to carcinoma *in situ*, and eventually to invasive cancer.

2. Some benign tumours. Commonly, benign tumours do not become malignant. However, there are some exceptions e.g.

i) Multiple villous adenomas of the large intestine have high incidence of developing adenocarcinoma.

ii) Neurofibromatosis (von Recklinghausen's disease) may develop into sarcoma.

3. Miscellaneous conditions. Certain inflammatory and hyperplastic conditions are prone to development of cancer, e.g.

i) Patients of long-standing ulcerative colitis are predisposed to develop colorectal cancer.

ii) Cirrhosis of the liver has predisposition to develop hepatocellular carcinoma.

iii) Chronic bronchitis in heavy cigarette smokers may develop cancer of the bronchus.

iv) Chronic irritation from jagged tooth or ill-fitting denture may lead to cancer of the oral cavity.

v) Squamous cell carcinoma developing in an old burn scar (Marjolin's ulcer).

C. Hormones and Cancer

Cancer is more likely to develop in organs and tissues which undergo proliferation under the influence of excessive hormonal stimulation. On cessation of hormonal stimulation, such tissues become atrophic. Hormone-sensitive tissues developing tumours are the breast, endometrium, myometrium, vagina, thyroid, liver, prostate and testis. Some examples of hormones influencing carcinogenesis in experimental animals and humans are given below:

1. OESTROGEN. Examples of oestrogen-induced cancers are as under:

i) In experimental animals. Induction of breast cancer in mice by administration of high-dose of oestrogen and reduction of the tumour development following oophorectomy is the most important example. Associated infection with mouse mammary tumour virus (MMTV, *Bittner milk factor*) has an added influence on the development of breast cancer in mice. Other cancers which can be experimentally induced in mice by oestrogens are squamous cell carcinoma of the cervix, connective tissue tumour of the myometrium, Leydig cell tumour of the testis in male mice, tumour of the kidney in hamsters, and benign as well as malignant tumours of the liver in rats.

ii) In humans. Women receiving oestrogen therapy and women with oestrogen-secreting granulosa cell tumour of the ovary have increased risk of developing endometrial carcinoma. Adenocarcinoma of the vagina is seen with increased frequency in adolescent daughters of mothers who had received oestrogen-therapy during pregnancy.

2. CONTRACEPTIVE HORMONES. The sequential types of oral contraceptives increase the risk of developing breast cancer. Other tumours showing a slightly increased frequency in women receiving contraceptive pills for long durations are benign tumours of the liver, and a few patients have been reported to have developed hepatocellular carcinoma.

3. ANABOLIC STEROIDS. Consumption of anabolic steroids by athletes to increase the muscle mass is not only unethical athletic practice but also increases the risk of developing benign and malignant tumours of the liver.

4. HORMONE-DEPENDENT TUMOURS. It has been shown in experimental animals that induction of hyperfunction of adenohypophysis is associated with increased risk of developing neoplasia of the target organs following preceding functional hyperplasia. There is tumour regression on removal of the stimulus for excessive hormonal secretion. A few examples of such phenomena are seen in humans:

i) *Prostatic cancer* usually responds to the administration of oestrogens.

ii) *Breast cancer* may regress with oophorectomy, hypophysectomy or on administration of male hormones.

iii) *Thyroid cancer* may slow down in growth with administration of thyroxine that suppresses the secretion of TSH by the pituitary.

CARCINOGENESIS: ETIOLOGY AND PATHOGENESIS OF CANCER

Carcinogenesis or oncogenesis or tumorigenesis means mechanism of induction of tumours (*pathogenesis of cancer*); agents which can induce tumours are called *carcinogens* (*etiology of cancer*). Since the time first ever carcinogen was identified, there has been ever-increasing list of agents implicated in etiology of cancer. There has been still greater accumulation in volumes of knowledge on pathogenesis of cancer, especially due to tremendous strides made in the field of molecular biology and genetics in the last decade.

The subject of etiology and pathogenesis of cancer is, therefore, discussed under the following 4 broad headings:

A. Molecular pathogenesis of cancer (genes and cancer)
B. Chemical carcinogens and chemical carcinogenesis
C. Physical carcinogens and radiation carcinogenesis
D. Biologic carcinogens and viral oncogenesis.

A. MOLECULAR PATHOGENESIS OF CANCER (GENES AND CANCER)

Basic Concept of Molecular Pathogenesis

The mechanism as to how a normal cell is transformed to a cancer cell is complex. At different times, attempts have been made to unravel this mystery by various mechanisms. In the last decade, there has been vast accumulation of literature to explain the pathogenesis of cancer at molecular level. The general concept of molecular mechanisms of cancer is briefly outlined below and diagrammatically shown in Fig. 8.6:

1. Monoclonality of tumours. There is strong evidence that most human cancers arise from a single clone of cells by genetic transformation or mutation. For example:

i) In a case of multiple myeloma (a malignant disorder of plasma cells), there is production of a single type of immunoglobulin or its chain as seen by monoclonal spike in serum electrophoresis.

ii) Due to inactivation of one of the two X-chromosomes in females (paternal or maternal derived), women are

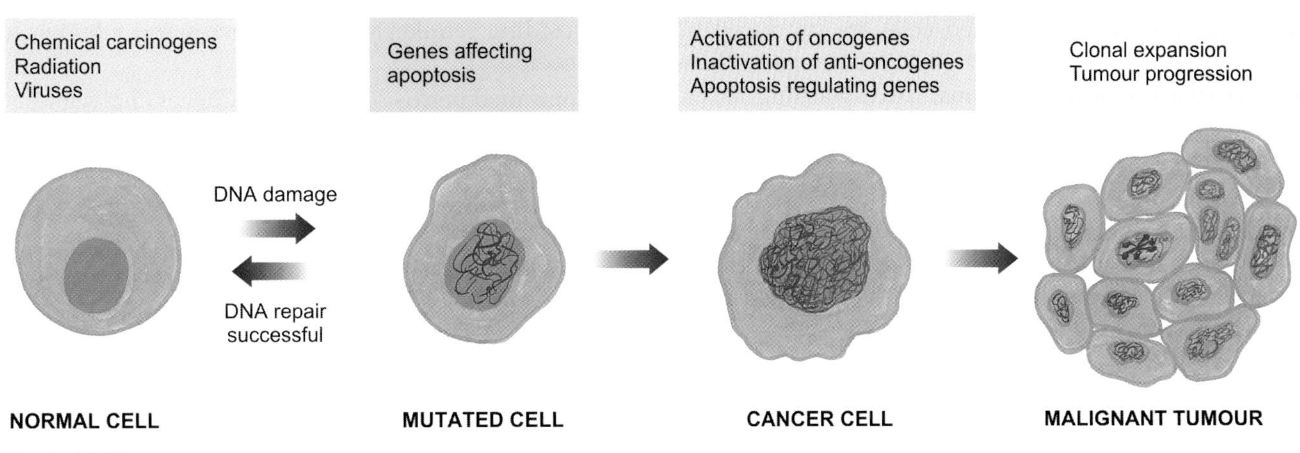

FIGURE 8.6

Schematic illustration to show molecular basis of cancer.

mosaics with two types of cell populations e.g. for glucose-6-phosphatase dehydrogenase (G6PD) isoenzyme A and B. It is observed that all the tumour cells in benign uterine tumours (leiomyoma) contain either A or B genotype of G6PD (i.e. the tumour cells are derived from a single progenitor clone of cell), while the normal myometrium is mosaic of both types of cells derived from A as well as B isoenzyme (Fig. 8.7).

2. Genetic theory of cancer. Cell growth of normal as well as abnormal types is under genetic control. In cancer, there is either abnormality in the genes of the cell, or there are normal genes with abnormal expression. The abnormality in genetic composition may be from an inherited or induced mutation (induced by etiologic carcinogenic agents namely: chemicals, viruses, radiation). The mutated cells transmit their characters to the next progeny of cells and result in cancer.

3. Genetic regulators of normal and abnormal mitosis. In normal cell growth, regulatory genes control mitosis as well as cell aging, terminating in cell death by apoptosis.

- **In normal cell growth,** there are 4 regulatory genes:

i) Proto-oncogenes are growth-promoting genes.

ii) Anti-oncogenes are growth-inhibiting or growth suppressor genes.

iii) Apoptosis regulatory genes control the programmed cell death.

iv) DNA repair genes are those normal genes which regulate the repair of DNA damage that has occurred during mitosis and also control the damage to proto-oncogenes and anti-oncogenes.

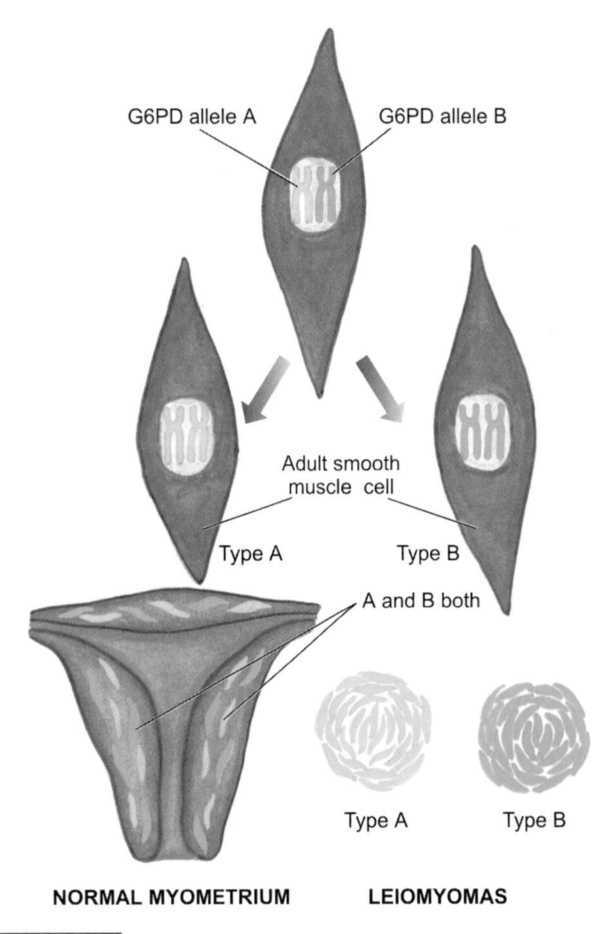

FIGURE 8.7

The monoclonal origin of tumour cells in uterine leiomyoma.

Chapter Eight

■ **In cancer,** the transformed cells are produced by abnormal cell growth due to genetic damage to these normal controlling genes. Thus, corresponding abnormalities are genetics, as under:

i) Activation of growth-promoting oncogenes causing transformation of cell (mutant form of normal proto-oncogene in cancer is termed *oncogene*). Gene products of oncogenes are called *oncoproteins.* Oncogenes are considered *dominant* since they appear inspite of presence of normal proto-oncogenes.

ii) Inactivation of cancer-suppressor genes (i.e. inactivation of anti-oncogenes) permitting the cellular proliferation of transformed cells. Anti-oncogenes are active in *recessive* form which mean that they are active only if both alleles are damaged.

iii) Abnormal apoptosis regulatory genes which may act as oncogenes or anti-oncogenes. Accordingly, these genes may be active in dominant or recessive form.

iv) Failure of DNA repair genes and thus inability to repair the DNA damage resulting in mutations.

4. Multi-step process of cancer growth and progression. Carcinogenesis is a gradual multi-step process involving many generations of cells. The various causes may act on the cell one after another (*multi-hit process*). The same process is also involved in further progression of the tumour. Ultimately, the cells so formed are genetically and phenotypically transformed cells having phenotypic features of malignancy—excessive growth, invasiveness and distant metastasis.

Chapter Eight

Cancer-related Genes and Cell Growth (Hallmarks of Cancer)

It is apparent from the above discussion that genes control the normal cellular growth, while in cancer these controlling genes are altered, typically by mutation. A large number of such cancer-associated genes have been described, each with a specific function in cell growth. Some of these genes are commonly associated in many tumours (e.g. *p53* or *TP53*), while others are specific to particular tumours. Therefore, it is considered appropriate to discuss the role of cancer-related genes with regard to their functions in cellular growth. Following are the *major genetic properties or hallmarks of cancer*:

1. Excessive and autonomous growth: Growth-promoting oncogenes.
2. Refractoriness to growth inhibition: Growth suppressing anti-oncogenes.
3. Escaping cell death by apoptosis: Genes regulating apoptosis and cancer.
4. Avoiding cellular aging: Telomeres and telomerase in cancer.
5. Continued perfusion of cancer: Cancer angiogenesis.
6. Invasion and distant metastasis: Cancer dissemination.
7. DNA damage and repair system: Mutator genes and cancer.
8. Cancer progression and tumour heterogeneity: Clonal aggressiveness.

These properties of cancer cells are described below in terms of molecular genetics and summed up in Fig. 8.8.

1. EXCESSIVE AND AUTONOMOUS GROWTH: GROWTH PROMOTING ONCOGENES

Mutated form of normal proto-oncogenes in cancer is called oncogenes. Oncogenes differ from 'normal genes' in following respects:

- mutation in the structure of gene;
- lacking the normal growth-promoting signals of proto-oncogenes; and
- they act by over-expression to promote autonomous and excessive cellular proliferation.

In general, activation of oncogenes in human tumours can occur by following mechanisms:

i) Point mutations and deletion. The most important example is *RAS* oncogene carried in many human tumours such as bladder cancer, pancreatic adenocarcinoma, cholangiocarcinoma.

ii) Chromosomal translocation. Mechanism of transfer of a portion of one chromosome to another is implicated in the pathogenesis of leukaemias and lymphomas e.g.

- Philadelphia chromosome seen in 95% cases of chronic myelogenous leukaemia in which *c-ABL* proto-oncogene on chromosome 9 is translocated to chromosome 22.
- In 75% cases of Burkitt's lymphoma, translocation of *c-MYC* proto-oncogene from its site on chromosome 8 to a portion on chromosome 14.

iii) Gene amplification. Chromosomal alterations that result in increase in the number of copies of a gene is found in some examples of solid human tumours e.g.

- Neuroblastoma having *n-MYC HSR* region.
- *ERB-B* in breast and ovarian cancer.

The steps in signal transduction for cell proliferation by oncogenes are discussed below in relation to mitosis in normal cell cycle:

i) Growth factors (GFs). These are polypeptides elaborated by many cells and normally act on another cell than the one which synthesised it to stimulate its

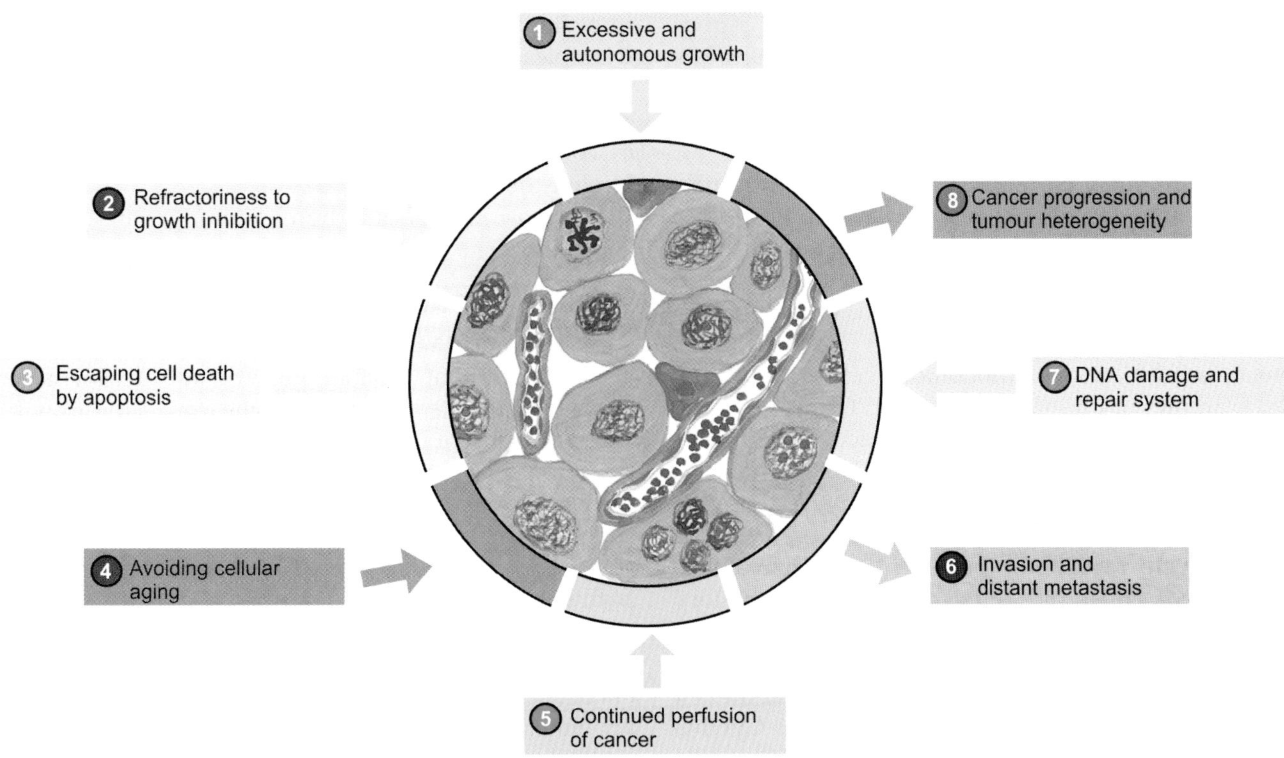

FIGURE 8.8

Schematic representation of major properties of cancer in terms of molecular carcinogenesis.

proliferation i.e. *paracrine action*. However, a cancer cell may synthesise a GF and respond to it as well; this way cancer cells acquire growth self sufficiency. The examples of such GFs are as under:

a) Platelet-derived growth factor (PDGF) in glioblastoma.

b) Transforming growth factor-α (TGF-α) is over-expressed in sarcomas.

c) *Fibroblast growth factor (FGF)* in cancer of the bowel and breast.

ii) Receptors for GFs. Many oncogenes encoding for GF receptors have been described which act more commonly by overexpression of normal GF than by mutation. For example:

a) ERB1 is an EGF receptor which acts by overexpression of normal GF receptor in squamous cell carcinoma.

b) HER2, also called *ERB2*, is another EGF receptor which is overexpressed in breast cancer and carcinoma of lungs, ovary, stomach.

iii) Signal transduction proteins. The normal signal transduction proteins which transduce signal from the GF receptors on the cell surface to the nucleus of the cell is mutated in some cancers. The examples of such oncogenes are as under:

a) Mutated RAS gene. This is the most common form of oncogene in human tumours. About a third of all human tumours carry mutated *RAS* gene (*RAS* for *Ra*t *S*arcoma gene where it was first described), seen in particular in carcinoma colon, lung and pancreas. Normally, the inactive form of *RAS* protein is GDP (guanosine diphosphate)-bound while the activated form is bound to guanosine triphosphate (GTP). GDP/GTP are homologous to G proteins and take part in signal transduction in a similar way just as G proteins act as 'on-off switch' for signal transduction. Normally, active *RAS* protein is inactivated by GTPase activity, while mutated *RAS* gene remains unaffected by GTPase and therefore, continues to signal the cell proliferation. Common mode of activation of *RAS* gene is by point mutation.

b) BCR-ABL hybrid gene. ABL gene is a non-GF receptor proto-oncogene having tyrosine kinase activity. *ABL* gene from its normal location on chromosome 9 is translocated to chromosome 22 where it fuses with *BCR* (breakpoint cluster region) gene and forms an *ABL-BCR* hybrid gene which is more potent in signal transduction pathway. *ABL-BCR* hybrid gene is seen in chronic myeloid leukaemia and some acute leukaemias.

iv) Nuclear regulatory molecules. The signal transduction pathway that started with GFs ultimately reaches the nucleus where it regulates DNA transcription. Out of various nuclear regulatory transcription proteins described, the most important is *MYC* gene, seen most commonly in human tumours. Normally *MYC* protein binds to the DNA and regulates the cell cycle by transcriptional activation and its levels fall immediately after cell enters the cell cycle. *MYC* oncogene, on the other hand, is associated with persistent or overexpression of *MYC* oncoproteins which, in turn, causes autonomous cell proliferation. The examples of tumours carrying *MYC* oncogene are:

a) Burkitt's lymphoma in which mutation in *MYC* gene is due to *translocation* t(8;14).

b) In cancer of lung, breast and colon, *MYC* gene is mutated due to *amplification*.

v) Cell cycle regulatory proteins. As discussed in Chapter 3, normally the cell cycle is under regulatory control of cyclins and cyclin-dependent kinases (CDKs) A, B, E and D. Cyclins are so named since they are cyclically synthesised during different phases of the cell cycle and their degradation is also cyclic. Cyclins activate as well as work together with CDKs, while many inhibitors of CDKs (CDKIs) are also known. Although all steps in the cell cycle are under regulatory controls, G1 → S phase is the most important checkpoint for regulation by oncogenes as well as anti-oncogenes (discussed below). Mutations in cyclins (in particular cyclin D) and CDKs (in particular CDK4) are most important growth promoting signals in cancers. The examples of tumours having such oncogenes are:

a) Overexpression of cyclin D in cancers of breast, liver and mantle cell lymphoma.

b) Amplification of CDK4 in malignant melanoma, glioblastoma and sarcomas.

Various oncogenes in human tumours are listed in Table 8.4.

2. REFRACTORINESS TO GROWTH INHIBITION: GROWTH SUPPRESSING ANTI-ONCOGENES

The mutation of normal growth suppressor anti-oncogenes results in removal of the brakes for growth; thus the inhibitory effect to cell growth is removed and the abnormal growth continues unchecked. In other words, mutated anti-oncogenes behave like growth-promoting oncogenes.

As compared to the signals and signal transduction pathways for oncogenes described above, the steps in mechanisms of action by growth suppressors are not as well understood. In general, the point of action by anti-oncogenes is also G1 → S phase transition and probably act either by inducing the dividing cell from the cell cycle to enter into G0 (resting) phase, or by acting in a way that the cell lies in the post-mitotic pool losing its dividing capability.

Major anti-oncogenes implicated in human cancers are as under (Table 8.5):

i) *RB* gene. *RB* gene is located on long arm (q) of chromosome 13. This is the first ever tumour suppressor

TABLE 8.4: Important Oncogenes, their Mechanism of Activation and Associated Human Tumours.

TYPE	ONCOGENE	ASSOCIATED HUMAN TUMOURS
1. Growth factors (GFs)		
	i) *PDGF*	Glioblastoma
	ii) *TGF-α*	Sarcomas
	iii) *FGF*	Ca bowel, breast
2. Receptors for GFs		
	i) *ERB B_1*	Squamous cell carcinoma
	ii) *HER_2 (α ERB_2)*	Ca breast, ovary, stomach, lungs
3. Signal transduction proteins		
	RAS	Common in 1/3rd human tumours, Ca lung, colon, pancreas
	BCR-ABL	CML, acute leukaemias
4. Nuclear regulatory molecules (Transcription proteins)	*MYC* (translocated)	Burkitt's lymphoma
	MYC (amplified)	Ca lungs, breast, colon
5. Cell cycle regulatory proteins		
	Cyclin D	Ca breast, liver, mantle cell lymphoma
	CDK4	Glioblastoma, melanoma, sarcomas

PDGF = platelet-derived growth factor; FGF = fibroblast growth factor; TGF-α = Transforming growth factor; CDK = cyclin-dependent kinase

Chapter Eight

TABLE 8.5: Important Tumour-suppressor Genes and Associated Human Tumours.

GENE	LOCATION	ASSOCIATED HUMAN TUMOURS
1. *RB*	Nucleus (q13)	Retinoblastoma, osteosarcoma
2. *TP53 (p53)*	Nucleus (p17)	Most human cancers, common in ca. lung, head and neck, colon, breast
3. *TGF–β*	Extracellular GF	Ca pancreas, colon, stomach
4. *APC*	Cytosol	Ca colon
5. Others		
i) WT 1 and 2	Nucleus	Wilms' tumour
ii) NF 1 and 2	Plasma membrane	Neurofibromatosis type 1 and 2
iii) BRCA 1 and 2	Nucleus	Ca breast, ovary

gene identified and thus has been amply studied. Normally, *RB* gene product is a nuclear transcription protein which is virtually present in every human cell. It exists in both an *active* and an *inactive* form. Active *RB* gene protein acts to inhibit the cell cycle at G1 → S phase. Stimulation of the cell by growth factors renders the *RB* gene protein inactive and thus permits the cell to cross G1 → S phase.

The mutant form of *RB* gene is involved in retinoblastoma, the most common intraocular tumour in young children. The tumour occurs in two forms: sporadic and inherited/familial. More than half the cases are sporadic affecting one eye; these cases have acquired simultaneous mutation in both the alleles in retinal cells after birth. In inherited cases, all somatic cells inherit one mutant *RB* gene from a carrier parent, while the other allele gets mutated later. The latter genetic explanation given by Knudson forms the basis of *two hit hypothesis* of inherited cancers. Besides retinoblastoma, children inheriting mutant *RB* gene have 200 times greater risk of development of other cancers in early adult life, most notably osteosarcoma; others are cancers of breast, colon and lungs.

ii) *TP53* gene (*p53*). Located on the short arm (p) of chromosome 17, *p53* gene (currently termed *TP53*) is normally a growth suppressor anti-oncogene.

The two major functions of *TP53* in the normal cell cycle are as under:

a) In blocking mitotic activity: TP53 inhibits the cyclins and CDKs and prevents the cell to enter G1 phase transiently. This breathing time in the cell cycle is utilised by the cell to repair the DNA damage.

b) In promoting apoptosis: *TP53* acts together with another anti-oncogene, *RB* gene, and identifies the genes that have damaged DNA which cannot be repaired by inbuilt system. *TP53* directs such cells to apoptosis by activating apoptosis-inducing *BAX* gene, and thus bringing the defective cells to an end. This process operates in the cell cycle at G1 and G2 phases before the cell enters the S or M phase.

Because of these significant roles in cell cycle, *TP53* is called as 'protector of the genome'.

In its mutated form, *TP53* stops to act as growth suppressor and instead acts like an oncogene, *c-onc*. Majority of human cancers have either a mutation in *TP53* or its expression is up- or down-regulated. Some common examples of human cancers having defective *TP53* are: cancers of lung, head and neck, colon and breast. Besides, mutated *TP53* is also seen in the sequential development stages of cancer from hyperplasia to carcinoma *in situ* and into invasive carcinoma.

Like in *RB* gene, defect in one of the two alleles of *TP53* gene either by inheritance or by mutation, renders the individual prone to a second hit on the other normal allele and thus predisposes such an individual to cancers of multiple organs (breast, bone, brain, sarcomas etc), termed *Li-Fraumeni syndrome.*

iii) Transforming growth factor-β (*TGF*-β). Normally, *TGF*-β is significant inhibitor of cell proliferation, mainly by its action on G1 phase of cell cycle. Its mutant form impairs the growth inhibiting effect and thus permits cell proliferation. Examples of mutated form of *TGF*-β are seen in cancers of pancreas, colon, stomach etc.

iv) Adenomatous polyposis coli (APC) gene. The *APC* gene is normally inhibitory to mitosis, which is done by a cytoplasmic protein, β-catenin. β-catenin normally blocks the signal to the nucleus for activating mitosis. In colon cancer, APC gene is lost and thus the cancer cells continue to undergo mitosis without the inhibitory influence of β-catenin.

v) Other anti-oncogenes. A few other tumour-suppressor genes having mutated germline in various tumours are as under:

a) Wilms' tumour (WT) gene: WT gene normally prevents neoplastic proliferation of cells in embryonic kidney.

Mutant form of WT-1 and 2 are seen in hereditary Wilms' tumour.

b) Neurofibroma (NF) gene: NF genes normally prevent proliferation of Schwann cells. Two mutant forms are described: *NF1* and *NF2* seen in neurofibromatosis type 1 and type 2.

c) BRCA 1 and BRCA 2 genes: These are breast *(BR)* cancer *(CA)* susceptibility genes, especially in inherited cases of breast cancer.

3. ESCAPING CELL DEATH BY APOPTOSIS: GENES REGULATING APOPTOSIS AND CANCER

Besides the role of mutant froms of growth-promoting oncogenes and growth-suppressing anti-oncogenes, another mechanism of tumour growth is by escaping apoptosis. Apoptosis in normal cell is guided by cell death receptor, CD95, resulting in DNA damage. Besides, there is role of some other pro-apoptotic factors (*BAD, BAX, BID* and *TP53*) and apoptosis-inhibitors (*BCL2, BCL-X*).

In cancer cells, the function of apoptosis is interfered due to mutations in the above genes which regulate apoptosis in the normal cell. The examples of tumours by this mechanism are as under:

a) ***BCL2* gene** is seen in normal lymphocytes, but its mutant form with characteristic translocation was first described in B-cell lymphoma and hence the name. It is also seen in many other human cancers such as that of breast, thyroid and prostate. Mutation in *BCL2* gene removes the apoptosis-inhibitory control on cancer cells, thus more live cells undergoing mitosis contributing to tumour growth.

b) ***CD95*** receptors are depleted in hepatocellular carcinoma and hence the tumour cells escape apoptosis.

4. AVOIDING CELLULAR AGING: TELOMERES AND TELOMERASE IN CANCER

As discussed in pathology of aging in Chapter 3, after each mitosis (cell doubling) there is progressive shortening of telomeres which are the terminal tips of chromosomes. Telomerase is the RNA enzyme that helps in repair of such damage to DNA and maintains normal telomere length in successive cell divisions. However, it has been seen that after repetitive mitosis for a maximum of 60 to 70 times, telomeres are lost in normal cells and the cells cease to undergo mitosis. Telomerase is active in normal stem cells but not in normal somatic cells.

Cancer cells in most malignancies have markedly upregulated telomerase enzyme, and hence telomere length is maintained. Thus, cancer cells avoid aging, mitosis does not slow down or cease, thereby immortalising the cancer cells.

5. CONTINUED PERFUSION OF CANCER: TUMOUR ANGIOGENESIS

Cancers can only survive and thrive if the cancer cells are adequately nourished and perfused, as otherwise they cannot grow further. Neovascularisation in the cancers not only supplies the tumour with oxygen and nutrients, but the newly formed endothelial cells also elaborate a few growth factors for progression of primary as well as metastatic cancer. The stimulus for angiogenesis is provided by the release of various factors:

i) Promoters of tumour angiogenesis include the most important *vascular endothelial growth factor (VEGF)* (released from genes in the parenchymal tumour cells) and *basic fibroblast growth factor (bFGF).*

ii) Anti-angiogenesis factors inhibiting angiogenesis include *thrombospondin-1* (also produced by tumour cells themselves), *angiostatin, endostatin and vasculostatin.* Mutated form of *TP53* gene in both alleles in various cancers results in removal of anti-angiogenic role of thrombospondin-1, thus favouring continued angiogenesis.

6. INVASION AND DISTANT METASTASIS: CANCER DISSEMINATION

One of the most important characteristic of cancers is invasiveness and metastasis. The mechanisms involved in the biology of invasion and metastasis are discussed already along with spread of tumours.

7. DNA DAMAGE AND REPAIR SYSTEM: MUTATOR GENES AND CANCER

Normal cells during complex mitosis suffer from minor damage to the DNA which is detected and repaired before mitosis is completed so that integrity of the genome is maintained. Similarly, small mutational damage to the dividing cell by exogenous factors (e.g. by radiation, chemical carcinogens etc) is also repaired. *TP53* gene is held responsible for detection and repair of DNA damage. However, if this system of DNA repair is defective as happens in some inherited mutations (mutator genes), the defect in DNA is passed to the next progeny of cells and cancer results.

The examples of mutator genes exist in the following inherited disorders associated with increased propensity to cancer:

i) Hereditary non-polyposis colon cancer (Lynch syndrome) is characterised by hereditary predisposition to develop colorectal cancer. It is due to defect in genes involved in DNA mismatch repair which results in accumulation of errors in the form of mutations in many genes.

ii) Ataxia telangiectasia (AT) has *ATM* (*M* for mutated) gene. These patients have multiple cancers besides other features such as cerebellar degeneration, immunologic derangements and oculo-cutaneous manifestations.

iii) Xeroderma pigmentosum is an inherited disorder in which there is defect in DNA repair mechanism. Upon exposure to sunlight, the UV radiation damage to DNA cannot be repaired. Thus, such patients are more prone to various forms of skin cancers.

iv) Bloom syndrome is an example of damage by ionising radiation which cannot be repaired due to inherited defect and the patients have increased risk to develop cancers, particularly leukaemia.

v) Hereditary breast cancer patients having mutated *BRCA1* and *BRCA2* genes carrying inherited defect in DNA repair mechanism. These patients are not only predisposed to develop breast cancer but also cancers of various other organs.

8. CANCER PROGRESSION AND HETEROGENEITY: CLONAL AGGRESSIVENESS

Another feature of note in biology of cancers is that with passage of time they become more aggressive; this property is termed *tumour progression*. Clinical parameters of cancer progression are: increasing size of the tumour, higher histologic grade (as seen by poorer differentiation and greater anaplasia), areas of tumour necrosis (i.e. tumour outgrows its blood supply), invasiveness and distant metastasis.

In terms of molecular biology, this attribute of cancer is due to the fact that with passage of time cancer cells acquire more and more *heterogeneity*. This means that though cancer cells remain monoclonal in origin, they acquire more and more mutations which in turn produce multiple-mutated subpopulations of more aggressive clones of cancer cells (i.e. heterogeneous cells) in the growth which have tendency to invade, metastasise and be refractory to hormonal influences. Some of these mutations in fact may kill the tumour cells as well.

The above properties of cancer cells are schematically illustrated in Fig. 8.9.

B. CHEMICAL CARCINOGENESIS

The first ever evidence of any cause for neoplasia came from the observation of Sir Percival Pott in 1775 that there was higher incidence of cancer of the scrotum in chimney-sweeps in London than in the general population. This invoked wide interest in soot and coal tar as possible carcinogenic agent and the possibility of other occupational cancers. The first successful experimental induction of cancer was produced by two Japanese workers (Yamagiwa and Ichikawa) in 1914 in the rabbit's skin by repeatedly painting with coal tar. Since then the list of chemical carcinogens which can experimentally induce cancer in animals and have epidemiological evidence in causing human neoplasia, is ever increasing.

Stages in Chemical Carcinogenesis

The induction of cancer by chemical carcinogens occurs after a delay—weeks to months in the case of experimental animals, and often several years in man. Other factors that influence the induction of cancer are the dose and mode of administration of carcinogenic chemical, individual susceptibility and various predisposing factors.

Basic mechanism of chemical carcinogenesis is by induction of mutation in the proto-oncogenes and anti-oncogenes. The phenomena of cellular transformation by chemical carcinogens (as also other carcinogens) is a progressive process involving 2 distinct sequential stages: initiation and promotion (Fig. 8.10).

1. INITIATION OF CARCINOGENESIS

Initiation is the first stage in carcinogenesis induced by initiator chemical carcinogens. The change can be produced by a single dose of the initiating agent for a short time, though larger dose for longer duration is more effective. The change so induced is sudden, irreversible and permanent. Chemical carcinogens acting as initiators of carcinogenesis can be grouped into 2 categories (Table 8.6):

I. Direct-acting carcinogens. These are a few chemical substances (e.g. alkylating agents, acylating agents) which can induce cellular transformation without undergoing any prior metabolic activation.

II. Indirect-acting carcinogens or procarcinogens. These require metabolic conversion within the body so as to become 'ultimate' carcinogens having carcinogenicity e.g. polycyclic aromatic hydrocarbons, aromatic amines, azo dyes, naturally-occurring products and others.

In either case, the following steps are involved in transforming 'the target cell' into 'the initiated cell':

a) Metabolic activation. Vast majority of chemical carcinogens are indirect-acting or procarcinogens requiring metabolic activation, while direct-acting carcinogens do not require this activation. The indirect-

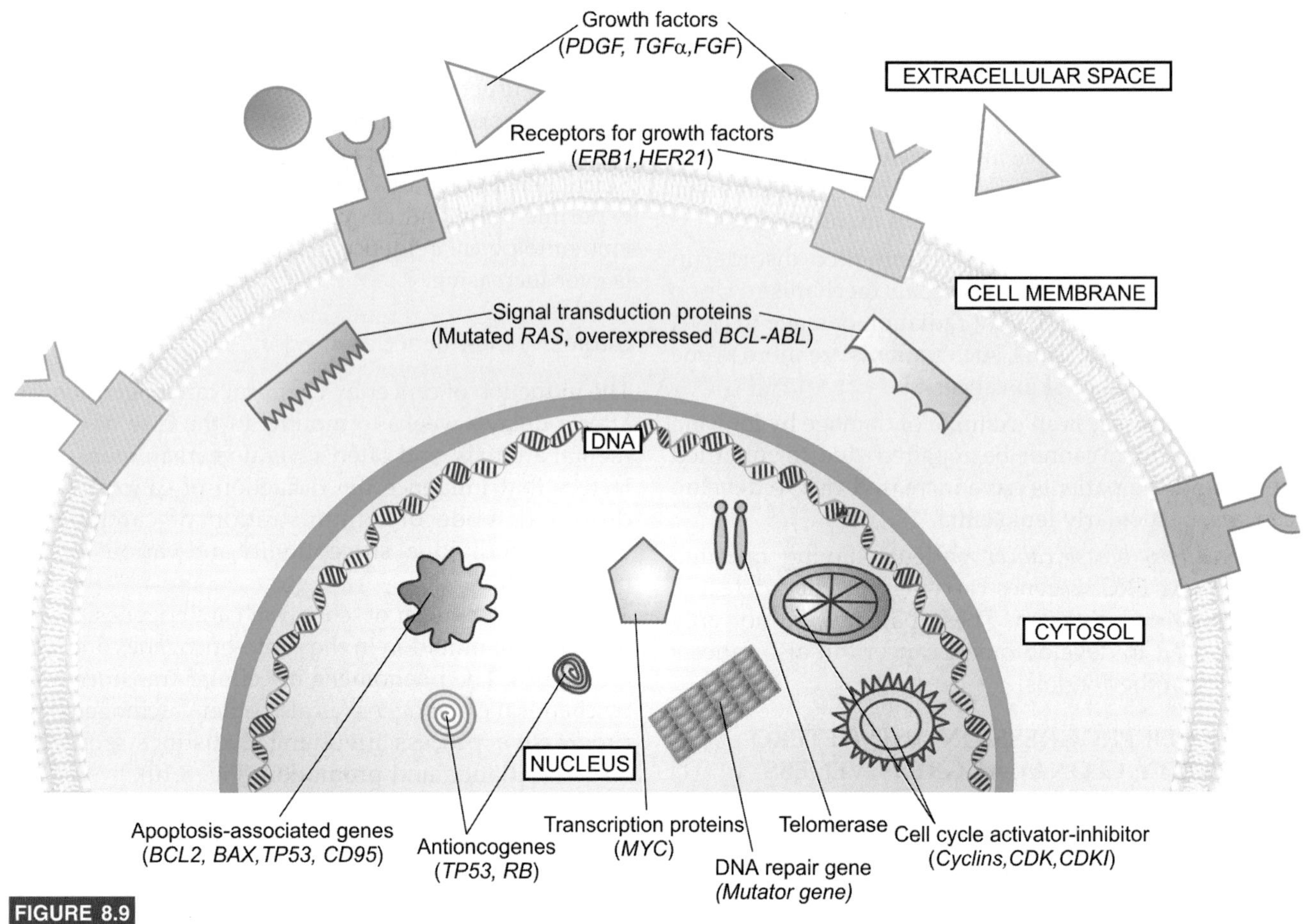

FIGURE 8.9

Schematic representation of activation-inactivation of cancer-associated genes in cell cycle.

acting carcinogens are activated in the liver by the mono-oxygenases of the cytochrome P-450 system in the endoplasmic reticulum. In some circumstances, the procarcinogen may be detoxified and rendered inactive metabolically.

In fact, following 2 requirements determine the carcinogenic potency of a chemical:

i) Balance between activation and inactivation reaction of the carcinogenic chemical.

ii) Genes that code for cytochrome P450-dependent enzymes involved in metabolic activation. For example, a genotype carrying susceptibility gene *CYP1A1* for the enzyme system has far higher incidence of lung cancer in light smokers as compared to those not having this permissive gene.

Besides these two, additional factors such as age, sex and nutritional status of the host also play some role in determining response of the individual to chemical carcinogen.

b) Reactive electrophiles. While direct-acting carcinogens are intrinsically electrophilic, indirect-acting substances become electron-deficient after metabolic activation i.e. reactive electrophiles. Following this step, both types of chemical carcinogens behave alike and their reactive electrophiles bind to electron-rich portions of other molecules of the cell such as DNA, RNA and other proteins.

c) Target molecules. The primary target of electrophiles is DNA, producing mutagenesis. The change in DNA may lead to 'the initiated cell' or some form of cellular enzymes may be able to repair the damage in DNA. The classic example of the latter situation as xeroderma pigmentosum, a precancerous condition, in which there is hereditary defect in DNA repair mechanism of the cell. The carcinogenic potential of a chemical can be tested *in vitro* by Ames' test for mutagenesis (described later).

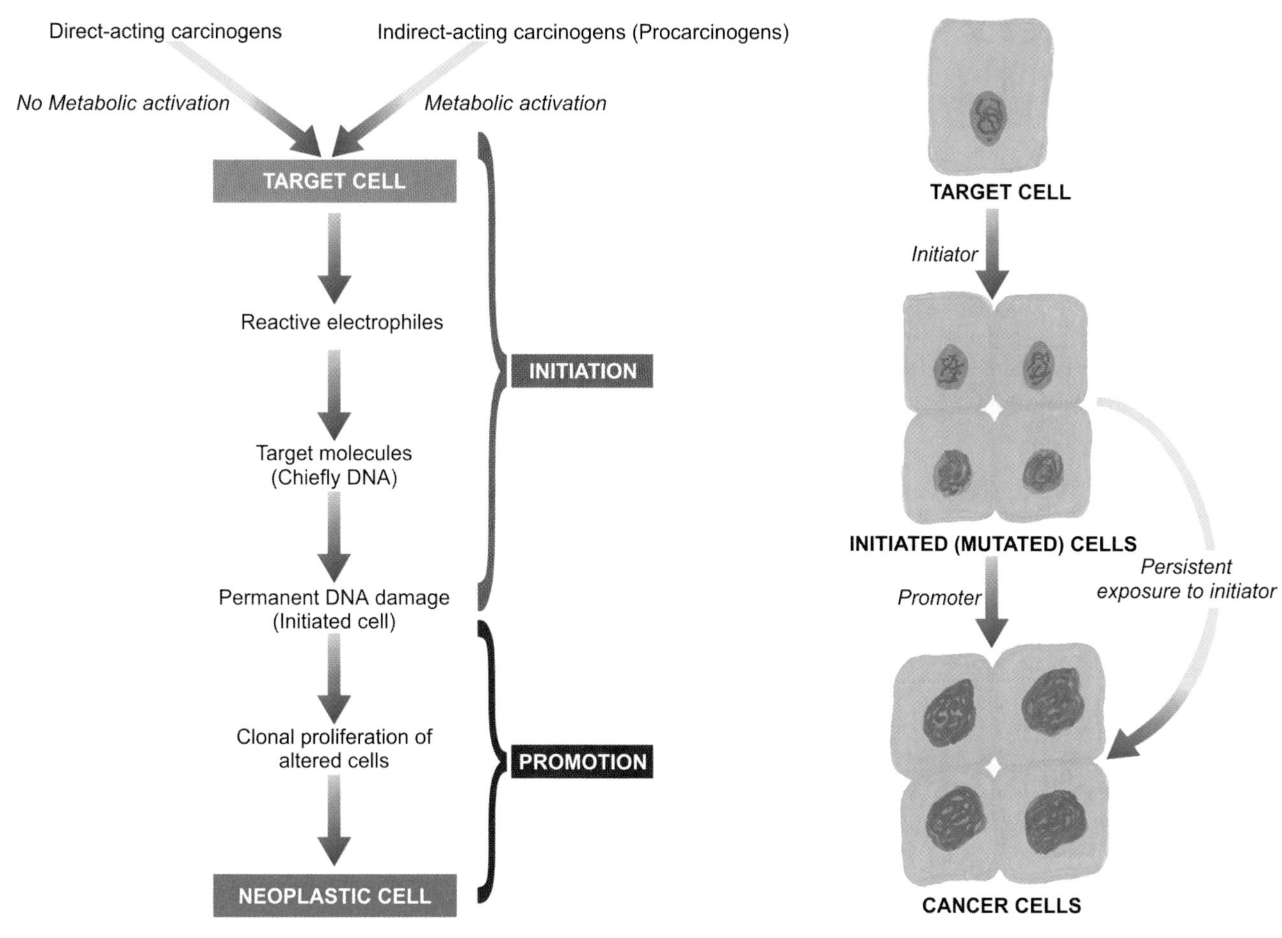

FIGURE 8.10

Sequential stages in chemical carcinogenesis (*left*) in evolution of cancer (*right*).

Any gene may be the target molecule in the DNA for the chemical carcinogen. However, on the basis of chemically induced cancers in experimental animals and epidemiologic studies in human beings, it has been observed that most frequently affected oncogene is *RAS* gene mutation and anti-oncogene (tumour suppressor) is *TP53* gene mutation.

d) The initiated cell. The unrepaired damage produced in the DNA of the cell becomes permanent and fixed only if the altered cell undergoes at least one cycle of proliferation. This results in transferring the change to the next progeny of cells so that the DNA damage becomes *permanent* and *irreversible*, which are the characteristics of the initiated cell, vulnerable to the action of promoters of carcinogenesis.

The stimulus for proliferation may come from regeneration of surviving cells, dietary factors, hormone-induced hyperplasia, viruses etc. A few examples are the occurrence of hepatocellular carcinoma in cases of viral hepatitis, association of endometrial hyperplasia with endometrial carcinoma, effect of oestrogen in breast cancer.

2. PROMOTION OF CARCINOGENESIS

Promotion is the next sequential stage in the chemical carcinogenesis. Promoters of carcinogenesis are substances such as phorbol esters, phenols, hormones, artificial sweeteners and drugs like phenobarbital. They differ from initiators in the following respects:

i) They do not produce sudden change.

ii) They require application or administration, as the case may be, *following* initiator exposure, for sufficient time and in sufficient dose.

iii) The change induced may be reversible.

iv) They do not damage the DNA *per se* and are thus not mutagenic but instead enhance the effect of direct-acting carcinogens or procarcinogens.

TABLE 8.6: Important Chemical Carcinogens.

	CARCINOGEN	TUMOUR
I.	***DIRECT-ACTING CARCINOGENS***	
a)	*Alkylating agents*	
	• Anti-cancer drugs (e.g. cyclophosphamide, chlorambucil, busulfan, melphalan, nitrosourea etc)	
	• β-propiolactone	• Lymphomas
	• Epoxides	• Leukaemias
b)	*Acylating agents*	
	• Acetyl imidazole	
	• Dimethyl carbamyl chloride	
II.	***INDIRECT-ACTING CARCINOGENS (PROCARCINOGENS):***	
a)	*Polycyclic, aromatic hydrocarbons (in tobacco, smoke, fossil fuel, soot, tar, minerals oil, smoked animal foods, industrial and atmospheric pollutants)*	• Lung cancer • Skin cancer
	• Anthracenes (benza-, dibenza-, dimethyl benza-)	• Cancer of oral cavity
	• Benzapyrene	• Sarcoma
	• Methylcholanthrene	
b)	*Aromatic amines and azo-dyes*	
	• β-naphthylamine	• Bladder cancer
	• Benzidine	
	• Azo-dyes (e.g. butter yellow, scarlet red etc)	• Hepatocellular carcinoma
c)	*Naturally-occurring products*	
	• Aflatoxin Bl	
	• Actinomycin D	
	• Mitomycin C	• Hepatocellular carcinoma
	• Safrole	
	• Betel nuts	
d)	*Miscellaneous*	
	• Nitrosamines and nitrosamides	• Gastric carcinoma
	• Vinyl chloride monomer	• Haemangiosarcoma of liver
	• Asbestos	• Bronchogenic carcinoma, mesothelioma
	• Arsenical compounds	• Epidermal hyperplasia, basal cell carcinoma
	• Metals (e.g. nickel, lead, cobalt, chromium etc)	• Lung cancer
	• Insecticides, fungicides (e.g. aldrin, dieldrin, chlordane etc)	• Cancer in experimental animals
	• Saccharin and cyclomates	

v) Tumour promoters act by further clonal proliferation and expansion of initiated (mutated) cells, and have reduced requirement of growth factor especially after *RAS* gene mutation.

It may be mentioned here that persistent and sustained application/exposure of the cell to initiator alone unassociated with subsequent application of promoter may also result in cancer. But the *vice versa* does not hold true since neither application of promoter alone, nor its application prior to exposure to initiator carcinogen, would result in transformation of target cell.

Carcinogenic Chemicals in Humans

The list of diverse chemical compounds which can produce cancer in experimental animals is a long one but only some of them have sufficient epidemiological evidence in human neoplasia.

Depending upon the mode of action of carcinogenic chemicals, they are divided into 2 broad groups: initiators and promoters (Table 8.6).

1. INITIATOR CARCINOGENS

Chemical carcinogens which can initiate the process of neoplastic transformation are further categorised into 2 subgroups—direct-acting and indirect-acting carcinogens or procarcinogens.

I. DIRECT-ACTING CARCINOGENS. These chemical carcinogens do not require metabolic activation and fall into 2 classes:

a) Alkylating agents. This group includes mainly various anti-cancer drugs (e.g. cyclophosphamide, chlorambucil, busulfan, melphalan, nitrosourea etc), β-propiolactone and epoxides. They are weakly carcinogenic and are implicated in the etiology of the lymphomas and leukaemias in human beings.

b) Acylating agents. The examples are acetyl imidazole and dimethyl carbamyl chloride.

II. INDIRECT-ACTING CARCINOGENS (PROCARCINOGENS). These are chemical substances which require prior metabolic activation before becoming potent 'ultimate' carcinogens. This group includes vast majority of carcinogenic chemicals. It includes the following 4 categories:

a) Polycyclic aromatic hydrocarbons. They comprise the largest group of common procarcinogens which, after metabolic activation, can induce neoplasia in many tissues in experimental animals and are also implicated in a number of human neoplasms. They cause different effects by various modes of administration e.g. by topical application may induce skin cancer, by subcutaneous injection may cause sarcomas, inhalation produces lung cancer, when introduced in different organs by parenteral/metabolising routes may cause cancer of that organ.

Main sources of polycyclic aromatic hydrocarbons are: combustion and chewing of tobacco, smoke, fossil fuel (e.g. coal), soot, tar, mineral oil, smoked animal foods, industrial and atmospheric pollutants. Important chemical compounds included in this group are: anthracenes (benza-, dibenza-, dimethyl benza-), benzapyrene and methylcholanthrene. The following examples have evidence to support the etiologic role of these substances:

- *Smoking:* There is 20 times higher incidence of lung cancer in smokers of 2 packs (40 cigarettes) per day for 20 years.
- *Skin cancer:* Direct contact of polycyclic aromatic hydrocarbon compounds with skin is associated with higher incidence of skin cancer. For example, the natives of Kashmir carry an earthen pot containing embers, the *kangri,* under their clothes close to abdomen for purposes of warmth, and skin cancer of the abdominal wall termed *kangri cancer* is common among them.
- *Tobacco and betel nut chewing:* Cancer of the oral cavity is more common in people chewing tobacco and betel nuts. The *chutta* is a cigar that is smoked in South India (in Andhra Pradesh) with the lighted end in the mouth (i.e. reversed smoking) and such individuals have higher incidence of cancer of the mouth.

b) Aromatic amines and azo-dyes. This category includes the following substances implicated in chemical carcinogenesis:

- *β-naphthylamine* in the causation of bladder cancer, especially in aniline dye and rubber industry workers.
- *Benzidine* in the induction of bladder cancer.
- *Azo-dyes* used for colouring foods (e.g. butter and margarine to give them yellow colour, scarlet red for colouring cherries etc) in the causation of hepatocellular carcinoma.

c) Naturally-occurring products. Some of the important chemical carcinogens derived from plant and microbial sources are aflatoxin B1, actinomycin D, mitomycin C, safrole and betel nuts. Out of these, aflatoxin B1 implicated in causing human hepatocellular carcinoma is the most important, especially when concomitant viral hepatitis B is present. It is derived from the fungus, *Aspergillus flavus,* that grows in stored grains and plants.

d) Miscellaneous. A variety of other chemical carcinogens having a role in the etiology of human cancer are as under:

- *Nitrosamines and nitrosamides* are involved in gastric carcinoma. These compounds are actually made in the stomach by nitrosylation of food preservatives.
- *Vinyl chloride monomer* derived from PVC (polyvinyl chloride) polymer in the causation of haemangiosarcoma of the liver.
- *Asbestos* in bronchogenic carcinoma and mesothelioma, especially in smokers.
- *Arsenical compounds* in causing epidermal hyperplasia and basal cell carcinoma.
- *Metals* like nickel, lead, cobalt chromium etc in industrial workers causing lung cancer.
- *Insecticides and fungicides* (e.g. aldrin, dieldrin, chlordane) in carcinogenesis in experimental animals.
- *Saccharin and cyclomates* in cancer in experimental animals.

2. PROMOTER CARCINOGENS

Promoters are chemical substances which lack the intrinsic carcinogenic potential but their application subsequent to initiator exposure helps the initiated cell to proliferate further. These include substances include phorbol esters, phenols, certain hormones and drugs.

i) Phorbol esters. The best known promoter in experimental animals is *TPA* (tetradecanoyl phorbol acetate) which acts by signal induction protein activation pathway.

ii) Hormones. Endogenous or exogenous oestrogen excess in promotion of cancers of endometrium and breast, prolonged administration of diethylstilbestrol in the etiology of postmenopausal endometrial carcinoma and in vaginal cancer in adolescent girls born to mothers exposed to this hormone during their pregnancy.
iii) Miscellaneous. e.g. dietary fat in cancer of colon, cigarette smoke and viral infections etc.

The feature of initiators and promoters are contrasted in Table 8.7.

Tests for Chemical Carcinogenicity

There are 2 main methods of testing chemical compound for its carcinogenicity:

1. EXPERIMENTAL INDUCTION. The traditional method is to administer the chemical compound under test to a batch of experimental animals like mice or other rodents by an appropriate route e.g. painting on the skin, giving orally or parenterally, or by inhalation. The chemical is administered repeatedly, the dose varied, and promoting agents are administered subsequently. After many months, the animal is autopsied and results obtained. However, all positive or negative tests cannot be applied to humans since there is sufficient species variation in susceptibility to particular carcinogen. Besides, the test is rather prolonged and expensive.

2. TESTS FOR MUTAGENICITY (AMES' TEST). A mutagen is a substance that can permanently alter the genetic composition of a cell. Ames' test evaluates the ability of a chemical to induce mutation in the mutant strain of *Salmonella typhimurium* that cannot synthesise histidine. Such strains are incubated with the potential carcinogen to which liver homogenate is added to supply enzymes required to convert procarcinogen to ultimate carcinogen. If the chemical under test is mutagenic, it will induce mutation in the mutant strains of *S. typhimurium* in the form of functional histidine gene, which will be reflected by the number of bacterial colonies growing on histidine-free culture medium (Fig. 8.11). Most of the carcinogenic chemicals tested positive in Ames' test are carcinogenic *in vivo*.

C. PHYSICAL CARCINOGENESIS

Physical agents in carcinogenesis are divided into 2 groups:

1. *Radiation,* both ultraviolet light and ionising radiation, is the most important physical agent. The role of radiation as carcinogenic agent is discussed below while its non-neoplastic complications are described in Chapter 3.

2. *Non-radiation* physical agents are the various forms of injury and are less important.

1. Radiation Carcinogenesis

Ultraviolet (UV) light and ionising radiation are the two main forms of radiation carcinogens which can induce cancer in experimental animals and are implicated in causation of some forms of human cancers. A property common between the two forms of radiation carcinogens is the appearance of mutations followed by a long period of latency after initial exposure, often 10-20 years or even later. Also, radiation carcinogens may act to enhance the effect of another carcinogen (co-carcinogens) and, like chemical carcinogens, may have sequential stages of initiation and promotion in their evolution. Ultraviolet light and ionising radiation differ in their mode of action as described below:

i) ULTRAVIOLET LIGHT. The main source of UV radiation is the sunlight; others are UV lamps and welder's arcs. UV light penetrates the skin for a few millimetres only so that its effect is limited to epidermis. The efficiency of UV light as carcinogen depends upon

TABLE 8.7: Contrasting Features of Initiator and Promoter Carcinogens.

FEATURE	INITIATOR	PROMOTER
1. *Mechanism*	Induction of mutation	Not mutagenic
2. *Dose*	Single for a short time	Repeated dose exposure, for a long time
3. *Response*	Sudden response	Slow response
4. *Change*	Permanent, irreversible	Change may be reversible
5. *Sequence*	Applied first, followed by promoter	Applied after prior exposure to initiator
6. *Effectivity*	Effective alone if exposed in large dose	Not effective alone
7. *Molecular changes*	Most common mutation of *RAS* oncogene, *TP53* anti-oncogene	Clonal expansion of mutated cells
8. *Examples*	Most chemical carcinogens, radiation	Hormones, phorbol esters

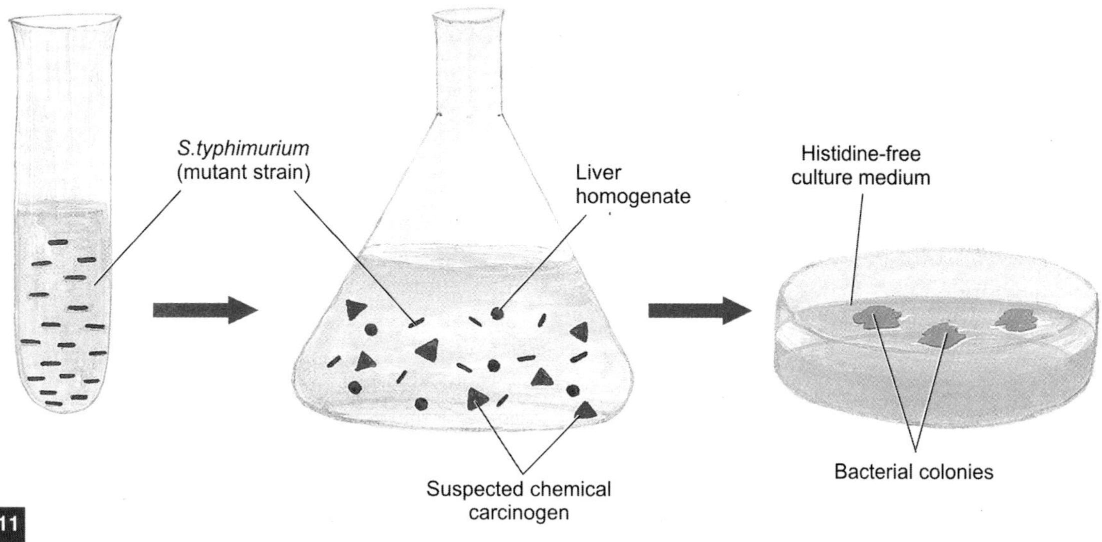

FIGURE 8.11

Schematic representation of the Ames' test.

the extent of light-absorbing protective melanin pigmentation of the skin. In humans, excessive exposure to UV rays can cause various forms of skin cancers—squamous cell carcinoma, basal cell carcinoma and malignant melanoma. In support of this is the epidemiological evidence of high incidence of these skin cancers in fair-skinned Europeans, albinos who do not tan readily, in people in Australia and New Zealand living close to the equator who receive more sunlight, and in farmers and outdoor workers due to the effect of actinic light radiation.

Mechanism. UV radiation may have various effects on the cells. The most important is induction of mutation; others are inhibition of cell division, inactivation of enzymes and sometimes causing cell death. The most important biochemical effect of UV radiation is the formation of pyrimidine dimers in DNA. Such UV-induced DNA damage in normal individuals is repaired, while in the predisposed persons who are excessively exposed to sunlight such damage remain unrepaired. The proof in favour of mutagenic effect of UV radiation comes from following recessive hereditary diseases characterised by a defect in DNA repair mechanism and associated with high incidence of cancers:

a) Xeroderma pigmentosum is predisposed to skin cancers at younger age (under 20 years of age).

b) Ataxia telangiectasia is predisposed to leukaemia.

c) Bloom's syndrome is predisposed to all types of cancers.

d) Fanconi's anaemia with increased risk to develop cancer.

Besides, like with other carcinogens, UV radiation also induces mutated forms of oncogenes (in particular *RAS* gene) and anti-oncogenes (*TP53* gene).

ii) IONISING RADIATION. Ionising radiation of all kinds like X-rays, α-, β- and γ-rays, radioactive isotopes, protons and neutrons can cause cancer in animals and in man. Most frequently, radiation-induced cancers are all forms of leukaemias (except chronic lymphocytic leukaemia); others are cancers of the thyroid (most commonly papillary carcinoma), skin, breast, ovary, uterus, lung, myeloma, and salivary glands (Fig. 8.12).The risk is increased by higher dose and with high LET (linear energy transfer) such as in neutrons and α-rays than with low LET as in X-rays and γ-rays. The evidence in support of carcinogenic role of ionising radiation is cited in the following examples:

a) Higher incidence of radiation dermatitis and subsequent malignant tumours of the skin was noted in X-ray workers and radiotherapists who did initial pioneering work in these fields before the advent of safety measures.

b) High incidence of osteosarcoma was observed in young American watch-working girls engaged in painting the dials with luminous radium who unknowingly ingested radium while using lips to point their brushes.

c) Miners in radioactive elements have higher incidence of cancers.

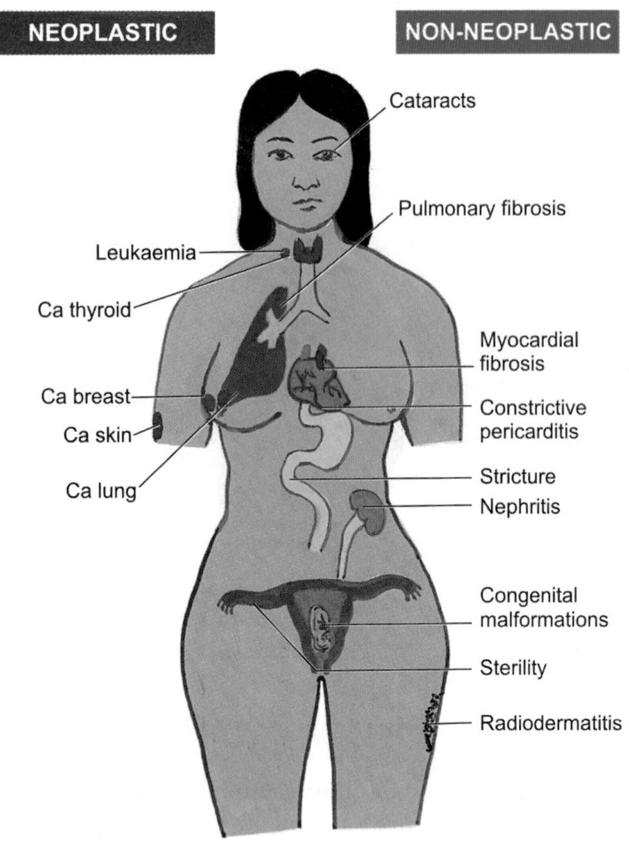

FIGURE 8.12

Neoplastic (left) and non-neoplastic complications (right) of ionising radiation.

d) Japanese atom bomb survivors of the twin cities of Hiroshima and Nagasaki after World War II have increased frequency of malignant tumours, notably acute and chronic myeloid leukaemias, and various solid tumours of breast, colon, thyroid and lung.

e) Accidental leakage at nuclear power plant in 1985 in Chernobyl (in former USSR, now in Ukraine) has caused long term hazardous effects of radioactive material to the population living in the vicinity.

f) It has been observed that therapeutic X-ray irradiation results in increased frequency of cancers, e.g. in patients of ankylosing spondylitis, in children with enlarged thymus, and in children irradiated *in utero* during investigations on the mother.

Mechanism. Radiation damages the DNA of the cell by one of the 2 possible mechanisms:

a) It may directly alter the cellular DNA.

b) It may dislodge ions from water and other molecules of the cell and result in formation of highly reactive free radicals that may bring about the damage.

Damage to the DNA resulting in mutagenesis is the most important action of ionising radiation. It may cause chromosomal breakage, translocation, or point mutation. The effect depends upon a number of factors such as type of radiation, dose, dose-rate, frequency and various host factors such as age, individual susceptibility, immune competence, hormonal influences and type of cells irradiated.

2. Non-radiation Physical Carcinogenesis

Mechanical injury to the tissues such as from stones in the gallbladder, stones in the urinary tract, and healed scars following burns or trauma, has been suggested as the cause of increased risk of carcinoma in these tissues but the evidence is not convincing. Asbestosis and asbestos-associated tumours of the lung are discussed in Chapter 15; the characteristic tumour being malignant mesothelioma of the pleura. Other examples of physical agents in carcinogenesis are the implants of inert materials such as plastic, glass etc in prostheses or otherwise, and foreign bodies observed to cause tumour development in experimental animals. However, tumorigenesis by these materials in humans is rare.

D. BIOLOGIC CARCINOGENESIS

The epidemiological studies on different types of cancers indicate the involvement of transmissible biologic agents in their development, chiefly *viruses.* Other biologic agents implicated in carcinogenesis are as follows:

- **Parasites** e.g. *Schistosoma haematobium* infection of the urinary bladder is associated with high incidence of squamous cell carcinoma of the urinary bladder in some parts of the world such as in Egypt. *Clonorchis sinensis,*the liver fluke, lives in the hepatic duct and is implicated in causation of cholangiocarcinoma.
- **Fungus** *Aspergillus flavus* grows in stored grains and liberates aflatoxin; its human consumption, especially by those with HBV infection, is associated with development of hepatocellular carcinoma.
- **Bacteria** *Helicobacter pylori,* a gram-positive spiral-shaped micro-organism, colonises the gastric mucosa and has been found in cases of chronic gastritis and peptic ulcer; its prolonged infection may lead to gastric lymphoma and gastric carcinoma.

However, the role of viruses in the causation of cancer is more significant. It has been estimated that about 20% of all cancers worldwide are virus-associated cancers. Therefore, biologic carcinogenesis is largely *viral carcinogenesis,* described below.

VIRAL CARCINOGENESIS

The association of oncogenic viruses with neoplasia was first observed by an Italian physician Sanarelli in 1889 who noted association between myxomatosis of rabbits with poxvirus. The contagious nature of the common human wart was first established in 1907. Since then, a number of viruses capable of inducing tumours (oncogenic viruses) in experimental animals, and some implicated in man, have been identified.

Oncogenic viruses can be transmitted by one of the 3 routes:

i) *Vertical transmission,* when the infection is genetically transmitted from infected parents to offsprings.

ii) *Horizontal transmission,* when the infection passes from one to another by direct contact as occurs in most contagious diseases.

iii) *By inoculation* as is done in experimental animals.

Based on their nucleic acid content, oncogenic viruses fall into 2 broad groups:

1. Those containing deoxyribonucleic acid are called *DNA oncogenic viruses.*
2. Those containing ribonucleic acid are termed *RNA oncogenic viruses.*

The two types of oncogenic viruses are described separately below, followed by their mechanisms of action. Most of the work is based on studies in experimental animals and only some have a role in human neoplasia.

DNA Oncogenic Viruses

DNA oncogenic viruses have direct access to the host cell nucleus and are incorporated into the genome of the host cell. DNA viruses are classified into 5 subgroups, each of which is capable of producing neoplasms in different hosts (Table 8.8). These are: Papovaviruses, Herpesviruses, Adenoviruses, Poxviruses and Hepadna viruses.

1. PAPOVAVIRUSES. This group consists of the papilloma virus including the human papilloma virus (HPV), polyoma virus and SV-40 (simian vacuolating) virus. These viruses have an etiologic role in a variety of benign and malignant neoplasms in animals and in humans:

i) Papilloma viruses. These viruses were the first to be implicated in the etiology of any human neoplasia. These viruses appear to replicate in the layers of stratified squamous epithelium. About 70 types of HPV have been identified, different types being implicated in cutaneous warts (benign squamous papillomas), genital warts (condyloma acuminata) and in squamous cell cancers. The following examples are cited to demonstrate their role in oncogenesis:

TABLE 8.8: DNA Oncogenic Viruses.

VIRUS	HOST	ASSOCIATED TUMOUR
1. *PAPOVAVIRUSES*		
Human papilloma virus	**Humans**	Cervical cancer and its precursor lesions, squamous cell carcinoma at other sites Skin cancer in epidermodysplasia verruciformis Papillomas (warts) on skin, larynx, genitals (genital warts)
Papilloma viruses	Cotton-tail rabbits Bovine	Papillomas (Warts) Alimentary tract cancer
Polyoma virus	Mice	Various carcinomas, sarcomas
SV-40 virus	Monkeys Hamsters **Humans**	Harmless Sarcoma ? Mesothelioma
2. *HERPESVIRUSES*		
Epstein-Barr virus	**Humans**	Burkitt's lymphoma Nasopharyngeal carcinoma
Human herpesvirus 8 (Kaposi's sarcoma herpesvirus)	**Humans**	Kaposi's sarcoma B cell lymphoma
Lucke' frog virus	Frog	Renal cell carcinoma
Marek's disease virus	Chickens	T-cell leukaemia-lymphoma
3. *ADENOVIRUSES*	Hamsters	Sarcomas
4. *POXVIRUSES*	Rabbits **Humans**	Myxomatosis Molluscum contagiosum, papilloma
5. *HEPADNAVIRUSES*		
Hepatitis B virus	**Humans**	Hepatocellular carcinoma

In humans—

- HPV was first detected as etiologic agent in common *skin warts* (squamous cell papillomas) by Shope in 1933; the condition is infectious. Current evidence supports implication of low risk HPV types 1,2, 4 and 7.
- Viral DNA of high risk HPV types 16 and 18 has been seen in 75-100% cases of *invasive cervical cancer* and its precursor lesions (carcinoma *in situ* and dysplasia) and is strongly implicated.
- HPV types 6 and 11 are involved in the etiology of genital warts or *condyloma acuminata.*
- HPVs are also involved in causation of *other squamous cell carcinomas* such as of anus, perianal region, vulva, penis and oral cavity.
- HPV is responsible for causing an uncommon condition, *epidermodysplasia verruciformis.* The condition is characterised by multiple skin warts and a genetic defect in the cell-mediated immunity. About one third of cases develop squamous cell carcinoma in the sun-exposed warts.
- Some strains of HPV are responsible for causing multiple *juvenile papillomas* of the larynx.

In animals—

- Benign warty lesions similar to those seen in humans are produced by different members of the papilloma virus family in susceptible animals such as in rabbits by cottontail rabbit papilloma virus, and in cattle by bovine papilloma virus (BPV).
- There is evidence to suggest the association of BPV and cancer of the alimentary tract in cattle.

ii) Polyoma virus. Polyoma virus occurs as a natural infection in mice.

- *In animals*—Polyoma virus infection is responsible for various kinds of carcinomas and sarcomas in immunodeficient (nude) mice and other rodents.
- *In humans*—Polyoma virus infection is not known to produce any human tumour but can cause progressive demyelinating leucoencephalopathy which is a fatal demyelinating disease.

iii) SV-40 virus. As the name suggests, simian vacuolating virus occurs in monkeys without causing any harm but can induce sarcoma in hamsters.

Recently, there is evidence of involvement of SV-40 infection in mesothelioma of the pleura.

2. HERPESVIRUSES. Primary infection of all the herpesviruses in man persists probably for life in a latent stage which can get reactivated later. Important members of herpesvirus family are Epstein-Barr virus, herpes simplex virus type 2 (HSV-2) and human herpes-virus 8 (HHV8), cytomegalovirus (CMV), Lucke's frog virus and Marek's disease virus. Out of these, Lucke's frog virus and Marek's disease virus are implicated in animal tumours only (renal cell carcinoma and T-cell leukaemia-lymphoma respectively). Earlier oncogenic role assigned to HSV-2 and CMV in human tumours has now been refuted. The other two—EBV and HHV are implicated in human tumours as follows.

EPSTEIN-BARR VIRUS (EBV). EBV infects human B-lymphocytes and stimulates them to proliferate. EBV is implicated in the following human tumours—Burkitt's lymphoma, anaplastic nasopharyngeal carcinoma, post-transplant lymphoproliferative disease, primary CNS lymphoma in AIDS patients, and Hodgkin's lymphoma. It is also shown to be the cause of infectious mononucleosis, a self-limiting disease in humans. The role of EBV in the first two human tumours is given below while others find mention elsewhere in relevant chapters.

Burkitt's lymphoma. Burkitt's lymphoma was initially noticed in African children by Burkitt in 1958 but is now known to occur in 2 forms—*African endemic form,* and *sporadic form* seen elsewhere in the world. The morphological aspects of the tumour are explained in Chapter 14, while oncogenesis is described here.

There is strong evidence linking Burkitt's lymphoma, a B-lymphocyte neoplasm, with EBV as observed from the following features:

a) Over 90% of Burkitt's lymphomas are EBV-positive in which the tumour cells carry the viral DNA.

b) 100% cases of Burkitt's lymphoma show elevated levels of antibody titers to various EBV antigens.

c) EBV has strong tropism for B lymphocytes. EBV-infected B cells grown in cultures are immortalised i.e. they continue to develop further along B cell-line to propagate their progeny in the altered form.

d) Though EBV infection is almost worldwide in all adults and is also known to cause self-limiting infectious mononucleosis, but the fraction of EBV-infected circulating B cells in such individuals is extremely small.

e) Linkage between Burkitt's lymphoma and EBV infection is very high in African endemic form of the disease and probably in cases of AIDS than in sporadic form of the disease.

However, a few observations, especially regarding sporadic cases of Burkitt's lymphoma, suggest that certain other supportive factors may be contributing. *Immunosuppression* appears to be one such most significant factor. The evidence in favour is as follows:

- The normal EBV-infected individuals as well as cases developing infectious mononucleosis are able to mount good immune response so that they do not develop Burkitt's lymphoma.

- In immunosuppressed patients such as in HIV infection and organ transplant recipients, there is marked reduction in body's T-cell immune response and higher incidence of this neoplasm.
- It is observed that malaria, which confers immunosuppressive effect on the host, is prevalent in endemic proportions in regions where endemic form of Burkitt's lymphoma is frequent. This supports the linkage of EBV infection and immunosuppression in the etiology of Burkitt's lymphoma.

Anaplastic nasopharyngeal carcinoma. This is the other tumour having close association with EBV infection. The tumour is prevalent in South-East Asia, especially in the Chinese, and in Eskimos. The morphology of nasopharyngeal carcinoma is described in Chapter 16. The evidence linking EBV infection with this tumour is as follows:

a) 100% cases of nasopharyngeal carcinoma carry DNA of EBV in tumour cells.

b) Individuals with this tumour have high titers of antibodies to various EBV antigens.

However, like in case of Burkitt's lymphoma, there may be some *co-factors* such as genetic susceptibility that account for the unusual geographic distribution.

HUMAN HERPESVIRUS 8 (HHV 8). It has been shown that infection with HHV 8 or Kaposi's sarcoma-associated herpesvirus (KSHV) is associated with Kaposi's sarcoma, a vascular neoplasm common in patients of AIDS. Compared to sporadic Kaposi's sarcoma, the AIDS-associated tumour is multicentric and more aggressive. HHV 8 has lymphotropism and is also implicated in causation of B cell lymphoma and multicentric variant of Castleman's disease.

3. ADENOVIRUSES. The human adenoviruses cause upper respiratory infections and pharyngitis.

- *In humans,* they are not known to be involved in any tumour.
- *In hamsters,* they may induce sarcomas.

4. POXVIRUSES. This group of oncogenic viruses is involved in the etiology of following lesions:

- *In rabbits*—poxviruses cause myxomatosis.
- *In humans*—poxviruses cause molluscum contagiosum and may induce squamous cell papilloma.

5. HEPADNAVIRUSES. *Hepatitis B virus (HBV)* is a member of hepadnavirus family. HBV infection in man causes an acute hepatitis and is responsible for a carrier state, which can result in some cases to chronic hepatitis progressing to hepatic cirrhosis, and onto hepatocellular carcinoma. These lesions and the structure of HBV are described in detail in Chapter 19. Suffice this to say here that there is strong epidemiological evidence linking HBV infection to development of hepatocellular carcinoma as evidenced by the following:

a) The geographic differences in the incidence of hepatocellular carcinoma closely match the variation in prevalence of HBV infection e.g. high incidence in Far-East and Africa.

b) Epidemiological studies in high incidence regions indicate about 200 times higher risk of developing hepatocellular carcinoma in HBV-infected cases as compared to uninfected population in the same area.

Posssible mechanism of hepatocellular carcinoma occurring in those harbouring long standing infection with HBV is chronic destruction of HBV-infected hepatocytes followed by continued hepatocyte proliferation. This process renders the hepatocytes vulnerable to the action of other risk factors such as to aflatoxin causing mutation and neoplastic proliferation.

More recent evidence has assigned an oncogenic role to another hepatotropic virus, hepatitis C virus (HCV), an RNA virus unrelated to HBV. HCV is implicated in about half the cases of hepatocellular carcinoma in much the same way as HBV.

RNA Oncogenic Viruses

RNA oncogenic viruses are retroviruses i.e. they contain the enzyme reverse transcriptase (RT), though all retroviruses are not oncogenic (Table 8.9). The enzyme, reverse transcriptase, is required for reverse transcription of viral RNA to synthesise viral DNA strands i.e. reverse of normal—rather than DNA encoding for RNA synthesis, viral RNA transcripts for the DNA by the enzyme RT present in the RNA viruses. RT is a DNA polymerase and helps to form complementary DNA (cDNA) that moves in to host cell nucleus and gets incorporated in to it.

Based on their activity to transform target cells into neoplastic cells, RNA viruses are divided into 3 subgroups—acute transforming viruses, slow transforming viruses, and human T-cell lymphotropic viruses (HTLV). The former two are implicated in inducing a variety of tumours in animals while HTLV is causative for human T-cell leukaemia and lymphoma.

In general, RNA viruses have 3 genes: *gag* gene (for group antigen), *pol* gene (that codes for polymerase enzyme), and *env* gene (for envelop protein), while acute transforming viruses have one a fourth gene *tat* gene that transforms the oncogene in the susceptible cell.

TABLE 8.9: RNA Oncogenic Viruses.

VIRUS	HOST	ASSOCIATED TUMOUR
1. *ACUTE TRANSFORMING VIRUSES*		
Rous sarcoma virus	Chickens	Sarcoma
Leukaemia-sarcoma virus	Avian, feline, bovine, primate	Leukaemias, sarcomas
2. *SLOW TRANSFORMING VIRUSES*		
	Mice, cats, bovine	Leukaemias, lymphomas
Mouse mammary tumour virus (Bittner milk factor)	Daughter mice	Breast cancer
3. *HUMAN T-CELL LYMPHOTROPIC VIRUS (HTLV)*		
HTLV-I	**Human**	Adult T-cell leukaemia lymphoma (ATLL)
HTLV-II	**Human**	T-cell variant of hairy cell leukaemia
4. *HEPATITIS C VIRUS*		
HCV	**Human**	Hepatocellular carcinoma

1. ACUTE TRANSFORMING VIRUSES. This group includes retroviruses which transform all the cells infected by them into malignant cells rapidly ('acute'). All the viruses in this group possess one or more viral oncogenes (*v-oncs*). All the members of acute transforming viruses discovered so far are defective viruses in which the particular *v-onc* has substituted other essential genetic material such as *gag, pol* and *env.* These defective viruses cannot replicate by themselves unless the host cell is infected by another 'helper virus'. Acute oncogenic viruses have not been detected in any human tumour so far, though they have been identified in tumours in different animals, e.g.

a) Rous sarcoma virus in chickens.

b) Leukaemia-sarcoma viruses of various types such as avian, feline, bovine and primate.

2. SLOW TRANSFORMING VIRUSES. These oncogenic retroviruses cause development of leukaemias and lymphomas in different species of animals (e.g. in mice, cats and bovine) and include the mouse mammary tumour virus (MMTV) that causes breast cancer in the daughter-mice suckled by the MMTV-infected mother via the causal agent in the mother's milk (*Bittner milk factor*). These viruses have long incubation period between infection and development of neoplastic transformation ('slow'). Slow transforming viruses cause neoplastic transformation by *insertional mutagenesis* i.e. viral DNA synthesised by viral RNA via reverse transcriptase is *inserted* or integrated near the proto-oncogenes of the host cell resulting in enhanced expression of proto-oncogenes as well as causes genetic damage (*mutagenesis*) to the host cell genome leading to neoplastic transformation.

3. HUMAN T-CELL LYMPHOTROPIC VIRUSES (HTLV). HTLV is a form of slow transforming virus but is described separately because of 2 reasons:

i) This is the only retrovirus implicated in human cancer.

ii) The mechanism of neoplastic transformation is different from slow transforming as well as from acute transforming viruses.

Four types of HTLVs are recognised—HTLV-I, HTLV-II, HTLV-III and HTLV-IV. It may be mentioned in passing here that the etiologic agent for AIDS, HIV, is also an HTLV (HTLV-III) as described in Chapter 4.

A link between HTLV-I infection and adult T-cell leukaemia-lymphoma syndrome (ATLL) has been identified while HTLV-II is implicated in causation of T-cell variant of hairy cell leukaemia. HTLV-I is transmitted through sexual contact, by blood, or to infants during breastfeeding. The highlights of this association and mode of neoplastic transformation are as under:

i) Epidemiological studies by tests for antibodies have shown that HTLV-I infection is endemic in parts of Japan and West Indies where the incidence of ATLL is high. The latent period after HTLV-I infection is, however, very long (20-30 years).

ii) The initiation of neoplastic process is similar to that for Burkitt's lymphoma except that HTLV-I has tropism for CD4+T lymphocytes as in HIV infection, while EBV of Burkitt's lymphoma has tropism for B lymphocytes.

iii) As in Burkitt's lymphoma, immunosuppression plays a supportive role in the neoplastic transformation by HTLV-I infection.

The underlying *molecular mechanism* of neoplastic transformation by HTLV-I infection differs from acute transforming viruses because it does not contain *v-onc*, and from other slow transforming viruses because it does not have fixed site of insertion for insertional mutagenesis.

The genome of HTLV-I contains *gag*, *pol* and *env* genes similar to other retroviruses but in addition it contains *tat* gene region also which stimulates neoplastic cell proliferation of T cells. Initially, this proliferation of T cells is polyclonal which then undergoes new mutations and leads to monoclonal T cell leukaemia-lymphoma. Chronic leukaemia retrovirus, HTLV-II, brings about transformation by 'promoter insertion' that produces oncogenesis by oncogenes and growth factors.

Mechanisms of Viral Oncogenesis

Mode of oncogenesis by DNA and RNA oncogenic viruses are different and are illustrated schematically in Fig. 8.13 and 8.14 respectively.

1. Mode of DNA viral oncogenesis. Host cells infected by DNA oncogenic viruses may have one of the following 2 results (Fig. 8.13):

i) Replication. The virus may replicate in the host cell with consequent lysis of the infected cell and release of virions.

ii) Integration. The viral DNA may integrate into the host cell DNA.

The latter event (integration) results in neoplastic transformation of the host cell, while the former (replication) brings about cell death but no neoplastic transformation. A feature essential for host cell transformation is the expression of virus-specific T-(transforming protein) antigens immediately after infection of the host cell by DNA oncogenic virus.

2. Mode of RNA viral oncogenesis. As the name suggests, RNA viruses or retroviruses contain two identical strands of RNA and the enzyme, reverse transcriptase. The steps involved in transformation of host cells by RNA oncogenic viruses are as under (Fig. 8.14):

i) Reverse transcriptase is RNA-dependent DNA synthetase that acts as a template to synthesise *a single strand of matching viral* DNA i.e. reverse of the normal in which DNA is transcribed into messenger RNA.

ii) The single strand of viral DNA is then copied by DNA dependent DNA synthetase to form another strand of complementary DNA resulting in *double-stranded viral* DNA or provirus.

iii) The provirus is then integrated into the DNA of the host cell genome and may transform the cell into *neoplastic cell*.

iv) Retroviruses are *replication-competent*. The host cells which allow replication of integrated retrovirus are called permissive cells. Non-permissible cells do not permit replication of the integrated retrovirus.

v) Viral replication begins after integration of the provirus into host cell genome. Integration results in transcription of proviral genes or progenes into messenger RNA which then forms *components of the virus particle*—virion core protein from *gag* gene, reverse transcriptase from *pol* gene, and envelope glycoprotein from *env* gene. The three components of virus particle are then assembled at the plasma membrane of the host cell and the virus particles released by budding off from the plasma membrane, thus completing the process of replication.

VIRUSES AND HUMAN CANCER: A SUMMARY

In man, epidemiological as well as circumstantial evidence has been accumulating since the discovery of contagious nature of common human wart (papilloma) in 1907 that cancer may have viral etiology. Presently, about 20% of all human cancers worldwide are believed to have 'virus association'. Aside from experimental evidence, the etiologic role of DNA and RNA viruses in a variety of human neoplasms has already been explained above. Here, a summary of different viruses implicated in human tumours is presented (Fig. 8.15):

Benign tumours. There are 2 conditions which are actually doubtful as tumours in which definite viral etiology is established. These are:

i) Human wart (papilloma) caused by human papilloma virus; and

ii) Molluscum contagiosum caused by poxvirus.

Malignant tumours. The following 8 human cancers have enough epidemiological, serological, and in some cases genomic evidence that viruses are implicated in their etiology:

i) *Burkitt's lymphoma* by Epstein-Barr virus.

ii) *Nasopharyngeal carcinoma* by Epstein-Barr virus.

iii) *Primary hepatocellular carcinoma* by hepatitis B virus and hepatitis C virus.

iv) *Cervical cancer* by high risk human papilloma virus types (HPV 16 and 18).

v) *Kaposi's sarcoma* by human herpes virus type 8 (HHV 8).

vi) *B cell lymphoma* by HHV8.

vii) *Adult T-cell leukaemia and lymphoma* by HTLV-I.

viii) *T-cell variant of hairy cell leukaemia* by HTLV-II.

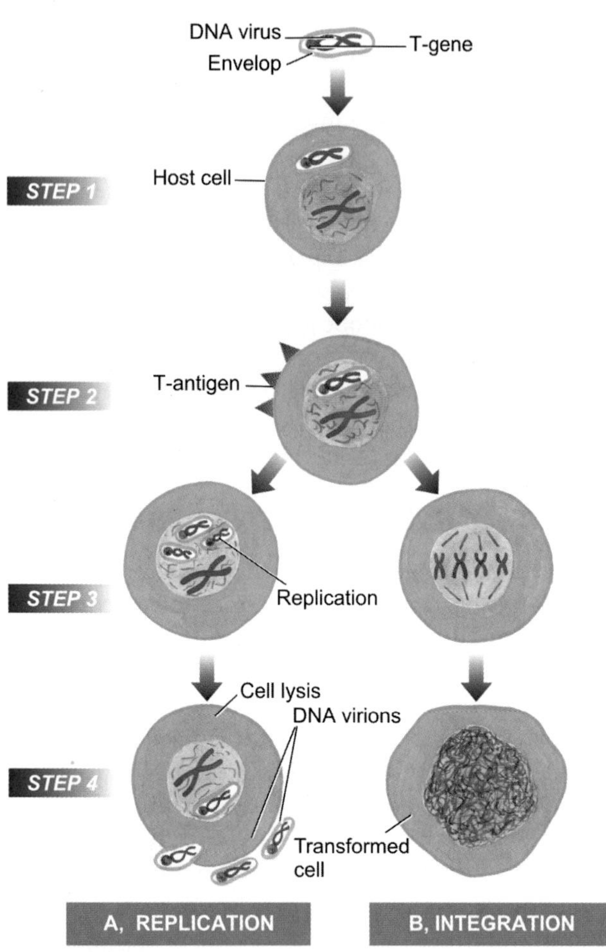

FIGURE 8.13

Replication and integration of DNA virus in the host cell.

A, Replication: *Step 1.* The DNA virus invades the host cell. *Step 2.* Viral DNA is incorporated into the host nucleus and T-antigen is expressed immediately after infection. *Step 3.* Replication of viral DNA occurs and other components of virion are formed. The new virions are assembled in the cell nucleus. *Step 4.* The new virions are released, accompanied by host cell lysis. B, Integration : *Steps 1 and 2* are similar as in replication. *Step 3.* Integration of viral genome into the host cell genome occurs which requires essential presence of functional T-antigen. *Step 4.* A 'transformed (neoplastic) cell' is formed.

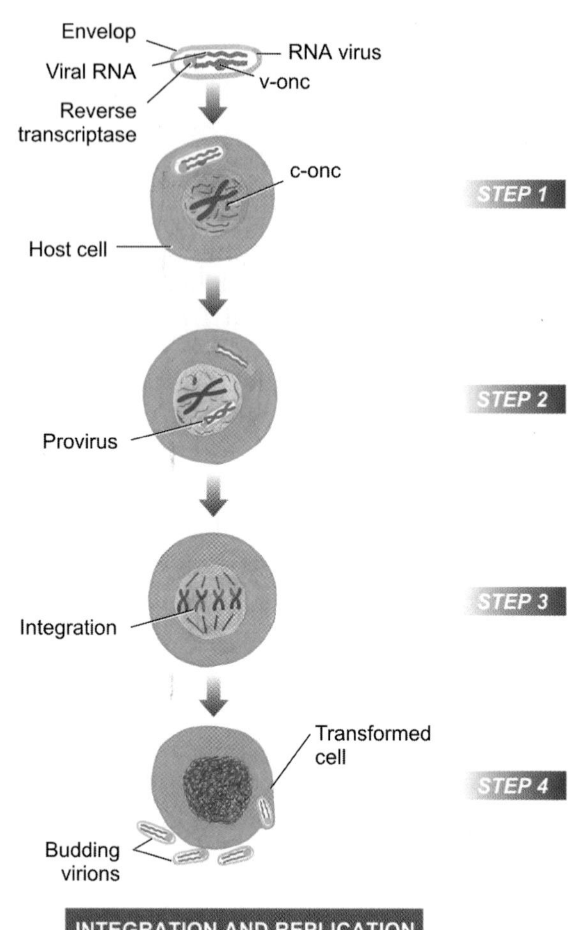

FIGURE 8.14

Integration and replication of RNA virus (retrovirus) in the host cell.

Step 1. The RNA virus invades the host cell. The viral envelope fuses with the plasma membrane of the host cell; viral RNA genome as well as reverse transcriptase are released into the cytosol. *Step 2.* Reverse transcriptase acts as template to synthesise single strand of matching viral DNA which is then copied to form complementary DNA resulting in double-stranded viral DNA (provirus). *Step 3.* The provirus is integrated into the host cell genome producing 'transformed host cell.' *Step 4.* Integration of the provirus brings about replication of viral components which are then assembled and released by budding.

CLINICAL ASPECTS OF NEOPLASIA

Two major aspects of clinical significance in assessing the course and management of neoplasia are: tumour-host inter-relationship (i.e. the effect of tumour on host and *vice versa*) and laboratory diagnosis of cancer.

TUMOUR-HOST INTER-RELATIONSHIP

The natural history of a neoplasm depends upon 2 features:

i) Effect of tumour on host
ii) Host response against tumour (Immunology of cancer)

EFFECT OFTUMOUR ON HOST

Malignant tumours produce more ill-effects than the benign tumours. The effects may be local, or generalised and more widespread.

1. LOCAL EFFECTS. Both benign and malignant tumours cause local effects on the host due to their size

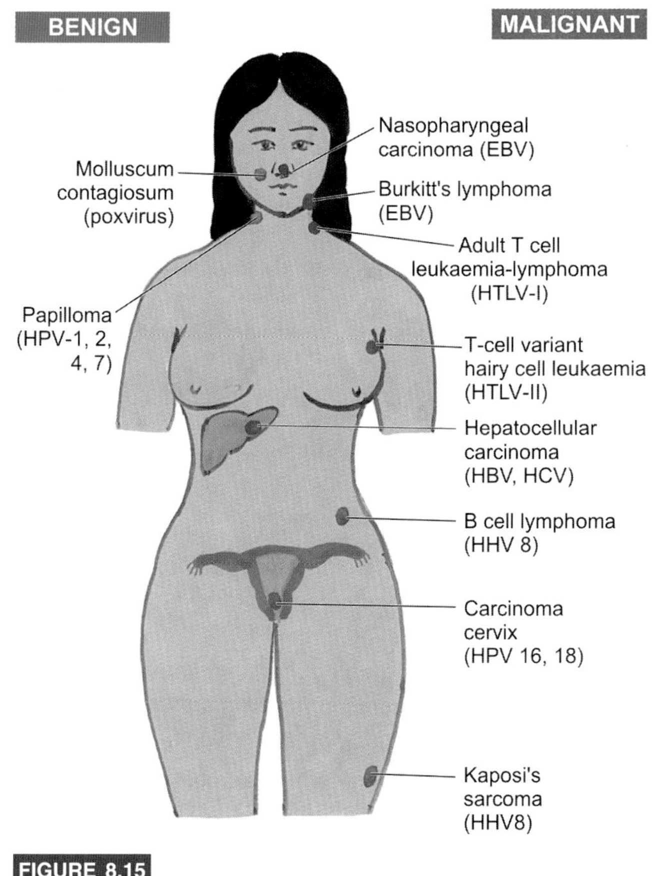

FIGURE 8.15

Viruses (in brackets) in human tumours.

or location. Malignant tumours due to rapid and invasive growth potential have more serious effects. Some of the local effects of tumours are as under:

i) Compression. Many benign tumours pose only a cosmetic problem. Some benign tumours, however, due to their critical location, have more serious consequences e.g. pituitary adenoma may lead to serious endocrinopathy; a small benign tumour in ampulla of Vater may lead to biliary obstruction.

ii) Mechanical obstruction. Benign and malignant tumours in the gut may produce intestinal obstruction.

iii) Tissue destruction. Malignant tumours, both primary and metastatic, infiltrate and destroy the vital structures.

iv) Infarction, ulceration, haemorrhage. Cancers have a greater tendency to undergo infarction, surface ulceration and haemorrhage than the benign tumours. Secondary bacterial infection may supervene. Large tumours in mobile organs (e.g. an ovarian tumour) may undergo torsion and produce infarction and haemorrhage.

2. CANCER CACHEXIA. Patients with advanced and disseminated cancers terminally have asthenia (emaciation), and anorexia, together referred to as cancer cachexia (meaning wasting). Exact mechanism of cachexia is not clear but it does not occur due to increased nutritional demands of the tumour. Possibly, cachectin or tumour necrosis factor α (TNF-α) and interleukin-1 derived from macrophages play a contributory role in cachexia. The various other causes include necrosis, ulceration, haemorrhage, infection, malabsorption, anxiety, pain, insomnia, hypermetabolism and pyrexia.

3. FEVER. Fever of unexplained origin may be presenting feature in some malignancies such as in Hodgkin's disease, adenocarcinoma kidney, osteogenic sarcoma and many other tumours. The exact mechanism of tumour associated fever is not known but probably the tumour cells themselves elaborate pyrogens.

4. PARANEOPLASTIC SYNDROMES. Paraneoplastic syndromes (PNS) are a group of conditions developing in patients with advanced cancer which are neither explained by direct and distant spread of the tumour, nor by the usual hormone elaboration by the tissue of origin of the tumour. About 10 to 15% of the patients with advanced cancer develop one or more of the syndromes included in the PNS. Rarely, PNS may be the earliest manifestation of a latent cancer.

The various clinical syndromes included in the PNS are as summarised in Table 8.10 and are briefly outlined below:

i) Endocrine syndrome. Elaboration of hormones or hormone-like substances by cancer cells of non-endocrine origin is called as ectopic hormone production. Some examples are given below:

a) *Hypercalcaemia.* Symptomatic hypercalcaemia unrelated to hyperparathyroidism is the most common syndrome in PNS. It occurs from elaboration of parathormone-like substance by tumours such as squamous cell carcinoma of the lung, carcinoma kidney, breast and adult T cell leukaemia lymphoma.

b) *Cushing's syndrome* About 10% patients of small cell carcinoma of the lung elaborate ACTH or ACTH-like substance producing Cushing's syndrome. In addition, cases with pancreatic carcinoma and neurogenic tumours may be associated with Cushing's syndrome.

c) *Polycythaemia.* Secretion of erythropoietin by certain tumours such as renal cell carcinoma, hepatocellular carcinoma and cerebellar haemangioma may cause polycythaemia.

d) *Hypoglycaemia.* Elaboration of insulin-like substance by fibrosarcomas, islet cell tumours of pancreas and mesothelioma may cause hypoglycaemia.

TABLE 8.10: Summary of Paraneoplastic Syndromes.

CLINICAL SYNDROME	UNDERLYING CANCER	MECHANISM
1. *ENDOCRINE SYNDROME:*		
i. Hypercalcaemia	Lung (sq. cell ca.), kidney, breast, Adult T-cell leukaemia-lymphoma	Parathromone-like protein vitamin D
ii. Cushing's syndrome	Lung (small cell carcinoma), pancreas, neural tumours	ACTH or ACTH-like substance
iii. Inappropriate anti-diuresis	Lung (small cell ca.), prostate, intracranial tumour	ADH or atrial natriuretic factor
iv. Hypoglycaemia	Pancreas (islet cell tumour), mesothelioma, fibrosarcoma	Insulin or insulin-like substance
v. Carcinoid syndrome	Bronchial carcinoid tumour, carcinoma pancreas, stomach	Serotonin, bradykinin
vi. Polycythaemia	Kidney, liver, cerebellar haemangioma	Erythropoietin
2. *NEUROMUSCULAR SYNDROMES:*		
i. Myasthenia gravis	Thymoma	Immunologic
ii. Neuromuscular disorders	Lung (small cell ca.), breast	Immunologic
3. *OSSEOUS, JOINT AND SOFT TISSUE:*		
i. Hypertrophic osteoarthropathy	Lung	Not known
ii. Clubbing of fingers	Lung	Not known
4. *HAEMATOLOGIC SYNDROMES:*		
i. Thrombophlebitis (Trousseau's phenomenon)	Pancreas, lung, GIT	Hypercoagulability
ii. Non-bacterial thrombotic endocarditis	Advanced cancers	Hypercoagulability
iii. Disseminated intravascular coagulation (DIC)	AML, adenocarcinoma	Chronic thrombotic phenomena
iv. Anaemia	Thymoma	Unknown
5. *GASTROINTESTINAL SYNDROMES:*		
i. Malabsorption	Lymphoma of small bowel	Hypoalbuminaemia
6. *RENAL SYNDROMES:*		
i. Nephrotic syndrome	Advanced cancers	Renal vein thrombosis, systemic amyloidosis
7. *CUTANEOUS SYNDROMES:*		
i. Acanthosis nigricans	Stomach, large bowel	Immunologic
ii. Seborrheic keratosis	Bowel	Immunologic
iii. Exfoliative dermatitis	Lymphoma	Immunologic
8. AMYLOIDOSIS:		
i. Primary	Multiple myeloma	Immunologic (AL protein)
ii. Secondary	Kidney, lymphoma, solid tumours	AA protein

ii) Neuromyopathic syndromes. About 5% of cancers are associated with progressive destruction of neurons throughout the nervous system without evidence of metastasis in the brain and spinal cord. This is probably mediated by immunologic mechanisms. The changes in the neurons may affect the muscles as well. The changes are: peripheral neuropathy, cortical cerebellar degeneration, myasthenia gravis syndrome, polymyositis.

iii) Effects on osseous, joints and soft tissue. e.g. hypertrophic osteoarthropathy and clubbing of fingers in cases of bronchogenic carcinoma by unknown mechanism.

iv) Haematologic and vascular syndrome. e.g. venous thrombosis (Trousseau's phenomenon), non-bacterial thrombotic endocarditis, disseminated intravascular coagulation (DIC), leukemoid reaction and normocytic normochromic anaemia occurring in advanced cancers.

Autoimmune haemolytic anaemia may be associated with B-cell tumours.

v) Gastrointestinal syndromes. Malabsorption of various dietary components as well as hypoalbuminaemia may be associated with a variety of cancers which do not directly involve small bowel.

vi) Renal syndromes. Renal vein thrombosis or systemic amyloidosis may produce nephrotic syndrome in patients with cancer.

vii) Cutaneous syndromes. Acanthosis nigricans characterised by the appearance of black warty lesions in the axillae and the groins may appear in the course of adenocarcinoma of gastrointestinal tract. Other cutaneous lesions in PNS include seborrheric dermatitis in advanced malignant tumours and exfoliative dermatitis in lymphomas and Hodgkin's disease.

viii) Amyloidosis. Primary amyloid deposits may occur in multiple myeloma whereas renal cell carcinoma and other solid tumours may be associated with secondary systemic amyloidosis.

HOST RESPONSE AGAINST TUMOUR (IMMUNE SURVEILLANCE OF CANCER)

It has long been thought that host defense mechanism in the form of immunological response exists so as to counter the growth and spread of cancer, *albeit*, more often partially. The following observations provide basis for this thinking:

1. Certain cancers evoke significant lymphocytic infiltrates composed of immunocompetent cells and such tumours have somewhat better prognosis e.g. medullary carcinoma breast, seminoma testis.
2. Rarely, a cancer may spontaneously regress partially or completely, probably under the influence of host defense mechanism. One such example is rare spontaneous disappearance of malignant melanoma from the primary site only to reappear as metastasis.
3. It is highly unusual to have primary and secondary tumours in the spleen due to its ability to destroy the growth and proliferation of tumour cells.
4. Immune surveillance exists is substantiated by increased frequency of cancers in immunodeficient host e.g. in AIDS patients, or in organ transplant recipients.

In an attempt to substantiate the above observations and to understand the underlying host defense mechanisms, experimental animal studies involving tumour transplants were carried out. The findings of animal experiments coupled with research on human cancers has led to the concept of immunology of cancer described below under the following headings:

1. Tumour antigens
2. Immune responses
3 Prospects of immunotherapy

1. TUMOUR ANTIGENS. It has been observed from experimental animal studies and in humans that following two types of tumour antigens encountered by cytotoxic T lymphocytes CTL, also called CD8+T cells:

i) Tumour-specific antigens (TSA) are located on tumour cells but are not present on normal cells. They are unique or specific antigens for particular tumour and not shared by normal cells. Therefore, TSAs are targets of attack by tumour-specific cytotoxic CD8+T lymphocytes. The examples are:

a) Testis specific antigen having MAGE genes.

b) Antigens responsible for mutational change in some tumours e.g. *TP53*, *RAS* gene, β-catenin etc.

c) Overexpressed antigens e.g. *HER2* protein in cancer of the breast, ovary.

d) Antigens from oncogenic viruses e.g. HPV, EBV.

e) Mucins associated antigens e.g. in cancers of the pancreas, breast, ovary.

f) Oncofoetal antigens e.g. α-foetoprotein, carcinoembryonic antigen in cancers of liver, colon.

ii) Tumour associated antigen (TAA) are present on tumour cells as well as on some normal cells. TAA are, thus, antigens shared by tumour cells and normal host cells from where the tumour originated. These antigens represent the stage at which the differentiation of tumour cells is arrested. The examples in this category are:

a) Tissue specific antigens such as melanocyte specific proteins.

b) Differentiation specific antigens e.g. CD10 in benign prostatic epithelium, prostate specific antigen (PSA) in carcinoma of prostate.

2. IMMUNE RESPONSES. The nature of host immune response to tumours demonstrated in animal studies and in patients with various types of cancers can be categorised as under:

i) Cell-mediated mechanism
ii) Humoral mechanism
iii) Inhibitory (regulatory) mechanism.

i) Cell-mediated mechanism. This is the main mechanism of destruction of tumour cells by the host. The following cellular responses can destroy the tumour cells and induce tumour immunity in humans:

a) *Specifically sensitised cytotoxic T lymphocytes (CTL)* i.e. CD8+ T cells which are directly cytotoxic requiring

Chapter Eight

contact between them and tumour cell. They specifically attack the virally induced cancers e.g. in Burkitt's lymphoma (EBV-induced), invasive squamous cell carcinoma (HPV-induced).

b) *Natural killer (NK) cells* are lymphocytes which destroy tumour cells without sensitisation, either directly or by antibody-dependent cellular cytotoxicity (ADCC). They are the first line of defense against tumour cells.

c) *Macrophages* are activated by interferon-γ secreted by T-cells and NK-cells, and therefore there is close collaboration of these lymphocytes with macrophages. Activated macrophages mediate cytotoxicity by production of oxygen free radicals or by tumour necrosis factor.

ii) Humoral mechanism. Humoral antibodies may act by complement activation or by antibody-dependent cytotoxicity by NK cells.

iii) Inhibitory (Regulatory) mechanism. In spite of host immune responses, most cancers grow relentlessly. This is due to some of the following controlling mechanisms:

a) During progression of the cancer, immunogenic cells may disappear.

b) Cytotoxic T-cells and NK-cells may play a self regulatory role.

c) Immunosuppression mediated by various acquired carcinogenic agents (viruses, chemicals, radiation).

d) Immunoinhibitory role of factors secreted by tumours e.g. transforming growth factor-β.

The mechanisms of these immune responses are schematically illustrated in Fig. 8.16.

3. PROSPECTS OF IMMUNOTHERAPY. Despite the existence of anti-tumour immune responses, the cancers still progress and eventually cause death of the host. The immune responses to be effective enough must eliminate the tumour cells more rapidly than their rate of proliferation and hence the role of boosting the immune response or immunotherapy.

i) Non-specific stimulation of the host immune response was initially attempted with BCG, *Corynebacterium parvum* and levamisole, but except slight effect in acute lymphoid leukaemia, it failed to have any significant influence in any other tumour.

ii) Specific stimulation of the immune system was attempted next by immunising the host with irradiated tumour cells but failed to yield desired results because if the patient's tumour within the body failed to stimulate effective immunity, the implanted cells of the same tumour are unlikely to do so.

iii) Current status of immunotherapy is focussed on following three main approaches:

a) *Cellular immunotherapy* consists of infusion of tumour-specific cytotoxic T cells which will increase the population of tumour-infiltrating lymphocytes. The patient's peripheral blood lymphocytes are cultured with interleukin-2 which generates lymphokine-activated killer cells having potent anti-tumour effect.

b) *Cytokine therapy* is used to build up specific and non-specific host defenses. These include: interleukin-2, interferon-α and -γ, tumour necrosis factor-α, and granulocyte-monocyte colony stimulating factor (GM-CSF).

c) *Monoclonal antibody therapy* is currently being tried as tumour cell toxin in the treatment of leukaemias and lymphomas.

DIAGNOSIS OF CANCER

When the diagnosis of cancer is suspected on clinical examination and on other investigations, it must be confirmed. The most certain and reliable method which has stood the test of time is the histological examination of biopsy, though recently many other methods to arrive at the correct diagnosis or confirm the histological diagnosis are available which are discussed in Chapter 2.

1. Histological Methods

These methods are based on microscopic examination of properly fixed tissue (excised tumour mass or open/needle biopsy from the mass), supported with complete clinical and investigative data. These methods are most valuable in arriving at the accurate diagnosis. The tissue must be fixed in 10% formalin for light microscopic examination and in glutaraldehyde for electron microscopic studies, while quick-frozen section and hormonal analysis are carried out on fresh unfixed tissues.

The histological diagnosis by either of these methods is made on the basis that cytological features of *benign tumours* resemble those of normal tissue and that they are unable to invade and metastasise, while *malignant tumours* are identified by lack of differentiation in cancer cells termed 'anaplasia' or 'cellular atypia' and may invade as well as metastasise. The light microscopic and ultrastructural characteristics of neoplastic cell have already been described in this chapter.

2. Cytological Methods

These are discussed in detail in Chapter 29.

Cytological methods for diagnosis consist of study of cells shed off into body cavities (exfoliative cytology) and study of cells by putting a fine needle introduced under vacuum into the lesion (fine needle aspiration cytology, FNAC).

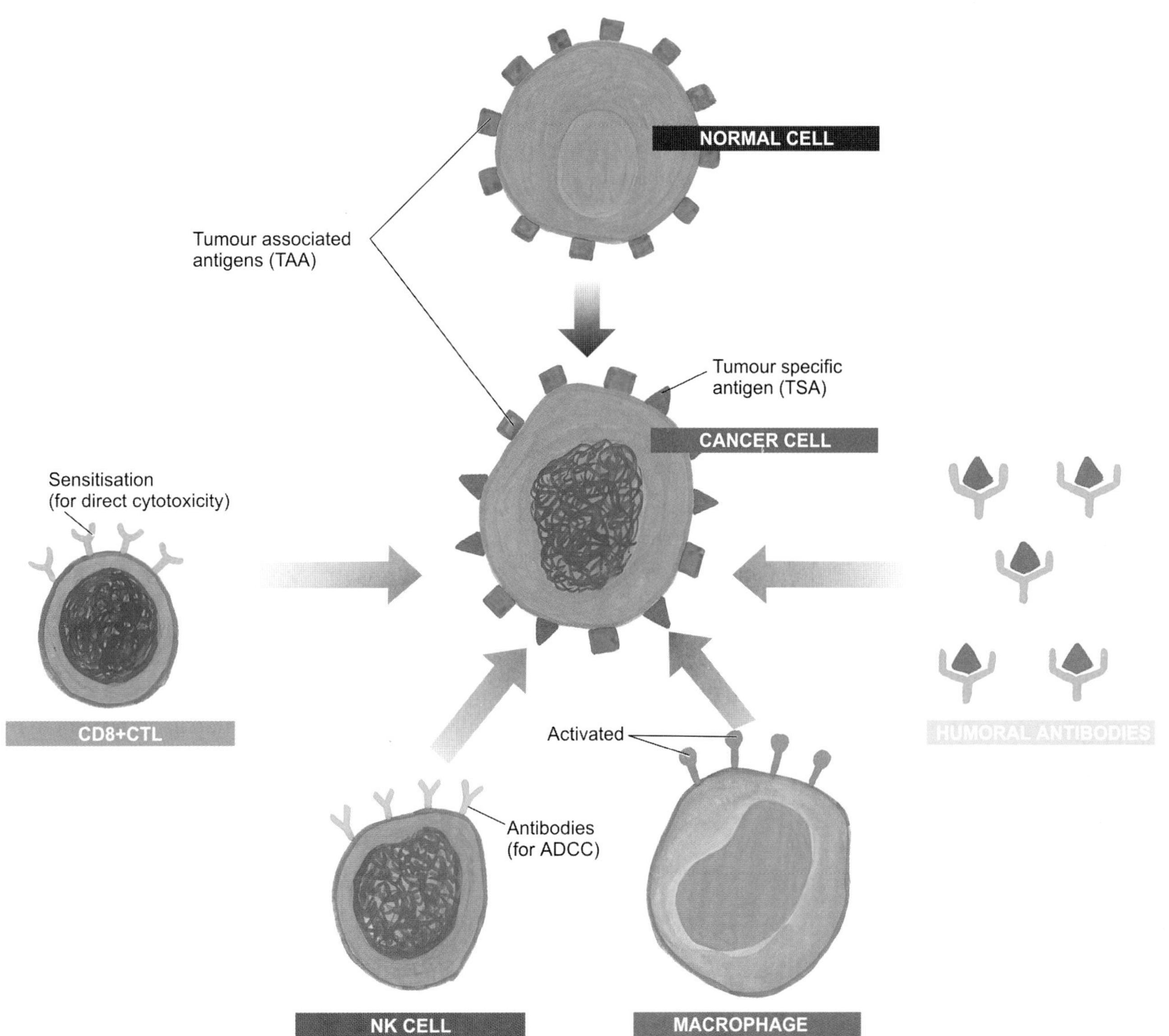

FIGURE 8.16

Schematic illustration of immune responses in cancer. For details see the text (CTL = cytotoxic T-lymphocyte; NK cell = natural killer cell; ADCC = antibody-dependent cellular cytotoxicity).

i) Exfoliative cytology. Cytologic smear (Papanicolaou Pap smear) method was initially employed for detecting dysplasia, carcinoma *in situ* and invasive carcinoma of the uterine cervix. However, its use has now been widely extended to include examination of sputum and bronchial washings; pleural, peritoneal and pericardial effusions; urine, gastric secretions, and CSF. The method is based on microscopic identification of the characteristics of malignant cells which are incohesive and loose and are thus shed off or 'exfoliated' into the lumen. However, a 'negative diagnosis' does not altogether rule out malignancy due to possibility of sampling error.

ii) Fine needle aspiration cytology (FNAC). Currently, cytopathology includes not only study of exfoliated cells but also materials obtained from superficial and deep-seated lesions in the body which do not shed off cells freely. The latter method consists of study of cells obtained by a fine needle introduced under vacuum into the lesion, so called *fine needle aspiration cytology (FNAC)*. The superficial masses can be aspirated under direct vision while deep-seated masses such as intra-abdominal, pelvic organs and retroperitoneum are frequently investigated by ultrasound (US) or computed tomography (CT) guided fine needle aspirations. The smears are fixed in 95% ethanol by wet fixation or may be air-dried unfixed. While Papanicolaou method of staining is routinely employed in most laboratories for *wet fixed smears*, others prefer H and E due to similarity in staining characteristics in the sections obtained by paraffin embedding. *Air-dried smears* are stained by May-Grunwald-Giemsa or Leishman stain. FNAC has a diagnostic reliability between 80-97% but it must not be substituted for clinical judgement or compete with an indicated histopathologic biopsy.

3. Histochemistry and Cytochemistry

Histochemistry and cytochemistry are additional diagnostic tools which help the pathologist in identifying the chemical composition of cells, their constituents and their products by special staining methods.

Though immunohistochemical techniques are more useful for tumour diagnosis (see below), histochemical and cytochemical methods are still employed for this purpose.

Some of the common examples are summarised in Table 8.11, while the subject is discussed at length in Chapter 2.

TABLE 8.11: Common Histochemical/Cytochemical Stains in Tumour Diagnosis.

SUBSTANCE	STAIN
1. *Basement membrane/collagen*	• Periodic acid-Schiff (PAS) • Reticulin • Van Gieson • Masson's trichrome
2. *Glycogen*	• PAS with diastase loss
3. *Glycoproteins, glycolipids (epithelial origin)*	• PAS with diastase persistence glycomucins
4. *Acid mucin (mesenchymal origin)*	• Alcian blue
5. *Mucin (in general)*	• Combined Alcian blue-PAS
6. *Argyrophilic/ argentaffin granules*	• Silver stains
7. *Cross striations*	• PTAH stain
8. *Enzymes*	• Myeloperoxidase • Acid phosphatase • Alkaline phosphatase
9. *Nucleolar organiser regions (NORs)*	• Colloidal silver stain

4. Immunohistochemistry

This is an immunological method of recognising a cell by one or more of its specific components in the cytoplasm, cell membrane or nucleus. These cell components (called antigens) combine with specific antibodies on the formalin-fixed paraffin sections or cytological smears. The complex of antigen-antibody on slide is made visible for light microscopic identification by either fluorescent dyes ('fluorochromes') or by enzyme system ('chromogens'). The specific antibody against a particular cellular antigen is now-a-days obtained by hybridoma technique for monoclonal antibody production. These monoclonal antibodies, besides being *specific* against antigen, are highly sensitive in detection of antigenic component, and, therefore, impart objectivity to the subjective tumour diagnosis made by the surgical pathologist.

Though the list of immunohistochemical stains is ever increasing, one important group of such antibody stains is directed against various classes of intermediate filaments which is useful in classification of poorly-differentiated tumours of epithelial or mesenchymal origin (Table 8.12). This subject is discussed already in Chapter 2.

TABLE 8.12: Intermediate Filaments and their Significance in Tumour Diagnosis.

INTERMEDIATE FILAMENT	TUMOUR
1. *Keratins*	Carcinomas, mesotheliomas, some germ cells tumours
2. *Vimentin*	Sarcomas, melanomas, lymphomas
3. *Desmin*	Myogenic tumours
4. *Neurofilaments (NF)*	Neural tumours
5. *Glial fibrillary acidic protein (GFAP)*	Glial tumours

5. Electron Microscopy

Ultrastructural examination of tumour cells offers selective role in diagnostic pathology. EM examination may be helpful in confirming or substantiating a tumour diagnosis arrived at by light microscopy and immunohistochemistry. A few general features of malignant tumour cells by EM examination are:

i) Cell junctions—their presence and type.
ii) Cell surface, e.g. presence of microvilli.

iii) Cell shape and cytoplasmic extensions.

iv) Shape of the nucleus and features of nuclear membrane.

v) Nucleoli—size and density.

vi) Cytoplasmic organelles—their number is generally reduced.

vii) Dense bodies in the cytoplasm.

viii) Any other secretory product in the cytoplasm e.g. melanosomes in melanoma and membrane-bound granules in endocrine tumours.

6. Tumour Markers (Biochemical Assays)

In order to distinguish from the preceding techniques of tumour diagnosis in which 'stains' are imparted on the tumour cells in section or smear, tumour markers are biochemical assays of products elaborated by the tumour cells in blood or other body fluids. It is, therefore, pertinent to keep in mind that many of these products are produced by normal body cells too, and thus the biochemical estimation of the product in blood reflects the total substance and not by the tumour cells alone. These methods, therefore, lack sensitivity as well as specificity and can only be employed for:

- *firstly,* as an adjunct to the pathologic diagnosis arrived at by other methods and not for primary diagnosis of cancer; and
- *secondly,* can be used for prognostic and therapeutic purposes.

Tumour markers include: cell surface antigens (or oncofoetal antigens), cytoplasmic proteins, enzymes, hormones and cancer antigens (Table 8.13). However, two of the best known examples of oncofoetal antigens secreted by foetal tissues as well as by tumours are alpha-foetoproteins (AFP) and carcinoembryonic antigens (CEA):

a) Alpha-foetoprotein (AFP): This is a glycoprotein synthesised normally by foetal liver cells. Their levels are elevated in hepatocellular carcinoma and non-seminomatous germ cell tumours of the testis. Certain non-neoplastic conditions also have increased levels of AFP e.g. in hepatitis, cirrhosis, toxic liver injury and pregnancy.

b) Carcino-embryonic antigen (CEA): CEA is also a glycoprotein normally synthesised in embryonic tissue of the gut, pancreas and liver. Their levels are high in cancers of the gastrointestinal tract, pancreas and breast. As in AFP, CEA levels are also elevated in certain non-neoplastic conditions e.g. in ulcerative colitis, Crohn's disease, hepatitis and chronic bronchitis.

7. Modern Aids in Tumour Diagnosis

In addition to the methods described above, some more modern diagnostic techniques have emerged for pathologic diagnosis but their availability as well as applicability are limited. These methods are discussed

TABLE 8.13: Important Tumour Markers.

MARKER	CANCER
1. *Oncofoetal antigens:*	
i. Alpha-foetoprotein (AFP)	Hepatocellular carcinoma, non-seminomatous germ cell tumours of testis
ii. Carcino-embryonic antigen (CEA)	Cancer of bowel, pancreas, breast
2. *Cytoplasmic proteins:*	
i. Immunoglobulins	Multiple myeloma, other gammopathies
ii. Prostate specific antigen (PSA)	Prostate carcinoma
3. *Enzymes:*	
i. Prostate acid phosphatase (PAP)	Prostatic carcinoma
ii. Neuron-specific enolase (NSE)	Neuroblastoma, oat cell carcinoma lung
4. *Hormones:*	
i. Human chorionic gonadotropin (HCG)	Trophoblastic tumours, non-seminomatous germ cell tumours of testis
ii. Calcitonin	Medullary carcinoma thyroid
iii. Catecholamines and vanillyl mandelic acid (VMA)	Neuroblastoma, pheochromocytoma
iv. Ectopic hormone production	Paraneoplastic syndromes
5. *Secreted cancer antigens:*	
i. CA-125	Ovary
ii. CA-15-3	Breast

in Chapter 2. Briefly, their role in tumour diagnosis is outlined below.

i) Flow cytometry. This is a computerised technique by which the detailed characteristics of individual tumour cells are recognised and quantified and the data can be stored for subsequent comparison too. Since for flow cytometry, single cell suspensions are required to 'flow' through the 'cytometer', it can be employed on blood cells and their precursors in bone marrow aspirates and body fluids, and sometimes on fresh-frozen unfixed tissue. The method employs either identification of cell surface antigen (e.g. in classification of leukaemias and lymphomas), or by the DNA content analysis (e.g. aneuploidy in various cancers).

ii) *In situ* hybridisation. This is a molecular technique by which nucleic acid sequences (cellular/viral DNA and RNA) can be localised by specifically-labelled nucleic acid probe directly in the intact cell (*in situ*) rather than by DNA extraction (see below). *In situ* hybridisation may be used for analysis of certain human tumours by the study of oncogenes aside from its use in diagnosis of viral infection.

iii) Molecular diagnostic techniques. The group of molecular biologic methods in the tumour diagnostic laboratory are a variety of DNA/RNA-based molecular techniques in which the DNA/RNA are extracted (compared from *in situ* above) from the cell and then analysed. These techniques are highly sensitive, specific and rapid and have revolutionised diagnostic pathology in neoplastic as well as non-neoplastic conditions (e.g. in infectious and inherited disorders, and in identity diagnosis). Molecular diagnostic techniques include: DNA analysis by Southern blot, RNA analysis by northern blot, and polymerase chain reaction (PCR). The molecular methods in tumour diagnosis can be applied in haematologic as well as non-haematologic malig–nancies by:

- analysis of molecular cytogenetic abnormalities;
- mutational analysis;
- antigen receptor gene rearrangement; and
- by study of oncogenic viruses at molecular level.

iv) DNA microarray analysis of tumours. Currently, it is possible to perform molecular profiling of a tumour by use of gene chip technology which allows measurement of levels of expression of several thousand genes (up-regulation or down-regulation) simultaneously. Fluorescent labels are used to code the cDNA synthesised by trigger from mRNA. The conventional DNA probes are substituted by silicon chip which contains the entire range of genes and high resolution scanners are used for the measurement.

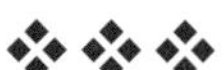

Environmental and Nutritional Diseases

9

INTRODUCTION

The subject of environmental hazards to health has assumed great significance in the modern world. In olden times, the discipline of 'tropical medicine' was of interest to the physician, largely due to contamination of air, food and water by infectious and parasitic organisms. Subsequently, the interest was focussed on 'geographic pathology' due to occurrence of certain environment-related diseases confined to geographic boundaries. Then emerged the knowledge of 'occupational diseases' caused by overexposure to a pollutant by virtue of an individual's occupation. Currently, the field of 'environmental pathology' encompasses all such diseases caused by progressive deterioration in the environment, most of which is man-made. In addition, is the related problem of over- and undernutrition.

Some of the important factors which have led to the alarming environmental degradation are as under:

1. Population explosion
2. Urbanisation of rural and forest land to accommodate the increasing numbers
3. Accumulation of wastes
4. Unsatisfactory disposal of radioactive waste
5. Industrial effluents and automobile exhausts.

But the above atmospheric pollutants appear relatively minor compared with *voluntary intake of three pollutants*—tobacco smoking, alcohol and intoxicant drugs. Attempts at prohibition of alcohol in some states in India or ban on smoking in some places have not been quite effective due to difficulty in implementation. Instead, prohibition has only resulted in off and on catastrophe of 'hooch tragedies' in some parts of this country due to illicit liquor consumption.

The present discussion on environmental and nutritional diseases is covered under the following groups:

1. *Environmental pollution:*
- Air pollution
- Tobacco smoking

2. *Chemical and drug injury:*
- Therapeutic (iatrogenic) drug injury
- Non-therapeutic toxic agents (e.g. alcohol, lead, carbon monoxide, drug abuse)
- Environmental chemicals

3. *Injury by physical agents:*
- Thermal and electrical injury
- Injury by ionising radiation

4. *Nutritional diseases:*
- Overnutrition (obesity)
- Undernutrition (starvation, protein energy malnutrition, vitamin deficiencies).

ENVIRONMENTAL POLLUTION

Any agent—chemical, physical or microbial, that alters the composition of environment is called pollutant. For survival of mankind, it is important to prevent depletion of ozone layer (O_3) in the outer space from pollutants such as chloroflurocarbons and nitrogen dioxide produced in abundance by day-to-day activities on our planet earth due to industrial effluent and automobile exhausts.

AIR POLLUTION

A vast variety of pollutants are inhaled daily some of which may cause trivial irritation to the upper respiratory pathways, while others may lead to acute or chronic injury to the lungs, and some are implicated in causation of lung cancer. Whereas some pollutants are prevalent in certain industries (such as coal dust, silica, asbestos), others are general pollutants present widespread in the ambient atmosphere (e.g. sulphur dioxide, nitrogen dioxide, carbon monoxide). The latter group of environmental pollutants is acted upon by sunlight to produce secondary pollutants such as ozone and free radicals capable of oxidant cell injury to respiratory passages. In highly polluted cities where coal consumption and automobile exhaust accumulate in the atmosphere, the air pollutants become visible as 'smog'. It has been reported that 6 out of 10 largest cities in India have such severe air pollution problem that the annual level of suspended particles is about three times higher than the WHO standards. An estimated 50,000 persons die prematurely every year due to high level of pollution in these cities, of which 7,500 in Delhi alone.

The adverse effects of air pollutants on lung depend upon a few variables that include:

- longer duration of exposure;
- total dose of exposure;
- impaired ability of the host to clear inhaled particles; and
- particle size of 1-5 μm capable of getting impacted in the distal airways to produce tissue injury.

Pneumoconiosis—the group of lung diseases due to occupational over-exposure to pollutants is discussed in Chapter 15.

TOBACCO SMOKING

Habits

Tobacco smoking is the most prevalent and preventable cause of disease and death. The harmful effects of smoking pipe and cigar are somewhat less. Long-term smokers of filter-tipped cigarettes appear to have 30-50% lower risk of development of cancer due to reduced inhalation of tobacco smoke constituents.

In India, a country of one billion people, a quarter (250 million) are tobacco users in one form or the other. Smoking *bidis* and chewing *pan masala, zarda* and *gutka* are more widely practiced than cigarettes (Fig. 9.1). Habit of smoking *chutta* (a kind of indigenous cigar) in which the lighted end is put in mouth is practiced in the Indian state of Andhra Pradesh and is associated with higher incidence of squamous cell carcinoma of hard palate. Another habit prevalent in Indian states of Uttar Pradesh and Bihar and in parts of Sri Lanka is chewing of tabacco alone or mixed with slaked lime as a bolus of *paan* kept in mouth for long hours which is the major cause of cancer of upper aerodigestive tract and oral cavity. *Hookah* smoking, in which tobacco smoke passes through a water-filled chamber which cools the smoke before it is inhaled by the smoker, is believed by some reports to deliver less tar and nicotine than cigarettes and hence fewer tobacco-related health consequences.

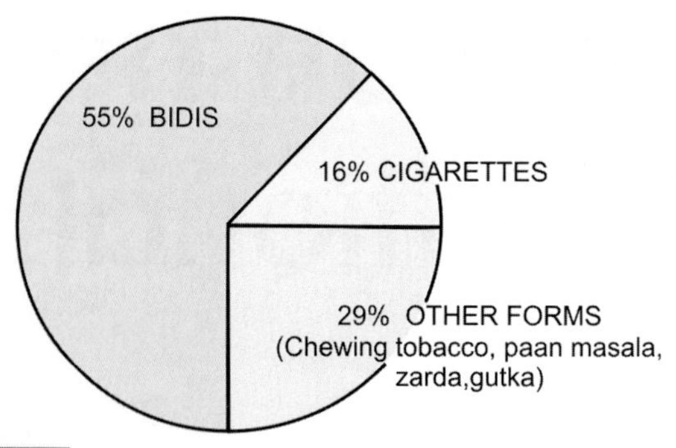

FIGURE 9.1

Consumption of tobacco in India as estimated by weight (*Source:* National Council of Applied Economic Research, New Delhi).

Besides the harmful effects of smoking on active smokers themselves, involuntary exposure of smoke to bystanders (passive smoking) is also injurious to health, particularly to infants and children.

Dose and Duration

The harmful effects of smoking are related to a variety of factors, the most important of which is dose of exposure expressed in terms of pack years. For example, one pack of cigarettes daily for 5 years means 5 pack years. It is estimated that a person who smokes 2 packs of cigarettes daily at the age of 30 years reduces his life by 8 years than a non-smoker. On cessation of smoking, the higher mortality slowly declines and the beneficial effect reaches the level of non-smokers after 20 or more of smoke-free years.

Tobacco-Related Diseases

Tobacco contains numerous toxic chemicals having adverse effects varying from minor throat irritation to carcinogenesis. Some of the important constituents of

TABLE 9.1: Major Constituents of Tobacco Smoke with Adverse Effects.

ADVERSE EFFECT	CONSTITUENTS
1. *Carcinogenesis*	• Tar • Polycyclic aromatic hydrocarbons • Nitrosamines
2. *Tumour promoters*	• Nicotine • Phenol
3. *Irritation and toxicity to respiratory mucosa*	• Formaldehyde Nitrogen oxide
4. *Reduced oxygen transport*	• Carbon monoxide

tobacco smoke with adverse effects are given in Table 9.1.

The major diseases accounting for higher mortality in tobacco smokers include, (in descending order of frequency):

i) Coronary heart disease;
ii) Cancer of the lung; and
iii) Chronic obstructive pulmonary disease (COPD).

Besides above, smokers suffer higher risk of development of a few other cancers and non-neoplastic conditions as illustrated in Fig. 9.2.

CORONARY HEART DISEASE. Cigarette smoking is one of the four major risk factors for myocardial infarction and acts synergistically with the other three—hypercholesterolaemia, hypertension and diabetes mellitus (Chapter 12). There is more severe, extensive and accelerated atherosclerosis of coronary arteries and aorta in smokers, possibly due to increased platelet aggregation and impaired lung function that causes reduced myocardial oxygen supply. Besides, the smokers have higher risk of development of atherosclerotic aortic aneurysm and Buerger's disease (thromboangiitis obliterans) affecting lower extremities (Chapter 11).

LUNG CANCER. This is the most common cancer in men throughout world and most frequent cancer in women too in the United States exceeding in incidence beyond that of breast cancer in that country. Cigarette smoking is strongly implicated in evolution of lung cancer as described in Chapter 15.

OTHER CANCERS. Besides lung cancer, smokers have higher risk of development of cancer of upper aerodigestive tract (lips, oral cavity, larynx, oesophagus), pancreas, urinary bladder and kidney.

NON-NEOPLASTIC DISEASES. These include the following:

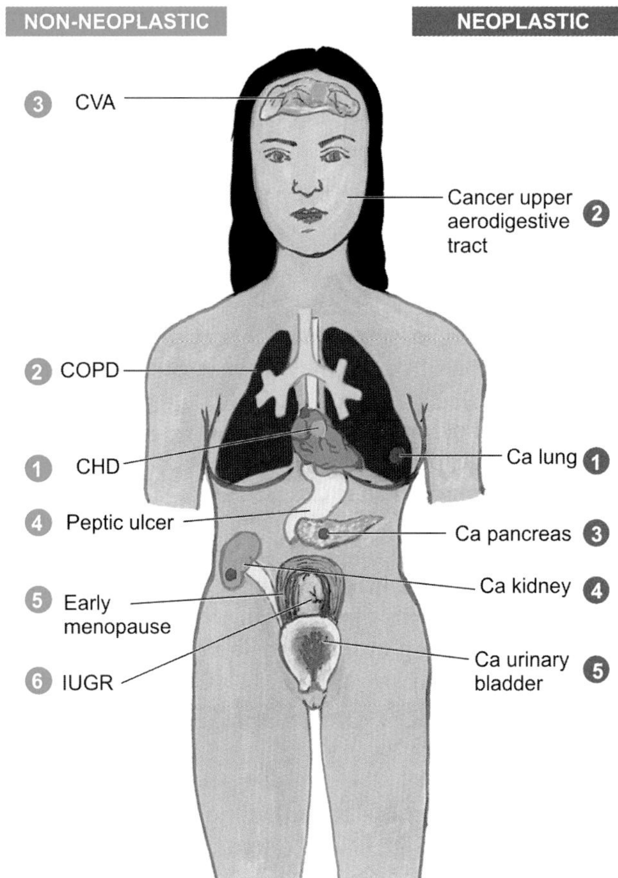

FIGURE 9.2

Major adverse effects of tobacco smoking. *Right side* shows smoking-related neoplastic diseases while *left side* indicates non-neoplastic diseases associated with smoking, numbered serially in order of frequency of occurrence.

i) Chronic obstructive pulmonary disease (COPD) that includes chronic bronchitis and emphysema as the most common.
ii) Peptic ulcer disease with 70% higher risk in smokers.
iii) Early menopause in smoker women.
iv) In smoking pregnant women, higher risk of lower birth weight of foetus, higher perinatal mortality and intellectual deterioration of newborn.

CHEMICAL AND DRUG INJURY

During life, each one of us is exposed to a variety of chemicals and drugs. These are broadly divided into the following three categories:

■ *Therapeutic (iatrogenic) agents* e.g. drugs, which when administered indiscrimately are associated with adverse effects.

- *Non-therapeutic agents* e.g. alcohol, lead, carbon monoxide, drug abuse.
- *Environmental chemicals* e.g. long-term or accidental exposure to certain man-made or naturally-occurring chemicals.

THERAPEUTIC (IATROGENIC) DRUG INJURY

Though the basis of patient management is rational drug therapy, adverse drug reactions do occur in 2-5% of patients. In general, the risk of adverse drug reaction increases with increasing number of drugs administered. Adverse effects of drugs may appear due to:

- overdose;
- genetic predisposition;
- exaggerated pharmacologic response;
- interaction with other drugs; and
- unknown factors.

It is beyond the scope of this book to delve into the list of drugs with their harmful effects. However, some of the common forms of iatrogenic drug injury and the offending drugs are outlined in Table 9.2.

TABLE 9.2: Iatrogenic Drug Injury.

ADVERSE EFFECT	OFFENDING DRUG
1. ***GASTROINTESTINAL TRACT***	
Gastritis, peptic ulcer	Aspirin, nonsteroidal anti-inflammatory drugs (NSAIDs)
Jejunal ulcer	Enteric-coated potassium tablets
Pancreatitis	Thiazide diuretics
2. ***LIVER***	
Cholestatic jaundice	Phenothiazines, tranquillisers, oral contraceptives
Hepatitis	Halothane, isoniazid
Fatty change	Tetracycline
3. ***NERVOUS SYSTEM***	
Cerebrovascular accidents	Anticoagulants, Oral contraceptives
Peripheral neuropathy	Vincristine, antimalarials
8th nerve deafness	Streptomycin
4. ***SKIN***	
Acne	Corticosteroids
Urticaria	Penicillin, sulfonamides
Exfoliative dermatitis, Stevens-Johnson syndrome	Penicillin, sulfonamides, phenyl butazone
Fixed drug eruptions	chemotherapeutic agents
5. ***HEART***	
Arrhythmias	Digitalis, propranalol
Congestive heart failure	Corticosteroids
Cardiomyopathy	Adriamycin
6. ***BLOOD***	
Aplastic anaemia	Chloramphenicol
Agranulocytosis, thrombocytopenia	Antineoplastic drugs
Immune haemolytic anaemia	Penicillin
Megaloblastic anaemia	Methotrexate
7. ***LUNGS***	
Alveolitis, interstitial pulmonary fibrosis	Anti-neoplastic drugs
Asthma	Aspirin, indomethacin
8. ***KIDNEYS***	
Acute tubular necrosis	Gentamycin, kanamycin
Nephrotic syndrome	Gold salts
Chronic interstitial nephritis, papillary necrosis	Phenacetin, salicylates
9. ***METABOLIC EFFECTS***	
Hypercalcaemia	Hypervitaminosis D, thiazide diuretics
Hepatic porphyria	Barbiturates
Hyperuricaemia	Anti-cancer chemotherapy
10. ***FEMALE REPRODUCTIVE TRACT***	
Cholelithiasis, thrombophlebitis, thromboembolism, benign liver cell adenomas	Long-term use of oral contraceptives
Vaginal adenosis, adenocarcinoma in daughters	Diethylstilbesterol by pregnant women
Foetal congenital anomalies	Thalidomide in pregnancy

NON-THERAPEUTICTOXIC AGENTS

ALCOHOLISM

Chronic alcoholism is defined as the regular imbibing of an amount of ethyl alcohol (ethanol) that is sufficient to harm an individual socially, psychologically or physically. It is difficult to give the number of 'drinks' after which the diagnosis of alcoholism can be made because of differences in individual susceptibility. However, adverse effects—acute as well as chronic, are related to the quantity of alcohol content imbibed and duration of consumption. Generally, 10 gm of ethanol is present in:

- a can of beer (or half a bottle of beer);
- 120 ml of neat wine; or
- 30 ml of 86° proof 43% liquor (small peg).

A daily consumption of 40 gm of ethanol (4 small pegs or 2 large pegs) is likely to be harmful but intake of 100 gm or more daily is certainly dangerous. Daily and heavy consumption of alcohol is more harmful than moderate social drinking since the liver, where ethanol is metabolised, gets time to heal.

Metabolism

Absorption of alcohol begins in the stomach and small intestine and appears in blood shortly after ingestion. Alcohol is then distributed to different organs and body fluids proportionate to the blood levels of alcohol. About 2-10% of absorbed alcohol is excreted via urine, sweat and exhaled through breath, the last one being the basis

Chapter Nine

of breath test employed by law-enforcement agencies for alcohol. Metabolism of alcohol is discussed in detail in Chapter 19, but in brief alcohol is metabolised in the liver by the following 3 pathways (Fig. 9.3):

- By the major rate-limiting pathway of alcohol dehydrogenase (ADH) in the cytosol, especially with low blood alcohol levels.
- Via microsomal P-450 system when the blood alcohol level is high.
- Minor pathway via catalase from peroxisomes.

In any of the three pathways, ethanol is biotransformed to toxic acetaldehyde in the liver and finally to carbon dioxide and water by acetyl coenzyme A.

Ill-Effects of Alcoholism

Alcohol consumption in moderation and socially acceptable limits is practiced mainly for its mood-altering effects. Heavy alcohol consumption in unhabituated person is likely to cause acute ill-effects on different organs. Though the diseases associated with alcoholism are discussed in respective chapters later, the spectrum of ill-effects are outlined below.

A. ACUTE ALCOHOLISM. The acute effects of inebriation are most prominent on the central nervous system but it also injures the stomach and liver.

1. Central nervous system. Alcohol acts as a CNS depressant; the intensity of effects of alcohol on the CNS are related to the quantity consumed and duration over which consumed, which are reflected by blood levels of alcohol:

- The initial effect of alcohol is on subcortical structures which is followed by disordered cortical function, motor ataxia and behavioural changes. These changes are apparent when blood alcohol levels do not exceed *100 mg/dl* which is the upper limit of sobriety in drinking as defined by law-enforcing agencies in most Western countries while dealing with cases of driving in drunken state.
- Blood levels of *100-200 mg/dl* are associated with depression of cortical centres, lack of coordination, impaired judgement and drowsiness.
- Stupor and coma supervene when blood alcohol levels are *about 300 mg/dl.*
- Blood levels of alcohol *above 400 mg/dl* can cause anaesthesia, depression of medullary centre and death from respiratory arrest.

However, chronic alcoholics develop CNS tolerance and adaptation and, therefore, can withstand higher blood levels of alcohol without such serious effects.

2. Stomach. Acute alcohol intoxication may cause vomiting, acute gastritis and peptic ulceration.

3. Liver. Acute alcoholic injury to the liver is explained in Chapter 19.

B. CHRONIC ALCOHOLISM. Chronic alcoholism produces widespread injury to organs and systems. Contrary to the earlier belief that chronic alcoholic injury

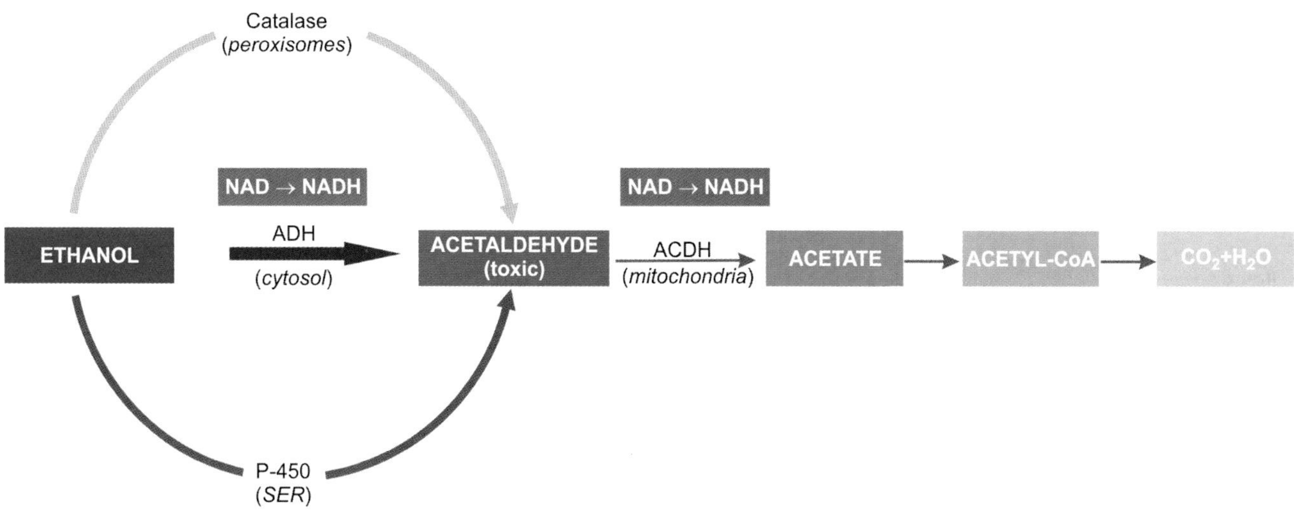

FIGURE 9.3

Metabolism of ethanol in the liver. Thickness and intensity of colour of arrow on left side of figure corresponds to extent of metabolic pathway followed (ADH-alcohol dehydrogenase; ACDH=hepatic acetaldehyde dehydrogenase; NAD=nicotinamide adenine dinucleotide; NADH=reduced NAD; NADP=nicotinamide adenine dinucleotide phosphate: NADPH=reduced NADP).

results from nutritional deficiencies, it is now known that most of the alcohol-related injury to different organs is due to toxic effects of alcohol and accumulation of its main toxic metabolite, acetaldehyde, in the blood. Other proposed mechanisms of tissue injury in chronic alcoholism is free-radical mediated injury and genetic susceptibility to alcohol-dependence and tissue damage.

Some of the more important organ effects in chronic alcoholism are as under (Fig 9.4):

1. **Liver.** Alcoholic liver disease and cirrhosis are the most common and important effects of chronic alcoholism (Chapter 19).

2. **Pancreas.** Chronic calcifying pancreatitis and acute pancreatitis are serious complications of chronic alcoholism.

3. **Gastrointestinal tract.** Gastritis, peptic ulcer and oesophageal varices associated with fatal massive bleeding may occur.

4. **Central nervous system.** Peripheral neuropathies and Wernicke-Korsakoff syndrome, cerebral atrophy, cerebellar degeneration and amblyopia (impaired vision) are seen in chronic alcoholics.

5. **Cardiovascular system.** Alcoholic cardiomyopathy and beer-drinkers' myocardiosis with consequent dilated cardiomyopathy may occur. Level of HDL (atherosclerosis-protective lipoprotein), however, has been shown to increase with moderate consumption of alcohol.

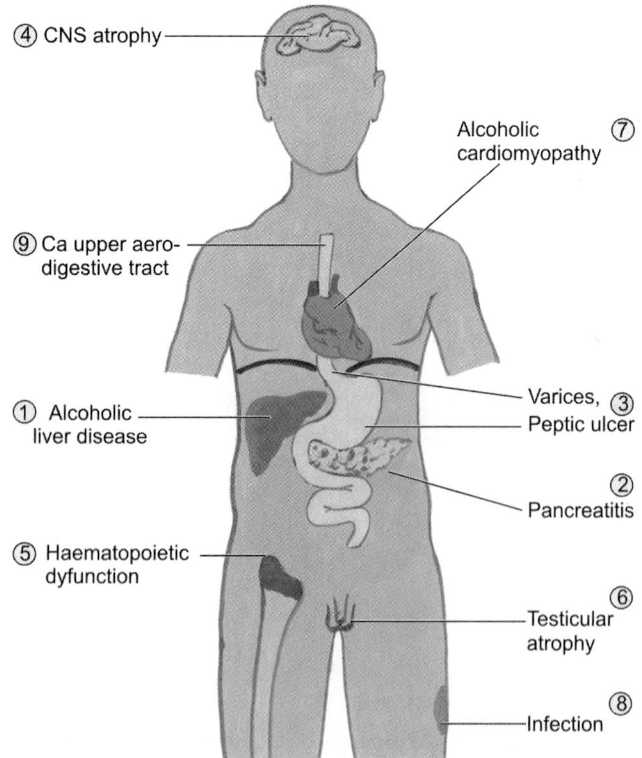

FIGURE 9.4

Complications of chronic alcoholism.

6. **Endocrine system.** In men, testicular atrophy, feminisation, loss of libido and potency, and gynaecomastia may develop. These effects appear to be due to lowering of testosterone levels.

7. **Blood.** Haematopoietic dysfunction with secondary megaloblastic anaemia and increased red blood cell volume may occur.

8. **Immune system.** Alcoholics are more susceptible to various infections.

9. **Cancer.** There is higher incidence of cancers of upper aerodigestive tract in chronic alcoholics but the mechanism is not clear.

LEAD POISONING

Lead poisoning may occur in children or adults due to accidental or occupational ingestion.

In children, the main sources are:

- Chewing of lead-containing furniture items, toys or pencils.
- Eating of lead paint flakes from walls.

In adults, the sources are:

- Occupational exposure to lead during spray painting, recycling of automobile batteries (lead oxide fumes), mining, and extraction of lead.
- Accidental exposure by contaminated water supply, house freshly coated with lead paint, and sniffing of lead-containing petrol (hence unleaded petrol introduced as fuel).

Lead is absorbed through the gastrointestinal tract or lungs. The absorbed lead is distributed in two types of tissues (Fig. 9.5):

a) *Bones, teeth, nails and hair* representing relatively harmless pool of lead. About 90% of absorbed lead accumulates in the developing metaphysis of bones in children and appears as areas of increased bone densities ('lead lines') on X-ray. Lead lines are also seen in the gingiva.

b) *Brain, liver, kidneys and bone marrow* accumulate the remaining 10% lead which is directly toxic to these organs. It is excreted via kidneys.

Lead toxicity occurs in the following organs predominantly:

1. **Nervous system:** The changes are as under:

- *In children,* lead encephalopathy; oedema of brain, flattening of gyri and compression of ventricles.

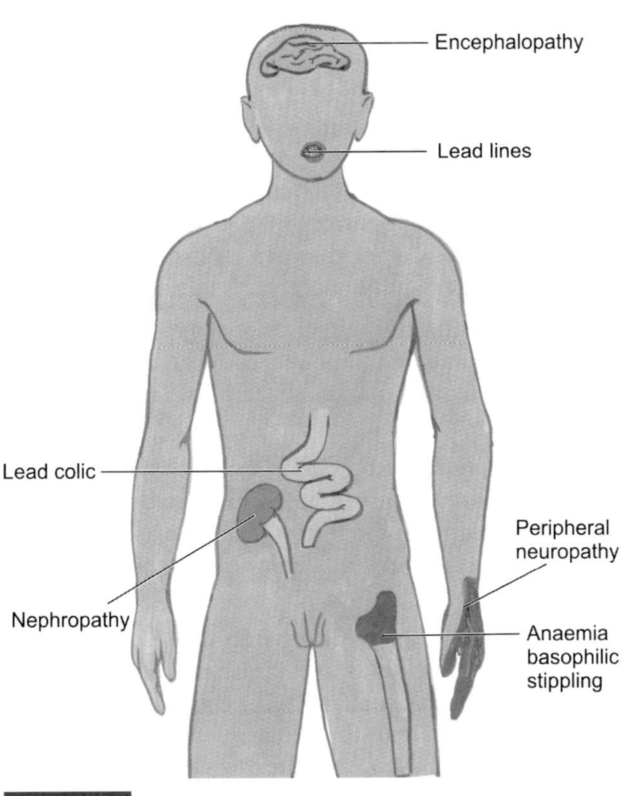

FIGURE 9.5

Complications of lead poisoning.

■ *In adults,* demyelinating peripheral motor neuropathy which typically affects radial and peroneal nerves resulting in wrist drop and foot drop respectively.

2. Haematopoietic system: The changes in blood are quite characteristic:

■ *Microcytic hypochromic anaemia* due to inhibition of two enzymes: delta-aminolevulinic acid dehydrogenase required for haem synthesis, and through inhibition of ferroketolase required for incorporation of ferrous iron into the porphyrin ring.

■ Prominent basophilic stippling of erythrocytes.

3. Kidneys: Lead is toxic to proximal tubular cells of the kidney and produces *lead nephropathy* characterised by accumulation of intranuclear inclusion bodies consisting of lead-protein complex in the proximal tubular cells.

4. Gastrointestinal tract: Lead toxicity in the bowel manifests as acute abdomen presenting as lead colic.

CARBON MONOXIDE POISONING

Carbon monoxide (CO) is a colourless and odourless gas produced by incomplete combustion of carbon. Sources of CO gas are:

■ automobile exhaust;
■ burning of fossil fuel in industries or at home; and
■ tobacco smoke.

CO is an important cause of accidental death due to systemic oxygen deprivation of tissues. This is because haemoglobin has about 200-times higher affinity for CO than for O_2 and thus varying amount of carboxyhaemoglobin is formed depending upon the extent of CO poisoning. Besides, carboxyhaemoglobin interferes with the release of O_2 from oxyhaemoglobin causing further aggravation of tissue hypoxia. Diagnosis of CO poisoning is, therefore, best confirmed by carboxyhaemoglobin levels in the blood.

CO poisoning may present in 2 ways:

■ **Acute CO poisoning** in which there is sudden development of brain hypoxia characterised by oedema and petechial haemorrhages.

■ **Chronic CO poisoning** presents with nonspecific changes of slowly developing hypoxia of the brain.

DRUG ABUSE

Drug abuse is defined as the use of certain drugs for the purpose of 'mood alteration' or 'euphoria' or 'kick' but subsequently leading to habit-forming, dependence and eventually addiction. Some of the commonly abused drugs and substances are as under:

1. *Marijuana* or *'pot'* is psychoactive substance most widely used. It is obtained from the leaves of the plant *Cannabis sativa* and contains tetrahydrocannabinol (THC). It may be smoked or ingested.

2. *Derivatives of opium* that includes heroin and morphine. Opioids are derived from the poppy plant. Heroin and morphine are self-administered intravenously or subcutaneously.

3. *CNS depressants* include barbiturates, tranquilisers and alcohol.

4. *CNS stimulants* e.g. cocaine and amphetamines.

5. *Psychedelic drugs* (meaning enjoyable perception-giving) e.g. LSD.

6. *Inhalants* e.g. glue, paint thinner, nail polish remover, aerosols, amyl nitrite.

It is beyond the scope of the present discussion to go into the pharmacologic actions of all these substances. However, apart from pharmacologic and physiologic actions of these street drugs, the most common complication is introduction of infection by parenteral use of many of these drugs. Sharing of needles by the drug-addicts accounts for high risk of most feared viral infections in them, AIDS and viral hepatitis (both HBV and HCV). A few common drug abuse-related infectious complications are:

1. At the site of injection—cellulitis, abscesses, ulcers, thrombosed veins
2. Thrombophlebitis
3. Bacterial endocarditis
4. High risk for AIDS
5. Viral hepatitis and its complications
6. Focal glomerulonephritis
7. Talc (foreign body) granuloma formation in the lungs.

ENVIRONMENTAL CHEMICALS

A large number of chemicals are found as contaminants in the ecosystem, food and water supply and find their way into the food chain of man. These substances exert their toxic effects depending upon their mode of absorption, distribution, metabolism and excretion. Some of the substances are directly toxic while others cause ill-effects via their metabolites. Environmental chemicals may have slow damaging effect or there may be sudden accidental exposure such as the Bhopal gas tragedy in India due to accidental leakage of methyl isocyanate (MIC) gas in December 1984.

Some of the common examples of environmental chemicals are given below:

1. Agriculture chemicals. Modern agriculture thrives on pesticides, fungicides, herbicides and organic fertilisers which may pose a potential acute poisoning as well as long-term hazard. The problem is particularly alarming in developing countries like India, China and Mexico where farmers and their families are unknowingly exposed to these hazardous chemicals during aerial spraying of crops.

- Acute poisoning by organophosphate insecticides is too well known as accidental or suicidal poison by inhibiting acetyl cholinesterase and sudden death.
- Chronic human exposure to low level agricultural chemicals is implicated in cancer, chronic degenerative diseases, congenital malformations and impotence but the exact cause-and-effect relationship is lacking.

According to the WHO estimates, about 7.5 lakh people are taken ill every year worldwide with pesticide poisoning, half of which occur in the third world countries due to use of hazardous pesticides which are otherwise banned in advanced countries. Pesticide residues in food items such as in fruits, vegetables, cereals, grains, pulses etc is of greatest concern. According to a country-wide study conducted by the Indian Council of Medical Research (ICMR), New Delhi, recently, it has been found that 82% of milk samples from 12 different Indian states contained residues of pesticides above the tolerance limit such as BHC and DDT which are widely used insecticides in India.

2. Volatile organic solvents. Volatile organic solvents and vapours are used in industry quite commonly and their exposure may cause acute toxicity or chronic hazard, often by inhalation than by ingestion. Such substances include methanol, chloroform, petrol, kerosene, benzene, ethylene glycol, toluene etc.

3. Metals. Pollution by occupational exposure to toxic metals such as mercury, arsenic, cadmium, iron, nickel and aluminium are important hazardous environmental chemicals.

4. Aromatic hydrocarbons. The halogenated aromatic hydrocarbons containing polychlorinated biphenyl which are contaminant in several preservatives, herbicides and antibacterial agents are a chronic health hazard.

5. Cyanide. Cyanide in the environment is released by combustion of plastic, silk and is also present in cassava and the seeds of apricots and wild cherries. Cyanide is a very toxic chemical and kills by blocking cellular respiration by binding to mitochondrial cytochrome oxidase.

6. Environmental dusts. These substances causing pneumoconioses are discussed in chapter 15 while those implicated in cancer are discussed in Chapter 8.

INJURY BY PHYSICAL AGENTS

THERMAL AND ELECTRICAL INJURY

Thermal and electrical burns, fall in body temperature below 35°C (hypothermia) and elevation of body temperature above 41°C (hyperthermia), are all associated with tissue injury.

- **Hypothermia** may cause focal injury as in frostbite, or systemic injury and death as occurs on immersion in cold water for varying time.
- **Hyperthermia** likewise, may be localised as in cutaneous burns, and systemic as occurs in fevers.
- **Thermal burns** depending upon severity are categorised into full thickness (third degree) and partial thickness (first and second degree). The most serious complications of burns are haemoconcentration, infections and contractures on healing.
- **Electrical burns** may cause damage by *firstly*, electrical dysfunction of the conduction system of the heart and death by ventricular fibrillation, and *secondly* by heat produced by electrical energy.

INJURY BY RADIATION

As discussed in the preceding chapter, the most important form of radiation injury is ionising radiation which has three types of effects on cells:

i) Somatic effects which cause acute cell killing.

ii) Genetic damage by mutations and therefore, causes genetic defects.

iii) Malignant transformation of cells (Chapter 8).

Ionising radiation is widely employed for diagnostic purpose as well as for radiotherapy of malignant tumours. Radiation-induced cell death is mediated by radiolysis of water in the cell with generation of toxic hydroxyl radicals (page 40). During radiotherapy, some normal cells coming in the field of radiation are also damaged. In general, radiation-induced tissue injury predominantly affects endothelial cells of small arteries and arterioles, causing necrosis and ischaemia.

Ionising radiation causes damage to the following major organs:

1. *Skin:* radiation dermatitis, cancer.
2. *Lungs:* interstitial pulmonary fibrosis.
3. *Heart:* myocardial fibrosis, constrictive pericarditis.
4. *Kidney:* radiation nephritis.
5. *Gastrointestinal tract:* strictures of small bowel and oesophagus.
6 *Gonads:* testicular atrophy in males and destruction of ovaries.
7. *Haematopoietic tissue:* pancytopenia due to bone marrow depression.
8. *Eyes:* cataract.

Besides ionising radiation, other form of harmful radiation is *solar (u.v.) radiation* which may cause acute skin injury as sunburns, chronic conditions such as solar keratosis and early onset of cataracts in the eyes. It may, however, be mentioned in passing here that electromagnetic radiation produced by microwaves (ovens, radars, diathermy) or ultrasound waves used for diagnostic purposes do not produce ionisation and thus are not known to cause any tissue injury.

NUTRITIONAL DISEASES

Nutritional status of a society varies according to the socioeconomic conditions. In the Western world, nutritional imbalance is more often a problem accounting for increased frequency of obesity, while in developing countries of Africa, Asia and South America, chronic malnutrition is a serious problem, particularly in children.

Before describing the nutritional diseases, it is essential to know the components of normal and adequate nutrition. The nutrients in diet can be grouped into essential and non-essential.

ESSENTIAL NUTRIENTS. There are 6 basic groups of essential nutrients. These are as under:

1. **Proteins.** Dietary proteins provide the body with amino acids for endogenous protein synthesis and are also a metabolic fuel for energy (1 g of protein provides 4 Kcal). *Eight essential amino acids* (isoleucine, leucine, lysine, methionine, phenylalanine, theonine, tryptophan and valine) as well as histidine must be supplied by dietary intake as these cannot be synthesised in the body.

2. **Fats.** Fats and fatty acids (in particular linolenic, linoleic and arachidonic acid) should comprise about 35% of diet with an increased ratio of poly-unsaturated to saturated fats so as to minimise the risk of atherosclerosis (1 g of fat yields 9 Kcal).

3. **Carbohydrates.** Dietary carbohydrates, though not essential, are the major source of dietary calories (1 g of carbohydrate provides 4 Kcal).

4. **Vitamins.** These are mainly derived from exogenous dietary sources and are essential for maintaining the normal structure and function of cells. Vitamin deficiencies result in individual deficiency syndromes, or may be part of a multiple deficiency state.

5. **Minerals.** A number of minerals like iron, calcium, phosphorus and certain trace elements (e.g. zinc, copper, selenium, iodine, chlorine, sodium, potassium, magnesium, manganese, cobalt, molybdenum etc) are essential for health. Their deficiencies result in a variety of lesions and deficiency syndromes.

6. **Water.** Water intake is essential to cover the losses in faeces, urine, exhalation and insensible loss so as to avoid under- or over-hydration.

NON-ESSENTIAL NUTRIENTS. Dietary fibre composed of cellulose, hemicellulose and pectin, though considered non-essential, are important due to beneficial effects in colonic cancer, diabetes, coronary artery disease, and in lowering the incidence of colonic cancer.

Pathogenesis of Deficiency Diseases

The nutritional deficiency disease develops when the essential nutrients are not provided to the cells adequately. The nutritional deficiency may be of 2 types:

1. **Primary deficiency.** This is due to either the lack or decreased amount of essential nutrients in diet.

2. **Secondary or conditioned deficiency.** Secondary or conditioned deficiency is malnutrition occurring as a result of the various factors. These are as under:

i) *Interference with ingestion* e.g. in gastrointestinal disorders, neuropsychiatric illness, anorexia, alcoholism, food allergy, pregnancy.

ii) *Interference with absorption* e.g. in hypermotility of the gut, achlorhydria, biliary disease.

iii) *Interference with utilisation* e.g. in liver dysfunction, malignancy, hypothyroidism.

iv) *Increased excretion* e.g. in lactation, perspiration, polyuria.

v) *Increased nutritional demand* e.g. in fever, pregnancy, lactation, hyperthyroidism.

Irrespective of the type of nutritional deficiency (primary or secondary), nutrient reserves in the tissues begin to get depleted, which initially result in biochemical alterations and eventually lead to functional and morphological changes in tissues and organs (Fig. 9.6).

In the following pages, a brief account of nutritional imbalance (viz. *obesity*) is followed by description of multiple or mixed deficiencies (viz. *starvation, protein-energy malnutrition*) and individual nutrient deficiencies (viz. *vitamin deficiencies*).

OBESITY

Dietary imbalance and overnutrition may lead to diseases like obesity. Aesthetic considerations aside, *obesity is defined as an excess of adipose tissue that imparts health risk; a body weight of 20% excess over ideal weight for age, sex and height is considered a health risk.*

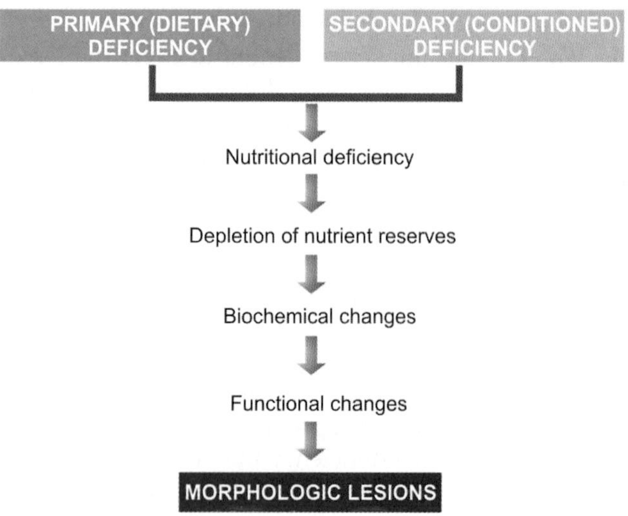

FIGURE 9.6

Schematic representation of pathogenesis of nutritional deficiency diseases.

ETIOLOGY. *Obesity results when caloric intake exceeds utilisation.* The imbalance of these two components can occur in the following situations:

1. *Inadequate pushing of oneself away from the dining table* causing overeating.
2. *Insufficient pushing of oneself out of the chair* leading to inactivity and sedentary life style.
3. *Genetic predisposition* to develop obesity.
4. *Diets largely derived from carbohydrates* and fats than protein-rich diet.
5. *Secondary obesity* may result following a number of underlying diseases such as hypothyroidism, Cushing's disease, insulinoma and hypothalamic disorders.

SEQUELAE OF OBESITY. Marked obesity is a serious health hazard and may predispose to a number of clinical disorders and pathological changes described below and illustrated in Fig. 9.7.

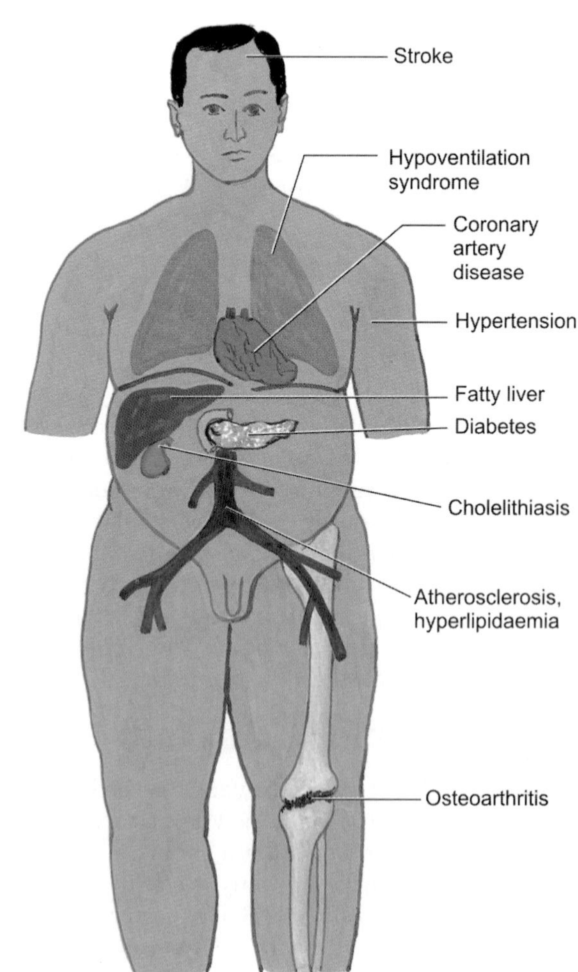

FIGURE 9.7

Major sequelae of obesity.

PATHOLOGIC CHANGES. Obesity is associated with increased adipose stores in the subcutaneous tissues, skeletal muscles, internal organs such as the kidneys, heart, liver and omentum; fatty liver is also more common in obese individuals. There is increase in both size and number of adipocytes i.e. there is hypertrophy as well as hyperplasia.

METABOLIC CHANGES. These are as under:

1. **Hyperinsulinaemia.** Increased insulin secretion is a feature of obesity. Many obese patients exhibit hyperglycaemia or frank diabetes despite hyperinsulinaemia. This is due to a state of insulin-resistance consequent to tissue insensitivity.

2. **Non-insulin dependent diabetes.** There is a strong association of non-insulin dependent diabetes mellitus with obesity. Obesity often exacerbates the diabetic state and in many cases weight reduction often leads to amelioration of diabetes.

3. **Hypertension.** A strong association between hypertension and obesity is observed which is perhaps due to increased blood volume. Weight reduction leads to significant reduction in systolic blood pressure.

4. **Hyperlipoproteinaemia.** The plasma cholesterol circulates in the blood as low density lipoprotein (LDL) containing most of the circulating triglycerides. Obesity is strongly associated with VLDL and mildly with LDL. Total blood cholesterol levels are also elevated in obesity.

5. **Atherosclerosis.** Obesity predisposes to development of atherosclerosis.

6. **Coronary artery disease and stroke.** As a result of atherosclerosis and hypertension, there is increased risk of myocardial infarction and stroke in obese individuals.

7. **Cholelithiasis.** There is six times higher incidence of gallstones in obese persons, mainly due to increased total body cholesterol.

8. **Hypoventilation syndrome (Pickwickian syndrome).** This is characterised by hypersomnolence, both at night and during day in obese individuals along with carbon dioxide retention, hypoxia, polycythaemia and eventually right-sided heart failure. (Mr Pickwick was a character, the fat boy, in Charles Dickens' *Pickwick Papers*. The term pickwickian syndrome was first used by Sir William Osler for the sleep-apnoea syndrome).

9. **Osteoarthritis.** These individuals are more prone to develop degenerative joint disease due to wear and tear following trauma to joints as a result of large body weight.

10. **Cancer.** Certain cancers such as of endometrium and breast seem to be related to obesity. Particularly implicated are the diets derived from animal fats and meats. However, a definite evidence in support of role of diet in cancer is lacking.

STARVATION

Starvation is a state of overall deprivation of nutrients. Its causes may be:

i) deliberate fasting—religious or political;
ii) famine conditions in a country or community; or
iii) secondary undernutrition such as due to chronic wasting diseases (infections, inflammatory conditions, liver disease), cancer etc. Cancer results in malignant cachexia as a result of which cytokines are elaborated e.g. tumour necrosis factor-α, elastases, proteases etc.

A starved individual has lax, dry skin, wasted muscles and atrophy of internal organs.

METABOLIC CHANGES. The following metabolic changes take place in starvation:

1. **Glucose.** *Glucose stores* of the body are sufficient for one day's metabolic needs only. During fasting state, insulin-independent tissues such as the brain, blood cells and renal medulla continue to utilise glucose while insulin-dependent tissues like muscle stop taking up glucose. This results in release of glycogen stores of the liver to maintain normal blood glucose level. Subsequently, hepatic gluconeogenesis from other sources such as breakdown of proteins takes place.

2. **Proteins.** Protein stores and the triglycerides of adipose tissue have enough energy for about 3 months in an individual. *Proteins* breakdown to release amino acids which are used as fuel for hepatic gluconeogenesis so as to maintain glucose needs of the brain. This results in nitrogen imbalance due to excretion of nitrogen compounds as urea.

3. **Fats.** After about one week of starvation, protein breakdown is decreased while *triglycerides* of adipose tissue breakdown to form glycerol and fatty acids. The fatty acids are converted into ketone bodies in the liver which are used by most organs including brain in place of glucose. Starvation can then continue till all the body fat stores are exhausted following which death occurs.

PROTEIN-ENERGY MALNUTRITION

The inadequate consumption of protein and energy as a result of primary dietary deficiency or conditioned deficiency may cause loss of body mass and adipose tissue, resulting in protein energy or protein calorie malnutrition (PEM or PCM). The primary deficiency is more frequent due to socioeconomic factors limiting the quantity and quality of dietary intake, particularly prevalent in the developing countries of Africa, Asia and

TABLE 9.3: Contrasting Features of Kwashiorkor and Marasmus.

FEATURE	KWASHIORKOR	MARASMUS
Definition	Protein deficiency with sufficient calorie intake	Starvation in infants with overall lack of calories
Clinical features (Fig. 9.8)	Occurs in children between 6 months and 3 years of age	Common in infants under 1 year of age
	Growth failure	Growth failure
	Wasting of muscles but preserved adipose tissues	Wasting of all tissues including muscles and adipose tissues
	Oedema, localised or generalised, present	Oedema absent
	Enlarged fatty liver	No hepatic enlargement
	Serum proteins low	Serum proteins low
	Anaemia present	Anaemia present
	'Flag sign'—alternate bands of light (depigmented) and dark (pigmented) hair	Monkey-like face, protuberant abdomen, thin limbs
Morphology	Enlarged fatty liver	No fatty liver
	Atrophy of different tissues and organs but subcutaneous fat preserved	Atrophy of different tissues and organs including subcutaneous fat

South America. The impact of deficiency is marked in infants and children.

The spectrum of *clinical syndromes* produced as a result of PEM includes the following:

1. *Kwashiorkor* which is related to protein deficiency though calorie intake may be sufficient.

2. *Marasmus* is starvation in infants occurring due to overall lack of calories.

The salient features of the two conditions are contrasted in Table 9.3. However, it must be remembered that mixed forms of kwashiorkor-marasmus syndrome may also occur.

DISORDERS OF VITAMINS

Vitamins are organic substances which can not be synthesised within the body and are essential for maintenance of normal structure and function of cells. Thus, these substances must be provided in the human diet. Most of the vitamins are of plant or animal origin so that they normally enter the body as constituents of ingested plant food or animal food. They are required in minute amounts in contrast to the relatively large amounts of essential amino acids and essential fatty acids. Vitamins do not play any part in production of energy.

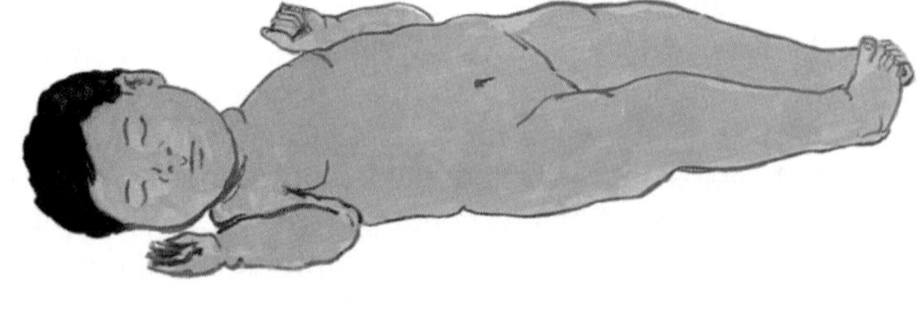

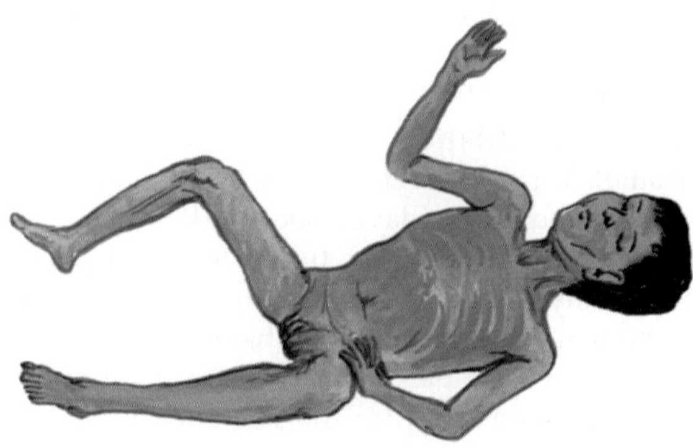

FIGURE 9.8
Two forms of PEM.

In the developing countries, *multiple deficiencies* of vitamins and other nutrients are common due to generalised malnutrition of dietary origin. In the developed countries, *individual vitamin deficiencies* are noted more often, particularly in children, adolescent, pregnant and lactating women, and in some due to poverty. However, secondary or conditioned deficiencies can occur in either case. Chronic alcoholism comprises an important cause of vitamin deficiency in the United States.

Vitamins are conventionally divided into 2 groups: fat-soluble and water-soluble.

1. Fat-soluble vitamins are vitamin A, D, E and K. They are absorbed from intestine in the presence of bile salts and intact pancreatic function. Their deficiencies occur more readily due to conditioning factors (*secondary deficiency*). Beside the deficiency syndromes of these vitamins, a state of *hypervitaminosis* due to excess of vitamin A and D also occurs.

2. Water-soluble vitamins are vitamin C and B complex group. These vitamins are more readily absorbed from small intestine. Deficiency of these vitamins is mainly due to *primary (dietary) factors.* Being water soluble, these vitamins are more easily lost due to cooking or processing of food.

Table 9.4 sums up the various clinical disorders produced by vitamin deficiencies.

FAT-SOLUBLE VITAMINS

Vitamin A (Retinol)

PHYSIOLOGY. Vitamin A or retinol is a fat soluble alcohol. It is available in diet in 2 forms:

TABLE 9.4: Vitamin Deficiencies.

VITAMINS	DEFICIENCY DISORDERS
I. FAT-SOLUBLE VITAMINS	
Vitamin A (Retinol)	Ocular lesions (night blindness, xerophthalmia, keratomalacia, Bitot's spots, blindness) Cutaneous lesions (xeroderma) Other lesions (squamous metaplasia of respiratory epithelium, urothelium and pancreatic ductal epithelium, subsequent anaplasia; retarded bone growth)
Vitamin D (Calcitriol)	Rickets in growing children Osteomalacia in adults Hypocalcaemic tetany
Vitamin E	Degeneration of neurons, retinal pigments, axons of peripheral nerves; denervation of muscles Reduced red cell life span Sterility in male and female animals
Vitamin K	Hypoprothrombinaemia (in haemorrhagic disease of newborn, biliary obstruction, malabsorption, anticoagulant therapy, antibiotic therapy, diffuse liver disease)
II. WATER-SOLUBLE VITAMINS	
Vitamin C (Ascorbic acid)	Scurvy (haemorrhagic diathesis, skeletal lesions, delayed wound healing, anaemia, lesions in teeth and gums)
Vitamin B Complex	
(i) Thiamine (Vitamin B_1)	Beriberi ('dry' or peripheral neuritis, 'wet' or cardiac manifestations, 'cerebral' or Wernicke-Korsakoff's syndrome)
(ii) Riboflavin (Vitamin B_2)	Ariboflavinosis (ocular lesions, cheilosis, glossitis, dermatitis)
(iii) Niacin (Nicotinic acid)	Pellagra (dermatitis, diarrhoea, dementia)
(iv) Pyridoxine (Vitamin B_6)	Vague lesions (convulsions in infants, dermatitis, cheilosis, glossitis, sideroblastic anaemia)
(v) Folate (Folic acid)	Megaloblastic anaemia
(vi) Cyanocobalamin (Vitamin B_{12})	Megaloblastic anaemia Pernicious anaemia

■ *As preformed retinol,* the dietary sources of which are animal-derived foods such as yolk of eggs, butter, whole milk, fish, liver, kidney.

■ *As provitamin precursor carotenoid,* which is derived from β-carotene-containing foods such as yellow plants and vegetables e.g. carrots, potatoes, pumpkins, mangoes, spinach. β-carotene can be absorbed intact or converted in the intestinal mucosa to form retinaldehyde which is subsequently reduced to retinol.

Retinol is stored in the liver cells and released for transport to peripheral tissues after binding to retinol-binding protein found in blood.

The **physiologic functions** of retinol are as follows:

1. *Maintenance of normal vision in reduced light.* This involves synthesis of rhodopsin, a light sensitive pigment in the rods and cones of retina, by oxidation of retinol. This pigment then transforms the radiant energy into nerve impulses.

2. *Maintenance of structure and function of specialised epithelium.* Retinol plays an important role in the synthesis of glycoproteins of the cell membrane of specialised epithelium such as mucus-secreting columnar epithelium in glands and mucosal surfaces, respiratory epithelium and urothelium.

3. *Maintenance of normal cartilaginous and bone growth.*

4. *Anti-proliferative effect.* Recently, it has been found that β-carotene by anti-oxidant action may cause regression of certain non-tumorous skin diseases, premalignant conditions and certain cancers.

LESIONS IN VITAMIN A DEFICIENCY. Nutritional deficiency of vitamin A is common in countries of South-East Asia, Africa, Central and South America whereas malabsorption syndrome may account for conditioned vitamin A deficiency in developed countries.

PATHOLOGIC CHANGES. Consequent to vitamin A deficiency following pathologic changes are seen (Fig. 9.9):

1. Ocular lesions. Lesions in the eyes are most obvious. *Night blindness* is usually the first sign of vitamin A deficiency. As a result of replacement metaplasia of mucus-secreting cells by squamous cells, there is dry and scaly scleral conjunctiva (*xerophthalmia*). The lacrimal duct also shows hyperkeratosis. Corneal ulcers may occur which may get infected and cause *keratomalacia. Bitot's spots* may appear which are focal triangular areas of opacities due to accumulation of keratinised epithelium. If these occur on cornea, they impede transmission of light. Ultimately, infection, scarring and opacities lead to *blindness.*

2. Cutaneous lesions. The skin develops papular lesions giving toad-like appearance (*xeroderma*). This is due to follicular hyperkeratosis and keratin plugging in the sebaceous glands.

3. Other lesions. These are as under:

i) *Squamous metaplasia of respiratory epithelium* of bronchus and trachea may predispose to respiratory infections.

ii) *Squamous metaplasia of pancreatic ductal epithelium* may lead to obstruction and cystic dilatation.

iii) *Squamous metaplasia of urothelium* of the pelvis of kidney may predispose to pyelonephritis and perhaps to renal calculi.

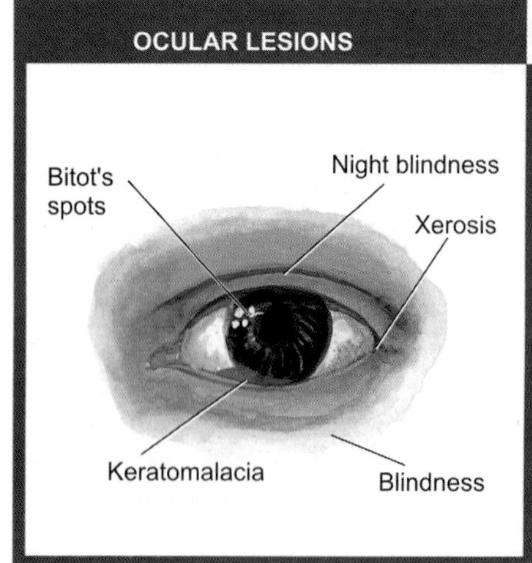

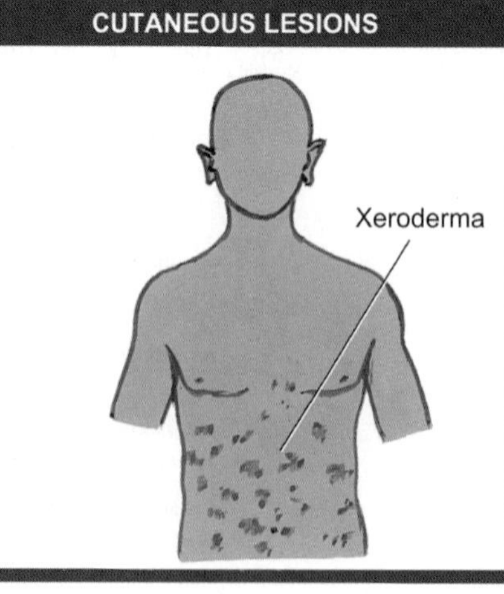

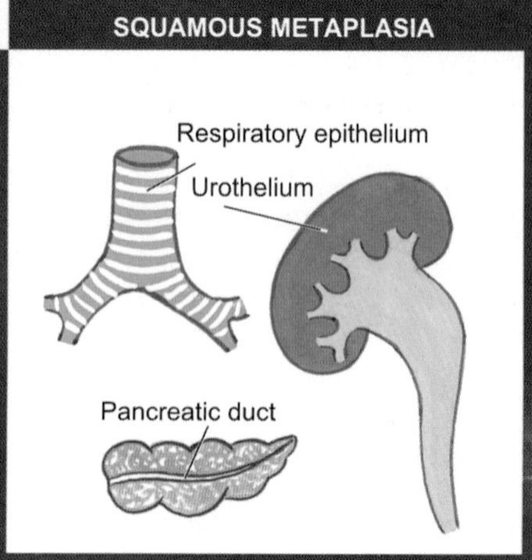

FIGURE 9.9

Lesions resulting from vitamin A deficiency.

iv) Long-standing metaplasia may cause progression to *anaplasia* under certain circumstances.
v) *Bone growth* in vitamin A deficient animals is retarded.

HYPERVITAMINOSIS A. Very large doses of vitamin A can produce toxic manifestations in children as well as in adults. These may be *acute or chronic.*

Acute toxicity. This results from a single large dose of vitamin A. The effects include neurological manifestations resembling brain tumour e.g. headache, vomiting, stupor, papilloedema.

Chronic toxicity. The clinical manifestations of chronic vitamin A excess are as under:
i) *Neurological* such as severe headache and disordered vision due to increased intracranial pressure.
ii) *Skeletal pains* due to loss of cortical bone by increased osteoclastic activity as well as due to exostosis.
iii) *Cutaneous involvement* may be in the form of pruritus, fissuring, sores at the corners of mouth and coarseness of hair.
iv) *Hepatomegaly* with parenchymal damage and fibrosis.
v) *Hypercarotenaemia* is yellowness of palms and skin due to excessive intake of β-carotene containing foods like carrots or due to inborn error of metabolism.

The effects of toxicity usually disappear on stopping excess of vitamin A intake.

Vitamin D (Calcitriol)

PHYSIOLOGY. This fat-soluble vitamin exists in 2 activated *sterol forms:*
- Vitamin D_2 or *calciferol;* and
- Vitamin D_3 or *cholecalciferol.*

The material originally described as vitamin D_1 was subsequently found to be impure mixture of sterols. Since vitamin D_2 and D_3 have similar metabolism and functions, they are therefore referred to as vitamin D.

There are 2 *main sources* of vitamin D:

i) Endogenous synthesis. 80% of body's need of vitamin D is met by endogenous synthesis from the action of ultraviolet light on 7-dehydrocholesterol widely distributed in oily secretions of the skin. The vitamin so formed by irradiation enters the body directly through the skin. Pigmentation of the skin reduces the beneficial effects of ultraviolet light.

ii) Exogenous sources. The other source of vitamin D is diet such as deep sea fish, fish oil, eggs, butter, milk, some plants and grains.

Irrespective of the source of vitamin D, it must be converted to its *active metabolites* (25-hydroxy vitamin D and 1,25-dihydroxy vitamin D or calcitriol) for being functionally active (Fig. 9.10).

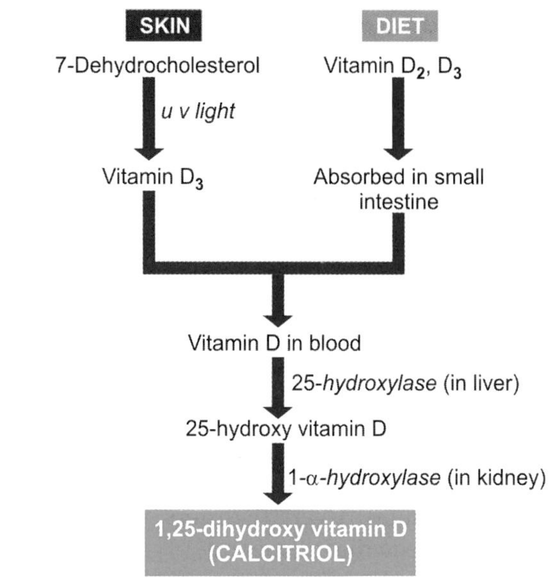

FIGURE 9.10
Normal metabolism of vitamin D.

1, 25-dihydroxy vitamin D (calcitriol) is 5-10 times more potent biologically than 25-hydroxy vitamin D. The production of calcitriol by the kidney is regulated by:
- plasma levels of calcitriol (hormonal feedback);
- plasma calcium levels (hypocalcaemia stimulates synthesis); and
- plasma phosphorus levels (hypophosphataemia stimulates synthesis).

The main storage site of vitamin D is the adipose tissue rather than the liver which is the case with vitamin A.

The main **physiologic functions** of the most active metabolite of vitamin D, calcitriol, are as follows:

1. Maintenance of normal plasma levels of calcium and phosphorus. The major essential function of vitamin D is to promote mineralisation of bone. This is achieved by the following actions of vitamin D:

i) *Intestinal absorption* of calcium and phosphorus is stimulated by vitamin D.

ii) *On bones.* Vitamin D is normally required for mineralisation of epiphyseal cartilage and osteoid matrix. However, in hypocalcaemia, vitamin D collaborates with parathyroid hormone and causes osteoclastic resorption of calcium and phosphorus from bone so as to maintain the normal blood levels of calcium and phosphorus.

iii) *On kidneys.* Vitamin D stimulates reabsorption of calcium at distal renal tubular level, though this function is also parathyroid hormone-dependent.

2. Immune regulation. Recently, vitamin D has been found to play an immune regulatory role due to the presence of receptors for a metabolite of vitamin D on activated lymphocytes and macrophages.

LESIONS IN VITAMIN D DEFICIENCY. Deficiency of vitamin D may result from:

i) reduced endogenous synthesis due to inadequate exposure to sunlight;

ii) dietary deficiency of vitamin D;

iii) malabsorption of lipids due to lack of bile salts such as in intrahepatic biliary obstruction, pancreatic insufficiency and malabsorption syndrome;

iv) derangements of vitamin D metabolism as occur in kidney disorders (chronic renal failure, nephrotic syndrome, uraemia), liver disorders (diffuse liver disease) and genetic disorders; and

v) resistance of end-organ to respond to vitamin D.

Deficiency of vitamin D from any of the above mechanisms results in:

1. rickets in growing children;
2. osteomalacia in adults; and
3. hypocalcaemic tetany due to neuromuscular dysfunction.

RICKETS. The primary defects in rickets are:

- interference with mineralisation of bone; and
- deranged endochondral and intramembranous bone growth.

The pathogenesis of lesions in rickets are better understood by contrasting them with sequence of changes in normal bone growth as outlined in Table 9.5.

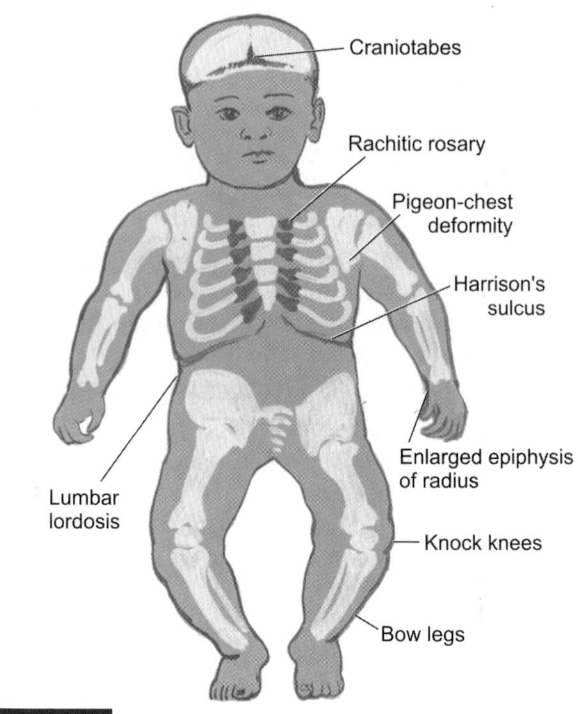

FIGURE 9.11
Lesions in rickets.

Rickets occurs in growing children from 6 months to 2 years of age. The disease has the following lesions and clinical characteristics (Fig. 9.11):

Skeletal changes. These are as under:

i) *Craniotabes* is the earliest bony lesion occurring due to small round unossified areas in the membranous

TABLE 9.5: Contrasting Features of Rickets with Normal Bone Growth.

NORMAL BONE GROWTH	RICKETS
I. ENDOCHONDRAL OSSIFICATION *(occurring in long tubular bones)*	
i. Proliferation of cartilage cells at the epiphyses followed by provisional mineralisation	i. Proliferation of cartilage cells at the epiphyses followed by inadequate provisional mineralisation
ii. Cartilage resorption and replacement by osteoid matrix	ii. Persistence and overgrowth of epiphyseal cartilage; deposition of osteoid matrix on inadequately mineralised cartilage resulting in enlarged and expanded costochondral junctions
iii. Mineralisation to form bone	iii. Deformed bones due to lack of structural rigidity
iv. Normal vascularisation of bone	iv. Irregular overgrowth of small blood vessels in disorganised and weak bone
II. INTRAMEMBRANOUS OSSIFICATION *(occurring in flat bones)*	
Mesenchymal cells differentiate into osteoblasts which develop osteoid matrix and subsequent mineralisation	Mesenchymal cells differentiate into osteoblasts with laying down of osteoid matrix which fails to get mineralised resulting in soft and weak flat bones

bones of the skull, disappearing within 12 months of birth. The skull looks square and box-like.

ii) *Harrison's sulcus* appears due to indrawing of soft ribs on inspiration.

iii) *Rachitic rosary* is a deformity of chest due to cartilaginous overgrowth at costochondral junction.

iv) *Pigeon-chest deformity* is the anterior protrusion of sternum due to action of respiratory muscles.

v) *Bow legs* occur in ambulatory children due to weak bones of lower legs.

vi) *Knock knees* may occur due to enlarged ends of the femur, tibia and fibula.

vii) *Lower epiphyses of radius may be enlarged.*

viii) *Lumbar lordosis* is due to involvement of the spine and pelvis.

Biochemical changes. These are as follows:

i) Lowered levels of active metabolites of vitamin D (25-hydroxy vitamin D and 1, 25-dihydroxy vitamin D).

ii) Plasma calcium levels are normal or slightly low.

iii) Plasma phosphate levels are lowered.

iv) Plasma alkaline phosphatase is usually raised due to osteoblastic activity.

Vitamin D-dependent rickets is an autosomal dominant disorder of vitamin D. The disease responds rapidly to administration of 1,25-dihydroxy vitamin D.

OSTEOMALACIA. Osteomalacia is the adult counterpart of rickets in which there is failure of mineralisation of the osteoid matrix. It may occur following dietary deficiency, poor endogenous synthesis of vitamin D, or as a result of conditioned deficiency.

PATHOLOGIC CHANGES. Due to deficiency of vitamin D, osteoid matrix laid down fails to get mineralised. In H and E stained microscopic sections, this is identified by widened and thickened osteoid seams (stained pink) and decreased mineralisation at the borders between osteoid and bone (stained basophilic). *von Kossa's stain* for calcium may be employed to mark out the wide seams of unstained osteoid while the calcified bone is stained black. In addition, there may be increased osteoclastic activity and fibrosis of marrow.

Clinical features. Osteomalacia is characterised by:

i) muscular weakness;
ii) vague bony pains;
iii) fractures following trivial trauma;
iv) incomplete or green-stick fractures; and
v) looser's zones or pseudofractures at weak places in bones.

Biochemical changes. These are:

i) normal or low serum calcium levels;
ii) plasma phosphate levels lowered; and
iii) raised serum alkaline phosphatase due to increased osteoblastic activity.

It may be worthwhile to note here that another chronic disorder of skeleton seen in elderly, *osteoporosis*, is clinically similar but biochemically different disease (Chapter 26).

HYPERVITAMINOSIS D. Very large excess of vitamin D may cause increased intestinal absorption of calcium and phosphorus, leading to hypercalcaemia, hyperphosphataemia and increased bone resorption. These changes may result in the following effects:

i) increased urinary excretion of calcium and phosphate;
ii) predisposition to renal calculi;
iii) osteoporosis; and
iv) widespread metastatic calcification, more marked in the renal tubules, arteries, myocardium, lungs and stomach.

Vitamin E (α-Tocopherol)

PHYSIOLOGY. Out of many naturally-occurring tocoferols, α-tocopherol is biologically the most active fat soluble compound. Vitamin E is found in most of the ordinary foods such as vegetables, grains, nuts and oils. It is absorbed from the intestine and transported in blood in the form of chylomicrons. It is stored in fat depots, liver and muscle.

The main physiologic function of vitamin E is its antioxidant activity. Vitamin E prevents the oxidative degradation of cell membranes containing phospholipids by its anti-oxidant property and scavenges free radicals formed by redox reaction in the body (Chapter 3) and thus maintains the integrity of the cell.

LESIONS IN VITAMIN E DEFICIENCY. The deficiency of vitamin E is mainly by conditioning disorders affecting its absorption and transport such as abetalipoproteinaemia, intra-and extrahepatic biliary cholestasis, cystic fibrosis of pancreas and malabsorption syndrome. Low birth weight neonates, due to physiologic immaturity of liver and bowel, may also develop vitamin E deficiency. Lesions of vitamin E deficiency are as follows:

1. *Neurons* with long axons develop degeneration in the posterior columns of spinal cord.
2. *Peripheral nerves* may also develop myelin degeneration in the axons.
3. *Skeletal muscles* may develop denervation.

4. *Retinal pigmentary degeneration* may occur.
5. *Red blood cells* deficient in vitamin E such as in premature infants have reduced life span.
6. In experimental animals, vitamin E deficiency can produce *sterility* in both male and female animals.

Vitamin K

PHYSIOLOGY. Vitamin K (*K for Koagulations in Danish*) exists in nature in *2 forms:*

- Vitamin K_1 or *phylloquinone,* obtained from exogenous dietary sources such as most green leafy vegetables; and
- Vitamin K_2 or *menadione,* produced endogenously by normal intestinal flora.

Like other fat-soluble vitamins, vitamin K is absorbed from the small intestine and requires adequate bile flow and intact pancreatic function.

The main physiologic function of vitamin K is in hepatic microsomal carboxylation reaction for vitamin K-dependent coagulation factors (most importantly factor II or prothrombin; others are factors VII, IX and X).

LESIONS IN VITAMIN K DEFICIENCY. Since vitamin K is necessary for the manufacture of prothrombin, its deficiency leads of *hypoprothrombinaemia* (Chapter 13). Estimation of plasma prothrombin, thus, affords a simple *in vitro* test for determining whether there is deficiency of vitamin K. Subjects with levels below 70% of normal should receive therapy with vitamin K.

Because most of the green vegetables contain vitamin K and that it can be synthesised endogenously, vitamin K deficiency is frequently a conditioned deficiency. The conditions which may bring about vitamin K deficiency are as follows:

1. **Haemorrhagic disease of newborn.** The newborn infants are deficient in vitamin K because of minimal stores of vitamin K at birth, lack of established intestinal flora for endogenous synthesis and limited dietary intake since breast milk is a poor source of vitamin K. Hence the clinical practice is to routinely administer vitamin K at birth.

2. **Biliary obstruction.** Bile is prevented from entering the bowel due to biliary obstruction so that this fat-soluble vitamin cannot be absorbed. Surgery on jaundiced patients, therefore, leads to marked tendency to bleeding.

3. **Malabsorption syndrome.** Patients suffering from malabsorption of fat develop vitamin K deficiency e.g. coeliac disease, sprue, pancreatic disease, hypermotility of bowel etc.

4. **Anticoagulant therapy.** Patients on warfarin group of anticoagulants have impaired biosynthesis of vitamin K-dependent coagulation factors.

5. **Antibiotic therapy.** The use of broad spectrum antibiotics and sulfa drugs reduces the normal intestinal flora.

6. **Diffuse liver disease.** Patients with diffuse liver disease (e.g. cirrhosis, amyloidosis of liver, hepatocellular carcinoma, hepatoblastoma) have hypoprothrombinaemia due to impaired synthesis of prothrombin. Administration of vitamin K to such patients is of no avail since liver, where prothrombin synthesis utilising vitamin K takes place, is diseased.

WATER-SOLUBLE VITAMINS

Vitamin C (Ascorbic Acid)

PHYSIOLOGY. Vitamin C exists in natural sources as L-ascorbic acid closely related to glucose. The major sources of vitamin C are citrus fruits such as orange, lemon, grape fruit and some fresh vegetables like tomatoes and potatoes. It is present in small amounts in meat and milk. The vitamin is easily destroyed by heating so that boiled or pasteurised milk may lack vitamin C. It is readily absorbed from the small intestine and is stored in many tissues, most abundantly in adrenal cortex.

The **physiologic functions** of vitamin C are due to its ability to carry out *oxidation-reduction reactions:*

$$\text{L-Ascorbic Acid} \rightleftharpoons \text{Dehydro L-Ascorbic acid} + 2H^+ + 2e$$

1. Ascorbic acid is required for hydroxylation of proline to form hydroxyproline which is an essential component of *collagen.*
2. Besides collagen, it is necessary for the *ground substance* of other mesenchymal structures such as osteoid, chondroitin sulfate, dentin and cement substance of vascular endothelium.
3. Vitamin C being a *reducing substance* has other functions such as:
   - hydroxylation of dopamine to norepinephrine;
   - maintenance of folic acid levels by preventing oxidation of tetrahydrofolate; and
   - role in iron metabolism in its absorption, storage and keeping it in reduced state.
4. Recently, vitamin C has been found to play a role in synthesis of neurotransmitters, neuropeptide hormone synthesis and in immune response.

LESIONS IN VITAMIN C DEFICIENCY. Vitamin C deficiency in the food or as a conditioned deficiency results in scurvy. The lesions and clinical manifestations of scurvy are seen more commonly at two peak ages: in early childhood and in the very aged. These are as under (Fig. 9.12):

1. **Haemorrhagic diathesis.** A marked tendency to bleeding is characteristic of scurvy. This may be due to deficiency of intercellular cement which holds together the cells of capillary endothelium. There may be haemorrhages in the skin, mucous membranes, gums, muscles, joints and underneath the periosteum.

2. **Skeletal lesions.** These changes are more pronounced in growing children. The most prominent change is the *deranged formation of osteoid matrix and not deranged mineralisation* (c.f. the pathological changes underlying rickets already described). Growing tubular bones as well as flat bones are affected. The epiphyseal ends of growing long bones have cartilage cells in rows which normally undergo provisional mineralisation. However, due to vitamin C deficiency, the next step of laying down of osteoid matrix by osteoblasts is poor and results in failure of resorption of cartilage. Consequently, mineralised cartilage under the widened and irregular epiphyseal plates project as *scorbutic rosary.* The skeletal changes are further worsened due to haemorrhages and haematomas under the periosteum and bleeding into the joint spaces.

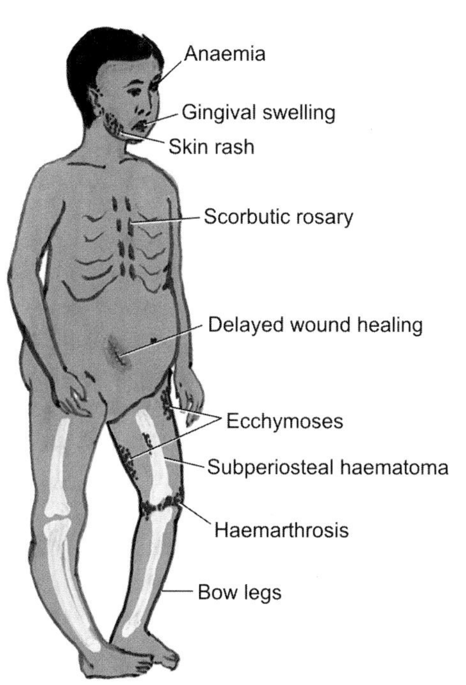

FIGURE 9.12

Lesions in scurvy.

3. **Delayed wound healing.** There is delayed healing of wounds in scurvy due to:
- deranged collagen synthesis;
- poor preservation and maturation of fibroblasts; and
- localisation of infections in the wounds.

4. **Anaemia.** Anaemia is common in scurvy. It may be the result of haemorrhage, interference with formation of folic acid or deranged iron metabolism. Accordingly, anaemia is most often normocytic normochromic type; occasionally it may be megaloblastic or even iron deficiency type.

5. **Lesions in teeth and gums.** Scurvy may interfere with development of dentin. The gums are soft and swollen, may bleed readily and get infected commonly.

6. **Skin rash.** Hyperkeratotic and follicular rash may occur in scurvy.

VITAMIN B COMPLEX

The term vitamin B was originally coined for a substance capable of curing beriberi (B from beriberi). Now, vitamin B complex is commonly used for *a group of essential compounds which are biochemically unrelated but occur together in certain foods* such as green leafy vegetables, cereals, yeast, liver and milk. Most of the vitamins in this group are involved in metabolism of proteins, carbohydrates and fats.

The principal members of vitamin B complex are thiamine (vitamin B_1), riboflavin (vitamin B_2) niacin (nicotinic acid), pyridoxine (vitamin B_6), folate (folic acid) and cyanocobalamin (vitamin B_{12}). Two other compounds—biotin and pantothenic acid, are also considered components of vitamin B complex but there is no definite evidence that any clinical disorder results from their deficiency.

Thiamine (Vitamin B_1)

PHYSIOLOGY. Thiamine hydrochloride is available in a variety of items of diet such as peas, beans, pulses, yeast, green vegetable roots, fruits, meat, pork, rice and wheat bran. The vitamin is lost in refined foods such as polished rice, white flour and white sugar. A few substances in the diet (strong tea, coffee) act as *antithiamines.* Since the vitamin is soluble in water, considerable amount of the vitamin is lost during cooking of vegetables. The vitamin is absorbed from the intestine either by passive diffusion or by energy-dependent transport. Reserves of vitamin B_1 are stored in skeletal muscles, heart, liver, kidneys and bones.

The main **physiologic function** of thiamine is in carbohydrate metabolism. Thiamine after absorption is phosphorylated to form thiamine pyrophosphate which is the functionally active compound. This compound acts as coenzyme for carboxylase so as to decarboxylate pyruvic acid, synthesises ATP and also participates in the synthesis of fat from carbohydrate.

LESIONS IN THIAMINE DEFICIENCY. Thiamine deficiency, primary or conditioned, leads to failure of complete combustion of carbohydrate and accumulation of pyruvic acid. This results in beriberi which produces lesions at 3 target tissues (peripheral nerves, heart and brain). Accordingly, beriberi is of 3 types:

- dry beriberi (*peripheral neuritis*);
- wet beriberi (*cardiac manifestations*), and
- cerebral beriberi (*Wernicke-Korsakoff's syndrome*).

It is worth-noting that lesions in beriberi are mainly located in the nervous system and heart. This is because the energy requirement of the brain and nerves is solely derived from oxidation of carbohydrates which is deranged in beriberi. Lesions in the heart appear to arise due to reduced ATP synthesis in beriberi which is required for cardiac functions.

The features of 3 forms of beriberi are as under:

1. Dry beriberi (peripheral neuritis). This is marked by neuromuscular symptoms such as weakness, paraesthesia and sensory loss. The nerves show polyneuritis, myelin degeneration and fragmentation of axons.

2. Wet beriberi (cardiac manifestations). This is characterised by cardiovascular involvement, generalised oedema, serous effusions and chronic passive congestion of viscera. The heart in beriberi is flabby (due to thin and weak myocardium), enlarged and globular in appearance due to dilatation of all the 4 chambers (Fig. 9.13).

Microscopic examination of heart shows hydropic degeneration of myocardial fibres, loss of striations, interstitial oedema and lymphocytic infiltration.

3. Cerebral beriberi (Wernicke-Korsakoff's syndrome). It consists of the following features:

i) *Wernicke's encephalopathy* occurs more often due to conditioned deficiencies such as in chronic alcoholism. It is characterised by degeneration of ganglia cells, focal demyelination and haemorrhage in the nuclei surrounding the region of ventricles and aqueduct.

Microscopic examination shows degeneration and necrosis of neurons, hypertrophy-hyperplasia of small blood vessels and haemorrhages.

ii) *Korsakoff's psychosis* results from persistence of psychotic features following brain haemorrhage in Wernicke's encephalopathy.

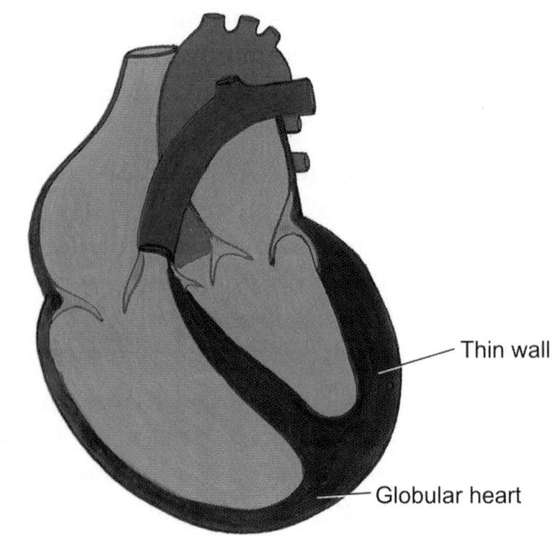

FIGURE 9.13

Wet (Cardiac) beriberi. Flabby, thin-walled, enlarged and globular appearance of the heart due to four-chamber dilatation.

Riboflavin (Vitamin B_2)

PHYSIOLOGY. Riboflavin used to be called 'yellow respiratory enzyme' (*flavus* = yellow), currently known as 'cytochrome oxidase enzyme' which is important in cellular respiration. The vitamin is usually distributed in plant and animal foods such as the liver, beaf, mutton, pork, eggs, milk and green vegetables. Like other water-soluble vitamins, it is rapidly absorbed from the bowel and stored in tissues like liver.

LESIONS IN RIBOFLAVIN DEFICIENCY. Lesions due to primary or conditioned deficiency of riboflavin (*ariboflavinosis*) are as follows:

1. *Ocular lesions* consist of vascularisation of normally avascular cornea due to proliferation of capillaries from limbus. Subsequently, conjunctivitis, interstitial keratitis and corneal ulcers may develop.
2. *Cheilosis* and *angular stomatitis* are characterised by occurrence of fissures and cracks at the angles of mouth.
3. *Glossitis* is development of red, cyanosed and shiny tongue due to atrophy of mucosa of tongue (*'bald tongue'*).
4 *Skin changes* appear in the form of scaly dermatitis resembling seborrheic dermatitis on nasolabial folds on face, scrotum and vulva.

Niacin (Nicotinic Acid)

PHYSIOLOGY. As with thiamine and riboflavin, niacin is also widely distributed in plant and animal foods such as the liver, kidney, meat, green vegetables and whole grain cereals. Niacin includes biologically active derivative *nicotinamide* which is essential for the formation of 2 oxidative coenzymes (*dehydrogenases*):

- NAD (nicotinamide adenine dinucleotide) which is required for dehydrogenation in the metabolism of fat, carbohydrates and proteins.
- NADP (nicotinamide adenine dinucleotide phosphate) which is essential for dehydrogenation in the hexose monophosphate shunt of glucose metabolism.

LESIONS IN NIACIN DEFICIENCY. Deficiency of niacin. causes pellagra, so named because of the rough skin of such patients (Italian *pelle agra* = rough skin). Pellagra may result from dietary deficiency in those who largely subsist on maize since niacin in maize is present in bound form and hence not absorbable. Since niacin can be endogenously synthesised from tryptophan, a diet deficient in this amino acid or disorders of tryptophan metabolism such as in carcinoid syndrome or Hartnup syndrome results in niacin deficiency.

Lesions in pellagra are characterised by *3D's:*

1 *Dermatitis:* The sun-exposed areas of skin develop erythema resembling sunburn. This may progress to chronic type of dermatitis with blister formation.

2. *Diarrhoea:* Lesions similar to those seen in skin may develop in mucous membrane of the alimentary tract resulting in glossitis, lesions in mouth, oesophagus, stomach and colon and cause diarrhoea, nausea, vomiting and burning sensation.

3. *Dementia:* Degeneration of neurons of the brain and of spinal tract results in neurological symptoms such as dementia, peripheral neuritis, ataxia and visual and auditary disturbances.

Pyridoxine (Vitamin B_6)

PHYSIOLOGY. Pyridoxine or vitamin B_6 is widely distributed in all animal and plant foods such as meat, liver, eggs, green vegetables and whole grain cereals. Pyridoxine exists in 3 closely related naturally-occurring substances—*pyridoxine, pyridoxal* and *pyridoxamine.* All of these can be converted into biologically active coenzyme, pyridoxal 5-phosphate.

The major **physiologic functions** of pyridoxine are related to:

- fat metabolism;
- protein metabolism;
- amino acid metabolism such as decarboxylation of amino acids, transmethylation of methionine, tryptophan metabolism and formation of melanin;
- transmission of neural impulses; and
- in the immune response.

LESIONS IN PYRIDOXINE DEFICIENCY. Vitamin B_6 deficiency may result from inadequate dietary intake or may result from secondary deficiency such as increased demand in pregnancy and lactation, chronic alcoholism and intake of certain drugs (e.g. isoniazid in the treatment of tuberculosis, penicillamine, oestrogen in oral contraceptives etc).

The **lesions** of pyridoxine deficiency are vague and include the following:

1. Convulsions in infants born to mothers who had been administered large doses of vitamin B_6 for hyperemesis gravidarum (pyridoxine dependence)
2. Dermatitis
3. Cheilosis and angular stomatitis
4. Glossitis (bald tongue)
5. Sideroblastic anaemia.

Folate (Folic Acid) and Cyanocobalamin (Vitamin B_{12})

Both these vitamins included in the B complex group are required for red cell formation. Their deficiency leads to megaloblastic anaemia which is described in Chapter 13.

In closing the discussion of vitamin B complex, it must be mentioned that many of the animal and plant foods contain vitamin B complex group of vitamins. Their deficiency, whether primary from poverty, ignorance etc, or secondary from conditioning factors like chronic alcoholism, is more frequently *multiple vitamin deficiency.* Hence, the clinical practice is to administer combination of these members of vitamin B complex.

TRACE ELEMENTS

Several minerals in trace amounts are essential for health since they form components of enzymes and cofactors for metabolic functions. Besides *calcium* and *phosphorus* required for vitamin D manufacture, others include: *iron, copper, iodine, zinc, selenium, manganese, nickel, chromium, molybdenum, fluorine.* However, out of these, the dietary deficiency of first five trace elements is associated with deficiency states which are discussed in detail in respective chapters later. These are:

i) *Iron:* Microcytic hypochromic anaemia.

ii) *Copper:* Muscle weakness, neurologic defect.

iii) *Iodine:* Goitre and hyperthyroidism.

iv) *Zinc:* Growth retardation, infertility.

v) *Selenium:* Myopathy, cardiomyopathy.

DIET AND CANCER

Before closing the discussion of environmental and nutritional pathology, it is worthwhile to sum up its relationship to carcinogenesis discussed in preceding chapter. There are three possible mechanisms on which the story of this relationship can be built up:

1. Dietary content of exogenous carcinogens:

i) The most important example in this mechanism comes from naturally-occurring carcinogen *aflatoxin* which is strongly associated with high incidence of hepatocellular carcinoma in those consuming grain contaminated with *Aspergillus flavus*.

ii) *Artificial sweeteners* (e.g. saccharine cyclomates), food additives and pesticide contamination of food are implicated as carcinogens derived from diet.

2. Endogenous synthesis of carcinogens or promoters:

i) In the context of etiology of *gastric carcinoma*, nitrites, nitrates and amines from the digested food are transformed in the body to carcinogens—nitrosamines and nitrosamides.

ii) In the etiology of *colon cancer*, low fibre intake and high animal-derived fats are implicated. High fat diet results in rise in the level of bile acids and their metabolites produced by intestinal bacteria which then act as carcinogens. The low fibre diet, on the other hand, does not provide adequate protection to the mucosa and reduces the stool bulk and thus increases the time the stools remain in the colon.

iii) In the etiology of *breast cancer*, epidemiologic studies have implicated the role of animal proteins, fats and obesity with as yet unsubstantiated evidence.

3. Inadequate protective factors: As already mentioned, some components of diet such as *vitamin C, A, E, selenium*, and *β-carotenes* have protective role against cancer. These substances in normal amounts in the body act as antioxidants and protect the cells against free radical injury but their role of supplementation in diet as prevention against cancer is unproven.

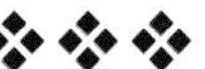

Genetic and Paediatric Diseases

10

GENETIC DISEASES—INTRODUCTION

The last chapter of General Pathology deals with the group of disorders affecting the foetus during intrauterine life (developmental as well as genetic) and paediatric age group. In the western countries, developmental and genetic birth defects constitute about 50% of total mortality in infancy and childhood, while in the developing and underdeveloped countries 95% of infant mortality is attributed to environmental factors such as poor sanitation and undernutrition.

For the purpose of convenience of discussion, genetic and paediatric diseases are covered under the following headings:

1 *Developmental defects:* Errors in morphogenesis

2. *Cytogenetic (Karyotypic) defects:* chromosomal abnormalities

3. *Single-gene defects:* Mendelian disorders

4. *Multifactorial inheritance disorders*

5. *Other paediatric diseases*

Though many of diseases included in the groups above have been discussed alongwith relevant chapters later, broad overview of these disorders is presented below.

DEVELOPMENTAL DEFECTS

Developmental defects are a group of abnormalities during foetal life due to errors in morphogenesis. The branch of science dealing with the study of developmental anomalies is called *teratology*. Certain chemicals, drugs, physical and biologic agents are known to induce such birth defects and are called *teratogens.* The morphologic abnormality or defect of an organ or anatomic region of the body so produced is called *malformation.*

Pathogenesis

The teratogens may result in one of the following outcome:

i) intrauterine death;
ii) intrauterine growth retardation;
iii) functional defects; and
iv) malformation.

The **effects** of teratogens in inducing developmental defects are related to the following factors:

■ *Variable individual susceptibility to teratogen:* All patients exposed to the same teratogen do not develop birth defect.

■ *Intrauterine stage at which patient is exposed to teratogen:* Most teratogens induce birth defects during the first trimester of pregnancy.

■ *Dose of teratogen:* Higher the exposure dose of teratogen, greater the chances of inducing birth defects.

■ *Specificity of developmental defect for specific teratogen:* A particular teratogen acts in a particular way and induces the same specific developmental defect.

Classification

Various developmental anomalies resulting from teratogenic effects are categorised as under:

Agenesis means the complete absence of an organ e.g. unilateral or bilateral agenesis of kidney.

Aplasia is the absence of development of an organ with presence of rudiment or anlage e.g. aplasia of lung with rudimentary bronchus.

Hypoplasia is incomplete development of an organ not reaching the normal adult size e.g. microglossia.

Atresia refers to incomplete formation of lumen in hollow viscus e.g. oesophageal atresia.

Developmental dysplasia is defective development of cells and tissues resulting in abnormal or primitive histogenetic structures e.g. renal dysplasia (*Developmental dysplasia* is different from *dysplasia* in relation to precancerous lesions discussed on page 62).

Dystraphic anomalies are the defects resulting from failure of fusion e.g. spina bifida.

Ectopia or heterotopia refers to abnormal location of tissue at ectopic site e.g. pancreatic heterotopia in the wall of stomach.

Examples of Developmental Defects

Some common clinically important examples are given below:

1. **Anencephaly-spina bifida complex.** This is the group of anomalies resulting from failure to fuse (dystraphy). While anencephaly results from failure of neural tube closure, spina bifida occurs from incomplete closure of the spinal cord and vertebral column, often in the lumbar region. The latter results in meningocele or meningomyelocele.

2. **Thalidomide malformations.** Thalidomide is the best known example of teratogenic drug used as a sedative by pregnant women in 1960s in England and Germany and resulted in high incidence of limb-reduction anomalies (phocomelia) in the newborns.

3. **Foetal hydantoin syndrome.** Babies born to mothers on anti-epileptic treatment with hydantoin have characteristic facial features and congenital heart defects.

4. **Foetal alcohol syndrome.** Ethanol is another potent teratogen. Consumption of alcohol by pregnant mother in first trimester increases the risk of miscarriages, still births, growth retardation and mental retardation in the newborn.

5. **TORCH complex.** Infection with TORCH group of organisms (Toxoplasma, Rubella, Cytomegalovirus, and Herpes simplex) during pregnancy is associated with multisystem anomalies and TORCH syndrome in the newborn (page 196).

6. **Congenital syphilis.** As discussed in Chapter 6, vertical transmission of syphilis from mother to foetus is characterised by Hutchinson's triad: interstitial keratitis, sensorineural deafness and deformed Hutchinson's teeth, alongwith saddle-nose deformity.

CYTOGENETIC (KARYOTYPIC) ABNORMALITIES

Human germ cells (ova and sperms) contain 23 chromosomes (haploid or N) while all the nucleated somatic cells of the human body contain 23 pairs of chromosomes (diploid or 2N)—44 autosomes and 2 sex chromosomes, being XX in females (46, XX) and XY in males (46, XY). The branch of science dealing with the study of human chromosomal abnormalities is called cytogenetics (discussed in Chapter 2).

In a female, one of the two X chromosomes (paternal or maternal derived) is inactivated during embryogenesis as stated in *Lyon hypothesis.* This inactivation is passed to all the somatic cells while the germ cells in the female remain unaffected i.e. ovary will always have active X chromosome. Such an inactive X chromosome in the somatic cells in females lies condensed in the nucleus and is called as *sex chromatin* seen specifically in the somatic cells in females. *Nuclear sexing* can be done for genetic female testing by preparing and staining the smears of squamous cells scraped from oral cavity, or by identifying the *Barr body* in the circulating neutrophils as drumstick appendage attached to one of the nuclear lobes (Fig. 10.1). A minimum of 30% cells positive for sex chromatin is indicative of genetically female composition.

Though chromosomes can be studied in any human nucleated cells, circulating lymphocytes are more often used for this purpose. The study is done by arresting the dividing cells in metaphase by colchicine and then spreading them on glass slide and staining them with Giemsa stain.

Karyotype is the photographic representation of the stained preparation of chromosomes.

Each chromosome is composed of a pair of identical double helix of chromosomal DNA called *chromatids.* The chromosomes are classified based on their length and location of the *centromere;* centromere is the point where the two chromatids cross each other (Fig. 10.2). The distal end of each chromosome is called telomere.

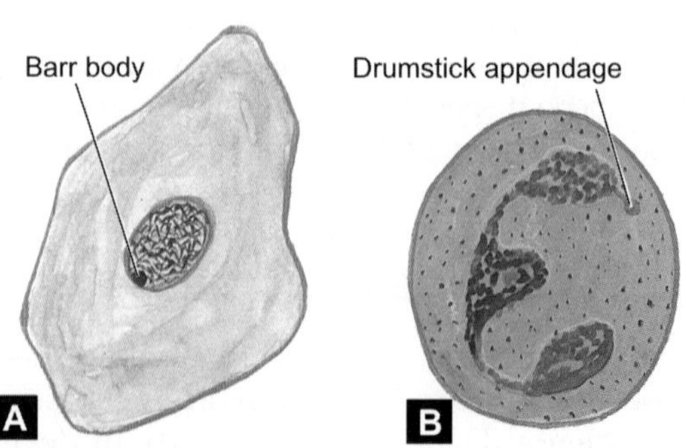

FIGURE 10.1

Nuclear sexing. A, sex chromatin as seen in scraped squamous cells from oral cavity. B, Barr body seen as drumstick appendage attached to a lobe of a circulating neutrophil.

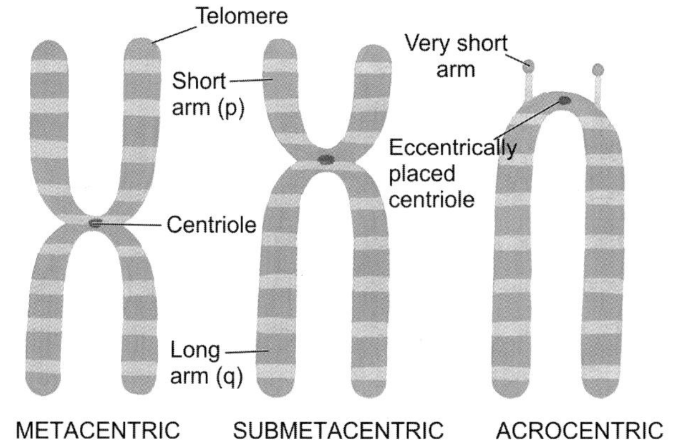

FIGURE 10.2

Classification of chromosomes based on size and location of centromere.

Based on centromeric location, they are classified into 3 groups:

- *Metacentric chromosomes* (numbers 1, 3, 16, 19, 20) are those in which the centromere is exactly in the middle.
- *Submetacentric chromosomes* (numbers 1, 3) in which the centromere divides the chromosomes into short arm (*p* arm; *petit* means short in French) and long arm (*q* arm; for letter next to p).
- *Acrocentric chromosomes* (numbers 13, 14, 15, 21, 22, and Y) have very short arm and the centromere is eccentrically located.

Based on length of chromosomes, they are divided into 7 groups—A to G, called *Denver classification* adopted at a meeting in Denver, Colorado in US.

Chromosomal banding techniques are employed for study of classes of chromosomes. Chromosomal bands are unique alternate dark and light staining patterns. Banding techniques include:

i) G-banding (Giemsa stain);
ii) Q-banding (quinacrine fluorescence stain);
iii) R-banding (reverse Giemsa staining); and
iv) C-banding (constitutive heterochromatin demonstration).

With these brief introductory comments, we can now turn to abnormalities of chromosomes which can be divided into 2 types:

1. Numerical abnormalities; and
2. Structural abnormalities.

Numerical Abnormalities

As mentioned above, normal karyotype of a human nucleated somatic cell is diploid or 2 N (46 chromosomes) while the germ cells have haploid or 1 N (23 chromosomes).

1. Polyploidy is the term used for the number of chromosomes which is a multiple of haploid number e.g. triploid or 3 N (69 chromosomes), tetraploid or 4 N (92 chromosomes). Polyploidy occurs normally in megakaryocytes and dividing liver cells. Polyploidy in somatic cells of conceptus results in spontaneous abortions.

2. Aneuploidy is the number of chromosomes which is not an exact multiple of haploid number e.g. hypodiploid or 2N-1 (45 chromosomes) monosomy, hyperdiploid or 2 N+1 (47 chromosomes) trisomy.

The most common mechanism of aneuploidy is **nondisjunction.** Nondisjunction is the failure of chromosomes to separate normally during cell division during first or second stage of meiosis, or in mitosis.

- *Nondisjunction during first meiotic division* stage will result in two gametes from both the parental chromosomes due to failure to separate while the other two gametes will have no chromosomes (nullisomic).
- *Nondisjunction during second meiotic division* stage results in one gamete with two identical copies of the same chromosome, one nullisomic gamete, and two gametes with normal chromosome number.
- *Nondisjunction during mitosis* results in mosaicism, meaning thereby that the individual has two or more types of cell lines derived from the same zygote. Mosaicism of mitotic nondisjunction of chromosomes occurs in cancers.
- *Anaphase lag* is a form of nondisjunction involving single pair of chromosomes in which one chromosome in meiosis or a chromatid in mitosis fails to reach the pole of dividing cell at the same time (i.e. it lags behind) and is left out of the nucleus of daughter cell. This results in one normal daughter cell and the other monosomic for the missing chromosome.

Three clinically important syndromes resulting from numerical aberrations of chromosomes due to nondisjunction are as under and their main clinical features are illustrated in Fig. 10.3:

- **Down's syndrome.** There is trisomy 21 in about 95% cases of Down's syndrome due to nondisjunction during meiosis in one of the parents. Down's syndrome is the most common chromosomal disorder and is the commonest cause of mental retardation. The incidence of producing offspring with Down's syndrome rises in mothers over 35 years of age.
- **Klinefelter's syndrome.** Klinefelter's syndrome is the most important example of sex chromosome trisomy.

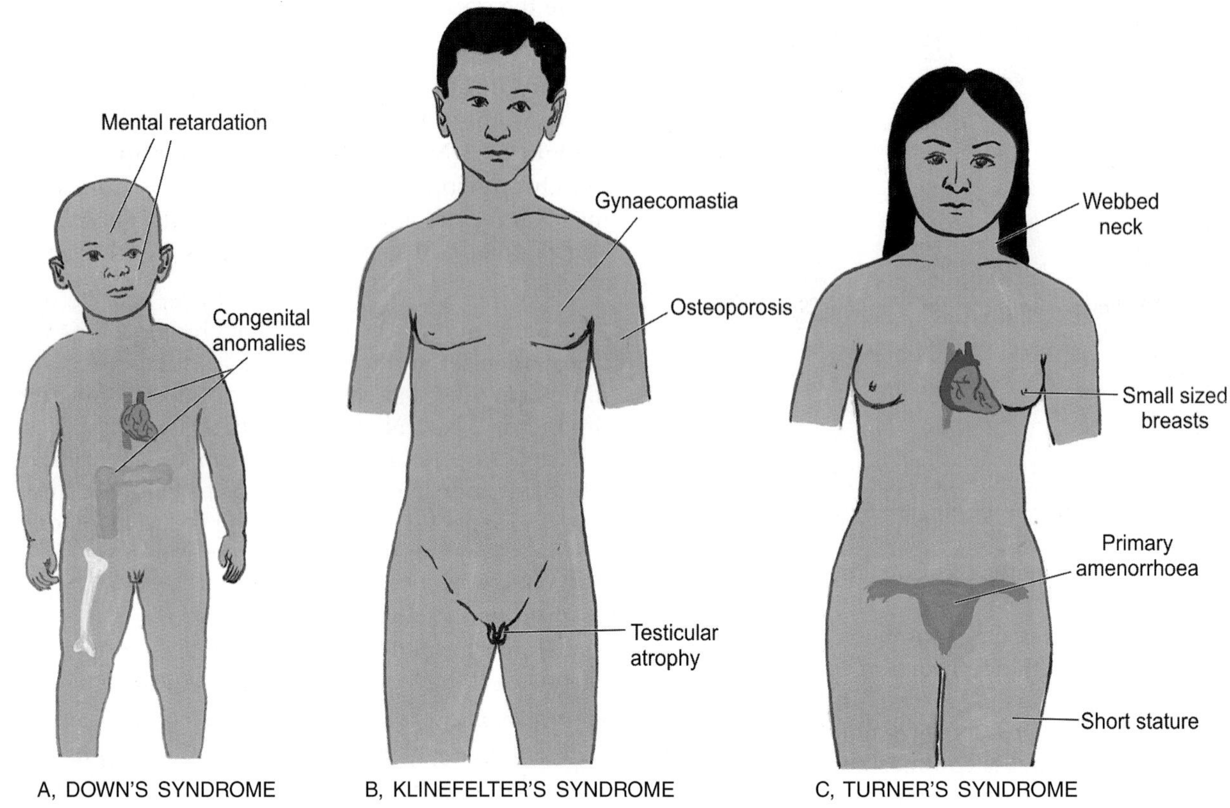

FIGURE 10.3

Clinical features of important forms of numerical chromosomal abnormalities.

About 80% cases have 47, XXY karyotype while others are mosaics. Typically, these patients have testicular dysgenesis. In general, sex chromosome trisomies are more common than trisomies of autosomes.

■ **Turner's syndrome.** Turner's syndrome is an example of monosomy (45, X0) most often due to loss of X chromosome in paternal meiosis.

Structural Abnormalities

During cell division (meiosis as well as mitosis), certain structural abnormalities of chromosomes may appear. These may occur during gametogenesis and then transmitted to all somatic cells and cause hereditary transmissible disorders, or may produce somatic cell mutations and result in changes varying from no effect to some forms of cancers. Structural abnormalities may be balanced or unbalanced.

■ *Balanced structural alteration means* no change in total number of genes or genetic material.

■ *Unbalanced structural alteration* refers to gene re-arrangement resulting in loss or gain of genetic material.

Some common forms of structural abnormalities are as under (Fig. 10.4):

TRANSLOCATIONS. Translocation means crossing over or exchange of fragment of chromosome which may occur between non-homologous or homologous chromosomes. There are two main types of translocations: reciprocal in about two-third and Robertsonian in one-third cases.

■ **Reciprocal translocation** is the exchange of genetic material between two non-homologous (heterologous) chromosomes without involving centromere (acentric). Such translocations occur due to single breaks in both the chromosomes and the exchange is detected by banding techniques. Reciprocal translocation may be balanced (without any loss of genetic material during the exchange) or unbalanced (with some loss of genetic material).

i) *Balanced reciprocal translocation* is more common and the individual is phenotypically normal e.g. translocation between long arm(q) of chromosomes 22 and long arm(q) of chromosome 9 written as 46, XX, t (9;22). This

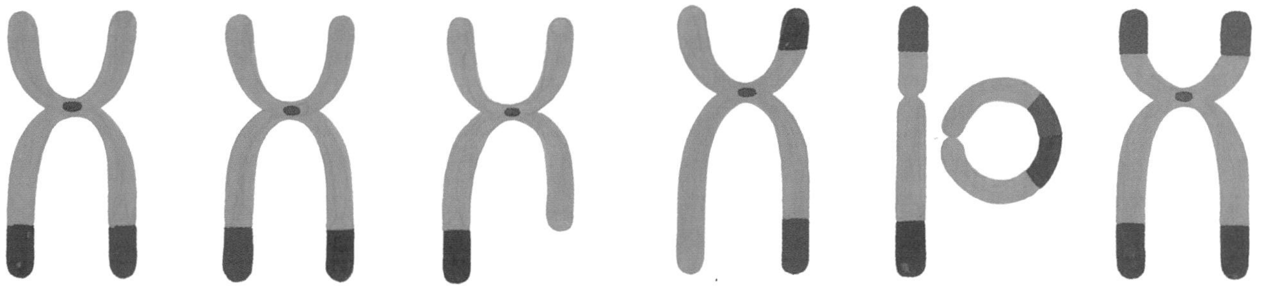

NORMAL | TRANSLOCATION | DELETION | INVERSION | RING FORMATION | ISOCHROMOSOME

FIGURE 10.4

Common structural abnormalities of human chromosomes.

translocation is termed Philadelphia chromosome seen in most cases of chronic myeloid leukaemia.

ii) *Unbalanced reciprocal translocations* are less common and account for repeated abortions and malformed children.

■ **Robertsonian translocation** is less common than reciprocal translocation. In this, there is fusion of two acrocentric chromosomes (having very short arms) at the centromere (centric fusion) with loss of short arms. The result of this fusion is one very large chromosome and the other very small one. Individuals born with Robertsonian translocation may be phenotypically normal but suffer from infertility and are at higher risk of producing malformed children in the next progeny.

DELETIONS. Loss of genetic material from the chromosome is called deletion. Deletion may be from the terminal or middle portion of the chromosome. The examples of deletion are: *cri du chat* (named after cry of infant like that of a cat) syndrome (deletion of short arm of chromosome 5) and several cancers with hereditary basis (e.g. retinoblastoma with deletion of long arm of chromosome 13, Wilms' tumour with deletion of short arm of chromosome 11).

INVERSION. Inversion is a form of rearrangement involving breaks of a single chromosome at two points. Inversion may be pericentric or paracentric, depending upon whether the rotation occurs at the centromere or at the acentric portion of the arm of chromosome. Inversions are not associated with any abnormality.

RING CHROMOSOME. A ring of chromosome is formed by a break at both the telomeric (terminal) ends of a chromosome followed by deletion of the broken fragment and then end-to-end fusion. The consequences of ring chromosome depend upon the amount of genetic material lost due to break.

ISOCHROMOSOME. When centromere rather than dividing parallel to the long axis, instead divides transverse to the long axis of chromosome, it results in either two short arms only or two long arms only called isochromosomes. The example involving isochromosome of X-chromosome is seen in some cases (15%) of Turner's syndrome.

SINGLE-GENE DEFECTS (MENDELIAN DISORDERS)

The classic laws of inheritance of characteristics or traits were outlined by Austrian monk Gregor Mendel in 1866 based on his observations of cross-breeding of red and white garden peas. Single-gene defects follow the classic mendelian patterns of inheritance and are also called mendelian disorders. These disorders are the result of mutation of a single gene of large effect.

MUTATIONS. The term mutation is applied to permanent change in the DNA of the cell. Mutations affecting germ cells are transmitted to the next progeny producing *inherited diseases,* while the mutations affecting somatic cells give rise to *various cancers* and *congenital malformations.* Presently, following types of mutations have been described:

i) **Point mutation** is the result of substitution of a single nucleotide base by a different base i.e. replacement of an amino acid by another e.g. in sickle cell anaemia there is point mutation by substitution of glutamic acid by valine in the polypeptide chain.

ii) **Stop codon or nonsense mutation** refers to a type of point mutation in which the protein chain is prematurely terminated or truncated.

iii) **Frameshift mutation** occurs when there is insertion or deletion of one or two base pairs in the DNA sequence e.g. in cystic fibrosis of pancreas.

iv) **Trinucleotide repeat mutation** is characterised by amplification of a sequence of three nucleotides.

Thus it can be surmised from above that single-gene defects are synonymous with various types of heritable mutations. Currently, approximately 5000 single-gene defects have been described—some major and others of minor consequence. While most of these disorders are discussed in relevant chapters later, the group of storage diseases (inborn errors of metabolism) is considered below.

The inheritance pattern of genetic abnormalities may be *dominant or recessive, autosomal or sex-linked. A dominant gene** produces its effects, whether combined with similar dominant or recessive gene. *Recessive genes* are effective only if both genes are similar. However, when both alleles of a gene pair are expressed in heterozygote state, it is called *codominant inheritance.* A single gene may express in multiple allelic forms known as *polymorphism.* Genes on Y-chromosome are determinant for testis and are not known to cause any sex-linked disorder. Therefore, all sex-linked disorders are, in fact, X-linked disorders.

Table 10.1 lists important examples of groups of genetic disorders: *autosomal* recessive (the largest group), codominant (intermediate), and dominant, and *sex-(X-) linked* recessive and dominant disorders.

TABLE 10.1: Important Examples of Mendelian Disorders (Single Gene Defects).

I. AUTOSOMAL RECESSIVE INHERITANCE
1. β-thalassaemia
2. Sickle cell anaemia
3. Haemochromatosis
4. Cystic fibrosis of pancreas
5. Albinism
6. Wilson's disease
7. Xeroderma pigmentosum
8. Inborn errors of metabolism (Lysosomal storage diseases, glycogenosis, alkaptonuria, phenylketonuria)

II. AUTOSOMAL CODOMINANT INHERITANCE
1. ABO blood group antigens
2. α 1-antitrypsin deficiency
3. HLA antigens

III. AUTOSOMAL DOMINANT INHERITANCE
1. Familial polyposis coli
2. Adult polycystic kidney
3. Hereditary spherocytosis
4. Neurofibromatosis (von Recklinghausen's disease)
5. Marfan's syndrome
6. von Willebrand's disease
7. Hereditary haemorrhagic telangiectasia
8. Acute intermittent porphyria
9. Familial hypercholesterolaemia
10. Osteogenesis imperfecta

IV. SEX-(X-) LINKED RECESSIVE INHERITANCE
1. Haemophilia A
2. G6PD deficiency
3. Diabetes insipidus
4. Chronic granulomatous disease
5. Colour blindness
6. Bruton's agammaglobulinaemia
7. Muscular dystrophies

V. SEX-(X-) LINKED DOMINANT INHERITANCE
1. Hypophosphataemic rickets
2. Incontinentia pigmenti

STORAGE DISEASES (INBORN ERRORS OF METABOLISM)

Storage diseases or inborn errors of metabolism are biochemically distinct groups of disorders occurring due to genetic defect in the metabolism of carbohydrates, lipids, and proteins resulting in intracellular accumulation of metabolites. These substances may collect within the cells throughout the body but most commonly affected organ or site is the one where the stored material is normally found and degraded. Since lysosomes comprise the chief site of intracellular digestion (autophagy as well as heterophagy), the material is naturally stored in the lysosomes, and hence the generic name 'lysosomal storage diseases'. Cells of mononuclear-phagocyte system are particularly rich in lysosomes; therefore, reticuloendothelial organs containing numerous phagocytic cells like the liver and spleen are most commonly involved in storage disease.

Based on the biochemical composition of the accumulated material within the cells, storage diseases are classified into distinct groups, each group containing a number of diseases depending upon the specific enzyme deficiency. A summary of major groups of storage diseases alongwith their respective enzyme deficiencies, major accumulating metabolites and the organs involved is presented in Table 10.2. A few general comments can be made about all storage diseases:

- All the storage diseases occur as a result of autosomal recessive, or sex-(X-) linked recessive genetic transmission.
- Most, but not all, of the storage diseases are lysosomal storage diseases. Out of the glycogen storage diseases, only type II (Pompe's disease) is due to lysosomal enzyme deficiency.

*A particular characteristic of an individual is determined by a pair of single *genes,* located at the same specific site termed *locus,* on a pair of homologous chromosomes. These paired genes are called *alleles* which may be *homozygous* when alike, and *heterozygous* if dissimilar. *Genotype* is the genetic composition of an individual while *phenotype* is the effect of genes produced.

TABLE 10.2: Storage Diseases (Inborn Errors of Metabolism).

DISEASE	ENZYME DEFICIENCY	ACCUMULATING METABOLITE	ORGANS INVOLVED
GLYCOGEN STORAGE DISEASE			
Type I (von Gierke's disease)	Glucose-6-phosphatase	Glycogen	Liver, kidney
Type II (Pompe's disease)	Acid-α-glucosidase (acid maltase)	Glycogen	Heart, skeletal muscle
Type III (Forbes'/Cori's disease)	Amylo-glucosidase (debrancher)	Limit dextrin	Heart, skeletal muscle
Type IV (Anderson's disease)	Amylo-trans-glucosidase (brancher)	Amylopectin	Liver
Type V (McArdle's disease)	Muscle phosphorylase	Glycogen	Skeletal muscle
Type VI (Hers' disease)	Liver phosphorylase	Glycogen	Liver
Type VII	Phosphofructokinase	Glycogen	Muscle
Type VIII	Phosphorylase kinase	Glycogen	Liver
MUCOPOLYSACCHARIDOSES (MPS)			
Type I to type VI MPS syndromes	Different lysosomal enzymes	Chondroitin sulphate, dermatan sulphate, heparan sulphate, keratan sulphate	Connective tissue, liver, spleen, bone marrow, lymph nodes, kidneys, heart, brain
SPHINGOLIPIDOSES (GANGLIOSIDOSES)			
GM1-gangliosidosis (infantile and juvenile types)	GM1 ganglioside-galactose	GM1-ganglioside	Liver, kidney, spleen, heart, brain
GM2-gangliosidosis (Tay-Sachs, Sandhoff's disease)	Hexosaminidase	GM2-ganglioside	Liver, kidney, spleen, heart, brain
SULFATIDOSES			
Metachromatic leucodystrophy	Aryl sulfatase A	Sulfatide	Brain, liver, spleen, heart, kidney
Krabbe's disease	Galactocerebrosidase	Galactocerebroside	Nervous system, kidney
Fabry's disease	α-Galactosidase	Ceramide	Skin, kidney, heart, spleen
Gaucher's disease	Glucocerebrosidase	Glucocerebroside	Spleen, liver, bone marrow
Niemann-Pick disease	Sphingomyelinase	Sphingomyelin	Spleen, liver, bone marrow, lymph nodes, lung

A few important forms of storage diseases are described below:

Glycogen Storage Diseases (Glycogenoses)

These are a group of inherited disorders in which there is defective glucose metabolism resulting in excessive intracellular accumulation of glycogen in various tissues. Based on specific enzyme deficiencies, glycogen storage diseases are divided into 8 main types designated by Roman numerals I to VIII (Table 10.2). However, based on pathophysiology, glycogen storage diseases can be divided into 3 main subgroups:

1. **Hepatic forms** are characterised by inherited deficiency of hepatic enzymes required for synthesis of glycogen for storage (e.g. von Gierke's disease or type I glycogenosis) or due to lack of hepatic enzymes necessary for breakdown of glycogen into glucose (e.g. type VI glycogenosis).

2. **Myopathic forms** on the other hand, are those disorders in which there is genetic deficiency of glycolysis to form lactate in the striated muscle resulting in accumulation of glycogen in the muscles (e.g. McArdle's disease or type V glycogenosis, type VII disease).

3. **Other forms** are those in which glycogen storage does not occur by either hepatic or myopathic mechanisms. In Pompe's disease or type II glycogenosis, there is lysosomal storage of glycogen, while in type IV there is deposition of abnormal metabolites of glycogen in the brain, heart, liver and muscles.

The prototypes of these three forms are briefly considered below.

VON GIERKE'S DISEASE I (TYPE I GLYCOGENOSIS). This condition is inherited as an autosomal recessive disorder due to deficiency of enzyme, glucose-6-phosphatase. In the absence of glucose-6-phosphatase, excess of normal type of glycogen accumulates in the liver and also results in hypoglycaemia due to reduced formation of free glucose from glycogen. As a result, fat is metabolised for energy requirement leading to hyperlipoproteinaemia and ketosis. Other changes due to deranged glucose metabolism are hyperuricaemia and accumulation of pyruvate and lactate.

The disease manifests clinically in infancy with failure to thrive and stunted growth. Most prominent feature is enormous hepatomegaly with intracytoplasmic and intranuclear glycogen. The kidneys are also enlarged and show intracytoplasmic glycogen in tubular epithelial cells. Other features include gout, skin xanthomas and bleeding tendencies due to platelet dysfunction.

POMPE'S DISEASE (TYPE II GLYCOGENOSIS). This is also an autosomal recessive disorder due to deficiency of a lysosomal enzyme, acid maltase, and is the only example of *lysosomal* storage disease amongst the various types of glycogenoses. Acid maltase is normally present in most cell types and is responsible for the degradation of glycogen. Its deficiency, therefore, results in accumulation of glycogen in many tissues, most often in the heart and skeletal muscle, leading to cardiomegaly and hypotonia.

McARDLE'S DISEASE (TYPE V GLYCOGENOSIS). The condition occurs due to deficiency of muscle phosphorylase resulting in accumulation of glycogen in the muscle (deficiency of liver phosphorylase results in type VI glycogenosis). The disease is common in 2nd to 4th decades of life and is characterised by painful muscle cramps, especially after exercise, and detection of myoglobinuria in half the cases.

Mucopolysaccharidoses (MPS)

Mucopolysaccharidoses are a group of six inherited syndromes numbered from MPS I to MPS VI. Each of these results from deficiency of specific lysosomal enzyme involved in the degradation of mucopolysaccharides or glycosaminoglycans, and are, therefore, a form of lysosomal storage diseases. Mucopolysaccharides which accumulate in the MPS are: chondroitin sulphate, dermatan sulphate, heparan sulphate and keratan sulphate. All these syndromes are autosomal recessive disorders except MPS II (Hunter's syndrome) which has X-linked recessive transmission.

Syndrome of MPS manifests in infancy or early childhood and involves multiple organs and tissues, chiefly connective tissues, liver, spleen, bone marrow, lymph nodes, kidneys, heart and brain. The mucopolysaccharides accumulate in mononuclear phagocytic cells, endothelial cells, intimal smooth muscle cells and fibroblasts. The material is finely granular and PAS-positive by light microscopy. By electron microscopy, it appears in the swollen lysosomes and can be identified biochemically as mucopolysaccharide.

Gaucher's Disease

This is an autosomal recessive disorder in which there is deficiency of lysosomal enzyme, glucocerebrosidase, which normally cleaves glucose from ceramide. This results in lysosomal accumulation of glucocerebroside (ceramide-glucose) in phagocytic cells of the body and sometimes in the neurons. The main sources of glucocerebroside in phagocytic cells are the membrane glycolipids of old leucocytes and erythrocytes, while the deposits in the neurons consist of gangliosides.

Clinically, 3 subtypes of Gaucher's disease are identified:

- **Type I or classic form** is the adult form of disease in which there is storage of glucocerebrosides in the phagocytic cells of the body, principally involving the spleen, liver, bone marrow, and lymph nodes. This is the most common type comprising 80% of all cases of Gaucher's disease.
- **Type II** is the infantile form in which there is progressive involvement of the central nervous system.
- **Type III** is the juvenile form of the disease having features in between type I and type II i.e. they have systemic involvement like in type I and progressive involvement of the CNS as in type II.

The clinical features depend upon the clinical subtype of Gaucher's disease. In addition to involvement of different organs and systems (splenomegaly, hepatomegaly, lymphadenopathy, bone marrow and cerebral involvement), a few other features include pancytopenia, or thrombocytopenia secondary to hypersplenism, bone pains and pathologic fractures.

Microscopy shows large number of characteristically distended and enlarged macrophages called *Gaucher cells* which are found in the spleen, liver, bone marrow and lymph nodes, and in the case of neuronal involvement, in the Virchow-Robin space. The cytoplasm of these cells is abundant, granular and fibrillar resembling crumpled tissue paper. They have mostly a single nucleus but occasionally may have two or three nuclei (Fig. 10.5, A). Gaucher cells are positive with PAS, oil red O, and Prussian-blue reaction indicating the nature of accumulated material as glycolipids admixed with haemosiderin. These cells often show erythrophagocytosis and are rich in acid phosphatase.

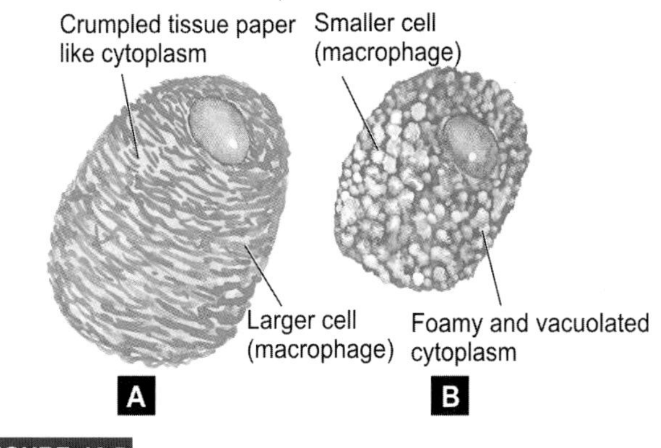

FIGURE 10.5

A, Typical Gaucher cell. B, Typical macrophage in Niemann-Pick disease.

Niemann-Pick Disease

This is also an autosomal recessive disorder characterised by accumulation of sphingomyelin and cholesterol. Majority of the cases (about 80%) have deficiency of sphingomyelinase which is required for cleavage of sphingomyelin, while a few cases probably result from deficiency of an activator protein.

The condition presents in infancy and is characterised by hepatosplenomegaly, lymphadenopathy and physical and mental underdevelopment. About a quarter of patients present with familial amaurotic idiocy with characteristic cherry-red spots in the macula of the retina (*amaurosis* = loss of vision without apparent lesion of the eye).

Microscopy shows storage of sphingomyelin and cholesterol within the lysosomes, particularly in the cells of mononuclear phagocyte system. The cells of Niemann-Pick disease are somewhat smaller than Gaucher cells and their cytoplasm is not wrinkled but is instead foamy and vacuolated which stains positively with fat stains (Fig. 10.5, B). These cells are widely distributed in the spleen, liver, lymph nodes, bone marrow, lungs, bowel and brain.

DISORDERS WITH MULTIFACTORIAL INHERITANCE

These are disorders which result from the combined effect of genetic composition and environmental influences. Some normal phenotypic characteristics have also multifactorial inheritance e.g. colour of hair, eye, skin, height and intelligence. Examples of disorders where environmental influences unmask the mutant genes are:

1. Cleft lip and cleft palate
2. Pyloric stenosis
3. Diabetes mellitus
4. Hypertension
5. Congenital heart disease
6. Coronary heart disease.

OTHER PAEDIATRIC DISEASES

As mentioned in the foregoing discussion, many diseases affecting infancy and childhood are genetic or developmental in origin. Here, we shall describe other diseases affecting the period from birth to puberty under the heading of paediatric diseases. This period is conventionally subdivided into 4 stages:

- *Neonatal period:* birth to first 4 weeks
- *Infancy:* first year of life
- *Early childhood:* 1-4 years
- *Late childhood:* 5-14 years

Each of these four stages has distinct anatomic, physiologic and immunologic development compared to adults and, therefore, has different groups of diseases unique to particular age groups. Before discussing these diseases affecting different age groups, a few general comments about these stages can be made:

1. Neonatal period is the period of continuation of dependent intrauterine foetal life to independent postnatal period. Therefore, this is the period of maximum risk to life due to perinatal causes (e.g. prematurity, low birth weight, perinatal infections, respiratory distress syndrome, birth asphyxia, birth trauma etc) and congenital anomalies. If adequate postnatal medical care is not provided, neonatal mortality is high. Neonatal mortality in first week after birth is about 10-times higher compared to second week, and shows improvement with every passing week at this stage.

2. In infancy, the major health problems are related to congenital anomalies, infections of lungs and bowel, and sudden infant death syndrome (often during sleep).

3. Young children from 1-4 years are exposed to higher risk of sustaining injuries, and manifest certain congenital anomalies. Some malignant tumours are peculiar to this age group.

4. Older children from 5-14 years too have higher risk of injuries from accidents and have other problems related to congenital anomalies and certain malignant tumours at this age.

Thus, hazardous effects of congenital anomalies are a common denominator for all age groups from birth to adolescence and have been discussed already. Tumours peculiar to infants and children are discussed alongwith discussion in related chapters of Systemic Pathology. However, a short note on general aspects of this subject is given below.

TUMOURS OF INFANCY AND CHILDHOOD

Tumours of infancy and childhood comprise 2% of all malignant tumours but they are the leading cause of death in this age group exceeded only by accidents. Benign tumours are more common than malignant neoplasms but they are generally of little immediate consequence. Another aspect requiring consideration here is the difficulty in differentiating benign tumours from tumour-like lesions discussed below.

HISTOGENESIS. Histogenetic evolution of tumours at different age groups takes place as under:

- Some tumours have probably evolved *in utero* and are apparent at birth or in immediate postnatal period. Such tumours are termed *developmental tumours.*
- Many other tumours originate in abnormally developed organs and organ rests; they become apparent subsequently and are termed *embryonic tumours.*
- In embryonic tumours, proliferation of embryonic cells occurs which *have not reached the differentiation stage* essential for specialised functions i.e. the cells proliferate as *undifferentiated or as partially differentiated* stem cells and an embryonal tumour is formed.
- Tumours of infancy and childhood have *some features of normal embryonic or foetal cells* in them which proliferate under growth promoting influence of oncogenes and suffer from mutations which make them appear morphologically malignant.
- Under appropriate conditions, these malignant embryonal cells may *cease to proliferate* and transform into non-proliferating mature differentiated cells e.g. a neonatal neuroblastoma may mature and differentiate into benign ganglioneuroma; foetal sacrococcygeal teratoma matures with age to adult tissues and is assigned better prognosis.

Thus, normal somatic cell maturation and neoplastic development in embryonal tumours represent two opposite ends of *ontogenesis,* with capability of some such tumours to mature and differentiate to turn benign from malignant.

Benign Tumours and Tumour-like Conditions

Many of the benign tumours seen in infancy and childhood are actually growth of displaced cells and masses of tissues and their proliferation takes place alongwith the growth of the child. Some of these tumours undergo a phase of spontaneous regression subsequently—a feature usually not seen in true benign tumours. While some consider such lesions as mere *'tumour-like lesions or malformations'*, others call them benign tumours. A few such examples are as under:

1. Hamartomas. Hamartomas are focal accumulations of cells normally present in that tissue but are arranged in an abnormal manner i.e. though present at normal site they do not reproduce normal architecture identical to adjacent tissues (page 198).

2. Choristoma (heterotopia). Choristoma or heterotopia is collection of normal cells and tissues at aberrant locations e.g. heterotopic pancreatic tissue in the wall of small bowel or stomach.

A list of common benign tumours and tumour-like lesions is presented in Table 10.3.

TABLE 10.3: Common Paediatric Benign Tumours and Tumour-like Lesions.

NOMENCLATURE	MAIN FEATURES
BENIGN TUMOURS	
i. Haemangioma	• Most common in infancy • Commonly on skin (e.g. port-wine stain) • May regress spontaneously
ii. Lymphangioma	• Cystic and cavernous type common • Located in skin or deeper tissues • Tends to increase in size after birth
iii. Sacrococcygeal teratoma	• Often accompanied with other congenital malformations • Majority (75%) are benign; rest are immature or malignant
iv. Fibromatosis	• Solitary (which generally behaves as benign) to multifocal (aggressive lesions)
TUMOUR-LIKE LESIONS/BENIGN TUMOURS	
i. Naevocellular naevi	• Very common lesion on the skin
ii. Liver cell adenoma	• Most common benign tumour of liver
iii. Rhabdomyoma	• Rare foetal and cardiac tumour

Malignant Tumours

Cancers of infancy and childhood differ from those in adults in the following respects:

1. Sites. Cancers of this age group more commonly pertain to haematopoietic system, neural tissue and soft tissues compared to malignant tumours in adults at sites such as the lung, breast, prostate, colon and skin.

2. Genetic basis. Many of paediatric malignant tumours have underlying genetic abnormalities.

3. Regression. Foetal and neonatal malignancies have a tendency to regress spontaneously or to mature.

4. Histologic feature. These tumours have unique histologic feature in having primitive or embryonal appearance rather than pleomorphic-anaplastic histologic appearance.

5. Management. Many of paediatric malignant tumours are curable by chemotherapy and/or radiotherapy but may develop second malignancy.

A few *generalisations* can be drawn about these cancers:

- In infants and children under 4 years of age: the most common malignant tumours are various types of *blastomas.*
- Children between 5 to 9 years of age: *haematopoietic malignancies* are more common.
- In the age range of 10-14 years (prepubertal age): *soft tissue and bony sarcomas* are the prominent tumours.

Based on these broad guidelines, classification of common paediatric malignant tumours at different age groups is presented in Table 10.4. These have been discussed in related chapters later.

TABLE 10.4: Common Paediatric Malignant Tumours.

SYSTEM	AGE < 4 YRS	AGE 5-9 YRS	AGE 10-14 YRS
1. *Haematopoietic*	Acute leukaemia —	Acute leukaemia Lymphoma	— Hodgkin's
2. *Blastomas*	Neuroblastoma Hepatoblastoma Retinoblastoma Nephroblastoma (Wilms'tumour)	Neuroblastoma Hepatocellular carcinoma	— Hepatocellular carcinoma
3. *Soft tissues*	Rhabdomyosarcoma	Soft tissue sarcoma	Soft tissue sarcoma
4. *Bony*	—	Ewing's sarcoma	Osteogenic sarcoma
5. *Neural*	CNS tumours	CNS tumours	—
6. *Others*	Teratoma	—	Thyroid cancer

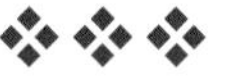

SECTION II

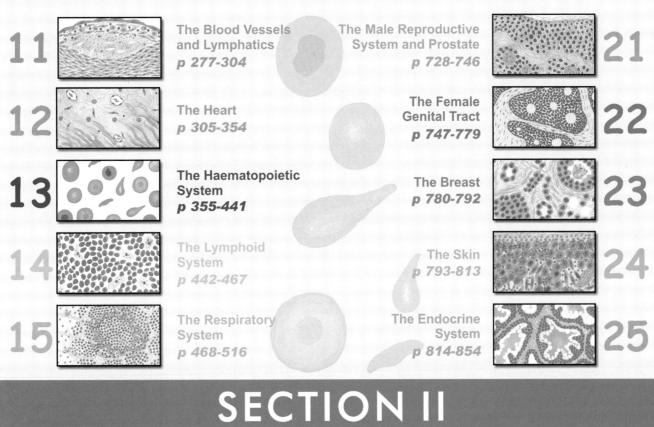

SYSTEMIC PATHOLOGY

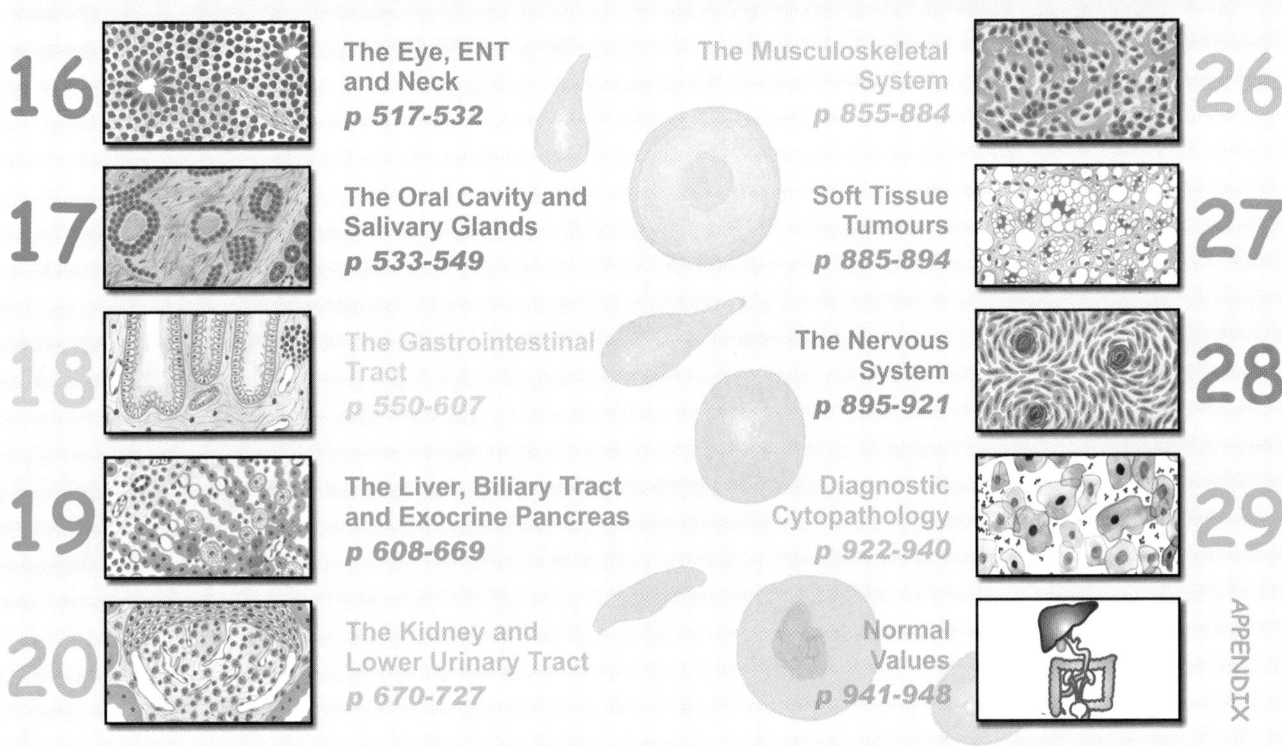

The Blood Vessels and Lymphatics

11

The blood vessels are closed circuits for the transport of blood from the left heart to the metabolising cells, and then back to the right heart. The blood containing oxygen, nutrients and metabolites is routed through arteries, arterioles, capillaries, venules and veins (Fig. 11.1). These blood vessels differ from each other in their structure and function.

ARTERIES

NORMAL STRUCTURE

Depending upon the calibre and certain histologic features, arteries are divided into 3 types: large (elastic) arteries, medium-sized (muscular) arteries and the smallest arterioles.

Histologically, all the arteries of the body have 3 layers in their walls: the tunica intima, the tunica media and the tunica adventitia. These layers progressively decrease with diminution in the size of the vessels.

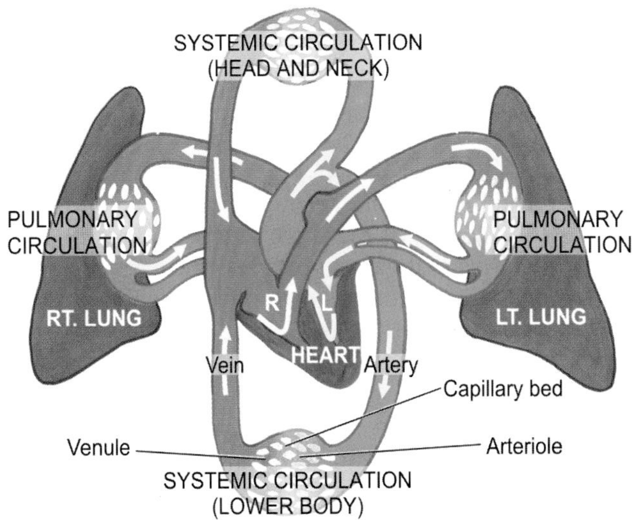

FIGURE 11.1

Systemic circulation in the body.

1. **Tunica intima.** This is the inner coat of the artery. It is composed of the lining endothelium, subendothelial connective tissue and bounded externally by internal elastic lamina.

■ The *endothelium* is a layer of flattened cells adjacent to the flowing blood. Narrow junctions exist between the adjoining endothelial cells through which certain materials pass. The integrity of the endothelial layer is of paramount importance in the maintenance of vascular functions since damage to it is the most important event in the initiation of thrombus formation at the site.

■ The *subendothelial tissue* consists of loose meshwork of connective tissue that includes myointimal cells, collagen, proteoglycans, elastin and matrix glycoproteins.

■ The *internal elastic lamina* is a layer of elastic fibres having minute fenestrations.

2. Tunica media. Tunica media is the middle coat of the arterial wall, bounded internally by internal elastic lamina and externally by external elastic lamina. This layer is the thickest and consists mainly of smooth muscle cells and elastic fibres. The *external elastic lamina* consisting of condensed elastic tissue is less well defined than the *internal elastic lamina.*

3. Tunica adventitia. The outer coat of arteries is the tunica adventitia. It consists of loose mesh of connective tissue and some elastic fibres that merge with the adjacent tissues. This layer is rich in lymphatics and autonomic nerve fibres.

The layers of arterial wall receive nutrition and oxygen from 2 sources:

1. The tunica intima and inner third of the media are nourished by *direct diffusion* from the blood present in the lumen.
2. The outer two-thirds of the media and the adventitia are supplied by *vasa vasora (i.e. vessels of vessels)*, the nutrient vessels arising from the parent artery.

As the calibre of the artery decreases, the three layers progressively diminish. Thus, there are structural variations in the three types of arteries:

■ The *large, elastic arteries* such as the aorta, innominate, common carotid, major pulmonary, and common iliac arteries have very high content of elastic tissue in the media and thick elastic laminae and hence the name.

■ The *medium-sized, muscular arteries* are the branches of elastic arteries. All the three layers of arterial wall are thinner than in the elastic arteries. The internal elastic lamina appears as a single wavy line while the external elastic lamina is less prominent. The media primarily consists of smooth muscle cells and some elastic fibres (Fig. 11.2).

■ The *arterioles* are the smallest branches with internal diameter 20-100 μm. Structurally, they consist of the three layers as in muscular arteries but are much thinner and cannot be distinguished. The arterioles consist of a layer of endothelial cells in the intima, one or two smooth muscle cells in the media and small amount of collagen and elastic tissue comprising the adventitia. The elastic laminae are virtually lost.

■ Capillaries are about the size of an RBC (7-8 μm) and have a layer of endothelium but no media. Blood from capillaries returns to the heart via *post-capillary venules* and thence into venules and then veins.

Diseases of arteries are discussed first which are divided into 3 major headings: arteriosclerosis, arteritis (vasculitis) and aneurysms. This is followed by brief outline of diseases of veins and lymphatics, while the vascular tumours are described at the end of the chapter.

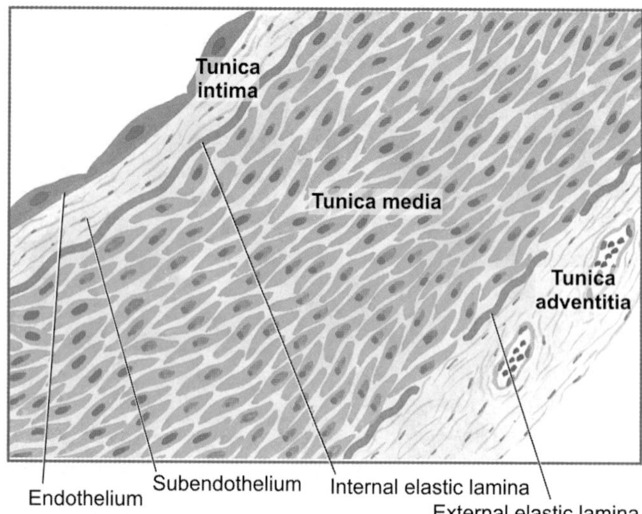

FIGURE 11.2

The structure of a medium-sized muscular artery.

ARTERIOSCLEROSIS

Arteriosclerosis is a general term used to include all conditions with thickening and hardening of the arterial walls. The following morphologic entities are included under arteriosclerosis:

I. Senile arteriosclerosis
II. Hypertensive arteriolosclerosis
III. Mönckeberg's arteriosclerosis (Medial calcific sclerosis)
IV. Atherosclerosis

The last-named, atherosclerosis, is the most common and most important form of arteriosclerosis; if not specified, the two terms are used interchangeably with each other.

SENILE ARTERIOSCLEROSIS

Senile arteriosclerosis is the thickening of media and intima of the arteries seen due to aging. The changes are non-selective and affect most of the arteries. These are possibly induced by stress and strain on vessel wall during life.

PATHOLOGIC CHANGES. The changes are as under:
1. *Fibroelastosis:* The intima and media are thickened due to increase in elastic and collagen tissue.
2. *Elastic reduplication:* The internal elastic lamina is split or reduplicated so that two wavy layers are seen.

Eventually, the fibrotic changes result in age-related elevation of systolic blood pressure.

HYPERTENSIVE ARTERIOLOSCLEROSIS

Hypertension is the term used to describe an elevation in blood pressure. Pathology of 3 forms of hypertension—systemic, pulmonary and portal, are discussed in detail with diseases of the kidneys (Chapter 20), lungs (Chapter 15) and liver (Chapter 19) respectively.

Arteriolosclerosis is the term used to describe 3 morphologic forms of vascular disease affecting arterioles and small muscular arteries. These are: hyaline arteriolosclerosis, hyperplastic arteriolosclerosis and necrotising arteriolitis. All the three types are common in hypertension but may occur due to other causes as well.

Hyaline Arteriolosclerosis

Hyaline sclerosis is a common arteriolar lesion that may be seen *physiologically* due to aging, or may occur *pathologically* in hypertensives and in diabetics. The lesions are more severe in patients with hypertension, especially in the kidneys (Chapter 20).

PATHOLOGIC CHANGES. The visceral arterioles are particularly involved. The vascular walls are thickened and the lumina narrowed or even obliterated. ***Microscopically,*** the thickened vessel wall shows structureless, eosinophilic, hyaline material in the intima and media (Fig. 11.3,A).

PATHOGENESIS. The exact pathogenesis is not known. However, the following hypotheses have been proposed:

i) The lesions result most probably from *leakage of components of plasma* across the vascular endothelium. This is substantiated by the demonstration of immunoglobulins, complement, fibrin and lipids in the lesions. The permeability of the vessel wall is increased, due to haemodyanamic stress in hypertension and metabolic stress in diabetes, so that these plasma components leak out and get deposited in the vessel wall.

ii) An alternate possibility is that the lesions may be due to *immunologic reaction.*

iii) Some have considered it to be *normal aging process* that is exaggerated in hypertension and diabetes mellitus.

Hyperplastic Arteriolosclerosis

The hyperplastic or proliferative type of arteriolosclerosis is a characteristic lesion of malignant hypertension; other causes include haemolytic-uraemic syndrome, scleroderma and toxaemia of pregnancy.

PATHOLOGIC CHANGES. The morphologic changes affect mainly the intima, especially of the interlobular arteries in the kidneys. Three types of intimal thickening may occur.

i) *Onion-skin lesion* consists of loosely-placed concentric layers of hyperplastic intimal smooth muscle cells like the bulb of an onion. The basement membrane is also thickened and reduplicated (Fig. 11.3, B).

ii) *Mucinous intimal thickening* is the deposition of amorphous ground substance, probably proteoglycans, with scanty cells.

iii) *Fibrous intimal thickening* is less common and consists of bundles of collagen, elastic fibres and hyaline deposits in the intima.

Severe intimal sclerosis results in narrowed or obliterated lumen. With time, the lesions become more and more fibrotic.

PATHOGENESIS. The pathogenesis of hyperplastic intimal thickening is unclear. Probably, the changes result following endothelial injury from systemic hypertension, hypoxia or immunologic damage leading to increased permeability. A healing reaction occurs in the form of proliferation of smooth muscle cells with fibrosis.

Necrotising Arteriolitis

In cases of severe hypertension and malignant hypertension, parts of small arteries and arterioles show changes of hyaline sclerosis and parts of these show necrosis, or necrosis may be superimposed on hyaline sclerosis. However, hyaline sclerosis may not be always present in the vessel wall.

PATHOLOGIC CHANGES. Besides the changes of hyaline sclerosis, the changes of necrotising arteriolitis include fibrinoid necrosis of vessel wall, acute inflammatory infiltrate of neutrophils in the adventitia. Oedema and haemorrhages often surround the affected vessels (Fig. 11.3,C).

PATHOGENESIS. Since necrotising arteriolitis occurs in vessels in which there is sudden and great elevation of pressure, the changes are said to result from direct physical injury to the vessel wall.

MÖNCKEBERG'S ARTERIOSCLEROSIS (MEDIAL CALCIFIC SCLEROSIS)

Mönckeberg's arteriosclerosis is calcification of the media of large and medium-sized muscular arteries,

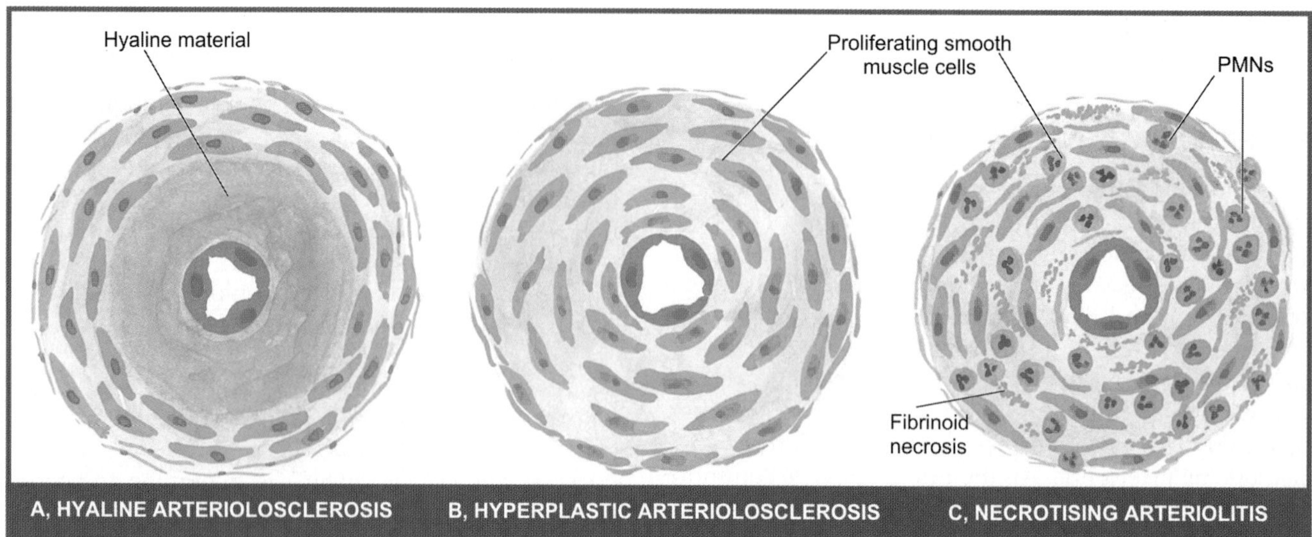

FIGURE 11.3

Diagrammatic representation of three forms of arteriolosclerosis, commonly seen in hypertension.

especially of the extremities and of the genital tract. The condition occurs as an age-related degenerative process, and therefore, an example of dystrophic calcification, commonly seen in the elderly individuals and has little or no clinical significance. However, medial calcification also occurs in some pathological states like pseudoxanthoma elasticum and in idiopathic arterial calcification of infancy.

PATHOLOGIC CHANGES. Medial calcification is often an incidental finding in X-rays of the affected sites. The deposition of calcium salts in the media produces pipestem-like rigid tubes without causing narrowing of the lumen.

Microscopically, Mönckeberg's arteriosclerosis is characterised by deposits of calcium salts in the media without associated inflammatory reaction while the intima and the adventitia are spared (COLOUR PLATE XIII: CL 49). Often, the coexistent changes of atherosclerosis are present altering the histologic appearance.

PATHOGENESIS. Pathogenesis of this condition is not known but it is considered as an age-related physiologic change due to prolonged effect of vasoconstriction.

ATHEROSCLEROSIS

Definition

Atherosclerosis is a specific form of arteriosclerosis affecting primarily the intima of large and medium-sized muscular arteries and is characterised by fibrofatty plaques or atheromas. The term atherosclerosis is derived from *athero-*(meaning porridge) referring to the soft lipid-rich material in the centre of atheroma, and *sclerosis* (scarring) referring to connective tissue in the plaques. Atherosclerosis is the commonest and the most important of the arterial diseases. Though any large and medium-sized artery may be involved in atherosclerosis, the most commonly affected are the aorta, the coronary and the cerebral arterial systems. Therefore, the major clinical syndromes resulting from ischaemia due to atherosclerosis are the myocardial infarcts (*heart attacks*) and the cerebral infarcts (*strokes*); other less common sequelae are peripheral vascular disease, aneurysmal dilatation due to weakened arterial wall, chronic ischaemic heart disease, ischaemic encephalopathy and mesenteric occlusion.

Etiology

Atherosclerosis is widely prevalent in industrialised countries. However, majority of the incidences quoted in the literature are based on the major clinical syndromes produced by it, the most important interpretation being that death from myocardial infarction is related to underlying atherosclerosis. Cardiovascular disease, mostly related to atherosclerotic coronary heart disease or ischaemic heart disease (IHD) is the most common cause of death in the developed countries of the world.

Extensive epidemiologic investigations on living populations have revealed a number of **risk factors**

TABLE 11.1: Risk Factors in Atherosclerosis.

I. MAJOR RISK FACTORS	II. MINOR RISK FACTORS
A) Constitutional	1. Environmental influences
1. Age	2. Obesity
2. Sex	3. Hormones:oestrogen deficiency, oral contraceptives
3. Genetic factors	
4. Familial and racial factors	4. Physical inactivity
B) Acquired	5. Stressful life
1. Hyperlipidaemia	6. Infections (*C.pneumoniae*, Herpesvirus, CMV)
2. Hypertension	
3. Diabetes mellitus	7. Homocystinuria
4. Smoking	8. Role of alcohol

which are associated with increased risk of developing clinical atherosclerosis. Often, these risk factors are acting in combination rather than singly.

These risk factors are divided into two groups (Table 11.1):

I. Major risk factors. These are further considered under 2 headings:

A) *Major constitutional risk factors:* These are non-modifiable major risk factors that includes: increasing age, male sex, genetic abnormalities, and familial and racial predisposition.

B) *Major acquired risk factors*: This includes major risk factors which can be controlled and includes: hyperlipidaemia, hypertension, diabetes mellitus and smoking.

II. Minor risk factors. This includes a host of factors whose role in atherosclerosis is minimal, and in some cases, even uncertain.

Apparently, a combination of etiologic risk factors have additive effect in producing the lesions of atherosclerosis.

MAJOR CONSTITUTIONAL RISK FACTORS

Age, sex and genetic influences do affect the appearance of lesions of atherosclerosis.

1. AGE. Atherosclerosis is an age-related disease. Though early lesions of atherosclerosis may be present in childhood, clinically significant lesions are found with increasing age. Fully-developed atheromatous plaques usually appear in the 4th decade and beyond. Evidence in support comes from the high death rate from IHD in this age group.

2. SEX. The incidence and severity of atherosclerosis are more in men than in women. The prevalence of atherosclerotic IHD is about three times higher in men in 4th decade than in women and the difference slowly declines with age but remains higher at all ages in men. The lower incidence of IHD in women, especially in premenopausal age, is probably due to high levels of oestrogen and high-density lipoproteins, both of which have anti-atherogenic influence.

3. GENETIC FACTORS. Genetic factors play a significant role in atherogenesis. Hereditary genetic derangements of lipoprotein metabolism predispose the individual to high blood lipid level and familial hypercholesterolaemia.

4. FAMILIAL AND RACIAL FACTORS: The familial predisposition to atherosclerosis may be related to other risk factors like diabetes, hypertension and hyperlipoproteinaemia. Racial differences too exist; Blacks have generally less severe atherosclerosis than Whites.

MAJOR ACQUIRED RISK FACTORS

There are four major acquired risk factors in atherogenesis—hyperlipidaemia, hypertension, cigarette smoking and diabetes mellitus.

1. HYPERLIPIDAEMIA. Virchow in 19th century first identified cholesterol crystals in the atherosclerotic lesions. Since then, extensive information on lipoproteins and their role in atherosclerotic lesions has been gathered. It is now well established that hypercholesterolaemia has directly proportionate relationship with atherosclerosis and IHD. The following evidences are cited in support of this:

i) The atherosclerotic plaques contain cholesterol and cholesterol esters, largely derived from the lipoproteins in the blood.

ii) The lesions of atherosclerosis can be induced in experimental animals by feeding them with diet rich in cholesterol.

iii) Individuals with hypercholesterolaemia due to various causes such as in diabetes mellitus, myxoedema, nephrotic syndrome, von Gierke's disease, xanthomatosis and familial hypercholesterolaemia have increased risk of developing atherosclerosis and IHD.

iv) Populations having hypercholesterolaemia have higher mortality from IHD. Dietary regulation and administration of cholesterol-lowering drugs have beneficial effect on reducing the risk of IHD.

The main lipids in blood are cholesterol (desirable normal 140-200 mg/dl, borderline high 240 mg/dl) and triglycerides (below 160 mg/dl). An elevation of serum cholesterol levels above 260 mg/dl in men and women between 30 and 50 years of age has three times higher risk of developing IHD as compared with people with serum cholesterol levels within normal limits. The concentration of cholesterol in the serum reflects the concentrations of different lipoproteins in the serum. The lipoproteins are divided into classes according to the density of solvent in which they remain suspended on centrifugation at high speed. The major classes of lipoprotein particles are *chylomicrons, very-low density lipoproteins (VLDL), low-density lipoproteins (LDL),* and *high-density lipoproteins (HDL).* Lipids are insoluble in blood and therefore are carried in circulation and across the cell membrane by carrier proteins called *apoproteins.* Apoprotein surrounds the lipid for carrying it, different apoproteins being named by letter A, B, C,D etc while their subfractions are numbered serially. The major fractions of lipoproteins and their varying effects on atherosclerosis and IHD are as under (Table 11.2):

- *Low-density lipoprotein (LDL)* is richest in cholesterol and has the maximum association with atherosclerosis.
- *Very-low-density lipoprotein (VLDL)* carries much of the triglycerides and has less marked effect than LDL.
- *High-density lipoprotein (HDL)* is protective 'good cholesterol' against atherosclerosis.

Many studies have demonstrated the harmful effect of diet containing larger quantities of saturated fats (e.g. in eggs, meat, milk, butter etc) which raise the plasma cholesterol level. This type of diet is consumed more often by the affluent societies who are at greater risk of developing atherosclerosis. On the contrary, a diet low in saturated fats and high in poly-unsaturated fats and having omega-3 fatty acids (e.g. in fish, fish oils etc) lowers the plasma cholesterol levels. Aside from lipid-rich diet, high intake of the total number of calories from carbohydrates, proteins, alcohol and sweets has adverse effects.

How hypercholesterolaemia and various classes of lipoproteins produce atherosclerosis is described under 'pathogenesis'.

2. HYPERTENSION. Hypertension is the other major risk factor in the development of atherosclerotic IHD and cerebrovascular disease. It acts probably by mechanical injury to the arterial wall due to increased blood pressure. A systolic pressure of over 160 mmHg or a diastolic pressure of over 95 mmHg is associated with five times higher risk of developing IHD than in people with blood pressure within normal range (140/90 mmHg or less).

3. SMOKING. The extent and severity of atherosclerosis are much greater in smokers than in non-smokers. Cigarette smoking is associated with higher risk of atherosclerotic IHD and sudden cardiac death. Men who smoke a pack of cigarettes a day are 3-5 times more likely to die of IHD than non-smokers. The increased risk and severity of atherosclerosis in smokers is due to reduced level of HDL and accumulation of carbon monoxide in the blood that produces carboxy-haemoglobin and eventually hypoxia in the arterial wall favouring atherosclerosis.

4. DIABETES MELLITUS. Clinical manifestations of atherosclerosis are far more common and develop at an early age in people with both insulin-dependent and non-insulin dependent diabetes mellitus. The risk of developing IHD is doubled, tendency to develop cerebrovascular disease is high, and frequency to develop gangrene of foot is about 100 times increased. The causes of increased severity of atherosclerosis are complex and numerous which include increased aggregation of platelets, increased LDL and decreased HDL.

MINOR RISK FACTORS

There are a number of less important and minor risk factors having some role in the etiology of atherosclerosis. These are as under:

1. Higher incidence of atherosclerosis in developed countries and low prevalence in underdeveloped countries, suggesting the role of *environmental influences.*
2. *Obesity,* if the person is overweight by 20% or more, is associated with increased risk.
3. Use of *exogenous hormones* (e.g oral contraceptives) by women or *endogenous oestrogen deficiency* (e.g. in post-menopausal women) has been shown to have increased risk of developing myocardial infarction or stroke.

TABLE 11.2: Fractions of Lipoproteins in Serum.

	CLASSES	SITES OF SYNTHESIS	NORMAL SERUM LEVELS	ROLE IN ATHEROSCLEROSIS
1.	*HDL cholesterol*	Liver, intestine	> 40 mg/dl	Protective
2.	*LDL cholesterol*	Liver	< 130 mg/dl	Maximum
3.	*VLDL triglycerides*	Intestine, liver	< 160 mg/dl	Less marked
4.	*Chylomicrons*	Liver, intestine, macrophage	—	Indirect

Chapter Eleven

4. *Physical inactivity* and lack of exercise are associated with the risk of developing atherosclerosis and its complications.
5. *Stressful life style,* termed as type A behaviour pattern, characterised by aggressiveness, competitive drive, ambitiousness and a sense of urgency, is associated with enhanced risk of IHD compared with type B behaviour of relaxed and happy-go-lucky type.
6. Recently role of *infections,* particularly of *Chlamydia pneumoniae* and viruses such as herpesvirus and cytomegalovirus, has been found in coronary atherosclerotic lesions. Possibly, infections may be acting in combination with some other factors.
7. Patients with *homocystinuria,* an uncommon inborn error of metabolism, have been reported to have early atherosclerosis and coronay artery disease.
8. Moderate consumption of *alcohol* appears to have slightly beneficial effect by raising the level of HDL cholesterol and by causing vasodilatation but the matter remains controversial.

Pathogenesis

As stated above, atherosclerosis is not caused by a single etiologic factor but is a multifactorial disease whose exact pathogenesis is still not known. A number of theories have been proposed since the times of Virchow.

■ ***Insudation hypothesis.*** The concept hypothesised by *Virchow in 1856* that atherosclerosis is a form of cellular proliferation of the intimal cells resulting from increased imbibing of lipids from the blood came to be called the *'lipid theory'*, currently known as *'response to injury hypothesis'* and is now-a-days the most widely accepted theory.

■ ***Encrustation hypothesis.*** The proposal put forth by *Rokitansky in 1852* that atheroma represented a form of encrustation on the arterial wall from the components in the blood forming thrombi composed of platelets, fibrin and leucocytes, was named as *'encrustation theory'* or *'thrombogenic theory'*. Since currently it is believed that encrustation or thrombosis is not the sole factor in atherogenesis but the components of thrombus (platelets, fibrin and leucocytes) have a role in atheromatous lesions, this theory has now been incorporated into the foregoing recent theory of response to injury.

Thus, there is no consensus regarding the origin and progression of lesion of atherosclerosis. The role of four key factors—arterial smooth muscle cells, endothelial cells, blood monocytes and hyperlipidaemia, is accepted by all. However, the areas of disagreement exist in the mechanism and sequence of events involving these factors in initiation, progression and complications of disease. Currently, pathogenesis of atherosclerosis is explained on the basis of the following two theories:

1. Reaction-to-injury hypothesis, first described in 1973, and modified in 1986 and 1993 by Ross.
2. Monoclonal theory, based on neoplastic proliferation of smooth muscle cells, postulated by Benditt and Benditt in 1973.

1. REACTION-TO-INJURY HYPOTHESIS. This theory is most widely accepted and incorporates aspects of two older historical theories of atherosclerosis—the lipid theory of Virchow and thrombogenic (encrustation) theory of Rokitansky.

■ The *original response to injury theory* was first described in 1973 according to which the initial event in atherogenesis was considered to be endothelial injury followed by smooth muscle cell proliferation so that the early lesions, according to this theory, consist of smooth muscle cells mainly.

■ The *modified response-to-injury hypothesis* described subsequently in 1993 implicates lipoprotein entry into the intima as the initial event followed by lipid accumulation in the macrophages (foam cells now) which according to modified theory, are believed to be the dominant cells in early lesions.

Both these theories—original and modified, have attracted support and criticism. However, following is the generally accepted role of key components involved in atherogenesis, diagrammatically illustrated in Fig. 11.4.

i) Endothelial injury. It has been known for many years that endothelial injury is the initial triggering event in the development of lesions of atherosclerosis. Actual endothelial denudation is not an essential requirement, but endothelial dysfunction may initiate the sequence of events. Numerous causes ascribed to endothelial injury in experimental animals are: mechanical trauma, haemodynamic forces, immunological and chemical mechanisms, metabolic agent as chronic hyperlipidaemia, homocystine, circulating toxins from systemic infections, viruses, hypoxia, radiation, carbon monoxide and tobacco products.

In man, two of the major risk factors which act together to produce endothelial injury are: *haemodynamic stress from hypertension and chronic hyperlipidaemia.* The role of haemodynamic forces in causing endothelial injury is further supported by the distribution of atheromatous plaques at points of bifurcation or branching of blood vessels which are under greatest shear stress.

ii) Intimal smooth muscle cell proliferation. Endothelial injury causes adherence, aggregation and platelet release reaction at the site of exposed subendothelial

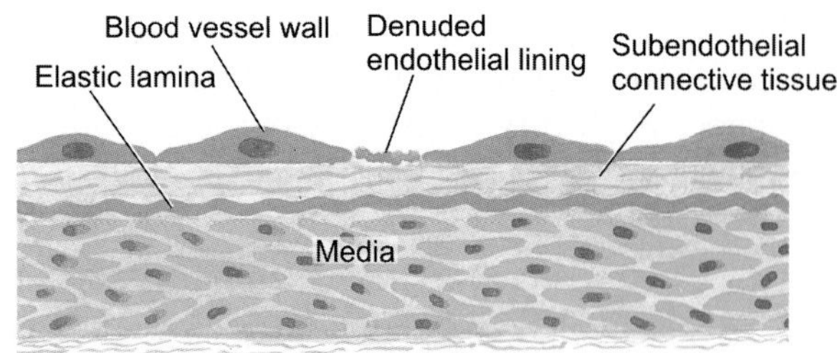

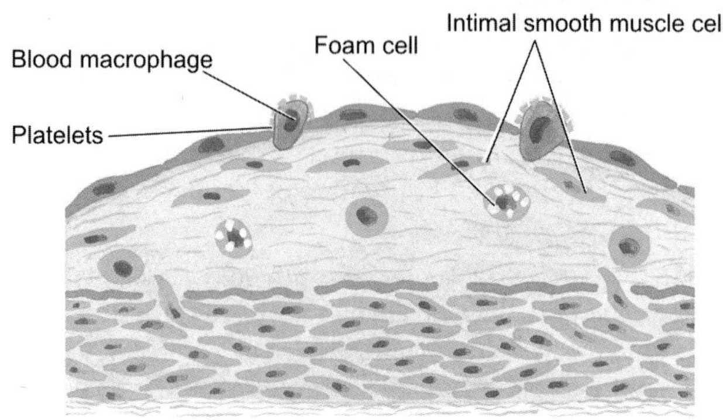

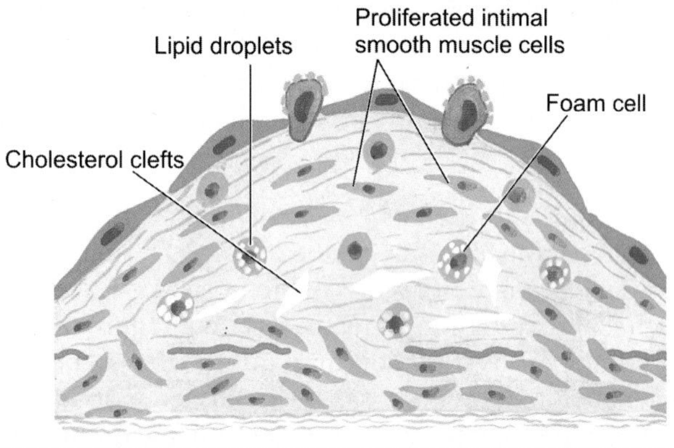

FIGURE 11.4

Diagrammatic representation of pathogenesis of atherosclerosis as explained by 'reaction-to-injury hypothesis.A, Endothelial injury. B, Adhesion of platelets and migration of blood monocytes from blood stream. C, Smooth muscle cell proliferation into the intima and ingrowth of new blood vessels.

connective tissue. Proliferation of intimal smooth muscle cells is stimulated by various mitogens released from platelets adherent at the site of endothelial injury and monocytes, the most important of which is platelet-derived growth factor *(PDGF)*; others are fibroblast growth factor *(FGF)*, and transforming growth factor-alpha (*TGF*-α). Smooth muscle cell proliferation is also facilitated by biomolecules such as nitric oxide and *endothelin* released from endothelial cells. Intimal proliferation of smooth muscle cells is accompanied by synthesis of matrix proteins—collagen, elastic fibre proteins and proteoglycans.

iii) Role of blood monocytes. Though blood monocytes do not possess receptors for normal LDL, LDL does appear in the monocyte cytoplasm to form foam cell by mechanism illustrated in Fig. 11.5. Plasma LDL on entry into the intima undergoes oxidation. The 'oxidised LDL' so formed in the intima performs the following all-important functions on monocytes and endothelium:

- *For monocytes,* oxidised LDL acts to attract, proliferate, immobilise and activate them as well as is readily taken up by scavenger receptor on the monocyte to transform it to a lipid-laden foam cell.
- For *endothelium,* oxidised LDL is cytotoxic.

Death of foam cell by apoptosis releases lipid to form lipid core of plaque.

iv) Role of hyperlipidaemia. As stated already, chronic hyperlipidaemia in itself may initiate endothelial injury and dysfunction by causing increased permeability.

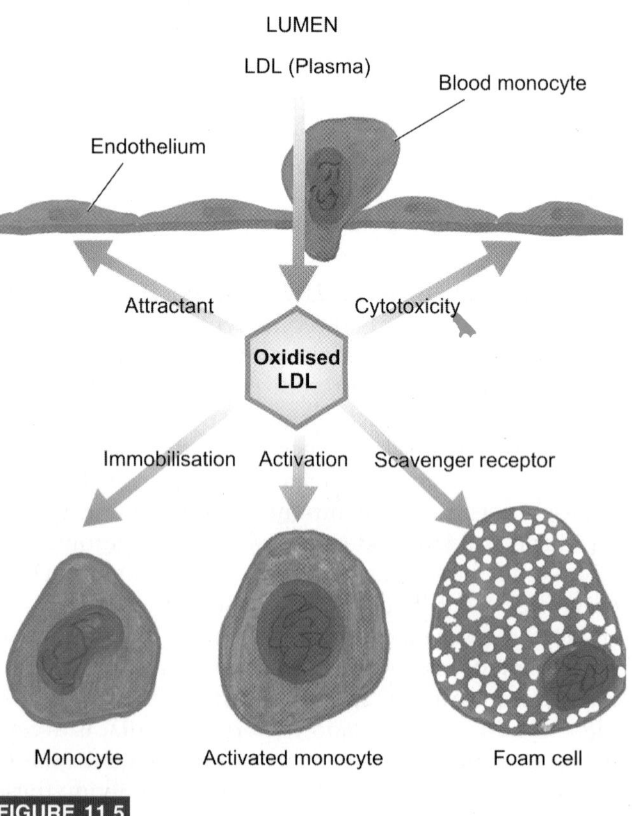

FIGURE 11.5

Mechanism of foam cell formation.

Chapter Eleven

Secondly, increased serum concentration of LDL and VLDL promotes formation of foam cells, while high serum concentration of HDL has anti-atherogenic effect.

v) Thrombosis. As apparent from the foregoing, endothelial injury exposes subendothelial connective tissue resulting in formation of small platelet aggregates at the site and causing proliferation of smooth muscle cells. This causes mild inflammatory reaction which together with foam cells is incorporated into the atheromatous plaque. The lesions enlarge by attaching fibrin and cells from the blood so that thrombus becomes a part of atheromatous plaque.

2. MONOCLONAL HYPOTHESIS. This hypothesis is based on the postulate that proliferation of smooth muscle cells is the primary event and that this proliferation is monoclonal in origin similar to cellular proliferation in neoplasms (e.g. in uterine leiomyoma, Chapter 8). The evidence cited in support of monoclonal hypothesis is the observation on proliferated smooth muscle cells in atheromatous plaques which have only one of the two forms of glucose-6-phosphate dehydrogenase (G6PD) isoenzymes, suggesting monoclonality in origin. The monoclonal proliferation of smooth muscle cells in atherosclerosis may be initiated by mutation caused by exogenous chemicals (e.g. cigarette smoke), endogenous metabolites (e.g. lipoproteins) and some viruses (e.g. Marek's disease virus in chickens, herpesvirus).

PATHOLOGIC CHANGES

Early lesions in the form of diffuse intimal thickening, fatty streaks and gelatinous lesions are often the forerunners in the evolution of atherosclerotic lesions (Fig. 11.6,A). However, the clinical disease states due to luminal narrowing in atherosclerosis are caused by fully developed atheromatous plaques and complicated plaques (Fig. 11.6,B, C).

1. FATTY STREAKS AND DOTS. Fatty streaks and dots on the intima by themselves are harmless but may be the precursor lesions of atheromatous plaques. They are seen in all races of the world and begin to appear in the first year of life. However, they are uncommon in older persons and are probably absorbed. They are especially prominent in the aorta and other major arteries, more often on the posterior wall than the anterior wall.

Grossly, the lesions may appear as flat or slightly elevated and yellow. They may be either in the form of small, multiple dots, about 1 mm in size, or in the form of elongated, beaded streaks.

Microscopically, fatty streaks lying under the endothelium are composed of closely-packed foam cells,

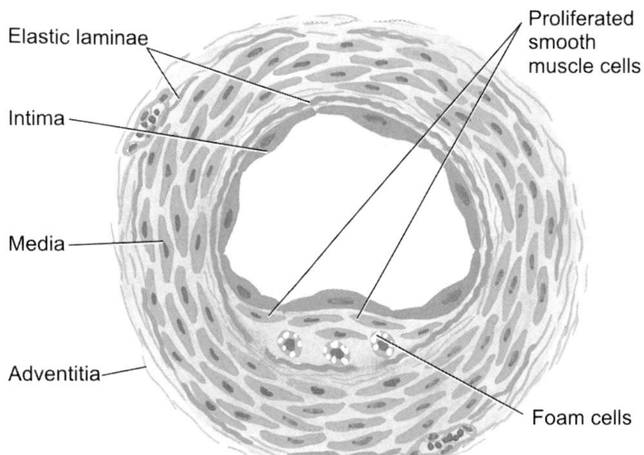

A, EARLY LESION

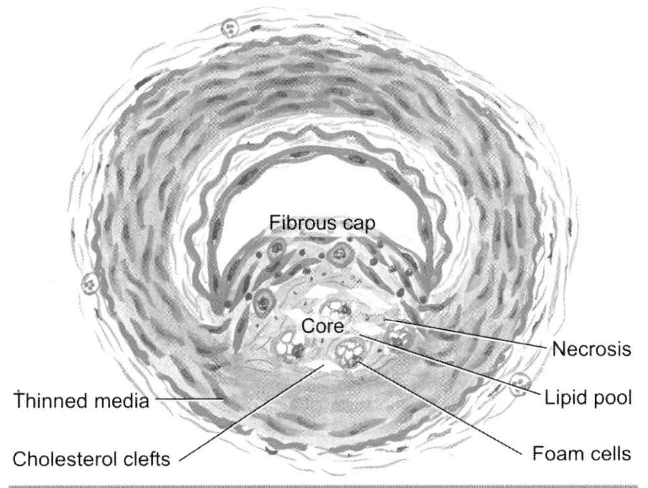

B, FULLY-DEVELOPED ATHEROMATOUS PLAQUE

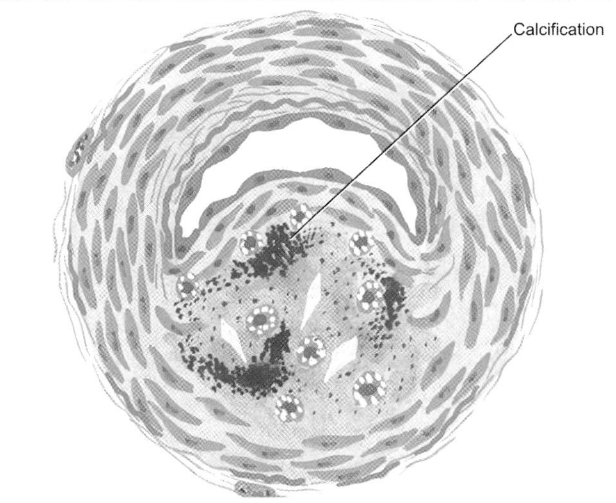

C, COMPLICATED PLAQUE

FIGURE 11.6

Evolution of lesions in atherosclerosis. For details, see the text.

Chapter Eleven

lipid-containing elongated smooth muscle cells and a few lymphoid cells. Small amount of extracellular lipid, collagen and proteoglycans are also present.

2. GELATINOUS LESIONS. Gelatinous lesions develop in the intima of the aorta and other major arteries in the first few months of life. Like fatty streaks, they may also be precursors of plaques. They are round or oval, circumscribed grey elevations, about 1 cm in diameter.

Microscopically, gelatinous lesions are foci of increased ground substance in the intima with thinned overlying endothelium.

3. ATHEROMATOUS PLAQUES. A fully developed atherosclerotic lesion is called atheromatous plaque, also called *fibrous plaque, fibrofatty plaque or atheroma.* Unlike fatty streaks, atheromatous plaques are selective in different geographic locations and races and are seen in advanced age. These lesions may develop from progression of early lesions of the atherosclerosis described above. *Most often and most severely affected is the abdominal aorta,* though smaller lesions may be seen in descending thoracic aorta and aortic arch. The major branches of the aorta around the ostia are often severely involved, especially the iliac, femoral, carotid, coronary, and cerebral arteries.

Grossly, atheromatous plaques are white to yellowish-white lesions, varying in diameter from 1-2 cm and raised on the surface by a few millimetres to a centimetre in thickness (Fig. 11.7,A). Cut section of the plaque reveals the luminal surface as a firm, white *fibrous cap* and a *central core* composed of yellow to yellow-white, soft, porridge-like material and hence the name atheroma.

Microscopically, the appearance of plaque varies depending upon the age of the lesion. However, the following features are invariably present (Fig. 11.7,B):

- The superficial luminal part of *fibrous cap* is covered by endothelium, and is composed of smooth muscle cells, dense connective tissue and extracellular matrix containing proteoglycans and collagen.
- The *cellular area* under the fibrous cap is comprised by a mixture of macrophages, foam cells, lymphocytes and a few smooth muscle cells which may contain lipid.
- The deeper *central soft core* consists of extracellular lipid material, cholesterol clefts, fibrin, necrotic debris and lipid-laden foam cells.
- In older and *more advanced lesions,* the collagen in the fibrous cap may be dense and hyalinised, smooth muscle cells may be atrophic and foam cells are fewer **(COLOUR PLATE XIII: CL 50).**

4. COMPLICATED PLAQUES. Various pathologic changes that occur in fully-developed atheromatous plaques are called the complicated lesions. These account for the most serious harmful effects of atherosclerosis and even death. These changes include

Chapter Eleven

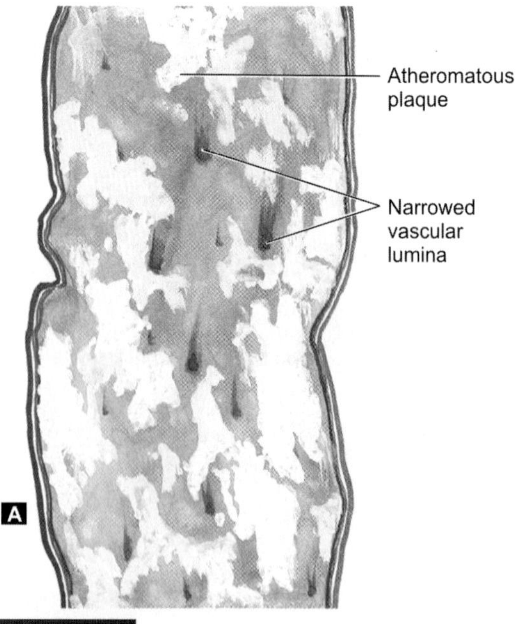

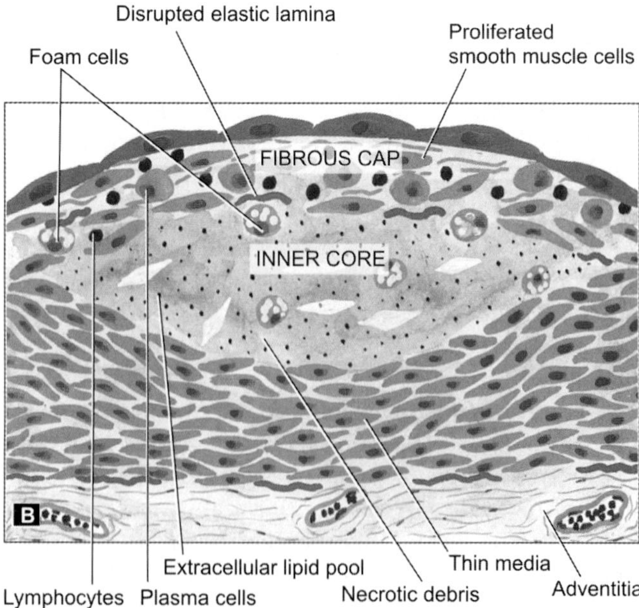

FIGURE 11.7

Structure of a fully-developed atheroma. A, Inner surface of opened abdominal aorta shows a variety of atheromatous lesions. While some are raised fibrous plaques, others are ulcerated with superimposed thrombosis. Orifices of some of the branches are narrowed by the atherosclerotic process. B, Diagrammatic view of the histologic appearance of a fully-developed atheroma.

calcification, ulceration, thrombosis, haemorrhage and aneurysmal dilatation. It is not uncommon to see more than one form of complication in a plaque.

i) Calcification. Calcification occurs more commonly in advanced atheromatous plaques, especially in the aorta and coronaries. The diseased intima cracks like an egg-shell when the vessel is incised and opened.

Microscopically, the calcium salts are deposited in the vicinity of necrotic area and in the soft lipid pool deep in the thickened intima (COLOUR PLATE XIII: CL 51). This form of atherosclerotic *intimal* calcification differs from Mönckeberg's medial calcific arteriosclerosis that affects only the tunica media (page 279).

ii) Ulceration. The layers covering the soft pultaceous material of an atheroma may ulcerate as a result of haemodynamic forces or mechanical trauma. This results in discharge of emboli composed of lipid material and debris into the blood stream, leaving a shallow, ragged ulcer with yellow lipid debris in the base of the ulcer. Occasionally, atheromatous plaque in a coronary artery may suddenly rupture into the arterial lumen forcibly and cause thromboembolic occlusion.

iii) Thrombosis. The ulcerated plaque and the areas of endothelial damage are vulnerable sites for formation of superimposed thrombi. These thrombi may get dislodged to become emboli and lodge elsewhere in the circulation, or may get organised and incorporated into the arterial wall as mural thrombi. Mural thrombi may become occlusive thrombi which may subsequently recanalise.

iv) Haemorrhage. Intimal haemorrhage may occur in an atheromatous plaque either from the blood in the vascular lumen through an ulcerated plaque, or from rupture of thin-walled capillaries that vascularise the atheroma from adventitial vasa vasorum. Haemorrhage is particularly a common complication in coronary arteries. The haematoma formed at the site contains numerous haemosiderin-laden macrophages.

v) Aneurysm formation. Though atherosclerosis is primarily an intimal disease, advanced lesions are associated with secondary changes in the media and adventitia. The changes in media include atrophy and thinning of the media and fragmentation of internal elastic lamina. The adventitia undergoes fibrosis and some inflammatory changes. These changes cause weakening in the arterial wall resulting in aneurysmal dilatation.

Based on progressive pathological changes and clinical correlation , American Heart Association (1995) has classified human atherosclerosis into 6 sequential types in ascending order of grades of lesions as shown in Table 11.3.

TABLE 11.3: American Heart Association Classification (1995) of Human Atherosclerosis.

TYPES	MAIN HISTOLOGY	MAIN PATHOGENESIS	AGE AT ONSET	CLINICAL
Type I: Initial lesions	Macrophages, occasional foam cell	Accumulation of lipoprotein	1st decade	Asymptomatic
Type II: Fatty streaks	Many layers of macrophages and foam cells	Accumulation of lipoprotein	1st decade	Asymptomatic
Type III: Intermediate lesions	Many lipid-laden cells and scattered extracellular lipid droplets	Accumulation of lipoprotein	3rd decade	Asymptomatic
Type IV: Atheromatous lesions	Intra-as well as extra-cellular lipid pool	Accumulation of lipid	3rd decade	Asymptomatic or manifest symptoms
Type V: Fibrofatty lesions	Fibrotic cap and lipid core (V a), may have calcification (V b)	Smooth muscle cell proliferation and increased collagen	4th decade	Asymptomatic or manifest symptoms
Type VI: Complicated lesions	Ulceration, haemorrhage, haematoma, thrombosis	Haemodynamic stress, thrombosis, haematoma	4th decade	Asymptomatic or manifest symptoms

Clinical Effects

The clinical effects of atherosclerosis depend upon the size and type of arteries affected. In general, the clinical effects result from the following:

1. Slow luminal narrowing causing ischaemia and atrophy.
2. Sudden luminal occlusion causing infarction necrosis.
3. Propagation of plaque by formation of thrombi and emboli.
4. Formation of aneurysmal dilatation and eventual rupture.

Large arteries affected most often are the aorta, renal, mesenteric and carotids, whereas the medium- and small-sized arteries frequently involved are the coronaries, cerebrals and arteries of the lower limbs. Accordingly, the symptomatic atherosclerotic disease involves most often the heart, brain, kidneys, small intestine and lower extremities (Fig. 11.8). The effects pertaining to these organs are described in relevant chapters later. Some of the important effects are listed below (Fig. 11.9):

i) *Aorta*—Aneurysm formation, thrombosis and embolisation to other organs.
ii) *Heart*—Myocardial infarction, ischaemic heart disease.
iii) *Brain*—Chronic ischaemic brain damage, cerebral infarction.
iv) *Small intestine*—Ischaemic bowel disease, infarction.
v) *Lower extremities*—Intermittent claudication, gangrene.

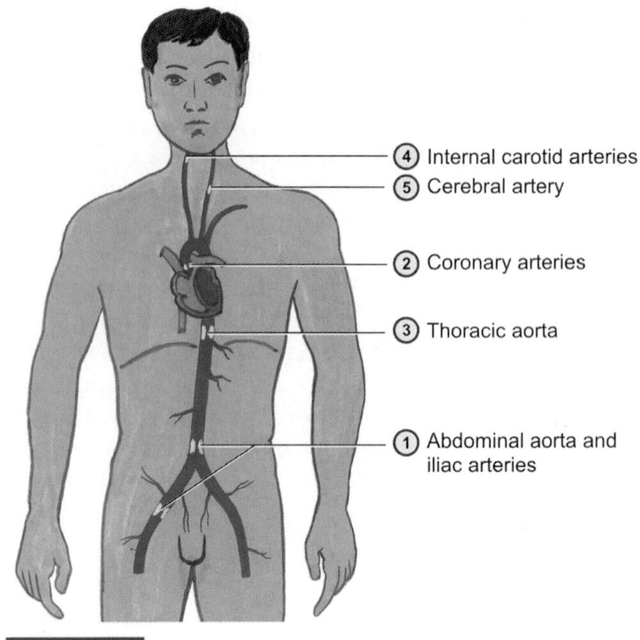

FIGURE 11.8

Major sites of atherosclerosis (serially numbered) in descending order of frequency.

ARTERITIS

Arteritis, angiitis and vasculitis are the common terms used for inflammatory process in an artery or an arteriole. It may occur following invasion of the vessel by infectious agents, or may be induced by non-infectious injuries such as chemical, mechanical, immunologic and radiation injury. The non-infectious group is more important than the infectious type. Accordingly, classification of arteritis based on this is given in Table 11.4.

I. INFECTIOUS ARTERITIS

Direct invasion of the artery by infectious agents, especially bacteria and fungi, causes infectious arteritis.

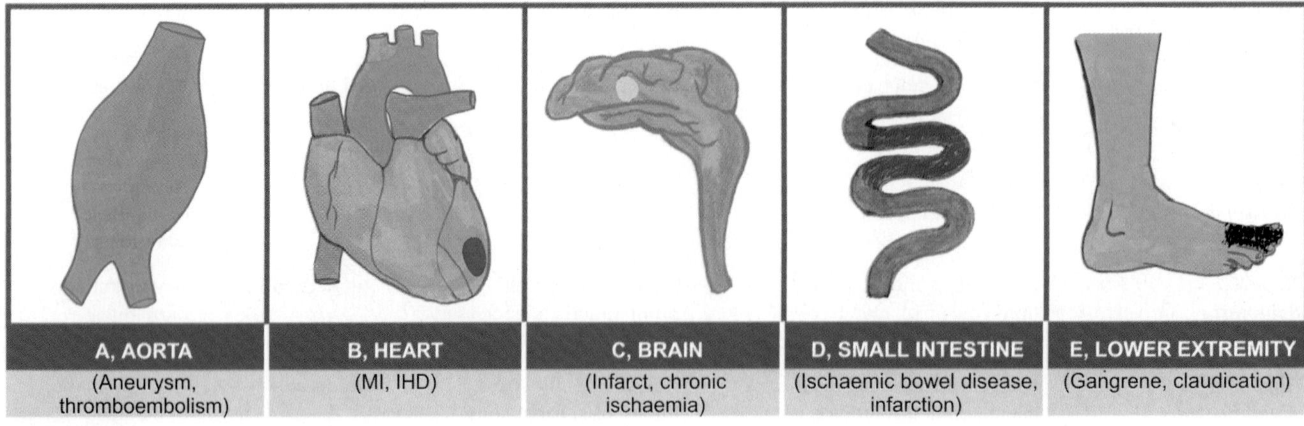

FIGURE 11.9

Major forms of symptomatic atherosclerotic disease.

TABLE 11.4: Classification of Vasculitis.

I. **Infectious arteritis:**
   1. Endarteritis obliterans
   2. Non-syphilitic infective arteritis
   3. Syphilitic arteritis

II. **Non-infectious arteritis:**
   1. Polyarteritis nodosa (PAN)
   2. Hypersensitivity (allergic, leucocytoclastic) vasculitis
   3. Wegener's granulomatosis
   4. Temporal (giant cell) arteritis
   5. Takayasu's arteritis (pulseless disease)
   6. Kawasaki's disease
   7. Buerger's disease (thromboangiitis obliterans)
   8. Miscellaneous vasculitis

It may be found in the vicinity of an infected focus like in tuberculosis, pneumonia, abscesses, etc. or less frequently may arise from haematogenous spread of infection such as in infective endocarditis, septicaemia, etc. Some common types are described below.

1. Endarteritis Obliterans

Endarteritis obliterans is not a disease entity but a pathologic designation used for non-specific inflammatory response of arteries and arterioles to a variety of irritants. It is commonly seen close to the lesions of peptic ulcers of the stomach and duodenum, tuberculous and chronic abscesses in the lungs, chronic cutaneous ulcers, chronic meningitis, and in post-partum and post-menopausal uterine arteries.

Macroscopically, the affected vessels may appear unaltered externally but on cross-section show obliteration of their lumina.

Microscopically, the obliteration of the lumen is due to concentric and symmetric proliferation of cellular fibrous tissue in the intima. Though the condition has suffix—*itis* attached to it, there is minimal or no inflammatory cell infiltrate.

2. Non-syphilitic Infective Arteritis

Various forms of invasions of the artery by bacteria, fungi, parasites or viruses, either directly or by haematogenous route, cause non-syphilitic infective arteritis.

Microscopically, the inflammatory infiltrate is present in the vessel wall. The vascular lumen may get occluded by thrombi and result in ischaemic necrosis of the affected tissue.

3. Syphilitic Arteritis

Syphilitic or luetic vascular involvement occurs in all stages of syphilis but is more prominent in the tertiary stage. The changes that are found in the syphilitic arteritis are seen within the arterial tissue (*syphilitic endarteritis*) and in the periarterial tissues (*syphilitic periarteritis*). Manifestations of the disease are particularly prominent at two sites—the aorta and the cerebral arteries.

SYPHILITIC AORTITIS. Syphilitic involvement of the ascending aorta and the aortic arch is the commonest manifestation of cardiovascular syphilis. It occurs in about 80% cases of tertiary syphilis. The preferential involvement of arch of aorta may be due to involvement of mediastinal lymph nodes in secondary syphilis through which the treponemes spread to the lymphatics around the aortic arch. The lesions diminish in severity in descending thoracic aorta and disappear completely at the level of the diaphragm.

Macroscopically, the affected part of the aorta may be dilated, and its wall somewhat thickened and adherent to the neighbouring mediastinal structures. Longitudinally opened vessels show intimal surface studded with pearly-white thickenings, varying from a few millimeters to a centimeter in diameter. These lesions are separated by wrinkled normal intima, giving it characteristic *tree-bark appearance.* Cut section of the lesion shows more firm and fibrous appearance than the atheromatous plaques. However, superimposed atherosclerotic lesions may be present.

Microscopically, the conspicuous features are as under (Fig. 11.10):

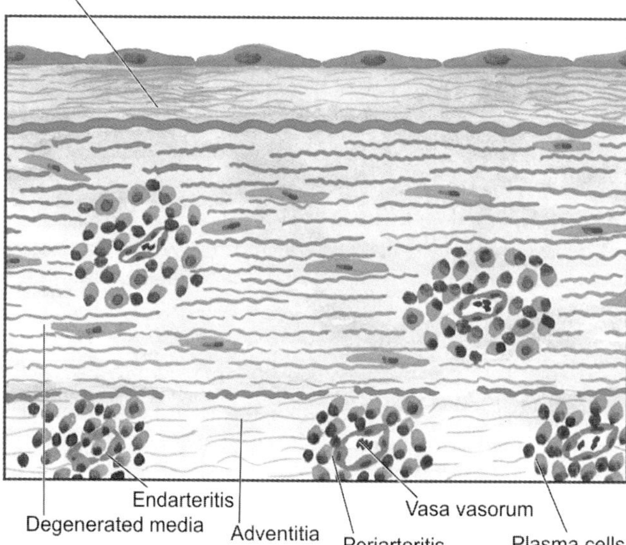

FIGURE 11.10

Syphilitic aortitis. There is endarteritis and periarteritis of the vasa vasorum in the media and adventitia. There is perivascular infiltrate of plasma cells, lymphocytes and macrophages.

■ Endarteritis and periarteritis of the vasa vasorum located in the media and adventitia.
■ Perivascular accumulation of plasma cells, lymphocytes and macrophages that may form miliary gummas which undergo necrosis and are replaced by scar tissue.
■ Intimal thickenings consist of dense avascular collagen that may undergo hyalinisation and calcification.

The *effects* of syphilitic aortitis may vary from trivial to catastrophic. These are as follows:

a) *Aortic aneurysm* may result from damage to the aortic wall (page 295).

b) *Aortic valvular incompetence* used to be considered an important sequela of syphilis but now-a-days rheumatic disease is considered more important cause for this. The aortic incompetence results from spread of the syphilitic process to the aortic valve ring.

c) *Stenosis of coronary ostia* is seen in about 20% cases of syphilitic aortitis and may lead to progressive myocardial fibrosis, angina pectoris and sudden death.

The features distinguishing syphilitic aortitis from aortic atheroma are given in Table 11.5.

CEREBRAL SYPHILITIC ARTERITIS (HEUBNER'S ARTERITIS). Syphilitic involvement of small and medium-sized cerebral arteries occurs during the tertiary syphilis. The changes may accompany syphilitic meningitis.

Macroscopically, the cerebral vessels are white, rigid and thick-walled.
Microscopically, changes of endarteritis and periarteritis similar to those seen in syphilitic aortitis are found. There is atrophy of muscle in the media and replacement by fibrosis. This results in ischaemic atrophy of the brain.

II. NON-INFECTIOUS ARTERITIS

This group consists of most of the important forms of vasculitis, more often affecting arterioles, venules and capillaries, and hence also termed as *small vessel vasculitis.* Their exact etiology is not known but available evidence suggests that many of them have immunologic origin. Serum from many of patients with vasculitis of immunologic origin show the presence of following immunologic features:

1. Anti-neutrophil cytoplasmic antibodies (ANCAs). Patients with immunologic vasculitis have autoantibodies in their serum against the cytoplasmic antigens of the neutrophils, macrophages and endothelial cells; these are called ANCAs. Neutrophil immunofluorescence is used to demonstrate their presence, of which two distinct patterns of ANCAs are seen:
■ *Cytoplasmic ANCA (c-ANCA) pattern* is specific for proteinase-3 (PR-3), a constituent of neutrophilic granules; this is seen in cases with active Wegener's granulomatosis.
■ *Perinuclear ANCA (p-ANCA) pattern* is specific for myeloperoxidase enzyme; this is noted in patients with microscopic polyarteritis nodosa and primary glomerular disease.

2. Anti-endothelial cell antibodies (AECAs). These antibodies are demonstable in cases of SLE, Kawasaki disease and Buerger's disease.

3. Pauci-immune vasculitis. While most cases of immunologic vasculitis have immune complex deposits in the vessel wall, there are some cases which do not have such immune deposits and are termed as cases of pauci-immune vasculitis (similar to pauci-immune glomerulonephritis, Chapter 20). Pathogenesis of lesions in these cases is explained by other mechanisms.

1. Polyarteritis Nodosa

Polyarteritis nodosa (PAN) is a necrotising vasculitis involving small and medium-sized muscular arteries of

TABLE 11.5: Contrasting Features of Syphilitic Aortitis and Aortic Atheroma.

FEATURES	SYPHILITIC AORTITIS	AORTIC ATHEROMA
1. *Sites*	Ascending aorta, aortic arch; absent below diaphragm	Progressive increase from the arch to abdominal aorta, more often at the bifurcation
2. *Macroscopy*	Pearly-white intimal lesions resembling tree-bark without fat in the core; ulceration and calcification often not found	Yellowish-white intimal plaques with fat in the core; ulceration and calcification in plaques common
3. *Microscopy*	Endarteritis and periarteritis of vasa vasorum, perivascular infiltrate of plasma cells and lymphocytes	Fibrous cap with deeper core containing foam cells, cholesterol clefts and soft lipid
4. *Effects*	Thoracic aortic aneurysm, incompetence of the aortic valve, stenosis of coronary ostia	Abdominal aortic aneurysm, aortic valve stenosis, stenosis of abdominal branches

multiple organs and tissues. 'Polyarteritis' is the preferred nomenclature over 'periarteritis' because inflammatory involvement occurs in all the layers of the vessel wall.

The disease occurs more commonly in adult males than females. Most commonly affected organs, in descending order of frequency of involvement, are the kidneys, heart, liver, gastrointestinal tract, muscle, pancreas, testes, nervous system and skin. The syndrome of PAN presents with varied symptoms pertaining to different organs. However, some usual clinical features are fever, malaise, weakness, weight loss, renal manifestations (albuminuria, haematuria and renal failure), vascular lesions in the alimentary tract (abdominal pain and melaena), peripheral neuritis and hypertension. The condition is believed to result from deposition of immune complexes and tumour-related antigens.

Macroscopically, the lesions of PAN involve segments of vessels, especially at the bifurcations and branchings, as tiny beaded nodules.

Microscopically, there are 3 sequential stages in the evolution of lesions in PAN:

i) *Acute stage*—There is fibrinoid necrosis in the centre of the nodule located in the media. An acute inflammatory response develops around the focus of fibrinoid necrosis. The inflammatory infiltrate is present in the entire circumference of the affected vessel (periarteritis) and consists chiefly of neutrophils and eosinophils, and some mononuclear cells. The lumen may show thrombi and the weakened wall may be the site of aneurysm formation.

ii) *Healing stage*—This is characterised by marked fibroblastic proliferation producing firm nodularity. The inflammatory infiltrate now consists mainly of lymphocytes, plasma cells and macrophages.

iii) *Healed stage*—In this stage, the affected arterial wall is markedly thickened due to dense fibrosis. The internal elastic lamina is fragmented or lost. Healed stage may contain haemosiderin-laden macrophages and organised thrombus.

However, it may be mentioned here that various stages of the disease may be seen in different vessels and even within the same vessel.

2. Hypersensitivity (Allergic, Leucocytoclastic) Vasculitis

Hypersensitivity vasculitis, also called as allergic or leucocytoclastic vasculitis or microscopic polyarteritis, is a group of clinical syndromes differing from PAN in having inflammatory involvement of venules, capillaries and arterioles. The tissues and organs most commonly involved are the skin, mucous membranes, lungs, brain, heart, gastrointestinal tract, kidneys and muscle. The condition results from immunologic response to an identifiable antigen that may be bacteria (e.g. streptococci, staphylococci, mycobacteria), viruses (e.g. hepatitis B virus, influenza virus, CMV), malarial parasite, certain drugs and chemicals. Hypersensitivity vasculitis includes clinicopathologic entities such as serum sickness, Henoch-Schönlein purpura, mixed cryoglobulinaemia, vasculitis associated with malignancy, and vasculitis associated with connective tissue diseases like rheumatoid arthritis and SLE.

Microscopically, the lesions characteristically involve smallest vessels, sparing medium-sized and larger arteries. Two histologic forms are described:

i) *Leucocytoclastic vasculitis,* characterised by fibrinoid necrosis with neutrophilic infiltrate in the vessel wall. Many of the neutrophils are fragmented. This form is found in vasculitis caused by deposits of immune complexes.

ii) *Lymphocytic vasculitis,* in which the involved vessel shows predominant infiltration by lymphocytes. This type is seen in vascular injury due to delayed hypersensitivity or cellular immune reactions.

3. Wegener's Granulomatosis

Wegener's granulomatosis is another form of necrotising vasculitis characterised by a *clinicopathologic triad* consisting of the following:

i) Acute necrotising granulomas of the upper and lower respiratory tracts involving nose, sinuses and lungs;

ii) focal necrotising vasculitis, particularly of the lungs and upper airways; and

iii) focal or diffuse necrotising glomerulonephritis.

A *limited form* of Wegener's granulomatosis is the same condition without renal involvement. As with PAN, the condition is more common in adult males and involves multiple organs and tissues. Most commonly involved organs are lungs, paranasal sinuses, nasopharynx and kidneys. Other involved organs are joints, skin, eyes, ears, heart and nervous system. Accordingly, clinical features are variable. Typical features include pneumonitis with bilateral infiltrates in the lungs (Chapter 15), chronic sinusitis, nasopharyngeal ulcerations (Chapter 16) and renal disease (Chapter 20). The etiology is not known but possibly the lesions occur due to the presence of circulating immune complexes.

This is supported by the observation of subepithelial immunoglobulin deposits on the glomerular basement membrane and induction of remission by immunosuppressive therapy. The serum of these patients shows C-ANCA positivity. Disseminated form of Wegener's granulomatosis differs from a related entity, *idiopathic lethal midline granuloma,* in the sense that the latter condition is highly destructive and progressively necrotic disease of the upper airways.

Histologically, the characteristic feature of Wegener's granulomatosis is the presence of necrotising granulomatous inflammation of the tissues and necrotising vasculitis with or without granulomas:

- The granulomas consist of fibrinoid necrosis with extensive infiltration by neutrophils, mononuclear cells, epithelioid cells, multinucleate giant cells and fibroblastic proliferation.
- The necrotising vasculitis may be segmental or circumferential.
- The renal lesions are those of focal or diffuse necrotising glomerulonephritis.

4. Temporal (Giant Cell) Arteritis

This is a form of granulomatous inflammation of medium-sized and large arteries. Preferential sites of involvement are the cranial arteries, especially the temporal, and hence the name. However, the aorta and other major arteries like common carotid, axillary, brachial, femoral and mesenteric arteries are also involved, and therefore, it is preferable to call the entity as *'giant cell arteritis'*. The patients are generally over the age of 70 years with slight female preponderance. The usual clinical manifestations are headache and blindness if ophthalmic artery is involved. An association with polymyalgia rheumatica has been observed. The cause of the condition remains unknown though there is suggestion of an T cell mediated immunologic reaction to some component of the arterial wall, especially against the damaged internal elastic lamina. Biopsy of the affected artery is not only of diagnostic value but also relieves the patient of painful symptoms.

Grossly, the affected artery is thickened, cord-like and the lumen is usually reduced to a narrow slit.
Histologically, the features include the following:
i) There is chronic granulomatous reaction, usually around the internal elastic lamina and typically involves the entire circumference of the vessel.
ii) Giant cells of foreign body or Langhans' type are found in two-third of cases.
iii) The internal elastic lamina is often fragmented.
iv) There is eccentric or concentric intimal cellular proliferation causing marked narrowing of the lumen. The narrowed lumen may contain thrombus.
v) Occasionally, only nonspecific inflammatory cell infiltrate consisting of neutrophils, lymphocytes and eosinophils is found throughout the arterial wall.

5. Takayasu's Arteritis (Pulseless Disease)

This is a form of granulomatous vasculitis affecting chiefly the aorta and its major branches and hence is also referred to as *aortic arch syndrome.* The disease affects chiefly young women and is typically characterised by absence of pulse in both arms and presence of ocular manifestations. Other features referable to ischaemic effects from thrombotic occlusion of vessels include myocardial infarction, congestive heart failure and neurologic deficits. The etiology of Takayasu's arteritis is not known but the autoimmune reaction to aortic tissue has been suggested as the possible cause.

Grossly, the aortic wall is irregularly thickened and intima wrinkled. The branches of major arteries coming off the aortic arch have obliterated lumina.
Histologically, the features are as under:
i) There is severe mononuclear inflammatory infiltrate involving the full thickness of the affected vessel wall.
ii) The inflammatory changes are more severe in the adventitia and media and there is perivascular infiltration of the vasa vasorum.
iii) Granulomatous changes in the media with central necrosis and Langhans' giant cells are found in many cases.
iv) Advanced lesions show extensive fibrosis of the media and adventitia causing thickening in the vessel wall.

6. Kawasaki's Disease

Also known by more descriptive name of *'mucocutaneous lymph node syndrome'*, it is an acute and subacute illness affecting mainly young children and infants. Kawasaki's disease is a febrile illness with mucocutaneous symptoms like erosions of oral mucosa and conjunctiva, skin rash and lymphadenopathy. The etiology is unknown; possible causes considered are infectious, genetic, toxic and immunological. The most characteristic finding is the presence of multiple aneurysms of the coronaries detected by angiography during life or observed at autopsy. Other vessels that may be involved are renal, mesenteric, hepatic and pancreatic arteries.

Histologically, the picture is of panarteritis resembling PAN, characterised by necrosis and inflammation of the entire thickness of the vessel wall. Therefore, some consider Kawasaki's disease as an infantile form of PAN.

7. Buerger's Disease (Thromboangiitis Obliterans)

Buerger's disease is a specific disease entity affecting chiefly small and medium-sized arteries and veins of the extremities and characterised by acute and chronic occlusive inflammatory involvement. The disease affects chiefly men under the age of 35 years who are heavy cigarette smokers. The symptom-complex consists of intermittent claudication due to ischaemia manifested by intense pain affecting the limbs, more commonly the legs. Eventually, gangrene of the affected extremities occurs requiring amputation.

ETIOPATHOGENESIS. Following possible mechanisms have been suggested:

- There is consistent association with heavy cigarette smoking. This has led to the hypothesis that *tobacco products* cause either direct endothelial damage leading to hypercoagulability and thrombosis, or it is a result in hypersensitivity to tobacco products. In support is the demonstration of anti-endothelial cell antibodies (AECAs).
- *Genetic factors* seem to play a role as the disease is has familial occurrence, has HLA association and is seen more commonly in persons from Israel, Japan and in India. An increased prevalence is seen in individuals with HLA-A9 and HLA-B5 antigens.

Macroscopically, the lesions are typically segmental affecting small and medium-sized arteries, especially of the lower extremities. Involvement of the arteries is often accompanied with involvement of adjacent veins and nerves. Fibrous tissue cuff generally surrounds these three structures. Mural thrombi are frequently present in the vessels.

Microscopically, the following changes are seen in different stages of the disease:

i) In *early stage*, there is infiltration by polymorphs in all the layers of vessels and there is invariable presence of mural or occlusive thrombosis of the lumen (Fig. 11.11). The appearance differs from atherosclerosis in having microabscesses in the thrombi, proliferation of endothelial cells, lack of lipid aggregates and presence of intact internal elastic lamina.

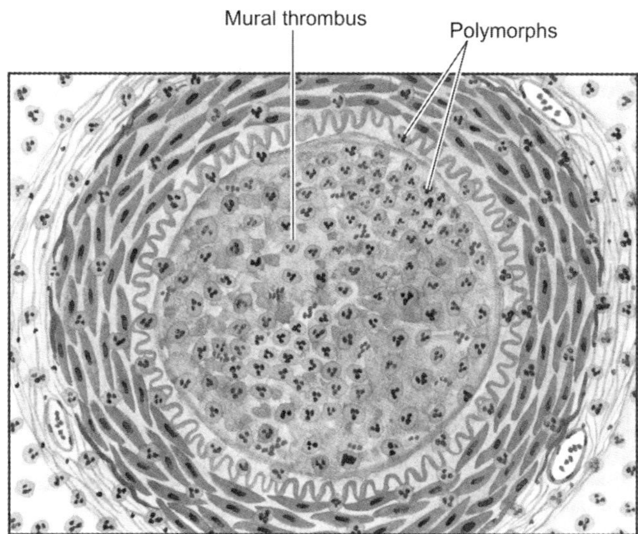

FIGURE 11.11

Buerger's disease (Thromboangiitis obliterans). There is acute panarteritis. The lumen is occluded by a thrombus containing microabscesses.

ii) In *advanced stage*, the cellular infiltrate is predominantly mononuclear and may contain an occasional epithelioid cell granuloma with Langhans' giant cells. The thrombi undergo organisation and recanalisation. In more chronic cases, marked fibrosis of the media is present.

8. Miscellaneous Vasculitis

Various connective tissue diseases (e.g. rheumatoid arthritis, ankylosing spondylitis and SLE), rheumatic fever, certain malignancies and Henoch-Schönlein purpura are associated with vasculitis. The type of vasculitis is generally of hypersensitivity or allergic angiitis as already explained but sometimes may resemble PAN.

- *Rheumatoid vasculitis* affects chiefly the small and medium-sized arteries of multiple visceral organs in patients who have rheumatoid nodules of long duration. Vasculitis in SLE affects mainly the small arteries of the skin.
- *Rheumatic vasculitis* involves the aorta, carotid and coronary arteries and the visceral vessels. Usually, fibrinoid change and perivascular inflammation are seen rather than typical Aschoff nodules (page 330).

Raynaud's Disease and Raynaud's Phenomenon

Raynaud's disease is not a vasculitis but is a functional vasospastic disorder affecting chiefly small arteries and arterioles of the extremities, occurring mainly in otherwise young healthy females. The disease affects most commonly the fingers and hands. The ischaemic effect is provoked primarily by cold but other stimuli such as emotions, trauma, hormones and drugs also seem to play a role. Clinically, the affected digits show *pallor*, followed by *cyanosis*, and then *redness*, corresponding to *arterial ischaemia*, *venostasis* and *hyperaemia* respectively. Long-standing cases may develop ulceration and necrosis of digits but occurrence of true gangrene is rare. The cause of the disease is unknown but probably occurs due to vasoconstriction mediated by autonomic stimulation of the affected vessels. Though usually no pathologic changes are observed in the affected vessels, long-standing cases may show endothelial proliferation and intimal thickening.

Raynaud's phenomenon differs from Raynaud's disease in having an underlying cause e.g. secondary to artherosclerosis, connective tissue diseases like scleroderma and SLE, Buerger's disease, multiple myeloma, pulmonary hypertension and ingestion of ergot group of drugs. Raynaud's phenomenon like Raynaud's disease, also shows cold sensitivity but differs from the latter in having structural abnormalities in the affected vessels. These changes include segmental inflammation and fibrinoid change in the walls of capillaries.

ANEURYSMS

DEFINITION

An aneurysm is defined as a permanent abnormal dilatation of a blood vessel occurring due to congenital or acquired weakening or destruction of the vessel wall. Most commonly, aneurysms involve large elastic arteries, especially the aorta and its major branches. Aneurysms can cause various ill-effects such as thrombosis and thromboembolism, alteration in the flow of blood, rupture of the vessel and compression of neighbouring structures.

CLASSIFICATION

Aneurysms can be classified on the basis of various features:

A. Depending upon the composition of the wall, these can be:

1 *True aneurysm* composed of all the layers of a normal vessel wall.

2. *False aneurysm* having fibrous wall and occurring often from trauma to the vessel.

B. Depending upon the shape, aneurysms can be of following types (Fig. 11.12):

1. *Saccular* having large spherical outpouching.
2. *Fusiform* having slow spindle-shaped dilatation.
3. *Cylindrical* with a continuous parallel dilatation.
4. *Serpentine or varicose* which has tortuous dilatation of the vessel.
5. *Racemose or circoid* having mass of intercommunicating small arteries and veins.

C. Based on pathogenetic mechanisms, aneurysms can be classified as under (Fig. 11.13):

1. *Atherosclerotic (arteriosclerotic) aneurysms* are the most common type,
2. *Syphilitic (luetic) aneurysms* found in the tertiary stage of the syphilis.
3. *Dissecting aneurysms (Dissecting haematoma)* in which the blood enters the separated or dissected wall of the vessel.
4. *Mycotic aneurysms* which result from weakening of the arterial wall by microbial infection.
5. *Berry aneurysms* which are small dilatations especially affecting the circle of Willis in the base of the brain (Chapter 28).

The three common types of aortic aneurysms—atherosclerotic, syphilitic and dissecting, are described below:

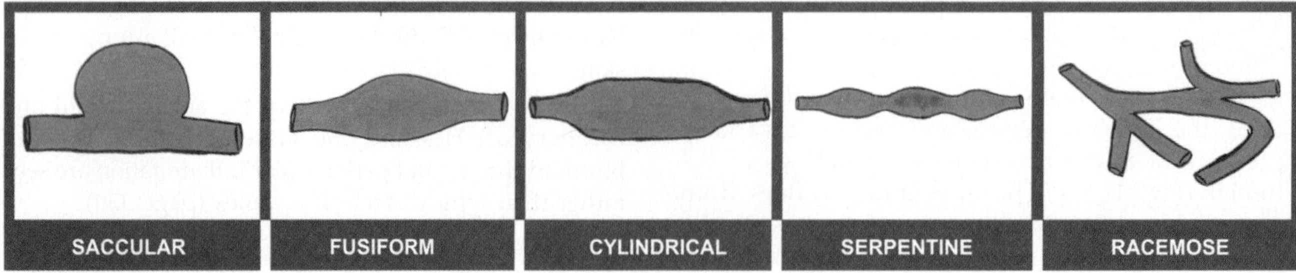

FIGURE 11.12

Common shapes of aneurysms of various types.

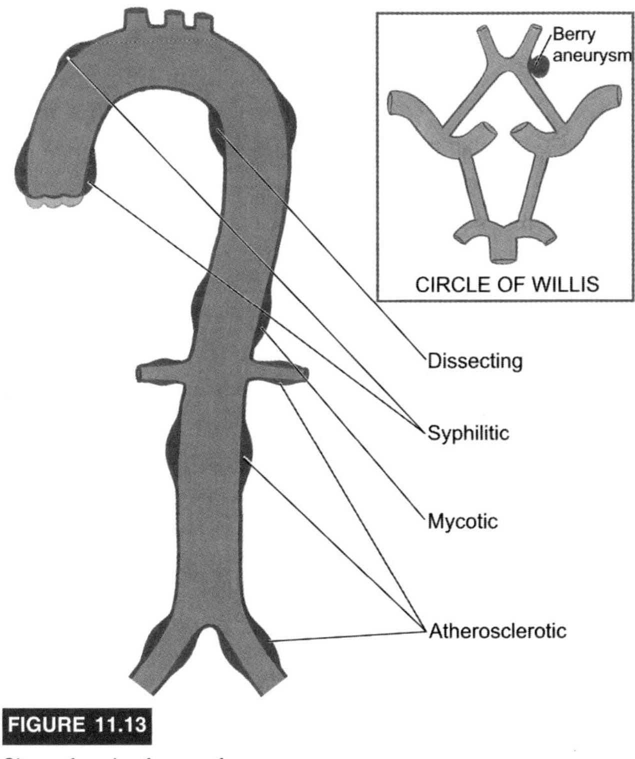

FIGURE 11.13

Sites of major forms of aneurysms.

Atherosclerotic Aneurysms

Atherosclerotic aneurysms are the most common form of aortic aneurysms. They are seen more commonly in males and the frequency increases after the age of 50 years when the incidence of complicated lesions of advanced atherosclerosis is higher. They are most common in the abdominal aorta, so much so that all forms of aneurysms of abdominal aorta (fusiform, cylindrical and saccular) should be considered atherosclerotic until proved otherwise. Other locations include thoracic aorta (essentially the ascending part and arch of aorta), iliac arteries and other large systemic arteries.

PATHOGENESIS. Obviously, severe atherosclerotic lesions are the basic problem which cause thinning and destruction of the medial elastic tissue resulting in atrophy and weakening of the wall. Since atherosclerotic lesions are most common and severe in abdominal aorta, atherosclerotic aneurysms occur most frequently here. In the thoracic aorta, besides atherosclerotic lesions, medial degeneration is another additional factor implicated in pathogenesis.

PATHOLOGIC CHANGES. Atherosclerotic aneurysms of the abdominal aorta are most frequently infra-renal, above the bifurcation of the aorta but may extend into common iliac arteries. They may be of variable size but are often larger than 5-6 cm in diameter. Atherosclerotic aneurysm is most frequently fusiform in shape and the lumen of aneurysm often contains mural thrombus (Figs. 11.12 and 11.13). ***Histologically,*** the wall of atherosclerotic aneurysm loses its normal arterial structure. Instead, there is predominance of fibrous tissue in the media and adventitia with mild chronic inflammatory reaction. The intima and inner part of the media show remnants of atheromatous plaques and mural thrombus.

EFFECTS. The clinical effects of atherosclerotic aneurysms are due to complications. These are as under:

1. **Rupture.** Rupture of the atherosclerotic aneurysm is the most serious and fatal complication. The risk of rupture depends upon the size and duration of the aneurysm and the blood pressure. Rupture of abdominal aneurysm may occur either into the peritoneum or into the retroperitoneum resulting in sudden and massive bleeding. Occasionally, there may be slow progressive leak from the aneurysm. A ruptured aneurysm is more likely to get infected.

2. **Compression.** The atherosclerotic aneurysm may press upon some adjacent structures such as compression of ureter and erosion on the vertebral bodies.

3. **Arterial occlusion.** Atherosclerotic aneurysms of the abdominal aorta may occlude the inferior mesenteric artery, or there may be development of occlusive thrombosis. However, collateral circulation develops slowly and is nearly always sufficient so as not to produce effects of ischaemia. Thromboembolism is rather common in abdominal aneurysms.

Syphilitic (Luetic) Aneurysms

Cardiovascular syphilis occurs in about 10% cases of syphilis. It causes arteritis—syphilitic aortitis and cerebral arteritis, both of which are already described in this chapter. One of the major complications of syphilitic aortitis is syphilitic or luetic aneurysm that develops in the tertiary stage of syphilis. It usually manifests after the age of 50 years and is more common in men. The predominant site of involvement is thoracic aorta, especially in the ascending part and arch of aorta. It may extend proximally into the aortic valve causing aortic incompetence and may lead to syphilitic heart disease. Less often, it may extend distally to involve abdominal aorta.

PATHOGENESIS. About 40% cases of syphilitic aortitis develop syphilitic aneurysms. The process begins from inflammatory infiltrate around the vasa vasorum of the adventitia, followed by endarteritis obliterans. This results in ischaemic injury to the media causing destruction of the smooth muscle and elastic tissue of the media and scarring. Since syphilitic aortitis involves the proximal aorta maximally, aortic aneurysm is found most frequently in the ascending aorta and in the aortic arch.

PATHOLOGIC CHANGES. Syphilitic aneurysms occurring most often in the ascending part and the arch of aorta are saccular in shape and usually 3-5 cm in diameter (Figs. 11.12 and 11.13). Less often, they are fusiform or cylindrical. The intimal surface is wrinkled and shows *tree-bark appearance.* When the aortic valve is involved, there is stretching and rolling of the valve leaflets producing valvular incompetence and left ventricular hypertrophy due to volume overload. This results in massively enlarged heart called 'cor bovinum'.

Histologically, the features of healed syphilitic aortitis are seen (page 289). The adventitia shows fibrous thickening with endarteritis obliterans of vasa vasorum. The fibrous scar tissue may extend into the media and the intima. Rarely, spirochaetes may be demonstrable in syphilitic aneurysm. Often, mural thrombus is found in the aneurysm.

EFFECTS. The clinical manifestations are found much more frequently in syphilitic aneurysms than in atherosclerotic aneurysms. The effects include the following:

1. Rupture. Syphilitic aneurysm is likely to rupture causing massive and fatal haemorrhage into the pleural cavity, pericardial sac, trachea and oesophagus.

2. Compression. The aneurysm may press on the adjacent tissues and cause symptoms such as on trachea causing dyspnoea, on oesophagus causing dysphagia, on recurrent laryngeal nerve leading to hoarseness; and erosion of vertebrae, sternum and ribs due to persistent pressure.

3. Cardiac dysfunction. When the aortic root and valve are involved, syphilitic aneurysm produces aortic incompetence and cardiac failure. Narrowing of the coronary ostia may further aggravate cardiac disease.

Dissecting Aneurysms and Cystic Medial Necrosis

The term dissecting aneurysm is applied for a dissecting haematoma in which the blood enters the separated (dissected) wall of the vessel and spreads for varying distance longitudinally. The most common site is the aorta and is an acute catastrophic aortic disease. The condition occurs most commonly in men in the age range of 50 to 70 years. In women, dissecting aneurysms may occur during pregnancy.

PATHOGENESIS. The pathogenesis of dissecting aneurysm is explained on the basis of weakened aortic media. Various conditions causing weakening in the aortic wall resulting in dissection are as under:

i) Hypertensive state. About 90% cases of dissecting aneurysm have hypertension which predisposes such patients to degeneration of the media in some questionable way.

ii) Non-hypertensive cases. These are cases in whom there is some local or systemic connective tissue disorder e.g.

a) *Marfan's syndrome,* an autosomal dominant disease with genetic defect in fibrillin which is a connective tissue protein required for elastic tissue formation.

b) Development of *cystic medial necrosis of Erdheim,* especially in old age.

c) *Iatrogenic trauma* during cardiac catheterisation or coronary bypass surgery.

d) *Pregnancy,* for some unknown reasons.

Once medial necrosis has occurred, haemodynamic factors, chiefly hypertension, cause tear in the intima and initiate the dissecting aneurysms. The media is split at its weakest point by the inflowing blood. An alternative suggestion is that the medial haemorrhage from the vasa vasorum occurs first and the intimal tear follows it. Further extension of aneurysm occurs due to entry of blood into the media through the intimal tear.

PATHOLOGIC CHANGES. Dissecting aneurysm differs from atherosclerotic and syphilitic aneurysms in having no significant dilatation. Therefore, it is currently referred to as *'dissecting haematoma'.* Dissecting aneurysm classically begins in the arch of aorta. In 95% of cases, there is a sharply-incised, transverse or oblique intimal tear, 3-4 cm long, most often located in the ascending part of the aorta. The dissection is seen most characteristically between the outer and middle third of the aortic media so that the column of blood in the dissection separates the *intima and inner two-third of the media* on one side from the *outer one-third of the media and the adventitia* on the other. The dissection extends proximally into the aortic valve ring as well as distally into the abdominal aorta (Fig. 11.14).

Occasionally, the dissection may extend into the branches of aorta like into the arteries of the neck,

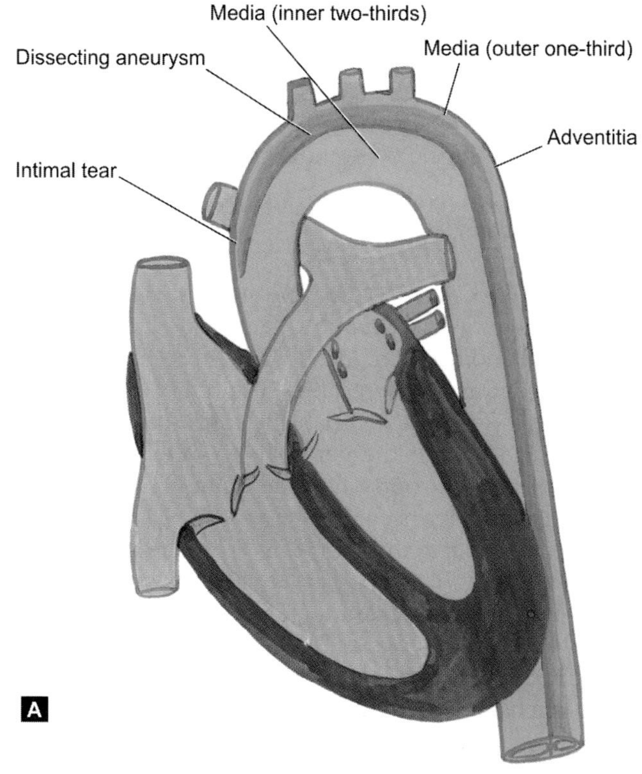

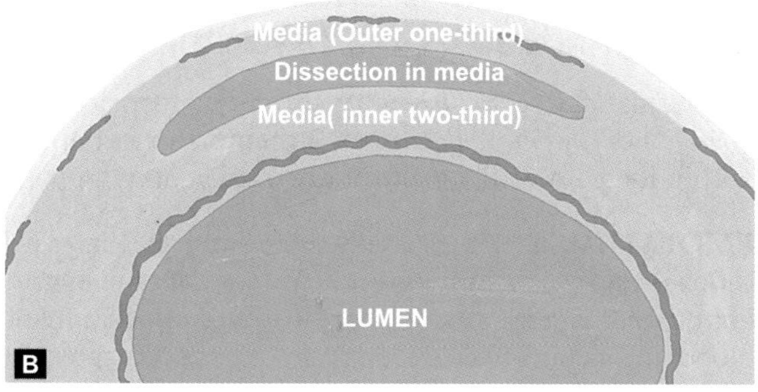

FIGURE 11.14

A. Dissecting aneurysm, (Type 1) beginning in the aortic arch and extending distally into the descending thoracic aorta as well as proximally into the ascending aorta. An intimal tear is seen in the arch. B, The cross-section shows dissection typically separating the intima and inner two-thirds of the media on *luminal* side, from the *outer* one-third of the media and the adventitia.

coronaries, renal, mesenteric and iliac arteries. The dissection may affect the entire circumference of the aortic media or a segment of it. In about 10% of dissecting aneurysms, a second intimal tear is seen in the distal part of the dissection so that the blood enters the false lumen through the proximal tear and re-enters the true lumen through the distal tear. If the patient survives, the false lumen may develop endothelial lining and *'double-barrel aorta'* is formed.

Depending upon the extent of dissecting aneurysms, three types are described:

Type I: Comprises 75% of cases, begins in the ascending aorta and extends distally for some distance.

Type II: Comprises 5% of cases and is limited to the ascending aorta.

Type III: Constitutes the remaining 20% cases and begins in the ascending thoracic aorta near the origin of subclavian artery.

Types I and II involving ascending aorta are also called as *group A dissection,* and type III not involving ascending aorta is referred to as *group B dissection.*

Histologically, the characteristic features of cystic medial necrosis are found. These are as under:

- Focal separation of the fibromuscular and elastic tissue of the media.
- Numerous cystic spaces in the media containing basophilic ground substance.
- Fragmentation of the elastic tissue.
- Increased fibrosis of the media.

EFFECTS. The classical clinical manifestation of a dissecting aneurysm is excruciating tearing pain in the chest moving downwards. The complications arising from dissecting aneurysms are as under:

1. **Rupture.** Haemorrhage from rupture of a dissecting aneurysm in the ascending aorta results in mortality in 90% of cases. Most often, haemorrhage occurs into the pericardium; less frequently it may rupture into thoracic cavity, abdominal cavity or retroperitoneum.

2. **Cardiac disease.** Involvement of the aortic valve results in aortic incompetence. Obstruction of coronaries results in ischaemia causing fatal myocardial infarction. Rarely, dissecting aneurysm may extend into the cardiac chamber.

3. **Ischaemia.** Obstruction of the branches of aorta by dissection results in ischaemia of the tissue supplied. Thus, there may be renal infarction, cerebral ischaemia and infarction of the spinal cord.

FIBROMUSCULAR DYSPLASIA

Fibromuscular dysplasia first described in 1976, is a non-atherosclerotic and non-inflammatory disease affecting arterial wall, most often renal artery. Though the process may involve intima, media or adventitia, medial fibroplasia is the most common.

*PATHOLOGIC CHANGES. **Grossly,*** the involvement is characteristically segmental—affecting vessel in a bead-like pattern with intervening uninvolved areas.

Microscopically, the beaded areas show collections of smooth muscle cells and connective tissue. There is often rupture and retraction of internal elastic lamina.

The main **effects** of renal fibromuscular dysplasia, depending upon the region of involvement, are renovascular hypertension and changes of renal atrophy.

VEINS

NORMAL STRUCTURE

The structure of normal veins is basically similar to that of arteries. The walls of the veins are thinner, the three tunicae (intima, media and adventitia) are less clearly demarcated, the elastic tissue is scanty and not clearly organised into internal and external elastic laminae. The media contains very small amount of smooth muscle cells with abundant collagen. All veins, except vena cavae and common iliac veins, have valves best developed in veins of the lower limbs. The valves are delicate folds of intima, located every 1-6 cm, often next to point of entry of a tributary vein. They prevent any significant retrograde venous blood flow.

VARICOSITIES

Varicosities are abnormally dilated and tortuous veins. The veins of lower extremities are involved most frequently, called *varicose veins.* The veins of other parts of the body which are affected are the lower oesophagus (*oesophageal varices,* Chapter 19), the anal region (*haemorrhoids,* Chapter 18) and the spermatic cord (*varicocele,* Chapter 21).

VARICOSE VEINS

Varicose veins are permanently dilated and tortuous superficial veins of the lower extremities, especially the long saphenous vein and its tributaries. About 10-12% of the general population develops varicose veins of lower legs, with the peak incidence in 4th and 5th decades of life. Adult females are affected more commonly than the males, especially during pregnancy. This is attributed to venous stasis in the lower legs because of compression on the iliac veins by pregnant uterus.

ETIOPATHOGENESIS. A number of etiologic and pathogenetic factors are involved in causing varicose veins. These are as follows:

i) Familial weakness of vein walls and valves is the most common cause.

ii) Increased intraluminal pressure due to prolonged upright posture e.g. in nurses, policemen, surgeons etc.

iii) Compression of iliac veins e.g. during pregnancy, intravascular thrombosis, growing tumour etc.

iv) Hormonal effects on smooth muscle.

v) Obesity.

vi) Chronic constipation.

PATHOLOGIC CHANGES. The affected veins, especially of the lower extremities, are dilated, tortuous, elongated and nodular. Intraluminal thrombosis and valvular deformities are often found.
Histologically, there is variable fibromuscular thickening of the wall of the veins due to alternate dilatation and hypertrophy. Degeneration of the medial elastic tissue may occur which may be followed by calcific foci. Mural thrombosis is commonly present which may get organised and hyalinised leading to irregular intimal thickening.

EFFECTS. Varicose veins of the legs result in venous stasis which is followed by congestion, oedema, thrombosis, stasis, dermatitis, cellulitis and ulceration. Secondary infection results in chronic varicose ulcers.

PHLEBOTHROMBOSIS AND THROMBOPHLEBITIS

The terms *'phlebothrombosis'* or thrombus formation in veins, and *'thrombophlebitis'* or inflammatory changes within the vein wall, are currently used synonymously.

ETIOPATHOGENESIS. Venous thrombosis that precedes thrombophlebitis is initiated by *triad* of changes: endothelial damage, alteration in the composition of blood and venous stasis. The factors that predispose to these changes are cardiac failure, malignancy, use of oestrogen-containing compounds, postoperative state and immobility due to various reasons.

PATHOLOGIC CHANGES. The most common locations for phlebothrombosis and thrombophlebitis are the deep veins of legs accounting for 90% of cases. Other locations are periprostatic venous plexus in males, pelvic veins in the females, and near the foci of infection in the abdominal cavity such as acute appendicitis, peritonitis, acute salpingitis and pelvic abscesses.
Grossly, the affected veins may appear normal or may be distended and firm. Often, a mural or occlusive thrombus is present.
Histologically, the thrombus that is attached to the vein wall induces inflammatory-reparative response

beginning from the intima and infiltrating into the thrombi. The response consists of mononuclear inflammatory cells and fibroblastic proliferation. In late stage, thrombus is either organised or resolved leading to a thick-walled fibrous vein.

EFFECTS. The clinical effects due to phlebothrombosis and thrombophlebitis may be local or systemic.

Local effects are oedema distal to occlusion, heat, swelling, tenderness, redness and pain.

Systemic effects are more severe and occur due to embolic phenomena, pulmonary thromboembolism being the most common and most important. Other systemic manifestations include bacteraemia and septic embolisation to brain, meninges, liver etc.

SpecialTypes of Phlebothrombosis

A few special variants of phlebothrombosis are considered below:

1. THROMBOPHLEBITIS MIGRANS. Thrombophlebitis migrans or migratory thrombophlebitis or Trousseau's syndrome is the term used for multiple venous thrombi that disappear from one site so as to appear at another site. The condition is not a morphologic entity but a clinical one, seen most often in disseminated visceral cancers (e.g. cancer of lungs, prostate, female reproductive tract, breast, pancreas and gastrointestinal tract) as part of paraneoplastic syndrome and is also found in nonbacterial thrombotic endocarditis.

2. PHLEGMASIA ALBA DOLENS. This term meaning 'painful white leg' refers to extensive swelling of the leg, occurring most frequently due to iliofemoral venous thrombosis. It occurs most often in women during late pregnancy or following delivery when the pregnant uterus causes pressure on the iliofemoral veins, or after extensive pelvic surgery. Development of pulmonary embolism may occur due to involvement of inferior vena cava.

3. PHLEGMASIA CERULEA DOLENS. This term meaning 'painful blue leg' refers to markedly swollen bluish skin with superficial gangrene. It is a serious complication of massive iliofemoral venous thrombosis and decreased arterial blood flow.

4. SUPERIOR VENA CAVAL SYNDROME. Superior vena caval syndrome refers to obstruction of the superior vena cava. The obstruction results most often from external compression or from thrombosis. Some of the common causes of superior vena caval syndrome are malignancy (especially lung cancer and lymphoma), syphilitic aortic aneurysm and tuberculous mediastinitis. Clinical features include dilated veins of neck and thorax, oedema of the face, neck and upper chest, visual disturbances and disturbed sensorium.

5. INFERIOR VENA CAVAL SYNDROME. Inferior vena caval syndrome is the obstruction of the inferior vena cava. Most often, obstruction results from thrombosis by extension from iliofemoral veins. Other causes of obstruction are external compression and neoplastic invasion. Clinical features are oedema of lower extremities, dilated leg veins and collateral venous channels in the lower abdomen

LYMPHATICS

NORMAL STRUCTURE

Lymphatic capillaries, lymphatic vessels and lymph nodes comprise the lymphatic system. Lymphatic capillaries resemble blood capillaries, and larger lymphatics are identical to veins. However, lymphatics lined by a single layer of endothelium have thin muscle in their walls than in veins of the same size and the valves are more numerous. Lymphatic capillaries and lymphatics form plexuses around tissues and organs. The walls of lymphatic capillaries are permeable to tissue fluid, proteins and particulate matter.

LYMPHANGITIS

Inflammation of the lymphatics or lymphangitis may be acute or chronic.

Acute lymphangitis occurs in the course of many bacterial infections. The most common organisms are (β-haemolytic streptococci and staphylococci). Acute lymphangitis is often associated with lymphadenitis.

> ***Grossly,*** the affected lymphatics are dilated and appear as cutaneous streaks.
> ***Microscopically,*** the dilated lumen contains acute inflammatory exudate, cell debris and clotted lymph. There is inflammatory infiltration into the perilymphatic tissues alongwith hyperaemia and oedema. Acute lymphangitis generally heals completely.

Chronic lymphangitis occurs due to persistent and recurrent acute lymphangitis or from chronic infections like tuberculosis, syphilis and actinomycosis.

> ***Histologically,*** there is permanent obstruction due to fibrosis of affected lymphatics called chronic lymphoedema.

LYMPHOEDEMA

Lymphoedema is swelling of soft tissues due to localised increase in the quantity of lymph (page 98). It may be primary (idiopathic) or secondary (obstructive).

I. PRIMARY (IDIOPATHIC) LYMPHOEDEMA. Lymphoedema occurring without underlying secondary cause is called primary or idiopathic lymphoedema. Its various types are as under:

1. Congenital lymphoedema. Congenital lymphoedema has further 2 subtypes—familial hereditary form (Milroy's disease) and non-familial (simple) form.

i) Milroy's disease is a form of congenital and familial oedema generally affecting one limb but at times may be more extensive and involve the eyelids and lips. The disease is inherited as an autosomal dominant trait and is often associated with other congenital anomalies. The condition results from developmental defect of lymphatic channels so that the affected tissue shows abnormally dilated lymphatics and the area shows honey-combed appearance. Recurrent infection of the tissue causes cellulitis and fibrosis of lymphatic vessels.

ii) Simple congenital lymphoedema is non-familial form with unknown etiology. It is often associated with Turner's syndrome and affects one member of the family. The pathologic changes are similar to those of Milroy's disease.

2. Lymphoedema praecox. This is a rare form of lymphoedema affecting chiefly young females. The oedema usually begins in the foot and progresses slowly upwards to involve the whole extremity. With passage of time, the affected area becomes rough and the oedema is non-pitting. The etiology is unknown but probably the condition is related to female reproductive system because of preponderance in females and aggravation during menses.

II. SECONDARY (OBSTRUCTIVE) LYMPHOEDEMA. This is the more common form of lymphoedema. The various causes of lymphatic obstruction causing lymphoedema are:

i) Lymphatic invasion by malignant tumour.

ii) Surgical removal of lymphatics e.g. in radical mastectomy.

iii) Post-irradiation fibrosis.

iv) Parasitic infestations e.g. in filariasis of lymphatics producing elephantiasis.

v) Lymphangitis causing scarring and obstruction.

Obstructive lymphoedema occurs only when the obstruction is widespread as otherwise collaterals develop. The affected area consists of dilatation of lymphatics distal to obstruction with increased interstitial fluid. With passage of time, there is inflammatory scarring and the lymphatics become fibrosed with enlargement of the affected part. Rupture of dilated large lymphatics may result in escape of milky chyle into the peritoneum (*chyloperitoneum*), into the pleural cavity (*chylothorax*), into pericardial cavity (*chylopericardium*) and into the urinary tract (*chyluria*).

TUMOURS ANDTUMOUR-LIKE LESIONS

Majority of benign vascular tumours are malformations or hamartomas. A hamartoma is a tumour-like lesion made up of tissues indigenous to the part but lacks the true growth potential of true neoplasms. However, there is no clear-cut distinction between vascular hamartomas and true benign tumours and are often described together. On the other hand, there are true vascular tumours which are of intermediate grade and there are frank malignant tumours.

A classification of vascular tumours and tumour-like conditions is given in Table 11.6.

TABLE 11.6: Tumours and Tumour-like Lesions of Blood Vessels and Lymphatics.

A. Benign Tumours and Hamartomas
1. Haemangioma
2. Lymphangioma
3. Glomus tumour (glomangioma)
4. Arteriovenous malformations

B. Intermediate Grade Tumours
Haemangioendothelioma

C. Malignant Tumours
1. Haemangiopericytoma
2. Angiosarcoma
3. Kaposi's sarcoma

A. BENIGNTUMOURS AND HAMARTOMAS

Haemangioma

Haemangiomas are quite common lesions, especially in infancy and childhood. The most common site is the skin of the face. Amongst the various clinical and histologic types, three important forms are described below.

CAPILLARY HAEMANGIOMA. These are the most common type. Clinically, they appear as small or large, flat or slightly elevated, red to purple, soft and lobulated lesions, varying in size from a few millimeters to a few centimeters in diameter. They may be present at birth or appear in early childhood. Strawberry birthmarks and 'port-wine mark' are some good examples. The common sites are the skin, subcutaneous tissue and mucous membranes of oral cavity and lips. Less common sites are internal visceral organs like liver, spleen and kidneys.

Histologically, capillary haemangiomas are well-defined but unencapsulated lobules. These lobules are composed of capillary-sized, thin-walled, blood-filled vessels. These vessels are lined by single layer of plump endothelial cells surrounded by a layer of pericytes (COLOUR PLATE XIII: CL 52). The vessels are separated by some connective tissue stroma (Fig. 11.15).

Many of the capillary haemangiomas regress spontaneously within a few years.

CAVERNOUS HAEMANGIOMA. Cavernous haemangiomas are single or multiple, discrete or diffuse, red to blue, soft and spongy masses. They are often 1 to 2 cm in diameter. They are most common in the skin (especially of the face and neck); other sites are mucosa of the oral cavity, stomach and small intestine, and internal viscera like the liver and spleen.

Histologically, cavernous haemangiomas are composed of thin-walled cavernous vascular spaces, filled partly or completely with blood. The vascular spaces are lined by flattened endothelial cells (COLOUR PLATE XIV: CL 53). They are separated by scanty connective tissue stroma (Fig. 11.16).

Cavernous haemangiomas rarely involute spontaneously.

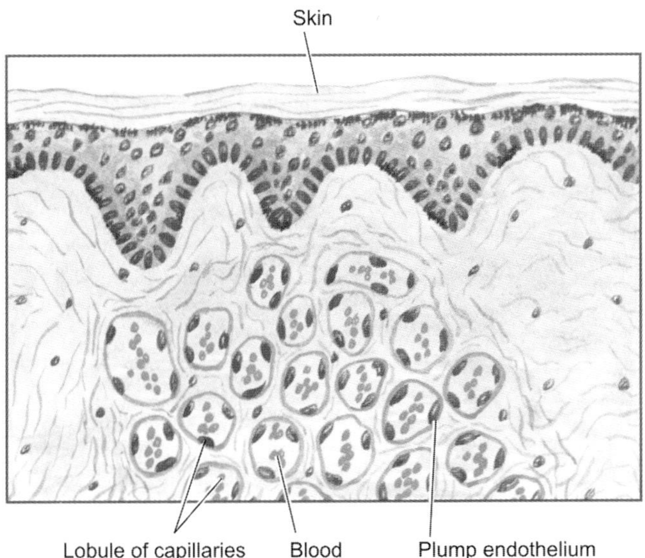

FIGURE 11.15

Capillary haemangioma of the skin. There are capillaries lined by plump endothelial cells and containing blood. The intervening stroma consists of scant connective tissue.

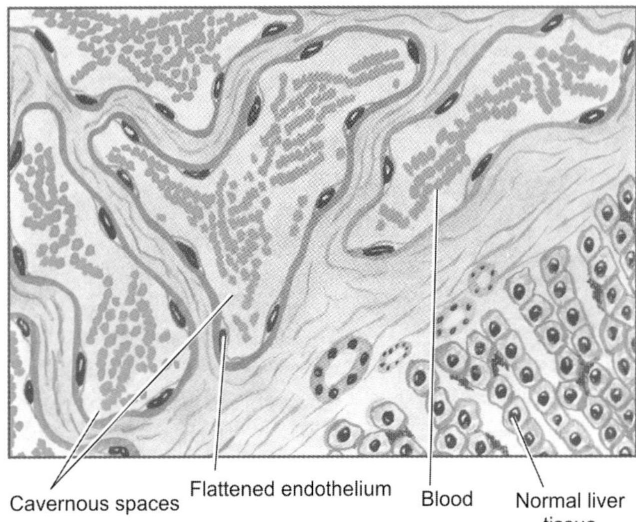

FIGURE 11.16

Cavernous haemangioma of the liver. The vascular spaces are large, dilated, many containing blood, and are lined by flattened endothelial cells. Scanty connective tissue stroma is seen between the cavernous spaces.

GRANULOMA PYOGENICUM. Granuloma pyogenicum is also referred to as *haemangioma of granulation tissue type.* True to its name, it appears as exophytic, red granulation tissue just like a nodule, commonly on the skin and mucosa of gingiva or oral cavity. *Pregnancy tumour* or *granuloma gravidarum* is a variant occurring on the gingiva during pregnancy and regresses after delivery. Granuloma pyogenicum often develops following trauma and is usually 1 to 2 cm in diameter.

Histologically, it shows proliferating capillaries similar to capillary haemangioma but the capillaries are separated by abundant oedema and inflammatory infiltrate, thus resembling inflammatory granulation tissue.

Lymphangioma

Lymphangiomas are lymphatic counterparts of vascular haemangiomas. Lymphangiomas are congenital lesions which are classified as capillary, cavernous and cystic hygroma. Combinations are also often seen.

CAPILLARY LYMPHANGIOMA. It is also called as lymphangioma simplex. It is a small, circumscribed, slightly elevated lesion measuring 1 to 2 cm in diameter. The common locations are the skin of head and neck, axilla and mucous membranes. Rarely, these may be found in the internal organs.

Histologically, capillary lymphangioma is composed of a network of endothelium-lined, capillary-sized spaces containing lymph and often separated by lymphoid aggregates.

CAVERNOUS LYMPHANGIOMA. It is more common than the capillary type. The common sites are in the region of head and neck or axilla. A large cystic variety called *cystic hygroma* occurs in the neck producing gross deformity in the neck.

Histologically, cavernous lymphangioma consists of large dilated lymphatic spaces lined by flattened endothelial cells and containing lymph. Scanty intervening stromal connective tissue is present (Fig. 11.17) (COLOUR PLATE XIV: CL 54). These lesions, though benign, are often difficult to remove due to infiltration into adjacent tissues.

Glomus Tumour (Glomangioma)

Glomus tumour is an uncommon true benign tumour arising from contractile glomus cells that are present in the arteriovenous shunts (Sucquet-Hoyer anastomosis). These tumours are found most often in the dermis of the fingers or toes under a nail; other sites are mucosa of the stomach and nasal cavity. These lesions are characterised by extreme pain. They may be single or multiple, small, often less than 1 cm in diameter, flat or slightly elevated, red-blue, painful nodules.

Histologically, the tumours are composed of small blood vessels lined by endothelium and surrounded by aggregates, nests and masses of glomus cells. The glomus cells are round to cuboidal cells with scanty cytoplasm. The intervening connective tissue stroma contains some non-myelinated nerve fibres (Fig. 11.18) (COLOUR PLATE XIV: CL 55).

4. Arteriovenous Malformations

An arteriovenous (AV) malformation is a communication between an artery and vein without an intervening capillary bed. It may be congenital or acquired type. Congenital AV malformations have thick-walled vessels with hyalinisation and calcification. Acquired AV malformations reveal mainly changes in the veins which are dilated and thick-walled.

B. INTERMEDIATE GRADE TUMOURS

Haemangioendothelioma

Haemangioendothelioma is a true tumour of endothelial cells, the behaviour of which is intermediate between a haemangioma and haemangiosarcoma. It is found most

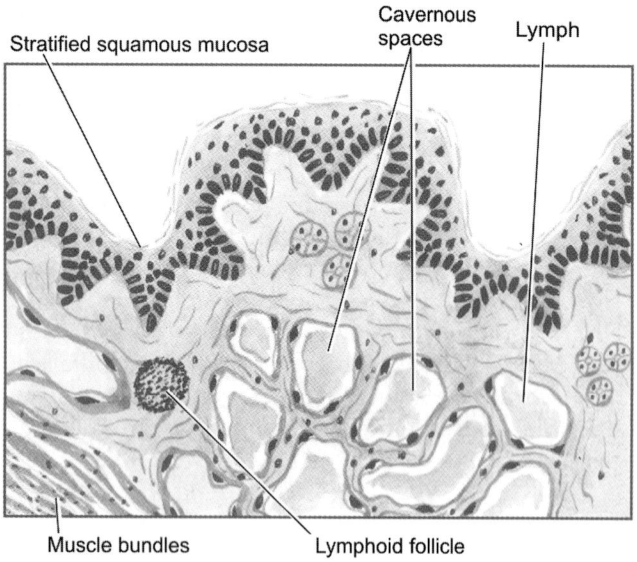

Stratified squamous mucosa
Cavernous spaces
Lymph
Muscle bundles
Lymphoid follicle

FIGURE 11.17

Cavernous lymphangioma of the tongue. Large cystic spaces lined by the flattened endothelial cells and containing lymph are present. Stroma shows scattered collection of lymphocytes.

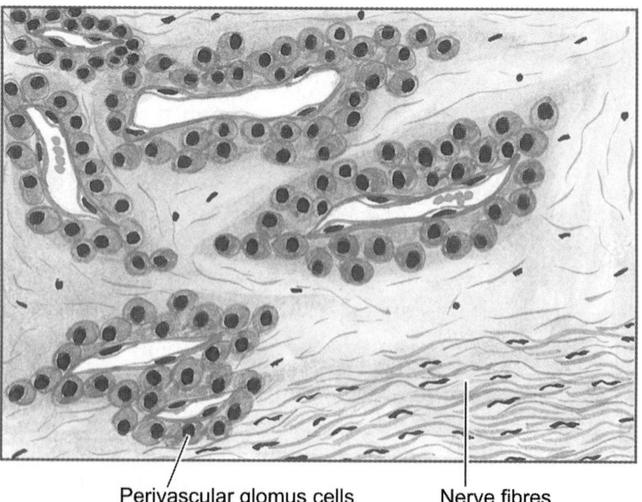

FIGURE 11.18

Glomus tumour. There are blood-filled vascular channels lined by endothelial cells and surrounded by nests and masses of glomus cells.

Chapter Eleven

often in the skin and subcutaneous tissue in relation to medium-sized and large veins, *Haemangioblastoma* is the term used for similar tumour occurring in the cerebellum (Chapter 28).

Grossly, the tumour is usually well-defined, grey-red, polypoid mass.
Microscopically, there is active proliferation of endothelial cells forming several layers around the blood vessels so that vascular lumina are difficult to identify. Reticulin stain delineates the pattern of cell proliferation inner to the basement membrane.

C. MALIGNANT TUMOURS

Haemangiopericytoma

Haemangiopericytoma is an uncommon tumour arising from pericytes. Pericytes are cells present external to the endothelial cells of capillaries and venules. This is a rare tumour that can occur at any site and at any age and may vary in size from 1 to 8 cm.

Microscopically, the tumour is composed of capillaries surrounded by spindle-shaped pericytes outside the capillary basement membrane forming whorled arrangement. Silver impregnation stain (i.e. reticulin stain) is employed to confirm the presence of pericytes outside the basement membrane of capillaries and to distinguish it from haemangioendothelioma.

Local recurrences are common and distant spread occurs in about 20% of cases.

Angiosarcoma

Also known as haemangiosarcoma and malignant haemangioendothelioma, it is a malignant vascular tumour occurring most frequently in the skin, subcutaneous tissue, liver, spleen, bone, lung and retroperitoneal tissues. It can occur in both sexes and at any age. *Hepatic angiosarcomas* are of special interest in view of their association with carcinogens like polyvinyl chloride, arsenical pesticides and radioactive contrast medium, thorotrast.

Grossly, the tumours are usually bulky, pale grey-white, firm masses with poorly-defined margins. Areas of haemorrhage, necrosis and central softening are frequently present.
Microscopically, the tumours may be well-differentiated masses of proliferating endothelial cells around well-formed vascular channels, to poorly-differentiated lesions composed of plump, anaplastic and pleomorphic cells in solid clusters with poorly identifiable vascular channels (COLOUR PLATE XIV: CL 56).

These tumours invade locally and may have distant metastases in lungs and other organs. *Lymphangiosarcoma* is a histologically similar tumour occurring in obstructive lymphoedema of long duration.

Kaposi's Sarcoma

Kaposi's sarcoma is a malignant angiomatous tumour, first described by Kaposi, Hungarian dermatologist, in 1872. However, the tumour has attracted greater attention more recently due to its frequent occurrence in patients with AIDS.

CLASSIFICATION. Presently, four forms of Kaposi's sarcoma are described:

1. Classic (European) Kaposi's sarcoma. This is the form which was first described by Kaposi. It is more common in men over 60 years of age of Eastern European descent. The disease is slow and appears as multiple, small, purple, dome-shaped nodules or plaques in the skin, especially on the legs. Involvement of visceral organs occurs in about 10% cases after many years.

2. African (Endemic) Kaposi's sarcoma. This form is common in equatorial Africa. It is so common in Uganda that it comprises 9% of all malignant tumours in men. It is found in younger age, especially in boys and in young men and has a more aggressive course than the classic form. The disease begins in the skin but grows rapidly to involve other tissues, especially lymph nodes and the gut.

3. Epidemic (AIDS-associated) Kaposi's sarcoma. This form is seen in about 30% cases of AIDS, especially in young male homosexuals than the other high risk groups. The cutaneous lesions are not localised to lower legs but are more extensively distributed involving mucous membranes, lymph nodes and internal organs early in the course of disease.

4. Kaposi's sarcoma in renal transplant cases. This form is associated with recipients of renal transplants who have been administered immunosuppressive therapy for a long time. The lesions may be localised to the skin or may have widespread systemic involvement.

PATHOGENESIS. The etiology of Kaposi's sarcoma is not clearly known.

■ Epidemiological studies have suggested a *viral association* implicating HIV and human herpesvirus 8

Chapter Eleven

(HSV 8, also called Kaposi's sarcoma HSV) . The excessive proliferation of mesenchymal spindle cells of vascular origin occurs due to cooperation between HIV-derived protein and angiogenic cytokines (e.g. oncostatin-M, and basic fibroblast growth factor). Higher incidence of Kaposi's sarcoma in male homosexuals is explained by increased secretion of cytokines by their activated immune system.

- Defective immunoregulation plays a role in its pathogenesis is further substantiated by observation of *second malignancy* (e.g. leukaemia, lymphoma and myeloma) in about one-third of patients with Kaposi's sarcoma.
- An *HLA association* with classic type of Kaposi's sarcoma has been observed, implying thereby the role of genetic factors in its etiology.
- *Growth factors* such as cytokines may be produced locally by implying an autocrine or paracrine mode of proferation of tumour cells.

PATHOLOGIC CHANGES. Pathologically, all forms of Kaposi's sarcoma are similar

Grossly, the lesions in the skin, gut and other organs form prominent, irregular, purple, dome-shaped plaques or nodules.

Histologically, the changes are nonspecific in *the early patch stage* and more characteristic in the *late nodular stage.*

- In the **early patch stage,** there are irregular vascular spaces separated by interstitial inflammatory cells and extravasated blood and haemosiderin.
- In the **late nodular stage,** there are slit-like vascular spaces containing red blood cells and separated by spindle-shaped, plump tumour cells. These spindle-shaped tumour cells are probably of endothelial origin (Fig. 11.19).

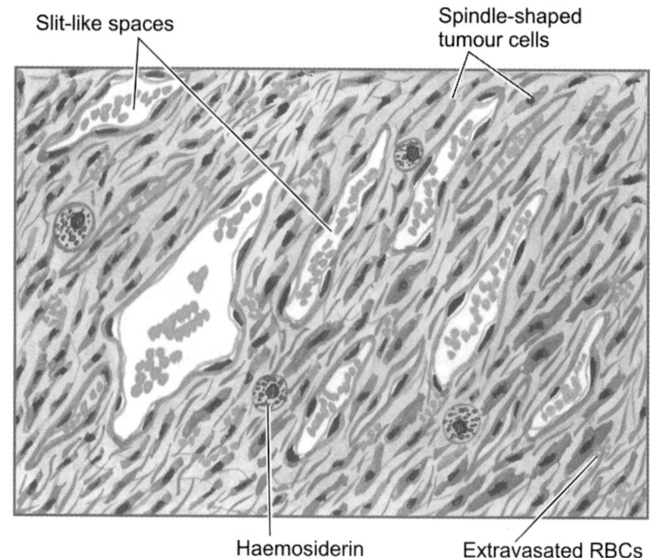

FIGURE 11.19

Kaposi's sarcoma in late nodular stage. There are slit-like blood-filled vascular spaces. Between them are present bands of plump spindle-shaped tumour cells.

CLINICAL COURSE. The clinical course and biologic behaviour of Kaposi's sarcoma is quite variable. The classic form of Kaposi's sarcoma is largely confined to skin and the course is generally slow and insidious with long survival. The endemic (African) and epidemic (AIDS-associated) Kaposi's sarcoma, on the other hand, has a rapidly progressive course, often with widespread cutaneous as well as visceral involvement, and high mortality.

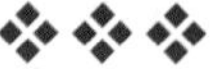

The Heart

12

NORMAL STRUCTURE

ANATOMY AND PHYSIOLOGY. The heart is a muscular pump that ejects blood into the vascular tree with sufficient pressure to maintain optimal circulation. The average weight of heart in an adult male is 300-350 gm while that of an adult female is 250-300 gm. It is divided into four chambers: a right and a left atrium both lying superiorly, and a right and a left ventricle both lying inferiorly and are larger. The atria are separated by a thin interatrial partition called *interatrial septum*, while the ventricles are separated by thick muscular partition called *interventricular septum.* The thickness of the right ventricular wall is 0.3 to 0.5 cm while that of the left ventricular wall is 1.3 to 1.5 cm. The blood in the heart chambers moves in a carefully prescribed pathway: venous blood from systemic circulation → right atrium → right ventricle → pulmonary arteries → lung → pulmonary veins → left atrium → left ventricle → aorta → systemic arterial supply (Fig. 12.1).

The transport of blood is regulated by cardiac valves: two loose flap-like atrioventricular valves, tricuspid on the right and mitral (bicuspid) on the left; and two semilunar valves with three leaflets each, the pulmonary and aortic valves, guarding the outflow tracts. The normal circumference of the valvular openings measures about 12 cm in tricuspid, 8.5 cm in pulmonary, 10 cm in mitral and 7.5 cm in aortic valve.

The wall of the heart consists mainly of the *myocardium* which is covered externally by thin membrane, the *epicardium* or visceral pericardium, and lined internally by another thin layer, the *endocardium.*

The **myocardium** is the muscle tissue of the heart composed of syncytium of branching and anastomosing, transversely striated muscle fibres arranged in parallel fashion.The space between myocardial fibres contains a rich capillary network and loose connective tissue. The myocardial fibres are connected to each other by irregular joints called as *intercalated* discs. They represent the apposed cell membranes of individual cells which

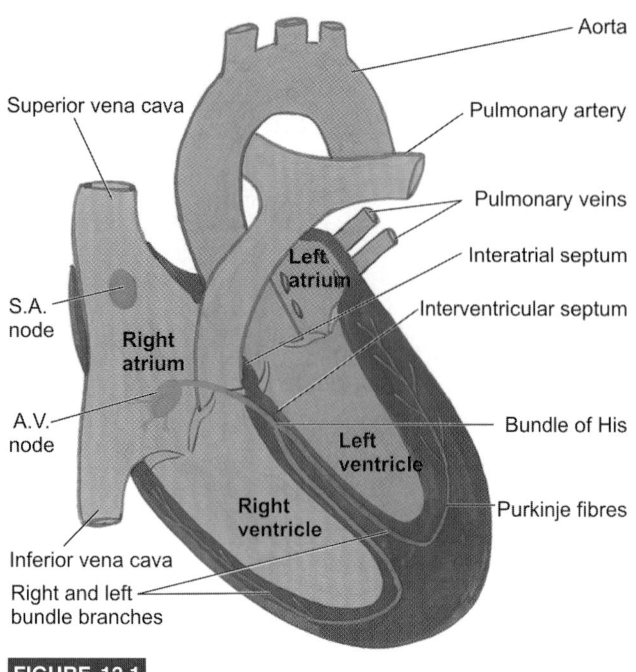

FIGURE 12.1

The normal structure of the heart.

act as tight junctions for free transport of ions and action potentials. The cardiac myocyte is very rich in mitochondria which is the source of large amount of ATP required for cardiac contraction. The cardiac muscle fibre has abundant sarcoplasmic reticulum corresponding to endoplasmic reticulum of other cells. Transverse lines divide each fibre into *sarcomeres* which act as structural and functional subunits. Each sarcomere consists of prominent central *dark A-band* attributed to thick myosin filaments and flanked on either side by *light I-bands* consisting of thin actin filament. The actin bands are in the form of twisted rods overlying protein molecules called *tropomyosin*. These protein molecules are of 3 types: *troponin-I, troponin-T, and troponin-C.* Troponin molecules respond to calcium ions in cyclical contraction-relaxation of myocardial fibres.

The **conduction system** of the heart located in the myocardium is responsible for regulating rate and rhythm of the heart. It is composed of specialised Purkinje fibres which contain some contractile myofilaments and conduct action potentials rapidly. The conduction system consists of 4 major components:

1. The *sinoatrial (SA) node* is located in the posterior wall of the right atrium adjacent to the point at which the superior vena cava enters the heart. It is also called cardiac pacemaker since it is responsible for determining the rate of contraction for all cardiac muscle.

2. The *atrioventricular (AV) bundle* conducts the impulse from the SA node to the AV node.

3. The *atrioventricular (AV) node* is located on the top of the interventricular septum and receives impulses from the SA node via AV bundle and transmits them to the bundle of His.

4. The *bundle of His* extends through the interventricular septum and divides into right and left bundle branches which arborise in the respective ventricular walls. These fibres transmit impulses from the AV node to the ventricular walls.

The **pericardium** consists of a closely apposed layer, *visceral pericardium or epicardium,* and an outer fibrous sac, the *parietal pericardium*. The two layers enclose a narrow pericardial cavity which is lined by mesothelial cells and normally contains 10-30 ml of clear, watery serous fluid. This fluid functions as lubricant and shock absorbant to the heart.

The **endocardium** is the smooth shiny inner lining of the myocardium that covers all the cardiac chambers, the cardiac valves, the chordae tendineae and the papillary muscles. It is lined by endothelium with connective tissue and elastic fibres in its deeper part.

The **valve cusps and semilunar leaflets** are delicate and translucent structures. The valves are strengthened by collagen and elastic tissue and covered by a layer of endothelium (valvular endocardium).

MYOCARDIAL BLOOD SUPPLY. The cardiac muscle, in order to function properly, must receive adequate supply of oxygen and nutrients. Blood is transported to myocardial cells by the coronary arteries which originate immediately above the aortic semilunar valve. Most of blood flow to the myocardium occurs during diastole. There are three major coronary trunks, each supplying blood to specific segments of the heart (Fig. 12.2):

1. The **anterior descending branch of the left coronary artery** supplies most of the apex of the heart, the anterior surface of the left ventricle, the adjacent third of the anterior wall of the right ventricle, and the anterior two-third of the interventricular septum.

2. The **circumflex branch of the left coronary artery** supplies the left atrium and a small portion of the lateral aspect of the left ventricle.

3. The **right coronary artery** supplies the right atrium, the remainder of the anterior surface of the right ventricle, the adjacent half of the posterior wall of the left ventricle and the posterior third of the interventricular septum.

There are 3 anatomic patterns of distribution of the coronary blood supply, depending upon which of the

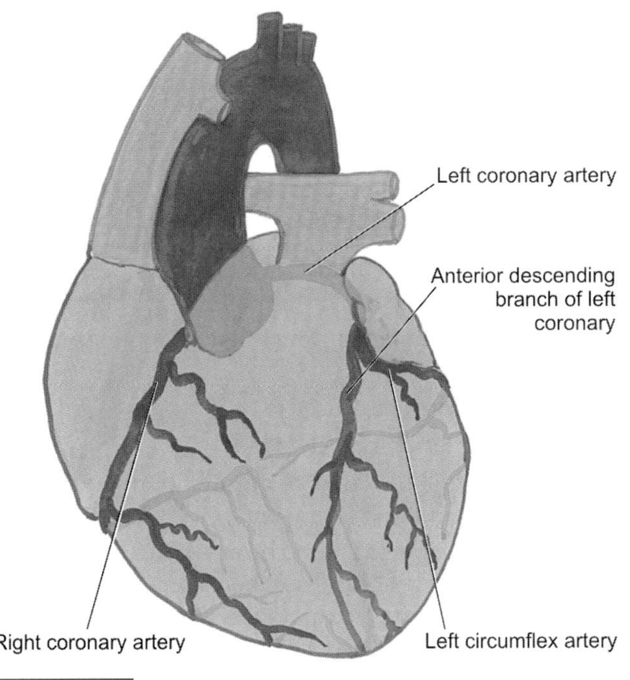

FIGURE 12.2

Distribution of blood supply to the heart.

coronary arteries crosses the crux. *Crux* is the region on the posterior surface of the heart where all the four cardiac chambers and the interatrial and interventricular septa meet. These patterns are as under:

■ **Right coronary artery preponderance** is the most common pattern. In this, right coronary artery supplies blood to the whole of right ventricle, the posterior half of the interventricular septum and a part of the posterior wall of the left ventricle by crossing the crux.

■ **Balanced cardiac circulation** is the next most frequent pattern. In this, the right and left ventricles receive blood supply entirely from right and left coronary arteries respectively. The posterior part of the interventricular septum is supplied by a branch of the right coronary while the anterior part is supplied by a branch of the left coronary artery.

■ **Left coronary preponderance** is the least frequent pattern. In this, the left coronary artery supplies blood to the entire left ventricle, whole of interventricular septum and also supplies blood to a part of the posterior wall of the right ventricle by crossing the crux.

Coronary veins run parallel to the major coronary arteries to collect blood after the cellular needs of the heart are met. Subsequently, these veins drain into the *coronary sinus*

PATTERNS AND CLASSIFICATION OF HEART DISEASES

For the purpose of pathologic discussion of heart diseases, they are categorised on the basis of *anatomic region involved* and *the functional impairment*. Accordingly, topics on heart diseases are discussed in this chapter under the following headings:

1. Heart failure
2. Congenital heart diseases
3. Ischaemic heart disease
4. Hypertensive heart disease
5. Cor pulmonale
6. Rheumatic fever and rheumatic heart disease
7. Non-rheumatic endocarditis
8. Valvular diseases and deformities
9. Myocardial disease
10. Pericardial disease
11. Tumours of the heart
12. Pathology of cardiac interventions.

It may be mentioned here that pattern of heart diseases in developing and developed countries is distinct due to difference in living standards. In children, valvular diseases are common all over the world, but in developing countries including India, infections, particularly rheumatic valvular disease, is the dominant cause compared to congenital etiology in affluent countries. On the other hand, ischaemic heart disease and hypertensive cardiomyopathy are the major heart diseases in adults in western populations.

HEART FAILURE

Definition

Heart failure is defined as the pathophysiologic state in which impaired cardiac function is unable to maintain an adequate circulation for the metabolic needs of the tissues of the body. It may be *acute* or *chronic*. The term congestive heart failure (CHF) is used for the chronic form of heart failure in which the patient has evidence of congestion of peripheral circulation and of lungs (Chapter 5). CHF is the end-result of various forms of serious heart diseases.

Etiology

Heart failure may be caused by one of the following factors, either singly or in combination:

1. INTRINSIC PUMP FAILURE. The most common and most important cause of heart failure is weakening of the ventricular muscle due to disease so that the heart fails to act as an efficient pump. The various diseases which may culminate in pump failure by this mechanisms are:

i) Ischaemic heart disease

ii) Myocarditis

iii) Cardiomyopathies

iv) Metabolic disorders e.g. beriberi

v) Disorders of the rhythm e.g. atrial fibrillation and flutter.

2. INCREASED WORKLOAD ON THE HEART. Increased mechanical load on the heart results in increased myocardial demand resulting in myocardial failure. Increased load on the heart may be in the form of pressure load or volume load.

i) Increased pressure load may occur in the following states:

a) Systemic and pulmonary arterial hypertension.

b) Valvular disease e.g. mitral stenosis, aortic stenosis, pulmonary stenosis.

c) Chronic lung diseases.

ii) Increased volume load occurs when a ventricle is required to eject more than normal volume of the blood resulting in cardiac failure. This is found in the following conditions:

a) Valvular insufficiency

b) Severe anaemia

c) Thyrotoxicosis

d) Arteriovenous shunts

e) Hypoxia due to lung diseases.

3. IMPAIRED FILLING OF CARDIAC CHAMBERS. Decreased cardiac output and cardiac failure may result from extra-cardiac causes or defect in filling of the heart:

a) Cardiac tamponade e.g. haemopericardium, hydropericardium

b) Constrictive pericarditis.

Types of Heart Failure

Heart failure may be acute or chronic, right-sided or left-sided, and forward or backward failure.

ACUTE AND CHRONIC HEART FAILURE. Depending upon whether the heart failure develops rapidly or slowly, it may be acute or chronic.

Acute heart failure. Sudden and rapid development of heart failure occurs in the following conditions:

i) Larger myocardial infarction

ii) Valve rupture

iii) Cardiac tamponade

iv) Massive pulmonary embolism

v) Acute viral myocarditis

vi) Acute bacterial toxaemia.

In acute heart failure, there is sudden reduction in cardiac output resulting in systemic hypotension but oedema does not occur and a state of cardiogenic shock and cerebral hypoxia develops.

Chronic heart failure. More often, heart failure develops slowly as observed in the following states:

i) Myocardial ischaemia from atherosclerotic coronary artery disease

ii) Multivalvular heart disease

iii) Systemic arterial hypertension

iv) Chronic lung diseases resulting in hypoxia and pulmonary arterial hypertension

v) Progression of acute into chronic failure.

In chronic heart failure, compensatory mechanisms like tachycardia, cardiac dilatation and cardiac hypertrophy try to make adjustments so as to maintain adequate cardiac output. This often results in well-maintained arterial pressure and there is accumulation of oedema.

LEFT-SIDED AND RIGHT-SIDED HEART FAILURE. Though heart as an organ eventually fails as a whole, but functionally, the left and right heart act as independent units. From clinical point of view, therefore, it is helpful to consider failure of the left and right heart separately. The clinical manifestations of heart failure result from the accumulation of excess fluid *upstream* to the left or right cardiac chamber whichever is initially affected (Fig. 12.3).

Left-sided heart failure. Left-sided heart failure is initiated by stress to the left heart. The major causes are:

i) Systemic hypertension

ii) Mitral or aortic valve disease (stenosis)

iii) Ischaemic heart disease

iv) Myocardial diseases e.g. cardiomyopathies, myocarditis.

v) Restrictive pericarditis.

The clinical manifestations of left-sided heart failure result from accumulation of fluid *upstream* in the lungs and from decreased left ventricular output. Accordingly, the major pathologic changes are as under:

i) Pulmonary congestion and oedema causing dyspnoea and orthopnoea (Chapter 5).

ii) Decreased left ventricular output causing hypoperfusion and diminished oxygenation of tissues e.g. in kidneys causing ischaemic acute tubular necrosis

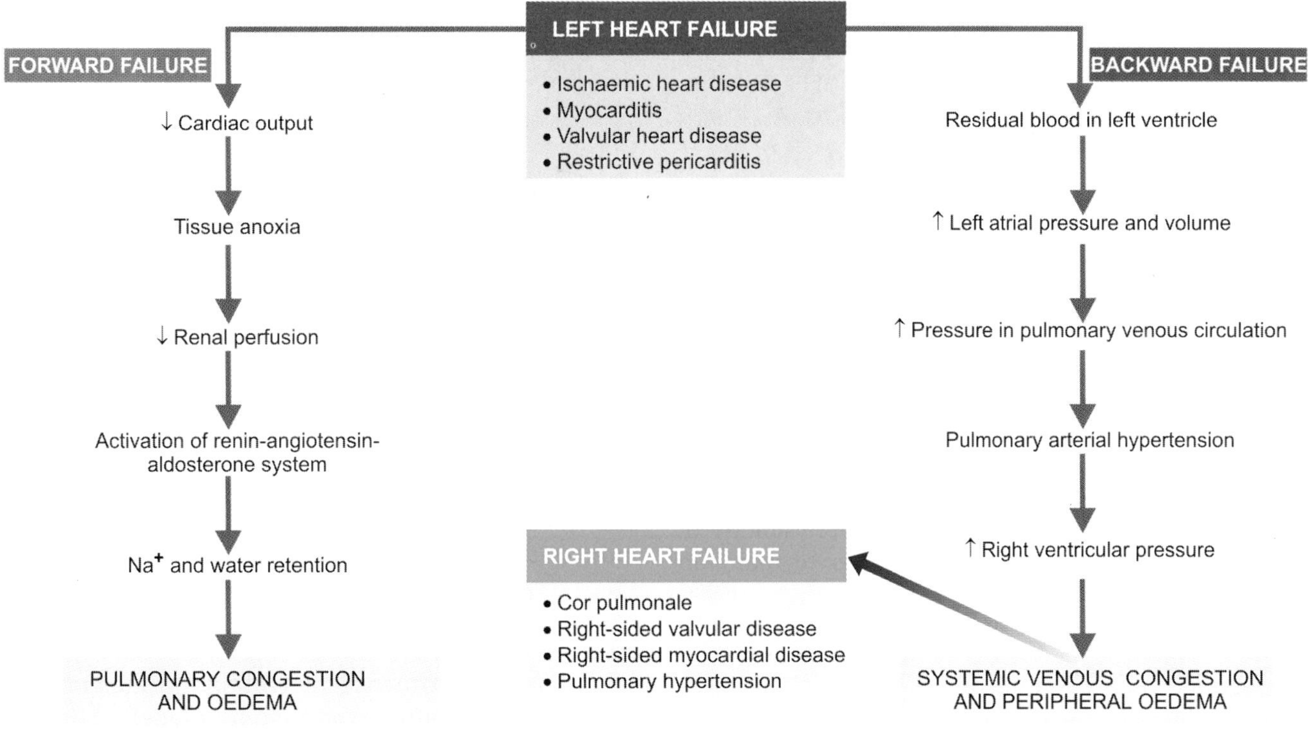

FIGURE 12.3

Schematic evolution of congestive heart failure and its effects.

(Chapter 20), in brain causing hypoxic encephalopathy (Chapter 28), and in skeletal muscles causing muscular weakness and fatigue.

Right-sided heart failure. Right-sided heart failure occurs more often as a consequence of left-sided heart failure. However, some conditions affect the right ventricle primarily, producing right-sided heart failure. These are as follows:

i) As a consequence of left ventricular failure.

ii) Cor pulmonale in which right heart failure occurs due to intrinsic lung diseases (Chapter 15).

iii) Pulmonary or tricuspid valvular disease.

iv) Pulmonary hypertension secondary to pulmonary thromboembolism.

v) Myocardial disease affecting right side.

vi) Congenital heart disease with left-to-right shunt.

Whatever be the underlying cause, the clinical manifestations of right-sided heart failure are *upstream* of the right heart such as systemic and portal venous congestion, and reduced cardiac output. Accordingly, the pathologic changes are as under:

i) Systemic venous congestion in different tissues and organs e.g. subcutaneous oedema on dependent parts, passive congestion of the liver, spleen, and kidneys (Chapter 5), ascites, hydrothorax, congestion of leg veins and neck veins.

ii) Reduced cardiac output resulting in circulatory stagnation causing anoxia, cyanosis and coldness of extremities.

In summary, in early stage the left heart failure manifests with features of pulmonary congestion and decreased left ventricular output, while the right heart failure presents with systemic venous congestion and involvement of the liver and spleen. CHF, however, combines the features of both left and right heart failure. A schematic summary of evolution of CHF is presented in Fig. 12.3.

BACKWARD AND FORWARD HEART FAILURE. The mechanism of clinical manifestations resulting from heart failure can be explained on the basis of mutually interdependent backward and forward failure.

Backward heart failure. According to this concept, either of the ventricles fails to eject blood normally, resulting in rise of end-diastolic volume in the ventricle and increase in volume and pressure in the atrium which is transmitted *backward* producing elevated pressure in the veins.

Forward heart failure. According to this hypothesis, clinical manifestations result directly from failure of the heart to pump blood causing diminished flow of blood to the tissues, especially diminished renal perfusion and activation of renin-angiotensin-aldosterone system.

Compensatory Mechanisms: Cardiac Hypertrophy and Dilatation

In order to maintain normal cardiac output , several compensatory mechanisms play a role. These include:

■ Compensatory enlargement in the form of *cardiac hypertrophy, cardiac dilatation, or both.*

■ *Tachycardia* (i.e. increased heart rate) due to activation of neurohumoral system e.g. release of norepinephrine and atrial natrouretic peptide, activation of renin-angiotensin-aldosterone mechanism.

According to *Starling's law* on pathophysiology of heart, the failing dilated heart, in order to maintain cardiac performance, increases the myocardial contractility and thereby attempts to maintain stroke volume. This is achieved by increasing the length of sarcomeres in dilated heart. Ultimately, however, dilatation decreases the force of contraction and leads to residual volume in the cardiac chambers causing volume overload and thus cardiac failure supervenes that ends in death (Fig. 12.4).

Cardiac Hypertrophy

Hypertrophy of the heart is defined as an increase in size and weight of the myocardium. It generally results from increased pressure load while increased volume load (e.g. valvular incompetence) results in hypertrophy with dilatation of the affected chamber due to regurgitation of the blood through incompetent valve. The atria may also undergo compensatory changes due to increased workload.

The basic factors that stimulate the hypertrophy of the myocardial fibres are not known. It appears that stretching of myocardial fibres in response to stress induces the cells to increase in length. The elongated fibres receive better nutrition and thus increase in size. Other factors which may stimulate increase in size of myocardial fibres are anoxia (e.g. in coronary atherosclerosis) and influence of certain hormones (e.g. catecholamines, pituitary growth hormone).

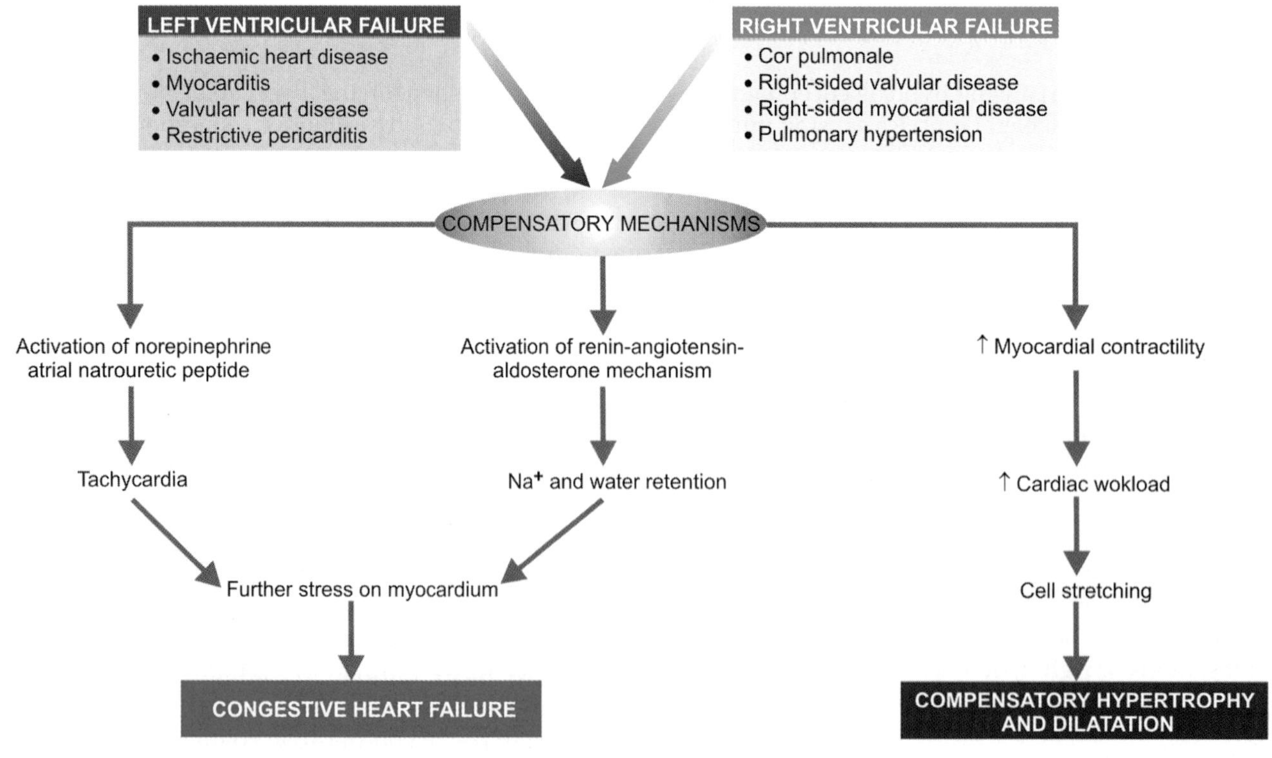

FIGURE 12.4

Schematic pathophysiology of compensatory mechanisms in cardiac failure.

CAUSES. Hypertrophy with or without dilatation may involve predominantly the left or the right heart, or both sides.

Left ventricular hypertrophy. The common causes of left ventricular hypertrophy are:

i) Systemic hypertension
ii) Aortic stenosis and insufficiency
iii) Mitral insufficiency
iv) Coarctation of the aorta
v) Occlusive coronary artery disease
vi) Congenital anomalies like septal defects and patent ductus arteriosus
vii) Conditions with increased cardiac output e.g. thyrotoxicosis, anaemia, arteriovenous fistulae.

Right ventricular hypertrophy. Most of the causes of right ventricular hypertrophy are due to pulmonary arterial hypertension. These are:

i) Pulmonary stenosis and insufficiency
ii) Tricuspid insufficiency
iii) Mitral stenosis and/or insufficiency
iv) Chronic lung diseases e.g. chronic emphysema, bronchiectasis, pneumoconiosis, pulmonary vascular disease etc.
v) Left ventricular hypertrophy and failure of the left ventricle.

Cardiac Dilatation

Quite often, hypertrophy of the heart is accompanied by cardiac dilatation. Stress leading to accumulation of excessive volume of blood in a chamber of the heart causes increase in length of myocardial fibres and hence cardiac dilatation as a compensatory mechanism.

CAUSES. Causes of accumulation of excessive volume of blood within the cardiac chambers may result in dilatation of the respective ventricles or both. These are:

i) Valvular insufficiency (mitral and/or aortic insufficiency in left ventricular dilatation, tricuspid and/or pulmonary insufficiency in right ventricular dilatation)
ii) Left-to-right shunts e.g. in VSD
iii) Conditions with high cardiac output e.g. thyrotoxicosis, arteriovenous shunt
iv) Myocardial diseases e.g. cardiomyopathies, myocarditis
v) Systemic hypertension.

PATHOLOGIC CHANGES. Hypertrophy of the myocardium without dilatation is referred to as *concentric,* and when associated with dilatation is called *eccentric* (Fig. 12.5). The weight of the heart is increased above the normal, often over 500 gm. However, excessive epicardial fat is not indicative of true hypertrophy.

Grossly, The thickness of the left ventricular wall (excluding trabeculae carneae and papillary muscles) above 15 mm is indicative of significant hypertrophy. In concentric hypertrophy, the lumen of the chamber is smaller than usual, while in eccentric hypertrophy the lumen is dilated. In pure hypertrophy, the papillary muscles and trabeculae carneae are rounded and enlarged, while in hypertrophy with dilatation these are flattened.

Microscopically, there is increase in size of individual muscle fibres. There may be multiple minute foci of degenerative changes and necrosis in the

Chapter Twelve

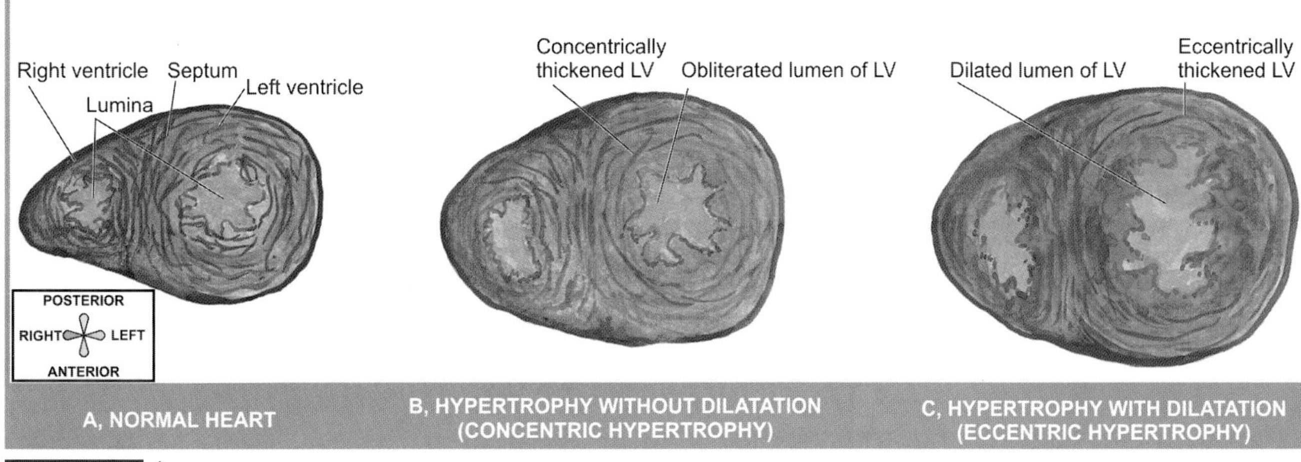

FIGURE 12.5

Transverse section through the ventricles showing left ventricular hypertrophy.

hypertrophied myocardium. These changes appear to arise as a result of relative hypoxia of the hypertrophied muscle as the blood supply is inadequate to meet the demands of the increased fibre size. Ventricular hypertrophy renders the inner part of the myocardium more liable to ischaemia.

Electron microscopy reveals increase in the number of myofilaments comprising myofibrils, mitochondrial changes and multiple intercalated discs which are active sites for the formation of new sarcomeres. Besides, the nucleic acid content determinations have shown increase in total RNA and increased ratio of RNA to DNA content of the hypertrophied myocardial fibres.

CONGENITAL HEART DISEASE

Congenital heart disease is the abnormality of the heart present from birth. It is the most common and important form of heart disease in the early years of life and is present in about 0.5% of newborn children. The incidence is higher in premature infants. The cause of congenital heart disease is unknown in majority of cases. It is attributed to multifactorial inheritance involving genetic and environmental influences. Other factors like rubella infection to the mother during pregnancy, drugs taken by the mother and heavy alcohol drinking by the mother have all been implicated in causing *in utero* injury resulting in congenital malformations of the heart.

CLASSIFICATION. Congenital anomalies of the heart may be either *shunts* (left-to-right or right-to-left), or defects causing *obstructions* to flow. However, complex anomalies involving *combinations* of shunts and obstructions are also often present.

A simple classification of important and common examples of these groups is given in Table 12.1.

TABLE 12.1: Classification of Congenital Heart Diseases.

I. MALPOSITIONS OF THE HEART	
II. SHUNTS (CYANOTIC CONGENITAL HEART DISEASE)	
A. Left-to-right shunts (Acyanotic or late cyanotic group)	
1. Ventricular septal defect (VSD)	(25-30%)
2. Atrial septal defect (ASD)	(10-15%)
3. Patent ductus arteriosus (PDA)	(10-20%)
B. Right-to-left shunts (Cyanotic group)	
1. Tetralogy of Fallot	(6-15%)
2. Transposition of great arteries	(4-10%)
3. Persistent truncus arteriosus	(2%)
4. Tricuspid atresia and stenosis	(1%)
III. OBSTRUCTIONS (OBSTRUCTIVE CONGENITAL HEART DISEASE)	
1. Coarctation of aorta	(5-7%)
2. Aortic stenosis and atresia	(4-6%)
3. Pulmonary stenosis and atresia	(5-7%)

I. MALPOSITIONS OFTHE HEART

Dextrocardia is the condition when the apex of the heart points to the right side of the chest. It may be accompanied by situs inversus so that all other organs of the body are also transposed in similar way and thus heart is in normal position in relation to them. However, isolated dextrocardia is associated with major anomalies of the heart such as transposition of the atria in relation to ventricles or transposition of the great arteries.

II. SHUNTS (CYANOTIC CONGENITAL HEART DISEASE)

A shunt may be left-to-right side or right-to-left side of the circulation.

A. Left-to-Right Shunts (Acyanotic or Late Cyanotic Group)

In conditions where there is shunting of blood from left-to-right side of the heart there is volume overload on the right heart producing pulmonary hypertension and right ventricular hypertrophy. At a later stage, the pressure on the right side is higher than on the left side creating late cyanotic heart disease. The important conditions included in this category are described below:

1. VENTRICULAR SEPTAL DEFECT (VSD). VSD is the most common congenital anomaly of the heart and comprises about 30% of all congenital heart diseases. The condition is recognised early in life. The smaller defects often close spontaneously, while larger defects remain patent and produce significant effects.

Depending upon the location of the defect, VSD may be of the following types:

1. In 90% of cases, the defect involves *membranous septum* and is very close to the bundle of His (Fig. 12.6).
2. The remaining 10% cases have VSD immediately below the pulmonary valve (*subpulmonic*), below the aortic valve (*subaortic*), or exist in the form of multiple defects in the muscular septum.

The ***effects*** of VSD are produced due to left-to-right shunt at the ventricular level, increased pulmonary flow and increased volume in the left side of the heart. These effects are:

i) Volume hypertrophy of the right ventricle.

ii) Enlargement and haemodynamic changes in the tricuspid and pulmonary valves.

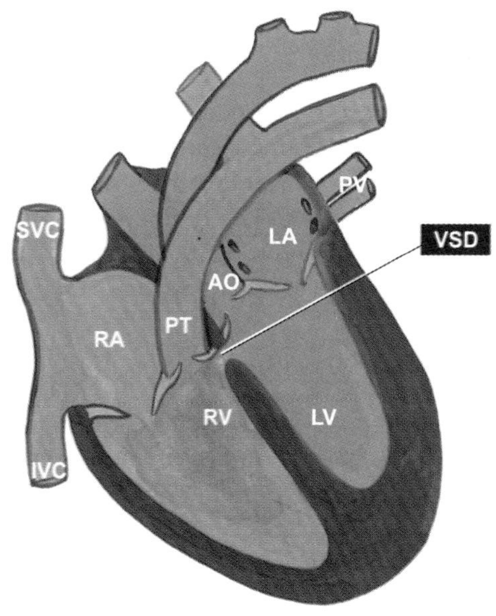

FIGURE 12.6

Ventricular septal defect, a schematic representation (LA = Left atrium; LV = Left ventricle; AO = Aorta; PV = Pulmonary valve; PT = Pulmonary trunk; RA = Right atrium; RV = Right ventricle; SVC = Superior vena cava; IVC = Inferior vena cava).

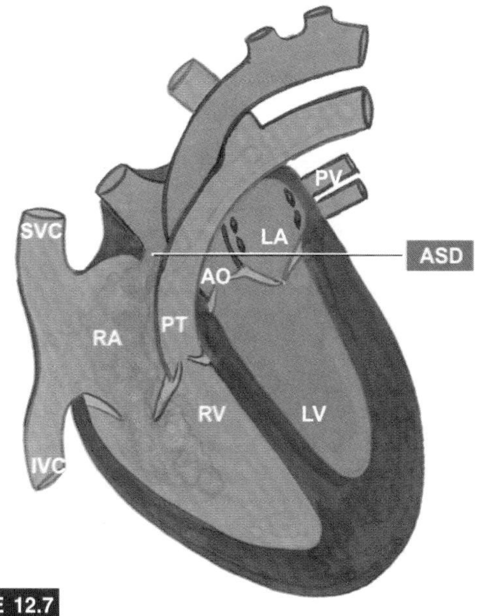

FIGURE 12.7

Atrial septal defect fossa ovalis type, a schematic representation (LA = Left atrium; LV = Left ventricle; PV = Pulmonary vein; AO = Aorta; PT = Pulmonary trunk; RA = Right atrium; RV = Right ventricle; SVC = Superior vena cava; IVC = Inferior vena cava).

iii) Endocardial hypertrophy of the right ventricle.

iv) Pressure hypertrophy of the right atrium.

v) Volume hypertrophy of the left atrium and left ventricle.

vi) Enlargement and haemodynamic changes in the mitral and aortic valves.

2. ATRIAL SEPTAL DEFECT (ASD). Isolated ASD comprises about 10% of congenital heart diseases. The condition remains unnoticed in infancy and childhood till pulmonary hypertension is induced causing late cyanotic heart disease and right-sided heart failure.

Depending upon the location of the defect, there are 3 types of ASD:

i) Fossa ovalis type or ostium secundum type is the most common form comprising about 90% cases of ASD. The defect is situated in the region of the fossa ovalis (Fig. 12.7).

ii) Ostium primum type comprises about 5% cases of ASD. The defect lies low in the interatrial septum adjacent to atrioventricular valves. There may be cleft in the aortic leaflet of the mitral valve producing mitral insufficiency.

iii) Sinus venosus type accounts for about 5% cases of ASD. The defect is located high in the interatrial septum near the entry of the superior vena cava.

The ***effects*** of ASD are produced due to left-to-right shunt at the atrial level with increased pulmonary flow. These effects are:

i) Volume hypertrophy of the right atrium and right ventricle.

ii) Enlargement and haemodynamic changes of tricuspid and pulmonary valves.

iii) Focal or diffuse endocardial hypertrophy of the right atrium and right ventricle.

iv) Volume atrophy of the left atrium and left ventricle.

v) Small-sized mitral and aortic orifices.

3. PATENT DUCTUS ARTERIOSUS (PDA). The ductus arteriosus is a normal vascular connection between the aorta and the bifurcation of the pulmonary artery. Normally, the ductus closes functionally within the first or second day of life. Its persistence after 3 months of age is considered abnormal. The cause for patency of ductus arteriosus is not known but possibly it is due to continued synthesis of PGE_2 after birth which keeps it patent as evidenced by association of PDA with

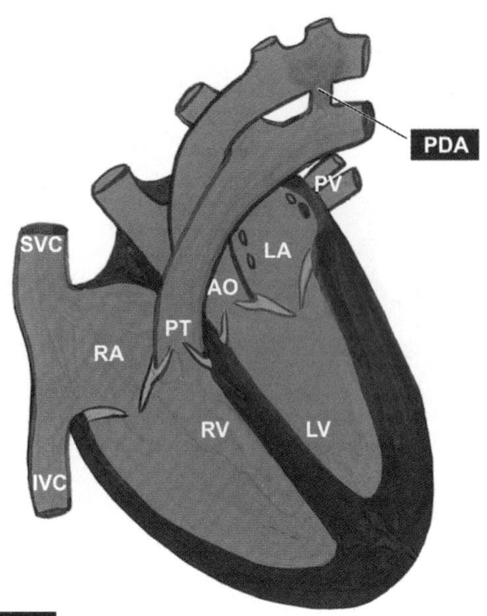

FIGURE 12.8

Patent ductus arteriosus, a schematic representation (LA = Left atrium; LV = Left ventricle; PT = Pulmonary trunk; PV = Pulmonary vein, AO = Aorta; RA = Right atrium; RV = Right ventricle; SVC = Superior vena cava; IVC = Inferior vena cava).

respiratory distress syndrome in infants and pharmacologic closure of PDA with administration of indomethacin to suppress PGE_2 synthesis. PDA constitutes about 10% of congenital malformations of the heart and great vessels. In about 90% of cases, it occurs as an isolated defect, while in the remaining cases it may be associated with other anomalies like VSD, coarctation of aorta and pulmonary or aortic stenosis. A patent ductus may be upto 2 cm in length and upto 1 cm in diameter (Fig. 12.8).

The ***effects*** of PDA on heart occur due to left-to-right shunt at the level of ductus resulting in increased pulmonary flow and increased volume in the left heart. These effects are as follows:

i) Volume hypertrophy of the left atrium and left ventricle.

ii) Enlargement and haemodynamic changes of the mitral and pulmonary valves.

iii) Enlargement of the ascending aorta.

B. Right-to-Left Shunts (Cyanotic Group)

In conditions where there is shunting of blood from right side to the left side of the heart, there is entry of poorly-oxygenated blood into systemic circulation resulting in early cyanosis. The examples described below are not pure shunts but are combinations of shunts with obstructions but are described here since there is functional shunting of blood from one to the other side of circulation.

1. TETRALOGY OF FALLOT. Tetralogy of Fallot is the most common cyanotic congenital heart disease, found in about 10% of children with anomalies of the heart. The four features of tetralogy are (Fig. 12.9):

i) Ventricular septal defect (VSD) *('shunt')*.

ii) Displacement of the aorta to right so that it overrides the VSD.

iii) Pulmonary stenosis *('obstruction')*.

iv) Right ventricular hypertrophy.

The severity of the clinical manifestations is related to two factors: extent of pulmonary stenosis and the size of VSD. Accordingly, there are two forms of tetralogy: cyanotic and acyanotic.

In **cyanotic tetralogy,** pulmonary stenosis is greater and the VSD is mild so that there is more resistance to the outflow of blood from right ventricle resulting in right-to-left shunt at the ventricular level and cyanosis. The ***effects*** on the heart are:

i) Pressure hypertrophy of the right atrium and right ventricle.

ii) Smaller and abnormal tricuspid valve.

iii) Smaller left atrium and left ventricle.

iv) Enlarged aortic orifice.

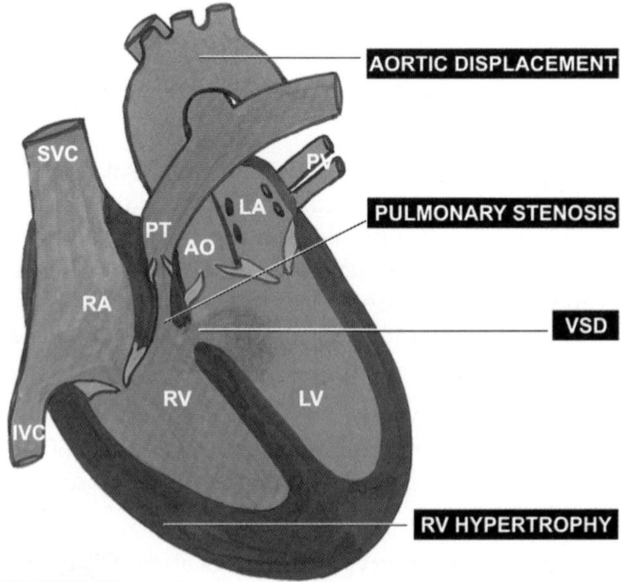

FIGURE 12.9

Tetralogy of Fallot, a schematic representation (LA = Left atrium; LV = Left ventricle; PT = Pulmonary trunk; PV = Pulmonary vein; AO = Aorta; RA = Right atrium; RV = Right ventricle; SVC = Superior vena cava; IVC = Inferior vena cava).

In **acyanotic tetralogy,** the VSD is larger and pulmonary stenosis is mild so that there is mainly left-to-right shunt with increased pulmonary flow and increased volume in the left heart but no cyanosis. The ***effects*** on the heart are:

i) Pressure hypertrophy of the right ventricle and right atrium.

ii) Volume hypertrophy of the left atrium and left ventricle.

iii) Enlargement of mitral and aortic orifices.

2. TRANSPOSITION OF GREAT ARTERIES. The term transposition is used for complex malformations as regards position of the aorta, pulmonary trunk, atrioventricular orifices and the position of atria in relation to ventricles. Accordingly, there are several forms of transpositions. The common ones are described below:

i) Regular transposition is the most common type. In this, the aorta which is normally situated to the right and posterior with respect to the pulmonary trunk, is instead displaced anteriorly and to right. In regular complete transposition, the aorta emerges from the right ventricle and the pulmonary trunk from the left ventricle so that there is cyanosis from birth.

ii) Corrected transposition is an uncommon anomaly. There is complete transposition of the great arteries with aorta arising from the right ventricle and the pulmonary trunk from the left ventricle, as well as transposition of the great veins so that the pulmonary veins enter the right atrium and the systemic veins drain into the left atrium. This results in a physiologically corrected circulation.

3. PERSISTENT TRUNCUS ARTERIOSUS. Persistent truncus arteriosus is a rare anomaly in which the arch that normally separates the aorta from the pulmonary artery fails to develop. This results in a single large common vessel receiving blood from the right as well as left ventricle. The orifice may have 3 to 6 cusps. There is often an associated VSD. There is left-to-right shunt and frequently early systemic cyanosis. The prognosis is generally poor.

4. TRICUSPID ATRESIA AND STENOSIS. Tricuspid atresia and stenosis are rare anomalies. There is often associated pulmonary stenosis or pulmonary atresia. In tricuspid atresia, there is absence of tricuspid orifice and instead there is a dimple in the floor of the right atrium. In tricuspid stenosis, the tricuspid ring is small and the valve cusps are malformed. In both the conditions, there is often an interatrial defect through which right-to-left shunt of blood takes place. Children are cyanotic since birth and live for a few weeks or months.

III. OBSTRUCTIONS (OBSTRUCTIVE CONGENITAL HEART DISEASE)

Congenital obstruction to blood flow may result from obstruction in the aorta due to narrowing (*coarctation of aorta*), obstruction to outflow from the left ventricle (*aortic stenosis and atresia*), and obstruction to outflow from the right ventricle (*pulmonary stenosis and atresia*).

1. COARCTATION OF AORTA. The word 'coarctation' means contracted or compressed. Coarctation of aorta is localised narrowing in any part of aorta, but the constriction is more often just distal to ductus arteriosus (*postductal or adult*), or occasionally proximal to the ductus arteriosus (*preductal or infantile type*) in the region of transverse aorta.

i) In **postductal or adult type,** the obstruction is just distal to the point of entry of ductus arteriosus which is often closed (Fig. 12.10). In the stenotic segment, the aorta is drawn in as if a suture has been tied around it. The aorta is dilated on either side of the constriction. The condition is recognised in adulthood, characterised by hypertension in the upper extremities, weak pulses and low blood pressure in the lower extremities and

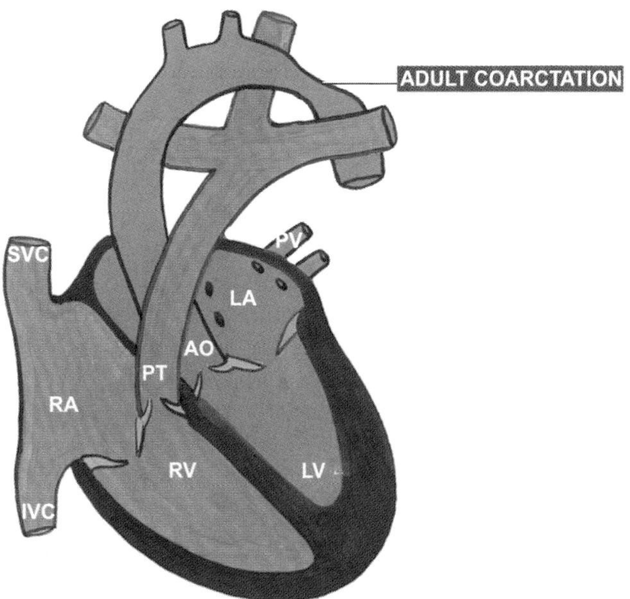

FIGURE 12.10

Postductal or adult type coarctation of the aorta, a schematic representation (LA = Left atrium; LV = Left ventricle; PT = Pulmonary trunk; PV = Pulmonary vein; AO = Aorta; RA = Right atrium; RV = Right ventricle; SVC = Superior vena cava; IVC = Inferior vena cava).

effects of arterial insufficiency such as claudication and coldness. In time, there is development of collateral circulation between pre-stenotic and post-stenotic arterial branches so that intercostal arteries are enlarged and palpable and may produce erosions on the inner surface of the ribs.

ii) In **preductal or infantile type,** the manifestations are produced early in life. The narrowing is proximal to the ductus arteriosus which usually remains patent. The narrowing is generally gradual and involves larger segment of the proximal aorta. There is often associated interatrial septal defect. Preductal coarctation results in right ventricular hypertrophy while the left ventricle is small. Cyanosis develops in the lower half of the body while the upper half remains unaffected since it is supplied by vessels originating proximal to the coarctation. Children with this defect have poor prognosis.

2. AORTIC STENOSIS AND ATRESIA. The most common congenital anomaly of the aorta is bicuspid aortic valve which does not have much functional significance but predisposes it to calcification (Chapter 11). Congenital aortic atresia is rare and incompatible with survival. Aortic stenosis may be acquired (e.g. in rheumatic heart disease, calcific aortic stenosis) or congenital. Congenital aortic stenosis may be of three types: valvular, subvalvular and supravalvular.

i) In **valvular stenosis,** the aortic valve cusps are malformed and are irregularly thickened. The aortic valve may have one, two or three such maldeveloped cusps.

ii) In **subvalvular stenosis,** there is thick fibrous ring under the aortic valve causing subaortic stenosis.

iii) In **supravalvular stenosis,** the most uncommon type, there is fibrous constriction above the sinuses of Valsalva.

In all these cases, there is pressure hypertrophy of the left ventricle and left atrium, and dilatation of the aortic root.

3. PULMONARY STENOSIS AND ATRESIA. Pulmonary stenosis is the commonest form of obstructive congenital heart disease comprising about 7% of all congenital heart diseases. It may occur as a component of tetralogy of Fallot or as an isolated defect. Pulmonary stenosis is caused by fusion of cusps of the pulmonary valve forming a diaphragm-like obstruction to the outflow of blood from the right ventricle and dilatation of the pulmonary trunk.

In **pulmonary atresia,** there is no communication between the right ventricle and lungs so that the blood bypasses the right ventricle through an interatrial septal defect. It then enters the lungs via patent ductus arteriosus.

ISCHAEMIC HEART DISEASE

Ischaemic heart disease (IHD) is defined as acute or chronic form of cardiac disability arising from imbalance between the myocardial supply and demand for oxygenated blood. Since narrowing or obstruction of the coronary arterial system is the most common cause of myocardial anoxia, the alternate term *'coronary artery disease (CAD)'* is used synonymously with IHD. IHD or CAD is the leading cause of death in most industrialised countries (about one-third of all deaths) and somewhat low incidence is observed in the developing countries. Men develop IHD earlier than women and death rates are also slightly higher for men than for women until the menopause.

ETIOPATHOGENESIS

IHD is invariably caused by disease affecting the coronary arteries, the most prevalent being atherosclerosis accounting for more than 90% cases, while other causes are responsible for less than 10% cases of IHD. Therefore, it is convenient to consider the etiology of IHD under three broad headings:

i) coronary atherosclerosis;
ii) superadded changes in coronary atherosclerosis; and
iii) non-atherosclerotic causes.

I. Coronary Atherosclerosis

Coronary atherosclerosis resulting in 'fixed' obstruction is the major cause of IHD in more than 90% cases. The general aspects of atherosclerosis as regards its etiology, pathogenesis and the gross and microscopic features of atherosclerotic lesions have already been dealt with at length in the preceding Chapter 11. Here, a brief account of the pathology of lesions in *atherosclerotic coronary artery disease* is presented.

1. Distribution. Atherosclerotic lesions in coronary arteries are distributed in one or more of the three major coronary arterial trunks, the highest incidence being in the anterior descending branch of the left coronary, followed in decreasing frequency, by the right coronary artery and still less in circumflex branch of the left coronary. About one-third of cases have *single-vessel disease,* most often left anterior descending arterial involvement; another one-third have *two-vessel disease,* and the remainder have *three major vessel disease.*

2. Location. Almost all adults show atherosclerotic plaques scattered throughout the coronary arterial system. However, significant stenotic lesions that may produce chronic myocardial ischaemia show more than 75% (three-fourth) reduction in the cross-sectional area of a coronary artery or its branch. The area of severest involvement is about 3 to 4 cm from the coronary ostia, more often at or near the bifurcation of the arteries, suggesting the role of haemodynamic forces in atherogenesis.

3. Fixed atherosclerotic plaques. The atherosclerotic plaques in the coronaries are more often eccentrically located bulging into the lumen from one side (COLOUR PLATE XIII: CL 50). Occasionally, there may be concentric thickening of the wall of the artery. Atherosclerosis produces gradual luminal narrowing that may eventually lead to 'fixed' coronary obstruction. The general features of atheromas of coronary arteries are similar to those affecting elsewhere in the body and may develop similar complications like calcification, coronary thrombosis, ulceration, haemorrhage, rupture and aneurysm formation.

II. Superadded Changes in Coronary Atherosclerosis

The attacks of *acute coronary syndromes,* namely acute myocardial infarction, unstable angina and sudden ischaemic death, are precipitated by certain changes superimposed on a pre-existing fixed coronary atheromatous plaque. These are as under:

1. Acute changes in chronic atheromatous plaque. Though chronic fixed obstructions are the most frequent cause of IHD, acute coronary episodes are often precipitated by sudden changes in chronic plaques such as plaque haemorrhage, fissuring, or ulceration that results in embolisation of atheromatous debris. Acute plaque changes are brought about by factors such as sudden coronary artery spasm, tachycardia, intraplaque haemorrhage and hypercholesterolaemia.

2. Coronary artery thrombosis. Transmural acute myocardial infarction is often precipitated by partial or complete coronary thrombosis. The initiation of thrombus occurs due to surface ulceration of fixed chronic atheromatous plaque, ultimately causing complete luminal occlusion. The lipid core of plaque, in particular, is highly thrombogenic. Small fragments of thrombotic material are then dislodged which are embolised to terminal coronary branches and cause microinfarcts of the myocardium.

3. Local platelet aggregation and coronary artery spasm. Some cases of acute coronary episodes are caused by local aggregates of platelets on the atheromatous plaque, short of forming a thrombus. The aggregated platelets release vasospasmic mediators such as thromboxane A_2 which may probably be responsible for coronary vasospasm in the already atherosclerotic vessel.

III. Non-atherosclerotic Causes

A number of other lesions may cause IHD in less than 10% of cases. These are as under:

1. Vasospasm. It has been possible to document vasospasm of one of the major coronary arterial trunks in patients with no significant atherosclerotic coronary narrowing which may cause angina or myocardial infarction.

2. Stenosis of coronary ostia. Coronary ostial narrowing may result from extension of syphilitic aortitis or from aortic atherosclerotic plaques encroaching on the opening.

3. Arteritis. Various types of inflammatory involvements of coronary arteries or small branches like in rheumatic arteritis, polyarteritis nodosa, thromboangiitis obliterans (Buerger's disease), Takayasu's disease, Kawasaki's disease, tuberculosis and other bacterial infections may contribute to myocardial damage.

4. Embolism. Rarely, emboli originating from elsewhere in the body may occlude the left coronary artery and its branches and produce IHD. The emboli may originate from bland thrombi, or from vegetations of bacterial endocarditis; rarely fat embolism and air embolism of coronary circulation may occur.

5. Thrombotic diseases. Another infrequent cause of coronary occlusion is from hypercoagulability of the blood such as in shock, polycythaemia vera, sickle cell anaemia and thrombotic thrombocytopenic purpura.

6. Trauma. Contusion of a coronary artery from penetrating injuries may produce thrombotic occlusion.

7. Aneurysms. Extension of dissecting aneurysm of the aorta into the coronary artery may produce thrombotic coronary occlusion. Rarely, congenital, mycotic and syphilitic aneurysms may occur in coronary arteries and produce similar occlusive effects.

8. Compression. Compression of a coronary from outside by a primary or secondary tumour of the heart may result in coronary occlusion.

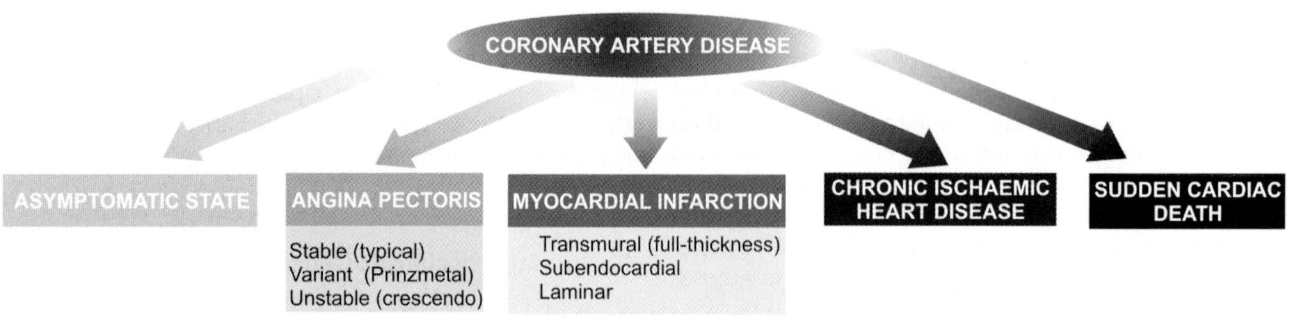

FIGURE 12.11

Spectrum of coronary ischaemic manifestations.

EFFECTS OF MYOCARDIAL ISCHAEMIA

Development of lesions in the coronaries is not always accompanied by cardiac disease. Depending upon the suddenness of onset, duration, degree, location and extent of the area affected by myocardial ischaemia, the range of changes and clinical features may vary from an asymptomatic state at one extreme to immediate mortality at another (Fig. 12.11):

A. *Asymptomatic state*

B. Angina pectoris (AP)

C. Acute myocardial infarction (AMI)

D. Chronic ischaemic heart disease (CIHD)/ Ischaemic cardiomyopathy/ Myocardial fibrosis

E. *Sudden cardiac death*

The term *acute coronary syndromes* include a triad of acute myocardial infarction, unstable angina and sudden cardiac death.

ANGINA PECTORIS

Angina pectoris is a clinical syndrome of IHD resulting from transient myocardial ischaemia. It is characterised by paroxysmal pain in the substernal or precordial region of the chest which is aggravated by an increase in the demand of the heart and relieved by a decrease in the work of the heart. Often, the pain radiates to the left arm, neck, jaw or right arm.

There are 3 overlapping clinical patterns of angina pectoris with some differences in their pathogenesis:

i) Stable or typical angina

ii) Prinzmetal's variant angina

iii) Unstable or crescendo angina

STABLE OR TYPICAL ANGINA. This is the most common pattern. Stable or typical angina is characterised by attacks of pain following physical exertion or emotional excitement and is relieved by rest. The pathogenesis of condition lies in *chronic stenosing coronary atherosclerosis* that cannot perfuse the myocardium adequately when the workload on the heart increases. During the attacks, there is depression of ST segment in the ECG due to poor perfusion of the subendocardial region of the left ventricle but there is no elevation of enzymes in the blood as there is no irreversible myocardial injury.

PRINZMETAL'S VARIANT ANGINA. This pattern of angina is characterised by pain at rest and has no relationship with physical activity. The exact pathogenesis of Prinzmetal's angina is not known. It may occur due to *sudden vasospasm* of a coronary trunk induced by coronary atherosclerosis, or may be due to release of humoral vasoconstrictors by mast cells in the coronary adventitia. ECG shows ST segment elevation due to transmural ischaemia. These patients respond well to vasodilators like nitroglycerin.

UNSTABLE OR CRESCENDO ANGINA. Also referred to as 'pre-infarction angina' or 'acute coronary insufficiency', this is the most serious pattern of angina. It is characterised by more frequent onset of pain of prolonged duration and occurring often at rest. It is thus indicative of an impending myocardial infarction. *Multiple factors* are involved in its pathogenesis which include: stenosing coronary atherosclerosis, complicated coronary plaques (e.g. superimposed thrombosis, haemorrhage, rupture, ulceration etc), platelet thrombi over atherosclerotic plaques and vasospasm of coronary arteries. More often, the lesions lie in a branch of the major coronary trunk so that collaterals prevent infarction.

ACUTE MYOCARDIAL INFARCTION

Acute myocardial infarction (AMI) is the most important consequence of coronary artery disease.

Many patients may die within the first few hours of the onset, while remainder suffer from effects of impaired cardiac function. A significant factor that may prevent or diminish the myocardial damage is the development of collateral circulation through anastomotic channels over a period of time. A regular and well-planned exercise programme is likely to encourage good collateral circulation.

INCIDENCE. In industrialised countries, MI accounts for 10-25% of all deaths. Due to the dominant etiologic role of coronary atherosclerosis in MI, the incidence of MI correlates well with the incidence of atherosclerosis in a geographic area.

Age. MI may virtually occur at all ages, though the incidence is higher in the elderly. About 5% of heart attacks occur in young people under the age of 40 years, particularly in those with major risk factors to develop atherosclerosis like hypertension, diabetes mellitus, cigarette smoking, familial hypercholesterolaemia etc.

Sex. Males throughout their life are at a significantly higher risk of developing MI as compared to females. Women during reproductive period have remarkably low incidence of MI, probably due to the protective influence of oestrogen. The use of oral contraceptives is associated with high risk of developing MI. After menopause, this sex difference gradually declines but the incidence of disease among women never reaches that among men of the same age.

ETIOPATHOGENESIS. The etiologic role of severe coronary atherosclerosis (more than 75% compromise of lumen) of one or more of the three major coronary arterial trunks in the pathogenesis of about 90% cases of acute MI is well documented by autopsy studies as well as by coronary angiographic studies. A few notable features in the etiology and pathogenesis of acute MI are considered below:

1. Mechanism of myocardial ischaemia. Myocardial ischaemia is brought about by one or more of the following mechanisms:

i) Diminised coronary blood flow e.g. in coronary artery disease, shock.

ii) Increased myocardial demand e.g. in exercise, emotions.

iii) Hypertrophy of the heart without simultaneous increase of coronary blood flow e.g. in hypertension, valvular heart disease.

2. Role of platelets. Rupture of an atherosclerotic plaque exposes the subendothelial collagen to platelets which undergo aggregation, activation and release reaction. These events contribute to the build-up of the platelet mass that may give rise to emboli or initiate thrombosis.

3. Complicated plaques. Two important complications in coronary atherosclerotic plaques which are frequently encountered are coronary thrombosis and haemorrhage (Chapter 11):

i) *Superimposed coronary thrombosis* is seen in about half the cases of acute MI. Infusion of intracoronary fibrinolysins in the first few hours of development of acute MI in such cases restores blood flow in the blocked vessel in majority of cases.

ii) *Intramural haemorrhage* is found in about one-third cases of acute MI. Haemorrhage and thrombosis may occur together in some cases.

4. Non-atherosclerotic causes. About 10% cases of acute MI are caused by non-atherosclerotic factors such as coronary vasospasm, arteritis, coronary ostial stenosis, embolism, thrombotic diseases, trauma and outside compression as already described.

5. Transmural *versus* subendocardial infarcts. There are some differences in the pathogenesis of the *transmural infarcts* involving the full thickness of ventricular wall and the *subendocardial (laminar) infarcts* affecting the inner subendocardial one-third to half. These are as under (Table 12.2, Fig. 12.12):

i) *Transmural (full thickness) infarcts* are the most common type seen in 95% cases. Critical coronary narrowing (more than 75% compromised lumen) is of great significance in the causation of such infarcts. Atherosclerotic plaques with superimposed thrombosis and intramural haemorrhage are significant in about 90% cases, and non-atherosclerotic causes in the remaining 10% cases.

ii) *Subendocardial (laminar) infarcts* have their genesis in reduced coronary perfusion due to coronary atherosclerosis but without critical stenosis (not necessarily 75% compromised lumen), aortic stenosis or haemorrhagic shock. This is because subendocardial myocardium is normally least well perfused by coronaries and thus is more vulnerable to any reduction in the coronary flow. Superimposed coronary thrombosis is frequently encountered in these cases too, and hence the beneficial role of fibrinolytic treatment in such patients.

TYPES OF INFARCTS. Infarcts have been classified in a number of ways by the physicians and the pathologists:

1. *According to the anatomic region of the left ventricle involved*, they are called anterior, posterior (inferior),

TABLE 12.2: Contrasting Features of Subendocardial and Transmural Infarcts.

	FEATURE	TRANSMURAL INFARCT	SUBENDOCARDIAL INFARCT
1.	*Definition*	Full-thickness, solid	Inner third to half, patchy
2.	*Frequency*	Most frequent (95%)	Less frequent
3.	*Distribution*	Specific area of coronary supply	Circumferential
4.	*Pathogenesis*	> 75% coronary stenosis	Hypoperfusion of myocardium
5.	*Coronary thrombosis*	Common	Rare
6.	*Epicarditis*	Common	None

lateral, septal and circumferential, and their combinations like anterolateral, posterolateral (or inferolateral) and anteroseptal.

2. *According to the degree of thickness of the ventricular wall involved,* infarcts are of two types (Fig. 12.12):

i) Full-thickness or transmural, when they involve the entire thickness of the ventricular wall.

ii) Subendocardial or laminar, when they occupy the inner subendocardial half of the myocardium.

3. *According to the age of infarcts,* they are of two types:

i) Newly-formed infarcts are called acute, recent or fresh.

ii) Advanced infarcts are called old, healed or organised.

LOCATION OF INFARCTS. Infarcts are most frequently located in the left ventricle. Right ventricle is less susceptible to infarction due to its thin wall, having less metabolic requirements and is thus adequately nourished by the thebesian vessels. Atrial infarcts, whenever present, are more often in the right atrium, usually accompanying the infarct of the left ventricle. Left atrium is relatively protected from infarction because it is supplied by the oxygenated blood in the left atrial chamber.

The region of infarction depends upon the area of obstructed blood supply by one or more of the three coronary arterial trunks. Accordingly, there are three regions of myocardial infarction (Fig. 12.13):

1. *Stenosis of the left anterior descending coronary artery* is the most common (40-50%). The region of infarction is the anterior part of the left ventricle including the apex and the anterior two-thirds of the interventricular septum.

2. *Stenosis of the right coronary artery* is the next most frequent (30-40%). It involves the posterior part of the left ventricle and the posterior one-third of the interventricular septum.

3. *Stenosis of the left circumflex coronary artery* is seen least frequently (15-20%). Its area of involvement is the lateral wall of the left ventricle.

PATHOLOGIC CHANGES. The gross and microscopic changes in the myocardial infarction vary according to the age of the infarct and are therefore described sequentially (Table 12.3).

Grossly, most infarcts occur singly and vary in size from 4 to 10 cm. As explained above, they are found most often in the left ventricle. Less often, there are multifocal lesions. The transmural infarcts, which by definition involve the entire thickness of the ventricular wall, usually have a thin rim of preserved subendocardial myocardium which is perfused directly by the blood in the ventricular chamber. The subendocardial infarcts which affect the inner subendocardial half of the myocardium produce less well-defined gross changes than the transmural infarcts. The sequence of macroscopic changes in all myocardial infarcts is as under:

1. *In 6 to 12 hours old infarcts,* no striking gross changes are discernible except that the affected myocardium is slightly paler and drier than normal. However, the early infarcts (3 to 6 hours old) can be detected by histochemical staining for *dehydrogenases* on unfixed slice of the heart. This consists of immersing a slice of unfixed heart in the solution of triphenyltetrazolium chloride (TTC) which imparts red brown colour to the normal heart muscle, while the area of infarcted muscle fails to stain due to lack of dehydrogenases. Another stain for viability of cardiac muscle is nitroblue tetrazolium (NBT) dye which imparts blue colour to unaffected cardiac muscle while infarcted myocardium remains unstained.

2. *By about 24 hours,* the infarct develops cyanotic, red-purple, blotchy areas of haemorrhage due to stagnation of blood.

3. *During the next 48 to 72 hours,* the infarct develops a yellow border due to neutrophilic infiltration and thus becomes more well defined.

4. *In 3-7 days,* the infarct has hyperaemic border while the centre is yellow and soft.

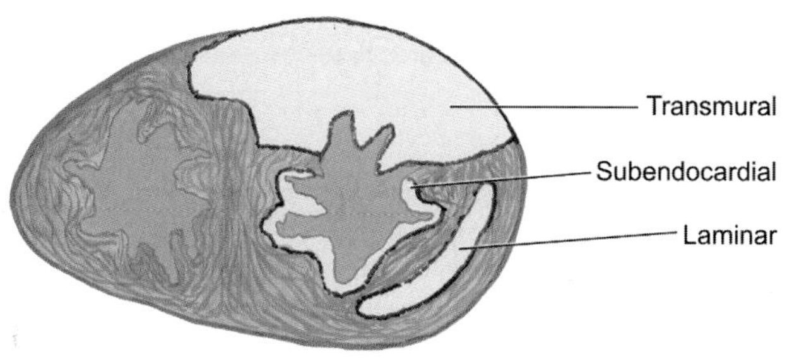

FIGURE 12.12

Diagrammatic representation of extent of myocardial infarction in the depth of myocardium.

5. *By 10 days,* the periphery of the infarct appears reddish-purple due to growth of granulation tissue. With the passage of time, further healing takes place; the necrotic muscle is resorbed and the infarct shrinks and becomes pale grey.

6. *By the end of 6 weeks,* the infarcted area is replaced by a thin, grey-white, hard, shrunken fibrous scar which is well developed in about 2 to 3 months. However, the time taken by an infarct to heal by fibrous scar may vary depending upon the size of the infarct and adequacy of collateral circulation.

Microscopically, the changes are similar in both transmural and subendocardial infarcts. As elsewhere in the body, myocardial ischaemia induces ischaemic coagulative necrosis of the myocardium which eventually heals by fibrosis. However, sequential light microscopic changes are observed as described below and illustrated in Fig. 12.15.

I. First week: The progression of changes takes place in the following way:

i) In the *first 6 hours* after infarction, usually no detectable histologic change is observed in routine light microscopy. However, some investigators have described stretching and waviness of the myocardial fibres within one hour of the onset of ischaemia.

ii) *After 6 hours,* there is appearance of some oedema fluid between the myocardial fibres. The muscle fibres at the margin of the infarct show vacuolar degeneration called myocytolysis.

iii) By *12 hours,* coagulative necrosis of the myocardial fibres sets in and neutrophils begin to appear at the margin of the infarct. Coagulative necrosis of fibres is characterised by loss of striations and intense eosinophilic, hyaline appearance and may show nuclear changes like karyolysis, pyknosis and karyorrhexis. Haemorrhages and oedema are present in the interstitium.

iv) During the *first 24 hours,* coagulative necrosis progresses further as evidenced by shrunken eosinophilic cytoplasm and pyknosis of the nuclei. The neutrophilic infiltrate at the margins of the infarct is slight (Fig. 12.14,A).

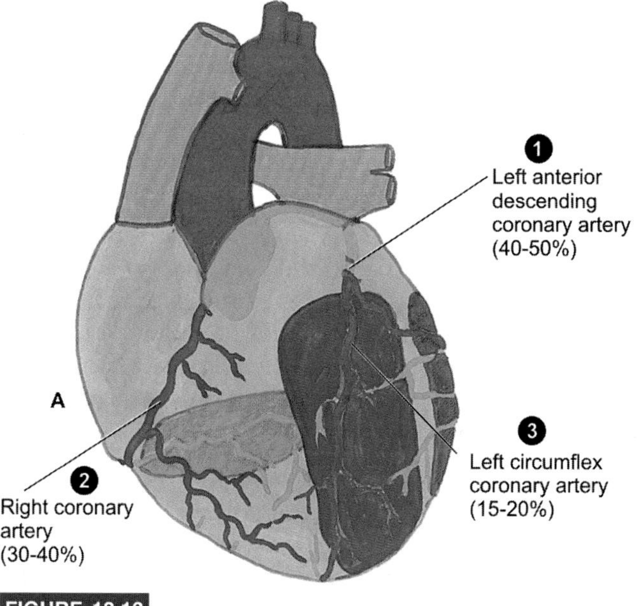

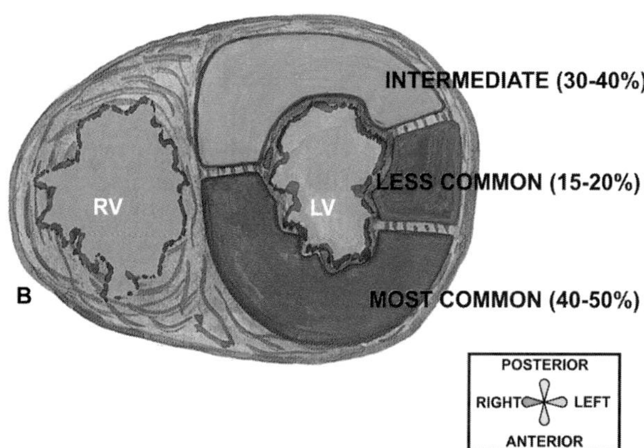

FIGURE 12.13

Common locations and the regions of involvement in myocardial infarction The figure shows region of myocardium affected by stenosis of three respective coronary trunks in descending order shown as: 1) left anterior descending coronary, 2) right coronary and 3) left circumflex coronary artery. A, As viewed from anterior surface. B, As viewed on transverse section at the apex of the heart.

TABLE 12.3: Sequential Pathologic Changes in Myocardial Infarction.

TIME	GROSS CHANGES	LIGHT MICROSCOPY
First week		
0-6 hours	No change or pale; TTC/ NBT test negative in infarcted area	No change; (?) stretching and waviness of fibres
6-12 hours	-do-	Coagulative necrosis begins; neutrophilic infiltration begins; oedema and haemorrhages present
24 hours	Cyanotic red-purple area of haemorrhage	Coagulative necrosis progresses; marginal neutrophilic infiltrate
48-72 hours	Pale, hyperaemic	Coagulative necrosis complete, neutrophilic infiltrate well developed
3-7th day	Hyperaemic border, centre yellow and soft	Neutrophils are necrosed and gradually disappear, beginning of resorption of necrosed fibres by macrophages, onset of fibrovascular response
Second week		
10th day	Red-purple periphery	Most of the necrosed muscle in a small infarct removed; fibrovascular reaction more prominent; pigmented macrophages, eosinophils, lymphocytes, plasma cells present
14th day	—	Necrosed muscle mostly removed; neutrophils disappear; fibrocollagenic tissue at the periphery
Third week	—	Necrosed muscle fibres from larger infarcts removed; more ingrowth of fibrocollagenic tissue
Fourth to sixth week	Thin, grey-white, hard, shrunken fibrous scar	Increased fibrocollagenic tissue, decreased vascularity; fewer pigmented macrophages, lymphocytes and plasma cells

v) During the *first 48 to 72 hours,* coagulative necrosis is complete with loss of nuclei. The neutrophilic infiltrate is well developed and extends centrally into the interstitium (Fig. 12.14,B).

vi) *In 3-7 days,* neutrophils are necrosed and gradually disappear. The process of resorption of necrosed muscle fibres by macrophages begins. Simultaneously, there is onset of proliferation of capillaries and fibroblasts from the margins of the infarct (Fig. 12.14,C) (COLOUR PLATE XV: CL 57).

2. **Second week:** The changes are as under:

i) By *10th day,* most of the necrosed muscle at the periphery of infarct is removed. The fibrovascular reaction at the margin of infarct is more prominent. Many pigmented macrophages containing yellow-brown lipofuscin (derived from breakdown of myocardial cells) and golden brown haemosiderin (derived from lysed erythrocytes in haemorrhagic areas) are seen. Also present are a few other inflammatory cells like eosinophils, lymphocytes and plasma cells.

ii) By the *end of the 2nd week,* most of the necrosed muscle in small infarcts is removed, neutrophils have almost disappeared, and newly laid collagen fibres replace the periphery of the infarct.

3. **Third week:** Necrosed muscle fibres from larger infarcts continue to be removed and replaced by ingrowth of newly formed collagen fibres. Pigmented macrophages as well as lymphocytes and plasma cells are prominent while eosinophils gradually disappear.

4. **Fourth to sixth week:** With further removal of necrotic tissue, there is increase in collagenous connective tissue, decreased vascularity and fewer pigmented macrophages, lymphocytes and plasma cells. Thus, at the end of 6 weeks, a contracted fibrocollagenic scar with diminished vascularity is formed. The pigmented macrophages may persist for a long duration in the scar, sometimes for years.

A summary of the sequence of gross and microscopic changes in myocardial infarction of varying duration is presented in Table 12.3.

SALVAGE IN EARLY INFARCTS AND REPERFUSION INJURY. In vast majority of cases of AMI, occlusive coronary artery thrombosis has been demonstrated superimposed on fibrofatty plaque. The ischaemic injury to myocardium is reversible if perfusion is restored within the first 20-30 minutes of onset of infarction, failing which irreversible ischaemic necrosis of myocardium sets in. The salvage

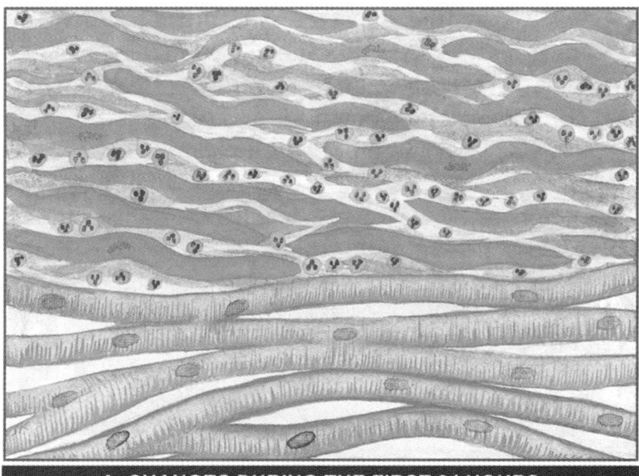

A, CHANGES DURING THE FIRST 24 HOURS

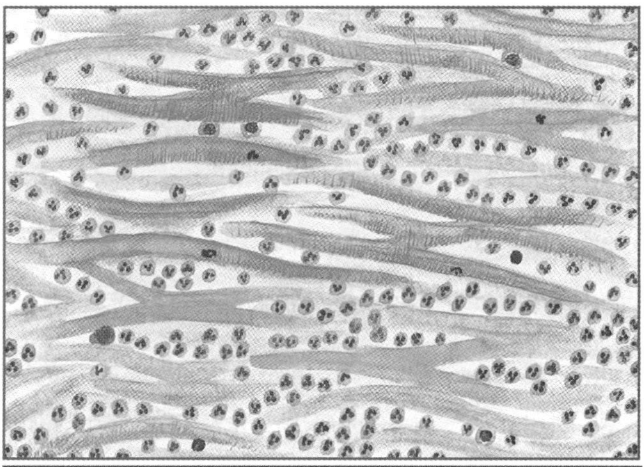

B, CHANGES DURING THE FIRST 48-72 HOURS

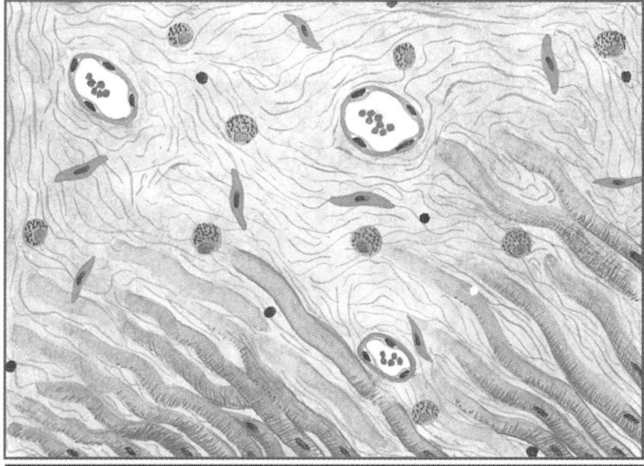

C, CHANGES BY THE END OF FIRST WEEK

FIGURE 12.14

Sequence of light microscopic changes in myocardial infarction.(For details, consult the text).

in early infarcts can be achieved by the following interventions:

1. Institution of *thrombolytic therapy* with thrombolytic agents such as streptokinase and tissue plasminogen activator.
2. *Percutaneous transluminal coronary angioplasty (PTCA).*
3. *Coronary artery stenting.*
4. *Coronary artery bypass surgery.*

However, attempt at reperfusion is fraught with the risk of ischaemic reperfusion injury (Chapter 3). Further myonecrosis during reperfusion is possible due to rapid influx of calcium ions and generation of toxic oxygen free radicals.

PATHOLOGIC CHANGES. Grossly, the myocardial infarct following reperfusion injury appears *haemorrhagic* rather than pale.

Microscopically, myofibres show *contraction band necrosis* which are transverse and thick eosinophilic bands.

CHANGES IN EARLY INFARCTS. By special techniques like electron microscopy, chemical and histochemical studies, changes can be demonstrated in early infarcts before detectable light microscopic alterations appear.

1. Electron microscopic changes. Changes by EM examination are evident in less than half an hour on onset of infarction. These changes are:

i) Disappearance of perinuclear glycogen granules within 5 minutes of ischaemia.

ii) Swelling of mitochondria in 20 to 30 minutes.

iii) Disruption of sarcolemma.

iv) Nuclear alterations like peripheral clumping of nuclear chromatin.

2. Chemical and histochemical changes. Analysis of tissues from early infarcts by chemical and histochemical techniques has shown a number of findings. These are:

i) Glycogen depletion in myocardial fibres within 30 to 60 minutes of infarction.

ii) Increase in lactic acid in the myocardial fibres.

iii) Loss of K^+ from the ischaemic fibres.

iv) Increase of Na^+ in the ischaemic cells.

v) Influx of Ca^{++} into the cells causing irreversible cell injury.

Based on the above observations and on leakage of enzymes from the ischaemic myocardium, alterations in the concentrations of various enzymes are detected in the blood of these patients.

DIAGNOSIS. The diagnosis of acute MI is made on the observations of 3 types of features—clinical features, ECG changes, and serum enzyme determinations.

1. **Clinical features.** Typically, AMI has a sudden onset. The following clinical features usually characterise a case of AMI.

i) *Pain:* Usually sudden, severe, crushing and prolonged, substernal or precordial in location, unrelieved by rest or nitroglycerin, often radiating to one or both the arms, neck and back.

ii) *Indigestion:* Pain is often accompanied by epigastric or substernal discomfort interpreted as 'heartburn' with nausea and vomiting.

iii) *Apprehension:* The patient is often terrified, restless and apprehensive due to great fear of death.

iv) *Shock:* Systolic blood pressure is below 80 mm Hg; lethargy, cold clammy limbs, peripheral cyanosis, weak pulse, tachycardia or bradycardia are often present.

v) *Oliguria:* Urine flow is usually less than 20 ml per hour.

vi) *Low grade fever:* Mild rise in temperature occurs within 24 hours and lasts upto one week, accompanied by leucocytosis and elevated ESR.

vii) *Acute pulmonary oedema:* Some cases develop severe pulmonary congestion due to left ventricular failure and develop suffocation, dyspnoea, orthopnoea and bubbling respiration.

2. **ECG changes.** The ECG changes are one of the most important parameters. Characteristic ECG changes include ST segment elevation, T wave inversion and appearance of wide deep Q waves (Fig. 12.15).

3. **Serum cardiac markers.** Certain proteins and enzymes are released into the blood from necrotic heart muscle after MI. Measurement of their levels in serum is helpful in making a diagnosis and plan management. Rapid assay of some more specific cardiac proteins is now available rendering the estimation of non-specific estimation of SGOT of historical importance only in current practice. Important myocardial markers in use nowadays are as under (Fig. 12.16):

i) *Creatine phosphokinase (CK) and CK-MB:* CK has three forms—

- CK-MM derived from skeletal muscle;
- CK-BB derived from brain and lungs; and
- CK-MB mainly from cardiac muscles and insignificant amount from extracardiac tissue.

Thus total CK estimation lacks specificity while elevation of CK-MB isoenzyme is considerably specific for myocardial damage. CK-MB has further 2 forms—CK-MB2 is the myocardial form while CK-MB1 is extracardiac form. A ratio of CK-MB2: CK-MB1 above 1.5 is highly sensitive for the diagnosis of acute MI after 4-6 hours of onset of myocardial ischaemia. CK-MB disappears from blood by 48 hours.

ii) *Lactic dehydrogenase (LDH).* Total LDH estimation also lacks specificity since this enzyme is present in various tissues besides myocardium such as in skeletal muscle, kidneys, liver, lungs and red blood cells. However, like CK, LDH too has two isoforms of which LDH-1 is myocardial-specific. Estimation of ratio of LDH-1: LDH-2 above 1 is reasonably helpful in making a diagnosis. LDH levels begin to rise after 24 hours, reach peak in 3 to 6 days and return to normal in 14 days.

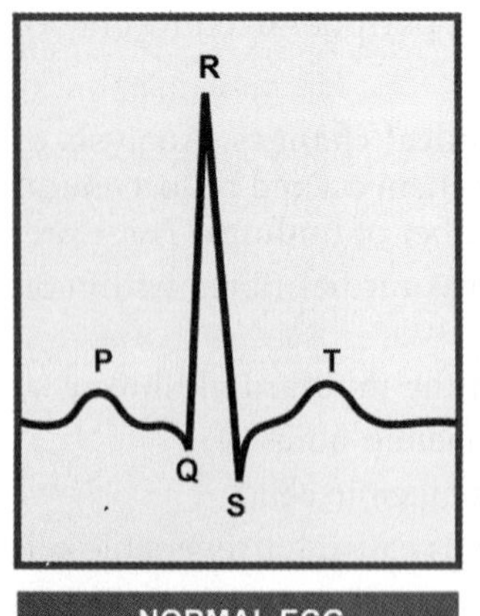

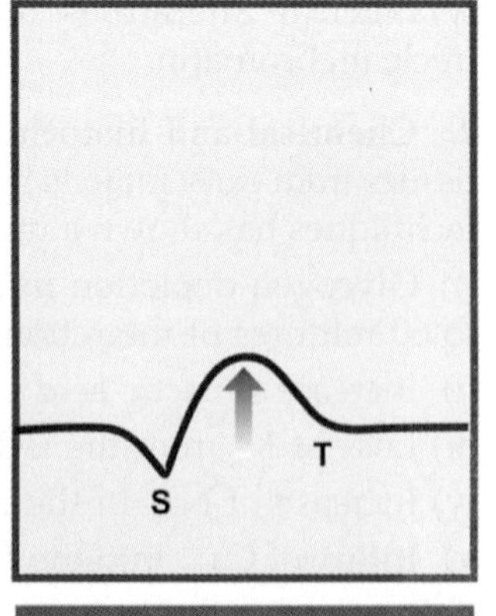

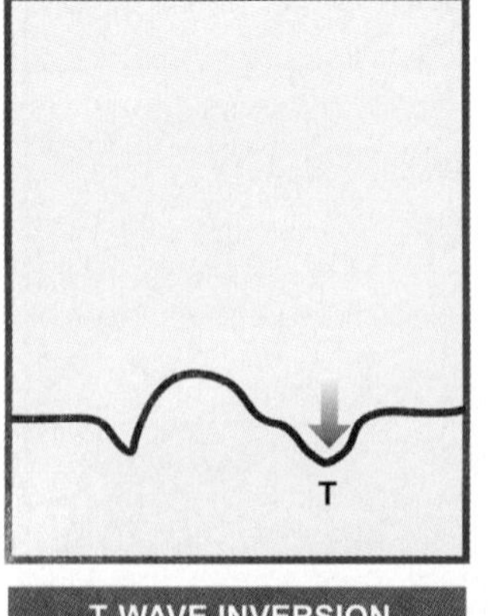

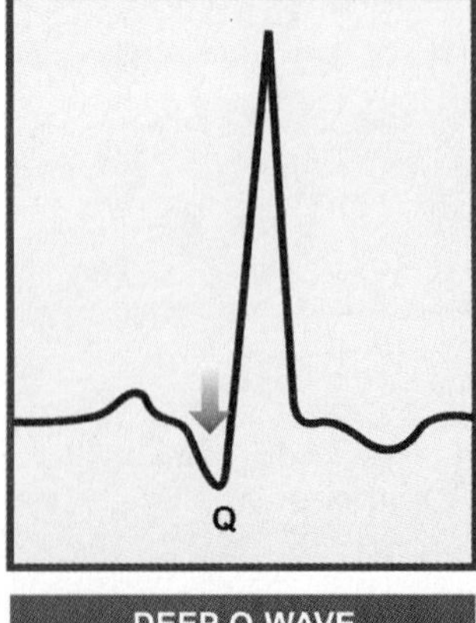

FIGURE 12.15

Some common ECG changes in acute myocardial infarction.

Chapter Twelve

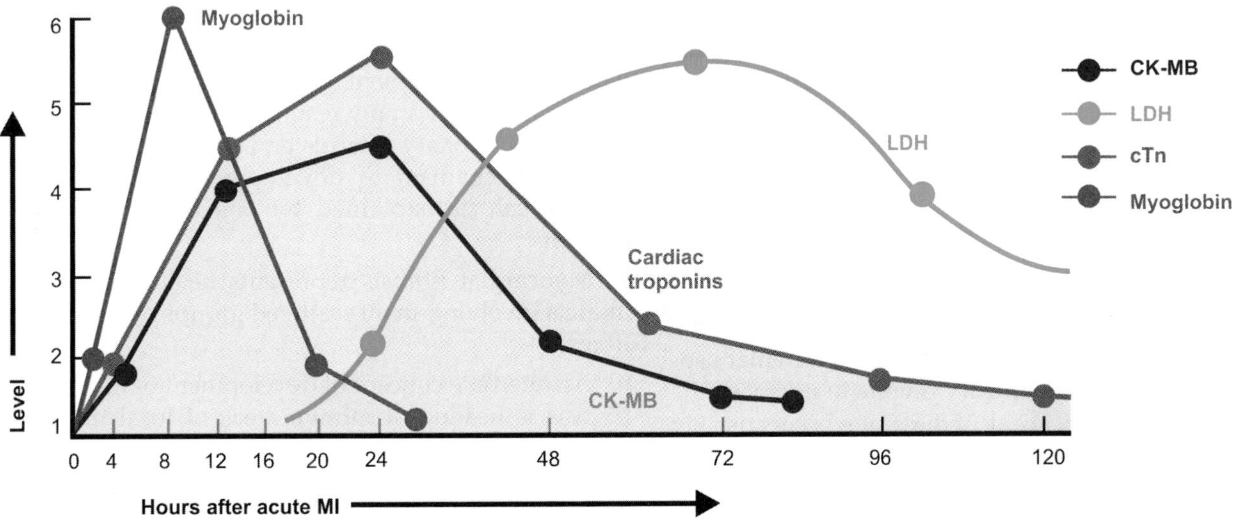

FIGURE 12.16

Time course of serum cardiac markers for the diagnosis of acute MI.

iii) *Cardiac-specific troponins (cTn):* Immunoassay of cTn recently as a new cardiac serum marker has rendered LDH estimation obsolete. Troponins are contractile muscle proteins present in human cardiac and skeletal muscle but cardiac troponins are specific for myocardium. There are two types of cTn:

- cardiac troponin T (cTnT); and
- cardiac troponin I (cTnI).

Both cTnT and cTnI are not found in the blood normally, but after myocardial injury their levels rise very high around the same time when CK-MB is elevated (i.e. after 4-6 hours). Both troponin levels remain high for much longer duration; cTnI for 7-10 days and cTnT for 10-14 days.

iv) *Myoglobin:* Though myoglobin is the first cardiac marker to become elevated after myocardial infarction, it lacks cardiac specificity and is excreted in the urine rapidly. Its levels, thus, return to normal within 24 hours of attack of acute MI.

COMPLICATIONS. Following an attack of acute MI, only 10-20% cases do not develop major complications and recover. The remainder 80-90% cases develop one or more major complications, some of which are fatal. The immediate mortality from acute MI (sudden cardiac death) is about 25%. The important complications which may develop following acute MI are as follows:

1. **Arrhythmias.** Arrhythmias are the most common form of complications in acute MI. These occur due to ischaemic injury or irritation to the conduction system, resulting in abnormal rhythm. Other causes of arrhythmias include leakage of K^+ from ischaemic muscle cells and increased concentration of lactate and free fatty acids in the tissue fluid. Arrhythmias may be in the form of sinus tachycardia or sinus bradycardia, atrial fibrillation, premature systoles, and the most serious ventricular fibrillation responsible for many sudden cardiac deaths.

2. **Congestive heart failure.** About half the patients with MI develop CHF which may be in the form of right ventricular failure, left ventricular failure or both. CHF is responsible for about 40% of deaths from acute MI. If the patient survives, healing may restore normal cardiac function but in some CHF may persist and require regular treatment later.

3. **Cardiogenic shock.** About 10% of patients with acute MI develop cardiogenic shock characterised by hypotension with systolic blood pressure of 80 mmHg or less for many days. Shock may be accompanied by peripheral circulatory failure, oliguria and mental confusion.

4. **Mural thrombosis and thromboembolism.** The incidence of thromboembolism from intracardiac thrombi and from thrombosis in the leg veins is 15-45% in cases of acute MI and is the major cause of death in 12% cases. Mural thrombosis in the heart develops due to involvement of the endocardium and subendocardium in the infarct and due to slowing of the heart rate. Mural

thrombi often form thromboemboli. Another source of thromboemboli is the venous thrombosis in the leg veins due to prolonged bed rest. Thromboemboli from either source may cause occlusion of the pulmonary, renal, mesenteric, splenic, pancreatic or cerebral arteries and cause infarcts in these organs.

5. **Rupture.** Rupture of heart occurs in upto 5% cases of acute MI causing death. Rupture occurs most often from the infarcted ventricular wall into the pericardial cavity causing haemopericardium and tamponade. Other sites of rupture are through interventricular septum and rupture of a papillary muscle in infarct of the left ventricle. Rupture at any of these sites occurs usually in the first week and is often fatal.

6. **Cardiac aneurysm.** Another 5% of patients of MI develop aneurysm, often of the left ventricle. It occurs in healed infarcts through thin, fibrous, non-elastic scar tissue. Cardiac aneurysms impair the function of the heart and are the common sites for mural thrombi. Rarely, calcification of the wall of aneurysm may occur.

7. **Pericarditis.** Sterile pericarditis appearing on about the second day is common over transmural infarcts. It is characterised by fibrinous pericarditis and may be associated with pericardial effusion. Often, it is of no functional significance and resolves spontaneously.

8. **Postmyocardial infarction syndrome.** About 3 to 4% of patients who suffered from acute MI develop postmyocardial infarction syndrome or *Dressler's syndrome* subsequently. It usually occurs 1 to 6 weeks after the attack of MI. It is characterised by pneumonitis. The symptoms are usually mild and disappear in a few weeks. The exact pathogenesis of this syndrome is not known. It may be due to autoimmune reaction as evidenced by circulating anti-heart antibodies in the serum of these patients. But these antibodies are also present in patients with MI who do not develop this syndrome.

CHRONIC ISCHAEMIC HEART DISEASE

Chronic ischaemic heart disease, ischaemic cardiomyopathy or myocardial fibrosis are the terms used for focal or diffuse fibrosis in the myocardium characteristically found in elderly patients of progressive IHD. Such small areas of fibrous scarring are commonly found in the heart of patients who have history of episodes of angina and attacks of MI some years back. The patients generally have gradually developing CHF due to decompensation over a period of years. Occasionally, serious cardiac arrhythmias or infarction may supervene and cause death.

ETIOPATHOGENESIS. In majority of cases, coronary atherosclerosis causes progressive ischaemic myocardial damage and replacement by myocardial fibrosis. A small percentage of cases may result from other causes such as emboli, coronary arteritis and myocarditis.

The mechanism of development of myocardial fibrosis can be explained by one of the following concepts:

i) Myocardial fibrosis represents healing of minute infarcts involving small scattered groups of myocardial fibres.

ii) An alternate concept of development of myocardial fibrosis is healing of minute areas of focal myocytolysis—the myocardial fibres in a small area undergo slow degeneration due to myocardial ischaemia. These fibres lose their myofibrils but nuclei remain intact. These foci are infiltrated by macrophages and eventually are replaced by proliferating fibroblasts and collagen.

PATHOLOGIC CHANGES. Grossly, the heart may be normal in size or hypertrophied. The left ventricular wall generally shows foci of grey-white fibrosis in brown myocardium. Healed scars of previous MI may be present. Valves of the left heart may be distorted, thickened and show calcification. Coronary arteries invariably show moderate to severe atherosclerosis.

Microscopically, the characteristic features are as follows (Fig. 12.17) (COLOUR PLATE XV: CL 58):

i) There are scattered areas of diffuse myocardial fibrosis, especially around the small blood vessels in the interstitial tissue of the myocardium.

ii) Intervening single fibres and groups of myocardial fibres show variation in fibre size and foci of myocytolysis.

iii) Areas of brown atrophy of the myocardium may also be present.

iv) Coronary arteries show atherosclerotic plaques and may have complicated lesions in the form of superimposed thrombosis.

SUDDEN CARDIAC DEATH

Sudden cardiac death is defined as sudden death within 24 hours of the onset of cardiac symptoms. The most important cause is coronary atherosclerosis; less commonly due to coronary vasospasm. Non-ischaemic causes for sudden cardiac death are: calcific aortic stenosis, myocarditis of various types, hypertrophic cardiomyopathy, mitral valve prolapse, endocarditis, and hereditary and acquired defects of the conduction

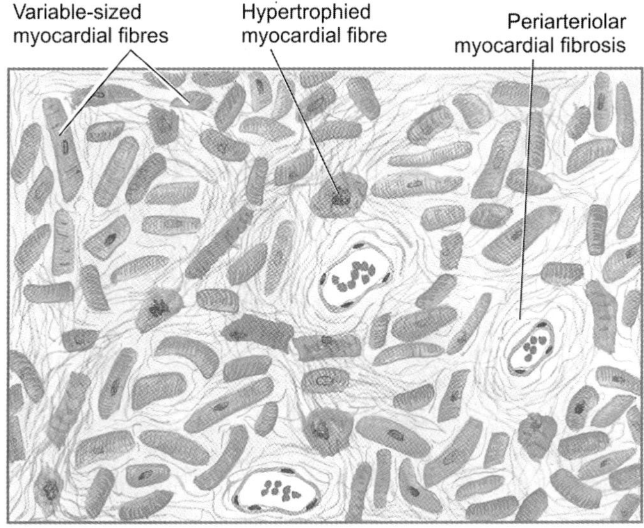

FIGURE 12.17

Chronic ischaemic heart disease. There is patchy myocardial fibrosis, especially around small blood vessels in the interstitium. The intervening single cells and groups of myocardial cells show myocytolysis.

system. The mechanism of sudden death by myocardial ischaemia is almost always by fatal arrhythmias, chiefly ventricular asystole or fibrillation.

PATHOLOGIC CHANGES. At autopsy, such cases reveal most commonly critical atherosclerotic coronary narrowing (more than 75% compromised lumen) in one or more of the three major coronary arterial trunks with superimposed thrombosis or plaque-haemorrhage. Healed and new myocardial infarcts are found in many cases.

Table 12.4 lists the important forms of coronary artery pathology in various types of IHD.

HYPERTENSIVE HEART DISEASE

Hypertensive heart disease or hypertensive cardiomyopathy is the disease of the heart resulting from systemic hypertension of prolonged duration and manifesting by left ventricular hypertrophy. Even mild hypertension (blood pressure higher than 140/90 mm Hg) of sufficient duration may induce hypertensive heart disease. It is the second most common form of heart disease after IHD. As already pointed out, hypertension predisposes to atherosclerosis. Therefore, most patients of hypertensive heart disease have advanced coronary atherosclerosis and may develop progressive IHD. Amongst the causes of death in hypertensive patients, cardiac decompensation leading to CHF accounts for about one-third of the patients; other causes of death are IHD, cerebrovascular stroke, renal failure following arteriolar nephrosclerosis, and dissecting aneurysm of the aorta.

PATHOGENESIS. The pathogenesis of systemic hypertension is discussed later (Chapter 20). Pathogenesis of left ventricular hypertrophy which is most commonly caused by systemic hypertension is described here.

Stimulus to hypertrophy of the left ventricle is pressure overload in systemic hypertension. The stress of pressure on the ventricular wall causes increased

TABLE 12.4: Lesions in Coronary Artery in Various Forms of IHD.

TYPES OF IHD	CORONARY LESION	MORPHOLOGY	CLINICAL EFFECTS
1. *Stable angina*	• Critical coronary narrowing (3/4th)	A, Normal	Nil
2. *Chronic IHD*	• Chronic progressive coronary atherosclerosis		
3. *Unstable (pre-infarction) angina*	• Plaque rupture, haemorrhage, ulceration • Mural thrombosis with thromboembolism	B, Severe, fixed 3/4th narrowing	Stable angina, CIHD
4. *Myocardial infarction*	• Plaque haemorrhage • Fissuring and ulceration • Complete mural thrombosis	C, Thrombosis with haemorrhage	Plaque haemorrhage, unstable angina
5. *Sudden ischaemic death*	• Severe multivessel disease • Acute changes in plaque • Thrombosis with thromboembolism	D, Occlusive thrombosis	Acute coronary syndromes

production of myofilaments, myofibrils, other cell organelles and nuclear enlargement. Since the adult myocardial fibres do not divide, the fibres are hypertrophied. However, the sarcomeres may divide to increase the cell width.

PATHOLOGIC CHANGES. Grossly, the most significant finding is marked hypertrophy of the heart, chiefly of the left ventricle (*see* Fig. 12.5). The weight of the heart increases to 500 gm or more (normal weight about 300 gm). The thickness of the left ventricular wall increases from its normal 13 to 15 mm upto 20 mm or more. The papillary muscles and trabeculae carneae are rounded and prominent. Initially, there is *concentric hypertrophy* of the left ventricle (without dilatation). But when decompensation and cardiac failure supervene, there is *eccentric hypertrophy* (with dilatation) with thinning of the ventricular wall and there may be dilatation and hypertrophy of right heart as well.

Microscopically, the features are not as prominent as macroscopic appearance. The changes include enlargement and degeneration of myocardial fibres with focal areas of myocardial fibrosis. In advanced cases, there may be myocardial oedema and foci of necrosis in the myocardium.

COR PULMONALE

Cor pulmonale (*cor* = heart; *pulmonale* = lung) or pulmonary heart disease is the disease of right side of the heart resulting from disorders of the lungs. It is characterised by right ventricular dilatation or hypertrophy, or both. Thus, cor pulmonale is the right-sided counterpart of the hypertensive heart disease described above.

Depending upon the rapidity of development, cor pulmonale may be acute or chronic:

- *Acute cor pulmonale* occurs following massive pulmonary embolism resulting in sudden dilatation of the pulmonary trunk, conus and right ventricle.
- *Chronic cor pulmonale* is more common and is often preceded by chronic pulmonary hypertension (Chapter 15). The various chronic lung diseases causing chronic pulmonary hypertension and subsequent cor pulmonale are:

i) chronic emphysema;
ii) chronic bronchitis;
iii) pulmonary tuberculosis;
iv) pneumoconiosis;
v) cystic fibrosis;
vi) hyperventilation in marked obesity (Pickwickian syndrome); and
vii) multiple organised pulmonary emboli.

PATHOGENESIS. Chronic lung diseases as well as diseases of the pulmonary vessels cause increased pulmonary vascular resistance and increased pulmonary blood pressure (pulmonary hypertension). Pulmonary hypertension causes pressure overload on the right ventricle and hence right ventricular enlargement. Initially, there is right ventricular hypertrophy, but as cardiac decompensation sets in and right heart failure ensues, dilatation of right ventricle occurs.

The sequence of events involved in the pathogenesis of cor pulmonale is summarised in Fig. 12.18.

PATHOLOGIC CHANGES. In *acute cor pulmonale,* there is characteristic ovoid dilatation of the right ventricle, and sometimes of the right atrium. In *chronic cor pulmonale,* there is increase in thickness of the right ventricular wall from its normal 3 to 5 mm upto 10 mm or more. Often, there is dilatation of the right ventricle too.

RHEUMATIC FEVER AND RHEUMATIC HEART DISEASE

DEFINITION

Rheumatic fever (RF) is a systemic, post-streptococcal, non-suppurative inflammatory disease, principally affecting the heart, joints, central nervous system, skin and subcutaneous tissues. The chronic stage of RF involves all the layers of the heart (pancarditis) causing major cardiac sequelae referred to as rheumatic heart disease (RHD). In spite of its name suggesting an acute arthritis migrating from joint to joint, it is now well known that it is the heart rather than the joints which

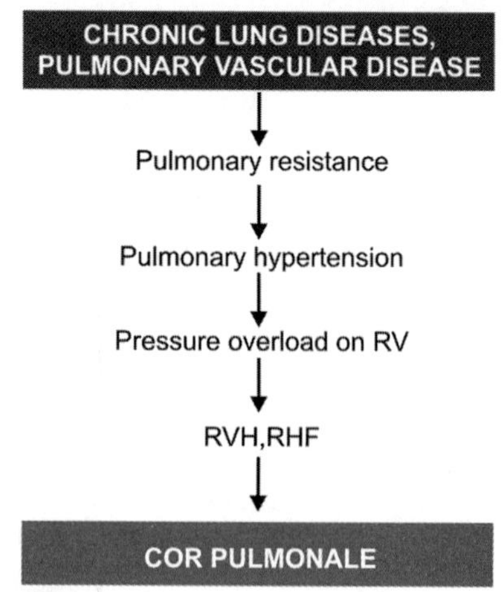

FIGURE 12.18

Pathogenesis of cor pulmonale (RVH= right ventricular hypertrophy, RHF= right heart failure).

is first affected. William Boyd years ago gave the dictum *'rheumatism licks the joint, but bites the whole heart'*.

INCIDENCE

The disease appears most commonly in children between the age of 5 to 15 years when the streptococcal infection is most frequent and intense. Both the sexes are affected equally, though some investigators have noted a slight female preponderance.

The geographic distribution, incidence and severity of RF and RHD are generally related to the frequency and severity of streptococcal pharyngeal infection. The disease is seen more commonly in poor socioeconomic strata of the society living in damp and overcrowded places which promote interpersonal spread of the streptococcal infection. Its incidence has declined in the developed countries as a result of improved living conditions and use of antibiotics in streptococcal infection. But it is still common in the developing countries of the world like in India, Pakistan, some Arab countries, parts of Africa and South America. In India, RHD and RF continue to a major public health problem. In a multicentric survey in school-going children by the Indian Council of Medical Research, an incidence of 1 to 5.5 per 1000 children has been reported.

ETIOPATHOGENESIS

After a long controversy, the etiologic role of preceding throat infection with β-haemolytic streptococci of group A in RF is now generally accepted. However, the mechanism of lesions in the heart, joints and other tissues is not by direct infection but by induction of hypersensitivity or autoimmunity. Thus, there are 2 types of evidences in the etiology and pathogenesis of RF and RHD: the *epidemiologic evidence* and the *immunologic evidence.*

A. EPIDEMIOLOGIC EVIDENCE. There is a body of clinical and epidemiological evidence to support the concept that RF occurs following infection of the throat and upper respiratory tract with β-haemolytic streptococci of Lancefield group A. These evidences are as under:

1. There is often a *history* of infection of the pharynx and upper respiratory tract with this microorganism about 2 to 3 weeks prior to the attack of RF. This period is usually the latent period required for sensitisation to the bacteria.
2. *Subsequent attacks* of streptococcal infection are generally associated with exacerbations of RF.
3. A higher incidence of RF has been observed after outbreaks and *epidemics* of streptococcal infection of throat in children from schools or in youngmen from training camps.
4. Administration of *antibiotics* leads to lowering of the incidence as well as severity of RF and its recurrences.
5. Cardiac lesions similar to those seen in RHD have been produced in experimental animals by *induction* of repeated infection with β-haemolytic streptococci of group A.
6. Patients with RF have *elevated titres* of antibodies to the antigens of β-haemolytic streptococci of group A such as antistreptolysin O (ASO) and S, antistreptokinase, antistreptohyaluronidase and anti- DNAase B.
7. *Socioeconomic factors* like poverty, poor nutrition, density of population, overcrowding in quarters for sleeping etc are associated with spread of infection, lack of proper medical attention, and hence higher incidence of RF.
8. The *geographic distribution* of the disease, as already pointed out, shows higher frequency and severity of the disease in the developing countries of the world where the living conditions are substandard and medical facilities are insufficient. Populations in these regions develop recurrent throat infections which remain untreated and have higher incidence of RF.
9. The role of *climate* in the development of RF has been reported by some workers. The incidence of the disease is higher in subtropical and tropical regions with cold, damp climate near the rivers and water-ways which favour the spread of infection.
10. The *individual susceptibility* to RF and familial incidence have been reported. The factors contributing to proneness to develop RF include adverse social conditions, presence of streptococcal carrier at home and, as yet unclear role of hereditary defect.

Despite all these evidences, only a small proportion of patients with streptococcal pharyngeal infection develop RF—the attack rate is less than 3%. There is a suggestion that a *concomitant virus* enhances the effect of streptococci in individuals who develop RF.

B. IMMUNOLOGIC EVIDENCE. It has ben observed that though throat of patients during acute RF contain streptococci, the clinical symptoms of RF appear after a delay of 2-3 weeks and the organisms can not be grown from the lesions in the target tissues. This has led to the concept that lesions are produced as a result of immune response by formation of autoantibodies against bacteria. A number of components of *Streptococcus* identify or cross-react with target human tissues in RHD i.e. cardiac muscle, valves, joints, skin, neurons etc. One such important component is *M-protein* identified as a surface protein of streptococcus which has various antigenic types, and hence corresponding antibodies in humans which target different tissues. The evidences in support are as under:

1. *Cell wall polysaccharide* of group A streptococcus forms antibodies which are reactive against cardiac valves. This is supported by observation of persistently elevated corresponding autoantibodies in patients who have cardiac valvular involvement than those without cardiac valve involvement.

2. *Hyaluronate capsule* of group A streptococcus is identical to human hyaluronate present in joint tissues and thus these tissues are the target of attack.

3. *Membrane antigens* of group A streptococcus react with sarcolemma of smooth and cardiac muscle, dermal fibroblasts and neurons of caudate nucleus.

PATHOLOGIC CHANGES

RF is generally regarded as an autoimmune focal inflammatory disorder of the connective tissues throughout the body. The *cardiac lesions* of RF in the form of pancarditis, particularly the valvular lesions, are its major manifestations. However, supportive connective tissues at other sites like the synovial membrane, periarticular tissue, skin and subcutaneous tissue, arterial wall, lungs, pleura and the CNS are all affected (*extracardiac lesions*).

A. Cardiac Lesions

The cardiac manifestations of RF are in the form of focal inflammatory involvement of the interstitial tissue of all the three layers of the heart, the so-called *pancarditis*. The pathognomonic feature of pancarditis in RF is the presence of distinctive *Aschoff nodules* or *Aschoff bodies*.

THE ASCHOFF NODULES OR BODIES. The Aschoff nodules or the Aschoff bodies are spheroidal or fusiform distinct tiny structures, 1-2 mm in size, occurring in the interstitium of the heart in RF and may be visible to naked eye. They are especially found in the vicinity of small blood vessels in the myocardium and endocardium and occasionally in the pericardium and the adventitia of the proximal part of the aorta. Lesions similar to the Aschoff nodules may be found in the extracardiac tissues.

Evolution of fully-developed Aschoff bodies involves 3 stages all of which may be found in the same heart at different stages of development. These are as follows:

1. Early (exudative or degenerative) stage. The earliest sign of injury in the heart in RF is apparent by *about 4th week* of illness. Initially, there is oedema of the connective tissue and increase in acid mucopolysaccharide in the ground substance. This results in separation of the collagen fibres by accumulating ground substance. Eventually, the collagen fibres are fragmented and disintegrated and the affected focus takes the appearance and staining characteristics of fibrin. This change is referred to as *fibrinoid degeneration*.

2. Intermediate (proliferative or granulomatous) stage. It is this stage of the Aschoff body which is pathognomonic of rheumatic conditions (Fig. 12.19). This stage is apparent in 4th to 13th week of illness. The early stage of fibrinoid change is followed by proliferation of cells that includes infiltration by lymphocytes (mostly T cells), plasma cells, a few neutrophils and the characteristic *cardiac histiocytes (Anitschkow cells)* at the margin of the lesion. Cardiac histiocytes or Anitschkow cells are present in small numbers in normal heart but their number is increased in the Aschoff bodies; therefore they are not characteristic of RHD. These are large mononuclear cells having central round nuclei and contain moderate amount of amphophilic cytoplasm. The nuclei are vesicular and contain prominent central chromatin mass which in longitudinal section appears serrated or caterpillar-like, while in cross-section the chromatin mass appears as a small rounded body in the centre of the vesicular nucleus, just like an owl's eye (Fig. 12.19, *inbox*). Some of these modified cardiac histiocytes become multinucleate cells containing 1 to 4 nuclei and are called *Aschoff cells* and are pathognomonic of RHD.

3. Late (healing or fibrous) stage. The stage of healing by fibrosis of the Aschoff nodule occurs in about *12 to 16 weeks* after the illness. The nodule becomes oval or fusiform in shape, about 200 μm wide and 600 μm long. The Anitschkow cells in the nodule become spindle-shaped with diminished cytoplasm and the nuclei stain solidly rather than showing vesicular character. These cells tend to be arranged in a palisaded manner. With passage of months and years, the Aschoff body becomes less cellular and the collagenous tissue is increased.

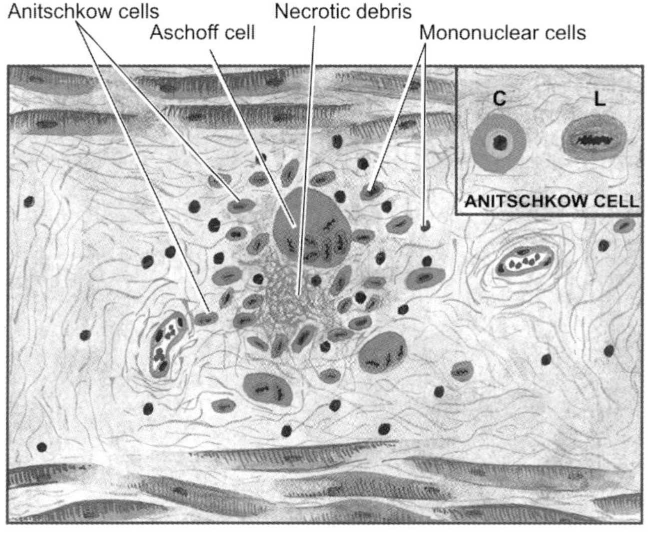

FIGURE 12.19

An Aschoff body (granulomatous stage) in the myocardium. *Inbox* shows Anitschkow cell in longitudinal section (L) with caterpillar-lie serrated nuclear chromatin, while cross-section (C) shows owl-eye appearance of central chromatin mass and perinuclear halo.

Eventually, it is replaced by a small fibrocollagenous scar with little cellularity, frequently located perivascularly.

RHEUMATIC PANCARDITIS. Although all the three layers of the heart are affected in RF, the intensity of their involvement is variable.

1. RHEUMATIC ENDOCARDITIS. Endocardial lesions of RF may involve the valvular and mural endocardium, causing *rheumatic valvulitis* and *mural endocarditis,* respectively. Rheumatic valvulitis is chiefly responsible for the major cardiac manifestations in chronic RHD.

RHEUMATIC VALVULITIS. ***Grossly,*** the valves in **acute RF** show thickening and loss of translucency of the valve leaflets or cusps. This is followed by the formation of characteristic, small (1 to 3 mm in diameter), multiple, warty *vegetations* or *verrucae,* chiefly along the line of closure of the leaflets and cusps. These tiny vegetations are almost continuous so that the free margin of the cusps or leaflets appears as a rough and irregular ridge. The vegetations in RF appear grey-brown, translucent and are firmly attached so that they are not likely to get detached to form emboli, unlike the friable vegetations of infective endocarditis (page 338).

Though all the four heart valves are affected, their frequency and severity of involvement varies: mitral valve alone being the most common site, followed in decreasing order of frequency, by combined mitral and aortic valve (Fig. 12.20). The tricuspid and pulmonary valves usually show infrequent and slight involvement. The higher incidence of vegetations on left side of the heart is possibly because of the greater mechanical stresses on the valves of the left heart, especially along the line of closure of the valve cusps (Fig. 12.21,A). The occurrence of vegetations on the atrial surfaces of the atrioventricular valves (mitral and tricuspid) and on the ventricular surface of the semilunar valves (aortic and pulmonary) further lends support to the role of mechanical pressure on the valves in the pathogenesis of vegetations.

The **chronic stage of RHD** is characterised by permanent deformity of one or more valves, especially the mitral (in 98% cases alone or along with other valves) and aortic. The approximate frequency of deformity of various valves is as under:

- Mitral alone=37% cases.
- Mitral+aortic=27% cases.
- Mitral+aortic+tricuspid=22% cases.
- Mitral+tricuspid=11% cases.

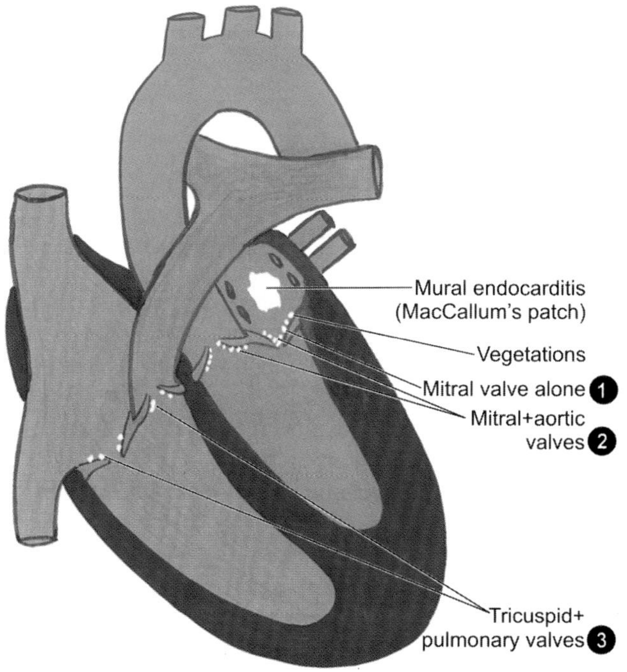

FIGURE 12.20

Schematic representation of the anatomic regions of involvement and location of vegetations in rheumatic endocarditis (both valvular and mural). Serial numbers 1, 2 and 3 are denoted for the frequency of valvular involvement.

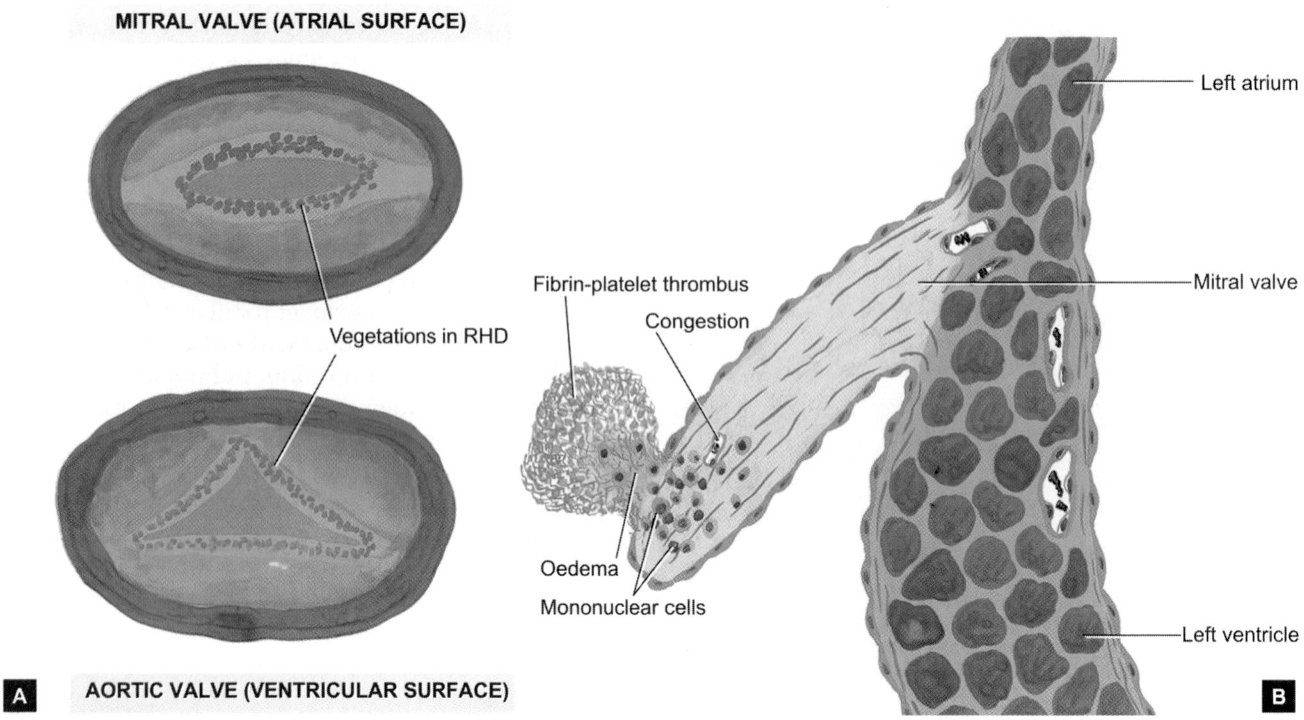

MITRAL VALVE (ATRIAL SURFACE)

Vegetations in RHD

A AORTIC VALVE (VENTRICULAR SURFACE)

Fibrin-platelet thrombus
Congestion
Oedema
Mononuclear cells
Left atrium
Mitral valve
Left ventricle
B

FIGURE 12.21

Rheumatic valvulitis. A, Location of vegetations on the valves of the left heart. The location of vegetations on mitral valve (above) is shown as viewed from the left atrium, while the vegetations on aortic valve (below) are shown as seen from the left ventricular surface. B, Microscopic structure of the rheumatic valvulitis and a vegetation on the cusp of mitral valve in sagittal section.

- Aortic alone=2%.
- Mitral+aortic+tricuspid+pulmonary=less than 1% cases.

Thus, mitral valve is almost always invoved in RHD. Gross appearance of chronic healed mitral valve in RHD is characteristically *'fish mouth'* or *'button hole'* stenosis. Mitral stenosis and insufficiency are commonly combined in chronic RHD; calcific aortic stenosis may also be found. These healed chronic valvular lesions in RHD occur due to diffuse fibrocollagenous thickening and calcification of the valve cusps or leaflets which cause adhesions between the lateral portions, especially in the region of the commissures. Thickening, shortening and fusion of the chordae tendineae further contribute to the chronic valvular lesions.

Microscopically, the inflammatory changes begin in the region of the valve rings (where the leaflets are attached to the fibrous annulus) and then extend throughout the entire leaflet, whereas vegetations are usually located on the free margin of the leaflets and cusps.

i) In the **early (acute) stage,** the histological changes are oedema of the valve leaflet, presence of increased number of capillaries and infiltration with lymphocytes, plasma cells, histiocytes with many Anitschkow cells and a few polymorphs. Occasionally, Aschoff bodies with central foci of fibrinoid necrosis and surrounded by palisade of cardiac histiocytes are seen, but more often the cellular infiltration is diffuse in acute stage of RF. Vegetations present at the free margins of cusps appear as eosinophilic, tiny structures mainly consisting of fibrin with superimposed platelet-thrombi and do not contain bacteria (Fig. 12.21,B).

ii) In the **healed (chronic) stage,** the vegetations have undergone organisation. The valves show diffuse thickening as a result of fibrous tissue with hyalinisation, and often calcification. Vascularisation of the valve cusps may still be evident in the form of thick-walled blood vessels with narrowed lumina. Typical Aschoff bodies are rarely seen in the valves at this stage.

RHEUMATIC MURAL ENDOCARDITIS. Mural endocardium may also show features of rheumatic carditis though the changes are less conspicuous as compared to valvular changes.

Grossly, the lesions are seen most commonly as *MacCallum's patch* which is the region of endocardial surface in the posterior wall of the left atrium just above the posterior leaflet of the mitral valve. MacCallum's patch appears as a map-like area of thickened, roughened and wrinkled part of the endocardium (Fig. 12.20).

Microscopically, the appearance of MacCallum's patch is similar to that seen in rheumatic valvulitis. The affected area shows oedema, fibrinoid change in the collagen, and cellular infiltrate of lymphocytes, plasma cells and macrophages with many Anitschkow cells. Typical Aschoff bodies may sometimes be found.

2. RHEUMATIC MYOCARDITIS. ***Grossly,*** in the *early (acute) stage*, the myocardium, especially of the left ventricle, is soft and flabby. In the *intermediate stage*, the interstitial tissue of the myocardium shows small foci of necrosis. Later, tiny pale foci of the Aschoff bodies may be visible throughout the myocardium.

Microscopically, the most characteristic feature of rheumatic myocarditis is the presence of distinctive Aschoff bodies. These diagnostic nodules are scattered throughout the interstitial tissue of the myocardium and are most frequent in the interventricular septum, left ventricle and left atrium. Derangements of the conduction system may, thus, be present. The Aschoff bodies are best identified in the intermediate stage when they appear as granulomas with central fibrinoid necrosis and are surrounded by palisade of Anitschkow cells and multinucleate Aschoff cells. There is infiltration by lymphocytes, plasma cells and some neutrophils. In the late stage, the Aschoff bodies are gradually replaced by small fibrous scars in the vicinity of blood vessels and the inflammatory infiltrate subsides. Presence of active Aschoff bodies along with old healed lesions is indicative of rheumatic activity.

3. RHEUMATIC PERICARDITIS. Inflammatory involvement of the pericardium commonly accompanies RHD.

Grossly, the usual finding is fibrinous pericarditis in which there is loss of normal shiny pericardial surface due to deposition of fibrin on its surface and accumulation of slight amount of fibrinous exudate in the pericardial sac. If the parietal pericardium is pulled off from the visceral pericardium, the two separated surfaces are shaggy due to thick fibrin covering them. This appearance is often likened to *'bread and butter appearance'* i.e. resembling the buttered surfaces of two slices in a sandwich when they are gently pulled apart. If fibrinous pericarditis fails to resolve and, instead, undergoes organisation, the two layers of the pericardium form fibrous adhesions resulting in chronic adhesive pericarditis.

Microscopically, fibrin is identified on the surfaces. The subserosal connective tissue is infiltrated by lymphocytes, plasma cells, histiocytes and a few neutrophils. Characteristic Aschoff bodies may be seen which later undergo organisation and fibrosis. Organisation of the exudate causes fibrous adhesions between the visceral and parietal surfaces of the pericardial sac and obliterates the pericardial cavity.

B. Extracardiac Lesions

Patients of the syndrome of acute rheumatism develop lesions in connective tissue elsewhere in the body, chiefly the joints, subcutaneous tissue, arteries, brain and lungs.

1. POLYARTHRITIS. Acute and painful inflammation of the synovial membranes of some of the joints, especially the larger joints of the limbs, is seen in about 90% cases of RF in adults and less often in children. As pain and swelling subside in one joint, others tend to get involved, producing the characteristic *'migratory polyarthritis'* involving two or more joints at a time.

Histologically, the changes are transitory. The synovial membrane and the periarticular connective tissue show hyperaemia, oedema, fibrinoid change and neutrophilic infiltration. Sometimes, focal lesions resembling Aschoff bodies are observed. A serous effusion into the joint cavity is commonly present.

2. SUBCUTANEOUS NODULES. The subcutaneous nodules of RF occur more often in children than in adult. These nodules are small (0.5 to 2 cm in diameter), spherical or ovoid and painless. They are attached to deeper structures like tendons, ligaments, fascia or periosteum and therefore often remain unnoticed by the patient. Characteristic locations are extensor surfaces of the wrists, elbows, ankles and knees.

Histologically, the subcutaneous nodules of RF are representative of giant Aschoff bodies of the heart. They consist of 3 distinct zones: a central area with fibrinoid changes, surrounded by a zone of histiocytes and fibroblasts forming a palisade arrangement, and the outermost zone of connective tissue which is infiltrated by non-specific chronic inflammatory cells and proliferating blood vessels.

It may be mentioned here that histologically similar but clinically different subcutaneous lesions appear in rheumatoid arthritis; they are larger, painful and tender and persist for months to years (Chapter 26).

3. ERYTHEMA MARGINATUM. This non-pruritic erythematous rash is characteristic of RF. The lesions occur mainly on the trunk and proximal parts of the extremities. The erythematous area develops central clearing and has slightly elevated red margins. The erythema is transient and migratory.

4. RHEUMATIC ARTERITIS. Arteritis in RF involves not only the coronary arteries and aorta but also occurs in arteries of various other organs such as renal, mesenteric and cerebral arteries. The lesions in the coronaries are seen mainly in the small intramyocardial branches.

Histologically, the lesions may be like those of hypersensitivity angiitis (Chapter 11), or sometimes may resemble polyarteritis nodosa. Occasionally, foci of fibrinoid necrosis or ill-formed Aschoff bodies may be present close to the vessel wall.

5. CHOREA MINOR. Chorea minor or Sydenham's chorea or Saint Vitus' dance is a delayed manifestation of RF as a result of involvement of the central nervous system. The condition is characterised by disordered and involuntary jerky movements of the trunk and the extremities accompanied by some degree of emotional instability. The condition occurs more often in younger age, particularly in girls.

Histologically, the lesions are located in the cerebral hemispheres, brainstem and the basal ganglia. They consist of small haemorrhages, oedema and perivascular infiltration of lymphocytes. There may be endarteritis obliterans and thrombosis of cortical and meningeal vessels.

6. RHEUMATIC PNEUMONITIS AND PLEURITIS. Involvement of the lungs and pleura occurs rarely in RF. Pleuritis is often accompanied with serofibrinous pleural effusion but definite Aschoff bodies are not present. In rheumatic pneumonitis, the lungs are large, firm and rubbery.

Histologically, the changes are oedema, capillary haemorrhages and focal areas of fibrinous exudate in the alveoli. Aschoff bodies are generally not found.

CLINICAL FEATURES

The first attack of acute RF generally appears 2 to 3 weeks after streptococcal pharyngitis, most often in children between the age of 5 to 15 years. With subsequent streptococcal pharyngitis, there is reactivation of the disease and similar clinical manifestations appear with each recurrent attack. The disease generally presents with migratory polyarthritis and fever. However, RF has widespread systemic involvement and no single specific laboratory diagnostic test is available. Therefore, for diagnosis, the following set of guidelines called *revised Jones' criteria* are followed:

A. **Major criteria** are:
1. Carditis
2. Polyarthritis
3. Chorea (Sydenham's chorea)
4. Erythema marginatum
5. Subcutaneous nodules

B. **Minor criteria** are:
1. Fever
2. Arthralgia
3. Previous history of RF
4. Laboratory findings of elevated ESR, raised C-reactive protein, and leucocytosis
5. ECG finding of prolonged PR interval.

C. Supportive evidence of preceding group A streptococcal infection: positive throat culture for group A streptococci, raised titres of streptococcal antibodies (antistreptolysin O and S, antistreptokinase, anti-streptohyaluronidase and anti DNAase B).

Clinical diagnosis of RF is made in a case with antecedent laboratory evidence of streptococcal throat infection in the presence of: any two of the major criteria, or occurrence of one major and two minor criteria.

If the heart is spared in a case of acute RF, the patient may have complete recovery without any sequelae. However, once the heart is involved, it is often associated with reactivation and recurrences of the disease. Myocarditis, in particular, is the most life-threatening due to involvement of the conduction system of the heart and results in serious arrhythmias. The long term sequelae or **stigmata** are the chronic valvular deformities, especially the mitral stenosis, as already explained on page 331. Initially, a state of compensation occurs, while later decompensation of the heart leads to full-blown cardiac failure. Currently, surgical replacement of the damaged valves can alter the clinical course of the disease.

The major **causes of death** in RHD are cardiac failure, bacterial endocarditis and embolism:

1. *Cardiac failure* is the most common cause of death from RHD. In young patients, cardiac failure occurs due to the chronic valvular deformities, while in older patients coronary artery disease may be superimposed on old RHD.

2. *Bacterial endocarditis* of both acute and subacute type may supervene due to inadequate use of antibiotics.

3. *Embolism* in RHD originates most commonly from mural thrombi in the left atrium and its appendages, in association with mitral stenosis. The organs most frequently affected are the brain, kidneys, spleen and lungs.

4. *Sudden death* may occur in RHD as a result of ball thrombus in the left atrium or due to acute coronary insufficiency in association with aortic stenosis.

NON-RHEUMATIC ENDOCARDITIS

Inflammatory involvement of the endocardial layer of the heart is called endocarditis. Though in common usage, if not specified endocarditis would mean inflammation of the valvular endocardium, several workers designate endocarditis on the basis of anatomic area of the involved endocardium such as: *valvular* for valvular endocardium, *mural* for inner lining of the lumina of cardiac chambers, *chordal* for the endocardium of the chordae tendineae, *trabecular* for the endocardium of trabeculae carneae, and *papillary* for the endocardium covering the papillary muscles. Endocarditis can be broadly grouped into *non-infective* and *infective* types (Table 12.5). Most types of endocarditis are characterised by the presence of 'vegetations' or 'verrucae' which have distinct features. A summary of the distinguishing features of the principal types of vegetations is presented in Table 12.7.

TABLE 12.5: Classification of Endocarditis.

A. NON-INFECTIVE
   1. Rheumatic endocarditis (page 331)
   2. Atypical verrucous (Libman-Sacks) endocarditis
   3. Non-bacterial thrombotic (cachectic, marantic) endocarditis

B. INFECTIVE
   1. Bacterial endocarditis
   2. Other infective types (tuberculous, syphilitic, fungal, viral, rickettsial)

ATYPICAL VERRUCOUS (LIBMAN-SACKS) ENDOCARDITIS

Libman and Sacks, two American physicians, described a form of endocarditis in 1924 that is characterised by sterile endocardial vegetations which are distinguishable from the vegetations of RHD and bacterial endocarditis.

ETIOPATHOGENESIS. Atypical verrucous endocarditis is one of the manifestations of 'collagen diseases'. Characteristic lesions of Libman-Sacks endocarditis are seen in *50% cases of acute systemic lupus erythematosus (SLE);* other diseases associated with this form of endocarditis are systemic sclerosis, thrombotic thrombocytopenic purpura (TTP) and other collagen diseases.

PATHOLOGIC CHANGES. Grossly, characteristic vegetations occur most frequently on the mitral and tricuspid valves. The vegetations of atypical verrucous endocarditis are small (1 to 4 mm in diameter), granular, multiple and tend to occur on both surfaces of affected valves, in the valve pockets and on the adjoining ventricular and atrial endocardium. The vegetations are sterile unless superimposed by bacterial endocarditis. Unlike vegetations of RHD, the healed vegetations of Libman-Sacks endocarditis do not produce any significant valvular deformity. Frequently, fibrinous or serofibrinous pericarditis with pericardial effusion is associated.

Microscopically, the verrucae of Libman-Sacks endocarditis are composed of fibrinoid material with superimposed fibrin and platelet thrombi. The endocardium underlying the verrucae shows characteristic histological changes which include fibrinoid necrosis, proliferation of capillaries and infiltration by histiocytes, plasma cells, lymphocytes, neutrophils and the pathognomonic *haematoxylin bodies of Gross* which are counterparts of LE cells of the blood. Similar inflammatory changes may be found in the interstitial connective tissue of the myocardium. The Aschoff bodies are never found in the endocardium or myocardium.

NON-BACTERIAL THROMBOTIC (CACHECTIC, MARANTIC) ENDOCARDITIS

Non-bacterial thrombotic, cachectic, marantic or terminal endocarditis or endocarditis simplex is an involvement of the heart valves by sterile thrombotic vegetations.

ETIOPATHOGENESIS. The exact pathogenesis of lesions in non-bacterial thrombotic endocarditis (NBTE) is not clear. These vegetations are found at autopsy in 0.5 to 5% of cases. The following diseases and conditions are frequently associated with their presence:

1. In patients dying of *chronic debilitating diseases* e.g. advanced cancer (in 50% case of NBTE), chronic tuberculosis, renal failure and chronic sepsis. Hence, the names such as 'cachectic', 'marantic' and 'terminal' endocarditis are used synonymously with NBTE. The underlying mechanism is increased blood coagulability or disseminated intravascular coagulation (DIC) syndrome which may develop as a terminal event in patients of cancer and other chronic wasting diseases.
2. Occurrence of these lesions in young and well-nourished patients is explained on the basis of *alternative hypothesis* such as allergy, vitamin C deficiency, deep vein thrombosis, and endocardial trauma (e.g. due to catheter in pulmonary artery and haemodynamic trauma to the valves).

PATHOLOGIC CHANGES. Grossly, the verrucae of NBTE are located on cardiac valves, chiefly the mitral, and less often aortic and tricuspid. These verrucae are usually small (1 to 5 mm in diameter), single or multiple, brownish and occur along the line of closure of the leaflets but are more friable than the vegetations of RHD. Organised and healed vegetations appear as fibrous nodules. Normal age-related appearance of tag-like appendage at the margin of the valve cusps known as 'Lambl's excrescences' is an example of such healed lesions. ***Microscopically,*** the vegetations in NBTE are composed of fibrin along with entangled RBCs , WBCs and platelets. Microorganisms are not seen.The underlying valve shows swollen collagen, fibrinoid change and capillary proliferation but does not show any inflammatory infiltrate.

Embolic phenomenon is seen in many cases of NBTE and results in infarcts in the brain, lungs, spleen and kidneys. The bland vegetations of NBTE on infection give rise to bacterial endocarditis.

BACTERIAL ENDOCARDITIS

DEFINITION. Bacterial endocarditis (BE) is serious infection of the valvular and mural endocardium caused by different forms of bacteria (other than tubercle bacilli and non-bacterial microorganisms) and is characterised by typical infected and friable vegetations. Depending upon the severity of infection, BE is subdivided into 2 clinical forms:

1. **Acute bacterial endocarditis (ABE)** is the fulminant and destructive acute infection of the endocardium by highly virulent bacteria in a previously normal heart and almost invariably runs a rapidly fatal course in a period of 2-6 weeks.

2. **Subacute bacterial endocarditis (SABE) or endocarditis lenta** (*lenta* = slow) is caused by less virulent bacteria in a previously diseased heart and has a gradual downhill course in a period of 6 weeks to a few months and sometimes years.

Although classification of bacterial endocarditis into acute and subacute forms has been largely discarded because the clinical course is altered by antibiotic treatment, still a few important distinguishing features are worth describing (Table 12.6). However, characteristics of the vegetations in the two forms of BE are difficult to distinguish.

INCIDENCE. Introduction of antibiotic drugs has helped greatly in lowering the incidence of BE as compared with its incidence in the pre-antibiotic era. Though BE may occur at any age, most cases of ABE as well as SABE occur over 50 years of age. Males are affected more often than females.

ETIOLOGY. All cases of BE are caused by *infection with microorganisms* in patients having certain predisposing factors.

A. **Infective agents.** About 90% cases of BE are caused by streptococci and staphylococci.

- *In ABE,* the most common causative organisms are virulent strains of staphylococci, chiefly *Staphylococcus aureus.* Others are pneumococci, gonococci, β-streptococci and enterococci.
- *In SABE,* the commonest causative organisms are the streptococci with low virulence, predominantly

TABLE 12.6: Distinguishing Features of Acute and Subacute Bacterial Endocarditis.

FEATURE	ACUTE	SUBACUTE
1. *Duration*	<6 weeks	>6 weeks
2. *Most common organisms*	*Staph. aureus,* β-streptococci	*Streptococcus viridans*
3. *Virulence of organisms*	Highly virulent	Less virulent
4. *Previous condition of valves*	Usually previously normal	Usually previously damaged
5. *Lesion on valves*	Invasive, destructive, suppurative	Usually not invasive or suppurative
6. *Clinical features*	Features of acute systemic infection	Splenomegaly, clubbing of fingers, petechiae

TABLE 12.7: Distinguishing Features of Vegetations in Major Forms of Endocarditis.

FEATURE	RHEUMATIC	LIBMAN-SACKS	NON-BACTERIAL THROMBOTIC	BACTERIAL
1. *Valves commonly affected*	Mitral alone; mitral and aortic combined	Mitral, tricuspid	Mainly mitral; less often aortic and tricuspid	Mitral; aortic; combined mitral and aortic
2. *Location on valve cusps or leaflets*	Occur along the line of closure, atrial surface of atrio-ventricular valves and ventricular surface of semilunar valves	Occur on both surfaces of valve leaflets or cusps, in the valve pockets	Occur along the line of closure	SABE more often on diseased valves: ABE on previously normal valves; location same as in RHD
3. *Macroscopy*	Small, multiple, warty, grey brown, translucent, firmly attached, generally produce permanent valvular deformity	Medium-sized, multiple, generally do not produce significant valvular deformity	Small but larger than those of rheumatic, single or multiple, brownish, firm, but more friable than those of rheumatic	Often large, grey-tawny to greenish, irregular, single or multiple, typically friable
4. *Microscopy*	Composed of fibrin with superimposed platelet thrombi and no bacteria, Adjacent and underlying endocardium shows oedema, proliferation of capillaries, mononuclear inflammatory infiltrate and occasional Aschoff bodies.	Composed of fibrinoid material with superimposed fibrin and platelet thrombi and no bacteria. The underlying endocardium shows fibrinoid necrosis, proliferation of capillaries and acute and chronic inflammatory infiltrate including the haematoxylin bodies of Gross.	Composed of degenerated valvular tissue, fibrin-platelets thrombi and no bacteria. The underlying valve shows swelling of collagen, fibrinoid change, proliferation of capillaries but no significant inflammatory cell infiltrate.	Composed of outer eosinophilic zone of fibrin and platelets, covering colonies of bacteria and deeper zone of non-specific acute and chronic inflammatory cells. The underlying endocardium may show abscesses in ABE and inflammatory granulation tissue in the SABE.

Streptococcus viridans, which forms part of normal flora of the mouth and pharynx. Other less common etiologic agents include other strains of streptococci and staphylococci (e.g. *Streptococcus bovis* which is the normal inhabitant of gastrointestinal tract, *Streptococcus pneumoniae,* and *Staphylococcus epidermidis* which is a commensal of the skin), gram-negative enteric bacilli (e.g. *E. coli, Klebsiella, Pseudomonas and Salmonella*), pneumococci, gonococci and *Haemophilus influenzae.*

B. Predisposing factors. There are 3 main factors which predispose to the development of both forms of BE:

1. conditions initiating transient bacteraemia, septicaemia and pyaemia;
2. underlying heart disease; and
3. impaired host defenses.

1. *Bacteraemia, septicaemia and pyaemia:* Bacteria gain entrance to the bloodstream causing transient and clinically silent bacteraemia in a variety of day-to-day procedures as well as from other sources of infection. Some of the common examples are:

i) Periodontal infections such as trauma from vigorous brushing of teeth, hard chewing, tooth extraction and other dental procedures.

ii) Infections of the genitourinary tract such as in catheterisation, cystoscopy, obstetrical procedures including normal delivery and abortions.

iii) Infections of gastrointestinal and biliary tract.

iv) Surgery of the bowel, biliary tract and genitourinary tracts.

v) Skin infections such as boils, carbuncles and abscesses.

vi) Upper and lower respiratory tract infections including bacterial pneumonias.

vii) Intravenous drug abuse.

viii) Cardiac catheterisation and cardiac surgery for implantation of prosthetic valves.

2. *Underlying heart disease:* SABE occurs much more frequently in previously diseased heart valves, whereas the ABE is common in previously normal heart.

Amongst the commonly associated underlying heart diseases are the following:

i) Chronic rheumatic valvular disease in about 50% cases.

ii) Congenital heart diseases in about 20% cases. These include VSD, subaortic stenosis, pulmonary stenosis, bicuspid aortic valve, coarctation of the aorta, and PDA.

iii) Other causes are syphilitic aortic valve disease, atherosclerotic valvular disease, floppy mitral valve, and prosthetic heart valves.

3. *Impaired host defenses:* All conditions in which there is depression of specific immunity, deficiency of complement and defective phagocytic function, predispose to BE. Following are some of the examples of such conditions:

i) Impaired specific immunity in lymphomas.

ii) Leukaemias.

iii) Cytotoxic therapy for various forms of cancers and transplant patients.

iv) Deficient functions of neutrophils and macrophages.

PATHOGENESIS. Bacteria on entering the bloodstream from any of the above-mentioned routes are implanted on the cardiac valves or mural endocardium. There are different hypotheses to explain the occurrence of bacterial implants on the valves:

1. The circulating bacteria are lodged much more frequently on *previously damaged valves* from diseases, chiefly RHD and congenital heart diseases, than on healthy valves.

2. Conditions producing *haemodynamic stress* on the valves are liable to cause damage to the endothelium, favouring the formation of platelet thrombi which get infected from circulating bacteria.

3. Another alternative hypothesis is the occurrence of *non-bacterial thrombotic endocarditis* from prolonged stress which is followed by bacterial contamination.

PATHOLOGIC CHANGES. The characteristic pathologic feature in both ABE and SABE is the presence of typical vegetations or verrucae on the valve cusps or leaflets, and less often, on mural endocardium.

Macroscopically, the lesions are found commonly on the valves of the left heart, most frequently on the mitral, followed in descending frequency, by the aortic, simultaneous involvement of both mitral and aortic valves, and quite rarely on the valves of the right heart. The vegetations in SABE are more often seen on previously diseased valves, whereas the vegetations of ABE are often found on previously normal valves. Like in RHD, the vegetations are often located on the atrial surface of atrioventricular valves and ventricular surface of the semilunar valves. They begin from the contact areas of the valve and may extend along the surface of the valves and on to the adjacent endocardium.

The *vegetations* of BE vary in size from a few millimeters to several centimeters, grey-tawny to greenish, irregular, single or multiple, and typically *friable.* They may appear flat, filiform, fungating or polypoid. The vegetations in ABE tend to be bulkier and globular than those of SABE and are located more often on previously normal valves, may cause ulceration or perforation of the underlying valve leaflet, or may produce myocardial abscesses (Fig. 12.22,A).

Microscopically, the vegetations of BE consist of 3 zones (Fig. 12.22,B):

i) The *outer layer or cap* consists of eosinophilic material composed of fibrin and platelets.

ii) Underneath this layer is the *basophilic zone* containing colonies of bacteria. However, bacterial component of the vegetations may be lacking in treated cases.

iii) The *deeper zone* consists of non-specific inflammatory reaction in the cusp itself, and in the case of SABE there may be evidence of repair **(COLOUR PLATE XV; CL 59).**

In the acute fulminant form of the disease, the inflammatory cell infiltrate chiefly consists of neutrophils and is accompanied with tissue necrosis and abscesses in the valve rings and in the myocardium. In the subacute form, there is healing by granulation tissue, mononuclear inflammatory cell infiltration and fibroblastic proliferation. Histological evidence of pre-existing valvular disease such as RHD may be present in SABE.

COMPLICATIONS AND SEQUELAE. Most cases of BE present with fever. The acute form of BE is characterised by high grade fever, chills, weakness and malaise while the subacute form of the disease has non-specific manifestations like slight fever, fatigue, loss of weight and flu-like symptoms. In the early stage, the lesions are confined to the heart, while subsequent progression of the disease leads to involvement of extracardiac organs. In general, severe complications develop early in ABE than in SABE. Complications and sequelae of BE are divided into cardiac and extracardiac (Fig. 12.23):

A. Cardiac complications. These include the following:

i) Valvular stenosis or insufficiency

ii) Perforation, rupture, and aneurysm of valve leaflets

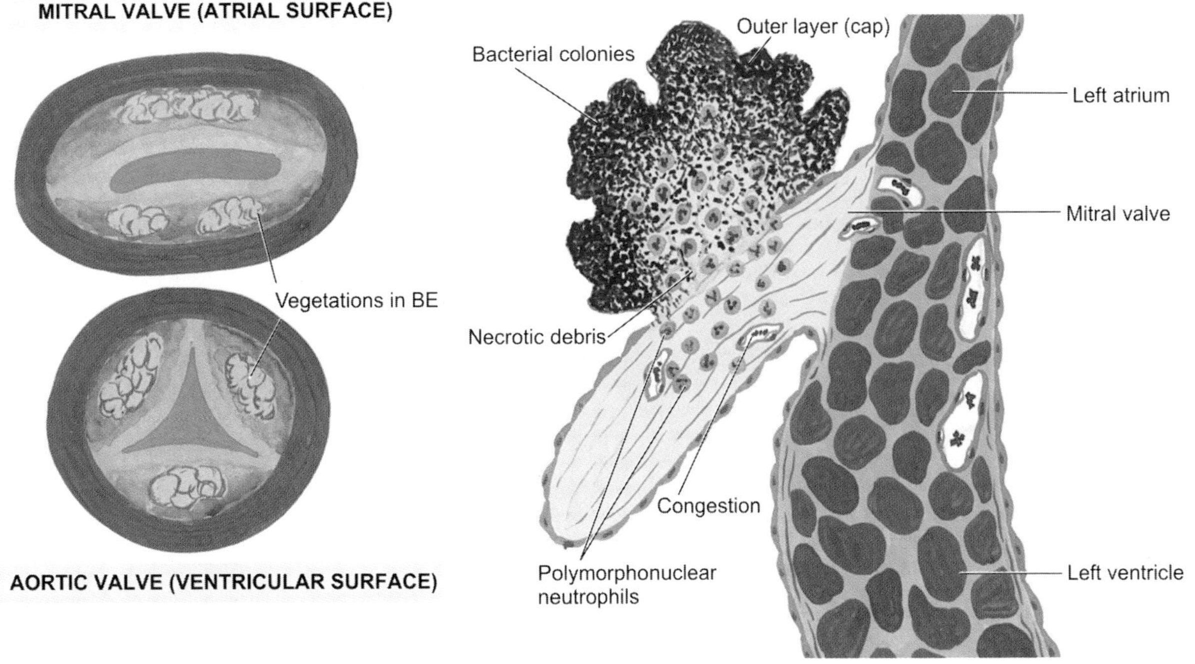

FIGURE 12.22

Bacterial endocarditis. A, Location of vegetations on the valves of the left heart. The vegetations are shown on the mitral valve (above) as viewed from the left atrium, while those on the aortic valve (below) are shown as seen from the left ventricle. B, Microscopic structure of a vegetation of BE on the surface of mitral valve in sagittal section.

iii) Abscesses in the valve ring

iv) Myocardial abscesses

v) Suppurative pericarditis

vi) Cardiac failure from one or more of the foregoing complications.

B. Extracardiac complications. Since the vegetations in BE are typically friable, they tend to get dislodged due to rapid stream of blood and give rise to embolism which is responsible for very common and serious extracardiac complications. These are as under:

i) Emboli originating from the *left side of the heart* and entering the systemic circulation affect organs like the spleen, kidneys, and brain causing infarcts, abscesses and mycotic aneurysms.

ii) Emboli arising from *right side of the heart* enter the pulmonary circulation and produce pulmonary abscesses.

iii) *Petechiae* may be seen in the skin and conjunctiva due to either emboli or toxic damage to the capillaries.

iv) In SABE, there are painful, tender nodules on the finger tips of hands and feet called *Osler's nodes,* while in ABE there is appearance of painless, non-tender subcutaneous maculopapular lesions on the pulp of the fingers called *Janeway's spots.* In either case, their origin is due to toxic or allergic inflammation of the vessel wall.

v) *Focal necrotising glomerulonephritis* is seen more commonly in SABE than in ABE. Occasionally diffuse glomerulonephritis may occur. Both these have their pathogenesis in circulating immune complexes (hypersensitivity phenomenon) (Chapter 20).

Treatment of BE with antibiotics in adequate dosage kills the bacteria but complications and sequelae of healed endocardial lesions may occur even after successful therapy. The *causes of death* are cardiac failure, persistent infection, embolism to vital organs, renal failure and rupture of mycotic aneurysm of cerebral arteries.

OTHER INFECTIVE ENDOCARDITIS

Besides BE, various other microorganisms may occasionally produce infective endocarditis. These include the following:

1. Tuberculous endocarditis. Though tubercle bacilli are bacteria, tuberculous endocarditis is described separate from the bacterial endocarditis due to specific granulomatous inflammation found in tuberculosis. It is characterised by presence of typical tubercles on the

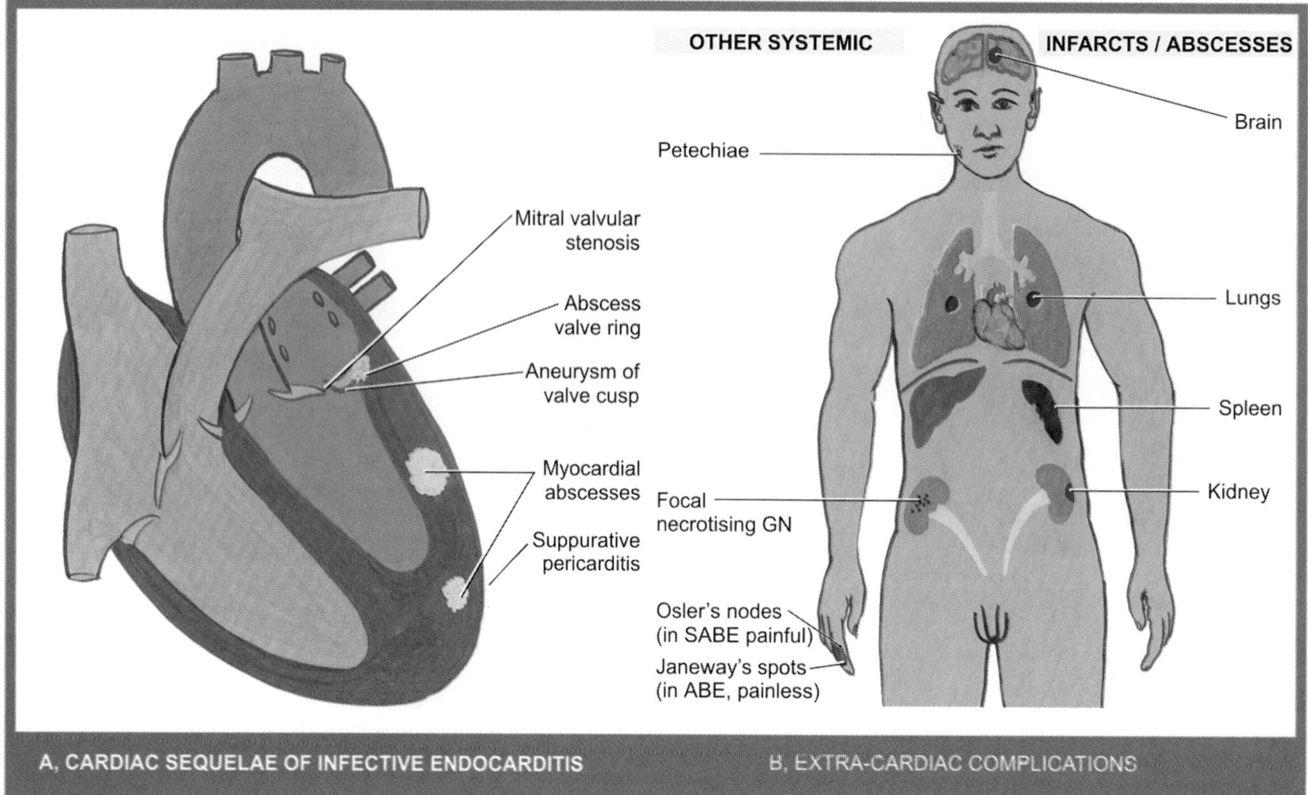

FIGURE 12.23

Complications and sequelae of infective endocarditis.

valvular as well as mural endocardium and may form tuberculous thromboemboli.

2. Syphilitic endocarditis. The endocardial lesions in syphilis have already been described in relation to syphilitic aortitis on page 289. The severest manifestation of cardiovascular syphilis is aortic valvular incompetence.

3. Fungal endocarditis. Rarely, endocardium may be infected with fungi such as from *Candida albicans, Histoplasma capsulatum, Aspergillus, Mucor*, coccidioidomycosis, cryptococcosis, blastomycosis and actinomycosis. Opportunistic fungal infections like candidiasis and aspergillosis are seen more commonly in patients receiving long-term antibiotic therapy, intravenous drug abusers and after prosthetic valve replacement.

4. Viral endocarditis. There is only experimental evidence of existence of this entity.

5. Rickettsial endocarditis. Another rare cause of endocarditis is from infection with rickettsiae in Q fever.

VALVULAR DISEASES AND DEFORMITIES

Valvular diseases are various forms of congenital and acquired diseases which cause valvular deformities. Many of them result in cardiac failure. Rheumatic heart disease is the most common form of acquired valvular disease. Valves of the left side of the heart are involved much more frequently than those of the right side of the heart. The mitral valve is affected most often, followed in descending frequency, by aortic valve, and combined mitral and aortic valves. The valvular deformities may be of 2 types: stenosis and insufficiency. *Stenosis* is the term used for failure of a valve to open completely during diastole resulting in obstruction to the forward flow of the blood. *Insufficiency or incompetence or regurgitation* is the failure of a valve to close completely during systole resulting in back flow or regurgitation of the blood.

The congenital valvular diseases have already been described (page 312). Various acquired valvular diseases that may deform the heart valves are listed below:

1. RHD, the commonest cause (page 328)
2. Infective endocarditis (page 336)
3. Non-bacterial thrombotic endocarditis (page 335)
4. Libman-Sacks endocarditis (page 335)
5. Syphilitic valvulitis (page 289)
6. Calcific aortic valve stenosis

7. Calcification of mitral annulus
8. Myxomatous degeneration (floppy valve syndrome)
9. Carcinoid heart disease.

The major forms of vegetative endocarditis involving the valves have already been described. Others alongwith the consequences of these valvular diseases in the form of stenosis and insufficiency of the heart valves are described below.

MITRAL STENOSIS

Mitral stenosis occurs in approximately 40% of all patients with RHD. About 70% of the patients are women. The latent period between the rheumatic carditis and development of symptomatic mitral stenosis is about two decades.

ETIOLOGY. Mitral stenosis is generally rheumatic in origin. Less common causes include bacterial endocarditis, Libman-Sacks endocarditis, endocardial fibroelastosis and congenital parachute mitral valve.

PATHOLOGIC CHANGES. The appearance of the mitral valve in stenosis varies according to the extent of involvement. Generally, the valve leaflets are diffusely thickened by fibrous tissue and/or calcific deposits, especially towards the closing margin. There are fibrous adhesions of mitral commissures and fusion and shortening of chordae tendineae. In less extensive involvement, the bases of the leaflets of mitral valve are mobile while the free margins have puckered and thickened tissue with narrowed orifice; this is called as *'purse-string puckering'*. The more advanced cases have rigid, fixed and immobile diaphragm-like valve leaflets with narrow, slit-like or oval mitral opening, commonly referred to as *'button-hole'* or *'fish-mouth'* mitral orifice (Fig. 12.24,B).

EFFECTS. In normal adults, the mitral orifice is about 5 cm^2. Symptomatic mitral stenosis develops if the valve opening is reduced to 1 cm^2 resulting in significant elevation of left atrial pressure from the normal of 12 mmHg to about 25 mmHg leading to dilatation of the left atrium. The elevated left atrial pressure, in turn, raises pressure in the pulmonary veins and capillaries, reducing the pulmonary function and causing exertional dyspnoea which is the chief symptom of mitral stenosis. The effects of mitral stenosis can thus be summarised as under:

1. Dilatation and hypertrophy of the left atrium.
2. Normal-sized or atrophic left ventricle due to reduced inflow of blood.
3. Pulmonary hypertension resulting from passive backward transmission of elevated left artial pressure which causes:
   i) chronic passive congestion of the lungs;
   ii) hypertrophy and dilatation of the right ventricle; and
   iii) dilatation of the right atrium when right heart failure supervenes.

MITRAL INSUFFICIENCY

Mitral insufficiency is caused by RHD in about 50% of patients but in contrast to mitral stenosis, pure mitral insufficiency occurs more often in men (75%). Subsequently, mitral insufficiency is associated with some degree of mitral stenosis.

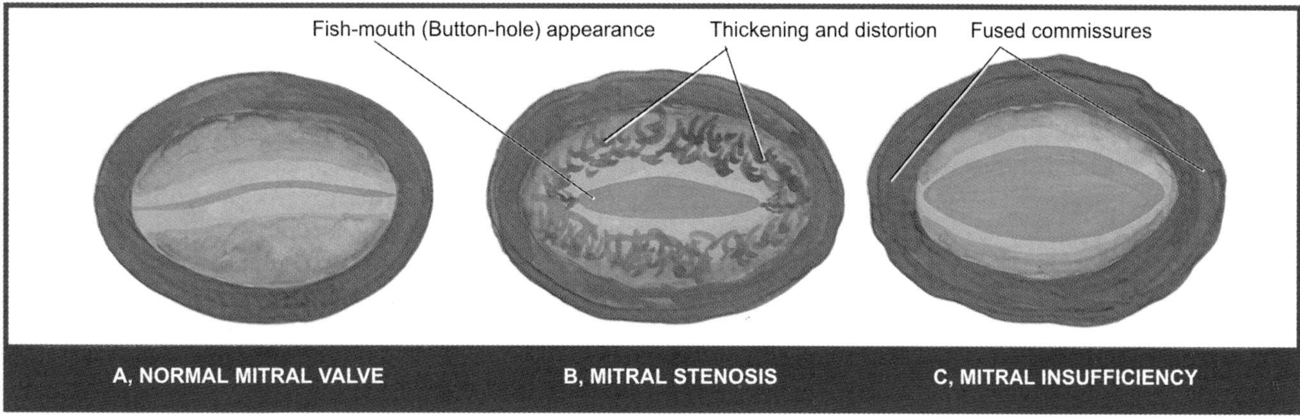

FIGURE 12.24

Mitral valve disease. Normal mitral valve (A) contrasted with mitral stenosis (B) and mitral insufficiency (C).

ETIOLOGY. All the causes of mitral stenosis may produce mitral insufficiency, RHD being the most common cause. In addition, mitral insufficiency may result from non-inflammatory calcification of mitral valve annulus (in the elderly), myxomatous transformation of mitral valve (floppy valve syndrome), rupture of a leaflet or of the chordae tendineae or of a papillary muscle. A few other conditions cause mitral insufficiency by dilatation of the mitral ring such as in myocardial infarction, myocarditis and left ventricular failure in hypertension.

PATHOLOGIC CHANGES. The appearance of the mitral valve in insufficiency varies according to the underlying cause. The rheumatic process produces rigidity, deformity and retraction of the valve leaflets and fusion of commissures as well as shortening and fusion of chordae tendineae (Fig. 12.24,C).

■ In *myxomatous degeneration* of the mitral valve leaflets (floppy valve syndrome) which is described on page 344, there is prolapse of one or both leaflets into the left atrium during systole.

■ In *non-inflammatory* calcification of mitral annulus seen in the aged, there is irregular, stony-hard, bead-like thickening in the region of mitral annulus without any associated inflammatory changes. It is thought to reflect degenerative changes of aging.

EFFECTS. The regurgitant mitral orifice produces progressive increase in left ventricular end-diastolic volume as well as pressure since the left ventricle cannot empty completely. This results in rise in left atrial pressure and dilatation. As a consequence of left atrial hypertension, pulmonary hypertension occurs resulting in pulmonary oedema and right heart failure. In symptomatic cases of mitral insufficiency, the major symptoms are related to decreased cardiac output (e.g. fatigue and weakness) and due to pulmonary congestion (e.g. exertional dyspnoea and orthopnoea) but the features are less well marked than in mitral stenosis. The effects of mitral insufficiency may be summarised as under:

1. Dilatation and hypertrophy of the left ventricle.
2. Marked dilatation of the left atrium.
3. Features of pulmonary hypertension such as:
   i) chronic passive congestion of the lungs;
   ii) hypertrophy and dilatation of the right ventricle; and
   iii) dilatation of the right atrium when right heart failure supervenes.

AORTIC STENOSIS

Aortic stenosis comprises about one-fourth of all patients with chronic valvular heart disease. About 80% patients of symptomatic aortic stenosis are males. It is of 2 main types: non-calcific and calcific type, the latter being more common.

1. Non-calcific aortic stenosis. The most common cause of non-calcific aortic stenosis is chronic RHD. Other causes are congenital valvular and subaortic stenosis and congenitally bicuspid aortic valve.

2. Calcific aortic stenosis. Calcific aortic stenosis is the more common type. Various causes have been ascribed to it. These include healing by scarring followed by calcification of aortic valve such as in RHD, bacterial endocarditis, *Brucella* endocarditis, Monckeberg's calcific aortic stenosis (page 279), healed congenital malformation and familial hypercholesterolaemic xanthomatosis.

PATHOLOGIC CHANGES. The aortic cusps show characteristic fibrous thickening and calcific nodularity of the closing edges. Calcified nodules are often found in the sinuses of Valsalva. In rheumatic aortic stenosis, the commissures are fused and calcified, while in non-rheumatic aortic stenosis there is no commissural fusion (Fig. 12.25,B).

EFFECTS. Aortic stenosis becomes symptomatic when the valve orifice is reduced to 1 cm^2 from its normal 3 cm^2. The symptoms appear many years later when the heart cannot compensate and the stenosis is quite severe. The major effect of aortic stenosis is obstruction to the outflow resulting in concentric hypertrophy of the left ventricle. Later, when cardiac failure supervenes, there is dilatation as well as hypertrophy of the left ventricle (eccentric hypertrophy).

The *three cardinal symptoms* of aortic stenosis are: exertional dyspnoea, angina pectoris and syncope. Exertional dyspnoea results from elevation of pulmonary capillary pressure. Angina pectoris usually results from elevation of pulmonary capillary pressure and usually develops due to increased demand of hypertrophied myocardial mass. Syncope results from accompanying coronary insufficiency. Sudden death may also occur in an occasional case of aortic stenosis.

AORTIC INSUFFICIENCY

About three-fourth of all patients with aortic insufficiency are males with some having family history of Marfan's syndrome.

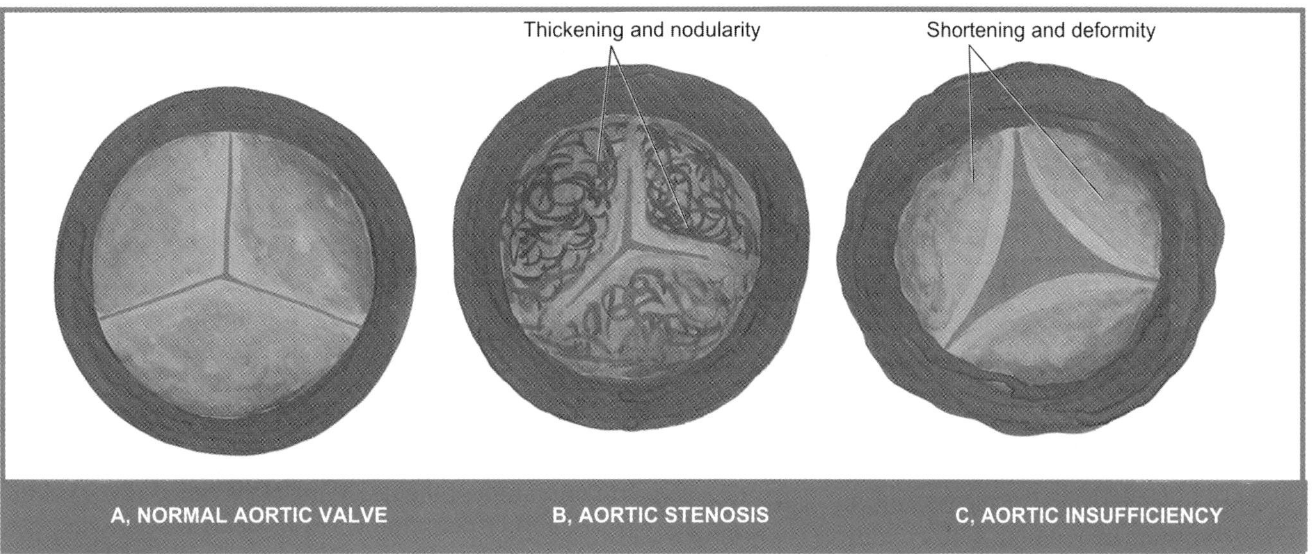

FIGURE 12.25

Aortic valve diseases. Normal aortic valve (A) contrasted with aortic stenosis (B) and aortic insufficiency (C).

ETIOLOGY. In about 75% of patients, the cause is chronic RHD. However, isolated aortic insufficiency is less often due to rheumatic etiology. Other causes include syphilitic valvulitis, infective endocarditis, congenital subaortic stenosis (congenitally bicuspid aortic valve), myxomatous degeneration of aortic valve (floppy valve syndrome), traumatic rupture of the valve cusps, dissecting aneurysm, Marfan's syndrome and ankylosing spondylitis.

PATHOLOGIC CHANGES. The aortic valve cusps are thickened, deformed and shortened and fail to close. There is generally distension and distortion of the ring (Fig. 12.25,C).

EFFECTS. As a result of regurgitant aortic orifice, there is increase of the left ventricular end-diastolic volume. This leads to hypertrophy and dilatation of the left ventricle producing massive cardiac enlargement so that the heart may weigh as much as 1000 gm. Failure of the left ventricle increases the pressure in the left atrium and eventually pulmonary hypertension and right heart failure occurs.

The characteristic physical findings in a patient of aortic insufficiency are awareness of the beatings of the heart, poundings in the head with each heartbeat, low diastolic and high pulse pressure, rapidly rising and collapsing water hammer pulse (Corrigan's pulse), booming 'pistol shot' sound over the femoral artery, and systolic and diastolic murmur heard over the femoral artery when it is lightly compressed (Durozier's sign). Sometimes, angina pectoris occurs due to increased myocardial demand or due to coronary insufficiency.

CARCINOID HEART DISEASE

ETIOLOGY. Carcinoid syndrome developing in patients with extensive hepatic metastases from a carcinoid tumour is characterised by cardiac manifestations in about half the cases (Chapter 18). The lesions are characteristically located in the valves and endocardium of the right side of the heart. The pathogenesis of the cardiac lesions is not certain. But in carcinoid tumour with hepatic metastasis, there is increased blood level of serotonin secreted by the tumour. The increased concentration of serotonin reaches the right side of the heart and causes the lesions but serotonin is inactivated on passage of the blood through the lungs and hence the left heart is relatively spared. In addition, high levels of bradykinin may play contributory role in carcinoid heart disease. However, chronic infusion of serotonin or bradykinin in experimental animals has not succeeded in producing cardiac lesions; hence the exact pathogenesis of carcinoid heart disease remains obscure.

PATHOLOGIC CHANGES. In majority of cases, the lesions are limited to the right side of the heart. Both pulmonary and tricuspid valves as well as the endocardium of the right chambers show characteristic cartilage-like fibrous plaques. Similar plaques may occur on the intima of the great veins, the coronary sinus and the great arteries. Occasionally, the lesions may be found on the left side of the heart.

EFFECTS. The thickening and contraction of the cusps and leaflets of the valves of the outflow tracts of the right heart result mainly in pulmonary stenosis and tricuspid regurgitation, and to a lesser extent, pulmonary regurgitation and tricuspid stenosis.

MYXOMATOUS DEGENERATION OF MITRAL VALVE (MITRAL VALVE PROLAPSE)

Myxomatous or mucoid degeneration of the valves of the heart is a peculiar condition occurring in young patients between the age of 20 and 40 years and is more common in women. The condition is common and seen in 5% of general adult population. The condition is also known by other synonyms like 'floppy valve syndrome' or 'mitral valve prolapse'.

ETIOLOGY. The cause of the condition is not known. Association with Marfan's syndrome has been observed in 90% of patients. Others have noted myxomatous degeneration in cases of Ehlers-Danlos syndrome and in myotonic dystrophy. A rheumatic or congenital etiology has been suggested by a few others. However, the myxomatous valvular changes seen in the aged patients are not related to this entity.

PATHOLOGIC CHANGES. Any cardiac valve may be involved but mitral valve is affected most frequently. The disease is usually most severe and most common in the posterior leaflet of the mitral valve. The affected leaflet is enlarged, thickened, opaque white, soft and floppy. Cut section of the valve reveals mucoid or myxoid appearance. A significant feature is the ballooning or aneurysmal protrusion of the affected leaflet and hence the name 'mitral valve prolapse' and 'floppy valve syndrome'. ***Microscopically,*** the enlarged cusp shows loose connective tissue with abundant mucoid or myxoid material between stellate cells.

EFFECTS. Usually the condition does not produce any symptoms or significant valvular dysfunction. The condition is recognised during life by the characteristic mid-systolic click followed by a systolic murmur due to mildly incompetent mitral valve caused by the mitral valve prolapse. Occasionally, complications may develop such as superimposed infective endocarditis, mitral insufficiency and arrhythmias. Rarely, sudden death from serious ventricular arrhythmias may occur.

MYOCARDIAL DISEASE

Involvement of the myocardium occurs in three major forms of diseases already discussed—ischaemic heart disease, hypertensive heart disease and rheumatic heart disease. There are two other broad groups of myocardial diseases considered here:

I. *Myocarditis* i.e. inflammatory involvement of the myocardium; and

II. *Cardiomyopathy* i.e. a non-inflammatory myocardial involvement with unknown (primary) or known (secondary) etiology.

MYOCARDITIS

Inflammation of the heart muscle is called myocarditis. It is a rather common form of heart disease that can occur at any age. Its exact incidence is difficult to ascertain as the histological examination has been confined to autopsy material only. Reports from different studies have estimated the incidence of myocarditis in 1 to 4% of all autopsies.

A number of classifications of myocarditis have been proposed in the past as follows:

- *Interstitial and parenchymatous type,* depending upon whether the inflammation is confined to interstitial tissue or the parenchyma;
- *Specific and non-specific type,* depending upon whether the inflammation is granulomatous or non-specific type; and
- *Acute, subacute and chronic type,* depending upon the duration of inflammatory response.

However, currently most commonly used is *etiologic classification* based upon the causative factors as shown in Table 12.8. According to this classification, myocarditis is divided into 4 main etiologic types described below.

I. INFECTIVE MYOCARDITIS

A number of infectious agents such as bacteria, viruses, protozoa, parasites, fungi, rickettsiae and spirochaetes may cause myocarditis by direct invasion or by their toxins. Some of the common forms are described below.

1. VIRAL MYOCARDITIS. A number of viral infections are associated with myocarditis. Some of the common examples are influenza, poliomyelitis, infectious mononucleosis, hepatitis, smallpox, chickenpox, measles, mumps, rubella, viral pneumonias, coxsackievirus and HIV infections. Cardiac involvement occurs in about 5% of viral infections. Viral myocarditis usually appears after a few days to a few weeks of

TABLE 12.8: Etiologic Classification of Myocarditis.

I. INFECTIVE MYOCARDITIS
1. Viral myocarditis
2. Suppurative myocarditis
3. Toxic myocarditis
4. Infective granulomatous myocarditis
5. Syphilitic myocarditis
6. Rickettsial myocarditis
7. Protozoal myocarditis
8. Helminthic myocarditis
9. Fungal myocarditis

II. IDIOPATHIC (FIEDLER'S) MYOCARDITIS
1. Diffuse type
2. Giant cell (idiopathic granulomatous) type

III. MYOCARDITIS IN CONNECTIVE TISSUE DISEASES
1. Rheumatoid arthritis
2. Lupus erythematosus
3. Polyarteritis nodosa
4. Dermatomyositis
5. Scleroderma

IV. MISCELLANEOUS TYPES OF MYOCARDITIS
1. Physical agents
2. Chemical agents
3. Drugs
4. Immunologic agents
5. Metabolic derangements

viral infections elsewhere in the body. The damage to the myocardium is caused either by direct viral cytotoxicity or by cell-mediated immune reaction. Regardless of the type of virus, the pathologic changes are similar.

Grossly, the myocardium is pale and flabby with dilatation of the chambers. There may be focal or patchy areas of necrosis.
Histologically, there are changes of acute myocarditis. Initially, there is oedema and infiltration of the interstitial tissue by neutrophils and lymphocytes. Later, there is necrosis of individual myocardial fibres and the infiltrate consists of lymphocytes and macrophages.

2. SUPPURATIVE MYOCARDITIS. Pyogenic bacteria, chiefly *Staphylococcus aureus* or *Streptococcus pyogenes*, which cause septicaemia and pyaemia may produce suppurative myocarditis. As already pointed out, acute bacterial endocarditis may sometimes cause bacterial myocarditis (page 338).

Grossly, There are either abscesses in the myocardium or there is diffuse myocardial involvement.
Microscopically, the exudate chiefly consists of neutrophils, admixed with lymphocytes, plasma cells and macrophages. There may be foci of myocardial degeneration and necrosis with areas of healing by fibrosis.

3. TOXIC MYOCARDITIS. A number of acute bacterial infections produce myocarditis by toxins e.g. in diphtheria, typhoid fever and pneumococcal pneumonia.

Grossly, the appearance is similar to that seen in viral myocarditis.
Histologically, there are small foci of coagulative necrosis in the muscle which are surrounded by non-specific acute and chronic inflammatory infiltrate.

Toxic myocarditis manifests clinically by cardiac arrhythmias or acute cardiac failure due to involvement of the conduction system. It may cause sudden death.

4. INFECTIVE GRANULOMATOUS MYOCARDITIS. Tuberculosis, brucellosis and tularaemia are some examples characterised by granulomatous inflammation in the myocardium. Sarcoidosis, though not a proved bacterial infection, has histological resemblance to other granulomatous myocarditis. Tuberculous myocarditis is rare and occurs either by haematogenous spread or by extension from tuberculous pericarditis. The condition must be distinguished from idiopathic granulomatous (giant cell) myocarditis (described later).

5. SYPHILITIC MYOCARDITIS. Syphilitic involvement of the myocardium may occur in 2 forms—a *gummatous lesion* consisting of granulomatous inflammation which is more common, and a *primary non-specific myocarditis* which is rare. The syphilitic gummas in the myocardium may be single or multiple and may be grossly discernible. The gummas may affect the conduction system of the heart.

6. RICKETTSIAL MYOCARDITIS. Myocarditis occurs quite frequently in scrub typhus (*R. tsutsugamushi*) and Rocky Mountain typhus fever caused by spotted *rickettsii.*

Microscopically, there is interstitial oedema and focal or patchy infiltration by inflammatory cells which include lymphocytes, plasma cells, macrophages, mast cells and eosinophils but necrosis and degeneration are generally not present.

7. PROTOZOAL MYOCARDITIS. Chagas' disease and toxoplasmosis are the two protozoal diseases causing myocarditis. Chagas' disease caused by *Trypanosoma cruzi* frequently attacks myocardium besides involving the skeletal muscle and the central nervous system. Toxoplasmosis caused by intracellular protozoan, *Toxoplasma gondii,* sometimes causes myocarditis in children and adults.

Microscopically, both these conditions show focal degeneration and necrosis of the myocardium, oedema and cellular infiltrate consisting of histiocytes, plasma cells, lymphocytes and a few polymorphs.The organisms are found in the muscle fibres.

8. HELMINTHIC MYOCARDITIS. *Echinococcus granulosus* and *Trichinella spiralis* are the two intestinal helminths which may cause myocarditis. *Echinococcus* rarely produces hydatid cyst in the myocardium while the larvae of *Trichinella* in trichinosis cause heavy inflammation in the myocardium as well as in the interstitial tissue.

9. FUNGAL MYOCARDITIS. Patients with immunodeficiency, cancer and other chronic debilitating diseases are more prone to develop fungal myocarditis. These include: candidiasis, aspergillosis, blastomycosis, actinomyosis, cryptococcosis, coccidioidomycosis and histoplasmosis.

II. IDIOPATHIC (FIEDLER'S) MYOCARDITIS

Idiopathic or Fiedler's myocarditis is an isolated myocarditis unaccompanied by inflammatory changes in the endocardium or pericardium and occurs without the usual apparent causes. The condition is rapidly progressive and causes sudden severe cardiac failure or sudden death.

Grossly, the heart is soft and flabby. The cardiac chambers are generally dilated and sometimes show hypertrophy. There are yellow-grey focal lesions throughout the myocardium. Mural thrombi are commonly present.

Histologically, two forms of idiopathic myocarditis are described: diffuse type and giant cell (idiopathic granulomatous) type.

i) Diffuse type is more common of the two. It is characterised by diffuse non-specific inflammatory infiltrate consisting of lymphocytes, plasma cells, macrophages, eosinophils and a few polymorphs in the interstitial tissue without formation of granulomas. Late stage shows healing by fibrosis.

ii) Giant cell type or idiopathic granulomatous type is characterised by formation of non-caseating granulomas consisting of macrophages, lymphocytes, plasma cells and multinucleate giant cells. The giant cells are of foreign body or Langhans' type or of myogenic origin. The granulomas do not show presence of acid-fast bacilli or spirochaetes. Some have suggested relationship of this condition with sarcoidosis but sarcoid granulomas are known to occur in the myocardium secondary to generalised sarcoidosis.

III. MYOCARDITIS IN CONNECTIVE TISSUE DISEASES

Inflammatory involvement of the myocardium occurs in a number of connective tissue diseases such as rheumatoid arthritis, lupus erythematosus, polyarteritis nodosa, dermatomyositis and scleroderma. The pathologic changes in the heart muscle are similar to the changes seen in other organs in these conditions as described elsewhere in relevant chapters.

IV. MISCELLANEOUS TYPES OF MYOCARDITIS

Apart from the three forms of myocarditis described above, the last group consists of myocarditis caused by a variety of agents—physical and chemical agents, drugs and metabolic derangements.

1. Physical agents. Physical agents like contusion of the myocardium, heatstroke, cardiac surgery and irradiation can initiate non-specific myocarditis. The features consist of an infiltrate of neutrophils, eosinophils and mononuclear cells and shows contraction-band necrosis of the myocardial fibres.

2. Chemical agents. Toxic chemicals such as arsenic, phosphorus and carbon monoxide cause focal areas of degeneration and necrosis of myocardial fibres and non-specific inflammatory reaction, chiefly consisting of lymphocytes and macrophages.

3. Drugs. Changes similar to those induced by chemical poisons are produced by certain drugs such as phenothiazine compounds, sulfonamides, catecholamines, and cytotoxic compounds.

4. Immunologic agents. Myasthenia gravis, Friedreich's ataxia, and progressive muscular dystrophies initiate a state of autoimmunisation against the myocardium resulting in focal myocardial degeneration and necrosis with secondary inflammatory reaction. Later, there may be myocardial fibrosis.

5. Metabolic derangements. Uraemia, hypokalaemia and shock are associated with degeneration and necrosis of the myocardial fibres, oedema of the interstitial tissue and non-specific inflammatory reaction.

CARDIOMYOPATHY

Cardiomyopathy literally means disease of the heart muscle but the term was originally coined to restrict its usage to *myocardial disease of unkown cause.* The WHO definition of cardiomyopathy also excludes heart muscle diseases of known etiologies. However, the term cardiomyopathy has been loosely used by various workers for myocardial diseases of known etiology as well e.g. alcoholic cardiomyopathy, amyloid cardiomyopathy, ischaemic cardiomyopathy etc. This controversy is resolved by classifying all cardiomyopathies into two broad groups:

a) *primary cardiomyopathy*; and

b) *secondary cardiomyopathy* i.e. myocardial disease with known underlying cause.

Based on these principles, a classification of cardiomyopathy and its subtypes is presented in Table 12.9.

A. PRIMARY CARDIOMYOPATHY

This is a group of myocardial diseases of unknown cause. It is subdivided into the following 3 pathophysiologic categories (Fig. 12.26):

1. Idiopathic dilated (congestive) cardiomyopathy.
2. Idiopathic hypertrophic cardiomyopathy.
3. Idiopathic restrictive or obliterative or infiltrative cardiomyopathy.

TABLE 12.9: Classification of Cardiomyopathies.

I. PRIMARY CARDIOMYOPATHY

1. Idiopathic dilated (or congestive) cardiomyopathy
2. Idiopathic hypertrophic cardiomyopathy
   i) Obstructive type
   ii) Non-obstructive type
3. Idiopathic restrictive (or obliterative or infiltrative) cardiomyopathy
   i) Cardiac amyloidosis
   ii) Endocardial fibroelastosis
   iii) Endomyocardial fibrosis
   iv) Löeffler's endocarditis (fibroplastic parietal endocarditis with peripheral blood eosinophilia)

II. SECONDARY CARDIOMYOPATHY

1. Nutritional disorders (e.g. alcoholic cardiomyopathy, beriberi heart disease)
2. Toxic chemicals (e.g. cobalt, arsenic, lithium, hydrocarbons)
3. Drugs (e.g. emetrine, cyclophosphamide, adriamycin, catecholamines)
4. Metabolic diseases (e.g. cardiac amyloidosis, haemochromatosis, glycogen storage diseases)
5. Neuromuscular diseases (e.g. Friedreich's ataxia, muscular dystrophies)
6. Infiltrations (e.g. leukaemia, carcinomas)
7. Connective tissue diseases (e.g. rheumatoid arthritis, lupus erythematosus, systemic sclerosis, dermatomyositis)

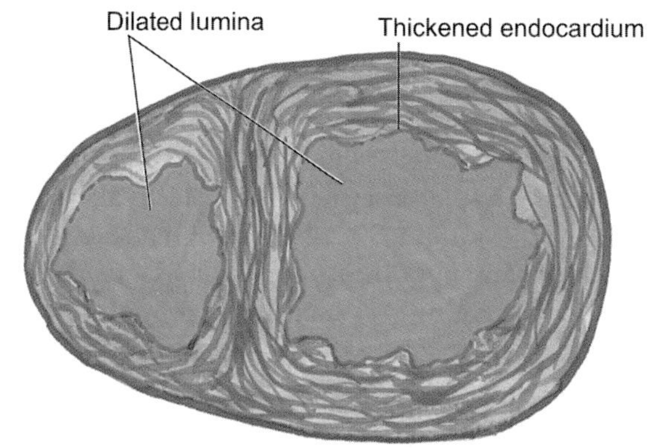

A, IDIOPATHIC DILATED CARDIOMYOPATHY

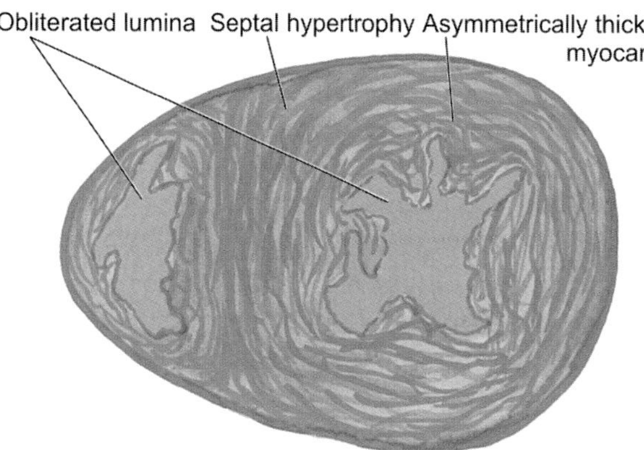

B, IDIOPATHIC HYPERTROPHIC CARDIOMYOPATHY

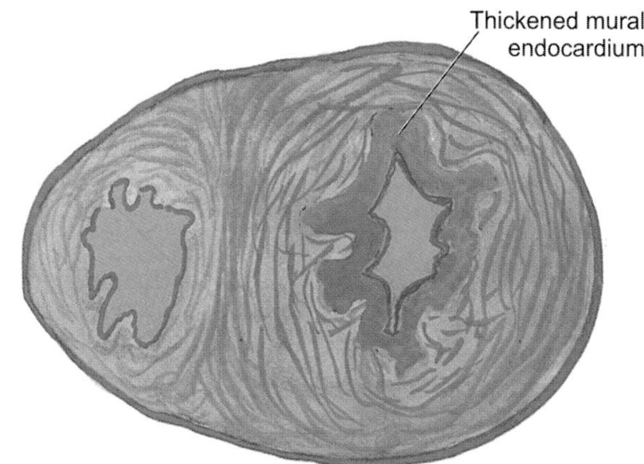

C, IDIOPATHIC RESTRICTIVE CARDIOMYOPATHY

FIGURE 12.26
The major pathophysiologic forms of idiopathic cardiomyopathies.

1. Idiopathic Dilated (Congestive) Cardiomyopathy

This type of cardiomyopathy is characterised by gradually progressive cardiac failure alongwith dilatation of all the four chambers of the heart. The condition occurs more often in adults and the average survival from onset to death is less than 5 years. Though the etiology is unknown, a few hypotheses based on associations with the following conditions have been proposed:

i) Possible association of *viral myocarditis* (especially coxsackievirus B) with dilated cardiomyopathy, due to presence of viral nucleic acids in the myocardium, has been noted.

ii) Association with *toxic damage* from cobalt and chemotherapy with doxorubicin and other anthracyclines is implicated in some cases.

iii) Role of *inherited mutations* has been emphasised lately. Mutations in certain sarcomere proteins such as cardiac troponin-T and β-myosin have been observed. Another mutation in cytoskeletal protein dystrophin gene on X-chromosome has been held responsible for muscular dystrophy as well as dilated cardiomyopathy.

iv) *Chronic alcoholism* has been found associated with dilated cardiomyopathy. It may be due to thiamine deficiency induced by alcohol and resulting in beri-beri heart disease (Chapter 9). This is referred to as 'alcoholic cardiomyopathy' and included by some workers as one of the subtypes of secondary cardiomyopathy. Another form of alcoholic cardiomyopathy is associated with consumption of large quantities of beer (beer drinkers' myocardiosis). Cobalt added to the beer so as to improve the appearance of foam is thought to cause direct toxic injury to the heart in this condition.

v) *Peripartum association* has been observed in some cases. Poorly-nourished women may develop this form of cardiomyopathy within a month before or after delivery.

PATHOLOGIC CHANGES. Grossly, the heart is enlarged and increased in weight (upto 1000 gm). The most characteristic feature is prominent dilatation of all the four chambers giving the heart typical globular appearance. Thickening of the ventricular walls even if present is masked by the ventricular dilatation (Fig. 12.26,A). The endocardium is thickened and mural thrombi are often found in the ventricles and atria. The cardiac valves are usually normal.

Microscopically, The endomyocardial biopsies or autopsy examination of the heart reveal non-specific and variable changes. There may be hypertrophy of some myocardial fibres and atrophy of others. Sometimes degenerative changes and small areas of interstitial fibrosis are found with focal mononuclear inflammatory cell infiltrate.

2. Idiopathic Hypertrophic Cardiomyopathy

This form of cardiomyopathy is known by various synonyms like asymmetrical hypertrophy, hypertrophic subaortic stenosis and Teare's disease. The disease occurs more frequently between the age of 25 and 50 years. It is often asymptomatic but becomes symptomatic due to heavy physical activity causing dyspnoea, angina, congestive heart failure and even sudden death. Though idiopathic, the following factors have been implicated:

i) *Autosomal dominant inheritance* of the disease is available in about half the cases suggesting genetic factors in its causation.

ii) *Inherited mutations* in genes encoding for sarcomere proteins have been reported in much larger number of cases of hypertrophic cardiomyopathy than those of dilated cardiomyopathy. Particularly implicated are the mutations in heavy and light chains of β-myosin, troponin-I and troponin-T. The condition may result from *myocardial ischaemia* resulting in fibrosis of the intramyocardial arteries and compensatory hypertrophy.

iii) *Other contributory factors* are: increased circulating level of catecholamines, myocardial ischaemia as a result of thickened vasculature of the myocardium and abnormally increased fibrous tissue in the myocardium due to hypertrophy.

PATHOLOGIC CHANGES. Grossly, the characteristic features are cardiac enlargement, increase in weight, normal or small ventricular cavities and myocardial hypertrophy. The hypertrophy of the myocardium is typically asymmetrical and affects the interventricular septum more than the free walls of the ventricles (Fig. 12.26,B). This asymmetric septal hypertrophy may be confined to the apical region of the septum (*non-obstructive type*) or may extend upto the level of the mitral valve causing obstruction to left ventricular outflow in the form of subaortic stenosis (*obstructive type*). The designation of *rhabdomyoma of the septum* was applied to this form of cardiomyopathy in the old literature.

Microscopically, the classical feature is the myocardial cell disorganisation in the ventricular septum. The bundles of myocardial fibres are irregularly and haphazardly arranged rather than the usual parallel pattern and are separated by bands of interstitial fibrous tissue. The individual muscle cells show hypertrophy and large prominent nuclei.

3. Idiopathic Restrictive (Obliterative or Infiltrative) Cardiomyopathy

This form of cardiomyopathy is characterised by restriction in ventricular filling due to reduction in the volume of the ventricles. It includes the following entities:

i) Cardiac amyloidosis
ii) Endocardial fibroelastosis
iii) Endomyocardial fibrosis
iv) Löeffler's endocarditis (Fibroplastic parietal endocarditis with peripheral blood eosinophilia).

I) CARDIAC AMYLOIDOSIS. Amyloidosis of the heart may occur in any form of systemic amyloidosis or may occur as isolated organ amyloidosis in amyloid of aging and result in subendocardial deposits (Chapter 4).

II) ENDOCARDIAL FIBROELASTOSIS. This is an unusual and uncommon form of heart disease occurring predominantly in infants and children under 2 years of age and less often in adults. The *infantile form* is clinically characterised by sudden breathlessness, cyanosis, cardiac failure and death whereas the symptoms in the *adult form* last for longer duration. The etiology of the condition remains obscure. However, a number of theories have been proposed. These are as under:

a) The infantile form is believed to be congenital in origin occurring due to the effect of intrauterine *endocardial anoxia.* The adult form may also be induced by anoxia-causing lesions such as anomalous coronary arteries, metabolic derangements influencing myocardial function etc.

b) It may occur due to *haemodynamic pressure overload* such as in congenital septal defects and coarctation of the aorta.

c) It may be an expression of *genetic disorder* as noticed in twins, triplets and siblings. Association of endocardial fibroelastosis with various congenital malformations in the heart or elsewhere further supports the genetic theory.

d) Some workers consider this disease a form of *connective tissue disorder.*

e) Certain factors causing *myocardial injury* may initiate the endocardial disease such as in thiamine deficiency (beri-beri heart disease) or from preceding idiopathic myocarditis.

f) *Lymphatic obstruction* of the heart has been suggested by some as the causative mechanism.

PATHOLOGIC CHANGES. ***Grossly,*** the characteristic feature is the diffuse or patchy, rigid, pearly-white thickening of the mural endocardium (Fig. 12.26,C). Left ventricle is predominantly involved, followed in decreasing frequency by left atrium, right ventricle and right atrium. Quite often, the valves, especially of the left heart, are affected. Some cases contain mural thrombi. Enlargement of the heart is present and is mainly due to left ventricular hypertrophy but the volume of the chamber is decreased.

Microscopically, the typical finding is the proliferation of the collagen and elastic tissue (fibroelastosis) comprising the thickened endocardium. The fibroelastosis generally does not extend into the subjacent myocardium. The lesion is devoid of inflammatory cells.

III) ENDOMYOCARDIAL FIBROSIS. This form of restrictive cardiomyopathy is a tropical condition prevalent in Africa, especially in Uganda and Nigeria, but some cases occur in South India, Sri Lanka, Malaysia and tropical South America. It is seen in children and young adults. The clinical manifestations consist of congestive heart failure of unknown cause just as in adult variety of endocardial fibroelastosis. The etiology of the condition remains obscure but the geographic distribution suggests the role of certain factors like malnutrition, viral infections and heavy consumption of banana (rich in serotonin).

PATHOLOGIC CHANGES. ***Grossly,*** endomyocardial fibrosis is characterised by fibrous scarring of the ventricular endocardium that extends to involve the inner third of the myocardium. The atrioventricular valve leaflets are often affected but the semilunar valves are uninvolved. Mural thrombi may be present. The heart may be normal-sized or hypertrophied but the volume of the affected chambers is diminished due to fibrous scarring.

Microscopically, the endocardium and parts of inner third of the myocardium show destruction of normal tissue and replacement by fibrous tissue. The condition differs from endocardial fibroelastosis in having mononuclear inflammatory cell infiltrate and lacking in elastic tissue. The superficial layer may show dense hyalinised connective tissue and even calcification.

IV) LÖEFFLER'S ENDOCARDITIS. Also known by the more descriptive term of 'fibroplastic parietal endocarditis with peripheral blood eosinophilia', the condition is considered by some as a variant of the entity described above, endomyocardial fibrosis. However, it differs from the latter in following respects:

a) There is generally a peripheral blood eosinophilic leucocytosis.

b) The inflammatory infiltrate in the endocardium and in the part of affected myocardium chiefly consists of eosinophils.

c) The condition has a worse prognosis.

B. SECONDARY CARDIOMYOPATHY

This is a group of myocardial diseases of known etiologies or having clinical associations. This, however, excludes well-defined entities such as ischaemic, hypertensive, valvular, pericardial, congenital and inflammatory involvements of the heart. The main entities included in this group are described elsewhere in the text and are listed below:

1. *Nutritional disorders e.g.* chronic alcoholism, thiamine deficiency causing beri-beri heart disease (Chapter 9).
2. *Toxic chemicals e.g.* cobalt, arsenic, lithium and hydrocarbons.
3. *Drugs* e.g. cyclophosphamide, adriamycin, catecholamines.
4. *Metabolic diseases e.g.* amyloidosis, haemochromatosis, glycogen storage diseases, hypo-and hyperthyroidism, hypo-and hyperkalaemia.
5. *Neuromuscular diseases e.g.* Friedreich's ataxia, muscular dystrophies.
6. *Infiltrations* e.g. from leukaemia and carcinoma.
7. *Connective tissue diseases e.g.* rheumatoid arthritis, systemic sclerosis, dermatomyositis, lupus erythematosus.

PERICARDIAL DISEASE

Diseases of the pericardium are usually secondary to, or associated with, other cardiac and systemic diseases. They are broadly of 2 types:

I. Pericardial fluid accumulations
II. Pericarditis

PERICARDIAL FLUID ACCUMULATIONS

Accumulation of fluid in the pericardial sac may be watery or pure blood. Accordingly, it is of 2 types: hydropericardium (pericardial effusion) and haemopericardium.

A. HYDROPERICARDIUM (PERICARDIAL EFFUSION). Accumulation of fluid in the pericardial cavity due to non-inflammatory causes is called hydropericardium or pericardial effusion. Normally, the pericardial cavity contains 30 to 50 ml of clear watery fluid. Considerable quantities of fluid (upto 1000 ml) can be accommodated in the pericardial cavity without seriously affecting the cardiac function if the accumulation is slow. But sudden accumulation of a smaller volume (upto 250 ml) may produce deficient diastolic filling of the cardiac chambers (cardiac tamponade). Pericardial effusion is detected by cardiac enlargement in the X-rays and by faint apex beat.

The various types of effusions and their causes are as follows:

1. **Serous effusions.** This is the most common type occurring in conditions in which there is generalised oedema e.g. in cardiac (in CHF), renal, nutritional and hepatic causes. The serous effusion is clear, watery, straw-coloured with specific gravity less than 1.015 (transudate). The serosal surface is smooth and glistening.

2. **Serosanguineous effusion.** This type is found following blunt trauma to chest and cardiopulmonary resuscitation.

3. **Chylous effusion.** Milky or chylous fluid accumulates in conditions causing lymphatic obstruction.

4. **Cholesterol effusion.** This is a rare type of fluid accumulation characterised by the presence of cholesterol crystals such as in myxoedema.

B. HAEMOPERICARDIUM. Accumulation of pure blood in the pericardial sac is termed haemopericardium. The condition must be distinguished from haemorrhagic pericarditis in which there is escape of small quantities of blood into the pericardial cavity. Massive and sudden bleeding into the sac causes compression of the heart leading to cardiac tamponade. The causes of haemopericardium are:

i) Rupture of the heart through a myocardial infarct.
ii) Rupture of dissecting aneurysm.
iii) Bleeding diathesis such as in scurvy, acute leukaemias, thrombocytopenia.
iv) Trauma following cardiopulmonary resuscitation or by laceration of a coronary artery.

PERICARDITIS

Pericarditis is the inflammation of the pericardial layers and is generally secondary to diseases in the heart or caused by systemic diseases. Primary or idiopathic pericarditis is quite rare. Based on the morphologic appearance, pericarditis is classified into acute and chronic types, each of which may have several etiologies. Acute and chronic pericarditis have further subtypes based on the character of the exudate (Table 12.10).

A. Acute Pericarditis

Acute bacterial and non-bacterial pericarditis are the most frequently encountered forms of pericarditis. These may have the following subtypes:

TABLE 12.10: Classification of Pericarditis.

A. ACUTE PERICARDITIS
1. Serous pericarditis
2. Fibrinous or serofibrinous pericarditis
3. Purulent or fibrinopurulent pericarditis
4. Haemorrhagic pericarditis

B. CHRONIC PERICARDITIS
1. Tuberculous pericarditis
2. Chronic adhesive pericarditis
3. Chronic constrictive pericarditis
4. Pericardial plaques (milk spots, soldiers' spots)

1. SEROUS PERICARDITIS. Acute pericarditis may be accompanied by accumulation of serous effusion which differs from transudate of hydropericardium in having increased protein content and higher specific gravity. Its various causes are as under:

i) Viral infection e.g. coxsackie A or B viruses, influenza virus, mumps virus, adenovirus and infectious mononucleosis.

ii) Rheumatic fever.

iii) Rheumatoid arthritis.

iv) Systemic lupus erythematosus.

v) Involvement of the pericardium by malignant tumour in the vicinity e.g. carcinoma lung, mesothelioma and mediastinal tumours.

vi) Tuberculous pericarditis in the early stage.

The fluid accumulation is generally not much and ranges from 50 to 200 ml but may rarely be large enough to cause cardiac tamponade.

Microscopically, the epicardial and pericardial surfaces show infiltration by some neutrophils, lymphocytes and histiocytes. The fluid usually resorbs with the resolution of underlying disease.

2. FIBRINOUS AND SEROFIBRINOUS PERICARDITIS. The response of the pericardium by fibrinous exudate is the most common type of pericarditis. Quite often, there is admixture of fibrinous exudate with serous fluid. The various causes of this type of pericarditis are:

i) Uraemia

ii) Myocardial infarction

iii) Rheumatic fever

iv) Trauma such as in cardiac surgery

v) Acute bacterial infections.

The amount of fluid accumulation is variable. The cardiac surface is characteristically covered by dry or moist, shaggy, fibrinous exudate which gives 'bread and butter' appearance (COLOUR PLATE XV: CL 60). Clinically, these cases manifest by friction rub. In less extensive cases of fibrinous or serofibrinous pericarditis, there is complete resorption of the exudate. In cases with advanced fibrinous exudate, pericarditis heals by organisation and develops fibrous adhesions resulting in adhesive pericarditis.

3. PURULENT OR FIBRINOPURULENT PERICARDITIS. Purulent or fibrinopurulent pericarditis is mainly caused by pyogenic bacteria (e.g. staphylococci, streptococci and pneumococci) and less frequently by fungi and parasites. The infection may spread to the pericardium by the following routes:

i) By direct extension from neighbouring inflammation e.g. in empyema of the pleural cavity, lobar pneumonia, infective endocarditis and mediastinal infections.

ii) By haematogenous spread.

iii) By lymphatic permeation.

iv) Direct implantation during cardiac surgery.

Generally, fibrinous or serofibrinous pericarditis precedes the development of purulent pericarditis. The amount of exudate is variable and is generally thick, creamy pus, coating the pericardial surfaces.

Microscopically, besides the purulent exudate on the pericardial surfaces, the serosal layers show dense infiltration by neutrophils. Purulent exudate generally does not resolve completely but instead heals by organisation resulting in adhesive or chronic constrictive pericarditis.

4. HAEMORRHAGIC PERICARDITIS. Haemorrhagic pericarditis is the one in which the exudate consists of admixture of an inflammatory effusion of one of the foregoing types alongwith blood. The causes are:

i) Neoplastic involvement of the pericardium

ii) Haemorrhagic diathesis with effusion

iii) Tuberculosis

iv) Severe acute infections

The outcome of haemorrhagic pericarditis is generally similar to that of purulent pericarditis.

B. Chronic Pericarditis

Chronic pericarditis is the term used for tuberculous pericarditis and the healed stage of one of the various forms of acute pericarditis already described. Included under this are: tuberculous pericarditis, chronic adhesive pericarditis, chronic constrictive pericarditis, and the pericardial plaques.

1. TUBERCULOUS PERICARDITIS. Tuberculous pericarditis is the most frequent form of granulomatous inflammation of the pericardium. The lesions may occur by one of the following mechanisms:

i) Direct extension from an adjacent focus of tuberculosis.

ii) By lymphatic spread e.g. from tracheobronchial lymph nodes, chronic pulmonary tuberculosis or infected pleura.

The exudate is slightly turbid, caseous or blood-stained with sufficient fibrin. Tubercles are generally visible on the pericardial surfaces and sometimes caseous areas are also visible to the naked eye.

Microscopically, typical tuberculous granulomas with caseation necrosis are seen in the pericardial wall. The lesions generally do not resolve but heal by fibrosis and calcification resulting in chronic constrictive pericarditis.

2. CHRONIC ADHESIVE PERICARDITIS. Chronic adhesive pericarditis is the stage of organisation and healing by formation of fibrous adhesions in the pericardium following preceding fibrinous, suppurative or haemorrhagic pericarditis. The process begins by formation of granulation tissue and neovascularisation. Subsequently, fibrous adhesions develop between the parietal and the visceral layers of the pericardium and obliterate the pericardial space (Fig. 12.27,A). Sometimes, fibrous adhesions develop between the parietal pericardium and the adjacent mediastinum and is termed as *adhesive mediastinopericarditis.* Chronic adhesive pericarditis differs from chronic constrictive pericarditis in not embarrassing the function of the heart. However, cardiac hypertrophy and dilatation may occur in severe cases due to increased workload.

3. CHRONIC CONSTRICTIVE PERICARDITIS. This is a rare condition characterised by dense fibrous or fibrocalcific thickening of the pericardium resulting in mechanical interference with the function of the heart and reduced cardiac output. The condition usually results from a long-standing preceding causes such as:

i) Tuberculous pericarditis

ii) Purulent pericarditis

iii) Haemopericardium

iv) Concato's disease (polyserositis)

v) Rarely, acute non-specific and viral pericarditis.

The heart is encased in 0.5 to 1 cm thick and dense collagenous scar which may be calcified. As a result, the heart fails to dilate during diastole. The dense fibrocollagenous tissue may cause narrowing of the openings of the vena cavae, resulting in obstruction to the venous return to the right heart and consequent right heart failure. In contrast to chronic adhesive pericarditis, hypertrophy and dilatation do not occur due to dense fibrous scarring. Instead, the heart size is normal or smaller (Fig. 12.27,B).

4. PERICARDIAL PLAQUES (MILK SPOTS, SOLDIERS' SPOTS). These are opaque, white, shining and well-circumscribed areas of organisation with fibrosis in the pericardium measuring 1 to 3 cm in diameter. They are seen most frequently on the anterior surface of the right ventricle. The exact cause is not known but they are generally believed to arise from healing of preceding pericarditis. The plaque-like lesions of pericardial thickenings are also termed *milk spots or soldiers' spots* as they were often found at autopsy in the soldiers in World War I who carried their shoulder bags causing pressure against the chest wall by the straps which produced chronic irritation of the pericardium.

TUMOURS OF THE HEART

Tumours of the heart are classified into primary and secondary, the latter being more common than the former.

PRIMARY TUMOURS

Primary tumours of the heart are quite rare, found in 0.04% of autopsies. In decreasing order of frequency, the benign tumours encountered in the heart are: myxoma, lipoma, fibroelastoma, rhabdomyoma, haemangioma and lymphangioma. The malignant tumours are still rarer, the important ones are: rhabdomyosarcoma, angiosarcoma and malignant mesothelioma. Out of all these, only myxoma of the heart requires elaboration.

MYXOMA. This is the most common primary tumour of the heart comprising about 50% of all primary cardiac tumours. Majority of them occur in the age range of 30 to 60 years. Myxomas may be located in any cardiac chamber or the valves, but 90% of them are situated in the left atrium.

Grossly, they are often single but may be multiple. They range in size from less than 1 to 10 cm, polypoid, pedunculated, spherical, soft and haemorrhagic masses resembling an organising mural thrombus. Some investigators actually consider them to be organising mural thrombi rather than true neoplasms.

Chapter Twelve

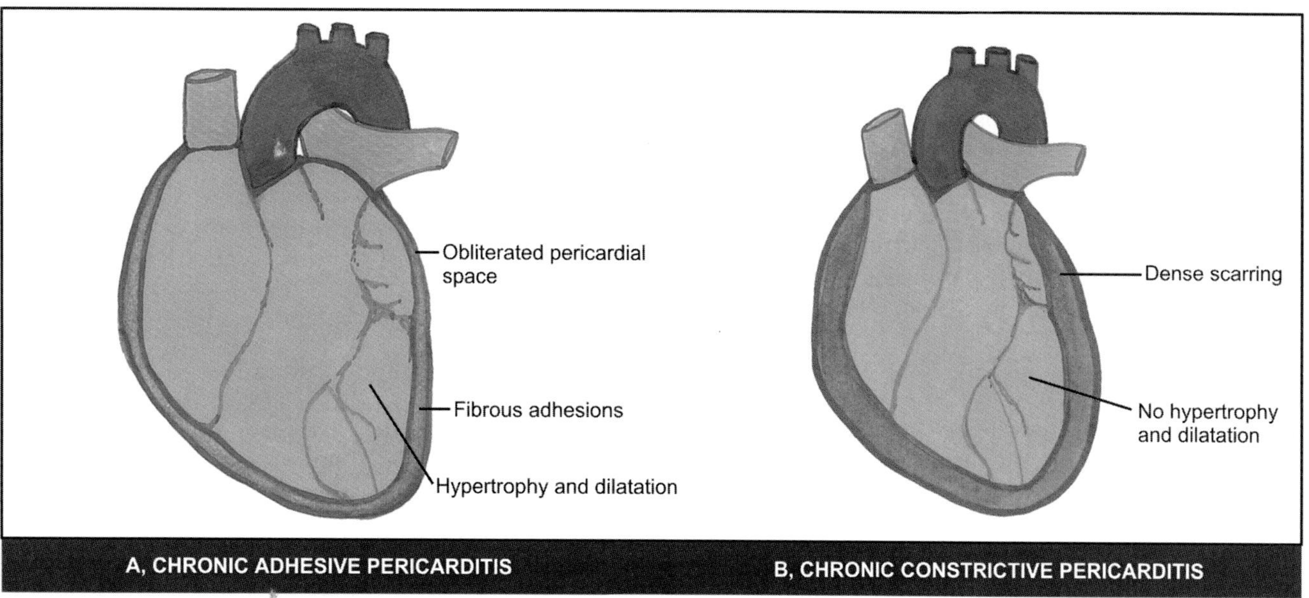

FIGURE 12.27

Appearance of the heart and the pericardium in chronic adhesive (A) and chronic constrictive pericarditis (B).

Microscopically, the tumour shows the following features:

i) There is abundant myxoid or mucoid intercellular stroma positive for mucin.

ii) The cellularity is sparse. The tumour cells are generally stellate-shaped, spindled and polyhedral, scattered in the stroma. Occasional multinucleate tumour giant cells are present.

iii) Numerous capillary-sized blood vessels are found and the tumour cells may be aggregated around them.

iv) A few lymphocytes, plasma cells and macrophages are seen.

v) Foci of haemorrhage and deposits of haemosiderin granules are often present.

SECONDARY TUMOURS

Metastatic tumours of the heart are more common than the primary tumours. About 10% cases with disseminated cancer have metastases in the heart. Most of these result from haematogenous or lymphatic spread. In descending order of frequency, primary sites of origin are: carcinoma of the lung, breast, malignant lymphoma, leukaemia and malignant melanoma. Occasionally, there may be direct extension of a primary intrathoracic tumour such as carcinoma of the lung into the pericardium and into the cardiac chambers.

PATHOLOGY OF CARDIAC INTERVENTIONS

Nowadays, with the development of surgical and non-surgical therapeutic interventions in coronary artery disease, it has been possible to study the pathology of native as well as grafted vessel and also the myocardium by endomyocardial biopsy.

ENDOMYOCARDIAL BIOPSY

Currently, it is possible to perform endomyocardial biopsy (EMB) for making a final histopathologic diagnosis in certain cardiac diseases. The main *indications* for EMB are: myocarditis, cardiac transplant cases, restrictive heart disease, infiltrative heart diseases such as in amyloidosis, storage disorders etc.

EMB is done by biopsy forceps introduced via cardiac catheter in to either of the ventricles but preferably right ventricle is biopsied for its relative ease and safety. The route for the catheter may be through internal jugular vein or femoral vein for accessing the right ventricle.

BALLOON ANGIOPLASTY

Balloon angioplasty is a non-surgical procedure that employs percutaneous insertion and manipulation of a balloon catheter into the occluded coronary artery. The balloon is inflated to dilate the stenotic artery which causes endothelial damage, plaque fracture, medial dissection and haemorrhage in the affected arterial wall. At this stage, unstable angioplasty is liable to be associated with acute coronary syndromes.

After 3-6 months of angioplasty, 30-40% cases of satisfactorily dilated vessel lumen are followed by restenosis. The restenosis is multifactorial in etiology that includes smooth muscle cell proliferation, extracellular matrix and local thrombosis. Currently, radioactive stents which emit low dose particles to inhibit smooth cell proliferation are also available.

CORONARY BYPASS GRAFTING

Autologous grafts are used to replace or bypass diseased coronary arteries. Most frequently used is autologous graft of saphenous vein which is reversed (due to valves in the vein) and transplanted, or left internal mammary artery may be used being in the operative area of the heart. Long-term follow-up of bypass surgery has yielded following observations on pathology of grafted vessel:

1. In a reversed saphenous vein graft, long-term luminal patency is 50% after 10 years. Pathologic changes which develop in grafted vein include thrombosis in early stage, intimal thickening and atherosclerosis with or without complicated lesions.
2. Internal mammary artery graft, however, has a patency of more than 90% after 10 years.
3. Atherosclerosis with superimposed complications may develop in native coronary artery distal to the grafted vessel as well as in the grafted vessel.

CARDIAC TRANSPLANTATION

Cardiac transplantation is done in end-stage cardiac diseases, most often in idiopathic cardiomyopathies. Worldwide, about 40,000 cardiac transplants have been carried out. The survival following heart transplants is reported as: 1 year in 85%, 5 years in 65 % and 10 years in 45% cases. Major complications are transplant rejection reaction and infections, particularly with *Toxoplasma gondii* and cytomegaloviruses. One of the main problems in cardiac transplant centres is the availability of donors.

The stem cell research in this area holds great promise for the future because then it would be possible to transplant transformed embryonic stem cells.

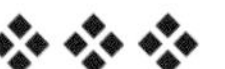

The Haematopoietic System

13

Chapter Thirteen

This section on disorders of the haematopoietic system is concerned with diseases of the blood and bone marrow. The account that follows here is arbitrarily divided into the following subsections for the purpose of convenience of discussion:

(1) bone marrow; (2) red blood cells; (3) white blood cells; (4) platelets and haemorrhagic diathesis; (5) blood groups and blood transfusion.

Broad outlines of the treatment of common haematological diseases are also included in the discussion below.

BONE MARROW

The pluripotent stem cells in the bone marrow give rise to two types of multipotent stem cells: *non-lymphoid stem cells* which differentiate in the bone marrow, and *lymphoid stem cells* which differentiate in the bone marrow and then migrate to the lymphoid tissues. The non-lymphoid stem cells form the circulating erythrocytes, granulocytes, monocytes and platelets. Monocytes on entering the tissues form a variety of phagocytic macrophages, both of which together constitute mononuclear-phagocyte system (Chapter 4). Lymphopoietic cells in the marrow undergo differentiation to form B and T lymphocytes of the immune system.

Circulating blood normally contains 3 main types of cells—the red cells (erythrocytes), the white cells (leucocytes) and the platelets (thrombocytes). These blood cells perform their respective physiologic functions: *erythrocytes* are largely concerned with oxygen transport, *leucocytes* play various roles in body defense against infection and tissue injury, while *thrombocytes* are primarily involved in maintaining integrity of blood vessels and in preventing blood loss. The life-span of these cells is variable—neutrophils have the blood life-span of 6-8 hours, followed by platelets with a life-span of 10 days, while the RBCs have the longest life-span of 90-120 days. The rates of production of these blood cells are normally regulated in healthy individuals in such a way so as to match the rate at which they are lost from circulation. Their concentration is normally maintained within well-defined limits unless the balance is disturbed due to some pathologic processes.

HAEMATOPOIESIS

In the human embryo, the *yolk sac* is the main site of haematopoiesis in the first few weeks of gestation. By about 3rd month, however, the *liver and spleen* are the main sites of blood cell formation and continue to do so until about 2 weeks after birth. Haematopoiesis commences in the *bone marrow* by 4th and 5th month and becomes fully active by 7th and 8th month so that at birth practically all the bones contain active marrow. During normal childhood and adult life, therefore, the marrow is the only source of new blood cells. However, during childhood, there is progressive fatty replacement throughout the long bones so that by adult life the haematopoietic marrow is confined to the central skeleton (vertebrae, sternum, ribs, skull, sacrum and pelvis) and proximal ends of femur, tibia and humerus (Fig. 13.1). Even in these haematopoietic areas, about 50% of the marrow consists of fat (Fig. 13.2). Non-haematopoietic marrow in the adult is, however, capable of reverting to active haematopoiesis in certain pathologic conditions. The spleen and liver can also resume their foetal haematopoietic role in certain pathologic conditions and is called *extramedullary haematopoiesis.*

In the bone marrow, the developing blood cells are situated outside the marrow sinuses, from where on maturation they enter the marrow sinuses, the marrow microcirculation and thence released into circulation.

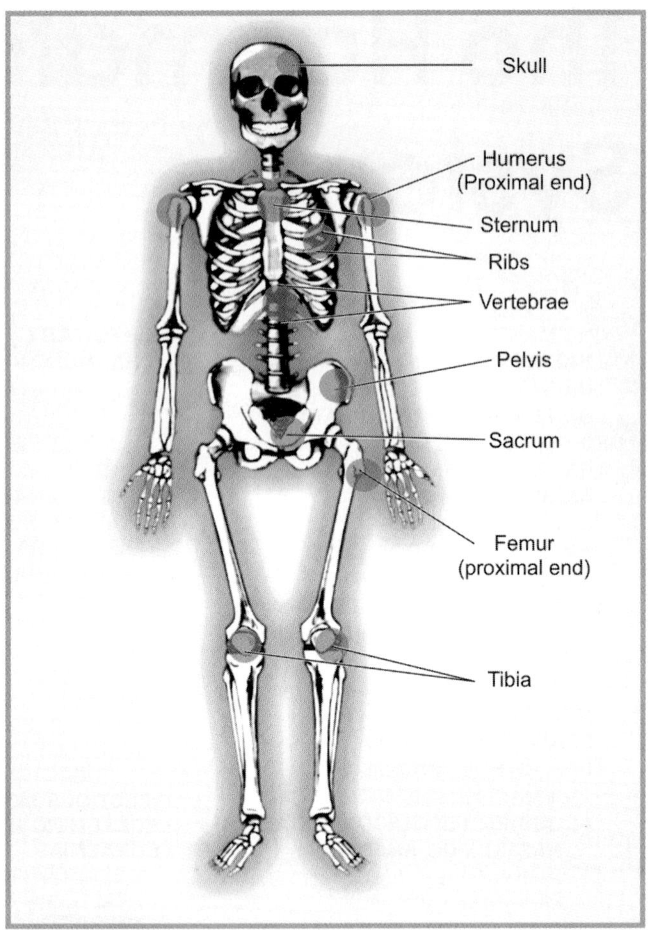

FIGURE 13.1

Sites of haematopoiesis in the bone marrow in the adult.

HAEMATOPOIETIC STEM CELLS

It is widely accepted that blood cells develop from a small population of common multipotent haematopoietic stem cells. The stem cells express a variety of cell surface proteins such as CD34 and adhesion proteins which help the stem cells to "home" to bone marrow when infused. The stem cells have the appearance of small or intermediate-sized lymphocytes and their presence in the marrow can be demonstrated by cell culture techniques by the growth of colony-forming units (CFU) pertaining to different cell lines. The stem cells have the capability of maintaining their progeny by self-replication. The bone marrow provides a suitable environment for growth and development of stem cells. For instance, if haematopoietic stem cells are infused intravenously into a suitably-prepared recipient, they seed the marrow successfully but do not thrive at other

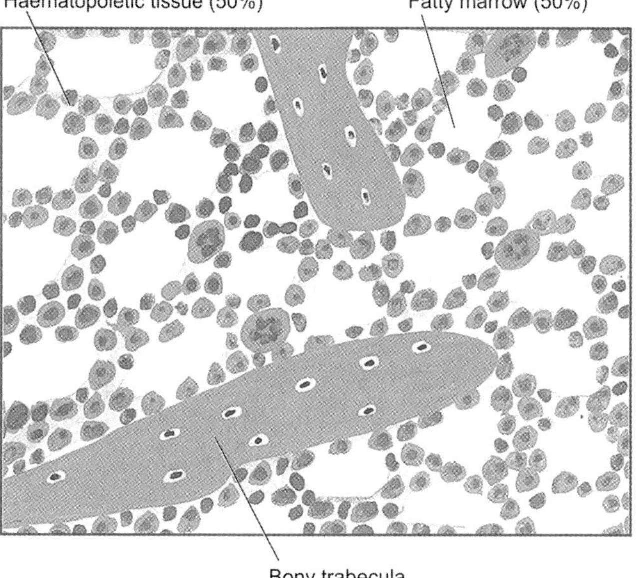

FIGURE 13.2

A normal bone marrow in an adult as seen in a section after trephine biopsy. Bony trabeculae support the marrow-containing tissue. Approximately 50% of the soft tissue of the bone consists of haematopoietic tissue and 50% is fatty marrow.

sites. This principle forms the basis of bone marrow transplantation performed for various haematologic diseases.

The stem cells, after a series of divisions, differentiate into two types of progenitors—*lymphoid* (immune system) stem cells, and *non-lymphoid or myeloid* (trilineage) stem cells. The former develop into T, B and null lymphocytes while the latter differentiate into 3 types of cell lines—granulocyte-monocyte progenitors (producing neutrophils, eosinophils, basophils and monocytes), erythroid progenitors (producing red cells), and megakaryocytes (as the source of platelets). The development of mature cells (*-poiesis*)—red cells (erythropoiesis), granulocytes (granulopoiesis), monocytes, lymphocytes (lymphopoiesis) and platelets (thrombopoiesis) are considered in detail later in relevant sections.

Myeloid haematopoiesis or myelopoiesis includes differentiation and maturation of granulocytes, monocytes, erythroid cells and megakaryocytes (Fig. 13.3). The differentiation and maturation of these cells from stem cell are regulated by endogenous glycoproteins called as *growth factors, cytokines and hormones.* These are:

- Erythropoietin
- Granulocyte colony-stimulating factor (G-CSF)
- Granulocyte-macrophage colony-stimulating factor (GM-CSF)
- Thrombopoietin

Each of these growth factors act on specific receptors for growth factor to initiate further cell events as shown schematically in Fig. 13.3.

BONE MARROW EXAMINATION

Examination of the bone marrow provides an invaluable diagnostic help in some cases, while in others it is of value in confirming a diagnosis suspected on clinical examination or on the blood film. A peripheral blood smear examination, however, must always precede bone marrow examination.

Bone marrow examination may be performed by two methods—*aspiration* and *trephine biopsy*. A comparison of the two methods is summarised in Table 13.1.

BONE MARROW ASPIRATION. The method involves suction of marrow via a strong, wide bore, short-bevelled needle fitted with a stylet and an adjustable guard in order to prevent excessive penetration; for instance Salah bone marrow aspiration needle (Fig. 13.4,A). Smears are prepared immediately from the bone marrow aspirate and are fixed in 95% methanol after air-drying. The usual Romanowsky technique is employed for staining and a stain for iron is performed routinely so as to assess the reticuloendothelial stores of iron.

The marrow film provides assessment of cellularity, details of developing blood cells (i.e. normoblastic or megaloblastic, myeloid, lymphoid, macrophages and megakaryocytic), ratio between erythroid and myeloid cells, storage diseases, and for the presence of cells foreign to the marrow such as secondary carcinoma, granulomatous conditions, fungi (e.g. histoplasmosis) and parasites (e.g. malaria, leishmaniasis, trypanosomiasis) (Fig. 13.4,C). Estimation of the proportion of cellular components in the marrow, however, can be provided by doing a differential count of at least 500 cells (myelogram, Table 13.2). In some conditions, the marrow cells can be used for more detailed special tests such as cytogenetics, microbiological culture, biochemical analysis, and immunological and cytological markers.

TREPHINE BIOPSY. Trephine biopsy is performed by a simple *Jamshidi trephine needle* by which a core of tissue from periosteum to bone marrow cavity is obtained (Fig. 13.4,B). The tissue is then fixed, decalcified and processed for histological sections and stained with haematoxylin and eosin and for reticulin. Trephine biospy is useful over aspiration since it provides an excellent view of the overall marrow architecture, cellularity, and presence or absence of infiltrates, but is less valuable than aspiration as far as individual cell morphology is concerned.

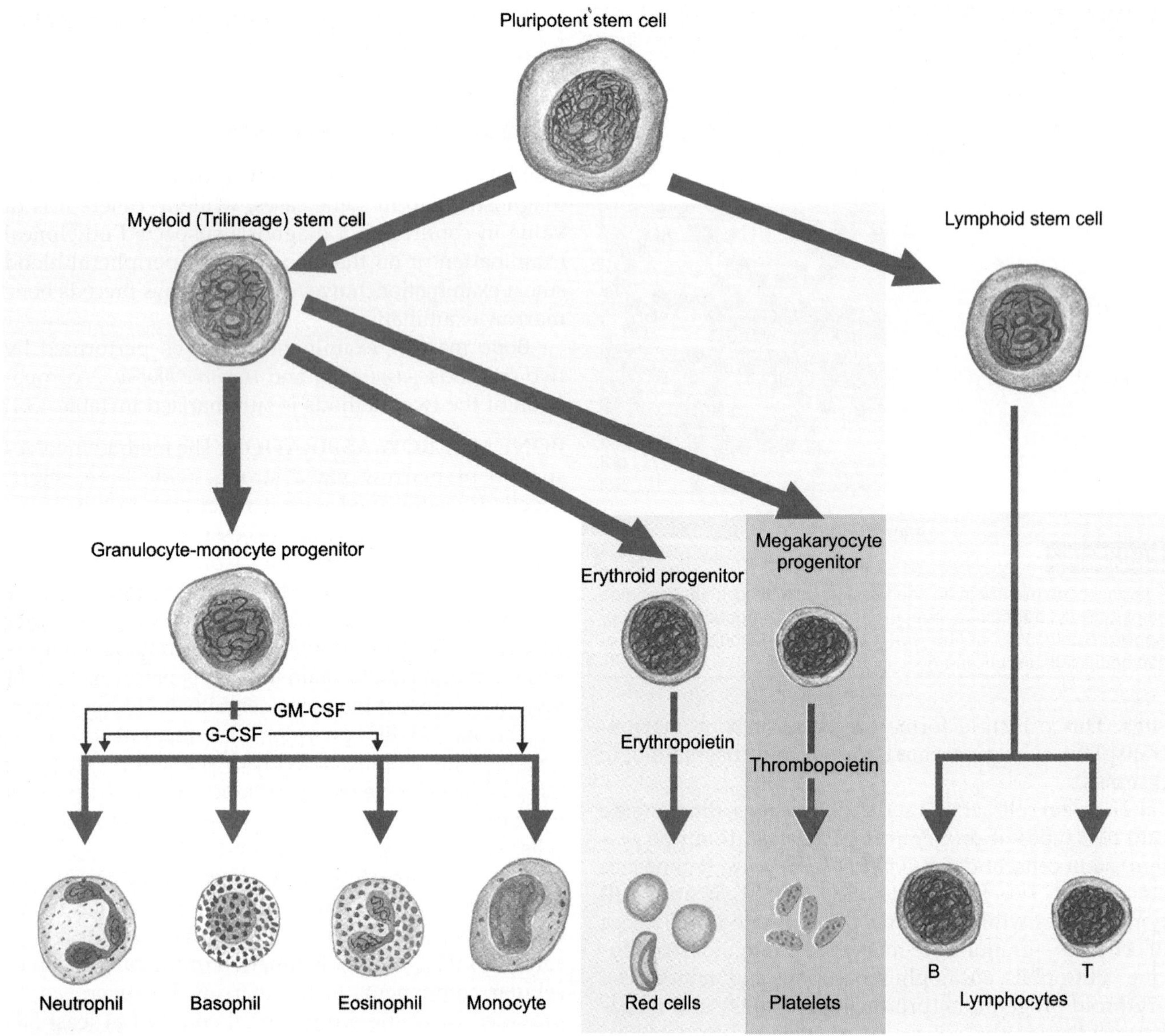

FIGURE 13.3

Schematic representation of differentiation of multipotent stem cells into blood cells.

RED BLOOD CELLS

ERYTHROPOIESIS

Although the stem cells which eventually form the mature erythrocytes of the peripheral blood cannot be recognised morphologically, there is a well-defined and readily recognisable lineage of nucleated red cells, the erythroid series, in the marrow.

Erythroid Series

These cells are as under (Fig. 13.5):

1. **PRONORMOBLAST.** The earliest recognisable cell in the marrow is a pronormoblast or proerythroblast. It is a large cell, 15-20 μm in diameter having deeply basophilic cytoplasm and a large central nucleus containing nucleoli. The deep blue colour of the cytoplasm is due to high content of RNA which is associated with active protein synthesis. As the cells mature, the nuclei lose their nucleoli and become smaller and denser, while the cytoplasm on maturation leads to replacement of dense blue colour progressively by pink-staining haemoglobin. Each pronormoblast undergoes 4-5 replications and forms 16-32 mature RBCs.

TABLE 13.1: Comparison of Bone Marrow Aspiration and Trephine Biopsy.

FEATURE	ASPIRATION	TREPHINE
1. *Site*	Sternum, posterior iliac crest; tibial head in infants	Posterior iliac crest
2. *Instrument*	Salah BM aspiration needle	Jamshidi trephine needle
3. *Stains*	Romanowsky, Perls' reaction for iron on smears	Haematoxylin and eosin, reticulin on tissue sections
4. *Time*	Within 1-2 hours	Within 1-7 days
5. *Morphology*	Better cellular morphology of aspiration smears but marrow architecture is indistinct	Better marrow architectural pattern but cell morphology is not as distinct since tissue sections are examined and not smears
6. *Indications*	Anaemias, suspected leukaemias, neutropenia thrombocytopenia, polycythaemia, myeloma, lymphomas, carcinomatosis, lipid storage diseases, granulomatous conditions, parasites, fungi, and unexplained enlargements of liver, spleen or lymph nodes.	Additional indications are: myelosclerosis, aplastic anaemia and in cases with 'dry tap' on aspiration.

2. **BASOPHILIC (EARLY) NORMOBLAST.** It is a round cell having a diameter of 12-16 μm with a large nucleus which is slightly more condensed than the pronormoblast and contains basophilic cytoplasm. Basophilic normoblast undergoes rapid proliferation.

3. **POLYCHROMATIC (INTERMEDIATE) NORMOBLAST.** Next maturation stage has a diameter of 12-14 μm. The nucleus at this stage is coarse and deeply basophilic. The cytoplasm is characteristically polychromatic i.e. contains admixture of basophilic RNA and acidophilic haemoglobin. The cell at this stage ceases to undergo proliferative activity.

4. **ORTHOCHROMATIC (LATE) NORMOBLAST.** The final stage in the maturation of nucleated red cells is the orthochromatic or late normoblast. The cell at this stage is smaller, 8-12 μm in diameter, containing a small and pyknotic nucleus with dark nuclear chromatin. The cytoplasm is characteristically acidophilic with diffuse basophilic hue due to the presence of large amounts of haemoglobin.

TABLE 13.2: Normal Adult Bone Marrow Counts (Myelogram).

Fat/cell ratio : 50:50
Myeloid/erythroid (M/E) ratio : 2-4:1 (mean 3:1)
Myeloid series: 30-45% (37.5%)
- Myeloblasts : 0.1-3.5%
- Promyelocytes: 0.5-5%

Erythroid series: 10-15% (mean 12.5%)
Megakaryocytes: 0.5%
Lymphocytes: 5-20%
Plasma cells: ≤ 3%
Reticulum cells: 0.1-2%

5. **RETICULOCYTE.** The nucleus is finally extruded from the late normoblast within the marrow and a reticulocyte results. The reticulocytes are juvenile red cells devoid of nucleus but contain ribosomal RNA so that they are still able to synthesise haemoglobin. A reticulocyte spends 1-2 days in the marrow and circulates for 1-2 days in the peripheral blood before maturing in the spleen, to become a biconcave red cell. The reticulocytes in the peripheral blood are distinguished from mature red cells by slightly basophilic hue in the cytoplasm similar to that of an orthochromatic normoblast. Reticulocytes can be counted in the laboratory by *vital staining* with dyes such as new methylene blue or brilliant cresyl blue. The reticulocytes by either of these staining methods contain deep blue reticulofilamentous material. While normoblasts are not normally present in human peripheral blood, reticulocytes are found normally in the peripheral blood. Normal range of reticulocyte count in health is 0.5-2.5% in adults and 2-6% in infants. Their percentage in the peripheral blood is a fairly accurate reflection of erythropoietic activity. Their proportion is increased in conditions of rapid red cell regeneration e.g. after haemorrhage, haemolysis and haematopoietic response of anaemia to treatment.

Erythropoietin

Erythropoietic activity is regulated by the hormone, erythropoietin, which is produced in response to anoxia. The principal site of erythropoietin production is the kidney though there is evidence of its extra-renal production in certain unusual circumstances. Its levels are, therefore, lowered in chronic renal diseases, while a case of renal cell carcinoma may be associated with its

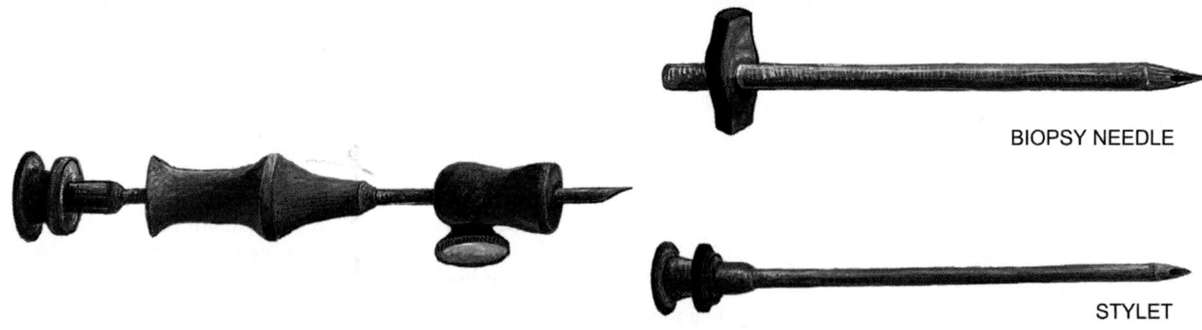

A, SALAH BONE MARROW ASPIRATION NEEDLE

B, JAMSHIDI TREPHINE NEEDLE

BONE MARROW ASPIRATION REPORT

No................ Date............................

Name ....Age....................Sex....................................

C.R.No/O.P.D. No....................................

Report.

Preparation/cellularity	:	Cellular preparation
M.E. ratio	:	Equal (Normal mean = 3:1)
Erythropoiesis	:	Micronormoblastic with inadequate haemoglobinisation
Myeloid cells	:	Normal in number, morphology and maturation
Megakaryocytes	:	Normal in number and morphology (Normal = 0.1-0.5%)
Plasma cells	:	Within normal limits (Normal = 0.1-3.5%)
Reticulum cells	:	Unremarkable (Normal = 0.3-0.9%)
Reticular iron	:	Grade zero (Normal = Grade III to IV)
Sideroblasts	:	None
Any other finding	:	Nil
Comments	:	IRON DEFICIENT ERYTHROPOIESIS

Signature

C, FORMAT OF BONE MARROW REPORT

FIGURE 13.4

The Salah bone marrow aspiration needle (A), Jamshidi trephine needle (B), and the format of a report (C) which can be provided by the haematologist examining the bone marrow aspirate smears.

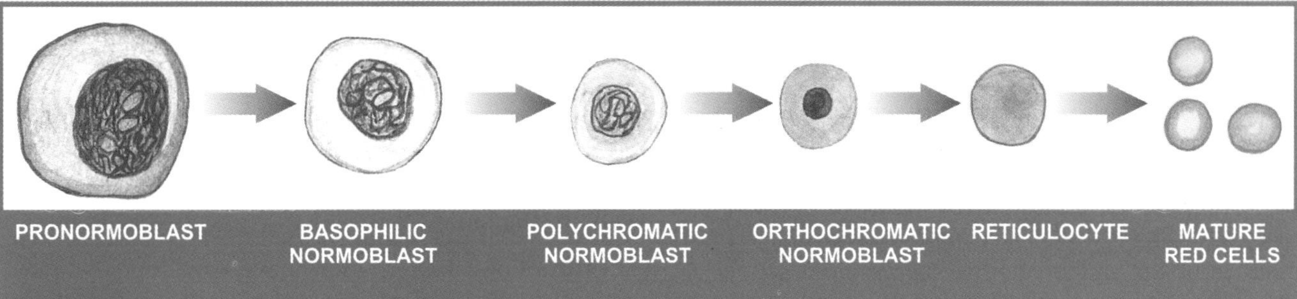

FIGURE 13.5

The erythroid series. There is progressive condensation of the nuclear chromatin which is eventually extruded from the cell at the late normoblast stage. The cytoplasm contains progressively less RNA and more haemoglobin.

enhanced production and erythrocytosis. Erythropoietin acts on the marrow at the various stages of morphologically unidentifiable as well as identifiable erythroid precursors.

There is an increased production of erythropoietin in various types of anaemias but in anaemia of chronic diseases (e.g. in infections and neoplastic conditions) there is no such enhancement of erythropoietin. In polycythaemia rubra vera, there is erythrocytosis but depressed production of erythropoietin. This is because of an abnormality of the stem cell class which is not under erythropoietin control.

The bioassay of erythropoietin in serum or urine is difficult due to quite low values. The alternative method for estimating erythropoietin concentration is *in vitro* method by induction of erythropoietin stimulation in mice.

The Red Cell

The mature erythrocytes of the human peripheral blood are non-nucleated cells and lack the usual cell organelles. The normal human erythrocyte is a biconcave disc, 7.2 μm in diameter, and has a thickness of 2.4 μm at the periphery and 1 μm in the centre. The biconcave shape renders the red cells quite flexible so that they can pass through capillaries whose minimum diameter is 3.5 μm. More than 90% of the weight of erythrocyte consist of haemoglobin. The life-span of red cells is 120 days.

NORMAL VALUES AND RED CELL INDICES. Range of *normal red cell* count in health is $5.5 \pm 1.0 \times 10^{12}$/L in men and $4.8 \pm 1.0 \times 10^{12}$/L in women. The *packed cell volume (PCV)* or *haematocrit* is the volume of erythrocytes per litre of whole blood indicating the proportion of plasma and red cells and ranges 0.47 ± 0.07 L/L (40-54%) in men and 0.42 ± 0.05 L/L (37-47%) in women. The *haemoglobin content* in health is 15.5 ± 2.5 g/dl (13-18 g/dl) in men and 14.0 ± 2.5 g/dl (11.5-16.5 g/dl) in women. Based on these normal values, a series of *absolute values* or red cell indices can be derived which have diagnostic importance. These are as under:

1. **Mean corpuscular volume (MCV) =**

$$\frac{\text{PCV in L/L}}{\text{RBC count/L}}$$

The normal value is 85 ± 8 fl (77-93 fl)*.

2. **Mean corpuscular haemoglobin (MCH) =**

$$\frac{\text{Hb/L}}{\text{RBC count/L}}$$

The normal range is 29.5 ± 2.5 pg (27-32 pg)*.

3. **Mean corpuscular haemoglobin concentration (MCHC) =**

$$\frac{\text{Hb/dl}}{\text{PCV in L/L}}$$

The normal value is 32.5 ± 2.5 g/dl (30-35 g/dl).

Since MCHC is independent of red cell count and size, it is considered to be of greater clinical significance as compared to other absolute values. It is low in iron deficiency anaemia but is usually normal in macrocytic anaemia.

RED CELL MEMBRANE. The red cell membrane is a trilaminar structure having a bimolecular lipid layer interposed between two layers of proteins. The important *proteins* in red cell membrane are band 3 protein (named on the basis of the order in which it migrates

*For conversions, the multiples used are as follows: 'deci (d) = 10^{-1}, milli (m) = 10^{-3}, micro (μ) = 10^{-6}, nano (n) = 10^{-9}, pico (p) = 10^{-12}, femto (f) = 10^{-15}

during electrophoresis), glycophorin and spectrin; important *lipids* are glycolipids, phospholipids and cholesterol; and *carbohydrates* form skeleton of erythrocytes having a lattice-like network which is attached to the internal surface of the membrane and is responsible for biconcave form of the erythrocytes.

A number of inherited disorders of the red cell membrane and cytoskeletal components produce abnormalities of the shape such as: *spherocytosis* (spherical shape from loss of part of the membrane), *ovalocytosis* (oval shape from loss of elasticity of cytoskeleton), *echinocytosis* (spiny processes from external surface due to metabolic abnormalities of red cells), and *stomatocytosis* (bowl-shaped red cells from expansion of inner membrane on one side).

NUTRITIONAL REQUIREMENTS FOR ERYTHROPOIESIS. New red cells are being produced each day for which the marrow requires certain essential substances. These substances are as under:

1. Metals. Iron is essential for red cell production because it forms part of the haem molecule in haemoglobin. Its deficiency leads to iron deficiency anaemia. Cobalt and manganese are certain other metals required for red cell production.

2. Vitamins. Vitamin B_{12} and folate are essential for biosynthesis of nucleic acids. Deficiency of B_{12} or folate causes megaloblastic anaemia. Vitamin C (ascorbic acid) plays an indirect role by facilitating the iron turnover in the body. Vitamin B_6 (pyridoxine), vitamin E (tocopherol) and riboflavin are the other essential vitamins required in the synthesis of red cells.

3. Amino acids. Amino acids comprise the globin component of haemoglobin. Severe amino acid deficiency due to protein deprivation causes depressed red cell production.

4. Hormones. As discussed above, erythropoietin plays a significant regulatory role in the erythropoietic activity. Besides erythropoietin, androgens and thyroxine also appear to be involved in the red cell production.

HAEMOGLOBIN. Haemoglobin consists of a basic protein, *globin*, and the iron-porphyrin complex, *haem*. The molecular weight of haemoglobin is 68,000. Normal adult haemoglobin (*HbA*) constitutes 96-98% of the total haemoglobin content and consists of four polypeptide chains, $\alpha_2\ \beta_2$. Small quantities of 2 other haemoglobins present in adults are: *HbF* containing $\alpha_2\ \gamma_2$ globin chains comprising 0.5-0.8% of total haemoglobin, and *HbA*$_2$ having $\alpha_2\ \delta_2$ chains and constituting 1.5-3.2% of total haemoglobin. Most of the haemoglobin (65%) is synthesised by the nucleated red cell precursors in the marrow, while the remainder (35%) is synthesised at the reticulocyte stage.

Synthesis of haem occurs largely in the mitochondria by a series of biochemical reactions summarised in Fig. 13.6. Coenzyme, pyridoxal-6-phosphate, derived from pyridoxine (vitamin B_6) is essential for the synthesis of

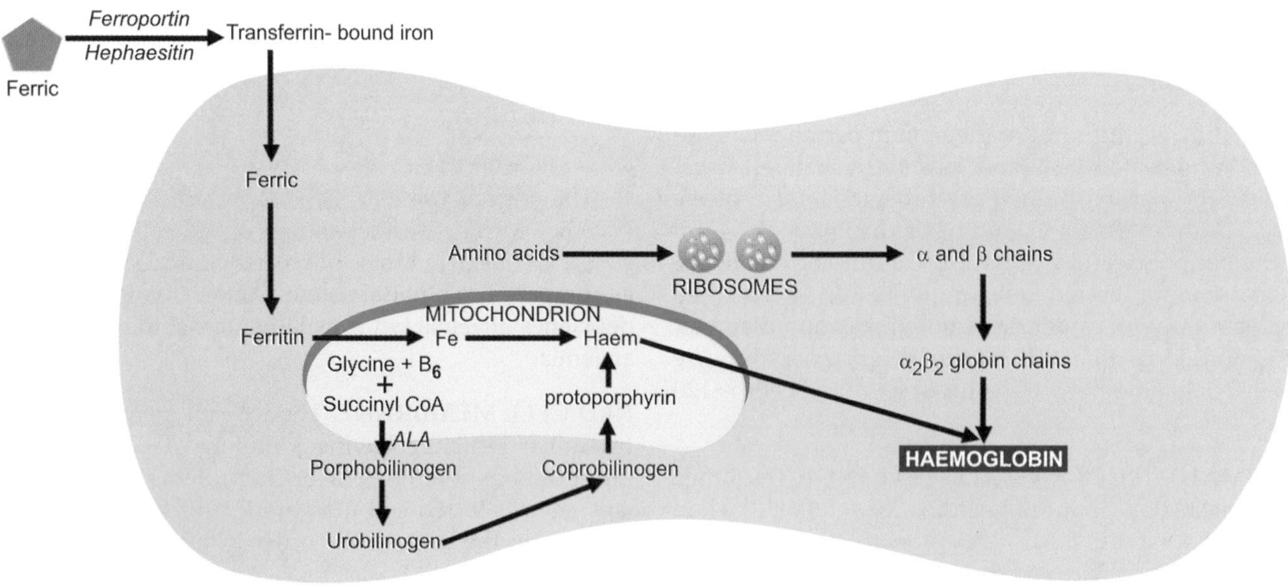

FIGURE 13.6

Schematic diagram of haemoglobin synthesis in the developing red cell.

amino levulinic acid (ALA) which is the first step in the biosynthesis of protoporphyrin. The reaction is stimulated by erythropoietin and inhibited by haem. Ultimately, protoporphyrin combines with iron supplied from circulating transferrin to form haem. Each molecule of haem combines with a globin chain synthesised by polyribosomes. A tetramer of 4 globin chains, each having its own haem group, constitutes the haemoglobin molecule (Fig. 13.7, A).

RED CELL FUNCTIONS. The essential function of the red cells is to carry oxygen from the lungs to the tissue and to transport carbon dioxide to the lungs. In order to perform these functions, the red cells have the ability to generate energy as ATP by anaerobic glycolytic pathway (Embden-Meyerhof pathway). This pathway also generates reducing power as NADH and NADPH by the hexose monophosphate (HMP) shunt.

1. Oxygen carrying. The normal adult haemoglobin, HbA, is an extremely efficient oxygen-carrier. The four units of tetramer of haemoglobin molecule take up oxygen in succession, which, in turn, results in stepwise rise in affinity of haemoglobin for oxygen. This is responsible for the *sigmoid shape* of the oxygen dissociation curve.

The oxygen affinity of haemoglobin is expressed in term of P_{50} value which is the oxygen tension (pO_2) at which 50% of the haemoglobin is saturated with oxygen. Pulmonary capillaries have high pO_2 and, thus, there is virtual saturation of available oxygen-combining sites of haemoglobin. The tissue capillaries, however, have relatively low pO_2 and, thus, part of haemoglobin is in deoxy state. The extent to which oxygen is released from haemoglobin at pO_2, in tissue capillaries depends upon 3 factors—the nature of globin chains, the pH, and the concentration of 2,3-biphosphoglycerate (2,3-BPG) as under (Fig 13.7, B).

- Normal adult haemoglobin (HbA) has *lower affinity for oxygen* than foetal haemoglobin and, therefore, releases greater amount of bound oxygen at pO_2 of tissue capillaries.
- A *fall in the pH* (acidic pH) lowers affinity of oxyhaemoglobin for oxygen, so called the Bohr effect, thereby causing enhanced release of oxygen from erythrocytes at the lower pH in tissue capillaries.
- A *rise in red cell concentration of 2,3-BPG,* an intermediate product of Embden-Meyerhof pathway, as occurs in anaemia and hypoxia, causes decreased affinity of HbA for oxygen. This, in turn, results in enhanced supply of oxygen to the tissue.

2. CO_2 transport. Another important function of the red cells is the CO_2 transport. In the tissue capillaries, the pCO_2 is high so that CO_2 enters the erythrocytes where much of it is converted into bicarbonate ions which diffuse back into the plasma. In the pulmonary

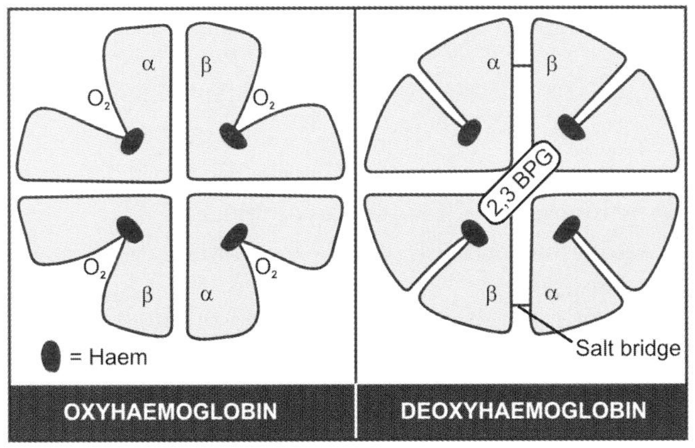

A, HAEMOGLOBIN MOLECULE

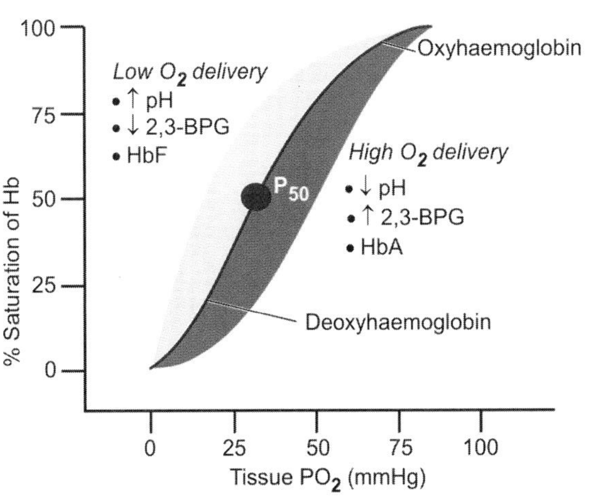

B, HB-DISSOCIATION CURVE

FIGURE 13.7

A, Normal adult haemoglobin molecule (HbA) consisting of α_2 β_2 globin chains, each with its own haem group in oxy and deoxy state. The haemoglobin tetramer can bind up to four molecules of oxygen in the iron containing sites of the haem molecules. As oxygen is bound, salt bridges are broken, and 2,3-BPG and CO_2 are expelled. B, Hb-dissociation curve. On dissociation of oxygen from Hb molecule i.e. on release of oxygen to the tissues, salt bridges are formed again, and 2,3-BPG and CO_2, bound. The shift of the curve to higher oxygen delivery is affected by acidic pH, increased 2,3-BPG and HbA molecule while oxygen delivery is less with high pH, low 2,3-BPG and HbF.

capillaries, the process is reversed and bicarbonate ions are converted back into CO_2. Some of the CO_2 produced by tissues is bound to deoxyhaemoglobin forming carbamino-haemoglobin. This compound dissociates in the pulmonary capillaries to release CO_2.

RED CELL DESTRUCTION. Red cells have a mean life-span of 120 days, after which red cell metabolism gradually deteriorates as the enzymes are not replaced. The destroyed red cells are removed mainly by the macrophages of the reticuloendothelial (RE) system of the marrow, and to some extent by the macrophages in the liver and spleen (Fig. 13.8). The breakdown of red cells liberates iron for recirculation via plasma transferrin to marrow normoblasts, and protoporphyrin which is broken down to bilirubin. Bilirubin circulates to the liver where it is conjugated to its diglucuronide which is excreted in the gut via bile and converted to stercobilinogen and stercobilin excreted in the faeces. Part of stercobilinogen and stercobilin is reabsorbed and excreted in the urine as urobilinogen and urobilin. A small fragment of protoporphyrin is converted to carbon monoxide and excreted in expired air from the lungs. Globin chains are broken down to amino acids and reused for protein synthesis in the body.

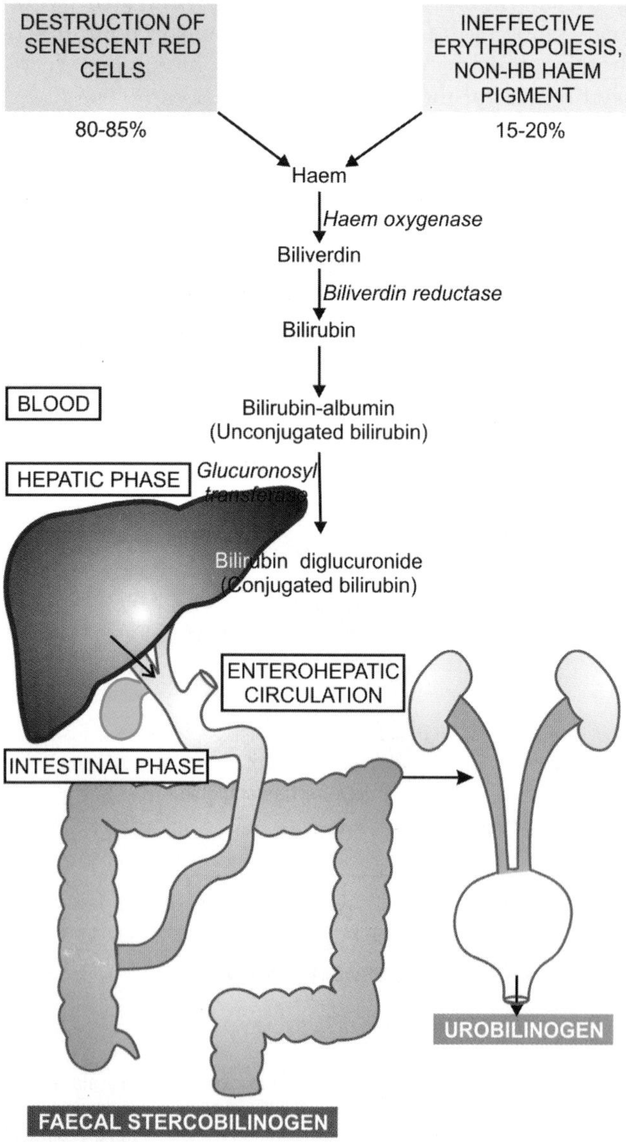

FIGURE 13.8

Normal red cell destruction in the RE system.

ANAEMIA—GENERAL CONSIDERATIONS

Anaemia is defined as a haemoglobin concentration in blood below the lower limit of the normal range for the age and sex of the individual. In adults, the lower extreme of the normal haemoglobin is taken as 13.0 g/dl for males and 11.5 g/dl for females. Newborn infants have higher haemoglobin level and, therefore, 15 g/dl is taken as the lower limit at birth, whereas at 3 months the lower level is 9.5 g/dl. Although haemoglobin value is employed as the major parameter for determining whether or not anaemia is present, the red cell counts, haematocrit (PCV) and absolute values (MCV, MCH and MCHC) provide alternate means of assessing anaemia.

Pathophysiology of Anaemia

Subnormal level of haemoglobin causes lowered oxygen-carrying capacity of the blood. This, in turn, initiates compensatory physiologic adaptations such as:

- increased release of oxygen from haemoglobin;
- increased blood flow to the tissues;
- maintenance of the blood volume; and
- redistribution of blood flow to maintain the cerebral blood supply.

Eventually, however, tissue hypoxia develops causing impaired functions of the affected tissues. The degree of functional impairment of individual tissues is variable depending upon their oxygen requirements. Tissues with high oxygen requirement such as the heart, CNS and the skeletal muscle during exercise, bear the brunt of clinical effects of anaemia.

Clinical Features of Anaemia

The haemoglobin level at which symptoms and signs of anaemia develop depends upon 4 main factors:

1. *The speed of onset of anaemia:* Rapidly progressive anaemia causes more symptoms than anaemia of slow onset as there is less time for physiologic adaptation.

2. *The severity of anaemia:* Mild anaemia produces no symptoms or signs but a rapidly developing severe anaemia (haemoglobin below 6.0 g/dl) may produce significant clinical features.

3. *The age of the patient*: The young patients due to good cardiovascular compensation tolerate anaemia quite well as compared to the elderly. The elderly patients develop cardiac and cerebral symptoms more prominently due to associated cardiovascular disease.

4. *The haemoglobin dissociation curve:* In anaemia, the affinity of haemoglobin for oxygen is depressed as 2,3-BPG in the red cells increases. As a result, oxyhaemoglobin is dissociated more readily to release free oxygen for cellular use, causing a shift of the oxyhaemoglobin dissociation curve to the right.

SYMPTOMS. In symptomatic cases of anaemia, the presenting features are: tiredness, easy fatiguability, generalised muscular weakness, lethargy and headache. In older patients, there may be symptoms of cardiac failure, angina pectoris, intermittent claudication, confusion and visual disturbances.

SIGNS. A few general signs common to all types of anaemias are as under:

1. **Pallor.** Pallor is the most common and characteristic sign which may be seen in the mucous membranes, conjunctivae and skin.

2. **Cardiovascular system.** A hyperdynamic circulation may be present with tachycardia, collapsing pulse, cardiomegaly, midsystolic flow murmur, dyspnoea on exertion, and in the case of elderly, congestive heart failure.

3. **Central nervous system.** The older patients may develop symptoms referable to the CNS such as attacks of faintness, giddiness, headache, tinnitus, drowsiness, numbness and tingling sensations of the hands and feet.

4. **Ocular manifestations.** Retinal haemorrhages may occur if there is associated vascular disease or bleeding diathesis.

5. **Reproductive system.** Menstrual disturbances such as amenorrhoea and menorrhagia and loss of libido are some of the manifestations involving the reproductive system in anaemic subjects.

6. **Renal system.** Mild proteinuria and impaired concentrating capacity of the kidney may occur in severe anaemia.

7. **Gastrointestinal system.** Anorexia, flatulence, nausea, constipation and weight loss may occur.

In addition to the general features, specific signs may be associated with particular types of anaemia which are described later together with discussion of specific types of anaemias.

Investigations of the Anaemic Subject

After obtaining the full medical history pertaining to different general and specific signs and symptoms, the patient is examined for evidence of anaemia. Special emphasis is placed on colour of the skin, conjunctivae, sclerae and nails. Changes in the retina, atrophy of the papillae of the tongue, rectal examination for evidence of bleeding, and presence of hepatomegaly, splenomegaly, lymphadenopathy and bony tenderness are looked for.

In order to confirm or deny the presence of anaemia, its type and its cause, the following plan of investigations is generally followed.

A. HAEMOGLOBIN ESTIMATION. The first and foremost investigation in any suspected case of anaemia is to carry out a haemoglobin estimation. Several methods are available but most reliable and accurate is the cyanmethaemoglobin (HiCN) method employing Drabkin's solution and a spectrophotometer. If the haemoglobin value is below the lower limit of the normal range for particular age and sex, the patient is said to be anaemic. In pregnancy, there is haemodilution and, therefore, the lower limit in normal pregnant women is less (10.5 g/dl) than in the non-pregnant state.

B. PERIPHERAL BLOOD FILM EXAMINATION. The haemoglobin estimation is invariably followed by examination of a peripheral blood film for morphologic features after staining it with the Romanowsky dyes (e.g. Leishman's stain, May-Grünwald-Giemsa's stain, Jenner-Giemsa's stain etc). The blood smear is evaluated in an area where there is neither rouleaux formation nor so thin as to cause red cell distortion. Such an area can usually be found towards the tail of the film, but not actually at the tail. The following abnormalities in erythroid series of cells are particularly looked for in a blood smear:

1. **Variation in size (Anisocytosis).** Normally, there is slight variation in diameter of the red cells from 6.7-7.7 μm (mean value 7.2 μm). Increased variation in size of the red cell is termed anisocytosis. Anisocytosis may be due to the presence of cells larger than normal (*macrocytosis*) or cells smaller than normal (*microcytosis*). Sometimes both microcytosis and macrocytosis are present (*dimorphic*).

- *Macrocytes* are classically found in megaloblastic anaemia; other causes are aplastic anaemia, other dyserythropoietic anaemias, chronic liver disease and in conditions with increased erythropoiesis.

- *Microcytes* are present in iron deficiency anaemia, thalassaemia and spherocytosis. They may also result from fragmentation of erythrocytes such as in haemolytic anaemia.

2. Variation in shape (Poikilocytosis). Increased variation in shape of the red cells is termed poikilocytosis. The nature of the abnormal shape determines the cause of anaemia. Poikilocytes are produced in various types of abnormal erythropoiesis e.g. in megaloblastic anaemia, iron deficiency anaemia, thalassaemia, myelosclerosis and microangiopathic haemolytic anaemia.

3. Inadequate haemoglobin formation (Hypochromasia). Normally, the intensity of pink staining of haemoglobin in a Romanowsky-stained blood smear gradually decreases from the periphery to the centre of the cell. Increased central pallor is referred to as *hypochromasia*. It may develop either from lowered haemoglobin content (e.g. in iron deficiency anaemia, chronic infections), or due to thinness of the red cells (e.g. in thalassaemia, sideroblastic anaemia). Unusually deep pink staining of the red cells due to increased haemoglobin concentration is termed *hyperchromasia* and may be found in megaloblastic anaemia, spherocytosis and in neonatal blood.

Chapter Thirteen

4. Compensatory erythropoiesis. A number of changes are associated with compensatory increase in erythropoietic activity. These are as under:

i) *Polychromasia* is defined as the red cells having more than one type of colour. Polychromatic red cells are slightly larger, generally stained bluish-grey and represent reticulocytes and, thus, correlate well with reticulocyte count.

ii) *Normoblastaemia* is presence of nucleated red cells in the peripheral blood film. A small number of normoblasts (or erythroblasts) may be normally found in cord blood at birth. They are found in large numbers in haemolytic disease of the newborn, other haemolytic disorders and in extramedullary erythropoiesis. They may also appear in the blood in various types of severe anaemias except in aplastic anaemia. Normoblastaemia may also occur after splenectomy.

iii) *Punctate basophilia* or *basophilic stippling* is diffuse and uniform basophilic granularity in the cell which does not stain positively with Perls' reaction (in contrast to Pappenheimer bodies which stain positively). Classical punctate basophilia is seen in aplastic anaemia, thalassaemia, myelodysplasia, infections and lead poisoning.

iv) *Howell-Jolly bodies* are purple nuclear remnants, usually found singly, and are larger than basophilic stippling. They are present in megaloblastic anaemia and after splenectomy.

5. Miscellaneous changes. In addition to the morphologic abnormalities of red cells described above, several other abnormal red cells may be found in different haematological disorders. Some of these are as follows (Fig. 13.9):

i) *Spherocytosis* is characterised by presence of spheroidal rather than biconcave disc-shaped red cells. Spherocytes are seen in hereditary spherocytosis, autoimmune haemolytic anaemia and in ABO haemolytic disease of the newborn.

ii) *Schistocytosis* is identified by fragmentation of erythrocytes. Schistocytes are found in thalassaemia, hereditary elliptocytosis, megaloblastic anaemia, iron deficiency anaemia, microangiopathic haemolytic anaemia and in severe burns.

iii) *Irregularly contracted red cells* are found in drug and chemical induced haemolytic anaemia and in unstable haemoglobinopathies.

iv) *Leptocytosis* is the presence of unusually thin red cells. Leptocytes are seen in severe iron deficiency and thalassaemia. *Target cell* is a form of leptocyte in which there is central round stained area and a peripheral rim of haemoglobin. Target cells are found in iron deficiency, thalassaemia, chronic liver disease, and after splenectomy.

v) *Sickle cells or drepanocytes* are sickle-shaped red cells found in sickle cell disease.

vi) *Crenated red cells* are the erythrocytes which develop numerous projections from the surface. They are present in blood films due to alkaline pH, presence of traces of fatty substances on the slides and in cases where the film is made from blood that has been allowed to stand overnight.

vii) *Acanthocytosis* is the presence of coarsely crenated red cells. Acanthocytes are found in large number in blood film made from splenectomised subjects, and in chronic liver disease.

viii) *Burr cells* are cell fragments having one or more spines. They are particularly found in uraemia.

ix) *Stomatocytosis* is the presence of stomatocytes which have central area having slit-like or mouth-like appearance. They are found in hereditary stomatocytosis, or may be seen in alcoholism.

x) *Ovalocytosis* or *elliptocytosis* is the oval or elliptical shape of red cells. Their highest proportion (79%) is

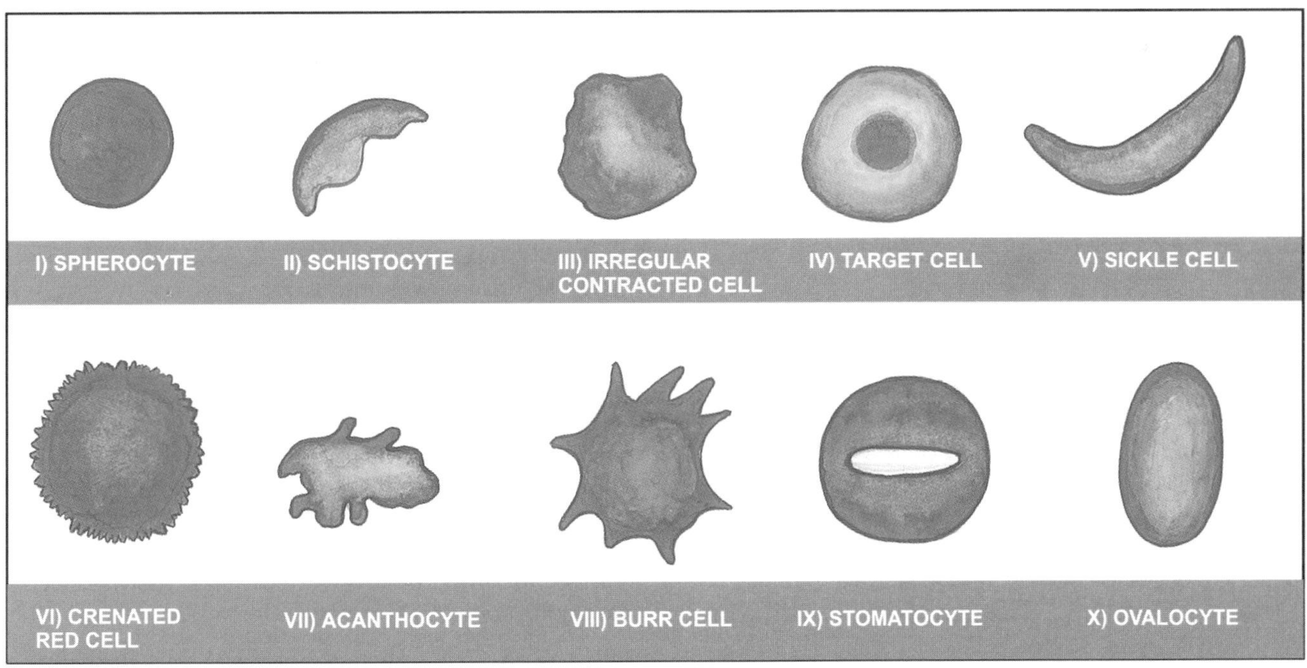

FIGURE 13.9

Some of the common morphologic abnormalities of red cells (The serial numbers in the illustrations correspond to the order in which they are described in the text).

seen in hereditary ovalocytosis and elliptocytosis; other conditions showing such abnormal shapes of red cells are megaloblastic anaemia and hypochromic anaemia.

C. RED CELL INDICES. An alternative method to diagnose and detect the severity of anaemia is by measuring the red cell indices.

- In iron deficiency and thalassaemia, MCV, MCH and MCHC are reduced.
- In anaemia due to acute blood loss and haemolytic anaemias, MCV, MCH and MCHC are all within normal limits.
- In megaloblastic anaemias, MCV is raised above the normal range.

D. LEUCOCYTE AND PLATELET COUNT. Measurement of leucocyte and platelet count helps to distinguish pure anaemia from pancytopenia in which red cells, granulocytes and platelets are all reduced. In anaemias due to haemolysis or haemorrhage, the neutrophil count and platelet counts are often elevated. In infections and leukaemias, the leucocyte counts are high and immature leucocytes appear in the blood.

E. RETICULOCYTE COUNT. Reticulocyte count (normal 0.5-2.5%) is done in each case of anaemia to assess the marrow erythropoietic activity. In acute haemorrhage and in haemolysis, the reticulocyte response is indicative of impaired marrow function.

F. ERYTHROCYTE SEDIMENTATION RATE. The ESR is a non-specific test used as a screening test for anaemia. It usually gives a clue to the underlying organic disease but anaemia itself may also cause rise in the ESR.

G. BONE MARROW EXAMINATION. Bone marrow aspiration is done in cases where the cause for anaemia is not obvious. The procedures involved for marrow aspiration and trephine biopsy and their relative advantages and disadvantages have already been discussed (page 359).

In addition to these general tests, certain specific tests are done in different types of anaemias which are described later under the discussion of specific anaemias.

Classification of Anaemias

Several types of classifications of anaemias have been proposed. Two of the widely accepted classifications are based on the pathophysiology and morphology (Table 13.3).

PATHOPHYSIOLOGIC CLASSIFICATION. Depending upon the pathophysiologic mechanism, anaemias are classified into 3 groups:

TABLE 13.3: Classification of Anaemias.

A. PATHOPHYSIOLOGIC

I. Anaemia due to increased blood loss
- a) Acute post-haemorrhagic anaemia
- b) Chronic blood loss

II. Anaemias due to impaired red cell production
- a) *Cytoplasmic maturation defects*
  1. Deficient haem synthesis: Iron deficiency anaemia
  2. Deficient globin synthesis: Thalassaemic syndromes
- b) *Nuclear maturation defects* Vitamin B_{12} and/or folic acid deficiency: Megaloblastic anaemia
- c) *Defect in stem cell proliferation and differentiation*
  1. Aplastic anaemia
  2. Pure red cell aplasia
- d) *Anaemia of chronic disorders*
- e) *Bone marrow infiltration*
- f) *Congenital anaemia*

III. Anaemias due to increased red cell destruction (Haemolytic anaemias) (Details in Table 13.10)
- A. *Extrinsic (extracorpuscular) red cell abnormalities*
- B. *Intrinsic (intracorpuscular) red cell abnormalities*

B. MORPHOLOGIC

I. Microcytic, hypochromic

II. Normocytic, normochromic

III. Macrocytic, normochromic

I. Anaemia due to blood loss. This is further of 2 types:

A. Acute post-haemorrhagic anaemia

B. Anaemia of chronic blood loss

II. Anaemia due to impaired red cell formation. A disturbance due to impaired red cell production from various causes may produce anaemia. These are as under:

A. *Cytoplasmic maturation defects*
1. Deficient haem synthesis: iron deficiency anaemia
2. Deficient globin synthesis: thalassaemic syndromes

B. *Nuclear maturation defects*

Vitamin B_{12} and/or folic acid deficiency: megaloblastic anaemia

C. *Haematopoietic stem cell proliferation and differentiation abnormality* e.g.
1. Aplastic anaemia
2. Pure red cell aplasia

D. *Bone marrow failure due to systemic diseases* (anaemia of chronic disorders) e.g.
1. Anaemia of inflammation/infections, disseminated malignancy
2. Anaemia in renal disease
3. Anaemia due to endocrine and nutritional deficiencies (hypometabolic states)
4. Anaemia in liver disease

E. *Bone marrow infiltration* e.g.
1. Leukaemias
2. Lymphomas
3. Myelosclerosis
4. Multiple myeloma

F. *Congenital anaemia* e.g.
1. Sideroblastic anaemia
2. Congenital dyserythropoietic anaemia

The term *hypoproliferative anaemias* is also used to denote impaired marrow proliferative activity and includes 2 main groups: hypoproliferation due to iron deficiency and that due to other hypoproliferative disorders; the latter category includes anaemia of chronic inflammation/infection, renal disease, hypometabolic states, and marrow damage.

III. Anaemia due to increased red cell destruction (haemolytic anaemias). This is further divided into 2 groups:
1. Intracorpuscular defect (hereditary and acquired).
2. Extracorpuscular defect (acquired haemolytic anaemias).

MORPHOLOGIC CLASSIFICATION. Based on the red cell size, haemoglobin content and red cell indices, anaemias are classified into 3 types:

1. Microcytic, hypochromic: MCV, MCH, MCHC are all reduced e.g. in iron deficiency anaemia and in certain non-iron deficient anaemias (sideroblastic anaemia, thalassaemia, anaemia of chronic disorders).

2. Normocytic, normochromic: MCV, MCH, MCHC are all normal e.g. after acute blood loss, haemolytic anaemias, bone marrow failure, anaemia of chronic disorders.

3. Macrocytic: MCV is raised e.g. in megaloblastic anaemia due to deficiency of vitamin B_{12} or folic acid.

With these general comments on anaemias, a discussion of the specific types of anaemias in the following pages.

ANAEMIA OF BLOOD LOSS

Depending upon the rate of blood loss due to haemorrhage, the effects of post-haemorrhagic anaemia appear.

ACUTE BLOOD LOSS. When the loss of blood occurs suddenly, the following events take place:

i) Immediate threat to life due to hypovolaemia which may result in shock and death.

ii) If the patient survives, shifting of interstitial fluid to intravascular compartment with consequent haemodilution with low haematocrit.

iii) Hypoxia stimulates production of erythropoietin resulting in increased marrow erythropoiesis.

Laboratory Findings

i) Normocytic and normochromic anaemia

ii) Low haematocrit

iii) Increased reticulocyte count in peripheral blood (10-15% after one week) reflecting accelerated marrow erythropoiesis.

CHRONIC BLOOD LOSS. When the loss of blood is slow and insidious, the effects of anaemia will become apparent only when the rate of loss is more than rate of production and the iron stores are depleted. This results in iron deficiency anaemia as seen in other clinical conditions discussed below.

HYPOCHROMIC ANAEMIA

Iron deficiency is the commonest cause of anaemia the world over. It is estimated that about 20% of women in child-bearing age group are iron deficient, while the overall prevalence in adult males is about 2%. It is the most important, though not the sole, cause of microcytic hypochromic anaemia in which all the three red cell indices (MCV, MCH and MCHC) are reduced and occurs due to defective haemoglobin synthesis. Hypochromic anaemias, therefore, are classified into 2 groups:

I. Hypochromic anaemia due to iron deficiency.

II. Hypochromic anaemias other than iron deficiency.

The latter category includes 3 groups of disorders—sideroblastic anaemia, thalassaemia and anaemia of chronic disorders.

IRON DEFICIENCY ANAEMIA

The commonest nutritional deficiency disorder present throughout the world is iron deficiency but its prevalence is higher in the developing countries. The factors responsible for iron deficiency in different populations are variable and are best understood in the context of normal iron metabolism.

Iron Metabolism

The amount of iron obtained from the diet should replace the losses from the skin, bowel and genitourinary tract. These losses together are about 1 mg daily in an adult male or in a non-menstruating female, while in a menstruating woman there is an additional iron loss of 0.5-1 mg daily. The iron required for haemoglobin synthesis is derived from 2 primary sources—ingestion of foods containing iron (e.g. leafy vegetables, beans, meats, liver etc) and recycling of iron from senescent red cells.

ABSORPTION. The average Western diet contains 10-15 mg of iron, out of which only 5-10% is normally absorbed. In pregnancy and in iron deficiency, the proportion of absorption is raised to 20-30%. Iron is absorbed mainly in the duodenum and proximal jejunum. *Iron from diet containing haem is better absorbed than non-haem iron.* Absorption of non-haem iron is enhanced by factors such as ascorbic acid (vitamin C), citric acid, amino acids, sugars, gastric secretions and hydrochloric acid. Iron absorption is impaired by factors like medicinal antacids, milk, pancreatic secretions, phytates, phosphates, ethylene diamine tetra-acetic acid (EDTA) and tannates contained in tea.

Non-haem iron is released as ferrous or ferric form but is absorbed almost exclusively as ferrous form; reduction when required takes place at the brush border by *ferrireductase*. Transport across the membrane is accomplished by divalent metal transporter 1 (DMT 1). Once inside the gut cells, ferric iron may be either stored as ferritin or further transported to transferrin by two vehicle proteins—*ferroportin* and *hephaestin*. The mechanism of dietary **haem iron** absorption is not quite clear yet. When the demand for iron is increased (e.g. during pregnancy, menstruation, periods of growth and various diseases), there is increased iron absorption, while excessive body stores of iron cause reduced intestinal iron absorption (see Fig. 13.13,A page 379).

DISTRIBUTION. In an adult, iron is distributed in the body as under:

1. **Haemoglobin**—present in the red cells, contains most of the body iron (65%).
2. **Myoglobin**—comprises a small amount of iron in the muscles (3.5%).
3. **Haem and non-haem enzymes**—e.g. cytochrome, catalase, peroxidases, succinic dehydrogenase and flavoproteins constitute a fraction of total body iron (0.5%).
4. **Transferrin-bound iron**—circulates in the plasma and constitutes another fraction of total body iron (0.5%).

All these forms of iron are in *functional form.*

5. **Ferritin and haemosiderin**—are the *storage forms* of excess iron (30%). They are stored in the mononuclear-phagocyte cells of the spleen, liver and bone marrow and in the parenchymal cells of the liver.

TRANSPORT. Iron is transported in plasma bound to a β-globulin, transferrin, synthesised in the liver. Transferrin-bound iron is made available to the marrow where the immature red cell precursors utilise iron for haemoglobin synthesis. Transferrin is reutilised after iron is released from it. A small amount of transferrin iron is delivered to other sites such as parenchymal cells of the liver. Normally, transferrin is about one-third saturated. But in conditions where transferrin-iron saturation is increased, parenchymal iron uptake is increased. Virtually, no iron is deposited in the mononuclear-phagocyte cells (RE cells) from the plasma transferrin-iron but instead these cells derive most of their iron from phagocytosis of senescent red cells. Storage form of iron (ferritin and haemosiderin) in RE cells is normally not functional but can be readily mobilised in response to increased demands for erythropoiesis. However, conditions such as malignancy, infection and inflammation interfere with the release of iron from iron stores causing ineffective erythropoiesis.

EXCRETION. The body is unable to regulate its iron content by excretion alone. The amount of iron lost per day is 0.5-1 mg which is independent of iron intake. This loss is nearly twice more (i.e. 1-2 mg/day) in menstruating women. Iron is lost from the body as a result of desquamation of epithelial cells from the gastrointestinal tract, from excretion in the urine and sweat, and loss via hair and nails. Iron excreted in the faeces mainly consists of unabsorbed iron and desquamated mucosal cells.

The daily iron cycle in the body is diagrammatically summarised in Fig. 13.10.

Pathogenesis

Iron deficiency anaemia develops when the supply of iron is inadequate for the requirement of haemoglobin synthesis. Initially, the negative iron balance is made good by mobilisation from the tissue stores so as to maintain haemoglobin synthesis. It is only after the tissue stores of iron are exhausted that the supply of iron to the marrow becomes insufficient for haemoglobin formation so that a state of iron deficiency anaemia develops. The development of iron deficiency depends upon one or more of the following factors:

1. Increased blood loss
2. Increased requirements
3. Inadequate dietary intake
4. Decreased intestinal absorption.

The relative significance of these factors varies with the age and sex of the patient (Table 13.4). Accordingly, certain groups of individuals at increased risk of developing iron deficiency can be identified (*see below*). In general, in developed countries the mechanism of iron deficiency is usually due to chronic occult blood loss, while in the underdeveloped countries poor intake of iron or defective absorption are responsible for iron deficiency anaemia.

Etiology

Iron deficiency anaemia is always secondary to an underlying disorder. Correction of the underlying cause, therefore, is essential part of its treatment. Based on the above-mentioned pathogenetic mechanisms, the following etiologic factors are involved in development of iron deficiency anaemia at different age and sex (Table 13.4):

1. FEMALES IN REPRODUCTIVE PERIOD OF LIFE. The highest incidence of iron deficiency anaemia is in women during their reproductive period of life. It may be from one or more of the following causes:

i) *Blood loss.* This is the most important cause of anaemia in women during child-bearing age group. Commonly, it is due to persistent and heavy menstrual blood loss such as occurs in various pathological states and due to insertion of IUCDs. Young girls at the onset of menstruation may develop mild anaemia due to blood loss. Significant blood loss may occur as a result of repeated miscarriages.

ii) *Inadequate intake.* Inadequate intake of iron is prevalent in women of lower economic status. Besides diet deficient in iron, other factors such as anorexia, impaired absorption and diminished bioavailability may act as contributory factors.

iii) *Increased requirements.* During pregnancy and adolescence, the demand of body for iron is increased. During a normal pregnancy, about 750 mg of iron may be siphoned off from the mother—about 400 mg to the foetus, 150 mg to the placenta, and 200 mg is lost at parturition and lactation. If several pregnancies occur at short intervals, iron deficiency anaemia certainly follows.

2. POST-MENOPAUSAL FEMALES. Though the physiological demand for iron decreases after cessation of menstruation, iron deficiency anaemia may develop in post-menopausal women due to chronic blood loss. Among the important causes are:

i) *Post-menopausal uterine bleeding* due to carcinoma of the uterus.

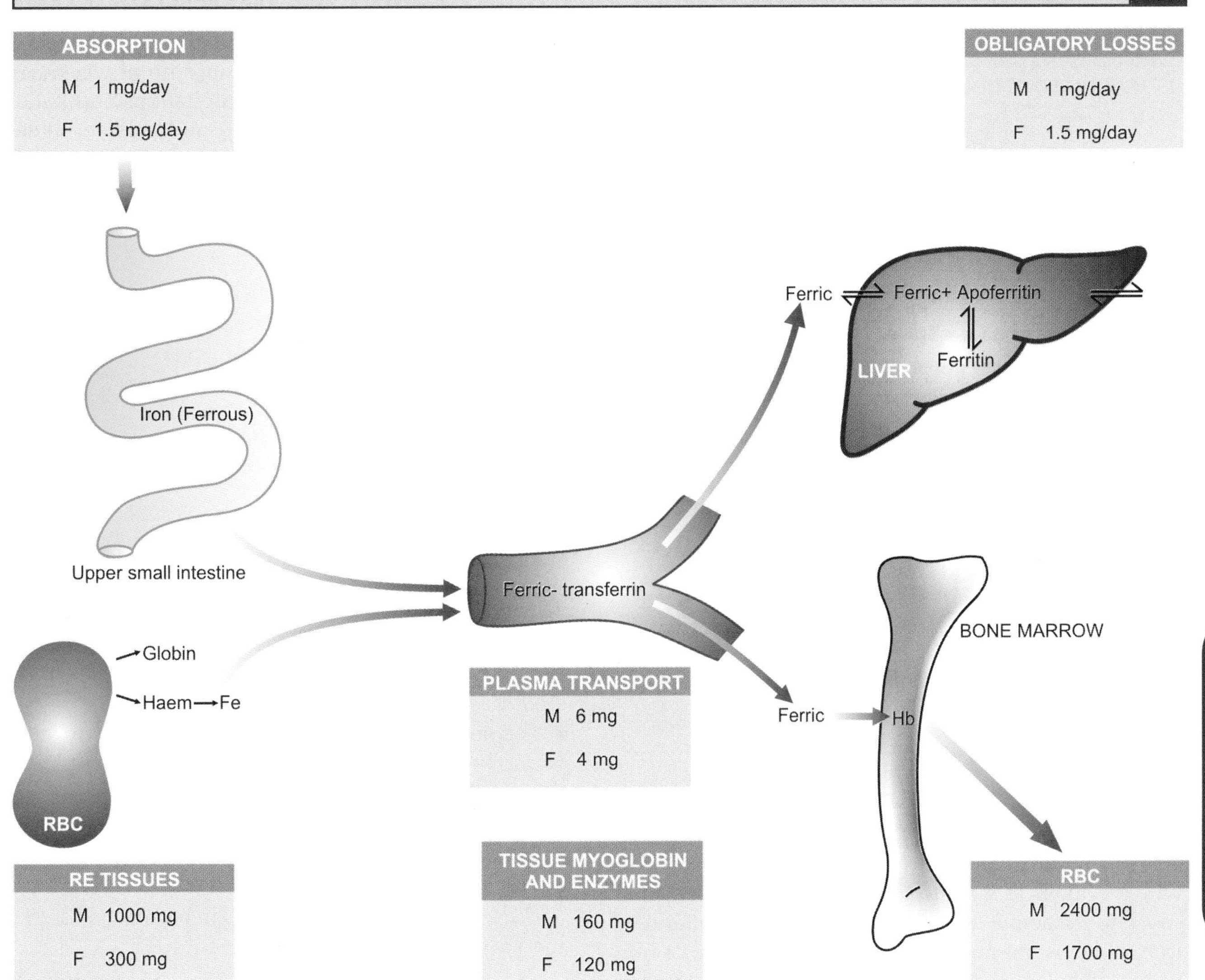

FIGURE 13.10

Daily iron cycle. Iron on absorption from upper small intestine circulates in plasma bound to transferrin and is transported to the bone marrow for utilisation in haemoglobin synthesis. The mature red cells are released into circulation, which on completion of their life-span of 120 days, die. They are then phagocytosed by RE cells and iron stored as ferritin and haemosiderin. Stored iron is mobilised in response to increased demand and used for haemoglobin synthesis, thus completing the cycle (M = males; F = females).

ii) *Bleeding from the alimentary tract* such as due to carcinoma of stomach and large bowel and hiatus hernia.

3. ADULT MALES. It is uncommon for adult males to develop iron deficiency anaemia in the presence of normal dietary iron content and iron absorption. The vast majority of cases of iron deficiency anaemia in adult males are due to chronic blood loss. The cause for chronic haemorrhage may lie at one of the following sites:

i) *Gastrointestinal tract* is the usual source of bleeding which may be due to peptic ulcer, haemorrhoids, hookworm infestation, carcinoma of stomach and large bowel, oesophageal varices, hiatus hernia, chronic aspirin ingestion and ulcerative colitis. Other causes in the GIT are malabsorption and following gastrointestinal surgery.

ii) *Urinary tract* e.g. due to haematuria and haemoglobinuria.

iii) *Nose* e.g. in repeated epistaxis.

iv) *Lungs* e.g. in haemoptysis from various causes.

TABLE 13.4: Etiology of Iron Deficiency Anaemia.

I. INCREASED BLOOD LOSS
1. *Uterine* e.g. excessive menstruation in reproductive years, repeated miscarriages, at onset of menarche, post-menopausal uterine bleeding.
2. *Gastrointestinal* e.g. peptic ulcer, haemorrhoids, hookworm infestation, cancer of stomach and large bowel, oesophageal varices, hiatus hernia, chronic aspirin ingestion, ulcerative colitis, diverticulosis.
3. *Renal tract* e.g. haematuria, haemoglobinuria.
4. *Nose* e.g. repeated epistaxis.
5. *Lungs* e.g. haemoptysis.

II. INCREASED REQUIREMENTS
1. Spurts of growth in infancy, childhood and adolescence.
2. Prematurity.
3. Pregnancy and lactation.

III. INADEQUATE DIETARY INTAKE
1. Poor economic status.
2. Anorexia e.g. in pregnancy.
3. Elderly individuals due to poor dentition, apathy and financial constraints.

IV. DECREASED ABSORPTION
1. Partial or total gastrectomy
2. Achlorhydria
3. Intestinal malabsorption such as in coeliac disease.

4. INFANTS AND CHILDREN. Iron deficiency anaemia is fairly common during infancy and childhood with a peak incidence at 1-2 years of age. The principal cause for anaemia at this age is increased demand of iron which is not met by the inadequate intake of iron in the diet. The normal full-term infant has sufficient iron stores for the first 4-6 months of life, while premature infants have inadequate reserves because iron stores from the mother are mainly laid down during the last trimester of pregnancy. Therefore, unless the infant is given supplemental feeding of iron or iron-containing foods, iron deficiency anaemia develops.

Clinical Features

As already mentioned, iron deficiency anaemia is much more common in women between the age of 20 and 45 years than in men; at periods of active growth in infancy, childhood and adolescence; and is also more frequent in premature infants. Initially, there are usually no clinical abnormalities. But subsequently, in addition to features of the underlying disorder causing the anaemia, the clinical consequences of iron deficiency manifest in 2 ways—anaemia itself and epithelial tissue changes.

1. ANAEMIA. The onset of iron deficiency anaemia is generally slow. The usual symptoms are of weakness, fatigue, dyspnoea on exertion, palpitations and pallor of the skin, mucous membranes and sclerae. Older patients may develop angina and congestive cardiac failure. Patients may have unusual dietary cravings such as pica. Menorrhagia is a common symptom in iron deficient women.

2. EPITHELIAL TISSUE CHANGES. Long-standing chronic iron deficiency anaemia causes epithelial tissue changes in some patients. The changes occur in the nails (koilonychia or spoon-shaped nails), tongue (atrophic glossitis), mouth (angular stomatitis), and oesophagus causing dysphagia from development of thin, membranous webs at the postcricoid area (Plummer-Vinson syndrome).

Laboratory Findings

The development of anaemia progresses in 3 stages:

- Firstly, *storage iron depletion* occurs during which iron reserves are lost without compromise of the iron supply for erythropoiesis.
- The next stage is *iron deficient erythropoiesis* during which the erythroid iron supply is reduced without the development of anaemia.
- The final stage is the development of *frank iron deficiency anaemia* when the red cells become microcytic and hypochromic.

The following laboratory tests can be used to assess the varying degree of iron deficiency (Fig. 13.11):

1. BLOOD PICTURE AND RED CELL INDICES. The degree of anaemia varies. It is usually mild to moderate but occasionally it may be marked (haemoglobin less than 6 g/dl) due to persistent and severe blood loss. The salient haematological findings in these cases are as under (COLOUR PLATE XVI: CL 61):

i) Haemoglobin. The essential feature is a fall in haemoglobin concentration up to a variable degree.

ii) Red cells. The red cells in the blood film are hypochromic and microcytic, and there is anisocytosis and poikilocytosis. Hypochromia generally precedes microcytosis. Hypochromia is due to poor filling of the red cells with haemoglobin so that there is increased central pallor. In severe cases, there may be only a thin rim of pink staining at the periphery. Target cells, elliptical forms and polychromatic cells are often present. Normoblasts are uncommon. RBC

	LABORATORY FINDINGS	NORMAL	IRON-DEFICIENCY ANAEMIA
BLOOD	RED CELL MORPHOLOGY	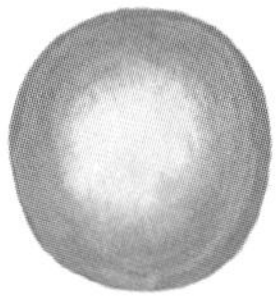 Normal red cell	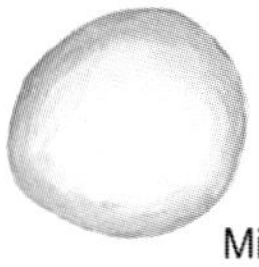 Microcytic hypochromic red cell
BLOOD	RED CELL INDICES	MCV, MCH, MCHC all normal	MCV ↓, MCH ↓, MCHC ↓
BONE MARROW	MARROW ERYTHROPOIESIS	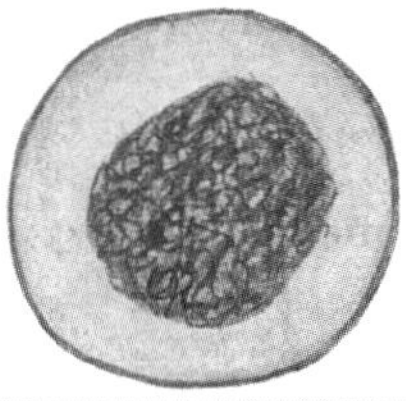 Normoblastic	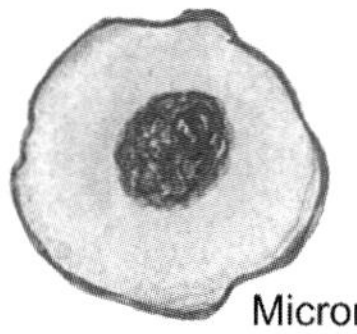 Micronormoblastic
BONE MARROW	MARROW IRON STORES	Normal	Deficient

FIGURE 13.11

Laboratory findings in iron deficiency anaemia.

count is below normal but is generally not proportionate to the fall in haemoglobin value. When iron deficiency is associated with severe folate or vitamin B_{12} deficiency, a *dimorphic* blood picture occurs with dual population of red cells—macrocytic as well as microcytic hypochromic.

iii) Reticulocyte count. The reticulocyte count is normal or reduced but may be slightly raised (2-5%) in cases after haemorrhage.

iv) Absolute values. The red cell indices reveal a diminished MCV (below 50 fl), diminished. MCH (below 15 pg) and diminished MCHC (below 20 g/dl).

v) Leucocytes. The total and differential white cell counts are usually normal.

vi) Platelets. Platelet count is usually normal but may be slightly to moderately raised in patients who have had recent bleeding.

2. BONE MARROW FINDINGS. Bone marrow examination is not essential in such cases routinely but is done in complicated cases so as to distinguish from other hypochromic anaemias. The usual findings are as follows:

i) Marrow cellularity. The marrow cellularity is increased due to erythroid hyperplasia (myeloid-erythroid ratio decreased).

ii) Erythropoiesis. There is normoblastic erythropoiesis with predominance of small polychromatic normoblasts (micronormoblasts). These normoblasts have a thin rim of cytoplasm around the nucleus and a ragged and irregular cell border. The *cytoplasmic maturation lags behind* so that the late normoblasts have pyknotic nucleus but persisting polychromatic cytoplasm (compared from megaloblastic anaemia in which the nuclear maturation lags behind, page 377).

iii) Other cells. Myeloid, lymphoid and megakaryocytic cells are normal in number and morphology.

iv) Marrow iron. Iron staining (Prussian blue reaction) carried out on bone marrow aspirate smear shows deficient reticuloendothelial iron stores and absence of siderotic iron granules from developing normoblasts.

3. BIOCHEMICAL FINDINGS. In addition to blood and bone marrow examination, the following biochemical tests are of value:

i) The *serum iron* level is low (normal 80-180 μg/dl); it is often under 50 μg/dl.

ii) *Total iron binding capacity (TIBC)* is high (normal 250-450 μg/dl) and rises to give less than 10% saturation (normal 33%). In anaemia of chronic disorders, serum iron as well as TIBC are reduced.

iii) The *serum ferritin* is very low (normal 150-2000 ng/dl) indicating poor tissue iron stores. The serum ferritin is raised in iron overload and is normal in anaemia of chronic disorders.

iv) The *red cell protoporphyrin* is very low (normal 20-40 μg/dl) due to its accumulation within the red cells as a result of insufficient iron supply to form haem.

Treatment

The management of iron deficiency anaemia consists of 2 essential principles: correction of disorder causing the anaemia, and correction of iron deficiency.

1. CORRECTION OF THE DISORDER. The underlying cause of iron deficiency is established after thorough check-up and investigations. Appropriate surgical, medical or preventive measures are instituted to correct the cause of blood loss.

2. CORRECTION OF IRON DEFICIENCY. The lack of iron is corrected with iron therapy as under:

i) Oral therapy. Iron deficiency responds very effectively to the administration of oral iron salts such as ferrous sulfate. One tablet containing 60 mg of elemental iron is administered thrice daily. Optimal absorption is obtained by giving iron fasting, but if side-effects occur (e.g. nausea, abdominal discomfort, diarrhoea) iron can be given with food or by using a preparation of lower iron content (e.g. ferrous gluconate containing 37 mg elemental iron). Oral iron therapy is continued long enough, both to correct the anaemia and to replenish the body iron stores. The response to oral iron therapy is observed by reticulocytosis which begins to appear in 3-4 days with a peak in about 10 days. Poor response to iron replacement may occur from various causes such as: incorrect diagnosis, non-compliance, continuing blood loss, bone marrow suppression by tumour or chronic inflammation, and malabsorption.

ii) Parenteral therapy. Parenteral iron therapy is indicated in cases who are intolerant to oral iron therapy, in GIT disorders such as malabsorption, or a rapid replenishment of iron stores is desired such as in women with severe anaemia a few weeks before expected date of delivery. Parenteral iron therapy is hazardous and expensive when compared with oral administration. The haematological response to parenteral iron therapy is no faster than the administration of adequate dose of oral iron but the stores are replenished much faster. Before giving the parenteral iron, total dose is calculated by a simple formula by multiplying the grams of haemoglobin below normal with 250 (250 mg of elemental iron is required for each gram of deficit haemoglobin). It may be given as a single intramuscular injection of iron dextran (imferon), or repeated injections of iron-sorbitol citrate (jectofer). The adverse effects include hypersensitivity or anaphylactoid reactions, haemolysis, hypotension, circulatory collapse, vomiting and muscle pain. A recently introduced preparation, iron gluconate, is given intravenously.

SIDEROBLASTIC ANAEMIA

The sideroblastic anaemias comprise a group of disorders of diverse etiology in which the nucleated erythroid precursors in the bone marrow, show characteristic 'ringed sideroblasts.'

Siderocytes and Sideroblasts

Siderocytes and sideroblasts are erythrocytes and normoblasts respectively which contain cytoplasmic granules of iron (Fig. 13.12).

SIDEROCYTES. These are red cells containing granules of non-haem iron. These granules stain positively with Prussian blue reaction as well as stain with Romanowsky dyes when they are referred to as *Pappenheimer bodies.* Siderocytes are normally not present in the human peripheral blood but a small number may appear following splenectomy. This is because the reticulocytes on release from the marrow are finally sequestered in the spleen to become mature red cells. In the absence of spleen, the final maturation step takes place in the peripheral blood and hence the siderocytes make their appearance in the blood after splenectomy.

SIDEROBLASTS. These are nucleated red cells (normoblasts) containing siderotic granules which stain positively with Prussian blue reaction. Depending upon

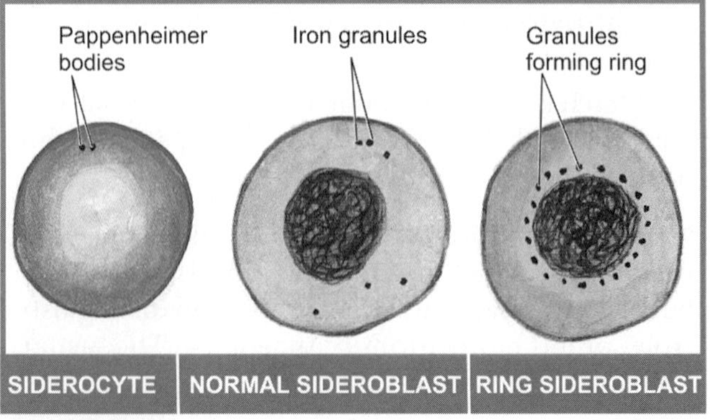

FIGURE 13.12

A siderocyte containing Pappenheimer bodies, a normal sideroblast and a ring sideroblast.

the number, size and distribution of siderotic granules, sideroblasts may be normal or abnormal (Fig. 13.12).

Normal sideroblasts contain a few fine, scattered cytoplasmic granules representing iron which has not been utilised for haemoglobin synthesis. These cells comprise 30-50% of normoblasts in the normal marrow but are reduced or absent in iron deficiency.

Abnormal sideroblasts are further of 2 types:

- *One type* is a sideroblast containing numerous, diffusely scattered, coarse cytoplasmic granules and are seen in conditions such as dyserythropoiesis and haemolysis. In this type, there is no defect of haem or globin synthesis but the percentage saturation of transferrin is increased.
- The other type is *ringed sideroblast* in which haem synthesis is disturbed as occurs in sideroblastic anaemias. Ringed sideroblasts contain numerous large granules, often forming a complete or partial ring around the nucleus. The ringed arrangement of these granules is due to the presence of iron-laden mitochondria around the nucleus.

Types of Sideroblastic Anaemias

Based on etiology, sideroblastic anaemias are classified into hereditary and acquired types. The acquired type is further divided into primary and secondary forms (Table 13.5).

I. HEREDITARY SIDEROBLASTIC ANAEMIA. This is a rare X-linked disorder associated with defective enzyme activity of *aminolevulinic acid (ALA) synthetase* required for haem synthesis. The affected males have moderate to marked anaemia while the females are carriers of the disorder and do not develop anaemia. The condition manifests in childhood or in early adult life.

II. ACQUIRED SIDEROBLASTIC ANAEMIA. The acquired sideroblastic anaemias are classified into primary and secondary types.

TABLE 13.5: Classification of Sideroblastic Anaemia.

I. HEREDITARY (CONGENITAL) SIDEROBLASTIC ANAEMIA

II. ACQUIRED SIDEROBLASTIC ANAEMIA

A. Primary (idiopathic, refractory) acquired sideroblastic anaemia

B. Secondary acquired sideroblastic anaemia

1. *Drugs, chemicals and toxins* e.g. isoniazid, cycloserine, chloramphenicol, cyclophosphamide, alcohol and lead.
2. *Haematological disorders* e.g. myelofibrosis, polycythaemia vera, acute leukaemia, myeloma, lymphoma and haemolytic anaemia.
3. *Miscellaneous* e.g. carcinoma, myxoedema, rheumatoid arthritis and SLE.

A. Primary acquired sideroblastic anaemia. Primary, idiopathic, or refractory acquired sideroblastic anaemia occurs spontaneously in middle-aged and older individuals of both sexes. The disorder has its pathogenesis in disturbed growth and maturation of erythroid precursors at the level of haematopoietic stem cell, possibly due to reduced activity of the enzyme, ALA synthetase. The anaemia is of moderate to severe degree and appears insidiously. The bone marrow cells commonly show chromosomal abnormalities, neutropenia and thrombocytopenia with associated bleeding diathesis. The spleen and liver may be either normal or mildly enlarged, while the lymph nodes are not enlarged. Unlike other types of sideroblastic anaemia, this type is regarded as a myelodysplastic disorder in the FAB (French-American-British) classification and thus, can be a preleukaemic disorder (page 404). About 10% of individuals with refractory acquired sideroblastic anaemia develop acute myelogenous leukaemia.

B. Secondary acquired sideroblastic anaemia. Acquired sideroblastic anaemia may develop secondary to a variety of drugs, chemicals, toxins, haematological and various other diseases.

1. *Drugs, chemicals and toxins:* Isoniazid, an anti-tuberculous drug and a pyridoxine antagonist, is most commonly associated with development of sideroblastic anaemia by producing abnormalities in pyridoxine metabolism. Other drugs occasionally causing acquired sideroblastic anaemia are: cycloserine, chloramphenicol and alkylating agents (e.g. cyclophosphamide). Alcohol and lead also cause sideroblastic anaemia. All these agents cause reversible sideroblastic anaemia which usually resolves following removal of the offending agent.
2. *Haematological disorders:* These include myelofibrosis, polycythaemia vera, acute leukaemia, myeloma, lymphoma and haemolytic anaemia.
3. *Miscellaneous:* Occasionally, secondary sideroblastic anaemia may occur in association with a variety of inflammatory, neoplastic and autoimmune diseases such as carcinoma, myxoedema, rheumatoid arthritis and SLE.

Laboratory Findings

Sideroblastic anaemias usually show the following haematological features:

1. There is generally moderate to severe degree of *anaemia.*
2. The *blood picture* shows hypochromic anaemia which may be microcytic, or there may be some normocytic red cells as well (dimorphic).

3. *Absolute values* (MCV, MCH and MCHC) are reduced in hereditary type but MCV is often raised in acquired type.

4. The *bone marrow examination* shows erythroid hyperplasia with usually macronormoblastic erythropoiesis. Marrow iron stores are raised and pathognomonic ring sideroblasts are present.

5. *Serum ferritin* levels are raised.

6. *Serum iron* is usually raised with almost complete saturation of TIBC.

7. There is increased *iron deposition* in the tissue.

Treatment

The treatment of secondary sideroblastic anaemia is primarily focussed on removal of the offending agent. No definite treatment is available for hereditary and idiopathic types of sideroblastic anaemias. However, pyridoxine is administered routinely to all cases of sideroblastic anaemia (200 mg per day for 2-3 months). Blood transfusions and other supportive therapy are indicated in all patients. More recently, clinical trials have been attempted by giving cytokines such as erythropoietin, colony-stimulating factor and interleukin-3.

Differential diagnosis of various types of hypochromic anaemias by laboratory tests is summarised in Table 13.6.

ANAEMIA OF CHRONIC DISORDERS

One of the commonly encountered anaemia is in patients of a variety of chronic systemic diseases in which anaemia develops secondary to disease process but there is no actual invasion of the bone marrow. A list of such chronic systemic diseases is given in Table 13.7. In general, the anaemia in chronic disorders is usually normocytic normochromic but can have mild degree of microcytosis and hypochromia unrelated to iron deficiency. The severity of anaemia is usually directly related to the primary disease process. The anaemia is corrected only if the primary disease is alleviated.

Pathogenesis

A number of factors may contribute to the development of anaemia in chronic systemic disorders, and in many conditions, the anaemia is complicated by other causes such as iron, B_{12} and folate deficiency, hypersplenism, renal failure with consequent reduced erythropoietic activity, endocrine abnormalities etc. However, in general, 2 factors appear to play significant role in the pathogenesis of anaemia in chronic disorders. These are: *defective red cell production* and *reduced red cell life-span.*

1. **Defective red cell production.** Though there is abundance of storage iron in these conditions but the amount of iron in developing erythroid cells in the marrow is subnormal. The mononuclear phagocyte system is hyperplastic and traps all the available free iron due to the activity of iron binding protein, lactoferrin. A defect in the transfer of iron from macrophages to the developing erythroid cells in the marrow leads to reduced availability of iron for haem synthesis despite adequate iron stores, elevating serum ferritin levels. The defect lies in suppression by cytokines at some stage in erythropoiesis e.g. TNF and IFN-β released in bacterial infections and tumours, IL-1 and IFN-γ released in patients of rheumatoid arthritis and autoimmune vasculitis.

2. **Reduced red cell life-span.** Slightly decreased survival of circulating red cells is also attributed to hyperplastic mononuclear phagocyte system.

TABLE 13.6: Laboratory Diagnosis of Hypochromic Anaemias.

TEST	IRON DEFICIENCY	CHRONIC DISORDERS	THALASSAEMIA	SIDEROBLASTIC ANAEMIA
1. *MCV, MCH, MCHC*	Reduced	Low normal-to-reduced	Very low	Very low (except MCV raised in aquired type)
2. *Serum iron*	Reduced	Reduced	Normal	Raised
3. *TIBC*	Raised	Reduced	Normal	Normal
4. *Serum ferritin*	Reduced	Raised	Normal	Raised (complete saturation)
5. *Marrow-iron stores*	Absent	Present	Present	Present
6. *Iron in normoblasts*	Absent	Absent	Present	Ring sideroblasts
7. *Hb electrophoresis*	Normal	Normal	Abnormal	Normal

TABLE 13.7: Anaemias Secondary to Chronic Systemic Disorders.

1. **ANAEMIA IN CHRONIC INFECTIONS/INFLAMMATION**
   a. *Infections e.g.* tuberculosis, lung abscess, pneumonia, osteomyelitis, subacute bacterial endocarditis, pyelonephritis.
   b. *Non-infectious inflammations* e.g. rheumatoid arthritis, SLE, vasculitis, dermatomyositis, scleroderma, sarcoidosis, Crohn's disease.
   c. *Disseminated malignancies* e.g. Hodgkin's disease, disseminated carcinomas and sarcomas.
2. **ANAEMIA OF RENAL DISEASE** e.g. uraemia, renal failure
3. **ANAEMIA OF HYPOMETABOLIC STATE** e.g. endocrinopathies (myxoedema, Addison's disease, hyperthyroidism, hypopituitarism, Addison's disease), protein malnutrition, scurvy and pregnancy, liver disease.

Laboratory Findings

The characteristic features of anaemia in these patients uncomplicated by other deficiencies are as under:

i) Haemoglobin. Anaemia is generally mild to moderate. A haemoglobin value of less than 8 g/dl suggests the presence of additional contributory factors.

ii) Blood picture. The type of anaemia in these cases is generally normocytic normochromic but may have slight microcytosis and hypochromia.

iii) Absolute values. Red cell indices indicate that in spite of normocytic normochromic anaemia, MCHC is slightly low.

iv) Reticulocyte count. The reticulocyte count is generally low.

v) Red cell survival. Measurement of erythrocyte survival generally reveals mild to moderate shortening of their life-span.

vi) Bone marrow. Examination of the marrow generally reveals normal erythroid maturation. However, the red cell precursors have reduced stainable iron than normal, while the macrophages in the marrow usually contain increased amount of iron. Cases of chronic infection often have myeloid hyperplasia and increase in plasma cells.

vii) Serum iron and TIBC. Both serum iron and TIBC are characteristically reduced in this group of anaemias (in contrast to iron deficiency where there is reduction in serum iron but no fall in TIBC, see Table 13.6).

viii) Serum ferritin. Serum ferritin levels are increased in these patients.

ix) Other plasma proteins. In addition, certain other plasma proteins called *'phase reactants'* are raised in patients with chronic inflammation, probably under the stimulus of interleukin-1 released by activated macrophages. These proteins include γ-globulin, C3, haptoglobin, α_1-antitrypsin and fibrinogen. Elevation of these proteins is responsible for raised ESR commonly present in these patients.

MEGALOBLASTIC ANAEMIA

The megaloblastic anaemias are disorders caused by impaired DNA synthesis and are characterised by a distinctive abnormality in the haematopoietic precursors in the bone marrow in which the *maturation of the nucleus is delayed relative to that of the cytoplasm.* Since cell division is slow but cytoplasmic development progresses normally, the nucleated red cell precursors tend to be larger which Ehrlich in 1880 termed *megaloblasts.* Megaloblasts are both morphologically and functionally abnormal with the result that the mature red cells formed from them and released into the peripheral blood are also abnormal in shape and size, the most prominent abnormality being *macrocytosis.*

The underlying defect for the asynchronous maturation of the nucleus is defective DNA synthesis due to deficiency of vitamin B_{12} (cobalamin) and/or folic acid (folate). Less common causes are interference with DNA synthesis by congenital or acquired abnormalities of vitamin B_{12} or folic acid metabolism. Before considering the megaloblastic anaemia, a brief account of vitamin B_{12} and folic acid metabolism is considered in order.

The salient nutritional aspects and metabolic functions of vitamin B_{12} and folic acid are summarised in Table 13.8.

Vitamin B_{12} Metabolism

BIOCHEMISTRY. Vitamin B_{12} or cobalamin is a complex organometallic compound having a cobalt atom situated within a corrin ring, similar to the structure of porphyrin from which haem is formed. In humans, there are 2 metabolically active forms of cobalamin—methyl-cobalamin and adenosyl-cobalamin, which act as coenzymes. The therapeutic vitamin B_{12} preparation is called cyanocobalamin.

SOURCES. The only dietary sources of vitamin B_{12} are foods of animal protein origin such as kidney, liver, heart, muscle meats, fish, eggs, cheese and milk. In contrast to folate, vegetables contain practically no vitamin B_{12}. Cooking has little effect on its activity. Vitamin B_{12} is synthesised in the human large bowel by micro-organisms but is not absorbed from this site and, thus, the humans are entirely dependent upon dietary

TABLE 13.8: Salient Features of Vitamin B_{12} and Folate Metabolism.

FEATURE	VITAMIN B_{12}	FOLATE
1. *Main foods*	Animal proteins only	Green vegetables, meats
2. *Cooking*	Little effect	Easily destroyed
3. *Daily requirements*	2-4 μg	100-200 μg
4. *Daily intake*	5-30 μg	100-500 μg
5. *Site of absorption*	Ileum	Duodenum and jejunum
6. *Mechanism of absorption*	Intrinsic factor	Conversion to methyl-THF
7. *Body stores*	2-3 mg (enough for 2-4 yrs)	10-12 mg (enough for 4 months)

sources. The average daily requirement for vitamin B_{12} is 2-4 μg.

ABSORPTION. After ingestion, vitamin B_{12} in food is released and forms a stable complex with gastric R-binder. R-binder is a form of glycoprotein found in various secretions (e.g. saliva, milk, gastric juice, bile), phagocytes and plasma. On entering the duodenum, the vitamin B_{12}-R-binder complex is digested releasing vitamin B_{12} which then binds to intrinsic factor (IF). The IF is a glycoprotein of molecular weight 50,000 produced by the parietal cells of the stomach and its secretion roughly parallels that of hydrochloric acid. The vitamin B_{12}-IF complex, on reaching the distal ileum, binds to the specific receptors on the mucosal brush border, thereby enabling the vitamin to be absorbed. The IF, therefore, acts as cell-directed carrier protein similar to transferrin. The receptor-bound vitamin B_{12}-IF complex is taken into the ileal mucosal cells where after several hours the IF is destroyed, vitamin B_{12} released and is transferred to another transport protein, transcobalamin (TC) II. The vitamin B_{12}-TC II complex is finally secreted into the portal circulation from where it is taken by the liver, bone marrow and other cells. There are 2 major vitamin B_{12} binding proteins—TC I and TC II, and a minor protein TC III. TC I is not essential for vitamin B_{12} transport but functions primarily as a storage protein while TC III is similar to TC II and binds a small amount of vitamin B_{12} (Fig. 13.13,B).

TISSUE STORES. Normally, the liver is the principal storage site of vitamin B_{12} and stores about 2 mg of the vitamin, while other tissues like kidney, heart and brain together store about 2 mg. The body stores of vitamin B_{12} are adequate for 2-4 years. Major source of loss is via bile and shedding of intestinal epithelial cells. A major part of the excreted vitamin B_{12} is reabsorbed in the ileum by the IF resulting in enterohepatic circulation.

FUNCTIONS. Vitamin B_{12} plays an important role in general cell metabolism, particulary essential for normal haematopoiesis and for maintenance of integrity of the nervous system. Vitamin B_{12} acts as a co-enzyme for 2 main biochemical reactions in the body:

- *Firstly, as methyl cobalamin (methyl B_{12})* in the methylation of homocysteine to methionine by methyl tetrahydrofolate (THF). The homocysteine-methionine reaction is closely linked to folate metabolism (Fig. 13.14):

$$\text{Homocysteine} \xrightarrow{\textit{Methyl } B_{12}} \text{Methionine}$$

When this reaction is impaired, folate metabolism is deranged and results in defective DNA synthesis responsible for megaloblastic maturation.

- *Secondly, as adenosyl cobalamin (adenosyl B_{12})* in propionate metabolism for the conversion of methyl malonyl co-enzyme A to succinyl co-enzyme A:

$$\text{Propionyl CoA} \longrightarrow \text{Methyl malonyl CoA} \xrightarrow{\textit{Adenosyl } B_{12}} \text{Succinyl CoA}$$

Lack of adenosyl B_{12} leads to large increase in the level of methyl malonyl CoA and its precursor, propionyl CoA. This results in synthesis of certain fatty acids which are incorporated into the neuronal lipids. This biochemical abnormality may contribute to the neurologic complications of vitamin B_{12} deficiency.

Folate Metabolism

BIOCHEMISTRY. Folate or folic acid, a yellow compound, is a member of water-soluble B complex vitamins with the chemical name of *pteroyl glutamic acid (PGA)*. Folic acid does not exist as such in nature but exists as folates in polyglutamate form (conjugated folates). For its metabolic action as co-enzyme, polyglutamates must be reduced to dihydro- and tetrahydrofolate forms.

SOURCES. Folate exists in different plants, bacteria and animal tissues. Its main dietary sources are fresh green leafy vegetables, fruits, liver, kidney, and to a lesser

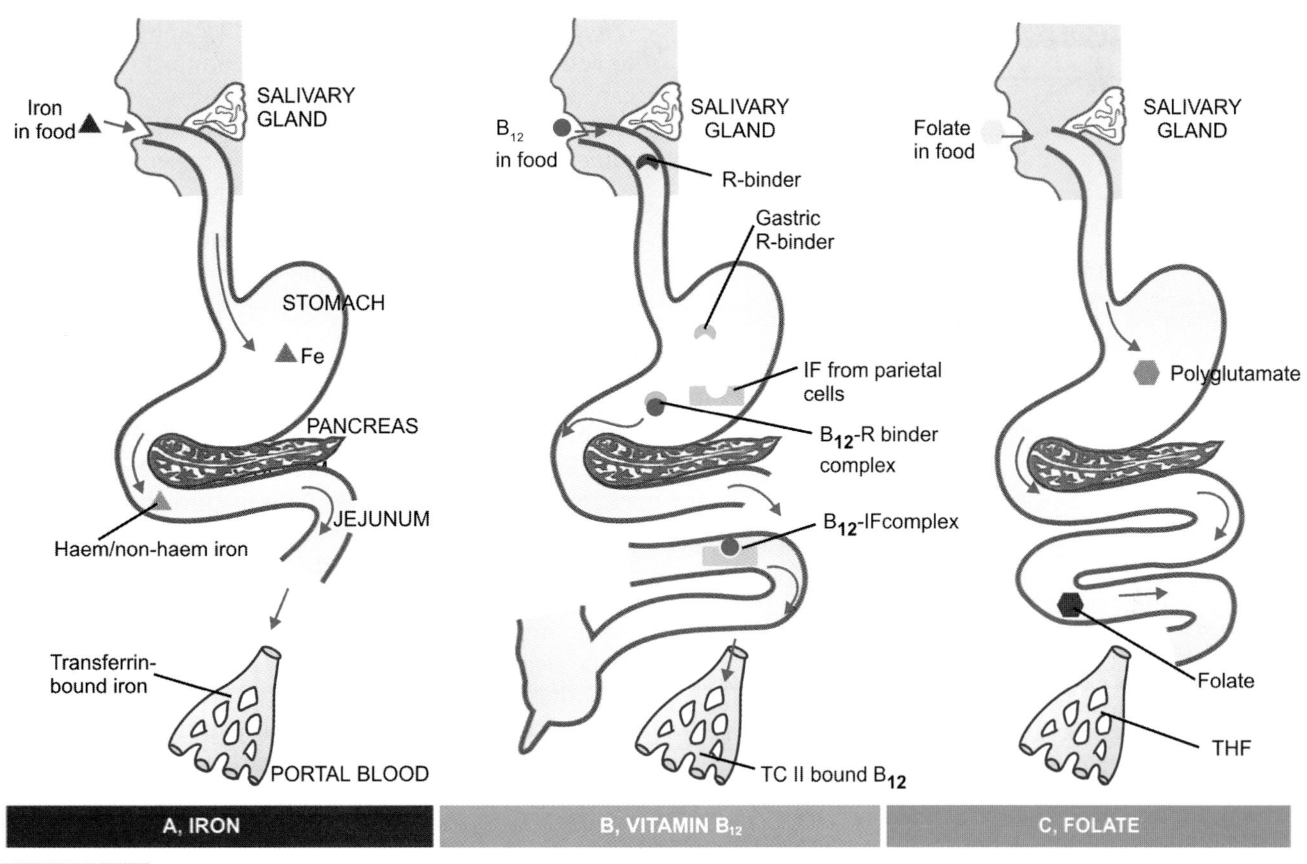

FIGURE 13.13

Contrasting pathways of absorption and transport of iron, vitamin B_{12} and folic acid.

extent, muscle meats, cereals and milk. Folate is labile and is largely destroyed by cooking and canning. Some amount of folate synthesised by bacteria in the human large bowel is not available to the body since its absorption takes place in the small intestine. Thus, humans are mainly dependent upon diet for its supply. The average daily requirement is 100-200 μg.

ABSORPTION AND TRANSPORT. Folate is normally absorbed from the duodenum and upper jejunum and to a lesser extent, from the lower jejunum and ileum. However, absorption depends upon the form of folate in the diet. Polyglutamate form in the foodstuffs is first cleaved by the enzyme, folate conjugase, in the mucosal cells to mono- and diglutamates which are readily assimilated. Synthetic folic acid preparations in polyglutamate form are also absorbed as rapidly as mono- and diglutamate form because of the absence of natural inhibitors. Mono- and diglutamates undergo further reduction in the mucosal cells to form tetrahydrofolate (THF), a monoglutamate. THF circulates in the plasma as methylated compound, methyl THF, bound to a protein. Once methyl THF is transported into the cell by a carrier protein, it is reconverted to polyglutamate (Fig. 13.13,C).

TISSUE STORES. The liver and red cells are the main storage sites of folate, largely as methyl THF polyglutamate form. The total body stores of folate are about 10-12 mg enough for about 4 months. Normally, folate is lost from the sweat, saliva, urine and faeces.

FUNCTIONS. Folate plays an essential role in cellular metabolism. It acts as a co-enzyme for 2 important biochemical reactions involving transfer of 1-carbon units (viz. methyl and formyl groups) to various other compounds. These reactions are as under:

- *Thymidylate synthetase reaction.* Formation of deoxy thymidylate monophosphate (dTMP) from its precursor form, deoxy uridylate monophosphate (dUMP).
- *Methylation of homocysteine to methionine.* This reaction is linked to vitamin B_{12} metabolism (Fig. 13.14).

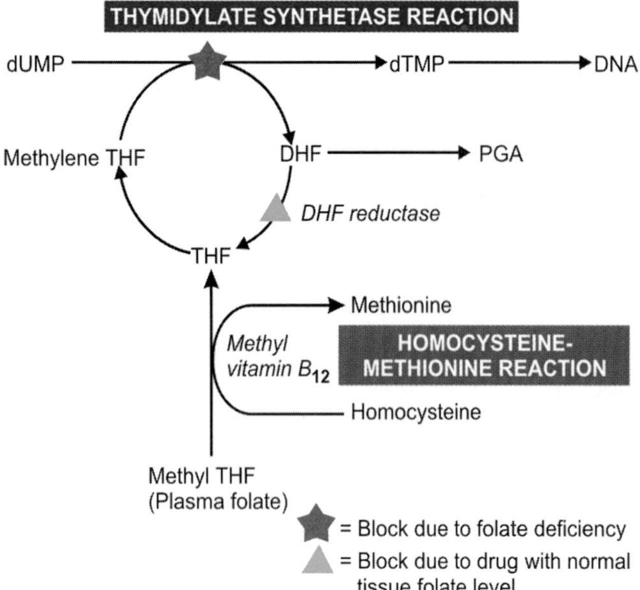

FIGURE 13.14

Biochemical basis of megaloblastic anaemia (THF = tetrahydrofolate; DHF = dihydrofolate; PGA = pteroyl glutamic acid; dUMP = deoxy uridylate monophosphate; dTMP = deoxy thymidylate monophosphate).

These biochemical reactions are considered in detail below together with biochemical basis of the megaloblastic anaemia.

Biochemical Basis of Megaloblastic Anaemia

The basic biochemical abnormality common to both vitamin B_{12} and folate deficiency is a block in the DNA synthesis pathway and that there is an inter-relationship between vitamin B_{12} and folate metabolism in the methylation reaction of homocysteine to methionine (Fig. 13.14).

As stated above, folate as co-enzyme methylene THF, is required for transfer of 1-carbon moieties (e.g. methyl and formyl) to form building blocks in DNA synthesis. These 1-carbon moieties are derived from serine or formiminoglutamic acid (FIGLU). Two of the important folate-dependent (1-carbon transfer) reactions for formation of building blocks in DNA synthesis are as under:

1. Thymidylate synthetase reaction. This reaction involves synthesis of deoxy thymidylate monophosphate (dTMP) from deoxy uridylate monophosphate (dUMP). The methyl group of dUMP → dTMP reaction is supplied by the co-enzyme, methylene-THF. After the transfer of 1-carbon from methylene-THF, dihydrofolate (DHF) is produced which must be reduced to active THF by the enzyme DHF-reductase before it can participate in further 1-carbon transfer reaction. Drugs like methotrexate (anti-cancer) and pyrimethamine (antimalarial) are inhibitory to the enzyme, DHF-reductase, thereby inhibiting the DNA synthesis.

2. Homocysteine-methionine reaction. Homocysteine is converted into methionine by transfer of a methyl group from methylene-THF. After transfer of 1-carbon from methylene-THF, THF is produced. This reaction requires the presence of vitamin B_{12} (methyl-B_{12}).

Deficiency of folate from any cause results in reduced supply of the coenzyme, methylene-THF, and thus interferes with the synthesis of DNA. Deficiency of vitamin B_{12} traps folate as its transport form, methyl-THF, thereby resulting in reduced formation of the active form, methylene-THF, needed for DNA synthesis. This is referred to as *methyl-folate trap hypothesis.* An alternative hypothesis of inter-relationship of B_{12} and folate is the *formate-saturation hypothesis.* According to this hypothesis, the active substrate is formyl-THF. Vitamin B_{12} deficiency results in reduced supply of formate to THF causing reduced generation of the active compound, formyl THF.

Etiology and Classification of Megaloblastic Anaemia

The etiology of megaloblastic anaemia varies in different parts of the world. As outlined in Table 13.9, megaloblastic anaemia is classified into 3 broad groups: vitamin B_{12} deficiency, folate deficiency, and other causes.

1. VITAMIN B_{12} DEFICIENCY. In Western countries, the deficiency of vitamin B_{12} is usually due to pernicious (Addisonian) anaemia. True vegetarians like in India and breast-fed infants have dietary lack of vitamin B_{12}. Gastrectomy by lack of intrinsic factor, and small intestinal lesions involving distal ileum where absorption of vitamin B_{12} occurs, may cause deficiency of the vitamin. Deficiency of vitamin B_{12} takes at least 2 years to develop when the body stores are totally depleted.

2. FOLATE DEFICIENCY. Folate deficiency is more often due to poor dietary intake. Other causes include malabsorption, excess folate utilisation such as in pregnancy and in various disease states, alcoholism, and excess urinary folate loss. Folate deficiency arises more rapidly than vitamin B_{12} deficiency since the body's stores of folate are relatively low which can last for up to 4 months only.

TABLE 13.9: Etiologic Classification of Megaloblastic Anaemia.

I. VITAMIN B_{12} DEFICIENCY

A. **Inadequate dietary intake** e.g. strict vegetarians, breast-fed infants.

B. **Malabsorption**

1. *Gastric causes:* pernicious anaemia, gastrectomy, congenital lack of intrinsic factor.
2. *Intestinal causes:* tropical sprue, ileal resection, Crohn's disease, intestinal blind loop syndrome, fish-tapeworm infestation.

II. FOLATE DEFICIENCY

A. **Inadequate dietary intake** e.g. in alcoholics, teenagers, infants, old age, poverty.

B. **Malabsorption** e.g. in tropical sprue, coeliac disease, partial gastrectomy, jejunal resection, Crohn's disease.

C. **Excess demand**

1. *Physiological:* pregnancy, lactation, infancy.
2. *Pathological :* malignancy, increased haematopoiesis, chronic exfoliative skin disorders, tuberculosis, rheumatoid arthritis.

D. **Excess urinary folate loss** e.g. in active liver disease, congestive heart failure.

III. OTHER CAUSES

A. **Impaired metabolism** e.g. inhibitors of dihydrofolate (DHF) reductase such as methotrexate and pyrimethamine; alcohol, congenital enzyme deficiencies.

B. **Unknown etiology** e.g. in Di Guglielmo's syndrome, congenital dyserythropoietic anaemia, refractory megaloblastic anaemia.

Patients with tropical sprue are often deficient in both vitamin B_{12} and folate. Combined deficiency of vitamin B_{12} and folate may occur from severe deficiency of vitamin B_{12} because of the biochemical inter-relationship with folate metabolism.

3. OTHER CAUSES. In addition to deficiency of vitamin B_{12} and folate, megaloblastic anaemias may occasionally be induced by other factors unrelated to vitamin deficiency. These include many drugs which interfere with DNA synthesis, acquired defects of haematopoietic stem cells, and rarely, congenital enzyme deficiencies.

Clinical Features

Deficiency of vitamin B_{12} and folate may cause the following clinical manifestations which may be present singly or in combination and in varying severity:

1. Anaemia. Macrocytic megaloblastic anaemia is the cardinal feature of deficiency of vitamin B_{12} and/or folate. The onset of anaemia is usually insidious and gradually progressive.

2. Glossitis. Typically, the patient has a smooth, beefy, red tongue.

3. Neurologic manifestations. Vitamin B_{12} deficiency, particularly in patients of pernicious anaemia, is associated with significant neurological manifestations in the form of subacute combined, degeneration of the spinal cord and peripheral neuropathy (Chapter 28), while folate deficiency may occasionally develop neuropathy only. The underlying pathologic process consists of demyelination of the peripheral nerves, the spinal cord and the cerebrum. Signs and symptoms include numbness, paraesthesia, weakness, ataxia, poor finger coordination and diminished reflexes.

4. Others. In addition to the cardinal features mentioned above, patients may have various other symptoms. These include: mild jaundice, angular stomatitis, purpura, melanin pigmentation, symptoms of malabsorption, weight loss and anorexia.

Laboratory Findings

The investigations of a suspected case of megaloblastic anaemia are aimed at 2 aspects:

A. *General laboratory investigations of anaemia* which include blood picture, red cell indices, bone marrow findings, and biochemical tests.

B. *Special tests* to establish the cause of megaloblastic anaemia as to know whether it is due to deficiency of vitamin B_{12} or folate.

Based on these principles, the following plan of investigations is followed:

A. General Laboratory Findings

These are as under (Fig. 13.15):

1. BLOOD PICTURE AND RED CELL INDICES. The estimation of haemoglobin, examination of a blood film and evaluation of absolute values are essential preliminary investigations.

i) Haemoglobin. The haemoglobin estimation reveals values below the normal range. The fall in haemoglobin concentration may be of a variable degree.

ii) Red cells. The red blood cell morphology in a blood film shows the characteristic macrocytosis. However, *macrocytosis* can also be seen in several other disorders such as: haemolysis, liver disease, alcoholism, hypothyroidism, aplastic anaemia, myeloproliferative disorders and reticulocytosis. In addition, the blood smear demonstrates marked anisocytosis, poikilocytosis and presence of macro-

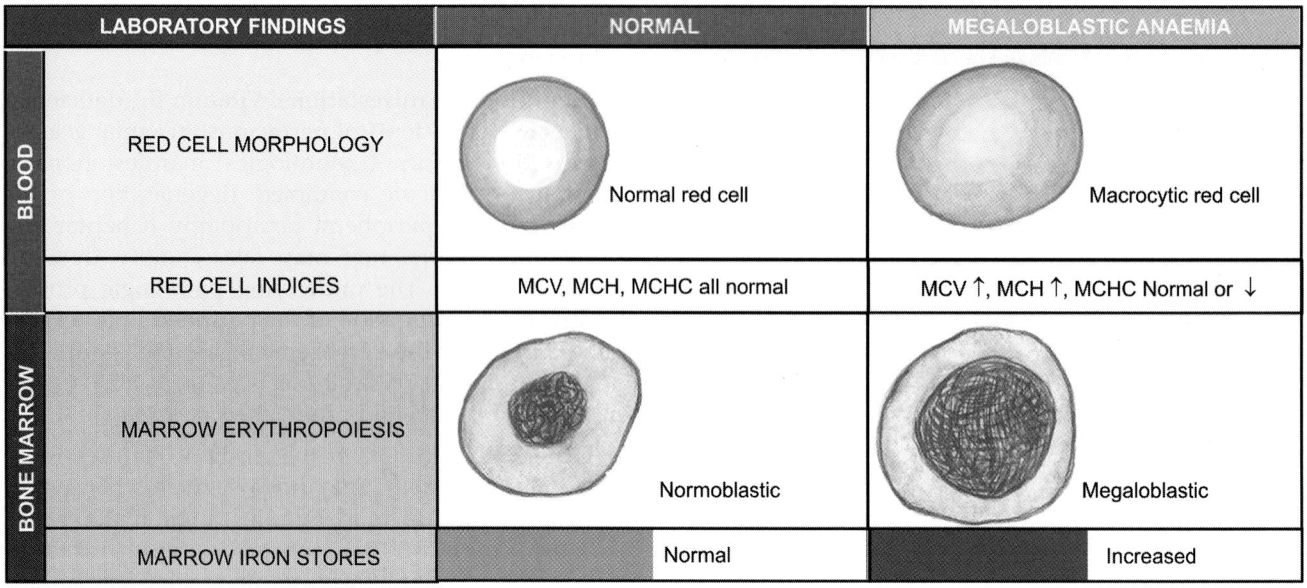

	LABORATORY FINDINGS	NORMAL	MEGALOBLASTIC ANAEMIA
BLOOD	RED CELL MORPHOLOGY	Normal red cell	Macrocytic red cell
BLOOD	RED CELL INDICES	MCV, MCH, MCHC all normal	MCV ↑, MCH ↑, MCHC Normal or ↓
BONE MARROW	MARROW ERYTHROPOIESIS	Normoblastic	Megaloblastic
BONE MARROW	MARROW IRON STORES	Normal	Increased

FIGURE 13.15

General laboratory findings in megaloblastic anaemia.

ovalocytes. Basophilic stippling and occasional normoblast may also be seen (COLOUR PLATE XVI: CL 62).

iii) Reticulocyte count. The reticulocyte count is generally low to normal in untreated cases.

iv) Absolute values. The red cell indices reveal an elevated MCV (above 120 fl) proportionate to the severity of macrocytosis, elevated MCH (above 50 pg) and normal or reduced MCHC.

v) Leucocytes. The total white blood cell count may be reduced. Presence of characteristic hypersegmented neutrophils (having more than 5 nuclear lobes) in the blood film should raise the suspicion of megaloblastic anaemia. An occasional myelocyte may also be seen.

vi) Platelets. Platelet count may be moderately reduced in severely anaemic patients. Bizarre forms of platelets may be seen.

2. BONE MARROW FINDINGS. The bone marrow examination is very helpful in the diagnosis of megaloblastic anaemia. Significant findings of marrow examination are as under:

i) Marrow cellularity. The marrow is hypercellular with a decreased myeloid-erythroid ratio.

ii) Erythropoiesis. The erythroid hyperplasia is due to characteristic megaloblastic erythropoiesis. *Megaloblasts* are abnormal, large, nucleated erythroid precursors, having nuclear-cytoplasmic asynchrony i.e. the nuclei are less mature than the development of cytoplasm. The nuclei are large, having fine, reticular and open chromatin that stains lightly, while the haemoglobinisation of the cytoplasm proceeds normally or at a faster rate i.e. *nuclear maturation lags behind that of cytoplasm* (compared from iron deficiency anaemia in which cytoplasmic maturation lags behind, page 373). Megaloblasts with abnormal mitoses may be seen. Features of ineffective erythropoiesis such as presence of degenerated erythroid precursors may be present.

iii) Other cells. Granulocyte precursors are also affected to some extent. Giant forms of metamyelocytes and band cells may be present in the marrow. Megakaryocytes are usually present in normal number but may occasionally be decreased and show abnormal morphology such as hypersegmented nuclei and agranular cytoplasm.

iv) Marrow iron. Prussian blue staining for iron in the marrow shows an increase in the number and size of iron granules in the erythroid precursors. Ring sideroblasts are, however, rare. Iron in the reticulum cells is increased.

3. BIOCHEMICAL FINDINGS. In addition to the general blood and marrow investigations and specific tests to determine the cause of deficiency (described below), the following biochemical abnormalities are observed in cases of megaloblastic anaemia:

i) There is rise in *serum unconjugated bilirubin and LDH* as a result of ineffective erythropoiesis causing marrow cell break down.

ii) The *serum iron and ferritin* may be normal or elevated.

B. Special Tests for Cause of Specific Deficiency

In evaluating a patient of megaloblastic anaemia, it is important to determine the specific vitamin deficiency by assay of vitamin B_{12} and folate.

TESTS FOR VITAMIN B_{12} DEFICIENCY. The normal range of vitamin B_{12} in serum is 200-900 pg/ml (or 200-900 ng/L). Values less than 100 pg/ml indicate clinically deficient stage. There are 3 types of tests to establish the vitamin B_{12} deficiency: serum vitamin B_{12} assay, radioisotope absorption test and serum enzyme levels.

1. SERUM VITAMIN B_{12} ASSAY. Assay of vitamin B_{12} blood can be done by 2 methods—microbiologic assay and radioassay.

i) Microbiological assay. This test is based on the principle that the serum sample to be assayed is added to a medium containing all other essential growth factors required for a vitamin B_{12}-dependent microorganism. The medium alongwith micro-organism is incubated and the amount of vitamin B_{12} determined turbimetrically which is then compared with the growth produced by a known amount of vitamin B_{12}. Several organisms have been used for this test such as *Euglena gracilis, Lactobacillus leichmannii, Escherichia coli* and *Ochromonas malhamensis. E. gracilis* is, however, considered more sensitive and accurate. The addition of antibiotics to the test interferes with the growth and yields false low result.

ii) Radioassay. Assays of serum B_{12} by radioisotope dilution (RID) and radioimmunoassay (RIA) have been developed. These tests are more sensitive and have the advantage over microbiologic assays in that they are simpler and more rapid, and the results are unaffected by antibiotics and other drugs which may affect the living organisms.

2. SCHILLING TEST (RADIOISOTOPE ABSORPTION TEST). Schilling test is done to detect vitamin B_{12} deficiency as well as to distinguish and detect lack of IF and malabsorption. The results of test also depend upon good renal function and proper urinary collection. The test is performed in 3 stages as under:

Stage I: Without IF. Oral dose of 0.5-2 μg of radioactively labelled vitamin B_{12} ('hot' B_{12}) is administered orally. After 2 hours, a large dose (4 mg) of unlabelled vitamin B_{12} ('cold' B_{12}) is given parenterally. The 'cold' B_{12} will saturate the serum as well as the tissue binding sites.

- In normal individuals, more than 7% of 1 μg of oral dose of 'hot' B_{12} is excreted in 24-hour urinary sample.
- Patients with IF deficiency excrete lower quantity of 'hot' B_{12} which is further confirmed by repeating the test as in stage II given below.

Stage II: With IF. If the 24-hour urinary excretion of 'hot' B_{12} is low, the test is repeated using the same procedure as in stage I but in addition high oral dose of IF is administered alongwith 'hot' B_{12}.

- If the 24-hour urinary excretion of 'hot' B_{12} is now normal, the low value in first stage of the test was due to IF deficiency.
- Patients with pernicious anaemia have abnormal test even after treatment with vitamin B_{12} due to IF deficiency. However, abnormal 24-hour urinary excretion of 'hot' B_{12} is further investigated in stage III for a cause in intestinal malabsorption of 'hot' B'_{12}.

Stage III: Test for malabsorption of vitamin B_{12}. Some patients absorb vitamin B_{12} in water as was stipulated in the original Schilling test. Currently, modified Schilling test employs the use of protein-bound vitamin B_{12}. In conditions causing malabsorption, the test is repeated after a course of treatment with antibiotics or anti-inflammatory drugs.

3. SERUM ENZYME LEVELS. Besides Schilling test, another way of distinguishing whether megaloblastic anaemia is due to cobalamine or folate is by serum determination of methylmalonic acid and homocysteine. Both are elevated in cobalamine deficiency, while in folate deficiency there is only elevation of homocysteine and not of methylmalonic acid.

TESTS FOR FOLATE DEFICIENCY. The normal range of serum folate is 6-12 ng/ml (6-12 μg/L). Values of 4 ng/ml or less are generally considered to be diagnostic of folate deficiency. Measurement of *formiminoglutamic acid (FIGLU) urinary excretion* after histidine load was used formerly for assessing folate status but it is less specific and less sensitive than the serum assays. Currently, there are 3 tests used to detect folate deficiency—urinary excretion of FIGLU, serum and red cell folate assay.

1. ***URINARY EXCRETION OF FIGLU.*** Folic acid is required for conversion of formiminoglutamic acid (FIGLU) to glutamic acid in the catabolism of histidine. Thus, on oral administration of histidine, urinary excretion of FIGLU is increased if folate deficiency is present.

2. ***SERUM FOLATE ASSAY.*** The folate in serum can be estimated by 2 methods—microbiological assay and radioassay.

i) Microbiological assay. This test is based on the principle that the serum folate acid activity is mainly due to the presence of a folic acid co-enzyme, 5-methyl THF, and that this compound is required for growth of the microorganism, *Lactobacillus casei.* The growth of *L. casei* is inhibited by addition of antibiotics.

ii) Radioassay. The principle and method of radioassay by radioisotope dilution (RID) test are similar to that for serum B_{12} assay. The test employs labelled pteroylglutamic acid or methyl-THF. Commercial kits are available which permit simultaneous assay of both vitamin B_{12} and folate.

3. ***RED CELL FOLATE ASSAY.*** Red cells contain 20-50 times more folate than the serum and that red cell folate assay is more reliable indicator of tissue stores of folate than serum folate assay. Both microbiological and radioassay methods can be used for estimation of red cell folate. Red cell folate values are decreased in patients with megaloblastic anaemia as well as in patients with pernicious anaemia.

Treatment

Most cases of megaloblastic anaemia need therapy with appropriate vitamin. This includes: hydroxycobalamin as intramuscular injection 1000 μg for 3 weeks and oral folic acid 5 mg tablets daily for 4 months. Severely-anaemic patients in whom a definite deficiency of either vitamin cannot be established with certainty are treated with both vitamins concurrently. Blood transfusion should be avoided since it may cause circulatory overload. Packed cells may, however, be infused slowly.

Treatment of megaloblastic anaemia is quite gratifying. Marrow begins to revert back to normal morphology within a few hours of initiating treatment and becomes normoblastic within 48 hours of start of treatment. Reticulocytosis appears within 4-5 days after therapy is started and peaks at day 7. Haemoglobin should rise by 2-3g/dl each fortnight. The peripheral neuropathy may show some improvement but subacute combined degeneration of the spinal cord is irreversible.

PERNICIOUS ANAEMIA

Pernicious anaemia (PA) was first described by Addison in 1855 as a chronic disorder of middle-aged and elderly individual of either sex in which intrinsic factor secretion ceases owing to atrophy of the gastric mucosa. The condition is, therefore, also termed Addisonian megaloblastic anaemia. The average age at presentation is 60 years but rarely it can be seen in children under 10 years of age (juvenile pernicious anaemia). PA is seen most frequently in individuals of northern European descent and American blacks and is uncommon in South Europeans and Orientals.

Pathogenesis

There is evidence to suggest that the atrophy of gastric mucosa in PA is caused by an autoimmune reaction against gastric parietal cells. The evidences in support of immunological abnormalities in pernicious anaemia are as under:

1. The incidence of PA is high in patients with *other autoimmune diseases* such as Graves' disease, myxoedema, thyroiditis, vitiligo, diabetes and idiopathic adrenocortical insufficiency.
2. Patients with PA have abnormal *circulating autoantibodies* such as anti-parietal cell antibody (90% cases) and anti-intrinsic factor antibody (50% cases).
3. *Relatives* of patients with PA have an increased incidence of the disease or increased presence of autoantibodies.
4. *Corticosteroids* have been reported to be beneficial in curing the disease both pathologically and clinically.
5. PA is more common in patients with *agammaglobulinaemia* supporting the role of cellular immune system in destruction of parietal cells.

PATHOLOGIC CHANGES The most characteristic pathologic finding in PA is gastric atrophy affecting the acid- and pepsin-secreting portion of the stomach and sparing the antrum (Chapter 18). Gastric epithelium may show cellular atypia. About 2-3% cases of PA develop carcinoma of the stomach. Other pathologic changes are secondary to vitamin B_{12} deficiency and include megaloblastoid alterations in the gastric and intestinal epithelium and neurologic abnormalities such as peripheral neuropathy and spinal cord damage.

Clinical Features

The disease has insidious onset and progresses slowly. The clinical manifestations are mainly due to vitamin B_{12} deficiency. These include: anaemia, glossitis, neurological abnormalities (neuropathy, subacute combined degeneration of the spinal cord, retrobulbar neuritis), gastrointestinal manifestations (diarrhoea, anorexia, weight loss, dyspepsia), hepatosplenomegaly, congestive heart failure and haemorrhagic manifestations.

Laboratory Findings

Laboratory examination of a case of PA reveals the following abnormalities:

1. *Hypergastrinaemia*
2. *Pentagastrinaemia*
3. *Haematologic findings* in blood and bone marrow are similar to those seen in megaloblastic anaemia discussed above.
4. *Biochemical alterations* reveal rise in serum bilirubin, LDH, haptoglobin, ferritin and iron. Serum folate is usually normal but red cell folate is almost always reduced.
5. *Schilling test* is abnormal due to IF deficiency as observed by low 24-hour urinary excretion of labelled vitamin B_{12} (page 383).
6. *Chromosomal abnormalities* are frequently present in bone marrow cells which disappear after therapy.

Treatment

Patients of PA are treated with vitamin B_{12} in the following way:

1. Replacement therapy with vitamin B_{12}.
2. Symptomatic and supportive therapy such as physiotherapy for neurologic deficits and occasionally blood transfusion.
3. Follow-up for early detection of cancer of the stomach.

Most of the abnormalities due to vitamin B_{12} deficiency can be corrected except the irreversible damage to the spinal cord. Corticosteroid therapy can improve the gastric lesion with a return of acid secretion but the higher incidence of gastric polyps and cancer of the stomach in these patients can only be detected by frequent follow-up.

HAEMOLYTIC ANAEMIAS

GENERAL ASPECTS

Definition and Classification

Haemolytic anaemias are defined as anaemias resulting from an increase in the rate of red cell destruction. Normally, effete red cells undergo lysis at the end of their life-span of 90-120 days within the cells of reticuloendothelial (RE) system in the spleen and elsewhere (extravascular haemolysis), and haemoglobin is not liberated into the plasma in appreciable amounts. The red cell life-span is shortened in haemolytic anaemia i.e. there is accelerated haemolysis. However, shortening of red cell life-span does not necessarily result in anaemia. In fact, compensatory bone marrow hyperplasia may cause 6-8-fold increase in red cell production without causing anaemia to the patient, so-called *compensated haemolytic disease.*

The premature destruction of red cells in haemolytic anaemia may occur by 2 mechanisms:

- **Firstly,** the red cells undergo lysis in the circulation and release their contents into plasma *(intravascular haemolysis).* In these cases the plasma haemoglobin rises substantially and part of it may be excreted in the urine *(haemoglobinuria).*
- **Secondly,** the red cells are taken up by cells of the RE system where they are destroyed and digested *(extravascular haemolysis).* In extravascular haemolysis, plasma haemoglobin level is, therefore, barely raised.

Extravascular haemolysis is more common than the former. One or more factors may be involved in the pathogenesis of various haemolytic anaemias.

Haemolytic anaemias are broadly classified into 2 main categories:

I. *Acquired haemolytic anaemias* caused by a variety of extrinsic environmental factors *(extracorpuscular).*

II. *Hereditary haemolytic anaemias* are usually the result of intrinsic red cell defects *(intracorpuscular).*

A simplified classification based on these mechanisms is given in Table 13.10 and diagrammatically represented in Fig. 13.16.

Features of Haemolysis

A number of clinical and laboratory features are shared by various types of haemolytic anaemias. These are briefly described below:

GENERAL CLINICAL FEATURES. Some of the general clinical features common to most congenital and acquired haemolytic anaemias are as under:

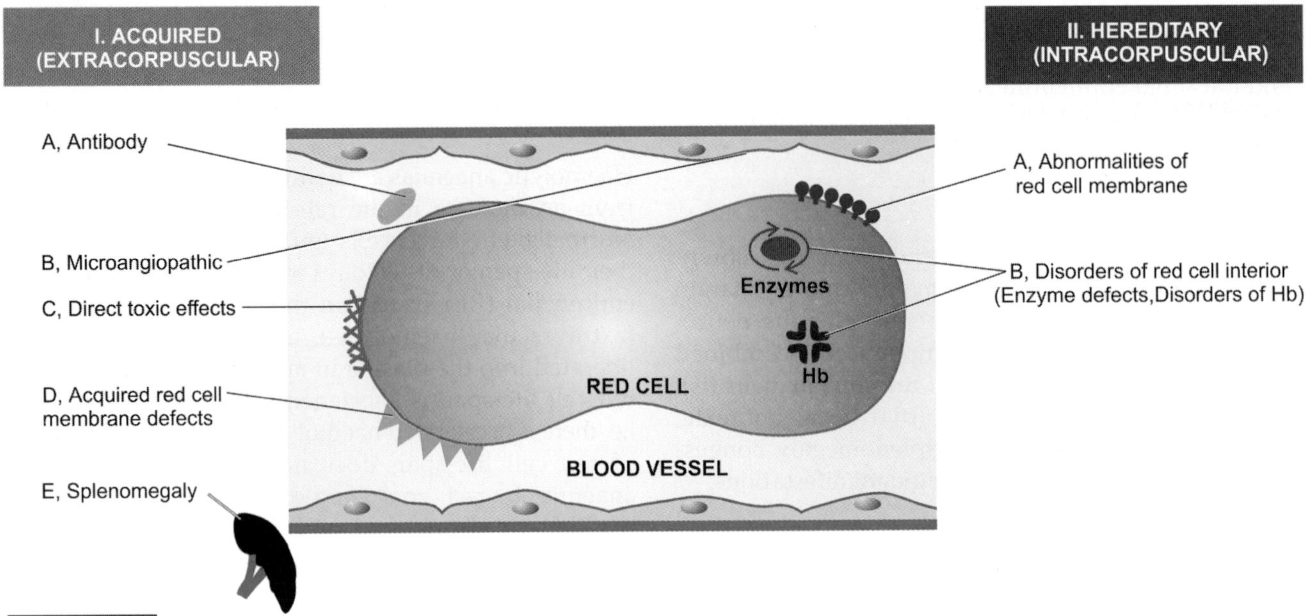

FIGURE 13.16

Diagrammatic representation of classification of haemolytic anaemias based on principal mechanisms of haemolysis.

1. Presence of pallor of mucous membranes.
2. Positive family history with life-long anaemia in patients with congenital haemolytic anaemia.
3. Mild fluctuating jaundice due to unconjugated hyperbilirubinaemia.
4. Urine turns dark on standing due to excess of urobilinogen in urine.
5. Splenomegaly is found in most chronic haemolytic anaemias, both congenital and acquired.
6. Pigment gallstones are found in some cases.

LABORATORY EVALUATION OF HAEMOLYSIS. The pathways by which haemoglobin derived from effete red cells is metabolised is already discussed on page 369. The investigations of a patient suspected to have haemolytic anaemia should provide answers to 3 vital questions:

1. Is there evidence of haemolysis?
2. What is the type of haemolytic mechanism?
3. What is the precise diagnosis?

And, if facilities are available, certain tests of scientific nature which are not normally required for making the diagnosis or predicting prognosis, may be carried out.

The laboratory findings are conveniently divided into the following 3 groups:

I. Tests of increased red cell breakdown. These include the following:

1. *Serum bilirubin*—unconjugated (indirect) bilirubin is raised.
2. *Urine urobilinogen* is raised but there is no bilirubinuria.
3. *Faecal stercobilinogen* is raised.
4. *Serum haptoglobin* (α-globulin binding protein) is reduced or absent.
5. *Plasma lactic dehydrogenase* is raised.
6. *Evidences of intravascular haemolysis* in the form of haemoglobinaemia, haemoglobinuria, methaemoglobinaemia and haemosiderinuria.

II. Tests of increased red cell production. These are as under:

1. *Reticulocyte count* reveals reticulocytosis which is generally early and is hence most useful initial test of marrow erythroid hyperplasia.
2. *Routine blood film* shows macrocytosis, polychromasia and presence of normoblasts.
3. *Bone marrow* shows erythroid hyperplasia with usually raised iron stores.
4. *X-ray of bones* shows evidence of expansion of marrow space, especially in tubular bones and skull.

III. Tests of damage to red cells. These include the following:

1. *Routine blood film* shows a variety of abnormal morphological appearances of red cells described on page 366 and illustrated in Fig. 13.9 already. A summary of contribution of morphology of RBCs in arriving at the diagnosis of haemolytic anaemia and its cause is given in Table 13.11.

TABLE 13.10: Classification of Haemolytic Anaemias.

I. ACQUIRED (EXTRACORPUSCULAR)

A. Antibody: Immunohaemolytic anaemias
1. Autoimmune haemolytic anaemia (AIHA)
   i) Warm antibody AIHA
   ii) Cold antibody AIHA
2. Drug-induced immunohaemolytic anaemia
3. Isoimmune haemolytic anaemia (page 440)

B. Mechanical trauma: Microangiopathic haemolytic anaemia

C. Direct toxic effects: Malaria, bacteria, infection and other agents

D. Acquired red cell membrane abnormalities: paroxysmal nocturnal haemoglobinuria (PNH)

E. Splenomegaly

II. HEREDITARY (INTRACORPUSCULAR)

A. Abnormalities of red cell membrane
1. Hereditary spherocytosis
2. Hereditary elliptocytosis (hereditary ovalocytosis)
3. Hereditary stomatocytosis

B. Disorders of red cell interior
1. *Red cell enzyme defects*
   i) Defects in the hexose monophosphate shunt: G6PD deficiency
   ii) Defects in the Embden-Meyerhof (or glycolytic) pathway: pyruvate kinase deficiency
2. *Disorders of haemoglobin*
   i) Structurally abnormal haemoglobins (haemoglobinopathies): sickle syndromes, other haemoglobinopathies
   ii) Reduced globin chain synthesis: thalassaemias

2. *Osmotic fragility* is increased.
3. *Autohaemolysis test* with or without addition of glucose.
4. *Coombs' antiglobulin test.*
5. *Electrophoresis* for abnormal haemoglobins.
6. *Estimation of HbA_2.*
7. *Estimation of HbF.*
8. *Tests for sickling.*
9. *Screening test for G6PD deficiency* and other enzymes (e.g. Heinz bodies test).

IV. Tests for shortened red cell life-span. A shortened red cell survival is best tested by ^{51}Cr labelling method. Normal RBC life-span of 120 days is shortened to 20-40 days in moderate haemolysis and to 5-20 days in severe haemolysis.

I. ACQUIRED (EXTRACORPUSCULAR) HAEMOLYTIC ANAEMIAS

Acquired haemolytic anaemias are caused by a variety of extrinsic factors, namely: antibody (immunohaemolytic anaemia), mechanical factors (microangiopathic haemolytic anaemia), direct toxic effect (in malaria, clostridial infection etc), splenomegaly, and certain acquired membrane abnormalities (paroxysmal nocturnal haemoglobinuria). These are discussed below:

A. IMMUNOHAEMOLYTIC ANAEMIAS

Immunohaemolytic anaemias are a group of anaemias occurring due to antibody production by the body against its own red cells. Immune haemolysis in these cases may be induced by one of the following three types of antibodies:

1. *Autoimmune haemolytic anaemia (AIHA)* characterised by formation of autoantibodies against patient's own red cells. Depending upon the reactivity of autoantibody, AIHA is further divided into 2 types:

i) 'Warm' antibody AIHA in which the autoantibodies are reactive at body temperature (37°C).

ii) 'Cold' antibody AIHA in which the autoantibodies react better with patient's own red cells at 4°C.

2. *Drug-induced immunohaemolytic anaemia.*

TABLE 13.11: Red Cell Morphologic Features in Various Types of Haemolytic Anaemias.

FEATURE	ETIOLOGY	TYPE OF HAEMOLYTIC ANAEMIA
1. *Spherocytes*	Loss of spectrin from membrane	Hereditary spherocytosis AIHA
2. *Target cells (Leptocytes)*	Increased ratio of surface area: volume	Thalassaemias Liver disease HbS disease HbC disease
3. *Schistocytes*	Traumatic damage to red cell membrane	Microangiopathy
4. *Sickle cells*	Polymerisation of HbS	Sickle syndromes
5. *Acanthocytes (Spur cells)*	Abnormality in membrane lipids	Severe liver disease
6. *Heinz bodies*	Precipitated Hb	Unstable Hb

Chapter Thirteen

3. *Isoimmune haemolytic anaemia* in which the antibodies are acquired by blood transfusions, pregnancies and haemolytic disease of the newborn.

An important diagnostic tool in all cases of immunohaemolytic anaemias is Coombs' antiglobulin test for detection of incomplete Rh-antibodies in saline directly (direct Coombs') or after addition of albumin (indirect Coombs').

Autoimmune Haemolytic Anaemia (AIHA)

'WARM' ANTIBODY AIHA

PATHOGENESIS. Warm antibodies reactive at body temperature and coating the red cells are generally IgG class antibodies and occasionally they are IgA. Little is known about the origin of these acquired red blood cell antibodies in AIHA but the mechanism of destruction of red cells coated with IgG is better understood. Human red cells coated with IgG antibodies are bound to the surface of RE cells, especially splenic macrophages. A part of the coated cell membrane is lost resulting in spherical transformation of the red cells (acquired spherocytosis). Red cells coated with IgG alongwith C3 on the surface further promote this red cell-leucocyte interaction, accounting for more severe haemolysis. The spleen is particularly efficient in trapping red cells coated with IgG antibodies. It is, thus, the major site of red cell destruction in warm antibody AIHA.

CLINICAL FEATURES. Warm antibody AIHA may occur at any age and in either sex. The disease may occur without any apparent cause (idiopathic) but about a quarter of patients develop this disorder as a complication of an underlying disease affecting the immune system, especially SLE, chronic lymphocytic leukaemia, lymphomas and certain drugs such as methyl DOPA, penicillin etc (Table 13.12).

TABLE 13.12: Conditions Predisposing to Autoimmune Haemolytic Anaemia (AIHA).

A. *Warm antibody AIHA*
   1. Idiopathic (primary)
   2. Lymphomas-leukaemias e.g. non-Hodgkin's lymphoma, CLL, Hodgkin's disease.
   3. Collagen vascular diseases e.g SLE
   4. Drugs e.g. methyl dopa, penicillin, quinidine group
   5. Post-viral

B. *Cold antibody AIHA*
   1. Cold agglutinin disease
      a) Acute: *Mycoplasma* infection, infectious mononucleosis
      b) Chronic: Idiopathic, lymphomas
   2. PCH (*Mycoplasma* infection, viral flu, measles, mumps, syphilis)

The disease tends to have remissions and relapses. The usual clinical features are:

1. Chronic anaemia of varying severity with remissions and relapses.
2. Splenomegaly.
3. Occasionally hyperbilirubinaemia.

Treatment of these cases consists of removal of the cause whenever present, corticosteroid therapy, and in severe cases blood transfusions. Splenectomy is the second line of therapy in this disorder.

LABORATORY FINDINGS. The haematological and biochemical findings in such cases are as under:

1. Mild to moderate chronic anaemia.
2. Reticulocytosis.
3. Prominent spherocytosis in the peripheral blood film.
4. Positive direct Coombs' (antiglobulin) test for presence of warm antibodies on the red cell, best detected at 37°C.
5. A positive indirect Coombs' (antiglobulin) test at 37°C may indicate presence of large quantities of warm antibodies in the serum.
6. Unconjugated (indirect) hyperbilirubinaemia.
7. Co-existent immune thrombocytopenia alongwith occasional venous thrombosis may be present (termed Evans' syndrome).
8. In more severe cases, haemoglobinaemia and haemoglobinuria may be present.

'COLD' ANTIBODY AIHA

PATHOGENESIS. Antibodies which are reactive in the cold (4°C) may induce haemolysis under 2 conditions: cold agglutinin disease and paroxysmal cold haemoglobinuria.

1. Cold agglutinin disease. In cold agglutinin disease, the antibodies are IgM type which bind to the red cells best at 4°C. These cold antibodies are usually directed against the *I* antigen on the red cell surface. Agglutination of red blood cells by IgM cold agglutinins is most profound at very low temperature but upon warming to 37°C or above, disagglutination occurs quickly. Haemolytic effect is mediated through fixation of C3 to the red blood cell surface and not by agglutination alone. Most cold agglutinins affect juvenile red blood cells.

The etiology of cold antibody remains unknown. It is seen in the course of certain infections (e.g. *Mycoplasma* pneumonia, infectious mononucleosis) and in lymphomas.

Chapter Thirteen

2. Paroxysmal cold haemoglobinuria (PCH). In PCH, the cold antibody is an IgG antibody (Donath-Landsteiner antibody) which is directed against *P* blood group antigen and brings about complement-mediated haemolysis. Attacks of PCH are precipitated by exposure to cold.

PCH is uncommon and may be seen in association with tertiary syphilis or as a complication of certain infections such as *Mycoplasma* pneumonia, flu, measles and mumps.

CLINICAL FEATURES. The clinical manifestations are due to haemolysis and not due to agglutination. These include:

1. Chronic anaemia which is worsened by exposure to cold.
2. Raynaud's phenomenon.
3. Cyanosis affecting the cold exposed regions such as tips of nose, ears, fingers and toes.
4. Haemoglobinaemia and haemoglobinuria occur on exposure to cold.

Treatment consists of keeping the patient warm and treating the underlying cause.

LABORATORY FINDINGS. The haematologic and biochemical findings are somewhat similar to those found in warm antibody AIHA except the thermal amplitude. These findings are:

1. Chronic anaemia.
2. Low reticulocyte count since young red cells are affected more.
3. Spherocytosis is less marked.
4. Positive direct Coombs' test for detection of C3 on the red cell surface but IgM responsible for C3 coating on red cells is not found.
5. The cold antibody titre is very high at 4°C and very low at 37°C (Donath-Landsteiner test). IgM class cold antibody has specificity for *I* antigen, while the rare IgG class antibody of PCH has *P* blood group antigen specificity.

Drug-induced Immunohaemolytic Anaemia

Drugs may cause immunohaemolytic anaemia by 3 different mechanisms:

1. α-METHYL DOPA TYPE ANTIBODIES. A small proportion of patients receiving α-methyl dopa develops immunohaemolytic anaemia which is identical in every respect to warm antibody AIHA described above.

2. PENICILLIN-INDUCED IMMUNOHAEMOLYSIS. Patients receiving large doses of penicillin or penicillin-type antibiotics develop antibodies against the red blood cell-drug complex which induces haemolysis.

3. INNOCENT BYSTANDER IMMUNOHAEMOLYSIS. Drugs such as quinidine form a complex with plasma proteins to which an antibody forms. This drug-plasma protein-antibody complex may induce lysis of bystanding red blood cells or platelets.

In each type of drug-induced immunohaemolytic anaemia, discontinuation of the drug results in gradual disappearance of haemolysis.

Isoimmune Haemolytic Anaemia

Isoimmune haemolytic anaemias are caused by acquiring isoantibodies or alloantibodies by blood transfusions, pregnancies and in haemolytic disease of the newborn. These antibodies produced by one individual are directed against red blood cells of the other. These conditions are considered on page 440.

B. MICROANGIOPATHIC HAEMOLYTIC ANAEMIA

Microangiopathic haemolytic anaemia is caused by abnormalities in the microvasculature. It is generally due to mechanical trauma to the red cells in circulation and is characterised by red cell fragmentation (schistocytosis). There are 3 different ways by which microangiopathic haemolytic anaemia results:

1. EXTERNAL IMPACT. Direct external trauma to red blood cells when they pass through microcirculation, especially over the bony prominences, may cause haemolysis during various activities e.g. in prolonged marchers, joggers, karate players etc. These patients develop haemoglobinaemia, haemoglobinuria *(march haemoglobinuria),* and sometimes myoglobinuria as a result of damage to muscles.

2. CARDIAC HAEMOLYSIS. A small proportion of patients who received prosthetic cardiac valves or artificial grafts develop haemolysis. This has been attributed to direct mechanical trauma to the red cells or shear stress from turbulent blood flow.

3. FIBRIN DEPOSIT IN MICROVASCULATURE. Deposition of fibrin in the microvasculature exposes the red cells to physical obstruction and eventual fragmentation of red cells and trapping of the platelets. Fibrin deposits in the small vessels may occur in the following conditions:

i) *Abnormalities of the vessel wall* e.g. in hypertension, eclampsia, disseminated cancers, transplant rejection, haemangioma etc.

ii) *Thrombotic thrombocytopenic purpura.*

iii) *Haemolytic-uraemic syndrome.*
iv) *Disseminated intravascular coagulation* (DIC)
v) Vasculitis in *collagen diseases.*

All these conditions are described in respective sections separately.

C. HAEMOLYTIC ANAEMIA FROM DIRECT TOXIC EFFECTS

Haemolysis may result from direct toxic effects of certain agents. These include the following examples:

1. *Malaria* by direct parasitisation of red cells (blackwater fever) **(COLOUR PLATE XVII: CL 68).**
2. *Bartonellosis* by direct infection of red cells by the microorganisms.
3. *Septicaemia* with *Clostridium welchii* by damaging the red cells.
4. *Other microorganisms* such as pneumococci, staphylococci and *Escherichia coli.*
5. *Copper* by direct haemolytic effect on red cells in Wilson's disease and patients on haemodialysis.
6. *Lead poisoning* shows basophilic stippling of red blood cells.
7. *Snake and spider bites* cause haemolysis by their venoms.
8. *Extensive burns.*

D. PAROXYSMAL NOCTURNAL HAEMOGLOBINURIA (PNH)

PNH is a rare acquired disorder of red cell membrane in which there is chronic intravascular haemolysis due to undue sensitivity of red blood cells to complement due to defective synthesis of a red cell membrane protein. The defect affects all the cells of myeloid progenitor lineage (RBCs, WBCs, platelets) suggesting a deficient haematopoiesis. The disorder generally presents in adult life.

PATHOGENESIS. PNH is considered as an acquired clonal disease of the cell membrane while normal clone also continues to proliferate. The defect in stem cells is a mutation affecting myeloid progenitor cells that normally is required for the biosynthesis of glycosyl phosphatidyl inositol (GPI) essential for anchoring of the cell; the mutant form of the gene is called PIG-A (phosphatidyl inositol glycan). Thus, as a result of mutation, there is partial or complete deficiency of anchor protein. Out of about 20 such proteins described so far, the lack of two of the proteins—*decay accelerating factor (DAF, CD55)* and a *membrane inhibitor of reactive lysis (MIRL, CD59)*, makes the RBCs sensitive to the lytic effect of complement.

CLINICAL AND LABORATORY FINDINGS. Clinical and laboratory findings are as under:

i) Haemolytic anaemia.
ii) Pancytopenia (mild granulocytopenia and thrombocytopenia frequent).
iii) Intermittent clinical haemoglobinuria; acute haemolytic episodes occur at night identified by passage of brown urine in the morning.
iv) Haemosiderinuria very common.
v) Venous thrombosis common complication.

The presence of inordinate sensitivity of red blood cells, leucocytes and platelets to complement in PNH can be demonstrated *in vitro* by *Ham's test* using red cell lysis at acidic pH or by sucrose haemolysis test.

About 20% cases of PNH may develop myeloproliferative or myelodysplastic disorder and some even develop acute myeloid leukaemia.

E. HAEMOLYTIC ANAEMIA IN SPLENOMEGALY

Haemolytic anaemia is common in splenic enlargement from any cause (Chapter 14). Normally, the spleen acts as a filter and traps the damaged red blood cells, destroys them and the splenic macrophages phagocytose the damaged red cells. A normal spleen poses no risk to normal red blood cells. But splenomegaly exaggerates the damaging effect to which the red cells are exposed. Besides haemolytic anaemia, splenomegaly is usually associated with pancytopenia. Splenectomy or reduction in size of spleen by appropriate therapy relieves the anaemia as well as improves the leucocyte and platelet counts.

II. HEREDITARY (INTRACORPUSCULAR) HAEMOLYTIC ANAEMIA

Hereditary haemolytic anaemias are usually the result of intracorpuscular defects. Accordingly, they are broadly classified into 2 groups (see Table 13.10):

- Those due to hereditary abnormalities of red cell membrane.
- Second are those with hereditay disorders of the interior of the red cells.

A. HEREDITARY ABNORMALITIES OF RED CELL MEMBRANE

The abnormalities of red cell membrane are readily identified on blood film examination. There are 3 important types of inherited red cell membrane defects: hereditary spherocytosis, hereditary elliptocytosis (hereditary ovalocytosis) and hereditary stomatocytosis.

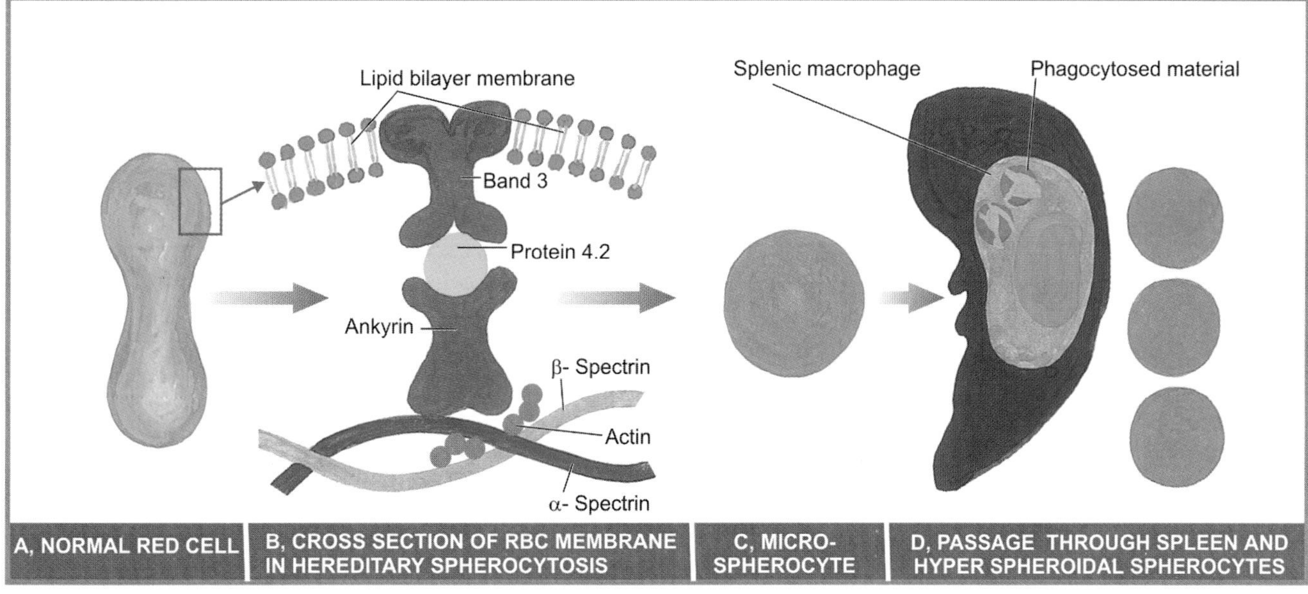

FIGURE 13.17

Diagrammatic representation of pathogenesis of hereditary spherocytosis. A, Normal red cell with biconcave surface and normal size. B, Red cell membrane as seen in cross section in hereditary spherocytosis. Mutations in membrane proteins—α-spectrin, β-spectrin and ankyrin, result in defect in anchoring of lipid bilayer of the membrane to the underlying cytoskeleton. C, This results in spherical contour and small size so as to contain the given volume of haemoglobin in the deformed red cell. D, During passage through the spleen, these rigid spherical cells lose their cell membrane further. This produces a circulating subpopulation of hyperspheroidal spherocytes while splenic macrophages in large numbers phagocytose defective red cells causing splenomegaly.

Hereditary Spherocytosis

Hereditary spherocytosis is a common type of hereditary haemolytic anaemia of autosomal dominant inheritance in which the red cell membrane is abnormal.

PATHOGENESIS. The molecular abnormality in hereditary spherocytosis is a defect in proteins which anchor the lipid bilayer to the underlying cytoskeleton. These protein abnormalities are as under and are schematically illustrated in Fig. 13.17:

1. **Spectrin deficiency.** Almost all cases have deficiency in the structural protein of the red cell membrane, spectrin. Spectrin deficiency correlates with the severity of anaemia. Mutation in spectrin by recessive inheritance called *α–spectrin* causes more severe form of anaemia, while mutation by dominant inheritance forming *β-spectrin* results in mild form of the disease.

2. **Ankyrin abnormality.** About half the cases of hereditary spherocytosis have defect in ankyrin, protein that binds protein 3 and spectrin. Homozygous state with recessive inheritance pattern have severe anaemia while heterozygotes with more common dominant inheritance pattern have milder anaemia.

Inherited mutation in spectrin or ankyrin causes defect in anchoring of lipid bilayer cell membrane. Red cells with such unstable membrane but with normal volume, when released in circulation, lose their membrane further, till they can accommodate the given volume. This results in formation of spheroidal contour and smaller size of red blood cells, termed *microspherocytes*. These deformed red cells are not flexible, unlike normal biconcave red cells. These rigid cells are unable to pass through the spleen, and in the process they lose their surface membrane further. This produces a subpopulation of *hyperspheroidal red cells* in the peripheral blood which are subsequently destroyed in the spleen.

CLINICAL FEATURES. The disorder may be clinically apparent at any age from infancy to old age and has equal sex incidence. The family history may be present. The major clinical features are as under:

1. *Anaemia* is usually mild to moderate.
2. *Splenomegaly* is a constant feature.
3. *Jaundice* occurs due to increased concentration of unconjugated (indirect) bilirubin in the plasma (also termed congenital haemolytic jaundice).

4. *Pigment gallstones* are frequent due to increased bile pigment production. Splenectomy offers the only reliable mode of treatment.

LABORATORY FINDINGS. The usual haematological and biochemical findings are as under (Fig. 13.18):

1. *Anaemia* of mild to moderate degree.
2. *Reticulocytosis,* usually 5-20%.
3. Blood film shows the characteristic abnormality of erythrocytes in the form of *microspherocytes.*
4. MCV is usually normal or slightly decreased but *MCHC* is increased.
5. Osmotic fragility test is helpful in testing the spheroidal nature of red cells which lyse more readily in solutions of low salt concentration i.e. *osmotic fragility is increased.*
6. *Autohaemolysis test* is similar to osmotic fragility test after incubation and shows increased spontaneous autohaemolysis (10-15% red cells) as compared to normal red cells (less than 4%). Autohaemolysis is correctable by addition of glucose.
7. *Direct Coombs' (antiglobulin) test* is negative so as to distinguish this condition from acquired spherocytosis of AIHA in which case it is positive.

Spherocytes may also be seen in blood film in acquired immune haemolytic anaemia and following red cell transfusion.

Hereditary Elliptocytosis (Hereditary Ovalocytosis)

Hereditary elliptocytosis or hereditary ovalocytosis is another autosomal dominant disorder involving red cell membrane protein *spectrin.* Some patients have an inherited defect in erythrocyte membrane protein 4.1 that interconnects spectrin with actin in the cytoskeleton. The disorder is similar in all respects to hereditary spherocytosis except that the blood film shows oval or elliptical red cells and is clinically a milder disorder than hereditary spherocytosis.

Acquired causes of elliptocytosis include iron deficiency and myeloproliferative disorders.

Hereditary Stomatocytosis

Stomatocytes are cup-shaped RBCs having one surface concave and the other side as convex. This causes a central slit-like or mouth-like appearance of red cells. The underlying defect is in membrane protein, *stomatin,* having autosomal dominant pattern of inheritance. The stomatocytes are swollen red cells (overhydrated red cells) due to increased permeability to sodium and potassium. The affected patients have mild anaemia and splenomegaly.

B. HEREDITARY DISORDERS OF RED CELL INTERIOR

Inherited disorders involving the interior of the red blood cells are classified into 2 groups:

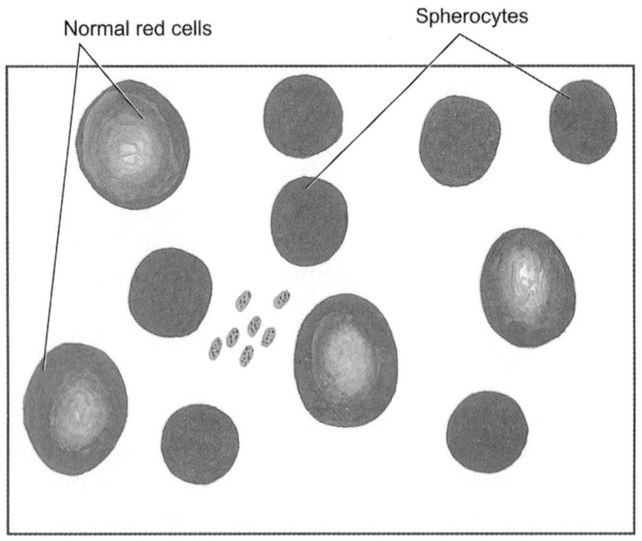

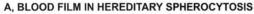

A, BLOOD FILM IN HEREDITARY SPHEROCYTOSIS

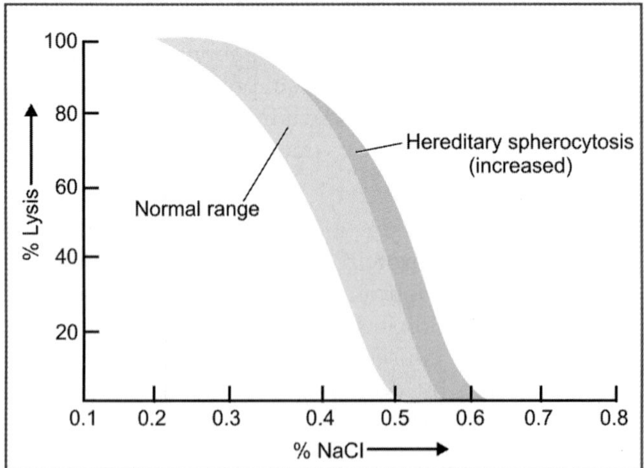

B, OSMOTIC FRAGILITY CURVE

FIGURE 13.18

Hereditary spherocytosis. A, Findings in peripheral blood film. B, Osmotic fragility test showing increased fragility.

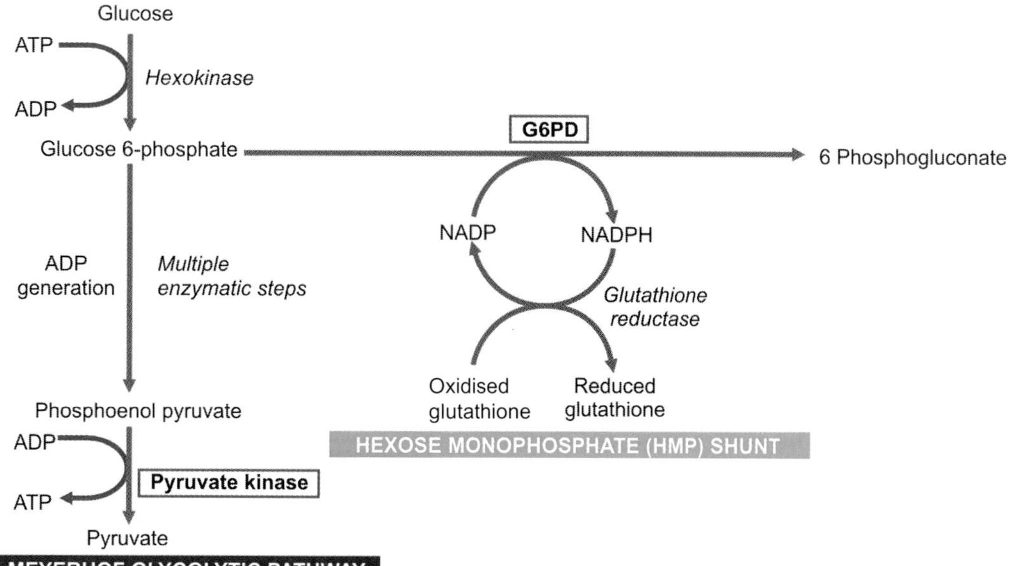

FIGURE 13.19

Abbreviated pathways of anaerobic glycolysis (Embden-Meyerhof) and hexose monophosphate (HMP) shunt in the metabolism of erythrocyte. The two red cell enzyme defects, glucose-6 phosphate dehydrogenase (G6PD) and pyruvate kinase, are shown bold.

1. Red cell enzyme defects: These cause defective red cell metabolism involving 2 pathways (Fig. 13.19):

i) *Defects in the hexose monophosphate shunt:* Common example is glucose-6-phosphate dehydrogenase (G6PD) deficiency.

ii) *Defects in the Embden-Meyerhof (glycolytic) pathway:* Example is pyruvate kinase (PK) deficiency.

2. Disorders of haemoglobin: These are divided into 2 subgroups:

i) *Abnormal haemoglobins (haemoglobinopathies):* Examples are sickle syndromes and other haemoglobinopathies.

ii) *Reduced globin chain synthesis:* Common examples are various types of thalassaemias.

These disorders are discussed below.

Red Cell Enzyme Defects

G6PD DEFICIENCY

Among the defects in hexose monophosphate shunt, the most common is G6PD deficiency. It affects millions of people throughout the world. The G6PD gene is located on the X chromosome and its deficiency is, therefore, a sex (X)-linked trait affecting males, while the females are carriers and are asymptomatic. Several variants of G6PD have been described. The normal G6PD variant is designated as type B but blacks have normally A+ (positive) type G6PD variant. The most common and significant clinical variant is A–(negative) type found in black males. Like the HbS gene, the A– type G6PD variant confers protection against malaria. Individuals with A–G6PD variant have shortened red cell life-span but without anaemia. However, these individuals develop haemolytic episodes on exposure to oxidant stress such as viral and bacterial infections, certain drugs (antimalarials, sulfonamides, nitrofurantoin, aspirin, vitamin K), metabolic acidosis and on ingestion of fava beans (favism).

PATHOGENESIS. Normally, the red blood cells are well protected against oxidant stress because of adequate generation of reduced glutathione via the hexose monophosphate shunt (Fig. 13.19). Individuals with inherited deficiency of G6PD, an enzyme required for hexose monophosphate shunt for glucose metabolism, fail to develop adequate levels of reduced glutathione in their red cells. This results in oxidation and precipitation of haemoglobin within the red cells forming Heinz bodies. Besides G6PD deficiency, deficiency of various other enzymes involved in the hexose monophosphate shunt may also infrequently cause clinical problems.

CLINICAL FEATURES. The clinical manifestations are those of an acute haemolytic anaemia within hours of exposure to oxidant stress. The haemolysis is, however, self-limiting even if the exposure to the oxidant is continued since it affects the older red cells only. Haemoglobin level may return to normal when the older population of red cells has been destroyed and only younger cells remain. Some patients may have only darkening of the urine from haemoglobinuria but more severely affected ones develop constitutional symptoms including jaundice. Treatment is directed towards the prevention of haemolytic episodes such as stoppage of offending drug. Blood transfusions are rarely indicated.

LABORATORY FINDINGS. These are as under:

1. During the period of acute haemolysis, there is rapid fall in haematocrit by 25-30%, features of intravascular haemolysis such as rise in plasma haemoglobin, haemoglobinuria, rise in unconjugated bilirubin and fall in plasma haptoglobin. Formation of Heinz bodies is visualised by means of supravital stains such as crystal violet, also called *Heinz body haemolytic anaemia.* However, Heinz bodies are not seen after the first one or two days since they are removed by the spleen, leading to the formation of 'bite cells' and fragmented red cells.

2. Between the crises, the affected patient generally has no anaemia. The red cell survival is, however, shortened.

The diagnosis of G6PD enzyme deficiency is made by one of the screening tests (e.g. methaemoglobin reduction test, fluorescent screening test, ascorbate cyanide screening test), or by direct enzyme assay on red cells.

PK DEFICIENCY

Pyruvate kinase (PK) deficiency is the only significant enzymopathy of the Embden-Meyerhof glycolytic pathway (Fig. 13.19). The disorder is inherited as an autosomal recessive pattern. Heterozygote state is entirely asymptomatic, while the homozygous individual presents during early childhood with anaemia, jaundice and splenomegaly.

LABORATORY FINDINGS: These are:

1. Normocytic and normochromic anaemia.
2. Reticulocytosis.
3. Blood film shows bizarre red cells.
4. Osmotic fragility is usually normal but after incubation it is increased.
5. Autohaemolysis is increased, but unlike hereditary spherocytosis, is not corrected by addition of glucose.
6. Direct specific enzyme assay on red cells is the only method of establishing the diagnosis.

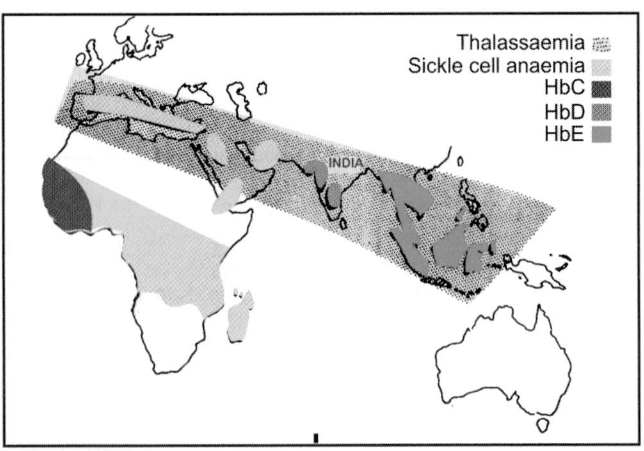

FIGURE 13.20

The geographic distribution of major haemoglobinopathies and thalassaemias. Thalassaemia and HbD are the haemoglobin disorders common in India.

Disorders of Haemoglobin

There are geographic variations in the distribution of various disorders of haemoglobin as shown in Fig. 13.20. These disorders are described below under 2 main headings: abnormal haemoglobins (haemoglobinopathies) and thalassaemias.

ABNORMAL HAEMOGLOBINS (HAEMOGLOBINOPATHIES)

SICKLE SYNDROMES

The most important and widely prevalent type of haemoglobinopathy is due to the presence of sickle haemoglobin (HbS) in the red blood cells. The red cells with HbS develop 'sickling' when they are exposed to low oxygen tension. Sickle syndromes have the highest frequency in black race and in Central Africa where *falciparum* malaria is endemic. Patients with HbS are relatively protected against *falciparum* malaria. Sickle syndromes occur in 3 different forms:

1. *As heterozygous state* for HbS: sickle cell trait (AS).
2. *As homozygous state* for HbS: sickle cell anaemia (SS).
3. *As double heterozygous states* e.g. sickle β-thalassaemia, sickle-C disease (SC), sickle-D disease (SD).

Heterozygous State: Sickle Cell Trait

Sickle cell trait is a benign heterozygous state of HbS in which only one abnormal gene is inherited. Patients with AS develop no significant clinical problems except when they become severely hypoxic and may develop sickle cell crises.

LABORATORY FINDINGS. These patients have no anaemia and have normal appearance of red cells. But in hypoxic crisis, sickle cell crises develop. The diagnosis is made by 2 tests:

1. *Demonstration of sickling* done under condition of reduced oxygen tension by an oxygen consuming reagent, sodium metabisulfite.
2. *Haemoglobin electrophoresis* reveals 35-40% of the total haemoglobin as HbS.

Homozygous State: Sickle Cell Anaemia

Sickle cell anaemia (SS) is a homozygous state of HbS in the red cells in which an abnormal gene is inherited from each parent. SS is a severely malignant disorder associated with protean clinical manifestations and decreased life expectancy.

PATHOGENESIS. Following abnormalities are observed (Fig. 13.21):

1. Basic molecular lesion: In HbS, basic genetic defect is the *single point mutation* in one amino acid out of 146 in haemoglobin molecule; there is *substitution of valine for glutamic acid* at the 6 residue position of the β-globin, producing Hb $\alpha_2\beta_2^s$.

2. Mechanism of sickling: During deoxygenation, the red cells containing HbS change from biconcave disc shape to an elongated crescent-shaped or sickle-shaped cell. This process termed *sickling* occurs both within the intact red cells and *in vitro* in free solution. The mechanism responsible for sickling upon deoxygenation of HbS-containing red cells is the polymerisation of deoxygenated HbS which aggregates to form elongated rod-like polymers. These elongated fibres align and distort the red cell into classic sickle shape.

3. Reversible-irreversible sickling: The oxygen-dependent sickling process is usually reversible. However, damage to red cell membrane leads to formation of irreversibly sickled red cells even after they are exposed to normal oxygen tension.

4. Factors determining rate of sickling: The following factors determine the rate at which the polymerisation of HbS and consequent sickling take place:

i) *Presence of non-HbS haemoglobins:* The red cells in patients of SS have predominance of HbS and a small part consists of non-HbS haemoglobins, chiefly HbF (2-20% of the total haemoglobin). HbF-containing red cells are protected from sickling while HbA-containing red cells participate readily in co-polymerisation with HbS.

ii) *Intracellular concentration of HbS.*

iii) *Total haemoglobin concentration.*

iv) *Extent of deoxygenation.*

v) *Acidosis and dehydration.*

vi) *Increased concentration of 2, 3-BPG in the red cells.*

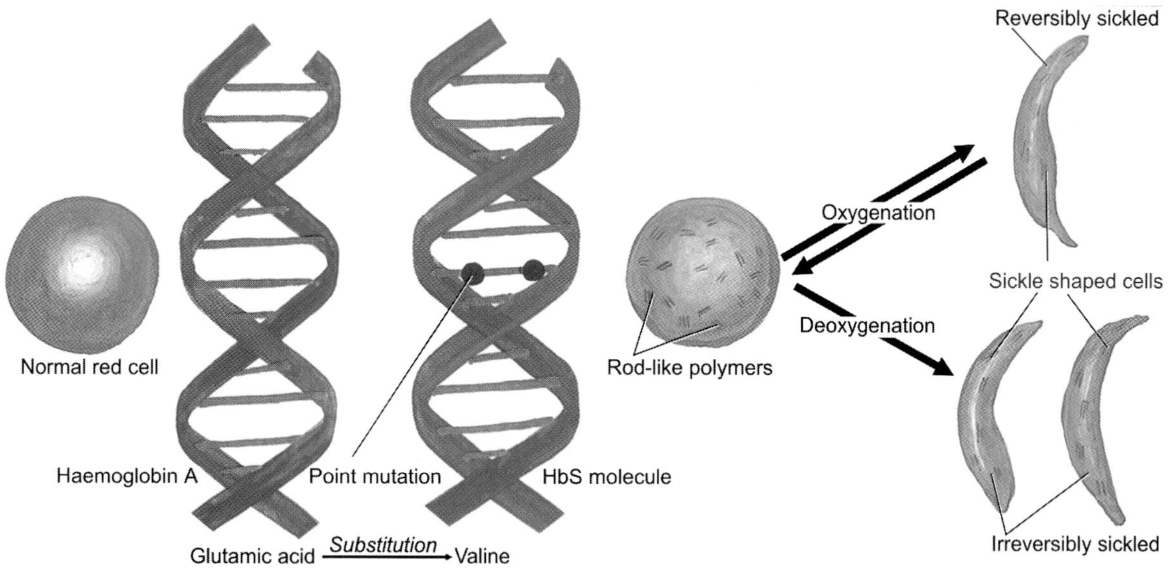

FIGURE 13.21

Pathogenesis of sickle cell anaemia. A, Basic molecular defect. B, Mechanism of polymerisation and consequent sickling of red cells containing HbS. C, Mechanism of sickling on oxygenation-deoxygenation.

CLINICAL FEATURES. The clinical manifestations of homozygous sickle cell disease are widespread. The symptoms begin to appear after 6th month of life when most of the HbF is replaced by HbS. Infection and folic acid deficiency result in more severe clinical manifestations. These features are as under:

1. **Anaemia.** There is usually severe chronic haemolytic anaemia (primarily extravascular) with onset of aplastic crisis in between. The symptoms of anaemia are generally mild since HbS gives up oxygen more readily than HbA to the tissues.

2. **Vaso-occlusive phenomena.** Patients of SS develop recurrent vaso-occlusive episodes throughout their lives due to obstruction to capillary blood flow by sickled red cells upon deoxygenation or dehydration. Vaso-obstruction affecting different organs and tissues results in infarcts which may be of 2 types:

i) *Microinfarcts* affecting particularly the abdomen, chest, back and joints and are the cause of recurrent painful crises in SS.

ii) *Macroinfarcts* involving most commonly the spleen (splenic sequestration, autosplenectomy), bone marrow (pains), bones (aseptic necrosis, osteomyelitis), lungs (pulmonary infections), kidneys (renal cortical necrosis), CNS (stroke), retina (damage) and skin (ulcers), and result in anatomic and functional damage to these organs.

3. **Constitutional symptoms.** In addition to the features of anaemia and infarction, patients with SS have impaired growth and development and increased susceptibility to infection due to markedly impaired splenic function.

LABORATORY FINDINGS. The diagnosis of SS is considered almost exclusively in a Negro patient with haemolytic anaemia. The laboratory findings in these cases are:

1. Moderate to severe anaemia (haemoglobin concentration 6-9 g/dl).
2. The blood film shows sickle cells and target cells and features of splenic atrophy such as presence of Howell-Jolly bodies.
3. A positive sickling test with a reducing substance such as sodium metabisulfite (described above).
4. Haemoglobin electrophoresis shows no normal HbA but shows predominance of HbS and 2-20% HbF.

Double Heterozygous States

Double heterozygous conditions involving combination of HbS with other haemoglobinopathies may occur. Most common among these are sickle-β-thalassaemia, sickle C disease (SC), and sickle D disease (SD). All these disorders behave like mild form of sickle cell disease. Their diagnosis is made by haemoglobin electrophoresis and separating the different haemoglobins.

OTHER HAEMOGLOBINOPATHIES

Besides sickle haemoglobin, about 400 structurally different abnormal human haemoglobins have been discovered in different parts of the world. Some of them are associated with clinical manifestations, while others are of no consequence. A few important and common variants are briefly described below:

HbC Haemoglobinopathy

HbC haemoglobinopathy is prevalent in West Africa and in American blacks. The molecular lesion in HbC is substitution of lysine for glutamic acid at β-6 globin chain position. The disorder of HbC may occur as benign homozygous HbC disease, or as asymptomatic heterozygous HbC trait, or as double heterozygous combinations such as sickle-HbC disease and HbC-β thalassaemia.

HbD Haemoglobinopathy

HbD occurs in North-West India, Pakistan and Iran. About 3% of Sikhs living in Punjab are affected with HbD haemoglobinopathy (called *HbD Punjab,* also known as *Hb-Los Angeles).* HbD Punjab arises from the substitution of glutamine for glutamic acid at β-121 globin chain position.

HbE Haemoglobinopathy

HbE is predominantly found in South-East Asia, India, Burma and Sri Lanka. HbE arises from the substitution of lysine for glutamic acid at β-26 globin chain position. Like other abnormal haemoglobins, HbE haemoglobinopathy may also occur as asymptomatic heterozygous HbE trait, compensated haemolytic homozygous HbE disease, or as double heterozygous states in combination with other haemoglobinopathies such as HbE-β thalassaemia and HbE-α thalassaemia.

Haemoglobin O-Arab Disease

Hb O-Arab disease was first identified in an Arab family but has now been detected in American blacks too. The homozygous form of the disease appears as mild haemolytic anaemia with splenomegaly.

Unstable-Hb Haemoglobinopathy

The unstable haemoglobins are those haemoglobin variants which undergo denaturation and precipitation within the red cells as Heinz bodies. These give rise to what is known as *congenital non-spherocytic haemolytic anaemia* or *congenital Heinz body haemolytic anaemia.* These disorders have either autosomal dominant inheritance or develop from spontaneous mutations. The unstable haemoglobins arise from either a single amino acid substitution in the globin chain or due to deletion of one or more amino acids within the β-globin chain so that the firm bonding of the haem group within the molecule is disturbed leading to formation of methaemoglobin and precipitation of globin chains as Heinz bodies.

Over 100 unstable haemoglobins have been described. They are named according to the place where they are encountered. For instance: Hb-Koln, Hb-Hammersmith, Hb-Zurich, Hb-Sydney, and so on. The diagnosis of unstable Hb disease is made by test for Heinz bodies and by haemoglobin electrophoresis.

THALASSAEMIA

DEFINITION AND CLASSIFICATION

The thalassaemias are a diverse group of hereditary disorders in which there is reduced rate of synthesis of one or more of the globin polypeptide chains. Thus, thalassaemias, unlike haemoglobinopathies which are qualitative disorders of haemoglobin, are *quantitative abnormalities of polypeptide globin chain synthesis.* Thalassaemias were first described in people of Mediterranean countries (North Africa, Southern Europe) from where it derives its name 'Mediterranean anaemia.' The Word *'thalassa'* in Greek means 'the sea' since the condition was found commonly in regions around the Mediterranean basin. It also occurs in the Middle East, India, South-East Asia and, in general in blacks (see Fig. 13.20).

Thalassaemias are genetically transmitted disorders. Normally, an individual inherits two β-globin genes located one each on two chromosomes 11, and two α-globin genes one each on two chromosomes 16, from each parent i.e. normal adult haemoglobin (HbA) is $\alpha_2 \beta_2$*. Depending upon whether the genetic defect or deletion lies in transmission of α- or β-globin chain genes, thalassaemias are classified into α- and β- thalassaemias. Thus, patients with α-thalassaemia have structurally normal α-globin chains but their production is impaired. Similarly, in β-thalassaemia, β-globin chains are structurally normal but their production is decreased. Each of the two main types of thalassaemias may occur as heterozygous (called α- *and β-thalassaemia minor* or *trait),* or as homogygous state (termed α- and β-*thalassaemia major).* The former is generally asymptomatic, while the latter is a severe congenital haemolytic anaemia.

A classification of various types of thalassaemias alongwith the clinical syndromes produced and salient laboratory findings are given in Table 13.13.

PATHOPHYSIOLOGY OF ANAEMIA IN THALASSAEMIA

A constant feature of all forms of thalassaemia is the presence of anaemia.

α-Thalassaemia: In α-thalassaemia major, the obvious cause of anaemia is the inability to synthesise adult haemoglobin, while in α-thalassaemia trait there is reduced production of normal adult haemoglobin.

β-Thalassaemia: In β-thalassaemia major, the most important cause of anaemia is premature red cell destruction brought about by erythrocyte membrane damage caused by the precipitated α-globin chains. Other contributory factors are: shortened red cell life-span, ineffective erythropoiesis, and haemodilution due to increased plasma volume. A deficiency of β-globin chains in β-thalassaemia leads to large excess of α-chains within the developing red cells. Part of these excessive α-chains are removed by pairing with γ-globin chains as HbF, while the remainder unaccompanied α-chains precipitate rapidly within the red cell as *Heinz bodies.* The precipitated α-chains cause cell membrane damage. During their passage through the splenic sinusoids, these red cells are further damaged and develop pitting due to removal of the precipitated aggregates. Thus, such red cells are irreparably damaged and are phagocytosed by the RE cells of the spleen and liver causing anaemia, hepatosplenomegaly, and excess of tissue iron stores. Patients with β-thalassaemia minor, on the other hand, have very mild ineffective erythropoiesis, haemolysis and shortening of red cell life-span.

α-THALASSAEMIA

MOLECULAR PATHOGENESIS. α-thalassaemias are disorders in which there is defective synthesis of α-globin chains resulting in depressed production of haemoglobins that contain α-chains i.e. HbA, HbA_2 and HbF. The α-thalassaemias are most commonly due to deletion of one or more of the α-chain genes located on short arm of chromosome 16. Since there is a pair of α-chain genes, the clinical manifestations of α-thalassaemia

*In a normal adult, distribution of haemoglobin is as under: HbA ($\alpha_2\beta_2$) = 95-98%, HbA_2 ($\alpha_2\delta_2$) (a minor variant of HbA) = 1.5-3.5%, HbF (α_2 γ_2) = less than 1%. But the level of HbF in children under 6 months is slightly higher.

Chapter Thirteen

TABLE 13.13: Classification of Thalassaemias.

TYPE	HB	HB-ELECTROPHORESIS	GENOTYPE	CLINICAL SYNDROME
α-Thalassaemias				
1. *Hydrops foetalis*	3-10 g/dl	Hb Barts (γ_4) (100%)	Deletion of four α-genes	Fatal *in utero* or in early infancy
2. *Hb-H disease*	2-12 g/dl	HbF (10%)	Deletion of three α-genes	Haemolytic anaemia
3. *α-Thalassaemia trait*	10-14 g/dl	Normal	Deletion of two α-genes	Microcytic hypochromic blood picture but no anaemia
β-Thalassaemias				
1. *β-Thalassaemia major*	< 5 g/dl	HbA (0-50%), HbF(50-98%)	$\beta^{thal}/\beta^{thal}$	Severe congenital haemolytic anaemia, requires blood transfusions
2. *β-Thalassaemia intermedia*	5-10 g/dl	Variable	Multiple mechanisms	Severe anaemia, but regular blood transfusions not required
3. *β-Thalassaemia minor*	10-12 g/dl	HbA_2 (4-9%) HbF (1-5%)	β^A/β^{thal}	Usually asymptomatic

depend upon the number of genes deleted. Accordingly, α-thalassaemias are classified into 4 types:

1. Four α-gene deletion: Hb Bart's hydrops foetalis.
2. Three α-gene deletion: HbH disease.
3. Two α-gene deletion: α-thalassaemia trait.
4. One α-gene deletion: α-thalassaemia trait (carrier).

Hb Bart's Hydrops Foetalis

When there is deletion of all the four α-chain genes (homozygous state) it results in total suppression of α-globin chain synthesis causing the most severe form of α-thalassaemia called Hb Bart's hydrops foetalis. Hb Bart's is a gamma globin chain tetramer (γ_4) which has high oxygen affinity leading to severe tissue hypoxia.

CLINICAL FEATURES. Hb Bart's hydrops foetalis is incompatible with life due to severe tissue hypoxia. The condition is either fatal *in utero* or the infant dies shortly after birth. If born alive, the features of severe Rh haemolytic disease are present (page 440).

LABORATORY FINDINGS. Infants with Hb Bart's hydrops foetalis born alive may have the following laboratory findings:

1. Severe anaemia (haemoglobin below 6g/dl).
2. Blood film show marked anisopoikilocytosis, hypochromia, microcytosis, polychromasia, basophilic stippling, numerous normoblasts and target cells.
3. Reticulocyte count is high.
4. Serum bilirubin level is elevated.
5. Haemoglobin electrophoresis shows 80-90% Hb-Bart's and a small amount of Hb-H and Hb-Portland but no HbA, HbA_2 or HbF.

HbH Disease

Deletion of three α-chain genes produces HbH which is a β-globin chain tetramer (β_4) and markedly impaired α-chain synthesis. HbH is precipitated as Heinz bodies within the affected red cells. An elongated α-chain variant of HbH disease is termed *Hb Constant Spring.*

CLINICAL FEATURES. HbH disease is generally present as a well-compensated haemolytic anaemia. The features are intermediate between that of β-thalassaemia minor and major. The severity of anaemia fluctuates and may fall to very low levels during pregnancy or infections. Majority of patients have splenomegaly and may develop cholelithiasis.

LABORATORY FINDINGS. These are:

1. Moderate anaemia (haemoglobin 8-9 g/dl).
2. Blood film shows severe microcytosis, hypochromia, basophilic stippling, target cells and normoblasts.
3. Mild reticulocytosis.
4. HbH inclusions as Heinz bodies can be demonstrated in mature red cells with brilliant cresyl blue stain.
5. Haemoglobin electrophoresis shows 2-4% HbH and the remainder consists of HbA, HbA_2 and HbF.

α-Thalassaemia Trait

The α-thalassaemia trait may occur by the following molecular pathogenesis:

■ By deletion of two of the four α-chain genes in homozygous form called *homozygous α-thalassaemia,* or in double heterozygous form termed *heterozygous α-thalassaemia.*

■ By deletion of a single α-chain gene causing heterozygous α-thalassaemia trait called *heterozygous α-thalassaemia.*

CLINICAL FEATURES. The α-thalassaemia trait due to two α-chain gene deletion is asymptomatic. It is suspected in a patient of refractory microcytic hypochromic anaemia in whom iron deficiency and β-thalassaemia minor have been excluded and the patient belongs to the high-risk ethnic group. One gene deletion α-thalassaemia trait is a silent carrier state.

LABORATORY FINDINGS. The patients of α-thalassaemia trait may have the following haematological findings:

1. Haemoglobin level normal or mildly reduced.
2. Blood film shows microcytic and hypochromic red cell morphology but no evidence of haemolysis or anaemia.
3. MCV, MCH and MCHC may be slightly reduced.
4. Haemoglobin electrophoresis reveals small amount of Hb-Bart's in neonatal period (1-2% in α-thalassaemia 2 and 5-6% in α-thalassaemia 1) which gradually disappears by adult life. HbA_2 is either normal or slightly decreased (contrary to the elevated HBA_2 levels in β-thalassaemia trait).

β-THALASSAEMIAS

MOLECULAR PATHOGENESIS. The β-thalassaemias are caused by decreased rate of β-chain synthesis resulting in reduced formation of HbA in the red cells. The molecular pathogenesis of the β-thalassaemias is more complex than that of α-thalassaemias. In contrast to α-thalassaemia, gene deletions rarely ever cause β-thalassaemia and is only seen in an entity called *hereditary persistence of foetal haemoglobin (HPFH).* Instead, most of β-thalassaemias arise from different types of mutations of β–globin gene resulting from single base changes. The symbol β° is used to indicate the complete absence of synthesis while $β^+$ denotes partial synthesis of the β-globin chains. More than 100 such mutations have been described affecting the preferred sites in the coding sequences e.g. in promoter region, termination region, splice junctions, exons, introns). Some of the important ones having effects on β-globin chain synthesis are as under (Fig. 13.22):

i) *Transcription defect:* Mutation affecting transcriptional promoter sequence causing reduced synthesis of β-globin chain. Hence the result is partially preserved synthesis i.e. *$β^+$ thalassaemia.*

ii) *Translation defect:* Mutation in the coding sequence causing stop codon (chain termination) interrupting β-globin messenger RNA. This would result in no synthesis of β-globin chain and hence *β° thalassaemia.*

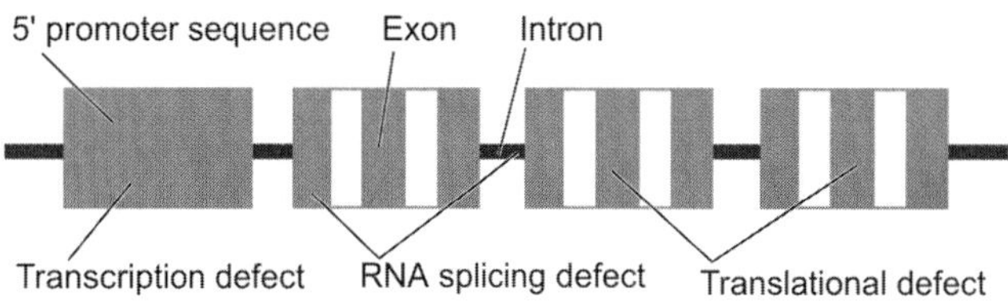

FIGURE 13.22

Schematic representation of sites of β-globin gene mutation in chromosome 11 giving rise to β-thalassaemia.

iii) *mRNA splicing defect:* Mutation leads to defective mRNA processing forming abnormal mRNA that is degraded in the nucleus. Depending upon whether part of splice site remains intact or is totally degraded, it may result in *$β^+$ thalassaemia or β° thalassaemia.*

Depending upon the extent of reduction in β-chain synthesis, there are 3 types of β-thalassaemia:

1. Homozygous form: β-Thalassaemia major. It is the most severe form of congenital haemolytic anaemia. It is further of 2 types (Fig. 13.23):

i) β° *thalassaemia major* characterised by complete absence of β-chain synthesis.

ii) $β^+$ *thalassaemia major* having incomplete suppression of β-chain synthesis.

2. β-Thalassaemia intermedia: It is β-thalassaemia of intermediate degree of severity that does not require regular blood transfusions. These cases are genetically heterozygous (β°/β or $β^+$/β).

3. Heterozygous form: β-Thalassaemia minor (trait). It is a mild asymptomatic condition in which there is moderate suppression of β-chain synthesis.

Besides β-thalassaemia minor, a few uncommon globin chain combinations resulting in β-thalassaemia trait are as under:

i) δβ-*thalassaemia minor* in which there is total absence of both β and δ chain synthesis and is characterised by elevated HbF level but unlike β-thalassaemia minor there is normal or reduced HbA_2 level.

ii) *Hb Lepore syndrome* characterised by nonhomologous fusion of β- and δ-genes forming an abnormal haemoglobin called Hb Lepore (named after a family called Lepore). There is total absence of normal β-chain synthesis.

An individual may inherit one β-chain gene from each parent and produce heterozygous, homozygous, or double heterozygous states. Statistically, 25% of

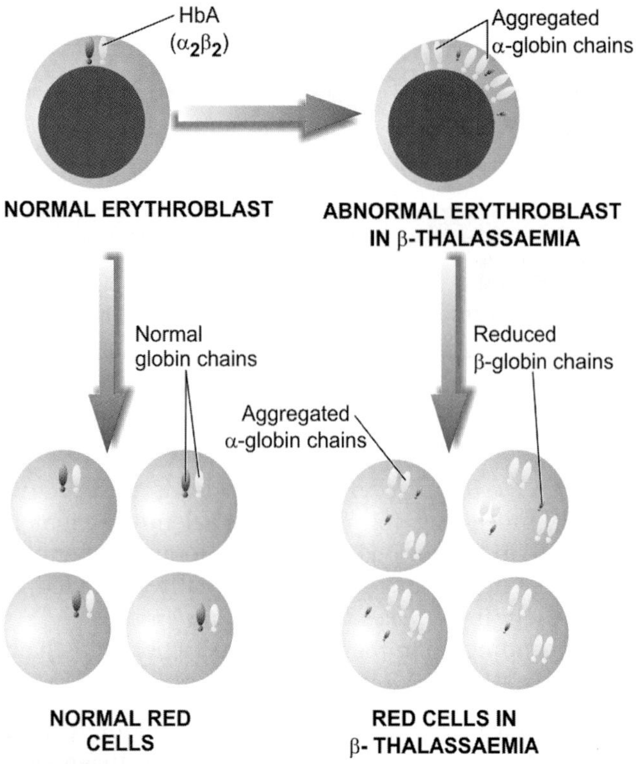

HbA ($\alpha_2\beta_2$)

Aggregated α-globin chains

NORMAL ERYTHROBLAST

ABNORMAL ERYTHROBLAST IN β-THALASSAEMIA

Normal globin chains

Reduced β-globin chains

Aggregated α-globin chains

NORMAL RED CELLS

RED CELLS IN β- THALASSAEMIA

FIGURE 13.23

Pathogenesis of β-thalassaemia major.

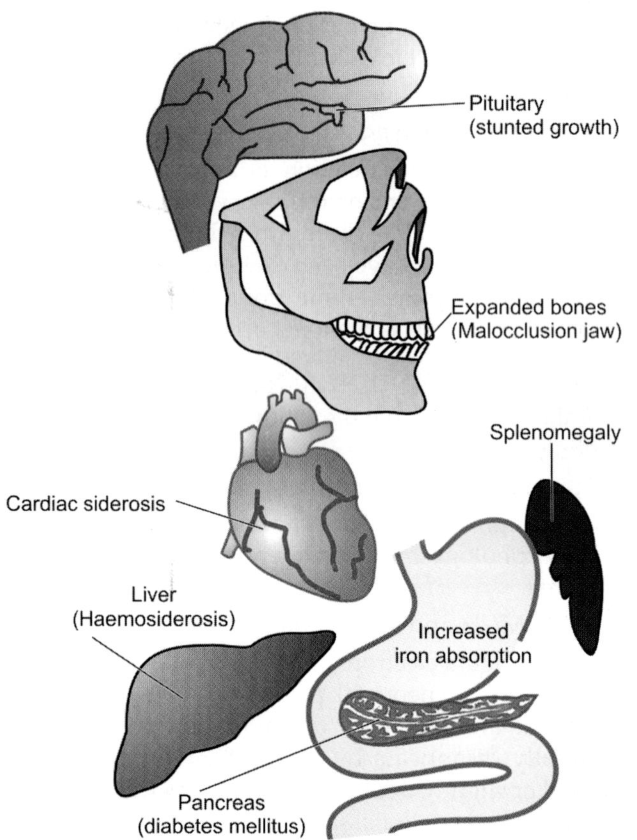

FIGURE 13.24

Major clinical features in β-thalassaemia major.

offsprings born to two heterozygotes (i.e. β-thalassaemia trait) will have the homozygous state i.e. β-thalassaemia major.

β-Thalassaemia Major

The β-thalassaemia major, also termed Mediterranean or Cooley's anaemia is the most common form of congenital haemolytic anaemia. More commonly, β-thalassaemia major is a homozygous state with either complete absence of β-chain synthesis (β° *thalassaemia major)* or only small amounts of β-chains are formed (β^+ *thalassaemia major).* These result in excessive formation of alternate haemoglobins, HbF ($\alpha_2\ \gamma_2$) and HbA_2 ($\alpha_2\ \delta_2$).

CLINICAL FEATURES. Clinical manifestations appear insidiously and are as under (Fig. 13.24):

1. Anaemia starts appearing within the first 4-6 months of life when the switch over from γ-chain to β-chain production occurs.
2. Marked hepatosplenomegaly occurs due to excessive red cell destruction, extramedullary haematopoiesis and iron overload.
3. Expansion of bones occurs due to marked erythroid hyperplasia leading to thalassaemic facies and malocclusion of the jaw.
4. Iron overload due to repeated blood transfusions causes damage to the endocrine organs resulting in slow rate of growth and development, delayed puberty, diabetes mellitus and damage to the liver and heart.

LABORATORY FINDINGS. The haematological investigations reveal the following findings (COLOUR PLATE XVI: CL 63):

1. *Anaemia,* usually severe.
2. *Blood film* shows severe microcytic hypochromic red cell morphology, marked anisopoikilocytosis, basophilic stippling, presence of many target cells, tear drop cells and normoblasts (Fig. 13.25,A).
3. *Serum bilirubin* (unconjugated) is generally raised.
4. *Reticulocytosis* is generally present.
5. *MCV, MCH and MCHC* are significantly reduced.
6. *WBC count is* often raised with some shift to left of the neutrophil series, with presence of some myelocytes and metamyelocytes.
7. *Platelet count* is usually normal but may be reduced in patients with massive splenomegaly.

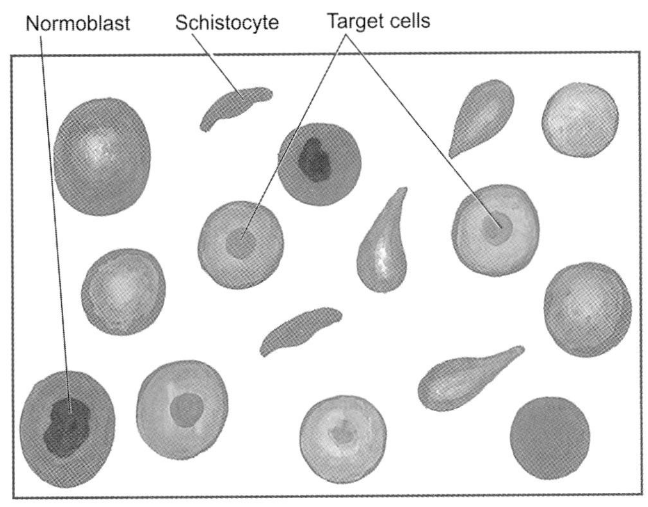

A, BLOOD FILM IN β-THALASSAEMIA MAJOR

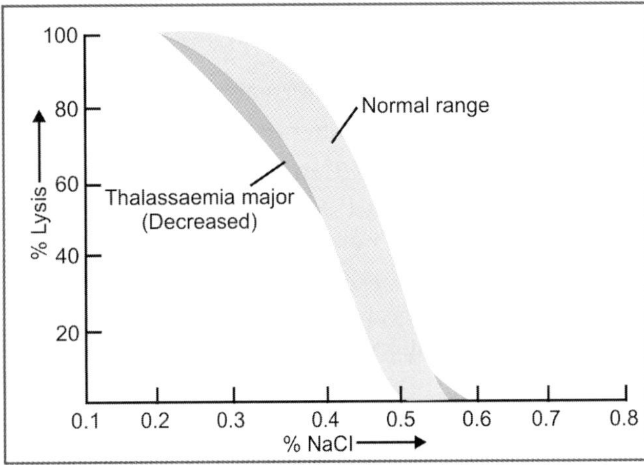

B, OSMOTIC FRAGILITY CURVE

FIGURE 13.25

Laboratory findings in β-thalassaemia major. A, Findings in peripheral blood film. B, Osmotic fragility test showing decreased fragility.

8. Osmotic fragility characteristically reveals increased resistance to saline haemolysis i.e. *decreased osmotic fragility* (Fig. 13.25,B).

9. *Haemoglobin electrophoresis* shows presence of increased amounts of HbF, increased amount of HbA_2, and almost complete absence or presence of variable amounts of HbA. The increased level of HbA_2 has not been found in any other haemoglobin abnormality except β-thalassaemia. The increased synthesis of HbA_2 is probably due to increased activity at both δ-chain loci.

10. *Bone marrow aspirate examination* shows normoblastic erythroid hyperplasia with predominance of intermediate and late normoblasts which are generally smaller in size than normal. Iron staining demonstrates siderotic granules in the cytoplasm of normoblasts, increased reticuloendothelial iron but ring sideroblasts are only occasionally seen.

Treatment

Treatment of β-thalassaemia major is largely supportive.

1. Anaemia is generally severe and patients require regular blood transfusions (4-6 weekly) to maintain haemoglobin above 8 g/dl.

2. In order to maintain increased demand of hyperplastic marrow, folic acid supplement is given.

3. Splenectomy is beneficial in children over 6 years of age since splenic sequestration contributes to shortened red cell life-span.

4. Prevention and treatment of iron overload is done by chelation therapy (desferrioxamine). Oral chelation with kelfer or deferiprone is also available now.

5. Bone marrow transplantation from HLA-matched donor is being done in many centres with fair success rate.

6. Some workers have found success with cord blood transfusion.

Since these patients require multiple blood transfusions, they are at increased risk of developing AIDS. In general, patients with β-thalassaemia major have short life expectancy and it is unusual for a patient with severe form of the disease to survive into adulthood. The biggest problem is iron overload and consequent myocardial siderosis leading to cardiac arrhythmias, congestive heart failure, and ultimately death.

β-Thalassaemia Minor

The β-thalassaemia minor or β-thalassaemia trait, a heterozygous state, is a common entity characterised by moderate reduction in β-chain synthesis.

CLINICAL FEATURES. Clinically, the condition is usually asymptomatic and the diagnosis is generally made when the patient is being investigated for a mild chronic anaemia. The spleen may be palpable.

LABORATORY FINDINGS. These are as under:

1. *Mild anaemia;* mean haemoglobin level is about 15% lower than in normal person for the age and sex.

2. *Blood film* shows mild anisopoikilocytosis, microcytosis and hypochromia, occasional target cells and basophilic stippling.
3. *Serum bilirubin* may be normal or slightly raised.
4. Mild *reticulocytosis* is often present.
5. *MCV, MCH and MCHC* may be slightly reduced.
6. Osmotic fragility test shows increased resistance to haemolysis i.e. *decreased osmotic fragility.*
7. *Haemoglobin electrophoresis* is confirmatory for the diagnosis and shows about two-fold increase in HbA_2 and a slight elevation in HbF (2-3%).

Treatment

Patients with β-thalassaemia minor do not require any treatment. But they should be explained about the genetic implications of the disorder, particularly to those of child-bearing age. If the two subjects of β-thalassaemia trait marry, there is a 25% chance of developing thalassaemia major in offsprings. Patients with β-thalassaemia minor have normal life expectancy but those who are treated under the mistaken diagnosis of iron deficiency may develop siderosis and its complications.

Prevention ofThalassaemia

Finally, since thalassaemia is an inheritable disease, its prevention is possible by making an antenatal diagnosis. This is done by chorionic villous biopsy or cells obtained by amniocentesis and DNA studied by PCR amplification technique for presence of genetic mutations of thalassaemias.

APLASTIC ANAEMIA AND OTHER PRIMARY BONE MARROW DISORDERS

'Bone marrow failure' is the term used for primary disorders of the bone marrow which result in impaired formation of the erythropoietic precursors and consequent anaemia. It includes the following disorders:
1. *Aplastic anaemia,* most importantly.
2. *Other primary bone marrow disroders* such as: myelophthisic anaemia, pure red cell aplasia, and myelodysplastic syndromes.

APLASTIC ANAEMIA

Aplastic anaemia is defined as pancytopenia (i.e. simultaneous presence of anaemia, leucopenia and thrombocytopenia) resulting from aplasia of the bone marrow. The underlying defect in all cases appears to be sufficient reduction in the number of haematopoietic pluripotent stem cells which makes them unable to divide and differentiate.

ETIOLOGY AND CLASSIFICATION. Based on the etiology, aplastic anaemia is classified into 2 main types: primary and secondary. The various causes that may give rise to both these types of aplastic anaemia are summarised in Table 13.14 and briefly considered below:

A. Primary aplastic anaemia. Primary type of aplastic anaemia includes 2 entities: a congenital form called Fanconi's anaemia and an immunologically-mediated acquired form.

1. *Fanconi's anaemia.* This has an autosomal recessive inheritance and is often associated with other congenital anomalies such as skeletal and renal abnormalities, and sometimes mental retardation.

2. *Immune causes.* In many cases, suppression of haematopoietic stem cells by immunologic mechanisms may cause aplastic anaemia. The observations in support of autoimmune mechanisms are the clinical response to immunosupppressive therapy and *in vitro* marrow culture experiments.

B. Secondary aplastic anaemia. Aplastic anaemia may occur secondary to a variety of industrial, physical, chemical, iatrogenic and infectious causes.

1. *Drugs.* A number of drugs are cytotoxic to the marrow and cause aplastic anaemia. The association of a drug with aplastic anaemia may be either predictably dose-related or an idiosyncratic reaction.

- *Dose-related aplasia* of the bone marrow occurs with antimetabolites (e.g. methotrexate), mitotic inhibitors (e.g. daunorubicin), alkylating agents (e.g. busulfan), nitroso urea and anthracyclines. In such cases, withdrawal of the drug usually allows recovery of the marrow elements.

TABLE 13.14: Causes of Aplastic Anaemia.

A. PRIMARY APLASTIC ANAEMIA
1. *Fanconi's anaemia (congenital)*
2. *Immunologically-mediated (acquired)*
B. SECONDARY APLASTIC ANAEMIA
1. *Drugs*
i) Dose-related aplasia e.g. with antimetabolites (methotrexate), mitotic inhibitors (daunorubicin), alkylating agents (busulfan), nitroso urea, anthracyclines.
ii) Idiosyncratic aplasia e.g. with chloramphenicol, sulfa drugs, oxyphenbutazone, phenylbutazone, chlorpromazine, gold salts.
2. *Toxic chemicals* e.g. benzene derivatives, insecticides, arsenicals.
3. *Infections* e.g. infectious hepatitis, EB virus infection, AIDS, other viral illnesses.
4. Miscellaneous e.g. association with SLE and therapeutic X-rays

■ *Idiosyncratic aplasia* is depression of the bone marrow due to qualitatively abnormal reaction of an individual to a drug when first administered. The most serious and most common example of idiosyncratic aplasia is associated with chloramphenicol. Other such common drugs are: sulfa drugs, oxyphenbutazone, phenylbutazone, chlorpromazine, gold salts etc.

2. *Toxic chemicals.* These include examples of industrial, domestic and accidental use of substances such as benzene derivatives, insecticides, arsenicals etc.

3. *Infections.* Aplastic anaemia may occur following viral hepatitis, Epstein-Barr virus infection, AIDS and other viral illnesses.

4. *Miscellaneous.* Lastly, aplastic anaemia has been reported in association with certain other illnesses such as SLE, and with therapeutic X-rays.

CLINICAL FEATURES. The onset of aplastic anaemia may occur at any age and is usually insidious. The clinical manifestations include the following:

1. Anaemia and its symptoms like mild progressive weakness and fatigue.
2. Haemorrhage from various sites due to thrombocytopenia such as from the skin, nose, gums, vagina, bowel, and occasionally in the CNS and retina.
3. Infections of the mouth and throat are commonly present.
4. The lymph nodes, liver and spleen are generally not enlarged.

LABORATORY FINDINGS. The diagnosis of aplastic anaemia is made by a thorough laboratory evaluation and excluding other causes of pancytopenia (Table 13.15). The following haematological features are found:

1. Anaemia. Haemoglobin levels are moderately reduced. The blood picture generally shows normocytic normochromic anaemia but sometimes macrocytosis may be present. The reticulocyte count is reduced or zero.

2. Leucopenia. The absolute granulocyte count is particularly low (below 1500/μl) with relative lymphocytosis. The neutrophils are morphologically normal but their alkaline phosphatase score is high.

3. Thrombocytopenia. Platelet count is always reduced.

4. Bone marrow aspiration. A bone marrow aspirate may yield a 'dry tap'. A trephine biopsy is generally essential for making the diagnosis which reveals patchy cellular areas in a hypocellular or aplastic marrow due to replacement by fat. There is usually a severe depression of myeloid cells, megakaryocytes and erythroid cells so that the marrow chiefly consists of lymphocytes and plasma cells.

TABLE 13.15: Causes of Pancytopenia.

I. Aplastic anaemia (Table 13.14)

II. Pancytopenia with normal or increased marrow cellularity e.g.

1. Myelodysplastic syndromes
2. Hypersplenism
3. Megaloblastic anaemia

III. Paroxysmal nocturnal haemoglobinuria (page 390)

IV. Bone marrow infiltrations e.g.

1. Haematologic malignancies (leukaemias, lymphomas, myeloma)
2. Non-haematologic metastatic malignancies
3. Storage diseases
4. Osteopetrosis
5. Myelofibrosis

Treatment

The patients of mild aplasia may show spontaneous recovery, while the management of severe aplastic anaemia is a most challenging task. In general, younger patients show better response to proper treatment. The broad outlines of the treatment are as under:

A. General management: It consists of the following:

1. Identification and elimination of the possible cause.
2. Supportive care consisting of blood transfusions, platelet concentrates, and treatment and prevention of infections.

B. Specific treatment: The specific treatment has been attempted with varying success and includes the following:

1. *Marrow stimulating agents* such as androgen may be administered orally.
2. *Immunosuppressive therapy* with agents such as anti-thymocyte globulin and anti-lymphocyte serum has been tried with 40-50% success rate. Very high doses of glucocorticoids or cyclosporine may yield similar responses. But splenectomy does not have any role in the management of aplastic anaemia.
3. *Bone marrow transplantation* is considered in severe cases under the age of 40 years where the HLA and mixed culture-matched donor is available. (*Other indications* for bone marrow transplantation are: acute leukaemias—AML in first remission and ALL in second

remission, thalassaemia major and combined immunodeficiency disease). Complications of bone marrow transplantation such as severe infections, graft rejection and graft-versus-host disease (GVHD) may occur (Chapter 4).

Severe aplastic anaemia is a serious disorder terminating in death within 6-12 months in 50-80% of cases. Death is usually due to bleeding and/or infection.

MYELOPHTHISIC ANAEMIA

Development of severe anaemia may result from infiltration of the marrow termed as myelophthisic anaemia. The causes for marrow infiltrations include (Table 13.15):

- Haematologic malignancies (e.g. leukaemia, lymphoma, myeloma),
- Metastatic deposits from non-haematologic malignancies (e.g. cancer breast, stomach, prostate, lung, thyroid),
- Advanced tuberculosis,
- Primary lipid storage diseases (Gaucher's and Niemann-Pick's disease).
- Osteopetrosis and myelofibrosis may rarely cause myelophthisis.

The type of anaemia in myelophthisis is generally normocytic normochromic with some fragmented red cells, basophilic stippling and normoblasts in the peripheral blood. Thrombocytopenia is usually present but the leucocyte count is increased with slight shift-to-left of myeloid cells i.e. a picture of *leucoerythroblastic reaction* consisting of immature myeloid cells and normoblasts is seen in the peripheral blood. Treatment consists of reversing the underlying pathologic process.

PURE RED CELL APLASIA

This is a rare syndrome involving a selective failure in the production of erythroid elements in the bone marrow but with normal granulopoiesis and megakaryocytopoiesis. Patients have normocytic normochromic anaemia with normal granulocyte and platelet count. Reticulocytes are markedly decreased or are absent.

Pure red cell aplasia exists in two forms: congenital and acquired.

- *Congenital red cell aplasia (Blackfan-Diamond syndrome)* is a rare chronic disorder of unknown etiology. The disorder is corrected by glucocorticoids and marrow transplantation.
- *Acquired red cell aplasia* is seen in middle-aged adults in association with some other diseases, most commonly thymoma; others are SLE, lymphoma, T-cell chronic lymphocytic leukaemia or even without any precipitating factor. Another treatable cause of pure red cell aplasia reported in children is chronic parvovirus B19 infection.In general, pure red cell aplasia probably results from selective cytotoxicity of marrow erythroblasts by complement-fixing IgG.

MYELODYSPLASTIC SYNDROMES

Myelodysplastic syndromes (MDS) or *preleukaemic syndromes* are a heterogeneous group of leukaemia-related conditions having abnormalities in development of different marrow elements in varying combinations. These conditions are, therefore, also termed as *dysmyelopoietic syndromes.* The various combinations of features include normocytic normochromic anaemia, presence of certain number of myeloblasts in the peripheral blood, neutropenia, thrombocytopenia and/or monocytosis. The bone marrow reveals disordered maturation of lymphoid, myeloid and megakaryocytic cells.

The *FAB (French-American-British) classification* divides myelodysplastic syndromes into the following 5 groups (Table 13.16):

1. Refractory anaemia (RA).
2. Refractory anaemia with ringed sideroblasts (primary acquired sideroblastic anaemia) (RARS).
3. Refractory anaemia with excess blasts (RAEB).
4. Chronic myelomonocytic leukaemia (CMML).
5. Refractory anaemia with excess of blasts in transformation (RAEB-t).

As per FAB classification, marrow may contain up to 30% myeloblasts in MDS and was considered as the dividing line for distinguishing cases of AML from MDS. However, as per recently described *WHO classification,* patients with blast count of 20-30% and labelled as RAEB-t (group 5 above) in FAB classification have prognosis similar to patients with blast count above 30% (i.e. AML cases). Thus, as per WHO classification, marrow blast count for making the diagnosis of AML has been revised and brought down to 20%. Patients with FAB category of RAEB-t are currently considered and treated as cases of AML and the term RAEB-t stands excluded from MDS according to the WHO classification.

MDS is found more frequently in older people (above 50 years of age). The etiology remains unknown but an association with chemotherapy or radiation has been observed in some cases. Many of the features are like those of acute leukaemia but the clinical course in myelodysplastic syndromes tends to be more chronic.

TABLE 13.16: French-American-British (FAB) Classification of Myelodysplastic Syndromes (MDS).

FINDINGS	RA	RARS	RAEB	CMML	RAEB-t
A. Incidence	28%	24%	23%	16%	9%
B. Peripheral Blood					
1. Haemoglobin	Low	Low	Low	Variable	Low
2. Myeloblasts	0-1%	0-1%	<5%	<5%	>5%
3. Monocytes	Rare	Rare	Rare	>1000/μl	Variable
C. Bone marrow					
1. Myeloblasts	<5%	<5%	5-20%	1-20%	20-30%
2. Ringed sideroblasts	±	>15%	±	±	±

Abbreviations: RA= refractory anaemia; RARS = refractory anaemia with ringed sideroblasts; RAEB = refractory anaemia with excess blasts; CMML= chronic myelomonocytic leukaemia; RAEB-t= refractory anaemia with excess blasts in transformation.

However, 5-20% patients actually evolve into frank acute myeloid leukaemia (with more than 30% blasts in the bone marrow), confirming their preleukaemic nature.

Survival in different subtypes ranges from 3-76 months, patients either succumbing to infections or developing into acute myeloid leukaemia. Patients with RA and RARS have a better prognosis while patients with RAEB and RAEB-t have a higher rate of leukaemic conversion and a shorter survival.

WHITE BLOOD CELLS

The leucocytes of the peripheral blood are of 2 main varieties, distinguished by the presence or absence of granules. These are: *granulocytes* and *nongranular leucocytes*. The granulocytes, according to the appearance of nuclei, are subdivided into polymorphonuclear leucocytes and monocytes. Depending upon the colour of granules, polymorphonuclear leucocytes are further of 3 types: neutrophils, eosinophils and basophils. The nongranular leucocytes are lymphocytes.

GRANULOPOIESIS

Site of Formation and Kinetics

All forms of granulocytes are produced in the bone marrow and are termed,*'myeloid series'*. These are: myeloblast (most primitive precursor), promyelocyte, myelocyte, metamyelocyte, band forms and segmented granulocyte (mature form). The myeloblast, promyelocyte and myelocyte form a *'proliferative or mitotic pool'*, while the latter series i.e. metamyelocyte, band forms and segmented granulocytes make up a *'mature or post-mitotic pool'*. It takes about 12 days for formation of mature granulocytes from the myeloblast. Normally the bone marrow contains more myeloid cells than the erythroid cells in the ratio of 2:1 to 15:1 (average 3:1), the largest proportion being that of metamyelocytes, band forms and segmented neutrophils.

Normally, the bone marrow storage compartment contains about 10-15 times the number of granulocytes found in the peripheral blood. Following their release from the bone marrow, granulocytes spend about 10 hours in the circulation before they move into the tissues, where they perform their function of phagocytosis. The blood pool of granulocytes consists of 2 components of about equal size—the *circulating pool* that is included in the blood count, and the *marginating pool* that is not included in the blood count. Granulocytes spend about 4-5 days in the tissues before they are either destroyed during phagocytosis or die due to senescence (Fig. 13.26). To control the various compartments of granulocytes, a 'feed-back system' exists between the circulating and tissue granulocytes on one side, and the marrow granulocytes on the other. The presence of a humoral regulatory substance, 'granulopoietin' analogous to erythropoietin has also been identified by *in vitro* studies of colony-forming units (CFU) and is characterised as G-CSF (granulocyte colony-stimulating factor) and GM-CSF (granulocyte-monocyte colony-stimulating factor).

The kinetics of monocytes is less well understood than that of other myeloid cells. Monocytes spend about 20-40 hours in the circulation after which they leave the blood to enter extravascular tissues where they perform their main function of active phagocytosis. The extravascular life-span of tissue macrophages which are the transformed form of blood monocytes, may vary from a few months to a few years.

Myeloid Series

The development of myeloid cells from myeloblast takes place in the following sequence (Fig. 13.26):

Chapter Thirteen

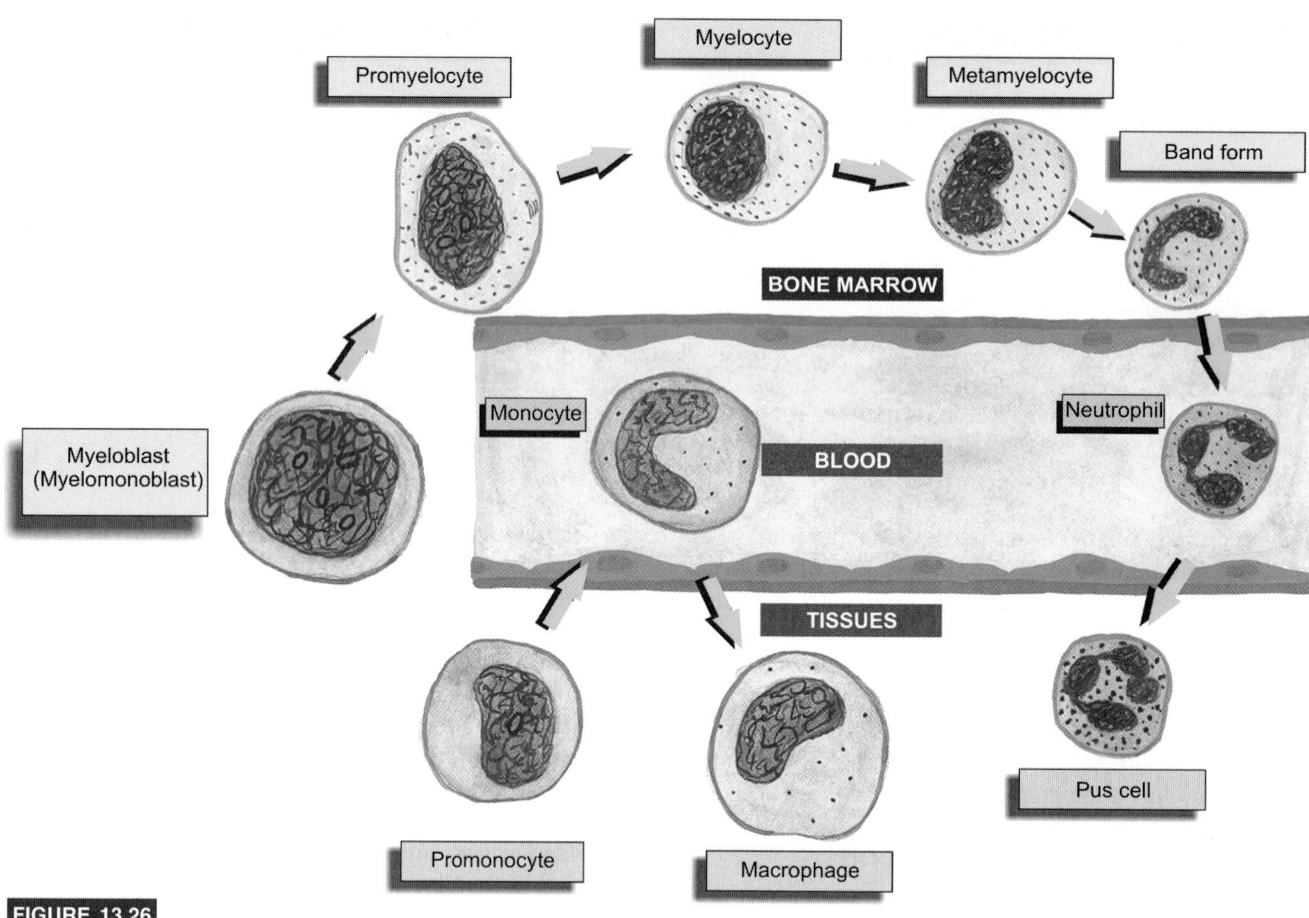

FIGURE 13.26

Granulopoiesis and the cellular compartments of myeloid cells in the bone marrow, blood and tissues.

1. MYELOBLAST. The myeloblast is the earliest recognisable precursor of the granulocytes, normally comprising about 2% of the total marrow cells. The myeloblast varies considerably in size (10-18 μm in diameter), having a large round to oval nucleus nearly filling the cell, has fine nuclear chromatin and contains 2-5 well-defined pale nucleoli. The thin rim of cytoplasm is deeply basophilic and devoid of granules. The myeloblasts of acute myeloid leukaemia may, however, show the presence of rod-like cytoplasmic inclusions called *Auer's rods* which represent abnormal derivatives of primary azurophilic granules.

The nuclei of successive stages during their development from myeloblast become progressively coarser and lose their nucleoli and the cytoplasm loses its blue colour. As the cells become mature the granules appear; firstly non-specific azurophilic granules appear which are followed by specific granules that differentiate the neutrophils, eosinophils and basophils.

2. PROMYELOCYTE. The promyelocyte is slightly larger than the myeloblast (12-18 μm diameter). It possesses a round to oval nucleus, having fine nuclear chromatin which is slightly condensed around the nuclear membrane. The nucleoli are present but are less prominent and fewer than those in the myeloblast. The main distinction of promyelocyte from myeloblast is in the cytoplasm which contains azurophilic (primary or non-specific) granules.

3. MYELOCYTE. The myelocyte is the stage in which specific or secondary granules appear in the cytoplasm, and accordingly, the cell can be identified at this stage as belonging to the neutrophilic, eosinophilic or basophilic myelocyte. Primary granules also persist at this stage but formation of new primary granules stops. The nucleus of myelocyte is eccentric, round to oval, having somewhat coarse nuclear chromatin and no visible nucleoli. The myeloid cells up to the myelocyte stage continue to divide and, therefore, comprise *mitotic or proliferative pool.*

4. METAMYELOCYTE. The metamyelocyte stage is 10-18 μm in diameter and is characterised by a clearly indented or horseshoe-shaped nucleus without nucleoli. The nuclear chromatin is dense and clumped. The cytoplasm contains both primary and secondary granules. The metamyelocytes are best distinguished from the monocytes by the clumped nuclear chromatin while the latter have fine chromatin.

5. **BAND FORMS.** Band form is juvenile granulocyte, 10-16 μm in diameter, characterised by further condensation of nuclear chromatin and transformation of nuclear shape into band configuration of uniform thickness.

6. **SEGMENTED GRANULOCYTES.** The mature polymorphonuclear leucocytes, namely: the neutrophils, eosinophils and basophils, are described later on page 408.

Monocyte-Macrophage Series

The monocyte-macrophage series of cells, though comprise a part of myeloid series alongwith other granulocytic series, but are described separately here in view of different morphologic stages in their maturation (Fig. 13.26).

1. **MONOBLAST.** The monoblast is the least mature of the recognisable cell of monocyte-macrophage series. It is very similar in appearance to myeloblasts except that it has ground-glass cytoplasm with irregular border and may show phagocytosis as indicated by the presence of engulfed red cells in the cytoplasm. However, differentiation from myeloblast at times may be difficult even by electron microscopy and, therefore, it is preferable to call the earliest precursor of granulocytic series as *myelomonoblast*.

2. **PROMONOCYTE.** The promonocyte is a young monocyte, about 20 μm in diameter and possesses a large indented nucleus containing a nucleolus. The cytoplasm is basophilic and contains no azurophilic granules but may have fine granules which are larger than those in the mature monocyte.

3. **MONOCYTE.** The mature form of monocytic series is described on page 411, while the transformed stages of these cells in various tissues (i.e. macrophages) are a part of RE system discussed in Chapter 4.

LYMPHOPOIESIS

Sites of Formation and Kinetics

The lymphocytes and the plasma cells are immunocompetent cells of the body. In man, the bone marrow and the thymus are the *primary lymphopoietic organs* where lymphoid stem cells undergo spontaneous division independent of antigenic stimulation. The *secondary or reactive lymphoid tissue* is comprised by the lymph nodes, spleen and gut-associated lymphoid tissue (GALT). These sites actively produce lymphocytes from the germinal centres of lymphoid follicles as a response to antigenic stimulation. Lymphocytes pass through a series of developmental changes in the course of their evolution into lymphocyte subpopulations and subsets. It includes migration of immature lymphocytes to other organs such as the thymus where locally-produced factors act on them.

Functionally, the lymphocytes are divided into T and B lymphocytes depending upon whether they are immunologically active in cell-mediated immunity or in humoral antibody response respectively. In man, the B cells are derived from the bone marrow stem cells, while in birds they mature in the bursa of Fabricius. After antigenic activation, the B cells proliferate and mature into plasma cells which secrete specific immunoglobulin antibodies. The T cells are also produced in the bone marrow and possibly in the thymus. The concept of T and B lymphocytes alongwith their subpopulations is discussed in Chapter 4.

Lymphoid Series

The maturation stages in production of lymphocytes are illustrated in Fig. 13.27 and are as under:

1. **LYMPHOBLAST.** The lymphoblast is the earliest identifiable precursor of lymphoid cells and is a rapidly dividing cell. It is a large cell, 10-18 μm in diameter, containing a large round to oval nucleus having slightly clumped or stippled nuclear chromatin. The nuclear membrane is denser and the number of nucleoli is fewer (1-2) as compared with those in myeloblast (2-5). The cytoplasm is scanty, basophilic and non-granular.

The distinguishing morphologic features between the myeloblast and lymphoblast are summarised in Table 13.17.

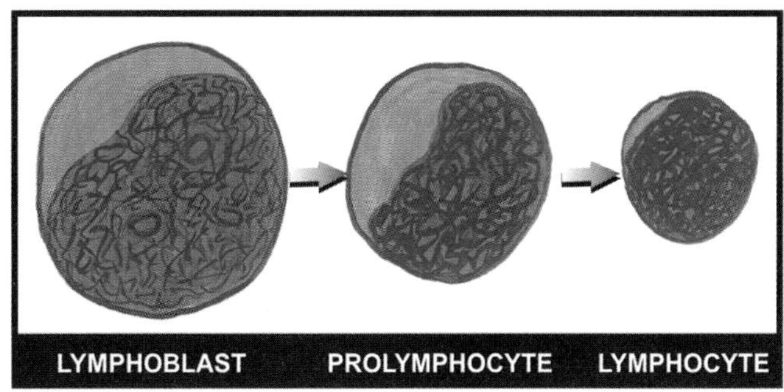

FIGURE 13.27
The formation of lymphoid series of cells.

Chapter Thirteen

TABLE 13.17: Morphologic Characteristics of the Blast Cells in Romanowsky Stains.

FEATURE	MYELOBLAST	LYMPHOBLAST
1. Size	10-18 μm	10-18 μm
2. Nucleus	Round or oval	Round or oval
3. Nuclear chromatin	Fine meshwork	Slightly clumped
4. Nuclear membrane	Very fine	Fairly dense
5. Nucleoli	2-5	1-2
6. Cytoplasm	Scanty, blue, agranular	Scanty, clear blue, agranular

2. **PROLYMPHOCYTE.** This stage is an intermediate stage between the lymphoblast and mature lymphocyte. These young lymphocytes are 9-18 μm in diameter, contain round to indented nucleus with slightly stippled or coarse chromatin and may have 0-1 nucleoli.

3. **LYMPHOCYTE.** The mature lymphocytes are described below.

MATURE LEUCOCYTES IN HEALTH AND DISEASE

Normally, only mature leucocytes namely: polymorphs, lymphocytes, monocytes, eosinophils and basophils, are found in the peripheral blood. The normal range of total and differential leucocyte count (TLC and DLC) in health in adults and children is given in Table 13.18. White cell count tends to be higher in infants and children than in adults. It also normally undergoes minor degree of diurnal variation with a slight rise in the afternoon. The total white cell count is normally high in pregnancy and following delivery, usually returning to normal within a week. The pathological variations in white cell values together with brief review of their morphology and functions are considered below (Fig. 13.28).

TABLE 13.18: Normal White Blood Cell Counts in Health.

	ABSOLUTE COUNT
TLC	
Adults	4,000–11,000/μl
Infants (Full term, at birth)	10,000–25,000/μl
Infants (1 year)	6,000–16,000/μl
Children (4–7 years)	5,000–15,000/μl
Children (8–12 years)	4,500–13,500/μl
DLC IN ADULTS	
Polymorphs (neutrophils) 40–75%	2,000–7,500/μl
Lymphocytes 20–50%	1,500–4,000/μl
Monocytes 2–10%	200–800/μl
Eosinophils 1–6%	40–400/μl
Basophils <1%	10–100/μl

Polymorphs (Neutrophils)

MORPHOLOGY. A polymorphonuclear neutrophil (PMN), commonly called polymorph or neutrophil, is 12-15 μm in diameter. It consists of a characteristic dense nucleus, having 2-5 lobes and pale cytoplasm containing numerous fine violet-pink granules. These granules contain several enzymes and are of 2 types:

Primary or azurophilic granules are large and coarse and appear early at the promyelocyte stage. These granules contain:

i) Myeloperoxidase(MPO) used as marker for PMNs(CD13 marker). MPO is involved in formation of hydrogen peroxide which is an important oxygen free radical.

ii) Hydrolases such as lysozymes, cathepsin, elastase and proteinase 3. MPO alongwith proteinase 3 is involved in ANCA-mediated vasculitis.

Secondary or specific granules are smaller and more numerous. These appear later at myelocyte stage, are MPO-negative and contain:

i) Lysozyme, type IV collagenase, lactoferrin.
ii) Alkaline phosphatase.
iii) Plasminogen activator.
iv) Leucocyte adhesion molecules.

The normal **functions** of neutrophils are as under:

1. *Chemotaxis* or cell mobilisation in which the cell is attracted towards bacteria or at the site of inflammation.
2. *Phagocytosis* in which the foreign particulate material is phagocytosed by actively motile neutrophils.
3. *Killing* of the microorganism is mediated by oxygen-dependent and oxygen-independent pathways (Chapter 3).

PATHOLOGIC VARIATIONS. Pathologic variations in neutrophils include variations in count, morphology and defective function.

Variation in count. An increase in neutrophil count *(neutrophil leucocytosis or neutrophilia)* or a decrease in count *(neutropenia)* may occur in various diseases.

Neutrophil leucocytosis. An increase in circulating neutrophils above 7,500/μl is the commonest type of leucocytosis and occurs most commonly as a response to acute bacterial infections. Some common causes of neutrophilia are as under:

1. *Acute infections, local or generalised,* especially by cocci but also by certain bacilli, fungi, spirochaetes, parasites and some viruses. For example: pneumonia, cholecystitis, salpingitis, meningitis, diphtheria, plague, peritonitis, appendicitis, actinomycosis, poliomyelitis, abscesses, furuncles, carbuncles, tonsillitis, otitis media, osteomyelitis etc.

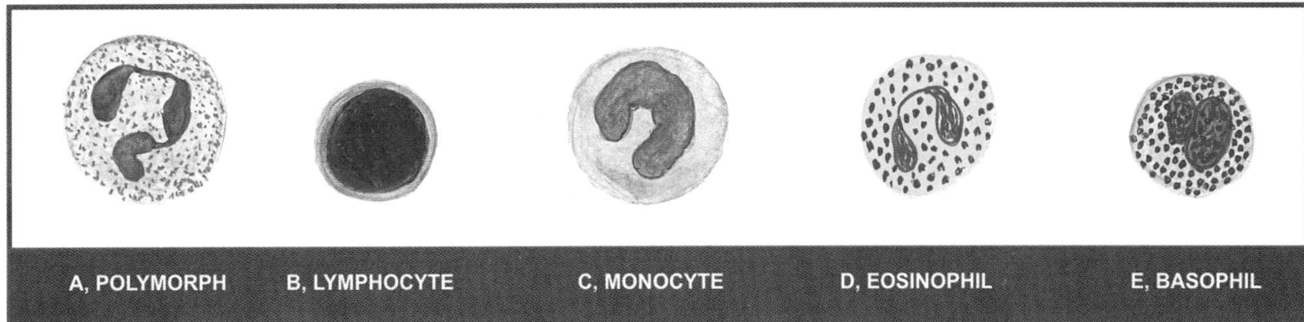

FIGURE 13.28

Morphology of normal mature leucocytes in peripheral blood.

2. *Other inflammations* e.g. tissue damage resulting from burns, operations, ischaemic necrosis (such as in MI), gout, collagen-vascular diseases, hypersensitivity reactions etc.
3. *Intoxication* e.g. uraemia, diabetic ketosis, eclampsia, poisonings by chemicals and drugs.
4. *Acute haemorrhage,* internal or external.
5. *Acute haemolysis.*
6. *Disseminated malignancies.*
7. *Myeloproliferative disorders* e.g. myeloid leukaemia, polycythaemia vera, myeloid metaplasia.
8. *Miscellaneous* e.g. following corticosteroid therapy, idiopathic neutrophilia.

Neutropenia. When the absolute neutrophil count falls below 2,500/μl, the patient is said to have neutropenia and is prone to develop recurrent infections. Some common causes of neutropenia (and hence leucopenia) are as follows:

1. *Certain infections* e.g. typhoid, paratyphoid, brucellosis, influenza, measles, viral hepatitis, malaria, kala-azar etc.
2. *Overwhelming bacterial infections* especially in patients with poor resistance e.g. miliary tuberculosis, septicaemia.
3. *Drugs, chemicals and physical agents* which induce aplasia of the bone marrow cause neutropenia, e.g. antimetabolites, nitrogen mustards, benzene, ionising radiation. Occasionally, certain drugs produce neutropenia due to individual sensitivity such as: anti-inflammatory (amidopyrine, phenylbutazone), antibacterial (chloramphenicol, cotrimoxazole), anticonvulsants, antithyroids, hypoglycaemics and antihistaminics.
4. *Certain haematological and other diseases* e.g. pernicious anaemia, aplastic anaemia, cirrhosis of the liver with splenomegaly, SLE, Gaucher's disease.
5. *Cachexia and debility.*
6. *Anaphylactoid shock.*
7. *Certain rare hereditary, congenital or familial disorders* e.g. cyclic neutropenia, primary splenic neutropenia, idiopathic benign neutropenia.

VARIATIONS IN MORPHOLOGY. Some of the common variations in neutrophil morphology are shown in Fig. 13.29. These are as under:

1. **Granules.** Heavy, dark staining, coarse toxic granules are characteristic of bacterial infections.

2. **Vacuoles.** In bacterial infections such as in septicaemia, cytoplasmic vacuolation may develop.

3. **Döhle bodies.** These are small, round or oval patches, 2-3 μm in size, in the cytoplasm. They are mostly seen in bacterial infections.

4. **Nuclear abnormalities.** These include the following:

i) *Sex chromatin* is a normal finding in 2-3% of neutrophils in female sex. It consists of a drumstick appendage of chromatin, about 1 μm across, and attached to one of the nuclear lobes by a thin chromatin strand. Their presence in more than 20% of PMNs is indicative of female sex chromosomes (Chapter 10).

ii) A *'shift-to-left'* is the term used for appearance of neutrophils with decreased number of nuclear lobes in the peripheral blood e.g. presence of band and stab forms and a few myelocytes in the peripheral blood. It is seen in severe infections, leucoerythroblastic reaction or leukaemia.

iii) A *'shift-to-right'* is appearance of hypersegmented (more than 5 nuclear lobes) neutrophils in the peripheral blood such as in megaloblastic anaemia, uraemia, and sometimes in leukaemia.

iv) *Pelger-Huët anomaly* is an inherited disorder in which majority of neutrophils have decreased number of

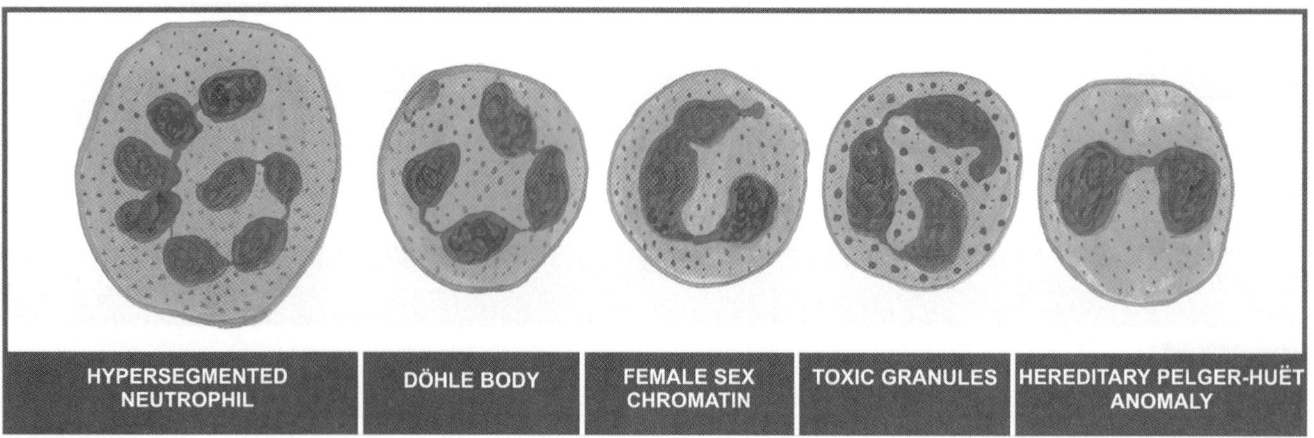

FIGURE 13.29

Common variations in neutrophil morphology.

nuclear segments (1-2) and coarsely staining chromatin. The nuclei appear rod-like, dumb-bell or spectacle-like.

DEFECTIVE FUNCTIONS. The following abnormalities in neutrophil function may sometimes be found:

1. **Defective chemotaxis** e.g. in a rare congenital abnormality called lazy-leucocyte syndrome; following corticosteroid therapy, aspirin ingestion, alcoholism, and in myeloid leukaemia.
2. **Defective phagocytosis** due to lack of opsonisation e.g. in hypogammaglobulinaemia, hypocomplementaemia, after splenectomy, in sickle cell disease.
3. **Defective killing** e.g. in chronic granulomatous disease, Chédiak-Higashi syndrome, myeloid leukaemias.

Lymphocytes

MORPHOLOGY. Majority of lymphocytes in the peripheral blood are *small* (9-12 μm in diameter) but *large* lymphocytes (12-16 μm in diameter) are also found. Both small and large lymphocytes have round or slightly indented nucleus with coarsely-clumped chromatin and scanty basophilic cytoplasm. Plasma cells are derived from B lymphocytes under the influence of appropriate stimuli. The nucleus of plasma cell is eccentric and has cart-wheel pattern of clumped nuclear chromatin. The cytoplasm is characteristically deeply basophilic with a pale perinuclear zone. Plasma cells are normally not present in peripheral blood but their pathological proliferation occurs in myelomatosis. Reactive lymphocytes (or Turk cells or plasmacytoid lymphocytes) are seen in certain viral infections and have sufficiently basophilic cytoplasm that they resemble plasma cells.

Functionally, there are 3 types of lymphocytes and possess distinct surface markers called clusters of differentiation (CD) which aid in identification of stage of their differentiation:

T lymphocytes i.e. thymus-dependent lymphocytes, which mature in the thymus and are also known as thymocytes. They are mainly involved in direct action on antigens and are therefore involved in *cell-mediated immune (CMI)* reaction by its subsets such as cytotoxic (killer) T cells (CD3+), CD8+ T cells, and *delayed hypersensitivity reaction* by CD4+ T cells.

B lymphocytes i.e. bone marrow-dependent or bursa-equivalent lymphocytes as well as their derivatives, plasma cells, are the source of specific immunoglobulin antibodies. They are, therefore, involved in *humoral immunity (HI) or circulating immune reactions.*

NK cells i.e. natural killer cells are those lymphocytes which morphologically have appearance of lymphocytes but do not possess functional features of T or B cells. As the name indicates they are identified with 'natural' or innate immunity and bring about direct 'killing' of microorganisms or lysis of foreign body.

PATHOLOGIC VARIATIONS. A rise in the absolute count of lymphocytes exceeding the upper limit of normal (above 4,000/μm) is termed *lymphocytosis,* while absolute lymphocyte count below 1,500/μm is referred to as *lymphopenia.*

Lymphocytosis. Some of the common causes of lymphocytosis are as under:

1. *Certain acute infections* e.g. pertussis, infectious mononucleosis, viral hepatitis, infectious lymphocytosis.
2. *Certain chronic infections* e.g. brucellosis, tuberculosis, secondary syphilis.
3. *Haematopoietic disorders* e.g. lymphatic leukaemias, lymphosarcoma, heavy chain disease.

4. *Relative lymphocytosis* is found in viral exanthemas, convalescence from acute infections, thyrotoxicosis, conditions causing neutropenia.

Lymphopenia. Lymphopenia is uncommon and occurs in the following conditions:
1. Most acute infections.
2. Severe bone marrow failure.
3. Corticosteroid and immunosuppressive therapy.
4. Widespread irradiation.

Monocytes

MORPHOLOGY. The monocyte is the largest mature leucocyte in the peripheral blood measuring 12-20 μm in diameter. It possesses a large, central, oval, notched or indented or horseshoe-shaped nucleus which has characteristically fine reticulated chromatin network. The cytoplasm is abundant, pale blue and contains many fine granules and vacuoles.

The main **functions** of monocytes are as under:
1. *Phagocytosis* of antigenic material or microorganisms.
2. Immunologic funtion as *antigen-presenting cells* and present the antigen to lymphocytes to deal with further.
3. As *mediator of inflammation*, they are involved in release of prostaglandins, stimulation of the liver to secrete acute phase reactants.

Tissue macrophages of different types included in RE system are derived from blood monocytes (Chapter 4).

PATHOLOGIC VARIATIONS. A rise in the blood monocytes above 800/ml is termed *monocytosis.* Some common causes of monocytosis are as follows:

1. *Certain bacterial infections* e.g. tuberculosis, subacute bacterial endocarditis, syphilis.
2. *Viral infections.*
3. *Protozoal and rickettsial infections* e.g. malaria, typhus, trypanosomiasis, kala-azar.
4. *Convalescence from acute infection.*
5. *Haematopoietic disorders* e.g. monocytic leukaemia, lymphomas, myeloproliferative disorders, multiple myeloma, lipid storage disease.
6. *Malignancies* e.g. cancer of the ovary, stomach, breast.
7. *Granulomatous diseases* e.g. sarcoidosis, inflammatory bowel disease.
8. *Collagen-vascular diseases.*

Eosinophils

MORPHOLOGY. Eosinophils are similar to segmented neutrophils in size (12-15 μm in diameter), and have coarse, deep red staining granules in the cytoplasm and have usually two nuclear lobes. Granules in eosinophils contain basic protein and stain more intensely for peroxidase than granules in the neutrophils. In addition, eosinophils also contain cell adhesion molecules, cytokines (IL-3, IL-5), and a protein that precipitates Charcot-Leyden crystals in lung tissues in asthmatic patients.

Eosinophils are involved in reactions to foreign proteins and to antigen-antibody reactions.

PATHOLOGIC VARIATIONS. An increase in the number of eosinophilic leucocytes above 400/μl is referred to as *eosinophilia* and below 40/μl is termed as *eosinopenia.*

Eosinophilia. The causes are:
1. Allergic disorders e.g. bronchial asthma, urticaria, angioneurotic oedema, hay fever, drug hypersensitivity.
2. *Parasitic infestations* e.g. trichinosis, echinococcosis, intestinal parasitism.
3. *Skin diseases* e.g. pemphigus, dermatitis herpetiformis, erythema multiforme.
4. *Löeffler's syndrome.*
5. *Pulmonary infiltration with eosinophilia* (PIE) syndrome.
6. *Tropical eosinophilia.*
7. *Haematopoietic diseases* e.g. CML, polycythaemia vera, pernicious anaemia, Hodgkin's disease, following splenectomy.
8. *Malignant diseases* with metastases.
9. *Irradiation.*
10. *Miscellaneous disorders* e.g. polyarteritis nodosa, rheumatoid arthritis, sarcoidosis.

Eosinopenia. Adrenal steroids and ACTH induce eosinopenia in man.

Basophils

MORPHOLOGY. Basophils resemble the other mature granulocytes but are distinguished by coarse, intensely basophilic granules which usually fill the cytoplasm and often overlie and obscure the nucleus.

The granules of basophils contain heparin, histamine and 5-HT. In the tissues these cells become *mast cells.* Mast cells or basophils on degranulation are associated with histamine release.

PATHOLOGIC VARIATIONS. Basophil leucocytosis or *basophilia* refers to an increase in the number of basophilic leucocytes above 100/μl. Basophilia is unusual and is found in the following conditions:
1. Chronic myeloid leukaemia
2. Polycythaemia vera

3. Myelosclerosis
4. Myxoedema
5. Ulcerative colitis
6. Following splenectomy
7. Hodgkin's disease
8. Urticaria pigmentosa.

INFECTIOUS MONONUCLEOSIS

Infectious mononucleosis (IM) or glandular fever is a benign, self-limiting lymphoproliferative disease caused by Epstein-Barr virus (EBV), one of the herpesviruses. Infection may occur from childhood to old age but the classical acute infection is more common in teenagers and young adults. The infection is transmitted by person-to-person contact such as by kissing with transfer of virally-contaminated saliva. Groups of cases occur particularly in young people living together in boarding schools, colleges, camps and military institutions. Primary infection in childhood is generally asymptomatic, while 50% of adults develop clinical manifestations. The condition is so common that by the age of 40, most people have been infected and developed antibodies. It may be mentioned here that EBV is oncogenic as well and is strongly implicated in the African (endemic) Burkitt's lymphoma and nasopharyngeal carcinoma as discussed in Chapter 8.

Pathogenesis

EBV, the etiologic agent for IM, is a B lymphotropic herpesvirus. The disease is characterised by fever, generalised lymphadenopathy, hepatosplenomegaly, sore throat, and appearance in blood of atypical 'mononucleosis cells'. The pathogenesis of these pathologic features is outlined below:

1. In a susceptible sero-negative host who lacks antibodies, the virus in the contaminated saliva *invades and replicates within epithelial cells* of the salivary gland and then enters B cells in the lymphoid tissues which possess receptors for EBV. The infection spreads throughout the body via the bloodstream or by infected B cells.

2. Viraemia and death of infected B cells causes an acute febrile illness and appearance of specific humoral antibodies which peak about 2 weeks after the infection and persist throughout life. The appearance of antibodies marks the *disappearance of virus from the blood.*

3. Though the viral agent has disappeared from the blood, the EBV-infected B cells continue to be present in the circulation as latent infection. *EBV-infected B cells undergo polyclonal activation and proliferation.* These cells perform two important roles which are the characteristic diagnostic features of IM:

i) They secrete *antibodies*—initially IgM but later IgG appears. IgM antibody is the heterophile anti-sheep antibody used for diagnosis of IM while IgG antibody persists for life and provides immunity against re-infection.

ii) They *activate T lymphocytes* of two types— CD8+ T lymphocytes and cytotoxic (suppressor) T cells. CD8+ T cells bring about killing of B cells while the cytotoxic T cells are pathognomonic atypical lymphocytes seen in blood in IM.

4. The proliferation of these cells is responsible for *generalised lymphadenopathy and hepatosplenomegaly.*

5. The *sore throat* in IM may be caused by either necrosis of B cells or due to viral replication within the salivary epithelial cells in early stage.

Besides the involvement of EBV in the pathogenesis of IM, its role in neoplastic transformation in nasopharyngeal carcinoma and Burkitt's lymphoma is discussed in Chapter 8 and diagrammatically depicted in Fig. 13.30.

Clinical Features

The incubation period of IM is 30-50 days in young adults, while children have shorter incubation period. A prodromal period of 3-5 days is followed by frank clinical features lasting for 1-3 weeks, and complete recovery after 2 months. The usual clinical features are as under:

1. During prodromal period (first 3-5 days), the symptoms are mild such as malaise, myalgia, headache and fatigue.

2. Frank clinical features (next 7-21 days), commonly are fever, sore throat and bilateral cervical lymphadenopathy. Less commonly, splenomegaly (50% patients), hepatomegaly (10% cases), transient erythematous maculopapular eruption on the trunk and extremities, and neurologic manifestations are found. Pneumonia and cardiac involvement are infrequent. One of the complications of IM is splenic rupture due to splenitis.

Laboratory Findings

The diagnosis of IM is made by characteristic haematologic and serologic findings.

1. Blood picture. The peripheral blood shows a moderate rise in total white cell count (10,000-20,000/μl) with an absolute lymphocytosis. The lymphocytosis is due to rise in normal as well as atypical

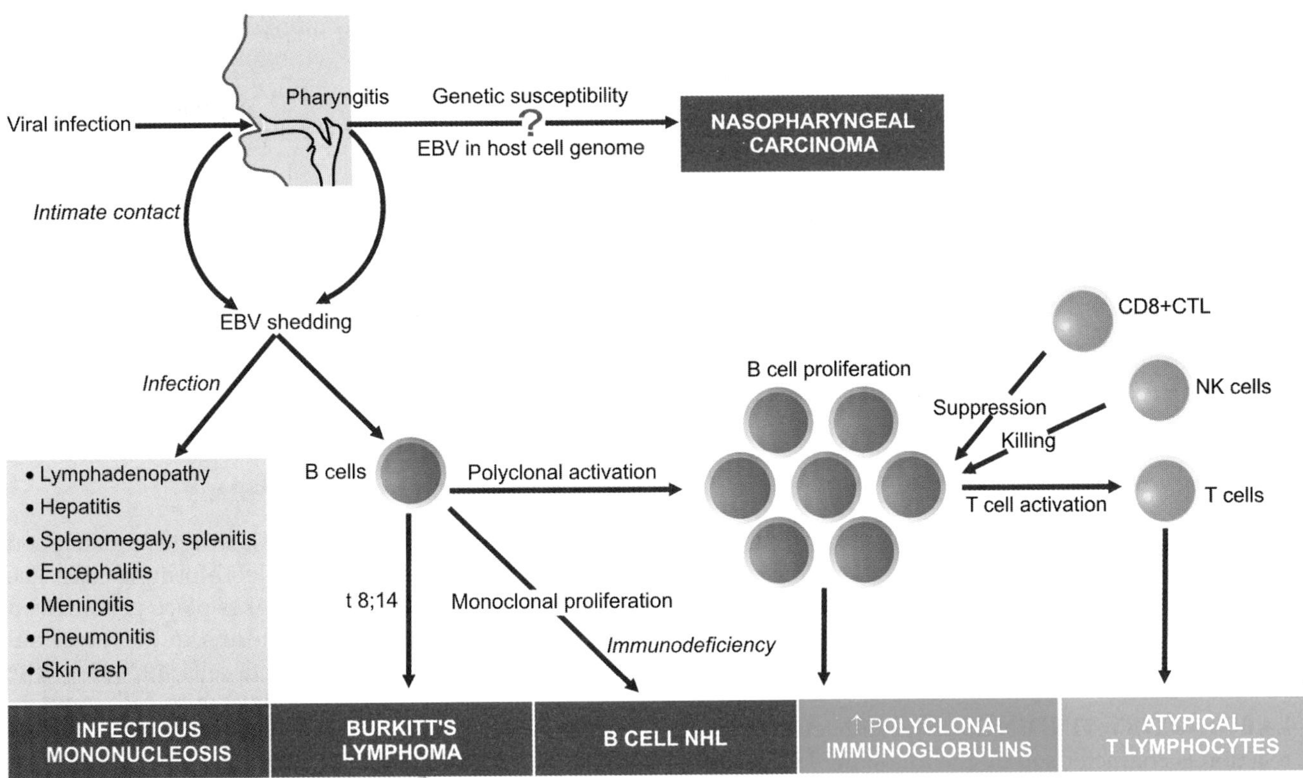

FIGURE 13.30

The role of EBV in the pathogenesis of infectious mononucleosis, nasopharyngeal carcinoma and Burkitt's lymphoma.

T lymphocytes. Essential to the diagnosis of IM is the presence of at least 10-12% *atypical T cells (or mononucleosis cells)* of the total lymphocytes in the peripheral blood. The mononucleosis cells are variable in appearance and are classed as Downey type I, II and III, of which Downey type I are found most frequently. These atypical T lymphocytes are usually of the size of large lymphocytes (12-16 μm diameter). The nucleus, rather than the usual round configuration, is oval, kidney-shaped or slightly lobate and contains relatively fine chromatin without nucleoli suggesting an immature pattern but short of leukaemic features. The cytoplasm is more abundant, basophilic and finely granular. The greatest number of atypical lymphocytes is found between 7th to 10th day of the illness and these cells may persist in the blood for up to 2 months.

2. Serologic diagnosis. The second characteristic laboratory finding is the demonstration of antibodies in the serum of infected patient. These are as under:

i) *Heterophile antibodies* against sheep red cells are found in the serum at high titer (Paul-Bunnell test) in 80-90% patients of IM, with a peak during the 2nd and 3rd week. Similar antibody is also produced in patients suffering from serum sickness and has to be distinguished by differential absorption studies. Heterophile antibody against ox and horse is also produced and is more specific. Heterophile antibody in the early stage is IgM but later IgA class antibody appears which persists throughout life.

ii) *Specific antibody for EBV antigen.* The appearance of specific EBV antibody in the first 2-3 weeks can also be demonstrated.

iii) *EBV antigen.* If viral diagnostic facilities are available, EBV antigen can also be demonstrated.

3. Other laboratory findings. In addition, abnormalities of the liver function test may be found in some cases. These include elevated serum levels of transaminases (SGOT and SGPT), rise in serum alkaline phosphatase and mild icterus.

LEUKAEMOID REACTIONS

Leukaemoid reaction is defined as a reactive excessive leucocytosis in the peripheral blood resembling that of leukaemia in a subject who does not have leukaemia.

In spite of confusing blood picture, the clinical features of leukaemia such as splenomegaly, lymphadenopathy and haemorrhages are usually absent and the features of underlying disorder causing the leukaemoid reaction are generally obvious.

Leukaemoid reaction may be myeloid or lymphoid; the former is much more common.

Myeloid Leukaemoid Reaction

CAUSES. The majority of leukaemoid reactions involve the granulocyte series. It may occur in association with a wide variety of diseases. These are as under:

1. *Infections* e.g. staphylococcal pneumonia, disseminated tuberculosis, meningitis, diphtheria, sepsis, endocarditis, plague, infected abortions etc.
2. *Intoxication* e.g. eclampsia, mercury poisoning, severe burns.
3. *Malignant diseases* e.g. multiple myeloma, myelofibrosis, Hodgkin's disease, bone metastases.
4. *Severe haemorrhage and severe haemolysis.*

LABORATORY FINDINGS. Myeloid leukaemoid reaction is characterised by the following laboratory features:

1. *Leucocytosis,* usually moderate, not exceeding 100,000/μl.
2. Proportion of *immature cells* mild to moderate, comprised by metamyelocytes, myelocytes (5-15%), and blasts fewer than 5% i.e. the blood picture simulates that of CML.
3. Infective cases may show *toxic granulation and Döhle bodies* in the cytoplasm of neutrophils.
4. *Neutrophil alkaline phosphatase (NAP) score* in the cytoplasm of mature neutrophils in leukaemoid reaction is characteristically high and is very useful to distinguish it from chronic myeloid leukaemia in doubtful cases.
5. *Cytogenetic studies* may be helpful in exceptional cases which reveal negative Philadelphia chromosome in myeloid leukaemoid reaction but positive in cases of CML.
6. *Additional features* include anaemia, normal-to-raised platelet count, myeloid hyperplasia of the marrow and absence of infiltration by immature cells in organs and tissues.

Lymphoid Leukaemoid Reaction

CAUSES. Lymphoid leukaemoid reaction may be found in the following conditions:

1. *Infections* e.g. infectious mononucleosis, cytomegalovirus infection, pertussis (whooping cough), chickenpox, measles, infectious lymphocytosis, tuberculosis.
2. *Malignant diseases* may rarely produce lymphoid leukaemoid reaction.

LABORATORY FINDINGS. The blood picture is characterised by the following findings:

1. Leucocytosis not exceeding 100,000/μl.
2. The differential white cell count reveals mostly mature lymphocytes simulating the blood picture found in cases of CLL.

LEUKAEMIAS

DEFINITION AND CLASSIFICATION

The leukaemias are a group of disorders characterised by malignant transformation of blood-forming cells. The proliferation of leukaemic cells takes place primarily in the bone marrow, and in certain forms, in the lymphoid tissues. Ultimately, the abnormal cells appear in the peripheral blood raising the total white cell count to high level. In addition, features of bone marrow failure (e.g. anaemia, thrombocytopenia, neutropenia) and involvement of other organs (e.g. liver, spleen, lymph nodes, meninges, brain, skin etc) occur.

In general, leukaemias are classified on the basis of cell types predominantly involved, into *myeloid* and *lymphoid,* and on the basis of natural history of the disease, into *acute* and *chronic.* Thus, the main types are: *acute myeloblastic leukaemia* and *acute lymphoblastic leukaemia* (AML and ALL), and *chronic myeloid leukaemia* and *chronic lymphocytic leukaemias* (CML and CLL); *hairy cell leukaemia* (HCL) is an unusual variant of lymphoid neoplasia.

Leukaemias account for 4% of all cancer deaths. Generally, acute leukaemias have a rapidly downhill course, whereas chronic leukaemias tend to have more indolent behaviour. The incidence of both acute and chronic leukaemias is higher in men than in women. ALL is primarily a disease of children and young adults, whereas AML occurs at all ages. CLL tends to occur in the elderly, while CML is found in middle age.

ETIOLOGY

The etiology of leukaemia is not known in most patients. However, a number of factors have been implicated.

1. GENETIC FACTORS. There is high concordance rate among identical twins if acute leukaemia develops in the first year of life. Families with excessive incidence of leukaemia have been identified. Acute leukaemia occurs with increased frequency with a variety of congenital disorders such as Down's, Bloom's, Klinefelter's and Wiskott-Aldrich's syndromes, Fanconi's anaemia and ataxia telangiectasia.

2. ENVIRONMENTAL FACTORS. Certain environmental factors are known to play a role in the etiology of leukaemia. These include the following:

i) Ionising radiation e.g. in individuals exposed to occupational radiation exposure, patients receiving radiation therapy, and Japanese survivors of the atomic bomb explosions. Radiation exposure is related to the development of CML, AML and ALL *but not to CLL or HCL.*

ii) Chemical carcinogens e.g. benzene and other aromatic hydrocarbons are associated with the development of AML.

iii) Certain drugs e.g. treatment with alkylating agents and other chemotherapeutic agents is associated with increased incidence of AML.

3. INFECTION. Induction of leukaemias in experimental animals by RNA viruses (retroviruses) has been studied for quite sometime but more recently viral etiology of adult T cell leukaemia-lymphoma (ATLL) by a human retrovirus called human T cell leukaemia-lymphoma virus I (HTLV-I) and HTLV II for T cell variant of hairy cell leukaemia has been established (Chapter 8).

PATHOGENESIS (LEUKAEMOGENESIS)

The leukaemia arises following *malignant transformation of a single clone of cells belonging to myeloid or lymphoid series, followed by proliferation of the transformed clone.* The evolution of leukaemia is multi-step process, and in many cases, acute leukaemia may develop after a pre-existing myelodysplastic or myeloproliferative disorder.

The salient features in the pathogenesis of leukaemias are as under:

- In acute leukaemia, the single most prominent characteristic of the leukaemic cells is a defect in maturation beyond the myeloblast or promyelocyte level in AML, and the lymphoblast level in ALL. However, it may be emphasised here that it is the *maturation defect* in leukaemic blasts rather than rapid proliferation of leukaemic cells responsible for causing acute leukaemia. In fact, the generation time of leukaemic blasts is somewhat prolonged rather than shortened.
- The leukaemic cells proliferate primarily in the bone marrow, circulate in the blood and *infiltrate into other tissues* such as lymph nodes, liver, spleen, skin, viscera and the central nervous system.
- The *mechanism of leukaemic transformation* is poorly understood. But the basic defect lies in the DNA, conferring a heritable malignant characteristic to the transformed cell and its progeny. A neoplastic phenotype may be induced by RNA viruses (e.g. HTLV-I) and causes insertional mutagenesis for which oncogenes may play a role as discussed in Chapter 8. A number of clonal cytogenetic abnormalities have been reported in association with the various forms of acute and chronic leukaemias. The most consistent chromosomal abnormality among these is Philadelphia (Ph) chromosome seen in 70-90% cases with CML, involving reciprocal translocation of parts of long arm of chromosome 22 to the long arm of chromosome 9 i.e. t(9;22) (Fig. 13.31).
- As the leukaemic cells accumulate in the bone marrow, they *suppress normal haematopoietic stem cells,* partly by physically replacing the normal marrow precursors. However, some patients with acute leukaemia have a hypocellular marrow indicating that marrow failure is not simply due to overcrowding by leukaemic cells but may inhibit normal haematopoiesis via cell-mediated or humoral mechanisms. Nevertheless, some normal haematopoietic stem cells do remain in the marrow which are capable of proliferating and

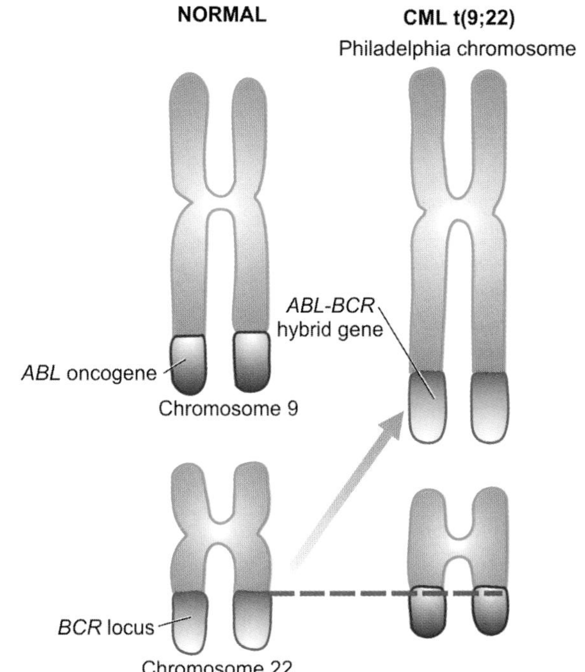

FIGURE 13.31

The Philadelphia (Ph) chromosome. There is reciprocal translocation of the part of the long arms of chromosome 22 to the long arms of chromosome 9 written as t(9;22).

restoring normal haematopoiesis after effective anti-leukaemic treatment.

ACUTE LEUKAEMIAS

Acute leukaemias are characterised by predominance of undifferentiated leucocyte precursors or leukaemic blasts. Acute leukaemias may be derived from the myeloid stem cells called *acute myeloblastic leukaemia (AML)*, or from the lymphoid stem cells termed *acute lymphoblastic leukaemia (ALL)*.

Recently, more definite criteria for diagnosis and classification of acute leukaemias have been laid down by a group of French, American and British haematologists commonly called the *FAB classification*. According to this system, a leukaemia is acute if the bone marrow consists of more than 30% blasts. FAB classification divides AML into 8 subtypes (M0 to M7) and ALL into 3 subtypes (L1 to L3) as shown in Table 13.19. Another classification called Revised European-American classification of Lymphoid neoplasms (REAL classification) has been formulated and includes lymphoid leukaemias (acute and chronic) and non-Hodgkin's lymphomas since they represent the counterparts of neoplastic cells in the bone marrow and lymphoid tissue (page 451). More recently, WHO classification for AML has been proposed which takes in to consideration cytogenetic and molecular abnormalities in different types.

Thus, the basis of these categorisation of leukaemias can be summed up as:

- *FAB classification* is based on *morphologic and cytochemical features.*
- *REAL classification* is based on *immunophenotypic features.*
- *WHO classification* is based on *cytogenetic and molecular features.*

Clinical Features

AML and ALL share many clinical features. In approximately 25% of patients with AML, a preleukaemic syndrome with anaemia and other cytopenias is usually present for a few months to years prior to the development of overt leukaemia.

TABLE 13.19: Revised FAB Classification of Acute Leukaemias.

FAB CLASS		PER CENT CASES	MORPHOLOGY	CYTOCHEMISTRY
ACUTE MYELOBLASTIC LEUKAEMIA (AML)				
M0:	*Minimally differentiated AML*	2	Blasts lack definite cytologic and cytochemical features but have myeloid lineage antigens	Myeloperoxidase –
M1:	*AML without maturation*	20	Myeloblasts predominate; few if any granules or Auer rods	Myeloperoxidase +
M2:	*AML with maturation*	30	Myeloblasts with promyelocytes predominate; Auer rods may be present	Myeloperoxidase +++
M3:	*Acute promyelocytic leukaemia*	5	Hypergranular promyelocytes; often with multiple Auer rods per cell	Myeloperoxidase +++
M4:	*Acute myelomonocytic leukaemia (Naegeli type)*	30	Mature cells of both myeloid and monocytic series in peripheral blood; myeloid cells resemble M2	Myeloperoxidase ++ Non-specific esterase +
M5:	*Acute monocytic leukaemia (Schilling type)*	10	Two subtypes: M5a shows poorly-differentiated monoblasts, M5b shows differentiated promonocytes and monocytes	Non-specific esterase ++
M6:	*Acute erythroleukaemia (Di Guglielmo's syndrome)*	<5	Erythroblasts predominate (>50%); myeloblasts and promyelocytes also increased	Erythroblasts:PAS + Myeloblasts: myeloperoxidase +
M7:	*Acute megakaryocytic leukaemia*	<5	Pleomorphic undifferentiated blasts predominate; react with antiplatelet antibodies	Platelet peroxidase +
ACUTE LYMPHOBLASTIC LEUKAEMIA (ALL)				
L1:	*Childhood-ALL (B-ALL, and T-ALL)*	More common in children	Homogeneous small lymphoblasts; scanty cytoplasm, regular round nuclei, inconspicuous nucleoli	PAS ± Acid phosphatase ±
L2:	*Adult-ALL (mostly T-ALL)*	More frequent in adults	Heterogeneous lymphoblasts; variable amount of cytoplasm, irregular or cleft nuclei, large nucleoli	PAS ± Acid phosphatase ±
L3:	*Burkitt type-ALL (B-ALL)*	Uncommon	Large homogeneous lymphoblasts; round nuclei, prominent nucleoli, cytoplasmic vacuolation	PAS – Acid phosphatase –

Clinical manifestations of acute leukaemias are divided into 2 groups: those *due to bone marrow failure*, and those *due to organ infiltration.*

I. DUE TO BONE MARROW FAILURE. These are as under:

1. *Anaemia* producing pallor, lethargy, dyspnoea.
2. *Bleeding manifestations* due to thrombocytopenia causing spontaneous bruises, petechiae, bleeding from gums and other bleeding tendencies.
3. *Infections* are quite common and include those of mouth, throat, skin, respiratory, perianal and other sites.
4. *Fever* is generally attributed to infections in acute leukaemia but sometimes no obvious source of infection can be found and may occur in the absence of infection.

II. DUE TO ORGAN INFILTRATION. The clinical manifestations of acute leukaemia are more often due to replacement of the marrow and other tissues by leukaemic cells. These features are as under:

1. *Pain and tenderness of bones* (e.g. sternal tenderness) are due to bone infarcts or subperiosteal infiltrates by leukaemic cells. These features are more frequent in children with ALL.
2. *Lymphadenopathy* and enlargement of the *tonsils* are more common in ALL.
3. *Splenomegaly* of moderate grade is common, especially in ALL. Splenic infarction, subcapsular haemorrhages, and rarely, splenic rupture may occur.
4. *Hepatomegaly* is frequently present due to leukaemic infiltration but the infiltrates usually do not interfere with the function of the liver.
5. *Leukaemic infiltration of the kidney* may be present and ordinarily does not interfere with its function unless secondary complications such as haemorrhage or blockage of ureter supervene.
6. *Gum hypertrophy* due to leukaemic infiltration of the gingivae is a frequent finding in myelomonocytic (M4) and monocytic (M5) leukaemias.
7. *Chloroma or granulocytic sarcoma* is a localised tumour-forming mass occurring in the skin or orbit due to local infiltration of the tissues by leukaemic cells. The tumour is greenish in appearance due to the presence of myeloperoxidase.
8. *Meningeal involvement* manifested by raised intracranial pressure, headache, nausea and vomiting, blurring of vision and diplopia are seen more frequently in ALL during haematologic remission. Sudden death from massive intracranial haemorrhage as a result of leucostasis may occur.
9. *Other organ infiltrations* include testicular swelling in ALL and mediastinal compression in T cell type ALL.

Laboratory Findings

The diagnosis of acute leukaemia is made by a combination of routine blood picture and bone marrow examination, coupled with cytochemical stains and certain biochemical investigations.

I. BLOOD PICTURE. Findings of routine haematologic investigations are as under (Fig. 13.32) (COLOUR PLATE XVI: CL 64):

1. Anaemia. Anaemia is almost always present in acute leukaemias. It is generally severe, progressive and normochromic in type. A moderate reticulocytosis up to 5% and a few nucleated red cells may be present.

2. Thrombocytopenia. The platelet count is usually moderately to severely decreased (below 50,000/μl) but occasionally it may be normal. Bleeding tendencies in acute leukaemia are usually correlated with the level of thrombocytopenia but most serious spontaneous haemorrhagic episodes develop in patients with fewer than 20,000/μl platelets. Acute promyelocytic leukaemia (M3) may be associated with a serious coagulation abnormality called disseminated intravascular coagulation (DIC).

3. White blood cells. The total WBC count ranges from subnormal-to-markedly elevated values. In 25% of patients, the total WBC count at presentation is reduced to 1,000-4,000 /μl. More often, however, there is progressive rise in white cell count which may exceed 100,000/μl in more advanced disease. The majority of leucocytes in the peripheral blood are blasts and there is often neutropenia due to marrow infiltration by leukaemic cells. Some patients present with pancytopenia and have a few blasts *(subleukaemic leukaemia)* or no blasts *(aleukaemic leukaemia)* in the blood. Both these conditions are nowadays included under *'myelodysplastic syndrome'* (page 404). The basic morphologic features of myeloblasts, lymphoblasts and monoblasts are described in Table 13.17. Typical characteristics of different forms of AML (M0 to M7) and ALL (L1 to L3) are given in Table 13.19. In some instances, the *identification of blast cells is greatly aided by the company they keep* i.e. by more mature and easily identifiable leucocytes in the company of blastic cells of myeloid or lymphoid series. It is usual to find some *'smear cells'* in the

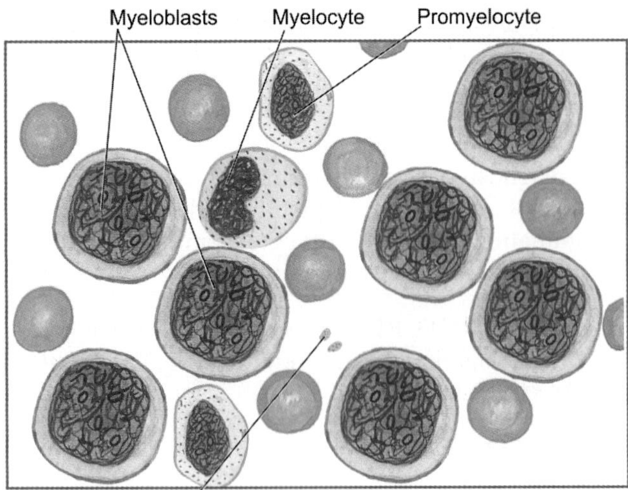

FIGURE 13.32

PBF findings in a case of acute myeloblastic leukaemia (AML).

peripheral blood which represent degenerated leucocytes, particularly in the case of ALL.

II. BONE MARROW EXAMINATION. An examination of bone marrow aspirate or trephine reveals the following features:

1. Cellularity. Typically, the marrow is hypercellular but sometimes a 'blood tap' or 'dry tap' occurs. A dry tap in acute leukaemia may be due to pancytopenia, but sometimes even when the marrow is filled with leukaemic cells they cannot be aspirated because the cells are adhesive and enmeshed in reticulin fibres. In such cases, trephine biopsy should be done.

2. Leukaemic cells. The bone marrow is generally tightly packed with leukaemic blast cells. The diagnosis of the type of leukaemic cells, according to FAB classification, is generally possible with routine Romanowsky stains but cytochemical stains may be employed as an adjunct to Romanowsky staining for determining the type of leukaemia. The essential criteria for diagnosis of acute leukaemia, as per FAB classification, is the presence of at least 30% blasts in the bone marrow. However, lately As per WHO classsification of leukaemias, these criteria have been revised upwards to 20% blasts in the marrow for labelling and treating a case as AML.

3. Erythropoiesis. Erythropoietic cells are reduced. Dyserythropoiesis, megaloblastic features and ring sideroblasts are commonly present.

4. Megakaryocytes. They are usually reduced or absent.

5. Cytogenetics. Chromosomal analysis of dividing leukaemic cells in the marrow shows karyotypic abnormalities in 75% of cases which may have a relationship to prognosis. WHO classification has recently emphasised on the categorisation of acute leukaemias on the basis of cytogenetic abnormalities. Two of the most consistent cytogenetic abnormalities in specific FAB groups are as under:

i) *M3* cases have t(15;17)(q22;q12).

ii) *M4Eo* (E for abnormal eosinophils in the bone marrow) cases have inv(16)(p13q22).

III. CYTOCHEMISTRY. Some of the commonly employed cytochemical stains, as an aid to classify the type of acute leukaemia, are listed below (also see Table 13.18):

1. Myeloperoxidase: Positive in immature myeloid cells containing granules and Auer rods but negative in M0 myeloblasts.

2. Sudan Black: Positive in immature cells in AML.

3. Periodic acid-Schiff (PAS): Positive in immature lymphoid cells and in erythroleukaemia (M6).

4. Non-specific esterase (NSE): Positive in monocytic series (M4 and M5).

5. Acid phosphatase: Focal positivity in leukaemic blasts in ALL and diffuse reaction in monocytic cells (M4 and M5).

IV. IMMUNOPHENOTYPING. AML cells express CD13 and CD33 antigens; M7 shows CD41 and CD42 positivity. However, for ALL the FAB classification given in Table 13.19 is based on morphologic features, currently as per REAL-WHO classification for all lymphoid malignancies (lymphoid leukaemias and lymphomas), lymphoid leukaemias (both ALL and CLL) are subdivided on the basis of immunologic features by identification as regards their B or T cell origin and cytogenetic abnormalities (*see* Table 14.3, page 451). According to this classification, ALL is redivided into pre-B ALL, T cell ALL and B cell ALL with distinct cytogenetic and immunologic features (Table 13.20).

V. OTHER INVESTIGATIONS. Other laboratory tests which may be of some help in classifying leukaemias are as under:

1. Serum muramidase. Serum levels of lysozyme (i.e. muramidase) are elevated in myelomonocytic (M4) and monocytic (M5) leukaemias.

TABLE 13.20: WHO-REAL Classification of ALL on the Basis of Immunologic and Cytogenetic Features.

SUBTYPE	INCIDENCE	MARKERS	FAB SUBTYPE	CYTOGENETIC ABNORMALITIES
Pre-B ALL	75%	CD10+ (90%), TdT+	L1, L2	t(9;22) i.e. Philadelphia+ALL
B cell ALL	5%	CD10+ (50%), TdT-	L3	t(8;14) (Burkitt's leukaemia)
T cell ALL	20%	CD10+ (30%), TdT+	L1, L2	14q11

(TdT= terminal deoxynucleotidyl transferase)

2. Serum uric acid. Because of rapidly growing number of leukaemic cells, serum uric acid level is frequently increased. The levels are further raised after treatment with cytotoxic drugs because of increased cell breakdown.

Treatment

The management of acute leukaemia involves the following aspects:

I. TREATMENT OF ANAEMIA AND HAEMORRHAGE. Anaemia and haemorrhage are managed by fresh blood transfusions and platelet concentrates. Patients with severe thrombocytopenia (platelet count below 20,000/μl) require regular platelet transfusions since haemorrhage is an important cause of death in these cases.

II. TREATMENT AND PROPHYLAXIS OF INFECTION. Neutropenia due to bone marrow replacement by leukaemic blasts and as a result of intensive cytotoxic therapy renders these patients highly susceptible to infection. The infections are predominantly bacterial but viral, fungal, and protozoal infections also occur. For prophylaxis against infection in such cases, the patient should be isolated and preferably placed in laminar airflow rooms. Efforts are made to reduce the gut and other commensal flora which are the usual source of infection. This is achieved by bowel sterilisation and by topical antiseptics. If these fail to achieve the desired results, systemic antibiotics and leucocyte concentrates are considered for therapy.

III. CYTOTOXIC DRUG THERAPY. The aims of cytotoxic therapy are firstly to induce remission, secondly to then continue the therapy to reduce the hidden leukaemic cell population by repeated courses of therapy. Most commonly, cyclic combinations of 2, 3 and 4 drugs are given with treatment-free intervals to allow the bone marrow to recover.

Treatment of AML. The most effective treatment of AML is a combination of 3 drugs: cytosine arabinoside, anthracyclines (daunorubicin, adriamycin) and 6-thioguanine. Another recent addition is amsacrine (m-AMSA) administered with cytosine arabinoside, with or without 6-thioguanine. Following remission-induction therapy, various drug combinations are given intermittently for maintenance.

As compared with ALL, remission rate with AML is lower (50-70%), often takes longer to achieve remission, and disease-free intervals are shorter. AML is most malignant of all leukaemias; median survival with treatment is 12-18 months.

Treatment of ALL. The most useful drugs in the treatment of ALL are combination of vincristine, prednisolone, anthracyclines (daunorubicin, adriamycin) and L-asparaginase. Other agents used are cytosine arabinoside and methotrexate. Though 90% of children with ALL show remission with this therapy, patients with T cell ALL and those with meningeal involvement carry a less favourable prognosis. Meningeal leukaemia is beyond the reach of most of the cytotoxic drugs used in the therapy of ALL. CNS prophylaxis in such cases is considered after the initial remission has been obtained and includes cranial irradiation and course of intrathecal methotrexate or cytosine arabinoside.

Mean survival in ALL with treatment in children without CNS prophylaxis is 33 months, while with CNS prophylaxis is 60 months or more. Adult (T cell) ALL, however, is as grave as AML and median survival is 12-18 months.

IV. BONE MARROW TRANSPLANTATION. Bone marrow transplantation from suitable allogenic or autologous donor (HLA and mixed lymphocytes culture-matched) is increasingly being used for treating young adults with AML in first remission, and in adult-ALL with relapses. The basic principle of marrow transplantation is to reconstitute the patient's haematopoietic system after total body irradiation and intensive chemotherapy have been given so as to kill the remaining leukaemic cells. Bone marrow transplantation has resulted in cure in about half the cases.

TABLE 13.21: Contrasting Features of AML and ALL.

FEATURE	AML	ALL
1. *Common age*	Adults between 15-40 years; comprise 20% of childhood leukaemias	Children under 15 years; comprise 80% of childhood leukaemias
2. *Physical findings*	Splenomegaly + Hepatomegaly + Lymphadenopathy + Bony tenderness + Gum hypertrophy +	Splenomegaly ++ Hepatomegaly ++ Lymphadenopathy ++ Bony tenderness + Meningeal involvement +
3. *Laboratory findings*	Low-to-high TLC; predominance of myeloblasts and promyelocytes in blood and bone marrow; thrombocytopenia moderate to severe.	Low-to-high TLC, predominance of lymphoblasts in blood and bone marrow; thrombocytopenia moderate to severe.
4. *Cytochemical stains*	Myeloperoxidase +, Sudan black +, NSE + in M4 and M5, acid phosphatase (diffuse) + in M4 and M5	PAS +, acid phosphatase (focal) +
5. *Specific therapy*	Cytosine arabinoside, anthracyclines (daunorubicin, adriamycin) and 6-thioguanine	Vincristine, prednisolone, anthracyclines and L-asparaginase
6. *Response to therapy*	Remission rate low, duration of remission shorter	Remission rate high, duration of remission prolonged
7. *Median survival*	12-18 months	Children without CNS prophylaxis 33 months, with CNS prophylaxis 60 months; adults 12-18 months

The salient differences between the two main forms of acute leukaemia are summarised in Table 13.21.

CHRONIC LEUKAEMIAS

Chronic leukaemias are those haematologic malignancies in which the predominant leukaemic cells are initially well-differentiated and easily recognisable as regards their cell type. Chronic leukaemias are divided into 2 main types: chronic myeloid (granulocytic) leukaemia (CML or CGL), and chronic lymphocytic leukaemia (CLL). Less common variants include: chronic eosinophilic, chronic basophilic, chronic monocytic, chronic neutrophilic and chronic lymphosarcoma cell leukaemias. An unusual chronic lymphoproliferative variant is hairy cell leukaemia (HCL). In general, chronic leukaemias have a better prognosis than the acute leukaemias. Currently CML has come to be classified alongwith other myeloproliferative syndromes due to common histogenesis from haematopoietic stem cells (described later). However, for the purpose of present discussion, CML is described here alongwith other chronic leukaemias.

CHRONIC MYELOID LEUKAEMIA (CML)

Chronic myeloid (myelogenous, granulocytic) leukaemia comprises about 20% of all leukaemias and its peak incidence is seen in 3rd and 4th decades of life. A distinctive variant of CML seen in children is called *juvenile CML*. Both the sexes are affected equally. The exact etiology is not known but an increased incidence of both AML and CML was observed years later in Japanese atomic bomb survivors implicating radiation in their etiology.

Clinical Features

The onset of CML is generally insidious. Some of the common presenting manifestations are as under:

1. Features of *anaemia* such as weakness, pallor, dyspnoea and tachycardia.
2. Symptoms due to *hypermetabolism* such as weight loss, lassitude, anorexia, night sweats.
3. *Splenomegaly* is almost always present and is frequently massive. In some patients, it may be associated with acute pain due to splenic infarction.
4. *Bleeding tendencies* such as easy bruising, epistaxis, menorrhagia and haematomas may occur.
5. Less *commonly,* features such as gout, visual disturbance, neurologic manifestations and priapism are present.
6. *Juvenile CML* is more often associated with lymph node enlargement than splenomegaly. Other features are frequent infections, haemorrhagic manifestations and facial rash.

Laboratory Findings

The diagnosis of CML is generally possible on blood picture alone. However, bone marrow, cytochemical stains and other investigations are of help.

I. BLOOD PICTURE. The typical blood picture in a case of CML at the time of presentation shows the following features (Fig. 13.33) **(COLOUR PLATE XVII: CL 65):**

1. Anaemia. Anaemia is usually of moderate degree and is normocytic normochromic in type. Occasional normoblasts may be present.

2. White blood cells. Characteristically, there is marked leucocytosis (approximately 200,000/μl or more at the time of presentation). The natural history of CML consists of 2 phases—chronic and blastic.

■ *The chronic phase of CML* begins as a myeloproliferative disorder and consists of excessive proliferation of myeloid cells of intermediate grade (i.e. myelocytes and metamyelocytes) and mature segmented neutrophils. Myeloblasts usually do not exceed 10% of cells in the peripheral blood and bone marrow. An increase in the proportion of basophils up to 10% is a characteristic feature of CML. A rising *basophilia* is indicative of impending blastic transformation. An *accelerated phase of CML* is also described in which there is progressively rising leucocytosis associated with thrombocytosis or thrombocytopenia and splenomegaly.

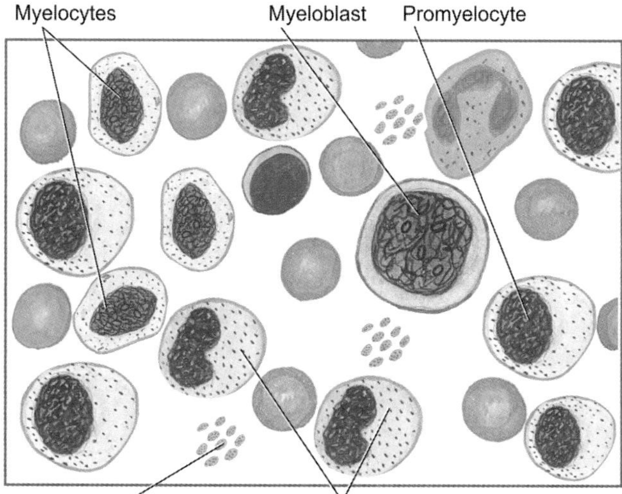

FIGURE 13.33

PBF findings in chronic myeloid leukaemia (CML).

■ *The blastic phase or blast crisis in CML* may be myeloid or lymphoid in origin. Myeloid blast crisis in CML is more common and resembles AML. However, unlike AML, Auer rods are never seen in myeloblasts of CML in blast crisis. *Lymphoid blast crisis* in CML having the characteristics of lymphoblasts such as presence of TdT and positivity for B cell markers (CD10, CD19) is seen in one-third cases of blastic phase in CML.

3. Platelets. The platelet count may be normal but is raised in about half the cases.

II. BONE MARROW EXAMINATION. Examination of marrow aspiration yields the following results:

1. Cellularity. Generally, there is hypercellularity with total or partial replacement of fat spaces by proliferating myeloid cells.

2. Myeloid cells. The myeloid cells predominate in the bone marrow with increased myeloid-erythroid ratio. The differential counts of myeloid cells in the marrow show similar findings as seen in the peripheral blood with predominance of myelocytes.

3. Erythropoiesis. Erythropoiesis is normoblastic but there is reduction in erythropoietic cells.

4. Megakaryocytes. Megakaryocytes are conspicuous but are usually smaller in size than normal.

5. Cytogenetics. Cytogenetic studies on blood and bone marrow cells show the characteristic chromosomal abnormality called Philadelphia (Ph) chromosome formed by reciprocal translocation between part of long arm of chromosome 22 and part of long arm of chromosome 9{(t(9;22)} seen in 70-90% cases with CML (*see* Fig. 13.31, page 415).

III. CYTOCHEMISTRY. The only significant finding on cytochemical stains is reduced scores of *neutrophil alkaline phosphatase (NAP)* which helps to distinguish CML from myeloid leukaemoid reaction in which case NAP scores are elevated (page 414). However, NAP scores in CML return to normal with successful therapy, corticosteroid administration and in infections.

IV. OTHER INVESTIGATIONS. A few other accompanying findings in cases of CML are:

1. Elevated serum B_{12} and vitamin B_{12} binding capacity.
2. Elevated serum uric acid (hyperuricaemia).

Treatment

Unless blastic crisis supervenes, the symptoms, physical findings and laboratory abnormalities of CML can be controlled by therapy, as outlined below:

Chronic phase. Patients with chronic phase of CML respond favourably to chemotherapy. The main chemotherapeutic agents used for chronic phase of CML are busulfan, cyclophosphamide (melphalan) and hydroxyurea. Besides chemotherapy, other forms of treatment include splenic irradiation, splenectomy, leucopheresis and bone marrow transplantation.

Effective chemotherapy results in eradication of Ph-positive cells. The median survival of chronic phase of CML with chemotherapy is 3-4 years.

Blast crisis. Acceleration of the disease is reflected by refractoriness to treatment which has been previously effective. Remissions of actual blastic phase of CML can be obtained by vincristine and prednisone or other combination chemotherapy regimens commonly employed for ALL.

Recently, it has been found that all cases of CML have an abnormally increased and dysregulated tyrosine kinase activity due to chimerism in *BCL-ABL* gene. This genetic abormality has been held responsible for proliferation of leukaemic cells in CML. This has helped in targetting the defect by specific therapy in the form of synthetic inhibitor of the *BCL-ABL* kinase called STI571that inhibits growth and proliferation of t(9;22)-bearing tumour cells.

The most common cause of death (in 80% cases) in CML is blastic transformation.

CHRONIC LYMPHOCYTIC LEUKAEMIA (CLL)

Chronic lymphocytic leukaemia constitutes about 25% of all leukaemias and is predominantly a disease of the elderly (over 50 years of age) with a male preponderance (male-female ratio 2:1). Currently, CLL is considered as part of the common lymphoid malignancy of mature B cells termed CLL/SLL i.e. CLL for cases with peripheral blood involvement while SLL for those without blood spread.

Clinical Features

The onset of disease is characteristically insidious. Common presenting manifestations are as under:

1. Features of *anaemia* such as gradually increasing weakness, fatigue and dyspnoea.
2. Enlargement of superficial *lymph nodes* is a very common finding. The lymph nodes are usually symmetrically enlarged, discrete and non-tender.
3. *Splenomegaly* and *hepatomegaly* are usual.
4. *Haemorrhagic manifestations* are found in case of CLL with thrombocytopenia.
5. *Infections,* particularly of respiratory tract, are common in CLL.
6. *Less common* are: mediastinal pressure, tonsillar enlargement, disturbed vision, and bone and joint pains.

Laboratory Findings

The diagnosis of CLL can usually be made on the basis of physical findings and blood smear examination (Fig. 13.34) (COLOUR PLATE XVII: CL 66):

I. BLOOD PICTURE. The findings of routine blood picture are as under:

1. Anaemia. Anaemia is usually mild to moderate and normocytic normochromic in type. Mild reticulocytosis may be present. About 20% cases develop a Coombs'-positive autoimmune haemolytic anaemia.

2. White blood cells. Typically, there is marked leucocytosis but less than that seen in CML (50,000-200,000/μl). Usually, more than 90% of leucocytes are mature small lymphocytes. Smear cells (degenerated forms) are present. The absolute neutrophil count is, however, generally within normal range. Granulocytopenia occurs in fairly advanced disease only.

3. Platelets. The platelet count is normal or moderately reduced.

II. BONE MARROW EXAMINATION. The typical findings are:

1. Increased lymphocyte count (25-95%).
2. Reduced myeloid precursors.
3. Reduced erythroid precursors.

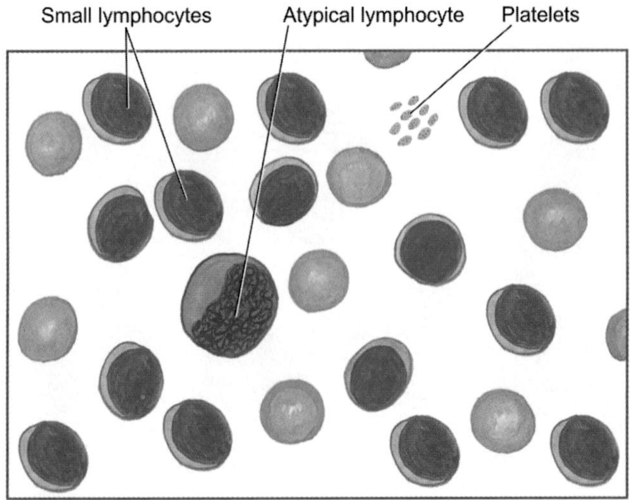

FIGURE 13.34
PBF findings in chronic lymphocytic leukaemia (CLL).

III. OTHER INVESTIGATIONS. These are:

1. *Erythrocyte rosette test* with mouse red cells is positive in more than 95% of cases indicating that CLL is a monoclonal B cell neoplasm.
2. *Positive pan-B-cell markers* e.g. CD19, CD20, CD23, surface immunoglobulins, monoclonal light chains (α or κ type).
3. *Serum immunoglobulin levels* are generally reduced.
4. *Coombs' test* is positive in 20% cases.

Treatment

Unlike other leukaemias, none of the available drugs and radiation therapy are capable of eradicating CLL and induce true complete remission. Treatment is, therefore, palliative and symptomatic, and with optimal management patient can usually lead a relatively normal life for several years. These approaches include: alkylating drugs (e.g. chlorambucil, cyclophosphamide), corticosteroids and radiotherapy. Splenectomy is indicated in cases of CLL with autoimmune haemolytic anaemia.

Prognosis is generally better than CML since *blastic transformation of CLL seldom occurs.* Rare T cell variant of CLL, however, runs a more malignant course. Prognosis generally correlates with the stage of disease as under:

Stage A: characterised by lymphocytosis alone, or with limited lymphadenopathy, has a good prognosis (median survival more than 10 years).

Stage B: having lymphocytosis with associated significant lymphadenopathy and hepatosplenomegaly has intermediate prognosis (median survival about 5 years).

Stage C: having lymphocytosis with associated anaemia and thrombocytopenia has a worse prognosis (median survival of less than 2 years).

HAIRY CELL LEUKAEMIA

Hairy cell leukaemia (HCL), is an unusual and uncommon form of chronic leukaemia in which there is presence of abnormal mononuclear cells with hairy cytoplasmic projections in the bone marrow, peripheral blood and spleen. These cells are best recognised under phase contrast microscopy but may also be visible in routine blood smears. These leukaemic 'hairy cells' have characteristically positive cytochemical staining for *tartrate-resistant acid phosphatase.* The controversy on the origin of hairy cells whether these cells represent neoplastic T cells, B cells or monocytes, is settled with the molecular analysis of these cells which assigns them *B cell origin* expressing CD19, CD20 and CD22 antigen. In addition to B cell markers, hairy cells are also positive for CD11, CD25 and CD103.

Hairy cell leukaemia occurs in the older males. It is characterised clinically by the manifestations due to infiltration of reticuloendothelial organs (bone marrow, liver and spleen) and, hence, its previous name as *leukaemic reticuloendotheliosis.* Patients have susceptibility to infection with *M. avium intercellulare.* Laboratory diagnosis is made by the presence of pancytopenia due to marrow failure and splenic sequestration, and identification of characteristic hairy cells in blood and bone marrow which are positive for tartrate-resistant acid phosphatase (TRAP).

The disease often runs a chronic course requiring supportive care. The mean survival is 4-5 years. Patients respond to splenectomy, α-interferon therapy and 2-chlorodeoxyadenosine (2-CDA).

OTHER MYELOPROLIFERATIVE DISORDERS

The myeloproliferative disorders are a group of neoplastic proliferation of multipotent haematopoietic stem cells. Besides their common stem cell origin, these disorders are closely related, occasionally leading to evolution of one entity into another during the course of the disease.

Myeloproliferative disorders include 4 disorders: chronic myeloid leukaemia (CML), polycythaemia vera, myeloid metaplasia with myelosclerosis, and essential thrombocytosis (or primary/idiopathic thrombocythaemia). The CML has already been discussed; other disorders are considered here.

POLYCYTHAEMIA VERA

DEFINITION AND ETIOLOGY. Polycythaemia vera (PV) is characterised by increased production of all myeloid elements resulting in pancytosis, elevated haemoglobin concentration and splenomegaly. The term 'polycythaemia vera' or 'polycythaemia rubra vera' is used for *primary or idiopathic polycythaemia* only. *Secondary polycythaemia or erythrocytosis* may occur due to several causes e.g. high altitude, cardiovascular disease, pulmonary disease with alveolar hypoventilation, heavy smoking, inappropriate increase in erythropoietin (renal cell carcinoma, hydronephrosis, hepatocellular carcinoma, cerebellar haemangioblastoma, massive uterine leiomyoma); sometimes relative or spurious polycythaemia may result from plasma loss such as in burns and in dehydration from vomiting or water deprivation. None of the secondary causes of polycythaemia are associated with splenic enlargement or increased leucocytes and platelets which are typical of PV.

In PV, unlike secondary polycythaemia, *the erythropoietin levels in serum and urine are reduced.* Thus, proliferation of haematopoietic cells in the bone marrow in PV is independent of the usual erythropoietin regulatory mechanism.

CLINICAL FEATURES. PV is a disease of late middle life and is slightly more common in males. The disease generally runs a chronic but slowly progressive course. Clinical features are the result of hyperviscosity, hypervolaemia, hypermetabolism and decreased cerebral perfusion. These are:

1. Headache, vertigo, tinnitus, visual alterations syncope or even coma.
2. Increased risk of thrombosis due to accelerated atherosclerosis.
3. Increased risk of haemorrhages due to increased blood volume and intrinsic platelet dysfunction e.g. epistaxis, peptic ulcer disease.
4. Splenomegaly producing abdominal fullness.
5. Pruritus, especially after a bath.
6. Increased risk of urate stones and gout due to hyperuricaemia.

LABORATORY FINDINGS. PV is diagnosed by the following haematologic findings:

1. Raised haemoglobin concentration (above 17.5 g/dl in males and 15.5 g/dl in females).
2. Erythrocytosis (above 6 million/μl in males and 5.5 million/μl in females).
3. Haematocrit (PCV) above 55% in males and above 47% in females.
4. Mild to moderate leucocytosis (15,000-25,000/μl) with basophilia and raised neutrophil alkaline phosphatase scores.
5. Thrombocytosis with defective platelet function.
6. Bone marrow examination reveals erythroid hyperplasia or panhyperplasia.
7. Cytogenetic abnormalities such as trisomy are found in 10% cases of PV.

TREATMENT. Therapy is aimed at maintaining normal blood counts. It includes *phlebotomy* (venesection) by blood letting; *cytotoxic myelosuppression* with busulfan, chlorambucil and cyclophosphamide; and in severe cases *intravenous administration of radioactive phosphorus* (^{32}P). Patients receiving phlebotomy alone may survive for 10-12 years. About 25% patients progress to myelofibrosis. A small proportion of patients develop secondary haematologic malignancies such as AML, non-Hodgkin's lymphoma and multiple myeloma. The majority of patients, however, die of vascular complications.

MYELOID METAPLASIA WITH MYELOFIBROSIS

DEFINITION AND ETIOLOGY. Myeloid metaplasia with myelofibrosis, also called agnogenic (of unknown origin) myeloid metaplasia, primary myelofibrosis and myelosclerosis, is characterised by proliferation of neoplastic stem cells at multiple sites outside the bone marrow (i.e. extramedullary haematopoiesis), especially in the liver and spleen. About 25% cases have a preceding history of polycythaemia. Secondary myelofibrosis, on the other hand, develops in association with certain well-defined marrow disorders, or are the result of toxic action of chemical agents or irradiation.

CLINICAL FEATURES. The disease begins in the late middle life and is gradual in onset. Both sexes are affected equally. The symptomatology includes the following:

1. Anaemia with constitutional symptoms such as fatigue, weakness and anorexia.
2. Massive splenomegaly producing abdominal discomfort, pain and dyspnoea.
3. Hepatomegaly is present in half the cases.
4. Petechial and other bleeding problems are found in about 20% cases.
5. Less common findings are lymphadenopathy, jaundice, ascites, bone pain and hyperuricaemia.

LABORATORY FINDINGS. These are as under:

1. *Mild anaemia* is usual except in cases where features of polycythaemia vera are coexistent.
2. *Leucocytosis* at the time of presentation but later there may be leucopenia.
3. *Thrombocytosis* initially but advanced cases show thrombocytopenia.
4. *Peripheral blood smear* shows bizarre red cell shapes, tear drop poikilocytes, basophilic stippling, nucleated red cells, immature leucocytes (i.e. leucoerythroblastic reaction), basophilia and giant platelet forms.
5. *Bone marrow aspiration* is generally unsuccessful and yields 'dry tap'. Examination of trephine biopsy shows focal areas of hypercellularity and increased reticulin network and variable amount of collagen in which clusters of megakaryocytes are seen well preserved.
6. *Extramedullary haematopoiesis* can be documented by liver biopsy or splenic aspiration.

ESSENTIAL THROMBOCYTOSIS

DEFINITION AND ETIOLOGY. Essential thrombocytosis or primary (idiopathic) thrombocythaemia is another myeloproliferative disorder characterised by markedly elevated platelet count in the absence of any recognisable stimulus. *Secondary or reactive thrombocytosis,* on the other hand, occurs in response to known stimuli such as: chronic infection, haemorrhage, postoperative state, chronic iron deficiency, malignancy, rheumatoid arthritis and postsplenectomy. Essential thrombocytosis represents an overproduction of platelets from megakaryocyte colonies without any added stimulus. Though an elevated platelet count is the dominant feature, other cell lines are also involved in the expansion of neoplastic clone.

CLINICAL FEATURES. The condition has an insidious onset and is more frequent in older people. Haemorrhagic and thrombotic events are common. These include:

1. Arterial or venous thrombosis.
2. Easy bruisability following minor trauma.
3. Spontaneous bleeding.
4. Transient ischaemic attack or frank stroke due to platelet aggregation in microvasculature of the CNS.

LABORATORY FINDINGS. The prominent laboratory features pertain to platelets. These include the following:

1. Sustained elevation in platelet count (above 400,000 μl).
2. Blood film shows many large platelets, megakaryocyte fragments and hypogranular forms.
3. Consistently abnormal platelet functions, especially abnormality in platelet aggregation.
4. Bone marrow examination reveals large number of hyperdiploid megakaryocytes and variable amount of increased fibrosis.

PLATELETS AND HAEMORRHAGIC DIATHESIS

THROMBOPOIESIS

Platelets are formed in the bone marrow by a process of fragmentation of the cytoplasm of megakaryocytes. Platelet production appears to be under the control of thrombopoietin, the nature and origin of which are not yet established. The stages in platelet production are: megakaryoblast, promegakaryocyte, megakaryocyte, and discoid platelets (Fig. 13.35).

MEGAKARYOBLAST. The earliest precursor of platelets in the bone marrow is megakaryoblast. It arises from haematopoietic stem cell by a process of differentiation.

PROMEGAKARYOCYTE. A megakaryoblast undergoes endo-reduplication of nuclear chromatin i.e. nuclear chromatin replicates repeatedly in multiples of two without division of the cell. Ultimately, a large cell containing up to 32 times the normal diploid content of nuclear DNA (polyploidy) is formed when further nuclear replication ceases and cytoplasm becomes granular.

MEGAKARYOCYTE. A mature megakaryocyte is a large cell, 30-90 μm in diameter, and contains 4-16 nuclear lobes having coarsely clumped chromatin. The cytoplasm is abundant, light blue in colour and contains red-purple granules. Platelets are formed from pseudopods of megakaryocyte cytoplasm which get detached into the blood stream. Each megakaryocyte may form up to 4000 platelets. The formation of platelets from the stem cell takes about 10 days.

PLATELETS. Platelets are small (1-4 μm in diameter), discoid, non-nucleate structures containing red-purple granules. The normal platelet count ranges from 150,000-400,000/μl and its life-span is 7-10 days. Newly-formed platelets spend 24-36 hours in the spleen before being released into circulation but splenic stasis does not cause any injury to the platelets normally.

The main **function** of platelets is in haemostasis which includes two closely linked processes:

1. Primary haemostasis is the term used for platelet plug formation at the site of injury. It is an immediate phenomenon appearing within seconds of injury and is responsible for cessation of bleeding from microvasculature. Primary haemostasis involves three steps: platelet adhesion, platelet granule release and platelet aggregation which are regulated by changes in membrane phospholipids, and calcium (Fig. 13.36). At molecular level, these important events are depicted diagrammatically in Fig. 13.37 and briefly outlined below:

- *Platelet adhesion:* Platelets adhere to collagen in the subendothelium due to presence of receptor on platelet surface, glycoprotein (Gp) Ia-IIa which is an integrin. The adhesion to the vessel wall is further stabilised by von Willebrand factor, an adhesion glycoprotein. This is achieved by formation of a link between von Willebrand factor and another platelet receptor, GpIb-IX complex.
- *Platelet release:* The adherent platelets release preformed granules that includes ADP, factor Va, thrombospondin, platelet-derived growth factor (PDGF),

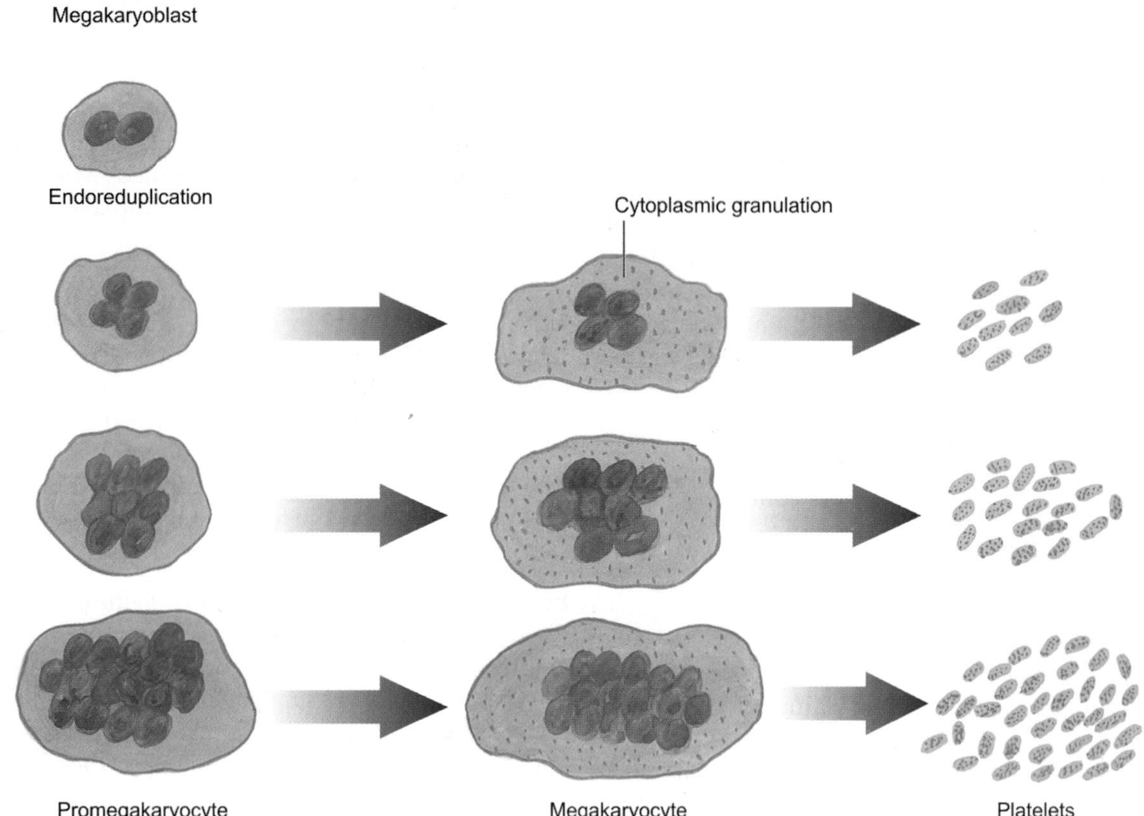

FIGURE 13.35
Thrombopoiesis.

von Willebrand factor (vWF), fibronectin, fibrinogen, heparinase and thromboxane A2 (Fig. 13.36).

■ *Platelet aggregation:* This process is mediated by fibrinogen which forms bridge between adjacent platelets via glycoprotein receptors on platelets, GpIIb-IIIa.

2. ***Secondary haemostasis*** involves plasma coagulation system resulting in fibrin plug formation and takes several minutes for completion. This is discussed in detail in Chapter 5.

HAEMORRHAGIC DIATHESIS (BLEEDING DISORDERS)

Bleeding disorders or haemorrhagic diatheses are a group of disorders characterised by defective haemostasis with abnormal bleeding. The tendency to bleeding may be *spontaneous* in the form of small haemorrhages into the skin and mucous membranes (e.g. petechiae, purpura, ecchymoses), or there may be excessive external or internal bleeding *following trivial trauma* and surgical procedure (e.g. haematoma, haemarthrosis etc).

The causes of haemorrhagic diatheses may or may not be related to platelet abnormalities. These causes are broadly divided into the following 4 groups:

I. Haemorrhagic diathesis due to vascular abnormalities.

II. Haemorrhagic diathesis related to platelet abnormalities.

III. Disorders of coagulation factors.

IV. Combination of all these as occurs in disseminated intravascular coagulation (DIC).

Before discussing the bleeding disorders, it is considered desirable to describe briefly the broad outlines of scheme of investigations to be carried out in such a case.

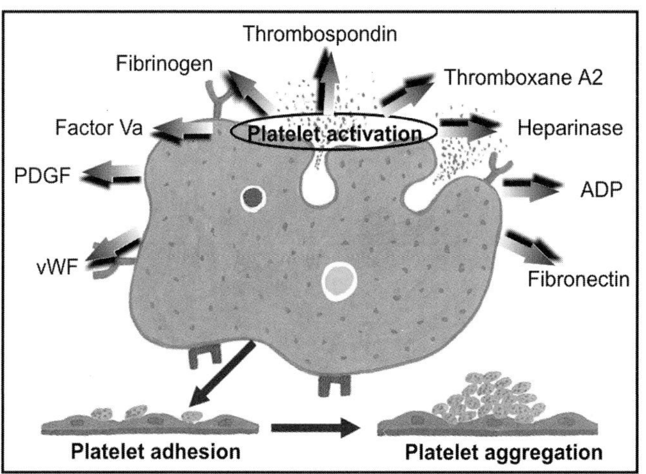

FIGURE 13.36

Main events in primary haemostasis—platelet adhesion, release (activation) and aggregation.

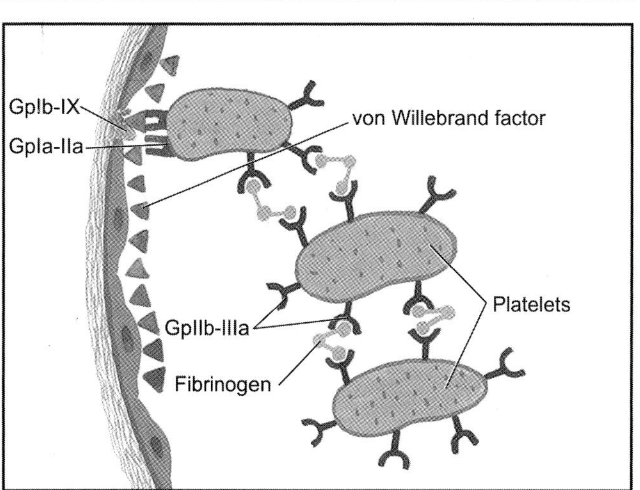

FIGURE 13.37

Molecular mechanisms in platelet adhesion and release reaction (Gp=glycoprotein).

INVESTIGATIONS OF HAEMOSTATIC FUNCTION

Normal haemostatic mechanism and thrombogenesis were discussed in Chapter 5. In general, the haemostatic mechanisms have 2 primary functions:

- To promote *local haemostasis* at the site of injured blood vessel.
- To ensure that the circulating blood remains in *fluid state* while in the vascular bed i.e. to prevent the occurrence of generalised thrombosis.

In order to perform these haemostatic functions, a delicate balance must exist among at least 5 components (Fig. 13.38): (i) blood vessel wall; (ii) platelets; (iii) plasma coagulation factors; (iv) inhibitors; and (v) fibrinolytic system.

Anything that interferes with any of these components results in defective haemostasis with abnormal bleeding. In order to establish a definite diagnosis in any case suspected to have abnormal haemostatic functions, the following scheme is followed:

A. Comprehensive *clinical evaluation,* including the patient's history, family history and details of the site, frequency and character of haemostatic defect.

B. Series of *screening tests* for assessing the abnormalities in various components involved in maintaining haemostatic balance.

C. *Specific tests* to pinpoint the cause.

A brief review of general principles of tests used to investigate haemostatic abnormalities is presented below and summarised in Table 13.22.

A. Investigations of Disordered Vascular Haemostasis

Disorders of vascular haemostasis may be due to increased vascular permeability, reduced capillary strength and failure to contract after injury. Tests of defective vascular function are as under:

1. BLEEDING TIME. This simple test is based on the principle of formation of haemostatic plug following a standard incision on the volar surface of the forearm and the time the incision takes to stop bleeding is measured. The test is dependent upon capillary function

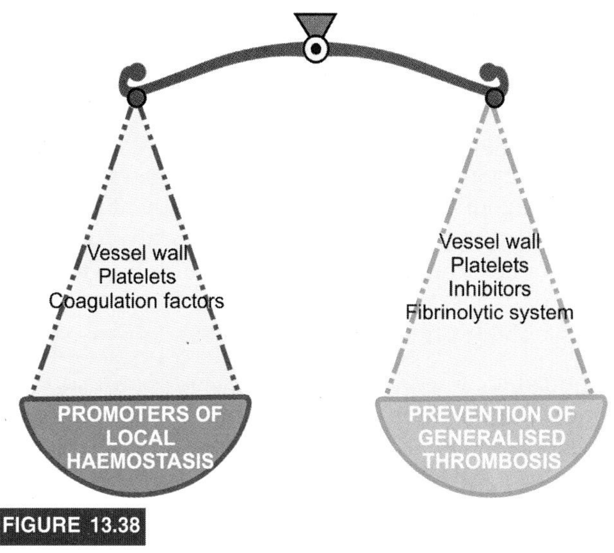

FIGURE 13.38

The Haemostatic balance.

TABLE 13.22: Screening Tests for Haemostasis (Coagulation Tests).

LABORATORY TEST	FACTOR/FUNCTION MEASURED	ASSOCIATED DISORDERS
1. ***Bleeding time***	Platelet function, vascular integrity	i) Qualitative disorders of platelets ii) von Willebrand's disease iii) Quantitative disorders of platelets iv) Acquired vascular disorders
2. ***Platelet count***	Quantification of platelets	i) Thrombocytopenia ii) Thrombocytosis
3. ***Prothrombin time***	Evaluation of extrinsic and common pathway (deficiency of factors I, II, V, VII, X)	i) Oral anticoagulant therapy ii) DIC iii) Liver disease
4. ***Partial thromboplastin time***	Evaluation of intrinsic and common pathway (deficiency of factors I, II, V, VIII, IX, X, XI, XII)	i) Parenteral heparin therapy ii) DIC iii) Liver disease
5. ***Thrombin time***	Evaluation of common pathway	i) Afibrinogenaemia ii) DIC iii) Parenteral heparin therapy

as well as on platelet number and ability of platelets to adhere to form aggregates. Normal range is 3-8 minutes. A prolonged bleeding time may be due to:

i) Thrombocytopenia.

ii) Disorders of platelet function.

iii) von Willebrand's disease.

iv) Vascular abnormalities (e.g. in Ehlers-Danlos syndrome).

v) Severe deficiency of factor V and XI.

2. HESS CAPILLARY RESISTANCE TEST (TOURNIQUET TEST). This test is done by tying sphygmomanometer cuff to the upper arm and raising the pressure in it between diastolic and systolic for 5 minutes. After deflation, the number of petechiae appearing in the next 5 minutes in 3 cm^2 area over the cubital fossa are counted. Presence of more than 20 petechiae is considered a positive test. The test is positive in increased capillary fragility as well as in thrombocytopenia.

B. Investigation of Platelets and Platelet Function

Haemostatic disorders are most commonly due to abnormalities in platelet number, morphology or function.

I. SCREENING TESTS. The screening tests carried out for assessing these are:

1. Peripheral blood platelet count.
2. Skin bleeding time.
3. Examination of fresh blood film to see the morphologic abnormalities of platelets.

II. SPECIAL TESTS. If these screening tests suggest a disorder of platelet function, the following platelet function tests may be carried out:

1. *Platelet adhesion tests* such as retention in a glass bead column, and other sophisticated techniques.
2. *Aggregation tests* which are turbidometric techniques using ADP, collagen or ristocetin.
3. *Granular content* of the platelets and their release can be assessed by electron microscopy or by measuring the substances released.
4. *Platelet coagulant activity* is measured indirectly by prothrombin consumption index.

C. Investigation of Blood Coagulation

The normal blood coagulation system consisting of intrinsic and extrinsic pathways and the common pathway is shown in Fig. 13.39.

I. SCREENING TESTS. Tests for blood coagulation system include a battery of screening tests. These are as under:

1. Whole blood coagulation time. The estimation of whole blood coagulation time done by various capillary and tube methods is of limited value since it is an insensitive and nonspecific test. Normal range is 4-9 minutes at 37°C.

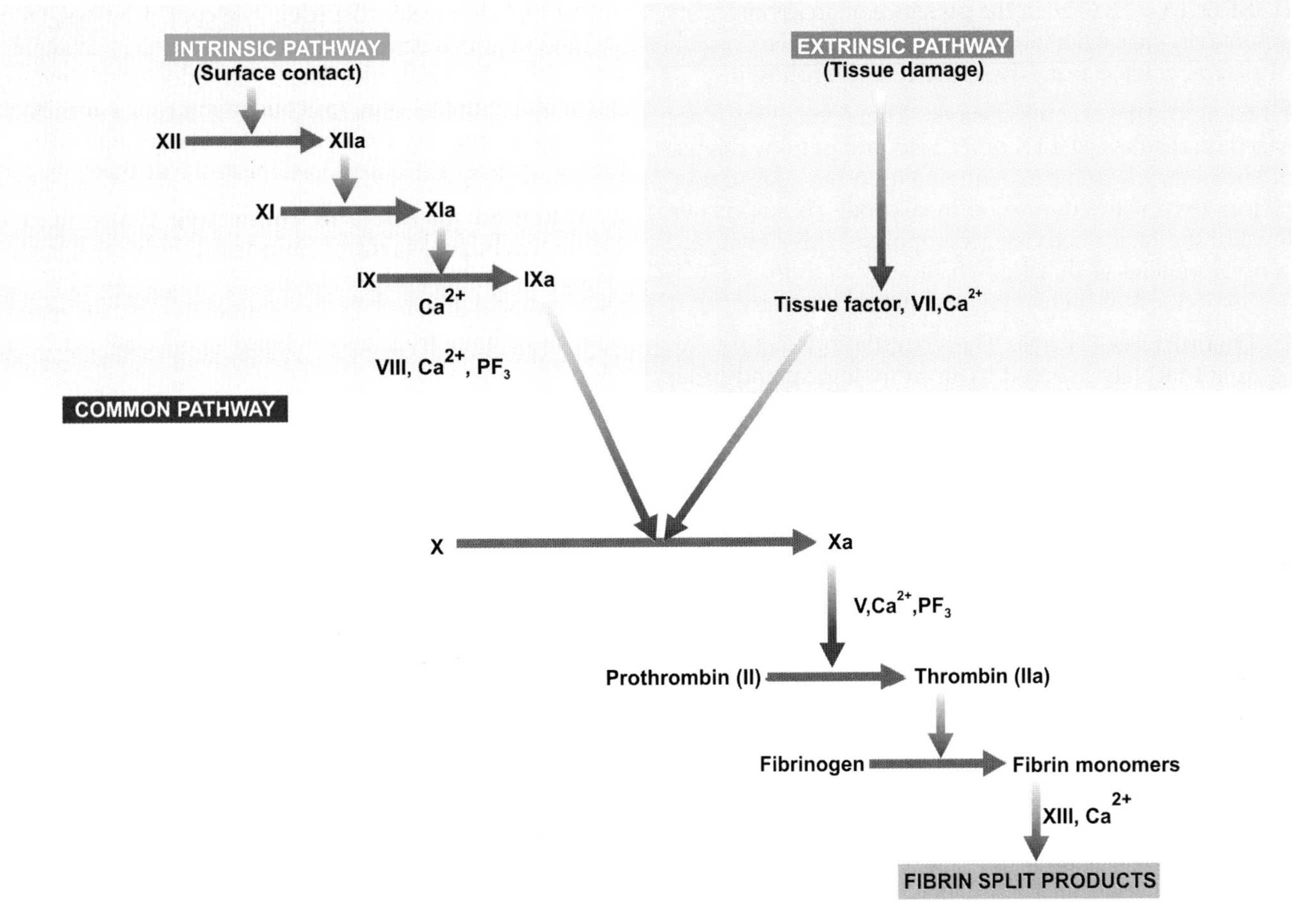

FIGURE 13.39
Pathways of blood coagulation.

2. Activated partial thromboplastin time (APTT) or partial thromboplastin time with kaolin (PTTK). This test is used to measure the intrinsic system factors (VIII, IX, XI and XII) as well as factors common to both intrinsic and extrinsic systems (factors X, V, prothrombin and fibrinogen). The test consists of addition of 3 substances to the plasma—calcium, phospholipid and a surface activator such as kaolin. The normal range is 30-40 seconds. The common causes of a prolonged PTTK (or APTT) are:

i) Parenteral administration of heparin.
ii) Disseminated intravascular coagulation.
iii) Liver disease.
iv) Circulating anticoagulants.

3. One-stage prothrombin time (PT). PT measures the extrinsic system factor VII as well as factors in the common pathway. In this test, tissue thromboplastin (e.g. brain extract) and calcium are added to the test. The normal PT in this test is 10-14 seconds. The common causes of prolonged one-stage PT are:

i) Administration of oral anticoagulant drugs.
ii) Liver disease, especially obstructive liver disease.
iii) Vitamin K deficiency.
iv) Disseminated intravascular coagulation.

4. Measurement of fibrinogen. The *screening tests* for fibrinogen deficiency are semiquantitative fibrinogen titre and thrombin time (TT). The normal value of thrombin time is under 20 seconds, while a fibrinogen titre in plasma dilution up to 32 is considered normal. The common causes for higher values in both these tests are:

i) Hypofibrinogenaemia (e.g. in DIC).
ii) Raised concentration of FDP.
iii) Presence of heparin.

II. SPECIAL TESTS. In the presence of an abnormality in screening tests, detailed investigations for the possible cause are carried out. These include the following:

1. Coagulation factor assays. These bioassays are based on results of PTTK or PT tests and employ the use of substrate plasma that contains all other coagulation factors except the one to be measured. The unknown level of the factor activity is compared with a standard control plasma with a known level of activity. Results are expressed as percentage of normal activity.

2. Quantitative assays. The coagulation factors can be quantitatively assayed by immunological and other chemical methods.

D. Investigation of Fibrinolytic System

Increased levels of circulating plasminogen activator are present in patients with hyperfibrinolysis. *Screening tests* done to assess these abnormalities in fibrinolytic system are:

1. Estimation of fibrinogen.
2. Fibrin degradation products (FDP) in the serum.
3. Ethanol gelation test.
4. Euglobin or whole blood lysis time.

More *specific tests* include: functional assays, immunological assays by ELISA, and chromogenic assays of plasminogen activators, plasminogen, plasminogen activator inhibitor, and FDP.

HAEMORRHAGIC DIATHESES DUE TO VASCULAR DISORDERS

Vascular bleeding disorders, also called non-thrombocytopenic purpuras or vascular purpuras, are normally mild and characterised by petechiae, purpuras or ecchymoses confined to the skin and mucous membranes. The pathogenesis of bleeding is poorly understood since majority of the standard screening tests of haemostasis including the bleeding time, coagulation time, platelet count and platelet function, are usually normal. Vascular purpuras arise from damage to the capillary endothelium, abnormalities in the subendothelial matrix or extravascular connective tissue that supports the blood vessels, or from formation of abnormal blood vessels.

Vascular bleeding disorders may be *inherited* or *acquired.*

A. Inherited Vascular Bleeding Disorders

A few examples of hereditary vascular disorders are given below:

1. Hereditary haemorrhagic telangiectasia (Osler-Weber-Rendu disease). This is an uncommon inherited autosomal dominant disorder. The condition begins in childhood and is characterised by abnormally telangiectatic (dilated) capillaries. These telangiectasias develop particularly in the skin, mucous membranes and internal organs and are the source of frequent episodes of bleeding from nose and gastrointestinal tract.

2. Inherited disorders of connective tissue matrix. These include Marfan's syndome, Ehlers-Danlos syndrome and pseudoxanthoma elasticum, all of which have inherited defect in the connective tissue matrix and, thus, have fragile skin vessels and easy bruising.

B. Acquired Vascular Bleeding Disorders

Several acquired conditions are associated with vascular purpuras. These are as under:

1. Henoch-Schönlein purpura. Henoch-Schönlein or anaphylactoid purpura is a self-limited type of hypersensitivity vasculitis occurring in children and young adults. Circulating immune complexes are deposited in the vessel wall consisting of IgA, C3 and fibrin, and in some cases, properdin suggesting activation of alternate complement pathway as the trigger event. The hypersensitivity vasculitis produces purpuric rash on the extensor surfaces of arms, legs and on the buttocks, as well as haematuria, colicky abdominal pain due to bleeding into the GIT, polyarthralgia and acute nephritis. In spite of these haemorrhagic features, all coagulation tests are normal.

2. Haemolytic-uraemic syndrome. Haemolytic-uraemic syndrome is a disease of infancy and early childhood in which there is bleeding tendency and varying degree of acute renal failure. The disorder remains confined to the kidney where hyaline thrombi are seen in the glomerular capillaries.

3. Simple easy bruising (Devil's pinches). Easy bruising of unknown cause is a common phenomenon in women of child-bearing age group.

4. Infection. Many infections cause vascular haemorrhages either by causing toxic damage to the endothelium or by DIC. These are especially prone to occur in septicaemia and severe measles.

5. Drug reactions. Certain drugs form antibodies and produce hypersensitivity (or leucocytoclastic) vasculitis responsible for abnormal bleeding.

6. Steroid purpura. Long-term steroid therapy or Cushing's syndrome may be associated with vascular purpura due to defective vascular support.

7. Senile purpura. Atrophy of the supportive tissue of cutaneous blood vessels in old age may cause senile atrophy, especially in the dorsum of forearm and hand.

Chapter Thirteen

8. Scurvy. Deficiency of vitamin C causes defective collagen synthesis which causes skin bleeding as well as bleeding into muscles, and occasionally into the gastrointestinal and genitourinary tracts.

HAEMORRHAGIC DIATHESES DUETO PLATELET DISORDERS

Disorders of platelets produce bleeding disorders by one of the following 2 mechanisms:

A. *Due to reduction in the number of platelets* i.e. various forms of thrombocytopenias.

B. *Due to defective platelet functions.*

A. THROMBOCYTOPENIAS

Thrombocytopenia is defined as a reduction in the peripheral blood platelet count below the lower limit of normal i.e. below 150,000/μl. Thrombocytopenia is associated with abnormal bleeding that includes spontaneous skin purpura and mucosal haemorrhages as well as prolonged bleeding after trauma. However, spontaneous haemorrhagic tendency becomes clinically evident only after severe depletion of the platelet count to level of about 20,000/μl.

Thrombocytopenia may result from 4 main groups of causes:

1. Impaired platelet production.
2. Accelerated platelet destruction.
3. Splenic sequestration.
4. Dilutional loss.

A list of causes of thrombocytopenia is given in Table 13.23. Three of the common and important causes—drug-induced thrombocytopenia, idiopathic thrombocytopenic purpura (ITP), and thrombotic thrombocytopenic purpura (TTP), are discussed below.

TABLE 13.23: Causes of Thrombocytopenia.

I. **IMPAIRED PLATELET PRODUCTION**

1. *Generalised bone marrow failure e.g.*

   Aplastic anaemia, leukaemia, myelofibrosis, megaloblastic anaemia, marrow infiltrations (carcinomas, lymphomas, multiple myeloma, storage diseases).

2. *Selective suppression of platelet production e.g.*

   Drugs (quinine, quinidine, sulfonamides, PAS, rifampicin, anticancer drugs, thiazide diuretics), alcohol intake.

II. **ACCELERATED PLATELET DESTRUCTION**

1. *Immunologic thrombocytopenias e.g.*

   ITP (acute and chronic), neonatal and post-transfusion (isoimmune), drug-induced, secondary immune 'thrombocytopenia (post-infection, SLE, AIDS, CLL, lymphoma).

2. *Increased consumption e.g.*

   DIC, TTP, giant haemangiomas, microangiopathic haemolytic anaemia.

III. **SPLENIC SEQUESTRATION**

   Splenomegaly

IV. **DILUTIONAL LOSS**

   Massive transfusion of old stored blood to bleeding patients.

Drug-induced Thrombocytopenia

Many commonly used drugs cause thrombocytopenia by depressing megakaryocyte production. In most cases, an immune mechanism by formation of drug-antibody complexes is implicated in which the platelet is damaged as an 'innocent bystander'. Drug-induced thrombocytopenia is associated with many commonly used drugs and includes: chemotherapeutic agents (alkylating agents, anthracyclines, antimetabolites), certain antibiotics (sulfonamides, PAS, rifampicin, penicillins), drugs used in cardiovascular diseases (digitoxin, thiazide diuretics), heparin and excessive consumption of ethanol.

Clinically, the patient presents with acute purpura. The platelet count is markedly lowered, often below 10,000/μl and the bone marrow shows normal or increased number of megakaryocytes. The immediate treatment is to stop or replace the suspected drug with instruction to the patient to avoid taking the offending drug in future. Occasional patients may require temporary support with glucocorticoids, plasmapheresis or platelet transfusions.

Idiopathic Thrombocytopenic Purpura (ITP)

Idiopathic thrombocytopenic purpura (ITP), also called immunologic thrombocytopenic purpura, is characterised by immunologic destruction of platelets and normal or increased megakaryocytes in the bone marrow.

PATHOGENESIS. On the basis of duration of illness, ITP is classified into acute and chronic forms, both of which have different pathogenesis.

Acute ITP. This is a self-limited disorder, seen most frequently in children following recovery from a viral illness (e.g. viral hepatitis, infectious mononucleosis, CMV infection) or an upper respiratory illness. The onset of acute ITP is sudden and thrombocytopenia is severe but recovery occurs within a few weeks to 6 months. The mechanism of acute ITP is by formation of *immune complexes* containing viral antigens, and by formation of *antibodies* against viral antigens which crossreact with platelets and lead to their immunologic destruction.

Chronic ITP. Chronic ITP occurs more commonly in adults, particularly in women of child-bearing age (20-40 years). The disorder develops insidiously and persists for several years. Though chronic ITP is idiopathic, similar immunologic thrombocytopenia may be seen in association with SLE, AIDS and autoimmune thyroiditis. The pathogenesis of chronic ITP is explained by formation of *anti-platelet autoantibodies,* usually by platelet-associated IgG humoral antibodies synthesised mainly in the spleen. These antibodies are directed against target antigens on the platelet glycoproteins, Gp IIb-IIIa and Gp Ib-IX complex. Some of the antibodies directed against platelet surface also interfere in their function. The mechanism of platelet destruction is similar to that seen in autoimmune haemolytic anaemias. Sensitised platelets are destroyed mainly in the spleen and rendered susceptible to phagocytosis by cells of the reticuloendothelial system.

CLINICAL FEATURES. The clinical manifestation of ITP may develop abruptly as in cases of acute ITP, or the onset may be insidious as occurs in majority of cases of chronic ITP. The usual manifestations are petechial haemorrhages, easy bruising, and mucosal bleeding such as menorrhagia in women, nasal bleeding, bleeding from gums, melaena and haematuria. Intracranial haemorrhage is, however, rare. Splenomegaly and hepatomegaly may occur in cases with chronic ITP but lymphadenopathy is quite uncommon in either type of ITP.

LABORATORY FINDINGS. The diagnosis of ITP can be suspected on clinical features after excluding the known causes of thrombocytopenia and is supported by the following haematologic findings (Fig. 13.40):

1. *Platelet count* is markedly reduced, usually in the range of 10,000-50,000/μl.
2. *Blood film* shows only occasional platelets which are often large in size.
3. *Bone marrow* shows increased number of megakaryocytes which have large non-lobulated single nuclei and may have reduced cytoplasmic granularity and presence of vacuoles (COLOUR PLATE XVII: CL 67).
4. With sensitive techniques, *anti-platelet IgG antibody* can be demonstrated on platelet surface or in the serum of patients.
5. *Platelet survival studies* reveal markedly reduced platelet life-span, sometimes less than one hour as against normal life-span of 7-10 days.

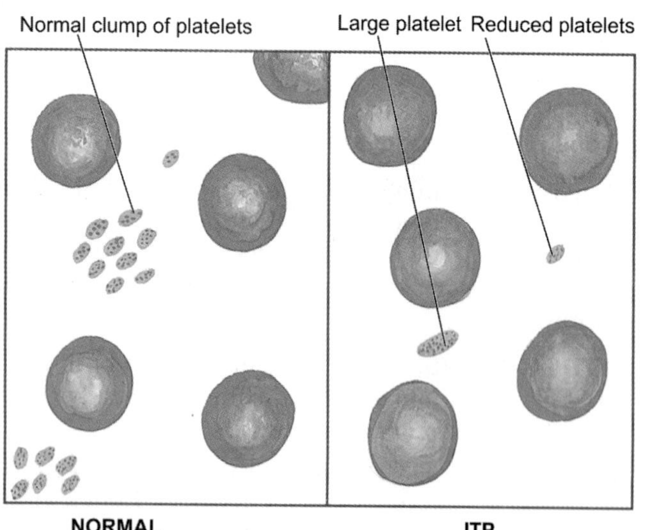

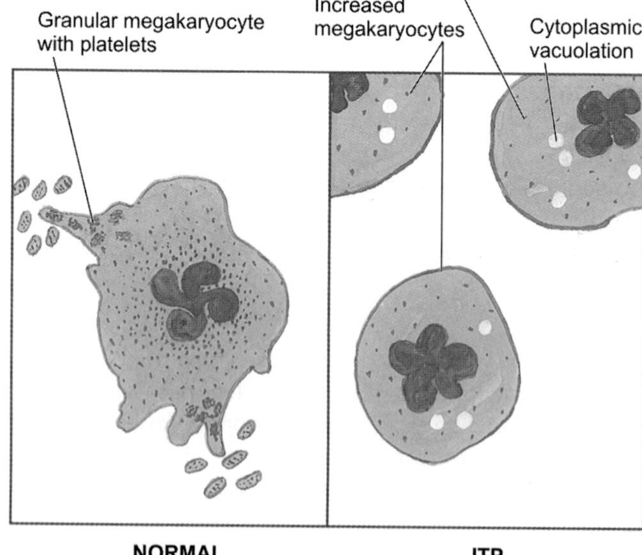

FIGURE 13.40

Laboratory findings of ITP contrasted with those found in a normal individual. A, Peripheral blood in ITP shows presence of reduced number of platelets which are often large. B, Bone marrow in ITP shows characteristically increased number of megakaryocytes with single non-lobulated nuclei and reduced cytoplasmic granularity and presence of vacuoles. The other cells in the peripheral blood and marrow are normal and are not included in the pictures here.

Treatment

Spontaneous recovery occurs in 90% cases of acute ITP, while only less than 10% cases of chronic ITP recover spontaneously. Treatment is directed at reducing the level and source of autoantibodies and reducing the rate of destruction of sensitised platelets. This is possible by corticosteroid therapy, immunosuppressive drugs (e.g. vincristine, cyclophosphamide and azathioprine) and splenectomy. The beneficial effects of splenectomy in chronic ITP are due to both removal of the major site of platelet destruction and the major source of auto-antibody synthesis. Platelet transfusions are helpful as a palliative measure only in patients with severe haemorrhage.

ThromboticThrombocytopenic Purpura (TTP)

Thrombotic thrombocytopenic purpura (TTP) is an uncommon but often fulminant and lethal disorder occurring in young adults. It is essentially characterised by triad of *thrombocytopenia, microangiopathic haemolytic anaemia and formation of hyaline fibrin microthrombi* within the microvasculature throughout the body. The intra-vascular microthrombi are composed predominantly of platelets and fibrin. The widespread presence of these platelet microthrombi is responsible for thrombocyto-penia due to increased consumption of platelets, micro-angiopathic haemolytic anaemia and protean clinical manifestations involving different organs and tissues throughout the body.

PATHOGENESIS. Unlike DIC, a clinicopathologically related condition, activation of the clotting system is not the primary event in formation of microthrombi. TTP is initiated by endothelial injury followed by release of von Willebrand factor and other procoagulant material from endothelial cells, leading to the forma-tion of microthrombi.The trigger for the endothelial injury comes from immunologic damage by diverse conditions such as in pregnancy, metastatic cancer, high-doze chemotherapy, HIV infection, and mitomycin C.

CLINICAL FEATURES. The clinical manifestations of TTP are due to microthrombi in the arterioles, capillaries and venules throughout the body. Besides features of thrombocytopenia and microangiopathic haemolytic anaemia, characteristic findings include fever, transient neurologic deficits and renal failure. The spleen may be palpable.

LABORATORY FINDINGS. The diagnosis can be made from the following findings:

1. Thrombocytopenia.
2. Microangiopathic haemolytic anaemia with negative Coombs' test.
3. Leucocytosis, sometimes with leukaemoid reaction.
4. Bone marrow examination reveals normal or slightly increased megakaryocytes accompanied with some myeloid hyperplasia.
5. Diagnosis is, however, established by examination of biopsy (e.g. from gingiva) which demonstrates typical microthrombi in arterioles, capillaries and venules, unassociated with any inflammatory changes in the vessel wall.

B. DISORDERS OF PLATELET FUNCTIONS

Defective platelet function is suspected in patients who show skin and mucosal haemorrhages and have prolonged bleeding time but a normal platelet count. These disorders may be hereditary or acquired.

1. Hereditary Disorders

Depending upon the predominant functional abnormality, inherited disorders of platelet functions are classified into the following 3 groups:

1. DEFECTIVE PLATELET ADHESION. These are as under:

i) *Bernard-Soulier syndrome* is an autosomal recessive disorder with inherited deficiency of a platelet membrane glycoprotein which is essential for adhesion of platelets to vessel wall.

ii) *In von Willebrand's disease,* there is defective platelet adhesion as well as deficiency of factor VIII (page 435).

2. DEFECTIVE PLATELET AGGREGATION. In *thrombasthenia (Glanzmann's disease),* there is failure of primary platelet aggregation with ADP or collagen due to inherited deficiency of two of platelet membrane glycoproteins.

3. DISORDERS OF PLATELET RELEASE REAC-TION. These disorders are characterised by normal initial aggregation of platelets with ADP or collagen but the subsequent release of ADP, prostaglandins and 5-HT is defective due to complex intrinsic deficiencies.

2. Acquired Disorders

Acquired defects of platelet functions include the following clinically significant examples:

1. ASPIRIN THERAPY. Prolonged use of aspirin leads to easy bruising and abnormal bleeding time. This is because aspirin inhibits the enzyme cyclooxygenase, and thereby suppresses the synthesis of prostaglandins which are involved in platelet aggregation as well as release reaction. The anti-platelet effect of aspirin is clinically made use of in preventing major thromboembolic disease in recurrent myocardial infarction.

2. OTHERS. Several other acquired disorders are associated with various abnormalities in platelet functions at different levels. These include: uraemia, liver disease, multiple myeloma, Waldenström's macroglobulinaemia and various myeloproliferative disorders.

COAGULATION DISORDERS

The physiology of normal coagulation is described in Chapter 5 together with relatively more common coagulation disorders of arterial and venous thrombosis and embolism. A deficiency of each of the thirteen known plasma coagulation factors has been reported, which may be inherited or acquired. In general, these coagulation disorders are uncommon as compared with other bleeding disorders. The type of bleeding in coagulation disorders is different from that seen in vascular and platelet abnormalities. Instead of spontaneous appearance of petechiae and purpuras, the plasma coagulation defects manifest more often in the form of large ecchymoses, haematomas and bleeding into muscles, joints, body cavities, GIT and urinary tract. For establishing the diagnosis, *screening tests for coagulation* (whole blood coagulation time, bleeding time, activated partial thromboplastin time and prothrombin time) are carried out, followed by *coagulation factor assays* as discussed already on page 427.

Disorders of plasma coagulation factors may have hereditary or acquired origin.

HEREDITARY COAGULATION DISORDERS. Most of the inherited plasma coagulation disorders are due to qualitative or quantitative defect in a single coagulation factor. Though defect of all the thirteen coagulation factors are reported, two of the most common inherited coagulation disorders are the sex-(X)-linked disorders—*classic haemophilia or haemophilia A* (due to inherited deficiency of factor VIII), and *Christmas disease or haemophilia B* (due to inherited deficiency of factor IX). Another common and related coagulation disorder, *von Willebrand's disease* (due to inherited defect of von Willebrand's factor), is also discussed here.

ACQUIRED COAGULATION DISORDERS. The acquired coagulation disorders, on the other hand, are usually characterised by deficiencies of multiple coagulation factors. The most common acquired clotting abnormalities are: vitamin K deficiency, coagulation disorder in liver diseases, fibrinolytic defects and disseminated intravascular coagulation (DIC).

The more common of the hereditary and acquired coagulation disorders are discussed below.

Classic Haemophilia (Haemophilia A)

Classic haemophilia or haemophilia A is the second most common hereditary coagulation disorder next to von Willebrand's disease occurring due to deficiency or reduced activity of factor VIII (anti-haemophilic factor). The disorder is inherited as a sex-(X-) linked recessive trait and, therefore, manifests clinically in males, while females are usually the carriers. However, occasional women carriers of haemophilia may produce factor VIII levels far below 50% and become symptomatic carriers, or rarely there may be true female haemophilics arising from consanguinity within the family (i.e. homozygous females). The chances of a proven carrier mother passing the abnormality onto her children is 50:50 for each son and 50:50 for each daughter. A haemophilic father will have normal sons as they inherit his Y chromosome only which does not carry the genetic abnormality.

The disease has been known since ancient times but Schönlein in 1839 gave this bleeder's disease its present name haemophilia. In 1952, it was found that haemophilia was not always due to deficiency of factor VIII as was previously thought but instead blood of some patients was deficient in factor IX (Christmas factor or plasma thromboplastin component). Currently, *haemophilia A (classic haemophilia)* is the term used for the disorder due to factor VIII deficiency, and *haemophilia B (Christmas disease)* for the disorder when factor IX is deficient.

The frequency of haemophilia varies in different races, the highest incidence being in populations of Britain, Northern Europe and Australia. Western literature reports give an overall incidence of haemophilia in 1 in 10,000 male births. Another interesting facet of the haemophilia which has attracted investigators and researchers is the occurrence of this disorder in the royal blood of Great Britain and some European royal families.

PATHOGENESIS. Haemophilia A is caused by quantitative reduction of factor VIII in 90% of cases, while 10% cases have normal or increased levels of factor VIII with reduced activity. Factor VIII is synthesised in hepatic parenchymal cells and regulates the activation of factor X in intrinsic coagulation pathway. Factor VIII circulates in blood complexed to another larger protein, von Willebrand's factor (vWF), which comprises 99% of the factor VIII-vWF complex. The genetic coding, synthesis and functions of vWF are different from those of factor VIII and are considered separately below under von Willebrand's disease. Normal haemostasis requires 25% factor VIII activity. Though occasional patients with 25% factor VIII level may develop bleeding, most symptomatic haemophilic patients have factor VIII levels below 5%.

CLINICAL FEATURES. Patients of haemophilia suffer from bleeding for hours or days after the injury. The clinical severity of the disease correlates well with plasma level of factor VIII activity. Haemophilic bleeding can involve any organ but occurs most commonly as recurrent painful haemarthroses and muscle haematomas, and sometimes as haematuria. Spontaneous intracranial haemorrhage and oropharyngeal bleeding are rare, but when they occur they are the most feared complications.

Symptomatic patients with bleeding episodes are treated with factor VIII replacement therapy, consisting of factor VIII concentrates or plasma cryoprecipitates. With the availability of this treatment, the life expectancy of even severe haemophilic patients was approaching normal but the occurrence of AIDS in multitransfused haemophilic patients has adversely affected the life expectancy.

LABORATORY FINDINGS. The following tests are abnormal:

1. Whole blood coagulation time is prolonged in severe cases only.
2. Prothrombin time is usually normal.
3. Activated partial thromboplastin time (APTT or PTTK) is typically prolonged.
4. Specific assay for factor VIII shows lowered activity. The diagnosis of *female carriers* is made by the findings of about half the activity of factor VIII, while the *manifest disease* is associated with factor VIII activity below 25%.

Christmas Disease (Haemophilia B)

Inherited deficiency of factor IX (Christmas factor or plasma thromboplastin component) produces Christmas disease or haemophilia B. Haemophilia B is rarer than haemophilia A; its estimated incidence is 1 in 100,000 male births. The inheritance pattern and clinical features of factor IX deficiency are indistinguishable from those of classic haemophilia but accurate laboratory diagnosis is critical since haemophilia B requires treatment with different plasma fraction. The usual screening tests for coagulation are similar to those in classic haemophilia but bioassay of factor IX reveals lowered activity.

The therapy in symptomatic haemophilia B consists of infusion of either fresh frozen plasma or a plasma enriched with factor IX. Besides the expected possibilities of complications of hepatitis, chronic liver disease and AIDS, the replacement therapy in factor IX deficiency may activate the coagulation system and cause thrombosis and embolism.

von Willebrand's Disease

DEFINITION AND PATHOGENESIS. von Willebrand's disease (vWD) is the most common hereditary coagulation disorder occurring due to qualitative or quantitative defect in von Willebrand's factor (vWF). Its incidence is estimated to be 1 in 1,000 individuals of either sex. The vWF comprises the larger fraction of factor VIII-vWF complex which circulates in the blood. Though the two components of factor VIII-vWF complex circulate together as a unit and perform the important function in clotting and facilitate platelet adhesion to subendothelial collagen, vWF differs from factor VIII in the following respects:

1. The *gene* for vWF is located at chromosome 12, while that of factor VIII is in X-chromosome. Thus, vWD is inherited as an autosomal dominant trait which may occur in either sex, while factor VIII deficiency (haemophilia A) is a sex (X-)-linked recessive disorder.
2. The vWF is *synthesised* in the endothelial cells, megakaryocytes and platelets but not in the liver cells, while the principal site of synthesis of factor VIII is the liver.
3. The main *function* of vWF is to facilitate the adhesion of platelets to subendothelial collagen, while factor VIII is involved in activation of factor X in the intrinsic coagulation pathway.

CLINICAL FEATURES. Clinically, the patients of vWD are characterised by spontaneous bleeding from mucous membranes and excessive bleeding from wounds. There are 3 major types of vWD:

Type I disease is the most common and is characterised by mild to moderate decrease in plasma vWF (50% activity). The synthesis of vWF is normal but the release of its multimers is inhibited.

Type II disease is much less common and is characterised by normal or near normal levels of vWF which is functionally defective.

Type III disease is extremely rare and is the most severe form of the disease. These patients have no detectable vWF activity and may have sufficiently low factor VIII levels.

Bleeding epidoses in vWD are treated with cryoprecipitates or factor VIII concentrates.

LABORATORY FINDINGS. These are :

1. Prolonged bleeding time.
2. Normal platelet count.
3. Reduced plasma vWF concentration.
4. Defective platelet aggregation with ristocetin, an antibiotic.
5. Reduced factor VIII activity.

Vitamin K Deficiency

Vitamin K is a fat-soluble vitamin which plays important role in haemostasis since it serves as a cofactor in the formation of 6 prothrombin complex proteins *(vitamin K-dependent coagulation factors)* synthesised in the liver: factor II, VII, IX, X, protein C and protein S. Vitamin K is obtained from green vegetables, absorbed in the small intestine and stored in the liver (Chapter 9). Some quantity of vitamin K is endogenously synthesised by the bacteria in the colon.

Vitamin K deficiency may present in the newborn or in subsequent childhood or adult life:

■ **Neonatal vitamin K deficiency.** Deficiency of vitamin K in the newborn causes haemorrhagic disease of the newborn. Liver cell immaturity, lack of gut bacterial synthesis of the vitamin and low quantities in breast milk, all contribute to vitamin K deficiency in the newborn and may cause haemorrhage on 2nd to 4th day of life. Routine administration of vitamin K to all newly born infants has led to disappearance of neonatal vitamin K deficiency.

■ **Vitamin K deficiency in children and adult.** There are 3 major causes of vitamin K deficiency in childhood or adult life:

1. Inadequate dietary intake.
2. Intestinal malabsorption.
3. Loss of storage site due to hepatocellular disease.

With the onset of vitamin K deficiency, the plasma levels of all the 6 vitamin K-dependent factors (prothrombin complex proteins) fall. This, in turn, results in prolonged PT and PTTK. Parenteral administration of vitamin K rapidly restores vitamin K levels in the liver.

Coagulation Disorders in Liver Disease

Since liver is the major site for synthesis and metabolism of coagulation factors, liver disease often leads to multiple haemostatic abnormalities. The liver also produces inhibitors of coagulation such as antithrombin III and protein C and S and plays a role in the clearance of activated factors and fibrinolytic enzymes. Thus, patients with liver disease may develop hypercoagulability and are predisposed to develop DIC and systemic fibrinolysis.

The major causes of bleeding in liver diseases are as under:

I. Anatomic lesions. These include:

1. Portal hypertension e.g. varices, splenomegaly with secondary thrombocytopenia.
2. Peptic ulceration.
3. Gastritis.

II. Hepatic dysfunctions, e.g.

1. Impaired hepatic synthesis of coagulation factors.
2. Impaired hepatic synthesis of coagulation inhibitors: protein C, protein S and antithrombin III.
3. Impaired absorption and metabolism of vitamin K.
4. Failure to clear activated coagulation factors causing DIC and systemic fibrinolysis.

III. Complications of therapy. These causes are:

1. Following massive transfusion leading to dilution of platelets and coagulation factors.
2. Infusion of activated coagulation proteins.
3. Following heparin therapy.

Many a times, the haemostatic abnormality in liver disease is complex but most patients have prolonged PT and PTTK, mild thrombocytopenia, normal fibrinogen level and decreased hepatic stores of vitamin K.

Fibrinolytic Defects

Normally, fibrinolysis consisting of plasminogen-plasmin and fibrin degradation products (FDPs) is an essential protective physiologic mechanism to limit the blood coagulation in the body. However, unchecked and excessive fibrinolysis may sometimes be the cause of bleeding. The causes of *primary pathologic fibrinolysis* leading to haemorrhagic defects are:

1. Deficiency of α_2-plasmin inhibitor following trauma or surgery.
2. Impaired clearance of tissue plasminogen activator such as in cirrhosis of liver.

At times, it may be difficult to distinguish primary pathologic fibrinolysis from secondary fibrinolysis accompanying DIC.

DISSEMINATED INTRAVASCULAR COAGULATION (DIC)

Disseminated intravascular coagulation (DIC), also termed defibrination syndrome or consumption

Chapter Thirteen

coagulopathy, is a complex thrombo-haemorrhagic disorder (intravascular coagulation and haemorrhage) occurring as a secondary complication in some systemic diseases.

ETIOLOGY. Although there are numerous conditions associated with DIC, most frequent causes are listed below:

1. **Massive tissue injury:** in obstetrical syndromes (e.g. abruptio placentae, amniotic fluid embolism, retained dead foetus), massive trauma, metastatic malignancies, surgery.

2. **Infections:** especially endotoxaemia, gram-negative and meningococcal septicaemia, certain viral infections, malaria, aspergillosis.

3. **Widespread endothelial damage:** in aortic aneurysm, haemolytic-uraemic syndrome, severe burns, acute glomerulonephritis.

4. **Miscellaneous:** snake bite, shock, acute intravascular haemolysis, heat stroke.

PATHOGENESIS. Although in each case, a distinct triggering mechanism has been identified, the sequence of events, in general, can be summarised as under (Fig. 13.41):

1. **Activation of coagulation.** The etiologic factors listed above initiate widespread activation of coagulation pathway by release of tissue factor.

2. **Thrombotic phase.** Endothelial damage from the various thrombogenic stimuli causes generalised platelet aggregation and adhesion with resultant deposition of small thrombi and emboli throughout the microvasculature.

3. **Consumption phase.** The early thrombotic phase is followed by a phase of consumption of coagulation factors and platelets.

4. **Secondary fibrinolysis.** As a protective mechanism, fibrinolytic system is secondarily activated at the site of intravascular coagulation. Secondary fibrinolysis causes breakdown of fibrin resulting in formation of FDPs in the circulation.

Pathophysiology of DIC is summed up schematically in Fig. 13.42.

CLINICAL FEATURES. There are 2 main features of DIC—*bleeding* as the most common manifestation, and *organ damage* due to ischaemia caused by the effect of widespread intravascular thrombosis such as in the kidney and brain. Less common manifestations include: microangiopathic haemolytic anaemia and thrombosis in larger arteries and veins.

LABORATORY FINDINGS. The laboratory manifestations include the following:

1. The platelet count is low.
2. Blood film shows the features of microangiopathic haemolytic anaemia. There is presence of schistocytes and fragmented red cells due to damage caused by trapping and passage through the fibrin thrombi.
3. Prothrombin time, thrombin time and activated partial thromboplastin time, are all prolonged.
4. Plasma fibrinogen levels are reduced due to consumption in microvascular coagulation.
5. Fibrin degradation products (FDPs) are raised due to secondary fibrinolysis.

BLOOD GROUPS AND BLOODTRANSFUSION

BLOOD GROUP ANTIGENS AND ANTIBODIES

The term *blood group* is applied to any well-defined system of red blood cell antigens which are inherited

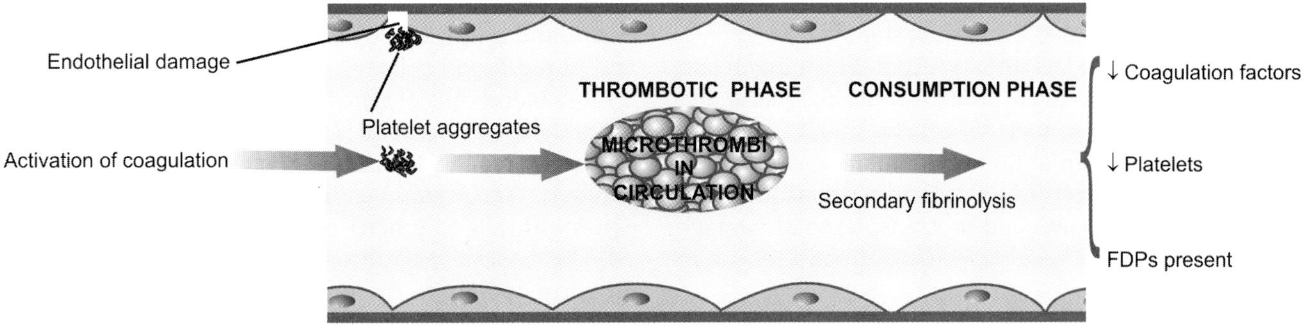

FIGURE 13.41

The pathogenesis of disseminated intravascular coagulation.

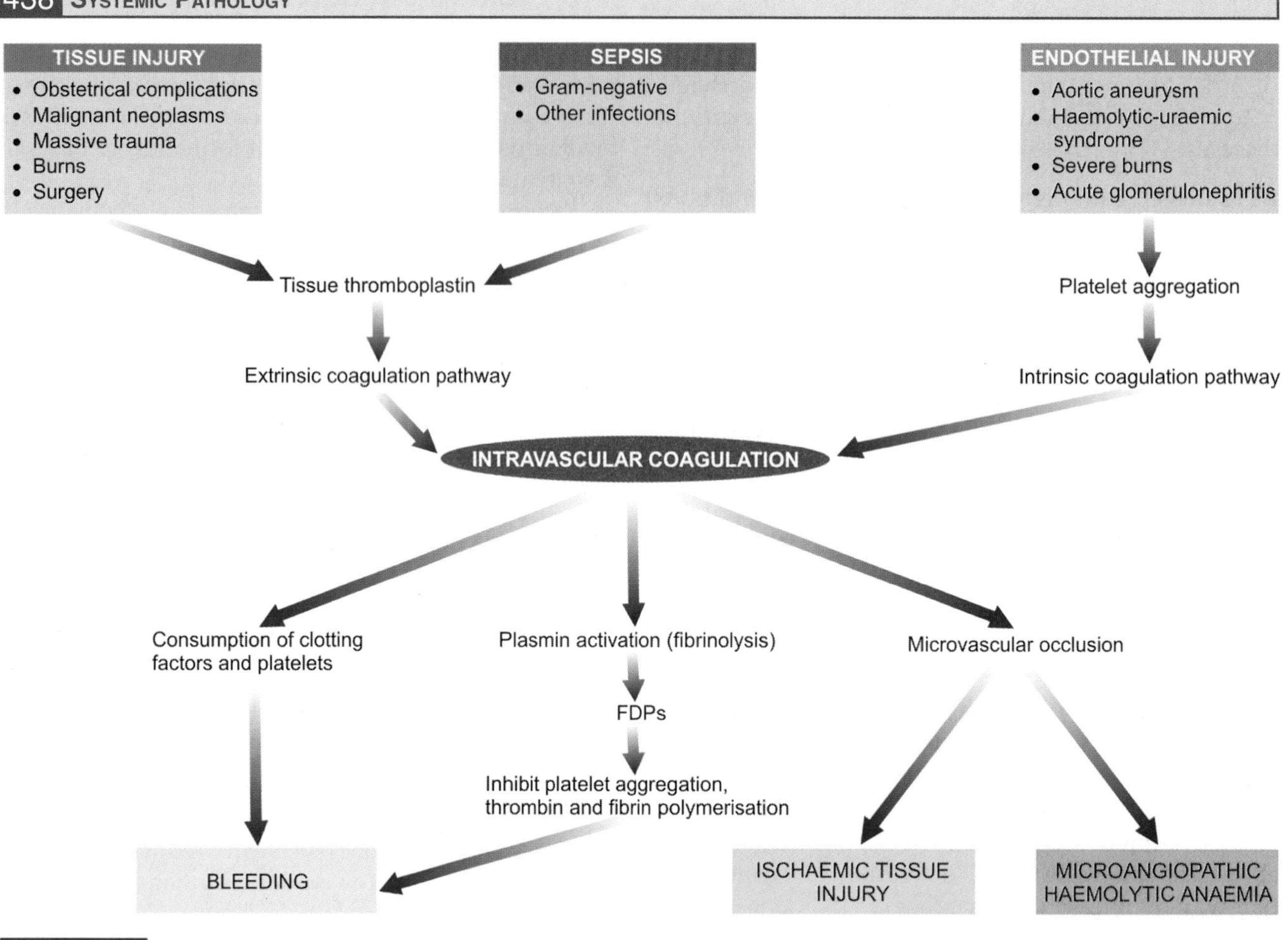

FIGURE 13.42

Pathophysiology of disseminated intravascular coagulation.

characteristics. Over 20 blood group systems having approximately 400 blood group antigens are currently recognised. The ABO and Rhesus (Rh) blood group systems are of major clinical significance. Other minor and clinically less important blood group systems are: Lewis system, P system, I system, MNS system, Kell and Duffy system, and Luthern system.

Individuals who lack the corresponding antigen and have not been previously transfused have *naturally-occurring antibodies* in their serum. The most important are anti-A and anti-B antibodies, usually of IgM class. *Immune antibodies,* on the other hand, are acquired in response to transfusion and by transplacental passage during pregnancy. These are warm antibodies, usually of IgG class.

ABO SYSTEM. This system consists of 3 major allelic genes: A,B and O, located on the long arm of chromosome 9. These genes control the synthesis of blood group antigens A and B. The serum of an individual contains naturally-occurring antibodies to A and/or B antigen, whichever antigen is lacking in the person's red cells (Table 13.24). Two subgroups of A—A_1 and A_2, and thus of AB also, A_1B and A_2B, are recognised but are of minor clinical significance. In routine practice, the ABO type is determined by testing the red blood cells with anti-A and anti-B and by testing the serum against A,B and O red blood cells.

Red blood cells of type O and A_2 have large amounts of another antigen called *H substance* which is genetically different from ABO but is a precursor of A and B antigens. An O group individual who inherits A or B genes but fails to inherit H gene from either parent is called O_h *phenotype or Bombay blood group.* In such rare individual, despite the presence of all the three antibodies in serum (anti-A, anti-B and anti-H), the red cells are not agglutinated by the antisera.

RHESUS SYSTEM. The Rhesus (Rh) blood group system was first discovered on human red cells by the

TABLE 13.24: The ABO Blood Groups.

BLOOD GROUP	ANTIGENS ON RED CELLS	NATURALLY-OCCURRING SERUM ANTIBODIES
AB	AB	None
A	A	Anti-B
B	B	Anti-A
O	O	Anti-A, Anti-B

use of antisera prepared by immunising rabbits with red cells from a Rhesus monkey. The Rh allelic genes are *C or c, D or d* and *E or e*, located on chromosome 1. One set of 3 genes is inherited from each parent giving rise to various complex combinations. The corresponding antigens are similarly named *Cc,Ee* and only *D* since no *d* antigen exists.

However, out of all these, *D* antigen is most strongly immunogenic and, therefore, clinically most important. In practice, Rh grouping is performed with anti-D antiserum. Individuals who are D-positive are referred to as *Rh-positive* and those who lack D antigen are termed *Rh-negative.*

Practically, there are no naturally-occurring Rh antibodies. All Rh antibodies in Rh-negative individuals are acquired from immunisation such as by transfusion and during pregnancy, resulting in fatal haemolytic transfusion reaction and haemolytic disease of the newborn (described later).

BLOOD TRANSFUSION

A pre-transfusion compatibility testing is essential prior to any blood transfusion. The procedure consists of the following:

1. ABO and Rh(D) grouping of the patient *(recipient).*
2. *Antibody screening* of the patient's serum to detect the presence of clinically significant antibodies.
3. Selecting the *donor* blood of the same ABO and Rh group.
4. *Cross-matching* the patient's serum against donor red cells to confirm donor-recipient compatibility.

The indications for blood transfusion are acute blood loss and various haematologic disorders considered already. In addition to the whole blood transfusion, the modern blood-banking techniques have made it possible to transfuse blood components such as packed red blood cells, platelets, white blood cell concentrates, plasma components and plasmapheresis in specific situations.

Complications of Blood Transfusion

A carefully prepared and supervised blood transfusion is quite safe. However, in 5-6% of transfusions, untoward complications occur, some of which are minor while others are more serious and at times fatal.

Transfusion reactions are generally classified into 2 types: *immune and non-immune.*

I. *Immunologic transfusion reactions* may be against red blood cells (haemolytic reactions), leucocytes, platelets or immunoglobulins.

II. *Non-immune transfusion reactions* include circulatory overload, massive transfusion, or transmission of an infectious agent.

These transfusion reactions are considered below.

I. IMMUNOLOGIC TRANSFUSION REACTIONS. These are as under:

1. Haemolytic transfusion reactions. Haemolytic transfusion reaction may be *immediate* or *delayed, intravascular* or *extravascular.*

■ The very rapid cell destruction associated with *intravascular haemolysis* is usually due to ABO incompatibility since both naturally-occurring antibodies, anti-A and anti-B, are capable of fixing complement. The symptoms include restlessness, anxiety, flushing, chest or lumbar pain, tachypnoea, tachycardia and nausea, followed by shock and renal failure.

■ *Extravascular haemolysis* is more often due to immune antibodies of the Rh system. The clinical manifestations are relatively less severe and usually consist of malaise and fever but shock and renal failure may rarely occur. Some patients develop delayed reactions in which the patient develops anaemia due to destruction of red cells in the RE system about a week after transfusion. Such delayed reactions are generally the result of previous transfusion or pregnancy (anamnestic reaction).

2. Other allergic reactions. Besides haemolytic transfusion reaction, others are:

i) *Febrile reaction* which its usually attributed to immunologic reaction against white blood cells, platelets, or IgA class immunoglobulins.

ii) Patients with antibodies against IgA molecule sometimes develop *anaphylactic shock* on transfusion of blood from other human subjects.

iii) *Allergic reactions* such as urticaria may occur.

iv) Transfusion-related *graft-versus-host disease* mediated by donor T lymphocytes may occur.

II. NONIMMUNE TRANSFUSION REACTIONS. This category includes the following adverse effects:

1. Circulatory overload. Circulatory overload resulting in pulmonary congestion and acute heart failure is the most important and most common complication that may result in death following transfusion. The risk of circulatory overload is particularly high in patients with chronic anaemia, and in infants and the elderly. The onset may be immediate, or may be delayed up to 24 hours.

2. Massive transfusion. When the volume of stored blood transfused to bleeding patients exceeds their normal blood volume, it results in dilutional thrombocytopenia and dilution of coagulation factors.

3. Transmission of infection. Many diseases can be transmitted by transfusion of an infected blood. These include: hepatitis (HBV, HCV), CMV infection, syphilis, malaria, toxoplasmosis, infectious mononucleosis, brucellosis and AIDS (HIV infection). The incidence increases in patients who receive multiple transfusions such as cases of haemophilia, thalassaemia major, acute leukaemias, acute severe haemorrhage etc. It is, therefore, mandatory that before transfusion, every unit of blood is screened for the serologic testing of HIV, HBV, HCV and syphilis and for the presence of malarial parasite.

4. Air embolism. Air embolism is unlikely to occur if the blood transfusion is carried out with plastic bags with negative pressure as is the usual practice now-a-days. A debilitated person may develop symptomatic air embolism even if a small volume (10-40 ml) makes its way into the circulation, whereas a healthy individual is at lesser risk.

5. Thrombophlebitis. The complication of thrombophlebitis is more commonly associated with venesection for blood transfusion, especially if it is done in the saphenous vein of the ankle rather than the veins of the arm. The risk of developing thrombophlebitis is further enhanced if the transfusion is continued longer than 12 hours at a single site.

6. Transfusion haemosiderosis. Post-transfusion iron overload with deposition of iron in the tissues of the body occurs after repeated transfusions in the absence of any blood loss e.g. in thalassaemia major and in severe chronic refractory anaemias. The body has no other means of getting rid of extra iron except iron excretion at the rate of 1 mg per day. A unit of whole blood (400 ml) contains about 250 mg of iron. After approximately 100 units, the liver, myocardium and endocrine glands are all damaged.

BLOOD COMPONENTS

Blood from donors is collected as whole blood in a suitable anticoagulant. Now-a-days it is a common practice to divide whole blood in to components which include: packed RBCs, platelets, fresh-frozen plasma (FFP) and cryoprecipitate.

The procedure consists of initial centrifugation at low speed to separate whole blood into two parts: *packed RBCs* and *platelet-rich plasma (PRP)*. Subsequently, PRP is centrifuged at high speed to yield two parts: *random donor platelets* and *FFP*. *Cryoprecipitates* are obtained by thawing of FFP followed by centrifugation. *Apheresis* is the technique of direct collection of large excess of platelets from a single donor.

The applications of these blood components in clinical use is briefly given below.

1. Packed RBCs. These are used to raise the oxygen-carrying capacity of blood and are used in normovolaemic patients of anaemia without cardiac disease. One unit of packed RBCs may raise haemoglobin by 1 g/dl.

2. Platelets. Transfusion of platelets is done in patients of thrombocytopenia who have haemorrhage. Optimally, platelet transfusions can be given to a patient with platelet count below 10,000/μl. Each unit of platelets can raise platelet count by 5,000 to 10,000/μl.

3. Fresh frozen plasma. FFP contains plasma proteins and coagulation factors that includes albumin, protein C and S and antithrombin. FFP transfusion in indicated in patients of coagulation failure and TTP. Each unit of FFP raises coagulation factors by about 2%.

4. Cryoprecipitate. Cryoprecipitate is a source of insoluble plasma proteins, fibrinogen, factor VIII and vWF. Indications for transfusion of cryoprecipitate are for patients requiring fibrinogen, factor VIII and vWF. Transfusion of single unit of cryoprecipitate yields about 80 IU of factor VIII.

HAEMOLYTIC DISEASE OF NEWBORN

Haemolytic disease of the newborn (HDN) results from the passage of IgG antibodies from the maternal circulation across the placenta into the circulation of the foetal red cells. Besides pregnancy, sensitisation of the mother may result from previous abortions and previous blood transfusion.

HDN can occur from incompatibility of ABO or Rh blood group system. ABO incompatibility is much more common but the HDN in such cases is usually mild, while Rh-D incompatibility results in more severe form of the HDN.

PATHOGENESIS. The pathogenesis of the two main forms of HDN is different.

HDN due to Rh-D incompatibility. Rh incompatibility occurs when a Rh-negative mother is sensitised to Rh-positive blood. This results most often from a Rh-positive foetus by passage of Rh-positive red cells across the placenta into the circulation of Rh-negative mother. Normally, during pregnancy very few foetal red cells cross the placenta but haemorrhage during parturition causes significant sensitisation of the mother. Sensitisation is more likely if the mother and foetus are ABO compatible rather than ABO incompatible. Though approximately 95% cases of Rh-HDN are due to anti-D, some cases are due to combination of anti-D with other immune antibodies of the Rh system such as anti-C and anti-E, and rarely anti-c alone.

It must be emphasised here that the risk of sensitisation of a Rh-negative woman married to Rh-positive man is small in first pregnancy but increases during successive pregnancies if prophylactic anti-D immunoglobulin is not given within 72 hours after the first delivery. If both the parents are Rh-D positive (homozygous), all the newborns will be Rh-D positive, while if the father is Rh-D positive (heterozygous), there is a 50% chance of producing a Rh-D negative child.

HDN due to ABO incompatibility. About 20% pregnancies with ABO incompatibility between the mother and the foetus develop the HDN. Naturally-occurring anti-A and anti-B antibodies' which are usually of IgM class do not cross the placenta, while immune anti-A and anti-B antibodies which are usually of IgG class may cross the placenta into foetal circulation and damage the foetal red cells. ABO HDN occurs most frequently in infants born to group O mothers who possess anti-A and/or anti-B IgG antibodies. ABO-HDN differs from Rh(D)-HDN, in that it occurs in first pregnancy, Coombs' (antiglobulin) test is generally negative, and is less severe than the latter.

CLINICAL FEATURES. The HDN due to Rh-D incompatibility in its *severest form* may result in intra-uterine death from *hydrops foetalis. Moderate disease* produces a baby born with severe anaemia and jaundice due to unconjugated hyperbilirubinaemia. When the level of unconjugated bilirubin exceeds 20 mg/dl, it may result in deposition of bile pigment in the basal ganglia of the CNS called *kernicterus* and result in permanent brain damage. *Mild disease,* however, causes only severe anaemia with or without jaundice.

LABORATORY FINDINGS. The haematologic findings in cord blood and mother's blood are as under:

1. *Cord blood* shows variable degree of anaemia, reticulocytosis, elevated serum bilirubin and a positive direct Coombs' test if the cord blood is Rh-D positive.
2. Mother's blood is Rh-D negative with high plasma titre of anti-D.

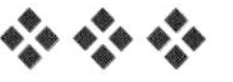

The Lymphoid System

14

The lymphoid system tissues consisting of peripheral lymphoid organs (lymph nodes, spleen, mucosa-associated lymphoid tissue—MALT, pharyngeal lymphoid tissue) and thymus are closely interlinked with the function of the bone marrow. B and T lymphocytes formed after differentiation from lymphopoietic precursor cells in the bone marrow undergo further maturation in peripheral lymphoid organs and thymus respectively. The discussion below pertains to diseases pertaining to lymph nodes, spleen and thymus.

LYMPH NODES

NORMAL STRUCTURE

The lymph nodes are bean-shaped or oval structures varying in length from 1 to 2 cm and form the part of lymphatic network distributed throughout the body. Each lymph node is covered by a connective tissue *capsule.* At the convex surface of the capsule several *afferent lymphatics* enter which drain into the peripheral *subcapsular sinus,* branch into the lymph node and terminate at the concavity (hilum) as a single *efferent lymphatic* vessel. These lymphatic vessels are lined by mononuclear phagocytic cells.

The inner structure of the lymph node is divided into a peripheral cortex and central medulla. The *cortex* consists of several rounded aggregates of lymphocytes called *lymphoid follicles.* The follicle has a pale-staining germinal centre surrounded by small dark-staining lymphocytes called the mantle zone. The deeper region of the cortex or *paracortex* is the zone between the peripheral cortex and the inner medulla. The *medulla* is predominantly composed of cords of plasma cells and some lymphocytes. The capsule and the structure within the lymph node are connected by supportive delicate reticulin framework (Fig. 14.1,A).

Functionally, the lymph node is divided into T and B lymphocyte zones:

- *B-cell zone* lies in the follicles in the cortex, the mantle zone and the interfollicular space, while *plasma cells* are also present in the interfollicular zone.
- *T-cell zone* is predominantly present in the medulla.

There are two main functions of the lymph node—to mount immune response in the body, and to perform the function of active phagocytosis for particulate material. Besides T and B-cells, the follicular centre has *dendritic histiocytes* and antigen presenting *Langerhans' histiocytes* (formerly together called tingible body macrophages due to engulfment of particulate material) and *endothelial cells.* The follicular centre is a very active zone where lymphocytes from peripheral blood continuously enter and leave, interact with macrophage-histiocytes and endothelial cells and undergo maturation and transformation. Lymphocytes and endothelial cells have surface molecules which interact and serve as 'addresses' so that endothelial cells can direct the lymphocytes; these molecules are appropriately termed as *addressins* or *homing receptors.* Peripheral blood B and T lymphocytes on entering the lymph node are stimulated immunologically which transforms them to undergo cytoplasmic and nuclear maturation which may be in the follicular centre or paracortex as per following sequence and schematically depicted in Fig. 14.1,B:

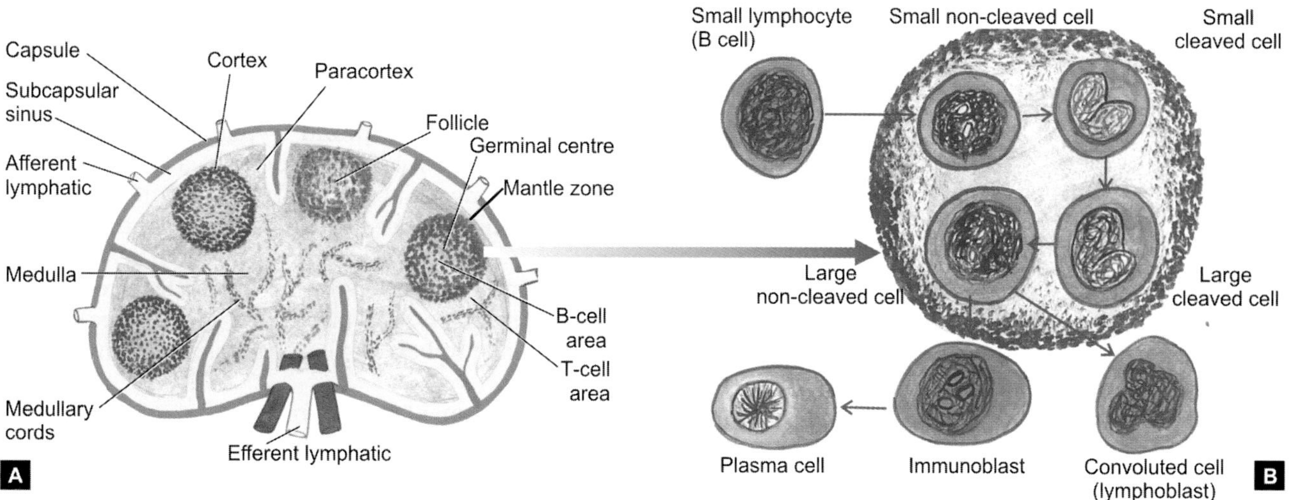

FIGURE 14.1

A, The anatomic structure and functional zones of a lymph node. B, Maturation of lymphoid cells in the follicle.

i) Follicular centre, small non-cleaved cells or centroblasts
ii) Follicular centre, small cleaved cells or centrocytes
iii) Follicular centre, large cleaved cells
iv) Follicular centre, large non-cleaved cells
v) Immunoblasts (in paracortex)
vi) Convoluted cells or lymphoblasts (in paracortex)
vii) Plasma cells

Lymph nodes are secondarily involved in a variety of systemic diseases, local injuries and infections, and are also the site for some important primary neoplasms. Many of these diseases such as tuberculosis, sarcoidosis, histoplasmosis, typhoid fever, viral infections etc have been considered elsewhere in the textbook alongwith description of these primary diseases. In the section of diseases of the lymph node that follows, the following topics are discussed:

1. Reactive lymphadenitis.
2. Malignant lymphomas.
3. Lymph node metastatic tumours.
4. Plasma cell disorders.
5. Langerhans' cell histiocytosis.

REACTIVE LYMPHADENITIS

Lymph nodes undergo reactive changes in response to a wide variety of stimuli which include microbial infections, drugs, environmental pollutants, tissue injury, immune-complexes and neoplasia. However, the most common causes of lymph node enlargement are inflammatory and immune reactions, aside from primary malignant neoplasms and metastatic tumour deposits. Those due to primary inflammatory reaction are termed *reactive lymphadenitis*, and those due to primary immune reactions are referred to as *lymphadenopathy*.

Reactive lymphadenitis is a nonspecific response and is categorised into acute and chronic types. In addition, a few variant lymphadenitis are also described below.

Acute Nonspecific Lymphadenitis

All kinds of acute inflammations may cause acute nonspecific lymphadenitis in the nodes draining the area of inflamed tissue. Most common causes are microbiologic infections or their breakdown products, and foreign bodies in the wound or into the circulation etc. Most frequently involved lymph nodes are: *cervical* (due to infections in the oral cavity), *axillary* (due to infection in the arm), *inguinal* (due to infection in the lower extremities), and *mesenteric* (due to acute appendicitis, acute enteritis etc).

Acute lymphadenitis is usually mild and transient but occasionally it may be more severe. Acutely inflamed nodes are enlarged, tender, and if extensively involved, may be fluctuant. The overlying skin is red and hot. After control of infection, majority of cases heal completely without leaving any scar. If the inflammation does not subside, acute lymphadenitis changes into chronic lymphadenitis.

PATHOLOGIC CHANGES. Grossly, the affected lymph nodes are enlarged 2-3 times their normal size and may show abscess formation if the involvement is extensive.

Microscopically, the sinusoids are congested, widely dilated and oedematous and contain numerous neutrophils. The lymphoid follicles are prominent with presence of many mitoses and phagocytosis. In more severe cases, necrosis may occur and neutrophil abscesses may form.

Chronic Nonspecific Lymphadenitis

Chronic nonspecific lymphadenitis, commonly called *reactive lymphoid hyperplasia,* is a common form of inflammatory reaction of draining lymph nodes as a response to antigenic stimuli such as repeated attacks of acute lymphadenitis and lymph from malignant tumours.

Depending upon the pattern in chronic nonspecific lymphadenitis, three types are distinguished, each having its own set of causes. These are: *follicular hyperplasia, paracortical hyperplasia* and *sinus histiocytosis.* However, mixed patterns may also be seen in which case one of the patterns predominates over the others.

PATHOLOGIC CHANGES. Grossly, the affected lymph nodes are usually enlarged, firm and non-tender.

Microscopically, the features of 3 patterns of reactive lymphoid hyperplasia are as under:

1. Follicular hyperplasia is the most frequent pattern, particularly encountered in children. Besides nonspecific stimulation, a few specific causes are: rheumatoid arthritis, toxoplasmosis, syphilis and AIDS. The microscopic features are as follows (COLOUR PLATE XVIII; CL 69).

i) There is marked enlargement and prominence of the germinal centres of lymphoid follicles (proliferation of B-cell areas) due to the presence of numerous mitotically active lymphocytes and proliferation of phagocytic cells containing phagocytosed material.

ii) Parafollicular and medullary regions are more cellular and contain plasma cells, histiocytes, and some neutrophils and eosinophils.

iii) There is hyperplasia of mononuclear phagocytic cells lining the lymphatic sinuses in the lymph node.

■ *Angiofollicular lymphoid hyperplasia* or *Castleman's disease* is a clinicopathologic variant of follicular hyperplasia. The condition may occur at any age and possibly has an association with Epstein-Barr virus infection. Two histologic forms are distinguished:

i) *Hyaline-vascular type* is more common (90% cases) and is characterised by the presence of hyalinised arterioles in small lymphoid follicles and proliferation of vessels in the interfollicular area.

ii) *Plasma cell form* is less common and is characterised by plasma cell hyperplasia and vascular proliferation in the interfollicular region.

2. Paracortical lymphoid hyperplasia is due to hyperplasia of T-cell-dependent area of the lymph node. Amongst the important causes are immunologic reactions caused by drugs (e.g. dilantin), vaccination, viruses (e.g. infectious mononucleosis) and autoimmune disorders. Its histologic features are:

i) Expansion of the paracortex (T-cell area) with increased number of T-cell transformed immunoblasts.

ii) Encroachment by the enlarged paracortex on the lymphoid follicles, sometimes resulting in their effacement.

iii) Hyperplasia of the mononuclear phagocytic cells in the lymphatic sinuses.

Variants of paracortical lymphoid hyperplasia are angio-immunoblastic lymphadenopathy, dermatopathic lymphadenopathy, dilantin lymphadenopathy and post-vaccinial lymphadenopathy.

■ *Angioimmunoblastic lymphadenopathy* is characterised by diffuse hyperplasia of immunoblasts rather than paracortical hyperplasia only, and there is proliferation of blood vessels. The condition occurs in elderly patients with generalised lymph node enlargement and hypergammaglobulinaemia.

■ *Dermatopathic lymphadenopathy* occurs in lymph node draining an area of skin lesion. Besides the hyperplastic paracortex, there is presence of dark melanin pigment within the macrophages in the lymph node.

3. Sinus histiocytosis or sinus hyperplasia is a very common type found in regional lymph nodes draining inflammatory lesions, or as an immune reaction of the host to a draining malignant tumour or its products. The hallmark of histologic diagnosis is the expansion of the sinuses by proliferating large histiocytes containing phagocytosed material. The presence of sinus histiocytosis in the draining lymph nodes of carcinoma such as in breast carcinoma has been considered by some workers to confer better prognosis in such patients due to good host immune response.

■ *Sinus histiocytosis with massive lymphadenopathy* is characterised by marked enlargement of lymph nodes, especially of the neck, in young adolescents. It is associated with characteristic clinical features of painless but massive lymphadenopathy with fever and leucocytosis and usually runs a benign and self-limiting course.

HIV-related Lymphadenopathy

HIV infection and AIDS have already been discussed in Chapter 4; here one of the frequent finding in early cases of AIDS, **persistent generalised lymphadenopathy (PGL),** is described. The presence of enlarged lymph nodes of more than 1 cm diameter at two or more extra-inguinal sites for more than 3 months without any other obvious cause is frequently the earliest symptom of primary HIV infection.

Histologically, the findings at biopsy of involved lymph node vary depending upon the stage of HIV infection:

1. *In the early stage* marked follicular hyperplasia is the dominant finding and reflects the polyclonal B-cell proliferation.
2. *In the intermediate stage,* there is a combination of follicular hyperplasia and follicular involution. However, adenopathic form of Kaposi's sarcoma too may develop at this stage (page 303).
3. *In the last stage,* there is decrease in the lymph node size indicative of prognostic marker of disease progression. Microscopic findings of node at this stage reveal follicular involution and lymphocyte depletion. At this stage, other stigmata of AIDS in the lymph node may also appear e.g. lymphoma, mycobacterial infection, toxoplasmosis, systemic fungal infections etc.

MALIGNANT LYMPHOMAS

Lymphomas are malignant tumours of lymphoreticular origin i.e. from lymphocytes and histiocytes and their precursor cells. Clinically and pathologically, lymphomas are quite heterogeneous. However, two distinct clinicopathologic groups are routinely distinguished:

I. *Hodgkin's lymphoma* or *Hodgkin's disease (HD)* characterised by pathognomonic presence of Reed-Sternberg cells. This group comprises about 25% of all cases of malignant lymphomas.

II. *Non-Hodgkin's lymphomas (NHL)* are more common and comprise the rest of cases.

Both these groups have further histopathologic subtypes and are considered separately below.

HODGKIN'S DISEASE

Hodgkin's disease (HD) primarily arises within the lymph nodes and involves the extranodal sites secondarily. The incidence of the disease has bimodal peaks—one in young adults between the age of 15 and 35 years and the other peak after 5th decade of life. The HD is more prevalent in young adult males than females. The classical diagnostic feature is the presence of *Reed-Sternberg (RS) cell (or Dorothy-Reed-Sternberg cell)* (described later).

Etiopathogenesis

The nature and origin of RS cells, which are the real neoplastic cells in HD, have been a matter of considerable debate. One main reason for this difficulty in their characterisation is that in HD, unlike most other malignancies, the number of neoplastic cells (i.e. RS cells) is very small (less than 5%) which are interspersed in the predominant reactive cells. However, it is still not clear what stimulates these lymphoid cells to undergo transformation. The following possible hypotheses are suggested:

1. EBV. For years, Epstein-Barr virus (EBV) has been implicated in the etiology of HD on the basis of epidemiologic and serologic studies. Recently, on the basis of molecular studies, genome of EBV has been identified in majority of cases of mixed cellularity type and some cases of nodular sclerosis HD.

2. Genetic etiology. It is suggested on the basis of observation of occurrence of HD in families and with certain HLA type. HD is 99 times more common in identical twin of an affected case compared with general population, implicating genetic origin strongly.

3. Cytokines. Presence of reactive inflammatory cells in the HD is due to secretion of cytokines from the RS cells e.g. IL-5 (growth factor for eosinophils), IL-13 (for autocrine stimulation of RS cells) and transforming growth factor-β (for fibrogenesis).

Classification

The diagnosis of HD requires accurate microscopic diagnosis by biopsy, usually from lymph node, and occasionally from other tissues. Unlike NHL, there is only one universally accepted classification of HD i.e. *Rye classification* adopted since 1966. Rye classification divides HD into the following 4 subtypes:

1. Lymphocyte-predominance type.
2. Nodular-sclerosis type.
3. Mixed-cellularity type.
4. Lymphocyte-depletion type.

More recently , however, according to the new WHO classification of all malignancies of lymphoid tissues (Harris et al, 1999) which takes into account clinical, morphologic, immunologic and genetic information, HD has been divided into 2 main groups:

I. Nodular lymphocyte-predominant HD (a new type).

II. Classic HD (includes all the 4 above subtypes in the Rye classification).

Central to the diagnosis of HD is the essential identification of *Reed-Sternberg cell* though this is not the sole criteria (see below).

The salient features of the 4 histologic subtypes of HD are summarised in Table 14.1.

Reed-Sternberg Cell

The diagnosis of Hodgkin's disease rests on identification of RS cells, though uncommonly similar cells can occur in infectious mononucleosis and other forms of lymphomas. Therefore, additional cellular and architectural features of the biopsy must be given due consideration for making the histologic diagnosis.

There are several morphologic variants of RS cells which characterise different histologic subtypes of HD (Fig. 14.2):

1. **Classic RS cell** is a large cell which has characteristically a bilobed nucleus appearing as mirror image of each other but occasionally the nucleus may be multilobed. Each lobe of the nucleus contains a prominent, eosinophilic, inclusion-like nucleolus with a clear halo around it, giving an owl-eye appearance. The cytoplasm of cell is abundant and amphophilic.

2. **Lacunar type RS cell** is smaller and in addition to above features has a pericellular space or lacuna in which it lies, which is due to artefactual shrinkage of the cell cytoplasm. It is characteristically found in nodular sclerosis variety of HD.

3. **Polyploid type (or popcorn or lymphocytic-histiocytic i.e. L and H) RS cells** are seen in lymphocyte predominance type of HD. This type of RS cell is larger with lobulated nucleus in the shape of popcorn.

4. **Pleomorphic RS cells** are a feature of lymphocyte depletion type. These cells have pleomorphic and atypical nuclei.

It may be mentioned here that in general the number of RS cells is inversely proportional to the number of lymphocytes in a particular histologic subtype of HD.

Immunophenotyping of RS cells reveals monoclonal lymphoid cell origin of RS cell from B-cells in most subtypes of Hodgkin's disease. RS cells in all types of Hodgkin's diseases, except in lymphocyte predominance type, express immunoreactivity for CD15 and CD30. RS cells in lymphocyte predominance type, however, are negative for both CD15 and CD30, but positive for CD20.

RS cells are invariably accompanied by variable number of *atypical Hodgkin cells* which are believed to be precursor RS cells but are not considered diagnostic of HD. Hodgkin cells are large mononuclear cells (rather than mirror image nuclei) having nuclear and cytoplasmic similarity to that of RS cell.

PATHOLOGIC CHANGES. Grossly, the affected lymph nodes initially remain discrete but later are matted together. The sectioned surface is homogeneous and fishflesh-like in *lymphocyte predominance type,* nodular due to scarring in *nodular sclerosis type,* and abundance of necrosis in *mixed cellularity* and *lymphocyte depletion types.* Hodgkin's disease of the liver, spleen and other organs forms spherical masses similar to metastatic carcinoma.

Microscopically, the criteria for diagnosis of histologic subtypes are as under:

I. CLASSIC HD

As per WHO classification, classic group of HD includes 4 types of HD of older Rye classification:

TABLE 14.1: Modified Rye Classification of Hodgkin's Disease.

HISTOLOGIC SUBTYPE	INCIDENCE	MAIN PATHOLOGY	RS CELLS	PROGNOSIS
I. CLASSIC HD				
Lymphocyte-predominance	5%	Proliferating lymphocytes, a few histiocytes	Few, classic and polyploid type, CD15–, CD30–, CD20+	Excellent
Nodular sclerosis	70%	Lymphoid nodules, collagen bands	Frequent, lacunar type, CD15+, CD30+	Very good
Mixed cellularity	22%	Mixed infiltrate	Numerous, classic type, CD15+, CD30+	Good
Lymphocyte-depletion (Diffuse fibrotic and reticular variants)	1%	Scanty lymphocytes, atypical histiocytes, fibrosis	Numerous, pleomorphic type, CD15+, CD30+	Poor
II. NODULAR LYMPHOCYTE-PREDOMINANT HD				
	2%	Proliferation of small lymphocytes, nodular pattern of growth	Sparse number of RS cells, CD45+, EMA+, CD15-, CD30-	Chronic relapsing, may transform into large B cell NHL

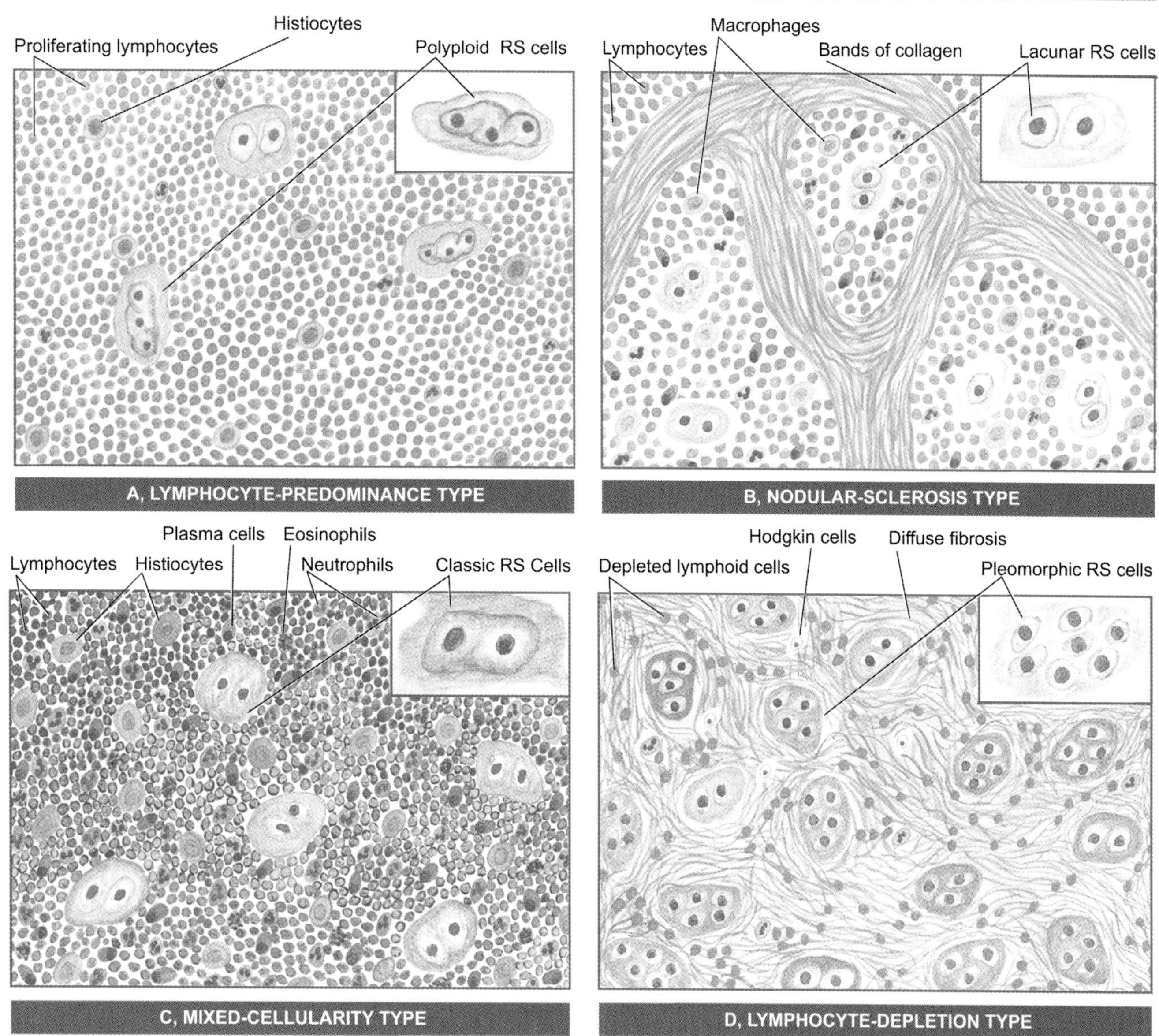

FIGURE 14.2

Microscopic features of 4 forms of Hodgkin's disease of lymph node. The inset on right side of each type shows the morphologic variant of RS cell seen more often in particular histologic type.

1. Lymphocyte-predominance type (Fig. 14.2,A). The lymphocyte-predominance type of HD is characterised by proliferation of small lymphocytes admixed with a varying number of histiocytes forming nodular or diffuse pattern.

i) *Nodular form* is characterised by replacement of nodal architecture by numerous large neoplastic nodules.

ii) *Diffuse form* does not have discernible nodules but instead there is diffuse proliferation of cells.

However, currently nodular form of lymphocyte predominent HD has been categorised separately due to its distinct immunophenotyping features and prognosis (discussed below).

For making the diagnosis, definite demonstration of RS cells is essential which are few in number, requiring a thorough search. In addition to typical RS cells, *polyploid variant* having polyploid, and twisted nucleus (popcorn-like) may be found in some cases. This type of HD usually does not show other cells like plasma cells, eosinophils and neutrophils, nor are necrosis or fibrosis seen.

2. Nodular-sclerosis type (Fig. 14.2,B). Nodular sclerosis is the most frequent type of HD, seen more commonly in women than in men. It is characterised by two essential features:

i) *Bands of collagen:* Variable amount of fibrous tissue is characteristically present in the involved lymph nodes. Occasionally, the entire lymph node may be replaced by dense hyalinised collagen.

ii) *Lacunar type RS cells:* Characteristic lacunar type of RS cells with distinctive pericellular halo are present. These cells appear lacunar due to the shrinkage of cytoplasm in formalin-fixed tissue. The pericellular halo is not seen if the tissue is fixed in Zenker's fluid.

In addition to these 2 characteristics, the nodules between the fibrous septa consist predominantly of lymphocytes and macrophages, sometimes with foci of necrosis.

3. Mixed-cellularity type (Fig. 14.2,C). This form of HD generally replaces the entire affected lymph nodes by heterogeneous mixture of various types of apparently normal cells. These include proliferating lymphocytes, histiocytes, eosinophils, neutrophils and plasma cells. Some amount of fibrosis and focal areas of necrosis are generally present. Typical RS cells are frequent (COLOUR PLATE XVIII: CL 71).

4. Lymphocyte-depletion type (Fig. 14.2,D). In this type of HD, the lymph node is depleted of lymphocytes. There are two variants of lymphocyte-depletion HD:

i) *Diffuse fibrotic variant* is hypocellular and the entire lymph node is replaced by diffuse fibrosis, appearing as homogeneous, fibrillar hyaline material. The area of hyalinosis contains some lymphocytes, atypical histiocytes (Hodgkin cells), and numerous typical and atypical (pleomorphic) RS cells.

ii) *Reticular variant* is much more cellular and consists of large number of atypical pleomorphic histiocytes, scanty lymphocytes and a few typical RS cells.

II. NODULAR LYMPHOCYTE-PREDOMINANT HD

This is a newly described entity which is distinct from the classic HD described above. This type was previously included in lymphocyte predominant type of HD. Its peculiarities are as under:

i) These cases of HD have a nodular growth pattern (similar to nodular sclerosis type).

ii) Like lymphocyte-predominant pattern of classic type, there is predominance of small lymphocyte with sparse number of RS cells.

iii) These cases of HD have distinctive immunophenotyping: CD45 positive, epithelial membrane (EMA) positive but negative for the usual markers for RS cells (CD15 and CD30 negative).

iv) Though generally it has a chronic relapsing course, but some cases of this type of HD may transform in to large B-cell NHL.

Clinical Features

Hodgkin's disease is particularly frequent among young and middle-aged adults. All histologic subtypes of HD, except the nodular sclerosis variety, are more common in males. The disease usually begins with superficial lymph node enlargement and subsequently spreads to other lymphoid and non-lymphoid structures.

1. Most commonly, patients present with painless, movable and firm *lymphadenopathy.* The cervical and mediastinal lymph nodes are involved most frequently. Other lymph node groups like axillary, inguinal and abdominal are involved sometimes.

2. Approximately half the patients develop *splenomegaly* during the course of the disease. *Liver enlargement* too may occur.

3. *Constitutional symptoms* (type B symptoms) are present in 25-40% of patients. The most common is low-grade fever with night sweats and weight loss. Other symptoms include fatigue, malaise, weakness and pruritus.

Other Laboratory Findings

Besides clinical and pathologic findings, there are some haematologic and immunologic abnormalities in HD.

Haematologic abnormalities:

1. A moderate, normocytic and normochromic *anaemia* is often present.
2. *Serum iron and TIBC* are low but marrow iron stores are normal or increased.
3. *Marrow infiltration* by the disease may produce marrow failure with leucoerythroblastic reaction.
4. *Routine blood counts* reveal moderate leukaemoid reaction. Cases with pruritus frequently show peripheral eosinophilia. Advanced disease is associated with absolute lymphopenia.
5 *Platelet count* is normal or increased.
6. *ESR* is invariably elevated.

Immunologic abnormalities:

1. There is progressive fall in immunocompetent T-cells with *defective cellular immunity.* There is reversal of CD4: CD8 ratio and anergy to routine skin tests.
2. *Humoral antibody production* is normal in untreated patients until late in the disease.

Staging

Following biopsy and histopathologic classification of HD, the extent of involvement of the disease (i.e. staging) is studied so as to select the proper treatment and assess the prognosis. *The Ann Arbor staging classification* takes into account both clinical and pathologic stage of the disease.

The suffix *A* or *B* are added to the above stages depending upon whether the three constitutional symptoms (fever, night sweats and unexplained weight loss exceeding 10% of normal) are absent (A) or present (B). The suffix *E* or *S* are used for extranodal involvement and splenomegaly respectively (Table 14.2).

For complete staging, a number of other *essential diagnostic studies* are recommended. These are as under:

1. Detailed physical examination including sites of nodal involvement and splenomegaly.
2. Chest radiograph to exclude mediastinal, pleural and lung parenchymal involvement.
3. CT scan of abdomen and pelvis.
4. Documentation of constitutional symptoms (B symptoms).
5. Laboratory evaluation of complete blood counts, liver and kidney function tests.
6. Bilateral bone marrow biopsy.
7. Finally, histopathologic documentation of the type of Hodgkin's disease.

More invasive investigations include *lymphangiography of lower extremities* and *staging laparotomy.* Staging laparotomy includes biopsy of selected lymph nodes in the retroperitoneum, splenectomy and wedge biopsy of the liver.

Prognosis

With use of aggressive radiotherapy and chemotherapy, the outlook for Hodgkin's disease has improved significantly. Although several factors affect the prognosis, two important considerations in evaluating its outcome are the *extent of involvement by the disease (i.e. staging)* and the *histologic subtype.*

■ With appropriate treatment, the overall 5 years survival rate for *stage I and II A* is as high as about 100%, while the advanced stage of the disease may have upto 50% 5-year survival rate.

■ Patients with *lymphocyte-predominance type* of HD tend to have localised form of the disease and have excellent prognosis.

■ The *nodular sclerosis* variety too has very good prognosis but those patients with larger mediastinal mass respond poorly to both chemotherapy and radiotherapy.

■ The *mixed cellularity type* occupies intermediate clinical position between the lymphocyte predominance and the lymphocyte-depletion type, but patients with disseminated disease and systemic manifestations do poorly.

■ The *lymphocyte-depletion type* is usually disseminated at the time of diagnosis and is associated with constitutional symptoms. These patients usually have the most aggressive form of the disease.

TABLE 14.2: Ann Arbor Staging Classification of Hodgkin's Disease.

Stage I (A or B)	I	Involvement of a single lymph node region.
	I_E	Involvement of a single extra-lymphatic organ or site.
Stage II (A or B)	II	Involvement of two or more lymph node regions on the same side of the diaphragm.
	II_E	(or) with localised contiguous involvement of an extranodal organ or site.
Stage III (A or B)	III	Involvement of lymph node regions on both sides of the diaphragm.
	III_E	(or) with localised contiguous involvement of an extranodal organ or site.
	III_S	(or) with involvement of spleen.
	III_{ES}	(or) both features of III_E and III_S.
Stage IV (A or B)	IV	Multiple or disseminated involvement of one or more extra-lymphatic organs or tissues with or without lymphatic involvement.

A = asymptomatic; B = presence of constitutional symptoms; E = extranodal involvement; S = splenomegaly

NON-HODGKIN'S LYMPHOMAS

Non-Hodgkin's lymphomas (NHL) are the malignant neoplasms of the immune system of the body and are more common than Hodgkin's lymphoma. The biologic and clinical behaviour of NHL are quite distinct from HD and thus the two are quite different diseases. NHL is most frequent in young adults (20-40 years). Its incidence is showing an upward trend due to increasing incidence of AIDS.

Majority of NHL arise in lymph nodes (65%) while the remaining 35% take origin in extranodal lymphoid tissues. However, all forms of NHL have potential to spread to other lymph nodes, liver, spleen and bone marrow. The involvement of bone marrow may be followed by spill over of NHL into the peripheral blood, and vice versa when lymphoid leukaemia originating in the bone marrow may spread to lymph nodes, creating an overlapping picture of lymphoid leukaemia and NHL. In such situations, it may become difficult to determine which appeared first in the affected patient.

Etiopathogenesis

Malignant lymphomas are considered as the clonal proliferation of immune cells. About 65% of NHL are of B-lymphocyte origin, 35% of T-lymphocytes, and less than 2% are histiocytic derivatives. The agents involved in inducing neoplastic transformation of these cells are poorly understood, but the following etiologic factors have been shown to have strong association with the development of NHL.

1. **Infections.** There is evidence to suggest that certain infections are involved in development of lymphomas:

i) Viral infections: Epstein-Barr virus (EBV) in endemic variety of Burkitt's lymphoma and post-transplant lymphoma, human-T-cell leukaemia virus type I (HTLV-I) in adult T-cell lymphoma-leukaemia, HIV in diffuse large B-cell lymphoma and Burkitt's lymphoma, hepatitis C virus in lymphoplasmacytic lymphoma, and human herpes virus 8 (HHV-8) in primary effusion lymphoma.

ii) Bacteria. Helicobacter pylori in MALT lymphoma of the stomach.

2. **Immunodeficiency diseases.** Various inherited and acquired immunodeficiency diseases including AIDS and iatrogenic immunosuppression induced by chemotherapy or radiation, are associated with subsequent development of lymphomatous transformation.

3. **Autoimmune disease association.** A few autoimmune diseases such as Sjögren's syndrome, non-tropical sprue, rheumatoid arthritis and SLE are associated with higher incidence of NHL.

4. **Chemical and drug exposure.** Long-term exposure to drugs such as phenytoin, radiation, prior chemotherapy and agriculture chemicals have all been associated with development of NHL. Patients treated for HD can develop NHL.

A number of cytogenetic abnormalities have been detected in cases of NHL, most important of which are chromosomal translocations involving antigen receptor genes, immunoglobulin genes, or overexpression of *BCL-2* protein.

Classification

Unlike Hodgkin's disease in which Rye classification is the only universally accepted classification since 1966 with some modifications, the pathologic classification of NHL has been difficult for both pathologists and clinicians. Several classifications have been described at different times adding further confusion. The widely used classification systems of NHL (in chronologic order) are: *Rappaport* (1966), *Lukes-Collins* (1974), *Working Formulations for clinical usage* (1982), REAL (1994), and WHO classification (1999). These classifications are given in Table 14.3 and briefly discussed below.

RAPPAPORT CLASSIFICATION. Rappaport in 1966 proposed a clinically relevant pathologic classification based on the following two main features:

1. *Low-power microscopy* of the overall pattern of the lymph node architecture.
2. *High-power microscopy* revealing the cytology of the neoplastic cells.

Based on these two features, Rappaport divided NHL into two major subtypes:

1. *Nodular or follicular lymphomas* which retain some of the features of normal lymph node in that the neoplastic cells form lymphoid 'nodules' rather than lymphoid follicles with germinal centres.
2. *Diffuse lymphomas,* on the other hand, are characterised by effacement of the normal lymph node architecture and there may be infiltration of neoplastic cells outside the capsule of the involved lymph node.

NHL was further classified according to the degree of differentiation of neoplastic cells into: *well-differentiated, poorly-differentiated,* and *histiocytic (large cells) types* of both nodular and diffuse lymphomas.

However, with the advent of modern immunologic methods, the following objections were raised regarding the applicability of Rappaport classification:

1. The term histiocytic lymphoma was found incorrect since almost all lymphomas were of lymphoid origin.
2. With the identification of T and B-cells and their subpopulations made possible, the Rappaport classification was found to be incomplete as regards the cell of origin of different subtypes of NHL.

LUKES-COLLINS CLASSIFICATION. Lukes and Collins in 1974 proposed a classification correlating the

TABLE 14.3: Classification of NHL.

RAPPAPORT CLASSIFICATION (1966)

A) Nodular NHL
1. Lymphocytic, well-differentiated
2. Lymphocytic, poorly-differentiated
3. Lymphocytic and histiocytic, mixed

B) Diffuse NHL
1. Lymphocytic, well-differentiated
2. Lymphocytic, poorly-differentiated
3. Lymphocytic and histiocytic, mixed
4. Histiocytic
5. Lymphoblastic
6. Diffuse undifferentiated, Burkitt's and non-Burkitt's

LUKES-COLLINS CLASSIFICATION (1974)

A) B-cell NHL
1. Small lymphocytic
2. Plasmacytoid lymphocytic
3. Follicular centre cell (small cleaved and large cleaved, small non-cleaved and large non-cleaved)
4. Immunoblastic

B) T-cell NHL
1. Small lymphocytic
2. Convoluted lymphocytic
3. Cerebriform lymphocytic
4. Immunoblastic

C) Histiocytic NHL

D) Undefined (U) NHL

WORKING FORMULATIONS FOR CLINICAL USAGE (1982)

I. Low-grade
- A) Small lymphocytic
- B) Follicular, predominantly small cleaved cell
- C) Follicular, mixed small and large cleaved cell

II. Intermediate-grade
- D) Follicular, predominantly large cell
- E) Diffuse, small cleaved cell
- F) Diffuse, mixed small and large cell
- G) Diffuse, large, cell

III. High-grade
- H) Large cell, immunoblastic
- I) Lymphoblastic
- J) Small non-cleaved cell (Burkitt's)

IV. Miscellaneous
1. Adult T-cell leukaemia/lymphoma
2. Cutaneous T-cell lymphoma
3. Histiocytic (Histiocytic medullary reticulosis)

REAL CLASSIFICATION (1994)

I. Leukaemias and lymphomas of B-cell origin (Pan-B CD19,20 positive)

A) Indolent B-cell malignancies
- i) Chronic lymphocytic leukaemia/small lymphocytic lymphoma
- ii) Hairy cell leukaemia
- iii) Follicular lymphomas (grade I small cleaved, grade II mixed small and large)
- iv) Lymphoplasmacytoid lymphoma/Waldenström's macroglobulinaemia
- v) Marginal zone lymphoma (lymphoma of mucosa-associated lymphoid tissue (MALT), splenic lymphoma)

B) Aggressive B-cell malignancies
- i) Diffuse large cell lymphoma
- ii) Follicular large cell lymphoma (grade III)
- iii) Mantle cell lymphoma
- iv) Burkitt's lymphoma
- v) Plasmacytoma/myeloma

II. Leukaemias and lymphomas of T-cell origin (CD2,7 positive)

a) Indolent T-cell malignancies
- i) T-CLL, T-prolymphocytic leukaemia
- ii) Cutaneous T-cell lymphoma (Sézary's syndrome, mycosis fungoides)

b) Aggressive T-cell malignancies
- i) Peripheral T-cell NHL
- ii) Angioimmunoblastic T-cell lymphoma
- iii) Intestinal T-cell lymphoma
- iv) Adult T-ALL

WHO CLASSIFICATION (1999)

I. B-cell neoplasms

Precursor B-cell malignancies:

Precursor B lymphoblastic leukaemia/lymphoma (precursor B-cell ALL)

Mature (Peripheral) B-cell malignancies:
1. B-cell CLL/SLL (chronic lymphocytic leukaemia/small lymphocytic lymphoma)
2. Plasma cell myeloma/plasmacytoma (page 459)
3. Extranodal marginal zone B-cell lymphoma, MALT type
4. Mantle cell lymphoma
5. Follicular lymphoma
6. Diffuse large B-cell lymphoma
7. Burkitt's lymphoma/Burkitt cell leukaemia
8. Other B-cell malignancies:
   - i) B-cell prolymphocytic leukaemia
   - ii) Hairy cell leukaemia
   - iii) Splenic marginal zone B-cell lymphoma
   - iv) Lymphoplasmacytic lymphoma
   - v) Nodal marginal zone lymphoma (Monocytoid B-cell lymphoma)

II. T-cell neoplasms

Precursor T-cell malignancies:

Precursor T lymphoblastic lymphoma/leukaemia (Precursor T-cell ALL)

Mature (Peripheral) T-cell malignancies:
1. Mycosis fungoides/Sézary syndrome
2. Adult T-cell lymphoma/leukaemia (HTLV-I +)
3. Anaplastic large T/null cell lymphoma, primary systemic type
4. Peripheral T-cell lymphoma, not otherwise specified
   - i) Angioimmunoblastic T-cell lymphoma
   - ii) Extranodal NK/T-cell lymphoma, nasal type
   - iii) Enteropathy-type T-cell lymphoma
   - iv) Hepatosplenic T-cell lymphoma
5. Other T-cell malignanies:
   - i) T-cell prolymphocytic leukaemia
   - ii) T-cell granular lymphocytic leukaemia
   - iii) Aggressive NK cell leukaemia

type of NHL with the immune system. Yet another modification of Lukes-Collins called *Kiel classification* appeared in 1981.

Employing immunologic markers for tumour cells, Lukes-Collins divided all malignant lymphomas into either B-cell or T-cell origin and rarely macrophages. The B and T-cell tumours are further subdivided on the basis of their light microscopic characteristics. The majority of NHL are B lymphocyte derivatives (about 65%) and arise from follicular centre cells (FCC). The FCC in the germinal centre undergo transformation to become large immunoblasts and pass through the four stages—*small cleaved cells* and *large cleaved cells, small non-cleaved cells* and *large non-cleaved cells.*

Though Lukes-Collins classification is immunologically correct, the classification is unclear about varying prognosis of different clinical types of NHL of either B-cell or T-cell origin.

WORKING FORMULATIONS FOR CLINICAL USAGE. This classification proposed in 1982 by a panel of experts from National Cancer Institute of the US incorporates the best features of all previous classification systems, and as the name implies, has strong clinical relevance. Based on the natural history of disease and long-term survival studies. Working Formulations divides all NHLs into 3 prognostic groups:

- *Low-grade NHL:* 5-year survival 50-70%;
- *Intermediate-grade NHL:* 5-year survival 35-45%; and
- *High-grade NHL:* 5-year survival 25-35%.

In this classification, no attempt is made to determine whether the tumour cells are B-cells, T-cells or macrophages. Each prognostic group includes a few morphologic subtypes, and lastly, a miscellaneous group is also described.

REAL CLASSIFICATION. International Lymphoma Study Group in 1994 has proposed another classification called *r*evised *E*uropean-*A*merican classification of *l*ymphoid neoplasms abbreviated as REAL classification. This classification is based on the hypothesis that all forms of lymphoid malignancies (NHLs as well as lymphoblastic leukaemias) represent malignant counterparts of normal population of immune cells (B-cells, T-cells and histiocytes) present in the lymph node and bone marrow. It is believed that lymphoid malignancies arise due to arrest at the various differentiation stages of B and T-cells since tumours of histiocytic origin are quite uncommon. Accordingly, it is considered essential to understand and correlate the differentiation stages of B and T-cells with various lymphoid malignancies (Fig. 14.3). REAL classification divides all lymphoid malignancies into two broad groups, each having further subtypes (Table 14.3):

- *Leukaemias and lymphomas of B-cell origin:* B-cell derivation comprises 80% cases of lymphoid leukaemias and 90% cases of NHLs. Based upon these phenotypic and genotypic features, B-cell neoplasms are of pre-B and mature B-cell origin. Based on their biologic behaviour, B-cell malignancies are further subclassified into indolent and aggressive. All these tumours express Pan-B (CD19) antigen besides other markers.
- *Leukaemias and lymphomas of T-cell origin:* T-cell malignancies comprise the remainder 20% cases of lymphoid leukaemia and 10% cases of NHLs. T-cell malignancies reflect the stages of T-cell ontogeny. Like B-cell malignancies, T-cell derivatives too are further categorised into indolent and aggressive T-cell malignancies. The most widely expressed T-cell antigens are CD2 and CD7.

WHO CLASSIFICATION. In 1999, the same group of workers (Harris et al) who described REAL classification revised their classification under the aegis of WHO. Although this classification has many similarities with REAL classification as regards identification of B and T cell types (Fig. 14.3), WHO classification has more classes. Besides, it takes into consideration clinicopathologic and immunologic profile of all lymphoid malignancies, and has a better clinical and therapeutic relevance.

PATHOLOGIC CHANGES

The diagnosis of NHL can only be reliably made on examination of lymph node biopsy.

Grossly, the affected group of lymph nodes are enlarged in majority of cases of NHL. Any lymph node group may be involved but most commonly affected are the cervical, supraclavicular and axillary groups. Less commonly at the time of diagnosis, there may be enlargement of lymphoid tissue elsewhere such as in the tonsils, spleen, stomach, bone etc. Initially, the lymph nodes are discrete and separate from one another but later the lymph nodes form a large matted mass due to infiltration into the surrounding connective tissue. Extranodal involvements produce either a discrete tumour or diffuse enlargement of the affected organ. The sectioned surface of the involved lymph nodes or extranodal organ involved appears grey-white and fishflesh-like. Thus, the gross appearance of Hodgkin's and non-Hodgkin's lymphoma is much the same.

Histologically, it is beyond the scope of the present text to describe the morphological details of all the

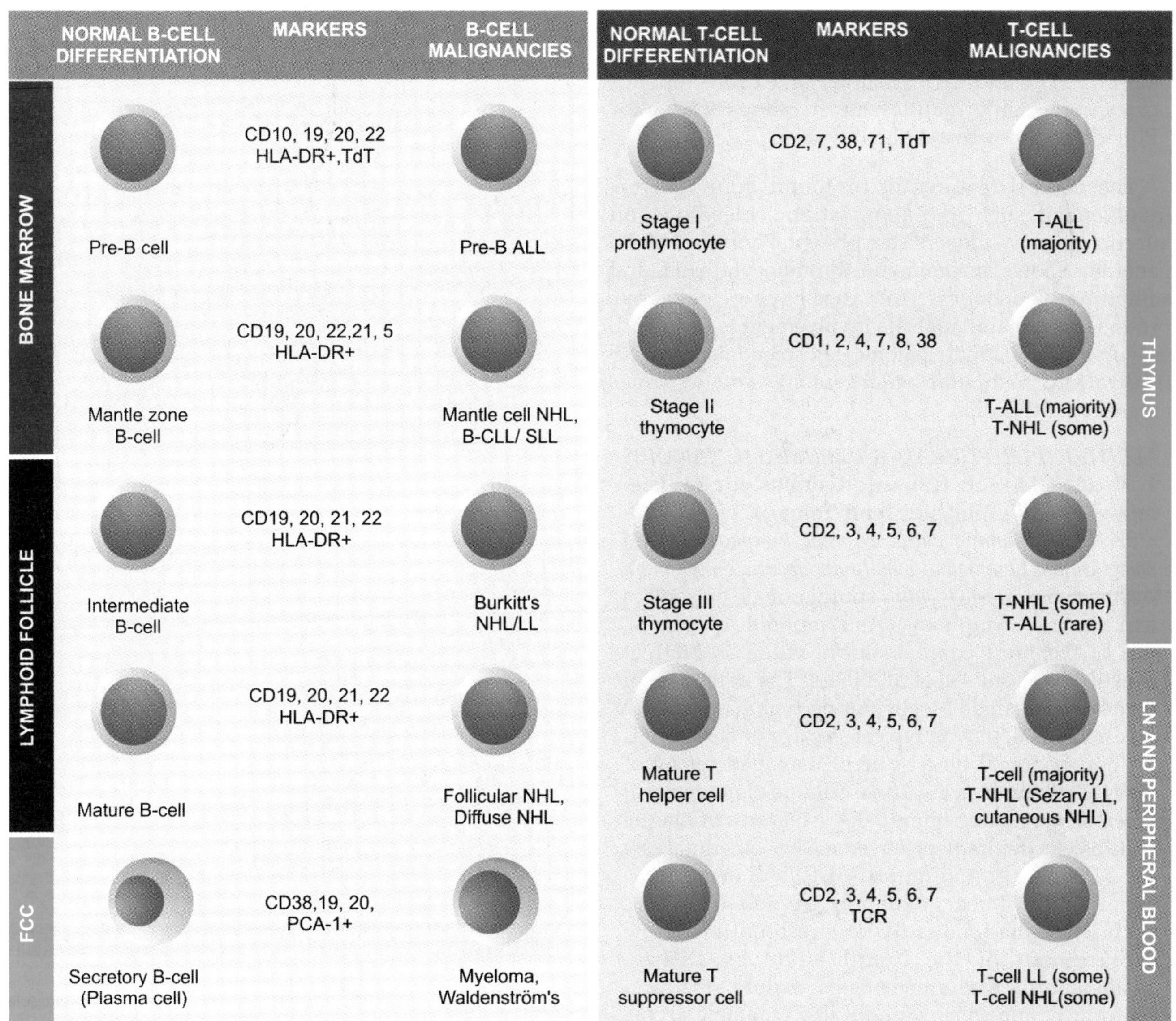

(PCA- Plasma cell antigen; TCR = T-cell receptor; FCC = Follicular centre B- cells, LN = Lymph node, LL = Lymphoid leukaemia)

FIGURE 14.3

Schematic representation of WHO-REAL classification. Various immunophenotypes of B and T-cell malignancies are correlated with normal immunophenotypic differentiation/maturation stages of B and T-cells in the bone marrow, lymphoid tissue, peripheral blood and thymus.

subtypes of NHL listed in Table 14.3 and Fig. 14.3 for which the reference works may be consulted. However, salient features of common clinicopathologic subtypes as per recent WHO classification are briefly outlined below. The synonyms in brackets in each subgroup of NHL described below (wherever counterpart subtypes applicable) correspond to the Rappaport, Lukes-Collins, and Working Formulation for Clinical Usage classification respectively.

I. B-CELL NEOPLASMS

PRECURSOR B-CELL MALIGNANCIES

Precursor B-cell lymphocytic leukaemia-lymphoma *(Diffuse lymphoblastic; Convoluted T-cell lymphoma; Lymphoblastic lymphoma).* This is the most common form of ALL in children; rarely presentation may be in the form of lymphoma in children or adults. The diagnosis is made by bone marrow biopsy which shows malignant cells of precursor B cell origin as demonstrated by immunophenotyping (CD10, 19, 20, 22, HLA-DR and TdT positive) and characteristic cytogenetic abnormalities, most often t(9;22) i.e. Philadelphia positive-ALL.

The clinical features of profound bone marrow involvement such as pallor, fatigue, bleeding and infections due to cytopenia are present. Peripheral blood generally shows anaemia and thrombocytopenia, and sometimes leucopenia. In cases having leukaemic presentation, extranodal site involvement is early such as lymphadenopathy, hepatomegaly, splenomegaly, CNS infiltration, testicular enlargement, and at times cutaneous infiltration.

MATURE (PERIPHERAL) B-CELL MALIGNANCIES

1. B-cell CLL/SLL (Chronic lymphocytic leukaemia—small lymphocytic lymphoma). *(Diffuse, well-differentiated lymphocytic; B-small lymphocytic and plasmacytoid lymphoma; Small lymphocytic lymphoma).* As the name implies, this subtype may present as leukaemia or lymphoma. As lymphoid leukaemia, this is the most common form, while as NHL it constitutes about 4% of all NHLs. The diagnosis of B-cell CLL is made by circulating lymphocytosis in excess of 4,000/μl with typical smudge or basket cells in the peripheral blood due to damaged nuclei of malignant lymphocytes. These cells are of monoclonal B-cell origin having immunologic features of mantle zone B-cells (typically positive for CD5; other markers are CD19, 20, 22 and for HLA-DR) and cytogenetic abnormalities (most commonly trisomy 12). Cases with lymphadenopathy at presentation show replacement of the lymph node by diffuse proliferation of well-differentiated, mature, small and uniform lymphocytes without any cytologic atypia or significant mitoses (Fig. 14.4,B) and having features of immunophenotype as for B-cell CLL.

B-cell CLL/SLL occurs more commonly in middle and older age groups. The condition may remain asymptomatic, or may present with nonspecific clinical features such as easy fatiguability, weight loss and anorexia. Patients frequently have hepatosplenomegaly, generalised lymphadenopathy, susceptibility to infections, autoimmune haemolytic anaemia and autoimmune thrombocytopenia. Generally, the course is indolent. However, some cases of SLL may transform into more aggressive diffuse large B-cell lymphoma, or may be associated with occurrence of an IgM monoclonal gammopathy called Waldenström's macroglobulinaemia (page 462).

2. Plasma cell myeloma/plasmacytoma. This entity is discussed separately later in this chapter.

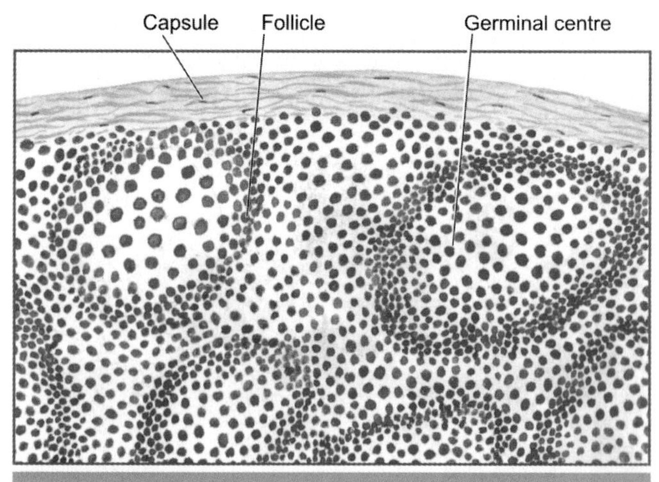

A, NORMAL LYMPH NODE

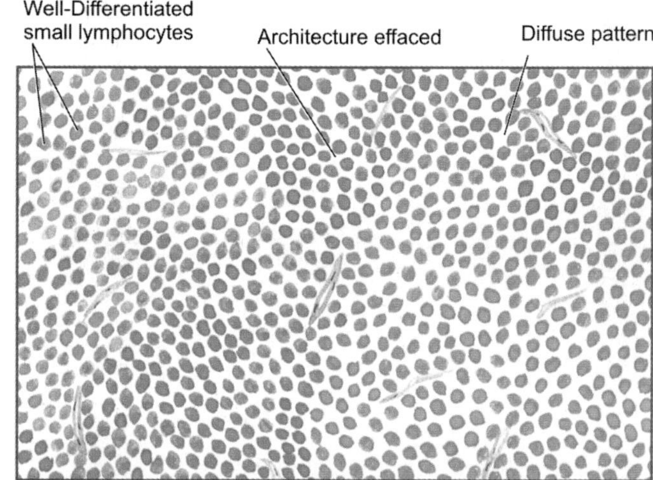

B, SMALL LYMPHOCYTIC LYMPHOMA(SLL/CLL)

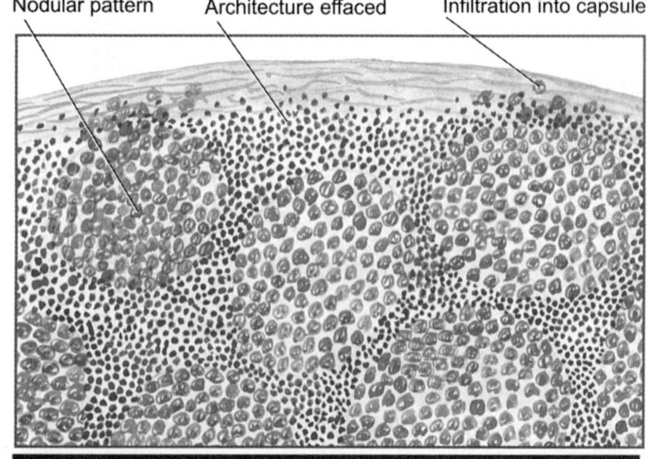

C, FOLLICULAR LYMPHOMA

FIGURE 14.4

Prototypes of non-Hodgkin's lymphoma.

Chapter Fourteen

3. Extranodal marginal zone B-cell lymphoma of MALT type. This type comprises about 8% of all NHLs. In the previous classification, it was included under SLL, but currently it is categorised separately for 2 reasons: etiologic association with *H. pylori* infection and occurrence at extranodal sites. Most frequent is gastric lymphoma of MALT type with its characteristic etiologic association with *H. pylori*; other extranodal sites for this subtype of NHL are intestine, orbit, lung, thyroid, salivary glands and CNS. Morphologically, it is characterised by diffuse infiltration by monoclonal small B lymphocytes which are negative for CD5.

Median age for this form of NHL is 60 years and often remains localised to the organ of origin but may infiltrate the regional lymph nodes. Rarely, it may be more aggressive and may metastasise, or transform into diffuse large B-cell lymphoma.

4. Mantle cell lymphoma. This subtype of NHL comprises about 6% of all NHLs. It was earlier included in SLL but has been identified as a separate subtype recently due to characteristic chromosomal translocation, t(11;14) and overexpression of *BCL-1* and surface immunoglobulins IgM and IgD protein. However, both SLL and mantle cell NHL are positive for CD5 antigen. Mantle cell lymphoma arises from B-cells of mantle zone of normal lymphoid follicle. The tumour cells show diffuse or nodular pattern of involvement in the lymph node and have somewhat indented nuclei.

Patients of mantle cell lymphoma are generally older males. The disease involves bone marrow, spleen, liver and bowel. It is more aggressive than other types of SLLs.

5. Follicular lymphoma *(Nodular, poorly-differentiated lymphocytic; Follicular centre cell, small/large cleaved lymphoma; Follicular, predominantly small/large cleaved cell lymphoma).* Follicular lymphomas comprise approximately 22% of all NHLs. Morphologically, as the name suggests, this form of follicular lymphoma is characterised by follicular or nodular pattern of growth. The nuclei of tumour cells may vary from predominantly small cleaved (or indented) to predominantly large cleaved variety (Fig. 14.4, C). The former is more common, has infrequent mitoses and the rate of growth slow (low grade), while the patients with large cell lymphoma have high proliferation and progress rapidly (high grade). In all follicular lymphomas, the tumour cells are positive for pan-B markers such as CD19 and CD20 along with expression of *BCL-2* protein (for distinction from normal germinal centre which is *BCL-2* negative). Cytogenetic studies show characteristic translocation t(14;18) in tumour cells.

The follicular lymphomas occur in older individuals, most frequently presenting with painless peripheral lymphadenopathy which is usually waxing and waning type. Bone marrow infiltration is typically paratrabecular. Peripheral blood involvement as occurs in SLL is uncommon in this variety. In contrast to diffuse lymphomas, extranodal involvement is also infrequent. About half the cases of low grade follicular lymphomas, during their indolent biologic course, may evolve into diffuse large B-cell lymphoma. Median survival for patients with low grade follicular lymphoma is 7-9 years.

6. Diffuse large B-cell lymphoma *(Diffuse poorly-differentiated lymphocytic/Diffuse histiocytic; Follicular centre cell, large, cleaved/non-cleaved diffuse lymphoma).* Diffuse large B-cell lymphoma is the most common comprising about 35% of all NHLs. This variety is the diffuse counterpart of follicular large cleaved cell lymphoma i.e. it is composed of large cleaved cells spread in a diffuse pattern. The cytoplasm in these tumour cells is pale and abundant while the nuclei have prominent 1-2 nucleoli (COLOUR PLATE XVIII: CL 70). Immunophenotypic markers for pan-B cells (CD19, CD20) are positive, besides overexpression of surface immunoglobulins (IgM, IgG and light chains) and of *BCL-2* protein.

Diffuse large B-cell lymphoma occurs in older patients with mean age of 60 years. It may present primarily as a lymph node disease or at extranodal sites. About half the cases have extranodal involvement at the time of presentation, particularly in the bone marrow and the alimentary tract. Primary diffuse large B-cell lymphoma of CNS may also occur.

A few subtypes of diffuse large B-cell lymphoma are described with distinct clinicopathologic settings:

- *Epstein-Barr virus (EBV)* infection has been etiologically implicated in diffuse large B-cell lymphoma in *immunosuppressed patients* of AIDS and organ transplant cases.
- *Human herpes virus type 8 (HHV-8)* infection along with presence of immunosuppression is associated with a subtype of diffuse large B-cell lymphoma presenting with effusion, termed *primary effusion lymphoma.*

■ *Mediastinal large B-cell lymphoma* is diagnosed in patients with prominent involvement of mediastinum, occurs in young females and frequently spreads to CNS and abdominal viscera.

In general, diffuse large B-cell lymphomas are aggressive tumours and disseminate widely.

7. Burkitt's lymphoma/leukaemia *(Diffuse undifferentiated Burkitt's and Non-Burkitt's; Follicular centre cell, small non-cleaved cell lymphoma; Small non-cleaved cell lymphoma).* Burkitt's lymphoma/leukaemia is an uncommon tumour in adults but comprises about 30% of childhood NHLs. Burkitt's leukaemia corresponds to L3 ALL of FAB grouping and is uncommon. Three subgroups of Burkitt's lymphoma are recognised: *African endemic, sporadic and immunodeficiency-associated,* but histologically all three are similar. The tumour cells are intermediate in size, non-cleaved, and homogeneous in size and shape. The nuclei are round to oval and contain 2-5 nucleoli. The cytoplasm is basophilic and contains lipid vacuolation. The tumour cells have a very high mitotic rate, and therefore high cell death. This feature accounts for presence of numerous macrophages in the background of this tumour containing phagocytosed tumour debris giving it a 'starry sky' appearance (Fig. 14.5).

■ *African endemic Burkitt's lymphoma* was first described in African children, predominantly presenting as jaw tumour that spreads to extranodal sites such as the bone marrow and meninges. The relationship of this tumour with oncogenic virus, Epstein-Barr virus (EBV), has been discussed in Chapter 8.

■ *Sporadic Burkitt's lymphoma* is a related tumour in which the tumour cells are similar to those of Burkitt's lymphoma but are more pleomorphic and may sometimes be multinucleated. Sporadic variety has a propensity to infiltrate the CNS and is more aggressive than true Burkitt's lymphoma.

■ *Immunodeficiency-associated Burkitt's lymphoma* includes cases seen in association with HIV infection.

Immunophenotypically, the tumour cells are positive for CD19 and CD10 and surface immunoglobulin IgM. Typical cytogenetic abnormalities in the tumour cells are t(8;22) involving *MYC* gene on chromosome 8, with overexpression of MYC protein ...ving transforming activity. Burkitt's lymphoma is ...h grade tumour and is the most rapidly ...sive human tumour.

...**ell malignancies.** Brief mention is made ...ther types of B-cell malignant tumours ...HO classification in Table 14.3:

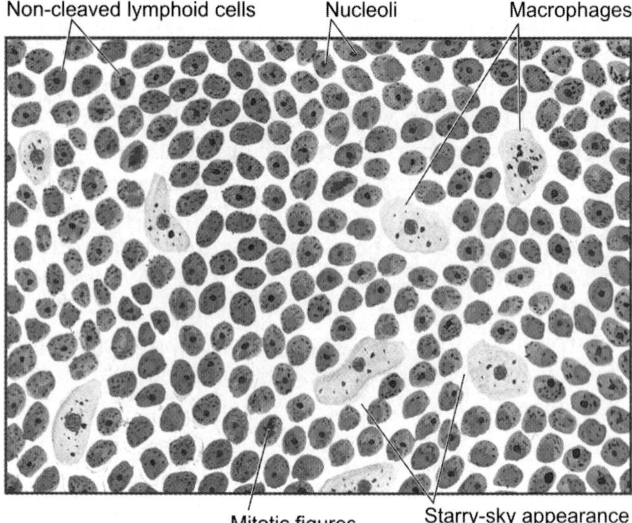

FIGURE 14.5

Burkitt's lymphoma. The tumour shows uniform cells having high mitotic rate. Scattered among the tumour cells are benign macrophages surrounded by a clear space giving 'stary sky' appearance.

i) B-cell prolymphocytic leukaemia is involvement of blood and bone marrow by large B lymphocytes having prominent nucleoli. These patients have leucocytosis with splenomegaly and lymphadenopathy.

ii) Hairy cell leukaemia is a rare B-cell malignancy characterised by presence of hairy cells in the blood and bone marrow and splenomegaly. The condition has already been discussed in Chapter 13.

iii) Splenic marginal zone lymphoma is another uncommon B-cell neoplasm in which the splenic white pulp is infiltrated by small monoclonal B lymphocytes. The condition has a slow and indolent behaviour.

iv) Lymphoplasmacytic lymphoma is tissue manifestation of Waldenström's macroglobulinaemia, discussed later in this chapter. There is infiltration by IgM-secreting monoclonal lymphoplasacytic cells into lymph nodes, spleen, bone marrow, and sometimes in the peripheral blood. Etiologic association of this form of lymphoma with hepatitis C virus infection has also been proposed.

v) Nodal marginal zone lymphoma (monocytoid B-cell lymphoma) is another uncommon subtype of aggressive NHL. At presentation, the patients often have disseminated disease, involving bone marrow and leukaemic picture.

II. T-CELL NEOPLASMS

PRECURSOR T-CELL MALIGNANCIES

Precursor T-cell lymphoblastic leukaemia/lymphoma. As the name implies, these cases may present as ALL or as lymphoma. Like precursor B-cell NHL, this subtype is also more common in children under 4 years of age. Since the precursor T-cells differentiate in the thymus, this tumour often presents as mediastinal mass and pleural effusion and progresses rapidly to develop leukaemia in the blood and bone marrow. Morphologically, precursor B and T-cell ALL/lymphoma are indistinguishable. However, immunophenotype of T-cell subtype is positive for CD2, CD7 and TdT.

Clinically, features of bone marrow failure are present which include anaemia, neutropenia and thrombocytopenia. Lymphadenopathy, hepatosplenomegaly and CNS involvement are frequent. Precursor T-cell lymphoma-leukaemia is, however, more aggressive than its B-cell counterpart.

MATURE (PERIPHERAL) T-CELL MALIGNANCIES

1. Mycosis fungoides/Sézary syndrome. Mycosis fungoides is a slowly evolving cutaneous T-cell lymphoma occurring in middle aged adult males. The condition is often preceded by eczema or dermatitis for several years (*premycotic stage*). This is followed by infiltration by CD4+T-cells in the epidermis and dermis as a plaque (*plaque stage*) and eventually as *tumour stage*. The disease may spread to viscera and to peripheral blood as a leukaemia characterised by Sézary cells having cerebriform nuclei termed as Sézary syndrome.

Mycosis fungoides/Sézary syndrome is an indolent NHL and has a median survival of 8 to 9 years.

2. Adult T-cell lymphoma/leukaemia (ATLL). This is an uncommon T-cell malignancy but has gained much prominence due to association with retrovirus, human T-cell lymphotropic virus-I (HTLV-I) (Chapter 8). The infection is acquired by blood transfusion, breast milk, sexual route or transplacentally. ATLL is observed in Japan, the Caribbean and parts of the US but is rare in rest of the world. The involved lymph nodes have proliferation of CD4 positive large atypical T-cells with indented nuclei, called 'flower cells', most prominent in the paracortical zone. The blood also shows large pleomorphic T-cell leukaemia.

The patients have usually widespread lymphadenopathy with leukaemia, hepatosplenomegaly and involvement of skin and leptomeninges. This disease has a fulminant course.

3. Anaplastic large T/Null cell lymphoma. This relatively newer entity is the T-cell counterpart of diffuse large B-cell lymphoma and was previously included under malignant histiocytosis or diagnosed as anaplastic carcinoma. There is diffuse infiltration of lymph nodes by anaplastic T-cells/null cells positive for CD30 (Ki 1). Cytogenetic abnormality consists of t(2;5). Involvement of skin occurs frequently and produces an indolent cutaneous large T/null cell lymphoma.

4. Peripheral T-cell lymphomas. This group includes a variety of aggressive T-cell lymphomas which are morphologically heterogeneous but have common immunotypic features of mature T-cells (CD4+, CD8+, or both). These are more common in young adults and often have bone marrow involvement at presentation. The subtypes of peripheral T-cell lymphomas include the following syndromes:

i) Angioimmunoblastic T-cell lymphoma is relatively more common subtype, comprising about 20% of all T-cell NHLs. The patients have profound constitutional symptoms (fever, weight loss, skin rash), generalised lymphadenopathy and polyclonal hypergammaglobulinaemia.

ii) Extranodal T/NK cell lymphoma of nasal type is involvement of upper airways by the monoclonal T-cells. The condition is quite aggressive and was earlier called as lethal midline granuloma or angiocentric lymphoma. The patients have haemophagocytic syndrome. During the course of the disease, blood and bone marrow may be involved producing leukaemic picture.

iii) Enteropathy type T-cell lymphoma is a rare aggressive lymphoma seen in association with untreated cases of gluten-sensitive enteropathy.

iv) Hepatosplenic T-cell lymphoma, unlike other lymphomas which occur as tumour masses, is characterised by sinusoidal infiltration of the liver, spleen and bone marrow by monoclonal T-cells. Systemic features are often present.

Clinical Features

Features pertaining to specific types of NHL have been given alongwith their morphologic description above. Some general clinical features common to most cases of NHL are as under:

1. Superficial lymphadenopathy. At presentation, there is painless, asymmetric enlargement of one or more groups of peripheral lymph nodes.

2. Constitutional symptoms. Fever, night sweats and more than 10% weight loss comprise the constitutional symptoms (type B symptoms) similar to those found in Hodgkin's disease.

3. Oropharyngeal involvement. Involvement of Waldeyer's ring is present in 5-10% of patients.

4. Abdominal disease. Enlargement of liver, spleen and mesenteric and retroperitoneal lymph nodes are found in some cases. Lymphomatous involvement of the GIT is the most common extranodal involvement after the bone marrow.

5. Other organs. Involvement of the skin or brain occurs in certain subtypes of NHL.

Other Laboratory Findings

In addition to clinical and histopathological findings, certain abnormal haematologic and immunologic findings are found in NHL.

Haematologic abnormalities:

1. Anaemia of normocytic normochromic type.
2. Advanced disease with marrow infiltration may show neutropenia, thrombocytopenia and leucoerythroblastic reaction.
3. Lymphosarcoma cell leukaemia (leukaemic conversion of NHL) occurs in some patients.
4. Marrow involvement by NHL is seen in 20% of cases.
5. Hyperuricaemia and hypercalcaemia occur late in the disease.

Immunologic abnormalities:

Immunologic studies reveal that majority of NHLs are of B lymphocyte origin. There may be associated monoclonal excess of immunoglobulins, usually IgG or IgM. Plasmacytoid lymphoma may produce excess of a heavy chain or a light chain.

Staging

The Ann Arbor staging system developed for Hodgkin's disease (page 449) is used for staging NHL too. This staging system depends upon the number and location of nodal and extranodal sites involved, and presence or absence of constitutional (B) symptoms. But the concept of staging is much less helpful in NHL than in Hodgkin's disease because the prognosis is not correlated with the anatomic site of involvement of the disease.

Prognosis

Low-grade lymphomas usually progress slowly and local radiotherapy brings about remission lasting for upto 10 years in 75% cases. More extensive disease is treated with combination chemotherapy and local radiotherapy. Children with lymphoblastic lymphoma and Burkitt's lymphoma respond extremely well to chemotherapy. Meningeal involvement is treated with irradiation of the brain. Patients with histiocytic lymphoma and T-cell leukaemia/lymphoma have an extremely poor prognosis.

The salient features to distinguish Hodgkin's disease and non-Hodgkin's lymphoma are summarised in Table 14.4.

LYMPH NODE METASTATICTUMOURS

The regional lymph nodes draining the site of a primary malignant tumour are commonly enlarged. This enlargement may be due to benign *reactive hyperplasia* or *metastatic tumour deposits.*

1. Benign reactive hyperplasia, as already discussed (page 443), is due to immunologic reaction by the lymph node in response to tumour-associated antigens. It may be expressed as sinus histiocytosis, follicular hyperplasia, plasmacytosis and occasionally may show non-caseating granulomas.

2. Metastatic deposits in regional lymph nodes occurs most commonly from carcinomas and malignant

TABLE 14.4: Contrasting Features of Hodgkin's Disease and Non-Hodgkin's Lymphoma.

	FEATURE	HODGKIN'S	NON-HODGKIN'S
1.	*Cell derivation*	B-cell mostly	90% B 10% T
2.	*Nodal involvement*	Localised, may spread to contiguous nodes	Disseminated nodal spread
3.	*Extranodal spread*	Uncommon	Common
4.	*Bone marrow involvement*	Uncommon	Common
5.	*Constitutional symptoms*	Common	Uncommon
6.	*Chromosomal defects*	Aneuploidy	Translocations, deletions
7.	*Spill-over*	Never	May spread to blood
8.	*Prognosis*	Better (75-85% cure)	Bad (30-40% cure)

melanoma. Sarcomas generally disseminate by the haematogenous route but uncommonly may metastasise to the regional lymph nodes. Metastatic tumour cells from the primary malignant tumour are drained via lymphatics into the subcapsular sinuses initially but subsequently the lymph node stroma is also invaded. The pushing margins of advancing metastatic tumour in stroma of lymph node is characteristically well demarcated. Areas of necrosis are frequent in metastatic carcinomas.

The morphologic features of primary malignant tumour are recapitulated in metastatic tumour in lymph nodes.

PLASMA CELL DISORDERS

The plasma cell disorders are characterised by abnormal proliferation of immunoglobulin-producing cells and result in accumulation of monoclonal immunoglobulin in serum and urine. The group as a whole is known by various synonyms such as *plasma cell dyscrasias, paraproteinaemias, dysproteinaemias and monoclonal gammopathies.* The group comprises the following four disease entities:

1. Multiple myeloma
2. Waldenström's macroglobulinaemia
3. Heavy chain disease
4. Primary amyloidosis (Chapter 4).

The feature common to all plasma cell disorders is the neoplastic proliferation of cells derived from B-lymphocyte lineage. Normally B lymphocytes have surface immunoglobulin molecules of both M and G heavy chains. Under normal circumstances, the B-cells are stimulated by exposure to surface immunoglobulin-specific antigen and mature to form IgG-producing plasma cells. However, in the plasma cell disorders, the control over this process is lost and results in abnormal production of immunoglobulin that appears in the blood and urine. These disorders differ from B-cell lymphomas in having monoclonal synthesis of immunoglobulins and lack of prominent lymphadenopathy. In addition to the rise in complete immunoglobulins, some plasma cell disorders synthesise excess of light chains (kappa or lambda), or heavy chains of a single class (alpha, gamma, or mu). Bence Jones proteins are free light chains present in blood and excreted in urine of some cases with plasma cell disorders.

After these brief general comments, we can now turn to the discussion of the specific plasma cell disorders.

MULTIPLE MYELOMA

Multiple myeloma is a multifocal malignant proliferation of plasma cells derived from a single clone of cells (i.e. monoclonal). The terms multiple myeloma and myeloma are used interchangeably. The tumour, its products (M component), and the host response result in the most important and most common syndrome in the group of plasma cell disorders that produces osseous as well as extraosseous manifestations. Multiple myeloma primarily affects the elderly (peak incidence in 5th-6th decades) and increases in incidence with age. It is rare under the age of 40 and is slightly more common in males.

Etiopathogenesis

Myeloma is a monoclonal proliferation of B-cells. The etiology of myeloma remains unknown. However, following factors have been implicated:
1. Radiation exposure.
2. Those exposed to petroleum products.
3. Farmers, wood workers, leather workers are more prone.

As regards its pathogenesis, following concepts have been proposed:

1. Genetic abnormalities. A variety of chromosomal alterations have been observed in cases of myeloma, out of which common ones are as under:

i) Translocation t(11;14)(q13;q32) is the most common.

ii) Overexpression of *MYC* or *RAS* genes in some cases.

iii) Mutation in p53 (TP53) and *RB* gene in some cases.

2. Role of growth factor. Interleukin (IL)-6 has been found to play role in B-cell proliferation in myeloma. Infection of the marrow macrophages with human herpes virus 8 with resultant release of viral IL-6 may be responsible for stimulation of neoplastic process in myeloma.

Pathologic Changes

Myeloma affects principally the bone marrow though in the course of the disease other organs are also involved. Therefore, the pathologic findings are described below under two headings—*osseous (bone marrow) lesions* and *extraosseous lesions.*

I. OSSEOUS (BONE MARROW) LESIONS. In more than 95% of cases, multiple myeloma begins in the bone marrow. In the majority of cases, the disease involves multiple bones. By the time the diagnosis is

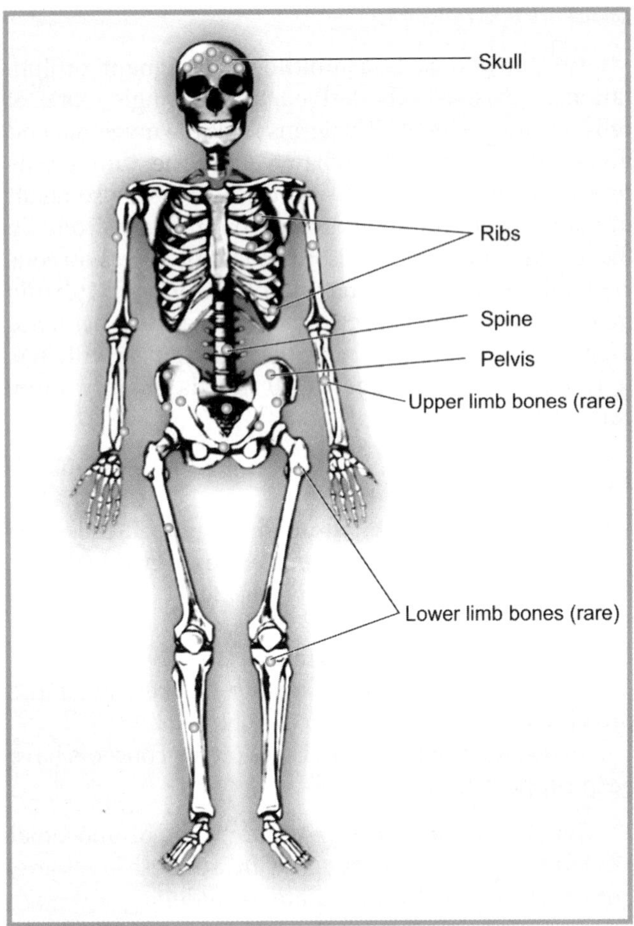

FIGURE 14.6

The major sites of lesions in multiple myeloma.

made, most of the bone marrow is involved. Most commonly affected bones are those with red marrow i.e. skull, spine, ribs and pelvis, but later long bones of the limbs are also involved (Fig. 14.6). The lesions of myeloma secrete osteoclast-stimulating factor resulting in rarefaction of the bones. The lesions begin in the medullary cavity, erode the cancellous bone and ultimately cause destruction of the bony cortex. Radiographically, these lesions appear as punched out, rounded, 1-2 cm sized defects in the affected bone.

Grossly, the normal bone marrow is replaced by soft, gelatinous, reddish-grey tumours. The affected bone usually shows focal or diffuse osteoporosis.

Microscopically, the diagnosis of multiple myeloma can be usually established by examining bone marrow aspiration from an area of bony rarefaction. However, if the bone marrow aspiration yields dry tap or negative results, biopsy of radiologically abnormal or tender site is usually diagnostic. The following features characterise a case of myeloma:

i) Cellularity: There is usually hypercellularity of the bone marrow.

ii) Myeloma cells: Myeloma cells constitute 15-30% of the marrow cellularity. These cells may form clumps or sheets, or may be scattered among the normal haematopoietic cells. Myeloma cells may vary in size from small, differentiated cells resembling normal plasma cells to large, immature and undifferentiated cells. Binucleate and multinucleate cells are sometimes present. The nucleus of myeloma cell is commonly eccentric similar to plasma cells but usually lacks the cart-wheel chromatin pattern seen in classical plasma cells. Nucleoli are frequently present. The cytoplasm of these cells is abundant and basophilic with perinuclear halo, vacuolisation and contains Russell bodies consisting of hyaline globules composed of synthesised immunoglobulin (Fig. 14.7) (COLOUR PLATE XVIII: CL 72).

In addition to multiple myeloma, *plasmacytosis* in the bone marrow can occur in some other disorders. These are: aplastic anaemia, rheumatoid arthritis, SLE, cirrhosis of liver, metastatic cancer and chronic inflammation. However, in all these conditions the plasma cells are mature and they do not exceed 10% of the total marrow cells.

II. EXTRAOSSEOUS LESIONS. Late in the course of disease, lesions at several extraosseous sites become evident. Some of the commonly involved sites are as under:

1. Blood. Approximately 50% of patients with multiple myeloma have a few atypical plasma cells in the blood. Other changes in the blood in myeloma are the presence of anaemia (usually normocytic normochromic type), marked red cell rouleaux formation due to hyperviscosity of blood, and an elevated ESR.

2. Myeloma kidney. Renal involvement in myeloma called myeloma nephrosis occurs in many cases (Chapter 20). The main mechanism of myeloma kidney is by filtration of light chain proteins (Bence Jones proteins) which are precipitated in the distal convoluted tubules in combination with Tamm-Horsfall proteins as tubular casts. The casts may be surrounded by some multinucleate giant-cells and a few inflammatory cells.

3. Myeloma neuropathy. Infiltration of the nerve trunk roots by tumour cells produces nonspecific

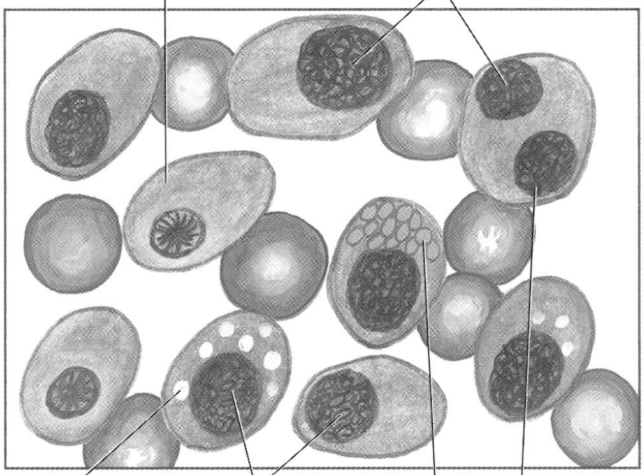

Plasma cells (cartwheel chromatin pattern)
Myeloma cells (Lack of cartwheel chromatin pattern)
Cytoplasmic vacuoles
Nucleoli
Russell bodies
Binucleate cell

FIGURE 14.7

Bone marrow aspirate in myeloma showing numerous plasma cells, many with abnormal features.

polyneuropathy. Pathologic fractures, particularly of the vertebrae may occur causing neurologic complications.

4. Systemic amyloidosis. Systemic primary generalised amyloidosis (AL amyloid) may occur in 10% cases of multiple myeloma and involve multiple organs and systems.

5. Liver, spleen involvement. Involvement of the liver and spleen by myeloma cells sufficient to cause hepatomegaly, and splenomegaly occurs in a small percentage of cases.

Clinical Features

The clinical manifestations of myeloma result from the effects of infiltration of the bones and other organs by neoplastic plasma cells and from immunoglobulin synthesis. The principal clinical features are as under :

1. *Bone pain* is the most common symptom. The pain usually involves the back and ribs. Pathological fractures may occur causing persistent localised pain. Bone pain results from the proliferation of tumour cells in the marrow and activation of osteoclasts which destroy the bones. Myeloma cells release osteoclast-activating factor (OAF) which is mediated by several cytokines, mainly TNF and IL-1.

2. *Susceptibility to infections* is the next most common clinical feature. Particularly common are bacterial infections such as pneumonias and pyelonephritis. The increased susceptibility to infection is related mainly to hypogammaglobulinaemia, and partly to granulocyte dysfunction and neutropenia.

3. *Renal failure* occurs in about 25% of patients, while renal pathology occurs in 50% of cases. Causes of renal failure in myeloma are hypercalcaemia, glomerular deposits of amyloid, hyperuricaemia and infiltration of the kidney by myeloma cells.

4. *Anaemia* occurs in majority of patients of myeloma and is related to marrow replacement by the tumour cells (myelophthisis) and inhibition of haematopoiesis.

5. *Bleeding tendencies* may appear in some patients due to thrombocytopenia, deranged platelet function and interaction of the M component with coagulation factors.

6. *Neurologic symptoms* occur in a minority of patients and are explained by hyperviscosity, cryoglobulins and amyloid deposits.

7. *Hyperviscosity syndrome* owing to hyperglobulinaemia may produce headache, fatigue, visual disturbances and haemorrhages.

8. *Biochemical abnormalities.* These include:

i) hypercalcaemia due to destruction of bone;

ii) hyperuricaemia from necrosis of tumour mass and from uraemia related to renal failure; and

iii) along with other globulins, there is increased β-2 microglobulins in urine and serum (considered as a single most important predictor of survival).

Diagnosis

The diagnosis of myeloma is made by classic *triad* of features:

1. marrow plasmacytosis of more than 10%;
2. radiologic evidence of lytic bony lesions; and
3. demonstration of serum and/or urine M component.

There is rise in the total serum protein concentration due to *paraproteinaemia.* Paraproteins are abnormal immunoglobulins or their parts circulating in plasma and excreted in urine. The most common paraprotein is *IgG* seen in two-third cases of myeloma, *IgA* in one-third, and rarely there may be *IgM* or *IgD* paraproteins, or various combinations. Though the commonest cause of paraproteinaemias is multiple myeloma, certain other conditions may also produce serum paraproteins such as:

- Waldenström's macroglobulinaemia;
- Benign monoclonal gammopathy;
- B-cell lymphomas;
- CLL;

- Light chain disease;
- Heavy chain disease; and
- Cryoglobulinaemia.

As a result of paraproteinaemia, normal serum immunoglobulins (IgG, IgA and IgM) and albumin are depressed. The paraprotein usually appears as a single narrow homogeneous *M-band* on the serum electrophoresis, most commonly in the region of γ-globulin (Fig. 14.8). About two-third cases of myeloma excrete Bence Jones (light chain) proteins in the urine, consisting of either kappa or lambda light chains, alongwith presence of Bence Jones paraproteins in the serum.

Two variants of myeloma which do not fulfil the criteria of classical triad are *solitary bone plasmacytoma* and *extramedullary plasmacytoma.* Both these are associated with M component in about a third of cases and occur in young individuals. Solitary bone plasmacytoma is a lytic bony lesion without marrow plasmacytosis. Extramedullary plasmacytoma involves most commonly the submucosal lymphoid tissue of nasopharynx or paranasal sinuses. Both variants have better prognosis than the classic multiple myeloma. *Plasma cell granuloma,* on the other hand, is an inflammatory condition having admixture of other inflammatory cells with mature plasma cells.

Prognosis

Treatment of multiple myeloma consists of systemic chemotherapy in the form of alkylating agents and symptomatic supportive care. The median survival is 2 years after the diagnosis is made. The terminal phase is marked by the development of pancytopenia, severe anaemia and sepsis.

WALDENSTRÖM'S MACROGLOBULINAEMIA

Waldenström's macroglobulinaemia is an uncommon malignant proliferation of monoclonal B lymphocytes which secrete IgM paraproteins called macroglobulins as they have high molecular weight. The condition is more common in men over 50 years of age and behaves clinically like a slowly progressive lymphoma.

ETIOPATHOGENESIS. Waldenström's macroglobulinaemia is a monoclonal proliferation of B-cells and is accompanied by IgM paraproteinaemia, but the exact etiology is not known. A possible relationship of IgM macroglobulin with myelin-associated glycoprotein which is lost in degenerating diseases has been suggested. The clinical evidence in favour is the appearance of peripheral neuropathy before the occurrence of macroglobulinaemia in some patients.

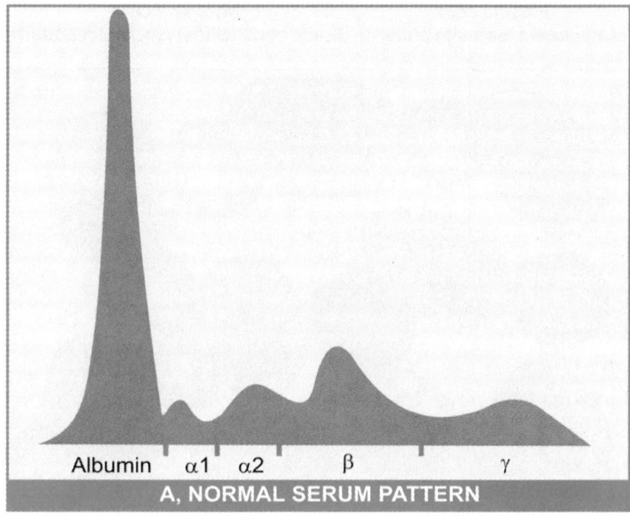

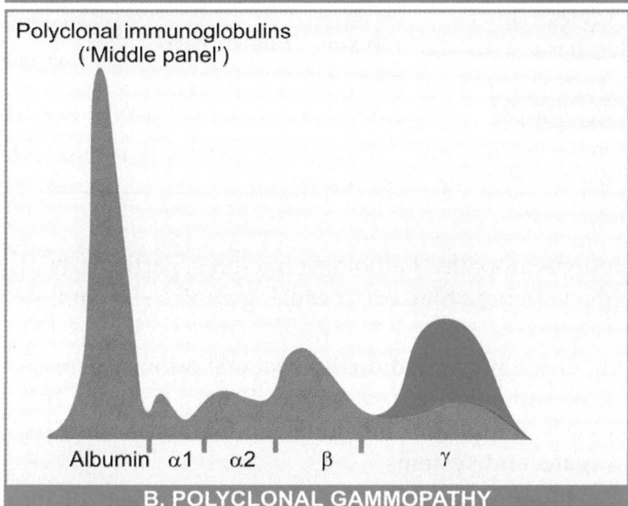

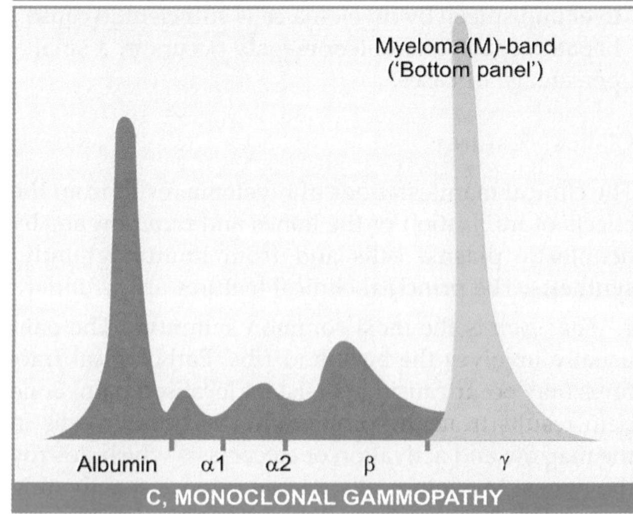

FIGURE 14.8

Serum electrophoresis showing normal serum pattern (A), as contrasted with that in polyclonal gammopathy (B) and in monoclonal gammopathy (C).

PATHOLOGIC CHANGES. Pathologically, the disease can be regarded as the hybrid between myeloma and small lymphocytic lymphoma.

■ *Like myeloma,* the disease involves the bone marrow, but unlike myeloma it usually does not cause extensive bony lesions or hypercalcaemia. The bone marrow shows pleomorphic infiltration by lymphocytes, plasma cells, lymphocytoid plasma cells, mast cells and histiocytes. Like in myeloma, serum M component is present.

■ *Unlike myeloma and more like small lymphocytic lymphoma,* enlargement of lymph nodes, spleen and liver due to infiltration by similar type of cells is present more frequently.

CLINICAL FEATURES. The clinical features of the disease are due to both infiltration by the disease and paraproteins in the blood.

1. *Hyperviscosity syndrome* is the major clinical manifestation. It results in visual disturbances, weakness, fatiguability, weight loss and nervous system symptoms. Raynaud's phenomenon may occur.
2. *Moderate organomegaly* in the form of lymphadenopathy, hepatomegaly and splenomegaly are frequently seen.
3. *Anaemia* due to bone marrow failure may be present.
4. *Bleeding tendencies* may occur due to interaction of macroglobulins with platelets and coagulation factors.

DIAGNOSIS. Unlike myeloma, there are no characteristic radiologic findings. The diagnosis rests on laboratory data. These are:

1. pleomorphic bone marrow infiltration;
2. raised total serum protein concentration;
3. raised serum monoclonal M component which is due to IgM paraprotein;
4. elevated ESR; and
5. normocytic normochromic anaemia.

PROGNOSIS. The management of the patients is similar to that of myeloma. Patients respond to chemotherapy with a median survival of 3-5 years.

HEAVY CHAIN DISEASES

Heavy chain diseases are rare malignant proliferations of B-cells accompanied by monoclonal excess of one of the heavy chains. Depending upon the type of excessive heavy chain, three types—γ, α and μ, of heavy chain diseases are distinguished.

GAMMA HEAVY CHAIN DISEASE. Also called Franklin's disease, it is characterised by excess of mostly γ_1-paraprotein, both in the serum and urine and is demonstrated as M component. Clinically, the condition may develop at any age and present with lymphadenopathy, splenomegaly, hepatomegaly, involvement of pharyngeal lymphoid tissue (Waldeyer's ring) and fever. Patients have rapidly downhill course due to severe and fatal infection.

ALPHA HEAVY CHAIN DISEASE. This is the commonest of heavy chain diseases characterised by α-heavy chains in the plasma which are difficult to demonstrate in electrophoresis due to rapid polymerisation. The patients present with bowel symptoms such as chronic diarrhoea, malabsorption and weight loss and may have enlargement of abdominal lymph nodes. Chemotherapy may induce long-term remissions.

MU HEAVY CHAIN DISEASE. This is the rarest heavy chain disease. The neoplastic B-cells produce μ heavy chains as well as κ light chains; the latter appear in the urine while the former do not. Another feature that distinguishes this type of heavy chain disease from the others is the presence of vacuoles in the malignant B lymphocytes. The course and prognosis are like those of leukaemia or lymphoma.

LANGERHANS' CELL HISTIOCYTOSIS

Langerhans' cell histiocytosis is a group of malignant proliferations of histiocytes and macrophages. Earlier, this group was referred to as histiocytosis-X and included three conditions: eosinophilic granuloma, Hand-Schüller-Christian disease and Letterer-Siwe syndrome. Now, it is known that:

■ *firstly,* histiocytosis-X are not proliferations of unknown origin (X-for unknown) but proliferating cells are in fact Langerhans' cells of marrow origin. Langerhans' cells are normally present mainly in the epidermis but also in some other organs; and

■ *secondly,* the three conditions included under histiocytosis-X are actually different expression of the same basic disorder. This has been made possible by demonstration of common antigens on these cells (positive for S-100 protein, CD1, CD 74 and HLA-DR) as well as by ultrastructural features of Langerhans' cell or Birbeck granules in the cytoplasm.

The three disorders included in the group are briefly considered below.

Eosinophilic Granuloma

Unifocal eosinophilic granuloma is more common (60%) than the multifocal variety which is often a component of Hand-Schüller-Christian disease (described below).

Most of the patients are children and young adults, predominantly males. The condition commonly presents as a solitary osteolytic lesion in the femur, skull, vertebrae, ribs and pelvis. The diagnosis requires biopsy of the lytic bone lesion.

Microscopically, the lesion consists largely of closely-packed aggregates of macrophages admixed with variable number of eosinophils. The macrophages contain droplets of fat or a few granules of brown pigment indicative of phagocytic activity. A few multinucleate macrophages may also be seen. The cytoplasm of a few macrophages may contain rod-shaped inclusions called *histiocytosis-X bodies.*

Clinically, unifocal eosinophilic granuloma is a benign disorder. The bony lesion remains asymptomatic until the erosion of the bone causes pain or fracture. Spontaneous fibrosis or healing may occur in some cases, while others may require curettage or radiotherapy.

Hand-Schüller-Christian Disease

A triad of features consisting of *multifocal bony defects, diabetes insipidus* and *exophthalmos* is termed Hand-Schüller-Christian disease. The disease develops in children under 5 years of age. The multifocal lytic bony lesions may develop at any site. Orbital lesion causes exophthalmos, while involvement of the hypothalamus causes diabetes insipidus. Multiple spherical lesions in the lungs are frequently present. Half the patients have involvement of the liver, spleen and lymph nodes.

Microscopically, the lesions are indistinguishable from those of unifocal eosinophilic granuloma.

Clinically, the affected children frequently have fever, skin lesions, recurrent pneumonitis and other infections. Though the condition is benign, it is more disabling than the unifocal eosinophilic granuloma. The lesions may resolve spontaneously or may require chemotherapy or radiation.

Letterer-Siwe Disease

Letterer-Siwe disease is an acute clinical syndrome of unknown etiology occurring in infants and children under three years of age. The disease is characterised by hepatosplenomegaly, lymphadenopathy, thrombocytopenia, anaemia and leucopenia. There is generalised hyperplasia of tissue macrophages in various organs.

Microscopically, the involved organs contain aggregates of macrophages which are pleomorphic and show nuclear atypia. The cytoplasm of these cells contains vacuoles and rod-shaped *histiocytosis-X bodies.*

Clinically, the child has acute symptoms of fever, skin rash, loss of weight, anaemia, bleeding disorders and enlargement of lymph nodes, liver and spleen. Cystic bony lesions may be apparent in the skull, pelvis and long bones. Intense chemotherapy helps to control Letterer-Siwe disease but intercurrent infections result in fatal outcome in many cases. The condition is currently regarded as an unusual form of malignant lymphoma.

SPLEEN

NORMAL STRUCTURE

The spleen is the largest lymphoid organ of the body. Under normal conditions, the average weight of the spleen is about 150 gm in the adult. Normally, the organ lies well protected by the 9th, 10th and 11th ribs in the upper left quadrant. The surface of the spleen is covered by a layer of peritoneum underneath which the organ is ensheathed by a thin *capsule.* From the capsule extend connective tissue *trabeculae* into the pulp of the organ and serve as supportive network. Blood enters the spleen by the splenic artery which divides into branches that penetrate the spleen via trabeculae. From the trabeculae arise small branches called *central arterioles.* Blood in the central arterioles empties partly into splenic venules and from there into splenic vein, but largely into vascular sinuses of the red pulp and thence into the splenic venous system.

Grossly, the spleen consists of homogeneous, soft, dark red mass called the *red pulp* and long oval grey-white nodules called the *white pulp (malpighian bodies).*

Microscopically, the red pulp consists of a network of thin-walled venous sinuses and adjacent blood spaces. The blood spaces contain blood cells, lymphocytes and macrophages and appear to be arranged in cords called *splenic cords* or *cords of Billroth.* The white pulp is made up of lymphocytes surrounding an eccentrically placed arteriole. The periarteriolar lymphocytes are mainly T-cells, while at other places the lymphocytes have a germinal centre composed principally of B-cells surrounded by densely packed lymphocytes.

The spleen is a lymphoreticular organ that performs at least the following four *functions:*

1. Like other lymphoid tissues, it is an organ of the immune system where B and T lymphocytes multiply and help in *immune responses.*
2. The spleen plays an active role in *sequestering* and removing normal and abnormal blood cells.

3. The vasculature of the spleen plays a role in *regulating portal blood flow.*
4. Under pathologic conditions, the spleen may become the site of *extramedullary haematopoiesis.*

The spleen is rarely the primary site of disease. Being the largest lymphoreticular organ, it is involved secondarily in a wide variety of systemic disorders which manifest most commonly as splenic enlargement (splenomegaly) described below. A few other systemic involvements such as splenic infarcts and chronic venous congestion (CVC) of spleen have already been considered in Chapter 5 of General Pathology (COLOUR PLATE V: CL 19).

SPLENOMEGALY

Enlargement of the spleen termed splenomegaly, occurs in a wide variety of disorders which increase the cellularity and vascularity of the organ. Many of the causes are exaggerated forms of normal splenic function. Splenic enlargement may occur as a result of one of the following pathophysiologic mechanisms:

I. Infections
II. Disordered immunoregulation
III. Altered splenic blood flow
IV. Lymphohaematogenous malignancies
V. Diseases with abnormal erythrocytes
VI. Storage diseases
VII. Miscellaneous causes.

Based on these mechanisms, an abbreviated list of causes of splenomegaly is given in Table 14.5. Most of these conditions have been discussed elsewhere.

The **degree of splenomegaly** varies with the disease entity:

- *Mild enlargement (upto 5 cm)* occurs in CVC of spleen in CHF, acute malaria, typhoid fever, bacterial endocarditis, SLE, rheumatoid arthritis and thalassaemia minor.
- *Moderate enlargement (upto umbilicus)* occurs in hepatitis, cirrhosis, lymphomas, infectious mononucleosis, haemolytic anaemia, splenic abscesses and amyloidosis.
- *Massive enlargement (below umbilicus)* occurs in CML, myeloid metaplasia with myelofibrosis, storage diseases, thalassaemia major, chronic malaria, leishmaniasis and portal vein obstruction.

Mild to moderate splenomegaly is usually symptomless, while a massively enlarged spleen may cause dragging sensation in the left hypochondrium. Spleen becomes palpable only when it is enlarged.

TABLE 14.5: Causes of Splenomegaly.

I. INFECTIONS
1. Malaria
2. Leishmaniasis
3. Typhoid
4. Infectious mononucleosis
5. Bacterial septicaemia
6. Bacterial endocarditis
7. Tuberculosis
8. Syphilis
9. Viral hepatitis
10. AIDS

II. DISORDERS OF IMMUNOREGULATION
1. Rheumatoid arthritis
2. SLE
3. Immune haemolytic anaemias
4. Immune thrombocytopenias
5. Immune neutropenias

III. ALTERED SPLENIC BLOOD FLOW
1. Cirrhosis of liver
2. Portal vein obstruction
3. Splenic vein obstruction
4. Congestive heart failure

IV. LYMPHO-HAEMATOGENOUS MALIGNANCIES
1. Hodgkin's disease
2. Non-Hodgkin's lymphomas
3. Multiple myeloma
4. Leukaemias
5. Myeloproliferative disorders (e.g. CML, polycythaemia vera, myeloid metaplasia with myelofibrosis)

V. DISEASES WITH ABNORMAL ERYTHROCYTES
1. Thalassaemias
2. Spherocytosis
3. Sickle cell disease
4. Ovalocytosis

VI. STORAGE DISEASES
1. Gaucher's disease
2. Niemann-Pick's disease

VII. MISCELLANEOUS
1. Amyloidosis
2. Primary and metastatic splenic tumours
3. Idiopathic splenomegaly

Grossly, an enlarged spleen is heavy and firm. The capsule is tense and thickened. The sectioned surface of the organ is firm with prominent trabeculae.

Microscopically, there is dilatation of sinusoids with prominence of splenic cords. The white pulp is

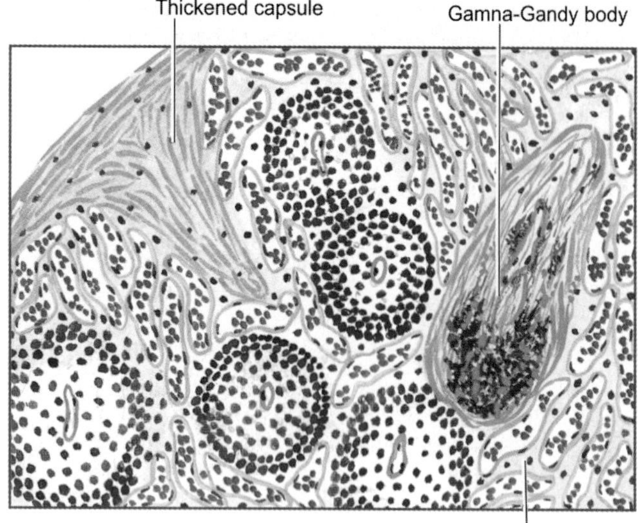

FIGURE 14.9

Microscopic characteristics in fibrocongestive splenomegaly. There is dilatation and congestion of splenic sinusoids with areas of haemorrhages and presence of Gamna-Gandy bodies. The trabeculae are prominent while the white pulp is atrophic.

atrophic while the trabeculae are thickened. Long-standing congestion may produce haemorrhages and *Gamna-Gandy bodies* resulting in *fibrocongestive splenomegaly,* also called *Banti's spleen* (Fig. 14.9) (COLOUR PLATE V: CL 19).

HYPERSPLENISM

The term hypersplenism is used for conditions which cause excessive removal of erythrocytes, granulocytes or platelets from the circulation. The mechanism for excessive removal could be due to increased sequestration of cells in the spleen by altered splenic blood flow or by production of antibodies against respective blood cells. The criteria for hypersplenism are as under:

1. Splenomegaly.
2. Splenic destruction of one or more of the cell types in the peripheral blood causing anaemia, leucopenia, thrombocytopenia, or pancytopenia.
3. Bone marrow cellularity is normal or hyperplastic.
4. Splenectomy is followed by improvement in the severity of blood cytopenia.

EFFECTS OF SPLENECTOMY

In view of the prominent role of normal spleen in sequestration of blood cells, splenectomy in a normal individual is followed by significant haematologic alterations. Induction of similar haematologic effects is made use in the treatment of certain pathologic conditions. For example, in autoimmune haemolytic anaemia or thrombocytopenia, the respective blood cell counts are increased following splenectomy. The blood changes following splenectomy are as under:

1. **Red cells:** There is appearance of target cells in the blood film. Howell-Jolly bodies are present in the red cells as they are no longer cleared by the spleen. Osmotic fragility test shows increased resistance to haemolysis. There may be appearance of normoblasts.
2. **White cells:** There is leucocytosis reaching its peak in 1-2 days after splenectomy. There is shift-to-left of the myeloid cells with appearance of some myelocytes.
3. **Platelets:** Within hours after splenectomy, there is rise in platelet count upto 3-4 times normal.

SPLENIC RUPTURE

The most common cause of splenic rupture or laceration is blunt trauma. The trauma may be direct or indirect. Non-traumatic or spontaneous rupture occurs in an enlarged spleen but almost never in a normal spleen. In acute infections, the spleen can enlarge rapidly to 2 to 3 times its normal size causing acute splenic enlargement termed *acute splenic tumour* e.g. in pneumonias, septicaemia, acute endocarditis etc. Some of the other common causes of spontaneous splenic rupture are splenomegaly due to chronic malaria, infectious mononucleosis, typhoid fever, splenic abscess, thalassaemia and leukaemias.

Rupture of spleen is an acute surgical emergency due to rapid blood loss and haemoperitoneum. Sometimes fragments of splenic tissue are autotransplanted within the peritoneal cavity and grow into tiny spleens there *(splenosis).*

TUMOURS

- **Primary tumours** of the spleen are extremely rare. The only notable benign tumours are haemangiomas and lymphangioma, while examples of primary malignant neoplasms are Hodgkin's disease and non-Hodgkin's lymphomas. Non-haematopoietic tumours of the spleen are rare.
- **Secondary tumours** occur late in the course of disease and represent haematogenous dissemination of the malignant tumour. Splenic metastases appear as multiple nodules. The most frequent primary sites include: lung, breast, prostate, colon and stomach. Rarely, direct extension from an adjacent malignant neoplasm may occur.

THYMUS

NORMAL STRUCTURE

The thymus gland is a complex lymphoreticular organ lying buried within the mediastinum. At birth, the gland weighs 10-35 gm and grows in size upto puberty, following which there is progressive involution in the elderly. In the adult, thymus weighs 5-10 gm.

The gland consists of right and left encapsulated lobes, joined together by fibrous connective tissue. Connective tissue septa pass inwards from the capsule and subdivide the lobe into large number of lobules. The histologic structure of the lobule shows *outer cortex* and *inner medulla.* Both cortex and medulla contain two types of cells: epithelial cells and lymphocytes (thymocytes).

- **The epithelial cells** are similar throughout the thymus gland. These cells have elongated cytoplasmic processes forming network in which thymocytes and macrophages are found. *Hassall's corpuscles* are distinctive structures within the medulla composed of onion skin-like concentrically arranged epithelial cells having central area of keratinisation.
- **Thymocytes** are predominantly present in the cortex. These cells include immature T lymphocytes in the cortex and mature T lymphocytes in the medulla. Well-developed B-cell lymphoid follicles with germinal centres are rare in thymus gland.

The main **function** of the thymus is in the cell-mediated immunity by T-cells and by secretion of thymic hormones such as *thymopoietin* and *thymosin-*α_1.

Thymic lesions are associated with diverse conditions which may be immunologic, haematologic or neoplastic. These can be broadly categorised into thymic hypoplasia and agenesis, thymic hyperplasia, thymoma, and thymus in myasthenia gravis (Chapter 26).

THYMIC HYPOPLASIA AND AGENESIS

Thymic hypoplasia and agenesis are acquired and congenital disorders respectively in which the gland is either unusually small or absent. These conditions are various types of hereditary (primary) immunodeficiency diseases such as DiGeorge's syndrome, severe combined immunodeficiency and reticular dysgenesis. Acquired hypoplasia occurs as an ageing phenomenon or may occur in the young due to severe stress, malnutrition, irradiation, therapy with cytotoxic drugs and glucocorticoids.

THYMIC HYPERPLASIA

Enlargement of the thymus or failure to involute produces thymic hyperplasia. Hyperplasia is usually associated with appearance of lymphoid follicles in the medulla of the thymus and is called *thymic follicular hyperplasia.* Most common cause of follicular hyperplasia of the thymus is myasthenia gravis. Less common causes are: Addison's disease, Graves' disease, rheumatoid arthritis, SLE, scleroderma and cirrhosis of liver.

THYMOMA

Most common primary tumour present in the antero-superior mediastinum is thymoma. Although thymus is a lymphoepithelial organ, the term thymoma is used for the tumour of epithelial origin. Most of the patients are adults. In about half the cases, thymoma remains asymptomatic and is accidentally discovered in X-rays. Other patients have associated conditions like myasthenia gravis or local symptoms such as cough, dyspnoea and chest pain.

PATHOLOGIC CHANGES. ***Grossly,*** the tumour is spherical, measuring 5-10 cm in diameter with an average weight of 150 gm. Sectioned surface is soft, yellowish, lobulated and may be either homogeneous or contain cysts due to the presence of haemorrhage and necrosis.

Microscopically, the tumour has a thick fibrous capsule from which extend collagenous septa into the tumour dividing it into lobules. The histology of lobule shows various patterns. The tumour consists of neoplastic epithelial cells and variable number of non-neoplastic lymphocytes. Thymoma may be of following types:

Benign thymoma is more common. It consists of epithelial cells which are similar to the epithelial cells in the medulla of thymus and hence also called as medullary thymoma.

Malignant thymoma is less common and is further of 2 types:

Type 1 is cytologically benign looking but aggressive and invades the mediastinal structures locally.

Type 2 is also called thymic carcinoma and has cytologic features of cancer. Further subtypes of epithelial malignancy may be squamous cell type (most common) and sometimes lymphoepithelial type.

Thymomas are known for their association with paraneoplastic syndrome. These include: myasthenia gravis (most common), hypogammaglobulinaemia, erythroid hypoplasia (pure red cell aplasia), peripheral T cell leukaemia, multiple myeloma, other autoimmune disease associations and other systemic malignancies.

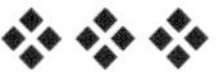

The Respiratory System

15

LUNGS

NORMAL STRUCTURE

ANATOMY. The normal *adult right lung* weighs 375 to 550 gm (average 450 gm) and is divided by two fissures into three lobes—the upper, middle and lower lobes. The weight of the normal *adult left lung* is 325 to 450 gm (average 400 gm) and has one fissure dividing it into two lobes—the upper and lower lobes, while the middle lobe is represented by the lingula. The airways of the lungs arise from the trachea by its division into right and left main bronchi which continue to divide and subdivide further so as to terminate into the alveolar sacs (Fig. 15.1).

The right main bronchus is more vertical so that aspirated foreign material tends to pass down to the right lung rather than to the left. The trachea, major bronchi and their branchings possess cartilage, smooth muscle and mucous glands in their walls, while the bronchioles have smooth muscle but lack cartilage as well as the mucous glands. Between the tracheal bifurcation and the smallest bronchi, about 8 divisions take place. The *bronchioles* so formed further undergo 3 to 4 divisions leading to the *terminal bronchioles* which are less than 2 mm in diameter. The part of the lung tissue distal to a terminal bronchiole is called an *acinus*. A cluster of about 5 acini supplied by terminal bronchioles and enclosed by visible fibrous septa is termed as the *pulmonary lobule*. An **acinus** consists of 3 parts:

1. Several (usually 3 to 5 generations) *respiratory bronchioles* originate from a terminal bronchiole.
2. Each respiratory bronchiole divides into several *alveolar ducts*.
3. Each alveolar duct opens into many *alveolar sacs (alveoli)* which are blind ends of the respiratory passages.

The lungs have double blood supply—oxygenated blood from the bronchial arteries and venous blood from the pulmonary arteries, and there is mixing of the blood to some extent. In case of blockage of one side of circulation, the supply from the other can maintain the vitality of pulmonary parenchyma. The bronchial veins drain the blood supplied by the bronchial arteries. The lungs have abundant intercommunicating lymphatics on the surface which drain into the subpleural plexus.

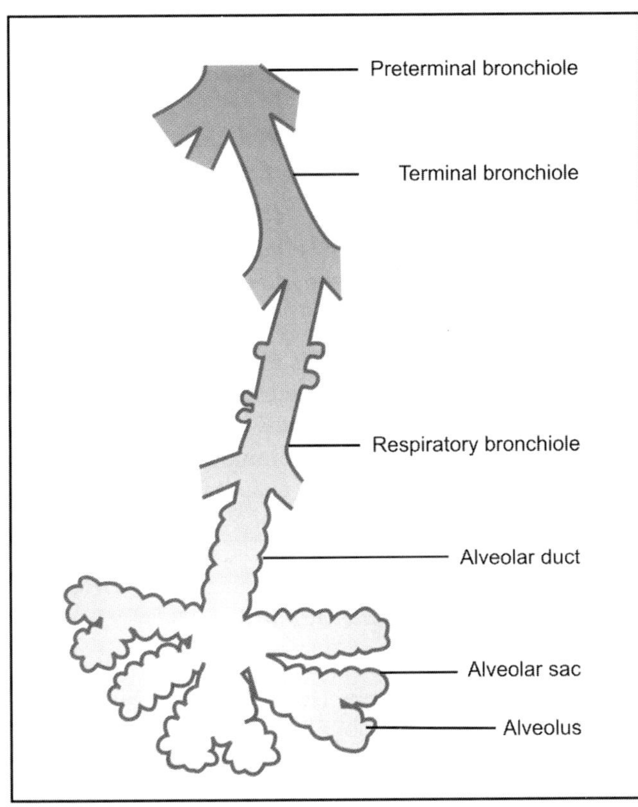

FIGURE 15.1

The structure of an acinus which is part of the lung distal to terminal bronchiole. It shows respiratory bronchiole, alveolar ducts and alveolar sacs.

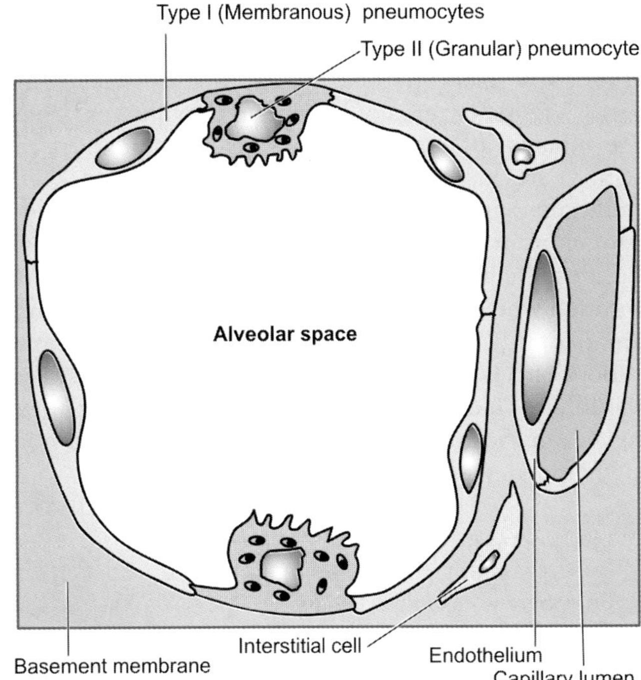

FIGURE 15.2

Histologic structure of alveolar wall (alveolar septa). It shows capillary endothelium, capillary basement membrane and scanty interstitial tissue and the alveolar lining cells (type I or membranous pneumocytes and type II or granular pneumocytes).

Hilar and tracheobronchial lymph nodes receive the lymph and drain into the thoracic duct.

HISTOLOGY. The bronchi and their subdivisions upto bronchioles are lined by pseudostratified columnar ciliated epithelial cells, also called *respiratory epithelium.* These cells are admixed with mucus-secreting goblet cells which decrease in number as the bronchioles are approached. The mucosa of bronchi contains numerous submucosal mucous glands and neuro-endocrine cells which are bronchial counterparts of the argentaffin cells of the alimentary tract (Chapter 18). The structure of bronchioles differs from that of bronchi and its subdivisions as well as from alveoli. They are lined by a single layer of pseudostratified columnar ciliated epithelium but no mucous cells and hence, unlike the bronchi, contain no mucus secretion on the surface. They contain some nonciliated Clara cells which secrete protein rich in lysozyme and immunoglobulins but unlike the alveoli contain no surfactant.

The **alveolar walls or alveolar septa** are the sites of exchange between the blood and air and have the following microscopic features (Fig. 15.2):

1. The *capillary endothelium* lines the anastomotic capillaries in the alveolar walls.
2. The capillary endothelium and the alveolar lining epithelial cells are separated by the *capillary basement membrane and some interstitial tissue.* The interstitial tissue consists of scanty amount of collagen, fibroblasts, fine elastic fibres, smooth muscle cells, a few mast cells and mononuclear cells.
3. The *alveolar epithelium* consists of 2 types of cells: *type I* or *membranous pneumocytes* are the most numerous covering about 95% of alveolar surface, and *type II* or *granular pneumocytes* project into the alveoli and are covered by microvilli. Type II pneumocytes are essentially reserve cells which undergo hyperplasia when type I pneumocytes are injured and are the source of pulmonary surfactant rich in lecithin. The main functions of coating of surfactant are to lower the surface tension of the alveolar lining cells and in maintaining the stability of the alveoli.
4. The *alveolar macrophages* belonging to mononuclear-phagocyte system are present either free in the alveolar spaces or are attached to the alveolar cells.
5. The *pores of Kohn* are the sites of alveolar connections between the adjacent alveoli and allow the passage of bacteria and exudate.

FUNCTIONS. The primary functions of lungs is oxygenation of the blood and removal of carbon dioxide. The respiratory tract is particularly exposed to infection as well as to the hazards of inhalation of pollutants from the inhaled air and cigarette smoke. There exists a natural mechanism of filtering and clearing of such pollutants through respiratory epithelium, tracheobronchial lymphatics and alveolar macrophages. Besides, the lungs are the only other organ after heart through which all the blood of the body passes during circulation. Therefore, cardiovascular diseases have serious effects on the lungs, and conversely, diseases of the lungs which interfere with pulmonary blood flow have significant effects on the heart and systemic circulation.

Diseases of the respiratory tract are studied under the following groups:

1. Paediatric lung disease (congenital and acquired)
2. Pulmonary vascular disease
3. Pulmonary infections
4. Chronic obstructive pulomonary disease
5. Chronic restrictive pulmonary disease
6. Tumours of lungs.

PAEDIATRIC LUNG DISEASE

A number of congenital anomalies (e.g. agenesis, hypoplasia, heterotopic tissue, vascular anomalies, tracheal and bronchial anomalies, congenital pulmonary overinflation or lobar emphysema, congenital cysts and bronchopulmonary sequestration) and certain neonatal acquired lung diseases, (broncho-pulmonary dysplasia, meconium aspiration syndrome, persistent foetal circulation, atelactasis, collapse and bronchiolitis) have been described. A few important conditions are discussed below.

CONGENITAL CYSTS

Developmental defects involving deficiency of bronchial or bronchiolar cartilage, elastic tissue and muscle result in congenital cystic disease of lungs. A single large cyst of this type occupying almost a lobe is called *pneumatocele.* Multiple small cysts are more common and give sponge-like appearance to the lung. The cysts are thin-walled and dilated and generally lined by flattened ciliated epithelium overlying a thin layer of supportive connective tissue. These cysts may contain air or may get infected and become abscesses. Cysts may rupture into bronchi producing haemoptysis, or into the pleural cavity giving rise to pneumothorax.

BRONCHOPULMONARY SEQUESTRATION

Sequestration is the presence of lobes or segments of lung tissue which are not connected to the airway system. The blood supply of the sequestered area is not from the pulmonary arteries but from the aorta or its branches. Sequestration may be intralobar or extralobar.

■ **Intralobar sequestration** is the sequestered bronchopulmonary mass within the pleural covering of the affected lung.

■ **Extralobar sequestration** is the sequestered mass of lung tissue lying outside the pleural investing layer such as in the base of left lung or below the diaphragm. The extralobar sequestration is predominantly seen in infants and children and is often associated with other congenital malformations.

NEONATAL RESPIRATORY DISTRESS SYNDROME (HYALINE MEMBRANE DISEASE)

Neonatal respiratory distress syndrome (RDS) or hyaline membrane disease (HMD) characterised by formation of pulmonary hyaline membrane is the most common and serious form of disease of the newborn infants. The condition begins with dyspnoea a few hours after birth with tachypnoea, hypoxia and cyanosis and in severe cases death occurs in a few hours. The milder cases, however, recover with adequate oxygen therapy by ventilator-assist methods in a few days. The mortality rate is high (20 to 30%) and is still higher in babies under 1 kg of body weight. Some who recover develop bronchopulmonary dysplasia later on.

ETIOLOGY. The neonatal RDS is primarily initiated by hypoxia, either shortly before birth or immediately afterward. The following clinical settings are commonly associated with neonatal RDS:

1. Preterm infants.
2. Infants born to diabetic mothers.
3. Delivery by caesarean section.
4. Infants born to mothers with previous premature infants.
5. Excessive sedation of the mother causing depression in respiration of the infant.
6. Birth asphyxia from various causes such as coils of umbilical cord around the neck.
7. Male preponderance (1.5 to 2 times) over female babies due to early maturation of female lungs.

Besides all these factors causing respiratory distress, a number of cases of neonatal RDS remain idiopathic. RDS may also occur in adults which is termed as *adult respiratory distress syndrome (ARDS)* and is discussed later (page 472).

PATHOGENESIS. *Entry of air into alveoli is essential for formation of HMD i.e. dead born infants do not develop HMD.* The basic defect in neonatal RDS is a deficiency of pulmonary surfactant, normally synthesised by type II alveolar cells. The production of surfactant is normally increased shortly before birth but in prematurity and in neonatal hypoxia from any of the foregoing causes, its synthesis is decreased. The main function of alveolar surfactant being lowering of alveolar surface tension, its deficiency leads to increased alveolar surface tension which in turn causes atelectasis. Atelectasis of the lungs results in hypoventilation, pulmonary hypoperfusion, ischaemic damage to capillary endothelium and necrosis of the alveolar cells, exudation of plasma proteins including fibrinogen into the alveoli and eventually formation of hyaline membrane containing largely fibrin.

The sequence of events is schematically illustrated in Fig. 15.3.

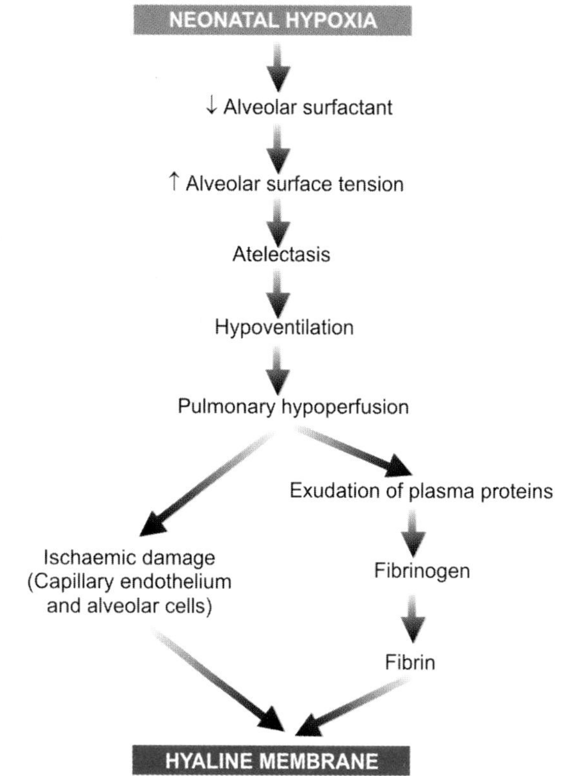

FIGURE 15.3

Schematic representation of sequence of events leading to the formation of hyaline membrane in neonatal respiratory distress syndrome.

PATHOLOGIC CHANGES. ***Grossly,*** the lungs are normal in size and reddish purple in colour. They are solid and airless so that they sink in water. ***Microscopically,*** the important features are as follows (Fig. 15.4) (COLOUR PLATE XIX: CL 73):

1. The presence of collapsed alveoli (atelectasis) alternating with dilated alveoli.
2. Formation of characteristic eosinophilic hyaline membranes lining the respiratory bronchioles, alveolar ducts and the proximal alveoli. The membrane is largely composed of fibrin admixed with cell debris derived from necrotic alveolar cells.
3. Vascular congestion, focal haemorrhages and dilatation of septal lymphatics.
4. Absence of inflammatory reaction.

BRONCHOPULMONARY DYSPLASIA

Bronchopulmonary dysplasia occurs as a complication in infants treated for neonatal RDS with oxygen and assisted ventilation. The toxicity of oxygen and barotrauma from high pressure of oxygen give rise to subacute or chronic fibrosing condition of the lungs termed bronchopulmonary dysplasia. The condition is clinically characterised by persistence of respiratory distress for upto 3 to 6 months.

Pathologically, there is organisation of hyaline membranes resulting in fibrous thickening of the alveolar walls, bronchiolitis, peribronchial fibrosis, and development of emphysema due to alveolar dilatation. Many bronchioles show squamous metaplasia.

ATELECTASIS AND COLLAPSE

Atelectasis in the newborn or *primary atelectasis* is defined as incomplete expansion of a lung or part of a lung, while pulmonary collapse or *secondary atelectasis* is the term used for reduction in lung size of a previously expanded and well-aerated lung. Obviously, the former occurs in newborn whereas the latter may occur at any age.

ATELECTASIS. Stillborn infants have total atelectasis, while the newborn infants with weak respiratory action develop incomplete expansion of the lungs and clinical atelectasis. The common causes are prematurity, cerebral birth injury, CNS malformations and intrauterine hypoxia.

Grossly, the lungs are small, dark blue, fleshy and non-crepitant

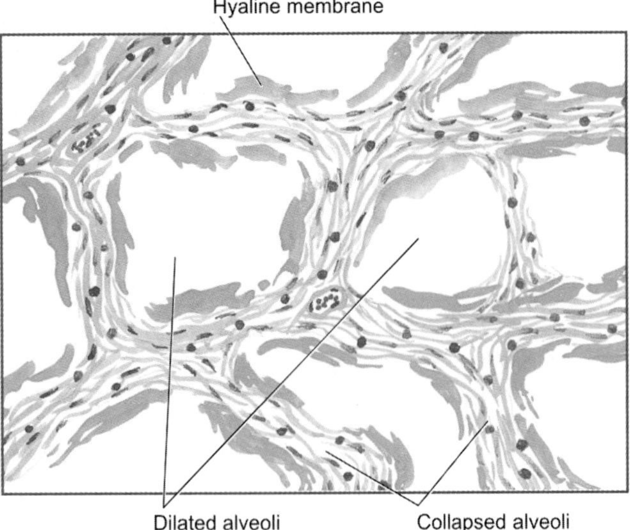

FIGURE 15.4

Histological appearance of hyaline membrane disease. There are alternate areas of collapsed and dilated alveolar spaces, many of which are lined by eosinophilic hyaline membranes.

Microscopically, the alveolar spaces in the affected area are small with thick interalveolar septa. The alveolar spaces contain proteinaceous fluid with a few epithelial squames and meconium. Scattered aerated areas of the lung are hyperinflated causing interstitial emphysema and pneumothorax.

COLLAPSE. Pulmonary collapse or secondary atelectasis in children and adults may occur from various causes such as compression, obstruction, contraction and lack of pulmonary surfactant. Accordingly, collapse may be of the following types:

1. Compressive collapse. Pressure from outside causes compressive collapse e.g. by massive pleural effusion, haemothorax, pneumothorax, intrathoracic tumour, high diaphragm and spinal deformities. Compressive collapse involves subpleural regions and affects lower lobes more than the central areas.

2. Obstructive/absorptive collapse. Obstruction of a bronchus or many bronchioles causes absorption of oxygen in the affected alveoli followed by collapse e.g. by viscid mucus secretions in bronchial asthma, chronic bronchitis, bronchiectasis, bronchial tumours and aspiration of foreign bodies. Obstructive collapse is generally less severe than the compressive collapse and is patchy.

3. Contraction collapse. This type occurs due to localised fibrosis in lung causing contraction followed by collapse.

BRONCHIOLITIS AND BRONCHIOLITIS OBLITERANS

Bronchiolitis and bronchiolitis obliterans are the inflammatory conditions affecting the small airways occurring predominantly in older paediatric age group and in quite elderly persons. A number of etiologic factors have been stated to cause this condition. These include viral infection (frequently adenovirus and respiratory syncytial virus), bacterial infection, fungal infection, inhalation of toxic gases (e.g. in silo-fillers' disease) and aspiration of gastric contents.

Microscopically, the lumina of affected bronchioles are narrow and occluded by fibrous plugs. The bronchiolar walls are inflamed and are infiltrated by lymphocytes and plasma cells. There are changes of interstitial pneumonitis and fibrosis in the alveoli around the affected bronchioles.

SUDDEN INFANT DEATH SYNDROME

Sudden infant death syndrome or crib death is an uncommon condition seen mainly in the western countries. It affects infants in the age group of 2 to 6 months. The condition is seen in premature babies born to mothers who have been smokers and indulged in drug abuse.

Pathologic findings at autopsy invariably show petechial haemorrhages in the upper respiratory airways and lungs.

PULMONARY VASCULAR DISEASE

As stated before, diseases of the heart affect the lungs and diseases of the lungs affect the heart. This is because of the peculiar characteristics of pulmonary vasculature. The pressure in the pulmonary arteries is much lower than in the systemic arteries. The pulmonary arterial system is thinner than the systemic arterial system. They are thin elastic vessels which can be easily distinguished from thick-walled bronchial arteries supplying the large airways and the pleura.

General diseases of vascular origin occurring in the lungs such as pulmonary oedema, pulmonary congestion, pulmonary embolism and pulmonary infarction, all of which have already been described in Chapter 5. Here, two specific forms of pulmonary vascular diseases—adult respiratory distress syndrome and pulmonary hypertension, will be discussed.

ADULT RESPIRATORY DISTRESS SYNDROME (ARDS)

Adult respiratory distress syndrome (ARDS) is known by various synonyms such as shock-lung syndrome, diffuse alveolar damage (DAD), acute alveolar injury, traumatic wet lungs and post-traumatic respiratory insufficiency. ARDS is a syndrome caused by diffuse alveolar capillary damage and clinically characterised by sudden and severe respiratory distress, tachypnoea, tachycardia, cyanosis and severe hypoxaemia that fails to respond to oxygen therapy and assisted ventilation unlike neonatal RDS described above. The condition was first recognised during World War II in survivors of non-thoracic injuries with shock. The chest radiographs of these patients show diffuse bilateral alveolar infiltrates which may progress.

ETIOLOGY. Diffuse alveolar damage in ARDS may occur from a number of causes. These are:

1. Shock due to sepsis, trauma, burns
2. Diffuse pulmonary infections, chiefly viral pneumonia
3. Pancreatitis
4. Oxygen toxicity
5. Inhalation of toxins and irritants e.g. smoke, war gases, nitrogen dioxide, metal fumes etc.
6. Narcotic overdose
7. Drugs e.g. salicylates, colchicine
8. Aspiration pneumonitis
9. Fat embolism
10. Radiation

PATHOGENESIS. The basic initiating event in the pathogenesis of ARDS is diffuse damage to the alveolocapillary wall by one of the injurious factors listed above.

The mechanism of acute injury depends upon the *imbalance between pro-inflammatory and anti-inflammatory cytokines.*

1. Activated pulmonay macrophages release *proinflammatory cytokines* such as interleukin (IL) 8, IL1, and tumour necrosis factor (TNF), while macrophage inhibitory factor (MIF) helps to sustain inflammation in the alveoli. Number of neutrophils in the alveoli is increased in acute injury; neutrophils on activation release products which cause active tissue injury e.g. proteases, platelet activating factor, oxidants and leukotrienes.

2. Besides the role of cytokines in acute injury, a few *fibrogenic cytokines* such as transforming growth factor-α (TGF-α) and platelet-derived growth factor (PDGF) play a role in repair process by stimulation of proliferation of fibroblast and collagen.

Injury to the capillary endothelium leads to increased vascular permeability. Injury to epithelial cells, especially to type 1 alveolar cells, causes necrosis of these cells. The net effect of injury to both capillary endothelium and alveolar epithelium is interstitial and intra-alveolar oedema, congestion, fibrin deposition and formation of hyaline membranes as seen in neonatal RDS describe above. As a result of lining of the alveoli with hyaline membranes, there is loss of surfactant causing collapse with pulmonary oedema called 'stiff lung'. There is an attempt at regeneration of alveolar cells by proliferation of type II alveolar cells. A stiff lung of ARDS may undergo complete recovery, or may undergo organisation by proliferation of interstitial cells leading to interstitial fibrosis or even death.

The sequence of events in the pathogenesis of ARDS is summarised in Fig. 15.5.

PATHOLOGIC CHANGES. Grossly, the lungs are characteristically stiff, congested and heavy.

Microscopically, the following features are evident:

1. Interstitial and intra-alveolar oedema.
2. Necrosis of alveolar epithelial cells with formation of hyaline membranes. The hyaline membranes are structurally similar to those of neonatal RDS i.e. they are chiefly composed of fibrin admixed with necrotic epithelial cells.
3. Congestion and intra-alveolar haemorrhages.
4. Changes of bronchopneumonia.
5. In organising stage, there may be interstitial fibrosis and regenerating flat alveolar epithelial cells lining the denuded alveoli.

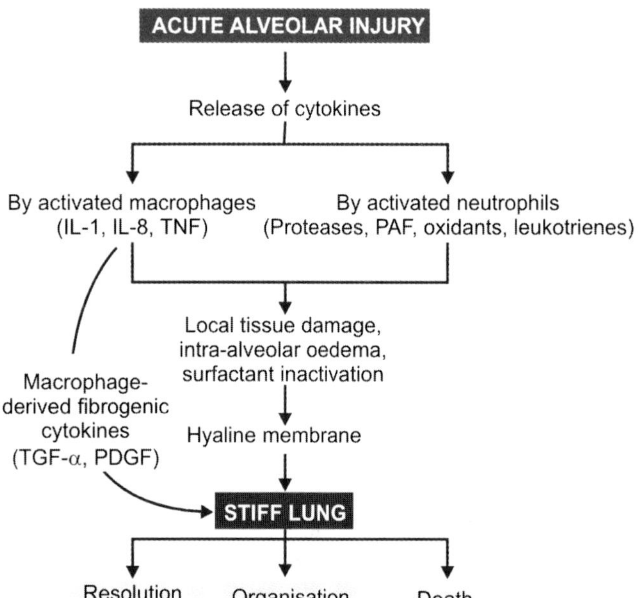

FIGURE 15.5

Pathogenesis of adult respiratory distress syndrome.

PULMONARY HYPERTENSION

Normally, the blood pressure in the pulmonary arterial circulation is much lower than the systemic blood pressure; it does not exceed 30/15 mmHg even during exercise (normally, blood pressure in the pulmonary veins is between 3 and 8 mmHg). Pulmonary hypertension is defined as a systolic blood pressure in the pulmonary arterial circulation above 30 mmHg. Pulmonary hypertension is broadly classified into 2 groups: primary (idiopathic) and secondary; the latter being more common.

Primary (Idiopathic) Pulmonary Hypertension

Primary or idiopathic pulmonary hypertension is an uncommon condition of unknown cause. The diagnosis can be established only after a thorough search for the usual causes of secondary pulmonary hypertension (discussed below). The patients are usually young females between the age of 20 and 40 years, or children around 5 years of age.

ETIOPATHOGENESIS. Though the etiology of primary pulmonary hypertension is unknown, a number of etiologic factors have been suggested to explain its pathogenesis:

1. A *neurohumoral vasoconstrictor mechanism* may be involved leading to chronic vasoconstriction that induces pulmonary hypertension.

2. The occurrence of disease in young females has prompted a suggestion that *unrecognised thromboemboli* or *amniotic fluid emboli* during pregnancy may play a role.

3. There is a suggestion that primary pulmonary hypertension may be a form of *collagen vascular disease.* This is supported by occurrence of Raynaud's phenomenon preceding the onset of this disease by a number of years in many patients, and association of the disease with SLE, scleroderma and rheumatoid arthritis.

4. *Pulmonary veno-occlusive disease* characterised by fibrous obliteration of small pulmonary veins is believed to be responsible for some cases of primary pulmonary hypertension, especially in children. Generally, this is considered to be a consequence of thrombosis or vasculitis.

5. *Ingestion of substances* like 'bush tea', oral contraceptives and appetite depressant agents like aminorex are believed to be related to primary pulmonary hypertension.

6. *Familial occurrence* has been reported in a number of cases.

Secondary Pulmonary Hypertension

When pulmonary hypertension occurs secondary to a recognised lesion in the heart or lungs, it is termed as secondary pulmonary hypertension. It is the more common type and may be encountered at any age, but more frequently over the age of 50 years.

ETIOPATHOGENESIS. Based on the underlying mechanism, causes of secondary pulmonary hypertension are divided into the following 3 groups:

A. Passive pulmonary hypertension. This is the commonest and is produced by diseases raising pressure in the pulmonary veins. These diseases are:

1. Mitral stenosis.
2. Chronic left ventricular failure (e.g. in severe systemic hypertension, aortic stenosis, myocardial fibrosis).

B. Hyperkinetic (Reactive) pulmonary hypertension. In this group are included causes in which the blood enters the pulmonary arteries in greater volume or at a higher pressure. These causes are:

1. Patent ductus arteriosus.
2. Atrial or ventricular septal defects.

C. Vaso-occlusive pulmonary hypertension. All such conditions which produce progressive diminution of the vascular bed in the lungs are included in this group. Vaso-occlusive causes may be further sub-divided into 3 types:

1. *Obstructive type,* in which there is block in the pulmonary circulation e.g.

i) Multiple emboli or thrombi
ii) Sickle cell disease
iii) Schistosomiasis

2. *Obliterative type,* in which there is reduction of pulmonary vascular bed by chronic parenchymal lung diseases e.g.

i) Chronic emphysema
ii) Chronic bronchitis
iii) Bronchiectasis
iv) Pulmonary tuberculosis
v) Pneumoconiosis

3. *Vasoconstrictive type,* in which there is widespread and sustained hypoxic vasoconstriction and alveolar hyperventilation leading to pulmonary hypertension e.g.

i) In residents at high altitude
ii) Pathologic obesity (Pickwickian disease)
iii) Upper airway disease such as tonsillar hypertrophy
iv) Neuromuscular diseases such as poliomyelitis
v) Severe kyphoscoliosis.

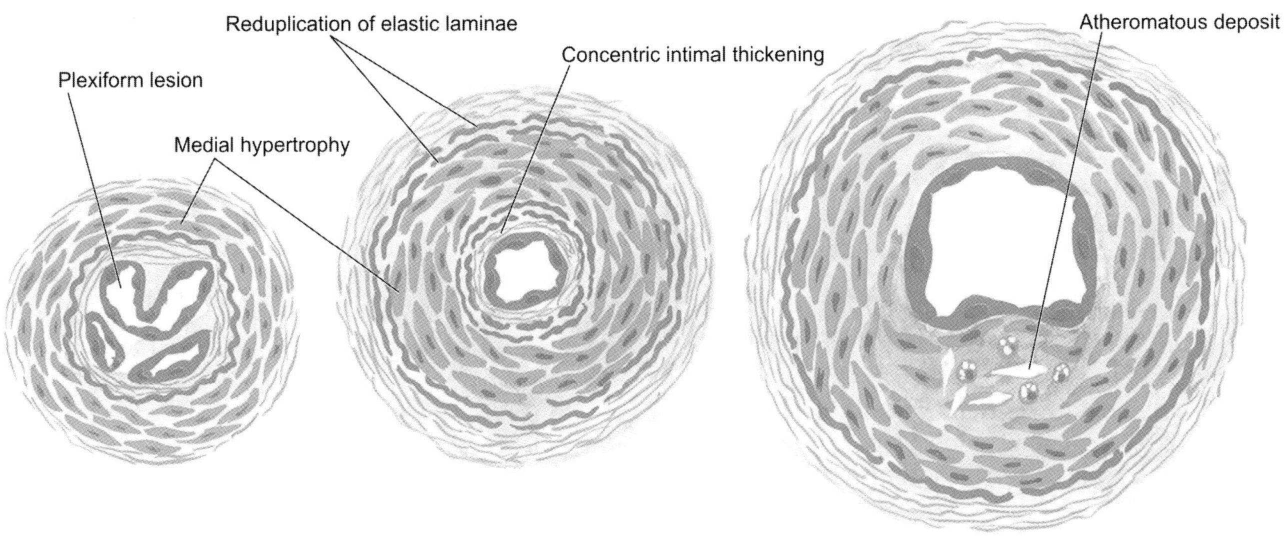

FIGURE 15.6

Histologic changes in the pulmonary arterial branches of different sizes in pulmonary hypertension.

PATHOLOGIC CHANGES. Irrespective of the type of pulmonary hypertension (primary or secondary), chronic cases invariably lead to cor pulmonale (Chapter 12). The pathologic changes are confined to the right side of the heart and pulmonary arterial tree in the lungs. There is hypertrophy of the right ventricle and dilatation of the right atrium. The vascular changes are similar in primary and secondary types and involve the entire arterial tree from the main pulmonary arteries down to the arterioles. These changes are as under (Fig. 15.6):

1. Arterioles and small pulmonary arteries: These branches show most conspicuous changes. These are:

i) Medial hypertrophy.

ii) Thickening and reduplication of elastic laminae.

iii) Plexiform pulmonary arteriopathy in which there is intraluminal tuft of capillary formation in dilated thin-walled arterial branches. These lesions are not so marked in secondary pulmonary hypertension.

2. Medium-sized pulmonary arteries:

i) Medial hypertrophy, which is not so marked in secondary pulmonary hypertension.

ii) Concentric intimal thickening.

iii) Adventitial fibrosis.

iv) Thickening and reduplication of elastic laminae.

3. Large pulmonary arteries:

i) Atheromatous deposits.

PULMONARY INFECTIONS

Acute and chronic pulmonary infections are common at all ages and are a frequent cause of death. They are generally caused by a wide variety of micro-organisms such as bacteria, viruses, fungi and mycoplasma. Important and common examples of acute pulmonary infectious diseases discussed here are *pneumonias, lung abscess* and *fungal infections,* while *pulmonary tuberculosis,* generally regarded as an example of chronic lung infections, is discussed in Chapter 6.

PNEUMONIAS

Pneumonia is defined as acute inflammation of the lung parenchyma distal to the terminal bronchioles which consist of the respiratory bronchiole, alveolar ducts, alveolar sacs and alveoli. The terms 'pneumonia' and 'pneumonitis' are often used synonymously for inflammation of the lungs, while 'consolidation' (meaning solidification) is the term used for macroscopic and radiologic appearance of the lungs in pneumonia.

PATHOGENESIS. The microorganisms gain entry into the lungs by one of the following four routes:

1. *Inhalation* of the microbes present in the air.
2. *Aspiration* of organisms from the nasopharynx or oropharynx.
3. *Haematogenous spread* from a distant focus of infection.
4. *Direct spread* from an adjoining site of infection.

The normal lung is free of bacteria because of the presence of a number of lung defense mechanisms at different levels such as nasopharyngeal filtering action, mucociliary action of the lower respiratory airways, the presence of phagocytosing alveolar macrophages and immunoglobulins. Failure of these defense mechanisms and presence of certain predisposing factors result in pneumonias. These conditions are as under:

1. Altered consciousness. The oropharyngeal contents may be aspirated in states causing unconsciousness e.g. in coma, cranial trauma, seizures, cerebrovascular accidents, drug overdose, alcoholism etc.

2. Depressed cough and glottic reflexes. Depression of effective cough may allow aspiration of gastric contents e.g. in old age, pain from trauma or thoraco-abdominal surgery, neuromuscular disease, weakness due to malnutrition, kyphoscoliosis, severe obstructive pulmonary diseases, endotracheal intubation and tracheostomy.

3. Impaired mucociliary transport. The normal protection offered by mucus-covered ciliated epithelium in the airways from the larynx to the terminal bronchioles is impaired or destroyed in many conditions favouring passage of bacteria into the lung parenchyma. These conditions are cigarette smoking, viral respiratory infections, immotile cilia syndrome, inhalation of hot or corrosive gases and old age.

4. Impaired alveolar macrophage function. Pneumonias may occur when alveolar macrophage function is impaired e.g. by cigarette smoke, hypoxia, starvation, anaemia, pulmonary oedema and viral respiratory infections.

5. Endobronchial obstruction. The effective clearance mechanism is interfered with in endobronchial obstruction from tumour, foreign body, cystic fibrosis and chronic bronchitis.

6. Leucocyte dysfunctions. Disorders of lymphocytes including congenital and acquired immunodeficiencies (e.g. AIDS, immunosuppressive therapy) and granulocyte abnormalities may predispose to pneumonia.

CLASSIFICATION. On the basis of the anatomic part of the lung parenchyma involved, pneumonias are traditionally classified into 3 main types:

1. Lobar pneumonia
2. Bronchopneumonia (or Lobular pneumonia)
3. Interstitial pneumonia

However, now that much is known about etiology and pathogenesis of pneumonias, current practice is to follow the etiologic classification (Table 15.1) which will be followed in the present discussion too.

TABLE 15.1: Etiologic Classification of Pneumonias.

A. BACTERIAL PNEUMONIA

I. Lobar pneumonia
II. Bronchopneumonia (Lobular pneumonia)

B. VIRAL AND MYCOPLASMAL PNEUMONIA (PRIMARY ATYPICAL PNEUMONIA)

C. OTHER TYPES OF PNEUMONIAS

1. *Pneumocystis carinii* pneumonia
II. *Legionella* pneumonia (Legionnaire's disease)
III. Aspiration (inhalation) pneumonia
IV. Hypostatic pneumonia
V. Lipid pneumonia

A. BACTERIAL PNEUMONIA

Bacterial infection of the lung parenchyma is the most common cause of pneumonia or consolidation of one or both the lungs. Two types of acute bacterial pneumonias are distinguished—lobar pneumonia and broncho-(lobular-) pneumonia, each with distinct etiologic agent and morphologic changes. Another type distinguished by some workers separately is *confluent pneumonia* which combines the features of both lobar and bronchopneumonia and involves larger (confluent) areas in both the lungs irregularly, while others consider this as a variant of bronchopneumonia.

1. Lobar Pneumonia

Lobar pneumonia is an acute bacterial infection of a part of a lobe, the entire lobe, or even two lobes of one or both the lungs.

ETIOLOGY. Based on the etiologic microbial agent causing lobar pneumonia, the following types are described:

1. Pneumococcal pneumonia. More than 90% of all lobar pneumonias are caused by *Streptococcus pneumoniae,* a lancet-shaped diplococcus. Out of various types, type *3-S. pneumoniae* causes particularly virulent form of lobar pneumonia. Pneumococcal pneumonia in majority of cases is community-acquired infection.

2. Staphylococcal pneumonia. *Staphylococcus aureus* causes pneumonia by haematogenous spread of infection from another focus or after viral infections.

3. Streptococcal pneumonia. β-haemolytic streptococci may rarely cause pneumonia such as in children after measles or influenza, in severely debilitated elderly patients and in diabetics.

4. Pneumonia by gram-negative aerobic bacteria. Less common causes of lobar pneumonia are gram-negative bacteria like *Haemophilus influenzae, Klebsiella pneumoniae (Friedlander's bacillus), Pseudomonas, Proteus* and

Escherichia coli, H. influenzae commonly causes pneumonia in children below 3 years of age after a preceding viral infection.

PATHOLOGIC CHANGES. Laennec's original description divides lobar pneumonia into 4 sequential pathologic phases: *stage of congestion* (initial phase), *red hepatisation* (early consolidation), *grey hepatisation* (late consolidation) and *resolution*. However, these classic stages seen in untreated cases are found much less often nowadays due to administration of antibiotics and improved medical care.

In lobar pneumonia, as the name suggests, part of a lobe, a whole lobe, or two lobes are involved, sometimes bilaterally. The lower lobes are affected most commonly. The sequence of pathologic changes described below represents the inflammatory response of lungs in bacterial infection.

1. STAGE OF CONGESTION: INITIAL PHASE (Fig. 15.7,A). The initial phase represents the early acute inflammatory response to bacterial infection and lasts for 1 to 2 days.

Grossly, the affected lobe is enlarged, heavy, dark red and congested. Cut surface exudes blood-stained frothy fluid.

Histologically, typical features of acute inflammatory response to the organisms are seen. These are as under:

i) Dilatation and congestion of the capillaries in the alveolar walls.

ii) Pale eosinophilic oedema fluid in the air spaces.

iii) A few red cells and neutrophils in the intra-alveolar fluid.

iv) Numerous bacteria demonstrated in the alveolar fluid by Gram's staining.

2. RED HEPATISATION: EARLY CONSOLIDATION (Fig. 15.7,B). This phase lasts for 2 to 4 days. The term hepatisation in pneumonia refers to liver-like consistency of the affected lobe on cut section.

Grossly, the affected lobe is red, firm and consolidated. The cut surface of the involved lobe is airless, red-pink, dry, granular and has liver-like consistency. The stage of red hepatisation is accompanied by serofibrinous pleurisy.

Histologically, the following features are observed (COLOUR PLATE XIX: CL 74):

i) The oedema fluid of the preceding stage is replaced by strands of fibrin.

ii) There is marked cellular exudate of neutrophils and extravasation of red cells.

iii) Many neutrophils show ingested bacteria.

iv) The alveolar septa are less prominent than in the first stage due to cellular exudation.

3. GREY HEPATISATION: LATE CONSOLIDATION (Fig. 15.7,C). This phase lasts for 4 to 8 days.

Grossly, the affected lobe is firm and heavy. The cut surface is dry, granular and grey in appearance with liver-like consistency. The change in colour from red to grey begins at the hilum and spreads towards the periphery. Fibrinous pleurisy is prominent.

Histologically, the following changes are present (COLOUR PLATE XIX: CL 75):

i) The fibrin strands are dense and more numerous.

ii) The cellular exudate of neutrophils is reduced due to disintegration of many inflammatory cells as evidenced by their pyknotic nuclei. The red cells are also fewer. The macrophages begin to appear in the exudate.

iii) The cellular exudate is often separated from the septal walls by a thin clear space.

iv) The organisms are less numerous and appear as degenerated forms.

4. RESOLUTION: (Fig. 15.7,D). This stage begins by 8th to 9th day if no chemotherapy is administered and is completed in 1 to 3 weeks. However, antibiotic therapy induces resolution on about 3rd day. Resolution proceeds in a progressive manner.

Grossly, the previously solid fibrinous constituent is liquefied by enzymatic action, eventually restoring the normal aeration in the affected lobe. The process of softening begins centrally and spreads to the periphery. The cut surface is grey-red or dirty brown and frothy, yellow, creamy fluid can be expressed on pressing. The pleural reaction may also show resolution but may undergo organisation leading to fibrous obliteration of pleural cavity.

Histologically, the following features are noted:

i) Macrophages are the predominant cells in the alveolar spaces, while neutrophils diminish in number. Many of the macrophages contain engulfed neutrophils and debris.

ii) Granular and fragmented strands of fibrin in the alveolar spaces are seen due to progressive enzymatic digestion.

iii) Alveolar capillaries are engorged.

iv) There is progressive removal of fluid content as well as cellular exudate from the air spaces, partly by expectoration but mainly by lymphatics, resulting in restoration of normal lung parenchyma with areation.

COMPLICATIONS. Since the advent of antibiotics, serious complications of lobar pneumonia are

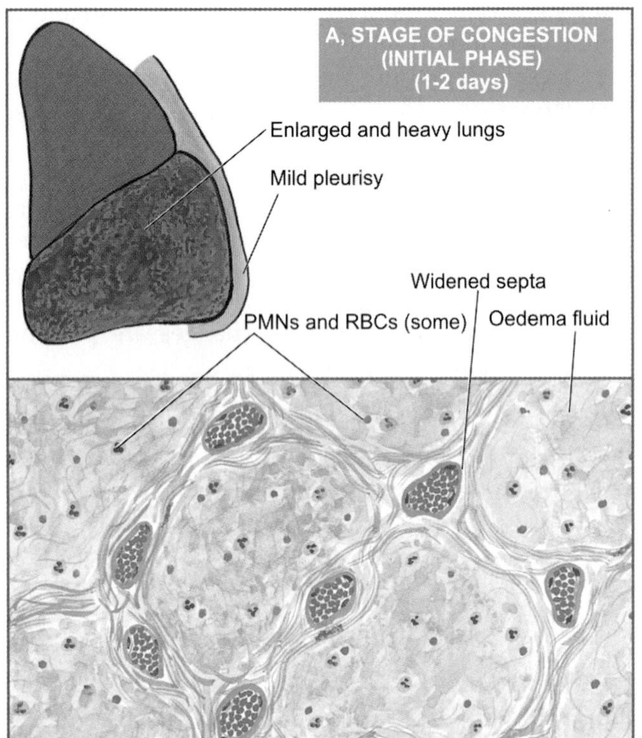

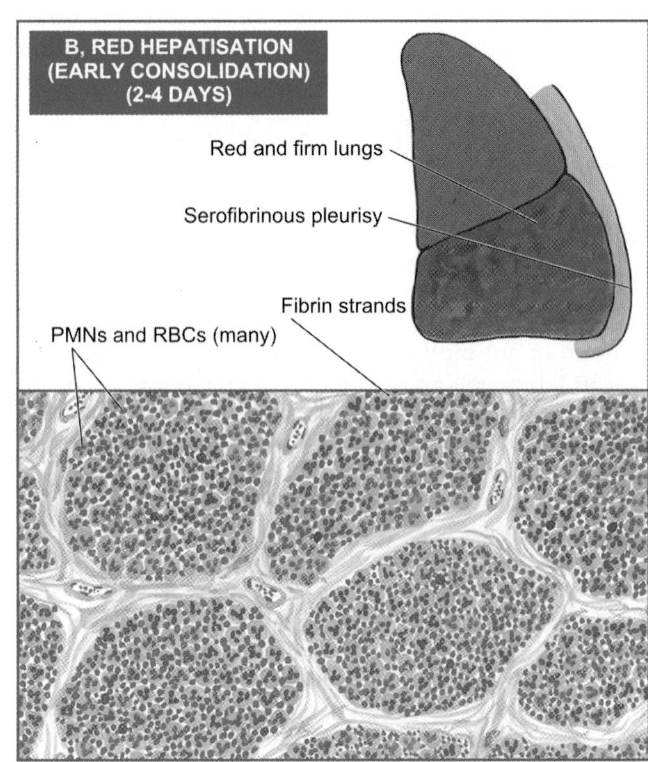

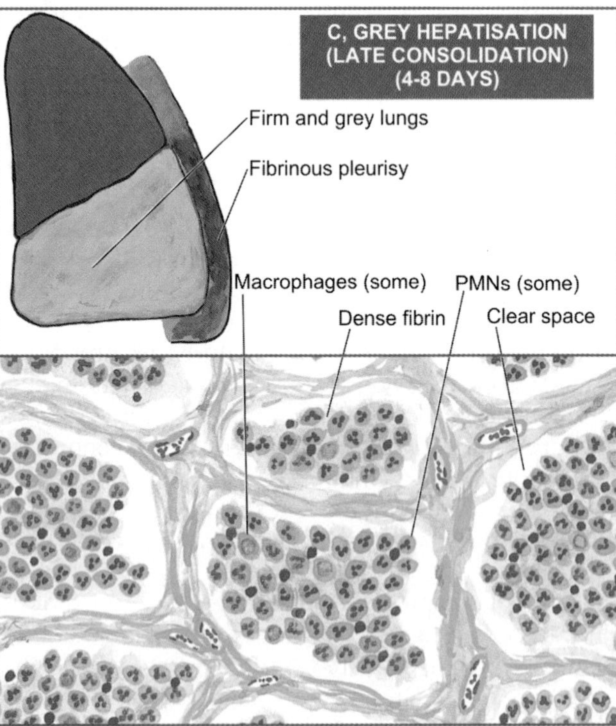

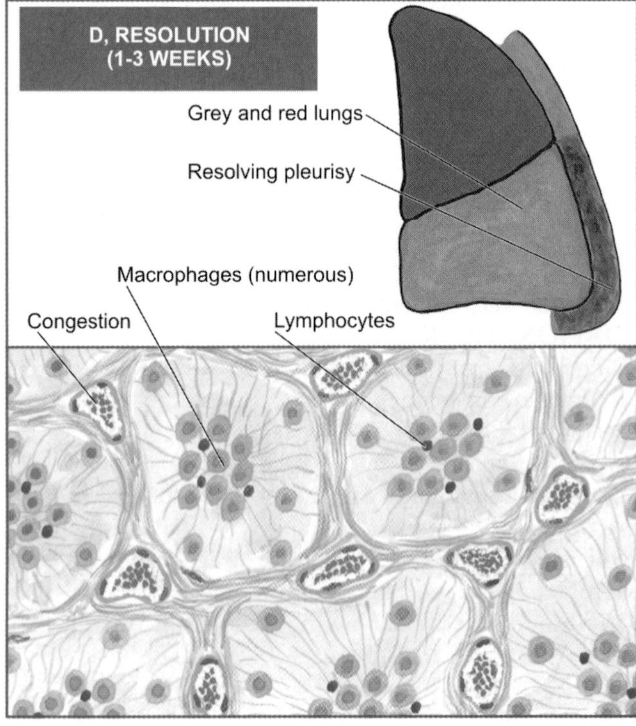

FIGURE 15.7

The four stages of lobar pneumonia, showing correlation of gross appearance of the lung with microscopic appearance in each stage. For details consult the text.

uncommon. However, they may develop in neglected cases and in patients with impaired immunologic defenses. These are as under:

1. **Organisation.** In about 3% of cases, resolution of the exudate does not occur but instead it is organised. There is ingrowth of fibroblasts from the alveolar septa resulting in fibrosed, tough, airless leathery lung tissue. This type of post-pneumonic fibrosis is called *carnification.*

2. **Pleural effusion.** About 5% of treated cases of lobar pneumonia develop inflammation of the pleura with effusion. The pleural effusion usually resolves but sometimes may undergo organisation with fibrous adhesions between visceral and parietal pleura.

3. **Empyema.** Less than 1% of treated cases of lobar pneumonia develop encysted pus in the pleural cavity termed empyema.

4. **Lung abscess.** A rare complication of lobar pneumonia is formation of lung abscess, especially when there is secondary infection by other organisms.

5. **Metastatic infection.** Occasionally, infection in the lungs and pleural cavity in lobar pneumonia may extend into the pericardium and the heart causing purulent pericarditis, bacterial endocarditis and myocarditis. Other forms of metastatic infection encountered rarely in lobar pneumonias are otitis media, mastoiditis, meningitis, brain abscess and purulent arthritis.

CLINICAL FEATURES. Classically, the onset of lobar pneumonia is sudden. The major symptoms are: shaking chills, fever, malaise with pleuritic chest pain, dyspnoea and cough with expectoration which may be mucoid, purulent or even bloody. The common physical findings are fever, tachycardia, and tachypnoea, and sometimes cyanosis if the patient is severely hypoxaemic. There is generally a marked neutrophilic leucocytosis. Blood cultures are positive in about 30% of cases. Chest radiograph may reveal consolidation. The culture of the organisms in the sputum and antibiotic sensitivity are most significant investigations for institution of specific antibiotics. The response to antibiotics is usually rapid with clinical improvement in 48 to 72 hours after the initiation of antibiotics.

II. Bronchopneumonia (Lobular Pneumonia)

Bronchopneumonia or lobular pneumonia is infection of the terminal bronchioles that extends into the surrounding alveoli resulting in patchy consolidation of the lung. The condition is particularly frequent at extremes of life (i.e. in infancy and old age), as a terminal event in chronic debilitating diseases and as a secondary infection following viral respiratory infections such as influenza, measles etc.

ETIOLOGY. The common organisms responsible for bronchopneumonia are staphylococci, streptococci, pneumococci, *Klebsiella pneumoniae, Haemophilus influenzae,* and gram-negative bacilli like *Pseudomonas* and coliform bacteria.

PATHOLOGIC CHANGES. Grossly, bronchopneumonia is identified by patchy areas of red or grey consolidation affecting one or more lobes, frequently found bilaterally and more often involving the lower zones of the lungs due to gravitation of the secretions (Fig. 15.8). On cut surface, these patchy consolidated lesions are dry, granular, firm, red or grey in colour, 3 to 4 cm in diameter, slightly elevated over the surface and are often centred around a bronchiole. These patchy areas are best picked up by passing the fingertips on the cut surface.

Histologically, the following features are observed (Fig. 15.9) (COLOUR PLATE XIX: CL 76):

i) Acute bronchiolitis.

ii) Suppurative exudate, consisting chiefly of neutrophils, in the peribronchiolar alveoli.

iii) Thickening of the alveolar septa by congested capillaries and leucocytic infiltration.

iv) Less involved alveoli contain oedema fluid.

COMPLICATIONS. The complications of lobar pneumonia may occur in bronchopneumonia as well.

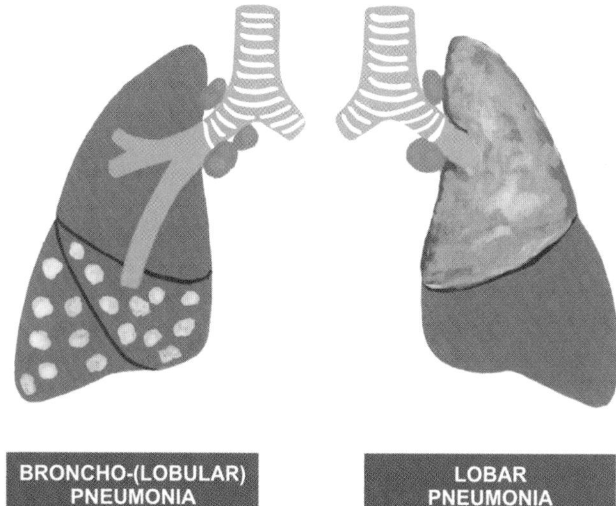

FIGURE 15.8

Gross appearance of bronchopneumonia contrasted with that of lobar pneumonia.

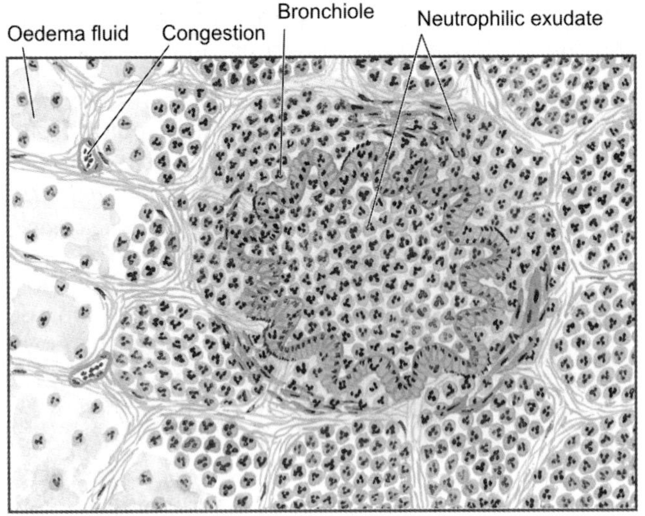

FIGURE 15.9

Microscopic appearance of bronchopneumonia. The bronchioles as well as the adjacent alveoli are filled with exudate consisting chiefly of neutrophils. The alveolar septa are thickened due to congested capillaries and neutrophilic infiltrate.

However, complete resolution of bronchopneumonia is uncommon. There is generally some degree of destruction of the bronchioles resulting in foci of bronchiolar fibrosis that may eventually cause bronchiectasis.

CLINICAL FEATURES. The patients of bronchopneumonia are generally infants or elderly individuals. There may be history of preceding bed-ridden illness, chronic debility, aspiration of gastric contents or upper respiratory infection. For initial 2 to 3 days, there are features of acute bronchitis but subsequently signs and symptoms similar to those of lobar pneumonia appear. Blood examination usually shows a neutrophilic leucocytosis. Chest radiograph shows mottled, focal opacities in both the lungs, chiefly in the lower zones.

The salient features of the two main types of bacterial pneumonias are contrasted in Table 15.2.

B. VIRAL AND MYCOPLASMAL PNEUMONIA (PRIMARY ATYPICAL PNEUMONIA)

Viral and mycoplasmal pneumonia is characterised by patchy inflammatory changes, largely confined to interstitial tissue of the lungs, without any alveolar exudate. Other terms used for these respiratory tract infections are *interstitial pneumonitis,* reflecting the interstitial location of the inflammation, and *primary atypical pneumonia,* atypicality being the absence of alveolar exudate commonly present in other pneumonias. Interstitial pneumonitis may occur in all ages. Most of the cases are mild and transient; exceptionally it may be severe and fulminant.

ETIOLOGY. Interstitial pneumonitis is caused by a wide variety of agents, the most common being *respiratory syncytial virus* (RSV). Others are *Mycoplasma pneumoniae* and many viruses such as influenza and parainfluenza

TABLE 15.2: Contrasting Features of Lobal Pneumonia and Bronchopneumonia.

FEATURE	LOBAR PNEUMONIA	BRONCHOPNEUMONIA
1. *Definition*	Acute bacterial infection of a part of a lobe of one or both lungs, or the entire lobe/s	Acute bacterial infection of the terminal bronchioles extending in to adjoining alveoli
2. *Age group*	More common in adults	Commoner at exteremes of age–infants and old age
3. *Predisposing factors*	More often affects healthy individuals	Preexisting diseases e.g. chronic debility, terminal illness, flu, measles
4. *Common etiologic agents*	Pneumococci, *Klebsiella pneuminae,* staphylococci, streptococci	Staphylococci, streptococci, Pseudomonas, *Haemophilus influenzae*
5. *Pathologic features*	Typical case passes through stages of congestion (1-2 days) , early (2-4 days) and late consolidation (4-8 days), followed by resolution (1-3 weeks)	Patchy consolidation with central granularity, alveolar exudation, thickened septa
6. *Investigations*	Neutrophilic leucocytosis, positive blood culture, X-ray shows consolidation	Neutrophilic leucocytosis, positive blood culture, X-ray shows mottled focal opacities
7 *Prognosis*	Better response to treatment, resolution common, prognosis good	Response to treatment variable, organisation may occur, prognosis poor
8. *Complications*	Less common; pleural effusion, empyema, lung abscess, organisation	Brochiectasis may occur; other complications same as for lobar pneumoina

Chapter Fifteen

viruses, adenoviruses, rhinoviruses, coxsackieviruses and cytomegaloviruses (CMV). Occasionally, psittacosis *(Chlamydia)* and Q fever *(Coxiella)* are associated with interstitial pneumonitis.

Infections of the respiratory tract with these organisms are quite common. In most cases, the infection remains confined to the upper respiratory tract presenting as common cold. Occasionally, it may extend lower down to involve the interstitium of the lungs. The circumstances favouring such extension of infection are malnutrition, chronic debilitating diseases and alcoholism.

PATHOLOGIC CHANGES. Irrespective of the etiologic agent, the pathologic changes are similar in all cases.

Grossly, depending upon the severity of infection, the involvement may be patchy to massive and widespread consolidation of one or both the lungs. The lungs are heavy, congested and subcrepitant. Sectioned surface of the lung exudes small amount of frothy or bloody fluid. The pleural reaction is usually infrequent and mild.

Histologically, hallmark of viral pneumonias is the interstitial nature of the inflammatory reaction. The microscopic features are as under (Fig. 15.10):

i) Interstitial inflammation: There is thickening of alveolar walls due to congestion, oedema and mononuclear inflammatory infiltrate comprised by lymphocytes, macrophages and some plasma cells.

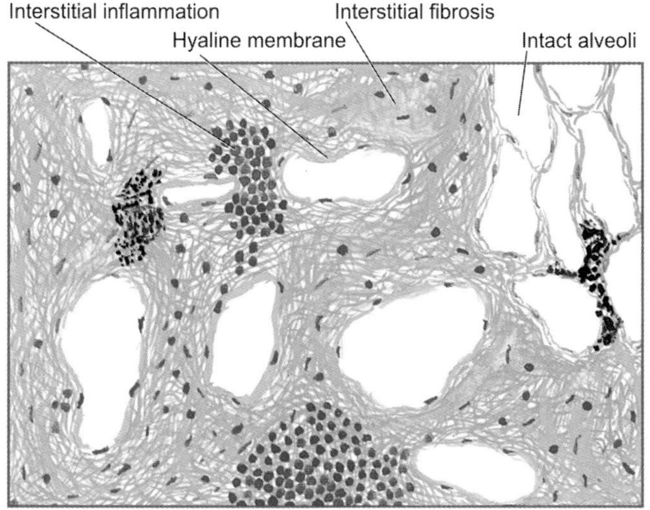

FIGURE 15.10

Microscopic appearance of interstitial pneumonitis (viral pneumonia). There are predominant inflammatory changes in the alveolar walls and pronounced interstitial fibrosis.

ii) Necrotising bronchiolitis: This is characterised by foci of necrosis of the bronchiolar epithelium, inspissated secretions in the lumina and mononuclear infiltrate in the walls and lumina.

iii) Reactive changes: The lining epithelial cells of the bronchioles and alveoli proliferate in the presence of virus and may form multinucleate giant cells and syncytia in the bronchiolar and alveolar walls. Occasionally, viral inclusions (intranuclear and/or intracytoplasmic) are found, especially in pneumonitis caused by CMV.

vi) Alveolar changes: In severe cases, the alveolar lumina may contain oedema fluid, fibrin, scanty inflammatory exudate and coating of alveolar walls by pink, hyaline membrane similar to the one seen in respiratory distress syndrome (page 470). Alveolar changes are prominent if bacterial infection supervenes.

COMPLICATIONS. The major complication of interstitial pneumonitis is superimposed bacterial infection and its complications. Most cases of interstitial pneumonitis recover completely. In more severe cases, there may be interstitial fibrosis and permanent damage.

CLINICAL FEATURES. Majority of cases of interstitial pneumonitis initially have upper respiratory symptoms with fever, headache and muscle-aches. A few days later appears dry, hacking, non-productive cough with retrosternal burning due to tracheitis and bronchitis. Chest radiograph may show patchy or diffuse consolidation. Cold agglutinin titres in the serum are elevated in almost half the cases of mycoplasmal pneumonia, 20% cases of adenovirus infection but absent in other forms of viral pneumonia. Isolation of the etiologic agent, otherwise, is difficult.

C. OTHERTYPES OF PNEUMONIAS

Some other types of pneumonias caused by *infective agents* (such as *Pneumocystis carinii* pneumonia and *Legionella* pneumonia) and certain *non-infective varieties* (e.g. aspiration pneumonia, hypostatic pneumonia and lipid pneumonia) are described here.

Table 15.3 lists the various etiologic types of pneumonias associated with HIV infection due to profound immunosuppression.

1. *Pneumocystis carinii* Pneumonia

Pneumocystis carinii, a protozoon widespread in the environment, causes pneumonia by inhalation of the organisms as an opportunistic infection in neonates and

TABLE 15.3: Etiologic Types of HIV-Infection Associated Pneumonias.

1. *Pneumocystis carinii*
2. Cytomegalovirus
3. *Mycobacterium avium-intracellulare*
4. *Mycobacterium tuberculosis*
5. *Streptococcus pneumoniae*
6. *Haemophilus influenzae*
7. Invasive aspergillosis
8. Invasive candidiasis

immunosuppressed people. Almost 100% cases of AIDS develop opportunistic infection, most commonly *Pneumocystis carinii* pneumonia. Other immunosuppressed groups are patients on chemotherapy for organ transplant and tumours, malnutrition, agammaglobulinaemia etc.

*PATHOLOGIC CHANGES. **Grossly,*** the affected parts of lung are consolidated, dry and grey. ***Microscopically,*** the features are as under:

i) Interstitial pneumonitis with thickening and mononuclear infiltration of the alveolar walls.
ii) Alveolar lumina contain pink frothy fluid.
iii) By Gomori's methenamine-silver (GMS) stain, the characteristic oval or crescentic cysts, about 5 μm in diameter and surrounded by numerous tiny black dot-like trophozoites of *P. carinii* are demonstrable in the frothy fluid.
iv) No significant inflammatory exudate is seen in the air spaces.

CLINICAL FEATURES. There is rapid onset of dyspnoea, tachycardia, cyanosis and non-productive cough. If untreated, it causes death in one or two weeks. Chest radiograph shows diffuse alveolar and interstitial infiltrate.

II. *Legionella* Pneumonia

Legionella pneumonia or legionnaire's disease is an epidemic illness caused by gram-negative bacilli, *Legionella pneumophila* that thrives in aquatic environment. It was first recognised following investigation into high mortality among those attending American Legion Convention in Philadelphia in July 1976. The epidemic occurs in summer months by spread of organisms through contaminated drinking water or in air-conditioning cooling towers. Impaired host defenses in the form of immunodeficiency, corticosteroid therapy, old age and cigarette smoking play important roles.

*PATHOLOGIC CHANGES. **Grossly,*** there are changes of widespread bronchopneumonia involving many lobes and there may be consolidation of the entire lung. Pleural effusion is frequently present. ***Histologically,*** the changes are not distinctive. The features commonly seen are:

i) Intra-alveolar exudate, initially of neutrophils but later composed mainly of macrophages.
ii) Alveolar septa show foci of hyperplasia of the lining epithelium and thrombosis of vessels in the septa.
iii) The organisms may be demonstrated in the macrophages by special stains or by immunofluorescent techniques.

CLINICAL FEATURES. The disease begins with malaise, headache and muscle-aches followed by high fever, chills, cough and tachypnoea. Systemic manifestations unrelated to pathologic changes in the lungs are seen due to bacteraemia and include abdominal pain, watery diarrhoea, proteinuria and mild hepatic dysfunction.

III. Aspiration (Inhalation) Pneumonia

Aspiration or inhalation pneumonia results from inhaling different agents into the lungs. These substances include food, gastric contents, foreign body and infected material from oral cavity. A number of factors predispose to inhalation pneumonia which include: unconsciousness, drunkenness, neurological disorders affecting swallowing, drowning, necrotic oropharyngeal tumours, in premature infants and congenital tracheo-oesophageal fistula. Some patients die immediately from asphyxiation or laryngospasm without developing pneumonia.

PATHOLOGIC CHANGES. Pathologic changes vary depending upon the particulate matter aspirated but in general right lung is affected more often due to direct path from the main bronchus:

1. Aspiration of small amount of **sterile foreign matter** such as acidic gastric contents produce *chemical pneumonitis.* It is characterised by haemorrhagic pulmonary oedema with presence of particles in the bronchioles. Patients rapidly develop cyanosis, dyspnoea, shock and bloody sputum and are often likely to die of cardiac failure. If the patient survives the acute episode, secondary bacterial infection is likely to occur.

2. **Non-sterile aspirate** causes widespread *bronchopneumonia* with multiple areas of necrosis and suppu-

ration. A granulomatous reaction with foreign body giant cells may surround the aspirated vegetable matter.

IV. Hypostatic Pneumonia

Hypostatic pneumonia is the term used for collection of oedema fluid and secretions in the dependent parts of the lungs in severely debilitated, bed-ridden patients. The accumulated fluid in the basal zone and posterior part of lungs gets infected by bacteria from the upper respiratory tract and sets in bacterial pneumonia. Hypostatic pneumonia is a common terminal event in the old, feeble, comatose patients.

V. Lipid Pneumonia

Another variety of noninfective pneumonia is lipid pneumonia. It is of 2 types: exogenous and endogenous.

1. **Exogenous lipid pneumonia.** This is caused by aspiration of a variety of oily materials. These are: inhalation of oily nasal drops, regurgitation of oily medicines from stomach (e.g. liquid paraffin), administration of oily vitamin preparation to reluctant children or to debilitated old patients.

2. **Endogenous lipid pneumonia.** Endogenous origin of lipids causing pneumonic consolidation is more common. The sources of origin are tissue breakdown following obstruction to airways e.g. obstruction by bronchogenic cancer, tuberculosis and bronchiectasis.

*PATHOLOGIC CHANGES. **Grossly,*** the exogenous type affects the right lung more frequently due to direct path from the main bronchus. Quite often, the lesions are bilateral. The affected part of the lungs is consolidated. Cut surface is characteristically 'golden yellow'.

Microscopically, the features are as under:

i) The lipid is finely dispersed in the cytoplasm of macrophages forming foamy macrophages within the alveolar spaces.

ii) There may be formation of cholesterol clefts due to liberation of cholesterol and other lipids.

iii) Formation of granulomas with foreign body giant cells may be seen around the large lipid droplets.

LUNG ABSCESS

Lung abscess is a localised area of necrosis of lung tissue with suppuration. It is of 2 types (Fig. 15.11):

- *Primary lung abscess* that develops in an otherwise normal lung. The commonest cause is aspiration of infected material.

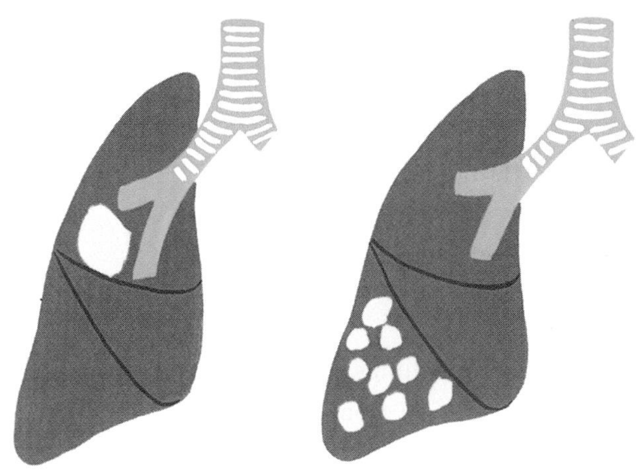

FIGURE 15.11

Common locations of lung abscess. A, primary lung abscess—mostly single, large, commonly due to aspiration, located most frequently in the lower part of right upper lobe or apex of right lower lobe. B, Secondary pulmonary abscesses—mostly multiple, small, most commonly post-pneumonic or following septic embolism.

- *Secondary lung abscess* that develops as a complication of some other disease of the lung or from another site.

ETIOPATHOGENESIS. The microorganisms commonly isolated from the lungs in lung abscess are streptococci, staphylococci and various gram-negative organisms. These are introduced into the lungs from one of the following mechanisms:

1. **Aspiration of infected foreign material.** A number of foreign materials such as food, decaying teeth, gastric contents, severely infected gingivae and teeth, and necrotic tissue from lesions in the mouth, upper respiratory tract or nasopharynx may be aspirated. This occurs particularly in favourable circumstances such as during sleep, unconsciousness, anaesthesia, general debility and acute alcoholism.

2. **Preceding bacterial infection.** Preceding bronchopneumonia in a debilitated patient may develop into lung abscess. Other infective conditions like tuberculosis, bronchiectasis and mycotic infections may occasionally result in formation of lung abscess.

3. **Bronchial obstruction.** An abscess may form distal to an obstructed bronchus such as from bronchial tumour or from impacted foreign body.

4. **Septic embolism.** Infected emboli originating from pyaemia, thrombophlebitis or from vegetative bacterial

endocarditis may be disseminated in the venous circulation and reach the right side of the heart from where they are lodged in the lung and result in multiple abscesses.

5. Miscellaneous. Rare causes of lung abscesses include:

i) Infection in pulmonary infarcts.

ii) Amoebic abscesses due to infection with *Entamoeba histolytica.*

iii) Trauma to the lungs.

iv) Direct extension from a suppurative focus in the mediastinum, oesophagus, subphrenic area or spine.

PATHOLOGIC CHANGES. Abscesses due to aspiration are more likely to be in right lung due to more vertical main bronchus and are frequently single. They are commonly located in the lower part of the right upper lobe or apex of right lower lobe (Fig. 15.11,A). Abscesses developing from preceding pneumonia and septic or pyaemic abscesses are often multiple and scattered throughout the lung (Fig. 15.11,B).

Grossly, abscesses may be of variable size from a few millimeters to large cavities, 5 to 6 cm in diameter. The cavity often contains exudate. An acute lung abscess is initially surrounded by acute pneumonia and has poorly-defined ragged wall. With passage of time, the abscess becomes chronic and develops fibrous wall.

Histologically, the characteristic feature is the destruction of lung parenchyma with suppurative exudate in the lung cavity. The cavity is initially surrounded by acute inflammation in the wall but later there is replacement by exudate of lymphocytes, plasma cells and macrophages. In more chronic cases, there is considerable fibroblastic proliferation forming a fibrocollagenic wall (COLOUR PLATE VII: CL 25).

CLINICAL FEATURES. The clinical manifestations are fever, malaise, loss of weight, cough, purulent expectoration and haemoptysis in half the cases. Clubbing of the fingers and toes appears in about 20% of patients. Secondary amyloidosis may occur in chronic long-standing cases.

FUNGAL INFECTIONS OF LUNG

Fungal infections of the lung are more common than tuberculosis in the United States of America. These infections in healthy individuals are rarely serious but in immunosuppressed individuals may prove fatal. Some of the common examples of fungal infections of the lung are briefly outlined below:

1. Histoplasmosis. It is caused by oval organism, *Histoplasma capsulatum,* by inhalation of infected dust or bird droppings. The condition may remain asymptomatic or may produce lesions similar to the Ghon's complex.

2. Coccidioidomycosis. Coccidioidomycosis is caused by *Coccidioides immitis* which are spherical spores. The infection in human beings is acquired by close contact with infected dogs. The lesions consist of peripheral parenchymal granuloma in the lung.

3. Cryptococcosis. It is caused by *Cryptococcus neoformans* which is round yeast having a halo around it due to shrinkage in tissue sections. The infection occurs from infection by inhalation of pigeon droppings. The lesions in the body may range from a small parenchymal granuloma in the lung to cryptococcal meningitis.

4. Blastomycosis. It is an uncommon condition caused by *Blastomyces dermatitidis.* The lesions result from inhalation of spores in the ground. Pathological features may present as Ghon's complex-like lesion, as a pneumonic consolidation, and as multiple skin nodules.

5. Aspergillosis. Aspergillosis is the most common fungal infection of the lung caused by *Aspergillus fumigatus.* The fungus exists as thin septate hyphae with dichotomous branching and grows best in cool, wet climate. The infection may result in *allergic bronchopulmonary aspergillosis, aspergilloma* and *necrotising bronchitis.* Immunocompromised persons develop more serious manifestations of aspergillus infection, especially in leukaemic patients on cytotoxic drug therapy. Extensive haematogenous spread of aspergillus infection may result in widespread changes in lung tissue due to arterial occlusion, thrombosis and infarction (COLOUR PLATE IX: CL 33).

6. Mucormycosis. Mucormycosis or phycomycosis is caused by *Mucor* and *Rhizopus.* The infection in the lung occurs in a similar way as in aspergillosis.The pulmonary lesions are especially common in patients of *diabetic ketoacidosis.*

7. Candidiasis. Candidiasis or moniliasis caused by *Candida albicans* is a normal commensal in oral cavity, gut and vagina but attains pathologic form in immunocompromised host. Angio-invasive growth of the organism may occur in the airways.

PULMONARY TUBERCULOSIS

The classical and most common example of chronic infection of the lungs is pulmonary tuberculosis. Pulmonary lesions caused by *Mycobacterium tuberculosis* and other mycobacteria have already been discussed alongwith general aspects of tuberculosis and other granulomatous inflammations in Chapter 6.

CHRONIC OBSTRUCTIVE PULMONARY DISEASE

Chronic obstructive pulmonary disease (COPD) or chronic obstructive airways disease (COAD) are commonly used clinical terms for a group of pathological conditions in which there is chronic, partial or complete, obstruction to the airflow at any level from trachea to the smallest airways resulting in functional disability of the lungs. The obstructive pulmonary disease must be distinguished from restrictive pulmonary disease (see Table 15.7). The following 4 entities are included in COPD:

I. Chronic bronchitis
II. Emphysema
III. Bronchial asthma
IV. Bronchiectasis

Chronic bronchitis and emphysema are quite common and often occur together. More recently, small airways disease involving inflammation of small bronchi and bronchioles (bronchiolitis) has been added to the group of COPD.

I. CHRONIC BRONCHITIS

Chronic bronchitis is a common condition defined clinically as persistent cough with expectoration on most days for at least three months of the year for two or more consecutive years. The cough is caused by oversecretion of mucus. In spite of its name, chronic inflammation of the bronchi is not a prominent feature. The condition is more common in middle-aged males than females; approximately 20% of adult men and 5% of adult women have chronic bronchitis, but only a minority of them develop serious disabling COPD or cor pulmonale. Quite frequently, chronic bronchitis is associated with emphysema.

ETIOPATHOGENESIS. The two most important etiologic factors responsible for majority of cases of chronic bronchitis are: cigarette smoking and atmospheric pollution. Other contributory factors are occupation, infection, familial and genetic factors.

1. Smoking. The most commonly identified factor implicated in causation of chronic bronchitis and in emphysema is heavy smoking. Heavy cigarette smokers have 4 to 10 times higher proneness to develop chronic bronchitis. Prolonged cigarette smoking appears to act on the lungs in a number of ways:

i) It impairs ciliary movement.

ii) It inhibits the function of alveolar macrophages.

iii) It leads to hypertrophy and hyperplasia of mucus-secreting glands.

iv) It causes considerable obstruction of small airways.

v) It stimulates the vagus and causes bronchoconstriction.

2. Atmospheric pollution. The incidence of chronic bronchitis is higher in industrialised urban areas where air is polluted. Some of the atmospheric pollutants which increase the risk of developing chronic bronchitis are sulfur dioxide, nitrogen dioxide, particulate dust and toxic fumes.

3. Occupation. Workers engaged in certain occupations such as in cotton mills (byssinosis), plastic factories etc are exposed to various organic or inorganic dusts which contribute to disabling chronic bronchitis in such individuals.

4. Infection. Bacterial, viral and mycoplasmal infections do not initiate chronic bronchitis but usually occur secondary to bronchitis. Cigarette smoke, however, predisposes to infection responsible for acute exacerbation in chronic bronchitis.

5. Familial and genetic factors. There appears to be a poorly-defined familial tendency and genetic predisposition to develop disabling chronic bronchitis. However, it is more likely that nonsmoker family members who remain in the air-pollution of home are significantly exposed to smoke (passive smoking) and hence have increased blood levels of carbon monoxide.

PATHOLOGIC CHANGES. Grossly, the bronchial wall is thickened, hyperaemic and oedematous. Lumina of the bronchi and bronchioles may contain mucus plugs and purulent exudate.

Microscopically, just as there is clinical definition, there is histologic definition of chronic bronchitis by increased Reid index. *Reid index* is the ratio between thickness of the submucosal mucous glands (i.e. hypertrophy and hyperplasia) in the cartilage-containing large airways to that of the total bronchial wall (Fig. 15.12). The increase in thickness can be quantitatively assessed by micrometer lens. The bronchial epithelium may show squamous metaplasia and dysplasia. There is little chronic inflammatory cell infiltrate. The non-cartilage containing small airways show goblet cell hyperplasia and intraluminal and peribronchial fibrosis.

CLINICAL FEATURES. There is considerable overlap of clinical features of chronic bronchitis and pulmonary emphysema (described later) as quite often the two coexist. The contrasting features of 'predominant

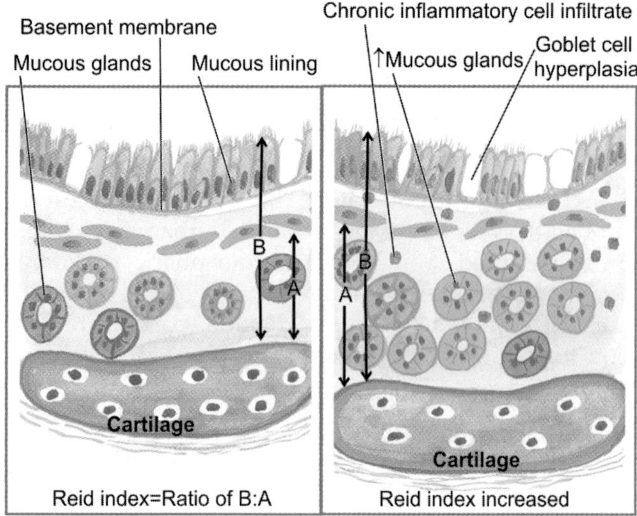

FIGURE 15.12

Diagrammatic representation of increased Reid's index in chronic bronchitis.

emphysema' and 'predominant bronchitis' are presented in Table 15.5. Some important features of 'predominant bronchitis' are as under:

1. Persistent cough with copious expectoration of long duration; initially beginning in a heavy smoker with 'morning catarrh' or 'throat clearing' which worsens in winter.
2. Recurrent respiratory infections are common.
3. Dyspnoea is generally not prominent at rest but is more on exertion.
4. Patients are called 'blue bloaters' due to cyanosis and oedema.
5. Features of right heart failure (cor pulmonale) are common.
6. Chest X-ray shows enlarged heart with prominent vessels.

II. EMPHYSEMA

The WHO has defined pulmonary emphysema as combination of permanent dilatation of air spaces distal to the terminal bronchioles and the destruction of the walls of dilated air spaces. *Thus, emphysema is defined morphologically, while chronic bronchitis is defined clinically.* Since the two conditions coexist frequently and show considerable overlap in their clinical features, it is usual to label patients as 'predominant emphysema' and 'predominant bronchitis' (see Table 15.5).

CLASSIFICATION. As mentioned in the beginning of this chapter, a lobule is composed of about 5 acini distal to a terminal bronchiole and that an acinus consists of 3 to 5 generations of respiratory bronchioles and a variable number of alveolar ducts and alveolar sacs (page 469). By strictly adhering to the WHO definition of pulmonary emphysema, it is classified, according to the portion of the acinus involved, into 5 types: centri-acinar, panacinar (panlobular), para-septal (distal acinar), irregular (para-cicatricial) and mixed (unclassified) emphysema. A number of other conditions to which the term 'emphysema' is losely applied are, in fact, examples of 'overinflation'. A classification based on these principles is outlined in Table 15.4. The morphologic appearance of the individual types is described later.

ETIOPATHOGENESIS. The commonest form of COPD is the combination of chronic bronchitis and pulmonary emphysema. Chronic bronchitis, however, does not always lead to emphysema nor all cases of emphysema have changes of chronic bronchitis. The association of the two conditions is principally linked to the common etiologic factors; most importantly, *tobacco smoke* and *air pollutants*. Other less significant contributory factors are occupational exposure, infection and somewhat poorly-understood familial and genetic influences. All these factors have already been discussed above.

However, the pathogenesis of the most significant event in emphysema, the *destruction of the alveolar walls*, is not linked to bronchial changes but is closely related to deficiency of serum alpha-1-antitrypsin (α1-protease inhibitor) commonly termed *protease-antiprotease hypothesis* detailed below.

Protease-antiprotease hypothesis. Alpha-1-antitrypsin (α-1-AT), also called α1-protease inhibitor (α-1-Pi), is a glycoprotein that forms the normal constituent of the α1-globulin fraction of the plasma proteins on serum

TABLE 15.4: Classification of 'True Emphysema' and 'Overinflation'.

A. TRUE EMPHYSEMA
1. Centriacinar (centrilobular) emphysema
2. Panacinar (panlobular) emphysema
3. Paraseptal (distal acinar) emphysema
4. Irregular (para-cicatricial) emphysema
5. Mixed (unclassified) emphysema

B. OVERINFLATION
1. Compensatory overinflation (compensatory emphysema)
2. Senile hyperinflation (aging lung, senile emphysema)
3. Obstructive overinflation (infantile lobar emphysema)
4. Unilateral translucent lung (unilateral emphysema)
5. Interstitial emphysema (surgical emphysema)

TABLE 15.5: Contrasting Salient Features of 'Predominant Bronchitis' and 'Predominant Emphysema'.

FEATURE	PREDOMINANT BRONCHITIS	PREDOMINANT EMPHYSEMA
1. *Age at diagnosis*	About 50 years	About 60 years
2. *Underlying pathology*	Hypertrophy of mucus-producing cells	Inflammatory narrowing of bronchioles and destruction of septal walls
3. *Dyspnoea*	Late, mild	Early, severe
4. *Cough*	Before dyspnoea starts	After dyspnoea starts
5. *Sputum*	Copious, purulent	Scanty, mucoid, less frequent
6. *Bronchial infections*	More frequent	Less frequent
7. *Respiratory insufficiency*	Repeated	Terminal
8. *Cyanosis*	Common ('blue-bloaters')	Rare ('pink-puffers')
9. *Lung capacity*	Normal	Increased (barrel-chest)
10. *Blood gas values*	$\downarrow pO_2$, $\downarrow pCO_2$, no compensatory hyperventilation	pO_2 and pCO_2 usually within normal limits due to compensatory hyperventilation
11. *Cor pulmonale*	Frequent	Rare and terminal
12. *Chest X-ray*	Large heart, prominent vessels	Small heart, hyperinflated lungs

electrophoresis. The single gene locus that codes for α-1-AT is located on the long arm of chromosome 15. It is normally synthesised in the liver and is distributed in the circulating blood, tissue fluids and macrophages. The normal function of α1-AT is to inhibit proteases and hence its name α1-protease inhibitor. The proteases (mainly elastases) are derived from neutrophils. Neutrophil elastase has the capability of digesting lung parenchyma but is inhibited from doing so by anti-elastase effect of α1-AT.

There are several known alleles of α1-AT which have an autosomal codominant inheritance pattern and are classified as normal (*PiMM*), deficient (*PiZZ*), null type (*Pi null null*) having no detectable level, and dysfunctional (*PiSS*) type having about half the normal level.

- The most common abnormal phenotype in classic α1-AT deficiency is *homozygous state PiZZ* resulting from a single amino acid substitution Glu → Lys which causes spontaneous polymerisation of α1-AT and inhibits its release from the liver. The remaining material of α1-AT in the liver causes hepatic cirrhosis (Chapter 19).
- Clinically significant deficiency is also associated with *homozygous Pi null null* and *heterozygous Pi nullZ*.
- The *heterozygote pattern* of *PiMZ* has intermediate levels which is not sufficient to produce clinical deficiency, but heterozygote individuals who smoke heavily have higher risk of developing emphysema.

The α1-AT deficiency develops in adults and causes pulmonary emphysema in smokers as well as in non-smokers, though the smokers become symptomatic about 15 years earlier than non-smokers. The other organ showing effects of α1-AT deficiency is liver which may develop obstructive jaundice early in infancy, and cirrhosis and hepatoma late in adulthood (Chapter 19).

The mechanism of alveolar wall destruction in emphysema by elastolytic action is based on the imbalance between proteases (chiefly *elastase)* and anti-proteases (chiefly *anti-elastase):*

- By decreased anti-elastase activity i.e. deficiency of α-1 antitrypsin.
- By increased activity of elastase i.e. increased neutrophilic infiltration in the lungs causing excessive elaboration of neutrophil elastase.

There are enough evidences to suggest that smoking promotes emphysema by both decreasing the amount of anti-elastase as well as by increasing the elastolytic protease in the lungs. These are as under:

1. Oxidant in cigarette smoke has inhibitory influence on α-1-antitrypsin thus lowering the level of anti-elastase activity.
2. Smokers have upto ten times more phagocytes and neutrophils in their lungs than nonsmokers. Thus they have very high elastase activity.

Pathogenesis of emphysema by protease-antiprotease mechanism is diagrammatically illustrated in Fig. 15.13.

PATHOLOGIC CHANGES. Emphysema can be diagnosed with certainty only by gross and histologic examination of sections of whole lung. The lungs

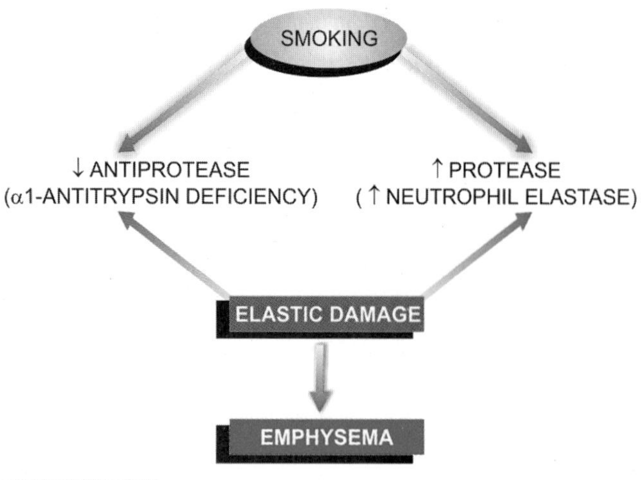

FIGURE 15.13

Pathogenesis of alveolar wall destruction in emphysema by protease-antiprotease mechanism.

should be perfused with formalin under pressure in inflated state to grade the severity of emphysema with naked eye.

Grossly, the lungs are voluminous, pale with little blood. The edges of the lungs are rounded. Mild cases show dilatation of air spaces visible with hand lens. Advanced cases show subpleural bullae and blebs bulging outwards from the surface of the lungs with rib markings between them. The *bullae* are air-filled cyst-like or bubble-like structures, larger than 1 cm in diameter (Fig. 15.14). They are formed by the rupture of adjacent air spaces while *blebs* are the result of rupture of alveoli directly into the subpleural interstitial tissue and are the common cause of spontaneous pneumothorax.

Microscopically, depending upon the type of emphysema, there is dilatation of air spaces and destruction of septal walls of part of acinus involved i.e. respiratory bronchioles, alveolar ducts and alveolar sacs. Changes of bronchitis may be present. Bullae and blebs when present show fibrosis and chronic inflammation of the walls.

CLINICAL FEATURES. Cases of 'predominant emphysema' develop clinical features after about one third of the pulmonary parenchyma is damaged which occurs most severely in panacinar emphysema. The age at the time of diagnosis is often a decade later (about 60 years) than the age for predominant bronchitis (about 50 years). Though there is considerable overlap between the clinical features of chronic bronchitis and emphysema, the following features generally characterise 'predominant emphysema':

1. There is long history of slowly increasing severe exertional dyspnoea.
2. Patient is quite distressed with obvious use of accessory muscles of respiration.
3. Chest is barrel-shaped and hyper-resonant.
4. Cough occurs late after dyspnoea starts and is associated with scanty mucoid sputum.
5. Recurrent respiratory infections are not frequent.
6. Patients are called 'pink puffers' as they remain well oxygenated and have tachypnoea.
7. Weight loss is common.
8. Features of right heart failure (cor pulmonale) and hypercapneic respiratory failure are the usual terminal events.
9. Chest X-ray shows small heart with hyperinflated lungs.

After these general comments about morphologic and clinical features of emphysema, the specific pathologic changes in individual types of 'emphysema' and 'overinflation' as classified in Table 15.4 are described below.

A. Morphology of Individual Types of Emphysema

1. CENTRIACINAR (CENTRILOBULAR) EMPHYSEMA. Centriacinar or centrilobular emphysema is one of the common types. It is characterised by initial

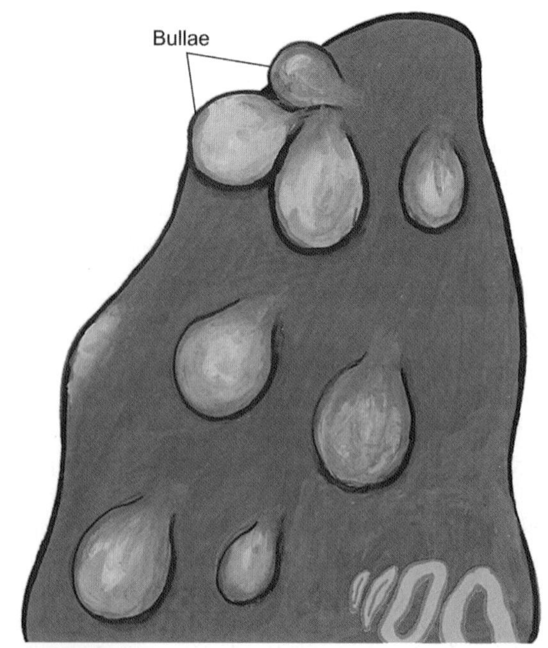

FIGURE 15.14

Bullous emphysema as seen on the external surface of the lung.

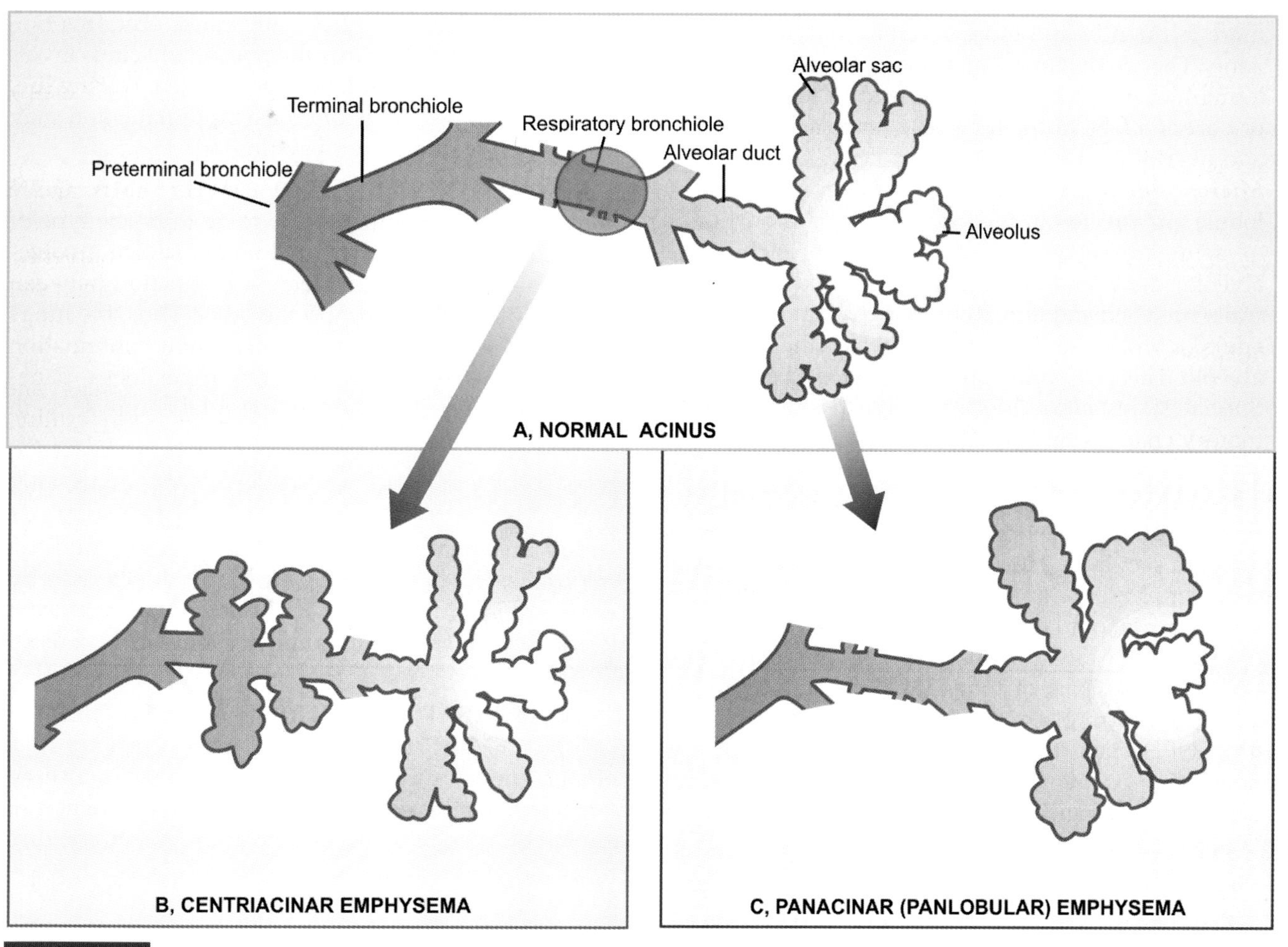

FIGURE 15.15

The anatomic regions of involvement in an acinus in major forms of emphysema.

involvement of respiratory bronchioles i.e. the central or proximal part of the acinus (Fig. 15.15,B). This is the type of emphysema that usually coexists with chronic bronchitis and occurs predominantly in smokers and in coal miners' pneumoconiosis (page 496).

Grossly, the lesions are more common and more severe in the upper lobes of the lungs. The characteristic appearance is obvious in cut surface of the lung. It shows distended air spaces in the centre of the lobules surrounded by a rim of normal lung parenchyma in the same lobule. The lobules are separated from each other by fine fibrous tissue septa. Large amount of black pigment is often present in the walls of emphysematous spaces. In more severe cases, distal parts of acini are also involved and the appearance may closely resemble panacinar emphysema.

Microscopically, there is distension and destruction of the respiratory bronchiole in the centre of lobules, surrounded peripherally by normal uninvolved alveoli. The terminal bronchioles supplying the acini show chronic inflammation and are narrowed (COLOUR PLATE XX: CL 77).

2. PANACINAR (PANLOBULAR) EMPHYSEMA. Panacinar or panlobular emphysema is the other common type. In this type, all portions of the acinus are affected but not of the entire lung (Fig. 15.15,C). Panacinar emphysema is most often associated with α1-antitrypsin deficiency in middle-aged smokers and is the one that produces the most characteristic anatomical changes in the lung in emphysema.

Grossly, in contrast to centriacinar emphysema, the panacinar emphysema involves lower zone of lungs more frequently and more severely than the upper zone. The involvement may be confined to a few lobules, or may be more widespread affecting a lobe or part of a lobe of the lung. The lungs are enlarged and overinflated.

Microscopically, usually all the alveoli within a lobule are affected to the same degree. All portions of acini are distended—respiratory bronchioles, alveolar ducts and alveoli, are all dilated and their walls stretched and thin. Ruptured alveolar walls and spurs of broken septa are seen between the adjacent alveoli. The capillaries are stretched and thinned. Special stains show loss of elastic tissue. Inflammatory changes are usually absent (Fig. 15.16).

3. PARASEPTAL (DISTAL ACINAR) EMPHYSEMA. This type of emphysema involves distal part of acinus while the proximal part is normal. Paraseptal or distal acinar emphysema is localised along the pleura and along the perilobular septa. The involvement is seen adjacent to the areas of fibrosis and atelectasis and involves upper part of lungs more severely than the lower. This form of emphysema is seldom associated with COPD but is the common cause of spontaneous pneumothorax in young adults. Grossly, the subpleural portion of the lung shows air-filled cysts, 0.5 to 2 cm in diameter.

4. IRREGULAR (PARA-CICATRICIAL) EMPHYSEMA. This is the most common form of emphysema, seen surrounding scars from any cause. The involvement is irregular as regards the portion of acinus involved as well as within the lung as a whole. During life, irregular emphysema is often asymptomatic and may be only an incidental autopsy finding.

5. MIXED (UNCLASSIFIED) EMPHYSEMA. Quite often, the same lung may show more than one type of emphysema. It is usually due to more severe involvement resulting in loss of clearcut distinction between one type of emphysema and the other. Thus, the lungs of an elderly smoker at autopsy may show continuation of centriacinar emphysema in the upper lobes, panacinar in the lower lobes, and paraseptal emphysema in the subpleural region.

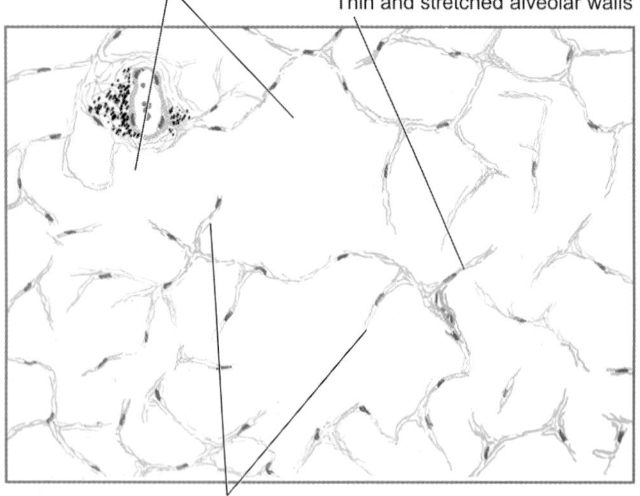

FIGURE 15.16

Panacinar (Panlobular) emphysema showing involvement of the entire lobules and whole of acinus.

B. Morphology of Types of Overinflation

Under this heading are covered a group of lung conditions of heterogeneous etiology characterised by overinflation of the parts of acini but without significant destruction of the walls and are sometimes loosely termed emphysema.

1. COMPENSATORY OVERINFLATION (COMPENSATORY EMPHYSEMA). When part of a lung or a lobe of lung is surgically removed, the residual lung parenchyma undergoes compensatory hyperinflation so as to fill the pleural cavity. Histologic examination shows dilatation of alveoli but no destruction of septal walls and hence the term compensatory overinflation is preferable over 'compensatory emphysema'.

2. SENILE HYPERINFLATION (AGING LUNG, SENILE EMPHYSEMA). In old people, the lungs become voluminous due to loss of elastic tissue, thinning and atrophy of the alveolar ducts and alveoli. The alveoli are thin-walled and distended throughout the lungs but there is no significant destruction of the septal walls and, therefore, preferable designation is 'senile hyperinflation' over 'senile emphysema.'

3. OBSTRUCTIVE OVERINFLATION (INFANTILE LOBAR EMPHYSEMA). Partial obstruction to the bronchial tree such as by a tumour or a foreign body causes overinflation of the region supplied by obstructed bronchus. Infantile lobar emphysema is a variant of obstructive overinflation occurring in infants in the first few days of life who develop respiratory distress or who have congenital hypoplasia of bronchial cartilage. In all such cases, air enters the lungs during inspiration but cannot leave on expiration resulting in ballooning up of the affected part of the lung.

4. UNILATERAL TRANSLUCENT LUNG (UNILATERAL EMPHYSEMA). This is a form of overinflation in which one lung or one of its lobes or segments of a lobe are radiolucent. The condition occurs in adults and there is generally a history of serious pulmonary infection in childhood, probably bronchiolitis obliterans. The affected lung is grossly overinflated. Microscopy shows overinflated alveoli and there is histologic evidence of preceding widespread bronchiolitis obliterans.

5. INTERSTITIAL EMPHYSEMA (SURGICAL EMPHYSEMA). The entry of air into the connective tissue framework of the lung is called interstitial or surgical emphysema. The usual sources of entry of air into stroma of the lung are rupture of alveoli or of larger airways. The causes are as under:

i) Violent coughing with bronchiolar obstruction e.g. in children with whooping cough, bronchitis, in patients with obstruction to the airways by foreign bodies, blood clots and exposure to irritant gases.

ii) Rupture of the oesophagus, trauma to the lung, or major bronchus and trachea.

iii) Entry of air through surgical incision.

iv) Fractured rib puncturing the lung parenchyma.

v) Sudden change in atmospheric pressure e.g. in decompression sickness.

The condition may affect patients of all ages. On rupture of alveoli, the leaked air enters the fibrous connective tissue of the alveolar walls from where it extends into the fibrous septa of the lung, into the mediastinum, the pleura, and even the subcutaneous tissues. Escape of air into the pleural cavity may cause pneumothorax. Collection of small quantities of air is generally harmless and is resorbed. However, extensive accumulation of air in surgical emphysema may produce impaired blood flow in the lungs. *Pneumo-mediastinum* may produce symptoms resembling myocardial infarction.

Histologically, the alveoli are distended but septal walls are not damaged; therefore it is not true emphysema. There are clear spaces of leaked out air in connective tissue septa.

III. BRONCHIAL ASTHMA

Asthma is a disease of airways that is characterised by increased responsiveness of the tracheobronchial tree to a variety of stimuli resulting in widespread spasmodic narrowing of the air passages which may be relieved spontaneously or by therapy. Asthma is an episodic disease manifested clinically by paroxysms of dyspnoea, cough and wheezing. However, a severe and unremitting form of the disease termed *status asthmaticus* may prove fatal.

Bronchial asthma is common and prevalent worldwide; in the United States about 4% of population is reported to suffer from this disease. It occurs at all ages but nearly 50% of cases develop it before the age of 10 years. In adults, both sexes are affected equally but in children there is 2:1 male-female ratio.

ETIOPATHOGENESIS AND TYPES. Based on the stimuli initiating bronchial asthma, two broad etiologic types are traditionally described: *extrinsic (allergic, atopic)* and *intrinsic (idiosyncratic, non-atopic) asthma.* A third type is a *mixed pattern* in which the features do not fit clearly into either of the two main types. The contrasting features of the two main types are summed up in Table 15.6.

1. Extrinsic (atopic, allergic) asthma. This is the most common type of asthma. It usually begins in childhood or in early adult life. Most patients of this type of asthma have personal and/or family history of preceding allergic diseases such as rhinitis, urticaria or infantile eczema. Hypersensitivity to various extrinsic antigenic substances or 'allergens' is usually present in these cases. Most of these allergens cause ill-effects by inhalation e.g. house dust, pollens, animal danders, moulds etc. Occupational asthma stimulated by fumes, gases and organic and chemical dusts is a variant of extrinsic asthma. There are increased levels of IgE in the serum and positive skin test with the specific offending inhaled antigen representing an IgE-mediated type I hypersensitivity reaction which includes an 'acute immediate response' and a late phase reaction':

- The *acute immediate response* is initiated by IgE-sensitised mast cells (tissue counterparts of circulating basophils) on the mucosal surface. Mast cells on degranulation release mediators like histamine, leukotrienes, prostaglandins, platelet activating factor and chemotactic factors for eosinophils and neutrophils. The net effects of these mediators are bronchoconstriction, oedema, mucus hypersecretion and accumulation of eosinophils and neutrophils.
- The *late phase reaction* follows the acute immediate response and is responsible for the prolonged manifestations of asthma. It is caused by excessive mobilisation of blood leucocytes that include basophils besides eosinophils and neutrophils. These result in further release of mediators which accentuate the above-mentioned effects. In addition, inflammatory injury is caused by neutrophils and by major basic protein (MBP) of eosinophils.

TABLE 15.6: Contrasting Features of the Two Major Types of Asthma.

FEATURE	EXTRINSIC ASTHMA	INTRINSIC ASTHMA
1. *Age at onset*	In childhood	In adult
2. *Personal/family history*	Commonly present	Absent
3. *Preceding allergic illness (atopy)*	Present (*e.g.* rhinitis, urticaria, eczema)	Absent
4. *Allergens*	Present (dust, pollens, danders etc)	None
5. *Drug hypersensitivity*	None	Present (usually to aspirin)
6. *Serum IgE levels*	Elevated	Normal
7. *Associated chronic bronchitis, nasal polyps*	Absent	Present
8. *Emphysema*	Unusual	Common

2. **Intrinsic (idiosyncratic, non-atopic) asthma.** This type of asthma develops later in adult life with negative personal or family history of allergy, negative skin test and normal serum levels of IgE. Most of these patients develop typical symptom-complex after an upper respiratory tract infection by viruses. Associated nasal polypi and chronic bronchitis are commonly present. There are no recognisable allergens but about 10% of patients become hypersensitive to drugs, most notably to small doses of aspirin (aspirin-sensitive asthma).

3. **Mixed type.** Many patients do not clearly fit into either of the above two categories and have mixed features of both. Those patients who develop asthma in early life have strong allergic component, while those who develop the disease late tend to be non-allergic. Either type of asthma can be precipitated by cold, exercise and emotional stress.

PATHOLOGIC CHANGES. The pathologic changes are similar in both major types of asthma. The pathologic material examined is generally autopsy of lungs in patients dying of status asthmaticus but the changes are expected to be similar in non-fatal cases.

Grossly, the lungs are overdistended due to over-inflation. The cut surface shows characteristic occlusion of the bronchi and bronchioles by viscid mucus plugs.

Microscopically, the following changes are observed:

1. The mucus plugs contain normal or degenerated respiratory epithelium forming twisted strips called *Curschmann's spirals* (Fig. 15.17,A).
2. The sputum usually contains numerous eosinophils and diamond-shaped crystals derived from eosinophils called *Charcot-Leyden crystals* (Fig. 15.17,B).
3. The bronchial wall shows thickened basement membrane of the bronchial epithelium, submucosal oedema and inflammatory exudate consisting of lymphocytes and plasma cells with prominence of eosinophils. There is hypertrophy of submucosal glands as well as of the bronchial smooth muscle.
4. Changes of bronchitis and emphysema may supervene, especially in intrinsic asthma.

CLINICAL FEATURES. Asthmatic patients suffer from episodes of acute exacerbations interspersed with symptom-free periods. Characteristic clinical features are paroxysms of dyspnoea, cough and wheezing. Most

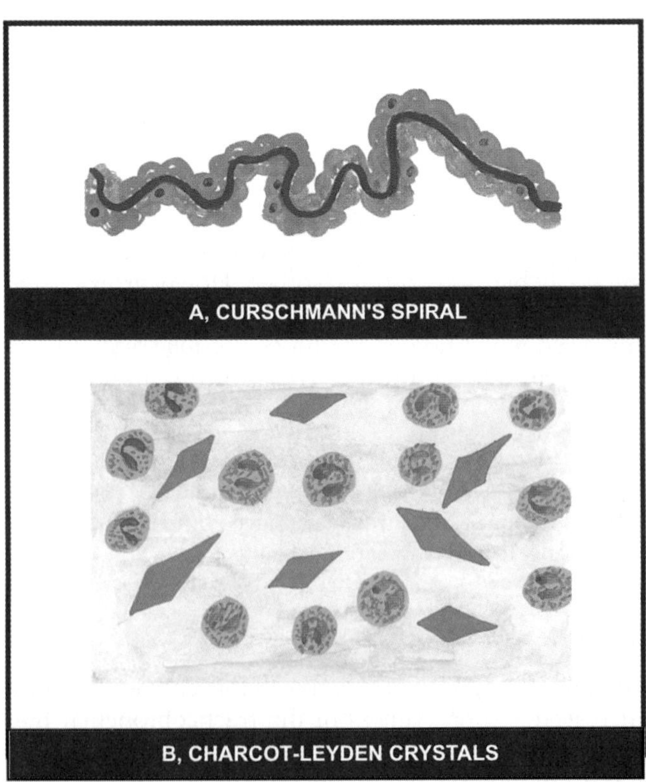

FIGURE 15.17

Curschmann's spiral (A) and Charcot-Leyden crystals (B) found in mucus plugs in patients with bronchial asthma.

attacks typically last for a few minutes to hours. When attacks occur continuously it may result in more serious condition called *status asthmaticus.* The clinical diagnosis is supported by demonstration of circulation eosinophilia and sputum demonstration of Curschmann's spirals and Charcot-Leyden crystals. More chronic cases may develop cor pulmonale.

IV. BRONCHIECTASIS

Bronchiectasis is defined as abnormal and irreversible dilatation of the bronchi and bronchioles (greater than 2 mm in diameter) developing secondary to inflammatory weakening of the bronchial walls. The most characteristic clinical manifestation of bronchiectasis is persistent cough with expectoration of copious amounts of foul-smelling, purulent sputum. Post-infectious cases commonly develop in childhood and in early adult life.

ETIOPATHOGENESIS. The origin of inflammatory destructive process of bronchial walls is nearly always a result of two basic mechanisms: obstruction and infection.

- *Endobronchial obstruction* by foreign body, neoplastic growth or enlarged lymph nodes causes resorption of air distal to the obstruction with consequent atelectasis and retention of secretions.
- *Infection* may be secondary to local obstruction and impaired systemic defense mechanism promoting bacterial growth, or infection may be a primary event i.e. bronchiectasis developing in suppurative necrotising pneumonia.

These 2 mechanisms—endobronchial obstruction and infection, are seen in a number of clinical settings. These are as under:

1. Hereditary and congenital factors. Several hereditary and congenital factors may result secondarily in diffuse bronchiectasis. These include:

i) *Congenital bronchiectasis* caused by developmental defect of the bronchial system.

ii) *Cystic fibrosis,* a generalised defect of exocrine gland secretions, results in obstruction, infection and bronchiectasis (Chapter 19).

iii) *Hereditary immune deficiency diseases* are often associated with high incidence of bronchiectasis.

iv) *Immotile cilia syndrome* that includes Kartagener's syndrome (bronchiectasis, situs inversus and sinusitis) is characterised by ultrastructural changes in the microtubules causing immotility of cilia of the respiratory tract epithelium, sperms and other cells. Males in this syndrome are often infertile (Chapter 21).

v) *Atopic bronchial asthma* patients have often positive family history of allergic diseases and may rarely develop diffuse bronchiectasis.

2. Obstruction. Post-obstructive bronchiectasis, unlike the congenital-hereditary forms, is of the localised variety, usually confined to one part of the bronchial system. The causes of endobronchial obstruction include foreign bodies, endobronchial tumours, compression by enlarged hilar lymph nodes and post-inflammatory scarring (e.g. in healed tuberculosis) all of which favour the development of post-obstructive bronchiectasis.

3. As secondary complication. *Necrotising pneumonias* such as in staphylococcal suppurative pneumonia and *tuberculosis* may develop bronchiectasis as a complication.

PATHOLOGIC CHANGES. The disease characteristically affects distal bronchi and bronchioles beyond the segmental bronchi.

Macroscopically, the lungs may be involved diffusely or segmentally. Bilateral involvement of lower lobes occurs most frequently. More vertical air passages of left lower lobe are more often involved than the right. The pleura is usually fibrotic and thickened with adhesions to the chest wall. The dilated airways, depending upon their gross or bronchographic appearance, have been subclassified into the following different types (Fig. 15.18):

i) *Cylindrical:* the most common type characterised by tube-like bronchial dilatation.

ii) *Fusiform:* having spindle-shaped bronchial dilatation.

iii) *Saccular:* having rounded sac-like bronchial distension.

iv) *Varicose:* having irregular bronchial enlargements.

Cut surface of the affected lobes, generally the lower zones, shows characteristic honey-combed appearance. The bronchi are extensively dilated nearly to the pleura, their walls are thickened and the lumina are filled with mucus or muco-pus. The intervening lung parenchyma is reduced and fibrotic (Fig. 15.19,A).

Microscopically, fully-developed cases show the following histologic features (Fig. 15.19,B) (COLOUR PLATE XX: CL 78).

i) The bronchial epithelium may be normal, ulcerated or may show squamous metaplasia.

ii) The bronchial wall shows infiltration by acute and chronic inflammatory cells and destruction of normal muscle and elastic tissue with replacement by fibrosis.

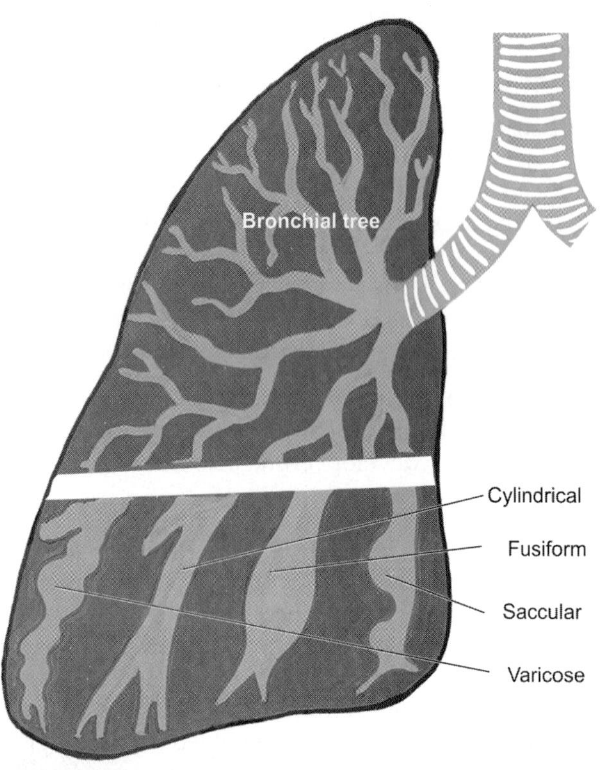

FIGURE 15.18

Types of bronchial dilatations in bronchiectasis.

iii) The intervening lung parenchyma shows fibrosis, while the surrounding lung tissue shows changes of interstitial pneumonia.

iv) The pleura in the affected area is adherent and shows bands of fibrous tissue between the bronchus and the pleura.

CLINICAL FEATURES. The clinical manifestations of bronchiectasis typically consist of chronic cough with foul-smelling sputum production, haemoptysis and recurrent pneumonia. Sinusitis is a common accompaniment of diffuse bronchiectasis. Development of clubbing of the fingers, metastatic abscesses (often to the brain), amyloidosis and cor pulmonale are late complications occurring in cases uncontrolled for years.

CHRONIC RESTRICTIVE PULMONARY DISEASE

The second large group of diffuse lung disease is 'chronic restrictive pulmonary disease' characterised by reduced expansion of lung parenchyma with decreased total lung capacity. This group of diseases must be distinguished from the foregoing COPD (Table 15.7).

Restrictive lung disease includes 2 types of conditions:

A. Restriction due to chest wall disorder. These causes are:

1. Kyphoscoliosis
2. Poliomyelitis
3. Severe obesity
4. Pleural diseases.

B. Restriction due to interstitial and infiltrative diseases. These are diseases characterised by non-infectious involvement of the interstitial connective tissue of lung parenchyma. The term 'infiltrative' is used here to denote the radiologic appearance of lungs in chest radiographs which show ground-glass shadows due to diffuse infiltration by small nodules or irregular lines. The conditions included in this group are as under:

I. Pneumoconiosis
II. Immunologic lung diseases
III. Collagen-vascular diseases
IV. Idiopathic pulmonary fibrosis
V. Sarcoidosis (Chapter 6).

The **pathogenesis** of the interstitial lung disease is explained by inflammatory reaction causing initial alveolitis in response to various stimuli. In alveolitis,

TABLE 15.7: Obstructive *versus* Restrictive Pulmonary Diseases.

FEATURE	OBSTRUCTIVE	RESTRICTIVE
1. *Airways*	Obstructed at any level from trachea to respiratory bronchiole	Reduced expansion of lung parenchyma
2. *Pulmonary function test*	Increased pulmonary resistance and obstruction of maximal expiratory airflow	Decreased total lung capacity
3. *X-ray chest*	Variable appearance depending upon the cause	Typically bilateral infiltrates giving ground-glass shadows
4. *Examples*	• Chronic bronchitis • Emphysema • Bronchial asthma • Bronchiectasis	• Chest cage disorders (e.g. kyphoscoliosis, poliomyelitis, severe obesity and pleural disease) • Interstitial and infiltrative diseases (e.g. pneumoconioses, idiopathic pulmonary fibrosis, immunologic lung diseases, collagen-vascular disease and sarcoidosis)

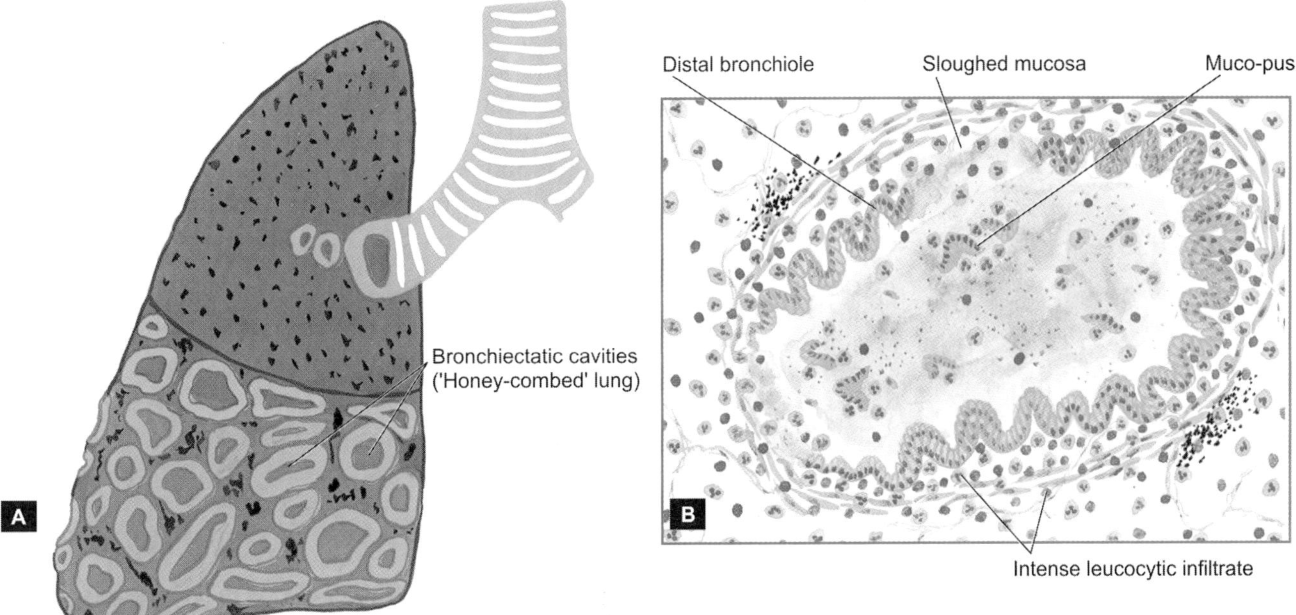

FIGURE 15.19

A, Sectioned surface of the lung showing bronchiectasis in the lower lobe. B, Microscopic appearance of a dilated distal bronchiole in bronchiectasis. The bronchial wall is thickened and infiltrated by acute and chronic inflammatory cells. The mucosa is sloughed off at places with exudate of muco-pus in the lumen.

there is accumulation of lymphocytes, macrophages, neutrophils and eosinophils, all of which result in inflammatory destruction of the pulmonary parenchyma followed by fibrosis. Eventually, there is widespread destruction of alveolar capillary walls resulting in end-stage lung or 'honeycomb lung'.

The *major clinical manifestations* of restrictive lung diseases are dyspnoea, tachypnoea and cyanosis, but no wheezing so characteristic of COPD.

After these general comments about the restrictive pulmonary disease, some common and important examples of infiltrative and interstitial lung diseases are described below.

I. PNEUMOCONIOSES

Pneumoconiosis is the term used for lung diseases caused by inhalation of dust, mostly at work. These diseases are, therefore, also called 'dust diseases' or 'occupational lung diseases'.

The type of lung disease varies according to the nature of inhaled dust. Some dusts are inert and cause no reaction and no damage at all, while others cause immunologic damage and predispose to tuberculosis or to neoplasia. The factors which determine the extent of damage caused by inhaled dusts are:

1. size and shape of the particles;
2. their solubility and physico-chemical composition;
3. the amount of dust retained in the lungs;
4. the additional effect of other irritants such as tobacco smoke; and
5. host factors such as efficiency of clearance mechanism and immune status of the host.

In general, most of the inhaled dust particles larger than 5 μm reach the terminal airways where they are ingested by alveolar macrophages. Most of these too are eliminated by expectoration but the remaining accumulate in alveolar tissue. Of particular interest are the particles smaller than 1 μm which are deposited in the alveoli most efficiently. Most of the dust-laden macrophages accumulated in the alveoli die leaving the dust, around which fibrous tissue is formed. Some macrophages enter the lymphatics and reach regional lymph nodes. The tissue response to inhaled dust may be one of the following three types:

- *Fibrous nodules* e.g. in coal-workers' pneumoconiosis and silicosis.
- *Interstitial fibrosis* e.g. in asbestosis.
- *Hypersensitivity reaction* e.g. in berylliosis.

A comprehensive list of various types of occupational lung diseases caused by inorganic (mineral) dusts

TABLE 15.8: Classification of Pneumoconioses.

AGENT	DISEASES
A. INORGANIC (MINERAL) DUSTS:	
1. ***Coal dust***	Simple coal-workers' pneumoconiosis Progressive massive fibrosis Caplan's syndrome
2. ***Silica***	Silicosis Caplan's syndrome
3. ***Asbestos***	Asbestosis Pleural diseases Tumours
4. ***Beryllium***	Acute berylliosis Chronic berylliosis
5. ***Iron oxide***	Pulmonary siderosis
B. ORGANIC (BIOLOGIC) DUSTS:	
1. ***Mouldy hay***	Farmer's lungs
2. ***Bagasse***	Bagassosis
3. ***Cotton, flax, hemp dust***	Byssinosis
4. ***Bird droppings***	Bird-breeders' (bird fancier's) lung
5. ***Mushroom compost dust***	Mushroom-workers' lung
6. ***Mouldy barley, malt dust***	Malt-workers' lung
7. ***Mouldy maple bark***	Maple-bark disease
8. ***Silage fermentation***	Silo-fillers' disease

and organic dusts is presented in Table 15.8. The more common examples of pneumoconioses are described here.

Coal-Workers' Pneumoconiosis

This is the commonest form of pneumoconiosis and is defined as the lung disease resulting from inhalation of coal dust particles, especially in coal miners engaged in handling soft bituminous coal for a number of years, often 20 to 30 years. It exists in 2 forms—a milder form of the disease called *simple coal workers' pneumoconiosis* and an advanced form termed *progressive massive fibrosis* (complicated coal-miners' pneumoconiosis). *Anthracosis,* on the other hand, is not a lung disease in true sense but is the common, benign and asymptomatic accumulation of carbon dust in the lungs of most urban dwellers due to atmospheric pollution and cigarette smoke. Anthracotic pigment is deposited in the macrophages in the alveoli and around the respiratory bronchioles and into the draining lymph nodes but does not produce any respiratory difficulty or radiologic changes.

PATHOGENESIS. Pathogenetically, it appears that anthracosis, simple coal-workers' pneumoconiosis and progressive massive fibrosis are different stages in the evolution of fully-developed coal-workers' pneumoconiosis. However, progressive massive fibrosis develops in a small proportion of cases (2-8%) of simple coal-workers' pneumoconiosis. A number of predisposing factors have been implicated in this transformation. These are:

1. Older age of the miners.
2. Severity of coal dust burden engulfed by macrophages.
3. Prolonged exposure (20 to 30 years) to coal dust.
4. Concomitant tuberculosis.
5. Additional role of silica dust.

Activation of alveolar macrophage plays the most significant role in the pathogenesis of progressive massive fibrosis by release of various mediators (Fig. 15.20,A):

i) *Free radicals* which are reactive oxygen species which damage the lung parenchyma.
ii) *Chemotactic factors* for various leucocytes (leukotrienes, TNF, IL-8 and IL-6) resulting in infiltration into pulmonary tissues by these inflammatory cells which on activation cause further damage.
iii) *Fibrogenic cytokines* such as IL-1, TNF and platelet derived growth factor (PDGF) which stimulate healing by fibrosis due to proliferation of fibroblasts at the damaged tissue site.

PATHOLOGIC CHANGES. In life, the pathologic changes in lung in coal-workers' pneumoconiosis are graded by radiologic appearance according to the size and extent of opacities. The pathologic findings at autopsy of lungs in the major forms of coal-workers' pneumoconiosis are considered below under 3 headings: simple coal-workers' pneumoconiosis, progressive massive fibrosis and rheumatoid pneumoconiosis (Caplan's syndrome).

SIMPLE COAL-WORKERS' PNEUMOCONIOSIS. ***Grossly,*** the lung parenchyma shows small, black focal lesions, measuring less than 5 mm in diameter and evenly distributed throughout the lung but have a tendency to be more numerous in the upper lobes. These are termed *coal macules,* and if palpable are called *nodules.* The air spaces around coal macules are dilated with little destruction of alveolar walls (Fig. 15.20,A). Though some workers have called it centrilobular emphysema of coal-miners (page 488), others prefer not to consider it emphysema because there is no significant destruction of alveolar walls. Similar

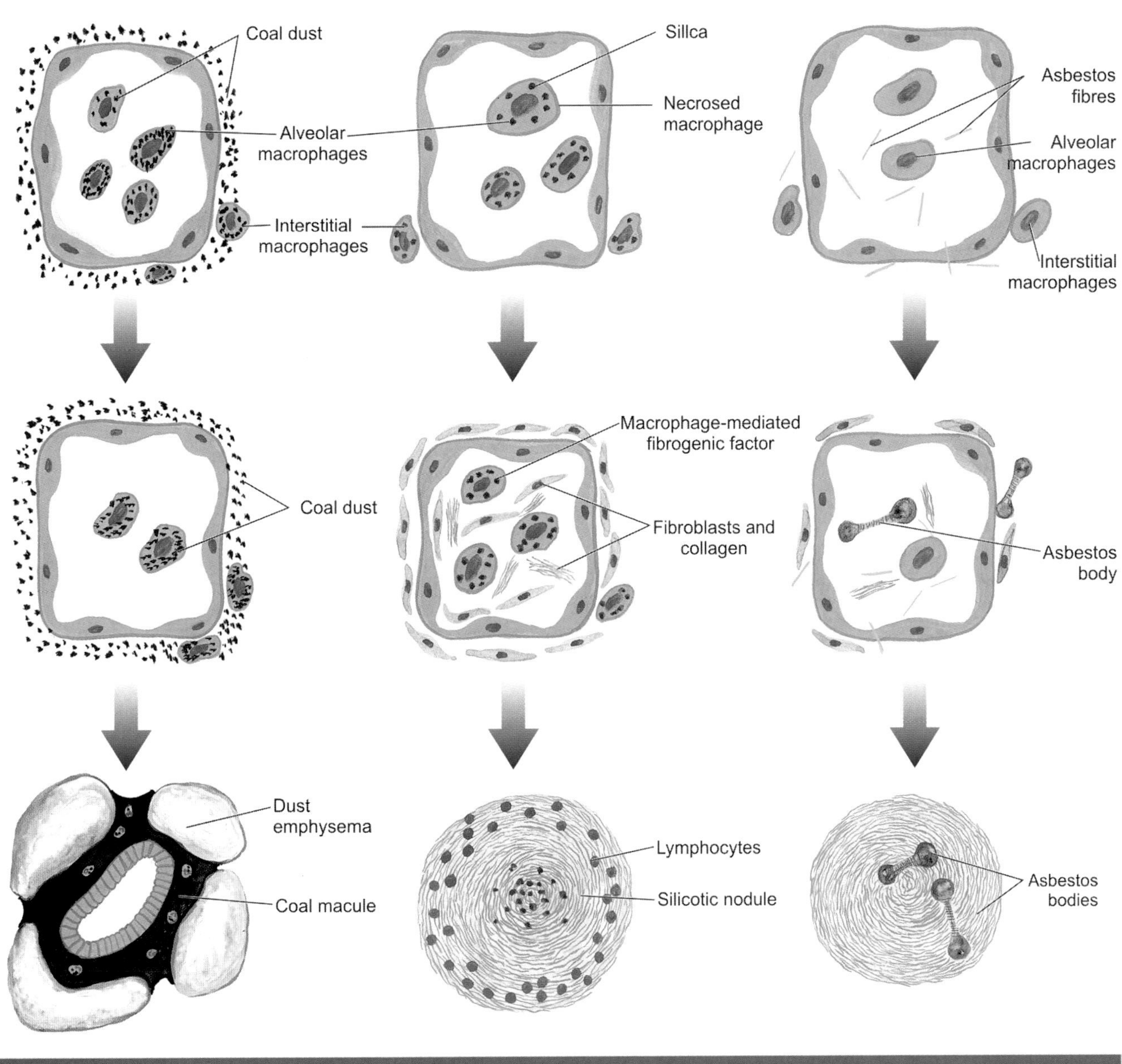

FIGURE 15.20

Pathogenesis of three common forms of pneumoconiosis. A, *Coal-workers' pneumoconiosis.* The macrophages phagocytose large amount of coal dust particles which are then passed into the interstitial tissue of lung and aggregate around respiratory bronchiole and cause focal dust emphysema. B, *Silicosis.* The tiny silica particles are toxic to macrophages. The dead macrophages release fibrogenic factor and eventually result in silicotic nodule. C, *Asbestosis.* Asbestos fibers initiate lot of interstitial fibrosis as well as form asbestos bodies.

blackish pigmentations are found on the pleural surface and in the regional lymph nodes (Fig. 15.21, A).

Histologically, the following features are seen (Fig. 15.22) (COLOUR PLATE II: CL 6):

1. Coal macules are composed of aggregates of dust-laden macrophages. These are present in the alveoli and in the bronchiolar and alveolar walls.
2. There is some increase in the network of reticulin and collagen in the coal macules.
3. Respiratory bronchioles and alveoli surrounding the macules are distended without significant destruction of the alveolar walls.

PROGRESSIVE MASSIVE FIBROSIS. *Grossly,* besides the coal macules and nodules of simple

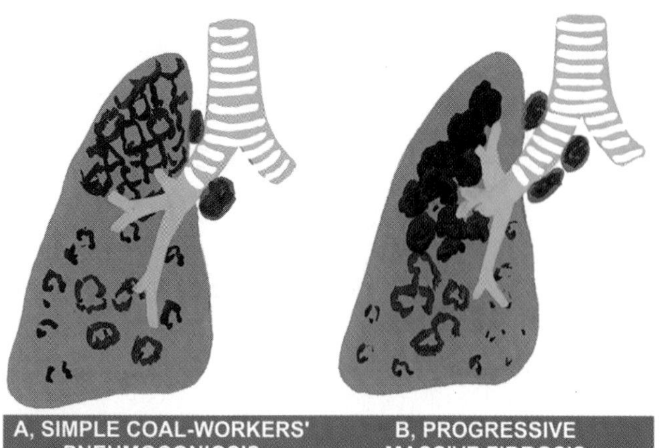

FIGURE 15.21

Macroscopic appearance of the lungs in simple coal-workers' pneumoconiosis (A) and progressive massive fibrosis (B).

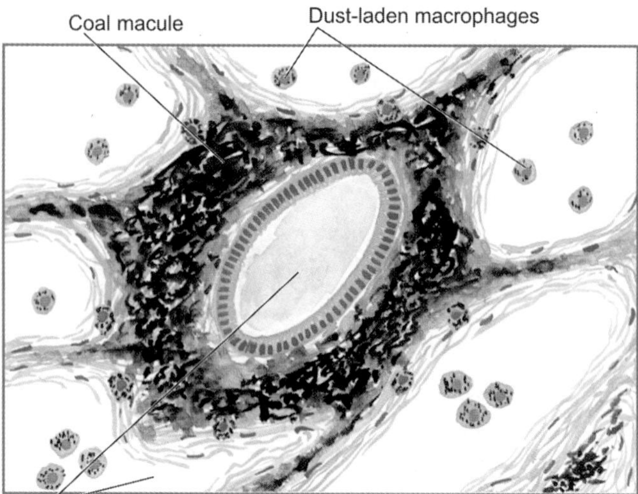

FIGURE 15.22

Histologic appearance of the lung in coal-workers' pneumoconiosis. A coal macule composed of aggregates of dust-laden macrophages is seen surrounding a respiratory bronchiole. The alveoli and respiratory bronchioles surrounding the coal macule are distended.

pneumoconiosis, there are larger, hard, black scattered areas measuring more than 2 cm in diameter and sometimes massive. They are usually bilateral and located more often in the upper parts of the lungs posteriorly. Sometimes, these masses break down centrally due to ischaemic necrosis or due to tuberculosis forming cavities filled with black semifluid resembling India ink. The pleura and the regional lymph nodes are also blackened and fibrotic (Fig. 15.21,B).

Histologically, the following features are present:

1. The fibrous lesions are composed almost entirely of dense collagen and carbon pigment.
2. The wall of respiratory bronchioles and pulmonary vessels included in the massive scars are thickened and their lumina obliterated.
3. There is scanty inflammatory infiltrate of lymphocytes and plasma cells around the areas of massive scars.
4. The alveoli surrounding the scars are markedly dilated.

Progressive massive fibrosis probably has immunological pathogenetic basis as described above.

RHEUMATOID PNEUMOCONIOSIS (CAPLAN'S SYNDROME). The development or rheumatoid arthritis in a few cases of coal-workers' pneumoconiosis, silicosis or absestosis is termed rheumatoid pneumoconiosis or Caplan's syndrome.

Grossly, the lungs have rounded, firm nodules with central necrosis, cavitation or calcification.

Histologically, the lung lesions are modified rheumatoid nodules with central zone of dust-laden fibrinoid necrosis enclosed by palisading fibroblasts and mononuclear cells.

The lung lesions in Caplan's syndrome have immunological basis for their origin as evidenced by detection of rheumatoid factor and antinuclear antibodies.

CLINICAL FEATURES. Simple coal-workers' pneumoconiosis is the mild form of disease characterised by chronic cough with black expectoration. The radiological findings of nodularities in the lungs appear after working for several years in coal mines. Progressive massive fibrosis is, however, a serious disabling condition manifested by progressive dyspnoea and chronic cough with jet-black sputum. Recurrent bacterial infections may produce purulent sputum. More advanced cases develop pulmonary hypertension and right ventricular hypertrophy (cor pulmonale). The radiological appearance may suggest tuberculosis or cancer. Tuberculosis and rheumatoid arthritis are more common in coal miners than the general population. Coal workers have increased risk of developing carcinomas of the stomach, probably due to swallowing of coal dust containing carcinogens. But bronchogenic carcinoma does not appear to be more common in coal-miners than in other groups.

Silicosis

Historically, silicosis used to be called 'knife grinders' lung. Silicosis is caused by prolonged inhalation of silicon dioxide, commonly called silica. Silica constitutes about one-fourth of earth's crust. Therefore, a number of occupations engaged in silceous rocks or sand and products manufactured from them are at increased risk. These include miners (e.g. of granite, sandstone, slate, coal, gold, tin and copper), quarry workers, tunnellers, sandblasters, grinders, ceramic workers, foundry workers and those involved in the manufacture of abrasives containing silica. Peculiar to India are the occupational exposure to pencil, slate and agate grinding industry carrying high risk of silicosis (agate = sort of very hard stone containing silica). According to a recent ICMR report, it is estimated that about 3 million workers in India are at high potential risk of silica exposure employed in a variety of occupations including construction workers. An infrequent acute form of silicosis called *accelerated silicosis* produces irregular fibrosis adjoining the alveoli which is filled with lipoproteinaceous exudate and resembles alveolar proteinosis (page 504). However, if not specified, silicosis refers to the common *chronic form* of the disease characterised by formation of small collagenous silicotic nodules.

PATHOGENESIS. Silicosis appears after prolonged exposure to silica dust, often a few decades. Besides, it depends upon a number of other factors such as total dose, duration of exposure, the type of silica inhaled and individual host factors. The mechanisms involved in the formation of silicotic nodules are not clearly understood. The following sequence of events has been proposed and schematically illustrated in Fig. 15.20, B:

1. Silica particles between 0.5 to 5 µm size on reaching the alveoli are taken by the macrophages which undergo necrosis. New macrophages engulf the debris and thus a repetitive cycle of *phagocytosis and necrosis* is set up.
2. Some silica-laden macrophages are carried to the respiratory bronchioles, alveoli and in the interstitial tissue. Some of the silica dust is transported to the subpleural and interlobar lymphatics and into the regional lymph nodes. The *cellular aggregates* containing silica become associated with lymphocytes, plasma cells, mast cells and fibroblasts.
3. Silica dust is *fibrogenic*. Crystalline form, particularly quartz, is more fibrogenic than non-crystalline form of silica.
4. As noted above, silica is *cytotoxic* and kills the macrophages which engulf it. The released silica dust activates viable macrophages leading to secretion of macrophage-derived growth factors such as interleukin-1 that favour fibroblast proliferation and collagen synthesis.
5. Simultaneously, there is *activation of T and B lymphocytes*. This results in increased serum levels of immunoglobulins (IgG and IgM), antinuclear antibodies, rheumatoid factor and circulating immune complexes as well as proliferation of T cells.

PATHOLOGIC CHANGES. Grossly, the chronic silicotic lung is studded with well-circumscribed, hard, fibrotic nodules, 1 to 5 mm in diameters. They are scattered throughout the lung parenchyma but are initially more often located in the upper zones of the lungs. These nodular lesions frequently have simultaneous deposition of coal-dust and may develop calcification. The pleura is grossly thickened and adherent to the chest wall. There may be similar fibrotic nodules on the pleura and within the regional lymph nodes. The nodular lesions are detectable as egg-shell shadows in chest X-rays. The lesions may undergo ischaemic necrosis and develop cavitation, or be complicated by tuberculosis and rheumatoid pneumoconiosis (Fig. 15.23).

Histologically, the following features are observed (Fig. 15.24):

1. The silicotic nodules are located in the region of respiratory bronchioles, adjacent alveoli, pulmonary arteries, in the pleura and the regional lymph nodes.
2. The *silicotic nodules* consist of central hyalinised material with scanty cellularity and some amount of dust. The hyalinised centre is surrounded by concentric laminations of collagen which is further enclosed by more cellular connective tissue, dust-filled macrophages and a few lymphocytes and plasma cells. Some of these nodules may have calcium deposits.
3. The collagenous nodules have cleft-like spaces between the lamellae of collagen which when examined polariscopically may demonstrate numerous birefringent particles of silica.
4. The severe and progressive form of the disease may result in coalescence of adjacent nodules and cause complicated silicosis similar to progressive massive fibrosis of coal-workers' pneumoconiosis (described above).
5. The intervening lung parenchyma may show hyperinflation or emphysema.
6. Cavitation when present may be due to ischaemic necrosis in the nodules, or may reveal changes of tuberculosis or rheumatoid pneumoconiosis (Caplan's syndrome), discussed already.

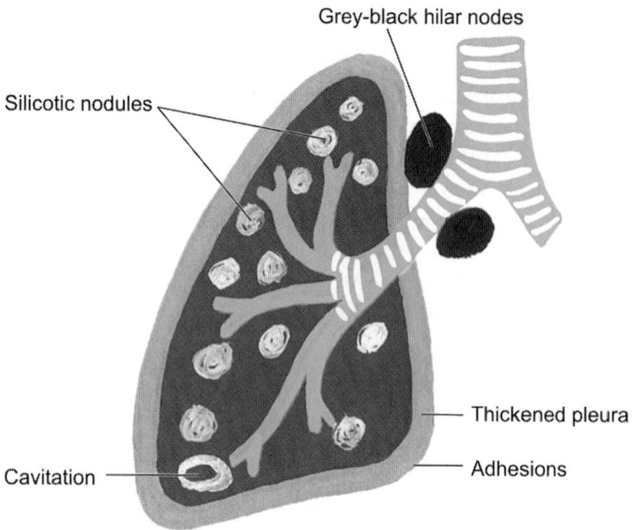

FIGURE 15.23

Macroscopic appearance of lung in silicosis.

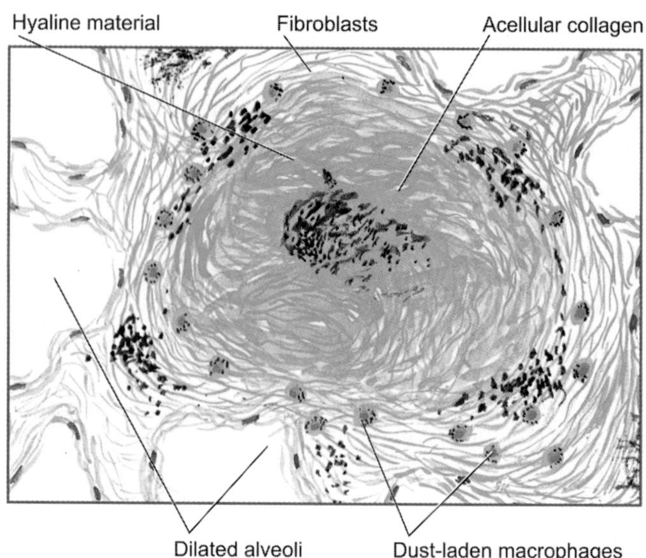

FIGURE 15.24

Microscopic picture of lung in silicosis. The silicotic nodule consists of hyaline centre surrounded by concentric layers of collagen which are further enclosed by fibroblasts and dust-laden macrophages. The intervening lung parenchyma shows dilated alveoli.

CLINICAL FEATURES. The functional effects of silicosis develop slowly and insidiously. The main presenting complaint is dyspnoea. In time, the patient may develop features of obstructive or restrictive pattern of disease. Other complications such as pulmonary tuberculosis, rheumatoid arthritis (Caplan's syndrome) and cor pulmonale may occur. The chest radiograph initially shows fine nodularity, while later there are larger and coalescent nodules. Silicosis does not carry increased risk of developing bronchogenic carcinoma.

Asbestos Disease

Asbestos as a mineral is known to mankind for more than 4000 years but its harmful effects have come to light during the last few decades. Asbestos is a Greek word meaning 'unquenchable'. In general, if *coal is lot of dust and little fibrosis, asbestos is little dust and lot of fibrosis.* Prolonged exposure for a number of years to asbestos dust produces three types of severe diseases: *asbestosis of lungs, pleural disease and tumours.* In nature, asbestos exists as long thin fibrils which are fire-resistant and can be spun into yarns and fabrics suitable for thermal and electrical insulation and has many applications in industries. Particularly at risk are workers engaged in mining, fabrication and manufacture of a number of products from asbestos such as asbestos pipes, tiles, roofs, textiles, insulating boards, sewer and water conduits, brake lining, clutch castings etc.

There are two major geometric forms of asbestos:

- *Serpentine* consisting of curly and flexible fibres. It includes the most common chemical form *chrysotile* (white asbestos) comprising more than 90% of commercially used asbestos.
- *Amphibole* consists of straight, stiff and rigid fibres. It includes the less common chemical forms *crocidolite* (blue asbestos), *amosite* (brown asbestos), *tremolite, anthophyllite* and *actinolyte.* However, the group of amphibole, though less common, is more important since it is associated with induction of malignant pleural tumours, particularly in association with crocidolite.

PATHOGENESIS. Overexposure to asbestos for more than a decade may produce asbestosis of the lung, pleural lesions and certain tumours. How asbestos causes all these lesions is not clearly understood but the following mechanisms have been suggested (Fig. 15.20,C):

1. The inhaled asbestos fibres are *phagocytosed by alveolar macrophages* from where they reach the interstitium. Some of the engulfed dust is transported via lymphatics to the pleura and regional lymph nodes.
2. The asbestos-laden macrophages release *chemoattractants* for neutrophils and for more macrophages, thus inciting cellular reaction around them.
3. Asbestos fibres are coated with glycoprotein and endogenous haemosiderin to produce characteristic beaded or dumbbell-shaped *asbestos bodies.*
4. All types of asbestos are *fibrogenic* and result in interstitial fibrosis. Fibroblastic proliferation may occur

via macrophage-derived growth factor such as interleukin-1. Alternatively, fibrosis may occur as a reparative response to tissue injury by lysosomal enzymes released from macrophages and neutrophils or by toxic free radicals.

5. A few *immunological abnormalities* such as antinuclear antibodies and rheumatoid factor have been found in cases of asbestosis but their role in the genesis of disease is not clear.

6. Asbestos fibres are *carcinogenic,* the most carcinogenic being crocidolite. There is high incidence of bronchogenic carcinoma in asbestosis which is explained on the basis of the role of asbestos fibres as tumour promoters or by causing cell death of the airways so that it is exposed to the carcinogenic effect of cigarette smoke. The development of pleural mesothelioma in these cases is probably by carrying of asbestos fibres via lymphatics to the pleura.

PATHOLOGIC CHANGES. As stated already, overexposure to asbestos is associated with 3 types of lesions: asbestosis, pleural disease and certain tumours.

A. ASBESTOSIS. The gross pulmonary fibrosis caused by asbestos exposure and histologic demonstration of asbestos bodies on asbestos fibres is termed asbestosis.

Grossly, the affected lungs are small and firm with cartilage-like thickening of the pleura. The sectioned surface shows variable degree of pulmonary fibrosis, especially in the subpleural areas and in the bases of lungs (Fig. 15.25). The advanced cases may show cystic changes.

Histologically, the following changes are observed:

1. There is non-specific interstitial fibrosis.
2. There is presence of characteristic *asbestos bodies* in the involved areas (Fig. 15.26). These are asbestos fibres coated with glycoprotein and haemosiderin and appear beaded or dumbbell-shaped. The coating stains positively for Prussian blue reaction.
3. There may be changes of emphysema in the pulmonary parenchyma between the areas of interstitial fibrosis.
4. The involvement of hilar lymph nodes in asbestosis is not as significant as in silicosis.

B. PLEURAL DISEASE. Pleural disease in asbestos exposure may produce one of the following 3 types of lesions:

1. Pleural Effusion. It develops in about 5% of asbestos workers and is usually serious type. Pleural effusion is generally accompanied by subpleural asbestosis.

2. Visceral pleural fibrosis. Quite often, asbestosis is associated with dense fibrous thickening of the visceral pleura encasing the lung.

3. Pleural plaques. Fibrocalcific pleural plaques are the most common lesions associated with asbestos exposure.

Grossly, the lesions appear as circumscribed, flat, small (upto 1 cm in diameter), firm or hard, bilateral nodules. They are seen more often on the posterolateral part of parietal pleura and on the pleural surface of the diaphragm.

Microscopically, they consist of hyalinised collagenous tissue which may be calcified so that they are visible on chest X-ray. Asbestos bodies are generally not found within the plaques.

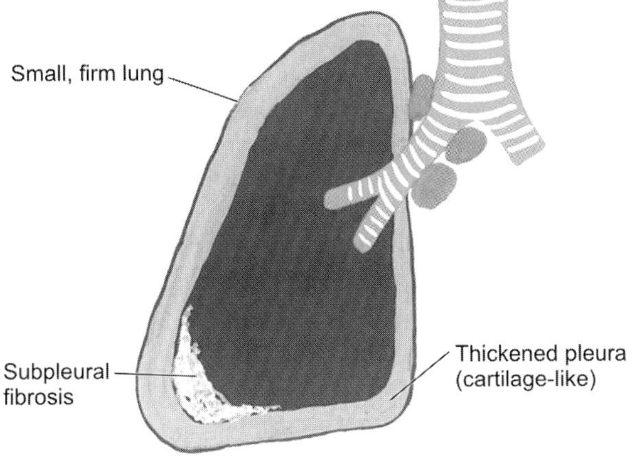

FIGURE 15.25

Macroscopic appearance of lung in asbestosis.

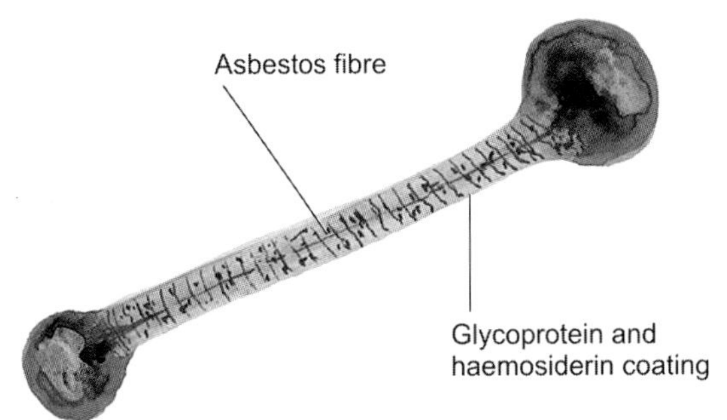

FIGURE 15.26

Microscopic appearance of asbestos body. An asbestos body is an asbestos fibre coated with glycoprotein and haemosiderin giving it beaded or dumbbell-shaped appearance with bulbous ends.

Chapter Fifteen

C. TUMOURS. Asbestos exposure predisposes to a number of cancers, most importantly bronchogenic carcinoma (page 505) and malignant mesothelioma (page 515). A few others are: carcinomas of oesophagus, stomach, colon, kidneys and larynx and various lymphoid malignancies.

1. Bronchogenic carcinoma is the most common malignancy in asbestos workers. Its incidence is 5 times higher in non-smoker asbestos workers than the non-smoker general population and 10 times higher in smoker asbestos workers than the other smokers.

2. Malignant mesothelioma is an uncommon tumour but association with asbestos exposure is present in 30 to 80% of cases with mesothelioma. The exposure need not be heavy because mesothelioma is known to develop in people living near asbestos plants or in wives of asbestos workers.

CLINICAL FEATURES. Asbestosis is a slow and insidious illness. The patient may remain asymptomatic for a number of years in spite of radiological evidence of calcific pleural plaques and parenchymatous changes. However, onset of interstitial fibrosis brings about dyspnoea with dry or productive cough. More advanced cases show development of Caplan's syndrome, pulmonary hypertension, cor pulmonale and various forms of cancers.

Berylliosis

Berylliosis is caused by heavy exposure to dust or fumes of metallic beryllium or its salts. Beryllium was used in the past in fluorescent tubes and light bulbs but currently it is principally used in nuclear and aerospace industries and in the manufacture of electrical and electronic equipments. Two forms of pulmonary berylliosis are recognised—*acute* and *chronic*.

ACUTE BERYLLIOSIS. Acute berylliosis occurs in individuals who are unusually sensitive to it and are heavily exposed to it for 2 to 4 weeks. The pulmonary reaction is in the form of an exudative chemical pneumonitis in which the alveoli are filled with protein-rich fluid with formation of hyaline membrane. The patient develops sudden dyspnoea, hyperapnoea and substernal pain. Most patients recover completely.

CHRONIC BERYLLIOSIS. Chronic berylliosis develops in individuals who are sensitised to it for a number of years, often after a delay of 20 or more years. The disease is a cell-mediated hypersensitivity reaction in which the metal beryllium acts as a hapten. The condition is characterised by development of non-caseating epithelioid granulomas like those of sarcoidosis. These granulomas are diffusely scattered throughout the lung parenchyma. The granulomas have giant cells which frequently contain 3 types of inclusions:

1. Birefringent crystals.
2. Concentrically-laminated haematoxyphilic Schaumann or conchoid bodies.
3. Acidophilic stellate-shaped asteroid bodies.

These inclusions are described in giant cells of granulomas in sarcoidosis too (Chapter 6). Similar sarcoid-like granulomas can occur in other organs such as in the liver, kidneys, spleen or lymph nodes in chronic berylliosis.

II. IMMUNOLOGIC LUNG DISEASE

Immunologic mechanisms play an important role in a number of lung diseases. These include the following important examples:

1. Bronchial asthma
2. Hypersensitivity (allergic) pneumonitis
3. Pulmonary eosinophilia
4. Goodpasture's syndrome
5. Pulmonary alveolar proteinosis

Bronchial Asthma

Though bronchial asthma is included in immunologic lung diseases, immunologic reactions are one of the mechanisms involved in its pathogenesis. Asthma has already been described under COPD (page 491).

Hypersensitivity (Allergic) Pneumonitis

Hypersensitivity pneumonitis are a group of immunologically-mediated interstitial lung diseases occurring in workers inhaling a variety of organic (biologic) antigenic materials. The condition may have an *acute* onset due to isolated exposure or may be *chronic* due to repeated low-dose exposure.

ETIOPATHOGENESIS. A list of important organic (biologic) dusts which may be inhaled to produce hypersensitivity pneumonitis is already given in Table 15.8. The immunologic mechanisms underlying hypersensitivity pneumonitis from any of these causes appear to be either type III immune-complex disease or type IV delayed-hypersensitivity reaction.

1. Farmers' lung is the classic example resulting from exposure to thermophilic actinomycetes generated by humid and warm mouldy hay.

2. Bagassosis occurs in individuals engaged in manufacture of paper and cardboard from sugarcane bagasse. Spores of thermophilic actinomycetes grow rapidly in mouldy sugarcane bagasse which are inhaled.

3. **Byssinosis** is an occupational lung disease occurring in workers exposed to fibres of cotton, flex and hemp for a number of years. The role of immunologic mechanisms in byssinosis is not as clear as in exposure to other organic dusts.

4. **Bird-breeders' (Bird-fanciers') lung** occurs in pigeon breeders, parrot breeders, chicken farmers and bird-fanciers who are exposed to bird-droppings and danders from their feathers.

5. **Mushroom-workers' lung** is found in mushroom cultivators exposed to mushroom compost dust.

6. **Malt-workers' lung** is seen in distillery and brewery workers who are exposed to mouldy barley and malt dust.

7. **Maple-bark disease** occurs in those involved in stripping of maple bark and inhale mouldy maple bark (maple tree is grown in northern hemisphere for timber and its leaf is the emblem of Canada).

8. **Silo-fillers' disease** occurs in individuals who enter the *silo* (silo is an airtight store-house of fodder for farm animals) in which toxic fumes of nitric oxide and nitrogen dioxide are formed due to fermentation of silage. The condition is generally rapidly fatal; less often it may lead to interstitial lung disease.

PATHOLOGIC CHANGES. The pathologic changes primarily involve the alveoli in contrast to bronchiolar involvement in asthma. The changes vary depending upon whether the biopsy is examined in early stage or in late stage.

- *In early stage,* the alveolar walls are diffusely infiltrated with lymphocytes, plasma cells and macrophages. A proportion of cases show granulomas consisting of histiocytes and giant cells of foreign body or Langhans' type.
- *In chronic cases,* the lungs show interstitial fibrosis with some inflammatory infiltrate. Honey-combing of the lung may be present.

CLINICAL FEATURES. The clinical features vary according to the stage. In acute cases, there is generally sudden attack of fever, myalgia, dyspnoea, cough and leucocytosis. In more chronic cases, there are signs of slowly progressive respiratory failure, dyspnoea and cyanosis as seen in other interstitial lung diseases.

Pulmonary Eosinophilia

Pulmonary eosinophilia, eosinophilic pneumonias or pulmonary infiltration with eosinophilia (PIE) syndrome are a group of immunologically-mediated lung diseases characterised by combination of 2 features:

- Infiltration of the lungs in chest radiographs; and
- Elevated eosinophil count in the peripheral blood.

ETIOPATHOGENESIS. PIE syndrome has a number of diverse causes and pathogenesis. These are as under:

1. **Löeffler's syndrome** is characterised by eosinophilia in the blood and typical wandering radiologic shadows, appearing in some part of the lung for a few days and then disappearing so as to appear somewhere else in the lung. The condition is generally self-limiting and mild, associated with slight fever and a few respiratory symptoms. The etiology is unknown.

2. **Tropical pulmonary eosinophilia** is caused by the passage of larvae of worms through the lungs e.g. in filariasis, ascariasis, strongyloidosis, toxocariasis and ancylostomiasis.

3. **Secondary chronic pulmonary eosinophilia** occurs secondary to adverse drug reactions; infection with fungi, bacteria, and helminths; allergic broncho-pulmonary aspergillosis and in association with asthma.

4. **Idiopathic chronic eosinophilic pneumonia** is characterised by prominent focal areas of consolidation of the lung. The condition is clinically diagnosed by excluding other known causes of pulmonary eosinophilia.

5. **Hypereosinophilic syndrome** is occurrence of eosinophilia of over 1500/μl for more than 6 months without any identifiable cause and without eosinophilic infiltrates in the lungs and other organs.

PATHOLOGIC CHANGES. The lesions in the lungs are similar in all cases.

Grossly, the lungs usually show patchy consolidation.

Microscopically, there is thickening of the alveolar walls by oedema and exudate, chiefly of eosinophils, and some lymphocytes and plasma cells. The alveolar lumina also contain eosinophils. Occasionally, small granulomas may be present.

Goodpasture's Syndrome

Goodpasture's syndrome is combination of necrotising haemorrhagic interstitial pneumonitis and rapidly progressive glomerulonephritis. The renal lesions of Goodpasture's syndrome are described in Chapter 20.

ETIOPATHOGENESIS. The condition results from immunologic damage produced by anti-basement membrane antibodies formed against antigens common to the glomerular and pulmonary basement membranes. The trigger for initiation of this autoimmune response is not clear; it could be virus infection, exposure to hydrocarbons and smoking.

*PATHOLOGIC CHANGES. **Grossly,*** the lungs are heavy with red-brown areas of consolidation.

Microscopically, the features vary according to the stage of the disease:

- *In acute stage,* there are focal areas of haemorrhages in the alveoli and focal necrosis in the alveolar walls.
- *In more chronic cases,* there is organisation of the haemorrhage leading to interstitial fibrosis and filling of alveoli with haemosiderin-laden macrophages.

CLINICAL FEATURES. The condition occurs commonly in 2nd or 3rd decades of life with preponderance in males. The pulmonary manifestations generally precede the renal disease. Most cases present with haemoptysis accompanied with dyspnoea, fatigue, weakness and anaemia. Renal manifestations soon appear which include haematuria, proteinuria, uraemia and progressive renal failure.

Pulmonary Alveolar Proteinosis

Pulmonary alveolar proteinosis is a rare chronic disease in which the distal airspaces of the lungs are filled with granular, PAS-positive, eosinophilic material with abundant lipid in it. The condition can occur at any age from infancy to old age.

ETIOPATHOGENESIS. The etiology and pathogenesis of alveolar proteinosis are unknown. A number of possibilities have been suggested:

- Since the alveolar material is combination of lipid and protein, it is not simply an overproduction of surfactant.
- Alveolar proteinosis may have an occupational etiology as seen in patients heavily exposed to silica.
- It may have an etiologic association with haematologic malignancies.
- There may be defective alveolar clearance of debris.

*PATHOLOGIC CHANGES. **Grossly,*** usually both lungs are involved, particularly the lower lobes. The lungs are heavier with areas of consolidation. Sectioned surface exudes abundant turbid fluid.

Histologically, the hallmark of the condition is presence of homogeneous, granular, eosinophilic material which stains brightly with PAS. Often, the material contains cholesterol clefts. There is no significant inflammatory infiltrate in the affected alveoli. Biochemically, the material consists of serum proteins of low molecular weight, cholesterol and phospholipids similar to surfactant. Electron microscopy reveals that the material consists of necrotic alveolar macrophages and desquamated alveolar epithelial cells.

CLINICAL FEATURES. The condition is manifested clinically by dyspnoea, cough, chest pain, pyrexia, fatigue and loss of weight. Chest X-ray shows confluent areas of consolidation. Occasionally, alveolar proteinosis may recover spontaneously but more often it is a fatal condition.

III. COLLAGEN-VASCULAR DISEASE

A number of collagen diseases may result in chronic interstitial fibrosis and destruction of blood vessels. These diseases are described in detail in Chapter 4 but the lung involvement in important forms of collagen diseases is briefly considered here.

1. SCLERODERMA (PROGRESSIVE SYSTEMIC SCLEROSIS). The lungs are involved in 80% cases of scleroderma. Interstitial pulmonary fibrosis is the most common form of pulmonary involvement. The disease usually involves the lower lobes and subpleural regions of the lungs and may lead to honey-combing of the lung. There is increased risk of development of cancer of the lung in pulmonary fibrosis in scleroderma.

2. RHEUMATOID ARTHRITIS. Pulmonary involvement in rheumatoid arthritis may result in pleural effusion, interstitial pneumonitis, necrobiotic nodules and rheumatoid pneumoconiosis (Caplan's syndrome, page 497). The parenchymatous lesions in rheumatoid arthritis are most commonly seen in the lower lobe. Necrobiotic nodules are the most specific manifestations of rheumatoid disease and closely resemble the subcutaneous nodules commonly found in rheumatoid arthritis.

3. SYSTEMIC LUPUS ERYTHEMATOSUS. Patients with systemic lupus erythematosus (SLE) commonly develop some form of lung disease during the course. The most common manifestation of SLE is pleurisy with small amount of pleural effusion that may contain LE cells. Other pulmonary lesions in SLE are interstitial pneumonitis, pulmonary haemorrhage and vasculitis.

4. SJÖGREN'S SYNDROME. Patients with Sjögren's syndrome often have rheumatoid arthritis and associated pulmonary changes. Involvement of the bronchial mucous gland by a process similar to that in the salivary glands can lead to inadequate bronchial clearance and repeated infections.

5. DERMATOMYOSITIS AND POLYMYOSITIS. Interstitial pneumonitis and interstitial fibrosis commonly accompany dermatomyositis and polymyositis.

6. WEGENER'S GRANULOMATOSIS. Wegener's granulomatosis is an inflammatory lesion having 4 components—granulomas of the upper respiratory tract, granulomas of the lungs, systemic vasculitis (page 291) and focal necrotising glomerulonephritis. *Localised or limited form* of the disease occurs in the lungs without involvement of other organs. Pulmonary involvement is in the form of single or multiple granulomas.

Microscopically, these granulomas have foci of fibrinoid necrosis and intense exudate of lymphocytes, plasma cells and macrophages with scattered multinucleate giant cells. Besides necrotising granulomas, there is associated vasculitis.

IV. IDIOPATHIC PULMONARY FIBROSIS

Diffuse interstitial fibrosis can occur as a result of a number of pathologic entities such as pneumoconiosis, hypersensitivity pneumonitis and collagen-vascular disease. However, in half the cases of diffuse interstitial fibrosis, no apparent cause or underlying disease is identifiable. Such cases are included under the entity *'idiopathic pulmonary fibrosis'* in the United States and *'cryptogenic fibrosing alveolitis'* in Britain. Some authors have termed the fully-developed condition as *'chronic interstitial pneumonitis'* or *'usual interstitial pneumonitis'* and distinguished it from the early stage of the disease called *'desquamative interstitial pneumonitis'*.

PATHOGENESIS. The pathogenesis of idiopathic pulmonary fibrosis is unknown and the condition is diagnosed by excluding all known causes of interstitial fibrosis. However, a few evidences point toward immunologic mechanism. These are:

1. High levels of autoantibodies such as rheumatoid factor and antinuclear antibodies.
2. Elevated titres of circulating immune complexes.
3. Immunofluorescent demonstration of the deposits of immunoglobulins and complement on the alveolar walls in biopsy specimens.

PATHOLOGIC CHANGES. The lung involvement in idiopathic pulmonary fibrosis is often bilateral and widespread.

Grossly, the lungs are firm, heavier with reduced volume. Honey-combing (i.e. enlarged, thick-walled air spaces) develops in parts of lung, particularly in the subpleural region.

Histologically, the changes vary according to the stage of the disease.

- **In early stage,** there is widening of the alveolar septa by oedema and cellular infiltrate by mononuclear inflammatory cells. The alveolar lining cells may show hyperplasia at places and are flattened at other places. There is often formation of hyaline membranes. The alveolar spaces contain exudate consisting of macrophages, lymphocytes and neutrophils. Many of the macrophages contain lamellar bodies derived from surfactant of the necrotic alveolar lining epithelial cells. Based on the observation of desquamative component in the cellular exudate, some authors label the early stage of idiopathic pulmonary fibrosis as *'desquamative interstitial pneumonitis'*.
- **In advanced stage,** there is organisation of the alveolar exudate and replacement fibrosis in the alveoli as well as in the interstitial septal wall with variable amount of inflammation. Eventually, there are small cystic areas (honey-comb lung) with alternating areas of fibrosis containing thick-walled and narrowed vessels. This stage is often referred to as *'chronic interstitial pneumonitis'* or *'usual interstitial pneumonitis'*.

CLINICAL FEATURES. Middle-aged males are affected more frequently. The usual features are of respiratory difficulty beginning with dry cough and slowly progressing dyspnoea. More advanced cases may develop clubbing of fingers and cor pulmonale. A rapidly progressive form of the idiopathic pulmonary fibrosis with death within 6 weeks to 6 months is termed Hamman-Rich syndrome.

TUMOURS OF LUNGS

A number of benign and malignant tumours occur in the lungs but the primary lung cancer, commonly termed bronchogenic carcinoma, is the most common (95% of all primary lung tumours). The lung is also the commonest site for metastasis from carcinomas and sarcomas. A histologic classification of various benign and malignant tumours of lungs as recommended by the World Health Organisation is given in Table 15.9.

BRONCHOGENIC CARCINOMA

Though the term bronchogenic carcinoma is commonly used for cancer of the lungs, it includes carcinomas having bronchial as well as bronchiolar origin.

INCIDENCE. Bronchogenic carcinoma is the most common primary malignant tumour in men in

TABLE 15.9: Histological Classification of Lung Tumours.

I. **EPITHELIAL TUMOURS**

A. **Benign**
1. Papilloma
2. Adenoma

B. **Dysplasia and carcinoma in situ**

C. **Malignant**
Bronchogenic carcinoma
1. Squamous cell (epidermoid) carcinoma
2. Small cell carcinoma
   i) Oat cell carcinoma
   ii) Intermediate cell carcinoma
   iii) Combined oat cell carcinoma
3. Adenocarcinoma
   i) Acinar adenocarcinoma
   ii) Papillary adenocarcinoma
   iii) Bronchiolo-alveolar carcinoma
   iv) Solid carcinoma with mucus formation
4. Large cell carcinoma
5. Adenosquamous carcinoma

Other carcinomas
1. Pulmonary neuroendocrine tumour (carcinoid tumour)
2. Bronchial gland carcinomas
   i) Adenoid cystic carcinoma
   ii) Mucoepidermoid carcinoma

II. **SOFT TISSUE TUMOURS**

(Fibroma, fibrosarcoma; leiomyoma, leiomyosarcoma; lipoma, chondroma, haemangioma, lymphangioma, granular cell myoblastoma)

III. **PLEURAL TUMOURS**

A. **Benign mesothelioma**
B. **Malignant mesothelioma**

IV. **MISCELLANEOUS TUMOURS**
1. Carcinosarcoma
2. Pulmonary blastoma
3. Malignant melanoma
4. Malignant lymphoma

V. **SECONDARY TUMOURS**

VI. **TUMOUR-LIKE LESIONS**
1. Hamartomas
2. Eosinophilic granuloma
3. Inflammatory pseudotumours

industrialised nations and accounts for nearly one-third of all cancer deaths in both sexes. Currently, the incidence in females in the United States has already exceeded breast cancer as a cause of death in women. Cancer of the lung is a disease of middle and late life with peak incidence in 5th to 7th decades, after which there is gradual fall in its incidence.

ETIOPATHOGENESIS. The high incidence of lung cancer is associated with a number of etiologic factors, most important of which is *cigarette smoking*.

1. Smoking. The most important factor for rise in the incidence of bronchogenic carcinoma is tobacco smoking. About 80% of lung cancer occurs in active smokers. A number of evidences support the positive relationship of lung cancer with tobacco smoking (see page 242):

i) Total dose: There is a direct statistical correlation between death rate from lung cancer and the total amount of cigarettes smoked e.g.

- An average regular smoker has 10 times greater risk of developing lung cancer than a non-smoker.
- The risk of smokers of more than 2 packs (40 cigarettes) per day for 20 years is 20 times greater.
- Cessation of smoking by a regular smoker results in gradual decline in the chances of developing lung cancer. After 10 years of abstinence from smoking, the risk is not greater than in a non-smoker.
- Pipe and cigar smokers, though have higher risk than non-smokers but are at lesser risk than cigarette smokers.

ii) Histologic alterations: The association of tobacco smoking is strongest for squamous cell carcinoma and small cell carcinoma of the lung. More than 90% of smokers have epithelial changes in the respiratory tract in the form of squamous metaplasia, dysplasia or carcinoma *in situ* (Fig. 15.27).

iii) Mechanism: How tobacco smoking causes lung cancer is not quite clear.

- Analysis of the tar from cigarette smoke has revealed a number of known carcinogens (e.g. polycyclic aromatic hydrocarbons, nitrosamines) and tumour promoters (e.g. phenol derivatives).
- In experimental animal studies, it has been possible to induce cancer by skin painting experiments with smoke-tar. However, it has not been possible to reproduce pattern of human respiratory tract cancer, probably because of the difficulty in reproducing human smoking methods in animals.

2. Atmospheric pollution. There is increased risk of developing bronchogenic carcinoma in nonsmokers living in industrialised and smoky cities than in the less polluted rural areas. It is possible that specific industrial pollutants may be at fault as evidenced by high rates for lung cancer in people living in the neighbourhood of petrochemical industries.

3. Occupational causes. There are number of well-established occupational causes of lung cancer. These

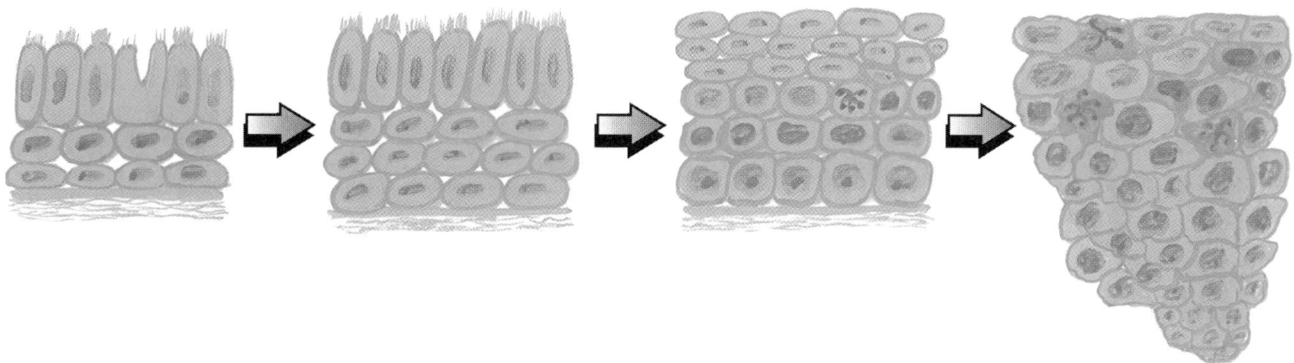

FIGURE 15.27

Schematic representation of sequential development of squamous cell carcinoma of the lung.

include workers exposed to asbestos, radiation of all types, bis-ethers, nickel, beryllium, arsenic, metallic iron and iron-oxide. Some industrial carcinogens and cigarette smoking have cocarcinogenic effect, particularly in uranium mines and asbestos workers.

4. Dietary factors. Susceptibility to respiratory cancers is increased in vitamin A deficiency. Smokers with low vitamin A intake have a greater risk of lung cancer than those with vitamin A-rich diet. The incidence of lung cancer is inversely related to socioeconomic level reflecting their dietary pattern.

5. Genetic factors. The risk of developing lung cancer in the relatives of lung cancer patients is two and half times greater than that in the general population. A few studies have suggested that ability to metabolise carcinogenic polycyclic aromatic hydrocarbons is under genetic control but the exact nature of genetic and familial influence is uncertain.

6. Chronic scarring. Peripheral adenocarcinomas occur more frequently in areas of chronic scarring caused by chronic inflammatory changes, old tuberculosis, asbestosis, chronic interstitial fibrosis, old infarcts and in scleroderma.

PATHOLOGIC CHANGES. Bronchogenic carcinoma can occur anywhere in the lung but the most common location is *hilar,* followed in descending frequency by *peripheral* type.

Grossly, these 2 main types show variation in appearance:

1. Hilar type (Fig. 15.28,A): Most commonly, the lung cancer arises in the main bronchus or one of its segmental branches in the hilar parts of the lung, more often on the right side. The tumour begins as a small roughened area on the bronchial mucosa at the bifurcation. As the tumour enlarges, it thickens the bronchial mucosa producing nodular or ulcerated surface. As the nodules coalesce, the carcinoma grows into a friable spherical mass, 1 to 5 cm in diameter, narrowing and occluding the lumen. The cut surface of the tumour is yellowish-white with foci of necrosis and haemorrhages which may produce cavitary lesions (Table 15.10 sums up a list of common conditions having *pulmonany cavitary lesions* or 'honeycomb lung' during the course of different lung diseases). It is common to find secondary changes in bronchogenic carcinoma of lung such as bronchopneumonia, abscess formation and bronchiectasis as a result of obstruction and intercurrent infections. The tumour soon spreads within the lungs by direct extension or by lymphatics, and to distant sites by lymphatic or haematogenous routes, as described later.

2. Peripheral type (Fig. 15.28,B): A small proportion of lung cancers, chiefly adenocarcinomas including bronchioloalveolar carcinomas, originate from a small peripheral bronchiole but the exact site of origin may not be discernible. The tumour may be a single nodule or multiple nodules in the periphery of the lung producing pneumonia-like consolidation of a

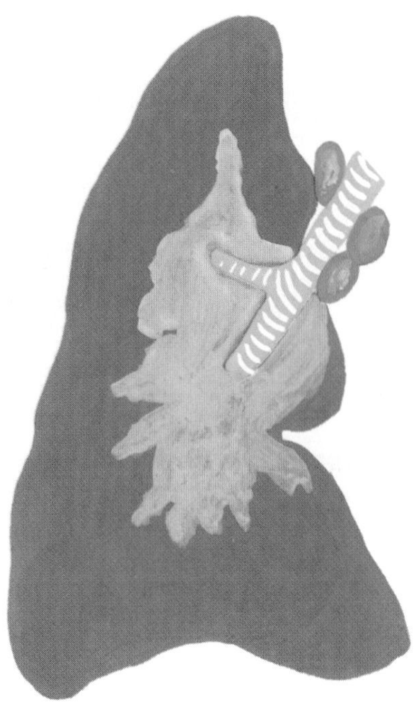

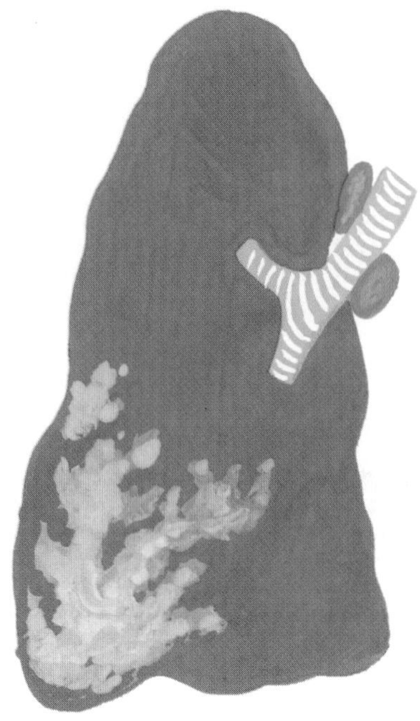

A, HILAR TYPE B, PERIPHERAL TYPE

FIGURE 15.28

The two main gross patterns of bronchogenic carcinoma.

large part of the lung. The cut surface of the tumour is greyish and mucoid.

Histologically, as per the World Health Organisation recommendations (see Table 15.9), bronchogenic carcinoma is divided into 5 main histologic types: squamous cell or epidermoid carcinoma (35-50%), small cell carcinoma (20-25%), adenocarcinoma (15-35%), large cell carcinoma (10-15%), and combined squamous cell carcinoma and adenocarcinoma (adenosquamous carcinoma, 1-3%). However, for therapeutic purposes, bronchogenic carcinoma can be classified into three groups:

1. Small cell carcinoma (20-25%)
2. Non-small cell carcinomas (70-75%) (includes squamous cell carcinoma, adenocarcinoma, and large cell carcinoma)
3. Combined/mixed patterns (5-10%).

The distinction between small cell and non-small cell carcinomas is important because the two not only differ in morphology, but there are major differences in immunophenotyping and response to treatment:

■ *Immunophenotyping:* Small cell carcinomas generally have mutations in *TP53* and *RB* gene while non-small cell carcinomas have more often inactivation of *p16/CDK/N2A* genes.

■ *Response to treatment:* Small cell carcinomas frequently have haemotogenous metastasis at the time of diagnosis and are treated by chemotherapy

TABLE 15.10: Conditions Producing Pulmonary Cavities (Honey-Comb Lung).

A. INFECTIONS
1. Pulmonary tuberculosis
2. Primary lung abscess (e.g. due to aspiration)
3. Secondary lung abscess (e.g. preceding pneumonia, pyaemia, sepsis)
4. Bronchiectasis
5. Fungal infections (e.g. aspergillosis, mucormycosis)
6. Actinomycosis
7. Nocardiosis

B. NON-INFECTIOUS CAUSES
1. Pneumoconiosis (e.g. simple coal-workers' pneumoconiosis, silicosis, asbestosis)
2. Bronchogenic carcinoma
3. Metastatic lung tumours
4. Wegener's granulomatosis
5. Pulmonary infarction
6. Congenital cysts
7. Idiopathic pulmonary fibrosis

with or without radiation rather than by surgery, while non-small cell carcinomas respond poorly to chemotherapy and are better treated by surgery.

The major differences in small cell and non-small cell carcinomas of the lung are summed up in Table 15.11.

By light microscopy, precise histologic classification of bronchogenic carcinoma is possible which is important because of prognostic and therapeutic considerations.

1. Squamous cell (epidermoid) carcinoma (Fig. 15.29): This is the most common type of bronchogenic carcinoma found more commonly in men, particularly with history of tobacco smoking. These tumours usually arise in a large bronchus and are prone to massive necrosis and cavitation. The tumour is diagnosed microscopically by identification of either intercellular bridges or keratinisation. The tumour may show varying histologic grades of differentiation such as well-differentiated, moderately-differentiated and poorly-differentiated (COLOUR PLATE XX: CL 79). Occasionally, a variant of squamous cell carcinoma, *spindle cell carcinoma,* having biphasic pattern of growth due to the presence of a component of squamous cell carcinoma and the

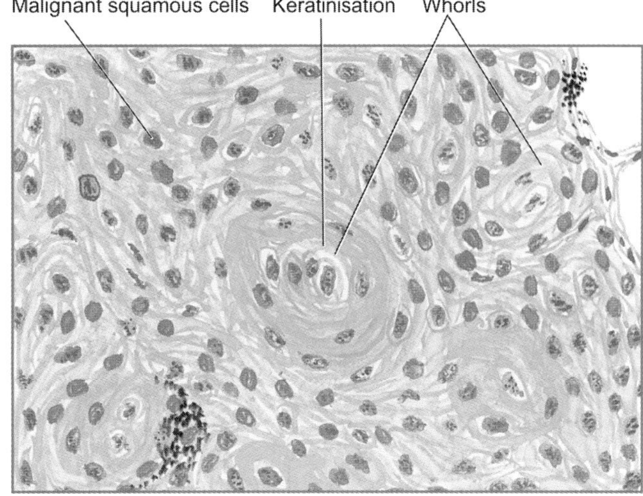

FIGURE 15.29

Squamous cell carcinoma of the lung. Islands of invading malignant squamous cells are seen. A few well-developed cell nests with keratinisation are evident.

TABLE 15.11: Comparison of Features of Small Cell and Non-small Cell Carcinoma of the Lung.

	FEATURE	SMALL CELL CARCINOMA	NON-SMALL CELL CARCINOMA
1.	***Etiologic relationship***	Strongly related to tobacco smoking	Smoking implicated, other factors: pollution, chronic scars, asbestos exposure
2.	***Morphology***		
	i) Pattern	Diffuse sheets	Squamous or glandular pattern
	ii) Nuclei	Hyperchromaic, fine chromatin	Pleomorphic, coarse chromatin
	iii) Nucleoli	Indistinct	Prominent
	iv) Cytoplasm	Scanty	Abundant
3.	***Neuroendocrine markers*** *(e.g. dense-core granules on EM, chromogranin, synaptophysin, neuron-specific enolase, CD56, CD57)*	Present	Absent
4.	***Epithelial markers*** *(e.g. epithelial membrane antigen, carcinoemebryonic antigen, cytokeratin)*	Present	Present
5.	***Mucin***	Absent	Present in adenocarcinoma
6.	***HLA, β2 microglobulin***	Absent to low	Present
7.	***Peptide hormone production***	Gastrin, ACTH, ADH, calcitonin	Parathormone
8.	***Genetic abnormalities***	3p allele loss, *RB* and *TP* 53 mutations	3p allele loss, *p16/CDKN2A* and *RAS* mutations
9.	***Treatment type***	Radiotherapy and/or chemotherapy	Surgical resection possible, limited response to radiotherapy and/or chemotherapy
10.	***Prognosis***	Poor	Better

other sarcoma-like spindle cell component, is found. Usually the spread of squamous cell carcinoma is more rapid than the other histologic types. Frequently, the edge of the growth and the adjoining uninvolved bronchi show squamous metaplasia, epithelial dysplasia and carcinoma *in situ*.

2. Small cell carcinoma: Small cell carcinomas are frequently hilar or central in location, have strong relationship to cigarette smoking and are highly malignant tumours. They are most often associated with ectopic hormone production because of the presence of neurosecretory granules in majority of tumour cells which are similar to those found in argentaffin or Kulchitsky cells normally found in bronchial epithelium. By immunohistochemistry, these tumour cells are positive for neuroendocrine markers: chromogranin, neuron-specific enolase (NSE) and synaptophysin. Small cell carcinomas have 3 subtypes:

i) *Oat cell carcinoma* (Fig. 15.30) is composed of uniform, small cells, larger than lymphocytes with dense, round or oval nuclei having diffuse chromatin, inconspicuous nucleoli and very sparse cytoplasm (*oat* = a form of grain). These cells are organised into cords, aggregates and ribbons or around small blood vessels forming pseudorosettes (COLOUR PLATE XX: CL 80).

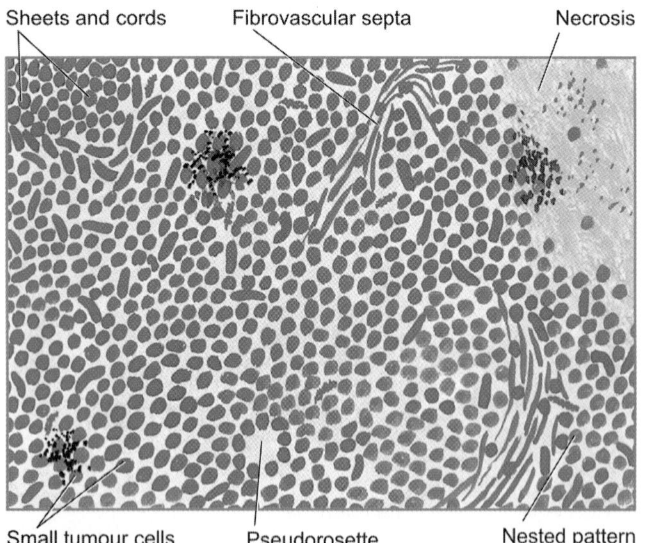

FIGURE 15.30

Oat cell carcinoma of the lung. The tumour cells are arranged in sheets, cords or aggregates and at places form pseudorosettes. The individual tumour cells are small, uniform, lymphocyte-like with scanty cytoplasm.

ii) *Small cell carcinoma, intermediate cell type* is composed of cells slightly larger than those of oat cell carcinoma and have similar nuclear characteristics but have more abundant cytoplasm. These cells are organised into lobules.

iii) *Combined oat cell carcinoma* is a tumour in which there is a definite component of oat cell carcinoma with squamous cell and/or adenocarcinoma.

3. Adenocarcinoma: Adenocarcinoma, also called *peripheral carcinoma* due to its location and *scar carcinoma* due to its association with areas of chronic scarring, is the most common bronchogenic carcinoma in women and is slow-growing. Adenocarcinoma is further subclassified into 4 types:

i) *Acinar adenocarcinoma* which has predominance of glandular structure and often occurs in the larger bronchi.

ii) *Papillary adenocarcinoma* which has a pronounced papillary configuration and is frequently peripherally located in the lungs and is found in relation to pulmonary scars (scar carcinoma).

iii) *Bronchiolo-alveolar carcinoma* (Fig. 15.31) is characterised by cuboidal to tall columnar and mucus-secreting epithelial cells growing along the existing alveoli and forming numerous papillary structures. Ultrastructurally, these tumour cells resemble Clara cells or less often type II pneumocytes.

iv) *Solid carcinoma* is a poorly-differentiated adenocarcinoma lacking acini, tubules or papillae but having mucus-containing vacuoles in many tumour cells.

4. Large cell carcinoma: These are undifferentiated carcinomas which lack the specific features by which they could be assigned into squamous cell carcinoma or adenocarcinoma. Large cell carcinomas are more common in men, have strong association with cigarette smoking and are highly malignant tumours. The tumour cells have large nuclei, prominent nucleoli, abundant cytoplasm and well-defined cell borders. Variants of large cell undifferentiated carcinomas include *giant cell carcinoma* with prominence of highly pleomorphic multinucleate cells and *clear cell carcinoma* composed of cells with clear or foamy cytoplasm without mucin.

5. Adenosquamous carcinoma: These are a small proportion of peripheral scar carcinomas having clear evidence of both keratinisation and glandular differentiation.

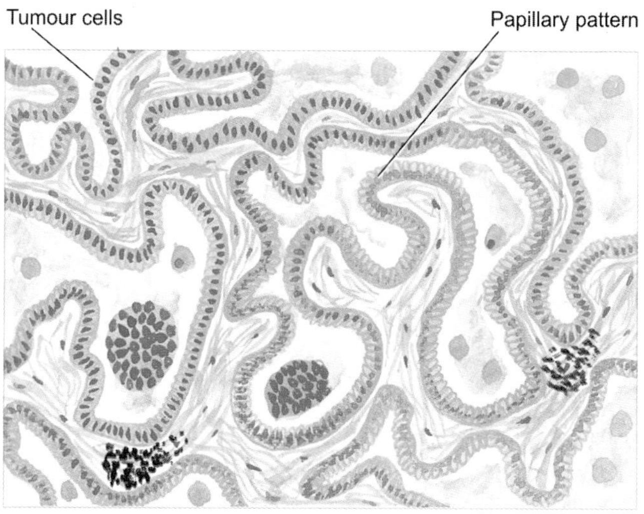

FIGURE 15.31

Bronchiolo-alveolar carcinoma. The alveolar walls are lined by cuboidal to tall columnar and mucin-secreting tumour cells with papillary growth pattern.

SPREAD. Bronchogenic carcinoma can invade the adjoining structures directly, or may spread by lymphatic and haematogenous routes.

1. Direct spread. The tumour extends directly by invading through the wall of the bronchus and destroys and replaces the peribronchial lung tissue. As it grows further, it spreads to the opposite bronchus and lung, into the pleural cavity, the pericardium and the myocardium and along the great vessels of the heart causing their constriction. Extension of the cancer located at the apex of the lung into the thoracic cage may involve brachial plexus and the sympathetic chain causing pain and sensory disturbances, so called *Pancoast's syndrome.*

2. Lymphatic spread. Initially, hilar lymph nodes are affected. Later, lymphatic metastases occur to the other groups leading to spread to mediastinal, cervical, supraclavicular and para-aortic lymph nodes. Invasion of the thoracic duct may produce chylous ascites.

3. Haematogenous spread. Distant metastases via blood stream are widespread and early. The sites affected, in descending order of involvement, are: the liver, adrenals, bones, pancreas, brain, opposite lung, kidneys and thyroid.

CLINICAL FEATURES. Symptoms of lung cancer are quite variable and result from local effects, effects due to occlusion of a bronchus, local and distant metastases and paraneoplastic syndromes. The additional diagnostic aids include radiologic examination of the chest, cytologic examination of the sputum and bronchial washings.

TABLE 15.12: Causes of Haemoptysis.

A. INFLAMMATORY

1. Bronchitis
2. Bronchiectasis
3. Tuberculosis
4. Lung abscess
5. Pneumonias

B. NEOPLASTIC

1. Primary and metastatic lung cancer
2. Bronchial adenoma

C. OTHERS

1. Pulmonary thromboembolism
2. Left ventricular failure
3. Mitral stenosis
4. Trauma
5. Foreign bodies
6. Primary pulmonary hypertension
7. Haemorrhagic diathesis

1. Local symptoms. Most common local complaints are cough, chest pain, dyspnoea and haemoptysis.

A list of various causes of haemoptysis is given in Table 15.12.

2. Bronchial obstructive symptoms. Occlusion of a bronchus may result in bronchopneumonia, lung abscess and bronchiectasis in the lung tissue distal to the site of obstruction and cause their attendant symptoms like fever, productive cough, pleural effusion and weight loss.

3. Symptoms due to metastases. Distant spread may produce varying features and sometimes these are the first manifestation of lung cancer. These include: superior vena caval syndrome, painful bony lesions, paralysis of recurrent nerve and other neurologic manifestations resulting from brain metastases.

4. Paraneoplastic syndromes. A number of paraneoplastic syndromes (page 233) are associated with lung cancer. These include the following:

i) ***Ectopic hormone production:*** Different hormonal syndromes are characteristic of different histologic types of lung cancer. Small cell carcinomas are associated most often with ectopic hormone production. The various hormones elaborated by lung cancer are:

a) ACTH, producing Cushing's syndrome.
b) ADH, inducing hyponatraemia.
c) Parathormone, causing hypercalcaemia.
d) Calcitonin, producing hypocalcaemia.

e) Gonadotropins, causing gynaecomastia.
f) Serotonin, associated with carcinoid syndrome.

ii) ***Other systemic manifestations:*** These include the following:

a) *Neuromuscular* e.g. polymyositis, myopathy, peripheral neuropathy and subacute cerebellar degeneration.

b) *Skeletal* e.g. clubbing and hypertrophic osteoarthropathy.

c) *Cutaneous* e.g. acanthosis nigricans and dermatomypathy.

d) *Cardiovascular* e.g. migratory thrombophlebitis (Trousseau's syndrome), nonbacterial thrombotic endocarditis.

e) *Haematologic* e.g. abnormalities in coagulation and leukaemoid reaction.

STAGING AND PROGNOSIS. The widely accepted clinical staging of lung cancer is according to the TNM classification, combining features of primary *T*umours, *N*odal involvement and distant *M*etastases. TNM staging divides all lung cancers into the following 4 stages:

Occult: Malignant cells in the broncho-pulmonary secretions but no evidence of primary tumour or metastasis.

Stage I: Tumour less than 3 cm, with or without ipsilateral nodal involvement, no distant metastasis.

Stage II: Tumour larger than 3 cm, with ipsilateral hilar lymph node involvement, no distant metastasis.

Stage III: Tumour of any size, involving adjacent structures, involving contralateral lymph nodes or distant metastasis.

In general, tumour size larger than 5 cm has worse prognosis. Symptomatic patients, particularly with systemic symptoms, fare far badly than the non-symptomatic patients. The overall prognosis of bronchogenic carcinoma is dismal; 5-year survival rate with surgery combined with radiotherapy or chemotherapy is about 9%. Adenocarcinoma and squamous cell carcinoma which are localised, are resectable and have a slightly better prognosis. *Small cell carcinoma has the worst prognosis* since surgical treatment is ineffective though the tumour is sensitive to radiotherapy and chemotherapy.

NEUROENDOCRINE TUMOURS (BRONCHIAL CARCINOID)

Bronchial carcinoids are tumours of low grade malignancy arising from neuroendocrine (Kulchitsky) cells of bronchial mucosa in common with cell of origin for small cell carcinomas described above. Formerly, they used to be classified as 'bronchial adenomas' but now it is known that these tumours are locally invasive and have the capacity to metastasise. Bronchial carcinoids tend to occur at a younger age than bronchogenic carcinoma, often appearing below the age of 40 years, and are not related to cigarette smoking.

PATHOLOGIC CHANGES. Bronchial carcinoids resemble their intestinal counterparts described in Chapter 18.

Grossly, bronchial carcinoids most commonly arise from a major bronchus and project into the bronchial lumen as a spherical polypoid mass, 3-4 cm in diameter. Less commonly, the tumour may grow into the bronchial wall and produce collar-button like lesion. The overlying bronchial mucosa is usually intact. Cut surface of the tumour is yellow-tan in colour.

Histologically, the tumour is composed of uniform cuboidal cells forming aggregates, trabeculae or ribbons separated by fine fibrous septa. The tumour cells have abundant, finely granular cytoplasm and oval central nuclei with clumped nuclear chromatin. Mitoses are rare and necrosis is uncommon. The secretory granules of bronchial carcinoids resemble those of other foregut carcinoids and stain positively with argyrophilic stains in which exogenous reducing agent is added for the reaction.

CLINICAL FEATURES. Most of the symptoms in bronchial carcinoids occur as a result of bronchial obstruction such as cough, haemoptysis, atelectasis and secondary infection. About 5-10% of bronchial carcinoids metastasise to the liver and these cases are capable of producing carcinoid syndrome (Chapter 18).

HAMARTOMA

Hamartoma is a tumour-like lesion composed of an abnormal admixture of pulmonary tissue components and is discovered incidentally as a coin-lesion in the chest-X-ray. Pulmonary hamartomas are of 2 types: chondromatous and leiomyomatous.

■ **Chondromatous hamartoma** is more common and usually asymptomatic. It forms a solitary, spherical mass, 2-5 cm in diameter, usually at the periphery of the lung. Typically, it shows nodules of cartilage associated with fibrous and adipose tissue admixed with bronchial epithelium.

■ **Leiomyomatous hamartoma** has a prominent smooth muscle component and bronchiolar structures.

They are frequently multiple, 1-2 mm in diameter and are more commonly located near the pleura.

METASTATIC LUNG TUMOURS

Secondary tumours of the lungs are more common than the primary pulmonary tumours. Metastases from carcinomas as well as sarcomas arising from anywhere in the body may spread to the lung by haematogenous or lymphatic routes, or by direct extension. Blood-borne metastases are the most common since emboli of tumour cells from any malignant tumour entering the systemic venous circulation are likely to be lodged in the lungs. Metastases are most common in the peripheral part of the lung forming single or multiple, discrete nodular lesions which appear radiologically as *'cannon-ball secondaries'*. Less frequently, the metastatic growth is confined to peribronchiolar and perivascular locations which is due to spread via lymphatics.

Most common sources of metastases in the lungs are: carcinomas of the bowel, breast, thyroid, kidney, pancreas, lung (ipsilateral or contralateral) and liver. Other tumours which frequently metastasise to the lungs are osteogenic sarcoma, neuroblastoma, Wilms' tumour, melanoma, lymphomas and leukaemias (COLOUR PLATE XII: CL 48).

PLEURA

NORMAL STRUCTURE

Visceral pleura covers the lungs and extends into the fissures while the parietal pleura limits the mediastinum and covers the dome of the diaphragm and inner aspect of the chest wall. The two layers between them enclose pleural cavity which contains less than 15 ml of clear serous fluid.

Microscopically, both the pleural layers are lined by a single layer of flattened mesothelial cells facing each other. Underneath the lining cells is a thin layer of connective tissue.

Diseases affecting the pleura are nearly always secondary to some other underlying disease. Broadly, they fall into inflammations, non-inflammatory pleural effusions, pneumothorax, and tumours.

INFLAMMATIONS

Inflammatory involvement of the pleura is commonly termed *pleuritis or pleurisy.* Depending upon the character of resultant exudate, it can be divided into serous, fibrinous and serofibrinous, suppurative or empyema, and haemorrhagic pleuritis.

1. SEROUS, FIBRINOUS AND SEROFIBRINOUS PLEURITIS. Acute inflammation of the pleural sac (acute pleuritis) can result in serous, serofibrinous and fibrinous exudate. Most of the causes of such pleuritis are infective in origin, particularly within the lungs, such as tuberculosis, pneumonias, pulmonary infarcts, lung abscess and bronchiectasis. Other causes include a few collagen diseases (e.g. rheumatoid arthritis and disseminated lupus erythematosus), uraemia, metastatic involvement of the pleura, irradiation of lung tumours and diffuse systemic infections (e.g. typhoid fever, tularaemia, blastomycosis and coccidioidomycosis).

Pleurisy causes pain in the chest on breathing and a friction rub is audible on auscultation. In most patients, the exudate is minimal and is resorbed resulting in resolution. Repeated attacks of pleurisy may result in organisation leading to fibrous adhesions and obliteration of the pleural cavity.

2. SUPPURATIVE PLEURITIS (EMPYEMA THORACIS). Bacterial or mycotic infection of the pleural cavity that converts a serofibrinous effusion into purulent exudate is termed suppurative pleuritis or empyema thoracis. The most common cause is direct spread of pyogenic infection from the lung. Other causes are direct extension from subdiaphragmatic abscess or liver abscess and penetrating injuries to the chest wall. Occasionally, the spread may occur by haematogenous or lymphatic routes.

In empyema, the exudate is yellow-green, creamy pus that accumulates in large volumes. Empyema is eventually replaced by granulation tissue and fibrous tissue. In time, tough fibrocollagenic adhesions develop which obliterate the cavity, and with passage of years, calcification may occur. The effect of these is serious respiratory difficulty due to inadequate pulmonary expansion.

3. HAEMORRHAGIC PLEURITIS. Haemorrhagic pleuritis differs from haemothorax in having inflammatory cells or exfoliated tumour cells in the exudate. The causes of haemorrhagic pleuritis are metastatic involvement of the pleura, bleeding disorders and rickettsial diseases.

NON-INFLAMMATORY PLEURAL EFFUSIONS

These include fluid collections in the pleural cavity such as hydrothorax, haemothorax and chylothorax.

1. HYDROTHORAX. Hydrothorax is non-inflammatory accumulation of serous fluid within the pleural cavities. Hydrothorax may be unilateral or bilateral depending upon the underlying cause. Occasionally, an effusion is limited to part of a pleural cavity by preexisting pleural adhesions.

The most common cause of hydrothorax, often bilateral, is congestive heart failure. Other causes are renal failure, cirrhosis of liver, Meig's syndrome (Chapter 22), pulmonary oedema and primary and secondary tumours of the lungs.

The non-inflammatory serous effusion in hydrothorax is clear and straw-coloured and has the characteristics of transudate with a specific gravity of under 1.012, protein content below 1 gm/dl and little cellular content.

If the fluid collection in pleural cavity is less than 300 ml (normal is less than 15 ml), no signs or symptoms are produced and may be apparent in chest X-ray in standing posture as obliterated costodiaphragmatic angle. If the pleural cavity contains abundant fluid, it imparts a characteristic opaque radiographic appearance to the affected side with deviation of trachea to the opposite side. In such cases, symptoms such as respiratory embarrassment and dyspnoea are produced which are promptly relieved on withdrawal of fluid.

2. HAEMOTHORAX. Accumulation of pure blood in the pleural cavity is termed as haemothorax. The most common causes of haemothorax are trauma to the chest wall or to the thoracic viscera and rupture of aortic aneurysm. It is important to remove the blood from the pleural cavity as early as possible. Otherwise the blood will clot and organise, resulting in fibrous adhesions and obliteration of the pleural cavity.

3. CHYLOTHORAX. Chylothorax is an uncommon condition in which there is accumulation of milky fluid of lymphatic origin into the pleural cavity. Chylothorax results most commonly from rupture of the thoracic duct by trauma or obstruction of the thoracic duct such as by malignant tumours, most often malignant lymphomas. Chylothorax is more often confined to the left side. Chylous effusion is milky due to high content of finely emulsified fats in the chyle.

PNEUMOTHORAX

An accumulation of air in the pleural cavity is called pneumothorax. It may occur in one of the three circumstances: spontaneous, traumatic and therapeutic.

i) Spontaneous pneumothorax occurs due to spontaneous rupture of alveoli in any form of pulmonary disease. Most commonly, spontaneous pneumothorax occurs in association with emphysema, asthma and tuberculosis. Other causes include chronic bronchitis in an old patient, bronchiectasis, pulmonary infarction and bronchial cancer. In young patients, recurrent spontaneous rupture of peripheral subpleural blebs may occur without any cause resulting in disabling condition termed *spontaneous idiopathic pneumothorax.*

ii) Traumatic pneumothorax is caused by trauma to the chest wall or lungs, ruptured oesophagus or stomach, and surgical operations of the thorax.

iii) Therapeutic (artificial) pneumothorax used to be employed formerly in the treatment of chronic pulmonary tuberculosis in which air was introduced into the pleural sac so as to collapse the lung and limit its respiratory movements.

The **effects** of pneumothorax due to any cause depend upon the amount of air collected in the pleural cavity. If the quantity of air in the pleura is small, it is resorbed. Larger volume of air collection in the pleural cavity causes dyspnoea and pain in the chest. Pneumothorax causes lung collapse and pulls the mediastinum to the unaffected side. Occasionally, the defect in the lungs is such that it acts as flap-valve and allows entry of air during inspiration but does not permit its escape during expiration, creating *tension pneumothorax* which requires urgent relief of pressure so as to relieve severe dyspnoea and circulatory failure.

TUMOURS OF PLEURA

Pleural tumours may be primary or secondary. In line with pulmonary tumours, the secondary tumours in the pleura are more common. The only important primary tumour of pleura is mesothelioma.

MESOTHELIOMA

Mesothelioma is an uncommon tumour arising from mesothelial lining of serous cavities, most often in pleural cavity, and rarely in peritoneal cavity and pericardial sac. Mesotheliomas are of 2 types—*benign (solitary) and malignant (diffuse).* The biologic behaviour of pleural mesotheliomas is usually predicted by their gross appearance—those forming solitary, discrete masses are generally benign, whereas those which grow diffusely are usually malignant.

Benign (Solitary) Mesothelioma

Benign or solitary mesothelioma is also called as pleural fibroma. *Asbestos exposure plays no role in etiology of benign mesothelioma.*

Grossly, it consists of a solitary, circumscribed, small, firm mass, generally less than 3 cm in diameter. Cut surface shows whorls of dense fibrous tissue.

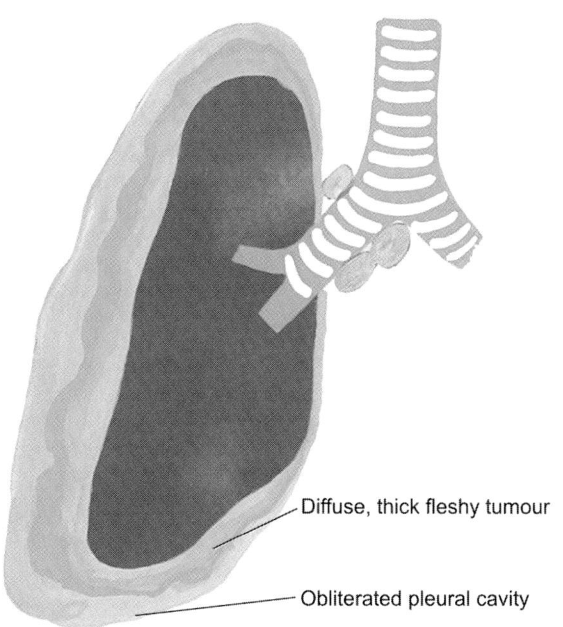

FIGURE 15.32

Malignant (diffuse) mesothelioma, gross appearance. The tumour is seen to form a thick, white, fleshy coat over the parietal and visceral surfaces.

Microscopically, the tumour is predominantly composed of whorls of collagen fibres and reticulin with interspersed fibroblasts. Rarely, mesothelial-lined clefts are seen in the tumour.

Benign mesothelioma causes no symptoms and is detected as an incidental radiologic finding. Sometimes the tumour is associated with systemic syndrome of osteoarthropathy or hypoglycaemia. Removal of the tumour is generally curative.

Malignant (Diffuse) Mesothelioma

Malignant or diffuse mesothelioma is rare. It is a highly malignant tumour associated with high mortality. The tumour is significant in view of its *recognised association with occupational exposure to asbestos* (particularly crocidolite) for a number of years, usually 20 to 40 years (page 501). About 90% of malignant mesotheliomas are asbestos-related. Mechanism of carcinogenicity by asbestos is not quite clear but it appears that prolonged exposure of amphibole type of asbestos is capable of inducing oncogenic mutation in the mesothelium. However, prolonged asbestos-exposure is considered more significant rather than heavy exposure as documented by occurrence of malignant mesothelioma in the family members of asbestos workers. Although combination of cigarette smoking and asbestos exposure greatly increases risk to develop bronchogenic carcinoma, there is no such extra increased risk of developing mesothelioma in asbestos workers who smoke. Recently, SV40 (simian vacuolating virus) antigen has also been implicated in the etiology of mesothelioma.

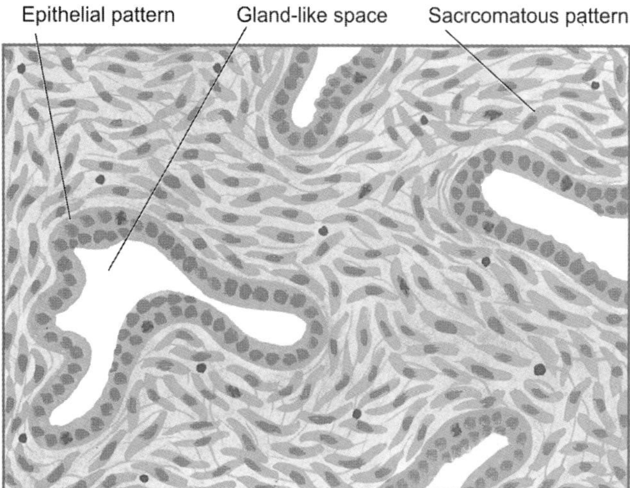

FIGURE 15.33

Malignant mesothelioma, showing biphasic pattern of growth.

Grossly, the tumour is characteristically diffuse, forming a thick, white, fleshy coating over the parietal and visceral surfaces (Fig. 15.32).

Microscopically, malignant mesothelioma may have epithelial, sarcomatoid or biphasic patterns.

i) Epithelial pattern resembles an adenocarcinoma, consisting of tubular and tubulo-papillary formations. The tumour cells are usually well-differentiated, cuboidal, flattened or columnar cells.

ii) Sarcomatoid pattern consists of spindle cell sarcoma resembling fibrosarcoma. The tumour cells are arranged in a storiform pattern with abundant collagen between them.

iii) Biphasic pattern shows mixed growth having epithelial as well as sarcomatoid pattern. Usually, there are slit-like or gland-like spaces lined by neoplastic mesothelial cells separated by proliferating spindle-shaped tumour cells (Fig. 15.33).

Asbestos bodies are found in the lungs of most patients with malignant mesothelioma of any histologic type.

Clinical manifestations include chest pain, dyspnoea, pleural effusion and infections. The tumour spreads rapidly by direct invasion into lung and by lymphatic spread into hilar lymph nodes and pericardium. Sometimes distant metastases, particularly to the liver, occur. The prognosis is poor; 50% of patients die within one year of diagnosis.

SECONDARY PLEURALTUMOURS

Metastatic malignancies in the pleura are more common than the primary tumours and appear as small nodules scattered over the lung surface. The most frequent primary malignant tumours metastasising to the pleura are of the lung and breast through lymphatics, and ovarian cancers via haematogenous route.

The Eye, ENT and Neck

16

EYE

NORMAL STRUCTURE

The structure of the eye is shown diagrammatically in Fig. 16.1. The *eyelids* are covered externally by skin and internally by *conjunctiva* which is reflected over the globe of the eye. The *lacrimal glands* which are compound racemose glands are situated at the outer upper angle of the orbit. The *globe of the eye* is composed of 3 layers: the cornea-sclera, choroid-iris, and retina.

The **cornea** consists of stratified epithelium which may be regarded as continuation of the conjunctiva over the cornea. The subepithelial stroma consists of fibrous connective tissue, and the posterior endothelium-lined thin elastic membrane called Descemet's membrane.

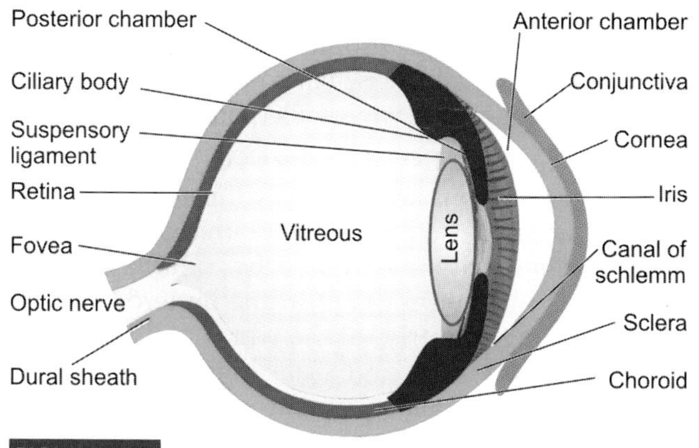

FIGURE 16.1
Schematic diagram of longitudinal section of the eyeball.

The **sclera** is composed of dense fibrous tissue which is thickest at the back of the eyeball.

The **choroid** is the vascular membrane in contact with the sclera. The choroid becomes thickened anteriorly forming ciliary body, ciliary processes and contains ciliary muscle.

The **iris** is the continuation of the choroid which extends in front of the lens. It is similar in structure to the choroid but contains pigment cells.

The **uveal tract** consists of 3 parts—the choroid and ciliary body posteriorly, and the iris anteriorly.

The **retina** is part of the central nervous system and corresponds in extent to the choroid which it lines internally. The retina is composed of a number of layers of cells and their synapses which are of 3 types—external photoreceptor cells (rods and cones), intermediate relay layer of bipolar cells, and internal layer of ganglion cells with their axons running into the central nervous system. The *central fovea* is a specially differentiated spot in the retina posteriorly which consists only of cones in the photoreceptor layer and the other layers are almost absent. *Macula lutea or yellow spot* surrounds the central fovea and though not as sensitive as central fovea, it is more so than the other parts of the retina. At the optic disc, the fibres of the nerve fibre layer of the retina pass into the optic nerve.

The **lens** is the biconvex mass of laminated transparent tissue with elastic capsule.

The **anterior chamber** is the space filled with the aqueous humour, and is bounded by the cornea in front and the iris behind, with anterior surface of the lens exposed in the pupil.

The **posterior chamber** containing aqueous humour is the triangular space between the back of the iris, the anterior surface of the lens and ciliary body forming its apex at the pupillary margin.

The **vitreous chamber** is the large space behind the lens containing gelatinous material, the vitreous humour.

The visual acuity which is the main *function* of the eye, depends upon a transparent focussing system comprised by the cornea, lens, transparent media consisting of aqueous and vitreous humours, and a normal retinal and neural conduction system. The cornea and lens receive their nutrient demands from the aqueous humour produced by the ciliary processes. The intraocular pressure is normally 15-20 mmHg and depends upon the rate of aqueous production and on the resistance in the outflow system.

CONGENITAL LESIONS

RETROLENTAL FIBROPLASIA (RETINOPATHY OF PREMATURITY). This is a developmental disorder occurring in premature infants who have been given oxygen-therapy at birth. The basic defect lies in the developmental prematurity of the retinal blood vessels which are extremely sensitive to high dose of oxygen-therapy. The peripheral retina is incompletely vascularised in such infants and exposure to oxygen results in vaso-obliteration. On stoppage of oxygen-therapy, vasoproliferation begins leading to neovascularisation, cicatrisation and retinal detachment.

RETINITIS PIGMENTOSA. Retinitis pigmentosa is a group of systemic and ocular diseases of unknown etiology, characterised by degeneration of the retinal pigment epithelium. The condition can have various inheritance patterns—autosomal dominant, autosomal recessive trait, or sex-linked recessive trait. The earliest clinical finding is night blindness due to loss of rods and may progress to total blindness.

Histologically, there is disappearance of rods and cones of the photoreceptor layer of the retina, degeneration of retinal pigment epithelium and ingrowth of glial membrane on the optic disc.

INFLAMMATORY CONDITIONS

Inflammatory conditions of the eye are designated according to the tissue affected. 'Uveitis' is the commonly used term for the ocular inflammation of the uveal tract which is the most vascular tissue of the eye. However, specific designation is used for the type of tissue of eye inflamed. Some of the important types are described below.

STYE (HORDEOLUM). Stye or 'external hordeolum' is an acute suppurative inflammation of the sebaceous glands of Zeis, the apocrine glands of Moll and the eyelash follicles. The less common 'internal hordeolum' is an acute suppurative inflammation of the meibomian glands.

CHALAZION. Chalazion is the chronic inflammatory process involving the meibomian glands. It occurs as a result of obstruction to the drainage of secretions. The inflammatory process begins with destruction of meibomian glands and duct and subsequently involves tarsal plate.

Histologically, the chalazion gives the appearance of a chronic inflammatory granuloma located in the tarsus and contains fat globules in the centre of the granulomas (COLOUR PLATE XXI: CL 81).

ENDOPHTHALMITIS. Endophthalmitis is an acute suppurative intraocular inflammation which may be of exogenous or endogenous origin. The exogenous agents may be bacteria, viruses or fungi introduced into the eye during an accidental or surgical perforating wound. The endogenous agents include opportunistic infections which may cause endophthalmitis via haematogenous route e.g. candidiasis, toxoplasmosis, nocardiosis, aspergillosis and cryptococcosis.

CONJUNCTIVITIS AND KERATOCONJUNCTIVITIS. Conjunctiva and cornea are constantly exposed to various types of physical, chemical, microbial (bacteria, fungi, viruses) and allergic agents and hence prone to develop acute, subacute and chronic inflammations. In the acute stage, there is corneal oedema and infiltration by inflammatory cells, affecting the transparency of the cornea. In the more chronic form of inflammation, there is proliferation of small blood vessels in the normally avascular cornea and infiltration by lymphocytes and plasma cells (pannus formation).

TRACHOMA AND INCLUSION CONJUNCTIVITIS. Both these conditions are caused by *Chlamydia* or TRIC agents. Trachoma is caused by *C. trachomatis* while inclusion conjunctivitis is caused by *C. oculogenitalis.* Trachoma is widely prevalent in the underdeveloped and developing countries of the world and is responsible for blindness on a large scale. In the early stage of infection, the trachoma agent that infects the conjunctival epithelium, can be recognised in the smears by the intracytoplasmic inclusion bodies formed by the proliferating microorganisms within the cells. Later, the conjunctiva thickens due to dense chronic inflammatory cell infiltrate alongwith lymphoid follicles and macrophages. The end-result is extensive corneal and conjunctival cicatrisation accounting for blindness in trachoma. Inclusion conjunctivitis, though caused by an organism closely related to trachoma agent, is a much less severe disease and causes mild keratoconjunctivitis.

GRANULOMATOUS UVEITIS. A number of chronic granulomatous conditions may cause granulomatous uveitis. These include bacteria (e.g. tuberculosis, leprosy, syphilis), viruses (e.g. CMV disease, herpes zoster), fungi (e.g. aspergillosis, blastomycosis, phycomycosis, histoplasmosis), and certain parasites (e.g. toxoplasmosis, onchocerciasis). Granulomatous uveitis is common in sarcoidosis as well.

SYMPATHETIC OPHTHALMIA (SYMPATHETIC UVEITIS). This is an uncommon condition in which there is bilateral diffuse granulomatous uveitis following penetrating injury to one eye. The condition probably results from an autosensitivity reaction to injured uveal tissue. It leads to a severe visual loss in both the eyes if not diagnosed and treated early.

Histologically, there is granulomatous uveal inflammation consisting of epithelioid cells and lymphocytes affecting both the eyes. There is no necrosis and no neutrophilic or plasma cell infiltration. If lens is also injured, it results in phacoanaphylactic endophthalmitis.

VASCULAR LESIONS

DIABETIC RETINOPATHY. Diabetic retinopathy is an important cause of blindness. It is related to the degree and duration of glycaemic control. The condition develops in more than 60% of diabetics 15 years or so after the onset of disease, and in about 2% of diabetics causes blindness. Other ocular complications of diabetes include glaucoma, cataract and corneal disease. Most cases of diabetic retinopathy occur over the age of 50 years. The risk is greater in type 1 diabetes mellitus (IDDM) than in type 2 diabetes mellitus, although in clinical practice there are more patients of diabetic retinopathy due to type 2 diabetes mellitus because of its higher prevalence. Women are more prone to diabetes as well as diabetic retinopathy. Diabetic retinopathy is directly correlated with Kimmelstiel-Wilson nephropathy (Chapter 20).

Histologically, two types of changes are described in diabetic retinopathy—background (non-proliferative) and proliferative retinopathy.

1. Background (non-proliferative) retinopathy. This is the initial retinal capillary microangiopathy. The following changes are seen:

i) Basement membrane shows varying thickness due to increased synthesis of basement membrane substance.

ii) Degeneration of pericytes and some loss of endothelial cells are found.

iii) Capillary microaneurysms appear which may develop thrombi and get occluded.

iv) 'Waxy exudates' accumulate in the vicinity of microaneurysms especially in the elderly diabetics because of hyperlipidaemia.

v) 'Dot and blot haemorrhages' in the deeper layers of retina are produced due to diapedesis of erythrocytes.

vi) Soft 'cotton-wool spots' appear on the retina which are microinfarcts of nerve fibre layers. 'Scotomas' appear from degeneration of nerve fibres and ganglion cells.

2. Proliferative retinopathy (retinitis proliferans). After many years, retinopathy becomes proliferative. Severe ischaemia and chronic hypoxia for long period leads to secretion of angiogenic factor by retinal cells and results in the following changes:

i) Neovascularisation of the retina at the optic disc.

ii) Friability of newly-formed blood vessels causes them to bleed easily and results in vitreous haemorrhages.

iii) Proliferation of astrocytes and fibrous tissue around the new blood vessels.

iv) Fibrovascular and gliotic tissue contracts to cause retinal detachment and blindness.

In addition to the changes on retina, severe diabetes may cause diabetic iridopathy with formation of adhesions between iris and cornea (peripheral anterior synechiae) and between iris and lens (posterior synechiae). Diabetics also develop cataract of the lens at an earlier age than the general population.

The pathogenesis of blindness in diabetes mellitus is schematically outlined in Fig. 16.2.

HYPERTENSIVE RETINOPATHY. In hypertensive retinopathy, the retinal arterioles are reduced in their diameter leading to retinal ischaemia. In acute severe hypertension as happens at the onset of malignant hypertension and in toxaemia of pregnancy, the vascular changes are in the form of spasms, while in chronic hypertension the changes are diffuse in the form of

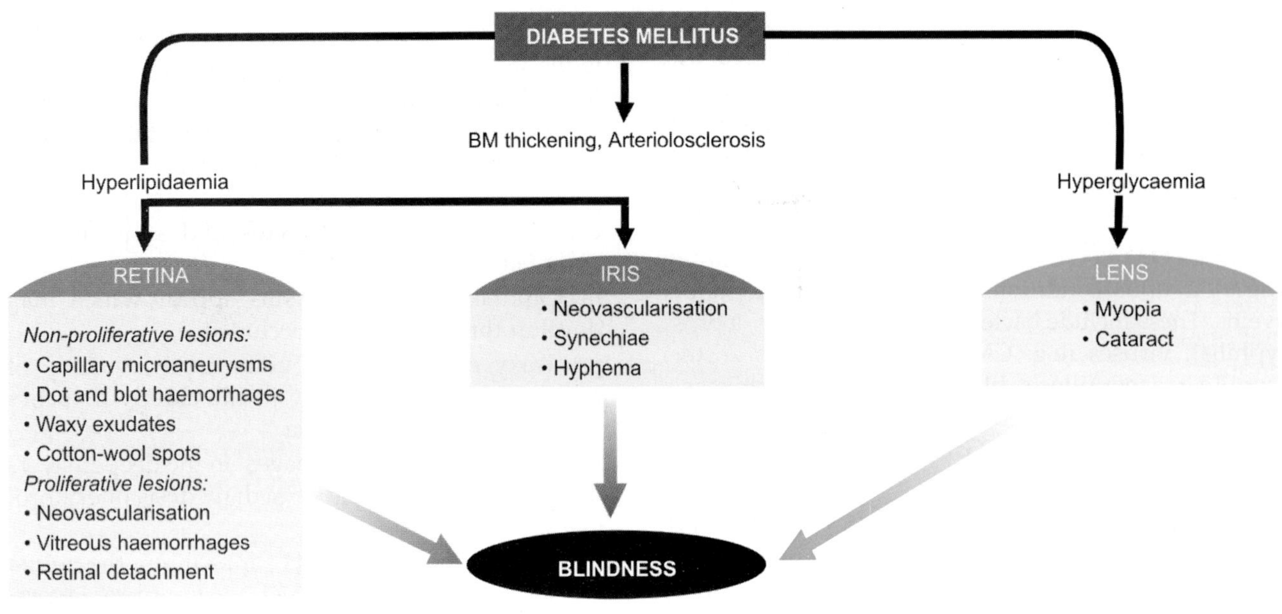

FIGURE 16.2

The effects of diabetes mellitus on eye in causing blindness.

onion-skin thickening of the arteriolar walls with narrowing of the lumina (page 279).

Features of hypertensive retinopathy include the following (Fig. 16.3):

i) Variable degree of arteriolar narrowing due to arteriolosclerosis.

ii) 'Flame-shaped' haemorrhages in the retinal nerve fibre layer.

iii) Macular star i.e. exudates radiating from the centre of macula.

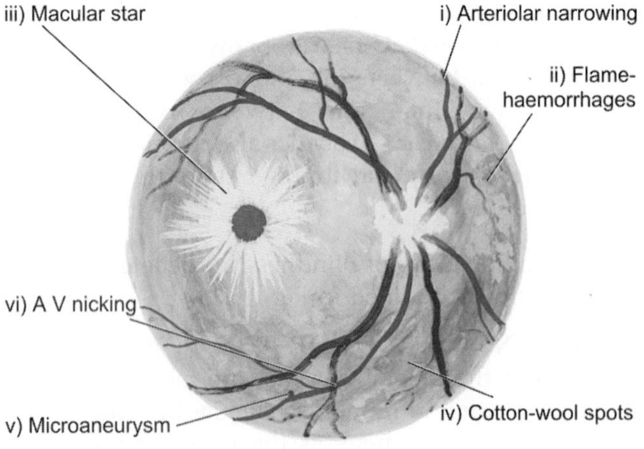

FIGURE 16.3

Ocular lesions in hypertension.

iv) Cotton-wool spots i.e. fluffy white bodies in the superficial layer of retina.

v) Microaneurysms.

vi) Arteriovenous nicking i.e. kinking of veins at sites where sclerotic arterioles cross veins.

vii) Hard exudates due to leakage of lipid and fluid into macula.

Hypertensive retinopathy is classified according to the severity of above lesions from grade I to IV. More serious and severe changes with poor prognosis occur in higher grades of hypertensive retinopathy. Malignant hypertension is characterised by necrotising arteriolitis and fibrinoid necrosis of retinal arterioles.

RETINAL INFARCTS. Infarcts of the retina may result from thrombosis or embolism in central artery of the retina, causing ischaemic necrosis of the inner two-third of the retina while occlusion of the posterior ciliary arteries causes ischaemia of the inner photoreceptor layer only. The usual causes of thrombosis and embolism are atherosclerosis, hypertension and diabetes. Occlusion of the central retinal vein produces haemorrhagic infarction of the entire retina.

MISCELLANEOUS CONDITIONS

PINGUECULA AND PTERYGIUM. Pinguecula is a degenerative condition of the collagen of the bulbar conjunctiva. Clinically, the condition appears as raised yellowish lesions on the interpalpebral bulbar conjunctiva of both eyes in middle-aged and elderly patients.

Histologically, there is characteristic basophilic degeneration of the subepithelial collagen of the conjunctiva. The overlying epithelium may show acanthosis, hyperkeratosis or dyskeratosis.

Pterygium is a lesion closely related to pinguecula but differs from the latter by being located at the limbus and often involves the cornea; hence the lesion is more important clinically.

SENILE MACULAR DEGENERATION. Age-related degeneration of the macular region of the retina is an important cause of bilateral central visual loss in the elderly people.

Histologically, in the early stage, there is irregular thickening of the Bruch's membrane that separates retinal pigment epithelium from the choroid, and there is degeneration of the photoreceptor and pigment epithelium. Later, there is ingrowth of capillaries into the choroid, exudation and haemorrhage under the retina which may eventually get organised and heal by fibrosis and result in permanent loss of central vision.

RETINAL DETACHMENT. Retinal detachment is the separation of the neurosensory retina from the retinal pigment epithelium. Normally, the rods and cones of the photoreceptor layer are interdigitated with projections of the retinal pigment epithelium, but the two can separate readily in many disease processes. There are 3 pathogenetic mechanisms of retinal detachment:

i) Pathologic processes in the vitreous or anterior segment, causing traction on the retina.

ii) Collection of serous fluid in the sub-retinal space from inflammation or tumour in the choroid.

iii) Accumulation of vitreous under the retina through a hole or a tear in the retina.

PHTHISIS BULBI. Phthisis bulbi is the end-stage of advanced degeneration and disorganisation of the entire eyeball in which the intraocular pressure is decreased and the eyeball shrinks. The causes of such end-stage blind eye are trauma, glaucoma and intraocular inflammations.

Histologically, there is marked atrophy and disorganisation of all the ocular structures, and markedly thickened sclera. Even osseous metaplasia may occur.

CATARACT. The cataract is the opacification of the normally crystalline lens. The various causes of cataract are : senility, congenital (e.g. rubella, galactosaemia), traumatic (e.g. penetrating injury, electrical injury) and metabolic (e.g. diabetes). The most common is, however, idiopathic senile cataract.

Histologically, the changes in the cataractous lens are similar irrespective of the underlying cause. The lens fibres undergo degeneration, fragmentation and liquefaction but the central nucleus remains intact because it is quite sclerotic.

GLAUCOMA. Glaucoma is a group of ocular disorders that have in common increased intraocular pressure. Glaucoma is one of the leading causes of blindness because of the ocular tissue damage produced by raised intraocular pressure. In almost all cases, glaucoma occurs due to impaired outflow of aqueous humour, though there is a theoretical possibility of increased production of aqueous by the ciliary body causing glaucoma. The obstruction to the aqueous flow may occur as a result of developmental malformations (**congenital glaucoma**); or due to complications of some other diseases such as uveitis, trauma, intraocular haemorrhage and tumours (**secondary glaucoma**); or may be **primary glaucoma** which is typically bilateral and is the most common type.

Primary glaucoma is of 2 main types—*primary open-angle* (chronic simple glaucoma) and *primary angle-closure* (acute congestive glaucoma). Primary open-angle glaucoma is more common type and is usually a genetically-determined disease. Primary angle-closure glaucoma occurs due to shallow anterior chamber and hence narrow angle causing blockage to aqueous outflow.

In all types of glaucoma, degenerative changes appear after some duration and eventually damage to the optic nerve and retina occurs.

PAPILLOEDEMA. Papilloedema is oedema of the optic disc resulting from increased intracranial pressure. This is due to anatomic continuation of the subarachnoid space of the brain around the optic nerve so that raised intracranial pressure is passed onto the optic disc area. In *acute papilloedema,* there is oedema, congestion and haemorrhage at the optic disc. In *chronic papilloedema,* there is degeneration of nerve fibres, gliosis and optic atrophy.

SJÖGREN'S SYNDROME. Sjögren's syndrome is characterised by triad of keratoconjunctivitis sicca, xerostomia (sicca syndrome) and rheumatoid arthritis. The condition occurs due to immunologically-mediated destruction of the lacrimal and salivary glands alongwith another autoimmune disease (Chapter 4).

MIKULICZ'S SYNDROME. This is characterised by inflammatory enlargement of lacrimal and salivary glands (Chapter 17). The condition may occur with Sjögren's syndrome, or with some diseases like sarcoidosis, leukaemia, lymphoma and macroglobulinaemia.

TUMOURS ANDTUMOUR-LIKE LESIONS

The eye and its adnexal structures are the site of a variety of benign and malignant tumours as well as tumour-like lesions. A brief list of such lesions is given in Table 16.1. The morphology of many of these tumours and tumour-like lesions is identical to similar lesions elsewhere in the body. However, a few examples peculiar to the eye are described below.

Inflammatory Pseudotumours

These are a group of inflammatory enlargements, especially in the orbit, which clinically look like tumours but surgical exploration and pathologic examination fail to reveal any evidence of neoplasm.

PATHOLOGIC CHANGES. Grossly, these lesions are circumscribed and sometimes have fibrous capsule. ***Microscopically,*** many of the lesions can be placed in well-established categories such as tuberculous, syphilitic, mycotic, parasitic, foreign-body granuloma etc, while others show non-specific histologic appearance having abundant fibrous tissue, lymphoid follicles and inflammatory infiltrate with prominence of eosinophils.

Sebaceous Carcinoma

This is the most frequent tumour of the eyelid next only to basal cell carcinoma, although it is very rare tumour elsewhere in the body. It arises either from the meibomian glands in the tarsus or from Zeis' glands of eyelash follicles. The tumour is seen more commonly in the upper eyelid (basal cell carcinoma is seen more frequently in the lower eyelid).

PATHOLOGIC CHANGES. Grossly, the tumour appears as a localised or diffuse swelling of the tarsus, or may be in the form of ulcerated or papillomatous tumour at the lid margin.
Microscopically, the tumour may show well-differentiated lobules of tumour cells with sebaceous differentiation, or may be poorly-differentiated tumour requiring confirmation by fat stains. These tumours can metastasise to the regional lymph nodes as well as to distant sites.

Uveal Malignant Melanoma

Malignant melanomas arising from neural crest-derived pigment epithelium of the uvea is the most common primary ocular malignancy in the white adults in North America and Europe.

TABLE 16.1: Tumours and Tumour-like Lesions of the Eye and Adnexal Structures.

	BENIGN	MALIGNANT
I.	**EYELID**	
	Squamous cell papilloma	Squamous cell carcinoma
	Basal cell papilloma	Basal cell carcinoma
	Sebaceous adenoma	Sebaceous adenocarcinoma
	Naevi	Malignant melanoma
II.	**CONJUNCTIVA-CORNEA**	
	Squamous cell papilloma	Squamous cell carcinoma
	Pseudoepitheliomatous hyperplasia	Mucoepidermoid carcinoma
	Naevi	Malignant melanoma
	Haemangioma	
III.	**LACRIMAL GLAND**	
	Pleomorphic adenoma	Carcinoma in pleomorphic adenoma
IV.	**ORBIT**	
	Glioma	Malignant glioma
	Inflammatory 'pseudotumour'	Malignant lymphoma
	Meningioma	Rhabdomyosarcoma
V.	**INTRAOCULAR**	
	Naevi	Malignant melanoma
	Neurofibroma	Retinoblastoma

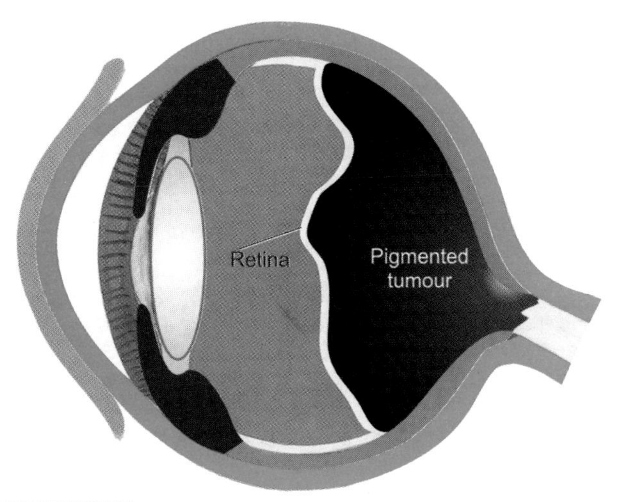

FIGURE 16.4

Choroidal melanoma appearing as a pigmented mass pushing the retina forward over it.

*PATHOLOGIC CHANGES. **Grossly,*** the malignant melanoma appears as a pigmented mass, most commonly in the posterior choroid, and less often in the ciliary body and iris. The mass projects into the vitreous cavity with retina covering it (Fig. 16.4). ***Microscopically,*** age-old classification of Callender (1931) which has prognostic significance is still followed with some modifications:

1. **Spindle A melanoma** is composed of uniform, spindle-shaped cells containing spindled nuclei. Nucleoli are indistinct and mitotic figures are rare. Tumours of this type have the most favourable prognosis (85% 10-year survival).

2. **Spindle B melanoma** is composed of larger and plump spindle-shaped cells with ovoid nuclei. Nucleoli are conspicuous and a few mitotic figures are present. These tumours carry slightly worse prognosis (80% 10-year survival).

3. **Epithelioid melanoma** consists of larger, irregular and pleomorphic cells with larger nuclei and abundant acidophilic cytoplasm. These tumours are the most malignant of the uveal melanomas and have poor prognosis (35% 10-year survival).

4. **Mixed cell type melanomas** have features of spindle cell type as well as of epithelioid cell type. These are more common tumours and carry an intermediate prognosis (45% 10-year survival).

In general, uveal malignant melanomas are usually slow-growing, late metastasising and have a better prognosis than malignant melanoma of the skin (Chapter 24). Uveal melanomas spread via haematogenous route and liver is eventually involved in 90% of cases. Various indicators of bad prognosis include large tumour size and epithelioid cell type.

Retinoblastoma

This is the most common malignant ocular tumour in children. It may be present at birth or recognised in early childhood before the age of 4 years. Retinoblastoma has some peculiar features. About 60% cases of retinoblastoma are sporadic and the remaining 40% are familial. Familial tumours are often multiple and multifocal and transmitted as an autosomal dominant trait by retinoblastoma susceptibility gene *(RB)* located on chromosome 13. Such individuals have a higher incidence of bilateral tumours and have increased risk of developing second primary tumour, particularly osteogenic sarcoma. Retinoblastoma may occur as a congenital tumour too. Clinically, the child presents with leukokoria i.e. white pupillary reflex.

*PATHOLOGIC CHANGES. **Grossly,*** the tumour characteristically appears as a white mass within the retina which may be partly solid and partly necrotic. The tumour may be *endophytic* when it protrudes into the vitreous, or *exophytic* when it grows between the retina and the pigment epithelium (Fig. 16.5). ***Microscopically,*** as the name implies, the tumour is composed of undifferentiated retinal cells with tendency towards formation of photo-receptor elements. In the better differentiated area, the tumour cells are characteristically arranged in rosettes. The rosettes may be of 2 types—*Flexner-Wintersteiner rosettes* characterised by small tumour cells arranged around a lumen with their nuclei away from the lumen, and *Homer-Wright rosettes* having radial arrangement of tumour cells around the central neurofibrillar structure (Fig. 16.6) (**COLOUR PLATE XXI: CL 82**). The tumour shows wide areas of necrosis and calcification and dissemination in all directions—into the vitreous, under the retina, into the optic nerve and even into the brain.

The tumour can spread widely via haematogenous route as well. Prognosis is determined by the extent of local invasion and distant metastasis.

Salient features of retinoblastoma are contrasted with those of uveal melanoma in Table 16.2.

Metastatic Tumours

Ocular metastatic tumours are quite common, choroid being the preferential site for metastasis. Common

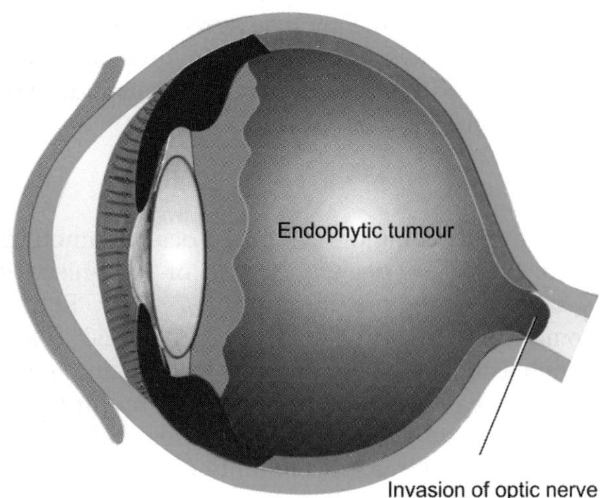

FIGURE 16.5

Retinoblastoma, showing white mass growing extensively within the posterior part of the eye.

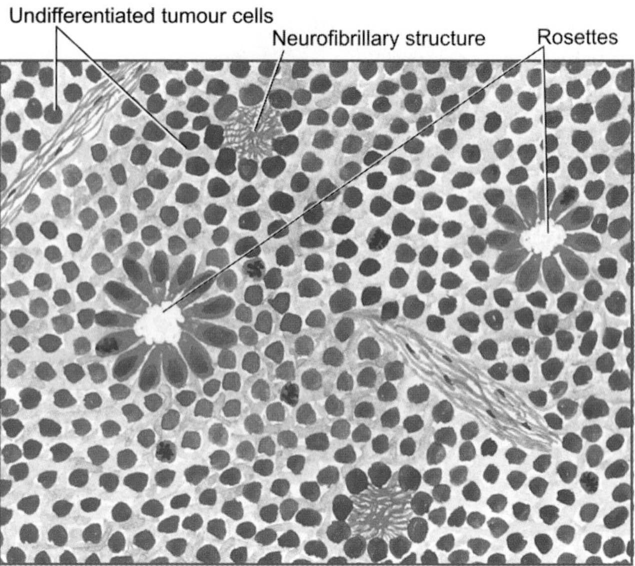

FIGURE 16.6

Retinoblastoma, showing undifferentiated retinal cells and the typical rosettes.

primary tumours that metastasise in the eye are cancers of the breast in women and lung in men. Involvement of the eye by leukaemia and malignant lymphoma is present in some cases.

EAR

NORMAL STRUCTURE

The ear is divided into 3 parts—the external, middle and inner ear.

The **external ear** comprises the auricle or pinna composed of cartilage, the external cartilaginous meatus and the external bony meatus. The external meatus is lined by stratified epithelium which is continued on to the external layer of the tympanic membrane. The tympanic membrane has middle layer of elastic fibrous tissue and the inner layer of mucous membrane and is supported around the periphery by the annulus.

The **middle ear** consists of 3 parts—the uppermost portion is the *attic,* the middle portion is *mesotympanum,* and the lowermost portion is the *hypotympanum.* Besides these, the middle ear has an opening, eustachian tube, the mastoid antrum and cells, and the three ossicles (the malleus, incus and stapes). The middle ear is lined by a single layer of flat ciliated and nonciliated epithelium.

The **inner ear** or labyrinth consists of bony capsule embedded in the petrous bone and contains the membranous labyrinth. The bony capsule consists of 3 parts—posteriorly three semicircular canals, in the middle is the vestibule, and anteriorly contains snail-like cochlea.

TABLE 16.2: Uveal Malignant Melanoma *versus* Retinoblastoma.

FEATURE	MELANOMA	RETINOBLASTOMA
1. *Inheritance*	Rare	About 40% cases
2. *Age*	>50 years	Birth to 4 years
3. *Race*	Common in Caucasians, uncommon in blacks	No predisposition
4. *Location*	Most commonly choroid	Retina
5. *Bilaterality*	Rare	Common (30%)
6. *Cell of origin*	Melanocytes	Retinal neurons
7. *Colour of tumour*	Grey black	Creamy
8. *Spread*	Haematogenous common, rarely via optic nerve	Common via both haematogenous and optic nerve

Besides the *function* of hearing, the stimulation of vestibular labyrinth can cause vertigo, nausea, vomiting and nystagmus.

INFLAMMATORY LESIONS

OTITIS MEDIA. This is the term used for inflammatory involvement of the middle ear. It may be acute or chronic. The usual source of infection is via the eustachian tube and the common causative organisms are *Streptococcus pneumoniae, Haemophilus influenzae* and β-*Streptococcus haemolyticus.* Otitis media may be suppurative, serous or mucoid. Acute suppurative otitis media (SOM) clinically presents as tense and hyperaemic tympanic membrane alongwith pain and tenderness and sometimes mastoiditis as well. Chronic SOM manifests clinically as draining ear with perforated tympanic membrane and partially impaired hearing. Serous or mucoid otitis media refers to non-suppurative accumulation of serous or thick viscid fluid in the middle ear. These collections of fluid are encountered more often in children causing hearing problems and occur due to obstruction of the eustachian tube.

RELAPSING POLYCHONDRITIS. This is an uncommon autoimmune disease characterised by complete loss of glycosaminoglycans resulting in destruction of cartilage of the ear, nose, eustachian tube, larynx and lower respiratory tract.

Histologically, the perichondral areas show acute inflammatory cell infiltrate and destruction and vascularisation of the cartilage. Late stage shows lymphocytic infiltration and fibrous replacement.

CHONDRODERMATITIS NODULARIS CHRONICA HELICIS. This condition involves the external ear superficially and presents as a 'painful nodule of the ear'. The skin in this location is in direct contact with the cartilage without protective subcutaneous layer.

Histologically, the nodule shows epithelial hyperplasia with degeneration of the underlying collagen, chronic inflammatory cell infiltrate, vascular proliferation and fibrosis.

MISCELLANEOUS CONDITIONS

CAULIFLOWER EAR. This is an acquired deformity of the external ear due to degeneration of cartilage as a result of repeated trauma as occurs in boxers and wrestlers.

Histologically, there is destruction of cartilage forming homogeneous matrix (chondromalacia) and fibrous replacement.

OTOSCLEROSIS. This is a dystrophic disease of labyrinth of the temporal bone. The footplate of stapes first undergoes fibrous replacement and is subsequently replaced by sclerotic bone. The exact etiology is not known but the condition has familial preponderance and autosomal dominant trait. It is seen more commonly in young males as a cause for sensori-neural type of deafness.

TUMOURS AND TUMOUR-LIKE LESIONS

Tumours and tumour-like conditions are relatively more common in the external than the middle and inner ear. The lesions seen in the external ear are similar to those seen in the skin e.g. *tumour-like lesions* such as epidermal cyst; *benign tumours* like naevi and squamous cell papilloma; and *malignant tumours* such as basal cell carcinoma, squamous cell carcinoma and malignant melanoma. However, tumours and tumour-like lesions which are specific to the ear are described below. These include: in the external ear—aural (otic) polyps and cerumen-gland tumours; in the middle ear—cholesteatoma (keratoma) and jugular paraganglioma (glomus jugulare tumour); and in the inner ear—acoustic neuroma.

AURAL (OTIC) POLYPS. Aural or otic polyps are tumour-like lesions arising from the middle ear as a complication of the chronic otitis media and project into the external auditory canal.

Histologically, they are composed of chronic inflammatory granulation tissue and are often covered by metaplastic squamous epithelium or pseudostratified columnar epithelium.

CERUMEN-GLAND TUMOURS. Tumours arising from cerumen-secreting apocrine sweat glands of the external auditory canal are cerumen-gland adenomas or cerumen-gland adenocarcinomas and are counterparts of sweat gland tumours (hideradenoma and adenocarcinoma) of the skin discussed in Chapter 24. Both these tumours may invade the temporal bone.

CHOLESTEATOMA (KERATOMA). This is a post-inflammatory 'pseudotumour' found in the middle ear or mastoid air cells. There is invariable history of acute or chronic otitis media. A marginal perforation is generally present through which the squamous epithelium enters the middle ear and results in exfoliation of squamous and formation of the keratin. Rarely, it may be a primary lesion arising from embryonal rests of squamous epithelium in the temporal bone.

Histologically, the lesion consists of cyst containing abundant keratin material admixed with cholesterol crystals and large number of histiocytes. In advanced cases, there may be pressure erosion of the bone.

JUGULAR PARAGANGLIOMA (GLOMUS JUGULARE TUMOUR, NON-CHROMAFFIN PARAGANGLIOMA). Tumours originating from parasympathetic ganglia are called 'paraganglioma' and are named according to the location of the tissue of origin. The one arising from glomus jugulare bodies of the middle ear (jugulotympanic bodies) is called jugular paraganglioma or chemodectoma or non-chromaffin paraganglioma and is the most common benign tumour of the middle ear. Histologically similar tumours are seen in the carotid bodies and vagus (Chapter 25).

Microscopically, the tumour cells containing neurosecretory granules are arranged in typical organoid pattern or nests. The tumour may extend locally to involve the skull and brain but may rarely metastasise.

ACOUSTIC NEUROMA (ACOUSTIC SCHWANNOMA). This is a tumour of Schwann cells of 8th cranial nerve (Chapter 28). It is usually located in the internal auditory canal and cerebellopontine angle. It is a benign tumour similar to other schwannomas but by virtue of its location and large size, may produce compression of the important neighbouring tissues leading to deafness, tinnitus, paralysis of 5th and 7th nerves, compression of the brainstem and hydrocephalus.

NOSE AND PARANASAL SINUSES

NORMAL STRUCTURE

The external nose and the septum are composed of bone and cartilage. On the lateral wall of the nasal cavity, there is a system of 3 ridges on each side known as conchae or turbinates—the inferior, middle and superior. The nasal accessory sinuses are air spaces in the bones of the skull and communicate with the nasal cavity. They are the frontal air sinus, maxillary air sinus and the anterior ethmoid air cells, comprising the *anterior group,* while posterior ethmoidal cells and sphenoidal sinus form the *posterior group.* The anterior group drains into the middle meatus while the posterior group drains into the superior meatus and the sphenoethmoidal recess. Nasal mucous membranes as well as the lining of the nasal sinus is by respiratory epithelium (pseudostratified columnar ciliated cells). Mucous and serous glands underlie the mucous membrane. Besides, the upper and middle turbinate processes and the upper third of the septum are covered with olfactory mucous membrane.

The main physiologic *functions* of the nose are smell, filtration, humidification and warming of the air being breathed.

INFLAMMATORY CONDITIONS

ACUTE RHINITIS (COMMON COLD). Acute rhinitis or common cold is the common inflammatory disorder of the nasal cavities that may extend into the nasal sinuses. It begins with rhinorrhoea, nasal obstruction and sneezing. Initially, the nasal discharge is watery, but later it becomes thick and purulent. The etiologic agents are generally adenoviruses that evoke catarrhal discharge. Chilling of the body is a contributory factor. Secondary bacterial invasion is common. The nasal mucosa is oedematous, red and thickened.

Microscopically, there are numerous neutrophils, lymphocytes, plasma cells and some eosinophils with abundant oedema.

ALLERGIC RHINITIS (HAY FEVER). Allergic rhinitis occurs due to sensitivity to allergens such as pollens. It is an IgE-mediated immune response consisting of an early acute response due to degranulation of mast cells, and a delayed prolonged response in which there is infiltration by leucocytes such as eosinophils, basophils, neutrophils and macrophages accompanied with oedema.

SINUSITIS. Acute sinusitis is generally a complication of acute or allergic rhinitis and rarely secondary to dental sepsis. The ostia are occluded due to inflammation and oedema and the sinuses are full. *'Mucocele'* is filling up of the sinus with mucus while *'empyema'* of the sinus occurs due to collection of pus. Acute sinusitis may become chronic due to incomplete resolution of acute inflammation and from damage to the mucous membrane. Sinusitis may rarely spread to produce osteomyelitis and intracranial infections.

NASAL POLYPS. Nasal polyps are pedunculated grape-like masses of tissue. They are the end-result of prolonged chronic inflammation causing polypoid thickening of the mucosa. They may be *allergic* or *inflammatory.* They are commonly bilateral and the middle turbinate is the common site. *Antrochoanal polyps* originate from the mucosa of the maxillary sinus and appear in the nasal cavity. Morphologically, nasal and antro-choanal polyps are identical.

Grossly, they are gelatinous masses with smooth and shining surface.

Microscopically, they are composed of loose oedematous connective tissue containing some mucous glands and varying number of inflammatory cells like lymphocytes, plasma cells and eosinophils. The polyps are covered by respiratory epithelium which may show squamous metaplasia.

RHINOSPORIDIOSIS. Rhinosporidiosis is caused by a fungus, *Rhinosporidium seeberi.* Typically it occurs in a nasal polyp but may be found in other locations like nasopharynx, larynx and conjunctiva. The disease is common in India and Sri Lanka.

Microscopically, besides the structure of inflammatory or allergic polyp, large number of organisms of the size of erythrocytes with chitinous wall are seen in the thick-walled *sporangia.* Each sporangium may contain a few thousand spores. On rupture of a sporangium, the spores are discharged into the submucosa or on to the surface of the mucosa. The intervening tissue consists of inflammatory granulation tissue (plasma cells, lymphocytes, histiocytes, neutrophils) while the overlying epithelium shows hyperplasia, focal thinning and occasional ulceration (Fig. 16.7) (COLOUR PLATE XXI: CL 83).

RHINOSCLEROMA. This is a chronic destructive inflammatory lesion of the nose and upper respiratory airways caused by diplobacilli, *Klebsiella rhinoscleromatis.* The condition is endemic in parts of Africa, America, South Asia and Eastern Europe. The condition begins as a common cold and progresses to atrophic stage, and then into the nodular stage characterised by small tumour-like submucosal masses.

Histologically, there is extensive infiltration by foamy histiocytes containing the organisms (Mikulicz cells) and other chronic inflammatory cells like lymphocytes and plasma cells.

GRANULOMAS. Many granulomatous inflammations may involve the nose. These include: tuberculosis, leprosy, syphilis, aspergillosis, mucormycosis, Wegener's granulomatosis and lethal midline granuloma.

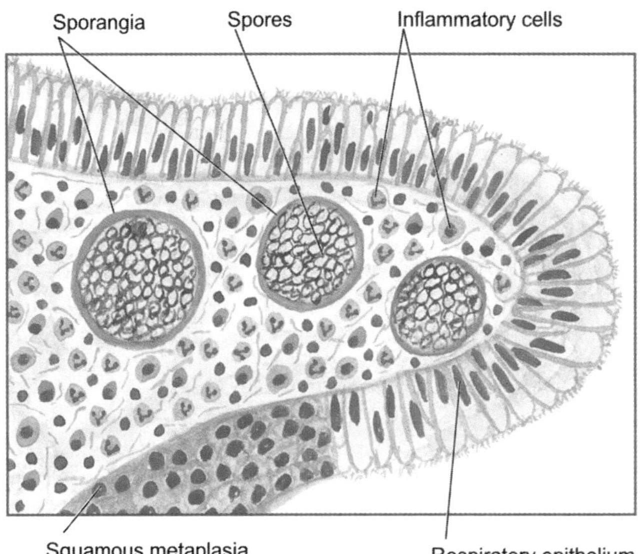

FIGURE 16.7

Rhinosporidiosis in a nasal polyp. The spores are present in sporangia as well as are intermingled in the inflammatory cell infiltrate.

1. **Tuberculosis or lupus** of the nose is uncommon and occurs secondary to pulmonary tuberculosis and usually produces ulcerative lesions on the anterior part of the septum of the nose.

2. **Leprosy** begins as a nodule that may ulcerate and perforate the septum.

3. **Syphilis** may involve the nose in congenital form causing destruction of the septum, or in acquired tertiary syphilis in the form of gummas perforating the septum. In either case, characteristic saddle-nose deformity occurs due to collapse of bridge of the nose.

4. **Aspergillosis** may involve the paranasal sinuses where the septate hyphae grow to form a mass called *aspergilloma.*

5. **Mucormycosis** is an opportunistic infection caused by *Mucorales* which are non-septate hyphae and involve the nerves and blood vessels.

6. **Wegener's granulomatosis** is a form of necrotising vasculitis with granuloma formation affecting the upper respiratory tract, lungs and kidneys. In 15-50% of cases, the condition may evolve into malignant lymphoma.

7. **Lethal midline granuloma or polymorphic reticulosis** is a rare and lethal lesion of the upper respiratory tract that causes extensive destruction of cartilage and necrosis of tissues and does not respond to antibiotic treatment. Besides the necrosis, lymphoid infiltrates of

pleomorphic and atypical cells admixed with small lymphocytes, plasma cells and macrophages are seen. Currently, the condition is considered to be a T cell lymphoma that may respond to chemotherapy and radiotherapy (page 457).

TUMOURS

The tumours of nose, nasal cavity and paranasal sinuses are uncommon. However, benign and malignant tumours of epithelial as well as mesenchymal origin can occur.

Benign Tumours

1. **CAPILLARY HAEMANGIOMA.** Capillary haemangioma of the septum of nose is a common benign lesion (COLOUR PLATE XIII: CL 52). If the surface is ulcerated and the lesion contains inflammatory cell infiltrate, it resembles inflammatory granulation tissue and is called *'haemangioma of granulation tissue type'* or *'granuloma pyogenicum'*.

2. **PAPILLOMAS.** Papillomas may occur in the nasal vestibule, nasal cavity and paranasal sinuses. They are mainly of 2 types—*fungiform papilloma* with exophytic growth, and *inverted papilloma* with everted growth. Each of these may be lined with various combinations of epithelia: respiratory, squamous and mucous type.

Malignant Tumours

1. **OLFACTORY NEUROBLASTOMA OR ESTHESIONEUROBLASTOMA.** It occurs over the olfactory mucosa as a polypoid mass that may invade the paranasal sinuses or skull. It is a highly malignant small cell tumour of neural crest origin that may, at times, be indistinguishable from other small cell malignancies like rhabdomyosarcoma, undifferentiated carcinoma, lymphoma or Ewing's sarcoma. Rosettes are found in about 10% of tumours.

2. **CARCINOMAS.** Majority of carcinomas of the nasal cavity and paranasal sinuses are squamous cell carcinomas. They are seen more commonly in the elderly with history of heavy smoking and severe chronic sinusitis, in nickel refinery workers and in wood workers. The tumour extends locally to involve the surrounding bone and soft tissues and also metastasises widely. Other types of malignancies found uncommonly in this location are: adenocarcinoma, adenoid cystic carcinoma, mucoepidermoid carcinoma, small cell carcinoma, lymphoma and malignant melanoma.

PHARYNX

NORMAL STRUCTURE

The pharynx has 3 parts—the nasopharynx, oropharynx (pharynx proper) and the laryngopharynx. The whole of pharynx is lined by stratified squamous epithelium. The lymphoid tissue of the pharynx is comprised by the tonsils and adenoids.

INFLAMMATORY CONDITIONS

LUDWIG'S ANGINA. This is a severe, acute streptococcal cellulitis involving the neck, tongue and back of the throat. The condition was more common in the pre-antibiotic era as a complication of compound fracture of the mandible and periapical infection of the molars. The condition often proves fatal due to glottic oedema, asphyxia and severe toxaemia.

VINCENT'S ANGINA. Vincent's angina is a painful condition of the throat characterised by local ulceration of the tonsils, mouth and pharynx. The causative organism is *Vincent's bacillus.* The condition may occur as an acute illness involving the tissues diffusely, or as chronic form consisting of ulceration of the tonsils.

DIPHTHERIA. Diphtheria is an acute communicable disease caused by *Corynebacterium diphtheriae.* It usually occurs in children and results in the formation of a yellowish-grey *pseudomembrane* in the mucosa of nasopharynx, oropharynx, tonsils, larynx and trachea. *C. diphtheriae* elaborates an exotoxin that causes necrosis of the epithelium which is associated with abundant fibrinopurulent exudate resulting in the formation of pseudomembrane. Absorption of the exotoxin in the blood may lead to more distant injurious effects such as myocardial necrosis, polyneuritis, parenchymal necrosis of the liver, kidney and adrenals. The constitutional symptoms such as fever, chills, malaise, obstruction of the airways and dyspnoea are quite marked. The condition has to be distinguished from the membrane of streptococcal infection.

TONSILLITIS. Tonsillitis caused by staphylococci or streptococci may be acute or chronic. *Acute tonsillitis* is characterised by enlargement, redness and inflammation. Acute tonsillitis may progress to acute follicular tonsillitis in which crypts are filled with debris and pus giving it follicular appearance. *Chronic tonsillitis* is caused by repeated attacks of acute tonsillitis in which case the tonsils are small and fibrosed. Acute tonsillitis may pass on to tissues adjacent to tonsils to form peritonsillar abscess or *quinsy.*

PERITONSILLAR ABSCESS (QUINSY). Peritonsillar abscess or quinsy occurs as a complication of acute tonsillitis. The causative organisms are staphylococci or streptococci which are associated with infection of the tonsils. The patient complains of acute pain in the throat, trismus, difficulty in speech and inability to swallow. The glands behind the angle of the mandible are enlarged and tender. Besides the surgical management of the abscess, the patient must be advised tonsillectomy because quinsy is frequently recurrent.

RETROPHARYNGEAL ABSCESS. Formation of abscess in the soft tissue between the posterior wall of the pharynx and the vertebral column is called retropharyngeal abscess. It occurs due to infection of the retropharyngeal lymph nodes. It is found in debilitated children. A chronic form of the abscess in the same location is seen in tuberculosis of the cervical spine *(cold abscess).*

TUMOURS

There are 3 main tumours of note in the pharynx—nasopharyngeal angiofibroma, nasopharyngeal carcinoma, and malignant lymphoma.

NASOPHARYNGEAL ANGIOFIBROMA. This is a peculiar tumour that occurs exclusively in adolescent males (10-20 years of age) suggesting the role of testosterone hormone in its production. Though a benign tumour of the nasopharynx, it may grow into paranasal sinuses, cheek and orbit but does not metastasise.

Microscopically, the tumour is composed of 2 components as the name suggests—numerous small endothelium-lined vascular spaces and the stromal cells which are myofibroblasts.

NASOPHARYNGEAL CARCINOMA. Nasopharyngeal carcinoma has 3 histologic variants:
i) Non-keratinising squamous cell carcinoma
ii) Keratinising squamous cell carcinoma
iii) Undifferentiated (transitional cell) carcinoma

Microscopically, non-keratinisng and keratinising squamous cell carcinomas are identical in morphology to typical tumours in other locations. The undifferentiated carcinoma, also called as transitional cell carcinoma, is characterised by masses and cords of cells which are polygonal to spindled and have large vesicular nuclei. A variant of undifferentiated carcinoma is *'lymphoepithelioma'* in which undifferentiated carcinoma is infiltrated by abundant non-neoplastic mature lymphocytes (COLOUR PLATE XXI: CL 84).

Nasopharyngeal carcinoma is a common cancer in South-East Asia, especially prevalent in people of Chinese descent under 45 years of age. Genetic susceptibility and role of Epstein-Barr virus are considered important factors in its etiology (page 229). In fact, EBV-genome is found virtually in all cases of nasopharyngeal carcinoma unlike Burkitt's lymphoma, another EBV-associated tumour. The primary tumour is generally small and undetected, while the metastatic deposits in the cervical lymph nodes may be large. The prognosis is usually fatal. Undifferentiated carcinoma is radiosensitive.

MALIGNANT LYMPHOMA. The lymphoid tissue of the nasopharynx and tonsils may be the site for development of malignant lymphomas which resemble similar tumours elsewhere in the body.

LARYNX

NORMAL STRUCTURE

The larynx is composed of cartilages which are bound together by ligaments and muscles and is covered by mucous membrane. The cartilages of the larynx are of 2 types—unpaired and paired.

The *unpaired laryngeal cartilages* are epiglottis, thyroid cartilage (Adam's apple) and cricoid cartilage.

The *paired cartilages* are the arytenoid cartilages which play important part in the movement of vocal cords.

The larynx as well as trachea are lined by respiratory epithelium, except over the true vocal cords and the epiglottis, which are lined by stratified squamous epithelium.

INFLAMMATORY CONDITIONS

ACUTE LARYNGITIS. This may occur as a part of the upper or lower respiratory tract infection. Atmospheric pollutants like cigarette smoke, exhaust fumes, industrial and domestic smoke etc predispose the larynx to acute bacterial and viral infections. *Streptococci* and *H. influenzae* cause acute epiglottitis which may be life-threatening. Acute laryngitis may occur in some other illnesses like typhoid, measles and influenza. Acute pseudomembranous (Diphtheric) laryngitis occurs due to infection with *C. diphtheriae.*

CHRONIC LARYNGITIS. Chronic laryngitis may occur from repeated attacks of acute inflammation, excessive smoking, chronic alcoholism or vocal abuse. The surface is granular due to swollen mucous glands. There may be extensive squamous metaplasia due to heavy smoking, chronic bronchitis and atmospheric pollution.

TUBERCULOUS LARYNGITIS. Tuberculous laryngitis occurs secondary to pulmonary tuberculosis. Typical caseating tubercles are present on the surface of the larynx.

ACUTE OEDEMA OF THE LARYNX. This hazardous condition is an acute inflammatory condition, causing swelling of the larynx that may lead to airway obstruction and death by suffocation. Acute laryngeal oedema may occur due to trauma, inhalation of irritants, drinking hot fluids or may be infective in origin.

TUMOURS

Both benign and malignant tumours occur in the larynx. The common examples of benign tumours are papillomas and polyps, while laryngeal carcinoma is an important example amongst malignant tumours.

LARYNGEAL PAPILLOMAS. These tumours are found more frequently in children between 1 and 6 years of age and are often multiple, while the adults have usually a single lesion. Multiple juvenile papillomas may undergo spontaneous regression at puberty. *Papova* group of viruses (human papilloma virus, HPV) have been implicated in the etiology of papillomas of the larynx.

Grossly, the lesions appear as warty growths on the true vocal cords.
Microscopically, papillomas are composed of finger-like papillae, each papilla contains fibrovascular core covered by stratified squamous epithelium.

LARYNGEAL POLYPS. Laryngeal polyps are seen mainly in adults and are found more often in heavy smokers and in individuals subjected to vocal abuse. Therefore, they are known by various synonyms like singers' nodes, preachers' node, and screamers' nodes. The patients have characteristic progressive hoarseness.

Grossly, it is a small lesion, less than 1 cm in diameter, rounded, smooth, usually sessile and polypoid swelling on the true vocal cords.
Microscopically, the nodules have prominent oedema with sparse fibrous tissue and numerous irregular and dilated vascular channels. Sometimes, the subepithelial basement membrane is thickened, resembling amyloid material.

LARYNGEAL CARCINOMA. Cancer of the larynx in 99% of cases is squamous cell carcinoma. Rarely, adenocarcinoma and sarcoma are encountered. Squamous carcinoma of the larynx occurs in males beyond 4th decade of life. Important etiologic factor is heavy smoking of cigarettes, cigar or pipe; other factors include excessive alcohol consumption, radiation and asbestos exposure. Carcinoma of the larynx is conventionally classified into *extrinsic* that arises or extends outside the larynx, and *intrinsic* that arises within the larynx. However, based on the anatomic location, laryngeal carcinoma is classified as under:

1. *Glottic* is the most common location, found in the region of true vocal cords and anterior and posterior commissures.
2. *Supraglottic* involving ventricles and arytenoids.
3. *Subglottic* in the walls of subglottis.
4. *Marginal zone* between the tip of epiglottis and aryepiglottic folds.
5. *Laryngo-(hypo-) pharynx* in the pyriform fossa, postcricoid fossa and posterior pharyngeal wall.

Grossly, the glottic carcinoma is the most common form and appears as a small, pearly white, plaque-like thickening that may be ulcerated or fungated.
Microscopically, keratinising and non-keratinising squamous carcinomas of varying grades are found. Generally, carcinoma of the supraglottic and subglottic regions tends to be more poorly-differentiated than the glottic tumour. Besides the keratinising and non-keratinising squamous carcinoma, 2 special varieties of squamous carcinoma in the larynx are: *verrucous carcinoma* which is a well-differentiated squamous carcinoma, and *spindle cell carcinoma* which has elongated tumour cells resembling sarcoma (pseudosarcoma).

Cervical lymph node metastasis of laryngeal carcinoma are found in a good proportion of cases at the time of diagnosis. Death from laryngeal cancer occurs due to local extension of growth into vital structures like trachea and carotid artery; other causes are bacterial infection, aspiration pneumonia, debility and disseminated metastases.

NECK

NORMAL STRUCTURE

The neck is the region from where important structures like oesophagus, trachea, carotid arteries, great veins and nerve trunks pass down. Besides, the neck has structures such as carotid body, sympathetic ganglia, larynx, thyroid, parathyroids and lymph nodes. Only the tumours and cysts of the neck are considered here while the lesions pertaining to other anatomic structures are described elsewhere in the textbook.

CYSTS OF NECK

The cysts of neck may be medial (midline) or lateral (Table 16.3).

I. Medial (Midline) Cervical Cysts

1. THYROGLOSSAL CYST. Thyroglossal cyst arises from the vestiges of thyroglossal duct that connects the foramen caecum at the base of the tongue with the normally located thyroid gland. The cyst is located in the midline, generally at the level of hyoid bone, and rarely at the base of the tongue.

Microscopically, the cyst is lined by respiratory and/ or stratified squamous epithelium.

2. MIDLINE DERMOID CYST. Dermoid cyst located in the midline of the neck occurs due to sequestration of dermal cells along the lines of closure of embryonic clefts. The cyst contains paste-like pultaceous material.

Microscopically, it is lined by epidermis and may contain skin adnexal structures.

II. Lateral Cervical Cysts

1. BRANCHIAL (LYMPHOEPITHELIAL) CYST. Branchial or lymphoepithelial cyst arises from incomplete closure of 2nd or 3rd branchial clefts. The cyst is generally located anterior to the sternocleidomastoid muscle near the angle of the mandible. The cyst is 1-3 cm in diameter and is filled with serous or mucoid material.

Microscopically, the cyst is lined by stratified squamous or respiratory epithelium, covering subepithelial lymphoid tissue aggregates or follicles with germinal centres.

TABLE 16.3: Cysts of the Neck.

I. *Medial (midline) cysts*
   1. Thyroglossal cyst
   2. Midline dermoid cyst

II. *Lateral cervical cysts*
   1. Branchial (lymphoepithelial) cyst
   2. Parathyroid cyst
   3. Cervical thymic cyst
   4. Cystic hygroma

2. PARATHYROID CYST. Parathyroid cyst is a lateral cyst of the neck usually located deep to the sternocleidomastoid muscle at the angle of the mandible. These may be microscopic cysts or larger. They are generally thin-walled, filled with clear watery fluid.

Microscopically, parathyroid cyst is lined by flattened cuboidal to low columnar epithelium and the cyst wall may contain any type of parathyroid cells.

3. CERVICAL THYMIC CYST. Cervical thymic cyst originates from cystic degeneration of Hassall's corpuscles. It is generally located in the left lateral side of the neck.

Microscopically, the cyst is lined by stratified squamous epithelium and the cyst wall may contain thymic structures.

4. CYSTIC HYGROMA. Cystic hygroma is a lateral swelling at the root of the neck, usually located behind the sternocleidomastoid muscle. It may be present congenitally or may manifest in the first 2 years of life. It is usually multilocular and may extend into the mediastinum and pectoral region.

Microscopically, cystic hygroma is a diffuse lymphangioma containing large cavernous spaces lined by endothelium and containing lymph fluid (page 301).

TUMOURS

Tumours of the neck may be primary or metastatic in cervical lymph nodes.

I. Primary Tumours

A few important examples of primary tumours in the neck are carotid body tumour, torticollis and malignant lymphomas.

1. CAROTID BODY TUMOUR (CHEMODECTOMA, CAROTID BODY PARAGANGLIOMA). Carotid body tumour arises in the carotid bodies which are situated at the bifurcation of the common carotid arteries. Carotid bodies are normally part of the chemoreceptor system and the cells of this system are sensitive to changes in the pH and arterial oxygen tension and are also the storage site for catecholamines. Histologically similar tumours are found in other parasympathetic ganglia represented by the vagus and glomus jugulare (jugulotympanic bodies, Chapter 25). Carotid body paragangliomas, as they are currently called, are rare tumours and occur between 3rd and 6th decades of life with slight female preponderance. A few (5%) are bilateral and some show familial incidence.

Grossly, they are small, firm, dark tan, encapsulated nodules.

Microscopically, well-differentiated tumour cells form characteristic organoid or alveolar pattern, as is the case with all other neuroendocrine tumours. The tumour cells contain dark neurosecretory granules containing catecholamines.

These tumours are mostly benign but recurrences are frequent and about 10% may metastasise widely.

2. TORTICOLLIS (FIBROMATOSIS COLLI, WRY NECK). This is a deformity in which the head is bent to one side while the chin points to the other side. The deformity may occur as congenital torticollis or may be an acquired form. The *acquired form* may occur secondary to fracture dislocation of the cervical spine, Pott's disease of the cervical spine, scoliosis, spasm of the muscles of neck, exposure to chill causing myositis, and contracture following burns or wound healing. The *congenital or primary torticollis* appears at birth or within the first few weeks of life as a firm swelling in the lower third of the sternocleidomastoid muscle. The etiology is unknown but about half the cases are associated with breech delivery.

Grossly, the muscle is contracted, shortened and fibrous.

Microscopically, abundant dense fibrous tissue separates the muscle fibres.

3. MALIGNANT LYMPHOMAS. Various forms of non-Hodgkin's lymphomas and Hodgkin's disease occur in the cervical lymph nodes which are described in Chapter 14.

II. Secondary Tumours

Cervical lymph nodes are common site for metastases of a large number of carcinomas. These include: squamous cell carcinoma of the lips, mouth, tongue, larynx and oesophagus; transitional cell carcinoma of the pharynx and nasopharynx; thoracic and abdominal cancers such as of stomach, lungs, ovaries, uterus and testis.

The Oral Cavity and Salivary Glands

17

ORAL SOFT TISSUES

NORMAL STRUCTURE

The oral cavity is the point of entry for digestive and respiratory tracts. The mucous membrane of the mouth consists of squamous epithelium covering vascularised connective tissue. The epithelium is keratinised over the hard palate, lips and gingiva, while elsewhere it is non-keratinised. Mucous glands (minor salivary glands) are scattered throughout the oral mucosa. Sebaceous glands are present in the region of the lips and the buccal mucosa only. Lymphoid tissue is present in the form of tonsils and adenoids.

The oral cavity is the site of numerous congenital and acquired diseases. Besides, many systemic diseases have oral manifestations. Some of the commonly occurring conditions are discussed here.

DEVELOPMENTAL ANOMALIES

1. FACIAL CLEFTS. *Cleft upper lip (harelip) and cleft palate,* alone or in combination, are the commonest developmental anomalies of the face. These occur from the failure of fusion of facial processes.

2. FORDYCE'S GRANULES. Fordyce's granules are symmetric, small, light yellow macular spots on the lips and buccal mucosa and represent collections of sebaceous glands. They remain undeveloped until puberty but occur quite commonly in adults.

3. LEUKOEDEMA. This is an asymptomatic condition occurring in children and is characterised by symmetric, grey-white areas on the buccal mucosa. ***Histologically,*** there is pronounced intracellular oedema. There is no increased malignant potential compared to leukoplakia discussed below.

4. DEVELOPMENTAL DEFECTS OF THE TONGUE. These are as under:

i) Macroglossia is the enlargement of the tongue, usually due to lymphangioma or haemangioma, and sometimes due to amyloid tumour.

ii) Microglossia and aglossia are rare congenital anomalies representing small-sized and absence of tongue respectively.

iii) Fissured tongue (scrotal, furrowed or grooved tongue) is a genetically-determined condition characterised by numerous small furrows or grooves on the dorsum of the tongue. It is often associated with mild glossitis.

iv) Bifid tongue is a rare condition occurring due to failure of the two lateral halves of the tongue to fuse in the midline.

v) Tongue tie occurs when the lingual fraenum is quite short, or when the fraenum is attached near the tongue tip.

vi) Hairy tongue is not a true developmental defect, but is mentioned here alongwith other similar conditions. The filiform papillae are hypertrophied and elongated. These 'hairs' are stained black, brown or yellowish-white by food, tobacco, oxidising agents or by oral flora.

MUCOCUTANEOUS LESIONS

Lesions of the oral mucosa occur in many diseases of the skin discussed in Chapter 24. Some of these are as under:

1. LICHEN PLANUS. Characteristically, oral lichen planus appears as interlacing network of whitening or keratosis on the buccal mucosa.

2. VESICULAR LESIONS. A number of vesicular or bullous diseases of the skin have oral lesions.

i) Pemphigus vulgaris. Vesicular oral lesions appear invariably in all cases at some time in the course of pemphigus vulgaris. In about half the cases oral lesions are the initial manifestations.

ii) Pemphigoid. Vesicles or bullae appear on oral mucosa as well as on conjunctiva in pemphigoid and are seen more often in older women.

iii) Erythema multiforme. Subepithelial vesicles may occur on the skin as well as mucosae.

iv) Stevens-Johnson syndrome is a rather fatal and severe form of erythema multiforme involving oral and other mucous membranes occurring following ingestion of sulfa drugs.

v) Epidermolysis bullosa is a hereditary condition having subepidermal bullae on the skin as well as has oral lesions.

INFLAMMATORY DISEASES

1. STOMATITIS. Inflammation of the mucous membrane of the mouth is called stomatitis. It can occur in the course of many different diseases.

i) Aphthous ulcers (Canker sores) is the commonest form of oral ulceration. The etiology is unknown but may be precipitated by emotional factors, stress, allergy, hormonal imbalance, nutritional deficiencies, gastrointestinal disturbances, trauma etc. The condition is characterised by painful oral ulcers, 1 cm or more in size. Recurrent *aphthae* may form a part of Behcet's syndrome and inflammatory bowel disease.

ii) Herpetic stomatitis is an acute disease occurring in infants and young children. It is the most common manifestation of primary infection with herpes simplex virus. The lesions are in the form of vesicles around the lips. Similar lesions may appear on the genital skin. Recurrent attacks occur due to stress, emotional upsets and upper respiratory infections.

iii) Necrotising stomatitis (Noma or Cancrum oris) occurs more commonly in poorly-nourished children like in kwashiorkor; infectious diseases such as measles; immunodeficiencies and emotional stress. The lesions are characterised by necrosis of the marginal gingiva and may extend on to oral mucosa, causing cellulitis of the tissue of the cheek. The condition may progress to gangrene of the cheek.

iv) Mycotic infections commonly involving the oral mucosa are actinomycosis and candidiasis.

- *Cervicofacial actinomycosis* is the commonest form of the disease developing at the angle of the mandible (Chapter 6).
- *Candidiasis (moniliasis or thrush)* is caused by *Candida albicans* which is a commensal in the mouth. It appears as an opportunistic infection in immunocompromised host. There are erythematous lesions on the palate and angular cheilitis.

2. GLOSSITIS. Acute glossitis characterised by swollen papillae occurs in eruptions of measles and scarlet fever. In **chronic glossitis,** the tongue is raw and red without swollen papillae and is seen in malnutrition such as in pellagra, ariboflavinosis and niacin deficiency. In iron deficiency anaemia, pernicious anaemia and sprue, there is *chronic atrophic glossitis* characterised by atrophied papillae and smooth raw tongue.

3. SYPHILITIC LESIONS. Oral lesions may occur in primary, secondary, tertiary and congenital syphilis (Chapter 6).

i) Extragenital chancre of *primary syphilis* occurs most commonly on the lips.

ii) Secondary syphilis shows maculopapular eruptions and mucous patches in the mouth.

iii) In the *tertiary syphilis,* gummas or diffuse fibrosis may be seen on the hard palate and tongue.

iv) Oral lesions of the *congenital syphilis* are fissures at the angles of mouth and characteristic peg-shaped notched Hutchinson's incisors (Chapter 6).

4. TUBERCULOUS LESIONS. Involvement of the mouth in tuberculosis is rare. The lesions are in the form of ulcers or elevated nodules.

5. HIV INFECTION. HIV infection of low grade as well as full-blown acquired immunodeficiency syndrome (AIDS) are associated with oral manifestations such as opportunistic infections, malignancy, hairy leukoplakia and others (Table 17.1). About half the cases of Kaposi's sarcoma have intraoral lesions as part of systemic involvement (Chapter 6).

PIGMENTARY LESIONS

Oral and labial melanotic pigmentation may be observed in certain systemic and metabolic disorders such as Addison's disease, Albright syndrome, Peutz-Jeghers syndrome and haemochromatosis. All types of pigmented naevi as well as malignant melanoma can occur in oral cavity. Exogenous pigmentation such as due to deposition of lead sulfide can also occur.

TUMOURS AND TUMOUR-LIKE LESIONS

Benign and malignant tumours of various types and also a number of tumour-like lesions and premalignant lesions are encountered in the oral soft tissues. A list of such lesions is presented in Table 17.2.

A. TUMOUR-LIKE LESIONS

A number of proliferative lesions arising from the oral tissues are tumour-like masses which clinically may resemble neoplasms. Some of these are as under:

TABLE 17.1: Oral Manifestations of AIDS.

A. OPPORTUNISTIC INFECTIONS		
Fungal	:	Candidiasis (oral thrush) Histoplasmosis Cryptococcosis
Bacterial	:	Dental caries and periodontitis Mycobacterial infections
Viral	:	Herpetic stomatitis Cytomegalovirus Human papilloma virus
B. TUMOURS		
		Kaposi's sarcoma Squamous cell carcinoma Non-Hodgkin's lymphoma
C. OTHERS		
	Hairy leukoplakia Recurrent aphthous ulcers	

TABLE 17.2: Classification of Tumours and Tumour-like Lesions of the Oral Soft Tissues.

A. TUMOUR-LIKE LESIONS
1. Fibrous growths
   (Fibroepithelial polyps, fibrous epulis, denture hyperplasia)
2. Pyogenic granuloma
3. Mucocele
4. Ranula
5. Dermoid cyst

B. BENIGN TUMOURS
1. Squamous papilloma
2. Haemangioma
3. Lymphangioma
4. Fibroma
5. Fibromatosis gingivae
6. Tumours of minor salivary glands
   (e.g. Pleomorphic adenoma)
7. Granular cell myoblastoma
8. Other rare benign tumours

C. PREMALIGNANT LESIONS
1. Hyperkeratotic leukoplakia
2. Dysplastic leukoplakia

D. MALIGNANT TUMOURS
1. Squamous cell (Epidermoid) carcinoma
2. Other malignant tumours

1. FIBROUS GROWTHS. Fibrous growths of the oral soft tissues are very common. These are not true tumours (unlike intraoral fibroma and papilloma), but are instead inflammatory or irritative in origin. A few common varieties are as under:

i) Fibroepithelial polyps occur due to irritation or chronic trauma. These are composed of reparative fibrous tissue, covered by a thin layer of stratified squamous epithelium.

ii) Fibrous epulis is a lesion occurring on the gingiva and is localised hyperplasia of the connective tissue following trauma or inflammation in the area.

iii) Denture hyperplasia occurs in edentulous or partly edentulous patients. The lesion is an inflammatory hyperplasia in response to local irritation by ill-fitting denture or an elongated tooth.

2. PYOGENIC GRANULOMA. This is an elevated, bright red swelling of variable size occurring on the lips, tongue, buccal mucosa and gingiva. It is a vaso-proliferative inflammatory lesion. *Pregnancy tumour* is a variant of pyogenic granuloma.

3. MUCOCELE. Also called mucous cyst, it is a cystic dilatation of the mucous glands of the oral mucosa.

The cyst often ruptures on distension and incites inflammatory reaction.

4. **RANULA.** It is a large mucocele located on the floor of the mouth. The cyst is lined by true epithelial lining.

5. **DERMOID CYST.** This tumour-like mass in the floor of the mouth represents a developmental malformation. The cyst is lined by stratified squamous epithelium. The cyst wall contains sebaceous glands, sweat glands, hair follicles and other mature tissues.

B. BENIGN TUMOURS

Different parts of the mouth have a variety of mesodermal tissues and keratinising and non-keratinising epithelium. Therefore, the majority of neoplasms arising from the oral tissues are just like their counterparts in other parts of the body. Some of the common benign tumours of the mouth are as under:

1. **SQUAMOUS PAPILLOMA.** Papilloma can occur anywhere in the mouth and has the usual papillary or finger-like projections.

Microscopically, each papilla is composed of vascularised connective tissue covered by squamous epithelium.

2. **HAEMANGIOMA.** Haemangioma can occur anywhere in the mouth; when it occurs on tongue it may cause macroglossia. It is most commonly capillary type, although cavernous and mixed types may also occur.

3. **LYMPHANGIOMA.** Lymphangioma may develop most commonly on the tongue producing macroglossia; on the lips producing macrocheilia, and on the cheek. *Cystic hygroma* is a special variety of lymphangioma occurring in children on the lateral side of neck.

Microscopically, lymphangioma is characterised by large lymphatic spaces lined by endothelium and containing lymph (Chapter 11).

4. **FIBROMA.** The true fibroma of mouth is relatively uncommon benign tumour and is more often a tumour-like lesion (discussed above).

Microscopically, fibroma is composed of collagenic fibrous connective tissue covered by stratified squamous epithelium.

5. **FIBROMATOSIS GINGIVAE.** This is a fibrous overgrowth of unknown etiology involving the entire gingiva. Sometimes the fibrous overgrowth is so much that the teeth are covered by fibrous tissue.

6. **TUMOURS OF MINOR SALIVARY GLANDS.** Minor salivary glands present in the oral cavity may sometimes be the site of origin of salivary tumours similar to those seen in the major salivary glands (page 545). Pleomorphic adenoma is a common example.

7. **GRANULAR CELL MYOBLASTOMA.** This is an unusual oral benign tumour, seen more often in the tongue.

Microscopically, the tumour is composed of large polyhedral cells with granular, acidophilic cytoplasm. The covering epithelium usually shows pronounced pseudoepitheliomatous hyperplasia.

8. **OTHER RARE BENIGN TUMOURS.** Some other rare benign tumours which can occur in the oral soft tissues are: neurilemmoma, neurofibroma, lipoma, giant cell granuloma, rhabdomyoma, leiomyoma, solitary plasmacytoma, osteoma, chondroma, naevi and vascular oral lesions seen in hereditary haemorrhagic telangiectasia (Osler-Rendu-Weber syndrome) and encephalofacial angiomatosis (Sturge-Weber syndrome).

C. ORAL LEUKOPLAKIA (WHITE LESIONS)

DEFINITION. Leukoplakia *(white plaque)* may be clinically defined as a white patch or plaque on the oral mucosa, exceeding 5 mm in diameter, which cannot be rubbed off nor can be classified into any other diagnosable disease. A number of other lesions are characterised by the formation of white patches listed in Table 17.3. However, from the pathologist's point of view, the term 'leukoplakia' is reserved for epithelial thickening which may range from completely benign to atypical and to premalignant cellular changes.

TABLE 17.3: Causes of White Lesions in the Oral Mucosa.

A. BENIGN
1. Fordyce's granules
2. Hairy tongue
3. Leukoedema
4. Lupus erythematosus
5. White sponge naevus

B. PREMALIGNANT
1. Leukoplakia
2. Oral lichen planus

C. MALIGNANT
Squamous cell carcinoma

Chapter Seventeen

INCIDENCE. It occurs more frequently in males than females. The lesions may be of variable size and appearance. The sites of predilection, in descending order of frequency, are: cheek mucosa, angles of mouth, alveolar mucosa, tongue, lip, hard and soft palate, and floor of the mouth. In about 4-6% cases of leukoplakia, carcinomatous change is reported. However, it is difficult to decide which white lesions may undergo malignant transformation, but speckled or nodular form is more likely to progress to malignancy. Therefore, it is desirable that all oral white patches be biopsied to exclude malignancy.

ETIOLOGY. The etiological factors are similar to those suggested for carcinoma of the oral mucosa. *It has the strongest association with the use of tobacco in various forms*, e.g. in heavy smokers (especially in pipe and cigar smokers) and improves when smoking is discontinued, and in those who chew tobacco as in paan, paan masaala, zarda, gutka etc. The condition is also known by other names such as *smokers keratosis* and *stomatitis nicotina*. Other etiological factors implicated are chronic friction such as with ill-fitting dentures or jagged teeth, and local irritants like excessive consumption of alcohol and very hot and spicy foods and beverages. A special variety of leukoplakia called *'hairy leukoplakia'* has been described in patients of AIDS and has hairy or corrugated surface but is not related to development of oral cancer.

PATHOLOGIC CHANGES. Grossly, the lesions of leukoplakia may appear white, whitish-yellow, or red-velvety of more than 5 mm diameter and variable in appearance. They are usually circumscribed, slightly elevated, smooth or wrinkled, speckled or nodular.

Histologically, leukoplakia is of 2 types:

1. **Hyperkeratotic type.** This is characterised by an orderly and regular hyperplasia of squamous epithelium with hyperkeratosis on the surface (COLOUR PLATE XXII: CL 85).

2. **Dysplastic type.** When the changes such as irregular stratification of the epithelium, focal areas of increased and abnormal mitotic figures, hyperchromatism, pleomorphism, loss of polarity and individual cell keratinisation are present, the lesion is considered as epithelial dysplasia. The subepithelial tissues usually show an inflammatory infiltrate composed of lymphocytes and plasma cells. The extent and degree of the epithelial changes indicate the degree of severity of the epithelial dysplasia.

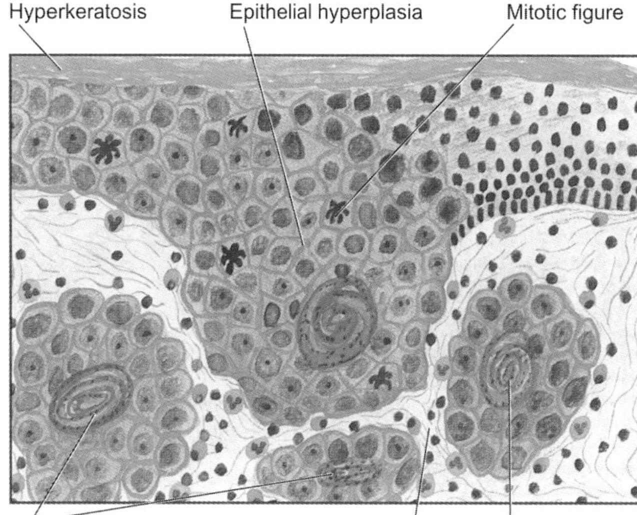

FIGURE 17.1

Oral mucosa showing epithelial dysplasia progressing to invasive squamous cell carcinoma. There is keratosis, irregular stratification, cellular pleomorphism, increased and abnormal mitotic figures and individual cell keratinisation, while a few areas show superficial invasive islands of malignant cells in the subepithelial soft tissues.

Usually, mild dysplasia may revert back to normal if the offending etiologic factor is removed, whereas severe dysplasia indicates that the case may progress to carcinoma. *Erythroplasia* is a form of dysplastic leukoplakia in which the epithelial atypia is more marked and thus has higher risk of developing malignancy. If the epithelial dysplasia is extensive so as to involve the entire thickness of the epithelium, the lesion is called carcinoma *in situ* which may progress to invasive carcinoma (Fig. 17.1).

D. MALIGNANT TUMOURS

Squamous Cell (Epidermoid) Carcinoma

Oral cancer is a disease with very poor prognosis because it is not recognised and treated when small and early.

INCIDENCE. Squamous cell (epidermoid) carcinoma comprises 90% of all oral malignant tumours and 5% of all human malignancies. The peak incidence in the UK and the USA is from 55 to 75 years of age, whereas in India it is from 40 to 45 years of age. Oral cancer is a very frequent malignancy in India, Sri Lanka and some Eastern countries, probably related to habits of betel-nut chewing and reversed smoking (Chapter 8). There is a definite male preponderance. It can occur anywhere in the mouth but certain sites are more commonly involved. These sites, in descending order of frequency,

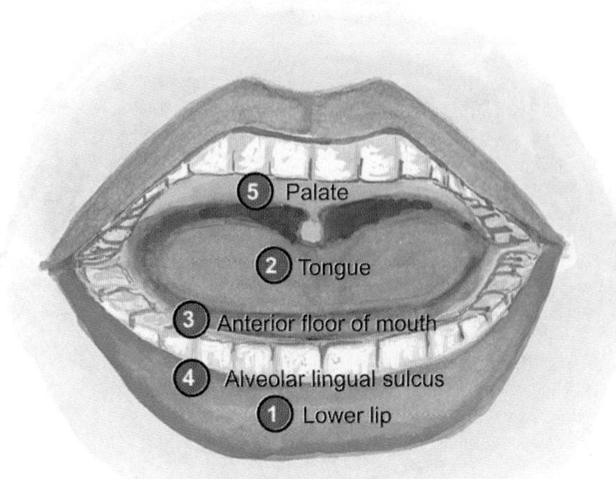

FIGURE 17.2

Frequency of occurrence of squamous cell carcinomas in the oral cavity.

are: the lips (more commonly lower), tongue, anterior floor of mouth, buccal mucosa in the region of alveolar lingual sulcus, and palate (Fig. 17.2).

ETIOLOGY. As with other forms of cancer, the etiology of squamous cell carcinoma is unknown. But a number of etiological factors have been implicated:

Strong association:

i) Tobacco smoking and tobacco chewing causing leukoplakia is the most important factor as discussed above.

ii) Chronic alcohol consumption.

iii) Human papilloma virus infection, particularly HPV 16, 18 and 33 types.

Weak association:

i) Chronic irritation from ill-fitting denture or jagged teeth.

ii) Submucosal fibrosis as seen in Indians consuming excess of chillies.

iii) Poor orodental hygiene.

iv) Nutritional deficiencies.

v) Exposure to sunlight (in relation to lip cancer).

vi) Exposure to radiation.

vii) Plummer-Vinson syndrome, characterised by atrophy of the upper alimentary tract.

*PATHOLOGIC CHANGES. **Grossly,*** squamous cell carcinoma of oral cavity may have the following types (Fig. 17.3):

i) Ulcerative type—is the most frequent type and is characterised by indurated ulcer and firm everted or rolled edges.

ii) Papillary or verrucous type—is soft and wartlike growth.

iii) Nodular type—appears as a firm, slow growing submucosal nodule.

iv) Scirrhous type—is characterised by infiltration into deeper structures.

All these types may appear on a background of leukoplakia or erythroplasia of the oral mucosa. Enlarged cervical lymph nodes may sometimes be present.

Histologically, squamous cell carcinoma ranges from well-differentiated keratinising carcinoma to highly-undifferentiated neoplasm (Chapter 24). Changes of epithelial dysplasia are often present in the surrounding areas of the lesion. Carcinoma of the lip and intraoral squamous carcinoma are usually always well-differentiated (Fig. 17.1) **(COLOUR PLATE X: CL 38).**

Carcinoma of the lip has a more favourable prognosis due to visible and easily accessible location and less frequent metastasis to the regional lymph nodes. However, intraoral squamous carcinomas have poor prognosis because they are detected late and metastasis to regional lymph nodes occur early, especially in the case of carcinoma of tongue and soft palate.

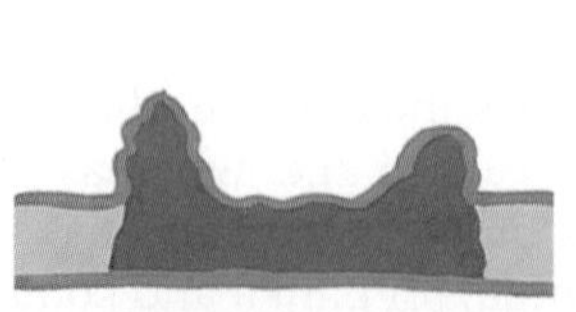

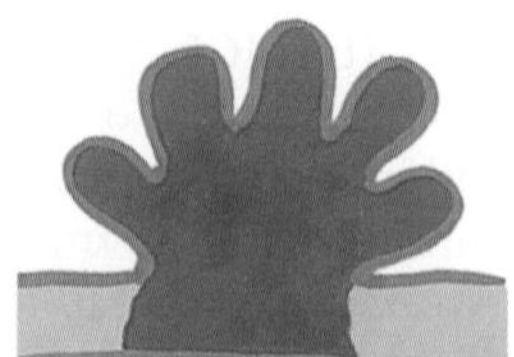

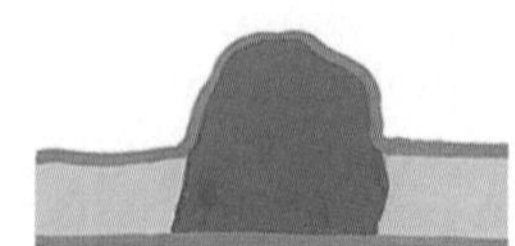

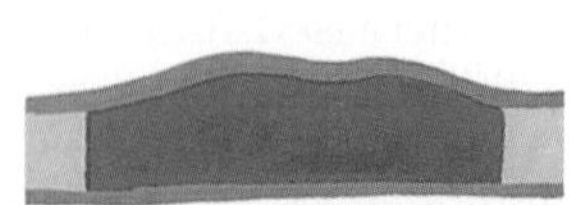

A, ULCERATIVE TYPE B, PAPILLARY (VERRUCOUS) TYPE C, NODULAR TYPE D, SCIRRHOUS TYPE

FIGURE 17.3

Squamous cell (Epidermoid) carcinoma of oral cavity, patterns of gross appearance.

Verrucous carcinoma, on the other hand, is composed of very well-differentiated squamous epithelium with minimal atypia and hence has very good prognosis.

OTHER MALIGNANT TUMOURS

Other less common malignant neoplasms which may be encountered in the oral cavity are: malignant melanoma, lymphoepithelial carcinoma, malignant lymphoma, malignant tumours of minor salivary glands, and various sarcomas like rhabdomyosarcoma, liposarcoma, alveolar soft part sarcoma, Kaposi's sarcoma and fibrosarcoma. Metastatic tumours can also occur in the soft tissues of the mouth.

TEETH AND PERIODONTAL TISSUES

Although care of the teeth belongs to the field of dental profession, the fully educated doctor should be familiar with certain principal diseases of teeth and periodontal tissues, especially about dental caries, periapical abscess and periodontitis, and common cysts and odontogenic tumours of the jaw. But first, a brief account of normal structure of these tissues.

NORMAL STRUCTURE

The teeth are normally composed of 3 calcified tissues, namely: enamel, dentine and cementum; and the pulp composed of connective tissue. The teeth are surrounded by the portion of oral mucosa called the gingiva or gum (Fig. 17.4).

Enamel in the outer covering of teeth composed almost entirely of inorganic material (as in bone) which can be demonstrated in ground sections only as it is lost in decalcified section.

Dentine lies under the enamel and comprises most of the tooth substance. It is composed of organic material in the form of collagen fibrils as well as inorganic material in the form of calcium phosphates as in bone. Dentine is composed of odontoblasts or dentine cells which are counterparts of osteocytes in bone but differ from the latter in having odontoblast processes.

Cementum is the portion of tooth which covers the dentine at the root of tooth and is the site where periodontal ligament is attached. Cementum is similar to bone in morphology and composition.

Dental pulp is inner to dentine and occupies the pulp cavity and root canal. It consists of connective tissue, blood vessels and nerves.

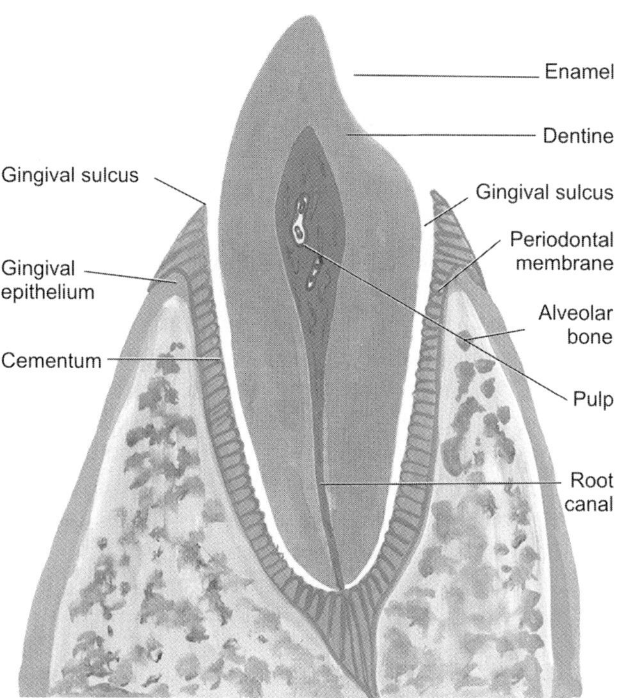

FIGURE 17.4
The normal structure of tooth embedded in the jaw.

DENTAL CARIES

Dental caries is the most common disease of dental tissues, causing destruction of the calcified tissues of the teeth.

ETIOPATHOGENESIS. Dental caries is essentially a disease of modern society, associated with diet containing high proportion of refined carbohydrates. It has been known for almost 100 years that mixture of sugar or bread with saliva in the presence of acidogenic bacteria of the mouth, especially streptococci, produces organic acids which can decalcify enamel and dentine. Enamel is largely composed of inorganic material which virtually disintegrates. Dentine contains organic material also which is left after decalcification. Bacteria present in the oral cavity cause proteolysis of the remaining organic material of dentine so that the process of destruction is complete. Diets rich in carbohydrates do not require much chewing and thus the soft and sticky food gets clung to the teeth rather than being cleared away, particularly in the areas of occlusal pits and fissures. 'Bacterial plaques' are formed in such stagnation areas. If these plaques are not removed by brushing or by vigorous chewing of fibrous foods, the process of tooth decay begins. There is evidence that consumption of water containing one part per million (ppm) fluoride is sufficient to reduce the rate of tooth decay in children.

PATHOLOGIC CHANGES. Caries occurs chiefly in the areas of pits and fissures, mainly of the molars and premolars, where food retention occurs, and in the cervical part of the tooth.

Macroscopically, the earliest change is the appearance of a small, chalky-white spot on the enamel which subsequently enlarges and often becomes yellow or brown and breaks down to form carious cavity. Eventually, the cavity becomes larger due to fractures of enamel. Once the lesion reaches enamel-dentine junction, destruction of dentine also begins. ***Microscopically,*** inflammation (pulpitis) and necrosis of pulp take place. There is evidence of reaction of the tooth to the carious process in the form of *secondary dentine,* which is a layer of odontoblasts laid down under the original dentine (Fig. 17.5).

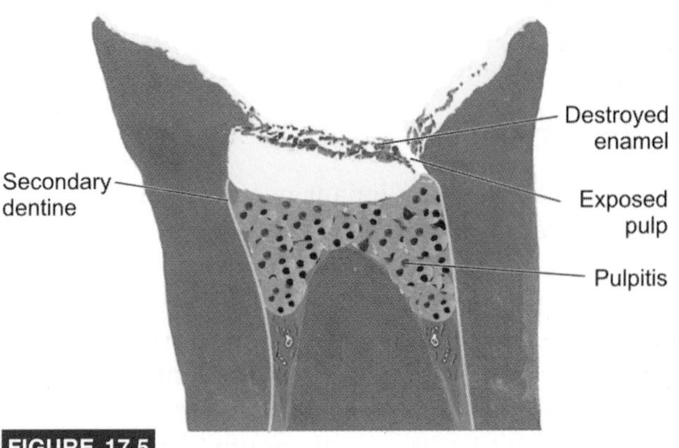

FIGURE 17.5

Dental caries. There is complete destruction of enamel, deposition of secondary dentine and evidence of pulpitis.

SEQUELAE OF CARIES. Carious destruction of dental hard tissues frequently produces pulpitis and other inflammatory lesions like apical granuloma and apical abscess. Other less common causes of these lesions are fracture of tooth and accidental exposure of pulp by the dentist.

1. **Pulpitis.** Pulpitis may be acute or chronic.

■ *Acute pulpitis* is accompanied by severe pain which may be continuous, throbbing or dull, and is accentuated by heat or cold. It is often accompanied by mild fever and leucocytosis.

■ *Chronic pulpitis* occurs when pulp is exposed widely. It is often not associated with pain. Chronically inflamed pulp tissue may protrude through the cavity forming polyp of the pulp. It may be partly covered by implanted squamous epithelium.

2. **Apical granuloma.** Pulpitis may lead to spread of infection through the apical foramen into the tissues surrounding the root of the tooth.

Histologically, there is chronic inflammatory reaction with formation of granulation tissue and inclusion of nests or strands of squamous epithelium derived from remnants of odontogenic epithelium normally present in the periodontal membrane. An apical granuloma may develop into a dental (radicular) cyst as discussed below.

3. **Apical abscess.** An apical granuloma or acute pulpitis may develop into apical abscess. Acute abscess is very painful, while pus in chronic abscess may escape through root canal and cause further complications like osteomyelitis, cellulitis, cerebral abscess, meningitis and cavernous sinus thrombosis.

PERIODONTAL DISEASE

Chronic inflammation and degeneration of the supporting tissues of teeth resulting in teeth loss is a common condition. Besides inflammation, two other diseases—leukaemia and scurvy, are associated with gingival swelling.

The inflammatory periodontal disease affects adults more commonly. Pregnancy, puberty and use of drugs like dilantin are also associated with periodontal disease more often. The disease begins as *chronic marginal gingivitis,* secondary to bacterial plaques around the teeth such as due to calculus (tartar) on the tooth surface, impacted food, uncontrolled diabetes, tooth-decay and ill-fitting dental appliances. The gingival sulcus acts as convenient site for lodgement of food debris and bacterial plaque leading to formation of periodontal pocket from which purulent discharge can be expressed by digital pressure.

Pathologically, chronic marginal gingivitis is characterised by heavy chronic inflammatory cell infiltrate, destruction of collagen, and epithelial hyperplasia so as to line the pocket. Untreated chronic marginal gingivitis slowly progresses to *chronic periodontitis* or *pyorrhoea* in which there is inflammatory destruction of deeper tissues. At this stage, progressive resorption of alveolar bone occurs and the tooth ultimately gets detached.

EPITHELIAL CYSTS OF JAW

The epithelium-lined cysts of dental tissue can have inflammatory or developmental origin. A classification of such cysts is given in Table 17.4.

A. INFLAMMATORY CYSTS

Radicular Cyst

Radicular cyst, also called as apical, periodontal or simply dental cyst, is the most common cyst originating from the dental tissues. It arises consequent to inflammation following destruction of dental pulp such as in dental caries, pulpitis, and apical granuloma. The epithelial cells of Mallasez, which normally lie in the periodontal ligament, proliferate within apical granuloma under the influence of inflammation, leading to the formation of an epithelium-lined cystic cavity. Most often, radicular cyst is observed at the apex of an erupted tooth and sometimes contains thick pultaceous material.

Histologically, the radicular cyst is lined by nonkeratinised squamous epithelium. Epithelial rete processes may penetrate the underlying connective tissues. Radicular cyst of maxilla may be lined by respiratory epithelium. The cyst wall is fibrous and contains chronic inflammatory cells (lymphocytes, plasma cells with Russell bodies and macrophages) hyaline bodies and deposits of cholesterol crystals which may be associated with foreign body giant cells (Fig. 17.6).

B. DEVELOPMENTAL CYSTS

1. Odontogenic Cysts

I) DENTIGEROUS (FOLLICULAR) CYST. Dentigerous cyst arises from enamel of an unerupted tooth.

TABLE 17.4: Classification of Epithelial Cysts of Jaw.

A. INFLAMMATORY
  - Radicular (apical, periodontal, dental) cyst

B. DEVELOPMENTAL
  1. **Odontogenic cysts**
     - (i) Dentigerous (follicular) cyst
     - (ii) Eruption cyst
     - (iii) Gingival cyst
     - (iv) Primordial cyst (odontogenic keratocyst)
  2. **Non-odontogenic and fissural cysts**
     - (i) Nasopalatine duct (Incisive canal, Median anterior maxillary) cyst
     - (ii) Nasolabial (nasoalveolar) cyst
     - (iii) Globulomaxillary cyst
     - (iv) Dermoid cyst

The mandibular third molars and the maxillary canines are most often involved. Dentigerous cysts are less common than radicular cysts and occur more commonly in children and young individuals. These cysts are more significant because of reported occurrence of ameloblastoma and carcinoma in them.

Histologically, dentigerous cyst is composed of a thin fibrous tissue wall lined by stratified squamous epithelium. Thus, the cyst may resemble radicular cyst, except that chronic inflammatory changes so characteristic of radicular cyst, are usually absent in dentigerous cyst (Fig. 17.7).

II) ERUPTION CYST. This is a cyst lying over the crown of an unerupted tooth and is lined by stratified squamous epithelium. It is thus a form of dentigerous cyst.

III) GINGIVAL CYST. It arises from the epithelial rests in the gingiva and is lined by keratinising squamous epithelium.

IV) PRIMORDIAL CYST (ODONTOGENIC KERATOCYST). Primordial cyst, like dentigerous cyst, also arises from tooth-forming epithelium. The common location is mandibular third molar.

Histologically, the cyst wall is thin and is lined by regular layer of keratinising stratified squamous epithelium. Inflammatory changes are normally absent. Primordial cysts have a marked tendency to recur (50%). Multiple primordial cysts occur in association with naevoid basal cell carcinoma syndrome.

2. Non-odontogenic and Fissural Cysts

I) NASOPALATINE DUCT (INCISIVE CANAL, MEDIAN, ANTERIOR MAXILLARY) CYST. This is the most common non-odontogenic (fissural) cyst and arises from the epithelial remnants of the nasopalatine duct.

Histologically, the cyst is lined by stratified squamous epithelium, respiratory epithelium, or both.

II) NASOLABIAL (NASOALVEOLAR) CYST. This cyst is situated in the soft tissues at the junction of median nasal, lateral nasal and maxillary processes, at the ala of the nose, and sometimes extending into the nostril.

Histologically, the cyst is lined by squamous or respiratory epithelium, or both.

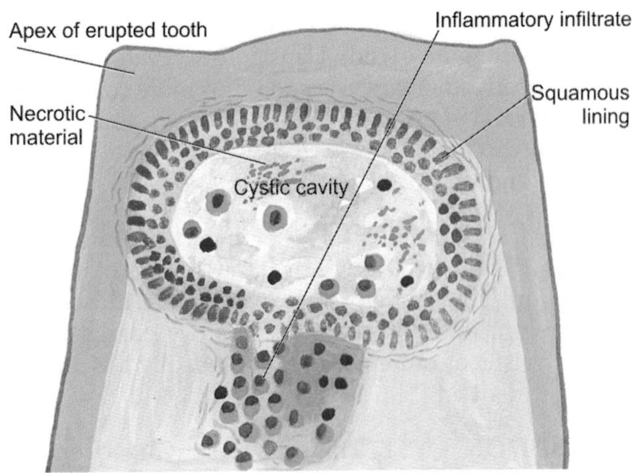

FIGURE 17.6

Dental (radicular) cyst. The cyst wall is composed of fibrous tissue and is lined by non-keratinised squamous epithelium. The cyst wall is densely infiltrated by chronic inflammatory cells, chiefly lymphocytes, plasma cells and macrophages.

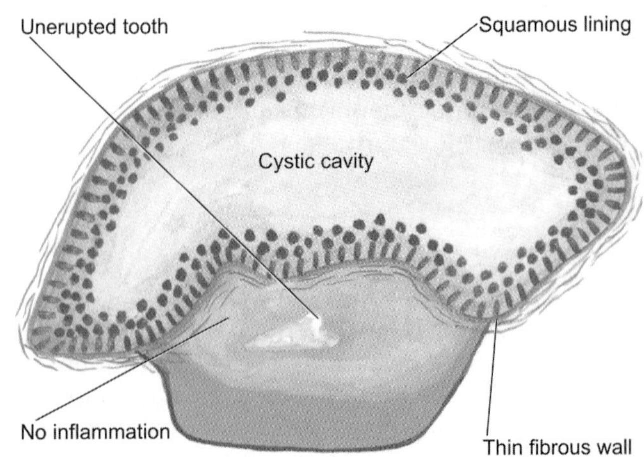

FIGURE 17.7

Dentigerous (Follicular) cyst. The cyst is composed of thin fibrous tissue wall and is lined by stratified squamous epithelium. A partly formed unerupted tooth is also seen in the wall. Inflammatory changes are conspicuously absent.

III) GLOBULOMAXILLARY CYST. This is an intraosseous cyst and is rare.

IV) DERMOID CYST. The dermoid cyst is common in the region of head or neck, especially in the floor of the mouth. The cyst arises from remains in the midline during closure of mandibular and branchial arches.

ODONTOGENIC TUMOURS

Odontogenic tumours are a group of uncommon lesions of jaw derived from the odontogenic apparatus. These tumours are usually benign but some have malignant counterparts. A brief classification modified from the WHO classification is presented in Table 17.5.

A. BENIGN ODONTOGENIC TUMOURS

Ameloblastoma

Ameloblastoma is the most common benign but locally invasive epithelial odontogenic tumour. It is commonest in the 3rd to 5th decades of life. Preferential sites are the mandible in the molar-ramus area and the maxilla. The tumour originates from dental epithelium of the enamel itself or its epithelial residues. Sometimes, the tumour may arise from the epithelial lining of a dentigerous cyst or from basal layer of oral mucosa. Radiologically, typical picture is of a multilocular destruction of bone. Rare instances of an extraosseous example, presence of an embedded tooth, or unilocular ameloblastoma can occur. Tumour with histologic resemblance to ameloblastoma can occur occasionally in the long bone, like adamantinoma of the tibia (Chapter 26).

Grossly, the tumour is greyish-white, usually solid, sometimes cystic, replacing and expanding the affected bone.

Histologically, ameloblastoma can show different patterns described below (COLOUR PLATE XXII: CL 86):

TABLE 17.5: Classification of Odontogenic Tumours.

A. BENIGN
- **a) Epithelial origin**
  1. Ameloblastoma
  2. Adenomatoid odontogenic tumour (Adeno-ameloblastoma)
  3. Calcifying epithelial odontogenic tumour
- **b) Mesenchymal origin**
  1. Odontogenic myxoma
  2. Odontogenic fibroma
  3. Cementoma
- **c) Mixed epithelial-mesenchymal origin**
  1. Ameloblastic fibroma
  2. Ameloblastic fibro-odontoma
  3. Complex odontomas

B. MALIGNANT
- **a) Epithelial origin**
  1. Malignant ameloblastoma
  2. Ameloblastic carcinoma
- **b) Mesenchymal origin**
  Ameloblastic fibrosarcoma

i) Follicular pattern is the most common. The tumour consists of follicles of variable size and shape and separated from each other by fibrous tissue. The structure of follicles is similar to that of enamel organ consisting of central area of stellate cells resembling stellate reticulum, and peripheral layer of cuboidal or columnar cells resembling epithelium. The central stellate areas may show cystic changes.

ii) Plexiform pattern is the next common pattern after follicular pattern. The tumour epithelium is seen to form irregular plexiform masses or network of strands. The stroma is usually scanty. Microcyst formation can occur in the stroma.

iii) Acanthomatous pattern is squamous metaplasia within the islands of tumour cells.

iv) Basal cell pattern of ameloblastoma is similar to basal cell carcinoma of the skin.

v) Granular cell pattern is characterised by appearance of acidophilic granularity in the cytoplasm of tumour cells.

Combination of more than one morphologic pattern may also be seen (Fig. 17.8).

Odontogenic Adenomatoid Tumour (Adeno-ameloblastoma)

This is a benign tumour seen more frequently in females in their 2nd decade of life. The tumour is commonly

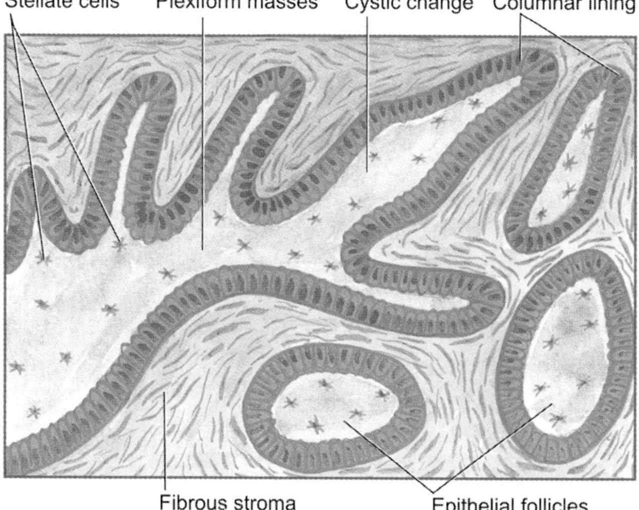

FIGURE 17.8

Ameloblastoma, follicular and plexiform patterns. Epithelial follicles are composed of central area of stellate cells and peripheral layer of cuboidal or columnar cells. Plexiform areas show irregular plexiform masses and network of strands of epithelial cells. A few areas show central cystic change.

associated with an unerupted tooth and thus closely resembles dentigerous cyst radiologically. Unlike ameloblastoma, adenomatoid odontogenic tumour is not invasive nor does it recur after enucleation.

Histologically, the lesion has extensive cyst formations. The wall of cyst contains scanty fibrous connective tissue in which are present characteristic tubule-like structures composed of epithelial cells and hence the name 'adenomatoid' (gland-like).

Calcifying Epithelial Odontogenic Tumour

This is a rare lesion which is locally invasive and recurrent like ameloblastoma. It is seen commonly in 4th and 5th decades and occurs more commonly in the region of mandible.

Histologically, the tumour consists of closely packed polyhedral epithelial cells having features of nuclear pleomorphism, giant nuclei and rare mitotic figures. The stroma is often scanty and appears homogeneous and hyalinised in which small calcified deposits are seen which are a striking feature of this tumour.

Odontogenic Myxoma (Myxofibroma)

Odontogenic myxoma is a locally invasive and recurring tumour.

Microscopically, it is characterised by abundant mucoid stroma and loose stellate cells in which are seen a few strands of odontogenic epithelium.

Ameloblastic Fibroma

This is a benign tumour consisting of epithelial and connective tissues derived from odontogenic apparatus. It resembles ameloblastoma but can be distinguished from it because ameloblastic fibroma occurs in younger age group (below 20 years) and the clinical behaviour is always benign.

Histologically, it consists of epithelial follicles similar to those of ameloblastoma, set in a very cellular connective tissue stroma.

Odontomas

Odontomas are hamartomas that contain both epithelial and mesodermal dental tissue components. There are 3 subtypes:

i) Complex odontoma is always benign and consists of enamel, dentine and cementum which are not differentiated, so that the structure of actual tooth is not identifiable.

ii) Compound odontoma is also benign and is comprised of differentiated dental tissue elements forming a number of denticles in fibrous tissue.

iii) Ameloblastic fibro-odontoma is a lesion that resembles ameloblastic fibroma with odontoma formation.

Cementomas

Cementomas are a variety of benign lesions which are characterised by the presence of cementum or cementum-like tissue. Five types of cementomas are described:

i) Benign cementoblastoma (true cementoma) is a solitary lesion of jaw, characterised by features comparable to those of osteoid osteoma and osteoblastoma.

ii) Cementifying fibroma consists of cellular fibrous tissue containing calcified masses of cementum-like tissue.

iii) Periapical cemental dysplasia (Periapical fibrous dysplasia) is most common and resembles cementifying fibroma except that it contains more fibrous tissue as well as cementum-like tissue.

iv) Multiple apical cementomas are found on the apical region of teeth and detected incidentally in postmenopausal women.

v) Gigantiform cementoma is a large lobulated mass of cementum-like tissue. Sometimes, there are multiple such masses in the jaw.

B. MALIGNANT ODONTOGENIC TUMOURS

Malignant odontogenic tumours are rare.

Odontogenic Carcinoma

i) *Malignant ameloblastoma* is the term used for the uncommon metastasising ameloblastoma.

ii) *Ameloblastic carcinoma* is the term employed for the ameloblastic tumour having cytologic features of malignancy in the primary tumour.

iii) *Primary intraosseous carcinoma* may develop within the jaw from the rests of odontogenic epithelium.

iv) Rarely, carcinomas may arise from the odontogenic epithelium lining the *odontogenic cysts.*

Odontogenic Sarcomas

The only example of odontogenic sarcoma is a rare ameloblastic fibrosarcoma. This tumour resembles ameloblastic fibroma but in this the mesodermal component is malignant (sarcomatous) whereas the ameloblastic epithelium remains differentiated and benign.

SALIVARY GLANDS

NORMAL STRUCTURE

There are two main groups of salivary glands—major and minor. The major salivary glands are the three paired glands: parotid, submandibular and sublingual. The minor salivary glands are numerous and widely distributed in the mucosa of oral cavity. The main duct of the parotid gland drains into the oral cavity opposite the second maxillary molar, while the ducts of submandibular and sublingual glands empty in the floor of the mouth. At times, heterotopic salivary gland tissue may be present in lymph nodes near or within the parotid gland.

Histologically, the salivary glands are tubuloalveolar glands and may contain mucous cells, serous cells, or both. The parotid gland is purely serous. The submandibular gland is mixed type but is predominantly serous, whereas the sublingual gland though also a mixed gland is predominantly mucous type. Similarly, minor salivary glands may also be serous, mucous or mixed type.

The secretory acini of the major salivary glands are drained by ducts lined by: low cuboidal epithelium in the intercalated portion, by tall columnar epithelium in the intralobular ducts, and by simpler epithelium in the secretory ducts.

The product of major salivary glands is *saliva* which performs various functions such as lubrication for swallowing and speech, and has enzyme amylase and antibacterial properties too.

SALIVARY FLOW DISTURBANCES

SIALORRHOEA (PTYALISM). Increased flow of saliva is termed sialorrhoea or ptyalism. It occurs commonly due to: stomatitis, teething, mentally retarded state, schizophrenia, neurological disturbances, increased gastric secretion and sialosis (i.e. uniform, symmetric, painless hypertrophy of salivary glands).

XEROSTOMIA. Decreased salivary flow is termed xerostomia. It is associated with the following conditions: Sjögren's syndrome, sarcoidosis, mumps parotitis, Mikulicz's syndrome, megaloblastic anaemia, dehydration, drug intake (e.g. antihistamines, antihypertensives, antidepressants).

SIALADENITIS

Inflammation of salivary glands, sialadenitis, may be acute or chronic, the latter being more common.

ETIOLOGY. Sialadenitis can occur due to the following causes:

1. Viral infections. The most common inflammatory lesion of the salivary glands particularly of the parotid glands, is mumps occurring in children of school-age. It is characterised by triad of pathological involvement—*epidemic parotitis (mumps), orchitis-oophoritis, and pancreatitis* (Fig. 17.9). Involvement of testis and pancreas may lead to their atrophy. Less commonly, cytomegalovirus infection may occur in parotid glands of infants and young children.

2. Bacterial and mycotic infections. Bacterial infections may cause acute sialadenitis more often. Sometimes there are recurrent attacks of acute parotitis when parotitis becomes chronic.

i) ***Acute sialadenitis.*** The causes are:

a) Acute infectious fevers

b) Acute postoperative parotitis (ascent of micro-organisms up the parotid duct from the mouth)

c) General debility

d) Old age

e) Dehydration.

ii) ***Chronic sialadenitis.*** This may result from the following causes:

a) Recurrent obstructive type. Recurrent obstruction due to calculi (sialolithiasis), stricture, surgery, injury etc may cause repeated attacks of acute sialadenitis by ascending infection and then chronicity.

b) Recurrent non-obstructive type. Recurrent mild ascending infection of the parotid gland may occur due to non-obstructive causes which reduce salivary secretion like due to intake of drugs causing hyposalivation (e.g. antihistamines, antihypertensives, antidepressants), effect of irradiation and congenital malformations of the duct system.

c) Chronic inflammatory diseases. Tuberculosis, actinomycosis and other mycoses may rarely occur in the salivary glands.

3. Autoimmune disease. Inflammatory changes are seen in salivary glands in 2 autoimmune diseases:

i) *Sjögren's syndrome* characterised by triad of dry eyes (keratoconjunctivitis sicca), dry mouth (xerostomia) and rheumatoid arthritis (Chapter 4).

ii) *Mikulicz's syndrome* is the combination of inflammatory enlargement of salivary and lacrimal glands with xerostomia.

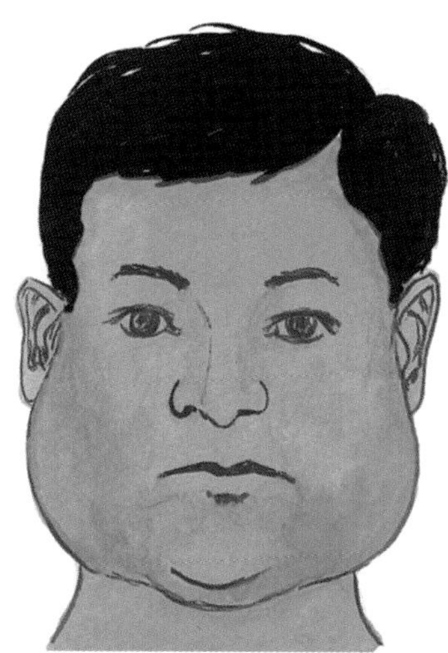

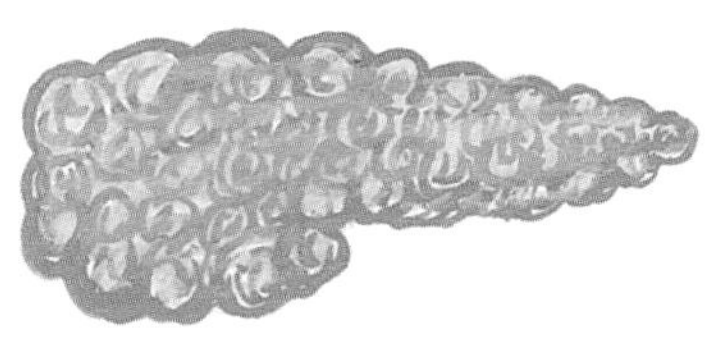

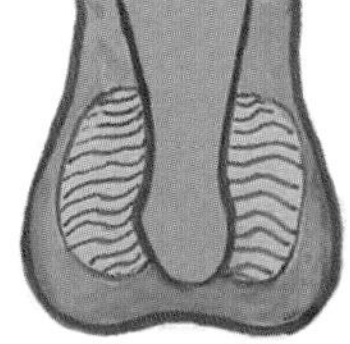

FIGURE 17.9
Lesions in mumps.

PATHOLOGIC CHANGES. Irrespective of the underlying etiology of sialadenitis, there is swelling of the affected salivary gland, usually restricted by the fibrous capsule. Acute stage is generally associated with local redness, pain and tenderness with purulent ductal discharge. Late chronic cases may be replaced by firm fibrous swelling.

Microscopically, *acute viral sialadenitis* in mumps shows swelling and cytoplasmic vacuolation of the acinar epithelial cells and degenerative changes in the ductal epithelium. There is interstitial oedema, fibrinoid degeneration of the collagen and dense infiltration by mononuclear cells (lymphocytes, plasma cells and macrophages). *Chronic and recurrent sialadenitis* is characterised by increased lymphoid tissue in the interstitium, progressive loss of secretory tissue and replacement by fibrosis.

TUMOURS OF SALIVARY GLANDS

The major as well as minor salivary glands can give rise to a variety of benign and malignant tumours (Table 17.6). The major glands, particularly the parotid glands (85%), are the most common sites. Majority of the

TABLE 17.6: Classification of Salivary Gland Tumours.

A. **BENIGN**

1. **Adenomas**
   i) Pleomorphic adenoma (Mixed tumour) (65-80%)
   ii) Monomorphic adenoma
      (a) Warthin's tumour (Papillary cystadenoma lymphomatosum, Adenolymphoma) (5-10%)
      (b) Oxyphil adenoma (Oncocytomas) (< 1%)
      (c) Other types (Myoepithelioma, Basal cell adenoma, Clear cell adenoma) (uncommon)
2. **Mesenchymal tumours (rare)**

B. **MALIGNANT**

1. Mucoepidermoid carcinoma (5-10%)
2. Malignant mixed tumour
   i) Carcinoma in pleomorphic adenoma (2%)
   ii) Carcinosarcoma (rare)
   iii) Metastasising mixed salivary tumour (rare)
3. Adenoid cystic carcinoma (cylindroma) (3-10%)
4. Acinic cell carcinoma (2-3%)
5. Adenocarcinoma (l-3%)
6. Epidermoid carcinoma (l-3%)
7. Undifferentiated carcinoma (<l%)
8. Miscellaneous (rare)

parotid gland tumour (65-85%) are benign, while in the other major and minor salivary glands 35-50% of the tumours are malignant. Most of the salivary gland tumours originate from the ductal lining epithelium and the underlying myoepithelial cells; a few arise from acini. Recurrent tumours of the parotid glands, due to their location, are often associated with facial palsy and obvious scarring following surgical treatment.

A. BENIGN SALIVARY GLAND TUMOURS

ADENOMAS

The adenomas of the salivary glands are benign epithelial tumours. They are broadly classified into 2 major groups—pleomorphic and monomorphic adenomas.

Pleomorphic Adenoma (Mixed Salivary Tumour)

This is the most common tumour of major (60-75%) and minor (50%) salivary glands. Pleomorphic adenoma is the commonest tumour in the parotid gland and occurs less often in other major and minor salivary glands. The tumour is commoner in women and is seen more frequently in 3rd to 5th decades of life. The tumour is solitary, smooth-surfaced but sometimes nodular, painless and slow-growing. It is often located below and in front of the ear (Fig. 17.10).

PATHOLOGIC CHANGES. Grossly, pleomorphic adenoma is a circumscribed, pseudoencapsulated, rounded, at times multilobulated, firm mass, 2-5 cm in diameter, with bosselated surface. The cut surface is grey-white and bluish, variegated, semitranslucent, usually solid but occasionally may show small cystic spaces. The consistency is soft and mucoid.

Microscopically, the pleomorphic adenoma is characterised by pleomorphic or 'mixed' appearance in which there are epithelial elements present in a matrix of mucoid, myxoid and chondroid tissue (Fig. 17.11):

■ **The epithelial component** may form various patterns like ducts, acini, tubules, sheets and strands of cells of ductal or myoepithelial origin. The ductal cells are cuboidal or columnar, and the underlying myoepithelial cells may be polygonal or spindle-shaped resembling smooth muscle cells. The material found in the lumina of duct-like structures is PAS-positive epithelial mucin. Focal areas of squamous metaplasia and keratinisation may be present. Immunohistochemically, the tumour cells are immunoreactive for epithelial (cytokeratin, EMA, CEA) as well as myoepithelial (actin, vimentin) antibodies.

■ **The mesenchymal elements** are present as loose connective tissue and as myxoid, mucoid and chondroid matrix, which simulates cartilage *(pseudocartilage)* but is actually connective tissue mucin. More recently, the matrix of the tumour has been characterised as a product of myoepithelial cells. However, true cartilage and even bone is observed in a small proportion of these tumours.

The epithelial and mesenchymal elements are intermixed and either of the two components may be dominant in any tumour (COLOUR PLATE XXII: CL 87).

PROGNOSIS. Pleomorphic adenoma is notorious for recurrences, sometimes after many years. The main factors responsible for the tendency to recur are incomplete surgical removal due to proximity to the facial nerve, multiple foci of tumour, pseudoencapsulation, and implantation in the surgical field. Although the tumour is entirely benign, under exceptionally rare circumstances, an ordinary pleomorphic adenoma may metastasise to distant sites which too will have benign appearance as the original tumour. However, actual malignant transformation can also occur in a pleomorphic adenoma *(vide infra).*

Monomorphic Adenomas

These are benign epithelial tumours of salivary glands without any evidence of mesenchyme-like tissues. Their various forms are as under:

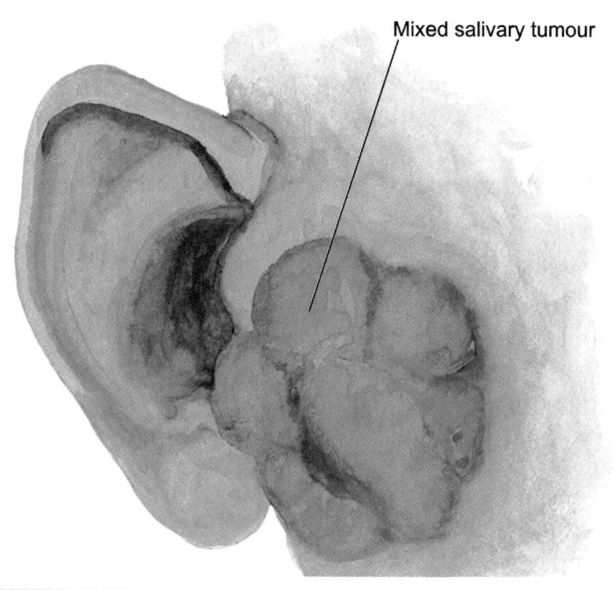

FIGURE 17.10

Pleomorphic adenoma (mixed salivary tumour) of the parotid gland.

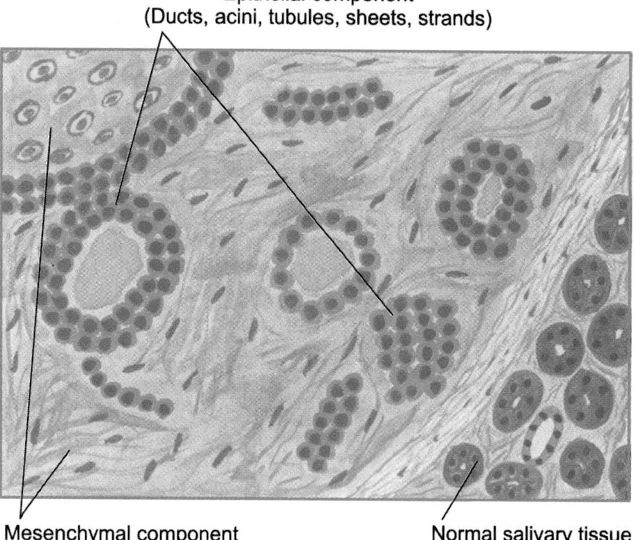

FIGURE 17.11

Pleomorphic adenoma, typical microscopic appearance. The epithelial element is comprised of ducts, acini, tubules, sheets and strands ot cuboidal and myoepithelial cells. These are seen randomly admixed with mesenchymal elements composed of pseudocartilage which is the matrix of myxoid, chondroid and mucoid material.

a) WARTHIN'S TUMOUR (PAPILLARY CYSTADENOMA LYMPHOMATOSUM, ADENOLYMPHOMA). It is a benign tumour of the parotid gland comprising about 8% of all parotid neoplasms, seen more commonly in men from 4th to 7th decades of life. Rarely, it may arise in the submandibular gland or in minor salivary glands. *Histogenesis* of the tumour has been much debated. Currently, most accepted theory is that the tumour develops from parotid ductal epithelium present in lymph nodes adjacent to or within parotid gland.

PATHOLOGIC CHANGES. Grossly, the tumour is encapsulated, round or oval with smooth surface. The cut surface shows characteristic slit-like or cystic spaces, containing milky fluid and having papillary projections.

Microscopically, the tumour shows 2 components: epithelial parenchyma and lymphoid stroma (Fig. 17.12) (COLOUR PLATE XXII: CL 88):

- **The epithelial parenchyma** is composed of glandular and cystic structures having papillary arrangement and lined by characteristic eosinophilic epithelium. Variants of epithelial patterns include presence of mucous goblet cells and sebaceous differentiation.
- **The lymphoid stroma** is .present under the epithelium in the form of prominent lymphoid tissue, often with germinal centres.

b) OXYPHIL ADENOMA (ONCOCYTOMA). It is a benign slow-growing tumour of the major salivary glands. The tumour consists of parallel sheets, acini or tubules of large cells with glandular eosinophilic cytoplasm (oncocytes) and hence the name.

c) OTHER TYPES OF MONOMORPHIC ADENOMAS. There are some uncommon forms of monomorphic adenomas:

i) Myoepithelioma is an adenoma composed exclusively of myoepithelial cells which may be arranged in tubular, alveolar or trabecular pattern.

ii) Basal cell adenoma is characterised by the type and arrangement of cells resembling basal cell carcinoma of the skin.

iii) Clear cell adenoma has spindle-shaped or polyhedral cells with clear cytoplasm.

MISCELLANEOUS BENIGN TUMOURS

A number of mesenchymal tumours can rarely occur in salivary glands. These include: fibroma, lipoma, neurilemmomas, neurofibroma, haemangioma and lymphangioma.

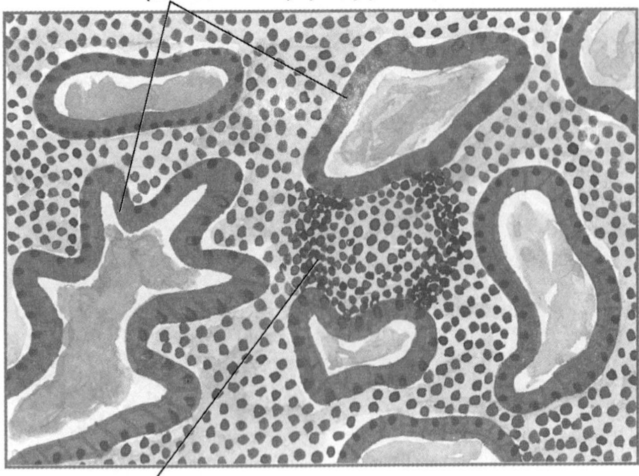

FIGURE 17.12

Warthin's tumour, showing eosinophilic epithelium forming glandular and papillary, cystic pattern with intervening stroma of lymphoid tissue.

B. MALIGNANT SALIVARY GLAND TUMOURS

Mucoepidermoid Carcinoma

The status of 'mucoepidermoid tumour' as an intermediate grade tumour in the previous classification has undergone upgradation to full-fledged mucoepidermoid carcinoma now having the following peculiar features:

- It is the most *common malignant* salivary gland tumour (both in the major and minor glands).
- The *parotid gland* amongst the major salivary glands and the minor salivary glands in the *palate* are the most common sites.
- The common age group affected is 30-60 years but it is also the most common malignant salivary gland tumour affecting *children and adolescents.*
- It is the most common example of *radiation-induced* malignant tumour, especially therapeutic radiation.

*PATHOLOGIC CHANGES. **Grossly,*** the tumour is usually circumscribed but not encapsulated. It varies in size from 1 to 4 cm.

Microscopically, the tumour is classified into low, intermediate and high grade depending upon the degree of differentiation and tumour invasiveness. The tumour is composed of combination of epidermoid cells and mucus-secreting cells (as the name implies) as also cells with intermediate differentiation between these two cell types and clear cells.

Malignant Mixed Tumour

Malignant mixed tumour comprises three distinct clinicopathologic entities:

- Carcinoma arising in benign mixed salivary gland tumour (carcinoma *ex* pleomorphic adenoma);
- Carcinosarcoma; and
- Metastasising mixed salivary tumour.

Carcinoma *ex* pleomorphic adenoma is more common while the other two are rare tumours. Approximately 2 to 5% of pleomorphic adenomas reveal areas of frank malignancy. The slow-growing adenoma may have been present for a number of years when suddenly it undergoes rapid increase in its size, becomes painful and the individual may develop facial palsy. Malignant transformation occurs in later age (6th decade) than the usual age for pleomorphic adenoma (4th to 6th decades). It may occur in primary tumour but more often occurs in its recurrences.

*PATHOLOGIC CHANGES. **Grossly,*** the tumour is poorly-circumscribed with irregular infiltrating margin. Cut section may show haemorrhages, necrosis and cystic degeneration.

Microscopically, besides the typical appearance of pleomorphic adenoma, malignant areas show cytologic features of carcinoma such as anaplasia, nuclear hyperchromatism, large nucleolisation, mitoses and evidence of invasive growth. All types of usual salivary gland carcinomas (described below) may develop in pleomorphic adenoma.

Adenoid Cystic Carcinoma (Cylindroma)

This is a highly malignant tumour due to its typical infiltrative nature, especially along the nerve sheaths. Adenoid cystic carcinoma is histologically characterised by cribriform appearance i.e. the epithelial tumour cells of duct-lining and myoepithelial cells are arranged in duct-like structures or masses of cells, having typical fenestrations or cyst-like spaces and hence the name 'adenoid cystic'.

Acinic Cell Carcinoma

This is a rare tumour composed of acinic cells resembling serous cells of normal salivary gland. These cells are arranged in sheets or acini and have characteristic basophilic granular cytoplasm. The degree of atypia may vary from a benign cytologic appearance to cellular features of malignancy.

Adenocarcinoma

Adenocarcinoma of the salivary gland does not differ from adenocarcinoma elsewhere in the body. It may have some variants such as mucoid adenocarcinoma, clear-cell adenocarcinoma and papillary cystadenocarcinoma.

Epidermoid Carcinoma

This rare tumour has features of squamous cell carcinoma with keratin formation and has intercellular bridges. The tumour commonly infiltrates the skin and involves the facial nerve early.

Undifferentiated Carcinoma

This highly malignant tumour consists of anaplastic epithelial cells which are too poorly differentiated to be placed in any other known category.

Miscellaneous MalignantTumours

Some rare malignant tumour of epithelial and mesenchymal origin are melanoma, sebaceous carcinoma, undifferentiated carcinoma, lymphoma, fibrosarcoma and leiomyosarcoma and are similar in morphology to such tumours elsewhere in the body. Besides, metastatic involvement of major salivary glands or the adjacent lymph nodes is common, especially from epidermoid carcinoma and malignant melanoma.

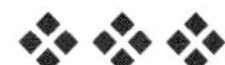

The Gastrointestinal Tract

18

OESOPHAGUS

NORMAL STRUCTURE

The oesophagus is a muscular tube extending from the pharynx to the stomach. In an adult, this distance measures 25 cm. However, from the clinical point of view, the distance from the incisor teeth to the gastro-oesophageal junction is about 40 cm. The region of proximal oesophagus at the level of cricopharyngeus muscle is called the *upper oesophageal sphincter,* while the portion adjacent to the anatomic gastro-oesophageal junction is referred to as *lower oesophageal sphincter.*

Histologically, the wall of the oesophagus consists of mucosa, submucosa, muscularis propria and adventitia/ serosa.

The **mucosa** is composed of non-keratinising stratified squamous epithelium overlying lamina propria. The basal layer of the epithelium may contain some melanocytes, argyrophil cells and Langerhans' cells. At the lower end of the oesophagus, there is sudden change from stratified squamous epithelium to mucin-secreting columnar epithelium for a distance of 0.5 to 1.5 cm; this is called the *junctional mucosa.*

The **submucosa** consists of loose connective tissue with sprinkling of lymphocytes, plasma cells, and occasional eosinophil and mast cell. Mucus-producing glands are scattered throughout the submucosa.

The **muscularis propria** is composed of 2 layers of smooth muscle—an inner circular coat and an outer longitudinal coat. The proximal portion of oesophagus contains skeletal muscle fibres from cricopharyngeus muscle. The parasympathetic nerve supply by the vagus nerve is in the form of extrinsic and intrinsic plexuses.

The **adventitia/serosa** is the outer covering of oesophagus. Serosa is present in intra-abdominal part of oesophagus only, while elsewhere the perioesophageal adventitia covers it.

The **major functions** of oesophagus are swallowing by peristaltic activity and to prevent the reflux of gastric contents into the oesophagus.

CONGENITAL ANOMALIES

Congenital anomalies of the oesophagus are uncommon and are detected soon after birth. Some of these are as under:

OESOPHAGEAL ATRESIA AND TRACHEO-OESOPHAGEAL FISTULA. In about 85% of cases, congenital atresia of the oesophagus is associated with tracheo-oesophageal fistula, usually at the level of tracheal bifurcation. For survival, the condition must be recognised and corrected surgically within 48 hours of birth of the newborn. Clinically, the condition is characterised by regurgitation of every feed, hypersalivation, attacks of cough and cyanosis. Death usually results from asphyxia, aspiration pneumonia and fluid-electrolyte imbalance. Morphologically, the condition is recognised by cord-like non-canalised segment of oesophagus having blind pouch at both ends.

OTHERS. Certain uncommon congenital anomalies of oesophagus are as follows:

- **Agenesis.** Congenital absence of oesophagus is quite rare and is incompatible with life.
- **Duplication of oesophagus.** This is another rare congenital abnormality in which there is double oesophagus.
- **Stenosis.** Oesophageal stenosis may occur as developmental anomaly or may follow oesophagitis. There is fibrous thickening of the oesophageal wall and atrophy of the mucularis propria.

MUSCULAR DYSFUNCTIONS

These are disorders in which there is motor dysfunction of the oesophagus, manifested clinically by dysphagia. These include achalasia, hiatus hernia, oesophageal diverticula, and webs and rings.

Achalasia (Cardiospasm)

Achalasia of the oesophagus is a neuromuscular dysfunction due to which the cardiac sphincter fails to relax during swallowing and results in progressive dysphagia and dilatation of the oesophagus *(mega-oesophagus).*

ETIOLOGY. The exact etiology is not known. It may be congenital. Emotional stress has been believed to contribute to the onset of the disease. Some investigators have demonstrated total absence of nerve fibres and ganglia of Auerbach's plexus in the terminal few centimetres of the oesophagus in achalasia. Chagas' disease, an epidemic parasitosis with *Trypansoma cruzi* has also been found to be associated with alterations of Auerbach's plexus.

PATHOLOGIC CHANGES. There is dilatation above the short contracted terminal segment of the oesophagus. Muscularis propria of the wall may be of normal thickness, hypertrophied as a result of obstruction, or thinned out due to dilatation. Secondary oesophagitis may supervene and cause oesophageal ulceration and haematemesis.

Hiatus Hernia

Hiatus hernia is the herniation or protrusion of the stomach through the oesophageal hiatus of the diaphragm. Oesophageal hiatal hernia is the cause of diaphragmatic hernia in 98% of cases. The condition is diagnosed radiologically in about 5% of apparently normal asymptomatic individuals. In symptomatic cases, especially the elderly women, the clinical features are heartburn (retrosternal burning sensation) and regurgitation of gastric juice into the mouth, both of which are worsened due to heavy work, lifting weights and excessive bending.

ETIOLOGY. The basic defect is the failure of the muscle fibres of the diaphragm that form the margin of the oesophageal hiatus. This occurs due to shortening of the oesophagus which may be congenital or acquired.

i) **Congenitally short oesophagus** may be the cause of hiatus hernia in a small proportion of cases.

ii) More commonly, it is **acquired** due to secondary factors which cause fibrous scarring of the oesophagus. These factors are:

a) Degeneration of muscle due to aging.

b) Increased intra-abdominal pressure such as in pregnancy, abdominal tumours etc.

c) Recurrent oesophageal regurgitation and spasm causing inflammation and fibrosis.

d) Increase in fatty tissue in obese people causing decreased muscular elasticity of diaphragm.

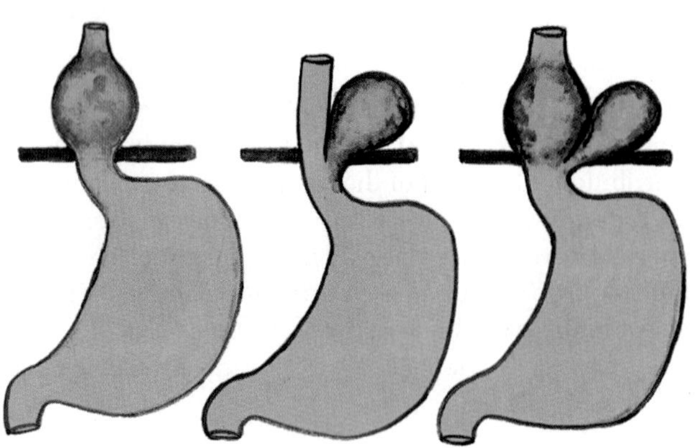

FIGURE 18.1

Patterns of hiatus hernia.

PATHOLOGIC CHANGES. There are 3 patterns in hiatus hernia (Fig. 18.1):

i) Sliding or oesophago-gastric hernia is the most common, occurring in 85% of cases. The herniated part of the stomach appears as supradiaphragmatic bell due to sliding up on both sides of the oesophagus.

ii) Rolling or para-oesophageal hernia is seen in 10% of cases. This is a true hernia in which cardiac end of the stomach rolls up para-oesophageally, producing an intrathoracic sac.

iii) Mixed or transitional hernia constitutes the remaining 5% cases in which there is combination of sliding and rolling hiatus hernia.

Oesophageal Diverticula

Diverticula are the outpouchings of oesophageal wall at the point of weakness. They may be congenital or acquired.

Congenital diverticula occur either at the upper end of the oesophagus or at the bifurcation of trachea.

Acquired diverticula may be of 2 types:

a) Pulsion (Zenker's) type—is seen in the region of hypopharynx and occurs due to oesophageal obstruction such as due to chronic oesophagitis, carcinoma etc. The mucosa and submucosa herniate through the weakened area or through defect in the muscularis propria.

b) Traction type—occurs in the lower third of oesophagus from contraction of fibrous tissue such as from pleural adhesions, scar tissue of healed tuberculous lesions in the hilum, silicosis etc.

Complications of diverticula include obstruction, infection, perforation, haemorrhage and carcinoma.

Oesophageal Webs and Rings

Radiological shadows in the oesophagus resembling 'webs' and 'rings' are observed in some patients complaining of dysphagia.

WEBS. Those located in the upper oesophagus, seen more commonly in adult women, and associated with dysphagia, iron deficiency anaemia and chronic atrophic glossitis (Plummer-Vinson syndrome) are called 'webs'.

RINGS. Those located in the lower oesophagus, not associated with iron-deficiency anaemia, nor occurring in women alone, are referred to as 'Schatzki's rings'.

PATHOLOGIC CHANGES. The rings and webs are transverse folds of mucosa and submucosa encircling the entire circumference, or are localised annular thickenings of the muscle (Fig. 18.2). These give characteristic radiological shadows.

HAEMATEMESIS OF OESOPHAGEAL ORIGIN

Massive haematemesis (vomiting of blood) may occur due to vascular lesions in the oesophagus. These lesions are as under:

1. OESOPHAGEAL VARICES. Oesophageal varices are tortuous, dilated and engorged oesophageal veins,

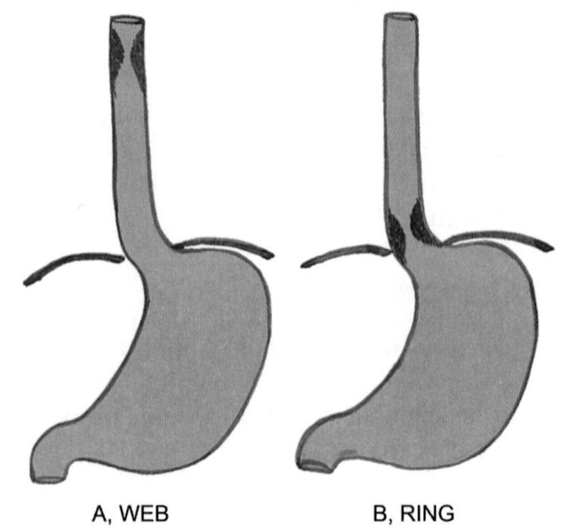

FIGURE 18.2

Oesophageal webs and rings.

seen along the longitudinal axis of oesophagus. They occur as a result of elevated pressure in the portal venous system, most commonly in cirrhosis of the liver (Chapter 19). Less common causes are: portal vein thrombosis, hepatic vein thrombosis (Budd-Chiari syndrome) and pylephlebitis. The lesions occur as a result of bypassing of portal venous blood from the liver to the oesophageal venous plexus. The increased venous pressure in the superficial veins of the oesophagus may result in ulceration and massive bleeding.

2. MALLORY-WEISS SYNDROME. In this condition, there is lacerations of mucosa at the gastro-oesophageal junction following minor trauma such as by vomiting, retching or vigorous coughing. Patients present with upper gastro-oesophageal bleeding.

3. RUPTURE OF THE OESOPHAGUS. Rupture of the oesophagus may occur following trauma, during oesophagoscopy, indirect injury (e.g. due to sudden acceleration and deceleration of the body) and spontaneous rupture (e.g. after overeating, extensive aerophagy etc).

4. OTHER CAUSES. Oesophageal haematemesis may also occur in the following conditions:

i) Bursting of aortic aneurysm into the lumen of oesophagus
ii) Vascular erosion by malignant growth in the vicinity
iii) Hiatus hernia
iv) Oesophageal cancer
v) Purpuras
vi) Haemophilia.

INFLAMMATORY LESIONS

Inflammation of the oesophagus, oesophagitis, occurs most commonly from reflux, although a number of other clinical conditions and infections may also cause oesophagitis as under:

Reflux (Peptic) Oesophagitis

Reflux of the gastric juice is the commonest cause of oesophagitis.

PATHOGENESIS. Gastro-oesophageal reflux, to an extent, may occur in normal healthy individuals after meals and in early pregnancy. However, in some clinical conditions, the gastro-oesophageal reflux is excessive, resulting in inflammation of the lower oesophagus. These conditions are as under:

i) Sliding hiatus hernia
ii) Chronic gastric and duodenal ulcers
iii) Nasogastric intubation
iv) Persistent vomiting
v) Surgical vagotomy
vi) Neuropathy in alcoholics, diabetics
vii) Oesophago-gastrostomy.

PATHOLOGIC CHANGES. ***Endoscopically,*** the demarcation between normal squamous and columnar epithelium at the junctional mucosa is lost. The affected distal oesophageal mucosa is red, erythematous, friable and bleeds on touch. In advanced cases, there are features of chronic disease such as nodularity, strictures, ulcerations and erosions.
Microscopically, the reflux changes in the distal oesophagus include basal cell hyperplasia and deep elongation of the papillae touching close to the surface epithelium. Inflammatory changes vary according to the stage of the disease. *In early stage,* mucosa and submucosa are infiltrated by some polymorphs and eosinophils; *in chronic stage,* there is lymphocytic infiltration and fibrosis of all the layers of the oesophageal wall.

Barrett's Oesophagus

This is a condition in which, following reflux oesophagitis, stratified squamous epithelium of the lower oesophagus is replaced by columnar epithelium (columnar metaplasia). The condition is seen more commonly in later age and is caused by factors producing gastro-oesophageal reflux disease (described above). Barrett's oesophagus is a premalignant condition evolving sequentially from Barrett's epithelium → dysplasia → carcinoma *in situ* → invasive adenocarcinoma.

PATHOLOGIC CHANGES. ***Endoscopically,*** the affected area is red and velvety. Hiatus hernia and peptic ulcer at squamo-columnar junction (Barrett's ulcer) are frequently associated.
Microscopically, the most common finding is the replacement of squamous epithelium by metaplastic columnar cells. Barrett's oesophagus may be composed of

- intestinal epithelium;
- fundic gastric glands; or
- cardiac mucous glands.

Other cells present in the glands may be Paneth cells, goblet cells, chief cells, parietal cells, mucus-secreting cells and endocrine cells.

Inflammatory changes, acute or chronic, are commonly accompanied. Dysplastic changes of the columnar epithelium or glands may be present. Long-standing cases of Barrett's oesophagus have 5-8% risk of developing adenocarcinoma of the oesophagus. Hence, there is need for follow-up of these cases by surveillance endoscopic biopsy.

Infective Oesophagitis

A number of opportunistic infections in immunosuppressed individuals can cause oesophagitis. Some of these agents are as follows:

i) Candida (Monilial) oesophagitis
ii) Herpes simplex (Herpetic oesophagitis)
iii) Cytomegalovirus
iv) Tuberculosis.

Other Causes of Oesophagitis

i) Intake of certain drugs (anticholinergic drugs, doxycycline, tetracycline)
ii) Ingestion of hot, irritating fluids
iii) Radiation
iv) Crohn's disease
v) Various vesiculobullous skin diseases.

TUMOURS OF OESOPHAGUS

Benign tumours of the oesophagus are uncommon and small in size (less than 3 cms). The epithelial benign tumours project as intraluminal masses arising from squamous epithelium (squamous cell papilloma), or from columnar epithelium (adenoma). The stromal or mesenchymal benign tumours are intramural masses such as leiomyoma and others like lipoma, fibroma, neurofibroma, rhabdomyoma, lymphangioma and haemangioma.

For all practical purposes, malignant tumours of the oesophagus are carcinomas because sarcomas such as leiomyosarcoma and fibrosarcoma occur with extreme rarity.

Carcinoma of Oesophagus

Carcinoma of the oesophagus is diagnosed late, after symptomatic oesophageal obstruction (dysphagia) has developed and the tumour has transgressed the anatomical limits of the organ. The tumour occurs more commonly in men over 50 years of age. Prognosis is dismal: with standard methods of therapy (surgical resection and/or irradiation), 70% of the patients die within one year of diagnosis. Five-year survival rate is 5-10%.

ETIOLOGY. Although exact etiology of carcinoma of the oesophagus is not known, a number of conditions and factors have been implicated as under:

1. Diet and personal habits:

i) Heavy smoking
ii) Alcohol consumption
iii) Intake of foods contaminated with fungus
iv) Nutritional deficiency of vitamins and trace elements

2. Oesophageal disorders:

i) Oesophagitis (especially Barrett's oesophagus in adenocarcinoma)
ii) Achalasia
iii) Hiatus hernia
iv) Diverticula
v) Plummer-Vinson syndrome.

3. Other factors:

i) *Race*—more common in the Chinese and Japanese than in Western races; more frequent in blacks than whites.
ii) *Family history*—association with tylosis (keratosis palmaris et plantaris).
iii) *Genetic factors*—predisposition with coeliac disease, epidermolysis bullosa, tylosis.

At molecular level, abnormality of *TP53* (earlier known as p53) tumour suppressor gene has been found associated with a number of above risk factors, notably with consumption of tobacco and alcohol, and in cases having proven Barrett's oesophagus.

PATHOLOGIC CHANGES. Carcinoma of the oesophagus is mainly of 2 types—squamous cell (epidermoid) and adenocarcinoma. The sites of predilection for each of these 2 forms is shown in Fig. 18.3.

SQUAMOUS CELL (EPIDERMOID) CARCINOMA. Squamous cell or epidermoid carcinoma comprises 90% of primary oesophageal cancers. It is exceeded in incidence by carcinoma colon, rectum and stomach amongst all the gastrointestinal cancers. The disease occurs in 6th to 7th decades of life and is more common in men than women. The sites of predilection are the three areas of oesophageal constrictions. Half of the squamous cell carcinomas of oesophagus occur in the middle third, followed by lower third, and the upper third of oesophagus in that order of frequency (Fig. 18.3).

Macroscopically, 3 types are recognised (Fig. 18.4):
i) *Polypoid fungating type*—is the most common form. It appears as a cauliflower-like friable mass protruding into the lumen.
ii) *Ulcerating type*—is the next common form. It looks grossly like a necrotic ulcer with everted edges.
iii) *Diffuse infiltrating type*—appears as an annular, stenosing narrowing of the lumen due to infiltration into the wall of oesophagus.

Chapter Eighteen

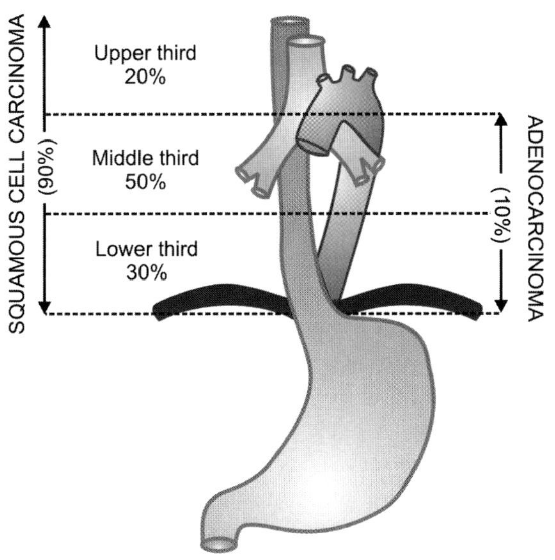

FIGURE 18.3

Carcinoma oesophagus—sites of predilection for squamous cell carcinoma and adenocarcinoma.

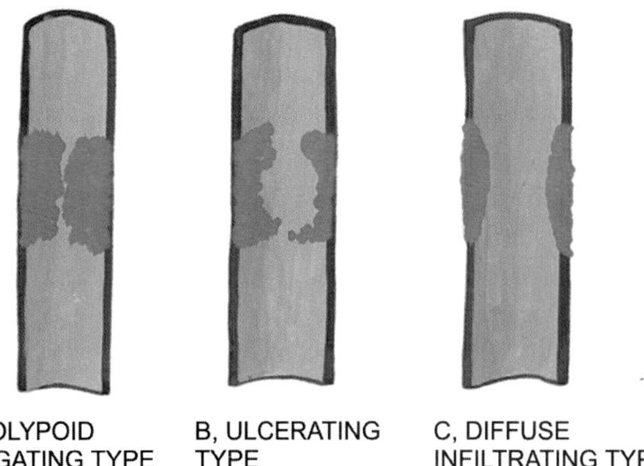

FIGURE 18.4

Macroscopic types of squamous cell carcinoma of the oesophagus.

Microscopically, majority of the squamous cell carcinomas of the oesophagus are well-differentiated or moderately-differentiated. Prickle cells, keratin formation and epithelial pearls are commonly seen. However, non-keratinising and anaplastic growth patterns can also occur (COLOUR PLATE X: CL 38). An exophytic, slow-growing, extremely well-differentiated variant, *verrucous squamous cell carcinoma,* has also been reported in the oesophagus.

ADENOCARCINOMA. Adenocarcinoma of the oesophagus constitutes less than 10% of primary oesophageal cancer. It occurs predominantly in men in their 4th to 5th decades. The common locations are lower and middle third of the oesophagus. These tumours have a strong and definite association with Barrett's oesophagus in which there are foci of gastric or intestinal type of epithelium.

Macroscopically, oesophageal adenocarcinoma appears as nodular, elevated mass in the lower oesophagus.

Microscopically, adenocarcinoma of the oesophagus can have 3 patterns:

i) *Intestinal type*—is the adenocarcinoma with a pattern similar to that seen in adenocarcinoma of intestine or stomach.

ii) *Adenosquamous type*—is the pattern in which there is an irregular admixture of adenocarcinoma and squamous cell carcinoma.

iii) *Adenoid cystic type*—is an uncommon variety and is akin to similar growth in salivary gland i.e. a cribriform appearance in an epithelial tumour.

The adenocarcinoma of the oesophagus must be distinguished from the adenocarcinoma of the gastric cardia. This is done by identifying normal oesophageal mucosa on distal as well as proximal margin of the tumour.

OTHER CARCINOMAS. Besides the two main histological types of oesophageal cancer, a few other varieties are occasionally encountered. These are as follow:

i) *Mucoepidermoid carcinoma* is a tumour having characteristics of squamous cell as well as mucus-secreting carcinomas.

ii) *Malignant melanoma* is derived from melanoblasts in the epithelium of the oesophagus.

iii) *Oat cell carcinoma* arises from argyrophil cells in the basal layer of the epithelium.

iv) *Undifferentiated carcinoma* is an anaplastic carcinoma which cannot be classified into any recognisable type of carcinoma.

v) *Carcinosarcoma* consists of malignant epithelial as well as sarcomatous components.

vi) *Secondary tumours* rarely occur in the oesophagus from carcinomas of the breast, kidney and adrenals.

SPREAD. The oesophageal cancer spreads locally as well as to distant sites.

i) Local spread. This is the most important mode of spread and is of great importance for surgical treatment. The local spread may occur in the transverse as well as longitudinal direction. The tumour may invade below into the stomach, above into the hypopharynx, into the trachea resulting in tracheo-oesophageal fistula, and may involve larynx causing hoarseness. The tumour may invade the muscular wall of the oesophagus and involve the mediastinum, lungs, bronchi, pleura and aorta.

ii) Lymphatic spread. Submucosal lymphatic permeation may lead to multiple satellite nodules away from the main tumour. Besides, the lymphatic spread may result in metastases to the cervical, para-oesophageal, tracheo-bronchial and subdiaphragmatic lymph nodes.

iii) Haematogenous spread. Blood-borne metastases from the oesophageal cancer are rare, probably because the death occurs early due to invasion of important structures by other modes of spread. However, metastatic deposits by haematogenous route can occur in the lungs, liver and adrenals.

STOMACH

NORMAL STRUCTURE

The stomach is 'gland with cavity', extending from its junction with lower end of the oesophagus (cardia) to its junction with the duodenum (pylorus). The *lesser curvature* is inner concavity on the right, while the *greater curvature* is the outer convexity on the left side of the stomach.

The stomach has 5 anatomical regions (Fig. 18.5):

1. **Cardia** is the oesophago-gastric junction and lacks the sphincter.

2. **Fundus** is the portion above the horizontal line drawn across the oesophago-gastric junction.

3. **Body** is the middle portion of the stomach between the fundus and the pyloric antrum.

4. **Pyloric antrum** is the distal third of the stomach.

5. **Pylorus** is the junction of distal end of the stomach with the duodenum. It has powerful sphincter muscle.

The mucosal folds in the region of the body and the fundus are loose (rugae), while the antral mucosa is somewhat flattened. *Gastric canal* is the relatively fixed portion of the pyloric antrum and the adjoining lesser curvature; it is the site for numerous pathological changes such as gastritis, peptic ulcer and gastric carcinoma.

The stomach receives its blood supply from the left gastric artery and the branches of the hepatic and splenic arteries with widespread anastomoses. Numerous gastric lymphatics which communicate freely with each other are also present. The innervation of the stomach is by the vagi and branches of the sympathetic which are connected with ganglia in the muscular and submucous layers.

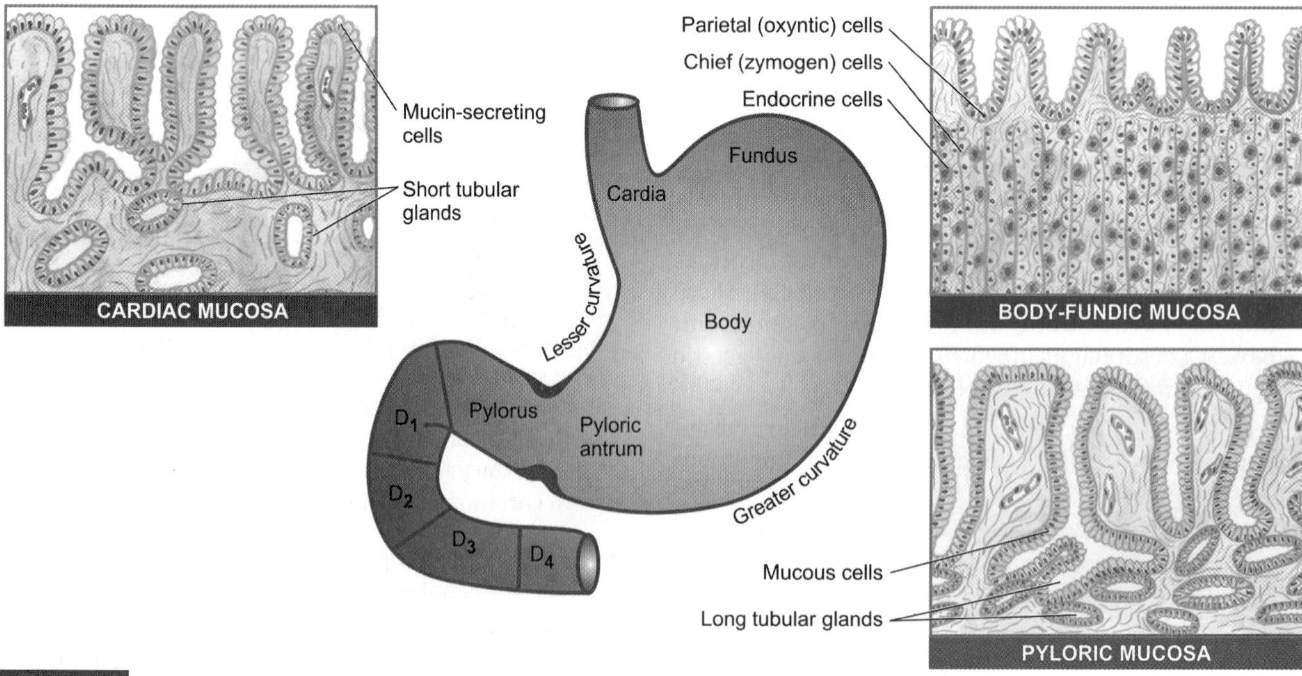

FIGURE 18.5

Anatomical subdivisions of the stomach correlated with histological appearance of gastric mucosa in different regions. D1, D2, D3 and D4 are the first to fourth parts of the duodenum.

Histologically, the wall of the stomach consists of 4 layers—serosa, muscularis, submucosa and mucosa.

1. Serosa is derived from the peritoneum which is deficient in the region of lesser and greater curvatures.

2. Muscularis consists of 3 layers of smooth muscle fibres—the outer longitudinal, the middle circular and the inner oblique. Nerve plexuses and ganglion cells are present between the longitudinal and circular layers of muscle. The pyloric sphincter is the thickened circular muscle layer at the gastroduodenal junction.

3. Submucosa is a layer of loose fibroconnective tissue binding the mucosa to the muscularis loosely and contains branches of blood vessels, lymphatics and nerve plexuses and ganglion cells.

4. Mucosa consists of 2 layers—superficial and deep. Between the two layers is the lamina propria composed of network of fibrocollagenic tissue with a few lymphocytes, plasma cells, macrophages and eosinophils. The mucosa is externally bounded by muscularis mucosae.

i) *THE SUPERFICIAL LAYER* consists of a single layer of surface epithelium composed of regular, mucin-secreting, tall columnar cells with basal nuclei. There is a very rapid turnover of these cells. These dip down at places to form crypts (or pits or foveolae).

- *Cardiac mucosa* is the transition zone between the oesophageal squamous mucosa and the oxyntic mucosa of the fundus and body with which it gradually merges.
- *Oxyntic mucosa* lines both gastric fundus and body.
- *Antral mucosa* lines the pyloric antrum.

ii) *THE DEEP LAYER* consists of glands that open into the bottom of the crypts. Depending upon the structure, these glands are of 3 types:

a) *Glands of the cardia* are simple tubular or compound tubulo-racemose, lined by mucin secreting cells. A few endocrine cells and occasional parietal and chief cells are also present.

b) *Glands of the body-fundus* are long, tubular and tightly packed which may be coiled or dilated. There are 4 types of cells present in the glands of body-fundic mucosa:

- *Parietal (Oxyntic) cells*—are the most numerous and line the superficial (upper) part of the glands. Parietal cells are triangular in shape, have dark-staining nuclei and eosinophilic cytoplasm. These cells are responsible for production of hydrochloric acid of the gastric juice and the blood group substances.
- *Chief (Peptic) cells*—are the dominant cells in the deeper (lower) parts of the glands. Their basal nuclei are large with prominent nucleoli and the cytoplasm is coarsely granular and basophilic. These cells secrete pepsin of the gastric juice.
- *Mucin-secreting neck cells*—are small and fewer. These cells are present in the region of the narrow neck of the gastric glands i.e. at the junction of the glands with the pits.
- *Endocrine (Kulchitsky or Enterochromaffin) cells*—are widely distributed in the mucosa of all parts of the alimentary tract and are described later (page 576).

c) *Glands of the pylorus* are much longer than the body-fundic glands. These are simple tubular glands which are often coiled. They are lined mainly by small, granular, mucin-secreting cells resembling neck cells and occasional parietal cells but no chief cells. Gastrin-producing G-cells are present predominantly in the region of antropyloric mucosa, with a small number of these cells in the crypts and Brunner's glands of the proximal duodenum.

The secretory products of the gastric mucosa are the *gastric juice* and the *intrinsic factor*, required for absorption of vitamin B_{12}. Gastric juice consists of hydrochloric acid, pepsin, mucin and electrolytes like Na^+, K^+, HCO'_3 and Cl^-. Hydrochloric acid is produced by the parietal (oxyntic) cells by the interaction of Cl′ ions of the arterial blood with water and carbon dioxide in the presence of the enzyme, carbonic anhydrase. The degree of gastric activity is correlated with the 'total parietal cell mass'. Injection of histamine can stimulate the production of acid component of the gastric juice, while the pepsin-secreting chief cells do not respond to histamine. Physiologically, the gastric secretions are stimulated by the food itself.

The **control of gastric secretions** chiefly occurs in one of the following 3 ways:

1. THE CEPHALIC PHASE—is stimulated by the sight, smell, taste or even thought of food. A neural reflex is initiated via branches of the vagus nerve that promotes the release of hydrochloric acid, pepsinogen and mucus.

2. THE GASTRIC PHASE—is triggered by the mechanical and chemical stimuli.

i) *The mechanical stimulation* comes from stretching of the wall of the stomach and conveying neural messages to the medulla for gastric secretion.

ii) *The chemical stimulation* is by digested proteins, amino acids, bile salts and alcohol which act on gastrin-producing G cells. The gastrin then passes into the blood stream and on return to the stomach promotes the release of gastric juice.

3. THE INTESTINAL PHASE—is triggered by the entry of protein-rich food in the small intestine. An intestinal hormone capable of stimulating gastric secretion is probably released into the blood stream.

GASTRIC ANALYSIS

In various diseases of the stomach, the laboratory tests to measure gastric secretions (consisting of gastric acid, pepsin, mucus and intrinsic factor) and serum gastrin are of particular significance (Table 18.1).

A. TESTS FOR GASTRIC SECRETIONS

1. Tests for Gastric Acid Secretions

The conventional fractional test meal (FTM) has been totally superseded by newer tests. These tests are based on the principle of measuring basal acid output (BAO) and maximal acid output (MAO) produced by the stomach under the influence of a variety of stimulants, and then comparing the readings of BAO and MAO with the normal values.

Quantitative analysis is performed after an overnight fast. The stomach is intubated and gastric secretion collected in 4 consecutive 15-minute intervals. This unstimulated, one-hour collection after titration for the acid concentration in it, is called BAO, expressed in mEq/hour. Subsequently, the stomach is stimulated to secrete maximal acid which is similarly collected for one hour and the acid content called as MAO, expressed in mEq/hour. Two highest 15-minute acid outputs are added and then multiplied by 2; this gives the peak acid output (PAO).

The tests for gastric acid secretion are named after the stimulants used for MAO. Some of the commonly used substances are as under:

TABLE 18.1: Gastric Analysis.

A. TESTS FOR GASTRIC SECRETIONS

1. *Tests for gastric acid secretions*
   - i) Histamine stimulation
   - ii) Histalog stimulation
   - iii) Pentagastrin (peptavlon) stimulation
   - iv) Insulin meal (Hollander test)
   - v) Tubeless analysis
2. *Tests for pepsin*
   Pepsin inhibitors
3. *Tests for mucus*
   Protein content of mucus
4. *Tests for intrinsic factor*

B. TESTS FOR GASTRIN

1. *Serum gastrin*
2. *Gastrin provocation tests*
   - i) Secretin test
   - ii) Calcium infusion test

i) HISTAMINE. Histamine was the first standard stimulant used for gastric acid secretion test. Subcutaneous injection of histamine phosphate (0.04 mg/kg body weight) is given with simultaneous administration of antihistaminic agent to prevent the untoward side-effects of histamine.

ii) HISTALOG (BETAZOLE). Subcutaneous injection of histalog (1-15 mg/kg body weight) is preferable over histamine due to fewer undesired side-effects and no need for administration of antihistaminic agent.

iii) PENTAGASTRIN (PEPTAVLON). Pentagastrin is currently the most preferred agent administered in the dose of 6 μg/kg body weight. Its activity is similar to gastrin.

iv) INSULIN MEAL (HOLLANDER TEST). This test is based on the fact that in a state of hypoglycaemia, direct vagal action on the parietal cell mass is responsible for acid secretion. Hypoglycaemia induced by intravenous insulin (15 IU soluble insulin) can be used as a test for evaluating the completeness of vagotomy. No increase in acid production should occur if the vagal resection is complete.

v) TUBELESS ANALYSIS. A resin-bound dye, diagnex blue, is given orally. The release of dye by the action of gastric acid and its appearance in the urine indicates the presence of gastric acid. The test can be repeated after giving stimulant of gastric secretion.

Significance

Normal value for BAO is 1.5-2.0 mEq/hour and for MAO is 12-40 mEq/hour. In gastric ulcer, the values of BAO and MAO are usually normal or slightly below normal.

Higher values are found in:

- duodenal ulcer,
- Zollinger-Ellison syndrome (gastrinoma); and
- anastomotic ulcer.

Low value or achlorhydria are observed in:

- pernicious anaemia (atrophic gastritis); and
- achlorhydria in the presence of gastric ulcer is highly suggestive of gastric malignancy.

2. Tests for Pepsin

Pepsin inhibitors are used for analysis of pepsin derived from pepsinogen for research purposes. The levels of pepsin are low in atrophic gastritis.

3. Tests for Mucus

Protein content of gastric mucus is measured, normal value being 1.8 mg/ml. The level is increased in chronic hypertrophic gastritis (Ménétrier's disease).

4. Test for Intrinsic Factor

Intrinsic factor (IF) is essential for vitamin B_{12} absorption from the small intestine. In its absence, the absorption of vitamin B_{12} is impaired as occurs in chronic atrophic gastritis and gastric atrophy. *The Schilling test* is used for evaluation of patients with suspected pernicious anaemia but can also be used as a diagnostic test for pancreatic insufficiency resulting in impaired absorption of vitamin B_{12} since gastric R-binder protein is not cleared from intrinsic factor due to reduced pancreatic proteolytic activity. The Schilling test is done in three stages and is discussed on page 383.

B. TESTS FOR GASTRIN

Circulating gastrin secreted by G-cells present in the antropyloric and proximal duodenal mucosa can be tested by the following methods:

1. Serum Gastrin Levels

Radioimmunoassay (RIA) is the commonly used method of measurement of serum gastrin levels. Normal fasting values are 20-150 pg/ml. The levels are high in:

- atrophic gastritis (with low gastric acid secretion);
- Zollinger-Ellison syndrome or gastrinoma (with high gastric acid secretion); and
- following surgery on the stomach.

2. Gastrin ProvocationTests

These tests are used to differentiate between hypergastrinaemia and gastric acid hypersecretion. These are as follows:

i) SECRETIN TEST. An intravenous injection of secretin (1 unit/kg body weight) is given. If the serum gastrin levels rise by more than 50% of basal value in 5-15 minutes, it is diagnostic of Zollinger-Ellison syndrome (gastrinoma). This rise does not occur in other conditions.

ii) CALCIUM INFUSION TEST. Intravenous infusion of calcium (5 mg/kg per hour) is given for 3 hour. Rise in serum gastrin levels by more than 50% of basal value is diagnostic of Zollinger-Ellison syndrome (gastrinoma).

CONGENITAL ANOMALIES

Pyloric Stenosis

Hypertrophy and narrowing of the pyloric lumen occurs predominantly in male children as a congenital defect *(infantile pyloric stenosis).* The *adult form* is rarely seen, either as a result of late manifestation of mild congenital anomaly or may be acquired type due to inflammatory fibrosis or invasion by tumours.

ETIOLOGY. The exact cause of *congenital (infantile)* pyloric stenosis is not known but it appears to have familial clustering and recessive genetic origin. The *acquired (adult)* pyloric stenosis is related to antral gastritis, and tumours in the region (gastric carcinoma, lymphoma, pancreatic carcinoma).

PATHOLOGIC CHANGES. Grossly and microscopically, there is hypertrophy as well as hyperplasia of the circular layer of muscularis in the pyloric sphincter accompanied by mild degree of fibrosis (Fig. 18.6).

CLINICAL FEATURES. The patient, usually a first born male infant 3 to 6 weeks old, presents with the following clinical features:

1. Vomiting, which may be projectile and occasionally contains bile or blood.
2. Visible peristalsis, usually noticed from left to right side of the upper abdomen.
3. Palpable lump, better felt after an episode of vomiting.
4. Constipation.
5. Loss of weight.

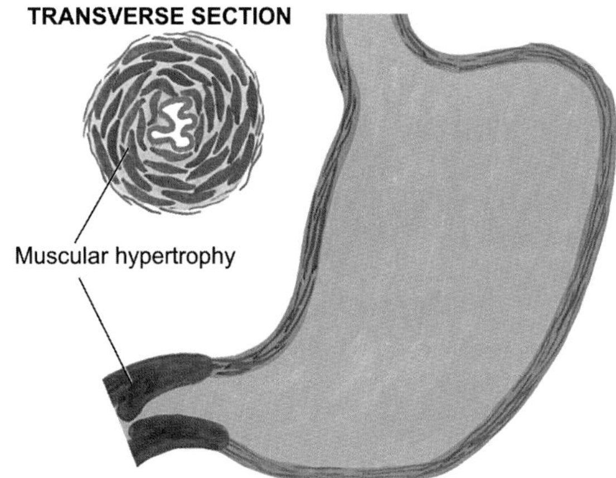

FIGURE 18.6

Pyloric stenosis, infantile type. Longitudinal and transverse section of stomach showing hypertrophy of the circular layer of the muscularis in the pyloric sphincter.

MISCELLANEOUS ACQUIRED CONDITIONS

Bezoars

Bezoars are foreign bodies in the stomach, usually in patients with mental illness who chew these substances. Some of the common bezoars are as follows:

- *Trichobezoars* composed of a ball of hair.
- *Phytobezoars* composed of vegetable fibres, seeds or fruit skin.
- *Trichophytobezoars* combining both hair and vegetable matter.

Acute Dilatation

Sudden and enormous dilatation of the stomach by gas or fluids due to paralysis of the gastric musculature may occur after abdominal operations, generalised peritonitis, and, in pyloric stenosis.

Gastric Rupture

The stomach may rupture rarely and prove fatal e.g. due to blunt trauma, external cardiac massage, ingestion of heavy meal or large quantity of liquid intake like beer.

INFLAMMATORY CONDITIONS

The two important inflammatory conditions of the stomach are *gastritis* and *peptic ulcer.* Rarely, stomach may be involved in tuberculosis, sarcoidosis and Crohn's disease.

GASTRITIS

The term 'gastritis' is commonly employed for any clinical condition with upper abdominal discomfort like indigestion or dyspepsia in which the specific clinical signs and radiological abnormalities are absent. The condition is of great importance due to its relationship with peptic ulcer and gastric cancer. Broadly speaking, gastritis may be of 2 types—acute and chronic. Chronic gastritis can further be of various types.

A simple classification of various types of gastritis is presented in Table 18.2.

TABLE 18.2: Classification of Gastritis.

A. ACUTE GASTRITIS		
1. Acute *H. pylori* gastritis		
2. Other acute infective gastritis (bacteria, viruses, fungi, parasites)		
3. Acute non-infective gastritis		
B. CHRONIC GASTRITIS		
1. Type A (autoimmune)	:	Body-fundic predominant
2. Type B (*H. pylori*-related) gastritis	:	Antral-predominant
3. Type AB (environmental)	:	Antral-body gastritis
4. Chemical (reflux) gastritis	:	Antral-body predominant
5. Uncommon forms of gastritis		

Acute Gastritis

Acute gastritis is a transient acute inflammatory involvement of the stomach, mainly mucosa.

ETIOPATHOGENESIS. A variety of etiologic agents have been implicated in the causation of acute gastritis. These are as follows:

1. Diet and personal habits:

- Highly spiced food
- Excessive alcohol consumption
- Malnutrition
- Heavy smoking

2. Infections:

- *Bacterial infections* e.g. *Helicobacter pylori,* diphtheria, salmonellosis, pneumonia, staphylococcal food poisoning.
- *Viral infections* e.g. viral hepatitis, influenza, infectious mononucleosis.

3. Drugs:

- Intake of drugs like non-steroidal anti-inflammatory drugs (NSAIDs), aspirin, cortisone, phenylbutazone, indomethacin, preparations of iron, chemotherapeutic agents.

4. Chemical and physical agents:

- Intake of corrosive chemicals such as caustic soda, phenol, lysol
- Gastric irradiation
- Freezing

5. Severe stress:

- Emotional factors like shock, anger, resentment etc.
- Extensive burns
- Trauma
- Surgery

The mucosal injury and subsequent acute inflammation in acute gastritis occurs by one of the following mechanisms:

1. *Reduced blood flow,* resulting in mucosal hypoperfusion due to ischaemia.

2. *Increased acid secretion* and its accumulation due to *H. pylori* infection resulting in damage to epithelial barrier.

3. *Decreased production of bicarbonate buffer.*

PATHOLOGIC CHANGES. Grossly, the gastric mucosa is oedematous with abundant mucus and haemorrhagic spots.

Microscopically, depending upon the stage, there is variable amount of oedema and infiltration by neutrophils in the lamina propria. In acute haemorrhagic and erosive gastritis, the mucosa is sloughed off and there are haemorrhages on the surface.

Chronic Gastritis

Chronic gastritis is the commonest histological change observed in biopsies from the stomach. The microscopic change is usually poorly correlated to the symptomatology, as the change is observed in about 35% of endoscopically normal mucosal biopsies. The condition occurs more frequently with advancing age; average age for symptomatic chronic gastritis being 45 years which corresponds well with the age incidence of gastric ulcer.

ETIOPATHOGENESIS. In the absence of clear etiology of chronic gastritis, a number of etiologic factors have been implicated. All the causative factors of acute gastritis described above may result in chronic gastritis too. Recurrent attacks of acute gastritis may result in chronic gastritis. Some additional causes are as under:

1. *Reflux of duodenal contents into the stomach,* especially in cases who have undergone surgical intervention in the region of pylorus.

2. Infection with *H. pylori* is strongly implicated in the etiology of chronic gastritis and is more common.

3. *Associated disease of the stomach and duodenum,* such as gastric or duodenal ulcer, gastric carcinoma.

4. *Chronic hypochromic anaemia,* especially associated with atrophic gastritis.

5. *Immunological factors* such as autoantibodies to gastric parietal cells in atrophic gastritis and autoantibodies against intrinsic factor.

The mechanism of chronic gastric injury by any of the etiologic agents is by cytotoxic effect of the injurious agent on the gastric mucosal epithelium, thus breaking the barrier and then inciting the inflammatory response.

CLASSIFICATION. Based on the type of mucosa affected (i.e. cardiac, body, pyloric, antral or transitional), a clinicopathologic classification has been proposed (Table 18.2).

1. Type A Gastritis (Autoimmune gastritis). Type A gastritis involves mainly the body-fundic mucosa. It is also called autoimmune gastritis due to the presence of circulating antibodies and is sometimes associated with other autoimmune diseases such as Hashimoto's thyroiditis and Addison's disease. As a result of the antibodies against parietal cells and intrinsic factor, there is depletion of parietal cells and impaired secretion of intrinsic factor. These changes may lead to significant gastric atrophy where intestinal metaplasia may occur, and a small proportion of these patients may develop pernicious anaemia. Due to depletion of gastric acid-producing mucosal area, there is hypo- or achlorhydria, and hyperplasia of gastrin-producing G cells in the antrum resulting in hypergastrinaemia.

2. Type B Gastritis (*H. pylori*-related). Type B gastritis mainly involves the region of antral mucosa and is more common. It is also called hypersecretory gastritis due to excessive secretion of acid, commonly due to infection with *H. pylori.* These patients may have associated peptic ulcer. Unlike type A gastritis, this form of gastritis has no autoimmune basis nor has association with other autoimmune diseases.

3. Type AB Gastritis (Environmental gastritis, Chronic atrophic gastritis). Type AB gastritis affects the mucosal region of A as well as B types (body-fundic and antral mucosa). This is the most common type of gastritis in all age groups. It is also called environmental gastritis because a number of as yet unidentified environmental factors have been implicated in its etiopathogenesis. Chronic atrophic gastritis is also used synonymously with type AB gastritis because in advanced stage, there is progression from chronic superficial gastritis to chronic atrophic gastritis, characterised by mucosal atrophy and metaplasia of intestinal or pseudopyloric type.

PATHOLOGIC CHANGES. Macroscopically, the features of all forms of gastritis are inconclusive. The gastric mucosa may be normal, atrophied, or oedematous.

Histologically, based on: i) the extent of inflammatory changes in the mucosa (i.e. superficial or deep); ii) the activity of inflammation (i.e. quiscent or active; acute or chronic); and iii) the presence of and type of metaplasia (i.e. intestinal or pseudo-pyloric), the following simple classification has been proposed:

1. Chronic superficial gastritis

2. Chronic atrophic gastritis
3. Gastric atrophy
4. Chronic hypertrophic gastritis (Ménétrier's disease)
5. Uncommon forms of chronic gastritis

Sydney system of recording of histologic changes in gastritis is more acceptable since it takes into account following multiple parameters:
i) Etiology (*H. pylori*, autoimmune, NSAIDs, infections).
ii) *Location* (pangastritis, predominant antral, predominant body-fundic).
iii) *Morphology* (depth of inflammation—superficial or deep, severity of inflammation, type of inflammation, atrophy, metaplasia).
iv) *Some special features* (e.g. granulomas, eosinophilic gastritis, erosions, necrosis, haemorrhages).

1. CHRONIC SUPERFICIAL GASTRITIS. As the name suggests there is inflammatory infiltrate consisting of plasma cells and lymphocytes in the superficial layer of the gastric mucosa, *but there are no histological changes in the deep layer of mucosa containing gastric glands.* Chronic superficial gastritis may resolve completely or may progress to chronic gastric atrophy.

H. pylori, a spiral-shaped bacteria, is found in almost all active cases of chronic superficial gastritis and about 65% of quiscent cases. The organism is identified on the epithelial layer on the luminal surface and does not invade the mucosa (Fig. 18.7, A). It is not seen on areas with intestinal metaplasia.

H. Pylori gastritis can be diagnosed by the following techniques:
i) *Invasive tests* based on endoscopic biopsy include:
a) histologic examination followed by Giemsa, Steiner silver or Warthin-Starry stains for identification of microorganism;
b) biopsy urease test which is quick and simple but not fully sensitive; and
c) culture of the microorganism that helps in determining specific antibiotic sensitivity.
ii) *Non-invasive tests* are:
a) serologic test which is cheap and convenient but may not be helpful in early follow-up cases; and
b) 14C urea breath test.

Although most patients of chronic superficial gastritis due to *H. pylori* remain asymptomatic, they may develop chronic atrophic gastritis, gastric atrophy, peptic ulcer disease and malignant transformation (Fig. 18.7,B).

2. CHRONIC ATROPHIC GASTRITIS. In this stage, *there is inflammatory cell infiltrate in the deeper layer of the mucosa and atrophy of the epithelial elements including destruction of the glands.* Two types of metaplasia are commonly associated with atrophic gastritis:

i) Intestinal metaplasia. Intestinal metaplasia is more common and involves antral mucosa more frequently. Characteristic histologic feature is the presence of intestinal type mucus-goblet cells; Paneth cells and endocrine cells may also be present. Parietal cells are very few or absent (Fig. 18.8). Intestinal

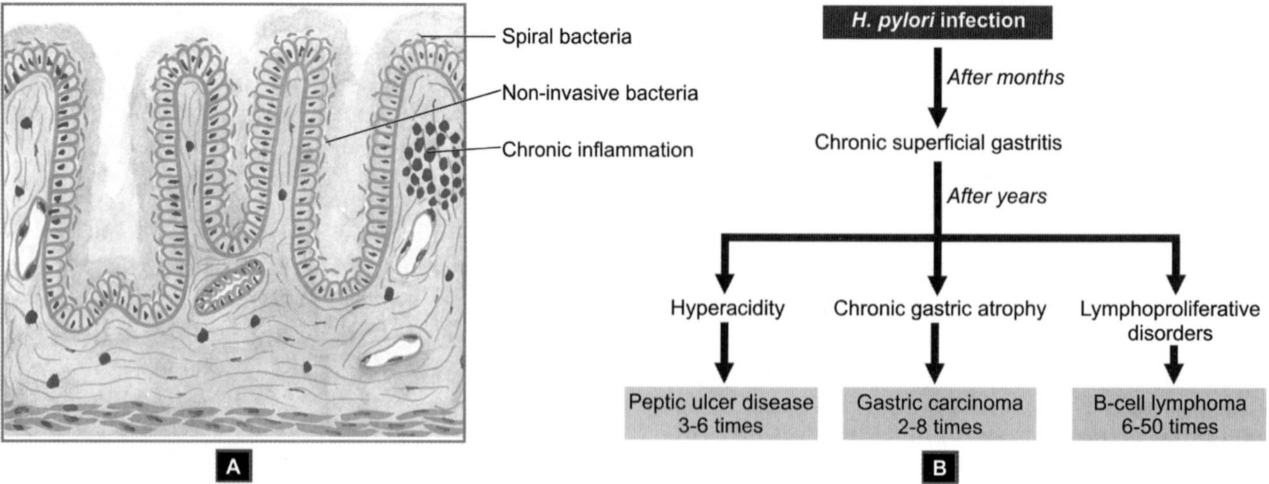

FIGURE 18.7

A, Histologic appearance of *H. pylori* chronic gastritis. B, Consequences of long-term *H. pylori* gastritis.

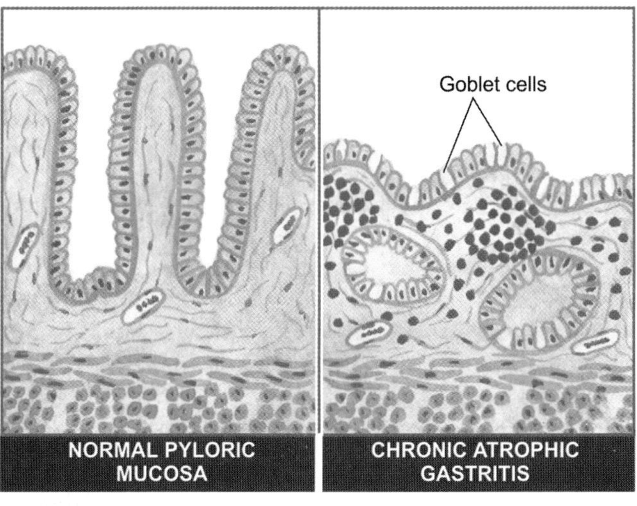

FIGURE 18.8

Chronic atrophic gastritis (right) contrasted with normal pyloric mucosa (left). There is marked gastric atrophy with disappearance of gastric glands and appearance of goblet cells (intestinal metaplasia).

metaplasia, focal or extensive, in atrophic gastritis is significant because its incidence is high in populations having high prevalence rate of gastric cancer like in Japan. However, areas of intestinal metaplasia are not colonised by *H. pylori*.

ii) Pseudopyloric metaplasia. It involves the body glands which are replaced by proliferated mucous neck cells, conforming in appearance to normal pyloric glands. Its significance is not known.

3. GASTRIC ATROPHY. In this, there is thinning of the gastric mucosa with loss of glands but no inflammation though lymphoid aggregates may be present.

4. CHRONIC HYPERTROPHIC GASTRITIS (MÉNÉTRIER'S DISEASE). This is an uncommon condition characterised pathologically by enormous thickening of gastric rugal folds resembling cerebral convolutions, affecting mainly the region of fundic-body mucosa and characteristically sparing antral mucosa. The patients present with dyspepsia, haematemesis, melaena or protein-losing enteropathy.

Histologically, the gastric pits are elongated and are tortuous. The mucosa is markedly thickened and parts of muscularis mucosae may extend into the thickened folds. Epithelium-lined cysts are commonly seen in the glandular layer. Inflammatory infiltrate is usually mild but lymphoid follicles may be present. The condition is considered significant in view of the risk of developing cancer.

5. UNCOMMON FORMS OF CHRONIC GASTRITIS. A few other types of gastritis which do not fit into the description of the types of gastritis described above are listed below:

i) Gastric candidiasis. Infection with *Candida albicans* may occur as an opportunistic infection in immunosuppressed and debilitated individuals.

ii) Eosinophilic gastritis. This condition is characterised by diffuse thickening of the pyloric antrum due to oedema and extensive infiltration by eosinophils in all the layers of the wall of antrum. Eosinophilic gastritis probably has an allergic basis.

iii) Chronic follicular gastritis. This is a variant of chronic atrophic gastritis in which numerous lymphoid follicles are present in the mucosa and submucosa of the stomach.

iv) Haemorrhagic (Erosive) gastritis. In this condition, there are superficial erosions and mucosal haemorrhages, usually following severe haematemesis. The causes for such erosions and haemorrhages are duodenal-gastric reflux, administration of non-steroidal anti-inflammatory drugs (NSAIDs), portal hypertension.

v) Granulomatous gastritis. Rarely, granulomas may be present in the gastric mucosa such as in tuberculosis, sarcoidosis, Crohn's disease, syphilis, various mycoses, and as a reaction to endogenous substance or foreign material.

PEPTIC ULCERS

Peptic ulcers are the areas of degeneration and necrosis of gastrointestinal mucosa exposed to acid-peptic secretions. Though they can occur at any level of the alimentary tract that is exposed to hydrochloric acid and pepsin, they occur most commonly (98-99%) in either the duodenum or the stomach in the ratio of 4:1. Each of the two main types may be acute or chronic.

Acute Peptic (Stress) Ulcers

Acute peptic ulcers or stress ulcers are multiple, small mucosal erosions, seen most commonly in the stomach but occasionally involving the duodenum.

ETIOLOGY. These ulcers occur following severe stress. The causes are as follows:

i) *Psychological stress*

ii) *Physiological stress* as in the following:

- Shock

- Severe trauma
- Septicaemia
- Extensive burns (Curling's ulcers in the posterior aspect of the first part of the duodenum).
- Intracranial lesions (Cushing's ulcers developing from hyperacidity following excessive vagal stimulation).
- Drug intake (e.g. aspirin, steroids, butazolidine, indomethacin).
- Local irritants (e.g. alcohol, smoking, coffee etc).

PATHOGENESIS. It is not clear how the mucosal erosions occur in stress ulcers because actual hypersecretion of gastric acid is demonstrable in only Cushing's ulcers occurring from intracranial conditions such as due to brain trauma, intracranial surgery and brain tumours. In all other etiologic factors, gastric acid secretion is normal or below normal. In these conditions, the possible hypotheses for genesis of stress ulcers are as under:

1. Ischaemic hypoxic injury to the mucosal cells.
2. Depletion of the gastric mucus 'barrier' rendering the mucosa susceptible to attack by acid-peptic secretions.

PATHOLOGIC CHANGES. ***Grossly,*** acute stress ulcers are multiple (more than three ulcers in 75% of cases). They are more common anywhere in the stomach, followed in decreasing frequency by occurrence in the first part of duodenum. They may be oval or circular in shape, usually less than 1 cm in diameter.

Microscopically, the stress ulcers are shallow and do not invade the muscular layer. The margins and base may show some inflammatory reaction depending upon the duration of the ulcers. These ulcers commonly heal by complete re-epithelialisation without leaving any scars. Complications such as haemorrhage and perforation may occur.

Chronic Peptic Ulcers (Gastric and Duodenal Ulcers)

If not specified, chronic peptic ulcers would mean gastric and duodenal ulcers, the two major forms of 'peptic ulcer disease' of the upper GI tract in which the acid-pepsin secretions are implicated in their pathogenesis. Peptic ulcers are common in the present-day life of the industrialised and civilised world.

Gastric and duodenal ulcers represent two distinct diseases as far as their etiology, pathogenesis and clinical features are concerned. However, pathological findings in both are similar and quite diagnostic. The contrasting features of both these conditions are described together below. A comparative summary of features of gastric and duodenal peptic ulcers is presented in Table 18.3.

INCIDENCE. Peptic ulcers are more frequent in middle-aged adults. The peak incidence for duodenal ulcer is 5th decade, while for gastric ulcer it is a decade later (6th decade). Duodenal as well as gastric ulcers are more common in males than in females. Duodenal ulcer is almost four times more common than gastric ulcer; the overall incidence of gastroduodenal ulcers being approximately 10% of the male population.

ETIOLOGY. The immediate cause of peptic ulcer disease is disturbance in normal protective mucosal 'barrier' by acid-pepsin, resulting in digestion of the mucosa. However, in contrast to duodenal ulcers, *the patients of gastric ulcer have low-to-normal gastric acid secretions, though true achlorhydria in response to stimulants never occurs in benign gastric ulcer.* Besides, 10-20% patients of gastric ulcer may have coexistent duodenal ulcer as well. Thus, the etiology of peptic ulcers possibly may not be explained on the basis of a single factor but is multifactorial. These factors are as under:

1. *Helicobacter pylori* gastritis. About 15-20% cases infected with *H. pylori* in the antrum develop duodenal ulcer in their life time while gastric colonisation by *H. pylori* never develops ulceration and remain asymptomatic. *H. pylori* can be identified in mucosal samples by histologic examination, culture, increased activity, and serology (IgG and IgA antibodies to *H. pylori)* (also *see* page 562).

2. Acid-pepsin secretions. There is conclusive evidence that some level of acid-pepsin secretion is essential for the development of duodenal as well as gastric ulcer. Peptic ulcers never occur in association with pernicious anaemia in which there are no acid and pepsin-secreting parietal and chief cells respectively.

3. Mucus secretion. Any condition that decreases the quantity or quality of normal protective mucus 'barrier' predisposes to the development of peptic ulcer.

4. Gastritis. Some degree of gastritis is always present in the region of gastric ulcer, though it is not clear whether it is the cause or the effect of ulcer. Besides, the population distribution pattern of gastric ulcer is similar to that of chronic gastritis.

5. Local irritants. Pyloric antrum and lesser curvature of the stomach are the sites most exposed for longer

TABLE 18.3: Distinguishing Features of Two Major Forms of Peptic Ulcers.

FEATURE	DUODENAL ULCER	GASTRIC ULCER
1. *Incidence*	i) Four times more common than gastric ulcers	Less common than duodenal ulcers
	ii) Usual age 25-50 years	Usually beyond 6th decade
	iii) More common in males than in females (4:1)	More common in males than in females (3.5:1)
2. *Etiology*	Most commonly as a result of *H. pylori* infection Other factors—hypersecretion of acid-pepsin, association with alcoholic cirrhosis, tobacco, hyperparathyroidism, chronic pancreatitis, blood group O, genetic factors	Gastric colonisation with *H. pylori* asymptomatic but higher chances of development of duodenal ulcer. Disruption of mucus barrier most important factor. Association with gastritis, bile reflux, drugs, alcohol, tobacco
3. *Pathogenesis*	i) Mucosal digestion from hyperacidity most significant factor	Usually normal-to-low acid levels; hyperacidity if present is due to high serum gastrin
	ii) Protective gastric mucus barrier may be damaged	Damage to mucus barrier significant factor
4. *Pathologic changes*	i) Most common in the first part of duodenum	Most common along the lesser curvature and pyloric antrum
	ii) Often solitary, 1-2.5 cm in size, round to oval, punched out	Grossly similar to duodenal ulcer
	iii) Histologically, composed of 4 layers—necrotic, superficial exudative, granulation tissue and cicatrisation	Histologically, indistinguishable from duodenal ulcer
5. *Complications*	Commonly haemorrhage, perforation, sometimes obstruction; malignant transformation never occurs	Perforation, haemorrhage and at times obstruction; malignant transformation in less than 1% cases
6. *Clinical features*	i) Pain-food-relief pattern	Food-pain pattern
	ii) Night pain common	No night pain
	iii) No vomiting	Vomiting common
	iv) Melaena more common than haematemesis	Haematemesis more common
	v) No loss of weight	Significant loss of weight
	vi) No particular choice of diet	Patients choose bland diet devoid of fried foods, curries etc.
	vii) Deep tenderness in the right hypochondrium	Deep tenderness in the midline in epigastrium
	viii) Marked seasonal variation	No seasonal variation
	ix) Occurs more commonly in people at greater stress	More often in labouring groups

periods to local irritants and thus are the common sites for occurrence of gastric ulcers. Some of the local irritating substances implicated in the etiology of peptic ulcers are heavily spiced foods, alcohol, cigarette smoking, unbuffered aspirin, non-steroidal anti-inflammatory drugs etc.

6. **Dietary factors.** Nutritional deficiencies have been regarded as etiologic factors in peptic ulcers e.g. occurrence of gastric ulcer in poor socioeconomic strata, higher incidence of duodenal ulcer in parts of South India. However, malnutrition does not appear to have any causative role in peptic ulceration in European countries and the U.S.

7. **Psychological factors.** Psychological stress, anxiety, fatigue and ulcer-type personality may exacerbate as well as predispose to peptic ulcer disease.

8. Genetic factors. People with blood group O appear to be more prone to develop peptic ulcers than those with other blood groups. Genetic influences appear to have greater role in duodenal ulcers as evidenced by their occurrence in families, monozygotic twins and association with HLA-B5 antigen.

9. Hormonal factors. Secretion of certain hormones by tumours is associated with peptic ulceration e.g. elaboration of gastrin by islet-cell tumour in Zollinger-Ellison syndrome, endocrine secretions in hyperplasia and adenomas of parathyroid glands, adrenal cortex and anterior pituitary.

10. Miscellaneous. Duodenal ulcers have been observed to occur in association with various other conditions such as alcoholic cirrhosis, chronic renal failure, hyperparathyroidism, chronic obstructive pulmonary disease, and chronic pancreatitis.

PATHOGENESIS. Although the role of various etiologic factors just described is well known in ulcerogenesis, two most important factors in peptic ulcer are:

- exposure of mucosa to gastric acid and pepsin secretion; and
- strong etiologic association with *H. pylori* infection.

There are distinct differences in the pathogenetic mechanisms involved in duodenal and gastric ulcers as under:

Duodenal ulcer. There is conclusive evidence to support the role of high acid-pepsin secretions in the causation of duodenal ulcers. Besides this, a few other noteworthy features in the pathogenesis of duodenal ulcers are as follows:

1. There is generally *hypersecretion of gastric acid* into the fasting stomach at night which takes place under the influence of vagal stimulation. There is high basal as well as maximal acid output (BAO and MAO) in response to various stimuli.

2. Patients of duodenal ulcer have *rapid emptying* of the stomach so that the food which normally buffers and neutralises the gastric acid, passes down into the small intestine, leaving the duodenal mucosa exposed to the aggressive action of gastric acid.

3. *Helicobacter* gastritis caused by *H. pylori* is seen in 95-100% cases of duodenal ulcers. The underlying mechanisms are as under:

i) *H. pylori*-infected mucosal epithelium releases *proinflammatory cytokines* such as IL-1, IL-6, IL-8 and tumour necrosis factor, all of which incite intense inflammatory reaction.

ii) Gastric *mucosal defense is broken* by bacterial elaboration of urease, protease, catalase and phospholipase.

iii) Epithelial injury is also induced by cytotoxin-associated gene protein *(CagA)*, while vacuolating cytotoxin *(VacA)* and *picB* induce elaboration of cytokines.

Gastric ulcer. The pathogenesis of gastric ulcer is mainly explained on the basis of impaired gastric mucosal defenses against acid-pepsin secretions. Some other features in the pathogenesis of gastric ulcer are as follows:

1. Hyperacidity may occur in gastric ulcer due to *increased serum gastrin* levels in response to ingested food in an atonic stomach.

2 However, many a patients of gastric ulcer have low-to-normal gastric acid levels. Ulcerogenesis in such patients is explained on the basis of damaging influence of *other factors* such as gastritis, bile reflux, cigarette smoke etc.

3. The normally protective *gastric mucus 'barrier'* against acid-pepsin is deranged in gastric ulcer. There is depletion in the quantity as well as quality of gastric mucus. One of the mechanisms for its depletion is colonisation of the gastric mucosa by *H. pylori* seen in 75-80% patients of gastric ulcer.

PATHOLOGIC CHANGES. Gross and microscopic changes in gastric and duodenal ulcers are similar and quite characteristic. *Gastric ulcers* are found predominantly along the lesser curvature in the region of pyloric antrum, more commonly on the posterior than the anterior wall. Most *duodenal ulcers* are found in the first part of the duodenum, usually immediate post-pyloric, more commonly on the anterior than the posterior wall. Uncommon locations include ulcer in the cardia, marginal ulcer and in the Meckel's diverticulum (Fig. 18.9).

Grossly, typical peptic ulcers are commonly solitary (80%), small (1-2.5 cm in diameter), round to oval and characteristically 'punched out'. Benign ulcers usually have flat margins in level with the surrounding mucosa. The mucosal folds converge towards the ulcer. The ulcers may vary in depth from being superficial (confined to mucosa) to deep ulcers (penetrating into the muscular layer). In about 10-20% of cases, gastric and duodenal ulcers are coexistent. Vast majority of the peptic ulcers are benign. *Chronic duodenal ulcer never turns malignant,* while chronic gastric ulcer may develop carcinoma in less

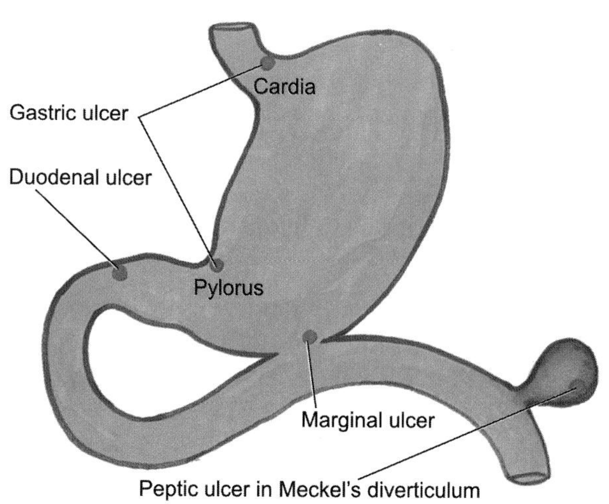

FIGURE 18.9

Distribution of peptic ulcers.

than 1% of cases. Malignant gastric ulcers are larger, bowl-shaped with elevated and indurated mucosa at the margin (Fig. 18.10).

Microscopically, chronic peptic ulcers have 4 histological zones (Fig. 18.11). From within outside, these are as under (COLOUR PLATE XXIII: CL 89):

1. *Necrotic zone*—lies in the floor of the ulcer and is composed of fibrinous exudate containing necrotic debris and a few leucocytes.
2. *Superficial exudative zone*—lies underneath the necrotic zone. The tissue elements here show coagulative necrosis giving eosinophilic, smudgy appearance with nuclear debris.
3. *Granulation tissue zone*—is seen merging into the necrotic zone. It is composed of nonspecific inflammatory infiltrate and proliferating capillaries.

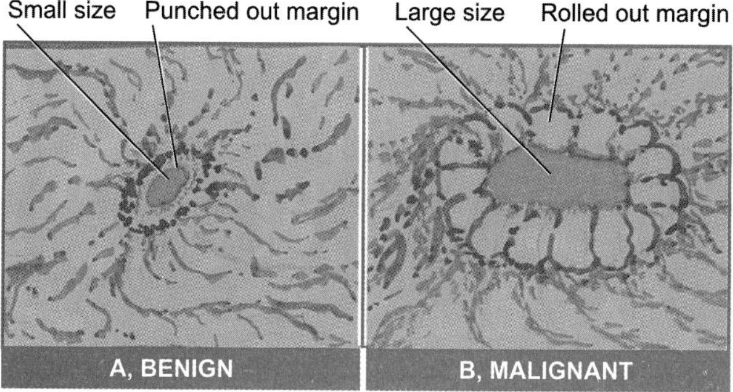

FIGURE 18.10

Chronic gastric ulcer (A) contrasted with malignant gastric ulcer (B).

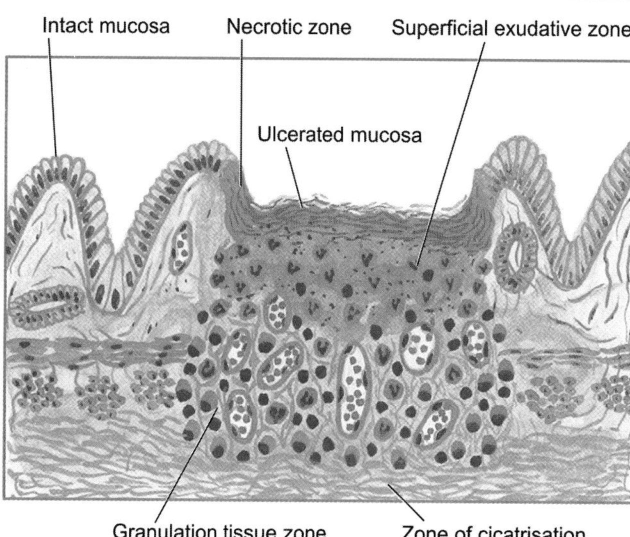

FIGURE 18.11

Chronic peptic ulcer. Histologic zones of the ulcer are illustrated in the diagram.

4. *Zone of cicatrisation*—is seen merging into thick layer of granulation tissue. It is composed of dense fibrocollagenic scar tissue over which granulation tissue rests. Thrombosed or sclerotic arteries may cross the ulcer which on erosion may result in haemorrhage.

COMPLICATIONS. Acute and subacute peptic ulcers usually heal without leaving any visible scar. However, healing of chronic, larger and deeper ulcers may result in complications. These are as follows:

1. Obstruction. Development of fibrous scar at or near the pylorus results in pyloric stenosis. In the case of healed duodenal ulcer, it causes duodenal stenosis. Healed ulcers along the lesser curvatures may produce 'hour glass' deformity due to fibrosis and contraction.

2. Haemorrhage. Minor bleeding by erosion of small blood vessels in the base of an ulcer occurs in all the ulcers and can be detected by testing the stool for occult blood. Chronic blood loss may result in iron deficiency anaemia. Severe bleeding may cause 'coffee ground' vomitus or melaena. A penetrating chronic ulcer may erode a major artery (e.g. left gastric, gastroduodenal or splenic artery) and cause a massive and severe hematemesis and sometimes death.

3. Perforation. A perforated peptic ulcer is an acute abdominal emergency. Perforation occurs more commonly in chronic duodenal ulcers than chronic gastric ulcers. Following sequelae may result:

i) On perforation the contents escape into the lesser sac or into the peritoneal cavity, causing *acute peritonitis.*

ii) Air escapes from the stomach and lies between the liver and the diaphragm giving the characteristic radiological appearance of *air under the diaphragm.*

iii) *Subphrenic abscess* between the liver and the diaphragm may develop due to infection.

iv) Perforation may extend to involve the *adjacent organs* e.g. the liver and pancreas.

4. **Malignant transformation.** The dictum *'cancers ulcerate but ulcers rarely cancerate'* holds true for most peptic ulcers. A chronic duodenal ulcer never turns malignant, while less than 1% of chronic gastric ulcers may transform into carcinoma.

CLINICAL FEATURES. Peptic ulcers are remitting and relapsing lesions. Their chronic and recurrent behaviour is summed up the saying: *'once a peptic ulcer patient, always a peptic ulcer patient.'* The two major forms of chronic peptic ulcers show variations in clinical features which are as follows:

1. **Age.** The peak incidence of duodenal ulcer is in 5th decade while that for gastric ulcer is a decade later.

2. **People at risk.** Duodenal ulcer occurs more commonly in people faced with more stress and strain of life (e.g. executives, leaders), while gastric ulcer is seen more often in labouring groups.

3. **Periodicity.** The attacks in gastric ulcers last from 2-6 weeks, with interval of freedom from 1-6 months. The attacks of duodenal ulcer, are classically worsened by *'work, worry and weather.'*

4. **Pain.** In gastric ulcer, epigastric pain occurs immediately or within 2 hours after food and never occurs at night. In duodenal ulcer, pain is severe, occurs late at night ('hunger pain') and is usually relieved by food.

5. **Vomiting.** Vomiting which relieves the pain is a conspicuous feature in patients of gastric ulcer. Duodenal ulcer patients rarely have vomiting but instead get heart-burn (retrosternal pain) and 'water brash' (burning fluid into the mouth).

6. **Haematemesis and melaena.** Haematemesis and melaena occur in gastric ulcers in the ratio of 60:40, while in duodenal ulcers in the ratio of 40:60. Both may occur together more commonly in duodenal ulcer than in gastric ulcer patients.

7. **Appetite.** The gastric ulcer patients, though have good appetite but are afraid to eat, while duodenal ulcer patients have very good appetite.

8. **Diet.** Patients of gastric ulcer commonly get used to a bland diet consisting of milk, eggs etc and avoid taking fried foods, curries and heavily spiced foods. In contrast, duodenal ulcer patients usually take all kinds of diets.

9. **Weight.** Loss of weight is a common finding in gastric ulcer patients while patients of duodenal ulcer tend to gain weight due to frequent ingestion of milk to avoid pain.

10. **Deep tenderness.** Deep tenderness is demonstrable in both types of peptic ulcers. In the case of gastric ulcer it is in the midline of the epigastrium, while in the duodenal ulcer it is in the right hypochondrium.

HAEMATEMESIS AND MELAENA OF GASTRIC ORIGIN

In continuity with the discussion on peptic ulcers which are the commonest cause of haematemesis and melaena, it is worthwhile listing various causes of haematemesis of gastric origin (causes of haematemesis of oesophageal origin are already given on page 552).

i) Chronic peptic ulcers (gastric as well as duodenal)
ii) Acute peptic ulcers (stress ulcers)
iii) Multiple gastric and duodenal erosions
iv) Carcinoma of the stomach
v) Peptic ulcer in Meckel's diverticulum
vi) Mallory-Weiss syndrome
vii) Anaemias
viii) Purpuras
ix) Haemophilia.

TUMOURS AND TUMOUR-LIKE LESIONS

The various types of tumour-like lesions (polyps) and benign and malignant tumours of the stomach are given in Table 18.4.

A. TUMOUR-LIKE LESIONS (POLYPS)

Tumour-like lesions are the polyps of the stomach which are of the following types:

Hyperplastic (Inflammatory) Polyps

Hyperplastic or inflammatory polyps are regenerative, non-neoplastic lesions which are the most common type (90%). They may be single or multiple and are more often located in the pyloric antrum.

Grossly, the lesions may be sessile or pedunculated, 1 cm or larger in size, smooth and soft. The surface may be ulcerated or haemorrhagic.

TABLE 18.4: Gastric Tumours and Tumour-like Lesions.

A. TUMOUR-LIKE LESIONS (POLYPS)
1. Hyperplastic (inflammatory) polyps
2. Hamartomatous polyps

B. BENIGN TUMOURS
1. *Epithelial*
Adenomas (adenomatous or neoplastic polyps)
2. *Non-epithelial*
Gastrointestinal spindle cell (stromal) tumours (GIST)

C. MALIGNANT TUMOURS
1. *Epithelial (90%)*
(i) Adenocarcinoma
(ii) Others
2. *Non-epithelial (2%)*
(i) Leiomyosarcoma
(ii) Leiomyoblastoma (epithelioid leiomyoma)
3. *Carcinoid tumour* (3%)
4. *Lymphoma (4%)*

Microscopically, they are composed of irregular hyperplastic glands, which may show cystic change. The lining epithelium is mostly superficial gastric type but antral glands, chief cells and parietal cells may be present. These lesions do not have cellular atypia and do not have malignant potential.

Hamartomatous Polyps

Hamartomatous polyps are not true neoplasms but are malformations. They are of various types such as gastric polyps of the Peutz-Jeghers syndrome (page 598), juvenile polyp, pancreatic heterotopia, heterotopia of Brunner's glands and inflammatory fibroid polyps (eosinophilic granulomatous polyps).

B. BENIGN TUMOURS

Benign tumours of the stomach are uncommon and usually incidental findings.

Adenomas (Adenomatous or Neoplastic Polyps)

Adenomas, also, referred to as adenomatous or neoplastic polyps, are true benign epithelial neoplasms and are much rarer in the stomach than in the large intestine. They are also found more often in the region of pyloric antrum. They are commonly associated with atrophic gastritis and pernicious anaemia. Morphologically, adenomatous polyps of the stomach resemble their counterparts in the large bowel and are described there (page 599).

Stromal Tumours

Stomach may be the site for occurrence of various uncommon benign tumours of stromal cell origin e.g. leiomyomas (being the most common); others are neurofibromas, schwannomas and lipomas. They are usually firm, circumscribed nodules, less than 4 cm in size and appear as submucosal nodules. They resemble in gross and microscopic appearance with their counterparts in other parts of the body.

Currently, the term *gastrointestinal stromal tumours (GISTs)* is used for a group of uncommon benign tumours composed of spindle cells or stromal cells but lacking the true phenotypic features of smooth muscle cells, neural cells or Schwann cells. They are uncommon but as compared to other sites in the GIT, are most common in the stomach. Their behaviour is generally benign but may be recurrent, aggressive or even metastasis may occur.

C. MALIGNANT TUMOURS

Gastric Carcinoma

INCIDENCE. Carcinoma of the stomach comprises more than 90% of all gastric malignancies and is the leading cause of cancer-related deaths in countries where its incidence is high. The highest incidence is between 4th to 6th decades of life and is twice more common in men than in women.

ETIOLOGY. A number of etiologic factors have been implicated in causation of gastric cancer. These are as under:

1. ***H. pylori* infection.** *H. pylori* infection of the stomach is an important risk factor for the development of gastric cancer. Epidemiologic studies throughout world have shown that a seropositivity with *H. pylori* is associated with 3 to 6 times higher risk of development of gastric cancer. It may be mentioned here that similar association of *H. pylori* infection exists with gastric lymphomas as well.

2. **Dietary factors.** Epidemiological studies suggest that dietary factors are most significant in the etiology of gastric cancer. The evidences in support of this are multifold:

i) Occurrence of gastric cancer in the region of gastric canal (i.e. along the lesser curvature and the pyloric antrum) where irritating foods exert their maximum effect.

ii) Populations consuming certain foodstuffs have high risk of developing gastric cancer e.g. ingestion of smoked foods, high intake of salt, pickled raw vegetables, high intake of carcinogens as nitrates in foods and drinking water, nitrites as preservatives for certain meats etc. However, intake of green leafy vegetables, citrus fruits and animal fats has been reported to have protective role in gastric cancer.

iii) Tobacco smoke, tobacco juice and consumption of alcohol have all been shown to have carcinogenic effect on gastric mucosa.

3. Geographical factors. There are geographic variations in the incidence of gastric cancer. Japan, Chile, Finland and Iceland have highest recorded death rate from gastric cancer, while the incidence is considerably low in the US, UK and Canada. The higher incidence in certain geographic locales is likely to be the result of environmental influences as observed from the finding of incidence of gastric cancer in the next generation of Japanese immigrants to the US which is comparable to that of native Americans.

4. Racial factors. Within the country, different ethnic groups may have variations in incidence of gastric cancer e.g. incidence is higher in Blacks, American Indians, Chinese in Indonesia, North Wales than other parts of Wales.

5. Genetic factors. Genetic influences have some role in the etiology of gastric cancer. Not more than 4% of patients of gastric cancer have a family history of this disease. Individuals with blood group A have higher tendency to develop gastric cancer (Recall that the peptic ulcer is more common in individuals with blood group O).

6. Pre-malignant changes in the gastric mucosa. There are some pre-cancerous conditions of gastric mucosa implicated in the etiology of gastric cancer. These are:

i) Hypo- or achlorhydria in atrophic gastritis of gastric mucosa.

ii) Adenomatous (neoplastic) polyps of the stomach.

iii) Chronic gastric ulcer (ulcer-cancer), and its association with achlorhydria.

iv) Stump carcinoma in patients who have undergone partial gastrectomy.

PATHOLOGIC CHANGES. Gastric carcinoma is most commonly located in the region of gastric canal (prepyloric region) formed by lesser curvature, pylorus and antrum. Other less common locations are the body, cardia and fundus (Fig. 18.12).

Before turning to classification of carcinoma of the stomach, it must be stated here that current

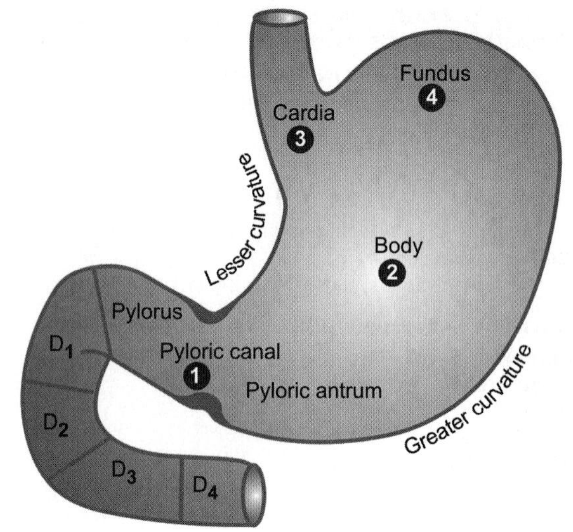

FIGURE 18.12

Distribution of gastric carcinoma in the anatomical subdivisions of the stomach. The serial numbers in the figure indicate the order of frequency of occurrence of gastric cancer.

studies indicate a pathogenetic evolution for all gastric carcinomas from an initial stage of *in situ* carcinoma confined to mucosal layers called early gastric carcinoma (EGC). EGC eventually penetrates the muscularis or beyond, resulting in advanced gastric carcinoma.

Based on this pathogenetic sequence, gastric carcinomas are broadly classified into 2 main groups:

I. *Early gastric carcinoma (EGC).*

II. *Advanced gastric carcinoma,* which has 5 further major gross subtypes:

i) Ulcerative carcinoma
ii) Fungating (Polypoid) carcinoma
iii) Scirrhous carcinoma (Linitis plastica)
iv) Colloid (Mucoid) carcinoma
v) Ulcer-cancer

In addition to the above classification, gastric carcinomas have been classified, *on the basis of extent of invasion,* into 2 groups:

I. *Expanding (formerly intestinal type) carcinomas* that grow laterally by an invasive margin. The tumour cells are in the form of cohesive clusters.

II. *Infiltrating (formerly diffuse type) carcinomas* have poorly-defined invasive border. The tumour cells are loose and invade singly or in small group.

These classifications are summarised in Fig. 18.13. The morphological features of various types are described below and illustrated in Fig. 18.15.

I. EARLY GASTRIC CARCINOMA (EGC) (Fig. 18.15,A). EGC is the term used to describe cancer

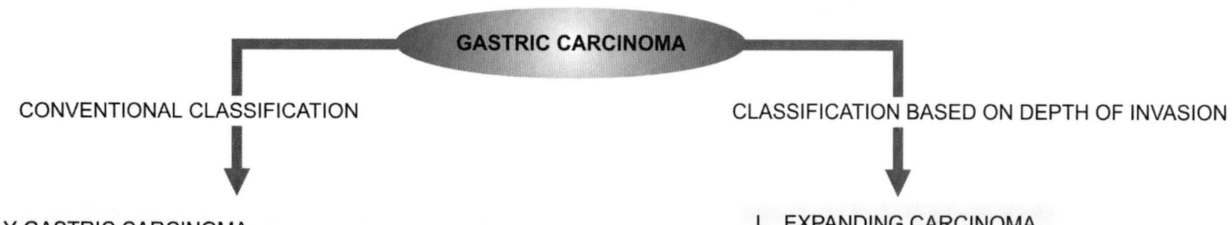

I. EARLY GASTRIC CARCINOMA
II. ADVANCED GASTRIC CARCINOMA

I. EXPANDING CARCINOMA
II. INFILTRATING CARCINOMA

Macroscopic subtype	*Main microscopic pattern*
i) Ulcerative carcinoma	Tubular adenocarcinoma
ii) Fungating (polypoid) carcinoma	Papillary adenocarcinoma
iii) Scirrhous carcinoma (linitis plastica)	Signet ring cell carcinoma
iv) Colloid (Mucoid) carcinoma	Mucinous adenocarcinoma
v) Ulcer-cancer	Adenocarcinoma, no specific types

FIGURE 18.13

Classifications of gastric carcinomas. A, Conventional classification, showing correlation of the macroscopic subtypes with the main histological patterns. B, Classification based on the depth of invasion by the tumour.

limited to the mucosa and submucosa. The diagnosis of this condition has been made possible by extensive work on histogenesis of gastric cancer by Japanese pathologists by the use of fibreoptic endoscope and gastrocamera. In Japan, EGC comprises 35% of newly-diagnosed cases of gastric cancer.

Grossly, the lesion of EGC may have 3 patterns—polypoid (protruded), superficial and ulcerated (Fig. 18.14):

Type I	:	Polypoid type
Type IIa	:	Superficial elevated
Type II b	:	Superficial flat
Type II c	:	Superficial depressed
Type III	:	Ulcerated type

Histologically, EGC is a typical glandular adenocarcinoma, usually well-differentiated type.

Prognosis of EGC after surgical resection is quite good; 5-year survival rate being 93-99%.

Early gastric carcinoma must be distinguished from certain related terms as under.

■ *Epithelial dysplasia* is cellular atypia seen in intestinal metaplasia such as in atrophic gastritis and pernicious anaemia.

■ *Carcinoma in situ* in the stomach is a state of severe cellular atypia or dysplasia, without invasion across the basement membrane of the glands.

II. ADVANCED GASTRIC CARCINOMA. When the carcinoma crosses the basement membrane into the muscularis propria or beyond, it is referred to as

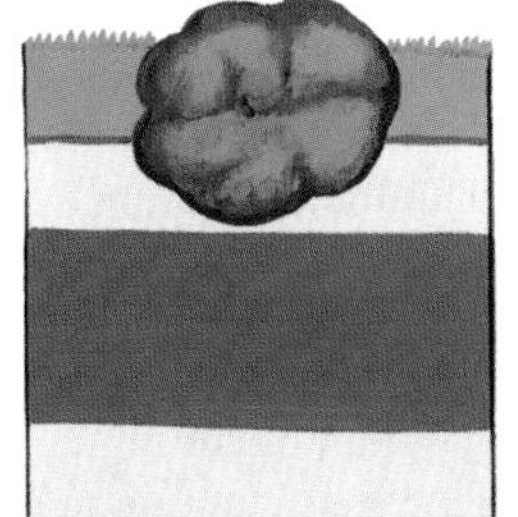
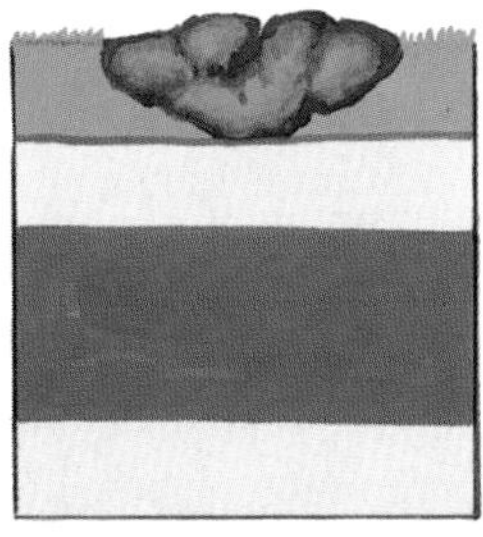
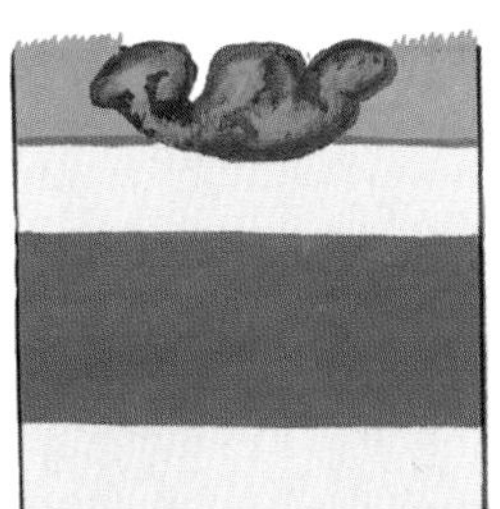
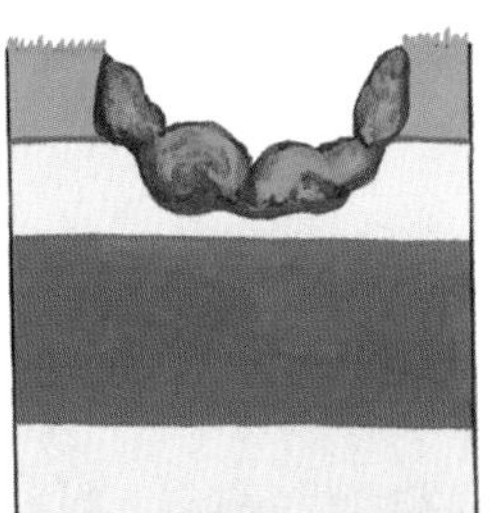
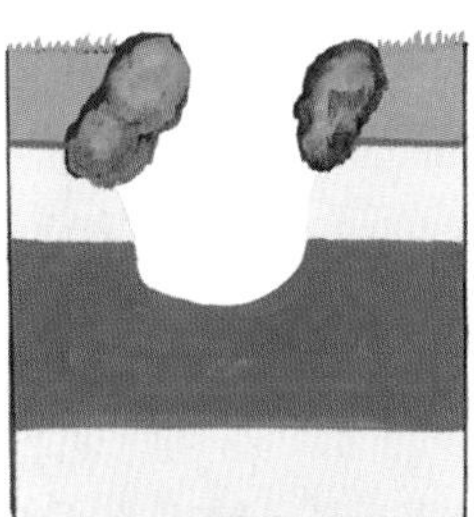

TYPE I	TYPE II a	TYPE II b	TYPE II c	TYPE III
Polypoid type	**Superficial elevated**	**Superficial flat**	**Superficial depressed**	**Ulcerated type**

FIGURE 18.14

Diagrammatic representation of gross patterns of early gastric carcinoma.

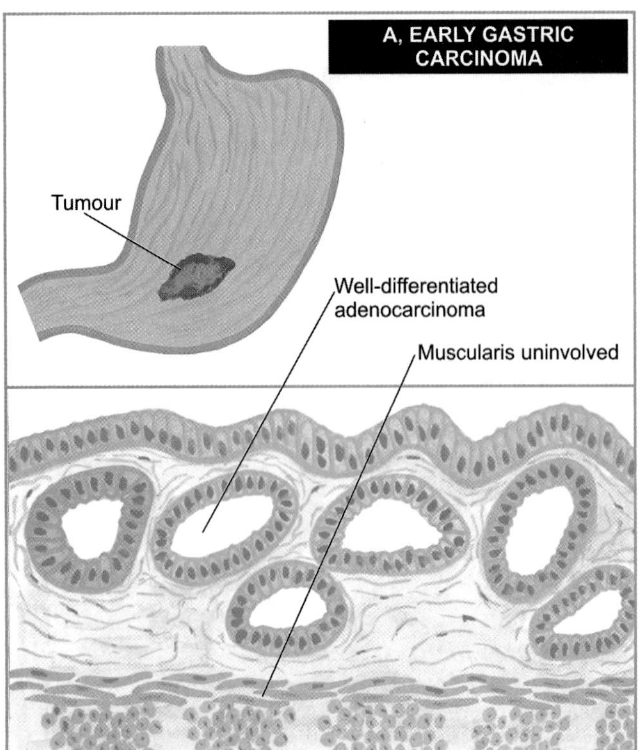

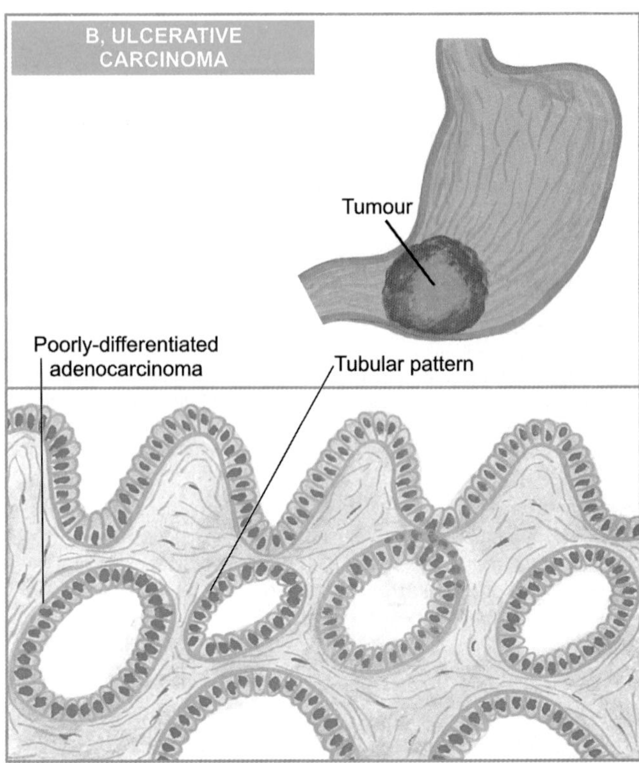

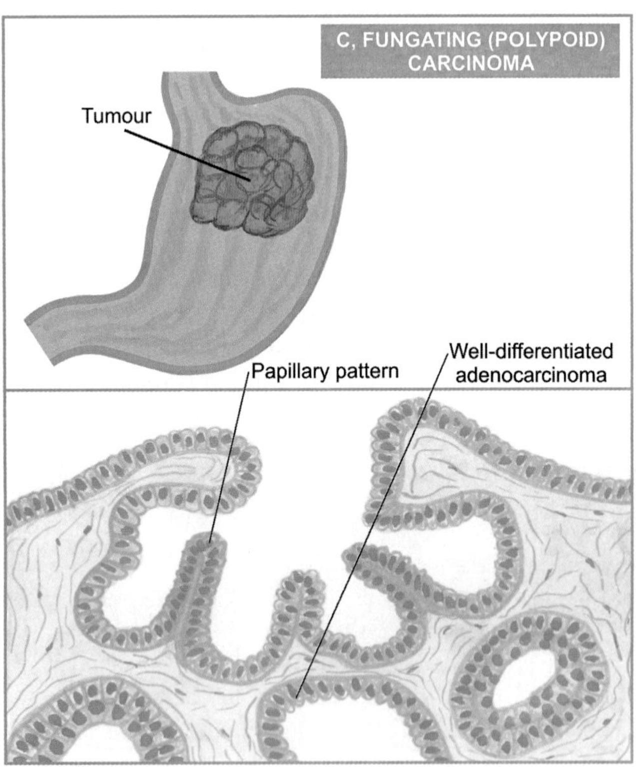

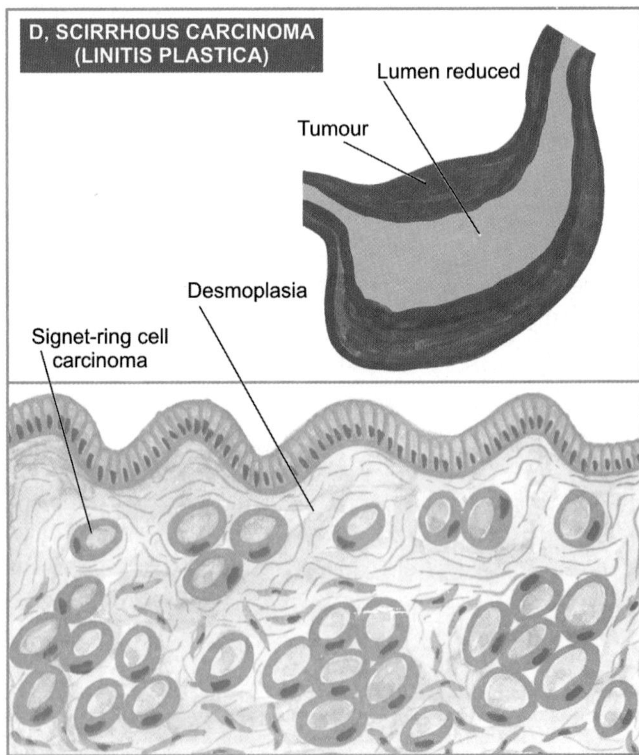

FIGURE 18.15

Gastric carcinoma, macroscopic subtypes and their corresponding dominant histological patterns.

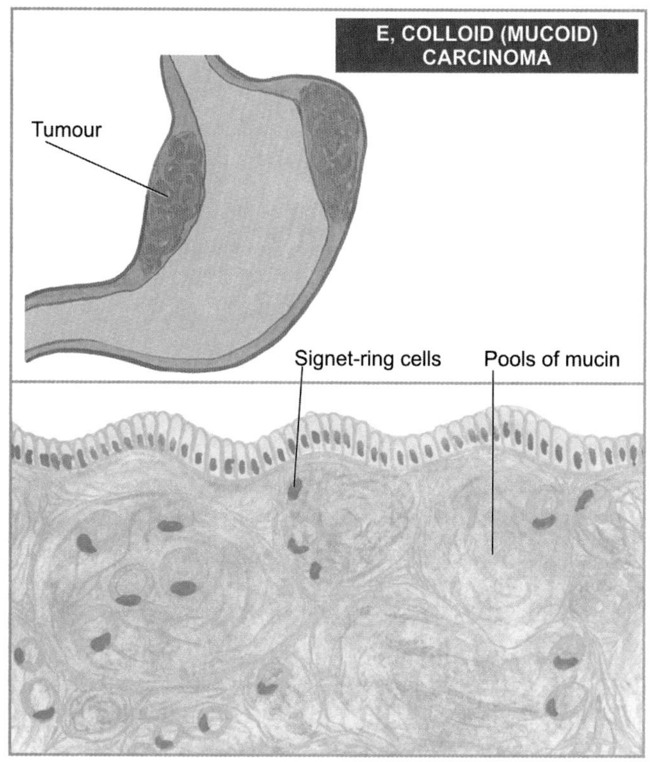

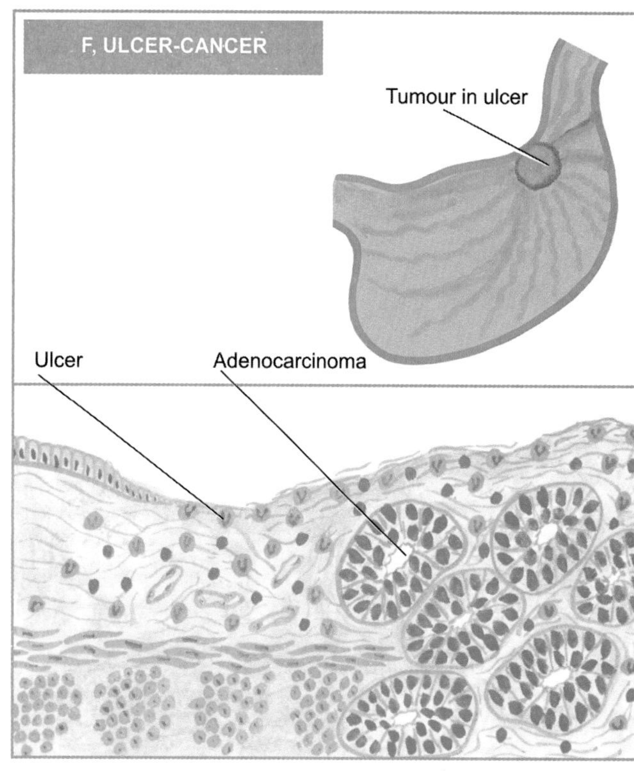

FIGURE 18.15 *contd...*

Gastric carcinoma, macroscopic subtypes and their corresponding dominant histological patterns.

advanced gastric carcinoma. Advanced gastric carcinoma has further 5 patterns (COLOUR PLATE XXV: CL 95, 96):

i) Ulcerative carcinoma (Fig. 18.15,B). This is the most common pattern. The tumour appears as a flat, infiltrating and ulcerative growth with irregular necrotic base and raised margin. It is seen more commonly in the region of gastric canal.

Histologically, ulcerative carcinomas are poorly-differentiated adenocarcinomas, which invade deeply into the stomach wall. Tubular and acinar patterns are seen more commonly.

ii) Fungating (polypoid) carcinoma (Fig. 18.15,C). The second common pattern is a cauliflower growth projecting into the lumen, similar to what is commonly seen in the large intestine. It is seen more often in the fundus. The tumour undergoes necrosis and infection commonly.

Histologically, fungating or polypoid carcinomas are well-differentiated adenocarcinomas, commonly papillary type.

iii) Scirrhous carcinoma (Linitis plastica) (Fig. 18.15,D). In this pattern, the stomach wall is thickened due to extensive desmoplasia giving the appearance as 'leather-bottle stomach' or 'linitis plastica'. The involvement may be localised to pyloric antrum, or diffuse affecting whole of the stomach from the cardia to pylorus. The lumen of the stomach is reduced. There are no ulcers but rugae are prominent.

Histologically, it may be an adenocarcinoma or signet-ring cell carcinoma, extensively infiltrating the stomach wall, but due to marked desmoplasia cancer cells may be difficult to find.

iv) Colloid (Mucoid) carcinoma (Fig. 18.15,E). This pattern is usually seen in the fundus. The tumour grows like masses having gelatinous appearance due to secretion of large quantities of mucus.

Histologically, mucoid carcinoma contains abundant pools of mucin in which are seen a small number of tumour cells, sometimes having signet-ring appearance.

v) Ulcer-cancer (Fig. 18.15,F). Development of cancer in chronic gastric ulcer is a rare occurrence (less than 1%). Majority of ulcer-cancers are malignant lesions from the beginning. For confirmation of cancer in a

TABLE 18.5: Differences between Benign and Malignant Gastric Ulcers.

FEATURE	BENIGN ULCER	MALIGNANT ULCER
1. ***Age***	Younger age	Older age
2. ***Sex***	Markedly common in males	Slightly common in males
3. ***Duration of symptoms***	Weeks to years	Weeks to months
4. ***Location***	Commonly lesser curvature of pylorus and antrum	Commonly greater curvature of pylorus and antrum
5. ***Gross features***		
a) *Size*	Small	Large
b) *Shape*	Regular	Irregular
c) *Mucosal folds*	Radiating	Interrupted
d) *Ulcer bed*	Haemorrhagic	Necrotic
6. ***Barium studies***	Punched out ulcer	Irregular filling defect
7. ***Acidity***	Usually normal-to-low	May be normal-to-even achlorhydria
8. ***Therapy***	Responds well to medical therapy	Usually does not respond to medical therapy

pre-existing gastric ulcer, the characteristic microscopic appearance of peptic ulcer should be demonstrable with one portion of the base or the margin of the ulcer showing carcinomatous changes. ***Histologically,*** ulcer-cancers are adenocarcinomas without any specific features. The differences between a benign and malignant gastric ulcer are summarised in Table 18.5 (*also see* Fig. 18.10).

SPREAD. Carcinoma of the stomach may spread by the following routes:

1. Direct spread. Direct spread by local extension is the most common feature of gastric carcinoma. The spread occurs mainly from the loose submucosal layer but eventually muscularis and serosa are also invaded. After the peritoneal covering of the stomach is involved, transcoelomic dissemination may occur in any other part of the peritoneal cavity but ovarian masses (one side or both-sided) occur more commonly, referred to as *Krukenberg tumours* (Chapter 22). Submucosal spread occurs more often upwards into the oesophagus due to continuity of the layers of stomach with those of oesophagus, while the spread downwards into the duodenum occurs less often due to the presence of pyloric sphincter and submucosal Brunner's glands. The tumour may directly involve other neighbouring structures and organs like lesser and greater omentum, pancreas, liver, common bile duct, diaphragm, spleen and transverse colon.

2. Lymphatic spread. Metastases to regional lymph nodes occur early, especially in the scirrhous carcinoma. The groups of lymph nodes involved are along the lesser and greater curvature around the cardia and suprapancreatic lymph nodes. Involvement of left supraclavicular lymph node, *Virchow* or *Troisier's sign,* is sometimes the presenting feature of gastric carcinoma.

3. Haematogenous spread. Blood spread of gastric carcinoma may occur to the liver, lungs, brain, bones, kidneys and adrenals. It occurs more commonly with the poorly-differentiated carcinoma.

The American Joint Committee on Cancer has developed *TNM staging* system for gastric carcinoma based on tumour invasion (T), lymph node involvement (N) and distant metastasis (M) into earliest stage T_{is} N_0 M_0 (intraepithelial tumour) to most advanced stage T_{any} N_{any} M_1.

CLINICAL FEATURES. Gastric carcinoma may have diverse presentations. The usual clinical features are:

i) Persistent abdominal pain
ii) Gastric distension and vomiting
iii) Loss of weight (cachexia)
iv) Loss of appetite (anorexia)
v) Anaemia, weakness, malaise.

The most common complication of gastric cancer is haemorrhage (in the form of haematemesis and/or melaena); others are obstruction, perforation and jaundice.

Gastric carcinoma remains undiagnosed until late when the symptoms appear. Therefore, the prognosis is generally poor; 5-year survival rate being 5-15% from the time of diagnosis of advanced gastric carcinoma. However, 5-year survival rate for early gastric carcinoma is far higher (93-99%) and hence the need for early diagnosis of the condition.

Other Carcinomas

Besides the various morphologic patterns of adenocarcinoma just described, other carcinomas that occur rarely in the stomach are: adenosquamous carcinoma, squamous cell carcinoma and undifferentiated carcinoma, all of which are morphologically similar to such tumours elsewhere.

Leiomyosarcoma

Leiomyosarcoma, though rare, is the commonest soft tissue sarcoma, the stomach being the more common site in the gastrointestinal tract.

Grossly, the tumour may be of variable size but is usually quite large, pedunculated and lobulated mass into the lumen.

Microscopically, leiomyosarcoma is characterised by high cellularity and presence of mitotic figures. Tumour is usually well-differentiated.

Leiomyoblastoma (Epithelioid Leiomyoma)

This is a rare tumour, the behaviour of which is intermediate between clearly benign and malignant tumour.

Grossly, the tumour is large, circumscribed and projects into the lumen.

Microscopically, it is characterised by round to polygonal cells with clear perinuclear halos. The number of mitoses determines the biological behaviour of the tumour.

CarcinoidTumour

Carcinoid tumours are rare in the stomach and are usually non-argentaffin type but argentaffinomas also occur. Their behaviour is usually malignant, They are described in detail on page 591.

Lymphomas of Gut

Primary gastrointestinal lymphomas are defined as lymphomas arising in the gut without any evidence of systemic involvement at the time of presentation.

Secondary gastrointestinal lymphomas, on the other hand, appear in the gut after dissemination from other primary site. Gastric lymphomas constitute over 50% of all bowel lymphomas; other sites being small and large bowel in decreasing order of frequency. Prognosis of primary gastric lymphoma is better than for intestinal lymphomas. Primary lymphoma of stomach is the most common malignant gastric tumour (4%) next to carcinoma.

Clinical manifestations of gastric lymphomas may be similar to gastric carcinoma. Age incidence for lymphomas of the gastrointestinal tract is usually lower than that for carcinoma (30-40 years as compared to 40-60 years in gastric carcinoma) and may occur even in childhood. Relationship with long-standing chronic *H. pylori* gastritis with lymphoid hyperplasia has been strongly suggested.

Grossly, gastric lymphomas have 2 types of appearances:

1. *Diffusely infiltrating type,* producing thickening of the affected gut wall, obliteration of mucosal folds and ulcerations. Cut section shows lesions in the mucosa and submucosa but in late stage whole thickness of the gut wall may be affected.

2. *Polypoid type,* which produces large protruding mass into the lumen with ulcerated surface.

Lymph node involvement may occur in either of the two patterns.

Microscopically gastric lymphomas are most often non-Hodgkin's lymphomas of the following types:

- *High-grade* large cell immunoblastic lymphoma being the most common.
- *Low-grade* small lymphocytic well-differentiated B-cell lymphoma referred to as *MALToma* is the next in frequency (arising from Mucosa Associated Lymphoid Tissue). The term *pseudolymphoma* is sometimes used for non-invasive stage of MALToma.

SMALL INTESTINE

NORMAL STRUCTURE

Anatomically, the small bowel includes the duodenum, jejunum and ileum and tends to become narrower throughout its course.

Histologically, the small bowel is identified by recognition of villi. The wall of the small intestine consists of 4 layers:

1. The **serosa** is the outer covering of the small bowel which is complete except over a part of the duodenum.

2. The **muscularis propria** is composed of 2 layers of smooth muscle tissue—outer thinner longitudinal and inner thicker circular layer. These muscles are functionally important for peristalsis. Between the two

layers of muscle lie ganglionated plexus, myenteric plexus of Auerbach.

3. The **submucosa** is composed of loose fibrous tissue with blood vessels and lacteals in it. It contains a gangliated plexus, Meissner's plexus, having fewer and smaller cells than the Auerbach's plexus.

4. The **mucosa** consists of glandular epithelium overlying the lamina propria composed of loose connective tissue and contains phagocytic cells and abundance of lymphoid cells (Peyer's patches in the ileum) and plasma cells. It is supported externally by thin layer of smooth muscle fibres, *muscularis mucosae.* The mucous membrane is thrown into folds or *plicae* which are more in the jejunum and less in the ileum, thus increasing the absorptive surface enormously. The absorptive surface is further increased by the intestinal villi. *Villi* are finger-like or leaf-like projections which contain 3 types of cells:

i) *SIMPLE COLUMNAR CELLS* which perform absorptive function due to the presence of brush border consisting of large number of microvilli.

ii) *GOBLET CELLS* which are mucus-secreting cells and are interspersed between the columnar cells.

iii) *ENDOCRINE CELLS.* These are scattered in the villi as well as are widely distributed throughout the gastrointestinal tract. These cells have various synonyms as under:

- *Kulchitsky cells,* after the name of its discoverer;
- *Enterochromaffin cells,* due to their resemblance to chromaffin cells of the adrenal medulla;
- *Argentaffin cells,* as the intracytoplasmic granules stain positively with silver salts by reduction reaction (argyrophil cells, on the other hand, require the addition of exogenous reducing substance for staining); and
- *Endocrine cells,* as these specialised cells are considered to be part of APUD cell system (having common properties as *A*mine content, amine *P*recursor *U*ptake and *D*ecarboxylation). APUD cells are considered to be of endodermal origin, while previously they were thought to be neural crest derivative. Other endocrine cells belonging to the APUD cell system are C-cells of the thyroid, chromaffin cells of the adrenal medulla, certain cells of the carotid body, bronchi, hypothalamus, pituitary and sympathetic ganglia.

Endocrine cells are heavily populated in the proximal small bowel as this is the most active site for absorption and secretory activities. They are sparse in the colon which is less active site for such functions.

The duodenum contains distinctively branched *Brunner's glands* present in the submucosa and going up to muscularis mucosae. The deeper layer of the mucosa of the small intestine elsewhere contains intestinal glands or *crypts of Lieberkuhn.* They are lined by columnar cells, goblet cells, endocrine cells and Paneth cells. Paneth cells are normally exclusively found in the small intestine and occasionally in the caecum. These cells are characterised by the presence of supranuclear granules rich in lysozyme.

The blood supply of the whole of small intestine, except the first part of the duodenum, is by the superior mesenteric artery which supplies blood by mesenteric arterial arcades and the straight arteries.

The main **function** of the small intestine is digestion and absorption so that ultimately nutrients passing into the blood stream are utilised by the cells in metabolism. The mucosal layer of the small intestine has remarkable capacity for regeneration and new lining is laid every 3-4 days.

CONGENITAL ANOMALIES

Intestinal Atresia and Stenosis

- **Intestinal atresia** is congenital absence of lumen, most commonly affecting the ileum or duodenum. The proximal segment has a blind end which is separated from distal segment freely, or the two segments are joined by a fibrous cord. The condition must be recognised early and treated surgically, as otherwise it is incompatible with life.

- **Intestinal stenosis** is congenital narrowing of the lumen affecting a segment of the small intestine. Intestinal segment above the level of obstruction is dilated and that below it is collapsed.

Meckel's Diverticulum

Meckel's diverticulum is the most common congenital anomaly of the gastrointestinal tract, occurring in 2% of population. It is more common in males. The anomaly is commonly situated on the antimesenteric border of the ileum, about 1 meter above the ileocaecal valve. Like other true diverticula, Meckel's diverticulum is an outpouching containing all the layers of the intestinal wall in their normal orientation (Fig. 18.16). It is almost always lined by small intestinal type of epithelium, though at times it may contain islands of gastric mucosa and ectopic pancreatic tissue. Embryologic origin of Meckel's diverticulum is from incomplete obliteration of vitellointestinal duct. (Other anomalies resulting from the remnants of vitellointestinal duct are vitelline sinus and vitelline cyst).

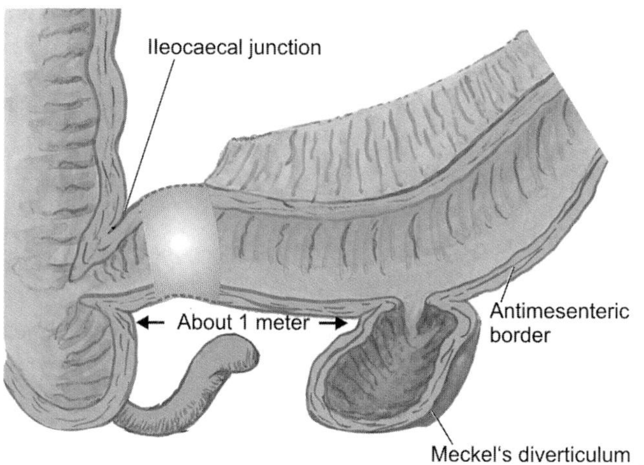

FIGURE 18.16
Meckel's diverticulum, common location and gross appearance.

The common *complications* of Meckel's diverticulum are perforation, haemorrhage and diverticulitis.

In addition to congenital Meckel's diverticulum, *acquired diverticula* also occur in the small intestine. These are commonly multiple (diverticulosis), frequently located on the mesenteric border, and are sometimes associated with malabsorption.

Intestinal Malrotation

Malrotation is a developmental abnormality of the midgut (i.e. the portion of intestine between the duodeno-jejunal flexure and the middle of transverse colon). Due to failure of normal rotation of midgut, the following consequences can occur:

i) Exomphalos i.e. intestinal eventration at the umbilicus.

ii) Misplacement of the caecum, appendix and ascending colon.

iii) Mobile caecum.

INTESTINAL OBSTRUCTION

Conditions which interfere with the propulsion of contents in the intestine are considered under the heading of intestinal obstruction. The causes of intestinal obstruction can be classified under the following 3 broad groups:

1. **Mechanical obstruction.** It can occur as a result of the following causes:

i) *Internal obstruction* (in the wall or the lumen) such as due to the following:

- Inflammatory strictures (e.g. Crohn's disease)
- Congenital stenosis, atresia, imperforate anus
- Tumours
- Meconium in mucoviscidosis
- Roundworms
- Gallstones, faecoliths, foreign bodies
- Ulceration induced by potassium chloride tablets prescribed to counter hypokalaemia.

ii) *External compression* such as from the following causes:

- Peritoneal adhesions and bands
- Strangulated hernias
- Intussusception
- Volvulus
- Intra-abdominal tumour.

2. **Neurogenic obstruction.** It occurs due to paralytic ileus i.e. paralysis of muscularis of the intestine as a result of shock after abdominal operation or by acute peritonitis

3. **Vascular obstruction.** Obstruction of the superior mesenteric artery or its branches may result in infarction causing paralysis. The causes are as under:

- Thrombosis
- Embolism
- Accidental ligation

Out of the various causes listed above, conditions producing external compression on the bowel wall are the most common cause of intestinal obstruction (80%). Some of these are described below.

Peritoneal Adhesions and Bands

Adhesions and bands in the peritoneum composed of fibrous tissue result following healing in peritonitis. Rarely, such fibrous adhesions and bands may be without any preceding peritoneal inflammation and are of congenital origin. In either case, peritoneal bands and adhesions result in partial or complete intestinal obstruction by outside pressure on the bowel wall.

Hernias

Hernia is protrusion of portion of a viscus through an abnormal opening in the wall of its natural cavity.

- **External hernia** is the protrusion of the bowel through a defect or weakness in the peritoneum.
- **Internal hernia** is the term applied for herniation that does not present on the external surface.

Two major factors involved in the formation of a hernia are as under:

i) *Local weakness* which may be congenital e.g. at the umbilicus, inguinal and femoral canals, and in surgical scars called 'incisional hernia'.

ii) *Increased intra-abdominal pressure* that is produced by coughing, straining and exertion.

Inguinal hernias are more common, followed in decreasing frequency, by femoral and umbilical hernias. Inguinal hernias may be:

- **direct** when hernia passes medial to the inferior epigastric artery and it appears through the external abdominal ring; and
- **indirect** when it follows the inguinal canal lateral to the inferior epigastric artery.

When the contents of hernia such as loop of intestine can be returned to the abdominal cavity, it is called *reducible.* When it is not possible to reduce hernia due to large contents or due to adhesions in the hernial sac, it is referred to as *irreducible.*

When the blood flow in the hernial sac is obstructed, it results in *strangulated hernia.* Obstruction to the venous drainage and arterial supply may result in infarction or gangrene of the affected loop of intestine. The gross and microscopic appearance of strangulated intestine is the same as that of infarction of intestine.

Intussusception

Intussusception is the telescoping of a segment of intestine into the segment below due to peristalsis. The telescoped segment is called the *intussusceptum* and lower receiving segment is called the *intussuscipiens.* The condition occurs more commonly in infants and young children, more often in the ileocaecal region when the portion of ileum invaginates into the ascending colon without affecting the position of the ileocaecal valve (Fig. 18.17). Less common forms are ileo-ileal and colo-colic intussusception.

In children, the cause is usually not known though enlargement of the lymphoid tissue in the terminal ileum has been suggested by some. In the case of adults, the usual causes are foreign bodies and tumours.

The main *complications* of intussusception are intestinal obstruction, infarction, gangrene, perforation and peritonitis.

Volvulus

Volvulus is the twisting of loop of intestine upon itself through 180° or more. This leads to obstruction of the intestine as well as cutting off of the blood supply to the affected loop. The usual causes are bands and adhesions (congenital or acquired) and long mesenteric attachment. The condition is more common in the sigmoid colon than the small bowel.

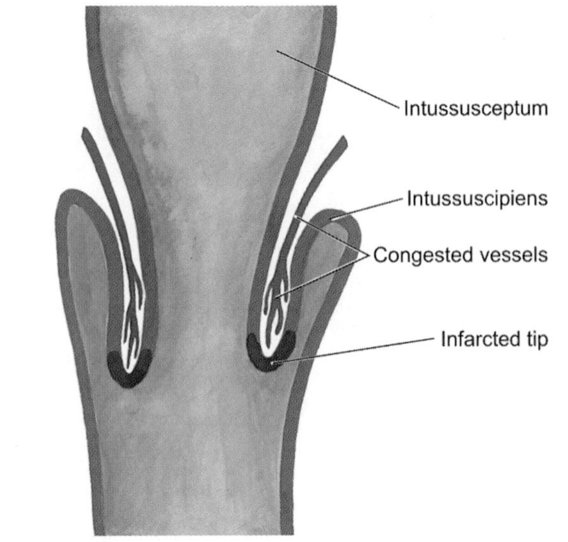

FIGURE 18.17

Ileocaecal intussusception.

ISCHAEMIC BOWEL DISEASE (ISCHAEMIC ENTEROCOLITIS)

Ischaemic lesions of the gastrointestinal tract may occur in the small intestine and/or colon; the latter is called *ischaemic colitis or ischaemic enterocolitis* and is commonly referred to as ischaemic bowel disease. In either case, the cause of ischaemia is compromised mesenteric circulation, while ischaemic effect is less likely to occur in the stomach, duodenum and rectum due to abundant collateral blood supply.

Depending upon the extent and severity of ischaemia, 3 patterns of pathologic lesions can occur:

1. *Transmural infarction,* characterised by transmural ischaemic necrosis and gangrene of the bowel.

2 *Mural infarction,* characterised by haemorrhagic gastroenteropathy (haemorrhage and necrosis). The ischaemic effect in mural infarction is limited to mucosa, submucosa and superficial muscularis, while mucosal infarction is confined to mucosal layers superficial to muscularis mucosae.

3. *Ischaemic stenosis,* due to chronic ischaemia causing fibrotic narrowing of the affected bowel.

These pathologic patterns are described below:

Transmural Infarction

Ischaemic necrosis of the full-thickness of the bowel wall is more common in the small intestine than the large intestine.

ETIOPATHOGENESIS. The common causes of transmural infarction of small bowel are as under:

i) *Mesenteric arterial thrombosis* such as due to the following:

- Atherosclerosis (most common)
- Aortic aneurysm
- Vasospasm
- Fibromuscular hyperplasia
- Invasion by the tumour
- Use of oral contraceptives
- Arteritis of various types

ii) *Mesenteric arterial embolism* arising from the following causes:

- Mural thrombi in the heart
- Endocarditis (infective and nonbacterial thrombotic)
- Atherosclerotic plaques
- Atrial myxoma

iii) *Mesenteric venous occlusion* is less common cause of full-thickness infarction of the bowel. The causes are as under:

- Intestinal sepsis e.g. appendicitis
- Portal venous thrombosis in cirrhosis of the liver
- Tumour invasion
- Use of oral contraceptives

iv) *Miscellaneous causes*:

- Strangulated hernia
- Torsion
- Fibrous bands and adhesions.

PATHOLOGIC CHANGES. Grossly, irrespective of the underlying etiology, infarction of the bowel is haemorrhagic (red) type (page 129). A varying length of the small bowel may be affected. In the case of colonic infarction, the distribution area of superior and inferior mesenteric arteries (i.e. *splenic flexure)* is more commonly involved. The affected areas becomes dark purple and markedly congested and the peritoneal surface is coated with fibrinous exudate. The wall is thickened, oedematous and haemorrhagic. The lumen is dilated and contains blood and mucus. In arterial occlusion, there is sharp line of demarcation between the infarcted bowel and the normal intestine (Fig. 18.18), whereas in venous occlusion the infarcted area merges imperceptibly into the normal bowel.

Microscopically, there is coagulative necrosis and ulceration of the mucosa and there are extensive submucosal haemorrhages. The muscularis is less severely affected by ischaemia. Subsequently, inflammatory cell infiltration and secondary infection occur, leading to gangrene of the bowel (Fig. 18.19).

The condition is clinically characterised by 'abdominal angina' in which the patient has acute abdominal pain, nausea, vomiting, and sometimes diarrhoea. The disease is rapidly fatal, with 50-70% mortality rate.

Mural and Mucosal Infarction (Haemorrhagic Gastroenteropathy, Membranous Colitis)

Mural and mucosal infarctions are limited to superficial layers of the bowel wall, sparing the deeper layer of the muscularis and the serosa. The condition is also referred to as *haemorrhagic gastroenteropathy,* and in the case of colon as *membranous colitis.*

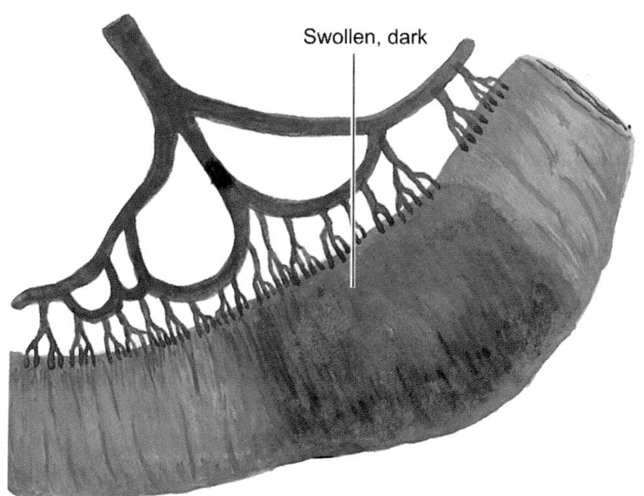

FIGURE 18.18

Haemorrhagic infarct of the small intestine. The infarcted area is swollen, dark in colour and coated with fibrinous exudate. A sharp line of demarcation separates infarcted area from the normal bowel.

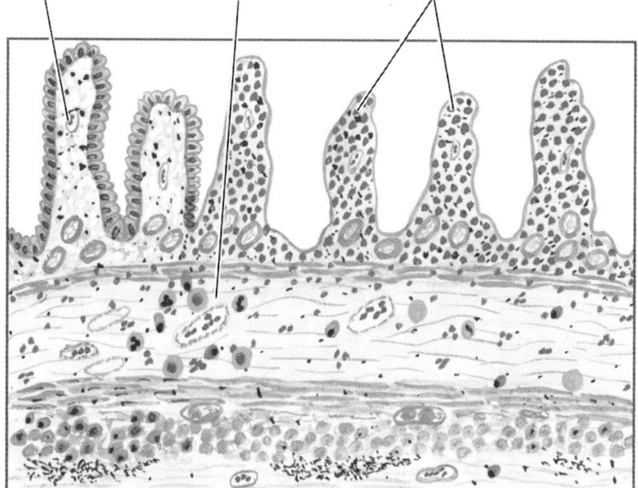

FIGURE 18.19

Infarct small intestine, microscopic appearance. The mucosa in the infarcted area shows coagulative necrosis and submucosal haemorrhages: muscularis is also partly affected. Inflammatory cell infiltration is marked at the line of demarcation between the infarcted and normal bowel.

ETIOPATHOGENESIS. Haemorrhagic gastroenteropathy results from conditions causing non-occlusive hypoperfusion (compared from transmural infarction which occurs from occlusive causes). These are as under:

- Shock
- Cardiac failure
- Infections
- Intake of drugs causing vasoconstriction e.g. digitalis, norepinephrine.

*PATHOLOGIC CHANGES. **Grossly,*** the lesions affect variable length of the bowel. The affected segment of the bowel is red or purple but without haemorrhage and exudation on the serosal surface. The mucosa is oedematous at places, sloughed and ulcerated at other places. The lumen contains haemorrhagic fluid.
Microscopically, there is patchy ischaemic necrosis of mucosa, vascular congestion, haemorrhages and inflammatory cell infiltrate. The changes may extend into superficial muscularis but deeper layer of muscularis and serosa are spared. Secondary bacterial infection may supervene resulting in pseudomembranous enterocolitis.

Clinically, as in transmural infarction, the features of abdominal pain, nausea, vomiting and diarrhoea are present, but the changes are reversible and curable. With adequate therapy, normal morphology is completely restored in superficial lesions, while deeper lesions may heal by fibrosis leading to stricture formation.

Ischaemic Stenosis

Although this condition affects primarily colon in the region of splenic flexure, it is described here due to its apparent pathogenetic relationship with ischaemic injury. The disease has 2 phases:

i) Ischaemic colitis—characterised by acute colonic necrosis as described above.

ii) Ischaemic stricture—occurring following segmental inflammation of the colon.

Grossly, there is fusiform or saccular external appearance. There is patchy and longitudinal mucosal ulceration.
Microscopically, the ulcerated areas of the mucosa show granulation tissue. The submucosa is characteristically thickened due to inflammation and fibrosis. The muscularis may also show inflammatory changes and patchy replacement by fibrosis. The blood vessels may show atheromatous emboli, organising thrombi and endarteritis obliterans.

NECROTISING ENTEROCOLITIS

Necrotising enterocolitis is an acute inflammation of the terminal ileum and ascending colon, occurring primarily in premature and low-birth-weight infants within the first week of life and less commonly in full-term infants.

ETIOLOGY. The condition has been considered as a variant of the spectrum of ischaemic bowel disease. Important factors in the etiology of this disorder, thus, are as follows:

1. Ischaemia
2. Hypoxia/anoxia of the bowel due to bypassing of blood from the affected area
3. Bacterial infection and endotoxins
4. Establishment of feeding
5. Infants fed on commercial formulae than breast-fed, implying the role of immunoprotective factors.

*PATHOLOGIC CHANGES. **Macroscopically,*** the affected segment of the bowel is dilated, necrotic, haemorrhagic and friable. Bowel wall may contain bubbles of air (pneumatosis intestinalis).
Microscopically, the changes are variable depending upon the stage. Initial changes are confined to mucosa and show oedema, haemorrhage and coagulative necrosis. A *pseudomembrane* composed of necrotic epithelium, fibrin and inflammatory cells may develop. As the ischaemic process extends to the subjacent layers, muscle layer is also involved and may lead to perforation and peritonitis.

In healed cases, stricture formation, malabsorption and short bowel syndrome are the usual complications.

INFLAMMATORY BOWEL DISEASE (CROHN'S DISEASE AND ULCERATIVE COLITIS)

DEFINITION. The term 'inflammatory bowel disease (IBD)' is commonly used to include 2 idiopathic bowel diseases having many similarities but the conditions usually have distinctive morphological appearance. These 2 conditions are Crohn's disease (regional enteritis) and ulcerative colitis:

1. Crohn's disease or Regional enteritis is an idiopathic chronic ulcerative IBD, characterised by transmural, non-caseating granulomatous inflammation, affecting most commonly the segment of terminal ileum and/or colon, though any part of the gastrointestinal tract may be involved.

2. Ulcerative colitis is an idiopathic form of acute and chronic ulcero-inflammatory colitis affecting chiefly the mucosa and submucosa of the rectum and descending colon, though sometimes it may involve the entire length of large bowel.

Both these disorders primarily affect the bowel but may have systemic involvement in the form of poly-arthritis, uveitis, ankylosing spondylitis, skin lesions and hepatic involvement. Both diseases can occur at any age but are more common in 2nd and 3rd decades of life. Females are affected slightly more often.

ETIOPATHOGENESIS. The exact etiology of IBD remains unknown. The following observations, however, point towards multifactorial etiopathogenesis:

1. Genetic factors. Genetic factors are implicated in the etiopathogenesis of IBD is supported by the following evidences:

i) There is about 3 to 20 times higher incidence of occurrence of IBD in first-degree relatives.

ii) There is approximately 50% chance of development of IBD (particularly Crohn's disease) in monozygotic twins.

iii) Genomic search has revealed that disease-associated loci of IBD are present in chromosomes 16, 12, 7, 3 and 1 although there are no consistent genetic abnormalities.

iv) HLA studies show that ulcerative colitis is more common in DR2-related genes while Crohn's disease is more common in DR5 DQ1alleles.

2. Immunologic factors. Defective immunologic regulation in IBD has been shown to play significant role in the pathogenesis of IBD:

i) *Defective regulation of immune suppression.* In a normal individual, there is lack of immune responsiveness to dietary antigens and commensal flora in the intestinal lumen. The mechanism responsible for this is by activation of CD4+ T cells secreting cytokines inhibitory to inflammation (IL-10, TGF-β) which suppress inflammation in the gut wall. In IBD, this immune mechanism of suppression of inflammation is defective and thus results in uncontrolled inflammation.

ii) *Transgenic mouse experimental model studies.* Gene 'knock out' studies on colitis in mice have revealed that multiple immune abnormalities may be responsible for IBD as under:

a) Deletion of inflammation inhibitory cytokines (e.g. IL-2, IL-10, TGF-β) or their receptors.

b) Deletion of molecules responsible for T cell recognition (e.g. T cell antigen receptors, MHC class II).

c) Interference with normal epithelial barrier function in the intestine (e.g. blocking N-cadherin, deletion of multi-drug resistance MDR gene).

iii) *Type of inflammatory cells.* In both types of IBD, activated CD4+ T cells are present in the lamina propria and in the peripheral blood. These cells either activate other inflammatory cells (e.g. macrophages and B cells), or recruit more inflammatory cells by stimulation of homing receptor on leucocytes and vascular endothelium. There are two main types of CD4+ T cells in IBD:

a) *TH1 cells* secrete proinflammatory cytokines IFN-γ and TNF which induce transmural granulomatous inflammation seen in Crohn's disease. IL-12 initiates TH1 cytokine pathway.

b) *TH2 cells* secrete IL-4, IL-5 and IL-13 which induce superficial mucosal inflammation characteristically seen in ulcerative colitis.

3. Microbial factors. There has been some evidence, though not clear-cut, that IBD may have infectious etiology. Though at different times, different microorganisms (bacteria, viruses, protozoa and fungi) have been implicated by different workers, currently attention is focused on the following three microbes:

i) *Mycobacterium paratuberculosis*: Seen in some patients of Crohn's disease but no confirmed association.

ii) *Measles virus:* Observation of parallel increase in incidence of Crohn's disease with use of measles vaccine in England but not substantiated elsewhere.

iii) *Helicobacter hepaticus:* Observation of inflammatory trigger by *H. hepaticus* to dysregulated immune system in experimental model but not seen in humans.

4. Psycosocial factors. It has been observed that individuals who are unduly sensitive, dependent on others and unable to express themselves, or some major life events such as illness or death in the family, divorce, interpersonal conflicts etc, suffer from irritable colon or have exacerbation of symptoms. Patients of IBD in the West have been found to suffer from greater functional impairment than the general population as assessed by *sickness impact profile* which is a measure of overall psychological and physical functioning.

PATHOLOGIC CHANGES. The morphologic features of Crohn's disease and ulcerative colitis are sufficiently distinctive so as to be classified separately. These features are presented below; the distinguishing features of the two conditions are summarised in Table 18.6.

CROHN'S DISEASE. Crohn's disease may involve any portion of the gastrointestinal tract but affects most commonly 15-25 cms of the terminal ileum which may extend into the caecum and sometimes into the ascending colon:

Grossly, characteristic feature is the multiple, well-demarcated segmental bowel involvement with intervening uninvolved 'skip areas'. The wall of the affected bowel segment is thick and hard, resembling a *'hose pipe'*. Serosa may be studded with minute granulomas. The lumen of the affected segment is markedly narrowed. The mucosa shows 'serpiginous ulcers', while intervening surviving mucosa is swollen giving 'cobblestone appearance'. There may be deep fissuring into the bowel wall (Fig. 18.20).

Histologically, the characteristic features are as follows (Fig. 18.21):

1. *Transmural inflammatory cell infiltrate consisting* of chronic inflammatory cells (lymphocytes, plasma cells and macrophages) is the classical microscopic feature.

TABLE 18.6: Distinguishing Features of Crohn's Disease and Ulcerative Colitis.

FEATURE	CROHN'S DISEASE	ULCERATIVE COLITIS
A. MACROSCOPIC FEATURES		
1. ***Distribution***	Segmental with skip areas	Continuous without skip areas
2. ***Location***	Commonly terminal ileum and/or ascending colon	Commonly rectum, sigmoid colon and extending upwards
3. ***Extent***	Usually involves the entire thickness of the affected segment of bowel wall	Usually superficial, confined to mucosal layers
4. ***Ulcers***	Serpiginous ulcers, may develop into deep fissures	Superficial mucosal ulcers without fissures
5. ***Pseudopolyps***	Rarely seen	Commonly present
6. ***Fibrosis***	Common	Rare
7. ***Shortening***	Due to fibrosis	Due to contraction of muscularis
B. MICROSCOPIC FEATURES		
1. ***Depth of inflammation***	Typically transmural	Mucosal and submucosal
2. ***Type of inflammation***	Non-caseating granulomas and infiltrate of mononuclear cells (lymphocytes, plasma cells and macrophages)	Crypt abscess and non-specific acute and chronic inflammatory cells (lymphocytes, plasma cells, neutrophils, eosinophils, mast cells)
3. ***Mucosa***	Patchy ulceration	Haemorrhagic mucosa with ulceration
4. ***Submucosa***	Widened due to oedema and lymphoid aggregates	Normal or reduced in width
5. ***Muscularis***	Infiltrated by inflammatory cells	Usually spared except in cases of toxic megacolon
6. ***Fibrosis***	Present	Usually absent
C. IMMUNOLOGIC FEATURES		
1. ***Lymphocyte type***	CD4+ TH1	CD4+ TH2
2. ***Cytokines***	INF-γ, TNF, IL-12	TGF-β, IL-4, IL-5, IL-13
3. ***ANCA-P antibodies***	Positive in a few	Positive in most
D. COMPLICATIONS		
1. ***Fistula formation***	Internal and external fistulae in 10% cases	Extremely rare
2. ***Malignant changes***	Rare	May occur infrequently in disease of more than 10 years'duration
3. ***Type of malignancy***	Lymphoma more than carcinoma	Carcinoma more than lymphoma
4. ***Fibrous strictures***	Common	Never

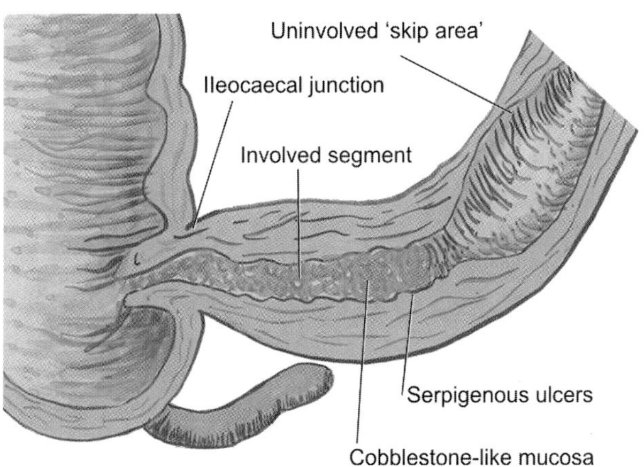

FIGURE 18.20

Crohn's disease of the terminal ileum. Grossly, the lesions are characteristically segmental with intervening uninvolved 'skip areas'. The bowel wall is thickened and the lumen narrowed, giving hose-pipe appearance. Serpiginous ulcers, some deep fissures and swollen intervening surviving mucosa giving 'cobblestone appearance', are present.

2. *Non-caseating, sarcoid-like granulomas* are present in all the layers of the affected bowel wall in 60% of cases and may even be seen in the regional lymph nodes.
3. There is *patchy ulceration* of the mucosa which may take the form of deep fissures, accompanied by inflammatory infiltrate of lymphocytes and plasma cells.
4. There is *widening of the submucosa* due to oedema and foci of lymphoid aggregates.
5. In more *chronic cases,* fibrosis becomes increasingly prominent in all the layers disrupting muscular layer.

Complications of Crohn's disease are as under:

1. *Malabsorption* due to impaired absorption of fat, vitamin B_{12}, proteins and electrolytes from the diseased small bowel.

2. *Fistula formation* may occur in long-standing cases. These may be internal fistulae between the loops of the intestine, or external fistulae such as enterocutaneous, rectal and anal fistulae.

3. *Stricture formation* may occur in chronic cases due to extensive fibrosis in the affected bowel wall.

4. *Development of malignancy* in the small intestine as a late complication of Crohn's disease is rarer than that in ulcerative colitis, but lymphoma may develop more often in Crohn's disease than adenocarcinoma (seen in some long-standing cases of ulcerative colitis).

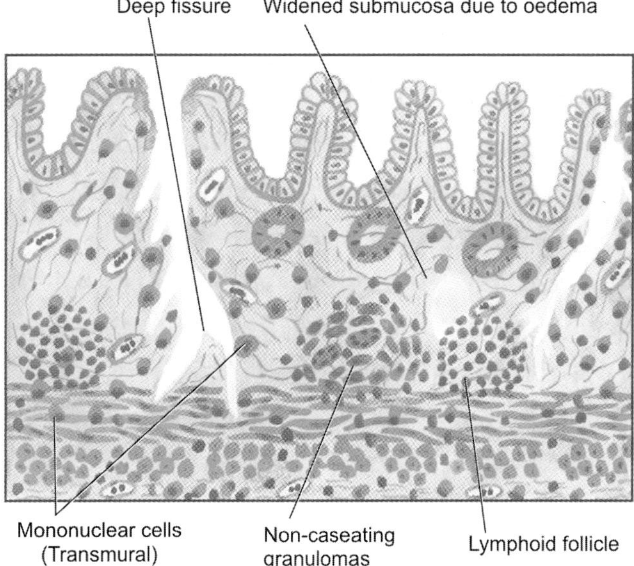

FIGURE 18.21

Crohn's disease of the ileum. The histological features present are: transmural chronic inflammatory cell infiltration, deep fissures into the bowel wall, submucosal widening due to oedema, some prominent lymphoid follicles and a few non-caseating epithelioid cell granulomas in the bowel wall.

ULCERATIVE COLITIS. Classically, ulcerative colitis begins in the rectum, and in continuity extends upwards into the sigmoid colon, descending colon, transverse colon, and sometimes may involve the entire colon. The colonic contents may rarely backflow into the terminal ileum in continuity, causing *'back-wash ileitis'* in about 10% of cases.

Grossly, the characteristic feature is the continuous involvement of rectum and colon without any uninvolved skip areas as seen in Crohn's disease. The appearance of colon may vary depending upon the stage and intensity of the disease because of remissions and exacerbations. Mucosa shows linear and superficial ulcers, usually not penetrating the muscular layer. The intervening intact mucosa may form inflammatory 'pseudopolyps.' The muscle layer is thickened due to contraction, producing shortening and narrowing of the affected colon with loss of normal haustral folds giving 'garden-hose appearance' (Fig. 18.22).

Histologically, ulcerative colitis because of remission and exacerbations, is characterised by alternating 'active disease process' and 'resolving colitis.' The changes in the 'active disease process' are as under (Fig. 18.23) (**COLOUR PLATE XXIII: CL 91**):

Chapter Eighteen

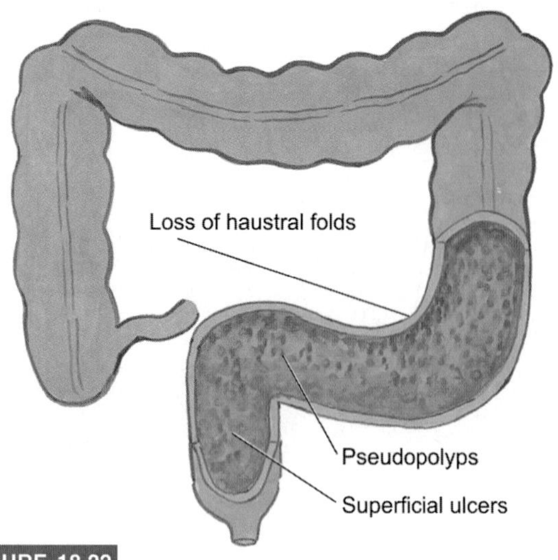

FIGURE 18.22

Ulcerative colitis. Continuous involvement of the rectum, sigmoid colon and descending colon are seen without any uninvolved skip areas. The ulcers are superficial with intervening inflammatory pseudopolyps. The lumen is narrow and the haustral folds are lost giving 'garden-hose appearance'.

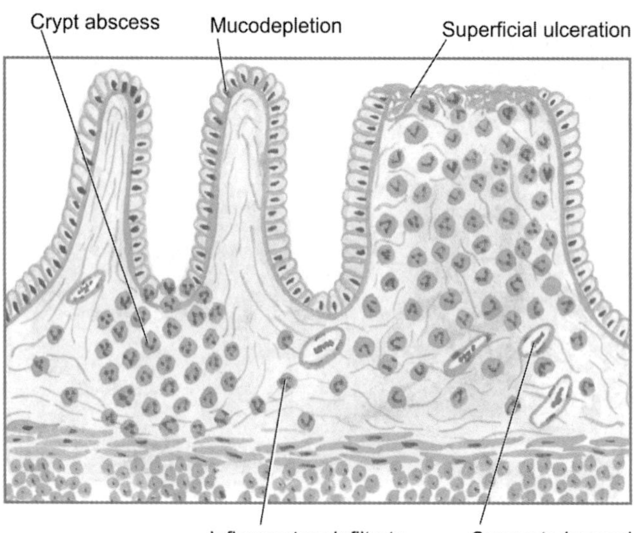

FIGURE 18.23

Ulcerative colitis in active phase. The microscopic features seen are superficial ulcerations, with mucosal infiltration by inflammatory cells and a 'crypt abscess'.

1. *Crypt distortion, cryptitis* and focal accumulations of neutrophils forming *crypt abscesses.*
2. *Marked congestion, dilatation and haemorrhages* from mucosal capillaries.
3. *Superficial mucosal ulcerations,* usually not penetrating into the muscle coat, except in severe cases, and is accompanied by nonspecific inflammatory cell infiltrate of lymphocytes, plasma cells, neutrophils, some eosinophils and mast cells in the lamina propria.
4. *Goblet cells* are markedly *diminished* in cases of active disease.
5. Areas of *mucosal regeneration and mucodepletion* of lining cells.
6. In long-standing cases, epithelial *cytologic atypia* ranging from mild to marked dysplasia and sometimes developing into carcinoma *in situ* and frank adenocarcinoma.

Complications of ulcerative colitis are as follows:

1. *Toxic megacolon (Fulminant colitis)* is the acute fulminating colitis in which the affected colon is thin-walled and dilated and is prone to perforation and faecal peritonitis. There is deep penetration of the inflammatory cell infiltrate into muscle layer which is disrupted.
2. *Perianal fistula* formation may occur rarely.
3. *Carcinoma* may develop in long-standing cases of ulcerative colitis of more than 10 years duration.
4. *Stricture formation* almost never occurs in ulcerative colitis.

OTHER INFLAMMATORY LESIONS OFTHE BOWEL

Besides the IBD, a variety of other acute and chronic inflammatory conditions affect small bowel (enteritis), large bowel (colitis), or both (enterocolitis); the last named being more common. Hence, all these conditions involving small bowel and/or large bowel are described together here for better correlation of features.

The various other forms of inflammations of the bowel (besides IBD) can be categorised broadly into *'infective enterocolitis'* and *'pseudomembranous enterocolitis.'*

INFECTIVE ENTEROCOLITIS

These are a group of acute and chronic inflammatory lesions of small intestine and/or colon caused by micro-organisms (bacteria, viruses, fungi, protozoa and helminths). All these are characterised by diarrhoeal syndromes. Pathogenetically speaking, these micro-organisms can cause enterocolitis by 2 mechanisms—by *enteroinvasive bacteria* producing ulcerative lesions, and by *enterotoxin-producing bacteria* resulting in non-ulcerative lesions.

A list of micro-organisms producing enterocolitis is presented in Table 18.7.

Some of the important forms are described below:

TABLE 18.7: Micro-organisms Causing Infective Enterocolitis.

A. **BACTERIAL ENTEROCOLITIS**

1. **Entero-invasive bacteria**
   (i) Tuberculosis
   (ii) Salmonella
   (iii) *Campylobacter jejuni*
   (iv) *Shigella*
   (v) *Escherichia coli*
   (vi) *Yersenia enterocolitica*
2. **Enterotoxin-producing bacteria**
   (i) *Vibrio cholerae*

B. **VIRAL ENTEROCOLITIS**

C. **FUNGAL ENTEROCOLITIS**
   (i) Candidiasis
   (ii) Mucormycosis

D. **PROTOZOAL AND METAZOAL INFESTATIONS**
   (i) *Giardia lamblia*
   (ii) *Entamoeba histolytica*
   (iii) *Balantidium coli*
   (iv) *Taenia solium*
   (v) *Ascaris lumbricoides*
   (vi) *Ancylostoma duodenale*
   (vii) *Strongyloides stercoralis*

Intestinal Tuberculosis

Intestinal tuberculosis can occur in 3 forms—primary, secondary and hyperplastic caecal tuberculosis.

1. PRIMARY INTESTINAL TUBERCULOSIS. Though an uncommon disease in the Western world, primary tuberculosis of the ileocaecal region is quite common in India. It used to occur by ingestion of unpasteurised cow's milk infected with *Mycobacterium bovis.* But now-a-days due to control of tuberculosis in cattle and pasteurisation of milk, virtually all cases of intestinal tuberculosis are caused by *M. tuberculosis.* The predominant changes are in the mesenteric lymph nodes without any significant intestinal lesion.

Grossly, the affected lymph nodes are enlarged, matted and caseous (tabes mesenterica). Eventually, there is healing by fibrosis and calcification (Fig. 18.24,A).

Microscopically, in the initial stage, there is primary complex or Ghon's focus in the intestinal mucosa as occurs elsewhere in primary tuberculous infection (Page 154). Subsequently, the mesenteric lymph nodes are affected which show typical tuberculous granulomatous inflammatory reaction with caseation necrosis. Tuberculous peritonitis may occur due to spread of the infection.

2. SECONDARY INTESTINAL TUBERCULOSIS. Swallowing of sputum in patients with active pulmonary tuberculosis may cause secondary intestinal tuberculosis, most commonly in the terminal ileum and rarely in the colon.

Grossly, the intestinal lesions are prominent than the lesions in regional lymph nodes as in secondary

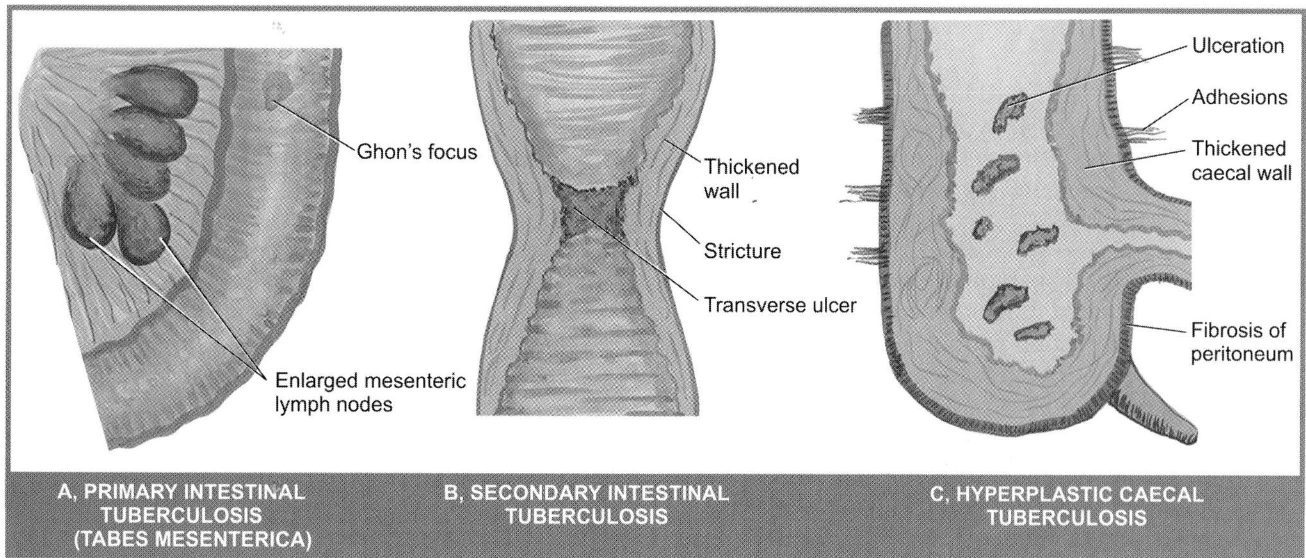

FIGURE 18.24

Intestinal tuberculosis, three patterns.

pulmonary tuberculosis. The lesions begin in the Peyer's patches or the lymphoid follicles with formation of small ulcers that spread through the lymphatics to form large ulcers which are *transverse to the long axis of the bowel,* (*c.f.* typhoid ulcers of small intestine, described below). These ulcers may be coated with caseous material. Serosa may be studded with visible tubercles. In advanced cases, transverse fibrous strictures and intestinal obstruction are seen (Fig. 18.24,B).

Histologically, the tuberculous lesions in the intestine are similar to those observed elsewhere i.e. presence of tubercles. Mucosa and submucosa show ulceration and the muscularis may be replaced by variable degree of fibrosis. Tuberculous peritonitis may be observed (COLOUR PLATE VII: CL 28).

3. **HYPERPLASTIC CAECAL TUBERCULOSIS.** This is a variant of secondary tuberculosis secondary to pulmonary tuberculosis.

Grossly, the caecum and/or ascending colon are thick-walled with mucosal ulceration. Clinically, the lesion is palpable and may be mistaken for carcinoma (Fig. 18.24,C).

Microscopically, the presence of caseating tubercles distinguishes the condition from Crohn's disease in which granulomas are non-caseating. Besides, bacteriological evidence by culture or animal inoculation and Mantoux test are helpful in differential diagnosis of the two conditions.

Enteric Fever

The term enteric fever is used to describe acute infection caused by *Salmonella typhi* (typhoid fever) or *Salmonella paratyphi* (paratyphoid fever). Besides these 2 salmonellae, *Salmonella typhimurium* causes food poisoning.

PATHOGENESIS. The typhoid bacilli are ingested through contaminated food or water. During the initial asymptomatic incubation period of about 2 weeks, the bacilli invade the lymphoid follicles and Peyer's patches of the small intestine and proliferate. Following this, the bacilli invade the blood stream causing bacteraemia, and the characteristic clinical features of the disease like continuous rise in temperature and 'rose spots' on the skin are observed. Immunological reactions (Widal's test) begin after about 10 days and peak titres are seen by the end of the third week. Eventually, the bacilli are localised in the intestinal lymphoid tissue (producing typhoid intestinal lesions), in the mesenteric lymph nodes (leading to haemorrhagic lymphadenitis), in the liver (causing foci of parenchymal necrosis), in the gall bladder (producing typhoid cholecystitis), and in the spleen (resulting in splenic reactive hyperplasia).

PATHOLOGIC CHANGES. The lesions are observed in the intestines as well as in other organs.

1. **INTESTINAL LESIONS.** ***Macroscopically,*** terminal ileum is affected most often, but lesions may be seen in the jejunum and colon. The Peyer's patches show oval typhoid ulcers with their *long axis along the length of the bowel,* (*c.f.* tuberculous ulcers of small intestine, described above). The base of the ulcers is black due to sloughed mucosa. The margins of the ulcers are slightly raised due to inflammatory oedema and cellular proliferation. There is never significant fibrosis and hence fibrous stenosis seldom occurs in healed typhoid lesions. The regional lymph nodes are invariably enlarged (Fig. 18.25,A).

Microscopically, there is hyperaemia, oedema and cellular proliferation consisting of phagocytic histiocytes (showing characteristic erythrophagocytosis), lymphocytes and plasma cells. Though enteric fever is an example of acute inflammation, neutrophils are invariably absent from the cellular infiltrate and this is reflected in the leucopenia with neutropenia and relative lymphocytosis in the peripheral blood (Fig. 18.25,B).

The main **complications** of the intestinal lesions of typhoid are perforation of the ulcers and haemorrhage.

2. **OTHER LESIONS.** Besides the intestinal involvement, various other organs and tissues showing pathological changes in enteric fever are as under:

i) *Mesenteric lymph nodes*—haemorrhagic lymphadenitis.
ii) *Liver*—foci of parenchymal necrosis.
iii) *Gallbladder*—typhoid cholecystitis.
iv) *Spleen*—splenomegaly with reactive hyperplasia.
v) *Kidneys*—nephritis.
vi) *Abdominal muscles*—Zenker's degeneration.
vii) *Joints*—arthritis.
viii) *Bones*—osteitis.
ix) *Meninges*—Meningitis.
x) *Testis*—Orchitis.

Persistence of organism in the gallbladder or urinary tract may result in passage of organisms in the faeces or urine creating a 'carrier state' which is a source of infection to others.

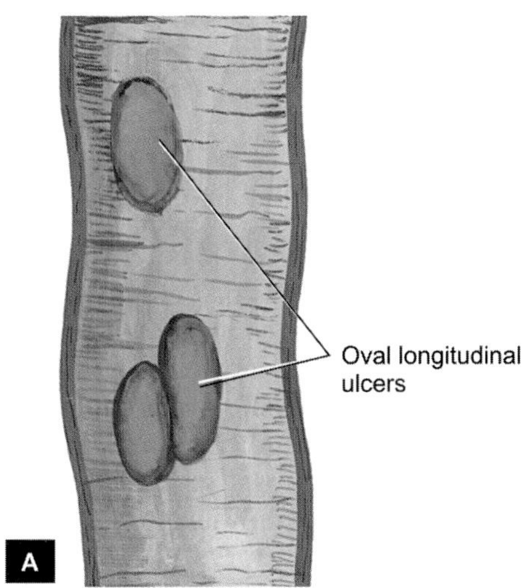

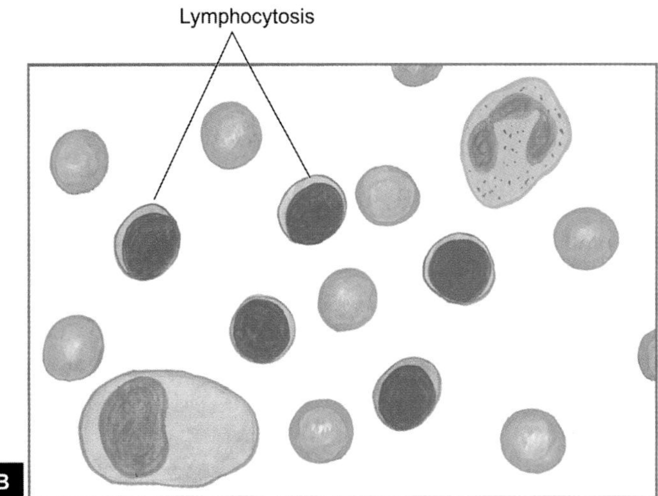

FIGURE 18.25

A, Typhoid ulcers in the small intestine appear characteristically oval with their long axis parallel to the long axis of the bowel. B, Blood picture in typhoid fever showing neutropenia and relative lymphocytosis.

Bacterial Food Poisoning

This is a form of acute bacterial illness that occurs following ingestion of food or water contaminated with bacteria other than those that cause specific acute intestinal infections like typhoid, paratyphoid, cholera or dysentery bacilli. The illness results from either bacterial invasion or bacterial toxigenic effect on the bowel.

The commonest causes of bacterial food poisoning resulting in enteritis or enterocolitis are as under:

1. **Staphylococcal food poisoning.** *Staphylococcus aureus* infection acquired from contaminated food produces either *mild food poisoning* by enterotoxins, or may cause more severe form of the illness called *pseudomembranous enterocolitis* described below. Staphylococcal food poisoning occurs due to liberation of enterotoxins by the bacteria.

2. **Clostridial food poisoning.** Infection with anaerobic organisms *Clostridium welchii,* following consumption of contaminated meat results in acute food poisoning (page 187). The illness occurs both by bacterial invasion as well as by toxins.

3. **Botulism.** This is a severe form of paralysing illness caused by ingestion of organism, *Clostridium botulinum,* which produces neurotoxin.

4. **Salmonella food poisoning (Salmonellosis).** This is an infection (and not caused by toxins) occurring due to food contaminated by *S. typhimurium* or *S. enteritidis.* The condition manifests with fever, vomiting, and diarrhoea. Death may result from depletion of water and electrolytes.

Dysenteries

The term 'dysentery' is used to mean diarrhoea with abdominal cramps, tenesmus and passage of mucus in the stools, from any cause. There are 2 main forms of dysenteries—bacillary and amoebic.

1. **BACILLARY DYSENTERY.** Bacillary dysentery is the term used for infection by *shigella* species: *S. dysenteriae, S. flexneri, S. boydii and S. sonnei.* Infection occurs by foeco-oral route and is seen with poor personal hygiene, in densely populated areas, and with contaminated food and water. The common housefly plays a role in spread of infection.

Macroscopically, the lesions are mainly found in the colon and occasionally in the ileum. Superficial transverse ulcerations of mucosa of the bowel wall occur in the region of lymphoid follicles but perforation is seldom seen. The intervening intact mucosa is hyperaemic and oedematous. Following recovery from the acute attack, complete healing usually takes place.

Microscopically, the mucosa overlying the lymphoid follicles is necrosed. The surrounding mucosa shows congestion, oedema and infiltration by neutrophils and lymphocytes. The mucosa may be covered by greyish-yellow *'pseudomembrane'* composed of fibrinosuppurative exudate.

The **complications** of bacillary dysentery are haemorrhage, perforation, stenosis, polyarthritis and iridocyclitis.

2. AMOEBIC DYSENTERY. This is due to infection by *Entamoeba histolytica.* It is more prevalent in the tropical countries and primarily affects the large intestine. Infection occurs from ingestion of cyst form of the parasite. The cyst wall is dissolved in the small intestine from where the liberated amoebae pass into the large intestine. Here, they invade the epithelium of the mucosa, reach the submucosa and produce the characteristic flask-shaped ulcers.

Macroscopically, early intestinal lesions appear as small areas of elevation on the mucosal surface. In advanced cases, typical flask-shaped ulcers having narrow neck and broad base are seen. They are more conspicuous in the caecum, rectum and in the flexures.

Microscopically, the ulcerated area shows chronic inflammatory reaction consisting of lymphocytes, plasma cells, macrophages and eosinophils. The trophozoites of *Entamoeba* are seen in the inflammatory exudate and are concentrated at the advancing margin of the lesion. Intestinal amoebae characteristically have ingested red cells in their cytoplasm. Oedema and vascular congestion are present in the area surrounding the ulcers.

Complications of intestinal amoebic ulcers are: amoebic liver abscess or amoebic hepatitis, perforation, haemorrhage and formation of amoeboma which is a tumour-like mass.

PSEUDOMEMBRANOUS ENTEROCOLITIS (ANTIBIOTIC-ASSOCIATED DIARRHOEA)

Pseudomembranous enterocolitis is a form of acute inflammation of colon and/or small intestine characterised by formation of *'pseudomembrane'* over the site of mucosal injury.

ETIOLOGY. Numerous studies have established the overgrowth of *Clostridium difficile* with production of its toxin in the etiology of antibiotic-associated diarrhoea culminating in pseudomembranous colitis. Oral antibiotics such as clindamycin, ampicillin and the cephalosporins are more often (20%) associated with antibiotic-associated diarrhoea, while development of pseudomembranous colitis may occur in 1-10% cases.

Pseudomembrane formation may also occur in various other conditions such as in:

- Staphylococcal enterocolitis
- Bacillary *(Shigella)* dysentery
- *Candida* enterocolitis

PATHOLOGIC CHANGES. Macroscopically, the lesions may be confined, to the large intestine or small intestine, or both may be involved. The mucosa of the bowel is covered by patchy, raised yellow-white plaques. Elsewhere, the mucosa is congested and may show small mucosal ulcerations.

Microscopically, the *'pseudomembrane'* is composed of network of fibrin and mucus, in which are entangled inflammatory cells and mucosal epithelial cells. There is focal necrosis of surface epithelial cells. The lamina propria contains inflammatory cell infiltrate, mainly neutrophils. The submucosa has congested capillaries and may show microthrombi. The inflammation spreads laterally rather than deeply.

MALABSORPTION SYNDROME

DEFINITION AND CLASSIFICATION

The malabsorption syndrome (MAS) is characterised by impaired intestinal absorption of nutrients especially of fat; some other substances are proteins, carbohydrates, vitamins and minerals. MAS is subdivided into 2 broad groups:

- **Primary MAS,** which is due to primary deficiency of the absorptive mucosal surface and of the associated enzymes.
- **Secondary MAS,** in which mucosal changes result secondary to other factors such as diseases, surgery, trauma and drugs.

Each of the two main groups has a number of causes listed in Table 18.8.

CLINICAL FEATURES

The clinical manifestations of MAS vary according to the underlying cause. However, some common symptoms are as follows:

1. Steatorrhoea (pale, bulky, foul-smelling stools)
2. Chronic diarrhoea
3. Abdominal distension
4. Barborygmi and flatulence
5. Anorexia
6. Weight loss
7. Muscle wasting
8. Dehydration
9. Hypotension
10. Specific malnutrition and vitamin deficiencies depending upon the cause.

TABLE 18.8: Classification of Malabsorption Syndrome.

I. PRIMARY MALABSORPTION
1. Coeliac sprue
2. Collagenous sprue
3. Tropical sprue
4. Whipple's disease
5. Disaccharidase deficiency
6. Allergic and eosinophilic gastroenteritis

II. SECONDARY MALABSORPTION

1. Impaired digestion
(i) Mucosal damage e.g. in tuberculosis, Crohn's disease, lymphoma, amyloidosis, radiation injury, systemic sclerosis
(ii) Hepatic and pancreatic insufficiency
(iii) Resection of bowel
(iv) Drugs e.g. methotrexate, neomycin, phenindione etc.

2. Impaired absorption
(i) Short or stagnant bowel (blind loop syndrome) from surgery or disease resulting in abnormal proliferation of microbial flora
(ii) Acute infectious enteritis
(iii) Parasitoses e.g. Giardia, Strongyloides, hookworms

3. Impaired transport
(i) Lymphatic obstruction e.g. in lymphoma tuberculosis, lymphangiectasia
(ii) Abetalipoproteinaemia

INVESTIGATIONS

When MAS is suspected on clinical grounds, the following investigations may be carried out to confirm it:

I. LABORATORY TESTS:

1. Tests for fat malabsorption:
i) Faecal analysis for fat content
ii) Microscopic analysis for faecal fat
iii) Blood lipid levels after a fatty meal
iv) Tests based on absorption of radioactive-labelled fat.

2. Tests for protein malabsorption:
i) Bile acid malabsorption
ii) Radioactive-labelled glycine breath test.
iii) Prothrombin time (vitamin K deficiency)
iv) Secretin and other pancreatic tests

3. Tests for carbohydrate malabsorption:
i) D-xylose tolerance test
ii) Lactose tolerance test
iii) Hydrogen breath test
iv) Bile acid breath test

4. Vitamin B_{12}, malabsorption:
i) Schilling test (page 383).

II. INTESTINAL BIOPSY:

Per-oral small intestinal biopsy employing Crosby-Kugler capsule is widely used for investigation and diagnosis of MAS. The biopsy should first be examined under dissecting microscope before histologic sectioning.

Normal villous (Fig. 18.26,A). Under the dissecting microscope, the normal jejunal mucosa has tall, slender, finger-shaped or leaf-shaped villi. It is lined by tall columnar absorptive epithelium and has scattered lymphocytes in the lamina propria.

Villous atrophy. Variable degree of flattening of intestinal mucosa in MAS is the commonest pathological change in mucosal pattern and is referred to as villous atrophy. It may be of 2 types—partial and subtotal/total type.

- *Partial villous atrophy* (Fig. 18.26,B) is the mild form of the lesion in which villi fuse with each other and thus become short and broad, commonly called as convolutions and irregular ridges. The epithelial cells show compensatory hyperplasia suggesting a turnover of these cells. Lamina propria shows increased cellular infiltrate, predominantly of plasma cells.

Partial villous atrophy is commonly found in children and adults with diarrhoea, parasitic infestations, Crohn's disease, ulcerative colitis and malabsorption due to drugs and radiation injury.

- *Subtotal/Total villous atrophy* (Fig. 18.26,C) is the severe form of the lesion in which there is flattening of mucosa due to more advanced villous fusion. The surface epithelium is cuboidal and there is increased plasma cell infiltrate in the lamina propria.

Subtotal and total villous atrophy is exhibited by a number of conditions such as nontropical sprue, tropical sprue, intestinal lymphomas, carcinoma, protein-calorie malnutrition etc.

IMPORTANT TYPES OF MAS

Coeliac Sprue (Non-tropical Sprue, Gluten-Sensitive Enteropathy, Idiopathic Steatorrhoea)

This is the most important cause of primary malabsorption occurring in temperate climates. The condition is characterised by significant loss of villi in the small intestine and thence diminished absorptive surface area. The condition occurs in 2 forms:

Childhood form, seen in infants and children and is commonly referred to as *coeliac disease.*

Adult form, seen in adolescents and early adult life and used to be called *idiopathic steatorrhoea.*

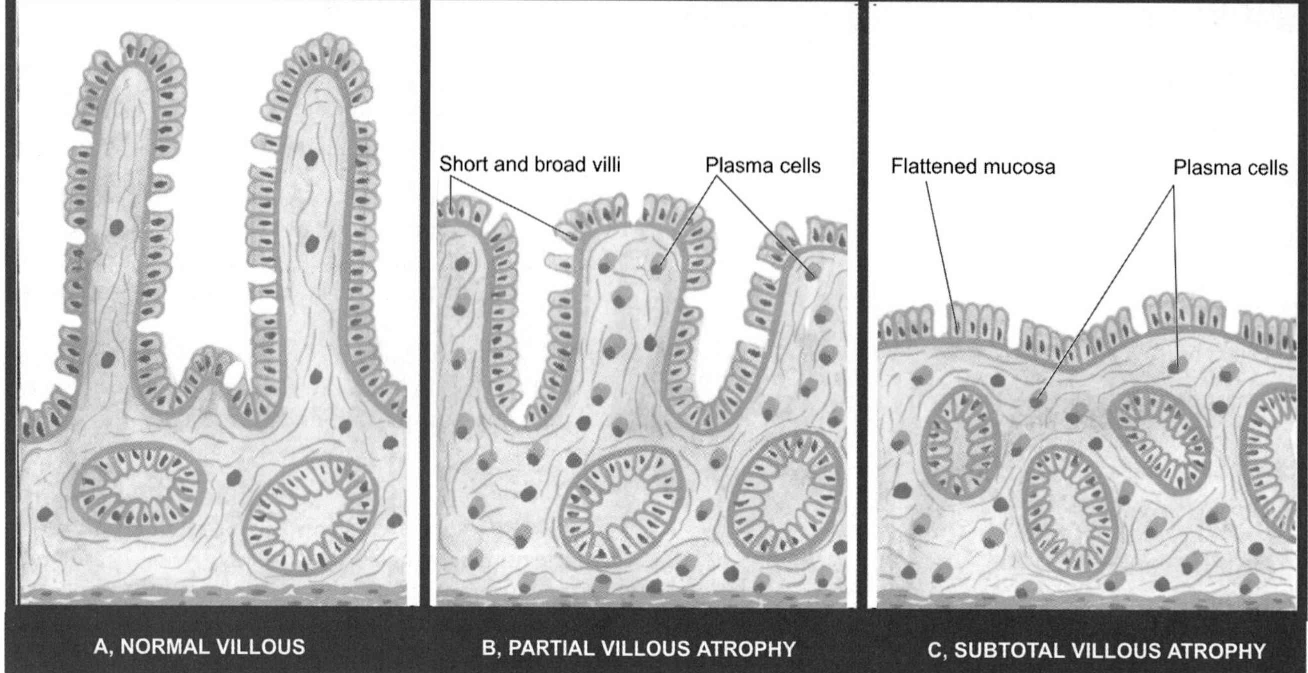

FIGURE 18.26

Jejunal biopsy appearance in malabsorption syndrome.

In either case, there is genetic abnormality resulting in sensitivity to gluten (a protein) and its derivative, gliadin, present in diets such as grains of wheat, barley and rye. The symptoms are usually relieved on elimination of gluten from the diet. The role of heredity is further supported by the observation of familial incidence and HLA association of the disease. Exact pathogenesis of the condition is not clear. However, following hypotheses are significant in causing mucosal cell damage:

1. *Hypersensitivity reaction* as evidenced by gluten-stimulated antibodies.
2. Toxic effect of gluten due to *inherited enzyme deficiency* in the mucosal cells.

PATHOLOGIC CHANGES. There are no differences in the pathological findings in children and adults. ***Histologically,*** there is variable degree of flattening of the mucosa, particularly of the upper jejunum, and to some extent of the duodenum and ileum. The surface epithelial cells are cuboidal or low columnar type. There may be *partial villous atrophy* which is replacement of normal villous pattern by convolutions, or *subtotal villous atrophy* characterised by flat mucosal surface. Lamina propria shows increased number of plasma cells and lymphocytes (COLOUR PLATE XXIII: CL 92).

The major sequela of long-term coeliac sprue is increased incidence of intestinal carcinoma in these cases.

Collagenous Sprue

This entity is regarded as the end-result of coeliac sprue in which the villi are totally absent *(total villous atrophy)* and there are unique and diagnostic broad bands of collagen under the basal lamina of surface epithelium. The condition is refractory to any treatment and the course is generally fatal. Some workers consider collagenous sprue as a variant of coeliac sprue without classifying it separately.

Tropical Sprue

This disease, as the name suggests, occurs in individuals living in or visiting tropical areas such as Caribbean countries, South India, Sri Lanka and Hong Kong. Pathogenesis of the condition is not clear but there is evidence to support enterotoxin production by some strains of *E. coli* which causes the intestinal injury. Severe cases are characterised by additional features such as macrocytic anaemia, glossitis and emaciation due to intestinal malabsorption of vitamin B_{12} and folate.

PATHOLOGIC CHANGES. Histologically, there is usually *partial villous atrophy* and sometimes *subtotal atrophy.*

The lesions are relieved by removal of the patient from the tropical area and by oral administration of antibiotics but gluten-free diet has no role in improvement.

Whipple's Disease (Intestinal Lipodystrophy)

This is an uncommon bacterial disease involving not only the intestines but also various other systems such as central nervous system, heart, blood vessels, skin, joints, lungs, liver, spleen and kidneys. The disease is more common in males in 4th to 5th decades of life. Patients may present with features of malabsorption or may have atypical presentation in the form of migratory polyarthritis, neurological disturbances and focal hyperpigmentation of the skin.

PATHOLOGIC CHANGES. Histologically, the affected tissues show presence of characteristic macrophages containing PAS-positive granules and rod-shaped micro-organisms (Whipple's bacilli). These macrophages are predominantly present in the lamina propria of the small intestine and mesenteric lymph nodes.

Patients respond very well to oral antibiotic therapy.

Protein-Losing Enteropathies

A number of disorders of the gastrointestinal tract are accompanied by excessive protein loss without concomitant increase in protein synthesis, thus resulting in hypoproteinaemia. These diseases are listed below:

i) Whipple's disease
ii) Crohn's disease
iii) Ulcerative colitis
iv) Sprue
v) Intestinal lymphangiectasia
vi) Ménétrier's disease (Hypertrophic gastritis).

SMALL INTESTINAL TUMOURS

For obscure reasons, benign as well as malignant tumours of the small bowel are surprisingly rare. Most common *benign tumours,* in descending order of frequency, are: leiomyomas, adenomas and vascular tumours (haemangioma, lymphangioma). Amongst the *malignant tumours,* the most frequently encountered, in descending frequency, are: carcinoid tumours, lymphomas (page 575) and adenocarcinoma. All these tumours are identical in morphology to those seen elsewhere in the alimentary tract. Carcinoid tumour, a peculiar neoplasm most common in the midgut, is described below.

Carcinoid Tumour (Argentaffinoma)

Carcinoid tumour or argentaffinoma is a generic term applied to tumours originating from endocrine cells (*synonyms:* argentaffin cells, Kulchitsky cells, enterochromaffin cells) belonging to APUD cell system and are therefore also called as apudomas (page 576). The endocrine cells are distributed throughout the mucosa of GI tract. These cells have secretory granules which stain positively with silver salts (argentaffin granules) or many stain after addition of exogenous reducing agent (non-argentaffin or argyrophil granules). Accordingly, carcinoid tumour may be argentaffin or argyrophil type. Depending upon the embryologic derivation of the tissues where the tumour is located, these are classified as foregut, midgut, and hindgut carcinoids.

- **Midgut carcinoids,** seen in terminal ileum and appendix are the most common (60-80%) and are more often argentaffin positive.
- **Hindgut carcinoids,** occurring in rectum and colon are more commonly argyrophil type, and comprise about 10-20% of carcinoids.
- **Foregut carcinoids,** located in the stomach, duodenum and oesophagus are also argyrophil type and are encountered as frequently as in the hindgut (10-20%).

Other uncommon locations are bronchus, trachea, gallbladder, and Meckel's diverticulum.

Appendix and terminal ileum, the two most common sites for carcinoids, depict variation in their age and sex incidence and biologic behaviour:

- **Appendiceal carcinoids,** occur more frequently in 3rd and 4th decades of life without any sex predilection, are often solitary and behave as locally malignant tumours.
- **Ileal carcinoids,** on the other hand, are seen more often in later age (7th decade) with female preponderance, are more commonly multiple and behave like metastasising carcinomas.

PATHOLOGIC CHANGES. Macroscopically, all carcinoids are small, button-like submucosal elevations with intact or ulcerated overlying mucosa. They are usually small; those larger than 2 cm are more often metastasising. Ileal and gastric carcinoids are commonly multiple, whereas appendiceal carcinoids commonly involve the tip of the organ and are

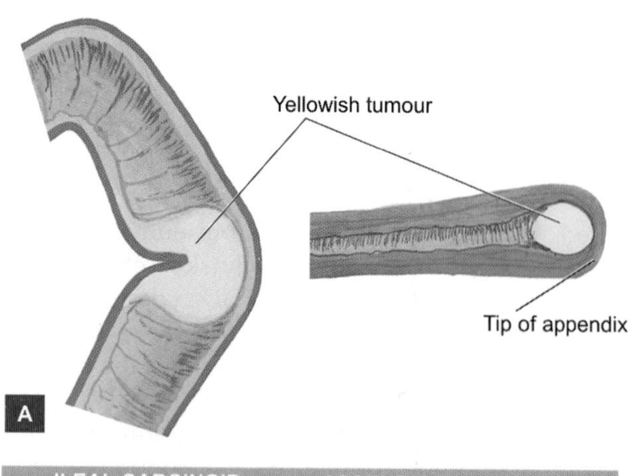

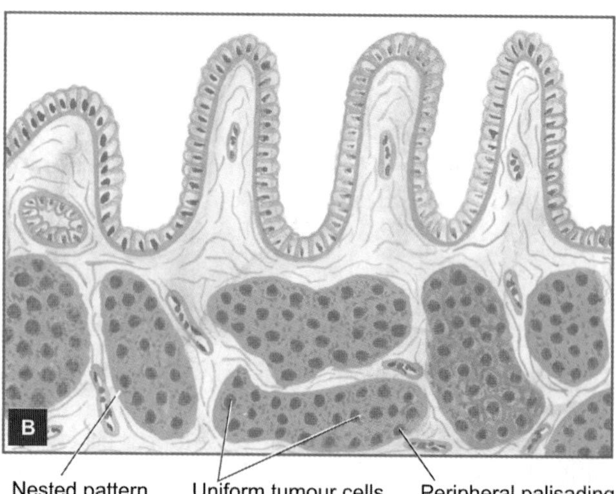

FIGURE 18.27

Carcinoid tumour. A, Gross appearance at common locations. B, Microscopic appearance showing solid masses and trabeculae of uniform, monotonous, small cells with palisading of the peripheral cells.

solitary (Fig. 18.27,A). Cut section of all the carcinoids is bright yellow.

Histologically, the tumour cells may be arranged in a variety of patterns—solid nests, sheets, cords, trabeculae and clusters, all of which show characteristic palisading of the peripheral cells. Acinar arrangement and rosettes are rarely seen. The tumour cells are classically small, monotonous, having uniform nuclei and poorly-defined cell boundaries (Fig. 18.27,B) (COLOUR PLATE XXIV: CL 94). The argentaffin carcinoids show eosinophilic granules in the cytoplasm which stain positively by the argentaffin reaction. Mitotic figures are rare. However, the cytologic features are a poor guide for distinguishing clinically benign from malignant behaviour of the tumour, but all carcinoids infiltrate the bowel wall.

CARCINOID SYNDROME. Carcinoid tumours that metastasise, especially to the liver, are sometimes associated with the carcinoid syndrome. The syndrome consists of the following features:

1. Intermittent attacks of flushing of the skin of face
2. Episodes of watery diarrhoea
3. Abdominal pain
4. Attacks of dyspnoea due to bronchospasm
5. Right-sided heart failure due to involvement of tricuspid and pulmonary valves and endocardium (page 343).

A number of *secretory products* in a functioning carcinoid tumour have been demonstrated:

i) 5-Hydroxytryptamine (5-HT, serotonin)
ii) 5-Hydroxytryptophan
iii) 5-Hydroxy-indole acetic acid (5-HIAA)
iv) Histamine
v) Kallikrein
vi) Bradykinin

However, 5-HT and its degradation product, 5-HIAA, are particularly significant in the production of *carcinoid syndrome.* 5-HT, a potent vasodilator and smooth muscle stimulant, is normally synthesised in the endocrine cells of the gut from dietary tryptophan. Tryptophan is first hydroxylated to 5-hydroxytryptophan, then decarboxylated to 5-HT and further oxidised to 5-HIAA by the monoamine oxidase in the liver cells. It is then excreted in the urine (Fig. 18.28). This capacity to synthesise 5-HT and 5-HIAA is markedly elevated in primary and hepatic metastatic carcinoids. Midgut carcinoids have rich decarboxylating enzymes and are thus able to produce large quantities of 5-HT and 5-HIAA, accounting for high frequency of carcinoid syndrome in them. Foregut and hindgut carcinoids, on the other hand, lack decarboxylating enzymes and, therefore, are less often associated with carcinoid syndrome.

APPENDIX

NORMAL STRUCTURE

Appendix is a vestigial organ which serves no useful purpose in man but instead becomes the site of trouble at times. It is like a diverticulum of the caecum, usually

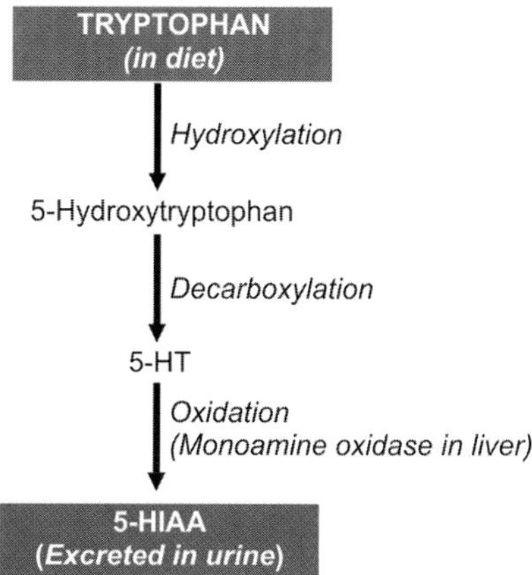

FIGURE 18.28

Biosynthesis of 5-HT and 5-HIAA in the production of carcinoid syndrome.

lying behind the caecum and varies in length from 4 to 20 cm (average 7 cm).

Histologically, appendix has four layers in its wall—*mucosa, submucosa, muscularis* and *serosa.* The mucosa has patchy distribution of crypts and the submucosa has abundant lymphoid tissue. Argentaffin and non-argentaffin endocrine cells are present in the base of mucosal glands just as in the small intestine. The muscularis of the appendix has two layers (inner circular and outer longitudinal) as elsewhere in the alimentary tract.

Two important diseases involving the appendix are appendicitis and appendiceal carcinoids.

APPENDICITIS

Acute inflammation of the appendix, acute appendicitis, is the most common acute abdominal condition confronting the surgeon. The condition is seen more commonly in older children and young adults, and is uncommon at the extremes of age. The disease is seen more frequently in the West and in affluent societies which may be due to variation in diet—a diet with low bulk or cellulose and high protein intake more often causes appendicitis.

ETIOPATHOGENESIS. The most common etiological factor is obstruction of the lumen that leads to increased intraluminal pressure. This presses upon the blood vessels to produce ischaemic injury which in turn favours the bacterial proliferation and hence acute appendicitis. The common causes of appendicitis are as under:

A. Obstructive:

1. Faecolith
2. Calculi
3. Foreign body
4. Tumour
5. Worms (especially *Enterobius vermicularis)*
6. Diffuse lymphoid hyperplasia, especially in children.

B. Non-obstructive:

1. Haematogenous spread of generalised infection
2. Vascular occlusion
3. Inappropriate diet lacking roughage.

PATHOLOGIC CHANGES. Macroscopically, the appearance depends upon the stage at which the acutely-inflamed appendix is examined. In *early acute appendicitis,* the organ is swollen and serosa shows hyperaemia. In well-developed acute inflammation called *acute suppurative appendicitis,* the serosa is coated with fibrinopurulent exudate and engorged vessels on the surface. In further advanced cases called *acute gangrenous appendicitis,* there is necrosis and ulcerations of mucosa which extend through the wall so that the appendix becomes soft and friable and the surface is coated with greenish-black gangrenous necrosis (Fig. 18.29,A).

Microscopically, the most important diagnostic histological criteria is the *neutrophilic infiltration of the muscularis.* In early stage, the other changes besides acute inflammatory changes, are congestion and oedema of the appendiceal wall. In later stages, the mucosa is sloughed off, the wall becomes necrotic, the blood vessels may get thrombosed and there may be neutrophilic abscesses in the wall. In either case, an impacted foreign body, faecolith, or concretion may be seen in the lumen (Fig. 18.29,B). Thus, there is good correlation between macroscopic and microscopic findings in acute appendicitis (COLOUR PLATE XXIII: CL 90).

CLINICAL COURSE. The patient presents with features of acute abdomen as under:

1. Colicky pain, initially around umbilicus but later localised to right iliac fossa
2. Nausea and vomiting
3. Pyrexia of mild grade
4. Abdominal tenderness
5. Increased pulse rate
6. Neutrophilic leucocytosis.

An attack of acute appendicitis predisposes the appendix to repeated attacks *(recurrent acute appendicitis)* and thus surgery has to be carried out. If appendicec-tomy is done at a later stage following acute attack

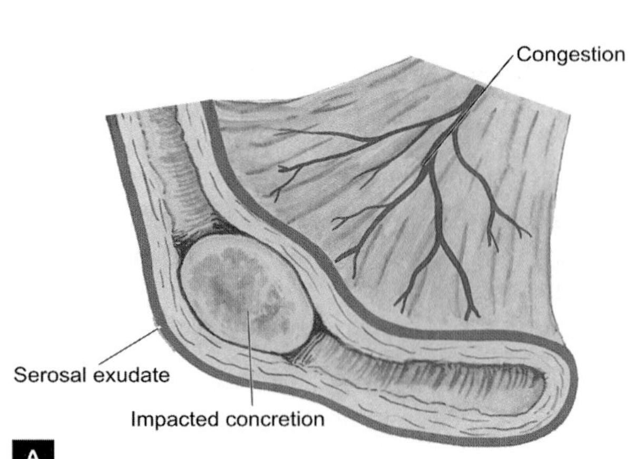

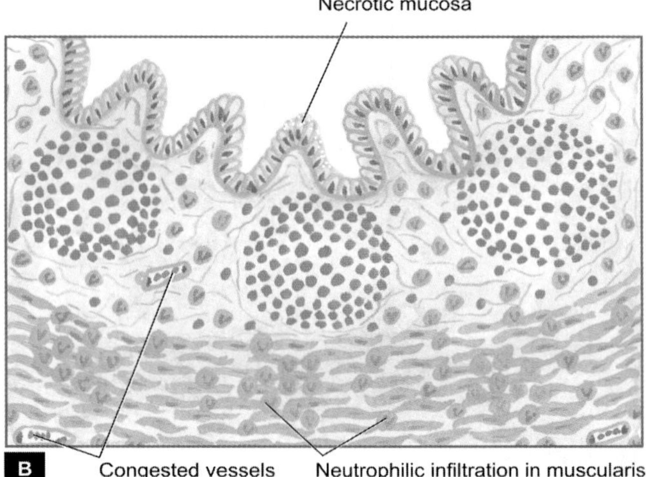

FIGURE 18.29

Acute appendicitis. A, Macroscopic appearance of longitudinally opened appendix showing impacted concretion in the lumen and exudate on the serosa. B, Microscopic appearance showing diagnostic neutrophilic infiltration into the muscularis. Other changes present are necrosis of mucosa and periappendicitis.

(interval appendicectomy), pathological changes of healing by fibrosis of the wall and chronic inflammation are observed.

COMPLICATIONS. If the condition is not adequately managed, the following complications may occur:

1. **Peritonitis.** A perforated appendix as occurs in gangrenous appendicitis may cause localised or generalised peritonitis.

2. **Appendix abscess.** This is due to rupture of an appendix giving rise to localised abscess in the right iliac fossa. This abscess may spread to other sites such as between the liver and diaphragm (subphrenic abscess), into the pelvis between the urinary bladder and rectum, and in the females may involve uterus and fallopian tubes.

3. **Adhesions.** Late complications of acute appendicitis are fibrous adhesions to the greater omentum, small intestine and other abdominal structures.

4. **Portal pylephlebitis.** Spread of infection into mesenteric veins may produce septic phlebitis and liver abscess.

5. **Mucocele.** Distension of distal appendix by mucus following recovery from an attack of acute appendicitis is referred to as mucocele. It occurs generally due to proximal obstruction but sometimes may be due to a benign or malignant neoplasm in the appendix. Extravasation of the mucus following rupture of mucocele gives rise to *pseudomyxoma peritonei.* An infected mucocele may result in formation of *empyema* of the appendix.

TUMOURS OF APPENDIX

Tumours of the appendix are quite rare. These include: carcinoid tumour (the most common), pseudomyxoma peritonei and adenocarcinoma.

CARCINOID TUMOUR. It is already described on page 591. Both argentaffin and argyrophil types are encountered, the former being more common.

Macroscopically, carcinoid tumour of the appendix is mostly situated near the tip of the organ and appears as a circumscribed nodule, usually less than 1 cm in diameter, involving the wall but metastases are rare.

Histologically, carcinoid tumour of the appendix resembles other carcinoids of the midgut.

PSEUDOMYXOMA PERITONEI. Pseudomyxoma peritonei is appearance of gelatinous mucinous material around the appendix which may be from benign mucinous cystadenoma of the ovary or mucin-secreting carcinoma of the appendix.

ADENOCARCINOMA. It is an uncommon tumour in the appendix and is morphologically similar to adenocarcinoma elsewhere in the alimentary tract.

LARGE INTESTINE

NORMAL STRUCTURE

The large bowel consists of 6 parts—the caecum, ascending colon, transverse colon, descending colon, sigmoid colon and rectum, and in all measures about 1.5 meters in length. The serosal surface of the large intestine except the rectum is studded with *appendices epiploicae* which are small, rounded collections of fatty tissue covered by peritoneum.

Histologically, the wall of large bowel consists of 4 layers as elsewhere in the alimentary tract—serosa, muscularis, submucosa and mucosa.

- The **mucosa** lacks villi and there is preponderance of goblet cells over columnar epithelial cells. The lymphoid tissue is less abundant than in the small bowel but lymphoid follicles are seen in the caecum and rectum.
- The **muscularis propria** of the large intestine is quite peculiar—the inner circular muscle layer ensheaths whole length of the intestine, while the outer longitudinal muscle layer is concentrated into 3 muscle bands called *taenia coli.* The length of outer muscle layer is shorter than the length of the intestine and therefore, it forms the *sacculations or haustra* of the large intestine. At the rectosigmoid junction, the three muscle bands fuse to form a complete covering.

The **blood supply** to the right colon is from the superior mesenteric artery which also supplies blood to the small bowel. The remaining portion of large bowel except the lower part of rectum receives blood supply from inferior mesenteric artery. The lower rectum is supplied by haemorrhoidal branches. The **innervation** of the large bowel consists of 3 plexuses of ganglion cells—*Auerbach's* or *myenteric plexus* lying between the two layers of muscularis, *Henle's plexus* lying in the deep submucosa inner to circular muscle layer, and *Meissner plexus* that lies in the superficial mucosa just beneath the muscularis mucosae. These are interconnected by non-myelinated nerve fibres.

Anal canal, 3-4 cm long tubular structure, begins at the lower end of the rectum, though is not a part of large bowel, but is included here to cover simultaneously lesions pertaining to this region. It is lined by keratinised or nonkeratinised stratified squamous epithelium. *Anal verge* is the junction between the anal canal and perineal skin, while *pectinate line* is the squamo-columnar junction between the anal canal and the rectum.

CONGENITAL MALFORMATIONS

Hirschsprung's Disease (Congenital Megacolon)

The term 'megacolon' is used for any form of marked dilatation of the entire colon or its segment and may occur as a congenital or acquired disorder. *Congenital form* characterised by congenital absence of ganglion cells in the bowel wall (enteric neurons) is called Hirschsprung's disease. As a result, the aganglionic segment remains contracted. Genetically, Hirschsprung's disease is a heterogeneous disorder as under:

1. Autosomal dominant inheritance with mutation in RET gene in some cases.
2. Autosomal recessive form with mutation in endothelin-B receptor gene in many other cases.

Clinically, the condition manifests shortly after birth with constipation, gaseous distension and sometimes with acute intestinal obstruction. Its frequency is 1 in 5,000 live-births, has familial tendency in about 4% of cases and has predilection for development in Down's syndrome. Pathogenesis lies in the failure of neuroblasts to migrate to the rectum which normally occurs at about 12 weeks of gestation. Depending upon the length of the segment affected by aganglionosis in Hirschsprung's disease, 4 patterns are recognised:

1. *Short segment (rectal and recto-sigmoid) disease* as the most common form.
2. *Long segment or subtotal colonic disease,* involving colon from rectosigmoid to the ileo-caecal valve.
3. *Total colonic aganglionosis.*
4. *Ultra-short segment disease.*

PATHOLOGIC CHANGES. Two types of biopsies may be done on infants suspected of having Hirschsprung's disease—full-thickness rectal biopsy, and suction biopsy that includes mucosa and submucosa.

Macroscopically, typical case of Hirschsprung's disease shows 2 segments—a *distal narrow segment* that is aganglionic and a *dilated proximal segment* that contains normal number of ganglion cells (Fig. 18.30).

Microscopically, the distal narrow segment shows total absence of ganglion cells of all the three plexuses (Auerbach's or myenteric plexus present between the two layers of muscularis, deep submucosal or Henle's plexus, and superficial mucosal or Meissner's plexus) and prominence of non-myelinated nerve fibres. Histochemical staining for acetylcholine esterase activity provides confirmation for identifying ganglion cells and nerve trunks.

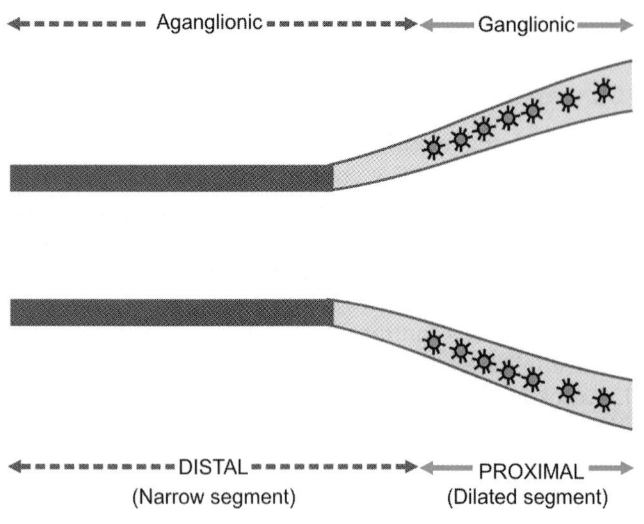

FIGURE 18.30

Hirschsprung's disease, diagrammatic representation of the pathologic changes.

The various causes of **acquired megacolon** are as under:

1. *Obstructive* e.g. due to tumour, post-inflammatory strictures.
2. *Endocrine* e.g. in myxoedema, cretinism.
3. *CNS disorders* e.g. spina bifida, paraplegia, parkinsonism.
4. *Psychogenic* e.g. emotional disturbances, psychiatric disorders.
5. *Chagas' disease* due to infection with *Trypanosoma cruzi* is the only example resulting in acquired loss of ganglion cells. In all other acquired causes listed above, the bowel innervation is normal.

COLITIS

Colitis may occur in isolation but more commonly involvement of small intestine is also present (enterocolitis). In view of the considerable overlapping of enteritis and colitis, these lesions have already been described under small intestine (page 578). Table 18.9 presents a classification of the various types of colitis/ enterocolitis.

TABLE 18.9: Classification of Colitis/Enterocolitis.

I. ISCHAEMIC BOWEL DISEASE

Ischaemic colitis ('Membranous' colitis)

II. INFLAMMATORY BOWEL DISEASE

1. Ulcerative colitis
2. Crohn's disease

III. OTHER INFLAMMATORY LESIONS

1. Infective enterocolitis (Dysenteries—bacillary, amoebic, other parasitic)
2. 'Pseudomembranous' enterocolitis (Antibiotic-associated diarrhoea)
3. Necrotising enterocolitis

MISCELLANEOUS LESIONS

Diverticulosis Coli

Diverticula are the outpouchings or herniations of the mucosa and submucosa of the colon through the muscle wall. *Diverticular disease,* as it is commonly known, is rare under 30 years of age and is seen more commonly as the age advances. Multiple diverticula of the colon are very common in the Western societies, probably due to ingestion of low-fibre diet but is seen much less frequently in tropical countries and in Japan. Diverticulosis is often asymptomatic and may be detected as an incidental finding at autopsy. However, a proportion of patients develop clinical symptoms such as low abdominal pain, distension, constipation and sometimes intermittent bleeding.

The etiologic role of the following 2 factors is generally accepted in the pathogenesis of diverticular disease of the colon:

1. *Increased intraluminal pressure* such as due to low fibre content of the diet causing hyperactive peristalsis and thereby sequestration, of mucosa and submucosa.
2. *Muscular weakness* of the colonic wall at the junction of the muscularis with submucosa.

PATHOLOGIC CHANGES. Grossly, diverticulosis is seen most commonly in the sigmoid colon (95%) but any other part of the entire colon may be involved. They may vary in number from a few to several hundred. They appear as small, spherical or flask-shaped outpouchings, usually less than 1 cm in diameter, commonly extend into appendices epiploicae and may contain inspissated faeces. They are connected to the intestinal lumen by a narrow neck.

Histologically, the flask-shaped structures extend from the intestinal lumen through the muscle layer. The colonic wall in the affected area is thin and is composed of atrophic mucosa, compressed submucosa and thin or deficient muscularis. However, muscularis propria in between the diverticular protrusions is hypertrophied. While diverticular disease may remain asymptomatic, inflammatory changes in the diverticula (diverticulitis) produce clinical symptoms.

The *complications* of diverticulosis and diverticulitis are perforation, haemorrhage, intestinal obstruction and fistula formation.

Melanosis Coli

Melanosis coli is a peculiar condition in which mucosa of the large intestine acquires brown-black coloration. The condition is said to occur in individuals who are habitual users of cathartics of anthracene type.

Macroscopically, the mucosal surface is intact and is pigmented brown-black.
Microscopically, large number of pigment-laden macrophages are seen in the lamina propria. The nature of this pigment is found to be both melanin and lipofuscin.

Haemorrhoids (Piles)

Haemorrhoids or piles are the varicosities of the haemorrhoidal veins. They are called *'internal piles'* if dilatation is of superior haemorrhoidal plexus covered over by mucous membrane, and *'external piles'* if they involve inferior haemorrhoidal plexus covered over by the skin. They are common lesions in elderly and pregnant women. They commonly result from increased venous pressure. The possible causes include the following:

1. Portal hypertension
2. Chronic constipation and straining at stool
3. Cardiac failure
4. Venous stasis of pregnancy
5. Hereditary predisposition
6. Tumours of the rectum.

Microscopically, thin-walled and dilated tortuous veins are seen under the rectal mucosa *(internal piles)* or anal skin *(external piles).* Secondary changes and complications that may occur include: thrombosis, haemorrhage, inflammation, scarring and strangulation *(prolapsed piles).*

Angiodysplasia

Angiodysplasia is a submucosal telangiectasia affecting caecum and right colon that causes recurrent acute and chronic haemorrhage. The condition is more common in the elderly past 6th decade. The pathogenesis is obscure but is possibly due to mechanical obstruction of the veins.

MISCELLANEOUS INFLAMMATORY CONDITIONS

■ **'Fistula-in-ano'** is a well known and common condition in which one or more fistulous tracts pass from the internal opening at the pectinate line through the internal sphincter on to the skin surface. The condition probably results from infection of the anal glands.

Histologically, nonspecific inflammatory changes are seen.

■ **'Anal fissure'** is an ulcer in the anal canal below the level of the pectinate line, mostly in midline and posteriorly. The common cause is trauma due to passage of hard stools, followed by chronic infection.

■ **'Solitary rectal ulcer syndrome'** is a condition characterised usually by solitary, at times multiple, rectal ulcers with prolapse of rectal mucosa and development of proctitis. The histological appearance is quite characteristic. Besides ulceration and inflammation of the rectal mucosa, lamina propria is occupied by spindle-shaped fibroblasts and smooth muscle cells. The condition is also called as *'localised form of colitis cystica profunda'* and must be differentiated from *'diffuse form of colitis cystica profunda'* seen in cases of ulcerative colitis. Submucosal cysts lined by foreign body giant cells and containing gas are also seen in *'pneumatosis cystoides intestinalis'*.

LARGE INTESTINAL POLYPS AND TUMOURS

Large bowel is the most common site for a variety of benign and malignant tumours, majority of which are of epithelial origin. Most of the benign tumours present clinically as polyps. A classification of polyps, alongwith benign tumours and malignant tumours, is presented in Table 18.10.

I. COLORECTAL POLYPS

A polyp is defined as any growth or mass protruding from the mucous membrane into the lumen. Polyps are much more common in the large intestine than in the small intestine and are more common in the rectosigmoid colon than the proximal colon. Polyps are broadly classified into 2 groups—non-neoplastic and neoplastic. Non-neoplastic polyps have further subtypes indicating their mode of origin. Neoplastic polyps, on the other hand, include epithelial tumours, both benign and malignant (Table 18.10).

A. NON-NEOPLASTIC POLYPS

Non-neoplastic polyps are more common and include the following 4 subtypes:

Hyperplastic (Metaplastic) Polyps

The hyperplastic or metaplastic polyps are the most common amongst all epithelial polyps, particularly in

TABLE 18.10: Polyps and Tumours of the Large Intestine.

I. COLORECTAL POLYPS

A. **Non-neoplastic polyps**

1. Hyperplastic (metaplastic) polyps
2. Hamartomatous polyps
   (i) Peutz-Jeghers polyps and polyposis
   (ii) Juvenile (Retention) polyps and polyposis
3. Inflammatory polyps (Pseudopolyps)
4. Lymphoid polyps

B. **Neoplastic polyps**

1. Adenoma
   (i) Tubular adenoma (Adenomatous polyp)
   (ii) Villous adenoma (villous papilloma)
   (iii) Tubulovillous adenoma (Papillary adenoma, villo-glandular adenoma)
2. Polypoid carcinoma

C. **Familial polyposis syndromes**

1. Familial polyposis coli (Adenomatosis)
2. Gardner's syndrome
3. Turcot's syndrome
4. Juvenile polyposis syndrome

II. OTHER BENIGN COLORECTAL TUMOURS
(Leiomyomas, leiomyoblastoma, neurilemmoma, lipoma and vascular tumours)

III. MALIGNANT COLORECTAL TUMOURS

A. **Carcinoma**

1. Adenocarcinoma
2. Other carcinomas
   (Mucinous adenocarcinoma, signet-ring cell carcinoma, adenosquamous carcinoma, undifferentiated carcinoma)

B. **Other malignant tumours**
(Leiomyosarcoma, malignant lymphoma, carcinoid tumours)

IV. TUMOURS OF THE ANAL CANAL

A. **Benign** (viral warts or condyloma acuminata)

B. **Malignant** (squamous cell carcinoma, basaloid carcinoma, mucoepidermoid carcinoma, adenocarcinoma, undifferentiated carcinoma, malignant melanoma)

the rectosigmoid. They are called *'hyperplastic'* because there is epithelial hyperplasia at the base of the crypts, and *'metaplastic'* as there are areas of cystic metaplasia. They may be seen at any age but are more common in the elderly (6th-7th decade).

*PATHOLOGIC CHANGES. **Grossly,*** hyperplastic polyps are generally multiple, sessile, smooth-surfaced and small (less than 0.5 cm).

Microscopically, they are composed of long and cystically dilated glands and crypts lined by normal epithelial cells. Their lining is partly flat and partly papillary. The luminal border of the lining epithelium is often serrated or saw-toothed.

Hyperplastic polyps are usually symptomless and have no malignant potential unless there is a coexistent adenoma.

Hamartomatous Polyps

These are tumour-like lesions composed of abnormal mixture of tissues indigenous to the part. They are further of 2 types:

I) PEUTZ-JEGHERS POLYPS AND POLYPOSIS. Peutz-Jeghers syndrome is autosomal dominant defect, characterised by hamartomatous intestinal polyposis and melanotic pigmentation of lips, mouth and genitalia. The polyps may be located in the stomach, small intestine or colon but are most common in the jejunum and ileum. The most common age is adolescence and early childhood.

*PATHOLOGIC CHANGES. **Grossly,*** these polyps are of variable size but are often large, multiple and pedunculated and more commonly situated in the small intestine.

Microscopically, the most characteristic feature is the tree-like branching of muscularis mucosae. The lining epithelium is by normal-appearing epithelial cells. The glands may show hyperplasia and cystic change (Fig. 18.31,A).

Peutz-Jeghers polyps do not undergo malignant transformation unless a coexistent adenoma is present. However, patients with Peutz-Jeghers syndrome are more prone to certain other cancers such as of pancreas, lung, breast, ovary and uterus.

II) JUVENILE (RETENTION) POLYPS. Juvenile or retention polyps, another form of hamartomatous polyps, occur more commonly in children below 5 years of age. Solitary juvenile polyps occur more often in the rectum, while juvenile polyposis may be present anywhere in the large bowel.

*PATHOLOGIC CHANGES. **Grossly,*** juvenile polyps are spherical, smooth-surfaced, about 2 cm in diameter and are often pedunculated.

Microscopically, the classical appearance is of cystically dilated glands containing mucus and lined by normal mucus-secreting epithelium. The stroma may show inflammatory cell infiltrate if there is chronic ulceration of the surface (Fig. 18.31,B) (COLOUR PLATE XXIV: CL 93).

Most cases, on becoming symptomatic in the form of rectal bleeding, are removed. In common with other non-neoplastic polyps, they are also not precancerous.

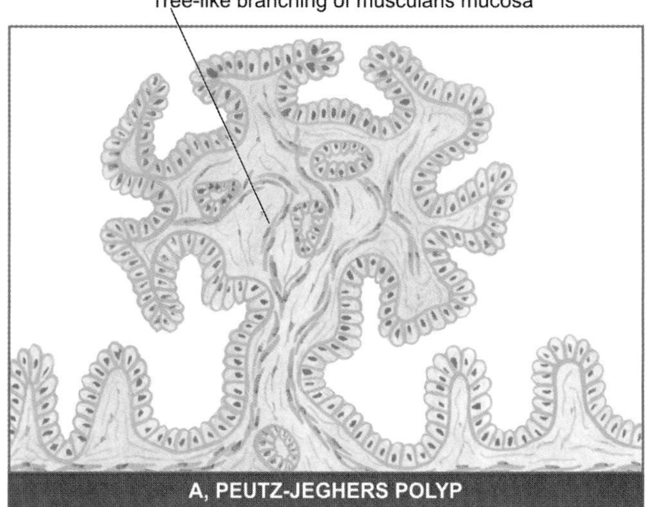

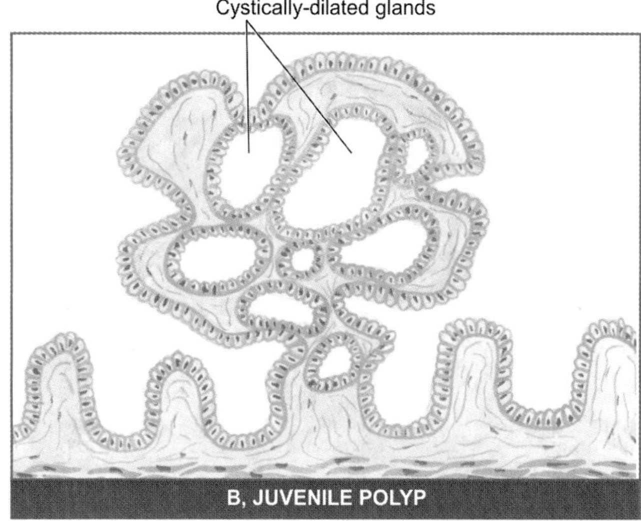

FIGURE 18.31

Two types of hamartomatous polyps.

Inflammatory Polyps (Pseudopolyps)

Inflammatory polyps or pseudopolyps appear due to re-epithelialisation of the undermined ulcers and overhanging margins in inflammatory bowel disease, most frequently in ulcerative colitis (colitis polyposa) and sometimes in Crohn's disease.

PATHOLOGIC CHANGES. Grossly, they are usually multiple, cylindrical to rounded overgrowths of mucosa and may vary from minute nodules to several centimeters in size.
Microscopically, the centre of inflammatory polyp consists of connective tissue core that shows some inflammatory cell infiltrate and is covered superficially by regenerating epithelial cells and some cystically-dilated glands.

These lesions have no malignant potential; carcinomas seen in long-standing cases of ulcerative colitis arise in the region of epithelial dysplasia and not from the polyps.

Lymphoid Polyps

Reactive hyperplasia of lymphoid tissue that is normally also more prominent in the rectum and terminal ileum, gives rise to localised or diffuse lymphoid polyps. Localised form occurs more often in the rectum in elderly, while diffuse form is seen at younger age and in children.

PATHOLOGIC CHANGES. Grossly, they are solitary or multiple, tiny elevated lesions.
Microscopically, they are composed of prominent lymphoid follicles with germinal centres located in the submucosa and mucosa, and are covered by epithelium that may be inflamed.

They are benign lesions and have to be distinguished from malignant lymphoma.

B. NEOPLASTIC POLYPS

Neoplastic polyps are benign (adenomas) and malignant (polypoid carcinomas) epithelial tumours. Adenomas have 3 main varieties (tubular, villous and tubulovillous), each of which represents a difference in the growth pattern of the same neoplastic process.

Tubular Adenoma (Adenomatous Polyp)

Tubular adenomas or adenomatous polyps are the most common neoplastic polyps (75%). They are common beyond 3rd decade of life and have slight male preponderance. They occur most often in the distal colon and rectum. They may be found singly as sporadic cases, or multiple tubular adenomas as part of familial polyposis syndrome with autosomal dominant inheritance pattern. Tubular adenomas may remain asymptomatic or may manifest by rectal bleeding.

PATHOLOGIC CHANGES. Grossly, adenomatous polyps may be single or multiple, sessile or pedunculated, vary in size from less than 1 cm to large, spherical masses with an irregular surface. Usually, the larger lesions have recognisable stalks.

Microscopically, the usual appearance is of benign tumour overlying muscularis mucosa and is composed of branching tubules which are embedded in the lamina propria. The lining epithelial cells are of large intestinal type with diminished mucus secreting capacity, large nuclei and increased mitotic activity (Fig. 18.32,A). However, tubular adenomas may show variable degree of cytologic atypia ranging from atypical epithelium restricted within the glandular basement membrane called as 'carcinoma *in situ*' to invasion into the fibrovascular stromal core referred to as frank 'adenocarcinoma'.

Malignant transformation is present in about 5% of tubular adenomas; the incidence being higher in larger adenomas.

Villous Adenoma (Villous Papilloma)

Villous adenomas or villous papillomas of the colon are much less common than tubular adenomas. The mean age at which they appear is 6th decade of life with approximatey equal sex incidence. They are seen most often in the distal colon and rectum, followed in decreasing frequency, by rest of the colon.

PATHOLOGIC CHANGES. Grossly, villous adenomas are round to oval exophytic masses, usually sessile, varying in size from 1 to 10 cm or more in diameter. Their surface may be haemorrhagic or ulcerated.

Microscopically, the characteristic histologic feature is the presence of many slender, finger-like villi, which appear to arise directly from the area of muscularis mucosae. Each of the papillae has fibrovascular stromal core that is covered by epithelial cells varying from apparently benign to anaplastic cells. Excess mucus secretion is sometimes seen (Fig. 18.32,B).

Villous adenomas are invariably symptomatic; rectal bleeding, diarrhoea and mucus being the common features. The presence of severe atypia, carcinoma *in situ* and invasive carcinoma are seen more frequently. Invasive carcinoma has been reported in 30% of villous adenomas.

Tubulovillous Adenoma (Papillary Adenoma, Villoglandular Adenoma)

Tubulovillous adenoma is an intermediate form of pattern between tubular adenoma and villous adenoma.

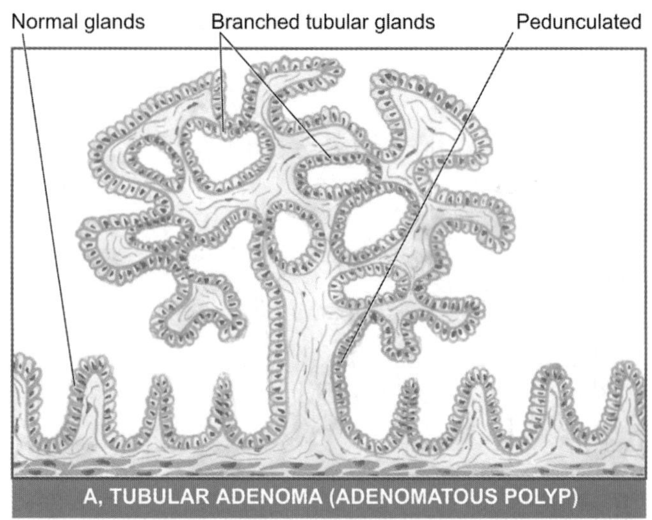

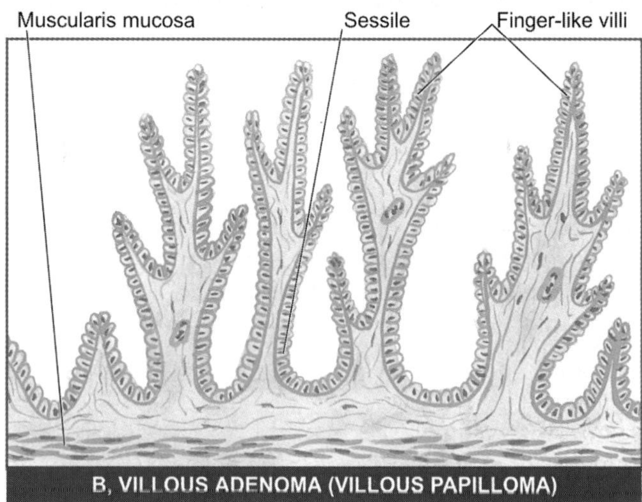

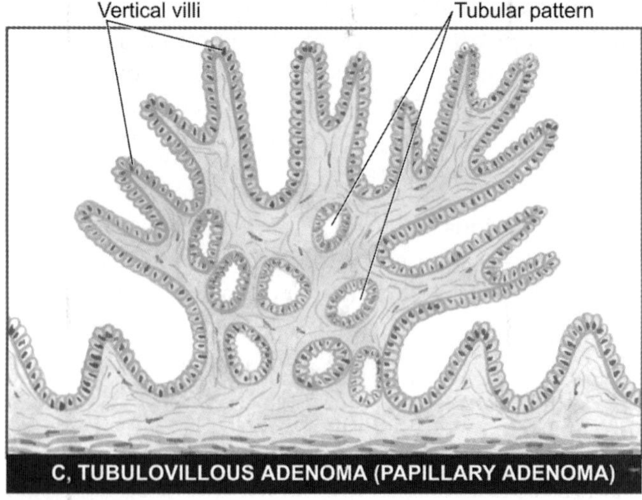

FIGURE 18.32

Adenomas (neoplastic polyps)—three main varieties.

It is also known by other names like papillary adenoma and villo-glandular adenoma. The distribution of these adenomas is the same as for tubular adenomas.

PATHOLOGIC CHANGES. Grossly, tubulovillous adenomas may be sessile or pedunculated and range in size from 0.5-5 cm.
Microscopically, they show intermediate or mixed pattern, characteristic vertical villi and deeper part showing tubular pattern (Fig. 18.32,C).

The behaviour of tubulovillous adenoma is intermediate between tubular and villous adenomas.

Polypoid Carcinoma

This pattern of carcinoma is described later on page 603.

C. FAMILIAL POLYPOSIS SYNDROMES

Familial polyposis syndromes are a group of disorders with multiple polyposis of the colon with autosomal dominant inheritance pattern. Important conditions included in familial polyposis are:

1. Familial polyposis coli (adenomatosis)
2. Gardner's syndrome
3. Turcot's syndrome
4. Juvenile polyposis syndrome

Some other conditions in which multiple polyposis of colon occur but do not have familial basis are Peutz-Jeghers syndrome (hamartomatous), Cronkhite-Canada syndrome (inflammatory), and nodular lymphoid hyperplasia. The familial polyposis syndromes are as follows.

Familial Polyposis Coli (Adenomatosis)

This hereditary disease is defined as the presence of more than 100 neoplastic polyps (adenomas) on the mucosal surface of the colon; the average number is about 1000. Adenomatosis can be distinguished from multiple adenomas in which the number of adenomas is fewer, not exceeding 100. The condition has autosomal dominant transmission and is due to germline mutations in *APC* gene which results in occurrence of hundreds of adenomas which progress to invasive cancer. The average age at diagnosis is 2nd and 3rd decades of life with equal incidence in both the sexes.

Grossly and microscopically, the commonest pattern is that of adenomatous polyps (tubular adenomas) discussed above.

The malignant potential of familial polyposis coli is very high. Colorectal cancer develops virtually in 100% of cases over a period of several years if not treated with colectomy. This subject of 'adenoma-carcinoma sequence' has been discussed again on page 602.

Gardner's Syndrome

Gardner's syndrome is combination of familial polyposis coli and certain extra-colonic lesions such as multiple osteomas (particularly of the mandible and maxilla), sebaceous cysts and connective tissue tumours. The number of polyps in Gardner's syndrome is generally fewer than in the familial polyposis coli but their clinical behaviour is identical.

Turcot's Syndrome

Turcot's syndrome is combination of familial polyposis coli and malignant neoplasms of the central nervous system.

Juvenile Polyposis Syndrome

Juvenile polyposis is appearance of multiple juvenile polyps in the colon, stomach and small intestine but their number is not as high as in familial polyposis coli. Family history in some cases may show autosomal dominant inheritance pattern, while it may be negative in others. They resemble the typical juvenile polyps as regards their age (under 5 years), sex distribution and morphology. They lack the malignant potential.

II. OTHER BENIGN TUMOURS

Some non-epithelial benign tumours that may rarely occur in large intestine are leiomyomas, leiomyoblastoma, neurilemmoma, lipoma and vascular tumours (haemangioma, lymphangioma).

III. MALIGNANT COLORECTAL TUMOURS

A. Colorectal Carcinoma

Colorectal cancer comprises 98% of all malignant tumours of the large intestine. It is the commonest form of visceral cancer, next only to lung cancer in the United States. The incidence of carcinoma of the large intestine rises with age; average age of patients is about 60 years. Cancer in the rectum is more common in males than females in the ratio of 2:1, while at other locations in the large bowel the overall incidence is equal for both sexes.

ETIOLOGY. As with most other cancers, etiology of colorectal carcinoma is not clear but a few etiological factors have been implicated, These are as under:

1. Geographic variations. The incidence of large bowel carcinoma shows wide variation throughout the world.

It is much more common in North America, Northern Europe than in South America, Africa and Asia. Colorectal cancer is generally thought to be a disease of affluent societies because its incidence is directly correlated with the socioeconomic status of the countries. In Japan, however, colon cancer is much less common than in the US but the incidence of rectal cancer is similar.

2. Dietary factors. Diet plays a significant part in the causation of colorectal cancer.

i) A low intake of vegetable fibre-diet leading to low stool bulk is associated with higher risk of colorectal cancer.

ii) Consumption of large amounts of fatty foods by populations results in excessive cholesterol and their metabolites which may be carcinogenic.

iii) Excessive consumption of refined carbohydrates that remain in contact with the colonic mucosa for prolonged duration changes the bacterial flora of the bowel, thus resulting in production of carcinogenic substances.

3. Adenoma-carcinoma sequence. There is strong evidence to suggest that colonic adenocarcinoma arises from pre-existing adenomas, referred to as adenoma-carcinoma sequence (Fig. 18.33). The following evidences are cited to support this hypothesis:

i) In a case with early invasive cancer, the surrounding tissue often shows *preceding changes* of evolution from adenoma → hyperplasia → dysplasia → carcinoma *in situ* → invasive carcinoma.

ii) *Incidence* of adenomas in a population is directly proportionate to the prevalence of colorectal cancer.

iii) The risk of adenocarcinoma colon declines with *endoscopic removal* of all identified adenomas.

iv) The peak incidence of adenomas generally *precedes* by some years to a few decades the peak incidence for colorectal cancer.

v) The risk of malignancy increases with the following *adenoma-related factors:*

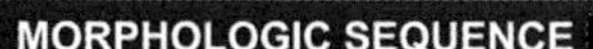

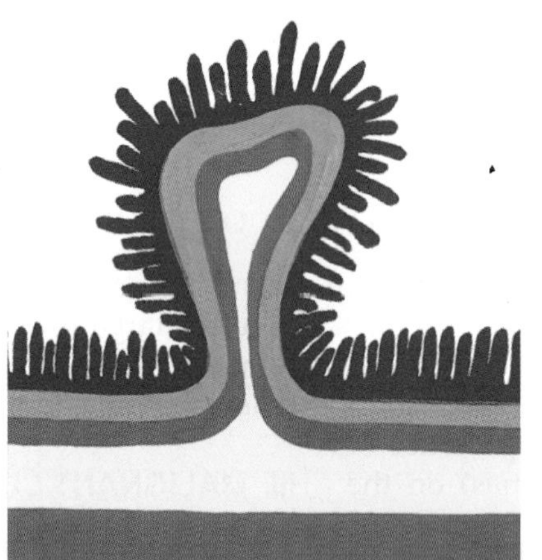

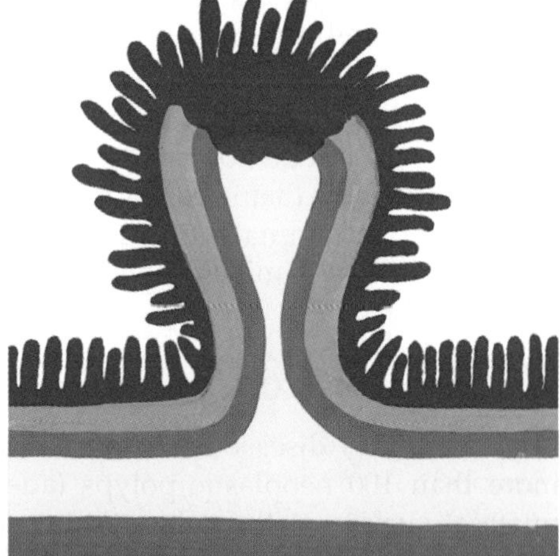

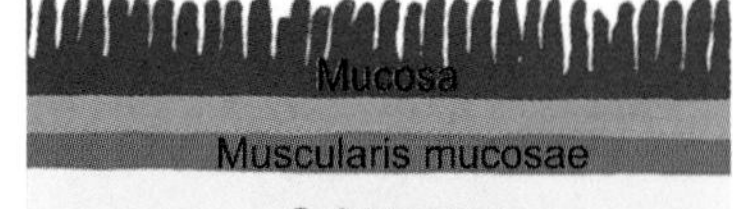

FIGURE 18.33

Schematic diagram of molecular and morphologic evolution of adenoma-carcinoma sequence.

a) *Number of adenomas*: familial polyposis syndromes almost certainly evolve into malignancy.
b) *Size of adenomas*: large size increases the risk.
c) *Type of adenomas*: greater villous component associated with higher prevalence.

4. Other diseases. Presence of certain pre-existing diseases such as inflammatory bowel disease (especially ulcerative colitis) and diverticular disease for long duration increases the risk of developing colorectal cancer subsequently. It may be recalled here that low fibre diet is implicated in the pathogenesis of diverticular disease as well.

GENETIC BASIS OF COLORECTAL CARCINOGENESIS. Studies by molecular genetics have revealed that there are sequential multistep mutations in evolution of colorectal cancer from adenomas by one of the following two mechanisms:

1. APC mutation/ β-catenin mechanism. This pathway of multiple mutations is generally associated with morphologically identifiable changes as described above in adenoma-carcinoma sequence. These changes are as under:

i) *Loss of tumour suppressor APC* (adenomatous polyposis coli) gene located on the long arm of chromosome 5 is present in 80% cases of sporadic colon cancer. Since the function of APC gene is linked to β-catenin, loss of *APC* gene results in translocation of β–catenin to the nucleus where it activates transcription of other genes, mainly *MYC* and cyclin D1, both of which stimulate cell proliferation.

ii) *Point mutation in K-RAS gene* follows loss of APC gene and is seen in 10 to 50% cases of adenoma-carcinoma.

iii) *Deletion of DCC gene* located on long arm of chromosome 18 (DCC for *d*eleted in *c*olorectal *c*ancer) in 60-70 % cases of colon cancer.

iv) *Loss of TP53 tumour suppressor gene* seen in 70-80% cases of colon cancer.

2. Microsatellite instability mechanism. In this pathway also, there are multiple mutations but of different genes, and unlike APC mutation/β–catenin mechanism there are no morphologically identifiable changes. This pathway accounts for 10-15% cases of colon cancer. Basic mutation is loss of DNA repair gene. This results in a situation in which repetitive DNA sequences (i.e. microsatellites) become unstable during replication cycle, termed microsatellite instability, which is the hallmark of this pathway. The significant DNA repair genes which are mutated in colon cancer as under:

i) *TGF-β receptor gene* which normally inhibits cell proliferation but in mutated form allows the uncontrolled proliferation of colonic epithelium in adenoma.

ii) *BAX gene* which normally causes apoptosis but a defect in it results in loss of apoptosis and dysregulated growth.

PATHOLOGIC CHANGES. *Distribution* of the primary colorectal cancer reveals that about 60% of the cases occur in the rectum, followed in descending order, by sigmoid and descending colon (25%), caecum and ileocaecal valve (10%); ascending colon, hepatic and splenic flexures (5%); and quite uncommonly in the transverse colon (Fig. 18.34).

Macroscopically, there are distinct differences between the growth on the right and left half of the colon (Fig. 18.35).

- The **right-sided growths** tend to be large, cauliflower-like, soft and friable masses projecting into the lumen *(fungating polypoid carcinoma).*
- **Growths in the left colon,** on the other hand, have napkin-ring configuration i.e. they encircle the bowel wall circumferentially with increased fibrous tissue forming annular ring, and have central ulceration on the surface with slightly elevated margins *(carcinomatous ulcers).*

These differences in right and left colonic growths are probably due to the liquid nature of the contents in the ascending colon leaving space for luminal

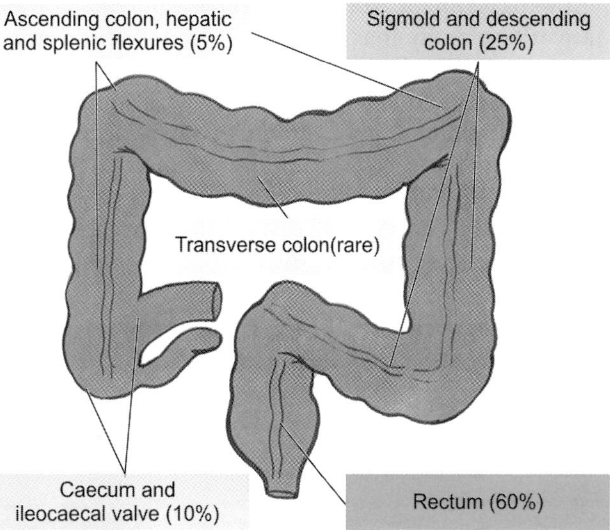

FIGURE 18.34

Distribution of the primary colorectal cancer.

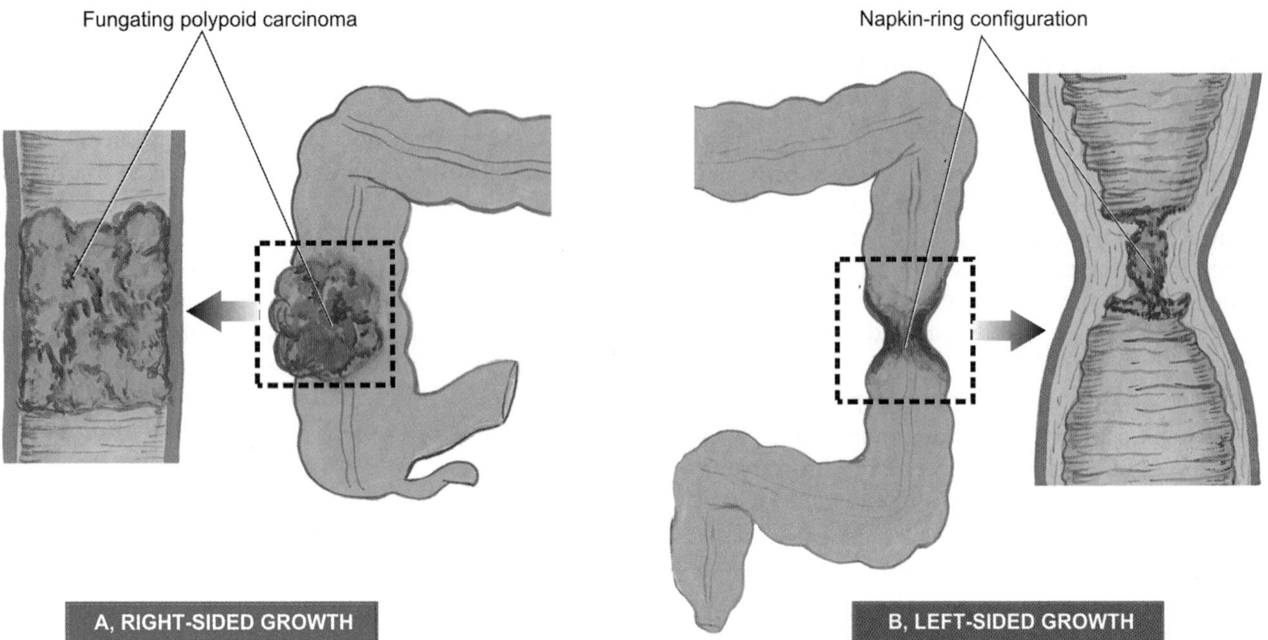

FIGURE 18.35

Macroscopic appearance of colorectal carcinoma. A, *Right-sided growth*—fungating polypoid carcinoma showing cauliflower-like growth projecting into the lumen. B, *Left-sided growth*—napkin-ring configuration with spread of growth into the bowel wall.

growth on right side, while the contents in left colon are more solid permitting the spread of growth into the bowel wall. However, early lesion in left as well as right colon are small, button-like areas of elevation.

Microscopically, the appearance of right and left-sided growths is similar. About 95% of colorectal carcinomas are adenocarcinomas of varying grades of differentiation, out of which approximately 10% are mucin-secreting colloid carcinomas (COLOUR PLATE XXIV: CL 95,96). The remaining 5% tumours include uncommon microscopic patterns like undifferentiated carcinoma, signet-ring cell carcinoma, and adeno-squamous carcinomas seen in more distal colon near the anus. The histologic grades indicating the degree of differentiation are: well-differentiated, moderately-differentiated and poorly-differentiated.

SPREAD. Carcinoma of the large intestine may spread by the following routes:

1. Direct spread. The tumour spreads most commonly by direct extension in both ways— *circumferentially* into the bowel wall as well as *directly* into the depth of the bowel wall to the serosa, pericolic fat, and sometimes into peritoneal cavity.

2. Lymphatic spread. Spread via lymphatics occurs rather commonly and involves, firstly the regional lymph nodes in the vicinity of the tumour, and then into other groups of lymph nodes like preaortic, internal iliac and the sacral lymph nodes.

TABLE 18.11: Staging and Prognosis of Colorectal Cancer (Duke's System as Modified by Astler-Coller).

STAGE		TNM	5-YEAR SURVIVAL	PATHOLOGIC FEATURES
A	I	T_1 No Mo	>90%	Cancer confined to mucosa only
B_1	II	T_2 No Mo	85%	Cancer extends into submucosa
B_2	II	T_3 No Mo	70-80%	Cancer extends into muscularis±serosa
C_1	III	Tx N_1 Mo	35-65%	Cancer involves muscularis+regional lymph nodes
C_2	III	Tx N_1 Mo	20-35%	Cancer extends into serosa+regional lymph nodes
D	IV	Tx Nx M_1	5%	Cancer with distant metastases

3. Haematogenous spread. Blood spread of large bowel cancer occurs relatively late and involves the liver, lungs, brain, bones and ovary.

CLINICAL FEATURES. Clinical symptoms in colorectal cancer appear after considerable time. These are as follows:

i) Occult bleeding (melaena)

ii) Change in bowel habits, more often in left-sided growth

iii) Loss of weight (cachexia)

iv) Loss of appetite (anorexia)

v) Anaemia, weakness, malaise.

The most common *complications* are obstruction and haemorrhage; less often perforation and secondary infection may occur. Aside from the diagnostic methods like stool test for occult blood, PR examination, proctoscopy, radiographic contrast studies and CT scan, recently the role of tumour-markers has been emphasised. Of particular importance is the estimation of carcinoembryonic antigen (CEA) level which is elevated in 100% cases of metastatic colorectal cancers, while it is positive in 20-40% of early lesions, and 60-70% of advanced primary lesions. However, the test may have prognostic significance only and is not diagnostic of colorectal cancer because it is positive in other cancers too such as of the lungs, breast, ovary, urinary bladder and prostate. CEA levels are elevated in some non-neoplastic conditions also like in ulcerative colitis, pancreatitis and alcoholic cirrhosis.

The **prognosis** of colorectal cancer depends upon a few variables:

i) Extent of the bowel involvement

ii) Presence or absence of metastases

iii) Histologic grade of the tumour

iv) Location of the tumour

The most important prognostic factor in colorectal cancer is, however, the stage of the disease at the time of diagnosis. Three staging systems are in use:

1. *Dukes' ABC staging* (modified Duke's includes stage D as well).

2. *Astler-Coller staging* which is a further modification of Duke's staging and is most widely used.

3. *TNM staging* described by American Joint committee is also used.

Table 18.11 and Fig. 18.36 sum up the features of staging classification and the overall 5-year survival rate in disease stage.

B. Other Colorectal Malignant Tumours

Aside from colorectal carcinoma, other malignant tumours which are encountered sometimes in the large bowel are leiomyosarcoma (page 575) and malignant lymphoma (page 575). Hindgut carcinoids may occur in the rectum and colon (page 591).

IV. TUMOURS OF THE ANAL CANAL

Epithelial tumours of the anal canal are uncommon and may be combination of several histological types. Amongst the *benign tumours* of the anal canal, multiple viral warts called as condyloma acuminata are the only tumours of note. *Malignant tumours* of the anal canal include the following:

1. Squamous cell carcinoma
2. Basaloid carcinoma
3. Mucoepidermoid carcinoma
4. Adenocarcinoma (rectal, of anal glands, within anorectal fistulas)
5. Undifferentiated carcinoma
6. Malignant melanoma

These tumours resemble in morphology with similar lesion elsewhere in the body.

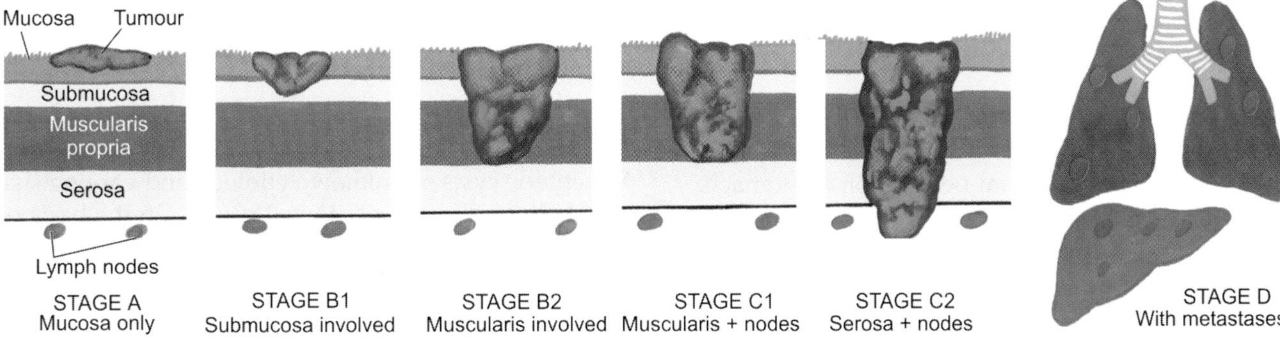

FIGURE 18.36

Pathologic staging according to Astler-Coller system. (Also see facing Table 18.11).

TABLE 18.12: Causes of Gastrointestinal (G.I.) Bleeding.

UPPER G.I. BLEEDING	SMALL INTESTINAL BLEEDING	LOWER G.I. BLEEDING
1. Oesophageal varices	Vascular ectasias	Inflammatory bowel disease (IBD)
2. Mallory-Weiss tear	Tumours(adenocarcinoma, lymphoma, leiomyoma)	Carcinoma colon
3. Haemorrhagic/erosive gastritis	NSAIDs	Carcinoma rectosigmoid
4. Duodenal ulcer	Meckel's diverticulum	Haemorroids
5. Gastric ulcer	Intussusception	Anal fissure
6. Cancer stomach	Crohn's disease	Diverticulosis

CAUSES OF GASTROINTESTINAL BLEEDING

Gastrointestinal bleeding from upper (haematemesis), middle (small intestinal) and lower (melaena) is a major presenting clinical feature of a variety of gastrointestinal diseases. Table 18.12 summarises the main causes of gastrointestinal bleeding.

PERITONEUM

NORMAL STRUCTURE

The peritoneal cavity is lined by a layer of surface mesothelium derived from mesoderm. The lining rests on vascularised subserosal fibrous tissue. Other structures topographically related to peritoneum are retroperitoneum, omentum, mesentery and umbilicus. These structures are involved in a variety of pathologic states but a few important conditions included below are inflammation (peritonitis), tumour-like lesions (idiopathic retroperitoneal fibrosis and mesenteric cysts) and tumours (primary and metastatic).

PERITONITIS

Inflammatory involvement of the peritoneum may result from chemical agents or bacteria.

1. **Chemical peritonitis** can be caused by the following:

- *Bile* extravasated due to trauma or diseases of the gallbladder.
- *Pancreatic secretions* released from pancreas in acute haemorrhagic pancreatitis.
- *Gastric juice* leaked from perforation of stomach.
- *Barium sulfate* from perforation of bowel during radiographic studies.

Chemical peritonitis is localised or generalised sterile inflammation of the peritoneum.

2. **Bacterial peritonitis** may be primary or secondary; the latter being more common.

Primary form is caused by streptococcal infection, especially in children. *Secondary* bacterial peritonitis may occur from the following disorders:

- Appendicitis
- Cholecystitis
- Salpingitis
- Rupture of peptic ulcer
- Gangrene of bowel
- Tuberculosis (specific inflammation).

Pathologic changes in bacterial peritonitis vary depending upon duration. It may be generalised or may get localised by omentum such as in appendiceal abscess following acute appendicitis. Depending upon duration, the fluid accumulation varies from serous, turbid, creamy to frankly suppurative. The fluid may eventually resolve or may heal by organisation with formation of fibrous adhesions.

IDIOPATHIC RETROPERITONEAL FIBROSIS

Also known as Ormond's disease or sclerosing retroperitonitis, this rare entity of unknown etiology is characterised by diffuse fibrous overgrowth and chronic inflammation. The condition is, therefore, more like inflammatory rather than of neoplastic origin. It may be associated with similar process in the mediastinum, sclerosing cholangitis and Riedel's thyroiditis and termed *multifocal fibrosclerosis.* Though idiopathic, the etiologic role of ergot derivative drugs and autoimmune reaction has been suggested.

MESENTERIC CYSTS

Mesenteric cysts of unknown etiology and varying size may be found in the peritoneal cavity. On the basis of their possible origin, they are of various types:

- *Chylous cyst* is a thin-walled cyst arising from lymph vessels and lined by endothelium.
- *Pseudocysts* are those which are formed following walled-off infection or pancreatitis.

■ *Neoplastic cysts* occur due to cystic change in tumours.

TUMOURS

Peritoneum may be involved in malignant tumours—primary and metastatic.

■ **Mesothelioma** is an example of primary peritoneal tumour (benign and malignant) and is similar in morphology as in pleural cavity (page 514).

■ **Intra-abdominal desmoplastic small cell tumour** is a recently described highly malignant tumour belonging to the group of other round cell or blue cell tumours such as small cell carcinoma lung, Ewing's sarcoma, rhabdomyosarcoma, neuroblastoma and others.

■ **Metastatic peritoneal tumours** are quite common and may occur from dissemination from any intra-abdominal malignancy.

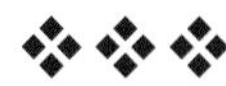

The Liver, Biliary Tract and Exocrine Pancreas

19

LIVER

NORMAL STRUCTURE

ANATOMY. The liver is the largest organ in the body weighing 1400-1600 gm in the males and 1200-1400 gm in the females. There are 2 main anatomical lobes—right and left, the right being about six times the size of the left lobe. The right lobe has quadrate lobe on its inferior surface and a caudate lobe on the posterior surface. The right and left lobes are separated anteriorly by a fold of peritoneum called the *falciform ligament*, inferiorly by the fissure for the *ligamentum teres*, and posteriorly by the fissure for the *ligamentum venosum* (Fig. 19.1).

The *porta hepatis* is the region on the inferior surface of the right lobe where blood vessels, lymphatics and common hepatic duct form the hilum of the liver. A firm smooth layer of connective tissue called *Glisson's capsule* encloses the liver and is continuous with the connective tissue of the porta hepatis forming a sheath around the structures in the porta hepatis. The liver has a double blood supply—the portal vein brings the venous blood from the intestines and spleen, and the hepatic artery coming from the coeliac axis supplies arterial blood to the liver. This dual blood supply provides sufficient protection against infarction in the liver. The portal vein and hepatic artery divide into branches to the right and left lobes in the porta. The right and left hepatic ducts also join in the porta to form the common hepatic duct. The venous drainage from the liver is into the right and left hepatic veins which enter the inferior vena cava. Lymphatics and the nerve fibres accompany the hepatic artery into their branchings and terminate around the porta hepatis.

HISTOLOGY. The hepatic parenchyma is composed of numerous hexagonal or pyramidal *classical lobules;* each with a diameter of 0.5 to 2 mm. Each classical lobule has a central tributary from the hepatic vein and at the periphery are 4 to 5 portal tracts or triads containing branches of bile duct, portal vein and hepatic artery. Cords of hepatocytes and blood-containing sinusoids radiate from the central vein to the peripheral portal

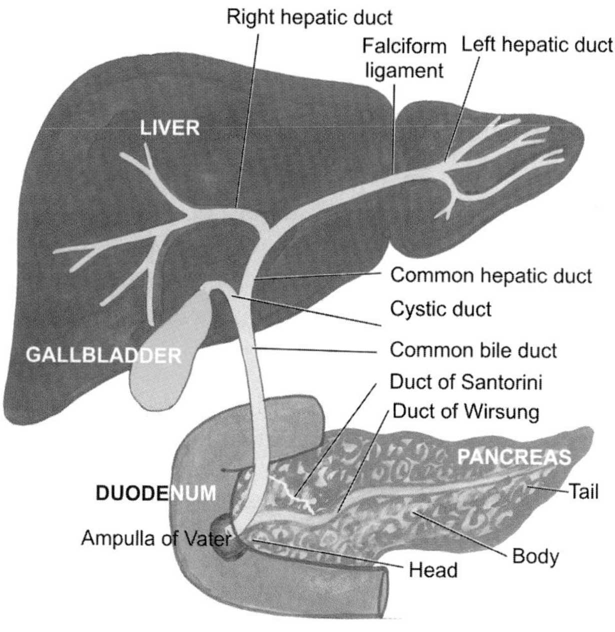

FIGURE 19.1

Anatomy of the liver and its relationship to the gallbladder, pancreas and duodenum.

triads. The *functioning lobule* or *liver acinus* as described by Rappaport has a portal triad in the centre and is surrounded at the periphery by portions of several classical lobules. However, in most descriptions on pathology of the liver, the term *lobule* is used in its classical form.

The blood supply to the liver parenchyma flows from the portal triads to the central veins. Accordingly, the hepatic parenchyma of liver lobule is divided into 3 zones (Fig. 19.2):

- **Zone 1** or the *periportal (peripheral) area* is closest to the arterial and portal blood supply and hence bears the brunt of all forms of toxic injury.
- **Zone 3** or the *centrilobular area* surrounds the central vein and is most remote from the blood supply and thus suffers from the effects of hypoxic injury.
- **Zone 2** is the intermediate *midzonal area.*

The **hepatocytes** are polygonal cells with a round single nucleus and a prominent nucleolus. The liver cells have a remarkable capability to undergo mitosis and regeneration. Thus it is not uncommon to find liver cells containing more than one nuclei and having polyploidy up to octoploidy. A hepatocyte has 3 surfaces: *one* facing the sinusoid and space of Disse, the *second* facing the canaliculus, and the *third* facing neighbouring hepatocytes.

The blood-containing *sinusoids* between cords of hepatocytes are lined by discontinuous endothelial cells and scattered flat Kupffer cells belonging to the reticuloendothelial system.

The *space of Disse* is the space between hepatocytes and sinusoidal lining endothelial cells. A few scattered fat storing *Ito cells* lie within the space of Disse.

The *portal triad or tract* besides containing portal vein radicle, the hepatic arteriole and bile duct, has a few mononuclear cells and a little connective tissue considered to be extension of Glisson's capsule. The portal triads are surrounded by a limiting plate of hepatocytes.

The *intrahepatic biliary system* begins with the bile canaliculi interposed between the adjacent hepatocytes. The bile canaliculi are simply grooves between the contact surfaces of the liver cells and are covered by microvilli. These canaliculi join at the periphery of the lobule to drain eventually into terminal bile ducts or ductules (canal of Hering) which are lined by cuboidal epithelium.

FUNCTIONS. The liver performs multifold functions. These are briefly listed below:

1. Manufacture and excretion of bile.
2. Manufacture of several major plasma proteins such as albumin, fibrinogen and prothrombin.
3. Metabolism of proteins, carbohydrates and lipids.
4. Storage of vitamins (A, D and B_{12}) and iron.

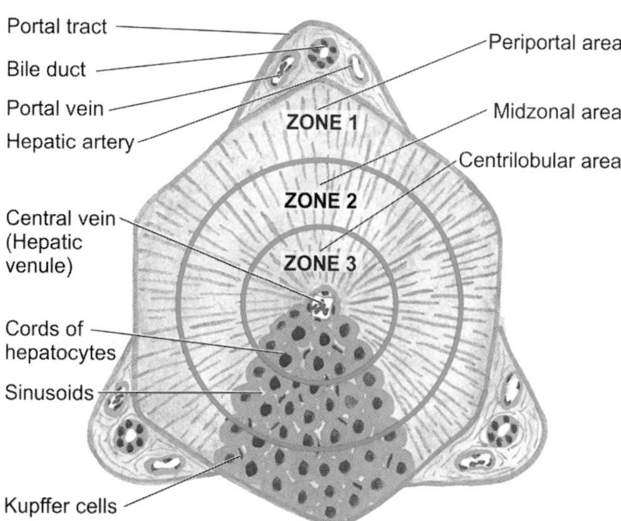

FIGURE 19.2

Histology of hepatic lobule. The hexagonal or pyramidal structure with central vein and peripheral 4 to 5 portal triads is termed the classical lobule. The functional divisions of the lobule into 3 zones are shown by circles.

5. Detoxification of toxic substances such as alcohol and drugs.

LIVER FUNCTION TESTS

In view of multiplicity and complexity of the liver functions, it is obvious that no single test can establish the disturbance in liver function. Thus a battery of liver function tests are employed for accurate diagnosis, to assess the severity of damage, to judge prognosis and to evaluate therapy. These tests are described below in relation to major liver functions.

I. TESTS FOR MANUFACTURE AND EXCRETION OF BILE

Bile is produced by the liver, stored in the gallbladder and secreted via biliary ducts into the duodenum. Bile consists of biliary phospholipids and primary and secondary bile acids. To understand the mechanisms underlying biliary pathology, it is important to understand normal bilirubin metabolism (page 613). In brief, jaundice will develop if bilirubin is excessively produced, or there is impaired hepatic uptake and conjugation of bilirubin, or it is insufficiently excreted into the duodenum. Tests employed to assess the synthesis and elimination of bilirubin pigment, urobilinogen and bile acids are outlined below:

1. **BILIRUBIN.** Bilirubin pigment can be detected in serum, faeces and urine.

i) **Serum bilirubin estimation** is based on *van den Bergh diazo reaction* by spectrophotometric method. Diazo reagent consists of diazotised sulfanilic acid. *Water-soluble conjugated* bilirubin gives *direct* van den Bergh reaction with diazo reagent within one minute, whereas *alcohol-soluble unconjugated* bilirubin is determined by *indirect* van den Bergh reaction. Addition of alcohol to the reaction mixture gives positive test for both conjugated and unconjugated bilirubin pigment. The unconjugated bilirubin level is then estimated by subtracting direct bilirubin value from this total value. The serum of normal adults contains less than 1 mg/dl of total bilirubin, out of which less than 0.25 mg/dl is conjugated bilirubin. Bilirubin level rises in diseases of hepatocytes, obstruction to biliary excretion into duodenum, in haemolysis, and defects of hepatic uptake and conjugation of bilirubin pigment such as in Gilbert's disease.

ii) In **faeces,** excretion of bilirubin is assessed by inspection of stools. Clay-coloured stool due to absence of faecal excretion of the pigment indicates obstructive jaundice.

iii) In **urine,** conjugated bilirubin can be detected by commercially available 'dipsticks', Fouchet's test, foam test or ictotest tablet method. Bilirubinuria does not occur in normal subjects nor is unconjugated bilirubin excreted in the urine. Bilirubinuria occurs only when there is raised level of conjugated bilirubin (filterable). Its excretion depends upon the level of conjugated bilirubin in plasma that is not protein-bound and is therefore available for glomerular filtration. Bilirubinuria appears in patients of hepatitis before the patient becomes jaundiced.

2. **UROBILINOGEN.** Urobilinogen is normally excreted in the urine. Its semiquantitative estimation in the urine can be done by preparing dilutions with Ehrlich's aldehyde reagent or by 'dipstick' method. An increase in urobilinogen in the urine is found in hepatocellular dysfunctions such as in alcoholic liver disease, cirrhosis and malignancy of the liver. It is also raised in haemolytic disease and in pyrexia. In cholestatic jaundice due to complete biliary obstruction, urobilinogen disappears from the urine.

3. **BROMSULPHALEIN EXCRETION.** Bromsulphalein (BSP) is a dye which is removed from circulation by the same mechanisms of binding, conjugation and excretion as bilirubin. BSP is injected intravenously and a sample of venous blood 45 minutes later is tested for percentage of injected dye remaining in the blood. The test is rarely performed nowadays because of the availability of enzyme estimations which are better indicators of hepatic dysfunction. Presently, the only value of BSP excretion test is in the diagnosis of Dubin-Johnson's syndrome (page 619).

4. **BILE ACIDS (BILE SALTS).** The primary bile acids (cholic acid and cheno-deoxycholic acid) are formed from cholesterol in the hepatocytes. These bile acids on secretion into the gut come in contact with colonic bacteria and undergo deconjugation with the production of secondary bile acids (deoxycholic acid and lithocholic acid). Most of these bile acids are reabsorbed through enterohepatic circulation and reach the liver. Only about 10% of the total bile acids are excreted in the faeces normally as unabsorbable toxic lithocholic acid.

Hepatobiliary diseases with cholestasis are associated with raised levels of serum bile acids which are responsible for producing itching (pruritus). These acids are excreted in the urine by active transport and passive diffusion and can be detected by simple methods as Hay's test and 'dipsticks'.

II. SERUM ENZYME ASSAYS

Determination of certain serum enzymes is considered useful in various types of liver injury, whether hepatocellular or cholestatic, as well as in quantifying liver damage. A combination of serum transaminases and alkaline phosphatase estimation is adequate to diagnose liver injury.

1. ALKALINE PHOSPHATASE. Serum alkaline phosphatase is produced by many tissues, especially bone, liver, intestine and placenta and is excreted in the bile. Most of the normal serum alkaline phosphatase (range 3-13 King-Armstrong units/dl or 25-85 IU/dl) is derived from bone. Elevation in activity of the enzyme can thus be found in diseases of bone, liver and in pregnancy. In the absence of bone disease and pregnancy, an elevated serum alkaline phosphatase levels generally reflect hepatobiliary disease. The greatest elevation (3 to 10 times normal) occurs in biliary tract obstruction. Slight to moderate increase is seen in parenchymal liver diseases such as in hepatitis and cirrhosis and in metastatic liver disease. It is possible to distinguish serum hepatic alkaline phosphatase from bony alkaline phosphatase by fractionation into isoenzymes but this is not routinely done.

2. γ-GLUTAMYL TRANSPEPTIDASE (γ-GT). The primary source of the enzyme, γ-GT, in serum is the liver. Its serum level parallels serum alkaline phosphatase and is used to confirm that the elevated serum alkaline phosphatase is of hepatobiliary origin. Besides its elevation in cholestasis and hepatocellular disease, the levels are high in patients with alcohol abuse even without liver disease.

3. TRANSAMINASES (AMINOTRANSFERASES). Assessment of liver cell necrosis is most frequently done by estimation of the following 2 serum enzymes:

i) Serum aspartate transaminase or AST (formerly glutamic oxaloacetic transaminase or SGOT): AST or SGOT is a *mitochondrial enzyme* released from heart, liver, skeletal muscle and kidney. Its normal serum level is 10-40 Karmen units/ml (0-35 IU).

ii) Serum alanine transaminase or ALT (formerly glutamic pyruvic transaminase or SGPT): ALT or SGPT is a *cytosolic enzyme* primarily present in the liver. Its normal serum level is 10-35 Karmen units/ml (0-35 IU).

Serum levels of SGOT and SGPT are increased on damage to the tissues producing them. Thus serum estimation of SGPT (ALT) which is fairly specific for liver tissue is of greater value in liver cell injury, whereas SGOT (AST) level may rise in acute necrosis or ischaemia of other organs such as the myocardium, besides liver cell injury.

Transaminase estimations are useful in the early diagnosis of viral hepatitis. Very high levels are seen in extensive acute hepatic necrosis such as in severe viral hepatitis and acute cholestasis. Alcoholic liver disease and cirrhosis are associated with mild to moderate elevation of transaminases.

4. OTHER SERUM ENZYMES. The determination of a few other serum enzymes is done sometimes but without any extra diagnostic advantage over the above mentioned enzyme assays. These are as under:

i) *5′-Nucleotidase* is another phosphatase derived from the liver. Its determination is useful to distinguish alkaline phosphatase of hepatic origin from that of bony tissue.

ii) *Lactic dehydrogenase (LDH)* is found to be elevated in serum of patients with metastatic liver involvement.

iii) *Choline esterase* synthesised by the liver is diminished in hepatocellular disease and malnutrition due to impaired synthesis.

III. TESTS FOR METABOLIC FUNCTIONS

The liver is the principal site of metabolism and synthesis of plasma proteins and amino acids, lipids and lipoproteins, carbohydrates and vitamins, besides detoxification of drugs and alcohol.

1. AMINO ACID AND PLASMA PROTEIN METABOLISM. Amino acids derived from the diet and from tissue breakdown are metabolised in the liver to ammonia and urea. A number of plasma proteins and immunoglobulins are synthesised on polyribosomes bound to the rough endoplasmic reticulum within the hepatocytes and discharged into plasma. Based on these metabolic functions of the liver, serum estimation of proteins, immunoglobulins and ammonia and aminoaciduria are employed to assess the liver cell damage.

i) Serum proteins. Liver cells synthesise albumin, fibrinogen, prothrombin, alpha-1-antitrypsin, haptoglobin, ceruloplasmin, transferrin, alpha fetoproteins and acute phase reactant proteins. The blood levels of these plasma proteins are decreased in extensive liver damage. Routinely estimated are total concentration of serum proteins (normal 5.5 to 8 gm/dl), serum albumin (normal 3.5 to 5.5 gm/dl), serum globulin (normal 2 to 3.5 gm/dl) and albumin/globulin (A/G) ratio (normal 1.5-3:1). Electrophoresis is used to determine the proportions of α_1, α_2, β and γ globulins. Due to the availability of protein electrophoresis, thymol turbidity and flocculation tests based on altered plasma protein components have been discontinued.

Hypoalbuminaemia may occur in liver diseases having significant destruction of hepatocytes. Hyperglobulinaemia may be present in chronic inflammatory disorders such as in cirrhosis and chronic hepatitis.

ii) Immunoglobulins. The levels of serum immunoglobulins produced by lymphocytes and plasma cells (IgG, IgM and IgA) show nonspecific abnormalities in liver diseases and represent inflammatory or immune response rather than liver cell dysfunction. IgA is the predominant immunoglobulin in bile and its level is raised in cirrhosis, IgG is markedly raised in chronic active hepatitis and IgM is markedly increased in primary biliary cirrhosis.

iii) Clotting factors. Hepatic synthetic function of several clotting factors can be assessed by a few simple coagulation tests. Prothrombin time and partial thromboplastin time, both of which reflect the activities of various clotting factors, are prolonged in patients with hepatocellular disease. Prothrombin time is dependent upon both hepatic synthesis of clotting factors and intestinal uptake of vitamin K, a fat soluble vitamin. Thus, obstruction of the bile duct and intrahepatic cholestasis which result in vitamin K deficiency due to impaired lipid absorption, are associated with prolonged prothrombin time. However, parenteral injection of vitamin K will normalise prothrombin time if the prolongation was due to obstruction, but there will be no improvement in prothrombin time if there is extensive hepatocellular disease.

iv) Serum ammonia. High blood levels of ammonia are found in acute fulminant hepatitis, cirrhosis and hepatic encephalopathy. The rise in serum ammonia is due to inability of severely damaged liver to convert ammonia to urea. Thus, urea synthesis is reduced in chronic liver disease.

2. LIPID AND LIPOPROTEIN METABOLISM. Lipids synthesised in the liver include cholesterol and cholesterol esters, phospholipids and triglycerides. These lipids are insoluble in water and are carried in circulation with three major types of lipoproteins which contain apoproteins. These are: high density lipoproteins (HDL), low density lipoproteins (LDL) and very low density lipoproteins (VLDL).

Blood lipids. Estimations of total serum cholesterol, triglycerides and lipoprotein fractions are frequently done in patients with liver disease.

- There is rise in total serum cholesterol in cholestasis, probably due to retention of cholesterol which is normally excreted in the bile (normal 130-230 mg/dl). Serum triglyceride is also elevated in cholestasis.
- Values are lowered in acute and chronic diffuse liver diseases and in malnutrition.

3. CARBOHYDRATE METABOLISM. The liver plays a central role in carbohydrate metabolism. Blood glucose level is lowered in fulminant acute hepatic necrosis. In chronic liver disease, there is impaired glucose tolerance and relative insulin resistance.

IV. IMMUNOLOGIC TESTS

Liver diseases are associated with various immunologic abnormalities which may be nonspecific immunologic reactions or may be antibodies against specific etiologic agents.

1. NONSPECIFIC IMMUNOLOGIC REACTIONS. These include the following:

i) *Smooth muscle antibody* to actin component of muscle is formed in certain hepatic disorders with hepatic necrosis. It appears that hepatocytes have a protein which is immunologically similar to actin.

ii) *Mitochondrial antibody* develops in patients with primary biliary cirrhosis.

iii) *Antinuclear antibody* is present in some patients of chronic hepatitis. The LE cell test may be positive in these cases.

2. ANTIBODIES TO SPECIFIC ETIOLOGIC AGENTS. These vary according to the etiologic agent causing the liver cell injury.

i) *Hepatitis B surface antigen (HBsAg)* can be demonstrated in cases of serum hepatitis. A confirmed positive test for HBsAg is definite proof of hepatitis B infection.

ii) *Hepatitis B core antibody (HBc)* can be detected in all patients with hepatitis B.

iii) *Hepatitis B e antigen (HBeAg)* can be found in chronic varieties of hepatitis B.

iv) *Amoeba antibodies* to *Entamoeba histolytica* develop in patients with amoebic liver abscess.

V. ANCILLARY DIAGNOSTICTESTS

In addition to laboratory tests described above, two ancillary tests which are invariably done by the physician are ultrasonography and percutaneous liver biopsy and/or FNAC.

1. ULTRASONOGRAPHY. Ultrasound (US) examination of the liver is indicated in the following situations:

i) Cholestasis of various etiologies to see the dilated intra- and extrahepatic canalicular tree.

ii) Space-occupying lesions (SOLs) within the liver to determine whether they are neoplasms or non-neoplastic cysts.

iii) To perform US-guided FNAC or liver biopsy.

2. FNAC AND/OR PERCUTANEOUS LIVER BIOPSY. Lastly, FNAC and percutaneous liver biopsy are employed to examine the microscopic changes of hepatic morphology in various diseases. Both these tests are done after evaluation of signs of obstruction since these are contraindicated in cholestasis. FNAC and liver biopsy are otherwise easily performed bedside tests of value. Their main indications are:

i) hepatocellular disease of unknown cause;

ii) suspected cases of chronic hepatitis;

iii) hepatomegaly of various etiologies;

iv) splenomegaly of unknown cause;

v) fever of unknown cause;and

vi) SOLs visualised in radiologic examination.

A summary of various liver function tests is given in Table 19.1.

JAUNDICE—GENERAL

Jaundice or icterus refers to the yellow pigmentation of the skin or sclerae by bilirubin (page 48). Bilirubin pigment has high affinity for elastic tissue and hence jaundice is particularly noticeable in tissues rich in elastin content. Jaundice is the result of elevated levels of bilirubin in the blood termed hyperbilirubinaemia. Normal serum bilirubin concentration ranges from 0.2-0.8 mg/dl, about 80% of which is unconjugated. Jaundice becomes clinically evident when the total serum bilirubin exceeds 2 mg/dl. A rise of serum bilirubin between the normal and 2 mg/dl is generally not accompanied by visible jaundice and is called *latent jaundice.*

Before considering the features and types of jaundice, it is essential to review the normal bilirubin metabolism.

NORMAL BILIRUBIN METABOLISM

Normal metabolism of bilirubin can be conveniently described under 4 main headings—source, transport, hepatic phase and intestinal phase as illustrated schematically earlier in Chapter 13 (see Fig. 13.8, page 364).

1. SOURCE OF BILIRUBIN. About 80-85% of the bilirubin is derived from the catabolism of haemoglobin present in senescent red blood cells. The destruction of effete erythrocytes at the end of their normal life-span of 120 days takes place in the reticuloendothelial system in the bone marrow, spleen and liver. The remaining 15-20% of the bilirubin comes partly from non-haemoglobin haem-containing pigments such as myoglobin, catalase and cytochromes, and partly from ineffective erythropoiesis. In either case, haem moiety is formed which is converted to biliverdin by microsomal haem oxygenase for which oxygen and NADPH are essential requirements. Bilirubin is formed from biliverdin by biliverdin reductase.

2. TRANSPORT OF BILIRUBIN. Bilirubin on release from macrophages circulates as unconjugated bilirubin in plasma tightly bound to albumin. Certain drugs such as sulfonamides and salicylates compete with bilirubin for albumin binding and displace bilirubin from albumin, thus facilitating bilirubin to enter into the brain in neonates and increase the risk of *kernicterus.* Bilirubin is found in body fluids in proportion to their albumin content such as in CSF, joint effusions, cysts etc.

3. HEPATIC PHASE. On coming in contact with the hepatocyte surface, unconjugated bilirubin is preferentially metabolised which involves 3 steps: hepatic uptake, conjugation and secretion in bile.

i) Hepatic uptake: Albumin-bound unconjugated bilirubin upon entry into the hepatocyte, is dissociated into bilirubin and albumin. The bilirubin gets bound to cytoplasmic protein *glutathione-S-transferase (GST)* (earlier called ligandin).

ii) Conjugation: Unconjugated bilirubin is not water-soluble but is alcohol-soluble and is converted into water-soluble compound by conjugation. Conjugation occurs in endoplasmic reticulum and involves conversion to bilirubin diglucuronide by the action of microsomal enzyme, *bilirubin- UDP-glucuronosyl transferase,* to mono- and diglucuronides (Fig. 19.3). The process of conjugation can be induced by drugs like phenobarbital.

Conjugated bilirubin is bound to albumin in two forms: reversible and irreversible. Reversible binding is similar to that of unconjugated bilirubin. However, when present in serum for a long time (e.g. in cholestasis, long-standing biliary obstruction, chronic active hepatitis), conjugated bilirubin is bound to albumin irreversibly and is termed *delta bilirubin* or *biliprotein.* This irreversible conjugated delta bilirubin is not excreted by the kidney, and remains detectable in serum for sufficient time after recovery from the diseases listed above.

iii) Secretion into bile: Conjugated (water soluble) bilirubin is rapidly transported directly into bile

TABLE 19.1: Liver Function Tests.

TESTS	SIGNIFICANCE
I. TESTS FOR MANUFACTURE AND EXCRETION OF BILE	
1. Bilirubin:	
i) Serum bilirubin	Increased in hepatocellular, obstructive and haemolytic disease, Gilbert's disease
ii) In faeces	Absent in biliary obstruction
iii) In urine	Conjugated bilirubinuria in patients of hepatitis
2. Urobilinogen:	Increased in hepatocellular and haemolytic diseases, absent in biliary obstruction
3. Bile acid (Bile salts):	Increased in serum and detectable in urine in cholestasis
II. SERUM ENZYME ASSAYS	
1. Alkaline phosphatase:	Increased in hepatobiliary disease (highest in biliary obstruction), bone diseases, pregnancy
2. γ-Glutamyl transpeptidase (γ-GT):	Rise parallels alkaline phosphatase but is specific for hepatobiliary diseases
3. Transaminases:	
i) SGOT (AST)	Increased in tissue injury to liver as well as to other tissues like in myocardial infarction
ii) SGPT (ALT)	Increase is fairly specific for liver cell injury
4. Other enzymes:	
i) 5'-Nucleotidase	Rise parallels alkaline phosphatase but more specific for diseases of hepatic origin
ii) Lactic dehydrogenase	Increased in tumours involving the liver
iii) Cholinesterase	Decreased in hepatocellular disease, malnutrition
III. TESTS FOR METABOLIC FUNCTIONS	
1. Amino acid and protein metabolism:	
i) Serum proteins (total, A/G ratio, protein electrophoresis)	Hypoalbuminaemia in hepatocellular diseases; hyperglobulinaemia in cirrhosis and chronic active hepatitis
ii) Immunoglobulins	Nonspecific alterations in IgA, IgG and IgM
iii) Clotting factors	Prothrombin time and partial thromboplastin time prolonged in patients with hepatocellular disease
iv) Serum ammonia	Increased in acute fulminant hepatitis, cirrhosis, hepatic encephalopathy
v) Aminoaciduria	In fulminant hepatitis
2. Lipid and lipoprotein metabolism:	
Blood lipids (total serum cholesterol, triglycerides and lipoprotein fractions)	Increased in cholestasis, decreased in acute and chronic diffuse liver disease and in malnutrition
3. Carbohydrate metabolism:	
Blood glucose and GTT	Decreased in hepatic necrosis
IV. IMMUNOLOGIC TESTS	
1. Nonspecific immunologic reactions:	
i) Smooth muscle antibody	In hepatic necrosis
ii) Mitochondrial antibody	In primary biliary cirrhosis
iii) Antinuclear antibody and LE cell test	In chronic active hepatitis
2. Antibodies to specific etiologic agents:	
i) Antibodies to hepatitis B (HBsAg, HBc, HBeAg)	In hepatitis B
ii) Amoeba antibodies	Amoebic liver abscess
V. ANCILLARY DIAGNOSTIC TESTS	
1. Ultrasound examination	Cholestasis of various etiologies; SOLs, US-guided-FNAC/liver biopsy
2. FNAC and/ or percutaneous liver biopsy	Unknown cause of hepatocellular disease, hepatomegaly and splenomegaly; long-standing hepatitis; PUO and SOLs of the liver

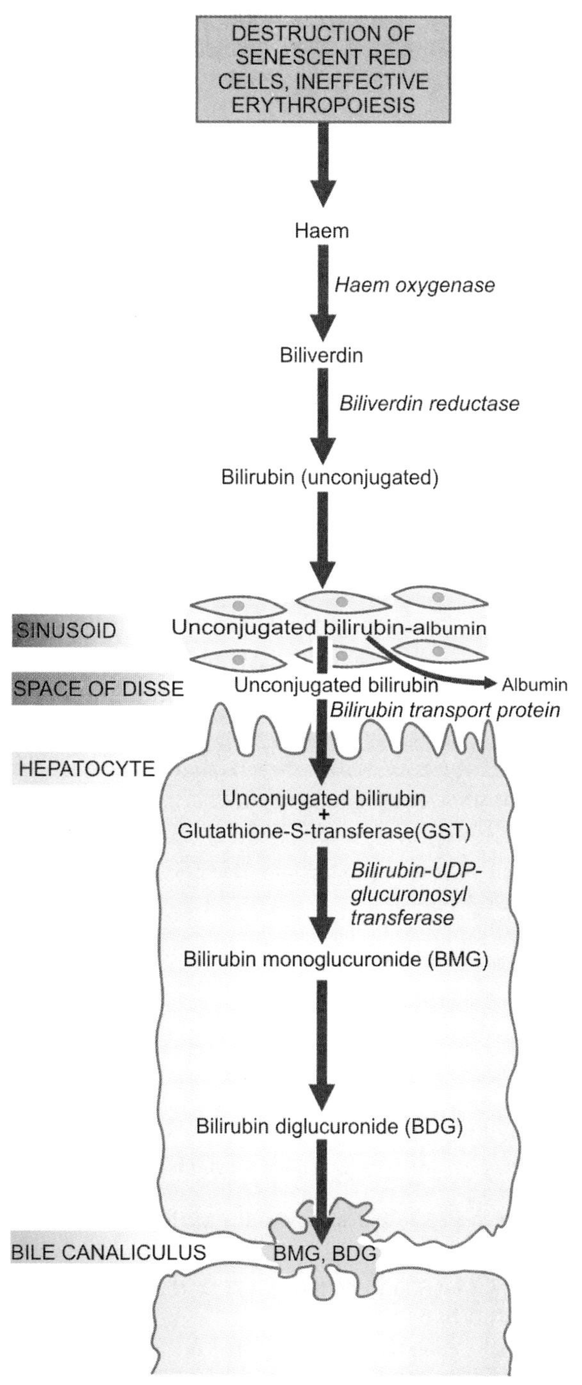

FIGURE 19.3

Schematic representation of hepatic phase of bilirubin transport.

canaliculi by energy-dependent process and then excreted into the bile.

4. INTESTINAL PHASE. Appearance of conjugated bilirubin in the intestinal lumen is followed by either direct excretion in the stool as stercobilinogen which imparts the normal yellow colour to stool, or may be metabolised to urobilinogen by the action of intestinal bacteria. Conjugated bilirubin is normally not reabsorbable whereas its metabolic product, urobilinogen, is reabsorbed from the small intestine and reaches enterohepatic circulation. Some of the absorbed urobilinogen in resecreted by the liver into the bile while the rest is excreted in the urine as urobilinogen.

The major differences between unconjugated and conjugated bilirubin are summarised in Table 19.2.

CLASSIFICATION AND FEATURES OF JAUNDICE

Based on pathophysiology, jaundice may result from one or more of the following mechanisms:

1. Increased bilirubin production
2. Decreased hepatic uptake
3. Decreased hepatic conjugation
4. Decreased excretion of bilirubin into bile

Accordingly, a simple classification of jaundice is to divide it into 3 predominant types: *pre-hepatic (haemolytic), hepatic,* and *post-hepatic cholestatic.* Hyperbilirubinaemia due to first three mechanisms is *mainly unconjugated* while the last variety yields *mainly conjugated* hyperbilirubinaemia. A simple test to determine whether hyperbilirubinaemia is of unconjugated or conjugated variety is to determine whether bilirubin is present in urine or not; its absence in urine suggests unconjugated hyperbilirubinaemia since unconjugated bilirubin is not filtered by the glomerulus. The presence of bilirubin in the urine is evidence of conjugated hyperbilirubinaemia.

Based on these mechanisms, the pathogenesis and main features of the two predominant forms of hyperbilirubinaemia are discussed below (Table 19.3).

Predominantly Unconjugated Hyperbilirubinaemia

This form of jaundice can result from the following three sets of conditions:

1. INCREASED BILIRUBIN PRODUCTION (HAEMOLYTIC, ACHOLURIC OR PREHEPATIC JAUNDICE). This results from excessive red cell destruction as occurs in intra- and extravascular haemolysis or due to ineffective erythropoiesis. There is increased release of haemoglobin from excessive breakdown of red cells that leads to overproduction of bilirubin. Hyperbilirubinaemia develops when the capacity of the liver to conjugate large amount of bilirubin is exceeded. In premature infants, the liver is deficient in enzyme necessary for conjugation while the rate of red cell destruction is high. This results in *icterus neonatorum*

TABLE 19.2: Major Differences between Unconjugated and Conjugated Bilirubin.

FEATURE	UNCONJUGATED BILIRUBIN	CONJUGATED BILIRUBIN
1. *Normal serum level*	More	Less (less than 0.25 mg/dl)
2. *Water solubility*	Absent	Present
3. *Affinity to lipids (alcohol solubility)*	Present	Absent
4. *Serum albumin binding*	High	Low
5. *van den Bergh reaction*	Indirect (Total minus direct)	Direct
6. *Renal excretion*	Absent	Present
7. *Bilirubin albumin covalent complex formation*	Absent	Present
8. *Affinity to brain tissue*	Present (Kernicterus)	Absent

which is particularly severe in haemolytic disease of the newborn due to maternal isoantibodies (Chapter 13). Since there is predominantly unconjugated hyperbilirubinaemia in such cases, there is danger of permanent brain damage in these infants from kernicterus when the serum level of unconjugated bilirubin exceeds 20 mg/dl.

Laboratory data in haemolytic jaundice, in addition to predominant unconjugated hyperbilirubinaemia, reveal normal serum levels of transaminases, alkaline phosphatase and proteins. Bile pigment being unconjugated type is absent from urine (acholuric jaundice). However, there is dark brown colour of stools due to excessive faecal excretion of bile pigment and increased urinary excretion of urobilinogen.

2. DECREASED HEPATIC UPTAKE. The uptake of bilirubin by the hepatocyte that involves dissociation of the pigment from albumin and its binding to cytoplasmic protein, GST or ligandin, may be deranged in certain conditions e.g. due to drugs, prolonged starvation and sepsis.

3. DECREASED BILIRUBIN CONJUGATION. This mechanism involves deranged hepatic conjugation due to defect or deficiency of the enzyme, glucuronosyl transferase. This can occur in certain inherited disorders of the enzyme (e.g. Gilbert's syndrome and Crigler-Najjar syndrome), or acquired defects in its activity (e.g. due to drugs, hepatitis, cirrhosis). However, hepatocellular damage causes deranged excretory capacity of the liver more than its conjugating capacity *(see below)*. The physiologic neonatal jaundice is also partly due to relative deficiency of UDP-glucuronosyl transferase in the neonatal liver and is partly as a result of increased rate of red cell destruction in neonates.

II. Predominantly Conjugated Hyperbilirubinaemia (Cholestasis)

This form of hyperbilirubinaemia is defined as failure of normal amounts of bile to reach the duodenum. Morphologically, cholestasis means accumulation of bile

TABLE 19.3: Pathophysiologic Classification of Jaundice.

I. PREDOMINANTLY UNCONJUGATED HYPERBILIRUBINAEMIA

1. Increased bilirubin production (Haemolytic, acholuric or prehepatic jaundice)
- Intra-and extravascular haemolysis
- Ineffective erythropoiesis

2. Decreased hepatic uptake
- Drugs
- Prolonged starvation
- Sepsis

3. Decreased bilirubin conjugation
- Hereditary disorders (e.g. Gilbert's syndrome, Crigler-Najjar syndrome)
- Acquired defects (e.g. drugs, hepatitis, cirrhosis)
- Neonatal jaundice

II. PREDOMINANTLY CONJUGATED HYPERBILIRUBINAEMIA (CHOLESTASIS)

1. Intrahepatic cholestasis (Impaired hepatic excretion)
- Hereditary disorders or *'pure cholestasis'* (e.g. Dubin-Johnson syndrome, Rotor's syndrome, fibrocystic disease of pancreas, benign familial recurrent cholestasis, intrahepatic atresia, cholestatic jaundice of pregnancy)
- Acquired disorders or *'hepatocellular cholestasis'* (e.g. viral hepatitis, drugs, alcohol-induced injury, sepsis, cirrhosis)

2. Extrahepatic cholestasis (Extrahepatic biliary obstruction)
- Mechanical obstruction (e.g. gallstones, inflammatory strictures, carcinoma head of pancreas, tumours of bile ducts, sclerosing cholangitis, congenital atresia of extrahepatic ducts)

in liver cells and biliary passages. The defect in excretion may be within the biliary canaliculi of the hepatocyte and in the microscopic bile ducts *(intrahepatic cholestasis or medical jaundice)*, or there may be mechanical obstruction to the extrahepatic biliary excretory apparatus *(extrahepatic cholestasis or obstructive jaundice)*. It is important to distinguish these two forms of cholestasis since extrahepatic cholestasis or obstructive jaundice is often treatable with surgery, whereas the intrahepatic cholestasis or medical jaundice cannot be benefitted by surgery but may in fact worsen by the operation. Prolonged cholestasis of either of the two types may progress to biliary cirrhosis (page 644).

1. INTRAHEPATIC CHOLESTASIS. Intrahepatic cholestasis is due to impaired hepatic excretion of bile and may occur from hereditary or acquired disorders.

i) Hereditary disorders producing intrahepatic obstruction to biliary excretion are characterised by *'pure cholestasis'* e.g. in Dubin-Johnson syndrome, Rotor syndrome, fibrocystic disease of pancreas, benign familial recurrent cholestasis, intrahepatic atresia and cholestatic jaundice of pregnancy.

ii) Acquired disorders with intrahepatic excretory defect of bilirubin are largely due to hepatocellular diseases and hence are termed *'hepatocellular cholestasis'* e.g. in viral hepatitis, alcoholic hepatitis, and drug-induced cholestasis such as from administration of chlorpromazine and oral contraceptives.

The **features** of intrahepatic cholestasis include: predominant conjugated hyperbilirubinaemia due to regurgitation of conjugated bilirubin into blood, bilirubinuria, elevated levels of serum bile acids and consequent pruritus, elevated serum alkaline phosphatase, hyperlipidaemia and hypoprothrombinaemia. 'Pure cholestasis' can be distinguished from 'hepatocellular cholestasis' by elevated serum levels of transaminases in the latter due to liver cell injury.

■ **Liver biopsy** in cases with intrahepatic cholestasis reveals milder degree of cholestasis than the extrahepatic disorders (Fig. 19.4,A). The biliary canaliculi of the hepatocytes are dilated and contain characteristic elongated green-brown *bile plugs*. The cytoplasm of the affected hepatocytes shows feathery degeneration. Canalicular bile stasis eventually causes proliferation of intralobular ductules followed by periportal fibrosis and produces a picture resembling biliary cirrhosis (page 644).

2. EXTRAHEPATIC CHOLESTASIS. Extrahepatic cholestasis results from mechanical obstruction to large bile ducts outside the liver or within the porta hepatis. The common causes are gallstones, inflammatory strictures, carcinoma head of pancreas, tumours of bile duct, sclerosing cholangitis and congenital atresia of extrahepatic ducts. The obstruction may be complete and sudden with eventual progressive obstructive jaundice, or the obstruction may be partial and incomplete resulting in intermittent jaundice.

The **features** of extrahepatic cholestasis (obstructive jaundice), like in intrahepatic cholestasis, are predominant conjugated hyperbilirubinaemia, bilirubinuria, elevated serum bile acids causing intense pruritus, high serum alkaline phosphatase and hyperlipidaemia.

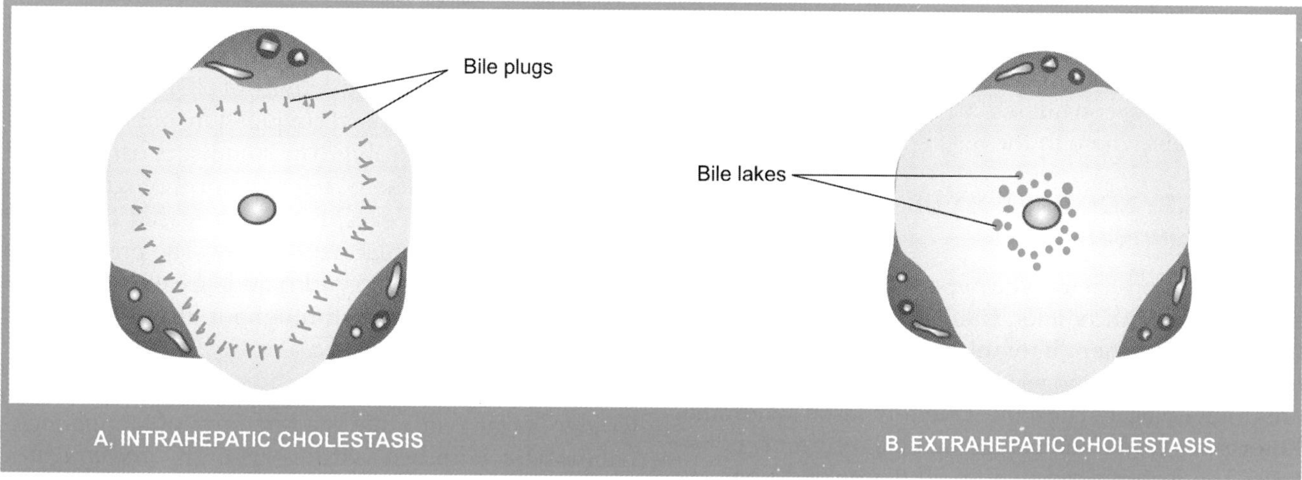

FIGURE 19.4

Salient features in morphology of liver in intra- and extrahepatic cholestasis. A, Intrahepatic cholestasis is characterised by elongated bile plugs in the canaliculi of hepatocytes at the periphery of the lobule. B, Extrahepatic cholestasis shows characteristic bile lakes due to rupture of canaliculi in the hepatocytes in the centrilobular area.

However, there are certain features which help to distinguish extrahepatic from intrahepatic cholestasis. In obstructive jaundice, there is malabsorption of fat-soluble vitamins (A,D,E and K) and steatorrhoea resulting in vitamin K deficiency. Prolonged prothrombin time in such cases shows improvement following parenteral administration of vitamin K, whereas hypoprothrombinaemia due to hepatocellular disease shows no such improvement in prothrombin time with vitamin K administration. The stools of such patients are clay-coloured due to absence of bilirubin metabolite, stercobilin, in faeces and there is virtual disappearance of urobilinogen from the urine. These patients may have fever due to high incidence of ascending bacterial infections (ascending cholangitis).

■ **Liver biopsy** in cases with extrahepatic cholestasis shows more marked changes of cholestasis (Fig. 19.4,B). Since the obstruction is in the extrahepatic bile ducts, there is progressive retrograde extension of bile stasis into intrahepatic duct system. This results in dilatation of bile ducts and rupture of canaliculi with extravasation of bile producing *bile lakes.* Since bile is toxic, the regions of bile lakes are surrounded by focal necrosis of hepatocytes. Stasis of bile predisposes to ascending bacterial infections with accumulation of polymorphs around the dilated ducts (ascending cholangitis). Eventually, there is proliferation of bile ducts and the appearance may mimic biliary cirrhosis (page 644).

NEONATAL JAUNDICE

Jaundice appears in neonates when the total serum bilirubin is more than 3 mg/dl. It may be the result of unconjugated or conjugated hyperbilirubinaemia; the former being more common. Important causes of neonatal jaundice are listed in Table 19.4. Some of these conditions are considered below, while others are discussed elsewhere in the relevant sections.

HEREDITARY NON-HAEMOLYTIC HYPERBILIRUBINAEMIAS

Hereditary non-haemolytic hyperbilirubinaemias are a small group of uncommon familial disorders of bilirubin metabolism when haemolytic causes have been excluded. The commonest is Gilbert's syndrome; others are Crigler-Najjar syndrome, Dubin-Johnson syndrome, Rotor's syndrome and benign familial recurrent cholestasis. The features common to all these conditions are presence of icterus but almost normal liver function tests and no well-defined morphologic changes except in Dubin-Johnson syndrome. Gilbert's syndrome and Crigler-Najjar syndrome are examples of *hereditary non-haemolytic unconjugated hyperbilirubinaemia,* whereas Dubin-Johnson syndrome, Rotor's syndrome and benign familial recurrent cholestasis are conditions with *hereditary conjugated hyperbilirubinaemia.* These conditions are briefly described below. Their distinguishing features are summarised in Table 19.5.

TABLE 19.4: Causes of Neonatal Jaundice.

A. Unconjugated hyperbilirubinaemia

1. Physiologic and prematurity jaundice
2. Haemolytic disease of the newborn and kernicterus (page 440)
3. Congenital haemolytic disorders (page 390)
4. Perinatal complications (e.g. haemorrhage, sepsis)
5. Gilbert's syndrome
6. Crigler-Najjar syndrome (type I and II)

B. Conjugated hyperbilirubinaemia

1. Hereditary (Dubin-Johnson syndrome, Rotor's syndrome)
2. Infections (e.g. hepatitis B, hepatitis C or non-A non-B hepatitis, rubella, coxsackievirus, cytomegalovirus, echovirus, herpes simplex, syphilis, toxoplasma, gram-negative sepsis)
3. Metabolic (e.g. galactosaemia, alpha-1-antitrypsin deficiency, cystic fibrosis, Niemann-Pick disease)
4. Idiopathic (neonatal hepatitis, congenital hepatic fibrosis)
5. Biliary atresia (intrahepatic and extrahepatic)
6. Reye's syndrome

Gilbert's Syndrome

This is the commonest of the familial, genetically-determined diseases of the liver affecting 2-5% of the population. Gilbert's syndrome is characterised by mild, benign, unconjugated hyperbilirubinaemia (serum bilirubin 1-5 mg/dl) which is not due to haemolysis. The condition is inherited as an autosomal dominant character. The defect in bilirubin metabolism is complex and appears to be reduced activity of UDP-glucuronosyl transferase with decreased conjugation, or an impaired hepatic uptake of bilirubin. The jaundice is usually mild and intermittent. There are no morphologic abnormalities in the liver except some increased lipofuscin pigment in centrilobular hepatocytes. The prognosis of patients with Gilbert's syndrome is excellent, though chronic jaundice persists throughout life.

Crigler-Najjar Syndrome

Crigler-Najjar syndrome is a rare form of familial non-haemolytic jaundice with very high *unconjugated hyperbilirubinaemia.* There are 2 forms of this condition: type I and type II.

Type I Crigler-Najjar syndrome. This is inherited as an autosomal recessive disorder. There is complete

TABLE 19.5: Contrasting Features of Major Hereditary Non-haemolytic Hyperbilirubinaemias.

FEATURE	GILBERT'S SYNDROME	TYPE 1 CRIGLER-NAJJAR SYNDROME	TYPE 2 CRIGLER-NAJJAR SYNDROME	DUBIN-JOHNSON SYNDROME	ROTOR SYNDROME
1. *Inheritance*	Autosomal dominant	Autosomal recessive	Autosomal dominant	Autosomal recessive	Autosomal recessive
2. *Predominant hyperbilirubinaemia*	Unconjugated	Unconjugated	Unconjugated	Conjugated	Conjugated
3. *Intensity of jaundice*	Mild (<5mg/dl)	Marked (>20 mg/dl)	Mild to moderate (<20 mg/dl)	Mild (<5 mg/dl)	Mild (< 5 mg/dl)
4. *Basic defect*	↓ UDP-glucuronosyl transferase activity	Absence of UDP-glucuronosyl transferase	↓ UDP-glucuronosyl transferase	Defect in canalicular excretion (Prolonged BSP excretion test)	Deranged hepatic uptake
5. *Hepatic morphology*	Normal (except slightly increased lipofuscin)	Normal (except mild canalicular stasis)	Normal	Greenish-black pigment	Normal
6. *Prognosis*	Excellent	Poor (due to kernicterus)	Good	Excellent	Excellent

absence of conjugating enzyme UDP-glucuronosyl transferase in the hepatocytes and hence no conjugated bilirubin is formed. There is extreme elevation of unconjugated bilirubin (usually more than 20 mg/dl) with high risk of developing permanent CNS damage from kernicterus. The prognosis is generally fatal, with death coming from kernicterus usually in the first year of life. There are no significant morphologic changes except some canalicular stasis.

Type II Crigler-Najjar syndrome. This is inherited as an autosomal dominant disease. There is deficiency of enzyme UDP-glucuronosyl transferase but not complete absence. Thus, unconjugated hyperbilirubinaemia is generally mild to moderate (usually less than 20 mg/dl). Occurrence of kernicterus is exceptional and patients respond well to phenobarbital therapy. There are no morphologic changes in the liver.

Dubin-Johnson Syndrome

Dubin-Johnson syndrome is autosomal recessive disorder characterised by predominant *conjugated hyperbilirubinaemia* (usually less than 5 mg/dl) with genetic defect in canalicular excretion of conjugated bilirubin. The condition differs from other forms of hereditary hyperbilirubinaemias in producing grossly greenish-black pigmented liver. The hepatocytes show dark-brown, melanin-like pigment in the cytoplasm, the exact nature of which is obscure but it is neither iron nor bile. Unrelated viral hepatitis mobilises the hepatic pigment of Dubin-Johnson syndrome leading to its excretion in urine but the pigment reappears after recovery from viral hepatitis. A prolonged BSP dye excretion test is diagnostic of Dubin-Johnson syndrome (page 610). The disease runs a benign course and does not interfere with life.

Rotor's Syndrome

This is another form of familial *conjugated hyperbilirubinaemia* with mild chronic jaundice but differs from Dubin-Johnson syndrome in having no brown pigment in the liver cells. The disease is inherited as an autosomal recessive character. Rotor's syndrome has an excellent prognosis.

NEONATAL HEPATITIS

Neonatal hepatitis, also termed giant cell hepatitis or neonatal hepatocellular cholestasis, is a general term used for the constant morphologic change seen in conjugated hyperbilirubinaemia as a result of known infectious and metabolic causes listed in Table 19.4, or may have an idiopathic etiology. The 'idiopathic' neonatal hepatitis is more common and accounts for 75% of cases. Though all the cases with either known etiologies or idiopathic type are grouped together under neonatal hepatitis, all of them are not necessarily inflammatory conditions, thus belying their nomenclature as 'hepatitis'. The condition usually presents in the first week of birth with jaundice, bilirubinuria, pale stools and high serum alkaline phosphatase.

PATHOLOGIC CHANGES. Irrespective of the etiology, there is morphologic similarity in all these cases. The histologic features are:
1. Loss of normal lobular architecture of the liver.
2. Presence of prominent multinucleate giant cells derived from hepatocytes.
3. Mononuclear inflammatory cell infiltrate in the portal tracts with some periportal fibrosis.
4. Haemosiderosis.
5. Cholestasis in small proliferated ductules in the portal tract and between necrotic liver cells.

BILIARY ATRESIAS

Biliary atresias, also called as *infantile cholangiopathies*, are a group of intrauterine developmental abnormalities of the biliary system. Though they are often classified as congenital, the abnormality of development in most instances is extraneous infection during the intrauterine development or shortly after birth that brings about inflammatory destruction of the bile ducts. The condition may, therefore, have various grades of destruction ranging from complete absence of bile ducts termed *atresia,* to reduction in their number called *paucity of bile ducts.*

Depending upon the portion of biliary system involved, biliary atresias may be extrahepatic or intrahepatic.

Extrahepatic Biliary Atresia

The extrahepatic bile ducts fail to develop normally so that in some cases the bile ducts are *absent* at birth, while in others the ducts may have been formed but start undergoing sclerosis in the perinatal period. It is common to have multiple defects and other congenital lesions. Extrahepatic biliary atresia is found in 1 per 10,000 livebirths. Cholestatic jaundice appears by the first week after birth. The baby has severe pruritus, pale stools, dark urine and elevated serum transaminases. In some cases, the condition is correctable by surgery, while in vast majority the atresia is not correctable and in such cases hepatic portoenterostomy (Kasai procedure) or hepatic transplantation must be considered. Death is usually due to intercurrent infection, liver failure, and bleeding due to vitamin K deficiency or oesophageal varices. Cirrhosis and ascites are late complications appearing within 2 years of age.

PATHOLOGIC CHANGES. Grossly, the liver is enlarged and dark green. The atretic segments of biliary system are reduced to cord-like structures.

Histologically, the condition must be distinguished from idiopathic neonatal hepatitis as surgical treatment is possible in extrahepatic biliary atresia but not in the latter. Besides, the α-1-antitrypsin deficiency also produces similar appearance in liver biopsy. The main histologic features are:
1. Inflammation and fibrous obliteration of the extrahepatic ducts with absence of bile in them.
2. Ductular proliferation and periductular inflammation.
3. Cholestasis and bile thrombi in the portal area.
4. Periportal fibrosis and later secondary biliary cirrhosis (page 645).
5. Transformation of hepatic parenchyma to neonatal (giant cell) hepatitis in 15% of cases.

Intrahepatic Biliary Atresia

Intrahepatic biliary atresia is characterised by biliary hypoplasia so that there is *paucity of bile ducts* rather than their complete absence. The condition probably has its origin in viral infection acquired during intrauterine period or in the neonatal period. Cholestatic jaundice usually appears within the first few days of birth and is characterised by high serum bile acids with associated pruritus, and hypercholesterolaemia with appearance of xanthomas by first year of life. Hepatic as well as urinary copper concentrations are elevated. In some cases, intrahepatic biliary atresia is related to α-1-antitrypsin deficiency.

PATHOLOGIC CHANGES. The microscopic features are:
1. Paucity of intrahepatic bile ducts.
2. Cholestasis.
3. Increased hepatic copper.
4. Inflammation and fibrosis in the portal area, eventually leading to cirrhosis.

REYE'S SYNDROME

Reye's syndrome is defined as an acute postviral syndrome of encephalopathy and fatty change in the viscera. The syndrome may follow almost any known viral disease but is most common after influenza A or B and varicella. Viral infection may act singly, or more often its effect is modified by certain exogenous factors such as by administration of salicylates, aflatoxins and insecticides. These effects cause mitochondrial injury and decreased activity of mitochondrial enzymes in the liver. This eventually leads to rise in blood ammonia and accumulation of triglycerides within hepatocytes.

Chapter Nineteen

The patients are generally children between 6 months and 15 years of age. Within a week after a viral illness, the child develops intractable vomiting and progressive neurological deterioration due to encephalopathy, eventually leading to stupor, coma and death. Characteristic laboratory findings are elevated blood ammonia, serum transaminases, bilirubin and prolonged prothrombin time.

*PATHOLOGIC CHANGES. **Grossly,*** the liver is enlarged and yellowish-orange.

Microscopically, the hepatocytes show small droplets of neutral fat in their cytoplasm (microvesicular fat). Similar fatty change is seen in the renal tubular epithelium and in the cells of skeletal muscles and heart. The brain shows oedema and sometimes focal necrosis of neurons.

HEPATIC FAILURE

Though the liver has a marked regenerative capacity and a large functional reserve, hepatic failure may develop from severe acute and fulminant liver injury with massive necrosis of liver cells *(acute hepatic failure)*, or from advanced chronic liver disease *(chronic hepatic failure)*. Acute hepatic failure develops suddenly with severe impairment of liver functions whereas chronic liver failure comes insidiously. The prognosis is much worse in acute hepatic failure than that in chronic liver failure.

ETIOLOGY. The two types of hepatic failure result from different causes:

- **Acute (fulminant) hepatic failure** occurs most frequently in severe viral hepatitis. Other causes are hepatotoxic drug reactions (e.g. anaesthetic agents, nonsteroidal anti-inflammatory drugs, anti-depressants), carbon tetrachloride poisoning, acute alcoholic hepatitis, mushroom poisoning and pregnancy complicated with eclampsia.
- **Chronic hepatic failure** is most often due to cirrhosis. Other causes include chronic active hepatitis, chronic cholestasis (cholestatic jaundice) and Wilson's disease.

MANIFESTATIONS. In view of the diverse functions performed by the liver, the syndrome of acute or chronic hepatic failure produces complex manifestations. The major manifestations are briefly discussed below.

1. Jaundice. Jaundice usually reflects the severity of liver cell damage since it occurs due to failure of liver cells to metabolise bilirubin. In acute failure such as in viral hepatitis, jaundice nearly parallels the extent of liver cell damage, while in chronic failure such as in cirrhosis jaundice appears late and is usually of mild degree.

2. Hepatic encephalopathy (Hepatic coma). Neuropsychiatric syndrome may complicate liver disease of both acute and chronic types. The features include disturbed consciousness, personality changes, intellectual deterioration, low slurred speech, flapping tremors, and finally, coma and death. The genesis of CNS manifestations in liver disease is considered to be by toxic products not metabolised by diseased liver. The toxic products may be ammonia and other nitrogenous substances from intestinal bacteria which reach the systemic circulation without detoxification in the damaged liver and thus damage the brain. Advanced cases of hepatic coma have poor prognosis but may respond favourably to hepatic transplantation.

3. Hyperkinetic circulation. All forms of hepatic failure are associated with a hyperkinetic circulation characterised by peripheral vasodilatation, increased splanchnic blood flow and increased cardiac output. There is increased splenic flow but reduced renal blood flow resulting in impaired renal cortical perfusion. These changes result in tachycardia, low blood pressure and reduced renal function.

4. Hepatorenal syndrome. The term hepatorenal syndrome is applied to patients of both acute and chronic hepatic failure who develop renal failure as well, in the absence of clinical, laboratory or morphologic evidence of other causes of renal dysfunction. The acute renal failure is usually associated with oliguria and uraemia but with good tubular function. The histology of kidney is virtually normal, suggesting functional defect for the renal failure. The pathogenesis of the syndrome is unclear but appears to be initiated by effective reduction of the renal blood flow (effective hypovolaemia) as a consequence of systemic vasodilatation and pooling of blood in portal circulation. The renal failure in the hepatorenal syndrome is reversible with improvement in hepatic function.

Diagnosis of hepatorenal syndrome should be made only after excluding other causes producing concomitant damage to both the organs, circulatory failure leading to acute tubular necrosis and other forms of reversible tubular damage.

5. Hepatopulmonary syndrome. The pulmonary changes in chronic hepatic failure such as in cirrhosis consist of pulmonary vasodilatation with intra-pulmonary arteriovenous shunting. This results in ventilation-perfusion inequality that may lead to impaired pulmonary function, clubbing of fingers and sometimes cyanosis.

6. Coagulation defects. Impaired synthesis of a number of coagulation factors by the diseased liver may result in coagulation disorders. These include disseminated intravascular coagulation (consumption coagulopathy), thrombocytopenia and presence of fibrin degradation products in the blood.

7. Ascites and oedema. Chronic liver failure due to cirrhosis may result in portal hypertension and ascites (page 651). Decreased synthesis of albumin by the liver resulting in hypoproteinaemia and consequent fall in plasma oncotic pressure, increased hydrostatic pressure due to portal hypertension and secondary hyperaldosteronism, contribute to the development of ascites and oedema in these patients.

8. Endocrine changes. Endocrine changes may be found in association with chronic hepatic failure. The changes are more common in alcoholic cirrhosis in active reproductive life. In the male, the changes are towards feminisation such as gynaecomastia and hypogonadism. In the female, the changes are less towards masculinisation but atrophy of gonads and breasts occurs. The underlying mechanism appears to be changed end-organ sensitiveness to sex hormones in cirrhosis.

9. Skin changes. In alcoholic cirrhosis *'arterial spiders'* having radiating small vessels from a central arteriole are frequent in the vascular region drained by superior vena cava such as in the neck, face, forearms and dorsum of hands. Less frequently, *palmar erythema,* especially in the hypothenar and thenar eminences and on the pulps of the fingers, is observed in chronic liver disease.

10. Foetor hepaticus. A sweetish pungent smell of the breath is found in severe cases of acute and chronic hepatocellular diseases. It appears to be of intestinal origin, possibly due to failure of the liver to detoxify sulfur-containing substances absorbed from the gut.

The major complications of hepatic failure are illustrated in Fig. 19.5.

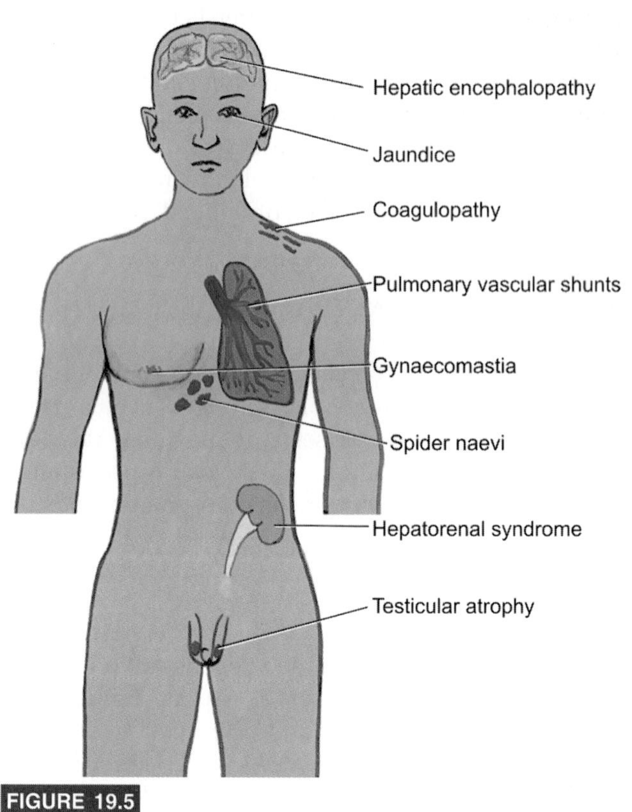

FIGURE 19.5
Complications of hepatic failure.

CIRCULATORY DISTURBANCES

Vascular disorders of general nature involving the liver such as chronic passive congestion and infarction have already been discussed in Chapter 5. Hepatic and portal venous obstruction and hepatic arterial obstruction are considered here.

I. HEPATIC VENOUS OBSTRUCTION

The central veins of lobules of the liver are tributaries of the hepatic veins. In the normal liver, there are no anastomoses between hepatic vein and portal vein but in cirrhotic liver there are such anastomoses. Normal pressure in the free hepatic vein is about 6 mmHg.

Two uncommon diseases produced by obstruction of the hepatic veins are Budd-Chiari syndrome (hepatic vein thrombosis) and hepatic veno-occlusive disease.

Budd-Chiari Syndrome (Hepatic Vein Thrombosis)

Budd-Chiari syndrome in its pure form consists of slowly developing thrombosis of the hepatic veins and the adjacent inferior vena cava, while some workers include hepatic veno-occlusive disease (described below) in this syndrome.

ETIOLOGY. The etiology of hepatic venous thrombosis in about a third of cases is unknown (idiopathic), while in the remaining cases various causes associated with increased thrombotic tendencies are attributed such as due to polycythaemia vera, paroxysmal nocturnal haemoglobinuria, oral contraceptives, pregnancy, post-partum state, intra-abdominal cancers (e.g. hepato-cellular carcinoma), chemotherapy, radiation and myelo-proliferative diseases. Formation of membranous webs, probably congenital or as a consequence of organised thrombosis, in the suprahepatic portion of inferior vena cava is another important cause.

PATHOLOGIC CHANGES. ***Grossly,*** the liver is enlarged, swollen, red-purple and has a tense capsule. ***Histologically,*** the changes in sudden hepatic vein occlusion are those of centrilobular congestion, necrosis and rupture of sinusoids into the space of Disse. In slowly developing thrombosis, the changes are more chronic and include fibrosing reaction in the centrilobular zone that may progress to cardiac cirrhosis.

CLINICAL FEATURES. Budd-Chiari syndrome is clinically characterised by either an acute form or chronic form depending upon the speed of occlusion.

- In the *acute form,* the features are abdominal pain, vomiting, enlarged liver, ascites and mild icterus.
- In the more usual *chronic form,* the patients present with pain over enlarged tender liver, ascites and other features of portal hypertension.

The acute form of illness leads to acute hepatic failure and death, whereas in chronic form the patient may live for months to a few years.

Hepatic Veno-occlusive Disease

Hepatic veno-occlusive disease consists of intimal thickening, stenosis and obliteration of the terminal central veins and medium-sized hepatic veins. The venous occlusion results in pathologic changes similar to those of Budd-Chiari syndrome and can be distinguished from the latter by demonstration of absence of thrombosis in the major hepatic veins.

The cause and stimulus for hepatic veno-occlusive disease are obscure. The condition is more widespread in countries such as Africa, India and certain other tropical countries where 'bush tea' (medicinal tea) is consumed that contains hepatotoxic alkaloids. More recently, the disease has been found in association with administration of antineoplastic drugs and immuno-suppressive therapy.

II. PORTAL VENOUS OBSTRUCTION

Obstruction of the portal vein may occur within the intrahepatic course or in extrahepatic site.

- **Intrahepatic cause** of portal venous occlusion is hepatic cirrhosis as the commonest and most important, followed in decreasing frequency by tumour invasion, congenital hepatic fibrosis and schistosomiasis.
- **Extrahepatic causes** of portal vein obstruction are intra-abdominal cancers, intra-abdominal sepsis, direct invasion by tumour, myeloproliferative disorders and upper abdominal surgical procedure followed by thrombosis.

The **effects** of portal venous obstruction depend upon the site of obstruction. The most important effect, irrespective of the site of occlusion or cause, is portal hypertension and its manifestations (page 651). If the obstruction is in the extrahepatic portal vein alongwith extension of occlusion into splenic vein, it may result in venous infarction of the bowel. Pylephlebitis may be followed by multiple pyaemic liver abscesses.

III. HEPATIC ARTERIAL OBSTRUCTION

Diseases from obstruction of the hepatic artery are uncommon. Rarely, accidental ligation of the main hepatic artery or its branch to right lobe may be followed by fatal infarction. Obstruction of the small intrahepatic arterial branches usually does not produce any effects because of good collateral circulation.

LIVER CELL NECROSIS

All forms of injury to the liver such as microbiologic, toxic, circulatory or traumatic, result in necrosis of liver cells. The extent of involvement of hepatic lobule in necrosis varies. Accordingly, liver cell necrosis is divided into 3 types: *diffuse* (submassive to massive), *zonal* and *focal.*

1. DIFFUSE (SUBMASSIVE TO MASSIVE) NECROSIS. When there is extensive and diffuse necrosis of the liver involving all the cells in groups of lobules, it is termed diffuse, or submassive to massive necrosis. It is most commonly caused by viral hepatitis or drug toxicity.

2. ZONAL NECROSIS. Zonal necrosis is necrosis of hepatocytes in 3 different zones of the hepatic lobule (page 609). Accordingly, it is of 3 types; each type affecting respective zone is caused by different etiologic factors:

i) Centrilobular necrosis is the commonest type involving hepatocytes in zone 3 (i.e. located around the central vein). Centrilobular necrosis is characteristic feature of ischaemic injury such as in shock and CHF since zone 3 is farthest from the blood supply. Besides, it also occurs in poisoning with chloroform, carbon tetrachloride and certain drugs.

ii) Midzonal necrosis is uncommon and involves zone 2 of the hepatic lobule. This pattern of necrosis is seen in yellow fever and viral hepatitis. In viral hepatitis, some of the necrosed hepatocytes of the mid-zone are transformed into acidophilic, rounded Councilman bodies.

iii) Periportal (peripheral) necrosis is seen in zone 1 involving the parenchyma closest to the arterial and portal blood supply. Since zone 1 is most well perfused, it is most vulnerable to the effects of circulating hepatotoxins e.g. in phosphorus poisoning and eclampsia.

3. **FOCAL NECROSIS.** This form of necrosis involves small groups of hepatocytes irregularly distributed in the hepatic lobule. Focal necrosis is most often caused by microbiologic infections. These include viral hepatitis, miliary tuberculosis, typhoid fever and various other forms of bacterial, viral and fungal infections. Focal necrosis may also occur in drug-induced hepatitis.

VIRAL HEPATITIS

The term viral hepatitis is used to describe infection of the liver caused by hepatotropic viruses. Currently there are 5 main varieties of these viruses and a sixth poorly-characterised virus, causing distinct types of viral hepatitis:

- *Hepatitis A virus (HAV),* causing a faecally-spread self-limiting disease;
- *Hepatitis B virus (HBV),* causing a parenterally transmitted disease that may become chronic;
- *Hepatitis C virus (HCV),* previously termed non-A, non-B (NANB) hepatitis virus involved chiefly in transfusion-related hepatitis;
- *Hepatitis delta virus (HDV)* which is sometimes associated as superinfection with hepatitis B infection;
- *Hepatitis E virus (HEV),* causing water-borne infection; and
- *Hepatitis G virus (HGV),* is a recently discovered parenterally transmitted hepatotropic virus.

All these human hepatitis viruses are RNA viruses except HBV which is a DNA virus.

Though a number of other viral diseases such as infection with Epstein-Barr virus (in infectious mononucleosis), arbovirus (in yellow fever), cytomegalovirus, herpes simplex and several others affect the liver but the changes produced by them are nonspecific and the term 'viral hepatitis' is strictly applied to infection of the liver by the hepatitis viruses.

ETIOLOGIC CLASSIFICATION

Based on the etiologic agent, viral hepatitis is currently classified into 6 etiologic types—hepatitis A, hepatitis B, hepatitis C, hepatitis D, hepatitis E and hepatitis G. The contrasting features of various types are presented in Table 19.6.

Hepatitis A

Infection with HAV causes hepatitis A (infectious hepatitis). Hepatitis A is responsible for 20-25% of clinical hepatitis in the developing countries of the world but the incidence is much lower in the developed countries. Hepatitis A is usually a benign, self-limiting disease and has an incubation period of 15-45 days. The disease occurs in epidemic form as well as sporadically. It is usually spread by faeco-oral route. Parenteral transmission is extremely rare. The spread is related to close personal contact such as in overcrowding, poor hygiene and poor sanitation. Most frequently affected age is 5-14 years; adults are often infected by spread from children.

HEPATITIS A VIRUS (HAV). The etiologic agent for hepatitis A, HAV, is a small, 27 nm diameter, icosahedral non-enveloped, single-stranded RNA virus. Viral genome has been characterised but only a single serotype has been identified. HAV infection can be transmitted to primates and the virus can be cultivated *in vitro.* Inactivation of viral activity can be achieved by boiling for 1 minute, by ultraviolet radiation on by contact with formaldehyde and chlorine. The virus is present in the liver cells, bile, stool and blood during the incubation period and in pre-icteric phase but viral shedding diminishes after the onset of jaundice. Chronic carriers have not been identified for HAV infection.

PATHOGENESIS. The mechanism by which HAV infection causes hepatitis A is poorly understood. An immunologic basis is suspected but the evidence in support is indirect in the form of immunologic markers but not direct demonstration of the etiologic agent in the affected hepatocytes. These markers are (Fig. 19.6):

1. *IgM anti-HAV antibody* appears in the serum at the onset of symptoms of acute hepatitis A.
2. *IgG anti-HAV antibody* is detected in the serum after IgM antibody and gives life-long protective immunity against reinfection with HAV.

Hepatitis B

Hepatitis B (serum hepatitis) caused by HBV infection has a longer incubation period (30-180 days) and is

TABLE 19.6: Features of Various Types of Hepatitis Viruses.

FEATURE	HEPATITIS A	HEPATITIS B	HEPATITIS C	HEPATITIS D	HEPATITIS E	HEPATITIS G
1. *Agent*	HAV	HBV	HCV	HDV	HEV	HGV
2. *Year identified*	1973	1965	1989	1977	1980	1995
3. *Viral particle*	27 nm	42 nm	30-60 nm	35-37 nm	32-34 nm	?
4. *Genome*	RNA, ss, linear	DNA, ss/ds	RNA, ss, linear circular	RNA, ss, circular	RNA, ss, linear	RNA, ss, linear
5. *Morphology*	Icosahedral non-enveloped	Double-shelled, enveloped	Enveloped	Enveloped, replication defective	Icosahedral, non-enveloped	?
6. *Spread*	Faeco-oral	Parenteral, close contact	Parenteral, close contact	Parenteral, close contact	Water-borne	Parenteral
7. *Incubation period*	15-45 days	30-180 days	20-90 days	30-50 days (In superinfection)	15-60 days	?
8. *Antigen(s)*	HAV	HBsAg HBcAg HBeAg HBxAg	HCV RNA C 100-3 C 33c NS5	HBsAg HDV	HEV	?
9. *Antibodies*	anti-HAV	anti-HBs anti-HBc anti-HBe	anti-HCV	anti-HBs anti-HDV	anti-HEV	?
10. *Severity*	Mild	Occasionally severe	Moderate	Occasionally severe	Mild	?
11. *Chronic hepatitis*	None	Occasional	Common	Common	None	?
12. *Carrier state*	None	<1%	<1%	1-10%	Unknown	1-2%
13. *Hepatocellular carcinoma*	No	+	+	±	None	?
14. *Prognosis*	Excellent	Worse with age	Moderate	Acute good; chronic poor	Good	?

ss= single-stranded; ss/ds= partially single-stranded partially double-stranded.

transmitted parenterally such as in recipients of blood and blood products, intravenous drug addicts, patients treated by renal dialysis and hospital workers exposed to blood, and by intimate physical contact such as from mother to child and sexually. The disease may occur at any age. HBV infection causes more severe form of illness that includes: acute hepatitis B, chronic hepatitis, progression to cirrhosis, fulminant hepatitis and an asymptomatic carrier stage. HBV plays some role in the development of hepatocellular carcinoma as discussed later (page 654).

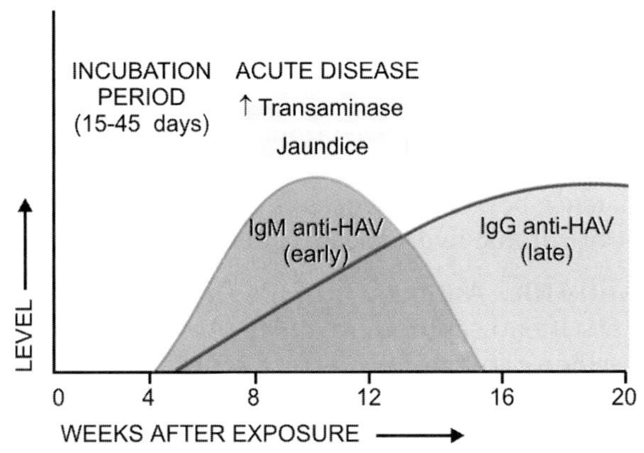

FIGURE 19.6

Sequence of appearance of antibodies to HAV.

HEPATITIS B VIRUS (HBV). The etiologic agent for hepatitis B, HBV, is a DNA virus which has been extensively studied. Electron microscopic studies on serum of patients infected with HBV show 3 forms of viral particles of 2 sizes—small (spheres and tubules/ filaments) and large (spheres) as under:

i) *Small particles* are most numerous and are in two forms: as 22 nm spheres, and as tubules 22 nm in diameter and 100 nm long. These are antigenically identical to envelope protein of HBV and represent excess of viral envelope protein referred as hepatitis B surface antigen (HBsAg).

ii) *Large particles,* 42 nm in diameter, are double-shelled spherical particles, also called as *Dane particles.* These are about 100 to 1000 times less in number in serum compared to small 22 nm particles and represent intact virion of HBV.

The genomic structure of HBV is quite compact and complex. The HBV DNA consists of 4 overlapping genes which encode for multiple proteins (Fig 19.7):

1. *S gene* codes for the major surface envelope protein, hepatitis B surface antigen (HBsAg). HBsAg is present on the outer surface of the large spherical particles as well as in small spherical and tubular structures. *Pre-S1 and pre-S2* regions of genome which are upstream of S gene, code for two other large proteins.

2. *P gene* is the largest and codes for DNA polymerase.

3. *C gene* codes for two nucleocapsid proteins, HBeAg and a core protein termed HBcAg.

4. *X gene* codes for HBxAg having a role in activation and transcription of viral and cellular genes and may actually contribute to carcinogenesis by binding with *TP53.*

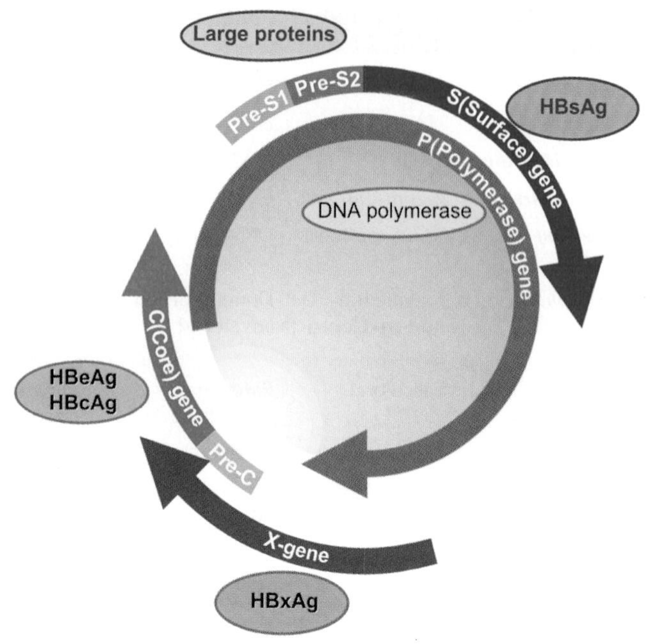

FIGURE 19.7
Genomic structure of Hepatitis B virus (Dane particle).

PATHOGENESIS. The evidence linking immunopathogenetic mechanism with hepatocellular damage is much stronger in HBV infection than with HAV infection. In support of immune pathogenesis is the demonstration of several immunological markers (serologic as well as viral), and molecular and morphologic evidence that hepatocytic damage is initiated by virus-infected CD8+T cytotoxic cells.

Serologic and viral markers. Various immunological markers indicative of presence of HBV infection can be demonstrated in the sera as well as in the hepatocytes of infected individuals. These are as under (Fig. 19.8):

1. HBsAg. In 1965, Blumberg and colleagues in Philadelphia found a lipoprotein complex in the serum of a multiple-transfused haemophiliac of Australian aborigine which was subsequently shown by them to be associated with serum hepatitis. This antigen was termed *Australia antigen* by them (In 1977, Blumberg was awarded the Nobel Prize for his discovery). The term Australia antigen is now used synonymous with hepatitis B surface antigen (HBsAg). HBsAg appears early in the blood after about 6 weeks of infection and its detection is an indicator of active HBV infection. It usually disappears in 3-6 months. Its persistence for more than 6 months implies a carrier state. HBsAg may also be demonstrated in the cell membrane of hepatocytes of carriers and chronic hepatitis patients by *Orcein staining* (orange positivity) but not in the hepatocytes during acute stage of illness.

2. Anti-HBs. Specific antibody to HBsAg in serum called anti-HBs appears late, about 3 months after the onset. Anti-HBs response may be both IgM and IgG type. The prevalence rate of anti-HBs ranges from 10-15%. In these individuals it persists for life providing protection against reinfection with HBV.

3. HBeAg. HBeAg derived from core protein is present transiently (3-6 weeks) during an acute attack. Its persistence beyond 10 weeks is indicative of development of chronic liver disease and carrier state.

4. Anti-HBe. Antibody to HBeAg called anti-HBe appears after disappearance of HBeAg. Seroconversion from HBeAg to anti-HBe during acute stage of illness is a prognostic sign for resolution of infection.

5. HBcAg. HBcAg derived from core protein cannot be detected in the blood. But HBcAg can be demonstrated in the nuclei of hepatocytes in carrier state and

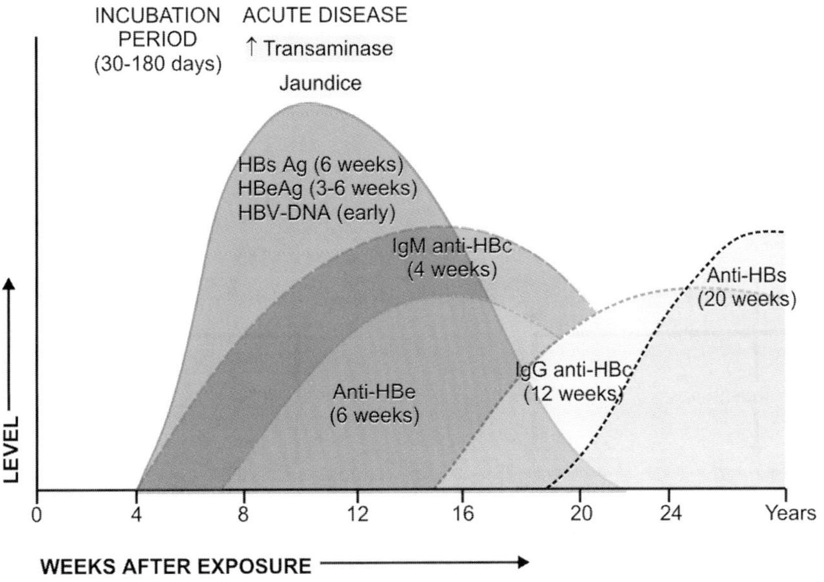

FIGURE 19.8

Sequence of serologic and viral markers in acute hepatitis B.

in chronic hepatitis patients by Orcein staining but not in the liver cells during acute stage.

6. Anti-HBc. Antibody to HBcAg called anti-HBc can, however, be detected in the serum of acute hepatitis B patients during pre-icteric stage. Anti-HBc may be IgM or IgG class antibody. IgM anti-HBc persists for 4-6 months and is followed later by IgG anti-HBc. Thus detection of high titre of IgM anti-HBc is indicative of recent acute HBV infection, while elevated level of IgG anti-HBc suggests HBV infection in the remote past.

7. HBV-DNA. Detection of HBV-DNA by molecular hybridisation using the Southern blot technique is the most sensitive index of hepatitis B infection. It is present in pre-symptomatic phase and transiently during early acute stage.

Hepatitis D

Infection with delta virus (HDV) in the hepatocyte nuclei of HBsAg-positive patients is termed hepatitis D. HDV is a defective virus for which HBV is the helper. Thus, hepatitis D develops when there is concomitant hepatitis B infection. HDV infection and hepatitis B may be simultaneous *(co-infection)*, or HDV may infect a chronic HBsAg carrier *(superinfection)* (Fig. 19.9):

- With **coinfection,** acute hepatitis D may range from mild to fulminant hepatitis but fulminant hepatitis is more likely in such simultaneous delta infection. Chronicity rarely develops in coinfection.
- With **superinfection,** (incubation period 30-35 days), chronic HBV infection gets worsened indicated by appearance of severe and fulminant acute attacks, progression of carrier stage to chronic delta hepatitis or acceleration towards cirrhosis. Hepatocellular carcinoma is, however, less common in HBsAg carriers with HDV infection.

HDV infection is worldwide in distribution though the incidence may vary in different countries. Endemic regions are Southern Europe, Middle-East, South India and parts of Africa. The high risk individuals for HDV infection are the same as for HBV infection i.e. intravenous drug abusers, homosexuals, transfusion recipients, and health care workers.

HEPATITIS DELTA VIRUS (HDV). The etiologic agent, HDV, is a small single-stranded RNA particle with a diameter of 36 nm. It is double-shelled—the outer shell consists of HBsAg and the inner shell consists of delta antigen provided by a circular RNA strand. It is highly infectious and can induce hepatitis in any HBsAg-positive host. HDV replication and proliferation takes place within the nuclei of liver cells. Markers for HDV infection include the following:

1. *HDV identification* in the blood and in the liver cell nuclei.

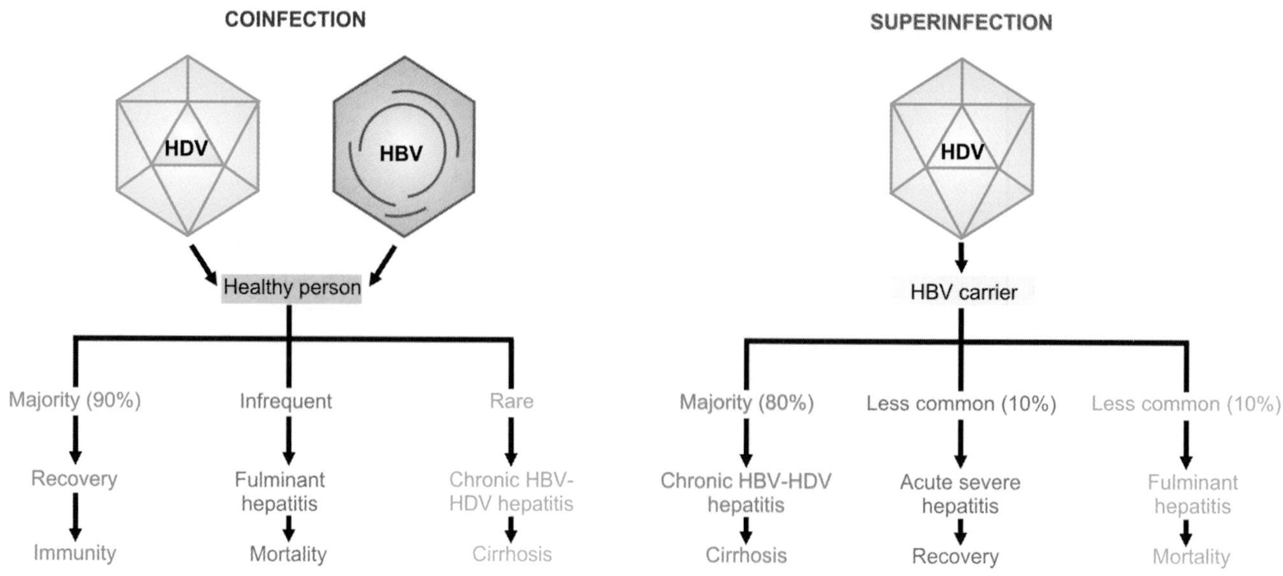

FIGURE 19.9

Consequences of coinfection *versus* superinfection in combined HDV-HBV infection.

2. *HDAg* detectable in the blood and on fixed liver tissue specimens.

3. *Anti-HD antibody* in acute hepatitis which is initially IgM type and later replaced by IgG type anti-HD antibody which persists for life to confer immunity against reinfection.

PATHOGENESIS. HDV, unlike HBV, is thought to cause direct cytopathic effect on hepatocytes. However, there are examples of transmission of HDV infection from individuals who themselves have not suffered from any attack of hepatitis, suggesting that it may not be always cytopathic. Thus, the exact mechanism remains unresolved.

Hepatitis C

The diagnosis of a third major category of hepatitis was earlier made after exclusion of infection with other known hepatitis viruses and was designated non-A, non-B (NANB) hepatitis. However, now this third type has been characterised and is called hepatitis C.

Hepatitis C infection is acquired by blood transfusions, blood products, haemodialysis, parenteral drug abuse and accidental cuts and needle-pricks in health workers. About 90% of post-transfusion hepatitis is of hepatitis C type. About 1-2% of volunteer blood donors and up to 5% of professional blood donors are carriers of HCV. Hepatitis C has an incubation period of 20-90 days (mean 50 days). Clinically, acute HCV hepatitis is milder than HBV hepatitis but HCV has a higher rate of progression to chronic hepatitis than HBV. Persistence of infection and chronic hepatitis are the key features of HCV. Occurrence of cirrhosis after 5 to 10 years and progression to hepatocellular carcinoma are other consequences of HCV infection. Currently, HCV is considered more important cause of chronic liver disease worldwide than HBV.

HEPATITIS C VIRUS (HCV). HCV is a single-stranded, enveloped RNA virus, having a diameter of 30-60 nm. HCV genome has about 3000 amino acids. The genomic organisation of HCV shows a 5′ terminal end, C (capsid) region and the envelope regions E1 and E2 in the exons (Fig. 19.10).

The viral proteins result in corresponding serologic and virologic markers for HCV infection as under (Fig. 19.11):

1. *Anti-HCV antibodies.* Three generations of anti-HCV IgG assays are available:

i) First generation antibodies are against C100-3 region proteins and appear 1 to 3 months after infection.

ii) Second generation antibodies are against C200 and C33c proteins and appear about one month earlier than the first generation.

iii) Third generation antibodies are against C22-3 and NS-5 region proteins and are detected even earlier.

2. *HCV-RNA.* HCV infection is, however, confirmed by HCV-RNA employing PCR technique which can be

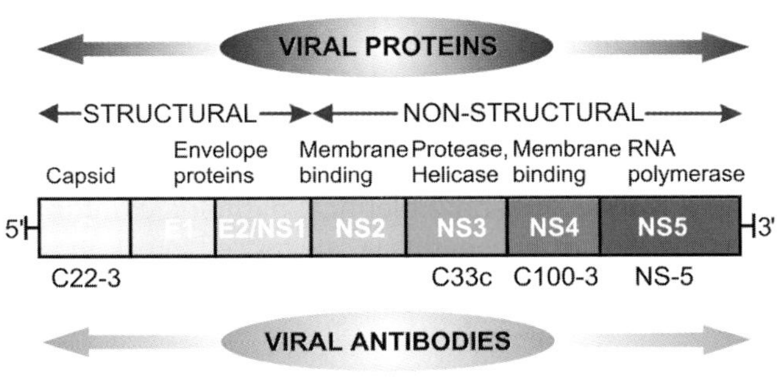

FIGURE 19.10

Diagrammatic structure of hepatitis C virus.

detected within a few days after exposure to HCV infection, much before appearance of anti-HCV and persists for the duration of HCV infection.

PATHOGENESIS. How HCV causes liver cell injury is not yet clearly established. HCV virions have not been identified in hepatocytes. Cell-mediated immune mechanism certainly play a role in hepatocytic injury due to HCV. Perhaps, HCV infection of lymphoid cells may play a role in immunologic injury to hepatocytes. In patients with chronic HCV hepatitis, HCV-specific CD4+ T cells and HLA-restricted CD8+ T cells have been identified. Viral and host crossreacting antibodies to liver and kidney microsomal antigen (anti-LKM) have been reported in a subset of patients that explains the association of autoimmune hepatitis and HCV hepatitis.

Hepatitis E

Hepatitis E is an enterically-transmitted virus, previously labelled as epidemic or enterically transmitted type of non-A non-B hepatitis. The infection occurs in young or middle-aged individuals, primarily in India, other Asian countries, Africa and central America.

The infection is generally acquired by contamination of water supplies such as after monsoon flooding. However, compared with HAV, secondary person-to-person infection does not occur with HEV. Thus HEV has some common epidemiologic features with HAV. HEV infection has a particularly high mortality in pregnant women but is otherwise a self-limited disease and has not been associated with chronic liver disease.

HEPATITIS E VIRUS (HEV). HEV is a single-stranded 32-34 nm, icosahedral non-enveloped virus. The virus has been isolated from stools, bile and liver of infected persons. Serologic markers for HEV include the following:

1. Anti-HEV antibodies of both IgM and IgG class.
2. HEV-RNA.

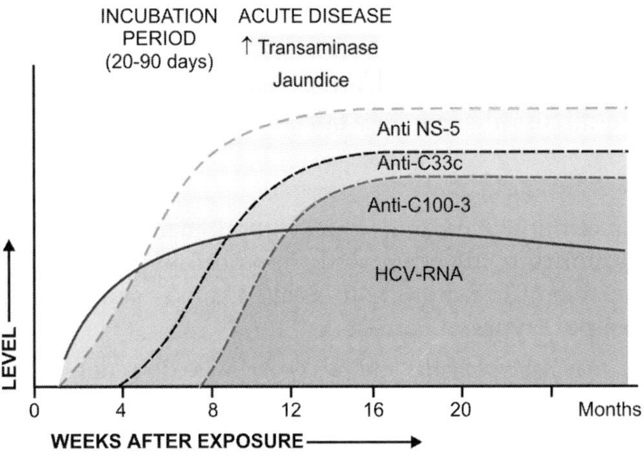

FIGURE 19.11

Sequence of serologic and viral markers of HCV infection.

However, testing for these markers for HEV is currently not available.

Hepatitis G

A virus distinct from the foregoing hepatitis viruses has been designated separately by two groups of workers as hepatitis G (HGV) and hepatitis F (HFV) virus. Like HCV, HGV is a blood-borne infection and may cause acute and chronic viral hepatitis.

HEPATITIS G VIRUS (HGV). HGV is a single-stranded RNA virus. At present HGV infection has been found in blood donors and is transmitted by blood transfusion. The virus has been identified by PCR amplification technique.

CLINICOPATHOLOGIC SPECTRUM

Among of the various etiologic types of hepatitis, evidence linking HBV and HCV infection with the spectrum of clinicopathologic changes is stronger than with other hepatotropic viruses. The typical pathologic changes of hepatitis by all hepatotropic viruses are virtually similar. HAV and HEV, however, do not have a carrier stage or cause chronic hepatitis. The various clinical patterns and pathologic consequences of different hepatotropic viruses can be considered under the following headings:

i) Carrier state
ii) Asymptomatic infection
iii) Acute hepatitis
iv) Chronic hepatitis
v) Fulminant hepatitis (Submassive to massive necrosis)

In addition, progression to cirrhosis (page 644) and association with hepatocellular carcinoma (page 654) are known to occur in certain types of hepatitis which are discussed separately later.

I. Carrier State

An asymptomatic individual without manifest disease, harbouring infection with hepatotropic virus and capable of transmitting it is called carrier state. There can be 2 types of carriers:

1. An *'asymptomatic healthy carrier'* who does not suffer from ill-effects of the virus infection.
2. An *'asymptomatic carrier with chronic disease'* capable of transmitting the organisms.

As stated before, hepatitis A and E do not produce the carrier state. Hepatitis B is responsible for the largest number of carriers in the world, while concomitant infection with HDV more often causes progressive disease rather than an asymptomatic carrier state. An estimated 2-3% of the general population are asymptomatic carriers of HCV. Data on HBV carrier state reveal role of 2 important factors rendering the individual more vulnerable to harbour the organisms—*early age at infection* and *impaired immunity.* Whereas approximately 10% of adults contracting hepatitis B infection develop carrier state, 90% of infected neonates fail to clear HBsAg from the serum within 6 months and become HBV carriers.

Clinical recognition of carrier state of HBV is more frequently done by detection of HBsAg in the serum and less often by other markers such as HBeAg, HBcAg and antibodies. Concomitant infection of HDV with HBV depends upon the demonstration of anti-HD.

PATHOLOGIC CHANGES. Carriers of HBV may or may not show changes on liver biopsy.

- *Healthy HBV carriers* may show no changes or minor hepatic change such as presence of finely granular, ground-glass, eosinophilic cytoplasm as evidence of HBsAg.
- *Asymptomatic carriers with chronic disease* may show changes of chronic hepatitis and even cirrhosis.

II. Asymptomatic Infection

These are cases who are detected incidentally to have infection with one of the hepatitis viruses as revealed by their raised serum transaminases or by detection of the presence of antibodies but are otherwise asymptomatic.

III. Acute Hepatitis

The most common consequence of all hepatotropic viruses is acute inflammatory involvement of the entire liver. In general, type A, B, C, D and E run similar clinical course and show identical pathologic findings.

Clinically, acute hepatitis is categorised into 4 phases: incubation period, pre-icteric phase, icteric phase and post-icteric phase.

1. Incubation period: It varies among different hepatotropic viruses: for hepatitis A it is about 4 weeks (15-45 days); for hepatitis B the average is 10 weeks (30-180 days); for hepatitis D about 6 weeks (30-50 days); for hepatitis C the mean incubation period is about 7 weeks (20-90 days), and for hepatitis E it is 2-8 weeks (15-60 days). The patient remains asymptomatic during incubation period but the infectivity is highest during the last days of incubation period.

2. Pre-icteric phase: This phase is marked by prodromal constitutional symptoms that include anorexia, nausea, vomiting, fatigue, malaise, distaste for smoking, arthralgia and headache. There may be low-grade fever preceding the onset of jaundice, especially in hepatitis A. The earliest laboratory evidence of hepatocellular injury in pre-icteric phase is the elevation of transaminases.

3. Icteric phase: The prodromal period is heralded by the onset of clinical jaundice and the constitutional symptoms diminish. Other features include dark-coloured urine due to bilirubinuria, clay-coloured stools due to cholestasis, pruritus as a result of elevated serum bile acids, loss of weight and abdominal discomfort due to enlarged, tender liver. The diagnosis is based on deranged liver function tests (e.g. elevated levels of serum bilirubin, transaminases and alkaline phosphatase; prolonged prothrombin time and hyperglobulinaemia) and serologic detection of hepatitis antigens and antibodies.

4. Post-icteric phase: The icteric phase lasting for about 1 to 4 weeks is usually followed by clinical and biochemical recovery in 2 to 12 weeks. The recovery phase is more prolonged in hepatitis B and hepatitis C. Up to 1% cases of acute hepatitis may develop severe form of the disease (fulminant hepatitis); and 5-10% of cases progress on to chronic hepatitis. Evolution into the carrier state (except in HAV and HEV infection) has already been described above.

PATHOLOGIC CHANGES. ***Grossly,*** the liver is slightly enlarged, soft and greenish.

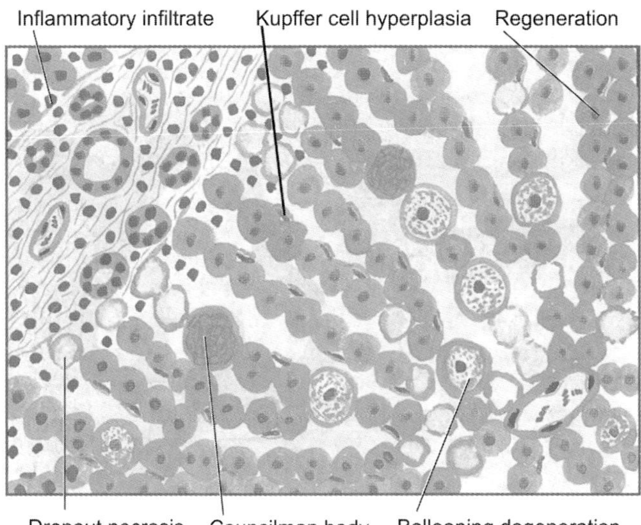

FIGURE 19.12

Acute viral hepatitis. The predominant histologic changes are: variable degree of necrosis of hepatocytes, most marked in zone 3 (centrilobular); and mononuclear cellular infiltrate, chiefly in zone 1 (portal area). Mild degree of liver cell necrosis is seen as ballooning degeneration while acidophilic Councilman bodies are indicative of more severe liver cell injury.

Histologically, the changes are as follows (Fig. 19.12) (COLOUR PLATE XXV: CL 97):

1. Hepatocellular injury: There may be variation in the degree of liver cell injury but it is most marked in zone 3 (centrilobular zone):

i) Mildly injured hepatocytes appear swollen with granular cytoplasm which tends to condense around the nucleus *(ballooning degeneration).*

ii) Others show acidophilic degeneration in which the cytoplasm becomes intensely eosinophilic, the nucleus becomes small and pyknotic and is eventually extruded from the cell, leaving behind necrotic, acidophilic mass called *Councilman body* or *acidophil body* by the process known as apoptosis.

iii) Another type of hepatocellular necrosis is *dropout necrosis* in which isolated or small clusters of hepatocytes undergo lysis.

iv) *Bridging necrosis* is a more severe form of hepatocellular injury in acute viral hepatitis and may progress to fulminant hepatitis or chronic hepatitis (page 633). Bridging necrosis is characterised by bands of necrosis linking portal tracts to central hepatic veins, one central hepatic vein to another, or a portal tract to another tract.

2. Inflammatory infiltrate: There is infiltration by mononuclear inflammatory cells, usually in the portal tracts, but may permeate into the lobules.

3. Kupffer cell hyperplasia: There is reactive hyperplasia of Kupffer cells many of which contain phagocytosed cellular debris, bile pigment and lipofuscin granules.

4. Cholestasis: Biliary stasis is usually not severe in viral hepatitis and may be present as intracytoplasmic bile pigment granules.

5. Regeneration: As a result of necrosis of hepatocytes, there is lobular disarray. Surviving adjacent hepatocytes undergo regeneration and hyperplasia. If the necrosis causes collapse of reticulin framework of the lobule, healing by fibrosis follows, distorting the lobular architecture.

The above histologic changes apply generally to viral hepatitis by various types of hepatotropic viruses and by HBV in particular. In general, it is not possible to distinguish histologically between viral hepatitis of various etiologies, the following morphologic features may help in giving an etiologic clue:

- **HAV hepatitis** is a panlobular involvement by heavy inflammatory infiltrate compared to other types.
- **HCV hepatitis** causes milder necrosis, with fatty change in hepatocytes, presence of lymphoid aggregates in the portal triads and degeneration of bile duct epithelium.

IV. Chronic Hepatitis

Chronic hepatitis is defined as continuing or relapsing hepatic disease for more than 6 months with symptoms alongwith biochemical, serologic and histopathologic evidence of inflammation and necrosis. Majority of cases of chronic hepatitis are the result of infection with hepatotropic viruses—hepatitis B, hepatitis C and combined hepatitis B and hepatitis D infection. However, some non-viral causes of chronic hepatitis include: Wilson's disease, α-1-antitrypsin deficiency, chronic alcoholism, drug-induced injury and autoimmune diseases. The last named gives rise to *autoimmune or lupoid hepatitis* which is characterised by positive serum autoantibodies (e.g. antinuclear, anti-smooth muscle and anti-mitochondrial) and a positive LE cell test but negative for serologic markers of viral hepatitis.

Until recent years, prediction of prognosis of chronic hepatitis used to be made on the basis of morphology which divided it into 2 main types—*chronic persistent* and *chronic active (aggressive) hepatitis*. A third form, *chronic lobular hepatitis* is distinguished separately by some as mild form of lobular inflammation without inflammation of portal tracts but these cases often recover completely. However, subsequent studies have revealed that morphologic subtypes do not necessarily correlate with the prognosis since the disease is not essentially static but may vary from mild form to severe and *vice versa*. Besides, two other factors which determine the vulnerability of a patient of viral hepatitis to develop chronic hepatitis are: *impaired immunity* and *extremes of age* at which the infection is first contracted.

Currently, chronic hepatitis is classified on the basis of etiology. The frequency and severity with which hepatotropic viruses cause chronic hepatitis varies with the organisms as under:

- *HCV* infection accounts for 40-60% cases of chronicity in adults. HCV infection is particularly associated with progressive form of chronic hepatitis that may evolve into cirrhosis.
- *HBV* causes chronic hepatitis in 90% of infected infants and in about 5% adult cases of hepatitis B.
- *HDV* superinfection on HBV carrier state may be responsible for chronic hepatitis in 10-40% cases.
- *HAV and HEV* do not produce chronic hepatitis.

PATHOLOGIC CHANGES. The pathologic features are common to both HBV and HCV infection and include the following lesions (Fig. 19.13).

1. Piecemeal necrosis. Piecemeal necrosis is defined as periportal destruction of hepatocytes at the limiting plate (*piecemeal* = piece by piece). Its features in chronic hepatitis are:

i) Necrosed hepatocytes at the limiting plate in periportal zone.

ii) Interface hepatitis due to expanded portal tract by infiltration of lymphocytes, plasma cells and macrophages.

iii) Expanded portal tracts are often associated with proliferating bile ductules as a response to liver cell injury.

2. Portal tract lesions. All forms of chronic hepatitis are characterised by variable degree of changes in the portal tract.

i) Inflammatory cell infiltration by lymphocytes, plasma cells and macrophages (triaditis).

ii) Proliferated bile ductules in the expanded portal tracts.

iii) Additionally, chronic hepatitis C may show lymphoid aggregates or follicles with reactive germinal centre and infiltration of inflammatory cells in the damaged bile duct epithelial cells.

3. Intralobular lesions. Generally, the architecture of lobule is retained in mild to moderate chronic hepatitis.

i) There are focal areas of necrosis and inflammation within the hepatic parenchyma.

ii) Scattered acidophilic bodies in the lobule.

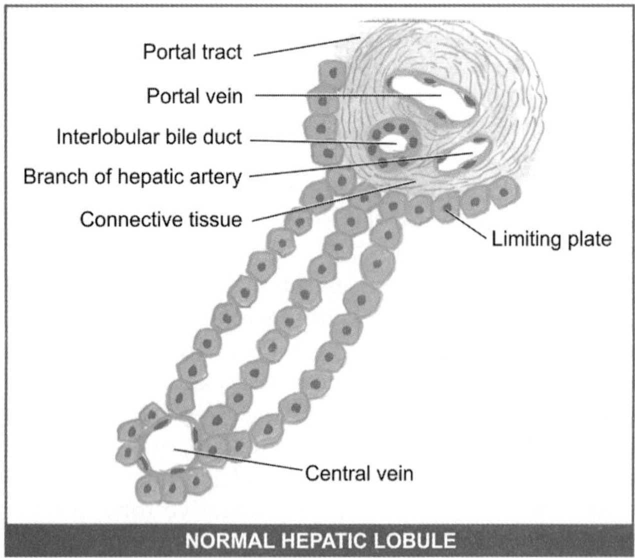

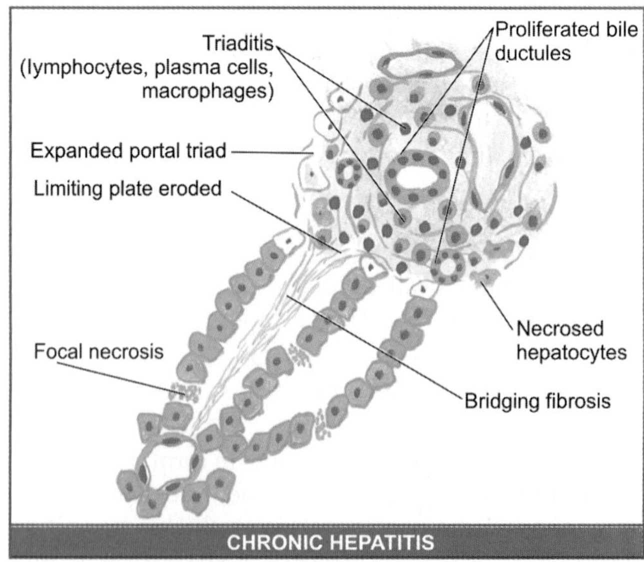

FIGURE 19.13

Diagrammatic representation of pathologic changes in chronic hepatitis.

iii) Kupffer cell hyperplasia.

iv) More severe form of injury shows bridging necrosis (i.e. bands of necrosed hepatocytes that may bridge portal tract-to-central vein, central vein-to-central vein, and portal tract-to-portal tract).

v) Regenerative changes in hepatocytes in cases of persistent hepatocellular necrosis.

vi) Cases of chronic hepatitis C show moderate fatty change.

vii) Cases of chronic hepatitis B show scattered ground-glass hepatocytes indicative of abundance of HBsAg in the cytoplasm.

4. Bridging fibrosis. The onset of fibrosis in chronic hepatitis from the area of interface hepatitis and bridging necrosis is a feature of irreversible damage.

i) At first, there is periportal fibrosis at the sites of interface hepatitis giving the portal tract stellate-shaped appearance.

ii) Progressive cases show bridging fibrosis connecting portal tract-to-portal tract or portal tract-to-central vein traversing the lobule.

iii) End stage of chronic hepatitis is characterised by dense collagenous septa destroying lobular architecture and forming nodules resulting in postnecrotic cirrhosis.

As prognostic indicator of chronic hepatitis, criteria have been evolved to classify chronic hepatitis by giving ***activity score*** (maximum score of 22; ranging from minimal/mild to moderate and severe) based on the following features:

- *periportal necrosis i.e. piecemeal necrosis and/or bridging necrosis* (ranging from score 0 as 'no necrosis' to score 10 as 'multilobular necrosis');
- *extent and depth of inflammation* (ranging from grade 0 as 'no inflammation' to grade 4 having 'marked portal inflammation'); and
- *extent and density of fibrosis* (ranging from score 0 as 'no fibrosis' to score 4 as 'cirrhosis').

A correlation of contemporary classification based on activity score and previous classification of chronic hepatitis is given in Table 19.7.

CLINICAL FEATURES. The clinical features of chronic hepatitis are quite variable ranging from mild disease to full blown picture of cirrhosis.

i) Mild chronic hepatitis shows only slight but persistent elevation of transaminases ('transaminitis') with fatigue, malaise and loss of appetite.

ii) Other cases may show mild hepatomegaly, hepatic tenderness and mild splenomegaly.

TABLE 19.7: Correlation of Older Classification and Activity Score in Chronic Hepatitis.

OLD CLASSIFICATION	ACTIVITY SCORE
Chronic persistent hepatitis	Mild activity, no or minimal fibrosis
Chronic lobular hepatitis	Mild to moderate activity, mild fibrosis
Chronic active hepatitis	Moderate to severe activity and fibrosis

iii) Laboratory findings may reveal prolonged prothrombin time, hyperbilirubinaemia, hyperglobulinaemia and markedly elevated alkaline phosphatase.

iv) Systemic features of circulating immune complexes due to HBV and HCV infection may produce features of immune complex vasculitis, glomerulonephritis and cryoglobulinaemia in a proportion of cases.

However, clinical features do not correlate with morphologic appearance of the liver biopsy. Some patients may have mild form of disease without progressing for several years while others may show rapid evolution into cirrhosis with its complications over a period of few years. Patients of long-standing HBV and HCV infection are known to evolve into hepatocellular carcinoma.

V. Fulminant Hepatitis (Submassive to Massive Necrosis)

Fulminant hepatitis is the most severe form of acute hepatitis in which there is rapidly progressive hepatocellular failure. Two patterns are recognised—*submassive necrosis* having a less rapid course extending up to 3 months; and *massive necrosis* in which the liver failure is rapid and fulminant occurring in 2-3 weeks.

Fulminant hepatitis of either of the two varieties can occur from viral and non-viral etiologies:

- *Acute viral hepatitis* accounts for about half the cases, most often from HBV and HCV; less frequently from combined HBV-HDV and rarely from HAV. However, HEV infection is a serious complication in pregnant women. In addition, herpesvirus can also cause serious viral hepatitis.
- *Non-viral causes* include acute hepatitis due to drug toxicity (e.g. acetaminophen, non-steroidal anti-inflammatory drugs, isoniazid, halothane and anti-depressants), poisonings, hypoxic injury and massive infiltration of malignant tumours into the liver.

The patients present with features of hepatic failure with hepatic encephalopathy (page 621). The mortality rate is high if hepatic transplantation is not undertaken.

PATHOLOGIC CHANGES. Grossly, the liver is small and shrunken, often weighing 500-700 gm. The capsule is loose and wrinkled. The sectioned surface shows diffuse or random involvement of hepatic lobes. There are extensive areas of muddy-red and yellow necrosis (previously called *acute yellow atrophy*) and patches of green bile staining.

Histologically, two forms of fulminant necrosis are distinguished—submassive and massive necrosis.

i) In **submassive necrosis,** large groups of hepatocytes in zone 3 (centrilobular area) and zone 2 (mid zone) are wiped out leading to a collapsed reticulin framework. Regeneration in submassive necrosis is more orderly and may result in restoration of normal architecture.

ii) In **massive necrosis,** the entire liver lobules are necrotic. As a result of loss of hepatic parenchyma, all that is left is the collapsed and condensed reticulin framework and portal tracts with proliferated bile ductules plugged with bile. Inflammatory infiltrate is scanty. Regeneration, if it takes place, is disorderly forming irregular masses of hepatocytes. Fibrosis is generally not a feature of fulminant hepatitis (Fig. 19.14).

The clinicopathologic course in two major forms of hepatitis, HBV and HCV, is summarised in Fig. 19.15.

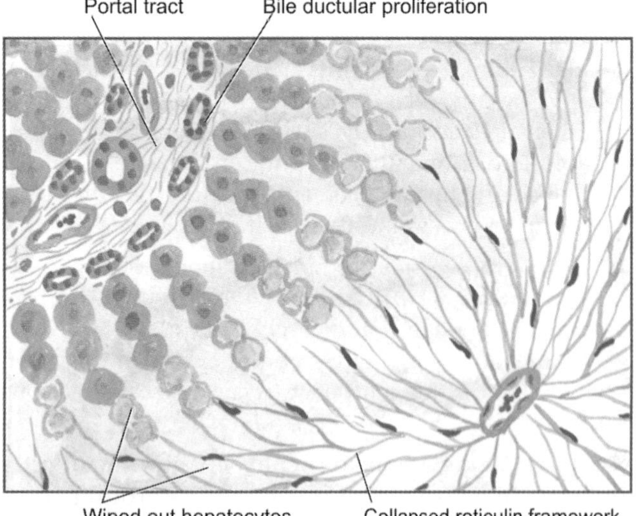

FIGURE 19.14

Fulminant hepatitis. There is complete wiping out of liver lobules with only collapsed reticulin framework left out in their place. There is no significant inflammation or fibrosis.

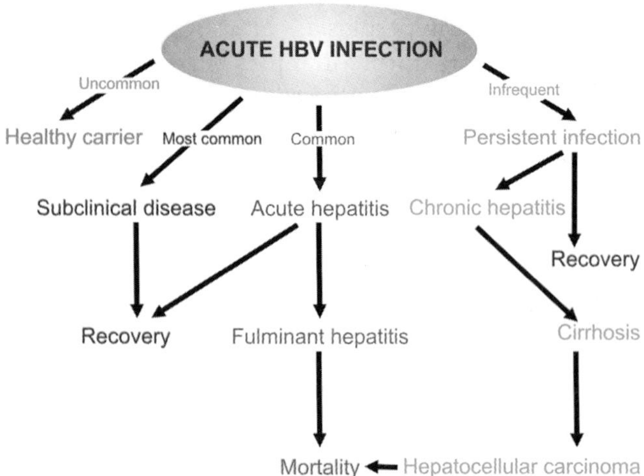

FIGURE 19.15

Clinicopathologic course of HBV and HCV infection.

IMMUNOPROPHYLAXIS AND HEPATITIS VACCINES

Best prophylaxis against the viral hepatitis remains prevention of its spread to the contacts after detection and identification of route by which infection is acquired such as from food or water contamination, sexual spread or parenteral spread. Of late, however, immunoprophylaxis and a few hepatitis vaccines have been developed and some more are under development. The principle underlying either of these two forms of prophylaxis is that the persons who develop good antibody response to the antigen of the hepatotropic virus following active infection are protected against the disease on reinfection. Thus, pre-testing of persons may be carried out so as to determine their antibody level. Immunoprophylaxis and hepatitis vaccination are unnecessary if the pre-testing for antibodies is positive.

1. Hepatitis A. Passive immunisation with immune globulin as well as active immunisation with a killed vaccine are available.

2. Hepatitis B. Earlier, only passive immunoprophylaxis with standard immune globulin was used. Later, active immunisation against HBsAg was introduced. Current recommendations include pre-exposure and post-exposure prophylaxis with recombinant hepatitis B vaccine:

■ *Pre-exposure prophylaxis* is done for individuals at high-risk e.g. health care workers, haemodialysis patients and staff, haemophiliacs, intravenous drug users etc. Three intramuscular injections of hepatitis vaccine at 0, 1 and 6 months are recommended.

■ *Post-exposure prophylaxis* is carried out for unvaccinated persons exposed to HBV infection and includes prophylaxis with combination of hepatitis B immune globulin and hepatitis B vaccine.

3. Hepatitis D. Hepatitis D infection can also be prevented by hepatitis B vaccine.

4. Hepatitis C. Currently, hepatitis C vaccine has yet not been feasible though antibodies to HCV envelope have been developed.

5. Hepatitis E. It is not certain whether immune globulin (like for HAV) prevents hepatitis E infection or not but a vaccine against HEV is yet to be developed.

OTHER INFECTIONS AND INFESTATIONS

Apart from viral hepatitis, the liver is affected by infections with bacteria, spirochaetes and fungi and is involved in some parasitic infestations. Some common examples of such conditions are described below.

CHOLANGITIS

Cholangitis is the term used to describe inflammation of the extrahepatic or intrahepatic bile ducts, or both. There are two main types of cholangitis—pyogenic and primary sclerosing. While primary sclerosing cholangitis is discussed later with biliary cirrhosis (page 646), pyogenic cholangitis is described below.

Pyogenic Cholangitis

Cholangitis occurring secondary to obstruction of a major extrahepatic duct causes pyogenic cholangitis. Most commonly, the obstruction is from impacted gallstone; other causes are carcinoma arising in the extrahepatic ducts, carcinoma head of pancreas, acute pancreatitis and inflammatory strictures in the bile duct. Bacteria gain entry to the obstructed duct and proliferate in the bile. Infection spreads along the branches of obstructed duct and reaches the liver, termed *ascending cholangitis.* The common infecting bacteria are enteric organisms such as *E.coli, Klebsiella* and *Enterobacter.*

PATHOLOGIC CHANGES. The affected ducts show small beaded abscesses accompanied by bile stasis along their course and larger abscesses within the liver. The abscesses are composed of acute inflammatory cells which in time are replaced by chronic inflammatory cells and enclosed by fibrous capsule.

PYOGENIC LIVER ABSCESS

Most liver abscesses are of bacterial (pyogenic) origin; less often they are amoebic, hydatid and rarely actinomycotic. Pyogenic liver abscesses are becoming uncommon due to improved diagnostic facilities and the early use of antibiotics. However, their incidence is higher in old age and in immunosuppressed patients such as in AIDS, transplant recipients and those on intensive chemotherapy.

Pyogenic liver abscesses are classified on the basis of the mode of entry. These are:

1. *Ascending cholangitis* through ascending infection in the biliary tract due to obstruction e.g. gallstones, cancer, sclerosing cholangitis and biliary strictures.
2. *Portal pyaemia* by means of spread of pelvic or gastrointestinal infection resulting in portal pylephlebitis or septic emboli e.g. from appendicitis, empyema of gallbladder, diverticulitis, regional enteritis, pancreatitis, infected haemorrhoids and neonatal umbilical vein sepsis.
3. *Septicaemia* through spread by hepatic artery.
4. *Direct infection* resulting in solitary liver abscess e.g. from adjacent perinephric abscess, secondary infection in amoebic liver abscess, metastasis and formation of haematoma following trauma.
5. *Iatrogenic causes* include liver biopsy, percutaneous biliary drainage and accidental surgical trauma.
6. *Cryptogenic* from unknown causes, especially in the elderly.

The commonest infecting organisms are gram-negative bacteria chiefly *E. coli;* others are *Pseudomonas, Klebsiella, Enterobacter* and a number of anaerobic organisms, bacteroides and actinomyces.

Liver abscesses are clinically characterised by pain in the right upper quadrant, fever, tender hepatomegaly and sometimes jaundice. Laboratory examination reveals leucocytosis, elevated serum alkaline phosphatase, hypoalbuminaemia and a positive blood culture.

PATHOLOGIC CHANGES. ***Grossly*** depending upon the cause for pyogenic liver abscess, they occur as single or multiple yellow abscesses, 1 cm or more in diameter, in an enlarged liver. A single abscess generally has a thick fibrous capsule. The abscesses are particularly common in right lobe of the liver (Fig. 19.16).

Microscopically, typical features of abscess are seen. There are multiple small neutrophilic abscesses with areas of extensive necrosis of the affected liver parenchyma. The adjacent viable area shows pus and blood clots in the portal vein, inflammation, congestion and proliferating fibroblasts. Direct extension from the liver may lead to subphrenic or pleuro-

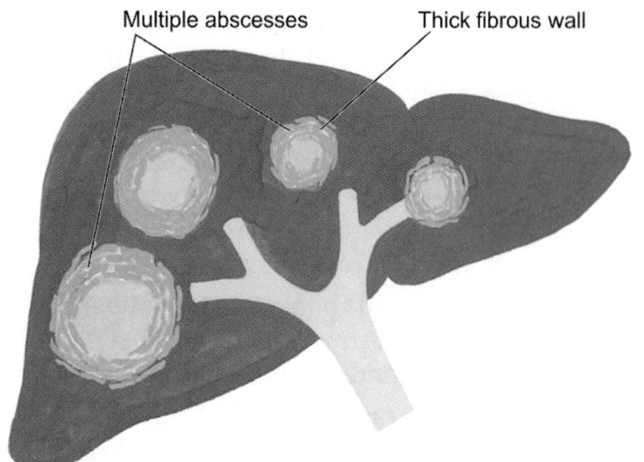

FIGURE 19.16
Macroscopic appearance of pyogenic abscesses in the liver.

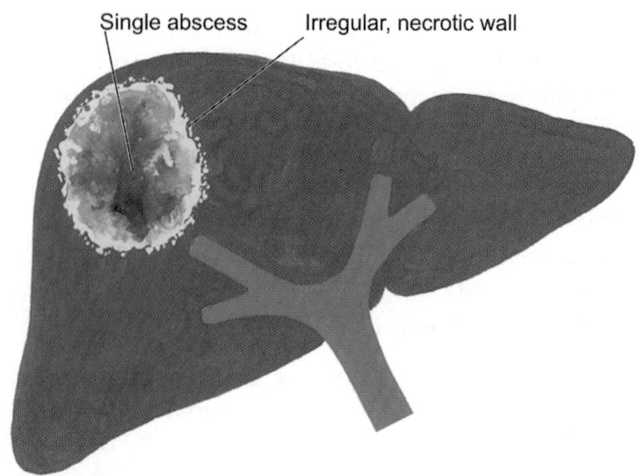

FIGURE 19.17
Amoebic liver abscess is commonly solitary and its wall is irregular and necrotic.

pulmonary suppuration or peritonitis. There may be small pyaemic abscesses elsewhere such as in the lungs, kidneys, brain and spleen.

AMOEBIC LIVER ABSCESS

Amoebic liver abscesses are less common than pyogenic liver abscesses and have many similar features. They are caused by the spread of *Entamoeba histolytica* from intestinal lesions. The trophozoite form of amoebae in the colon invade the colonic mucosa forming flask-shaped ulcers (page 194) from where they are carried to the liver in the portal venous system. Amoebae multiply and block small intrahepatic portal radicles resulting in infarction necrosis of the adjacent liver parenchyma.

The patients, generally from tropical and subtropical countries, may give history of amoebic dysentery in the past. Cysts of *E. histolytica* in stools are present in only 15% of patients of hepatic amoebiasis. Intermittent low-grade fever, pain and tenderness in the liver area are common presenting features. A positive haemagglutination test is quite sensitive and useful for diagnosis of amoebic liver abscess.

PATHOLOGIC CHANGES. Grossly, amoebic liver abscesses are usually solitary and more often located in the right lobe in the posterosuperior portion. Amoebic liver abscess may vary greatly in size but is generally of the size of an orange. The centre of the abscess contains large necrotic area having reddish-brown, thick pus resembling anchovy or chocolate sauce. The abscess wall consists of irregular shreds of necrotic liver tissue (Fig. 19.17).

Histologically, the necrotic area consists of degenerated liver cells, leucocytes, red blood cells, strands of connective tissue and debris. Amoebae are most easily found in the liver tissue at the margin of abscess. PAS-staining is employed to confirm the trophozoites of *E. histolytica.*

HEPATICTUBERCULOSIS

Tuberculosis of the liver occurs as a result of miliary dissemination from primary complex or from chronic adult pulmonary tuberculosis. The diagnosis is possible by liver biopsy. The patients may have unexplained fever, jaundice, hepatomegaly or hepatosplenomegaly. There may be elevated serum alkaline phosphatase levels and hyperglobulinaemia.

PATHOLOGIC CHANGES. The basic lesion is the epithelioid cell granuloma characterised by central caseation necrosis with destruction of the reticulin framework and peripheral cuff of lymphocytes. Ziehl-Neelsen staining for AFB or culture of the organism from the biopsy tissue is confirmatory. Rare lesions consist of tuberculous cholangitis and tuberculous pylephlebitis.

HYDATID DISEASE (ECHINOCOCCOSIS)

Hydatid disease occurs as a result of infection by the larval cyst stage of the tapeworm, *Echinococcus granulosus.* The dog is the common definite host, while man, sheep and cattle are the intermediate hosts. The dog is infected by eating the viscera of sheep containing hydatid cysts. The infected faeces of the dog contaminate grass and farmland from where the ova are ingested by sheep, pigs and man. Thus, man can acquire infection by handling dogs as well as by eating contaminated vegetables. The ova ingested by man are liberated from the chitinous wall by gastric juice and pass through the intestinal mucosa from where they are carried to the liver by portal venous system. These are trapped in the hepatic sinusoids where they eventually develop into hydatid cyst. About 70% of hydatid cysts develop in the liver which acts as the first filter for ova. However, ova which pass through the liver enter the right side of the heart and are caught in the pulmonary capillary bed and form pulmonary hydatid cysts. Some ova which enter the systemic circulation give rise to hydatid cysts in the brain, spleen, bone and muscles.

The disease is common in sheep-raising countries such as Australia, New Zealand and South America. The *uncomplicated hydatid cyst* of the liver may be silent or may produce dull ache in the liver area and some abdominal distension.

Complications of hydatid cyst include its rupture (e.g. into the peritoneal cavity, bile ducts and lungs), secondary infection and hydatid allergy due to sensitisation of the host with cyst fluid. The diagnosis is made by peripheral blood eosinophilia, radiologic examination and serologic tests such as indirect haemagglutination test and Casoni skin test.

PATHOLOGIC CHANGES. Hydatid cyst grows slowly and may eventually attain a size over 10 cm in diameter in about 5 years. *E. granulosus* generally causes unilocular hydatid cyst while *E. multilocularis* results in multilocular or alveolar hydatid disease in the liver.

The cyst wall is composed of 3 distinguishable zones—outer *pericyst*, intermediate characteristic *ectocyst* and inner *endocyst* (Fig. 19.18,A,B) (COLOUR PLATE IX: CL 36):

1. **Pericyst** is the outer host inflammatory reaction consisting of fibroblastic proliferation, mononuclear cells, eosinophils and giant cells, eventually developing into dense fibrous capsule which may even calcify.
2. **Ectocyst** is the intermediate layer composed of characteristic acellular, chitinous, laminated hyaline material.
3. **Endocyst** is the inner germinal layer bearing daughter cysts (brood-capsules) and scolices projecting into the lumen.

Hydatid sand is the grain-like material composed of numerous scolices present in the hydatid fluid. Hydatid fluid, in addition, contains antigenic proteins so that its liberation into circulation gives rise to pronounced eosinophilia or may cause anaphylaxis.

CHEMICAL AND DRUG INJURY

HEPATIC DRUG METABOLISM. The liver plays a central role in the metabolism of a large number of organic and inorganic chemicals and drugs which gain access to the body by inhalation, injection, or most commonly, via the intestinal tract. The main drug metabolising system resides in the microsomal fraction of the smooth endoplasmic reticulum of the liver cells via

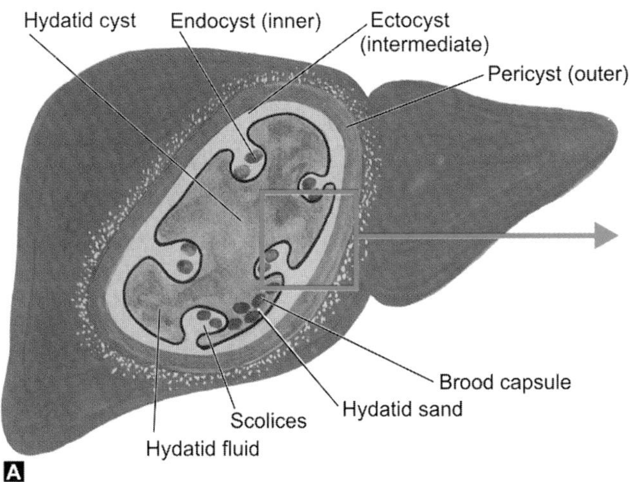

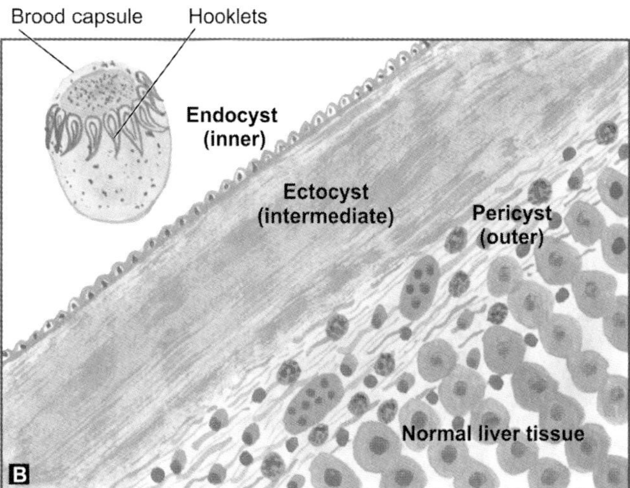

FIGURE 19.18

A, Hydatid cyst in the liver. B, Microscopy shows three layers in the wall of hydatid cyst.

P-450 cytochrome and cytochrome reductase enzyme systems. Other steps involved in the drug metabolism are its conjugation with an endogenous molecule, its active transport from the hepatocytes and ultimately its excretion in the bile or in urine depending upon the molecular weight of the substance. A number of risk factors predispose an individual to hepatic drug injury such as pre-existing liver disease, aging, female sex and genetic inability to perform a particular biotransformation.

HEPATOTOXICITY. Toxic liver injury produced by drugs and chemicals may virtually mimic any form of naturally-occurring liver disease. In fact, any patient presenting with liver disease or unexplained jaundice is thoroughly questioned about history of drug intake or exposure to chemicals. Hepatotoxicity from drugs and chemicals is the commonest form of iatrogenic disease. Severity of hepatotoxicity is greatly increased if the drug is continued after symptoms develop.

Among the various *inorganic compounds* producing hepatotoxicity are arsenic, phosphorus, copper and iron. *Organic agents* include certain naturally-occurring plant toxins such as pyrrolizidine alkaloids, mycotoxins and bacterial toxins. The synthetic group of organic compounds are a large number of medicinal agents. In addition, exposure to hepatotoxic compounds may be occupational, environmental or domestic that could be accidental, homicidal or suicidal ingestion.

In general, drug reactions affecting the liver are divided into two main classes:

1. Direct or predictable, when the drug or one of its metabolites is either directly toxic to the liver or it lowers the host immune defense mechanism. The adverse effects occur in most individuals who consume them and their hepatotoxicity is dose-dependent e.g. carbon tetrachloride.

2. Indirect or unpredictable or idiosyncratic, when the drug or one of its metabolites acts as a hapten and induces hypersensitivity in the host. The hepatotoxicity by this group does not occur regularly in all individuals and the effects are usually not dose-related e.g. acetaminophen.

A simplified clinicopathologic classification of important hepatic drug reactions and the agents causing them is presented in Table 19.8. The changes produced by hepatotoxic agents may vary from mild, which are diagnosed only by elevated serum transaminases, to instances of massive necrosis and death. The pathologic changes by hepatotoxins include 2 large categories:

1 *Acute liver disease* characterised by cholestasis, hepatocellular necrosis, fatty change, granulomatous reaction or vascular disease.

2. *Chronic liver disease* characterised by variable degree of fibrosis, cirrhosis or neoplasia.

As such, the pathologic changes induced by hepatotoxins are indistinguishable from the respective disease states.

CIRRHOSIS

Cirrhosis of the liver is a diffuse disease having the following 4 features:

TABLE 19.8: Classification of Hepatic Drug Reactions.

PATHOLOGIC CHANGES	AGENTS
A. Acute liver disease	
1. Zonal necrosis	Carbon tetrachloride Acetaminophen Halothane
2. Massive necrosis	Halothane Acetaminophen Methyl dopa
3. Fatty change	Tetracycline Salicylates Methotrexate Ethanol
4. Hepatitis	Methyl dopa Isoniazid Halothane Ketoconazole
5. Granuloma formation	Sulfonamides Methyl dopa Quinidine Allopurinol
6. Cholestasis	Sex hormones (including oral contraceptives) Chlorpromazine Nitrofurantoin
7. Veno-occlusive disease	Cytotoxic drugs
8. Hepatic/portal vein thrombosis	Oral contraceptives
B. Chronic liver disease	
1. Fibrosis-cirrhosis	Methotrexate
2. Focal nodular hyperplasia	Vinyl chloride Vitamin A Sex hormones
3. Adenoma	Sex hormones
4. Hepatocellular carcinoma	Sex hormones

Chapter Nineteen

1. It involves the entire liver.
2. The normal lobular architecture of hepatic parenchyma is disorganised.
3. There is formation of nodules separated from one another by irregular bands of fibrosis.
4. It occurs following hepatocellular necrosis of varying etiology so that there are alternate areas of necrosis and regenerative nodules.

However, regenerative nodules are not essential for diagnosis of cirrhosis since biliary cirrhosis and haemochromatosis have little regeneration. The fibrosis once developed is irreversible.

In the Western world, cirrhosis of the liver is one of the ten leading causes of death.

PATHOGENESIS

Irrespective of the etiology, cirrhosis in general is initiated by hepatocellular necrosis. Continued destruction of hepatocytes causes collapse of normal lobular hepatic parenchyma followed by *fibrosis* around necrotic liver cells and proliferated ductules and there is formation of compensatory *regenerative nodules.*

FIBROGENESIS. The mechanism of fibrosis that may be portal-central, portal-portal, or both, is by increased synthesis of all types of collagen and increase in the number of collagen-producing cells. Development of fibrosis leads to proliferation of fat-storing Ito cells underlying the sinusoidal epithelium which become transformed into myofibroblasts and fibrocytes. Besides collagen, two glycoproteins, fibronectin and laminin, are deposited in excessive amounts in area of liver cell damage. The nature of factors acting as stimulants for fibrosis is not clearly known, but possible candidate mediators are lymphokines and monokines.

REGENERATIVE NODULE. The cause of compensatory proliferation of hepatocytes to form regenerative nodules is obscure. Possibly, growth factors, chalones and hormonal imbalance, play a role in regeneration.

CLASSIFICATION

Cirrhosis can be classified on the basis of morphology and etiology (Table 19.9).

A. MORPHOLOGIC CLASSIFICATION. There are 3 morphologic types of cirrhosis—micronodular, macronodular and mixed. Each of these forms may have an active and inactive form.

■ An *active form* is characterised by continuing hepatocellular necrosis and inflammatory reaction, a process that closely resembles chronic hepatitis.

■ An *inactive form,* on the other hand, has no evidence of continuing hepatocellular necrosis and has sharply-defined nodules of surviving hepatic parenchyma without any significant inflammation.

1. Micronodular cirrhosis. In micronodular cirrhosis, the nodules are usually regular and small, *less than 3 mm* in diameter. There is diffuse involvement of all the hepatic lobules forming nodules by thick fibrous septa which may be portal-portal, portal-central, or both. The micronodular cirrhosis includes etiologic types of alcoholic cirrhosis, nutritional cirrhosis and Laennec's cirrhosis and represents impaired capacity for regrowth as seen in alcoholism, malnutrition, severe anaemia and old age.

2. Macronodular cirrhosis. In this type, the nodules are of variable size and are generally *larger than 3 mm* in diameter. The pattern of involvement is more irregular than in micronodular cirrhosis, sparing some portal tracts and central veins, and more marked evidence of regeneration. Macronodular cirrhosis corresponds to post-necrotic or post-hepatitic cirrhosis of the etiologic classification.

3. Mixed cirrhosis. In mixed type, some parts of the liver show micronodular appearance while other parts show macronodular pattern. All the portal tracts and central veins are not involved by fibrosis but instead some of them are spared. Mixed pattern is a kind of incomplete expression of micronodular cirrhosis.

B. ETIOLOGIC CLASSIFICATION. Based on the cause for cirrhosis, the etiologic categories of cirrhosis are given in Table 19.9.

The individual etiologic types, in conjunction with morphologic categories, are discussed later.

SPECIFIC TYPES OF CIRRHOSIS

Alcoholic Liver Disease and Cirrhosis

Alcoholic liver disease is the term used to describe the spectrum of liver injury associated with acute and chronic alcoholism. There are three stages in alcoholic liver disease: *alcoholic steatosis (fatty liver), alcoholic hepatitis* and *alcoholic cirrhosis.* Though the relationship of these three patterns of liver injury is controversial, available evidence suggests that an alcoholic who continues to drink, progresses from fatty liver to alcoholic hepatitis, and eventually to alcoholic cirrhosis in more than 10 years. On the other hand, there is experimental evidence that fatty change by itself does not lead to the development of cirrhosis, but alcoholic hepatitis in some cases appears to be the forerunner of alcoholic cirrhosis.

TABLE 19.9: Classification of Cirrhosis.

A. MORPHOLOGIC	B. ETIOLOGIC
I. Micronodular (nodules less than 3 mm)	1. Alcoholic cirrhosis (the most common, 60-70%)
II. Macronodular (nodules more than 3 mm)	2. Post-necrotic cirrhosis (10%)
III. Mixed	3. Biliary cirrhosis (5-10%)
	4. Pigment cirrhosis in haemochromatosis (5%)
	5. Cirrhosis in Wilson's disease
	6. Cirrhosis in α-1-antitrypsin deficiency
	7. Cardiac cirrhosis
	8. Indian childhood cirrhosis (ICC)
	9. Miscellaneous forms of cirrhosis
	10. Cryptogenic cirrhosis

Before discussing the features of alcoholic liver disease and cirrhosis, a brief outline of ethanol metabolism is outlined below and is discussed earlier in (page 244).

ETHANOL METABOLISM. One gram of alcohol gives 7 calories. But alcohol cannot be stored and must undergo obligatory oxidation, chiefly in the liver. Thus, these empty calories make no contribution to nutrition other than to give energy.

Ethanol after ingestion and absorption from the small bowel circulates through the liver where about 90% of it is oxidised to acetate by a *two-step enzymatic process* involving two enzymes: *alcohol dehydrogenase (ADH)* present in the cytosol, and *acetaldehyde dehydrogenase (ALDH)* in the mitochondria of hepatocytes (Fig. 19.19). The remaining 10% of ethanol is oxidised elsewhere in the body.

First step: Ethanol is catabolised to acetaldehyde in the liver by the following three pathways, one major and two minor:

i) *In the cytosol,* by the major rate-limiting pathway of alcohol dehydrogenase (ADH).

ii) *In the smooth endoplasmic reticulum,* via microsomal P-450 oxidases (also called microsomal ethanol oxidising system, MEOS), where only part of ethanol is metabolised.

iii) *In the peroxisomes,* minor pathway via catalase such as H_2O_2.

Acetaldehyde is toxic and may cause membrane damage and cell necrosis. Simultaneously, the cofactor nicotinamide-adenine dinucleotide (NAD) which is a hydrogen acceptor, is reduced to NADH.

Second step: The second step occurs in the mitochondria where acetaldehyde is converted to acetate with ALDH acting as a co-enzyme. Most of the acetate on leaving the liver is finally oxidised to carbon dioxide and water, or converted by the citric acid cycle to other compounds including fatty acids. Simultaneously, the same cofactor, NAD, is reduced to NADH resulting in *increased NADH: NAD redox ratio* which is the basic biochemical alteration occurring during ethanol metabolism. A close estimate of NADH:NAD ratio is measured by the ratio of its oxidised and reduced metabolites in the form of *lactate-pyruvate ratio* and *β-hydroxy butyrate-acetoacetate ratio.*

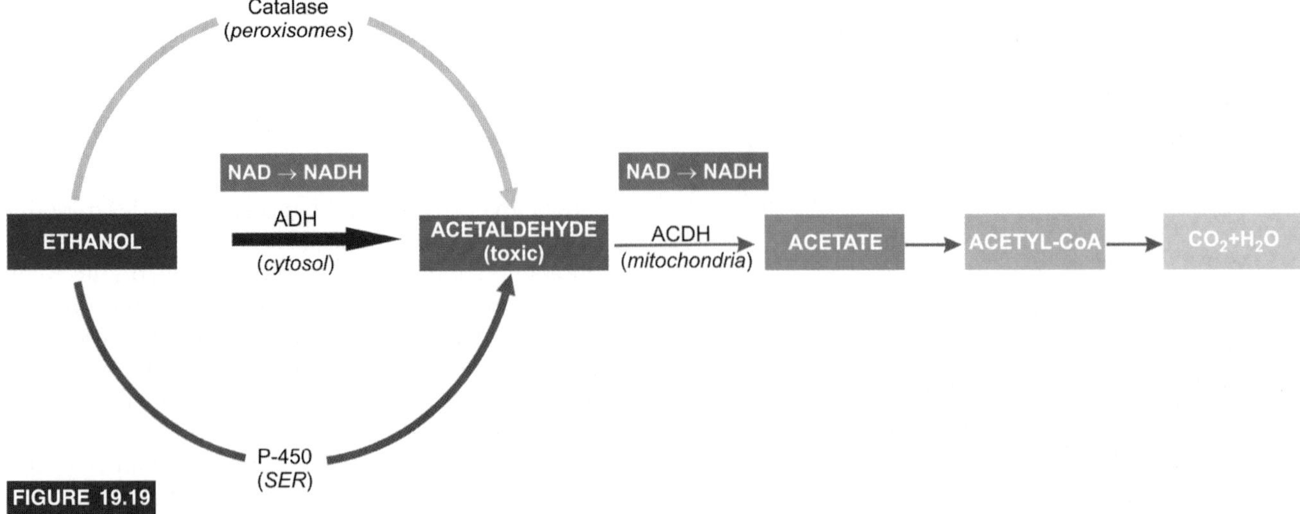

FIGURE 19.19

Metabolism of ethanol in the liver. Thickness and intensity of colour of arrows on left side of figure corresponds to extent of metabolic pathway followed (ADH-alcohol dehydrogenase; ACDH=hepatic acetaldehyde dehydrogenase; NAD=nicotinamide adenine dinucleotide; NADH=reduced NAD; NADP=nicotinamide adenine dinucleotide phosphate: NADPH=reduced NADP).

ETIOLOGY. All those who indulge in alcohol abuse do not develop liver damage. The incidence of cirrhosis among alcoholics at autopsy is about 10-15%. Why some individuals are predisposed to alcoholic cirrhosis is not clearly known, but a few factors have been implicated. These are as under:

1. **Drinking patterns.** Most epidemiologic studies have attributed alcoholic cirrhosis to chronic alcoholism. The quantity and duration of drinking necessary to cause cirrhosis is largely unknown but it is generally agreed that continued daily imbibing of more than 80 gm of any type of alcoholic beverage for at least 10 years is likely to result in alcoholic cirrhosis. Liver injury is related to the alcoholic content only and not to the type of alcoholic beverage consumed. Intermittent drinking for long duration is less harmful since the liver is given chance to recover.

2. **Malnutrition.** Absolute or relative malnutrition of proteins and vitamins is regarded as a contributory factor in the evolution of cirrhosis. The combination of chronic alcohol ingestion and impaired nutrition leads to alcoholic liver disease and not malnutrition *per se.* It appears that calories derived from alcohol displace other nutrients leading to malnutrition and deficiency of vitamins in alcoholics. Additional factors contributing to malnutrition in alcoholics are chronic gastritis and pancreatitis. The evidence in favour of synergistic effect of malnutrition in chronic alcoholism comes from clinical and morphologic improvement in cases of alcoholic cirrhosis on treatment with protein-rich diets.

3. **Infections.** Intercurrent bacterial infections are common in cirrhotic patients and may accelerate the course of the disease. Lesions similar to alcoholic cirrhosis may develop in non-alcoholic patients who have had viral infections in the past.

4. **Genetic factors.** The rate of ethanol metabolism is under genetic control. It is chiefly related to altered rates of elimination of ethanol due to genetic polymorphism for the two main enzyme systems, MEOS (microsomal P-450 oxidases) and alcohol dehydrogenase (ADH). Various HLA histocompatibility types have been associated with susceptibility of different populations to alcoholic liver damage but no single genotype has been identified yet.

PATHOGENESIS. The liver injury due to alcohol consumption culminating in morphologic lesions of alcoholic steatosis (fatty liver), alcoholic hepatitis and alcoholic cirrhosis is explained on the basis of the following mechanisms:

1. **Hepatotoxicity by ethanol.** There is some evidence to suggest that ethanol ingestion for a period of 8-10 days regularly may cause direct hepatotoxic effect on the liver and produce fatty change. Ethanol is directly toxic to microtubules, mitochondria and membrane of hepatocytes.

2. **Hepatotoxicity by ethanol metabolites.** The major hepatotoxic effects of ethanol are exerted by its metabolites, chiefly acetaldehyde. Acetaldehyde levels in blood are elevated in chronic alcoholics. Acetaldehyde is extremely toxic and can cause cytoskeletal and membrane damage and bring about hepatocellular necrosis.

3. **Free radicals.** Oxidation of ethanol by the cytochrome-450 oxidases (MEOS) leads to generation of free radicals which attack the membrane and proteins.

4. **Increased redox ratio.** Marked increase in the NADH:NAD redox ratio in the hepatocytes results in increased redox ratio of lactate-pyruvate, leading to lactic acidosis. This altered redox potential has been implicated in a number of metabolic consequences such as in fatty liver, collagen formation, occurrence of gout, impaired gluconeogenesis and altered steroid metabolism.

5. **Retention of liver cell water and proteins.** Alcohol is inhibitory to secretion of newly-synthesised proteins by the liver leading to their retention in the hepatocytes. Water is simultaneously retained in the cell in proportion to the protein and results in swelling of hepatocytes resulting in hepatomegaly in alcoholics.

6. **Hypoxia.** Chronic ingestion of alcohol results in increased oxygen demand by the liver resulting in a hypoxic state which causes hepatocellular necrosis in centrilobular zone (zone 3). Redox changes are also more marked in zone 3.

7. **Increased liver fat.** The origin of fat in the body was discussed on (page 44). In chronic alcoholism, there is rise in the amount of fat available to the liver which could be from exogenous (dietary) sources, excess mobilisation from adipose tissue or increased lipid synthesis by the liver itself. This may account for lipid accumulation in the hepatocytes.

8. **Immunological mechanism.** Cell-mediated immunity is impaired in alcoholic liver disease. Ethanol causes direct immunologic attack on hepatocytes. In a proportion of cases, alcohol-related liver cell injury continues unabated despite cessation of alcohol consumption which is attributed to immunologic mechanisms. Immunological mechanism may also explain the genesis of Mallory's alcoholic hyalin though more favoured hypothesis for its origin is the aggregation of intermediate filaments of prekeratin type due to alcohol-induced disorganisation of cytoskeleton.

9. **Fibrogenesis and inflammation.** The mechanisms of fibrosis and inflammatory response in alcoholic liver disease are uncertain but the possible mediators are lymphokines and monokines. The major stimulus for fibrogenesis is cell necrosis. All forms of collagen are increased and there is increased transformation of fat-storing Ito cells into myofibroblasts and fibrocytes. Leukotrienes which are important mediators of inflammation are produced by alcohol-damaged hepatocytes resulting in inflammatory reaction in the affected areas.

PATHOLOGIC CHANGES. Three types of morphologic lesions are described in alcoholic liver disease—alcoholic steatosis (fatty liver), alcoholic hepatitis and alcoholic cirrhosis.

1. **ALCOHOLIC STEATOSIS (FATTY LIVER).** The morphologic changes in fatty change in liver have already been described on page 45 and are briefly considered here.

Grossly, the liver is enlarged, yellow, greasy and firm with a smooth and glistening capsule.

Microscopically, the features consist of initial *microvesicular* droplets of fat in the hepatocyte cytoplasm followed by more common and pronounced feature of *macrovesicular* large droplets of fat displacing the nucleus to the periphery (Fig. 19.20). *Fat cysts* may develop due to coalescence and rupture of fat-containing hepatocytes. Less often, *lipogranulomas* consisting of collection of lymphocytes, macrophages and some multinucleate giant cells may be found.

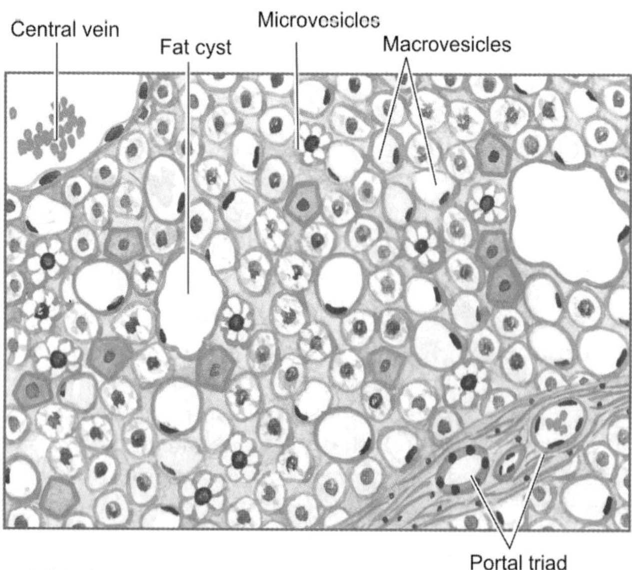

FIGURE 19.20

Fatty liver (alcoholic steatosis). Most of the hepatocytes are distended with large lipid vacuoles with peripherally displaced nuclei.

2. **ALCOHOLIC HEPATITIS.** Alcoholic hepatitis develops acutely, usually following a bout of heavy drinking. Repeated episodes of alcoholic hepatitis superimposed on pre-existing fatty liver are almost certainly a forerunner of alcoholic cirrhosis.

Histologically, the features of alcoholic hepatitis are as follows (Fig. 19.21) (COLOUR PLATE XXV: CL 98).

i) Hepatocellular necrosis: Single or small clusters of hepatocytes, especially in the centrilobular area (zone 3), undergo ballooning degeneration and necrosis.

ii) Mallory bodies or alcoholic hyalin: These are eosinophilic, intracytoplasmic inclusions seen in perinuclear location within swollen and ballooned hepatocytes. They represent aggregates of cytoskeletal intermediate filaments (prekeratin). They can be best visualised with connective tissue stains like Masson's trichrome and chromophobe aniline blue, or by the use of immunoperoxidase methods. Mallory bodies are highly suggestive of, but not specific for, alcoholic hepatitis since Mallory bodies are also found in certain other conditions such as: primary biliary cirrhosis, Indian childhood cirrhosis, cholestatic syndromes, Wilson's disease, intestinal bypass surgery, focal nodular hyperplasia and hepatocellular carcinoma.

iii) Inflammatory response: The areas of hepatocellular necrosis and regions of Mallory bodies are associated with an inflammatory infiltrate, chiefly consisting of polymorphs and some scattered

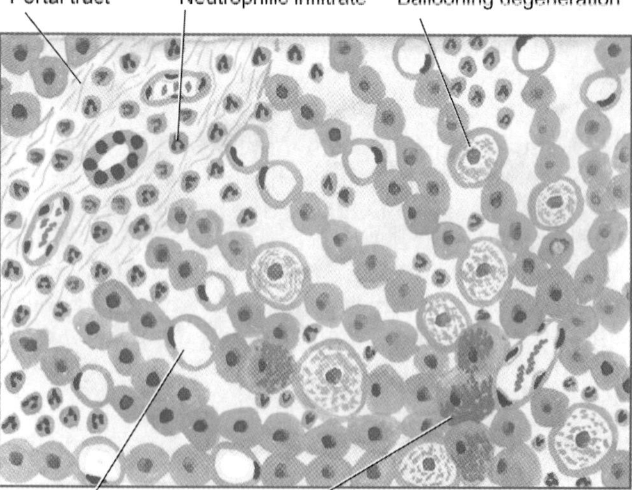

FIGURE 19.21

Alcoholic hepatitis. Liver cells show ballooning degeneration and necrosis with some containing Mallory's hyalin. Fatty change and clusters of neutrophils are also present.

mononuclear cells. In more extensive necrosis, the inflammatory infiltrate is more widespread and may involve the entire lobule.

iv) Fibrosis: Most cases of alcoholic hepatitis are accompanied by pericellular and perivenular fibrosis, producing a web-like or chickenwire-like appearance. This is also termed as *creeping collagenosis.*

3. ALCOHOLIC CIRRHOSIS. Alcoholic cirrhosis is the most common form of lesion, constituting 60-70% of all cases of cirrhosis. A multitude of terms have been used for this type of cirrhosis such as *Laennec's cirrhosis, portal cirrhosis, hobnail cirrhosis, nutritional cirrhosis, diffuse cirrhosis* and *micronodular cirrhosis.*

Macroscopically, alcoholic cirrhosis classically begins as micronodular cirrhosis (nodules less than 3 mm diameter), the liver being large, fatty and weighing usually above 2 kg (Fig. 19.22). Eventually over a span of years, the liver shrinks to less than 1 kg in weight, becomes nonfatty, having macronodular cirrhosis (nodules larger than 3 mm in diameter), resembling post-necrotic cirrhosis. The nodules of the liver due to their fat content are tawny-yellow, on the basis of which Laennec in 1818 introduced the term *cirrhosis* first of all (from Greek *kirrhos* = tawny). The surface of liver in alcoholic cirrhosis is studded with diffuse nodules which vary little in size, producing hobnail liver (because of the resemblance of the surface with the sole of an old-fashioned shoe having short nails with heavy heads). On cut section, spheroidal or angular nodules of fibrous septa are seen.

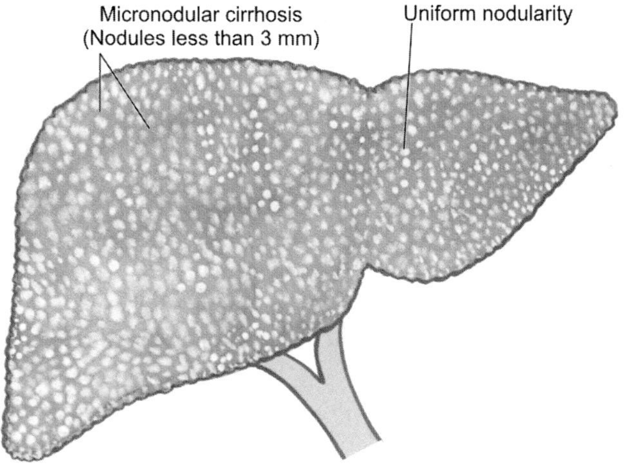

FIGURE 19.22

Alcoholic cirrhosis, showing the typical micronodular pattern in gross specimen.

Microscopically, alcoholic cirrhosis is a progressive alcoholic liver disease. Its features include the following (Fig. 19.23) (COLOUR PLATE XXV: CL 99):

i) Lobular architecture: No normal lobular architecture can be identified and central veins are hard to find.

ii) Fibrous septa: The fibrous septa that divide the hepatic parenchyma into nodules are initially delicate and extend from central vein to portal regions, or portal tract to portal tract, or both. As the fibrous scarring increases with time, the fibrous septa become dense and more confluent.

iii) Hepatic parenchyma: The hepatocytes in the islands of surviving parenchyma undergo slow proliferation forming regenerative nodules having disorganised masses of hepatocytes. The hepatic parenchyma within the nodules shows extensive fatty change early in the disease. But as the fibrous septa become more thick, the amount of fat in hepatocytes is reduced. Thus, there is an inverse relationship between the amount of fat and the amount of fibrous scarring in the nodules.

iv) Necrosis, inflammation and bile duct proliferation: The etiologic clue to diagnosis in the form of Mallory bodies is hard to find in a fully-developed alcoholic cirrhosis. The fibrous septa usually contain sparse infiltrate of mononuclear cells with some bile duct proliferation. Bile stasis and increased cytoplasmic haemosiderin deposits due to enhanced

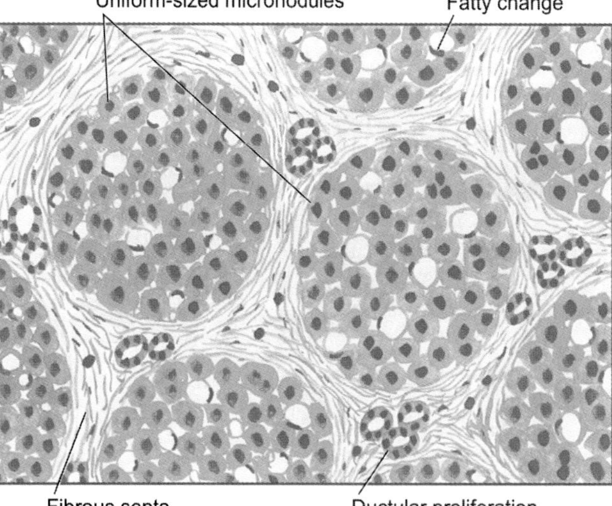

FIGURE 19.23

Alcoholic cirrhosis, microscopic appearance. It shows nearly uniform-sized micronodules, devoid of central veins and having thick fibrous septa dividing them. There is minimal inflammation and some reactive bile duct proliferation in the septa.

iron absorption in alcoholic cirrhosis are some other noticeable findings.

LABORATORY DIAGNOSIS. The clinical manifestations and complications of cirrhosis in general are described on page 650. The laboratory findings in the course of alcoholic liver disease may be quite variable and liver biopsy is necessary in doubtful cases. Progressive form of the disease, however, generally presents the following biochemical and haematological alterations:

1. Elevated transaminases: increase in SGOT (AST) is more than that of SGPT (ALT).
2. Rise in serum γ-glutamyl transpeptidase (γ-GT).
3. Marked elevation in serum alkaline phosphatase.
4. Hyperbilirubinaemia.
5. Hypoproteinaemia with reversal of albumin-globulin ratio.
6. Prolonged prothrombin time and partial thromboplastin time.
7. Anaemia.

Post-necrotic Cirrhosis

Post-necrotic cirrhosis, also termed *post-hepatitic cirrhosis, macronodular cirrhosis* and *coarsely nodular cirrhosis,* is characterised by large and irregular nodules with broad bands of connective tissue and occurring most commonly after previous viral hepatitis.

ETIOLOGY. Based on epidemiologic and serologic studies, the following factors have been implicated in the etiology of post-necrotic cirrhosis.

1. Viral hepatitis. About 25% of patients give history of recent or remote attacks of acute viral hepatitis followed by chronic hepatitis. Most common association is with hepatitis B and C but hepatitis A is not known to evolve into cirrhosis.

2. Drugs and chemical hepatotoxins. A small percentage of cases may have origin from toxicity due to chemicals and drugs such as phosphorus, carbon tetrachloride, mushroom poisoning, acetaminophen and α-methyl dopa.

3. Others. Certain infections (e.g. brucellosis), parasitic infestations (e.g. clonorchiasis), metabolic diseases (e.g. Wilson's disease or hepatolenticular degeneration) and advanced alcoholic liver disease may produce a picture of post-necrotic cirrhosis.

4. Idiopathic. After all these causes have been excluded, a group of cases remain in which the etiology is unknown.

PATHOLOGIC CHANGES. Typically, post-necrotic cirrhosis is macronodular type.

Grossly, the liver is usually small, weighing less than 1 kg, having distorted shape with irregular and coarse scars and nodules of varying size (Fig. 19.24). Sectioned surface shows scars and nodules varying in diameter from 3 mm to a few centimeters.

Microscopically, the features are as follows (Fig. 19.25) (COLOUR PLATE XXV: CL 100):

1. Lobular architecture: The normal lobular architecture of hepatic parenchyma is not completely lost. Instead, uninvolved portal tracts and central veins in the hepatic lobules can still be seen in some parts of surviving parenchyma.

2. Fibrous septa: The fibrous septa dividing the variable-sized nodules are generally thick.

3. Necrosis, inflammation and bile duct proliferation: Active liver cell necrosis is usually inconspicuous. Fibrous septa contain prominent mononuclear inflammatory cell infiltrate which may even form follicles. Often there is extensive proliferation of bile ductules derived from collapsed liver lobules.

4. Hepatic parenchyma: Liver cells vary considerably in size and multiple large nuclei are common in regenerative nodules. Fatty change may or may not be present in the hepatocytes.

CLINICAL FEATURES. Besides the general clinical features described on page 650, post-necrotic cirrhosis is seen as frequent in women as in men, especially in the younger age group. Like in alcoholic cirrhosis, the patients may remain asymptomatic or may present with prominent signs and symptoms of chronic active hepatitis (page 631). Splenomegaly and hypersplenism are other prominent features. The results of haematologic and liver function test are similar to those of alcoholic cirrhosis. Out of the various types of cirrhosis, post-necrotic cirrhosis, especially when related to hepatitis B and C virus infection in early life, is most frequently associated with hepatocellular carcinoma.

Biliary Cirrhosis

Biliary cirrhosis is defined as a chronic disorder characterised by clinical, biochemical and morphological features of long-continued cholestasis of intrahepatic or extrahepatic origin. Accordingly, biliary cirrhosis is of 2 main types:

- *Primary biliary cirrhosis* in which the destructive process of unknown etiology affects intrahepatic bile ducts.
- *Secondary biliary cirrhosis* resulting from prolonged mechanical obstruction of the extrahepatic biliary passages.

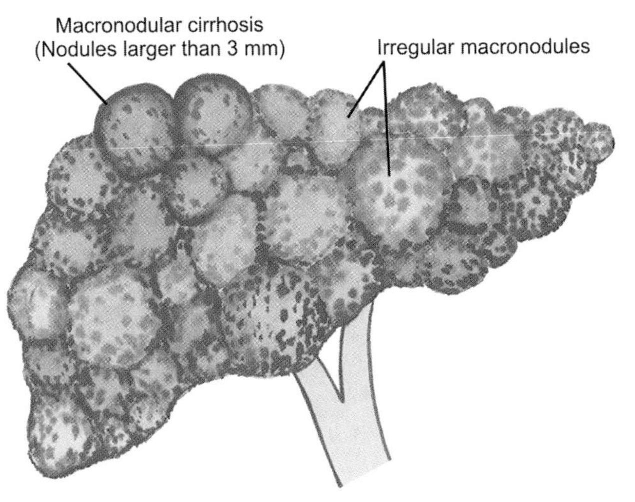

FIGURE 19.24

Post-necrotic cirrhosis, showing the typical irregular macronodular pattern in a small, distorted and irregularly scarred liver.

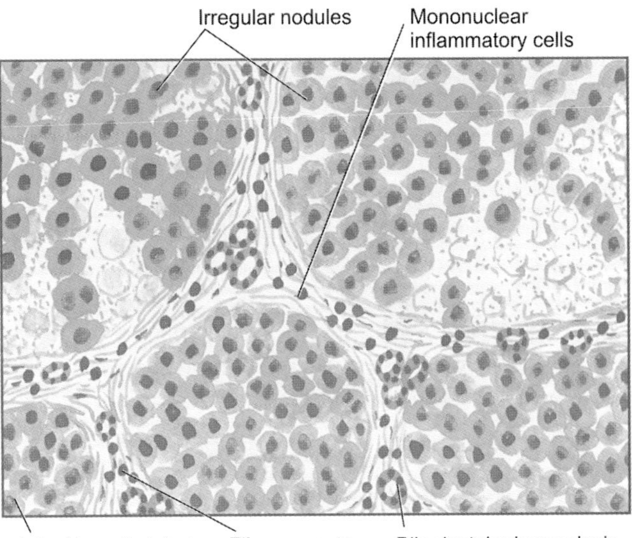

FIGURE 19.25

Post-necrotic cirrhosis, microscopic appearance. Fibrous septa dividing the hepatic parenchyma into nodules are thick and contain prominent mononuclear inflammatory cell infiltrate and bile ductular hyperplasia. A few intact hepatic lobules remain.

■ In addition, a third cause for biliary cirrhosis is *primary sclerosing cholangitis* discussed at the end of this discussion.

ETIOLOGY. The etiology of the two forms of biliary cirrhosis is distinctive:

A. Primary biliary cirrhosis. The etiology of this type remains unknown. However, a few observations have been made to unfold its possible etiology:

1. The condition is predominant in middle-aged women (male: female ratio = 1:9) and has led to the suggestion of a possible *endocrine origin.*
2. *Familial incidence* has been observed suggesting the role of some genetic influence and certain HLA types.
3. There is *elevated cholesterol* level with appearance of xanthoma and xanthelasma. Hepatomegaly and chronic liver disease are late features of the disease.
4. However, presently the most widely accepted hypothesis is *autoimmune origin* of the disease. In support are the following observations:

■ increased incidence of associated autoimmune diseases (e.g. scleroderma, Sjögren's syndrome, CREST syndrome, and autoimmune thyroiditis),

■ circulating anti-mitochondrial antibody of IgG class detected in more than 90% cases;

■ elevated levels of immunoglobulins, particularly of IgM;

■ increased levels of circulating immune complexes;

■ decreased number of circulating T-cells; and

■ accumulation of T cells around bile ducts.

B. Secondary biliary cirrhosis. Most cases of secondary biliary cirrhosis result from prolonged obstruction of extrahepatic biliary passages (page 617). These causes include:

1. Extrahepatic cholelithiasis, most common
2. Biliary atresia
3. Cancer of biliary tree and of head of pancreas
4. Postoperative strictures with superimposed ascending cholangitis.

PATHOLOGIC CHANGES. Grossly, in both primary and secondary biliary cirrhosis, the liver is initially enlarged and greenish-yellow in appearance, but later becomes smaller, firmer and coarsely micronodular. ***Microscopically,*** the features of intra- and extrahepatic cholestasis corresponding to primary and secondary biliary cirrhosis respectively have already been discussed on (page 617). The salient features of the two forms of biliary cirrhosis are as under:

A. Primary biliary cirrhosis: The diagnostic histologic feature is a chronic, non-suppurative, destructive cholangitis involving intrahepatic bile ducts. The disease evolves through the following 4 histologic states:

Stage I: There are *florid bile duct lesions* confined to portal tracts. The changes in the affected area consist of destruction of bile ducts, presence of bile plugs, infiltration with acute and chronic inflammatory cells and sometimes formation of granulomas and lymphoid follicles.

Stage II: There is *ductular proliferation.* The ductal involvement is quite widespread with very few normal bile ducts. The inflammatory infiltrate too extends beyond the portal tracts into surrounding hepatic parenchyma. Periportal Mallory bodies may be present.

Stage III: This stage is characterised by *fibrous scarring* interconnecting the portal areas. There is diminished inflammatory infiltrate and reduced number of bile ducts.

Stage IV: Well-formed *micronodular pattern* of cirrhosis develops in a period of a few years (Fig. 19.26).

B. Secondary biliary cirrhosis: Prolonged obstruction of extrahepatic bile ducts may produce the following histologic changes:

1. *Bile stasis,* degeneration and focal areas of centrilobular necrosis of hepatocytes.
2. Proliferation, dilatation and rupture of bile ductules in the portal area with formation of *bile lakes.*
3. *Cholangitis,* sterile or pyogenic, with accumulation of polymorphs around the bile ducts.
4. *Progressive expansion* of the portal tract by fibrosis and evolution into micronodular cirrhosis.

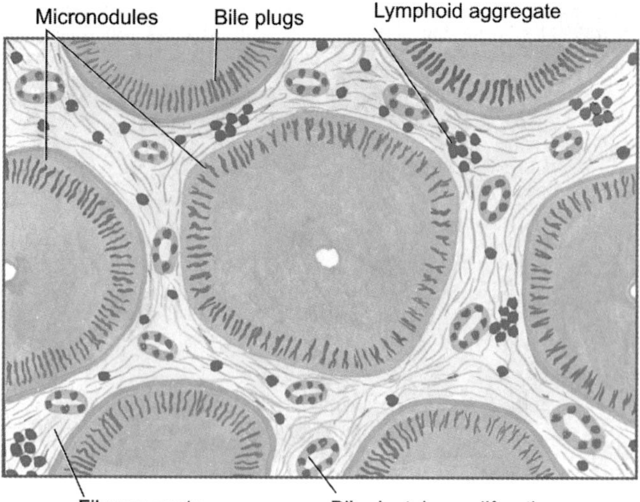

FIGURE 19.26

Primary biliary cirrhosis, diagrammatic representation. There are fibrous scars dividing the hepatic parenchyma into the micronodules. The fibrous septa contain prominent lymphoid infiltrate and proliferated bile ducts. Many of the hepatocytes contain elongated bile plugs.

CLINICAL FEATURES. Clinical features of primary and secondary biliary cirrhosis are variable:

- **Primary biliary cirrhosis** may remain asymptomatic for months to years. Symptoms develop insidiously. Basically, it is a cholestatic disorder. The patients present with persistent pruritus, dark urine, pale stools, steatorrhoea, jaundice and skin pigmentation. The earliest laboratory finding is a markedly elevated serum alkaline phosphatase level. Elevation of serum lipids is accompanied by appearance of periorbital xanthelasma and xanthomas over joints. Death usually results from hepatic failure, variceal bleeding, intercurrent infections and concomitant development of cancers of liver and breast.

- The diagnosis of **secondary biliary cirrhosis** is considered in patients with previous history of gallstones, biliary tract surgery or clinical features of ascending cholangitis.

PRIMARY SCLEROSING CHOLANGITIS. Primary or idiopathic sclerosing cholangitis is characterised by progressive, inflammatory, sclerosing and obliterative process affecting mainly extra-hepatic, and sometimes intrahepatic ducts as well. The disease occurs in 3rd to 5th decade of life with two fold preponderance in males.

ETIOLOGY. Though idiopathic, the condition coexists with the following:

1. Inflammatory bowel disease, particularly idiopathic.
2. Multifocal fibrosclerosis syndromes
3. AIDS.

PATHOLOGIC CHANGES. Grossly, there is characteristic beading of intra- and extrahepatic bile ducts due to irregular strictures and dilatation.

Microscopically, the changes include:

1. *Fibrosing cholangitis* with lymphocytic infiltrate around bile ducts with segmental involvement.
2. *Periductal fibrosis* with eventual obliteration of lumen of affected bile ducts.
3. *Intervening bile ducts* are dilated, tortuous and inflamed.
4. Late cases show *cholestasis* and full blown picture of biliary cirrhosis.

Clinically, the patients may remain asymptomatic or may show features of cholestatic jaundice (raised alkaline phosphatase, pruritus, fatigue). Late cases show manifestations of chronic liver disease.

The features of three main types of intrahepatic disorders leading to biliary cirrhosis are summarised in Table 19.10.

TABLE 19.10: Contrasting Features of Major Forms of Biliary Cirrhosis.

FEATURE	PRIMARY BILIARY CIRRHOSIS	SECONDARY BILIARY CIRRHOSIS	PRIMARY SCLEROSING CHOLANGITIS
1. *Etiology*	Possibly autoimmune; association with other autoimmune diseases	Extrahepatic biliary obstruction; biliary atresia	Possibly autoimmune; association with inflammatory bowel disease
2. *Age and sex*	Middle-aged women Male: Female=1:9	Any age and either sex	Middle age Male: Female=2:1
3. *Laboratory tests*	↑ Alkaline phosphatase ↑ Conjugated bilirubin Autoantibodies present	↑ Alkaline phosphatase ↑ Conjugated bilirubin	↑ Alkaline phosphatase ↑ Conjugated bilirubin Hypergammaglobulinaemia
4. *Pathologic changes*	Chronic destructive Cholangitis of intrahepatic bile ducts	Bile stasis in bile ducts, and sterile or pyogenic cholangitis	Fibrosing cholangitis with periductal fibrosis

Pigment Cirrhosis in Haemochromatosis

Haemochromatosis is an iron-storage disorder in which there is excessive accumulation of iron in parenchymal cells with eventual tissue damage and functional insufficiency of organs such as the liver, pancreas, heart and pituitary gland. The condition is characterised by a triad of features—*micronodular pigment cirrhosis, diabetes mellitus* and *skin pigmentation.* On the basis of the last two features, the disease has also come to be termed as *'bronze diabetes'*. Males predominate and manifest earlier since women have physiologic iron loss delaying the effects of excessive accumulation of iron. Haemochromatosis exists in 2 main forms:

1. *Idiopathic (primary, genetic) haemochromatosis* is an autosomal recessive disorder of excessive accumulation of iron associated with susceptible gene, linked to HLA-A3 complex on chromosome 6.
2. *Secondary (acquired) haemochromatosis* is gross iron overload with tissue injury arising secondary to other diseases such as thalassaemia, sideroblastic anaemias, alcoholic cirrhosis or multiple transfusions.

ETIOPATHOGENESIS. A general discussion of iron metabolism and iron excess states is given on page 47.

Normally, the body iron content is 3-4 gm which is maintained in such a way that intestinal mucosal absorption of iron is equal to its loss. This amount is approximately 1 mg/day in men and 1.5 mg/day in menstruating women. In haemochromatosis, however, this amount goes up to 4 mg/day or more, as evidenced by elevated serum iron (normal about 125 μg/dl) and increased serum transferrin saturation (normal 30%).

■ In **idiopathic haemochromatosis,** the primary mechanism of disease appears to be the genetic basis in which the defect may either lie at the intestinal mucosal level causing excessive iron absorption, or at the postabsorption excretion level leading to excessive accumulation of iron. The excess iron in primary haemochromatosis is deposited mainly in the cytoplasm of parenchymal cells of organs such as the liver, pancreas, spleen, heart and endocrine glands. Tissue injury results from iron-laden lysosomes of parenchymal cells and lipid peroxidation of cell organelles by excess iron.

■ In **secondary haemochromatosis,** there is excessive accumulation of iron due to acquired causes like ineffective erythropoiesis, defective haemoglobin synthesis, multiple blood transfusions and enhanced absorption of iron due to alcohol consumption. The last-named phenomenon is observed in *Bantu siderosis* affecting South African Bantu tribals who consume large quantities of home-brew prepared in iron vessels. Cases of secondary haemochromatosis have increased iron storage within the reticuloendothelial system and liver. However, the magnitude of the iron excess in secondary haemochromatosis is generally insufficient to cause tissue damage.

PATHOLOGIC CHANGES. Excessive deposit of iron in organs and tissues is ferritin and haemosiderin, both of which appear as golden-yellow pigment granules in the cytoplasm of affected parenchymal cells and haemosiderin stains positively with Prussian blue reaction. The organs most frequently affected are the liver and pancreas, and to a lesser extent, the heart, endocrine glands, skin, synovium and testis.

■ In the **liver,** excess of pigment accumulates in the hepatocytes, and less often Kupffer cells and in bile duct epithelium. The deposits in the initial stage may be prominent in the periportal liver cells alongwith increased fibrosis in the portal zone. But eventually, micronodular cirrhosis develops. The deposits may produce grossly chocolate-brown colour of the liver and nodular surface.

■ In the **pancreas,** pigmentation is less intense and is found in the acinar and islet cells. The deposits in pancreas produce diffuse interstitial fibrosis and atrophy of parenchymal cells leading to occurrence of diabetes mellitus.

CLINICAL FEATURES. The major clinical manifestations of haemochromatosis include skin pigmentation, diabetes mellitus, hepatic and cardiac dysfunction, arthropathy and hypogonadism. Characteristic bronze pigmentation is the presenting feature in about 90% of cases. Demonstration of excessive parenchymal iron stores is possible by measurement of serum iron, determination of percent saturation of transferrin, measurement of serum ferritin concentration, estimation of chelatable iron stores using chelating agent (e.g. desferrioxamine), and finally, by liver biopsy. Occurrence of hepatocellular carcinoma is a late complication of haemochromatosis-induced cirrhosis.

Cirrhosis in Wilson's Disease

Wilson's disease, also termed by a more descriptive designation of *hepatolenticular degeneration,* is an autosomal recessive inherited disease of copper metabolism, characterised by toxic accumulation of copper in many tissues, chiefly the liver, brain and eye. These accumulations lead to the *triad* of features:

1. Cirrhosis of the liver.
2. Bilateral degeneration of the basal ganglia of the brain.
3. Greenish-brown pigmented rings in the periphery of the cornea (Kayser-Fleischer rings).

The disease manifests predominantly in children and young adults (5-30 years). Initially, the clinical manifestations are referable to liver involvement such as jaundice and hepatomegaly *(hepatic form)* but later progressive *neuropsychiatric changes* and *Kayser-Fleischer rings* in the cornea appear.

PATHOGENESIS. The pathogenesis of Wilson's disease is best understood when compared with normal copper metabolism.

■ **Normally,** dietary copper is more than body's requirement. Excess copper so absorbed through the stomach and duodenum is transported to the liver where it is incorporated into α_2-globulin to form ceruloplasmin, which is excreted by the liver via bile normally. Most of the plasma copper circulates as ceruloplasmin. Only minute amount of copper is excreted in the urine normally.

■ **In Wilson's disease,** the initial steps of dietary absorption and transport of copper to the liver are normal but copper accumulates in the liver rather than being excreted by the liver. The underlying defect in chromosome 13 is a mutation in ATP7B gene, the normal hepatic copper-excreting gene. Eventually, capacity of hepatocytes to store copper is exceeded and copper is released into circulation which then gets deposited in extrahepatic tissues such as the brain, eyes and others. However, increased copper in the kidney does not produce any serious renal dysfunction.

Biochemical abnormalities in Wilson's disease include the following:

1 *Decreased serum ceruloplasmin* (due to impaired synthesis of apoceruloplasmin in damaged liver and defective mobilisation of copper from hepatocellular lysosomes).

2. *Increased hepatic copper* in liver biopsy (due to excessive accumulation of copper in the liver).

3. *Increased urinary excretion* of copper.

4. However, *serum copper levels* are of no diagnostic help and may vary from low-to-normal-to-high depending upon the stage of disease.

PATHOLOGIC CHANGES. The **liver** shows varying grades of changes that include fatty change, acute and chronic active hepatitis, submassive liver necrosis and macronodular cirrhosis. Mallory bodies are present in some cases. Copper is usually deposited in the periportal hepatocytes in the form of reddish granules in the cytoplasm or as reddish cytoplasmic coloration, stainable by rubeanic acid or rhodamine stains for copper.

Involvement of basal ganglia in **brain** is in the form of toxic injury to neurons, in the **cornea** as greenish-brown deposits of copper in Descemet's membrane, and in the **kidney** as fatty and hydropic change.

Cirrhosis in α-1-Antitrypsin Deficiency

Alpha-1-antitrypsin deficiency is an autosomal codominant condition in which the homozygous state produces liver disease (cirrhosis), pulmonary disease (emphysema), or both (page 486). α-1-antitrypsin is a glycoprotein normally synthesised in the rough endoplasmic reticulum of the hepatocytes and is the most potent protease inhibitor (Pi). A single autosomal dominant gene coding for α-1-antitrypsin is located on long arm of chromosome 14 that codes for immunoglobulin light chains too. Out of 24 different alleles labelled alphabetically, PiMM is the most common normal phenotype, while the most frequent abnormal phenotype in α-1-antitrypsin deficiency leading to liver and/or lung disease is PiZZ in homozygote form. Other phenotypes in which liver disease occurs are PiSS and Pi-null in which serum α-1-antitrypsin value is nearly totally deficient. Intermediate phenotypes, PiMZ and PiSZ persons are predisposed to develop hepatocellular carcinoma.

The patients may present with respiratory disease due to the development of emphysema, or may develop liver dysfunction, or both. At birth or in neonates, the features of cholestatic jaundice of varying severity may appear. In adolescence, the condition may evolve into hepatitis or cirrhosis which is usually well compensated.

PATHOLOGIC CHANGES. Pulmonary changes in α-1-antitrypsin deficiency in the form of emphysema are described in Chapter 15. The hepatic changes vary according to the age at which the deficiency becomes apparent. At birth or in neonates, the histologic features consist of neonatal hepatitis that may be acute or 'pure' cholestasis. Micronodular or macronodular cirrhosis may appear in childhood or in adolescence in which the diagnostic feature is the presence of intracellular, acidophilic, PAS-positive globules in the periportal hepatocytes. Ultrastructurally, these globules consist of dilated rough endoplasmic reticulum.

Cardiac Cirrhosis

Cardiac cirrhosis is an uncommon complication of severe right-sided congestive heart failure of long-standing duration (page 107). The common causes culminating in cardiac cirrhosis are cor pulmonale, tricuspid insufficiency or constrictive pericarditis. The pressure in the right ventricle is elevated which is transmitted to the liver via the inferior vena cava and hepatic veins. The patients generally have enlarged and tender liver with mild liver dysfunction. Splenomegaly occurs due to simple passive congestion.

PATHOLOGIC CHANGES. Grossly, the liver is enlarged and firm with stretched Glisson's capsule. ***Histologically,*** in acute stage, the hepatic sinusoids are dilated and congested with haemorrhagic necrosis of centrilobular hepatocytes *(central haemorrhagic necrosis)*. Severe and more prolonged heart failure results in delicate fibrous strands radiating from the central veins. These fibrous strands may form interconnections leading to cardiac cirrhosis and regenerative nodules.

Indian Childhood Cirrhosis

Indian childhood cirrhosis (ICC) is an unusual form of cirrhosis seen in children between the age of 6 months and 3 years in rural, middle class, Hindus in India and in parts of South-East Asia and the Middle-East. There is no role of viral infection in its etiology. Instead, a combination of some common toxic effects and inherited abnormality of copper metabolism has been suggested. Death occurs due to hepatic failure within a year of diagnosis.

PATHOLOGIC CHANGES. Five histologic types of ICC have been distinguished of which type II is the most common. This form is characterised by the following features:

i) Liver cell injury ranging from ballooning degeneration to significant damage to hepatocytes.

ii) Prominent Mallory bodies in some hepatocytes without fatty change.

iii) Neutrophilic and sometimes alongwith lymphocytic infiltrate.

iv) Creeping pericellular fibrosis which may eventually lead to fine micro-macro-nodular cirrhosis.

v) There is significant deposition of copper and copper-associated proteins in hepatocytes, often more than what is seen in Wilson's disease.

Thus, the picture resembles acute alcoholic hepatitis but without the fatty change and with greatly impaired regeneration. There is marked increase in hepatic copper since the milk consumed by such infants is often boiled and stored in copper vessels in India. The condition has to be distinguished from Wilson's disease.

Miscellaneous Forms of Cirrhosis

In addition to the various types of cirrhosis just described, a few other uncommon types are sometimes distinguished. These include the following:

1. **Metabolic disorders** e.g. in galactosaemia, hereditary fructose intolerance, glycogen storage diseases.

2. **Infectious diseases** e.g. in brucellosis, schistosomiasis, syphilis (hepar lobatum) and toxoplasma infection.

3. **Gastrointestinal disorders** e.g. in inflammatory bowel disease, cystic fibrosis of the pancreas and intestinal bypass surgery for obesity.

4. **Infiltrative diseases** e.g. in sarcoidosis.

Cryptogenic Cirrhosis

Finally, when all the known etiologic types of cirrhosis have been excluded, there remain patients with cirrhosis in whom the cause is unknown. These cases are grouped under a waste-basket diagnosis of cryptogenic cirrhosis (*crypto* = concealed).

NON-CIRRHOTIC PORTAL FIBROSIS

Non-cirrhotic portal fibrosis (NCPF) is a group of congenital and acquired diseases in which there is localised or generalised hepatic fibrosis without nodular regenerative activity and there is absence of clinical and functional evidence of cirrhosis. Besides, the patients of NCPF are relatively young as compared to those of cirrhosis and develop repeated bouts of haematemesis in the course of disease. One of the types associated with increased portal fibrosis without definite cirrhosis is seen in *idiopathic(primary) portal hypertension with splenomegaly,* reported from India and Japan. Another variant is *congenital hepatic fibrosis* seen in polycystic disease of the liver. The type common in India, particularly in young males, is related to *chronic arsenic ingestion* in drinking water and intake of orthodox medicines. It could also be due to portal vein thrombosis leading to intimal sclerosis of portal vein branches.

PATHOLOGIC CHANGES. Grossly, the liver is small, fibrous and shows prominent fibrous septa on both external as well as on cut surface forming irregular islands in the liver.

Histologically, the salient features are as under:
i) Standing out of portal tracts due to their fibrous thickening without significant inflammation.
ii) Obliterative sclerosis of portal vein branches in the portal tracts (obliterative portovenopathy).

CLINICAL MANIFESTATIONS AND COMPLICATIONS OF CIRRHOSIS

The range of clinical features in cirrhosis varies widely, from an asymptomatic state to progressive liver failure and death. The onset of disease is insidious. In general, the features of cirrhosis are more marked in the alcoholic form than in other varieties. These include weakness, fatiguability, weight loss, anorexia, muscle wasting, and low grade fever due to hepatocellular necrosis or some latent infection. Advanced cases develop a number of complications which are as follows:

1. *Portal hypertension* and its major effects such as ascites, splenomegaly and development of collaterals (e.g. oesophageal varices, spider naevi etc) as discussed below.
2. *Progressive hepatic failure* and its manifestations as described already (page 621).
3. Development of *hepatocellular carcinoma,* more often in post-necrotic cirrhosis (HBV and HCV more often) than following alcoholic cirrhosis (page 654).
4. *Chronic relapsing pancreatitis,* especially in alcoholic liver disease (page 668).
5. *Steatorrhoea* due to reduced hepatic bile secretion.
6. *Gallstones* usually of pigment type, are seen twice more frequently in patients with cirrhosis than in general population.
7. *Infections* are more frequent in patients with cirrhosis due to impaired phagocytic activity of reticulo-endothelial system.
8. *Haematologic derangements* such as bleeding disorders and anaemia due to impaired hepatic synthesis of coagulation factors and hypoalbuminaemia are present.
9. *Cardiovascular complications* such as atherosclerosis of coronaries and aorta and myocardial infarction are more frequent in cirrhotic patients.
10. *Musculoskeletal abnormalities* like digital clubbing, hypertrophic osteoarthropathy and Dupuytren's contracture are more common in cirrhotic patients.
11. *Endocrine disorders.* In males these consist of feminisation such as gynaecomastia, changes in pubic hair pattern, testicular atrophy and impotence, whereas in cirrhotic women amenorrhoea is a frequent abnormality.
12. *Hepatorenal syndrome* leading to renal failure may occur in late stages of cirrhosis (page 621).

The ultimate *causes of death* are hepatic coma, massive gastrointestinal haemorrhage from oesophageal varices (complication of portal hypertension), intercurrent infections, hepatorenal syndrome and development of hepatocellular carcinoma.

PORTAL HYPERTENSION

Increase in pressure in the portal system usually follows obstruction to the portal blood flow anywhere along its course. Portal veins have no valves and thus obstruction anywhere in the portal system raises pressure in all the veins proximal to the obstruction. However, unless proved otherwise, portal hypertension means obstruction to the portal blood flow by cirrhosis of the liver. The normal portal venous pressure is quite low (10-15 mm saline). Portal hypertension occurs when the portal pressure is above 30 mm saline. Measurement of *intrasplenic pressure* reflects pressure in the splenic vein; the

TABLE 19.11: Major Causes of Portal Hypertension.

A. INTRAHEPATIC
1. Cirrhosis
2. Metastatic tumours
3. Budd-Chiari syndrome
4. Hepatic veno-occlusive disease
5. Diffuse granulomatous diseases
6. Extensive fatty change

B. POSTHEPATIC
1. Congestive heart failure
2. Constrictive pericarditis
3. Hepatic veno-occlusive disease
4. Budd-Chiari syndrome

C. PREHEPATIC
1. Portal vein thrombosis
2. Neoplastic obstruction of portal vein
3. Myelofibrosis
4. Congenital absence of portal vein

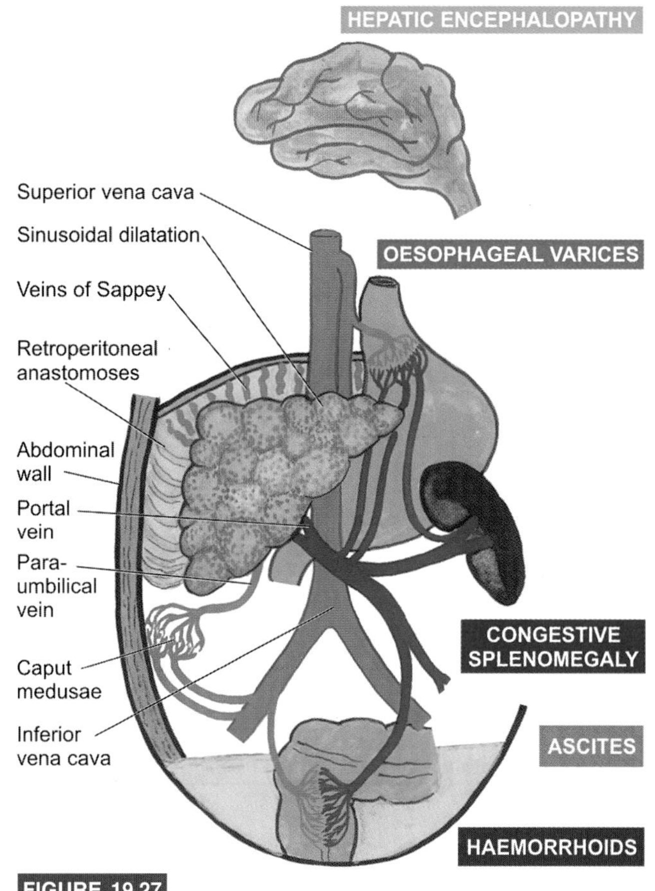

FIGURE 19.27

Major clinical consequences of portal hypertension.

percutaneous transhepatic pressure provides a measure of pressure in the main portal vein; and wedged hepatic *venous pressure* represents sinusoidal pressure. Measurement of these pressures helps in localising the site of obstruction and classifying the portal hypertension.

CLASSIFICATION. Based on the site of obstruction to portal venous blood flow, portal hypertension is categorised into 3 main types—*intrahepatic, posthepatic* and *prehepatic* (Table 19.11). Rare cases of idiopathic portal hypertension showing non-cirrhotic portal fibrosis are encountered as discussed above.

1. Intrahepatic portal hypertension. Cirrhosis is by far the commonest cause of portal hypertension. Other less frequent intrahepatic causes are metastatic tumours, non-cirrhotic nodular regenerative conditions, hepatic venous obstruction (Budd-Chiari syndrome), veno-occlusive disease, schistosomiasis, diffuse granulomatous diseases and extensive fatty change. In cirrhosis and other conditions, there is obstruction to the portal venous flow by fibrosis, thrombosis and pressure by regenerative nodules. About 30-60% patients of cirrhosis develop significant portal hypertension.

2. Posthepatic portal hypertension. This is uncommon and results from obstruction to the blood flow through hepatic vein into inferior vena cava. The causes are neoplastic occlusion and thrombosis of the hepatic vein or of the inferior vena cava (including Budd-Chiari syndrome). Prolonged congestive heart failure and constrictive pericarditis may also cause portal hypertension by transmitting the elevated pressure through the hepatic vessels into the portal vein.

3. Prehepatic portal hypertension. Blockage of portal flow before portal blood reaches the hepatic sinusoids results in prehepatic portal hypertension. Such conditions are thrombosis and neoplastic obstruction of the portal vein before it ramifies in the liver, myelofibrosis, and congenital absence of portal vein.

MAJOR SEQUELAE OF PORTAL HYPERTENSION. Irrespective of the mechanisms involved in the pathogenesis of portal hypertension, there are 4 major clinical consequences—*ascites, varices* (collateral channels or portosystemic shunts), *splenomegaly* and *hepatic encephalopathy* (Fig. 19.27).

1. Ascites. Ascites is the accumulation of excessive volume of fluid within the peritoneal cavity. It frequently accompanies cirrhosis and other diffuse liver diseases. The development of ascites is associated with haemodilution, oedema and decreased urinary output.

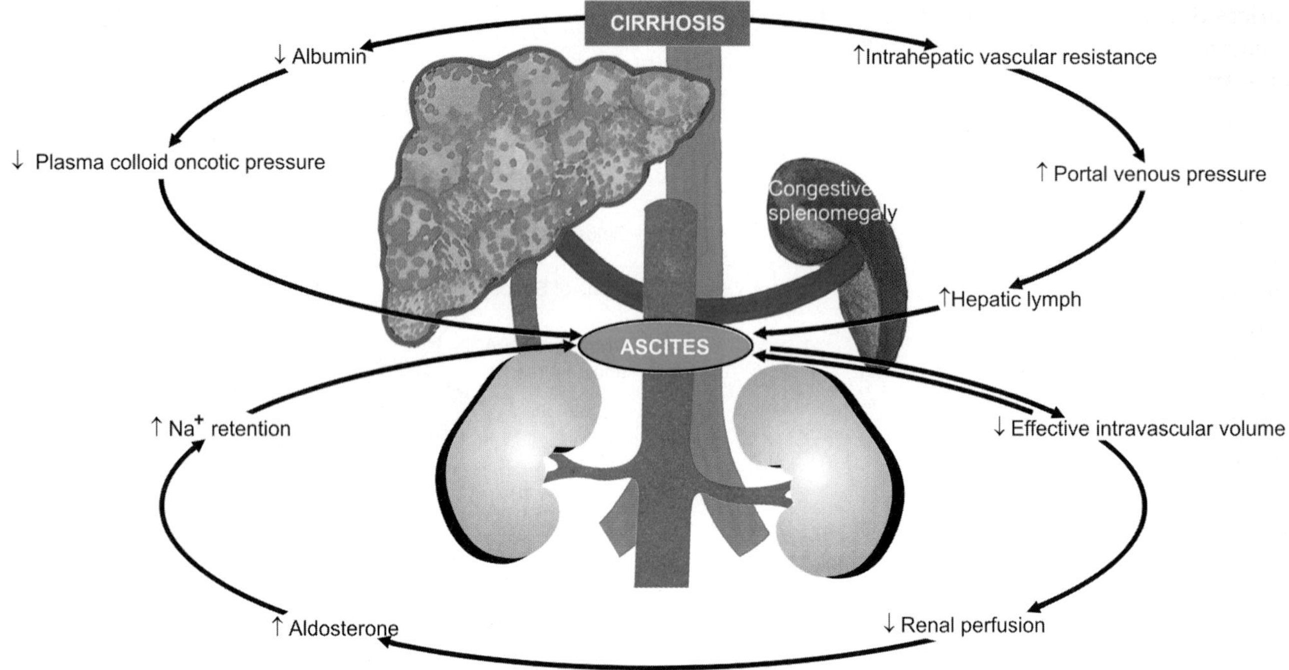

FIGURE 19.28

Mechanisms of ascites formation in cirrhosis.

Ascitic fluid is generally transudate with specific gravity of 1.010, protein content below 3 gm/dl and electrolyte concentrations like those of other extracellular fluids. It may contain a few mesothelial cells and mononuclear cells. But presence of neutrophils is suggestive of secondary infection and red blood cells in ascitic fluid points to disseminated intra-abdominal cancer.

Pathogenesis. The ascites becomes clinically detectable when more than 500 ml of fluid has accumulated in the peritoneal cavity. The mechanisms involved in its formation were discussed in Chapter 5. Briefly, the systemic and local factors favouring ascites formation are as under (Fig. 19.28):

A. SYSTEMIC FACTORS:

i) *Decreased plasma colloid oncotic pressure.* There is hypoalbuminaemia from impaired hepatic synthesis of plasma proteins including albumin, as well as from loss of albumin from the blood plasma into the peritoneal cavity. Hypoalbuminaemia, in turn, causes reduced plasma oncotic pressure and leads to loss of water into extravascular space.

ii) *Hyperaldosteronism.* In cirrhosis, there is increased aldosterone secretion by the adrenal gland, probably due to reduced renal blood flow, and impaired hepatic metabolism and excretion of aldosterone.

iii) *Impaired renal excretion.* Reduced renal blood flow and excessive release of antidiuretic hormone results in renal retention of sodium and water and impaired renal excretion.

B. LOCAL FACTORS:

i) *Portal hypertension.* Portal venous pressure is not directly related to ascites formation but portal hypertension in combination with other factors contributes to the formation and localisation of the fluid retention in the peritoneal cavity.

ii) *Increased hepatic lymph formation.* Obstruction of hepatic vein such as in Budd-Chiari syndrome and increased intra-sinusoidal pressure found in cirrhotic patients stimulates hepatic lymph formation that oozes through the surface of the liver.

2. Varices (Collateral channels or Porto-systemic shunts). As a result of rise in portal venous pressure and obstruction in the portal circulation within or outside the liver, the blood tends to bypass the liver and return to the heart by development of porto-systemic collateral channels (or shunts or varices). These varices develop at sites where the systemic and portal circulations have common capillary beds. The principal sites are as under:

i) Oesophageal varices: The development of oesophago-gastric varices which is frequently manifested by massive haematemesis is the most important consequence of portal hypertension (page 552).

ii) Haemorrhoids: Development of collaterals between the superior, middle and inferior haemorrhoidal veins resulting in haemorrhoids is another common accompaniment. Bleeding from haemorrhoids is usually not as serious a complication as haematemesis from oesophageal varices.

iii) Caput medusae: Anastomoses between the portal and systemic veins may develop between the hilum of the liver and the umbilicus along the paraumbilical plexus of veins resulting in abdominal wall collaterals. These appear as dilated subcutaneous veins radiating from the umbilicus and are termed caput medusae (named after the snake-haired *Medusa).*

iv) Retroperitoneal anastomoses: In the retroperitoneum, portocaval anastomoses may be established through the veins of Retzius and the veins of Sappey.

3. Splenomegaly. The enlargement of the spleen in prolonged portal hypertension is called congestive splenomegaly (page 465). The spleen may weigh 500-1000 gm and is easily palpable. The spleen is larger in young people and in macronodular cirrhosis than in micronodular cirrhosis.

4. Hepatic encephalopathy. Porto-systemic venous shunting may result in a complex metabolic and organic syndrome of the brain characterised by disturbed consciousness, neurologic signs and flapping tremors. Hepatic encephalopathy is particularly associated with advanced hepatocellular disease such as in cirrhosis (page 621).

HEPATIC TUMOURS AND TUMOUR-LIKE LESIONS

The liver is the site for benign tumours, tumour-like lesions, and both primary and metastatic malignant tumours. However, metastatic tumours are much more common than primary tumours and tumour-like lesions. Primary hepatic tumours may arise from *hepatic cells, bile duct epithelium,* or *mesodermal structures* (Table 19.12). But first, brief comments on tumour-like lesions occurring in the liver are given below.

TUMOUR-LIKE LESIONS

These include cysts in the liver and focal nodular hyperplasia.

TABLE 19.12: Classification of Primary Hepatic Tumours.

BENIGN	MALIGNANT
A. Hepatocellular tumours	
Hepatocellular (liver cell) adenoma	Hepatocellular (liver cell) carcinoma Hepatoblastoma (Embryoma)
B. Biliary tumours	
Bile duct adenoma (Cholangioma)	Cholangiocarcinoma Combined hepatocellular and cholangiocarcinoma Cystadenocarcinoma
C. Mesodermal tumours	
Haemangioma	Angiosarcoma Embryonal sarcoma

Hepatic Cysts

Cysts in the liver may be single or multiple. They are mainly of 3 types—congenital, simple (nonparasitic) and hydatid *(Echinococcus)* cysts.

1. CONGENITAL CYSTS. These are uncommon. They are usually small (less than 1 cm in diameter) and are lined by biliary epithelium. They may be single, or occur as polycystic liver disease, often associated with polycystic kidney. On occasions, these cysts have abundant connective tissue and numerous ducts, warranting the designation of *congenital hepatic fibrosis.*

2. SIMPLE (NON-PARASITIC) CYSTS. Simple cysts are solitary non-parasitic cysts seen more frequently in middle-aged women. The cyst is usually large (up to 20 cm in diameter), lying underneath the Glisson's capsule and filled with serous fluid. The cyst produces a palpable mass and may be associated with jaundice.

Histologically, the cyst wall is composed of compact fibrous tissue and is lined by low columnar to cuboid epithelium and occasionally by squamous lining.

3. HYDATID (ECHINOCOCCUS) CYSTS. Hydatid cyst has already been discussed on page 636.

Focal Nodular Hyperplasia

Grossly, Focal nodular hyperplasia is a well-demarcated tumour-like nodule occurring underneath the Glisson's capsule. The nodules may be single or multiple, measuring about 5 cm in diameter. It may be tan-yellow or bile-stained. The sectioned surface shows a central fibrous scar.

Histologically, it is composed of collagenous septa radiating from the central fibrous scar which separate nodules of normal hepatocytes without portal triads or central hepatic veins. The fibrous septa contain prominent lymphocytic infiltrate.

The *etiology* of focal nodular hyperplasia is not known but these lesions are more common in women taking oral contraceptives.

BENIGN HEPATIC TUMOURS

These are uncommon and some of them are incidental autopsy findings. These include hepatocellular (liver cell) adenoma, bile duct adenoma (cholangioma) and haemangioma.

Hepatocellular (Liver Cell) Adenoma

Adenomas arising from hepatocytes are rare and are reported in women in reproductive age group in association with use of oral contraceptives, sex hormone therapy and with pregnancy. The tumour presents as intrahepatic mass that may be mistaken for hepatocellular carcinoma and may rupture causing severe intraperitoneal haemorrhage.

*PATHOLOGIC CHANGES. **Grossly,*** the tumour usually occurs singly but about 10% are multiple. It is partly or completely encapsulated and slightly lighter in colour than adjacent liver or may be bile-stained. The tumours vary from a few centimetres up to 30 cm in diameter. On cut section, many of the tumours have varying degree of infarction and haemorrhage.

Histologically, liver cell adenomas are composed of sheets and cords of hepatocytes which may be normal-looking or may show slight variation in size and shape but no mitoses. The hepatocytes in adenomas contain greater amount of glycogen than the surrounding liver cells and may sometimes show fatty change. Hepatocellular adenomas lack portal tracts and bile ducts but bile canaliculi containing bile-plugs may be present. Numerous blood vessels are generally present in the tumour which may be thrombosed. Thrombosis leads to infarction and may result in rupture with intraperitoneal haemorrhage.

Bile Duct Adenoma (Cholangioma)

Intrahepatic or extrahepatic bile duct adenoma is a rare benign tumour. The tumour may be small, composed of acini lined by biliary epithelium and separated by variable amount of connective tissue, or are larger cystadenomas having loculi lined by biliary epithelium.

Haemangioma

Haemangioma is the commonest benign tumour of the liver. Majority of them are asymptomatic and discovered incidentally. Rarely, a haemangioma may rupture into the peritoneal cavity.

*PATHOLOGIC CHANGES. **Grossly,*** haemangiomas appear as solitary or multiple, circumscribed, red-purple lesions, commonly subcapsular and varying from a few millimetres to a few centimetres in diameter. They are commonly cavernous type giving the sectioned surface a spongy appearance.

Histologically, haemangioma of the liver shows characteristic large, cavernous, blood-filled spaces, lined by a single layer of endothelium and separated by connective tissue (see Fig. 11.16). Some haemangiomas may undergo progressive fibrosis and may later get calcified (COLOUR PLATE XIV: CL 53).

MALIGNANT HEPATIC TUMOURS

Among the primary malignant tumours of the liver, hepatocellular (liver cell) carcinoma accounts for approximately 85% of all primary malignant tumours, cholangiocarcinoma for about 5-10%, and infrequently mixed pattern is seen. The remainder are rare tumours that include hepatoblastoma, haemangiosarcoma (angiosarcoma) and embryonal sarcoma. Hepatic haemangiosarcoma and embryonal sarcoma resemble in morphology with their counterparts elsewhere in the body.

Hepatocellular Carcinoma

Hepatocellular or liver cell carcinoma (HCC), sometimes termed hepatoma, is the most common primary malignant tumour of the liver. The tumour shows marked geographic variations in incidence which is closely related to hepatitis B virus infection in the region. Whereas the prevalence of HCC is less than 1% of all autopsies in the United States and Europe, the incidence in Africa and South-East Asia is 2-8%. HCC is the leading malignant tumour in South-East Asia. Liver cell cancer is 4-6 times more common in males than in females. The peak incidence occurs in 5th to 6th decades of life but in high incidence areas where HBV infection is prevalent, it occurs a decade or two earlier. The tumour supervenes on cirrhosis, usually post-necrotic macronodular type, in 70-80% of cases.

ETIOPATHOGENESIS. A number of etiologic factors are implicated in the etiology of HCC, most important being *HBV and HCV infection, and association with cirrhosis.*

1. **Relation to HBV infection.** Genesis of HCC is linked to prolonged infection with HBV. The evidence in support is both epidemiologic and direct.

i) The incidence of HBsAg positivity is higher in HCC patients. For example, in Taiwan, HBsAg-positive carriers have more than 200 times greater risk of developing HCC than HBsAg-negative patients, particularly when the infection is acquired in early life.

ii) In African and Asian patients, 95% cases of HCC have anti-HBc.

iii) There is more direct evidence of integration of HBV-DNA genome in the genome of tumour cells of HCC.

2. **Relation to HCV infection.** More recent evidence points to long-standing HCV infection as a major factor in the etiology of HCC. The evidences in support are as under:

i) In developed countries where higher incidence of HCC was earlier attributed to endemic infection (e.g. in Japan) has shown a remarkable shift to HCV infection. However, in less developed countries HBV is still the predominant etiologic factor in the pathogenesis of HCC.

ii) The patients having anti-HCV and anti-HBc antibodies together have three times higher risk of developing HCC than in those with either antibody alone.

iii) It is also possible that HBV and HCV infection act synergistically to predispose to HCC.

3. **Relation to cirrhosis.** Cirrhosis of all etiologic types is more commonly associated with HCC but the most frequent association is with macronodular post-necrotic cirrhosis. The mechanism of progression to HCC appears to be chronic regenerative activity in cirrhosis, or that the damaged liver in cirrhosis is rendered vulnerable to carcinogenic influences. *Liver cell dysplasia* identified by cellular enlargement, nuclear hyperchromatism and multinucleate cells, is found in 60% of cirrhotic livers with HCC and in only 10% of non-cirrhotic livers.

4. **Relation to alcohol.** It has been observed that alcoholics have about four-fold increased risk of developing HCC. It is possible that alcohol may act as co-carcinogen with HBV infection, but alcohol does not appear to be a hepatic carcinogen *per se.*

5. **Mycotoxins.** An important mycotoxin, aflatoxin B1, produced by a mould *Aspergillus flavus,* can contaminate stored grains or groundnuts, especially in less developed countries. Aflatoxin B1 is carcinogenic; it may act as a co-carcinogen with hepatitis B or may suppress the cellular immune response.

6. **Chemical carcinogens.** A number of chemical carcinogens can induce liver cancer in experimental animals. These include butter-yellow and nitrosamines used as common food additives.

7. **Miscellaneous factors.** Limited role of various other factors in HCC has been observed. These include:

i) haemochromatosis;

ii) α-1-antitrypsin deficiency;

iii) prolonged immunosuppressive therapy in renal transplant patients;

iv) other types of viral hepatitis;

v) tobacco smoking; and

vi) parasitic infestations such as clonorchiasis and schistosomiasis.

Pathogenesis of hepatocellular carcinoma can be explained on the basis of genetic mutations induced by one of the above major etiologic factors. In many cases, this mutated gene has been identified as inactivation of tumour suppressor oncogene *TP53* by HBV that results in disruption of normal growth control. In this regards, the role of X-protein (HBxAg) generated from X-gene of HBV has been found to contribute to carcinogenesis by binding to *TP53.*

PATHOLOGIC CHANGES. Macroscopically, the HCC may form one of the following 3 patterns of growth, in decreasing order of frequency (Fig. 19.29):

i) *Expanding type:* Most frequently, it forms a *single,* yellow-brown, *large mass,* most often in the right lobe of the liver with central necrosis, haemorrhage and occasional bile-staining. It may be deceptively encapsulated.

ii) *Multifocal type:* Less often, *multifocal, multiple masses,* 3-5 cm in diameter, scattered throughout the liver are seen.

iii) *Infiltrating (Spreading) type:* Rarely, the HCC forms diffusely infiltrating tumour mass.

Microscopically, the tumour cells in the typical HCC resemble hepatocytes but vary with the degree of differentiation, ranging from well-differentiated to highly anaplastic lesions. Most of the HCC have trabecular growth pattern. The tumour cells have a tendency to invade and grow along blood vessels. Thus important diagnostic features are the *patterns of tumour cells* and their *cytologic features* (**COLOUR PLATE XXVI: CL 101**):

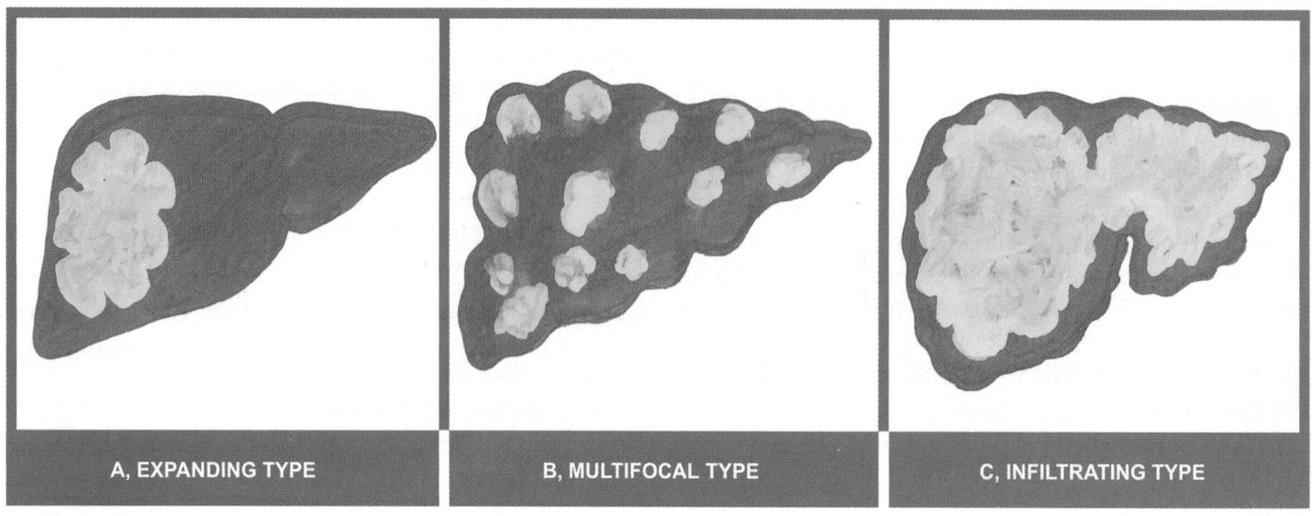

FIGURE 19.29

Macroscopic patterns of hepatocellular carcinoma.

1. Histologic patterns: These include the following:
i) *Trabecular or sinusoidal pattern* is the most common. The trabeculae are made up of 2-8 cell wide layers of tumour cells separated by vascular spaces or sinusoids which are endothelium-lined (Fig. 19.30).
ii) *Pseudoglandular or acinar pattern* is seen sometimes. The tumour cells are disposed around central cystic space formed by degeneration and breakdown in solid trabeculae.
iii) *Compact pattern* resembles trabecular pattern but the tumour cells form large solid masses with inconspicuous sinusoids.
iv) *Scirrhous pattern* is characterised by more abundant fibrous stroma.

2 Cytologic features: The typical cytologic features in the HCC consist of cells resembling hepatocytes having vesicular nuclei with prominent nucleoli. The cytoplasm is granular and eosinophilic but becomes increasingly basophilic with increasing malignancy. Aside from these features, a few other cytologic variants are: pleomorphism, bizarre giant cell formation, spindle-shaped cells, tumour cells with clear cytoplasm, presence of bile within dilated canaliculi, and intracytoplasmic Mallory's hyalin.

FIBROLAMELLAR CARCINOMA. A clinicopathologic variant of the HCC is fibrolamellar carcinoma of the liver found in young people of both sexes. The tumour forms a single large mass which may be encapsulated and occurs in the absence of cirrhosis.

Histologically, the tumour is composed of eosinophilic polygonal cells (oncocytes) forming cords and nests which are separated by bands of fibrous stroma.

The prognosis of fibrolamellar carcinoma is better than other forms of HCC.

CLINICAL FEATURES. Hepatic cancer may remain undetected initially because it often occurs in patients with underlying cirrhosis. The usual features consist of hepatomegaly with palpable mass in the liver, right upper quadrant pain or tenderness, and less often, jaundice, fever and haemorrhage from oesophageal varices. Ascites with RBCs and malignant cells is found in about half the patients. Rarely, systemic endocrine manifestations such as hypercalcaemia, hypoglycaemia, gynaecomastia and acquired porphyria are encountered.

Laboratory findings yield nonspecific results like anaemia, markedly elevated serum alkaline phosphatase as found in cirrhosis, and high serum alpha-foetoprotein (AFP) which is also found elevated in yolk sac tumour, cirrhosis, chronic hepatitis, massive liver necrosis and normal pregnancy. Very high levels of AFP (above 500 ng/ml) are observed in 70-80% cases of HCC. An abnormal type of prothrombin, des-γ-carboxy prothrombin, is also elevated and correlates well with AFP levels.

SPREAD. The HCC can have both intrahepatic and extrahepatic spread which faithfully reproduces the structure of the primary tumour.

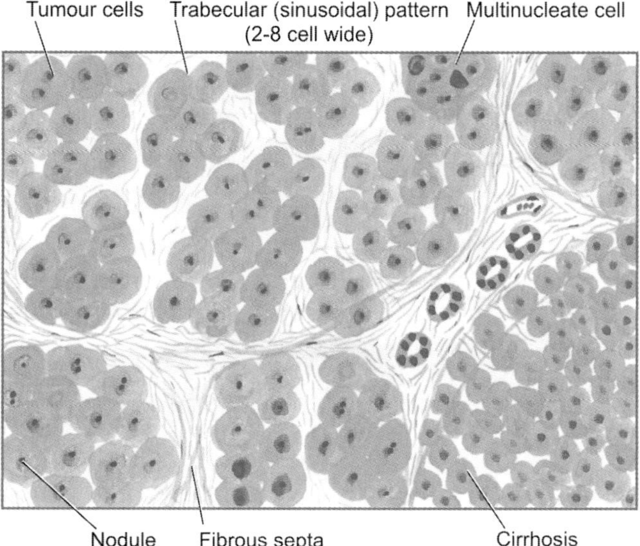

FIGURE 19.30

Hepatocellular carcinoma, typical microscopic pattern. The tumour cells resembling hepatocytes show pleomorphism and are seen forming 2-8 cell wide trabeculae which are separated by endothelium-lined sinusoidal spaces.

- **Intrahepatic spread** occurs by haematogenous route and forms multiple metastases in the liver.
- **Extrahepatic spread** occurs via hepatic or portal veins to different sites, chiefly to lungs and bones, and by lymphatic route to regional lymph nodes at the porta hepatis and to mediastinal and cervical lymph nodes.

The causes of death from the HCC are cachexia, massive bleeding from oesophageal varices, and liver failure with hepatic coma.

Cholangiocarcinoma

Cholangiocarcinoma is the designation used for carcinoma arising from bile duct epithelium within the liver *(peripheral cholangiocarcinoma)*. Carcinomas arising from the large hilar ducts *(hilar cholangiocarcinoma)* and from extrahepatic ducts are termed *bile duct carcinomas* (page 665). None of the etiologic factors related to HCC have any role in the genesis of cholangiocarcinoma. However, the etiological factors involved in it are exposure to radio-opaque dye thorotrast, anabolic steroids, clonorchiasis and fibrocystic disease. The tumour affects older people and the clinical features are those of HCC but with prominence of jaundice.

*PATHOLOGIC CHANGES. **Grossly,*** the tumour is firm to hard and whitish.

Microscopically, the tumour has glandular structure. The tumour cells resemble biliary epithelium but without bile secretion. They form various patterns such as tubular, ductular or papillary. The stroma consists of fibrous tissue with little or no capillary formation. Occasionally, mucinous, signet-ring and adenosquamous type of patterns are found. An uncommon variant is combined hepatocellular-cholangiocarcinoma.

Hepatoblastoma (Embryoma)

Hepatoblastoma is a rare malignant tumour arising from primitive hepatic parenchymal cells. It presents before the age of 2 years as progressive abdominal distension with anorexia, failure to thrive, fever and jaundice. It is more common in boys. The concentration of serum AFP is high. The tumour grows rapidly and causes death by haemorrhage, hepatic failure or widespread metastases.

*PATHOLOGIC CHANGES, **Grossly,*** the tumour is circumscribed and lobulated mass measuring 5-25 cm in size, having areas of cystic degeneration, haemorrhage and necrosis.

Microscopically, hepatoblastoma consists of 2 components:

i) Epithelial component contains 2 types of cells—*'embryonal' hepatocytes* are small with dark-staining, hyperchromatic nuclei and scanty cytoplasm, and *'foetal' hepatocytes* are larger with more cytoplasm that may be granular or clear. The epithelial cells are organised in trabeculae, ribbons or rosettes.

ii) Mesenchymal component includes fibrous connective tissue, cartilage and osteoid of variable degree of maturation. Extramedullary haematopoiesis is a frequent accompaniment.

Secondary HepaticTumours

Metastatic tumours in the liver are more common than the primary hepatic tumours. Most frequently, they are blood-borne metastases, irrespective of whether the primary tumour is drained by portal vein or systemic veins. Most frequent primary tumours metastasising to the liver, in descending order of frequency, are those of stomach, breast, lungs, colon, oesophagus, pancreas, malignant melanoma and haematopoietic malignancies. Sarcomas rarely metastasise to the liver. Occasionally, metastatic involvement may be present in the absence of obvious evidence of primary tumour. Aside from general features of disseminated malignancy such as anorexia, cachexia and anaemia, the patients have hepatomegaly with nodular free margin. There is little hepatic dysfunction until late in the course of hepatic metastatic disease.

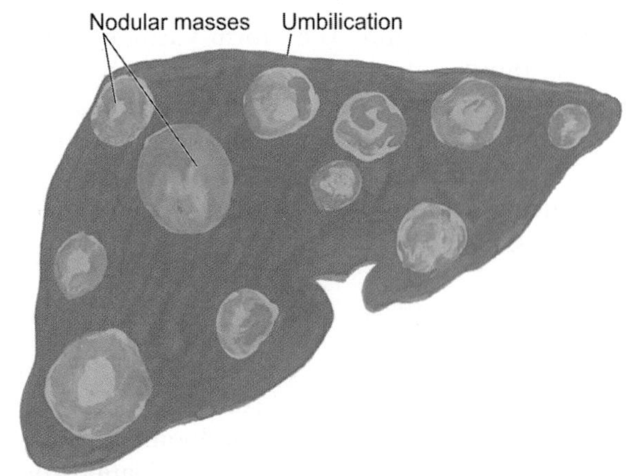

FIGURE 19.31

Metastatic tumour deposits in the liver from malignant melanoma as seen on sectioned surface. Characteristic features include multiple, variable-sized, nodular masses, often under the capsule, producing umbilication on the surface.

PATHOLOGIC CHANGES. ***Grossly,*** most metastatic carcinomas form multiple, spherical, nodular masses which are of variable size. Liver is enlarged and heavy, weighing 5 kg or more. The tumour deposits are white, well-demarcated, soft or haemorrhagic. The surface of the liver shows characteristic umbilication due to central necrosis of nodular masses (Fig. 19.31). ***Histologically,*** the metastatic tumours generally reproduce the structure of the primary lesions.

BILIARY SYSTEM

NORMAL STRUCTURE

ANATOMY. The gallbladder is a pear-shaped organ, 9 cm in length and has a capacity of approximately 50 ml. It consists of the *fundus, body* and *neck* that tapers into the cystic duct. The two hepatic ducts from right and left lobes of the liver unite at the porta hepatis to form the common hepatic duct which is joined by the cystic duct from the gallbladder to form the common bile duct. The common bile duct enters the second part of the duodenum posteriorly. In about 70% of cases, it is joined by the main pancreatic duct to form the combined opening in the duodenum *(ampulla of Vater).* In 30% cases, the common bile duct and the pancreatic duct open separately into the duodenum (*see* Fig. 19.1). The common bile duct in its duodenal portion is surrounded by longitudinal and circular muscles derived from the duodenum forming *sphincter of Oddi.*

HISTOLOGY. ***Histologically,*** the gallbladder, unlike the rest of gastrointestinal tract, lacks the muscularis mucosae and submucosa. The wall of the gallbladder is composed of the following 4 layers:

1. **Mucosal layer:** It has a single layer of tall columnar epithelium which is thrown into permanent folds that are larger and more numerous in the neck of the gallbladder. Beneath the epithelium is delicate lamina propria that contains capillaries, and in the region of the neck, a few acinar glands are present.

2. **Smooth muscle layer:** External to the lamina propria are smooth muscle bundles in layers—inner longitudinal, middle oblique, and outer circular.

3. **Perimuscular layer:** Outer to the muscle layer is a zone of fibrous connective tissue with some interspersed fat cells.

4. **Serosal layer:** The perimuscular layer is covered by serosa on the peritoneal surface of the gallbladder. The peritoneum covers the gallbladder except in the region of gallbladder fossa where it is embedded in the liver.

The *extrahepatic bile ducts* are also lined by tall columnar epithelium that overlies the lamina propria. It is surrounded by dense layer of fibromuscular tissue. The ducts which lie between the lobules of the liver and receive bile from the canaliculi are lined by cuboidal or flattened cells.

FUNCTIONS. The main function of the gallbladder is to store and concentrate the bile secreted by the liver and then deliver it into the intestine for digestion and absorption of fat. The concentrating ability of the gallbladder is due to its absorptive mucosal surface that has numerous folds. Normally, the liver secretes approximately 500 ml of bile per day and the gallbladder concentrates it 5-10 times. The motility, concentration and relaxation of the gallbladder are under the influence of a peptide hormone, cholecystokinin, released from neuroendocrine cells of the duodenum and jejunum.

CONGENITAL ANOMALIES

Several uncommon congenital anomalies of the biliary system have been described. These include: agenesis, duplication and heterotopic tissue. However, *congenital cystic lesions* of the bile ducts (as also of the liver) are more frequently being diagnosed. These conditions include: congenital intrahepatic biliary dilatation (Caroli's disease), choledochal cysts, polycystic liver disease and congenital hepatic fibrosis. They are found in various combinations and are usually inherited. All of them may be complicated by malignant change.

CHOLELITHIASIS (GALLSTONES)

Gallstones are formed from constituents of the bile (viz. cholesterol, bile pigments and calcium salts) alongwith other organic components. Accordingly, the gallstones commonly contain cholesterol, bile pigment and calcium salts in varying proportions. They are usually formed in the gallbladder, but sometimes may develop within extrahepatic biliary passages, and rarely in the larger intrahepatic bile duct.

RISK FACTORS. The incidence of gallstones varies markedly in different geographic areas, age, sex, diet and various other risk factors. These factors which largely pertain to cholesterol stones can be summed up in the old saying that gallstones are common in 4F's—*'fat, female, fertile (multipara)* and *forty'*. Some of the risk factors in lithogenesis are explained below:

1. **Geography.** Gallstones are quite prevalent in almost the entire Western world. American Indians have the highest known prevalence. Black Africans and populations in the Eastern world are relatively free of cholelithiasis.

2. **Genetic factors.** There is increased frequency of gallstones in first-degree relatives of patients with cholelithiasis. Patients of gallstones disease have increased secretion of dietary cholesterol in bile than in non-gallstone patients inspite of high-cholesterol diet.

3. **Age.** There is steady increase in the prevalence of gallstones with advancing age which may be related to increased cholesterol content in the bile. The incidence increases above the age of 40 and presentation is usually in the 50s and 60s.

4. **Sex.** Gallstones are twice more frequent in women than in men. In the United States, autopsy series have shown gallstones in about 20% of women and 8% of men above the age of 40. The incidence is higher in multiparous women than in nulliparous women.

5. **Drugs.** Women on oestrogen therapy or on birth control pills have higher incidence of gallstones. This is considered to be due to production of more lithogenic bile as a result of cholestatic effect of oestrogen. Similar is the influence of clofibrate used for lowering blood cholesterol.

6. **Obesity.** Obesity is associated with increased cholesterol synthesis and excretion resulting in higher incidence of gallstones in obese patients.

7. **Diet.** Deficiency of dietary fibre content is linked to higher prevalence of gallstones. A moderate consumption of alcohol, however, seems to protect against gallstones.

8. **Gastrointestinal diseases.** Certain gastrointestinal disorders such as Crohn's disease, ileal resection, ileal bypass surgery etc are associated with interruption in enterohepatic circulation followed by gallstone formation.

9. **Factors in pigment gallstones.** All the above factors apply largely to cholesterol stones. Pigment stones, whether pure or mixed type, are more frequently associated with haemolytic anaemias which lead to increased content of unconjugated bilirubin in the bile. Pigment stones are also more frequent in cirrhosis and hepatocellular disease.

PATHOGENESIS. The mechanism of gallstone formation or lithogenesis is explained separately below under 2 headings: firstly for cholesterol, mixed gallstones and biliary sludge, and, secondly for pigment gallstones as under:

PATHOGENESIS OF CHOLESTEROL, MIXED GALLSTONES AND BILIARY SLUDGE. Cholesterol is essentially insoluble in water and can be solublised by another lipid. Normally, cholesterol and phospholipids (lecithin) are secreted into bile as 'bilayered vesicles' but are converted into 'mixed miscelles' by addition of bile acids, the third constituent. If there is excess of cholesterol compared to the other two constituents, unstable cholesterol-rich vesicles remain behind which aggregate and form cholesterol crystals. Formation of such lithogenic (stone-forming) bile is explained by the following mechanisms (Fig. 19.32):

1. **Supersaturation of bile:** Several etiologic factors listed above favour increased secretion of cholesterol in the presence of normal bile acids and lecithin in the

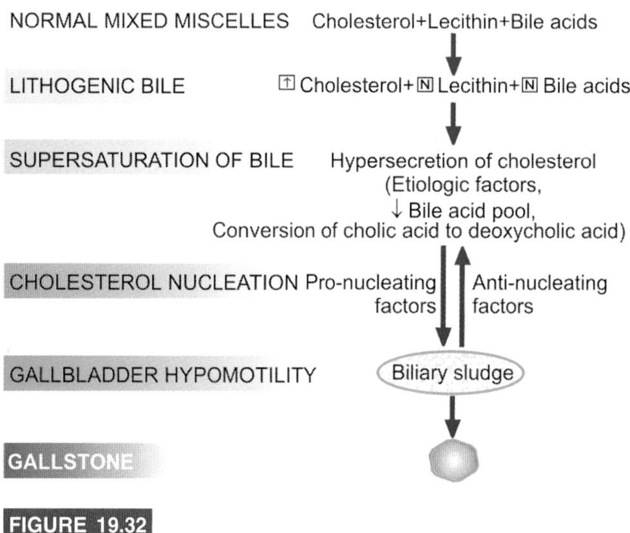

FIGURE 19.32

Schematic pathogenesis of gallstone formation.

bile as the major mechanism for initiation of gallstone formation. Two other disturbances which may contribute to supersaturation of the bile with cholesterol are as under:

i) *Reduced bile acid pool*: This causes rapid loss of the available bile acids into the small intestine and then into the colon, resulting in supersaturation of the bile with cholesterol.

ii) *Increased conversion of cholic acid to deoxycholic acid:* This causes increased secretion of deoxycholate in the bile which is associated with hypersecretion of cholesterol into the bile.

Although supersaturation of the bile with cholesterol is an important pre-requisite for lithogenesis, this in itself is not sufficient for cholesterol precipitation.

2. Cholesterol nucleation. Initiation of cholesterol stones occurs by nucleation of cholesterol monohydrate crystals. Accelerated nucleation of cholesterol monohydrate may occur either from pro-nucleating factors or from deficiency of anti-nucleating factors:

i) *Pro-nucleating factors* are mucin and non-mucin glycoproteins secreted by epithelial cells of the gallbladder.

ii) *anti-nucleating factors* are apolipoproteins AI and AII, and some glycoproteins.

Cholesterol monohydrate nucleation probably occurs in the mucin gel layer of the gallbladder followed by continued addition and precipitation of more crystals resulting in solid state crystals.

3. Gallbladder hypomotility. Normally, the gallbladder is capable of emptying and clearing any sludge or debris which might initiate stone formation. This takes place under the influence of *cholecystokinin* secreted from small intestine. However, the motility of gallbladder may be impaired due to decrease in cholecystokinin receptors in the gallbladder resulting in stasis of biliary sludge and lithogenesis. A defect in gallbladder emptying has been found to play a role in recurrence of gallstone formation in patients who undergo biliary lithotripsy.

PATHOGENESIS OF PIGMENT GALLSTONES. The mechanism of pigment stone formation is explained on the basis of following factors:

i) Chronic haemolysis resulting in increased level of unconjugated bilirubin in the bile.

ii) Alcoholic cirrhosis.

iii) Chronic biliary tract infection e.g. by parasitic infestations of the biliary tract such as by *Clonorchis sinensis* and *Ascaris lumbricoides.*

iv) Demographic and genetic factors e.g. in rural setting and prevalence in Asian countries.

TYPES OF GALLSTONES. As stated before, gallstones contain cholesterol, bile pigment and calcium carbonate, either in pure form or in various combinations. Accordingly, gallstones are of 3 major types—*pure gallstones, mixed gallstones* and *combined gallstones.* Mixed gallstones are the most common (80%) while pure and combined gallstones comprise 10% each. In general, gallstones are formed most frequently in the gallbladder but may occur in extrahepatic as well as intrahepatic biliary passages. Gallbladders containing pure stones show no significant inflammatory reaction, whereas chronic cholecystitis is invariably present in gallbladders with mixed and combined gallstones. Presence of calcium salts renders gallstones radio-opaque, while cholesterol stones appear as radiolucent filling defects in the gallbladder.

The salient features of various types of gallstones are summarised in Table 19.13 and presented below:

1. Pure gallstones. They constitute about 10% of all gallstones. They are further divided into 3 types according to the component of bile forming them. These are as under **(COLOUR PLATE XXVI: CL 103):**

i) Pure cholesterol gallstones: They are usually solitary, oval and fairly large (3 cm or more) filling the gallbladder. Their surface is hard, smooth, whitish-yellow and glistening. On cut section, the pure cholesterol stone shows radiating glistening crystals. It may result in deposition of cholesterol within the mucosal macrophages of the gallbladder producing *cholesterolosis* which is an asymptomatic condition. Pure cholesterol stones are radiolucent but 10-20% of them have calcium carbonate in them which renders them opaque.

ii) Pure pigment gallstones: These stones composed primarily of bile pigment, calcium bilirubinate, and contain less than 20% cholesterol. They are generally multiple, jet-black and small (less than 1 cm in diameter). They have mulberry like external surface. They are soft and can be easily crushed. The gallbladder usually appears uninvolved.

iii) Pure calcium carbonate gallstones: They are rare. Calcium carbonate gallstones are usually multiple, grey-white, small (less than 1 cm in diameter), faceted and fairly hard due to calcium content. They, too, do not produce any change in the gallbladder wall.

2. Mixed gallstones. Mixed gallstones are the most common (80%) and contain more than 50% cholesterol monohydarate plus an admixture of calcium salts, bile pigments and fatty acids. They are always multiple, multifaceted so that they fit together and vary in size from as tiny as sand-grain to 1 cm or more in diameter. On section, they have distinct laminated structure with alternating dark pigment layer and pale-white layer revealing different combinations of cholesterol, bilirubin pigment and calcium carbonate, laid down in layers at different times (COLOUR PLATE XXVI: CL 104). Mixed gallstones are invariably accompanied by chronic cholecystitis.

3. **Combined gallstones.** They comprise about 10% of all gallstones. Combined gallstones are usually solitary, large and smooth-surfaced. It has a *pure gallstone nucleus* (cholesterol, bile pigment or calcium carbonate) and outer shell of mixed gallstone; or a *mixed gallstone nucleus* with pure gallstone shell, (COLOUR PLATE XXVI: CL 104). Combined gallstones, too, are associated with chronic cholecystitis.

CLINICAL MANIFESTATIONS AND COMPLICATIONS. In about 50% cases, gallstones cause no symptoms and may be diagnosed by chance during investigations for some other condition *(silent gallstones).* The future course in such asymptomatic silent cases is controversial, most surgeons advocating cholecystectomy while physicians advising watchful waiting. Follow-up studies, however, show that only about 10% of such cases develop symptoms. Symptomatic gallstone disease appears only when complications develop. These are as under:

1. **Cholecystitis.** The relationship between cholelithiasis and cholecystitis is well known but it is not certain which of the two comes first. The patients with gallstones develop symptoms due to cholecystitis which include typical biliary colic precipitated by fatty meal, nausea, vomiting, fever alongwith leucocytosis and high serum bilirubin.

2. **Choledocholithiasis.** Gallstones may pass down into the extrahepatic biliary passages and the small bowel, or less often they may be formed in the biliary tree. Patients with gallstone in the common bile duct frequently develop pain and obstructive jaundice. Fever may develop due to bacterial ascending cholangitis.

3. **Mucocele.** Mucocele or hydrops of the gallbladder is distension of the gallbladder by clear, watery mucinous secretion resulting from impacted stones in the neck of the gallbladder.

4. **Biliary fistula.** An uncommon complication of cholelithiasis is formation of fistulae between one part of the biliary system and the bowel, and rarely between the gallbladder and the skin.

5. **Gallstone ileus.** A gallstone in the intestine may be passed in the faeces without causing symptoms. Occasionally, however, gallstones in the intestine may cause intestinal obstruction called gallstone ileus.

6. **Gallbladder cancer.** There is a small and doubtful risk of development of cancer of the gallbladder in cases with cholelithiasis (page 664).

CHOLECYSTITIS

Cholecystitis or inflammation of the gallbladder may be acute, chronic, or acute superimposed on chronic. Though chronic cholecystitis is more common, acute cholecystitis is a surgical emergency.

Acute Cholecystitis

In many ways, acute cholecystitis is similar to acute appendicitis. The condition usually begins with obstruction, followed by infection later.

ETIOPATHOGENESIS. Based on the initiating mechanisms, acute cholecystitis occurs in two types of situations—*acute calculous* and *acute acalculous cholecystitis.*

■ **Acute calculous cholecystitis.** In 90% of cases, acute cholecystitis is caused by obstruction in the neck of the gallbladder or in the cystic duct by a gallstone. The commonest location of impaction of a gallstone is in Hartmann's pouch. Obstruction results in distension of the gallbladder followed by acute inflammation which is initially due to chemical irritation. Later, however, secondary bacterial infection, chiefly by *E. coli* and *Streptococcus faecalis,* supervenes.

■ **Acute acalculous cholecystitis.** The remaining 10% cases of acute cholecystitis do not contain gallstones. In such cases, a variety of causes have been assigned such as previous nonbiliary surgery, multiple injuries, burns, recent childbirth, severe sepsis, dehydration, torsion of the gallbladder and diabetes mellitus. Rare causes include primary bacterial infection like salmonellosis and cholera and parasitic infestations.

PATHOLOGIC CHANGES. Except for the presence or absence of calculi, the two forms of acute cholecystitis are morphologically similar.

Grossly, the gallbladder is distended and tense. The serosal surface is coated with fibrinous exudate with congestion and haemorrhages. The mucosa is bright red. The lumen is filled with pus mixed with green bile. In calculous cholecystitis, a stone is generally impacted in the neck or in the cystic duct. When

TABLE 19.13: Features of Gallstones.

TYPE	FREQUENCY	COMPOSITION	GALLBLADDER CHANGES	APPEARANCE
1. *Pure gallstones*	10%	i) Cholesterol	Cholesterolosis	Solitary, oval, large, smooth, yellow-white; on C/S radiating glistening crystals
		ii) Bile pigment	No change	Multiple, small, jet-black, mulberry-shaped; on C/S soft black
		iii) Calcium carbonate	No change	Multiple, small, grey-white, faceted; C/S hard
2. *Mixed gallstones*	80%	Cholesterol, bile pigment and calcium carbonate in varying combination	Chronic cholecystitis	Multiple, multifaceted, variable size, on C/S laminated alternating dark-pigment layer and pale-white layer
3. *Combined gallstones*	10%	Pure gallstone nucleus with mixed gallstone shell, or mixed gallstone nucleus with pure gallstone shell	Chronic cholecystitis	Solitary, large, smooth; on C/S central nucleus of pure gallstone with mixed shell or vice versa

obstruction of the cystic duct is complete, the lumen is filled with purulent exudate and the condition is known as *empyema of the gallbladder.*

Microscopically, wall of the gallbladder shows marked inflammatory oedema, congestion and neutrophilic exudate. There may be frank abscesses in the wall and gangrenous necrosis with rupture into the peritoneal cavity *(gangrenous cholecystitis).*

CLINICAL FEATURES. The patients of acute cholecystitis of either type have similar clinical features. They present with severe pain in the upper abdomen with features of peritoneal irritation such as guarding and hyperaesthesia. The gallbladder is tender and may be palpable. Fever, leucocytosis with neutrophilia and slight jaundice are generally present. Early cholecystectomy within the first three days has a mortality of less than 0.5% and risk of complications such as perforation, biliary fistula, recurrent attacks and adhesions is avoided. However, medical treatment brings about resolution in a fairly large proportion of cases though chances of recurrence of attack persist.

Chronic Cholecystitis

Chronic cholecystitis is the commonest type of clinical gallbladder disease. There is almost constant association of chronic cholecystitis with cholelithiasis.

ETIOPATHOGENESIS. The association of chronic cholecystitis with mixed and combined gallstones is virtually always present. However, it is not known what initiates the inflammatory response in the gallbladder wall. Possibly, supersaturation of the bile with cholesterol predisposes to both gallstone formation and inflammation. In some patients, repeated attacks of mild acute cholecystitis result in chronic cholecystitis.

PATHOLOGIC CHANGES. Grossly, the gallbladder is generally contracted but may be normal or enlarged. The wall of the gallbladder is thickened which on cut section is grey-white due to dense fibrosis or may be even calcified. The mucosal folds may be intact, thickened, or flattened and atrophied. The lumen commonly contains multiple mixed stones or a combined stone (Fig. 19.33).

Histologically, the features are as under (Fig. 19.34) (COLOUR PLATE XXVI: CL 102):

1. Thickened and congested mucosa but occasionally mucosa may be totally destroyed.
2. Penetration of the mucosa deep into the wall of the gallbladder up to muscularis layer to form *Rokitansky-Aschoff sinuses.*
3. Variable degree of chronic inflammatory reaction, consisting of lymphocytes, plasma cells and macrophages, present in the lamina propria and subserosal layer.
4. Variable degree of fibrosis in the subserosal and subepithelial layers.

A few morphologic variants of chronic cholecystitis are considered below:

- **Cholecystitis glandularis,** when the mucosal folds fuse together due to inflammation and result in formation of crypts of epithelium buried in the gallbladder wall.
- **Porcelain gallbladder** is the pattern when the gallbladder wall is calcified and cracks like an egg-shell.

TABLE 19.13: Gallstones (continued).

MORPHOLOGY

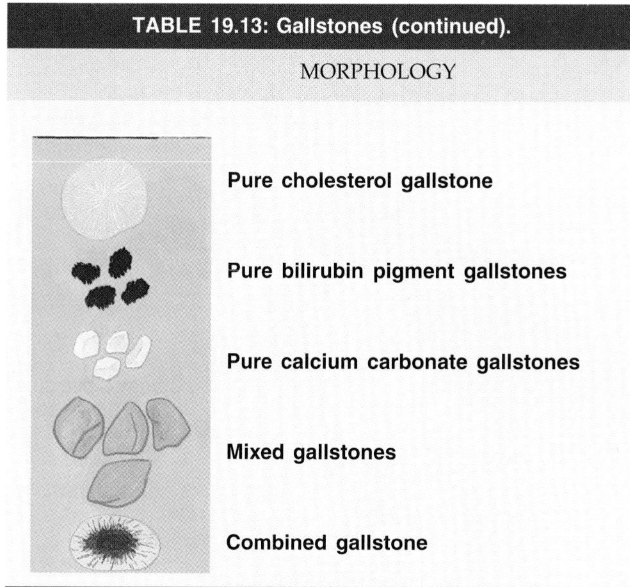

Figure facing Table 19.13

- **Acute on chronic cholecystitis** is the term used for the morphologic changes of acute cholecystitis superimposed on changes of chronic cholecystitis.

CLINICAL FEATURES. Chronic cholecystitis has ill-defined and vague symptoms. Generally, the patient—*a fat, fertile, female of forty or fifty,* presents with abdominal distension or epigastric discomfort, especially after a fatty meal. There is a constant dullache in the right hypochondrium and epigastrium and tenderness over the right upper abdomen. Nausea and flatulence are common. Biliary colic may occasionally occur due to passage of stone into the bile ducts. Cholecystography usually allows radiologic visualisation of the gallstones.

TUMOURS OF BILIARY SYSTEM

Tumours of the biliary tract include benign and malignant tumours and carcinoid of the biliary tract.

BENIGN TUMOURS

Benign tumours such as papilloma, adenoma, adenomyoma, fibroma, lipoma, myxoma, and haemangioma have been described in the biliary tract but all of them are exceedingly rare. *Adenomyoma* is more common benign tumour than the rest. All these tumours resemble their counterparts in morphology elsewhere in the body.

MALIGNANT TUMOURS

Carcinoma of the gallbladder and carcinoma of the bile ducts and ampulla of Vater are among the more frequent malignant tumours of the biliary tract.

Carcinoma of the Gallbladder

Primary carcinoma of the gallbladder is more prevalent than other cancers of the extrahepatic biliary tract. Like cholelithiasis and cholecystitis, it is more frequent in

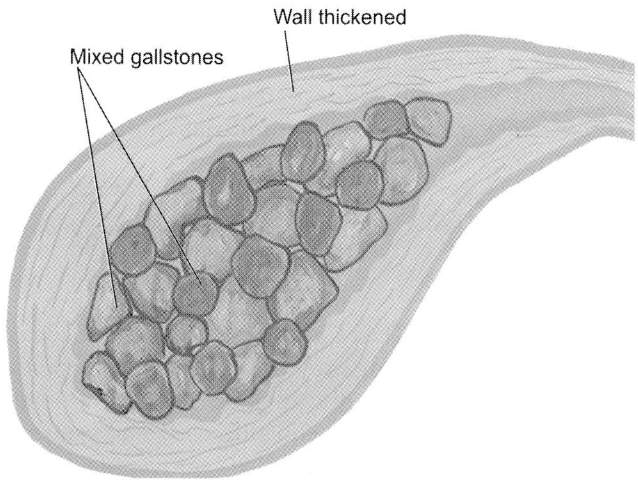

FIGURE 19.33

Chronic cholecystitis with cholelithiasis (mixed gallstones). The wall of the gallbladder is thickened and the lumen is packed with well-fitting, multiple, multi-faceted, mixed gallstones.

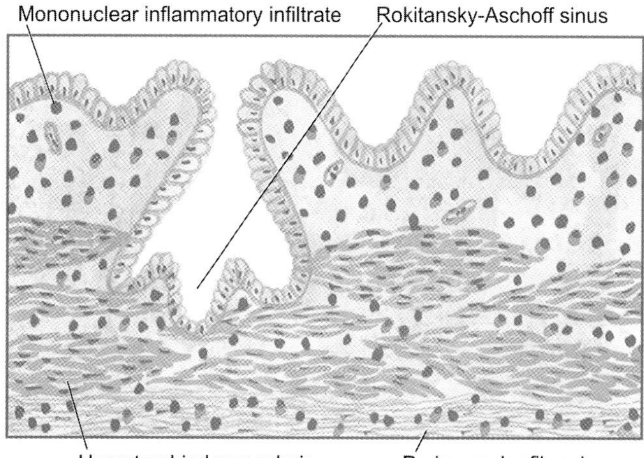

FIGURE 19.34

Chronic cholecystitis, microscopic appearance. There is penetration of epithelium-lined spaces into the gallbladder wall (Rokitansky-Aschoff sinus) in an area. There is subepithelial and subserosal fibrosis and hypertrophy of muscularis. Mononuclear inflammatory cell infiltrate is present in subepithelial and subserosal layers.

women than in men with a peak incidence in 7th decade of life. It is usually slow-growing and may remain undetected until the time it is widely spread and rendered inoperable.

ETIOLOGY. A number of etiologic factors have been implicated.

1. Cholelithiasis and cholecystitis. The most significant association of cancer of the gallbladder is with cholelithiasis and cholecystitis, though there is no definite evidence of causal relationship. Cholelithiasis and cholecystitis are present in about 75% cases of gallbladder cancer. But, on the other hand, the incidence of documented gallbladder cancer in the presence of cholelithiasis and cholecystitis is about 0.5% only. Porcelain gallbladdder is particularly likely to become cancerous.

2. Chemical carcinogens. A number of chemical carcinogens structurally similar to naturally-occurring bile acids have been considered to induce gallbladder cancer. These include methyl cholanthrene, various nitrosamines and pesticides. Workers engaged in rubber industry have higher incidence of gallbladder cancer.

3. Genetic factors. There is higher incidence of cancer of the gallbladder in certain populations living in the same geographic region suggesting a strong genetic component in the disease. Japanese immigrants and Native Americans of the South-Western America have increased frequency while American Indians and Mexicans have lower incidence.

4. Miscellaneous. Patients who have undergone previous surgery on the biliary tract have higher incidence of subsequent gallbladder cancer. Patients with inflammatory bowel disease (ulcerative colitis and Crohn's disease) have high incidence of gallbladder cancer.

PATHOLOGIC CHANGES. The commonest site is the fundus, followed next in frequency by the neck of the gallbladder (Fig. 19.35).

Grossly, cancer of the gallbladder is of 2 types—infiltrating and fungating type.

1. *Infiltrating type* appears as an irregular area of diffuse thickening and induration of the gallbladder wall. It may have deep ulceration causing direct invasion of the gallbladder wall and liver bed. On section, the gallbladder wall is firm due to scirrhous growth.
2. *Fungating type* grows like an irregular, friable, papillary or cauliflower-like growth into the lumen as well as into the wall of the gallbladder and beyond.

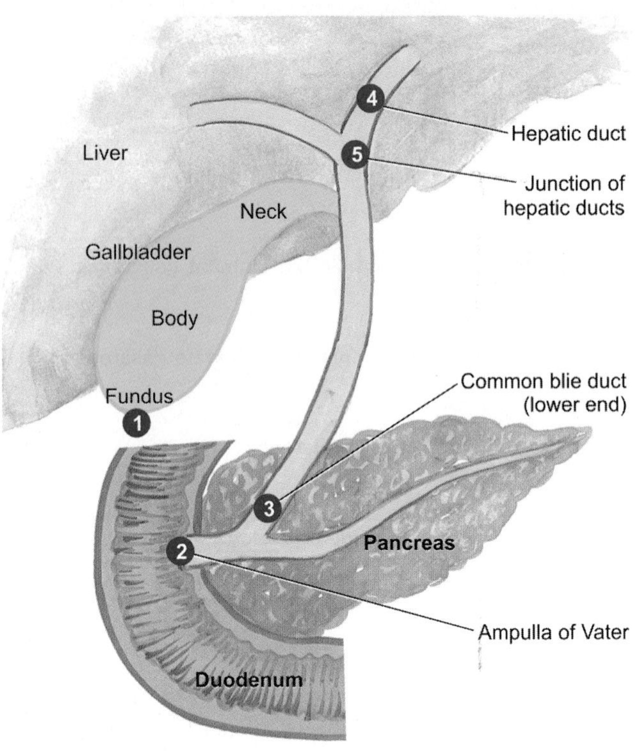

FIGURE 19.35
Frequency of cancer in the biliary system.

Histologically, the following patterns are observed:

1. Most gallbladder cancers are *adenocarcinomas* (90%). They may be papillary or infiltrative, well-differentiated or poorly-differentiated. Most are non-mucin secreting but some are colloid carcinomas forming mucus pools.
2. About 5% of gallbladder cancers are *squamous cell carcinomas* arising from squamous metaplastic epithelium.
3. A few cases show both squamous and adenocarcinoma pattern of growth called *adenosquamous carcinoma.*

CLINICAL FEATURES. Carcinoma of the gallbadder is slow-growing and causes symptoms late in the course of disease. Quite often, the diagnosis is made when gallbladder is removed for cholelithiasis. The symptomatic cases have pain, jaundice, noticeable mass, anorexia and weight loss. In such case, the growth has usually invaded the liver and other adjacent organs and has metastasised to regional lymph nodes and more distant sites such as the lung, peritoneum and gastrointestinal tract.

Carcinoma of Extrahepatic Bile Ducts and Ampulla of Vater

This is an infrequent neoplasm but is more common than the rare benign tumours of the biliary tract. Unlike other diseases of the biliary passages, it is more common in males with peak incidence in 6th decade of life.

ETIOLOGY. There is no association between bile duct carcinoma and gallstones. Bile duct cancers are associated with a number of other conditions such as ulcerative colitis, sclerosing cholangitis, parasitic infestations of the bile ducts with *Fasciola hepatica* (liver fluke), *Ascaris lumbricoides* and *Clonorchis sinensis.*

PATHOLOGIC CHANGES. Extrahepatic bile duct carcinoma may arise anywhere in the biliary tree but the most frequent sites, in descending order of frequency, are: the ampulla of Vater, lower end of common bile duct, hepatic ducts, and the junction of hepatic ducts to form common bile duct (Fig. 19.35).

Grossly, bile duct carcinoma is usually small, extending for 1-2 cm along the duct, producing thickening of the affected duct.

Histologically, the tumour is usually well-differentiated adenocarcinoma which may or may not be mucin-secreting. Perineural invasion is frequently present.

CLINICAL FEATURES. Obstructive jaundice is the usual presenting feature which is characterised by intense pruritus. Pain, steatorrhoea, weight loss and weakness may be present. The tumour usually metastasises to the regional lymph nodes.

EXOCRINE PANCREAS

NORMAL STRUCTURE

The human pancreas, though anatomically a single organ, histologically and physiologically has 2 distinct parts—the *exocrine* and *endocrine parts.* The endocrine part of the gland is dealt with in Chapter 25 while the exocrine gland is considered here. The whole of pancreas, exocrine and endocrine, is embryologically derived from the foregut endoderm.

ANATOMY. The pancreas lies obliquely in the concavity of the duodenum as an elongated structure about 15 cm in length and 100 gm in weight (*see* Fig. 19.1). It is subdivided into 3 topographic zones:

1. The *head* lying in the concavity of the duodenum and the *uncinate process* projecting from the head.
2. The *body* comprises the main part of the gland.
3. The *tail* is the thin, tapering part of the gland towards the hilum of the spleen.

HISTOLOGY. The exocrine pancreas constitutes 80 to 85% of the total gland, while the endocrine pancreas comprises the remaining part.

The exocrine part is divided into rhomboid lobules separated by thin fibrous tissue septa containing blood vessels, lymphatics, nerves and ducts. Each lobule is composed of numerous acini. The acini are lined by pyramid-shaped columnar epithelial cells. These secretory epithelial cells have microvilli projecting into the lumen from their surface. The apical portions of these cells contain zymogen granules in their cytoplasm, while the basal region is deeply basophilic and free of zymogen granules. The zymogen granules are membrane-bound sacs which fuse with the plasma membrane and are then released into the lumina of the acini. The secretions are carried from the acini by fine ductal branches into the small ducts in the lobules and eventually into the main pancreatic duct. The main pancreatic duct is formed by fusion of the ventral duct with the dorsal duct; the latter also called the *duct of Wirsung,* provides the main drainage for pancreatic secretions into the duodenum. The pancreatic secretions are delivered into the second part of the duodenum either by a combined opening of the pancreatic and bile ducts in the ampulla of Vater, or less often both open separately into the duodenum. Occasionally, the proximal part of the dorsal duct persists as the *duct of Santorini.*

FUNCTIONS. The main functions of the exocrine pancreas is the alkaline secretion of digestive enzymes prominent among which are trypsin, chymotrypsin, elastase, amylase, lipase and phospholipase.

DEVELOPMENTAL ANOMALIES

The significant developmental anomalies of the pancreas are ectopic or aberrant pancreatic tissue in Meckel's diverticulum (page 576), anomalies of the ducts, and cystic fibrosis. Only the last named requires elaboration here.

Cystic Fibrosis

Cystic fibrosis of the pancreas or fibrocystic disease is a hereditary disorder characterised by viscid mucous secretions in all the exocrine glands of the body *(mucoviscidosis)* and associated with increased concentrations of electrolytes in the eccrine glands. The terms 'cystic fibrosis' and 'fibrocystic disease' are preferable over 'mucoviscidosis' in view of the main pathologic change of fibrosis produced as a result of obstruction of the passages by viscid mucous secretions. The disease is transmitted as an *autosomal recessive trait* with apparent clinical features in homozygotes only. The genetic defect appears to lie in chromosome 7. It is quite common in the whites (1 per 2000 livebirths). The clinical manifestations may appear at birth or later in adolescence and pertain to multiple organs and systems such as pancreatic insufficiency, intestinal obstruction, steatorrhoea, malnutrition, hepatic cirrhosis and respiratory complications.

PATHOLOGIC CHANGES. Depending upon the severity of involvement and the organs affected, the pathologic changes are variable. Most of the changes are produced as a result of obstruction by viscid mucous.

1. Pancreas. The pancreas is almost invariably involved in cystic fibrosis.

Grossly, pancreatic lobules are ovoid rather than rhomboid. Fatty replacement of the pancreas and grossly visible cysts may be seen.

Microscopically, the lobular architecture of pancreatic parenchyma is maintained. There is increased interlobular fibrosis. The acini are atrophic and many of the acinar ducts contain laminated, eosinophilic concretions. Rarely, inflammation, fat necrosis and cyst formation may be seen. The islet tissue (endocrine pancreas) generally remains intact. Atrophy of the exocrine pancreas may cause impaired fat absorption, steatorrhoea, intestinal obstruction and avitaminosis A.

2. Liver. The bile canaliculi are plugged by viscid mucous which may cause diffuse fatty change, portal fibrosis and ductular proliferation. More severe involvement may cause biliary cirrhosis (page 644).

3. Respiratory tract. Changes in the respiratory passages are seen in almost all typical cases of cystic fibrosis. The viscid mucous secretions of the submucosal glands of the respiratory tract cause obstruction, dilatation and infection of the airways. The changes include chronic bronchitis, bronchiectasis, bronchiolitis, bronchiolectasis, peribronchiolar pneumonia and inflammatory nasal polyps.

4. Salivary glands. Pathologic changes in the salivary glands are similar to those in pancreas and include obstruction of the ducts, dilatation, fibrosis and glandular atrophy.

5. Sweat glands. Hypersecretion of sodium and chloride in the sweat observed in these patients may be reflected pathologically by diminished vacuolation of the cells of eccrine glands.

PANCREATITIS

Pancreatitis is inflammation of the pancreas with acinic cell injury. It is classified into acute and chronic forms both of which are two distinct entities.

Acute Pancreatitis

Acute pancreatitis is an acute inflammation of the pancreas presenting clinically with 'acute abdomen'. The severe form of the disease associated with macroscopic haemorrhages and fat necrosis in and around the pancreas is termed *acute haemorrhagic pancreatitis* or *acute pancreatic necrosis.* The condition occurs in adults between the age of 40 and 70 years and is commoner in females than in males.

The onset of acute pancreatitis is sudden, occurring after a bout of alcohol or a heavy meal. The patient presents with abdominal pain, vomiting and collapse and the condition must be differentiated from other diseases producing acute abdomen such as acute appendicitis, perforated peptic ulcer, acute cholecystitis, and infarction of the intestine following sudden occlusion of the mesenteric vessels. Characteristically, there is elevation of *serum amylase* level within the first 24 hours and of *serum lipase* level after 3 to 4 days; the latter being more specific for pancreatic disease. Glucosuria occurs in 10% of cases.

ETIOLOGY. The two leading causes associated with acute pancreatitis are *alcoholism* and *cholelithiasis,* both of which are implicated in more than 80% of cases. Less common causes of acute pancreatitis include trauma, ischaemia, shock, extension of inflammation from the adjacent tissues, blood-borne bacterial infection, viral infections, certain drugs (e.g. thiazides, sulfonamides, oral contraceptives), hypothermia, hyperlipoproteinaemia and hypercalcaemia from hyperparathyroidism. Rarely, *familial pancreatitis* is encountered. In a proportion of cases of acute pancreatitis, the etiology remains unknown *(idiopathic pancreatitis).*

PATHOGENESIS. The destructive changes in the pancreas are attributed to the liberation and activation of pancreatic enzymes. Though more than 20 enzymes are secreted by exocrine pancreas, 3 main groups of enzymes which bring about destructive effects on the pancreas are as under:

1. *Proteases* such as trypsin and chymotrypsin play the most important role in causing proteolysis. Trypsin also activates the kinin system by converting prekallikrein

to kallikrein, and thereby the clotting and complement systems are activated. This results in inflammation, thrombosis, tissue damage and haemorrhages found in acute haemorrhagic pancreatitis.

2. *Lipases and phospholipases* degrade lipids and membrane phospholipids.

3. *Elastases* cause destruction of the elastic tissue of the blood vessels.

The activation and release of these enzymes is brought about by one of the following mechanisms:

1. *Acinic cell damage* caused by the etiologic factors such as alcohol, viruses, drugs, ischaemia and trauma result in release of the intracellular enzymes.

2. *Duct obstruction* caused by cholelithiasis, chronic alcoholism and other obstructing lesions is followed by leakage of pancreatic enzymes from the ductules into the interstitial tissue.

3. *Block in exocytosis* of pancreatic enzymes occurring from nutritional causes results in activation of these intracellular enzymes by pancreatic lysosomal hydrolases.

PATHOLOGIC CHANGES. Macroscopically, in the early stage, the pancreas is swollen and oedematous. Subsequently, in a day or two, the characteristic variegated appearance of grey-white pancreatic necrosis, chalky-white fat necrosis and blue-black haemorrhages are seen. In typical case, the peritoneal cavity contains blood-stained ascitic fluid and white flecks of fat necrosis in the omentum, mesentry and peripancreatic tissue. The resolved lesions show areas of fibrosis, calcification and ductal dilatation.

Microscopically, the following features in varying grades are noticeable:

1. Necrosis of pancreatic lobules and ducts.
2. Necrosis of the arteries and arterioles with areas of haemorrhages.
3. Fat necrosis.
4. Inflammatory reaction, chiefly by polymorphs, around the areas of necrosis and haemorrhages.

COMPLICATIONS. A patient of acute pancreatitis who survives may develop a variety of systemic and local complications.

Systemic complications. These are:

1. Chemical and bacterial peritonitis.
2. Endotoxic shock.
3. Acute renal failure.

Local sequelae. These result after widespread involvement of the pancreas. These are:

1. Pancreatic abscess.
2. Pancreatic pseudocyst.
3. Duodenal obstruction.

Mortality in acute pancreatitis is high (20-30%). Patients succumb to hypotensive shock, infection, acute renal failure, and DIC.

Chronic Pancreatitis

Chronic pancreatitis or *chronic relapsing pancreatitis* is the progressive destruction of the pancreas due to repeated mild and subclinical attacks of acute pancreatitis. Most patients present with recurrent attacks of severe abdominal pain at intervals of months to years. Weight loss and jaundice are often associated. Later manifestations include associated diabetes mellitus and steatorrhoea. Abdominal radiographs show calcification in the region of pancreas and presence of pancreatic calculi in the ducts.

ETIOLOGY. Most cases of chronic pancreatitis are caused by the same factors as for acute pancreatitis. Thus, most commonly, chronic pancreatitis is related to *chronic alcoholism* with protein-rich diet, and less often to *biliary tract disease. Familial hereditary pancreatitis,* though uncommon, is more frequently chronic than the acute form. Other rare causes of chronic pancreatitis are hypercalcaemia, hyperlipidaemia and developmental failure of fusion of dorsal and ventral pancreatic ducts.

PATHOGENESIS. Acute haemorrhagic pancreatitis seldom develops into chronic pancreatitis, but instead develops pancreatic pseudocysts following recovery. Pathogenesis of alcoholic and non-alcoholic chronic pancreatitis is explained by different mechanisms:

1. Chronic pancreatitis due to *chronic alcoholism* accompanied by a high-protein diet results in increase in protein concentration in the pancreatic juice which obstructs the ducts and causes damage.

2. *Non-alcoholic cases* of chronic pancreatitis seen in tropical countries (tropical chronic pancreatitis) result from protein-calorie malnutrition. Genetic factors play a role in some cases of chronic pancreatitis.

PATHOLOGIC CHANGES. Macroscopically, the pancreas is enlarged, firm and nodular. The cut surface shows a smooth grey appearance with loss of normal lobulation. Foci of calcification and tiny pancreatic concretions to larger visible stones are frequently found. Pseudocysts may be present.

Microscopically, depending upon the stage of development, the following changes are seen:

1. Obstruction of the ducts by fibrosis in the wall and protein plugs or stones in the lumina.
2. Squamous metaplasia and dilatation of some inter- and intralobular ducts.
3. Chronic inflammatory infiltrate around the lobules as well as the ducts.
4. Atrophy of the acinar tissue with marked increase in interlobular fibrous tissue.
5. Islet tissue is involved in late stage only.

COMPLICATIONS. Late stage of chronic pancreatitis may be complicated by diabetes mellitus, pancreatic insufficiency with steatorrhoea and malabsorption and formation of pancreatic pseudocysts (Fig. 19.36).

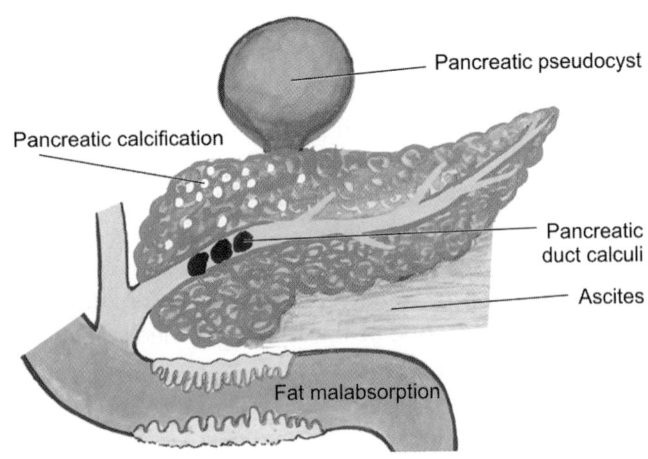

FIGURE 19.36
Complications of chronic pancreatitis.

TUMOURS ANDTUMOUR-LIKE LESIONS

Tumour-like masses of the exocrine pancreas include *congenital cystic disease* (involving the pancreas, liver and kidney) and *pancreatic pseudocysts.* True pancreatic tumours are classified into *benign* (e.g. serous cystadenoma, fibroma, lipoma and adenoma) and *malignant* (i.e. carcinoma of the pancreas). Out of all these, only two pancreatic lesions—pseudocyst and carcinoma of the pancreas, are common and are discussed below.

Pancreatic Pseudocyst

Pancreatic pseudocyst is a localised collection of pancreatic juice, necrotic debris and haemorrhages. It develops following either acute pancreatitis or trauma. The patients generally present with abdominal mass producing pain, intraperitoneal haemorrhage and generalised peritonitis.

PATHOLOGIC CHANGES. Grossly, the pseudocyst may be present within or adjacent to the pancreas. Usually it is solitary, unilocular, measuring up to 10 cm in diameter with thin or thick wall (Fig. 19.36). ***Microscopically,*** the cyst wall is composed of dense fibrous tissue with marked inflammatory reaction. There is evidence of preceding haemorrhage and necrosis in the form of deposits of haemosiderin pigment, calcium and cholesterol crystals. The lumen of the cyst contains serous or turbid fluid. The cyst does not show any epithelial lining.

Carcinoma of Pancreas

Pancreatic cancer is the term used for cancer of the exocrine pancreas. It is one of the common cancers, particularly in the Western countries and Japan. In the United States, cancer of the pancreas is the second most common cancer of the alimentary tract after colorectal cancer, and accounts for 5% of all cancer deaths in that country. It is commoner in males than in females and the incidence increases progressively after the age of 50 years.

ETIOLOGY. A significant increase in the incidence of pancreatic cancer has been observed in the UK and US during the last 50 years. Little is known about etiology of pancreatic cancer. However, following factors have been implicated in its etiology:

1. *Smoking:* Heavy cigarette smokers have higher incidence than the non-smokers. However, it is not known whether tobacco metabolites have a direct carcinogenic effect on the pancreas or by some other unknown mechanism.
2. *Diet and obesity:* Diet with high total caloric value and high consumption of animal proteins and fats is related to higher incidence of pancreatic cancer. Obesity is a risk factor for pancreatic cancer.
3. *Chemical carcinogens:* Individuals exposed to β naphthylamine, benzidine and nitrosamines have higher incidence of cancer of the pancreas.
4. *Diabetes mellitus:* Patients of long-standing diabetes mellitus have a higher incidence.
5. *Chronic pancreatitis* patients are at increased risk.

However, excessive consumption of alcohol or coffee, and cholelithiasis are not risk factors for pancreatic cancer. A mutation in *RAS* gene has been found in more than 85% cases of cancer of the pancreas.

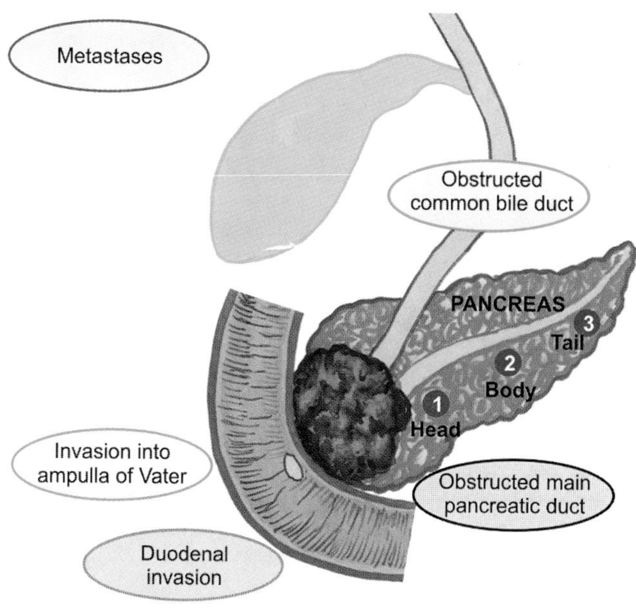

FIGURE 19.37

Distribution of carcinoma of the pancreas (numbered serially) and its major effects

PATHOLOGIC CHANGES. The most common location of pancreatic cancer is the head of pancreas (70%), followed in decreasing frequency, by the body and the tail of pancreas, (Fig. 19.37).

Grossly, carcinoma of the head of pancreas is generally small, homogeneous, poorly-defined, grey-white mass without any sharp demarcation between the tumour and the surrounding pancreatic parenchyma. The tumour of the head extends into the ampulla of Vater, common bile duct and duodenum, producing obstructive biliary symptoms and jaundice early in the course of illness. Carcinomas of the body and tail of the pancreas, on the other hand, are fairly large and irregular masses and frequently infiltrate the transverse colon, stomach, liver, spleen and regional lymph nodes (Fig. 19.37).

Microscopically, most pancreatic carcinomas arise from the ductal epithelium which normally comprises less than 4% of total pancreatic cells, whereas carcinoma of the acini constitutes less than 1% of pancreatic cancers. The following histologic patterns of pancreatic carcinoma are seen:

1. *Well-differentiated adenocarcinoma,* both mucinous and non-mucin secreting type, is the most common pattern. Perineural invasion is commonly present and is diagnostic of malignancy.
2. *Adenoacanthoma* consisting of glandular carcinoma and benign squamous elements is seen in a proportion of cases.
3. Rarely, peculiar *tumour giant cell formation* is seen with marked anaplasia, pleomorphism and numerous mitoses.
4 *Acinar cell carcinoma* occurs rarely and reproduces the pattern of acini in normal pancreas.

CLINICAL FEATURES. Clinical symptoms depend upon the site of origin of the tumour. Generally, the following features are present:

1. *Obstructive jaundice.* more often and early in the course of disease in cases with carcinoma head of the pancreas (80%), and less often in cancer of the body and tail of the pancreas. It is characterised by: dark urine, clay-like stools, pruritus, and very high serum alkaline phosphatase.

2. *Other features.* These include: abdominal pain, anorexia, weight loss, cachexia, weakness and malaise, nausea and vomiting, and migratory thrombophlebitis (Trousseau's syndrome), GI bleeding and splenomegaly.

The prognosis of pancreatic cancer is dismal: median survival is 6 months from the time of diagnosis. Approximately 10% patients survive 1 year and the 5-year survival is poor 1 to 2%.

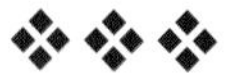

The Kidney and Lower Urinary Tract

20

KIDNEY

NORMAL STRUCTURE

ANATOMY. The kidneys are bean-shaped paired organs, each weighing about 150 gm in the adult male and about 135 gm in the adult female. The hilum of the kidney is situated at the midpoint on the medial aspect where the artery, vein, lymphatics and ureter are located. The kidney is surrounded by a thin fibrous capsule which is adherent at the hilum.

Cut surface of the kidney is made up of well-demarcated *peripheral cortex and inner medulla* (Fig. 20.1). The cortex is 1.2 to 1.5 cm in thickness and shows faint striations called *medullary rays* formed by the collecting tubules, ascending limbs and straight portions of the proximal convoluted tubules. The medulla is composed of several cone-shaped renal pyramids, the apex of each of which called the *papilla* is related to a calyx. Cortical tissue that extends into the space between adjacent pyramids is called the *renal column (septa) of Bertin.* The pelvis is the funnel-shaped, dilated proximal part of the ureter formed by the union of 2 to 3 *major calyces,* each of which is further subdivided into 3 to 4 minor calyces into which the papillae project.

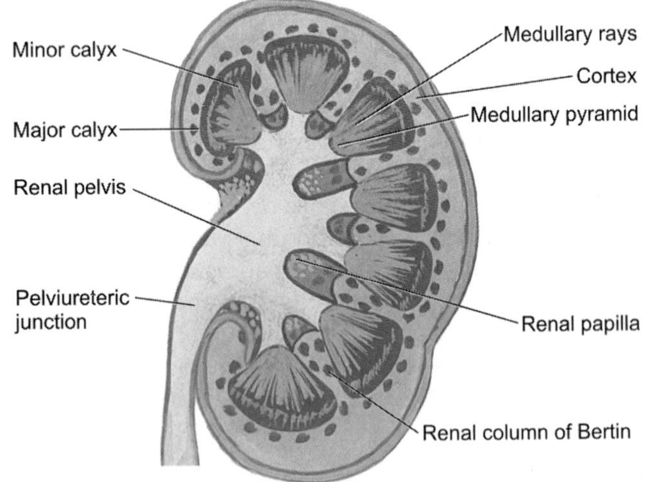

FIGURE 20.1

Macroscopic appearance of the kidney.

HISTOLOGY. The parenchyma of each kidney is composed of approximately one million microstructures called nephrons. A nephron, in turn, consists of 5 major parts, each having a functional role in the formation of urine: the glomerular capsule (glomerulus and Bowman's capsule), the proximal convoluted tubule (PCT), the loop of Henle, the distal convoluted tubule (DCT), and the collecting ducts. From point of view of diseases of the kidneys, 4 components of renal parenchyma require further elaboration : renal vasculature, glomeruli, tubules and interstitium.

1. Renal vasculature. Each kidney is supplied with blood by a main *renal artery* which arises from the aorta at the level of the 2nd lumbar vertebra. It usually divides into *anterior and posterior divisions* at the hilum although occasionally these divisions may even arise directly from the aorta. The anterior and posterior divisions divide into *segmental branches* from which interlobar arteries arise which course between the lobes. Along their course, they give off the *arcuate arteries* which arch between the cortex and medulla. The arcuate arteries, in turn, give off *interlobular arteries* which lie in the cortex perpendicular to the capsular surface in the part overlying the pyramids and, therefore, are also called *straight arteries* (Fig. 20.2). It is from the interlobular arteries that the *afferent arterioles* take their origin, each one supplying a single glomerulus. From the glomerulus emerge the efferent arterioles. Up to this stage, the arteries and arterioles are end-vessels. The efferent arterioles leaving the glomerulus supply *peritubular capillary plexus* which anastomoses with the capillary plexus of another nephron.

The juxtamedullary glomeruli, however, give off a series of parallel vessels called *vasa recta* which descend to the inner medulla supplying the loop of Henle and collecting ducts and anastomose at all levels throughout the medulla with the ascending vasa recta. These drain into *arcuate veins* and then into the veins that accompany the corresponding arteries and finally through a single renal vein into the inferior vena cava (Fig. 20.3). Lymphatic drainage likewise occurs through lymphatics associated with the intrarenal vasculature leaving the kidney at the hilum and draining to lateral aortic lymph nodes.

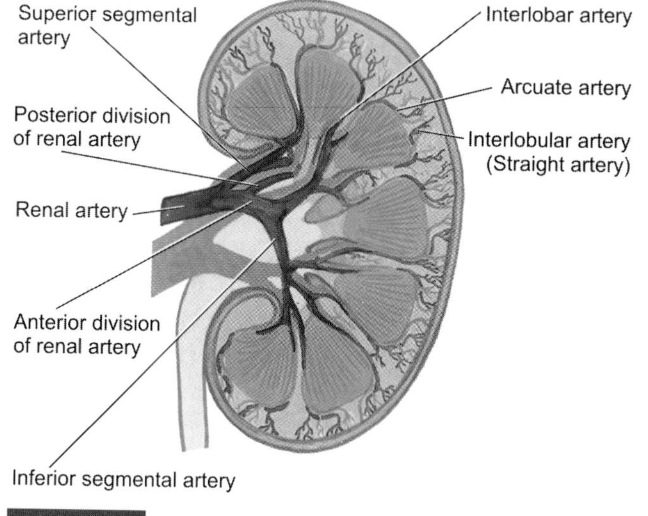

FIGURE 20.2

Arterial blood supply in the kidney.

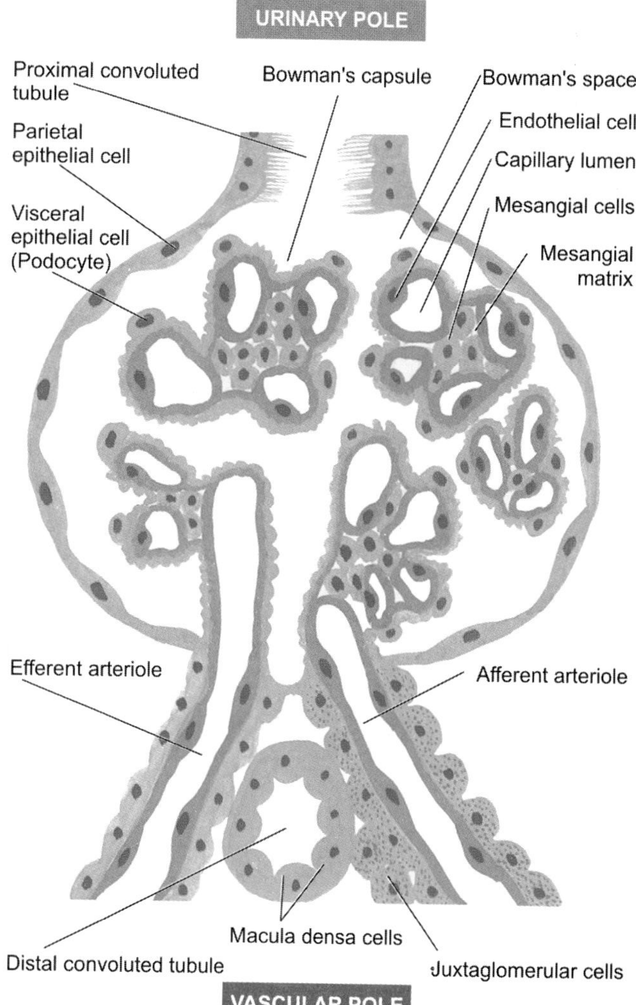

FIGURE 20.3

A schematic illustration of the structure of a nephron and associated blood supply.

The following important derivations can be made from the peculiarities of the renal vasculature:

i) The renal cortex receives about 90% of the total renal blood supply and that the pressure in the glomerular capillaries is high. Therefore, renal cortex is more prone to the effects of hypertension.

ii) The renal medulla, on the other hand, is poorly perfused and any interference in blood supply to it results in medullary necrosis.

iii) The divisions and subdivisions of the renal artery up to arterioles are end-arteries and have no anasto-

Chapter Twenty

moses. Thus, occlusion of any of the branches results in infarction of the renal parenchyma supplied by it.

iv) Since the tubular capillary beds are derived from the efferent arterioles leaving the glomeruli, diseases affecting the blood flow through glomerular tuft have significant effects on the tubules as well.

2. **Glomerulus.** The glomerulus consists of invagination of the blind end of the proximal tubule and contains a *capillary tuft* fed by the afferent arteriole and drained by efferent arteriole. The capillary tuft is covered by visceral epithelial cells (podocytes) which are continuous with those of the parietal epithelium at the *vascular pole.* The transition to proximal tubular cells occurs at the *urinary pole* of the glomerulus. The visceral and parietal epithelial cells are separated by the urinary space or *Bowman's space,* into which glomerular filtrate passes (Fig. 20.4).

Subdivisions of capillaries derived from the afferent arterioles result in the formation of *lobules* of which there are not more than eight within a glomerulus. Each lobule of a glomerular tuft consists of a centrilobular supporting stalk composed of mesangium containing *mesangial cells* and *mesangial matrix.* The mesangium is continuous at the hilum with the *lacis cells* of the juxtaglomerular apparatus. Besides their role as supportive cells, mesangial cells are involved in the production of mesangial matrix and glomerular basement membrane; they function in endocytosis of leaked macromolecules and also possibly in the control of glomerular blood flow through contractile elements present in these cells.

The major *function* of glomerulus is complex filtration from the capillaries to the urinary space. The barrier to glomerular filtration consists of the following 3 components (Fig. 20.5):

i) Fenestrated endothelial cells lining the capillary loops.

ii) Glomerular basement membrane (GBM) on which the endothelial cells rest and consists of 3 layers—the central lamina densa, bounded by lamina rara interna and lamina rara externa.

iii) Filtration slit pores between the foot processes of the visceral epithelial cells (podocytes) external to GBM.

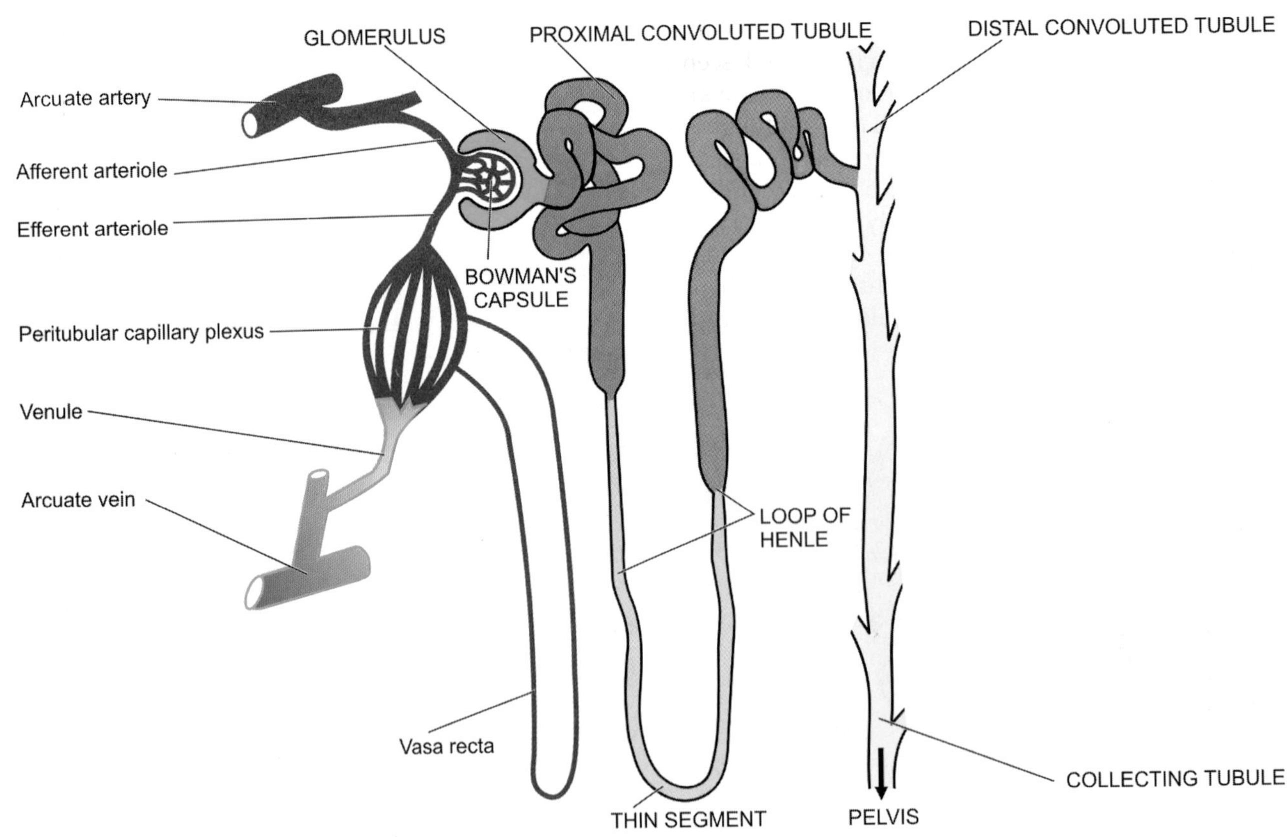

FIGURE 20.4

Structure of a glomerulus.

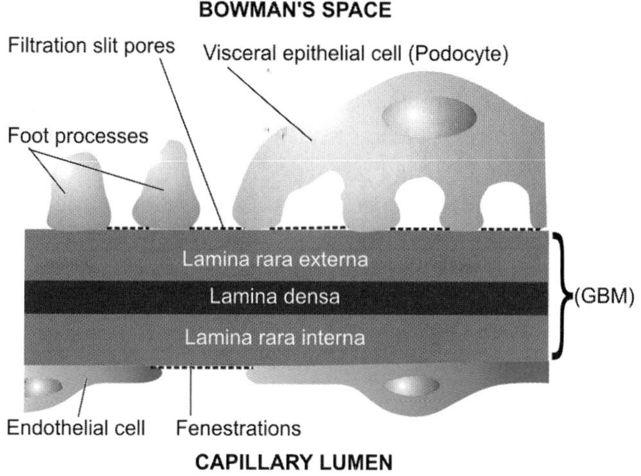

FIGURE 20.5

Ultrastructure of glomerular filtration barrier.

The barrier to filtration of macromolecules of the size and molecular weight of albumin and larger depends upon the following:

- A normal lamina densa.
- Maintenance of negative charge on both lamina rarae.
- A healthy covering of glomerular epithelial cells.

Juxtaglomerular apparatus. The juxtaglomerular apparatus (JGA) is situated at the vascular pole of the glomerulus and is made up of 3 parts (Fig. 20.4):

i) The *juxtaglomerular cells* are modified granular smooth muscle cells in the media of the afferent arteriole and contain the hormone, renin.

ii) The *macula densa* is comprised by specialised region of the distal tubule when it returns to the vascular pole of its parent glomerulus. The tubular cells here are taller and narrower than elsewhere with the nuclei lying close together.

iii) The *lacis cells* or *non-granular cells* occupy the space between the macula densa and the arterioles and merge with the glomerular mesangium.

The JGA is intimately concerned with sodium metabolism and is the principal source of renin production. The mechanism of the release of renin and its role in hypertension are discussed on page 710.

3. Tubules. The tubules of the kidney account for the greatest amount of the renal parenchyma. The structure of renal tubular epithelium varies in different parts of the nephron and is correlated with the functional capacity of that part of the tubule (Fig. 20.3).

i) Proximal convoluted tubule (PCT). This is the first part arising from the glomerulus and is highly specialised part functionally. It is lined by cuboidal cells with a brush border composed of microvilli and contains numerous mitochondria, Golgi apparatus and endoplasmic reticulum. The major functions of PCT are: *active reabsorption* of filtered sodium, potassium, glucose, amino acids, proteins, phosphate, calcium and uric acid, and *passive reabsorption* of 80% of filtered water.

ii) Loop of Henle. The PCT drains into the straight part of loop of Henle that consists of thin, descending and ascending limbs and the actual loop, all of which are found in the medulla. They are lined by a flattened type of epithelium. The thin ascending limb continues as thick ascending limb in the medullary rays. In cross section, the thick ascending limb is nearly of the same size as that of PCT and the lining cells are columnar. The major function of loop of Henle is *active reabsorption* of sodium and chloride, and *passive diffusion* of water resulting in urinary concentration.

iii) Distal convoluted tubule (DCT). The DCT represents a transition from thick ascending limb from the point where the ascending limb meets the vascular pole of the glomerulus of its origin, to the early collecting ducts. The lining cells are cuboidal which are lower than those of PCT. The epithelial cells at the point of beginning of DCT are taller, narrower and more closely packed to form the macula densa of JGA as already described. The DCT further contributes to urinary concentration and acidification, while the macula densa of JGA is the source of renin and has a role in sodium metabolism.

iv) Collecting ducts. The system of collecting ducts is the final pathway by which urine reaches the tip of renal papilla. The cells lining the collecting ducts are cuboidal but lack the brush border.

4. Interstitium. In health, the renal cortical interstitium is scanty and consists of a small number of fibroblast-like cells. But the medullary interstitium is more plentiful and contains stellate interstitial cells which are considered to produce an anti-hypertensive agent and are involved in the metabolism of prostaglandins.

RENAL FUNCTION TESTS

In general, the kidney performs the following vital functions in the body:

1. *Excretion of waste products* resulting from protein metabolism.

2. *Regulation of acid-base balance* by excretion of H^+ ions (acidification) and bicarbonate ions.

3. *Regulation of salt-water balance* by hormones secreted both intra- and extra-renally.

4. *Formation of renin and erythropoietin* and thereby playing a role in the regulation of blood pressure and erythropoiesis respectively.

In order to assess renal function, a number of tests have been devised which give information regarding the following parameters:

a) Renal blood flow
b) Glomerular filtration
c) Renal tubular function
d) Urinary outflow unhindered by any obstruction.

Renal function tests are broadly divided into 4 groups (Table 20.1):

1. Urine analysis.
2. Concentration and dilution tests.
3. Blood chemistry.
4. Renal clearance tests.

In addition, renal biopsy is performed to confirm the diagnosis of renal disease. Renal biopsy is ideally fixed in alcoholic Bouin's solution and examined morphologically supported by special stains and further studies as under:

1. *Periodic acid-Schiff* stain for highlighting glomerular basement membrane.
2. *Silver impregnation* to outline the glomerular and tubular basement membrane.
3. *Immunofluorescence* to localise the antigens, complements and immunoglobulins.
4. *Electron microscopy* to see the ultrastructure of glomerular changes.

TABLE 20.1: Renal Function Tests.

1. **Urine analysis:**
   i) Physical examination (output, colour, specific gravity, pH, osmolality)
   ii) Chemical constituents (protein, glucose, red cells, haemoglobin)
   iii) Bacteriologic examination
   iv) Microscopy
2. **Concentration and dilution tests:**
   i) Concentration test (fluid deprivation test)
   ii) Dilution test (excess fluid intake test)
3. **Blood chemistry:**
   i) Urea
   ii) Blood urea nitrogen (BUN)
   iii) Creatinine
4. **Renal clearance test:**
   i) Inulin or mannitol clearance test
   ii) Creatinine clearance
   iii) Urea clearance
   iv) Para-aminohippuric acid (PAH) clearance

1. URINE ANALYSIS. The simplest diagnostic tests for renal function is the physical, chemical, bacteriologic and microscopic examination of the urine.

i) The *physical examination* includes 24-hour urinary output, colour, specific gravity and osmolality.

ii) The *chemical tests* are carried out to detect the presence of protein, glucose, red cells and haemoglobin to assess the permeability of glomerular membrane. A number of convenient dipstick tests are available for testing these chemical substances and pH. These consist of paper strips impregnated with appropriate reagents and indicator dyes.

ii) The *bacteriologic examination* of the urine is done by proper and aseptic collection of midstream specimen of urine.

iv) *Urine microscopy* is undertaken on a fresh unstained sample. Various components observed on microscopic examination of urine in renal disease are red cells, pus cells, epithelial cells, crystals and urinary casts.

The casts are moulded into cylindrical shapes by passage along tubules in which they are formed. They are the result of precipitation of proteins in the tubule that includes not only albumin but also the tubular secretion of the *Tamm Horsfall protein*. The latter is a high molecular weight glycoprotein normally secreted by ascending loop of Henle and DCT and probably has body defence function normally. Its secretion is increased in glomerular and tubular diseases. Casts may be *hyaline type* consisting of only proteins indicating a non-inflammatory etiology of glomerular filtration of proteins, *leucocyte casts* inflammatory in origin, or *red cell casts* from haematuria.

2. CONCENTRATION AND DILUTION TESTS. Concentration and dilution tests are designed to evaluate functional capacity of the renal tubules. The ability of the nephron to concentrate or dilute urine is dependent upon both functional activity of the tubular cells in the renal medulla and the presence of antidiuretic hormone (ADH). Failure to achieve adequate urinary concentration can be due to either defects within the renal medulla *(nephrogenic diabetes insipidus)*, or due to the lack of ADH *(central diabetes insipidus)*.

Traditionally, urinary concentration is determined by specific gravity of the urine (normal range 1.003 to 1.030, average 1.018) which in cases of tubular disease remains constant at approximately 1.010 regardless of changing levels of plasma hydration. However, determination of urinary specific gravity provides only a rough estimate of osmolarity of the urine. The tubular disease can be diagnosed in its early stage by *water deprivation* (concentration) or *water excess* (dilution) tests.

i) In **concentration test,** an artificial fluid deprivation is induced in the patient for more than 20 hours. If the nephron is normal, water is selectively reabsorbed resulting in excretion of urine of high solute concentration (specific gravity of 1.025 or more). However, if the tubular cells are nonfunctional, the solute concentration of the urine will remain constant regardless of stress of water deprivation.

ii) In **dilution test,** an excess of fluid is given to the patient. Normally, renal compensation should result in excretion of urine with high water content and lower solute concentration (specific gravity of 1.003 or less). If the renal tubules are diseased, the concentration of solutes in the urine will remain constant irrespective of the excess water intake.

3. **BLOOD CHEMISTRY.** Impairment of renal function results in elevation of end-products of protein metabolism. This includes increased accumulation of certain substances in the blood, chiefly urea (normal range 20-40 mg/dl), blood urea nitrogen (BUN) (normal range 10-20 mg/dl) and creatinine (normal range 0.5-1.5 mg/dl). An increase of these end-products in the blood is called *azotaemia.*

High levels of creatinine are associated with high levels of *β2-microglobulin* in the serum as well as urine, a low-molecular weight protein filtered excessively in the urine due to glomerular disease or due to increased production by the liver.

4. **RENAL CLEARANCE TESTS.** A clearance test is employed to assess the rate of glomerular filtration and the renal blood flow. The rate of this filtration can be measured by determining the excretion rate of a substance which is filtered through the glomerulus but subsequently is neither reabsorbed nor secreted by the tubules. The glomerular filtration rate (normal 120 ml/minute in an average adult) is usually equal to clearance of that substance and is calculated from the following equation:

$$C = \frac{UV}{P} \text{ where}$$

C is the clearance of the substance in ml/ minute;
U is the concentration of the substance in the urine;
P is the concentration of the substance in the plasma; and
V is the volume of urine passed per minute.

The substances which are used for clearance tests include inulin, mannitol, creatinine and urea.

i) In **inulin or mannitol clearance tests,** an intravenous infusion of the substance inulin or mannitol is given to maintain constant plasma concentration and accurately timed urine samples are collected. Inulin, a mixture of fructose polymers, is considered the ideal substance for the clearance test since it is filtered from the glomerulus and is excreted unchanged in the urine.

ii) In **creatinine clearance test,** there is no need of intravenous infusion of creatinine since creatinine is normally released into plasma by muscle metabolism and a very small fraction of this substance is secreted by the tubules. The clearance of creatinine is determined by collecting urine over 24 hour period and a blood sample is withdrawn during the day. In spite of disadvantages like poor reproducibility and secretion of creatinine by the tubules, the 'endogenous' creatinine clearance test is easy and routinely employed method of estimating GFR.

iii) In **urea clearance test,** the sensitivity is much less than the creatinine or inulin clearance because plasma concentration of urea is affected by a number of factors (e.g. dietary protein, fluid intake, infection, trauma, surgery, and corticosteroids) and is partly reabsorbed by the tubules. Like in creatinine clearance, there is no need for intravenous infusion of urea.

iv) **Para-aminohippuric acid (PAH) clearance test** is employed to measure renal blood flow (unlike the preceding tests which measure GFR). PAH when infused intravenously is both filtered at the glomerulus as well as secreted by the tubules and its clearance is measured by determining its concentration in arterial blood and urine. Normally, renal blood flow is about 1200 ml per minute in an average adult.

PATHOPHYSIOLOGY OF RENAL DISEASE (RENAL FAILURE)

Traditionally, diseases of the kidneys are divided into 4 major groups according to the predominant involvement of corresponding morphologic components:

1. *Glomerular diseases:* These are most often immunologically-mediated and may be acute or chronic.
2. *Tubular diseases:* These are more likely to be caused by toxic or infectious agents and may be acute or chronic.
3. *Interstitial diseases:* These are likewise commonly due to toxic or infectious agents and quite often involve interstitium as well as tubules (tubulo-interstitial diseases).
4. *Vascular diseases:* These include changes in the nephron as a consequence of increased intra-glomerular pressure such as in hypertension or impaired blood flow.

In addition, other diseases described in this chapter include: congenital anomalies, obstructive uropathy (including urolithiasis) and tumours of the kidneys.

The major morphologic involvements of the kidneys in the initial stage is confined to one component (glomeruli, tubules, interstitium or blood vessels), but eventually all components are affected leading to *end-stage kidneys.*

Regardless of cause, renal disease usually results in the evolution of one of the two major pathological syndromes: *acute renal failure* and *chronic renal failure.* The term *'azotaemia'* is used for biochemical abnormality characterised by elevation of the blood urea nitrogen (BUN) and creatinine levels, while *'uraemia'* is defined as association of these biochemical abnormalities with clinical signs and symptoms. The pathophysiological aspects of acute and chronic renal failure are briefly discussed below.

Acute Renal Failure (ARF)

Acute renal failure (ARF) is a syndrome characterised by rapid onset of renal dysfunction, chiefly oliguria or anuria, and sudden increase in metabolic waste-products (urea and creatinine) in the blood with consequent development of uraemia.

ETIOPATHOGENESIS. The causes of ARF may be classified as pre-renal, intra-renal and post-renal in nature.

1. **Pre-renal causes.** Pre-renal diseases are those which cause sudden decrease in blood flow to the nephron. Renal ischaemia ultimately results in functional disorders or depression of GFR, or both. These causes include inadequate cardiac output and hypovolaemia or vascular disease causing reduced perfusion of the kidneys.

2. **Intra-renal causes.** Intra-renal disease is characterised by disease of renal tissue itself. These include vascular disease of the arteries and arterioles within the kidney, diseases of glomeruli, acute tubular necrosis due to ischaemia, or the effect of a nephrotoxin, acute tubulointerstitial nephritis and pyelonephritis.

3. **Post-renal causes.** Post-renal disease is characteristically caused by obstruction to the flow of urine anywhere along the renal tract distal to the opening of the collecting ducts. This may be caused by a mass within the lumen or from wall of the tract, or from external compression anywhere along the tract—ureter, bladder neck or urethra.

It is important to note that ARF originating in pre- and post-renal disease, such as by renal ischaemia or renal infection eventually leads to intra-renal disease. Thus, full-blown ARF reflects some degree of nephron damage.

CLINICAL FEATURES. The clinical features will depend to a large extent on the underlying cause of ARF and on the stage of the disease at which the patient presents. However, one of the following three major patterns usually emerge:

1. **Syndrome of acute nephritis.** This is most frequently associated with acute post-streptococcal glomerulonephritis and rapidly progressive glomerulonephritis. Renal dysfunction results from extensive proliferation of epithelial cells in the glomeruli with consequent mild increase in glomerular permeability and decrease in GFR. The characteristic features are: mild proteinuria, haematuria, oedema and mild hypertension. Fluid retention in acute nephritis syndrome appears to be due to both diminished GFR and increased salt and water reabsorption in distal nephron.

2. **Syndrome accompanying tubular pathology.** When the ARF is caused by destruction of the tubular cells of the nephron as occurs in acute tubular necrosis (page 703), the disease typically progresses through 3 characteristic stages from oliguria to diuresis to recovery.

i) *Oliguric phase:* The initial oliguric phase lasting on an average from 7 to 10 days is characterised by urinary output of less than 400 ml per day. The decline in formation of the urine leads to accumulation of waste products of protein metabolism in the blood and resultant azotaemia, metabolic acidosis, hyperkalaemia, hypernatraemia and hypervolaemia due to secondary effects of circulatory overload and pulmonary oedema. The specific gravity of the urine is low but the concentration of sodium in urine tends to be elevated.

ii) *Diuretic phase:* With the onset of healing of tubules, there is improvement in urinary output. This is believed to occur due to drawing of water and sodium by preceding high levels of creatinine and urea as they move through the nephron so as to be excreted. Since tubular cells have not regained normal functional capacity, the urine is of low or fixed specific gravity.

iii) *Phase of recovery:* Full recovery with healing of tubular epithelial cells occurs in about half the cases, while others terminate in death. The process of healing may take up to one year with restoration of normal tubular function.

3. **Pre-renal syndrome.** The ARF occurring secondary to disorders in which neither the glomerulus nor the tubules are damaged, results in pre-renal syndrome. Most typically, this pattern is seen in marginal ischaemia caused by renal arterial obstruction, hypovolaemia, hypotension or cardiac insufficiency. Due to depressed

renal blood flow, there is decrease in GFR causing oliguria, azotaemia (elevation of BUN and creatinine) and possible fluid retention and oedema. Since the tubular cells are functioning normally, the nephron retains its ability to concentrate the glomerular filtrate according to the adaptive needs.

Chronic Renal Failure (CRF)

Chronic renal failure is a syndrome characterised by progressive and irreversible deterioration of renal function due to slow destruction of renal parenchyma, eventually terminating in death when sufficient number of nephrons have been damaged. Acidosis is the major problem in CRF with development of biochemical azotaemia and clinical uraemia syndrome.

ETIOPATHOGENESIS. All chronic nephropathies can lead to CRF. The diseases leading to CRF can generally be classified into two major groups: *those causing glomerular pathology,* and *those causing tubulointerstitial pathology.* Though this classification is useful to facilitate study, the disease rarely remains confined to either glomeruli or tubulointerstitial tissue alone. In the final stage of CRF, all parts of the nephron are involved.

1. Diseases causing glomerular pathology. A number of glomerular diseases associated with CRF have their pathogenesis in immune mechanisms (page 685). Glomerular destruction results in changes in filtration process and leads to development of the nephrotic syndrome characterised by proteinuria, hypoalbuminaemia and oedema. The important examples of chronic glomerular diseases causing CRF are covered under two headings: primary and systemic.

i) *Primary glomerular pathology:* The major cause of CRF is chronic glomerulonephritis, usually initiated by various types of *glomerulonephritis* such as membranous glomerulonephritis, membranoproliferative glomerulonephritis, lipoid nephrosis (minimal change disease) and anti-glomerular basement membrane nephritis.

ii) *Systemic glomerular pathology:* Certain conditions originate outside the renal system but induce changes in the nephrons secondarily. Major examples of this type are systemic lupus erythematosus, serum sickness nephritis and diabetic nephropathy.

2. Diseases causing tubulointerstitial pathology. Damage to tubulointerstitial tissues results in alterations in reabsorption and secretion of important constituents leading to excretion of large volumes of dilute urine. Tubulointerstitial diseases can be categorised according to initiating etiology into 4 groups: vascular, infectious, toxic and obstructive.

i) *Vascular causes:* Long-standing primary or essential hypertension produces characteristic changes in renal arteries and arterioles referred to as nephrosclerosis (page 711). Nephrosclerosis causes progressive renal vascular occlusion terminating in ischaemia and necrosis of renal tissue.

ii) *Infectious causes:* A good example of chronic renal infection causing CRF is chronic pyelonephritis. The chronicity of process results in progressive damage to increasing number of nephrons leading to CRF.

iii) *Toxic causes:* Some toxic substances induce slow tubular injury, eventually culminating in CRF. The most common example is intake of high doses of analgesics such as phenacetin, aspirin and acetaminophen (chronic analgesic nephritis). Other substances that can cause CRF after prolonged exposure are lead, cadmium and uranium.

iv) *Obstructive causes:* Chronic obstruction in the urinary tract leads to progressive damage to the nephron due to fluid back-pressure. The examples of this type of chronic injury are stones, blood clots, tumours, strictures and enlarged prostate.

CLINICAL FEATURES. Regardless of the initiating cause, CRF evolves progressively through 4 stages:

1. Decreased renal reserve. At this stage, damage to renal parenchyma is marginal and the kidneys remain functional. The GFR is about 50% of normal, BUN and creatinine values are normal and the patients are usually asymptomatic except at times of stress.

2. Renal insufficiency. At this stage, about 75% of functional renal parenchyma has been destroyed. The GFR is about 25% of normal accompanied by elevation in BUN and serum creatinine. Polyuria and nocturia occur due to tubulointerstitial damage. Sudden stress may precipitate uraemic syndrome.

3. Renal failure. At this stage, about 90% of functional renal tissue has been destroyed. The GFR is approximately 10% of normal. Tubular cells are essentially nonfunctional. As a result, the regulation of sodium and water is lost resulting in oedema, metabolic acidosis, hypocalcaemia, and signs and symptoms of uraemia.

4. End-stage kidney. The GFR at this stage is less than 5% of normal and results in complex clinical picture of uraemic syndrome with progressive primary (renal) and secondary systemic (extra-renal) symptoms.

Clinical manifestations of full-blown CRF culminating in uraemic syndrome are thus described under 2 main headings: primary (renal) uraemic manifestations and secondary (systemic or extra-renal) uraemic manifestations.

A. Primary uraemic (renal) manifestations. Primary symptoms of uraemia develop when there is slow and progressive deterioration of renal function. The resulting imbalances cause the following manifestations:

1. **Metabolic acidosis.** As a result of renal dysfunction, acid-base balance is progressively lost. Excess of hydrogen ions occurs, while bicarbonate level declines in the blood, resulting in metabolic acidosis. The clinical symptoms of metabolic acidosis include: compensatory Kussmaul breathing, hyperkalaemia and hypercalcaemia.

2. **Hyperkalaemia.** A decreased GFR results in excessive accumulation of potassium in the blood since potassium is normally excreted mainly in the urine. Hyperkalaemia is further worsened by metabolic acidosis. The clinical features of hyperkalaemia are: cardiac arrhythmias, weakness, nausea, intestinal colic, diarrhoea, muscular irritability and flaccid paralysis.

3. **Sodium and water imbalance.** As GFR declines, sodium and water cannot pass sufficiently into Bowman's capsule leading to their retention. Release of renin from juxtaglomerular apparatus further aggravates sodium and water retention. The main symptoms referable to sodium and water retention are: hypervolaemia and circulatory overload with congestive heart failure.

4. **Hyperuricaemia.** Decreased GFR results in excessive accumulation of uric acid in the blood.

Uric acid crystals may be deposited in joints and soft tissues resulting in gout.

5. **Azotaemia.** The waste-products of protein metabolism fail to be excreted resulting in elevation in the blood levels of urea, creatinine, phenols and guanidines causing biochemical abnormality, azotaemia. The secondary manifestations of uraemia are related to toxic effects of these metabolic waste-products.

B. Secondary uraemic (extra-renal) manifestations. A number of extra-renal systemic manifestations develop secondarily following fluid-electrolyte and acid-base imbalances. These include the following:

1. **Anaemia.** Decreased production of erythropoietin by diseased kidney results in decline in erythropoiesis and anaemia. Besides, gastrointestinal bleeding may further aggravate anaemia.

2. **Integumentary system.** Deposit of urinary pigment such as urochrome in the skin causes sallow-yellow colour. The urea content in the sweat as well as in the plasma rises. On evaporation of the perspiration, urea remains on the facial skin as powdery *'uraemic frost'*.

3. **Cardiovascular system.** Fluid retention secondarily causes cardiovascular symptoms such as increased workload on the heart due to the hypervolaemia and eventually congestive heart failure.

4. **Respiratory system.** Hypervolaemia and heart failure cause pulmonary congestion and pulmonary oedema due to back pressure. Radiologically, uraemic pneumonitis shows characteristic central, butterfly-pattern of oedema and congestion in the chest radiograph.

5. **Digestive system.** Azotaemia directly induces mucosal ulcerations in the lining of the stomach and intestines. Subsequent bleeding can aggravate the existing anaemia. Gastrointestinal irritation may cause nausea, vomiting and diarrhoea.

6. **Skeletal system.** The skeletal manifestations of renal failure are referred to as *renal osteodystrophy* (Chapter 26). Two major types of skeletal disorders may occur:

i) *Osteomalacia* occurs from deficiency of a form of vitamin D which is normally activated by the kidney (page 257). Since vitamin D is essential for absorption of calcium, its deficiency results in inadequate deposits of calcium in bone tissue.

ii) *Osteitis fibrosa* occurs due to elevated levels of parathormone. How parathormone excess develops in CRF is complex. As the GFR is decreased, increasing levels of phosphates accumulate in the extracellular fluid which, in turn, cause decline in calcium levels. Decreased calcium level triggers the secretion of parathormone which mobilises calcium from bone and increases renal lubular reabsorption of calcium thereby conserving it. However, if the process of resorption of calcium phosphate from bone continues for sufficient time, hypercalcaemia may be induced with deposits of excess calcium salts in joints and soft tissues and weakening of bones (renal osteodystrophy).

CONGENITAL MALFORMATIONS

Approximately 10% of all persons are born with potentially significant malformations of the urinary system. These range in severity from minor anomalies which may not produce clinical manifestations to major anomalies which are incompatible with extrauterine life. About half of all patients with malformations of the kidneys have coexistent anomalies either elsewhere in the urinary tract or in other organs.

Malformations of the kidneys are classified into 3 broad groups:

I. **Abnormalities in amount of renal tissue.** These include: anomalies with deficient renal parenchyma (e.g.

unilateral or bilateral renal hypoplasia) or with excess renal tissue (e.g. renomegaly, supernumerary kidneys).

II. Anomalies of position, form and orientation. These are: renal ectopia (pelvic kidney), renal fusion (horseshoe kidney) and persistent foetal lobation.

III. Anomalies of differentiation. This group consists of the more important and common morphologic forms covered under the heading of *'cystic diseases of the kidney'* described in detail below.

CYSTIC DISEASES OF KIDNEY

Cystic lesions of the kidney may be *congenital or acquired, non-neoplastic or neoplastic.* Majority of these lesions are congenital non-neoplastic. Cystic lesions in the kidney may occur at any age, extending from foetal (detected on ultrasonography) to old age. Their clinical presentation may include: abdominal mass, infection, respiratory distress (due to accompanied pulmonary hypoplasia), haemorrhage, and neoplastic transformation.

Potter divided developmental renal cystic lesions into three types—I, II and III. A simple classification including all cystic lesions of the kidney is given in Table 20.2 and Fig. 20.6. Non-neoplastic lesions are discussed below while neoplastic cystic lesions of the kidney are described later (page 718).

I. Renal Cystic Dysplasia

The term 'renal cystic dysplasia' or Potter type II is used for defective renal differentiation with persistence of structures in the kidney not represented in normal nephrogenesis such as presence of undifferentiated mesenchyme containing smooth muscle or cartilage and immature collecting ducts. Renal dysplasia is thus diagnosed on the basis of histologic features. The condition is fairly common in the newborn and infants.

The pathogenesis of renal dysplasia is unknown. Since renal dysplasia is commonly associated with obstructive abnormalities of the ureter and lower urinary tract, it is hypothesised that the condition results from intrauterine obstruction and disorganised metanephrogenic differentiation.

TABLE 20.2: Classification of Cystic Lesions of the Kidney.

A. NON-NEOPLASTIC CYSTIC LESIONS
- I. **Renal cystic dysplasia (Potter type II)**
- II. **Polycystic kidney disease (PKD)**
  1. Adult (autosomal dominant) polycystic kidney disease (ADPKD) (Potter type III)
  2. Infantile (autosomal recessive) polycystic kidney disease (ARPKD) (Potter type I)
- III. **Glomerulocystic kidney disease**
- IV. **Medullary cystic disease**
  1. Medullary sponge kidney (MSK)
  2. Nephronophthiasis-medullary cystic disease complex
- V. **Simple renal cysts**
- VI. **Acquired renal cysts**
- VII. **Para-renal cysts**

B. NEOPLASTIC CYSTIC LESIONS
- I. **Cystic nephroma (page 718)**
- II. **Cystic partially-differentiated nephroblastoma (CPDN)**
- III. **Multifocal cystic change in Wilms' tumour (page 721)**

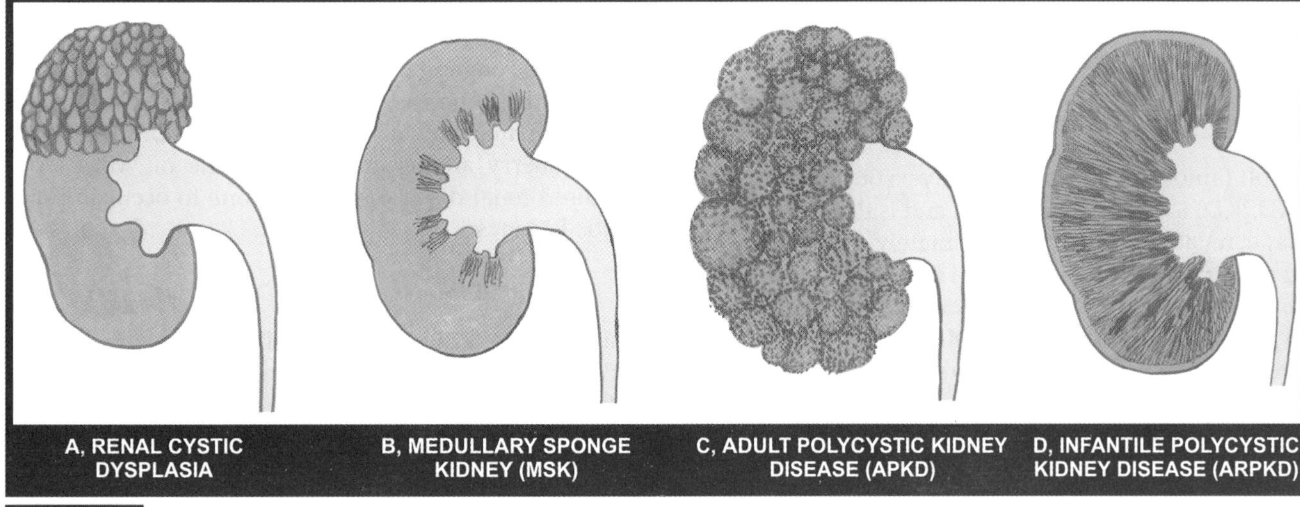

FIGURE 20.6

Cystic diseases of kidney.

PATHOLOGIC CHANGES. Renal dysplasia may be unilateral or bilateral. The dysplastic process may involve the entire renal mass or a part of it.

Grossly, the dysplastic kidney is almost always cystic. The kidney is replaced by disorderly mass of multiple cysts that is not reniform but resembles a bunch of grapes. No normal renal parenchyma is recognisable, and calyces and pelvis are not present. The ureter is invariably abnormal, being either absent or atretic.

Histologically, the characteristic feature is the presence of undifferentiated mesenchyme that contains smooth muscle or cartilage. The cysts are dilated tubules lined by flattened epithelium surrounded by concentric layers of connective tissue. Glomeruli are scanty or absent.

CLINICAL FEATURES. Unilateral renal dysplasia is frequently discovered in newborn or infants as a flank mass. Often, renal dysplasia is associated with other congenital malformations and syndromes such as ventricular septal defect, tracheo-esophageal fistula, lumbosacral meningomyelocele and Down's syndrome.

The prognosis of unilateral renal dysplasia following removal of the abnormal kidney is excellent while bilateral renal dysplasia results in death in infancy.

II. Polycystic Kidney Disease

Polycystic disease of the kidney (PKD) is a disorder in which major portion of the renal parenchyma is converted into cysts of varying size. The disease occurs in two forms:

A. An *adult type* inherited as an *autosomal dominant* disease; and

B. An *infantile type* inherited as an *autosomal recessive* disorder.

A. ADULT POLYCYSTIC KIDNEY DISEASE

Adult (autosomal dominant) polycystic kidney disease (ADPKD) is relatively common and is the cause of end-stage renal failure in approximately 10% of haemodialysis patients. The pattern of inheritance is *autosomal dominant* having high penetrance with variable expressivity. Family history of renal disease may be present. The condition occurs due to mutation in chromosome 16. The true adult polycystic renal disease is always bilateral and diffuse. Though the kidneys are abnormal at birth, renal function is retained, and symptoms appear in adult life, mostly between the age of 30 and 50 years.

PATHOLOGIC CHANGES. Grossly, kidneys in ADPKD are always bilaterally enlarged, usually symmetrically, heavy (weighing up to 4 kg) and cystic. The cut surface shows cysts throughout the renal parenchyma varying in size from tiny cysts to 4-5 cm in diameter (Fig. 20.7,A). The contents of the cysts vary from clear straw-yellow fluid to reddish-brown material. The renal pelvis and calyces are present but are greatly distorted by the cysts. The cysts, however, do not communicate with the pelvis of the kidney—a feature that helps to distinguish polycystic kidney from hydronephrotic kidney on sectioned surface (page 716).

Histologically, the cysts arise from all parts of nephron. It is possible to find some cysts containing recognisable glomerular tufts reflecting their origin from Bowman's capsule, while others have epithelial lining like that of distal or proximal tubules or collecting ducts. The intervening tissue between the cysts shows some normal renal parenchyma. With advancement of age of the patient, acquired lesions such as pyelonephritis, nephrosclerosis, fibrosis and chronic inflammation are increasingly seen.

CLINICAL FEATURES. The condition may become clinically apparent at any age but most commonly manifests in 3rd to 5th decades of life. The most frequent and earliest presenting feature is a dull-ache in the lumbar regions. In others, the presenting complaints are haematuria or passage of blood clots in urine, renal colic, hypertension, urinary tract infections and progressive CRF with polyuria and proteinuria.

About a third of patients with adult polycystic kidney disease have cysts of the liver (Chapter 19). Other associated congenital anomalies seen less frequently are cysts in the pancreas, spleen, lungs and other organs. Approximately 15% of patients have one or more intracranial berry aneurysms of the circle of Willis. Any acquired renal disease is more prone to occur in polycystic kidneys.

B. INFANTILE POLYCYSTIC KIDNEY DISEASE

The infantile (autosomal recessive) form of polycystic kidney disease (ARPKD) is distinct from the adult form. Infantile polycystic kidney disease is rare. It is transmitted as an *autosomal recessive* trait and the family history of similar disease is usually not present. The condition occurs due to a mutation in chromosome 6. It is invariably bilateral. The age at presentation may be

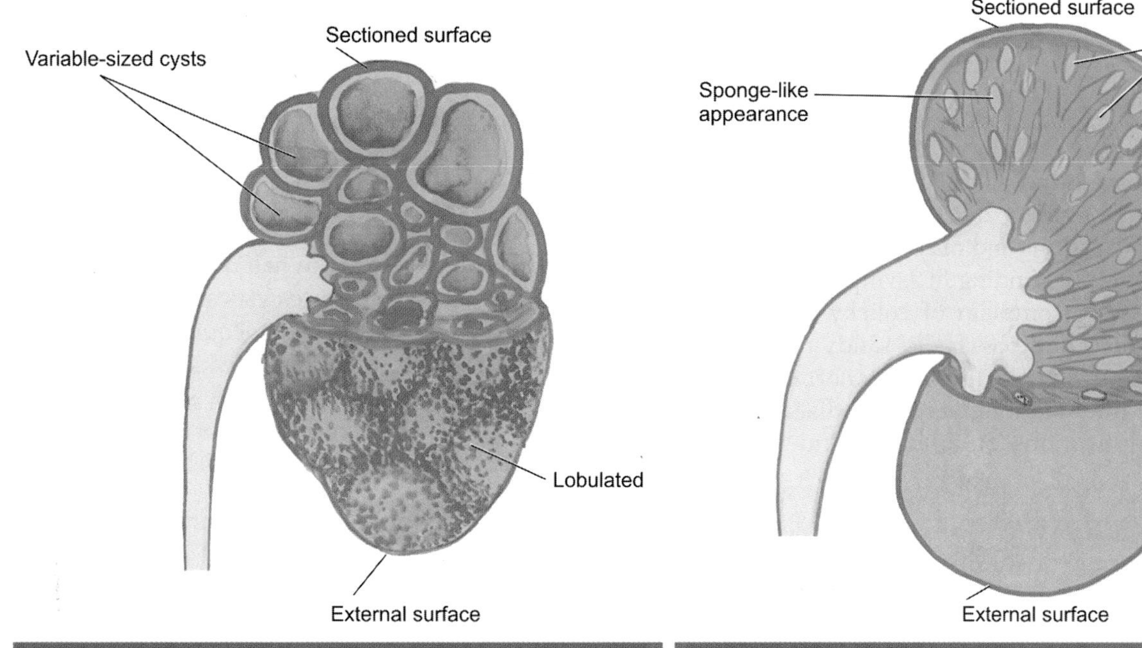

FIGURE 20.7

Macroscopic appearance of polycystic kidney disease.

perinatal, neonatal, infantile or juvenile, but frequently serious manifestations are present at birth and result in death from renal failure in early childhood.

PATHOLOGIC CHANGES. Grossly, the kidneys are bilaterally enlarged with smooth external surface and retained normal shape. Cut surface reveals small, fusiform or cylindrical cysts formed from dilatation of collecting tubules which extend radially to the outer cortex. This gives the sectioned surface of the kidney *sponge-like appearance* (Fig. 20.7,B). No normal renal parenchyma is grossly recognised. Pelvis, calyces and ureters are normal.

Histologically, the total number of nephrons is normal but all the collecting tubules show cylindrical or saccular dilatations and are lined by cuboidal to low columnar epithelium. Many of the glomeruli are also cystically dilated.

CLINICAL FEATURES. The clinical manifestations depend on age of the child. In severe form, the gross bilateral cystic renal enlargement may interfere with delivery. In infancy, renal failure may manifest early. Almost all the cases of infantile polycystic kidney disease have associated multiple epithelium-lined cysts in the liver or proliferation of portal bile ductules. In older children, these associated hepatic changes develop into what is termed *congenital hepatic fibrosis* which may lead to portal hypertension and splenomegaly.

III. Glomerulocystic Kidney Disease

Many cystic diseases of kidney may have both glomerular as well as tubular cysts e.g. in renal cystic dysplasia, ADPKD. In glomerulocystic kidney disease, exclusive glomerular cysts appear due to dilatation of Bowman's space.

PATHOLOGIC CHANGES. Grossly, there is marked bilateral enlargement of kidneys. Cut surface shows tiny cysts, 2-3 mm in size.

Microscopically, glomerular cysts are lined by flattened to cuboidal epithelium and have compressed glomerular tuft.

IV. Medullary Cystic Disease

Cystic disease of the renal medulla has two main types:

A. *Medullary sponge kidney,* a relatively common and innocuous condition; and

B. *Nephronophthiasis-medullary cystic disease complex,* a common cause of chronic renal failure in juvenile age group.

A. MEDULLARY SPONGE KIDNEY

Medullary sponge kidney consists of multiple cystic dilatations of the papillary ducts in the medulla. The condition occurs in adults and may be recognised as an incidental radiographic finding in asymptomatic cases, or the patients may complain of colicky flank pain, dysuria, haematuria and passage of sandy material in the urine. Renal function remains largely normal or may be mildly impaired in long-standing disease with secondary complications of infection and calculus formation.

PATHOLOGIC CHANGES. Grossly, the kidneys may be enlarged, normal or shrunken in size depending upon the extent of secondary pyelonephritis. On cut surface, the characteristic feature is the presence of several, small (less than 0.5 cm diameter), cystically dilated papillary ducts, which may contain spherical calculi.

Microscopically, the cysts are lined by tall columnar, cuboidal, transitional or squamous epithelium. Renal cortex may show secondary pyelonephritis but cortical cysts are never a component of medullary sponge kidney.

B. NEPHRONOPHTHIASIS-MEDULLARY CYSTIC DISEASE COMPLEX

This form of medullary cystic disease, also called *juvenile nephronophthiasis or uraemic sponge kidney,* is a progressive renal disease that makes its appearance in childhood. Familial occurrence is common and both patterns of inheritance occur, recessive transmission being more common than dominant transmission. The clinical manifestations are due to impaired urinary concentration consequent upon the medullary lesions and consist of polyuria, polydipsia and enuresis. Other features include renal osteodystrophy, growth retardation, anaemia and progressive renal failure leading to uraemia.

PATHOLOGIC CHANGES. Grossly, the kidneys are moderately reduced in size and granular and have narrow cortices. Cut surface reveals minute cysts, majority of which are present at the cortico-medullary junction.

Microscopically, the cysts are lined by flattened or cuboidal epithelium. There is widespread nonspecific chronic inflammatory infiltrate and interstitial fibrosis. Many glomeruli are hyalinised but tubular atrophy is more pronounced due to marked thickening of tubular basement membrane.

V. Simple Renal Cysts

Simple renal cysts are a very common postmortem finding. They are seen in about half of all persons above the age of 50 years. Since these cysts are rare in infants and children, they appear to be acquired rather than congenital lesions. Simple cysts of the kidneys are rarely responsible for symptoms. However, symptoms may result from rupture, haemorrhage or infection. The association between simple cysts and hypertension is common.

PATHOLOGIC CHANGES. Grossly, simple renal cysts are usually solitary but may be multiple. They are commonly located in the cortex. Their size varies from a few millimeters to 10 cm in diameter. The wall of cyst is characteristically yellowish-white and translucent. The cyst usually contains clear straw-coloured fluid which may become rust-coloured due to haemorrhage.

Microscopically, the lining of the cyst is by flattened epithelium. The cyst wall contains variable amount of collagenised fibrous tissue which may occasionally have deposits of haemosiderin or calcium salts.

VI. Acquired Renal Cysts

A number of acquired conditions give rise to renal cysts. These include the following:

1. Patients with end-stage renal disease on prolonged dialysis (dialysis-associated cystic disease).
2. Hydatid (echinococcal) cyst.
3. Tuberculosis of the kidney.
4. Cystic degeneration in carcinoma of kidney.
5. Traumatic intrarenal haematoma.
6. Drug-induced cystic disease in experimental animals.

VII. Pararenal Cysts

Cysts occurring adjacent to a kidney are termed pararenal cysts. These include the following:

1. Pyelocalyceal cysts
2. Hilar lymphangiectatic cysts
3. Retroperitoneal cysts
4. Perinephric pseudocysts from trauma.

GLOMERULAR DISEASES

DEFINITION AND CLASSIFICATION

Glomerular diseases encompass a large and clinically significant group of renal diseases. Glomerulonephritis (GN) or Bright's disease is the term used for diseases that primarily involve the renal glomeruli. It is convenient to classify glomerular diseases into 2 broad groups:

I. *Primary glomerulonephritis* in which the glomeruli are the predominant site of involvement.

II. *Secondary glomerular diseases* include certain systemic and hereditary diseases which secondarily affect the glomeruli.

Though this division is widely followed, it is somewhat arbitrary since many primary forms of glomerulonephritis have systemic effects, and many systemic diseases may initially present with glomerular involvement. Many classifications of different types of glomerulonephiritis have been described, but most widely accepted classification is based on clinical presentation and pathologic changes in the glomeruli given in Table 20.3.

TABLE 20.3: Clinicopathologic Classification of Glomerular Diseases.

I. Primary Glomerulonephritis
1. Acute GN
   i) Post-streptococcal
   ii) Non-streptococcal
2. Rapidly progressive GN
3. Minimal change disease
4. Membranous GN
5. Membrano-proliferative GN
6. Focal proliferative GN
7. Focal segmental glomerulosclerosis (FSGS)
8. IgA nephropathy
9. Chronic glomerulonephritis

II. Secondary Systemic Glomerular Diseases
1. Lupus nephritis (SLE)
2. Diabetic nephropathy
3. Amyloidosis (page 90)
4. Polyarteritis nodosa (page 290)
5. Wegener's granulomatosis (page 291)
6. Goodpasture's syndrome (page 503)
7. Henoch-Schönlein purpura (page 430)
8. Systemic infectious diseases (*bacterial* e.g. bacterial endocarditis, syphilis, leprosy; *viral* e.g. HBV, HCV, HIV; *parasitic* e.g. falciparum malaria, filariasis)
9. Idiopathic mixed cryoglobulinaemia

III. Hereditary Nephritis
1. Alport's syndrome
2. Fabry's disease
3. Nail-patella syndrome

CLINICAL MANIFESTATIONS

The clinical presentation of glomerular disease is quite variable but in general four features—proteinuria, haematuria, hypertension and disturbed excretory function, are present in varying combinations depending upon the underlying condition. A firm diagnosis, however, can be established by examination of renal biopsy under light, electron and immunofluorescence microscopy.

A number of clinical syndromes are recognised in glomerular diseases. The following are six major glomerular syndromes commonly found in different glomerular diseases:

- nephritic and nephrotic syndromes;
- acute and chronic renal failure;
- asymptomatic proteinuria and haematuria.

These are briefly described below.

I. ACUTE NEPHRITIC SYNDROME. This is the acute onset of haematuria, proteinuria, hypertension, oedema and oliguria following an infective illness about 10 to 20 days earlier.

1. The **haematuria** is generally slight giving the urine smoky appearance and erythrocytes are detectable by microscopy or by chemical testing for haemoglobin. Appearance of red cell casts is another classical feature of acute nephritic syndrome.

2. The **proteinuria** is mild (less than 3 gm per 24 hrs) and is usually non-selective *(nephritic range proteinuria).*

3. **Hypertension** is variable depending upon the severity of the glomerular disease but is generally mild.

4. **Oedema** in nephritic syndrome is usually mild and results from sodium and water retention (page 99).

5. **Oliguria** is variable and reflects the severity of glomerular involvement.

The underlying causes of acute nephritic syndrome may be primary glomerulonephritic diseases (classically acute glomerulonephritis and rapidly progressive glomerulonephritis) or certain systemic diseases (Table 20.4).

II. NEPHROTIC SYNDROME Nephrotic syndrome is a group of diseases having different pathogenesis and characterised by clinical findings of massive proteinuria, hypoalbuminaemia, oedema, hyperlipidaemia, lipiduria, and hypercoagulability.

1. **Heavy proteinuria** (protein loss of more than 3 gm per 24 hrs) is the chief characteristic of nephrotic syndrome *(nephrotic range proteinuria).* In children, protein loss is correspondingly less. A small amount of protein (20 to 150 mg/day) normally passes through

TABLE 20.4: Causes of Acute Nephritic Syndrome.

I. Primary Glomerulonephritis
1. Acute GN
   i) Post-streptococcal
   ii) Non-streptococcal
2. Rapidly progressive GN
3. Membranoproliferative GN
4. Focal GN
5. IgA nephropathy

II. Systemic Diseases
1. SLE
2. Polyarteritis nodosa
3. Wegener's granulomatosis
4. Henoch-Schonlein purpura
5. Cryoglobulinaemia

the glomerular filtration barrier and is reabsorbed by the tubules. But in case of increased glomerular permeability to plasma proteins, excess of protein is filtered out exceeding the capacity of tubules for reabsorption and, therefore, appears in the urine. Another feature of protein loss is its 'selectivity'. A *highly-selective proteinuria* consists mostly of loss of low molecular weight proteins, while a *poorly-selective proteinuria* is loss of high molecular weight proteins in the urine. In nephrotic syndrome, proteinuria mostly consists of loss of albumin (molecular weight 66,000) in the urine.

2. Hypoalbuminaemia is produced primarily consequent to urinary loss of albumin, and partly due to increased renal catabolism and inadequate hepatic synthesis of albumin. Often, the plasma albumin level is 1 to 3 gm/dl (normal 3.5 to 5.5 gm/dl) and there is reversed albumin-globulin ratio. The concentration of other proteins in the plasma such as immunoglobulins, clotting factors and antithrombin may fall rendering these patients more vulnerable to infections and thrombotic and thromboembolic complications.

3. Oedema in nephrotic syndrome appears due to fall in colloid osmotic pressure consequent upon hypoalbuminaemia. Sodium and water retention further contribute to oedema. Nephrotic oedema is usually peripheral but in children facial oedema may be more prominent (page 99).

4. Hyperlipidaemia is a frequent accompaniment of nephrotic syndrome. The exact mechanism of its genesis is not clear. It is hypothesised that the liver faced with the stress of massive protein synthesis in response to heavy urinary protein loss, also causes increased synthesis of lipoproteins. There are increased blood levels of total lipids, cholesterol, triglycerides, VLDL and LDL but decrease in HDL. Low blood level of HDL is partly due to its loss in the urine.

5. Lipiduria occurs following hyperlipidaemia due to excessive leakiness of glomerular filtration barrier.

6. Hypercoagulability. Patients with nephrotic syndrome may develop spontaneous arterial or venous thrombosis, renal vein thrombosis and pulmonary embolism as a result of various factors. These include: increased urinary loss of antithrombin III, hyperfibrinogenaemia due to increased synthesis in the liver, decreased fibrinolysis, increased platelet aggregation and altered levels of protein C and S.

The causes of nephrotic syndrome are diverse and are listed in Table 20.5. The morphology of individual types is described later. But it must be mentioned here that:

- in *children*, primary glomerulonephritis is the cause in majority of cases of the nephrotic syndrome, most frequently *lipoid nephrosis (65%); and*

TABLE 20.5: Causes of Nephrotic Syndrome.

I. Primary Glomerulonephritis
1. Minimal change disease *(most common in children)*
2. Membranous GN *(most common in adults)*
3. Membranoproliferative GN
4. Focal segmental glomerulosclerosis
5. Focal GN
6. IgA nephropathy

II. Systemic Diseases
1. Diabetes mellitus
2. Amyloidosis
3. SLE

III. Systemic Infections
1. Viral infections (HBV, HCV, HIV)
2. Bacterial infections (bacterial endocarditis, syphilis, leprosy)
3. Protozoa and parasites (*P. falciparum* malaria, filariasis)

IV. Hypersensitivity Reactions
1. Drugs (heavy metal compounds like gold and mercury, other drugs like penicillamine, trimethadione and tolbutamide, heroin addiction)
2. Bee stings, snake bite, poison ivy

V. Malignancy
1. Carcinomas
2. Myeloma
3. Hodgkin's disease

VI. Pregnancy
Toxaemia of pregnancy

VII. Circulatory Disturbances
1. Renal vein thrombosis
2. Constrictive pericarditis

VIII. Hereditary Diseases
1. Alport's disease
2. Fabry's disease
3. Nail-patella syndrome

■ *in adults,* on the other hand, systemic diseases (diabetes, amyloidosis and SLE) are more frequent causes of nephrotic syndrome. The most common primary glomerular disease in adults is *membranous glomerulonephritis* (40%).

III. ACUTE RENAL FAILURE. As already described above, acute renal failure (ARF) is characterised by rapid decline in renal function. ARF has many causes including glomerular disease, principally rapidly progressive GN and acute diffuse proliferative GN.

IV. CHRONIC RENAL FAILURE. Glomerular causes of chronic renal failure (CRF) have already been described above. These cases have advanced renal impairment progressing over years and is detected by significant proteinuria, haematuria, hypertension and azotaemia. Such patients generally have small contracted kidneys as a result of chronic glomerulonephritis.

V. ASYMPTOMATIC PROTEINURIA. Presence of proteinuria unexpectedly in a patient may be unrelated to renal disease (e.g. exercise-induced, extreme lordosis and orthostatic proteinuria), or may indicate an underlying mild glomerulonephritis. Association of asymptomatic haematuria, hypertension or impaired renal function with asymptomatic proteinuria should raise strong suspicion of underlying glomerulonephritis.

VI. ASYMPTOMATIC HAEMATURIA. Asymptomatic microscopic haematuria is common in children and young adolescents and has many diverse causes such as diseases of the glomerulus, renal interstitium, calyceal system, ureter, bladder, prostate, urethra, and underlying bleeding disorder, congenital abnormalities of the kidneys or neoplasia. Glomerular haematuria is indicated by the presence of red blood cells, red cell casts and haemoglobin in the urine. Glomerular haematuria is frequently associated with asymptomatic proteinuria.

PATHOGENESIS OF GLOMERULAR INJURY

Most forms of primary GN and many of the secondary glomerular diseases in human beings have immunologic pathogenesis. This view is largely based on immunofluorescence studies of GN in humans which have revealed glomerular deposits of immunoglobulins and complement in patterns that closely resemble those of experimental models. Non-immunologic mechanisms, however, play some role in certain forms of glomerular damage as discussed later.

The consequences of injury at different sites within the glomerulus in various glomerular diseases can be assessed when compared with the normal physiologic role of the main cells involved i.e. *endothelial, mesangial, visceral epithelial,* and *parietal epithelial cells* as well as of the *GBM* (Table 20.6).

Immunologic mechanisms underlying glomerular injury are primarily *antibody-mediated* (immune-complex disease). There is evidence to suggest that *cell-mediated immune reactions* in the form of delayed type hypersensitivity can also cause glomerular injury. In addition, a few secondary mechanisms and some non-immunologic mechanisms are involved in the pathogenesis of some forms of glomerular diseases in human beings (Table 20.7).

I. IMMUNOLOGIC MECHANISMS

Experimental studies and observations in man have revealed that immunologic mechanisms, most importantly antigen-antibody complexes, underlie most forms of glomerular injury. The general principles of these mechanisms in different forms of glomerular diseases are discussed below, while more specific features are described under the specific types of GN.

A. Antibody-Mediated Glomerular Injury

1. IMMUNE COMPLEX DISEASE. Majority of cases of glomerular disease result from deposits of immune

TABLE 20.6: Relationship of Physiologic Role of Glomerular Components with Consequences in Glomerular Injury.

	COMPONENT	PHYSIOLOGIC FUNCTION	CONSEQUENCE OF INJURY	RELATED GLOMERULAR DISEASE
1.	*Endothelial cells*	i) Maintain glomerular perfusion	Vasoconstriction	Acute renal failure
		ii) Prevent leucocyte adhesion	Leucocyte infiltration	Focal/diffuse proliferative GN
		iii) Prevent platelet aggregation	Intravascular microthrombi	Thrombotic microangiopathies
2.	*Mesangial cells*	Control glomerular filtration	Proliferation and increased matrix	Membranoproliferative GN
3.	*Visceral epithelial cells*	Prevent plasma protein filtration	Proteinuria	Minimal change disease, FSGS
4.	*GBM*	Prevents plasma protein filtration	Proteinuria	Membranous GN
5.	*Parietal epithelial cells*	Maintain Bowman's space	Crescent formation	RPGN

TABLE 20.7: Pathogenetic Mechanisms in Glomerular Diseases.

MECHANISM	RELATED GLOMERULAR DISEASE
I. IMMUNOLOGIC MECHANISMS	
A. *Antibody-mediated glomerular injury*	
1. Immune-complex disease	Immune-complex mediated GN (Acute diffuse proliferative GN, membranous GN, membranoproliferative GN, IgA nephropathy; secondary glomerular disease in SLE, malaria etc.)
2. Anti-glomerular basement membrane (Anti-GBM) disease	Goodpasture's disease
3. Alternate pathway disease	Membranoproliferative GN type II
4. Other mechanisms (anti-neutrophil cytoplasmic antibodies ANCA, anti-endothelial cell antibodies AECA)	Focal segmental GS
B. *Cell-mediated glomerular injury*	Pauci-immune GN (type III RPGN)
C. *Secondary pathogenetic mechanisms*	Mediate glomerular injury in various primary and secondary glomerular diseases
II. NON-IMMUNOLOGIC MECHANISMS	
1. Metabolic	Diabetic nephropathy, Fabry's disease
2. Haemodynamic	Hypertensive nephrosclerosis, FSGS
3. Deposition	Amyloid nephropathy
4. Infectious	HIV-nephropathy, immune-complex GN in SABE
5. Drugs	NSAIDs-associated minimal change disease
6. Inherited	Alport's syndrome, nail-patella syndrome

complexes (antigen-antibody complexes). The immune complexes are represented by *irregular or granular glomerular deposits* of immunoglobulins (IgG, IgM and IgA) and complement (mainly C3). Based on the experimental models and studies in human beings, the following 3 patterns of glomerular deposits of immune complexes in various glomerular diseases have been observed (Fig. 20.8):

i) *Exclusive mesangial deposits* are characterised by very mild form of glomerular disease.

ii) *Extensive subendothelial deposits* along the GBM are accompanied by severe hypercellular sclerosing glomerular lesions.

iii) *Subepithelial deposits* are seen between the outer surface of the GBM and the podocytes.

Deposits may be located at one or more of the above sites in any case of glomerular injury.

It was widely believed earlier that glomerular deposits result from circulating immune complexes. Now, it has been shown that glomerular deposits are formed by one of the following two mechanisms:

i) Local immune complex deposits. Formation of glomerular deposits of immune complex *in situ* occurs as a result of combination of antibodies with autologous non-basement membrane antigens or nonglomerular antigens planted on glomeruli. Currently, this mechanism is considered responsible for most cases of immune complex GN. Classic experimental model of *in situ* immune complex GN is *Heymann nephritis* (autologous immune complex nephritis) induced in rats by immunising animals with homologous preparations of proximal tubular brush border. The rats develop antibodies to brush border antigens and thereby membranous GN that closely resembles human membranous GN. The examples of *planted nonglomerular antigens* are cationic proteins, lectins, DNA, bacterial products (e.g. a protein of group A streptococci), viral and parasitic products and drugs.

ii) Circulating immune complex deposits. This mechanism used to be considered very important for glomerular injury but now it is believed that circulating immune complexes cause glomerular damage under certain circumstances only. These situations are: their presence in high concentrations for prolonged periods, or when they possess special properties that cause their binding to glomeruli, or when host mechanisms are defective and fail to eliminate immune complexes. The antigens evoking antibody response may be endogenous (e.g. in SLE) or may be exogenous (e.g. Hepatitis B virus, *Treponema pallidum, Plasmodium falciparum* and various tumour antigens). The antigen-antibody complexes are formed in the circulation and then trapped in the glomeruli where they produce glomerular injury after combining with complement.

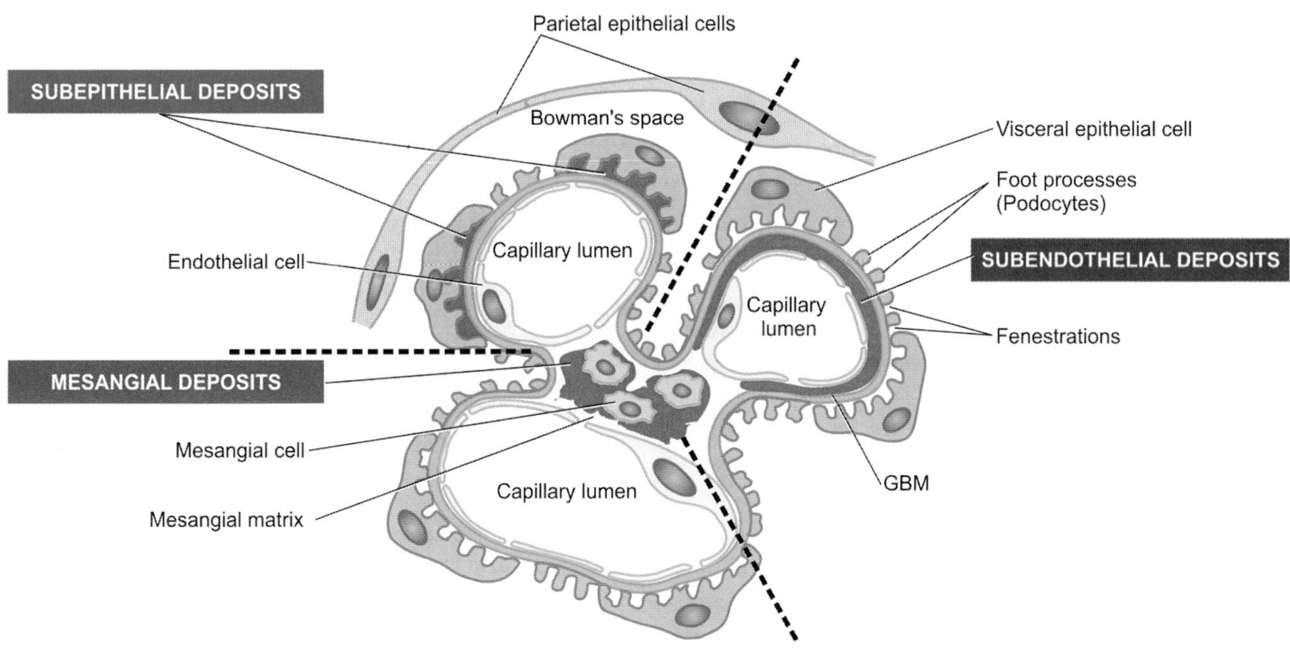

FIGURE 20.8

Electron microscopic appearance of a portion of glomerular lobule, showing three patterns of irregular or granular glomerular deposits in immune-complex disease.

Immune complex GN is observed in the following human diseases:

i) *Primary GN* e.g. acute diffuse proliferative GN, membranous GN, membranoproliferative GN, IgA nephropathy and some cases of rapidly progressive GN and focal GN.

ii) *Systemic diseases* e.g. glomerular disease in SLE, malaria, syphilis, hepatitis, Henoch-Schonlein purpura and idiopathic mixed cryoglobulinaemia.

2. ANTI-GBM DISEASE. Less than 5% cases of human GN are associated with anti-GBM antibodies. The constituent of GBM acting as antigen appears to be a component of collagen IV of the basement membrane. The experimental model of anti-GBM disease is *Masugi nephritis* (nephrotoxic serum nephritis) produced in rats by injection of heterologous antibodies against GBM prepared in rabbits by immunisation with rat kidney tissue.

Anti-GBM disease is classically characterised by *interrupted linear deposits* of anti-GBM antibodies (mostly IgG; rarely IgA and IgM) and complement (mainly C3) along the glomerular basement membrane. These deposits are detected by immunofluorescence microscopy or by electron microscopy.

Anti-GBM disease is characteristically exemplified by glomerular injury in Goodpasture's syndrome in some cases of rapidly progressive GN. About half to two-third of the patients with renal lesions in Goodpasture's syndrome have pulmonary haemorrhage mediated by cross-reacting autoantibodies against alveolar basement membrane (page 503).

3. ALTERNATE PATHWAY DISEASE. As apparent from the above mechanisms, the complement system, in particular C3, contributes to glomerular injury in most forms of GN. Deposits of C3 are associated with the early components C1, C2 and C4 which are evidence of classic pathway activation of complement. But in alternate pathway activation, there is decreased serum C3 level, decreased serum levels of factor B and properdin, normal serum levels of C1, C2 and C4 but C3 and properdin are found deposited in the glomeruli without immunoglobulin deposits, reflecting activation of alternate pathway of complement. Such patients have circulating anti-complementary nephritic factor called C3NeF which is an IgG antibody and acts as an autoantibody to the alternate C3 convertase and enhances alternate pathway activity.

The deposits in alternate pathway disease are characteristically electron-dense under electron microscopy, glomerular lesions in such cases are referred to as *dense-deposit disease.*

Alternate pathway disease occurs in most cases of type II membranoproliferative GN, some patients of rapidly progressive GN, acute diffuse proliferative GN, IgA nephropathy and in SLE.

4. OTHER MECHANISMS OF ANTIBODY-MEDIATED INJURY. A few autoantibodies have been implicated in some patients of focal segmental glomerulosclerosis and few other types of GN. These antibodies include the following:

i) Anti-neutrophil cytoplasmic antibodies (ANCA). About 40% cases of rapidly progressive GN are deficient in immunoglobulins in glomeruli and are positive for ANCA against neutrophil cytoplasmic antigens in their circulation. ANCA causes endothelial injury by generation of reactive oxygen radicals.

ii) Anti-endothelial cell antibodies (AECA). Autoantibodies against endothelial antigens have been detected in circulation in several inflammatory vasculitis and glomerulonephritis. These antibodies increase the adhesiveness of leucocytes to endothelial cells.

B. Cell-mediated Glomerular Injury (Delayed-type Hypersensitivity)

Recent evidence suggests that cell-mediated immune reactions may be involved in causing glomerular injury, particularly in cases with deficient immunoglobulins (e.g. in pauci-immune type glomerulonephritis in RPGN). Cytokines and other mediators released by activated T cells stimulate cytotoxicity, recruitment of more leucocytes and fibrogenesis. CD4+ T lymphocytes recruit more macrophages while CD8+ cytotoxic T lymphocytes and natural killer cells cause further glomerular cell injury by antibody-dependent cell toxicity. Soluble factor derived from T lymphocytes is implicated in proteinuria in minimal change disease focal GS.

However, cell-mediated injury, is yet less clear than antibody-mediated glomerular injury.

C. Secondary Pathogenetic Machanisms (Mediators of Immunologic Injury)

Secondary pathogenetic mechanisms are a number of mediators of immunologic glomerular injury operating in man and in experimental models. These include the following:

1. NEUTROPHILS. Neutrophils are conspicuous in certain forms of glomerular disease such as in acute diffuse proliferative GN, and may also be present in membranoproliferative GN and lupus nephritis. Neutrophils can mediate glomerular injury by activation of complement as well as by release of proteases, arachidonic acid metabolites and oxygen-derived free radicals. These agents cause degradation of GBM and cell injury.

2. MONONUCLEAR PHAGOCYTES. Many forms of human and experimental proliferative GN are associated with glomerular infiltration by monocytes and macrophages. Accumulation of mononuclear phagocytes is considered an important constituent of hypercellularity in these forms of GN aside from proliferation of mesangial and endothelial cells. Activated macrophages release a variety of biologically active substances which take part in glomerular injury.

3. COMPLEMENT SYSTEM. The pathogenetic role of classical and alternate pathway of activation of complement has already been highlighted above. Besides the components of complement which mediate glomerular injury via neutrophils already mentioned, C5b9 is capable of inducing damage to GBM directly.

4. PLATELETS. Platelet aggregation and release of mediators play a role in the evolution of some forms of GN. Increased intrarenal platelet consumption has been found to occur in some forms of glomerular disease.

5. MESANGIAL CELLS. There is evidence to suggest that mesangial cells present in the glomeruli may be stimulated to produce mediators of inflammation and take part in glomerular injury.

6. COAGULATION SYSTEM. The presence of fibrin in early crescents in certain forms of human and experimental GN suggests the role of coagulation system in glomerular damage. Fibrinogen may leak into Bowman's space and act as stimulus for cell proliferation. Crescents usually transform into scar tissue under the influence of fibronectin which is regularly present in crescents in human glomerular disease.

II. NON-IMMUNOLOGIC MECHANISMS

Though most forms of GN are mediated by immunologic mechanisms, a few examples of glomerular injury by non-immunologic mechanisms are found. These are:

1. *Metabolic glomerular injury* e.g. in diabetic nephropathy (due to hyperglycaemia), Fabry's disease (due to sialdosis).
2. *Haemodynamic glomerular injury* e.g. systemic hypertension, intraglomerular hypertension in FSGS.
3. *Deposition diseases* e.g. amyloidosis.

4. *Infectious diseases* e.g. HBV, HCV, HIV, *E. coli*-derived nephrotoxin.
5. *Drugs* e.g. minimal change disease due to NSAIDs.
6. *Inherited glomerular diseases* e.g. Alport's syndrome, nail-patella syndrome.

The evolution of end-stage renal failure is explained on the basis of adaptive glomerular hypertrophy of unaffected glomeruli that results in increased glomerular blood flow and increased glomerular capillary pressure inducing intraglomerular hypertension. These events lead to increased deposition of mesangial matrix and proliferation of mesangial cells, endothelial and epithelial cell injury, and eventually to progressive glomerulosclerosis and end-stage renal failure.

SPECIFIC TYPES OF GLOMERULAR DISEASES

Classification of different forms of glomerular diseases is already presented in Table 20.2. Features of individual types are described below and a summary of major forms of primary glomerulonephritis is given in Table 20.9 at the end of this discussion.

I. PRIMARY GLOMERULONEPHRITIS

Acute Glomerulonephritis
(Synonyms: Acute Diffuse Proliferative GN, Diffuse Endocapillary GN)

Acute GN is known to follow acute infection and characteristically presents as acute nephritic syndrome. Based on etiologic agent, acute GN is subdivided into 2 main groups: acute post-streptococcal GN and acute non-streptococcal GN, the former being more common.

ACUTE POST-STREPTOCOCCAL GN

Acute post-streptococcal GN is fairly common form of GN, seen most commonly in children 6 to 16 years of age but adolescents and adults may also be affected. The onset of disease is generally sudden after 1-2 weeks of streptococcal infection, most frequently of the throat (e.g. streptococcal pharyngitis) and sometimes of the skin (e.g. streptococcal impetigo).

ETIOPATHOGENESIS. The relationship between streptococcal infection and this form of GN is now well established. Particularly nephritogenic are types 12,4,1 and Red Lake of group A β-haemolytic streptococci (compare the etiologic agent with that of RHD, page 329). The glomerular lesions appear to result from deposition of immune complexes in the glomeruli. The evidences cited in support are as under:

i) There is *epidemiological* evidence of preceding streptococcal sore throat or skin infection about 1-2 weeks prior to the attack.

ii) The *latent period* between streptococcal infection and onset of clinical manifestations of the disease is compatible with the period required for building up of antibodies.

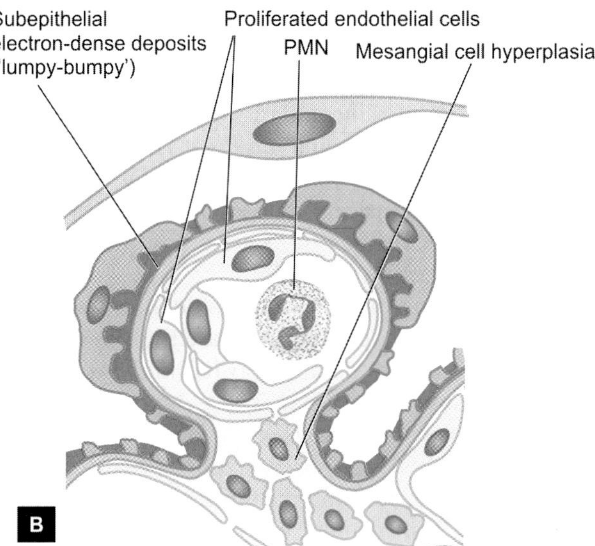

FIGURE 20.9

Acute post-streptococcal GN. A, light microscopic appearance. There is increased cellularity due to proliferation of mesangial cells, endothelial cells and some epithelial cells and infiltration of the tuft by neutrophils and monocytes. B, Electron microscopic appearance of a portion of glomerular lobule, showing characteristic electron-dense irregular deposits or 'humps' on the epithelial side of the GBM.

iii) Streptococcal infection may be identified by *culture* or may be inferred from elevated titres of *antibodies* against streptococcal antigens. These include:

- anti-streptolysin O (ASO);
- anti-deoxyribonuclease B (anti-DNAse B);
- anti-streptokinase (ASKase);
- anti-nicotinyl adenine dinucleotidase (anti-NADase); and
- anti-hyaluronidase (AHase).

iv) There is usually *hypocomplementaemia* indicating involvement of complement in the glomerular deposits.

v) More recently, it has been possible to identify antigenic component of streptococci which is cytoplasmic antigen, *endostreptosin.*

PATHOLOGIC CHANGES. Grossly, the kidneys are symmetrically enlarged, weighing one and a half to twice the normal weight. The cortical as well as sectioned surface show petechial haemorrhages giving the characteristic appearance of flea-bitten kidney.

Light microscopic findings are as under (COLOUR PLATE XXVII: Cl. 105):

i) Glomeruli—The glomeruli are affected diffusely. They are enlarged and hypercellular. The diffuse hypercellularity of the tuft is due to proliferation of mesangial, endothelial and occasionally epithelial cells *(acute proliferative lesions)* as well as by infiltration of leucocytes, chiefly polymorphs and sometimes monocytes (*acute exudative lesion,* Fig. 20.9,A). There may be small deposits of fibrin within the capillary lumina and in the mesangium.

ii) Tubules—Tubular changes are not very striking. There may be swelling and hyaline droplets in tubular cells, and tubular lumina may contain red cell casts.

iii) Interstitium—There may be some degree of interstitial oedema and leucocytic infiltration.

iv) Vessels—Changes in arteries and arterioles are seldom present in acute GN.

Electron microscopic findings, aside from confirming the light microscopic findings, are the characteristic electron-dense irregular deposits *('humps')* on the epithelial side of the GBM. These deposits represent the immune complexes (Fig. 20.9,B).

Immunofluorescence microscopy reveals that the irregular deposits along the GBM consist principally of IgG and complement C3.

CLINICAL FEATURES. Typically, the patient is a young child, presenting with acute nephritic syndrome (page 683), having sudden and abrupt onset following an episode of sore throat 1-2 weeks prior to the development of symptoms. The features include microscopic or intermittent haematuria, red cell casts, mild non-selective proteinuria (less than 3 gm per 24 hrs), hypertension, periorbital oedema and variably oliguria. Less often, the presentation may be as nephrotic syndrome. In adults, the features are atypical and include sudden hypertension, oedema and azotaemia. Development of hypertension in either case is a poor prognostic sign.

Prognosis varies with the age of the patient. Children almost always (95%) recover completely with reversal of proliferative glomerular changes. Complications arise more often in adults and occasionally in children. These include development of rapidly progressive GN, chronic GN, uraemia and chronic renal failure.

ACUTE NON-STREPTOCOCCAL GN

About one-third cases of acute GN are caused by organisms other than haemolytic streptococci. These include other bacteria (e.g. staphylococci, pneumococci, meningococci, *Salmonella* and *Pseudomonas),* viruses (e.g. hepatitis B virus, mumps, infectious mononucleosis and varicella), parasitic infections (e.g. malaria, toxoplasmosis and schistosomiasis) and syphilis. The appearance of renal biopsy by light microscopy, EM and immunofluorescence microscopy is similar to that seen in acute post-streptococcal GN. The prognosis of non-streptococcal GN is not as good as that of streptococcal GN.

Rapidly Progressive Glomerulonephritis *(Synonyms; RPGN, Crescentic GN, Extracapillary GN)*

RPGN presents with an acute reduction in renal function resulting in acute renal failure in a few weeks or months. It is characterised by formation of 'crescents' *(crescentic GN)* outside the glomerular capillaries *(extracapillary GN). 'Crescents'* are formed from the proliferation of parietal epithelial cells lining Bowman's capsule with contribution from visceral epithelial cells and the invading mononuclear cells. The stimulus for crescent formation appears to be the presence of fibrin in the capsular space. RPGN occurs most frequently in adults, with a slight male preponderance. Prognosis of RPGN in general is dismal.

ETIOPATHOGENESIS. A number of primary glomerular and systemic diseases are characterised by formation of crescents. Based on the etiologic agents and pathogenetic mechanism, patients with RPGN are divided into 3 groups (Table 20.8):

- RPGN in systemic diseases (anti-GBM type);

TABLE 20.8: Distinguishing Features of Three Main Categories of Rapidly Progressive Glomerulonephritis.

FEATURE	TYPE I RPGN (ANTI-GBM DISEASE)	TYPE II RPGN (IMMUNE COMPLEX DISEASE)	TYPE III RPGN (PAUCI-IMMUNE GN)
1. *Clinical syndrome*	Nephritic	Nephritic	Nephritic
2. *Pathogenetic type*	Anti-GBM	Immune-complex	Pauci-immune
3. *Immunofluorescence*	Linear Ig and C3	Granular Ig and C3	Sparse or absent Ig and C3
4. *Serologic markers*			
i) *Serum C3 level*	Normal	Low-to-normal	Normal
ii) *Anti-GBM antibody*	Positive	Negative	Negative
iii) *ANCA*	Negative	Negative	Positive
5. *Underlying cause*	Idiopathic Goodpasture's syndrome, SLE, vasculitis, Wegener's granulomatosis, Henoch-Schonlein purpura	Idiopathic Post-infectious (post-streptococcal GN)	Idiopathic Polyarteritis nodosa, Wegener's granulomatosis

- post-infectious RPGN (immune-complex type); and
- pauci-immune RPGN.

There are three main serologic markers in RPGN:

i) serum C3 level,
ii) anti-GBM antibody; and
iii) anti-neutrophil cytoplasmic antibody (ANCA)

Type I RPGN: Anti-GBM disease. A number of systemic diseases such as Goodpasture's syndrome, SLE, vasculitis, Wegener's granulomatosis, Henoch-Schonlein purpura and idiopathic mixed cryoglobulinaemia are associated with crescentic GN. Goodpasture's syndrome is the characteristic example of anti-GBM disease and is described below:

Goodpasture's syndrome. Goodpasture's syndrome is characterised by acute renal failure due to RPGN and pulmonary haemorrhages (page 503). The condition is more common in males in 3rd decade of life. The disease results from damage to the glomeruli by anti-GBM antibodies which cross-react with alveolar basement membrane and hence, produce renal as well as pulmonary lesions. The evidences in support are the characteristic linear deposits of anti-GBM antibodies consisting of IgG and complement along the GBM, detection of circulating anti-GBM antibodies and induction of glomerular lesions with injection of anti-GBM antibodies experimentally in monkeys. Pulmonary lesions can be experimentally induced if the lungs are previously injured by viral or bacterial infection or exposed to hydrocarbons. The Goodpasture's antigen appears to be a component of collagen type IV.

Type II RPGN: Immune complex disease. A small proportion of cases of post-streptococcal GN, particularly in adults and sometimes of non-streptococcal origin, develop RPGN. The evidences in support of post-infectious RPGN having immune complex pathogenesis are granular deposits of immune complexes of IgG and C3 along the glomerular capillary walls, lowering of blood complement levels and demonstration of circulating complexes.

Type III RPGN: Pauci-immune GN. These include cases of Wegener's granulomatosis and microscopic polyarteritis nodosa. The pathogenesis of pauci-immune GN is yet not fully defined. However, majority of these patients are ANCA-positive, implying a defect in humoral immunity. Serum complement levels are normal and anti-GBM antibody is negative. There is little or no glomerular immune deposit (i.e. pauci-immune).

PATHOLOGIC CHANGES. ***Grossly,*** the kidneys are usually enlarged and pale with smooth outer surface *(large white kidney).* Cut surface shows pale cortex and congested medulla.

Light Microscopic findings vary according to the cause but in general following features are present (COLOUR PLATE XXVII: CL 106):

i) Glomeruli—Irrespective of the underlying etiology, all forms of RPGN show pathognomonic *'crescents'* on the inside of Bowman's capsules. These are collections of pale-staining polygonal cells which commonly tend to be elongated. Eventually, crescents obliterate the Bowman's space and compress the glomerular tuft. Fibrin deposition is invariably present alongside crescents. Besides the crescents, glomerular tufts may show increased cellularity as a

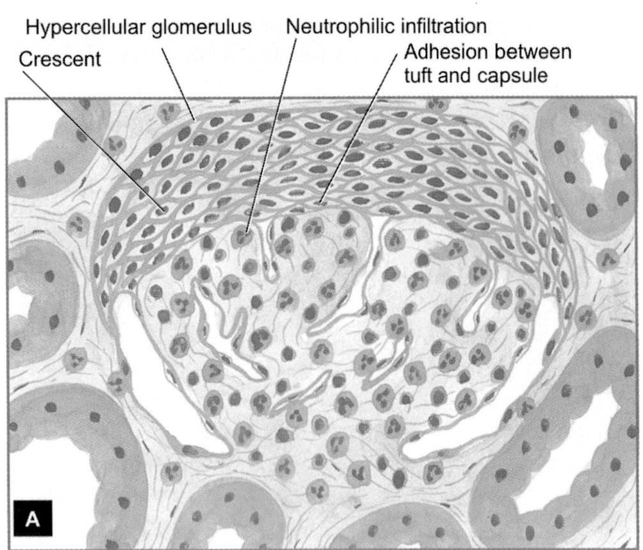

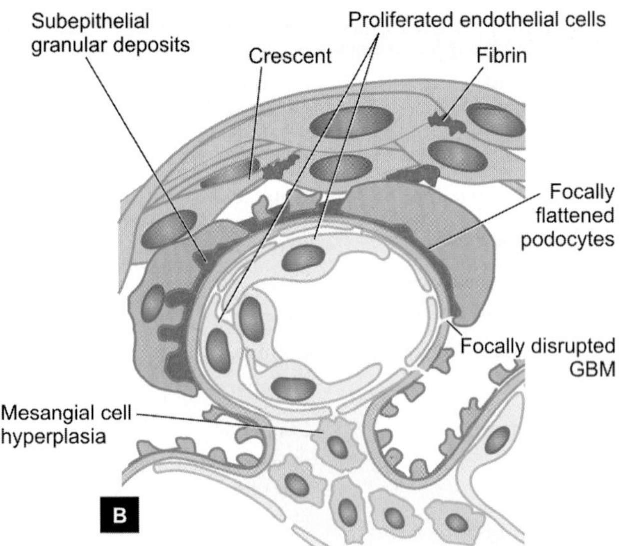

FIGURE 20.10

A, Post-infectious RPGN, light microscopic appearance. There are crescents in Bowman's space forming adhesions between the glomerular tuft and Bowman's capsule. The tuft shows hypercellularity and leucocytic infiltration. B, Electron microscopic appearance of a portion of glomerular lobule, showing epithelial crescent formation and subepithelial granular deposits.

result of proliferation of endothelial and mesangial cells and leucocytic infiltration (Fig. 20.10). Fibrin thrombi are frequently present in the glomerular tufts.

ii) Tubules—Tubular epithelial cells may show hyaline droplets. Tubular lumina may contain casts, red blood cells and fibrin.

iii) Interstitium—The interstitium is oedematous and may show early fibrosis. Inflammatory cells, usually lymphocytes and plasma cells, are commonly distributed in the interstitial tissue.

iv) Vessels—Arteries and arterioles may show no change, but cases associated with hypertension usually show severe vascular changes.

Electron microscopic findings vary according to the type of RPGN. Post-infectious RPGN cases show electron-dense subepithelial granular deposits similar to those seen in acute GN, while cases of RPGN in Goodpasture's syndrome show characteristic linear deposits along the GBM.

Immunofluorescence microscopy shows:

- linear pattern of RPGN in Goodpasture's syndrome (type I RPGN), containing IgG accompanied by C3 along the capillaries
- granular pattern of post-infectious RPGN (type II RPGN) consisting of IgG and C3 along the capillary wall; and
- scanty or no deposits of immunoglobulin and C3 in pauci-immune GN (type III RPGN).

CLINICAL FEATURES. Generally, the features of post-infectious RPGN are similar to those of acute GN, presenting as acute renal failure. The patients of Goodpasture's syndrome may present as acute renal failure and/or associated intrapulmonary haemorrhage producing recurrent haemoptysis. Prognosis of all forms of RPGN is poor. However, post-infectious cases have somewhat better outcome and may show recovery.

Minimal Change Disease
(Synonyms: MCD, Lipoid Nephrosis, Foot Process Disease, Nil Deposit Disease)

Minimal change disease (MCD) is a condition in which the nephrotic syndrome is accompanied by no apparent change in glomeruli by light microscopy. Its other synonyms, lipoid nephrosis and foot process disease, are descriptive terms for fatty changes in the tubules and electron microscopic appearance of flattened podocytes respectively. Minimal change disease accounts for 80% cases of nephrotic syndrome in children under 16 years of age with preponderance in boys (ratio of boys to girls 2:1).

ETIOPATHOGENESIS. The etiology of MCD remain elusive. However, following two groups have been identified:

i) Idiopathic (majority of cases).

ii) Cases associated with systemic diseases (Hodgkin's disease, HIV infection) and drug therapy (e.g. NSAIDs, rifampicin, interferon-α).

The following features point to possible immunologic pathogenesis for MCD:

i) Absence of deposits by electron microscopy.

ii) Normal circulating levels of complement but presence of circulating immune complexes in many cases.

iii) Universal satisfactory response to steroid therapy.

iv) Evidence of increased suppressor T cell activity with elaboration of cytokines (interleukin-8, tumour necrosis factor) which probably cause foot process flattening.

v) Recent detection of a mutation in nephrin gene in cases of congenital MCD has focused attention on genetic basis.

The Nephrotic syndrome in MCD *in children* is characterised by *selective proteinuria* containing mainly albumin, and minimal amounts of high molecular weight proteins such as α2-macroglobulin. The basis for selective proteinuria appears to be:

i) reduction of normal negative charge on GBM (page 673) due to loss of heparan sulfate proteoglycan from the GBM; and

ii) change in the shape of epithelial cells producing foot process flattening due to reduction of sialoglycoprotein cell coat.

Adults having MCD, however, have *non-selective proteinuria,* suggesting more extensive membrane permeability defect.

PATHOLOGIC CHANGES. Grossly, the kidneys are of normal size and shape.

By light microscopy, the findings are as under:

i) Glomeruli—The most characteristic feature is no apparent abnormality in the glomeruli except for slight increase in the mesangial matrix at the most.

ii) Tubules—There is presence of fine lipid vacuolation and hyaline droplets in the cells of proximal convoluted tubules and, hence, the older name of the condition as 'lipoid nephrosis'.

iii) Interstitium—There may be oedema of the interstitium.

iv) Vessels—Blood vessels do not show any significant change (minimal change).

By electron microscopy, the most characteristic feature of the disease is identified which is diffuse flattening of foot processes of the visceral epithelial cells (podocytes) and, hence, the name foot process disease (Fig. 20.11). Unlike other forms of GN, no deposits are seen and the GBM is normal.

By immunofluorescence microscopy, no deposits of complement or immunoglobulins are recognised (nil deposit disease).

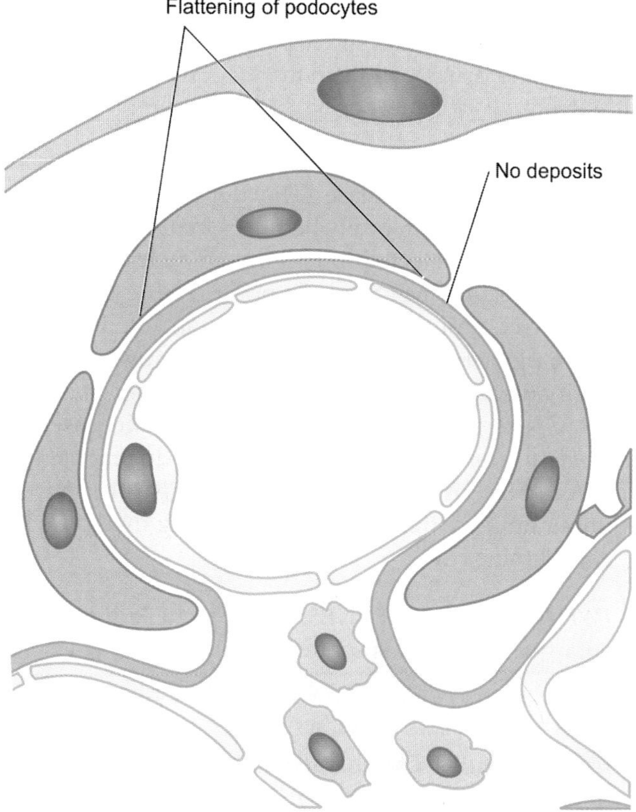

FIGURE 20.11

Minimal change disease, EM appearance of a portion of glomerular lobule showing comparison of normal area *(left)* with diseased area *(right).* There is diffuse fusion or flattening of foot processes of visceral epithelial cells (podocytes). The GBM is normal and there are no deposits.

CLINICAL FEATURES. The classical presentation of MCD is of fully-developed nephrotic syndrome with massive and *highly selective proteinuria,* but hypertension is unusual. Most frequently, the patients are children under 16 years (peak incidence at 6-8 years of age).

The onset may be preceded by an upper respiratory infection, atopic allergy or immunisation.

The disease characteristically responds to steroid therapy. In spite of remissions and relapses, long-term prognosis is very good and most children become free of albuminuria after several years.

Membranous Glomerulonephritis
(Synonym: Epimembranous Nephropathy)

Membranous GN is characterised by wide-spread thickening of the glomerular capillary wall and is the most common cause of nephrotic syndrome in adults. In about 15% of cases, membranous GN is *secondary* to an underlying condition (e.g. SLE, malignancies, infections such as chronic hepatitis B and C, syphilis, malaria and drugs), while in the majority of cases (85%) it is truly *idiopathic*.

ETIOPATHOGENESIS. *Idiopathic membranous GN* is an immune complex disease. The deposits of immune complex are formed locally because circulating immune complexes are detected in less than a quarter of cases. Since leucocytic infiltration is not a feature of membranous GN, damage to the GBM is mediated directly by complement. While nephritogenic antigen against which autoantibodies are formed in *idiopathic membranous* GN is not known yet, the antigen in cases of *secondary membranous GN* is either an endogenous (e.g. DNA in SLE) or exogenous one (e.g. hepatitis B virus, tumour antigen, treponema antigen, drug therapy with penicillamine).

PATHOLOGIC CHANGES. Grossly, the kidneys are enlarged, pale and smooth.

Light microscopy shows the following findings (COLOUR PLATE XXVII: CL 107):

i) Glomeruli—The characteristic finding is diffuse thickening of the glomerular capillary walls with all the glomeruli being affected more or less uniformly. As the disease progresses, the deposits are incorporated into enormously thickened basement membrane, producing 'duplication' of GBM which is actually formation of a new basement membrane. These basement membrane changes are best appreciated by silver impregnation stains (black colour) or by periodic acid-Schiff stain (pink colour). There is no cellular proliferation in the glomerular tufts (Fig. 20.12.A).

ii) Tubules—The renal tubules remain normal except in the early stage when lipid vacuolation of the proximal convoluted tubules may be seen.

iii) Interstitium—The interstitium may show fine fibrosis and scanty chronic inflammatory cells.

iv) Vessels—In the early stage, vascular changes are not prominent, while later hypertensive changes of arterioles may occur.

Electron microscopy shows electron-dense deposits situated in the epithelial side of the GBM. The basement membrane material protrudes between deposits as *'spikes'* (Fig. 20.12,B).

Immunofluorescence microscopy reveals granular deposits of immune complexes consisting of IgG associated with complement C3. In secondary cases of membranous GN the relevant antigen such as hepatitis B or tumour antigen may be seen.

CLINICAL FEATURES. The presentation in majority of cases is insidious onset of nephrotic syndrome in an adult. The proteinuria is usually of *non-selective* type. In addition, microscopic haematuria and hypertension may be present at the onset or may develop during the course of the disease. The changes in membranous GN are

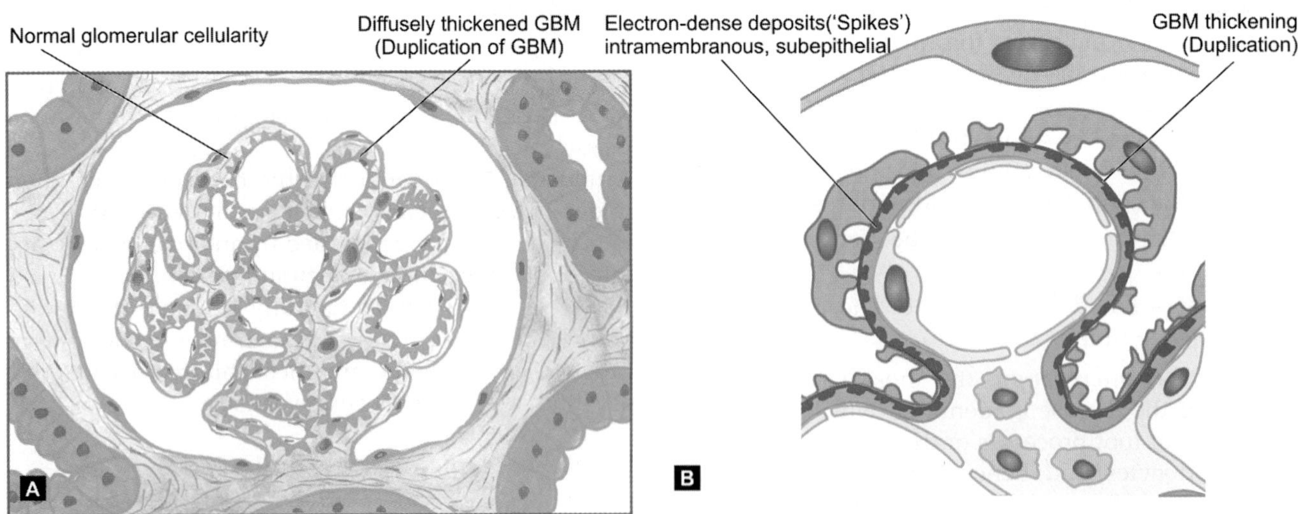

FIGURE 20.12

Membranous GN. A, Light microscopic appearance, showing normal glomerular cellularity but the capillary walls are diffusely thickened due to duplication of the GBM. B, Electron microscopic appearance of a portion of glomerular lobule. There are subepithelial deposits of electron-dense material so that the basement membrane material protrudes between these deposits.

irreversible in majority of patients. Progression to impaired renal function and end-stage renal disease with progressive azotaemia occurs in approximately 50% cases within a span of 2 to 20 years. Renal vein thrombosis has been found to develop in patients with membranous GN due to hypercoagulability. The role and beneficial effects of steroid therapy with or without the addition of immunosuppressive drugs is debatable.

Membranoproliferative Glomerulonephritis *(Synonyms: MPGN, Mesangiocapillary GN)*

Membranoproliferative GN is another important cause of nephrotic syndrome in children and young adults. As the name implies, it is characterised by two histologic features—increase in cellularity of the mesangium associated with increased lobulation of the tuft, and irregular thickening of the capillary wall.

ETIOPATHOGENESIS. Etiology of MPGN is unknown though in some cases there is evidence of preceding streptococcal infection. Based on ultrastructural, immunofluorescence and pathogenetic mechanisms, three types of MPGN are recognised:

- **Type I or classic form** is an example of immune complex disease and comprises more than 70% cases. It is characterised by immune deposits in the subendothelial position. Immune-complex MPGN is seen in association with systemic immune-complex diseases (e.g. SLE, mixed cryoglobulinaemia, Sjögren's syndrome), chronic infections (e.g. bacterial endocarditis, HIV, hepatitis B and C) and malignancies (e.g. lymphomas and leukaemias).

- **Type II or dense deposit disease** is the example of alternate pathway disease (page 687) and constitutes about 30% cases. The capillary wall thickening is due to the deposition of electron-dense material in the lamina densa of the GBM. Type II MPGN is an autoimmune disease in which patients have IgG autoantibody termed C3 nephritic factor.Type II cases have an association with partial lipodystrophy, an unusual condition of unknown pathogenesis characterised by symmetrical loss of subcutaneous fat from the upper half of the body.

- **Type III** is rare and shows features of type I MPGN and membranous nephropathy in association with systemic diseases or drugs.

PATHOLOGIC CHANGES. Grossly and by light microscopy, all the three types of MPGN are similar.

Grossly, the kidneys are usually pale in appearance and firm in consistency.

By light microscopy, the features are as under:

i) Glomeruli—Glomeruli show highly characteristic changes. They are enlarged with accentuated lobular pattern. The enlargement is due to variable degree of mesangial cellular proliferation and increase in mesangial matrix. The GBM is considerably thickened, which with silver stains shows two basement membranes with a clear zone between them. This is commonly referred to as *'double contour', splitting, or 'tram track'* appearance (Fig. 20.13,A).

ii) Tubules—Tubular cells may show vacuolation and hyaline droplets.

iii) Interstitium—There may be scattered chronic inflammatory cells and some finely granular foam cells in the interstitium.

iv) Vessels—Vascular changes are prominent in cases in which hypertension develops.

By electron microscopy and immunofluorescence microscopy, the changes are different in the three types of MPGN (Fig. 20.13,B):

Type I: It shows *electron-dense deposits* in subendothelial location conforming to immune-complex character of the disease. These deposits reveal positive fluorescence for C3 and slightly fainter staining for IgG.

Type II: The hallmark of type II MPGN is the presence of *dense amorphous deposits* within the lamina densa of the GBM and in the mesangium. Immunofluorescence studies reveal the universal presence of C3 and properdin in the deposits but the immunoglobulins are usually absent.

Type III: This rare form has *electron-dense deposits* within the GBM as well as in subendothelial and subepithelial regions of the GBM. Immunofluorescence studies show the presence of C3, IgG and IgM.

CLINICAL FEATURES. Clinically, there are many similarities between the main forms of MPGN. The most common age at diagnosis is between 15 and 20 years. Approximately 50% of the patients present with nephrotic syndrome; about 30% have asymptomatic proteinuria; and 20% have nephritic syndrome at presentation. The proteinuria is non-selective. Haematuria and hypertension are frequently present. Hypocomplementaemia is a common feature. With time, majority of patients progress to renal failure, while some continue to have proteinuria, haematuria and hypertension with stable renal function.

Prognosis of type I is relatively better and majority of patients survive without clinically significant impairment of GFR, while type II cases run a variable clinical course.

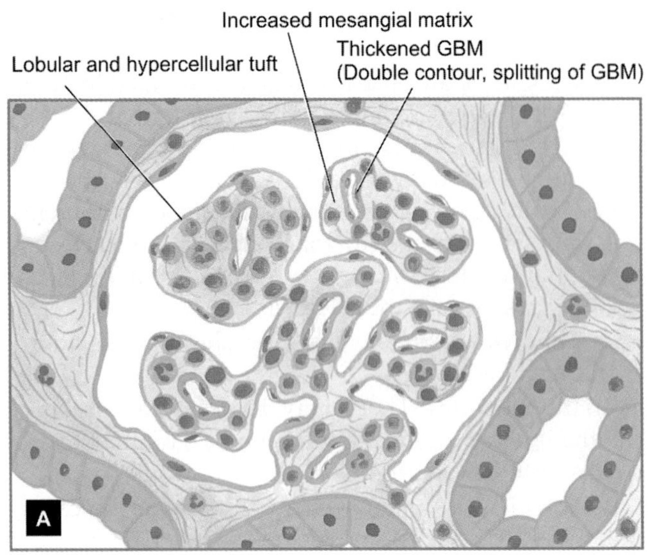

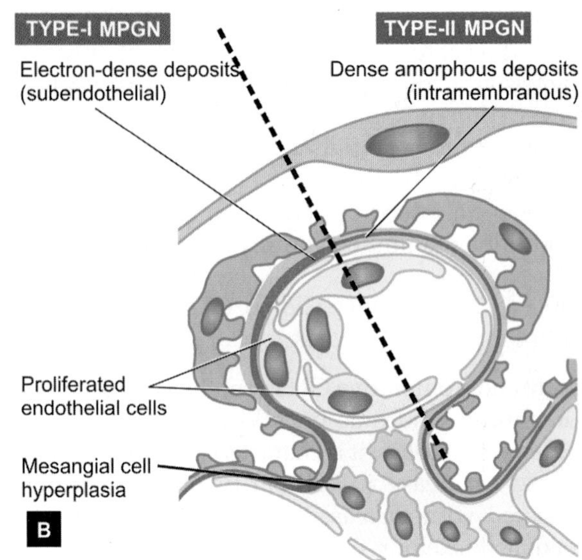

FIGURE 20.13

Membranoproliferative GN. A, Light microscopic appearance. The glomerular tufts show lobulation and mesangial hypercellularity. There is increase in the mesangial matrix between the capillaries. There is widespread thickening of the GBM. B, Electron microscopic appearance of a portion of glomerular lobule showing features of type I (left half) and type II (right half) MPGN. Type I (classic form) shows the characteristic subendothelial electron-dense deposits, while type II (dense deposit disease) is characterised by intramembranous dense deposits.

Focal Glomerulonephritis *(Synonyms: Focal Segmental GN, Mesangial Proliferative GN)*

Focal GN is characterised by pathologic changes in certain number of glomeruli *(focal),* and often confined to one or two lobules of the affected glomeruli *(segmental),* while other glomeruli are normal. Focal GN is, thus, a pathologic diagnosis.

ETIOPATHOGENESIS. It may occur under following diverse clinical settings:

- As an early manifestation of a number of *systemic diseases* such as SLE, Henoch-Schonlein purpura, subacute bacterial endocarditis, Wegener's granulomatosis, and polyarteritis nodosa, Goodpasture's syndrome.
- As a component of a known *renal disease* such as in IgA nephropathy.
- As a primary *idiopathic* glomerular disease unrelated to systemic or other renal disease.

The diverse settings under which focal GN is encountered make it unlikely that there are common etiologic agents or pathogenetic mechanisms. However, the observation of mesangial deposits of immunoglobulins and complement suggest immune complex disease and participation of the mesangium.

PATHOLOGIC CHANGES. By light microscopy, the single most important feature in focal GN is the abnormality seen in certain number of glomeruli and generally confined to one or two lobules of the affected glomeruli i.e. *focal and segmental glomerular involvement* (Fig. 20.14,A). The pathologic change most frequently consists of focal and segmental cellular proliferation of mesangial cells and endothelial cells but sometimes necrotising changes can be seen. The condition must be distinguished from focal and segmental glomerulosclerosis (discussed below).

By immunofluorescence microscopy, widespread mesangial deposits of immunoglobulins (mainly IgA with or without IgG), complement (C3) and fibrin are demonstrated in most cases of focal GN.

CLINICAL FEATURES. The clinical features vary according to the condition causing it. Haematuria is one of the most common clinical manifestation. Proteinuria is frequently mild to moderate but hypertension is uncommon.

Focal Segmental Glomerulosclerosis *(Synonyms: Focal Sclerosis, Focal Hyalinosis)*

Focal segmental glomerulosclerosis (FSGS) is a condition in which there is sclerosis and hyalinosis of some glomeruli and portions of their tuft (less than 50% in a

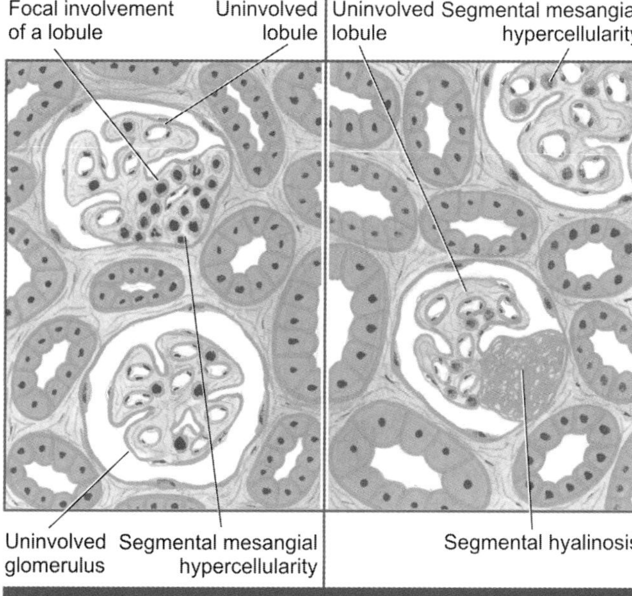

FIGURE 20.14

A, Focal GN. The characteristic feature is the cellular proliferation in some glomeruli and in one or two lobules of the affected glomeruli i.e. focal and segmental proliferative change. B, Focal segmental glomerulosclerosis. The features are focal and segmental involvement of the glomeruli by sclerosis and hyalinosis and mesangial hypercellularity.

tissue section), while the other glomeruli are normal by light microscopy i.e. involvement is focal and segmental. The incidence of FSGS has increased over the last decades and is currently responsible for about one-third cases of nephrotic syndrome in the adults.

ETIOPATHOGENESIS. FSGS was previously believed to be a variant of MCD with accentuation of epithelial damage in the form of hyalinosis and sclerosis. Currently, the condition is divided into 3 groups:

i) Idiopathic type. This group comprises majority of cases. It is found in children and young adults with presentation of nephrotic syndrome. It differs from minimal change disease in having non-selective proteinuria, in being steroid-resistant, and may progress to chronic renal failure. Immunofluorescence microscopy reveals deposits of IgM and C3 in the sclerotic segment.

ii) With superimposed primary glomerular disease. There may be cases of FSGS with superimposed MCD or IgA nephropathy. Those associated with MCD show good response to steroid therapy and progression to chronic renal failure may occur after a long time.

iii) Secondary type. This group consists of focal segmental sclerotic lesions as a secondary manifestation of certain diseases such as HIV, diabetes mellitus, reflux nephropathy, heroin abuse and analgesic nephropathy. Infection with HIV, particularly in blacks, has been found associated with a variant of FSGS which is characterised by *collapsing sclerosis*.

The hallmark of pathogenesis of FSGS is injury to visceral epithelial cells that results in disruption of visceral epithelial cells and resultant nephron loss.

*PATHOLOGIC CHANGES. **By light microscopy,*** depending upon the severity of the disease, variable number of glomeruli are affected focally and segmentally, while others are normal. The affected glomeruli show solidification or *sclerosis* of one or more lobules of the tuft. *Hyalinosis* refers to collection of eosinophilic, homogeneous, PAS-positive, hyaline material present on the inner aspect of a sclerotic peripheral capillary loop. Mesangial hypercellularity is present in appreciable number of cases (Fig. 20.14,B).

HIV-associated nephropathy in FSGS is characterised by focal sclerosis that may be segmental or global, having collapsed capillaries in the tuft. Besides glomerular changes, there is interstitial fibrosis and infiltration by mononuclear leucocytes, and tubular epithelial cell atrophy and degeneration.

By electron microscopy, diffuse loss of foot processes as seen in minimal change disease is evident but, in addition, there are electron-dense deposits in the region of hyalinosis and sclerosis which are believed to be immune complexes.

By Immunofluorescence microscopy, the deposits in the lesions are shown to contain IgM and C3.

CLINICAL FEATURES. The condition may affect all ages including children and has male preponderance. The most common presentation is in the form of nephrotic syndrome with heavy proteinuria. Haematuria and hypertension tend to occur more frequently than in minimal change disease. Evidence of renal failure may be present at the onset.

IgA Nephropathy
(Synonyms: Berger's Disease, IgA GN)

IgA nephropathy is another common form of glomerulopathy worldwide and is characterised by aggregates of IgA, deposited principally in the mesangium. The condition was first described by Berger, a French physician in 1968. (Not to be confused with

Buerger's disease or thromboangiitis obliterans described by an American pathologist in 1908 and discussed on page 293).

ETIOPATHOGENESIS. The etiology of IgA nephropathy remains unclear:

i) It is idiopathic in most cases.

ii) Seen as part of Henoch-Schonlein purpura.

iii) Association with chronic inflammation in various body systems (e.g. chronic liver disease, inflammatory bowel disease, interstitial pneumonitis, leprosy, dermatitis herpetiformis, uveitis, ankylosing spondylitis, Sjögren's syndrome, monoclonal IgA gammopathy).

Pathogenesis of IgA nephropathy is explained on the basis of following mechanisms:

i) In view of exclusive mesangial deposits of IgA and elevated serum levels of IgA and IgA-immune complexes, IgA nephropathy has been considered to arise from *entrapment* of these complexes in the mesangium.

ii) There is absence of early components of the complement but presence of C3 and properdin in the mesangial deposits, which point towards activation of *alternate complement pathway.*

iii) Since there is close association between mucosal infections (e.g. of the respiratory, gastrointestinal or urinary tract), it is suggested that IgA deposited in the mesangium could be due to increased *mucosal secretion of IgA.*

iv) HLA-B35 association has been reported in some cases. Another possibility is *genetically-determined* abnormality of the immune system producing an increase in circulating IgA.

PATHOLOGIC CHANGES. By light microscopy, the pattern of involvement varies. These include: focal proliferative GN, focal segmental glomerulosclerosis, membranoproliferative GN, and rarely RPGN.
By electron microscopy, finely granular electron-dense deposits are seen in the mesangium.
By immunofluorescence microscopy, the diagnosis is firmly established by demonstration of mesangial deposits of IgA, with or without IgG, and usually with C3 and properdin.

CLINICAL FEATURES. The disease is common in children and young adults. The clinical picture is usually characterised by recurrent bouts of haematuria that are often precipitated by mucosal infections. Mild proteinuria is usually present and occasionally nephrotic syndrome may develop.

Chronic Glomerulonephritis
(Synonym: End-Stage Kidney)

Chronic GN is the final stage of a variety of glomerular diseases which result in irreversible impairment of renal function. The conditions which may progress to chronic GN, in descending order of frequency, are as under:

i) Rapidly progressive GN (90%)
ii) Membranous GN (50%)
iii) Membranoproliferative GN (50%)
iv) Focal segmental glomerulosclerosis (50%)
v) IgA nephropathy (40%)
vi) Acute post-streptococcal GN (1%)

However, about 20% cases of chronic GN are *idiopathic* without evidence of preceding GN of any type.

PATHOLOGIC CHANGES. Grossly, the kidneys are usually small and contracted weighing as low as 50 gm each. The capsule is adherent to the cortex. The cortical surface is generally diffusely granular (Fig. 20.15,A). On cut section, the cortex is narrow and atrophic, while the medulla is unremarkable.
Microscopically, the changes vary greatly depending upon the underlying glomerular disease. In general, the following changes are seen (Fig. 20.15,B).

i) Glomeruli—Glomeruli are reduced in number and most of those present show completely hyalinised tufts, giving the appearance of acellular, eosinophilic masses which are PAS-positive. Evidence of underlying glomerular disease may be present.

ii) Tubules—Many tubules completely disappear and there may be atrophy of tubules close to scarred glomeruli. Tubular cells show hyaline-droplets, degeneration and tubular lumina frequently contain eosinophilic, homogeneous casts.

iii) Interstitium—There is fine and delicate fibrosis of the interstitial tissue and varying number of chronic inflammatory cells are often seen.

iv) Vessels—Advanced cases which are frequently associated with hypertension show conspicuous arterial and arteriolar sclerosis.

Patients of end-stage kidney disease on dialysis show a variety of dialysis associated changes that include acquired cystic disease (page 682), occurrence of adenomas and adenocarcinomas of the kidney, calcification of tufts and deposition of calcium oxalate crystals in tubules.

CLINICAL FEATURES. The patients are usually adults. The terminal stage of chronic GN is characterised by hypertension, uraemia and progressive deterioration of

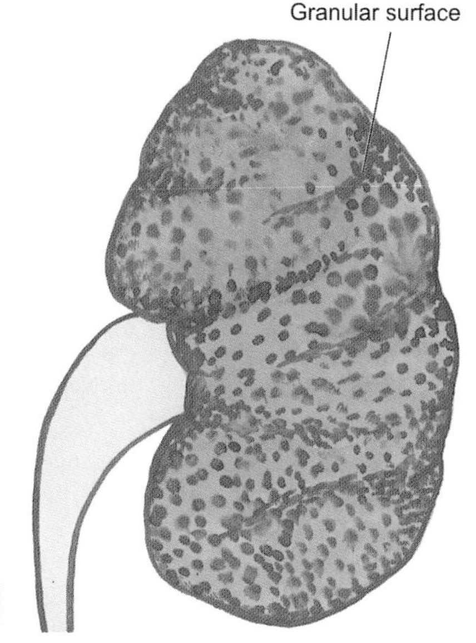

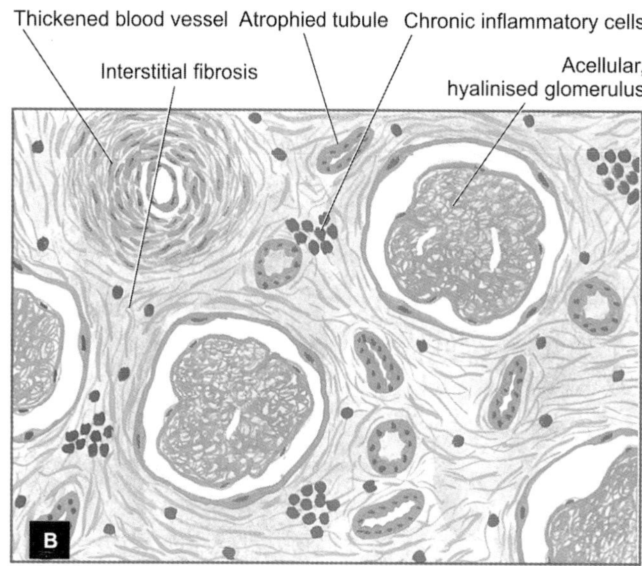

FIGURE 20.15

End-stage kidney (Chronic glomerulonephritis). A, Gross appearance showing diffusely granular cortical surface. B, Light microscopy shows acellular and completely hyalinised glomerular tufts, a hyalinised and thickened blood vessel and fine interstitial fibrosis with a few chronic inflammatory cells.

renal function. Besides the primary changes due to chronic renal failure, there are a variety of systemic manifestations of uraemia (page 678). These patients eventually die if they do not receive a renal transplant.

The salient features of various types of primary glomerulonephritis are summarised in Table 20.9.

II. SECONDARY GLOMERULAR DISEASES

Glomerular involvement may occur secondary to certain systemic diseases or a few hereditary diseases. In some of these, renal involvement may be the initial presentation, while in others clinical evidence of renal disease appears long after other manifestations have appeared. A list of these conditions has already been given in Table 20.2. The important examples are described below.

Lupus Nephritis

Renal manifestations of systemic lupus erythematosus (SLE) are termed lupus nephritis. Other clinical manifestations, etiology and pathogenesis of this multi-system autoimmune disease are described on page 77. The incidence of renal involvement in SLE ranges from 40 to 75%. The two cardinal clinical manifestations of lupus nephritis are proteinuria and haematuria. In addition, hypertension and casts of different types such as red cell casts, fatty casts and leucocyte casts in the urinary sediment are found.

PATHOLOGIC CHANGES. According to the WHO, six patterns of mutually-merging renal lesions are seen in lupus nephritis:

Class I: Minimal lesions. On light microscopy, these cases do not show any abnormality. But examination by electron microscopy and immunofluorescence microscopy shows deposits within the mesangium which consist of IgG and C3.

Class II: Mesangial lupus nephritis. These cases have mild clinical manifestations. By light microscopy, there is increase in the number of mesangial cells and of mesangial matrix. Ultrastructural and immunofluorescence studies reveal granular mesangial deposits of IgG and C3; sometimes IgA and IgM are also present in the deposits.

Class III: Focal segmental lupus nephritis. This is characterised by focal and segmental proliferation of endothelial and mesangial cells, together with infiltration by macrophages and sometimes neutrophils. Haematoxylin bodies of Gross may be present. Subendothelial and subepithelial deposits of IgG, often with IgM or IgA and C3, are seen.

Class IV: Diffuse proliferative lupus nephritis. In this type, all the morphologic manifestations of lupus are present in most advanced form. This is the most

TABLE 20.9: Comparative Features of Major Forms of Primary Glomerulonephritis.

TYPE	CLINICAL FEATURES	PATHOGENESIS	PATHOLOGY		
			LM	EM	IFM
1. *Acute GN*	Acute nephrotic syndrome	Immune complex disease (local or circulating)	Diffuse proliferation, leucocytic infiltration	Subepithelial deposits ('humps')	Irregular IgG, C3
2. *RPGN*	Acute renal failure	i) Type I: anti-GBM type ii) Type II: immune complex type iii) Type III: pauci-immune RPGN	Proliferation, crescents	i) Linear deposits along GBM ii) Subepithelial deposits iii) No deposits	i) Linear IgG, C3 ii) Granular IgG, C3 iii) Negative
3. *Minimal change disease*	Nephrotic syndrome (highly selective proteinuria)	Reduction of normal negative charge on GBM ?Cell-mediated mechanism	Normal glomeruli, lipid vacuolation in tubules	Loss of foot processes, no deposits	Negative
4. *Membranous GN*	Nephrotic syndrome	Immune complex disease (local)	Diffuse thickening of capillary wall	Subepithelial deposits ('spikes')	Granular IgG, C3
5. *Membrano-proliferative GN*	Nephrotic syndrome	Type I: immune complex disease Type II: dense deposit disease (alternate pathway activation) Type III: rare, with systemic diseases and drugs	Lobular proliferation of mesangial cells, increased mesangial matrix, double contour of GBM	Type I: Subendothelial deposits Type II: Dense intramembranous deposits Type III: Subendothelial and subepithelial deposits	Type I: IgG, C3 Type II: C3 properdin Type III: C3 IgG, IgM
6. *Focal GN*	Variable, haematuria common	Variable, possibly immune complex disease	Focal and segmental proliferation	Mesangial deposits	IgA ± IgG, C3 and fibrin
7. *Focal Segmental glomerulo-sclerosis*	Nephrotic syndrome	i) Idiopathic ii) With superimposed primary glomerular disease iii) Secondary type	Focal and segmental sclerosis and hyalinosis	Loss of foot processes, electron dense deposits in regions of sclerosis and hyalinosis	IgM, C3
8. *IgA nephropathy*	Recurrent haematuria, mild proteinuria	Unknown, possibly alternate pathway disease	Variable, commonly focal proliferative GN	Mesangial electron-dense deposits	IgA ± IgG, C3, properdin
9. *Chronic GN*	Chronic renal failure	Variable	Hyalinised glomeruli	Variable	Variable

GN = glomerulonephritis; LM = light microscopy; EM = electron microscopy; IFM = immunofluorescence microscopy.

severe and the most common form of lupus nephritis. There is diffuse proliferation of endothelial, mesangial, and sometimes epithelial cells, involving most or all glomeruli. Electron microscopy shows large electron-dense deposits in the mesangium and in the subendothelial region which on immunofluorescence are positive for IgG; sometimes also for IgA or IgM, and C3.

Class V: Membranous lupus nephritis. These lesions resemble those of idiopathic membranous GN. These consist of diffuse thickening of glomerular capillary wall on light microscopy and show subendothelial deposits of immune complexes containing IgG, IgM and C3 on ultrastructural studies.

Class VI: Sclerosing lupus nephritis. This is end-stage kidney of SLE, akin to chronic GN. Most glomeruli are sclerosed and hyalinised and there may be remnants of preceding lesions.

Diabetic Nephropathy

Renal involvement is an important complication of diabetes mellitus. End-stage kidney with renal failure accounts for deaths in more than 10% of all diabetics. Renal complications are more severe, develop early and more frequently in type 1 (i.e. insulin-dependent) diabetes mellitus (30-40% cases) than in type 2 (non-insulin-dependent) diabetics (about 20% cases). A variety of clinical syndromes are associated with diabetic nephropathy that includes asymptomatic proteinuria, nephrotic syndrome, progressive renal failure and hypertension. Cardiovascular disease is 40 times more common in patients of end-stage renal disease in diabetes mellitus than in non-diabetics and more diabetics die from cardiovascular complications than from uraemia.

PATHOLOGIC CHANGES. Diabetic nephropathy is the term that encompasses 4 types of renal lesions in diabetes mellitus: diabetic glomerulosclerosis, vascular lesions, diabetic pyelonephritis and tubular lesions (Armanni-Ebstein lesions).

1. DIABETIC GLOMERULOSCLEROSIS. Glomerular lesions in diabetes mellitus are particularly common and account for majority of abnormal findings referable to the kidney.

Pathogenesis of these lesions in diabetes mellitus is explained by following sequential changes: hyperglycaemia → glomerular hypertension → renal hyperperfusion → deposition of proteins in the mesangium → glomerulosclerosis → renal failure. In addition, cellular infiltration in renal lesions in diabetic glomerular lesions is due to growth factors, particularly transforming growth factor-β. Strict control of blood glucose level and control of systemic hypertension in these patients retards progression to diabetic nephropathy.

Glomerulosclerosis in diabetes may take one of the 2 forms: diffuse or nodular lesions (COLOUR PLATE XXVII: CL 108).

i) Diffuse glomerulosclerosis. Diffuse glomerular lesions are the most common. There is involvement of all parts of glomeruli. The pathologic changes consist of thickening of the GBM and diffuse increase in mesangial matrix with mild proliferation of mesangial cells. Various exudative lesions such as capsular hyaline drops and fibrin caps may also be present (Fig. 20.16,A) *Capsular drop* is an eosinophilic hyaline thickening of the parietal layer of Bowman's capsule and bulges into the glomerular space. *Fibrin cap* is homogeneous, brightly eosinophilic material appearing on the wall of a peripheral capillary of a lobule.

ii) Nodular glomerulosclerosis. Nodular lesions of diabetic glomerulosclerosis are also called as *Kimmelstiel-Wilson (KW) lesions* or *intercapillary glomerulosclerosis.* These lesions are specific for juvenile-onset diabetes or islet cell antibody-positive diabetes mellitus. The pathologic changes consist of one or more nodules in a few or many glomeruli. *Nodule* is an ovoid or spherical, laminated, hyaline, acellular mass located within a lobule of the glomerulus. The nodules are surrounded peripherally by glomerular capillary loops which may have normal or thickened GBM (Fig. 20.16,B). The nodules are PAS-positive and contain lipid and fibrin. As the nodular lesions enlarge, they compress the glomerular capillaries and obliterate the glomerular tuft. As a result of glomerular and arteriolar involvement, renal ischaemia occurs leading to tubular atrophy and interstitial fibrosis and grossly small, contracted kidney.

2. VASCULAR LESIONS. ***Atheroma*** of renal arteries is very common and severe in diabetes mellitus. ***Hyaline arteriolosclerosis*** (Chapter 11) affecting the afferent and efferent arterioles of the glomeruli is also often severe in diabetes. These vascular lesions are responsible for renal ischaemia that results in tubular atrophy and interstitial fibrosis.

3. DIABETIC PYELONEPHRITIS. Poorly-controlled diabetics are particularly susceptible to bacterial infections. Papillary necrosis (necrotising papillitis) (page 714) is an important complication of diabetes that may result in acute pyelonephritis. Chronic pyelonephritis is 10 to 20 times more common in diabetics than in others.

4. TUBULAR LESIONS (ARMANNI-EBSTEIN LESIONS). In untreated diabetics who have extremely high blood sugar level, the epithelial cells of the proximal convoluted tubules develop extensive glycogen deposits appearing as vacuoles. These are called Armanni-Ebstein lesions. The tubules return to normal on control of hyperglycaemic state.

Hereditary Nephritis

A group of hereditary diseases principally involving the glomeruli are termed hereditary nephritis. These include the following:

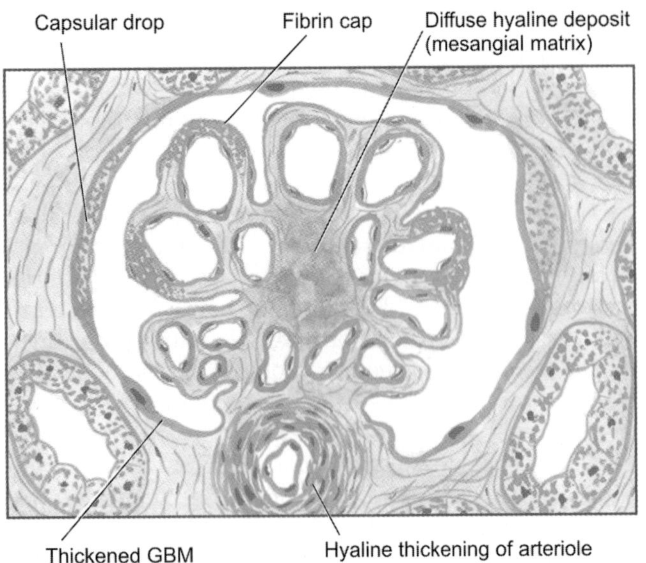

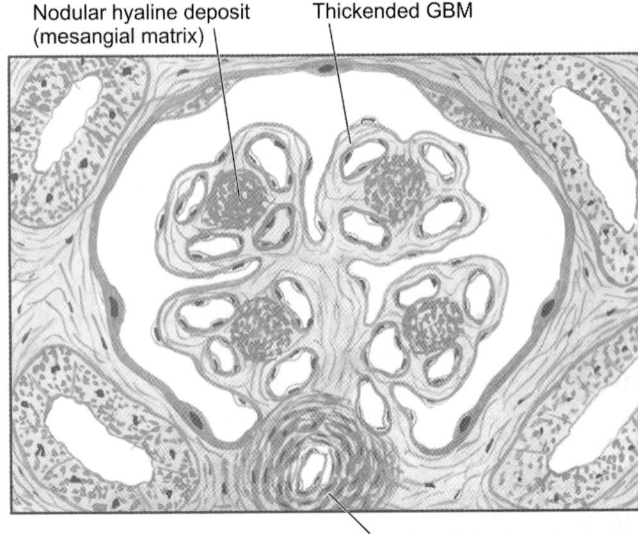

A, DIFFUSE GLOMERULOSCLEROSIS | B, NODULAR GLOMERULOSCLEROSIS

FIGURE 20.16

Diabetic glomerulosclerosis, microscopic appearance. *A, Diffuse lesions.* The characteristic features are diffuse involvement of the glomeruli showing thickening of the GBM and diffuse increase in the mesangial matrix with mild proliferation of mesangial cells and exudative lesions (fibrin caps and capsular drops). *B, Nodular lesion (Kimmelstiel-Wilson Lesion).* There are one or more hyaline nodules within the lobules of glomeruli, surrounded peripherally by glomerular capillaries with thickened walls.

1. Alport's syndrome
2. Fabry's disease
3. Nail-patella syndrome

1. Alport's syndrome. Out of various hereditary nephritis, Alport's syndrome is relatively more common and has been extensively studied. This is an X-linked dominant disorder having mutation in α–5 chain of type IV collagen located on X-chromosome. It affects males more severely than females. The syndrome consists of sensori-neural deafness and ophthalmic complications (lens dislocation, posterior cataracts and corneal dystrophy) associated with hereditary nephritis. The condition is slowly progressive, terminating in end-stage kidney in the 2nd to 3rd decades of life. The common presenting features are persistent or recurrent haematuria accompanied by erythrocyte casts, proteinuria and hypertension.

By ***light microscopy,*** the glomeruli have predominant involvement and show segmental proliferation of mesangial cells with increased mesangial matrix and occasional segmental sclerosis. Another prominent feature is the presence of *lipid-laden foam cells* in the interstitium. As the disease progresses, there is increasing sclerosis of glomeruli, tubular atrophy and interstitial fibrosis.

Electron microscopy reveals characteristic basement membrane splitting or lamination in the affected parts of glomeruli.

Immunofluorescence studies fail to show deposits of immunoglobulins or complement components.

2. Fabry's disease, another hereditary nephritis is characterised by accumulation of neutral glycosphingolipids in lysosomes of glomerular, tubular, vascular and interstitial cells.

3. Nail-patella syndrome or osteonychodysplasia is a rare hereditary disease having abnormality in α-1 chain of collagen V on chromosome 9 associated with multiple osseous defects of elbows, knees and nail dysplasia. About half the cases develop nephropathy.

TUBULAR DISEASES

Acute tubular necrosis is the pathologic entity that affects exclusively renal tubules. Many other diseases involve the tubules secondarily, or the tubular involvement is accompanied by interstitial involvement as well and are described later under the heading of 'tubulo-interstitial diseases.'

ACUTETUBULAR NECROSIS

Acute tubular necrosis (ATN) is the term used for acute renal failure (ARF) resulting from destruction of tubular epithelial cells. ATN is the most common and most important cause of ARF characterised by sudden cessation of renal function. Various other causes of ARF (pre-renal, intra-renal and post-renal) as well as the clinical syndrome accompanying ATN (oliguric phase, diuretic phase and phase of recovery) are described already on page 676. Two forms of ATN—ischaemic and toxic, are distinguished on etiology and morphology but both have a somewhat common pathogenesis.

Pathogenesis of ATN

The pathogenesis of both types of ATN resulting in ARF is explained on the basis of the following sequential mechanism:

- *Tubular damage* in ischaemic ATN is initiated by arteriolar vasoconstriction induced by renin-angiotensin system, while in toxic ATN by direct damage to tubules.
- This is followed by *tubular obstruction* by desquamated epithelium and casts in the lumina or by interstitial oedema.
- This causes *increased intratubular pressure* resulting in damage to tubular basement membrane.
- Due to increased intratubular pressure, there is *tubular rupture.*
- This leads to *back-leakage* of tubular fluid into the interstitium which increases interstitial pressure.
- Increased interstitial pressure causes *compression of tubules and blood vessels* and hence further accentuates ischaemia and necrosis.

Ischaemic ATN

Ischaemic ATN, also called tubulorrhectic ATN, lower nephron nephrosis, or shock kidney, occurs due to hypoperfusion of the kidneys resulting in focal damage to the tubules.

ETIOLOGY. Ischaemic ATN is more common than toxic ATN and accounts for more than 80% cases of tubular injury. Ischaemia may result from a variety of causes such as:

1. Shock (post-traumatic, surgical, burns, dehydration, obstetrical and septic type).
2. Crush injuries.
3. Non-traumatic rhabdomyolysis induced by alcohol, coma, muscle disease or extreme muscular exertion (myoglobinuric nephrosis).
4. Mismatched blood transfusions, black-water fever (haemoglobinuric nephrosis).

PATHOLOGIC CHANGES. Grossly, the kidneys are enlarged and swollen. On cut section, the cortex is often widened and pale, while medulla is dark.
Histologically, predominant changes are seen in the tubules, while glomeruli are normal. Interstitium shows oedema and mild chronic inflammatory cell infiltrate. Tubular changes are as follows (Fig. 20.17,A):
1. Dilatation of the proximal and distal convoluted tubules.
2. Focal tubular necrosis at different points along the nephron.
3. Flattened epithelium lining the tubules suggesting epithelial regeneration.
4. Eosinophilic hyaline casts or pigmented haemoglobin and myoglobin casts in the tubular lumina.
5. Disruption of tubular basement membrane adjacent to the cast (tubulorrhexis).

Prognosis of ischaemic ATN depends upon the underlying etiology. In general, cases that follow severe trauma, surgical procedures, extensive burns and sepsis have much worse outlook than the others.

Toxic ATN

Toxic or nephrotoxic ATN occurs as a result of direct damage to tubular cells by ingestion, injection or inhalation of a number of toxic agents.

ETIOLOGY. The toxic agents causing toxic ATN are as under:

1. General poisons such as mercuric chloride, carbon tetrachloride, ethylene glycol, mushrooms and insecticides.
2. Heavy metals (mercury, lead, arsenic, phosphorus and gold).
3. Drugs such as sulfonamides, certain antibiotics (gentamycin, cephalosporin), anaesthetic agents (methoxyflurane, halothane), barbiturates, salicylates.
4. Radiographic contrast material.

PATHOLOGIC CHANGES. Poisoning with mercuric chloride provides the best example that produces widespread and readily discernible tubular necrosis *(acute mercury nephropathy).*
Grossly, the kidneys are enlarged and swollen. On cut section, the cortex is pale and swollen, while the medulla is slightly darker than normal.

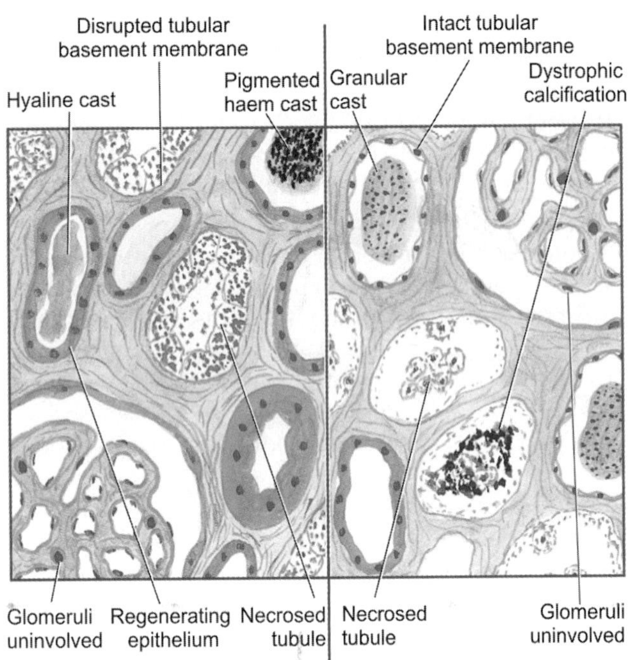

FIGURE 20.17

Acute tubular necrosis (ATN), patterns of tubular damage. A, Ischaemic ATN—There is focal necrosis along the nephron involving proximal convoluted tubule (PCT) as well as distal convoluted tubule (DCT). The affected tubules are dilated, their lumina contain casts (hyaline or pigmented haem) and the affected regions are lined by regenerating thin and flat epithelium. B, Toxic ATN—There is extensive necrosis of epithelial cells involving predominantly proximal convoluted tubule (PCT) diffusely. The necrosed cells are desquamated into the tubular lumina and may undergo dystrophic calcification. The tubular lumina contain casts (granular) and the regenerating flat epithelium lines the necrosed tubule.

Histologically, the appearance varies according to the cause of toxic ATN but, in general, involves the segment of tubule diffusely (unlike ischaemic ATN where the involvement of nephron is focal). In mercuric chloride poisoning, the features are as follows (Fig. 20.17,B):

1. Epithelial cells of mainly proximal convoluted tubules are necrotic and desquamated into the tubular lumina.
2. The desquamated cells may undergo dystrophic calcification.
3. Tubular basement membrane is generally intact.
4. The regenerating epithelium, which is flat and thin with few mitoses, may be seen lining the tubular basement membrane.

Prognosis of toxic ATN is good if there is no serious damage to other organs such as heart and liver.

TUBULOINTERSTITIAL DISEASE

The term tubulointerstitial nephritis is used for inflammatory process that predominantly involves the renal interstitial tissue and is usually accompanied by some degree of tubular damage. A number of primary glomerular, tubular, vascular and obstructive diseases are secondarily associated with interstitial reaction. However, the term *interstitial nephritis* is reserved for those cases where there is no primary involvement of glomeruli, tubules or blood vessels. The older nomenclature, interstitial nephritis, is currently used synonymously with *tubulointerstitial nephritis or tubulointerstitial nephropathy.*

A number of bacterial and non-bacterial, acute and chronic conditions may produce tubulointerstitial nephritis and are listed in Table 20.10. The important and common examples among these are discussed below.

Acute Pyelonephritis

Acute pyelonephritis is an acute suppurative inflammation of the kidney caused by pyogenic bacteria.

ETIOPATHOGENESIS. Most cases of acute pyelonephritis follow infection of the lower urinary tract. The most common pathogenic organism in urinary tract infection (UTI) is *Escherichia coli* (in 90% of cases), followed in decreasing frequency, by *Enterobacter, Klebsiella, Pseudomonas* and *Proteus.* The bacteria gain entry into the urinary tract, and thence into the kidney by one of the two routes: ascending infection and haematogenous infection (*see* Fig. 20.18):

1. **Ascending infection.** This is the most common route of infection. The common pathogenic organisms are

TABLE 20.10: Tubulointerstitial Diseases.

A. Infective

1. Acute pyelonephritis
2. Chronic pyelonephritis
3. Tuberculous pyelonephritis
4. Other infections (viruses, parasites etc)

B. Non-infective

1. Acute hypersensitivity interstitial nephritis
2. Analgesic abuse (phenacetin) nephropathy
3. Myeloma nephropathy
4. Balkan nephropathy
5. Urate nephropathy
6. Gout nephropathy
7. Radiation nephritis
8. Transplant rejection (page 81)
9. Nephrocalcinosis
10. Idiopathic interstitial nephritis

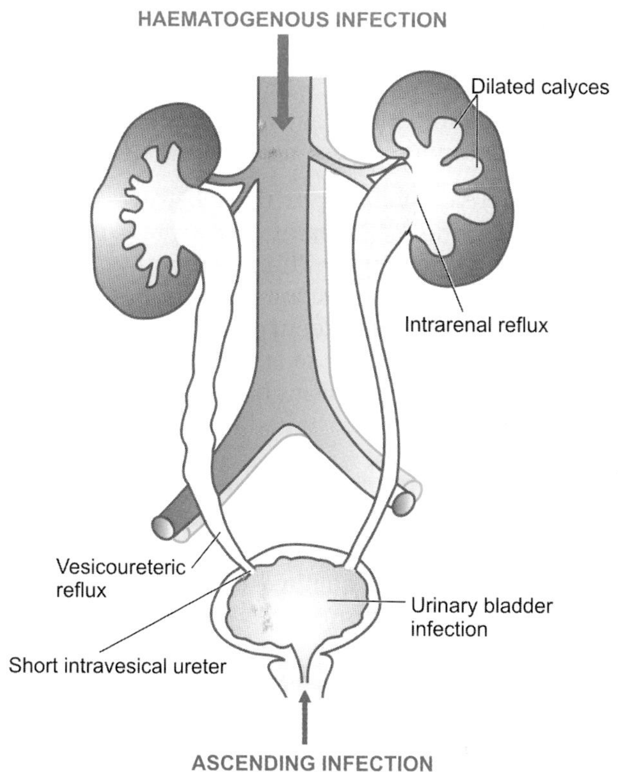

FIGURE 20.18

Pathogenesis of reflux nephropathy.

inhabitants of the colon and may cause faecal contamination of the urethral orifice, especially in females in reproductive age group. This has been variously attributed to shorter urethra in females liable to faecal contamination, hormonal influences facilitating bacterial adherence to the mucosa, absence of prostatic secretions which have antibacterial properties, and urethral trauma during sexual intercourse. The last named produces what is appropriately labelled as *'honeymoon pyelitis'*. Ascending infection may occur in a normal individual but the susceptibility is increased in patients with diabetes mellitus, pregnancy, urinary tract obstruction or instrumentation. Bacteria multiply in the urinary bladder and produce asymptomatic bacteriuria found in many of these cases. After having caused urethritis and cystitis, the bacteria in a small proportion of cases ascend further up into the ureters against the flow of urine, extend into the renal pelvis and then the renal cortex. The role of vesico-ureteral reflux is primarily of importance in the pathogenesis of chronic pyelonephritis but not in acute pyelonephritis.

2. Haematogenous infection. Less often, acute pyelonephritis may result from blood-borne spread of infection. This occurs more often in patients with obstructive lesions in the urinary tract, and in debilitated or immunosuppressed patients.

PATHOLOGIC CHANGES. ***Grossly,*** well-developed cases of acute pyelonephritis show enlarged and swollen kidney that bulges on section. The cut surface shows small, yellow-white abscesses with a haemorrhagic rim. These abscesses may be several millimetres across and are situated mainly in the cortex. ***Microscopically,*** acute pyelonephritis is characterised by extensive acute inflammation involving the interstitium and causing destruction of the tubules. Generally, the glomeruli and renal blood vessels show considerable resistance to infection and are spared. The acute inflammation may be in the form of large number of neutrophils in the interstitial tissue and bursting into tubules, or may form focal neutrophilic abscesses in the renal parenchyma.

CLINICAL FEATURES. Classically, acute pyelonephritis has an acute onset with chills, fever, loin pain, lumbar tenderness, dysuria and frequency of micturition. Urine will show bacteria in excess of 100,000/ml, pus cells and pus cell casts in the urinary sediment. Institution of specific antibiotics, after identification of bacteria by culture followed by sensitivity test, eradicates the infection in majority of patients.

COMPLICATIONS. Complications of acute pyelonephritis are encountered more often in patients with diabetes mellitus or with urinary tract obstruction. There are 3 important complications of acute pyelonephritis. These are as under:

1. Papillary necrosis. Papillary necrosis or necrotising papillitis develops more commonly in analgesic abuse nephropathy and in sickle cell disease but may occur as a complication of acute pyelonephritis as well. It may affect one or both kidneys.

Grossly, the necrotic papillae are yellow to grey-white, sharply-defined areas with congested border and resemble infarction. The pelvis may be dilated. ***Microscopically,*** necrotic tissue is separated from the viable tissue by a dense zone of polymorphs. The necrotic area shows characteristic coagulative necrosis as seen in renal infarcts.

2. Pyonephrosis. Rarely, the abscesses in the kidney in acute pyelonephritis are extensive, particularly in cases with obstruction. This results in inability of the abscesses to drain and this transforms the kidney into a multilocular sac filled with pus called as pyonephrosis or renal carbuncle.

3. Perinephric abscess. The abscesses in the kidney may extend through the capsule of the kidney into the perinephric tissue and form perinephric abscess.

Chronic Pyelonephritis

Chronic pyelonephritis is a chronic tubulointerstitial disease resulting from repeated attacks of inflammation and scarring.

ETIOPATHOGENESIS. Depending upon the etiology and pathogenesis, two types of chronic pyelonephritis are described—reflux nephropathy and obstructive pyelonephritis.

1. Reflux nephropathy. Reflux of urine from the bladder into one or both the ureters during micturition is the major cause of chronic pyelonephritis. *Vesicoureteric reflux* is particularly common in children, especially in girls, due to congenital absence or shortening of the intravesical portion of the ureter so that ureter is not compressed during the act of micturition. Reflux results in increase in pressure in the renal pelvis so that the urine is forced into renal tubules which is eventually followed by damage to the kidney and scar formation (Fig. 20.18). Vesicoureteric reflux is more common in patients with urinary tract infection, whether symptomatic or asymptomatic, but reflux of sterile urine can also cause renal damage.

2. Obstructive pyelonephritis. Obstruction to the outflow of urine at different levels predisposes the kidney to infection (page 714). Recurrent episodes of such obstruction and infection result in renal damage and scarring. Rarely, recurrent attacks of acute pyelonephritis may cause renal damage and scarring.

The two major mechanisms of chronic pyelonephritis are diagrammatically illustrated in Fig. 20.19.

PATHOLOGIC CHANGES. Grossly, the kidneys show rather characteristic appearance. The kidneys are usually small and contracted (weighing less than 100 gm) showing unequal reduction so as to distinguish it from other forms of contracted kidney. The surface of the kidney is irregularly scarred; the capsule can be stripped off with difficulty due to adherence to scars. These scars are of variable size and show characteristic U-shaped depressions on the cortical surface. There is generally dilatation of pelvis and blunted calyces (Fig. 20.20).

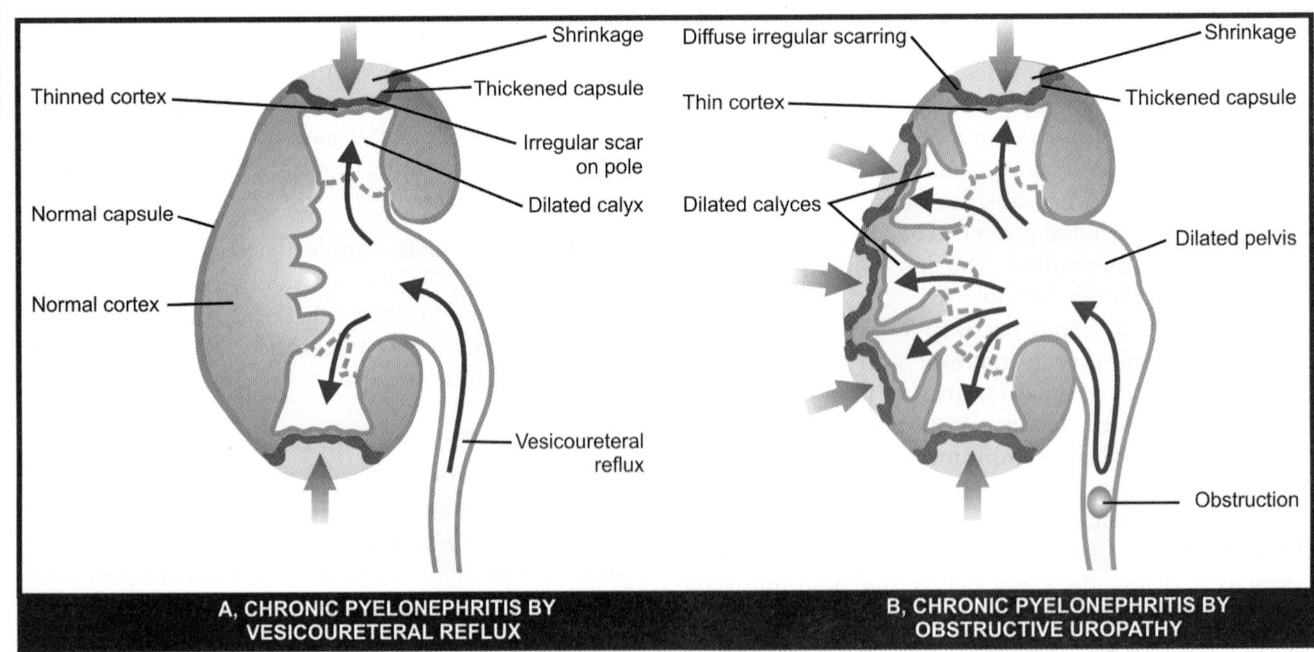

FIGURE 20.19

The two major types of chronic pyelonephritis. A, *Vesicoureteric reflux* causing infection of peripheral papillae and consequent scars at the poles of the kidney. B, *Obstructive pyelonephritis* due to obstruction of the urinary tract causing high pressure backflow of urine and infection of all the papillae and consequent diffuse scarring of the kidney and thinning of the cortex.

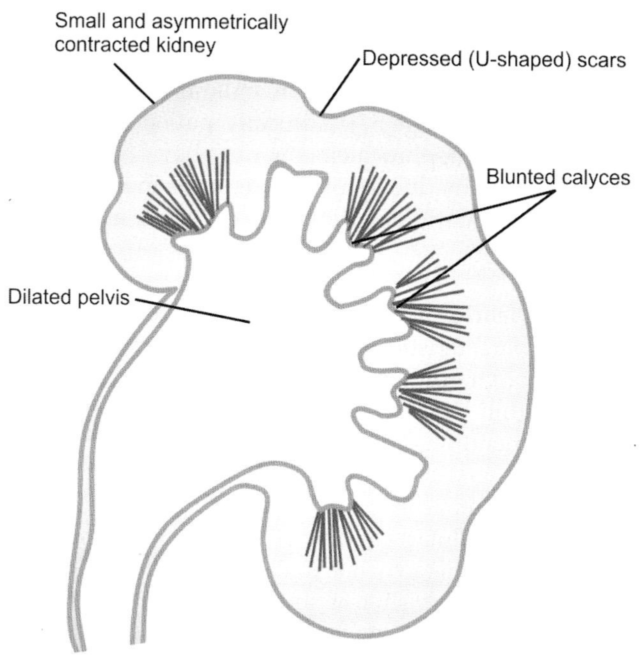

FIGURE 20.20

Chronic pyelonephritis, gross appearance. The kidney is asymmetrically small and contracted with characteristic U-shaped depressed scars on the cortical surface. There is dilatation of renal pelvis and blunted calyces.

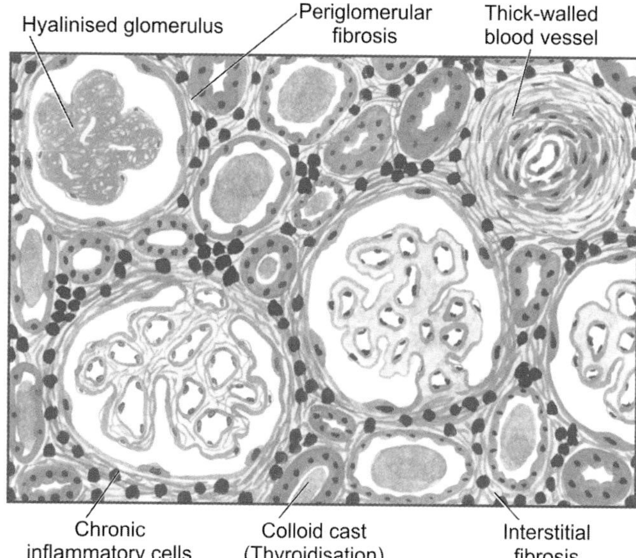

FIGURE 20.21

Chronic pyelonephritis, microscopic picture. The scarred area shows atrophy of some tubules and dilatation of others which contain colloid casts (thyroidisation). The tubules are surrounded by abundant fibrous tissue and chronic interstitial inflammatory reaction. The blood vessels included are thick-walled and the glomeruli show periglomerular fibrosis.

Microscopically, predominant changes are seen in interstitium and tubules (Fig. 20.21) (COLOUR PLATE XXVIII; CL 109):

i) Interstitium—There is chronic interstitial inflammatory reaction, chiefly composed of lymphocytes, plasma cells and macrophages with pronounced interstitial fibrosis. *Xanthogranulomatous pyelonephritis* is an uncommon variant characterised by collection of foamy macrophages admixed with other inflammatory cells and giant cells.

ii) Tubules—The tubules show varying degree of atrophy and dilatation. Dilated tubules may contain eosinophilic colloid casts producing thyroidisation of tubules. A few tubules may contain neutrophils.

iii) Pelvicalyceal system—The renal pelvis and calyces are dilated. The walls of pelvis and calyces show marked chronic inflammation and fibrosis. Lymphoid follicles with germinal centres may be present in the pelvicalyceal walls.

iv) Blood vessels—Blood vessels entrapped in the scarred areas show obliterative endarteritis. There may be changes of hypertensive hyaline arteriolosclerosis.

v) Glomeruli—Though glomerular tuft in the scarred area is usually intact, there is often periglomerular fibrosis. In advanced cases, there may be hyalinisation of glomeruli.

CLINICAL FEATURES. Chronic pyelonephritis often has an insidious onset. The patients present with clinical picture of chronic renal failure or with symptoms of hypertension. Sometimes, the patients may present with features of acute recurrent pyelonephritis with fever, loin pain, lumbar tenderness, dysuria, pyouria, bacteriuria and frequency of micturition. Diagnosis is made by intravenous pyelography (IVP). Culture of the urine may give positive results.

Tuberculous Pyelonephritis

Tuberculosis of the kidney occurs due to haematogenous spread of infection from another site, most often from the lungs. Less commonly, it may result from ascending infection from tuberculosis of the genitourinary system such as from epididymis or Fallopian tubes. The renal lesions in tuberculosis may be in the form of tuberculous pyelonephritis or appear as multiple miliary tubercles.

PATHOLOGIC CHANGES. Grossly, the lesions in tuberculous pyelonephritis are often bilateral, usually involving the medulla with replacement of the papillae by caseous tissue. Obstruction may result in tuberculous pyonephrosis in which thinned out renal parenchyma surrounds dilated pelvis and calyces filled with caseous material.

Histologically, typical granulomatous reaction is seen. Acid-fast bacilli can often be demonstrated in the lesions.

CLINICAL FEATURES. Most patients are young to middle-aged adults. The clinical presentation is extremely variable but it should always be considered as a possibility in a patient in whom there is persistent sterile pyouria, microscopic haematuria and mild proteinuria after effective antibiotic therapy for urinary tract infection. The diagnosis rests on identification of *M. tuberculosis* by repeated culture of urine on L.J. media.

Myeloma Nephropathy

Renal involvement in multiple myeloma (Chapter 14) is referred to as myeloma nephropathy or myeloma kidney. Functional renal impairment in multiple myeloma is a common manifestation, developing in about 50% of patients. The pathogenesis of myeloma kidney is related to excess filtration of Bence Jones proteins through the glomerulus, usually *kappa* (κ) light chains. These light chain proteins are precipitated in the distal convoluted tubules in combination with Tamm-Horsfall proteins, the urinary glycoproteins. The precipitates form tubular casts which are eosinophilic and often laminated. These casts may induce peritubular interstitial inflammatory reaction. Not all light chains are nephrotoxic and their toxicity occurs under acidic pH of the tubular fluid.

PATHOLOGIC CHANGES. Grossly, the kidneys may be normal or small and shrunken.

Histologically, there are some areas of tubular atrophy while many other tubular lumina are dilated and contain characteristic bright pink laminated casts. These casts are surrounded by peritubular interstitial inflammatory reaction including the presence of nonspecific inflammatory cells and some multinucleate giant cells induced by tubular casts.

Nephrocalcinosis

Nephrocalcinosis is a diffuse deposition of calcium salts in renal tissue in a number of renal diseases, in hypercalcaemia, hyperphosphataemia and renal tubular acidosis. Most commonly, it develops as a complication of severe hypercalcaemia such as due to hyperparathyroidism, hypervitaminosis D, excessive bone destruction in metastatic malignancy, hyperthyroidism, excessive calcium intake such as in milk-alkali syndrome and sarcoidosis (page 57). Clinically, patients of hypercalcaemia and nephrocalcinosis may have renal colic, band keratopathy due to calcium deposits in the cornea, visceral metastatic calcification, polyuria and renal failure.

Pathologically, nephrocalcinosis due to hypercalcaemia characteristically shows deposition of calcium in the tubular epithelial cells in the basement membrane, within the mitochondria and the cytoplasm. These concretions may produce secondary tubular atrophy, interstitial fibrosis and nonspecific chronic inflammation in the interstitium. As the calcification occurs intracellularly, radiological evidence is usually not present until fairly late in the disease. The calcium deposits are first visible as small opacities in the renal papillae.

RENAL VASCULAR DISEASES

Renal blood vessels which enormously perfuse the kidney are affected secondarily in majority of renal diseases. Renal blood flow is controlled by systemic and local haemodynamic, hormonal and intrinsic intrarenal mechanisms. Diseases which disturb these controlling mechanisms give rise to primary renal vascular lesions. These diseases are as under:

I. Most importantly, *hypertensive vascular disease* and its consequent renal manifestations in the form of benign and malignant nephrosclerosis.

II. *Thrombotic microangiopathy.*

III. *Renal cortical necrosis.*

IV. *Renal infarcts.*

Renal infarcts are already described in Chapter 5; other conditions are discussed here.

I. HYPERTENSIVE VASCULAR DISEASE

An elevated arterial blood pressure is a major health problem, particularly in developed countries. A persistent and sustained high blood pressure has damaging effects on the heart (e.g. hypertensive heart disease, Chapter 12), brain (e.g. cerebrovascular accident, Chapter 28) and kidneys (benign and malignant nephrosclerosis).

Definition and Classification

Arterial or systemic hypertension in a patient is defined clinically as *'borderline'* if the systolic blood pressure is more than 140 mm Hg, and diastolic pressure is above 90 mm Hg (currently labelled as *mild hypertension*), and *'hypertensive'* when the elevation of systolic and diastolic pressure exceeds 160 and 95 mm Hg respectively (now termed as *moderate hypertension*). The diastolic pressure is often considered more significant. However, blood pressure varies with many factors such as age of the patient, exercise, emotional disturbances like fear and anxiety. Therefore, it is important to measure blood pressure at least twice during two separate examinations under least stressful conditions. A clinically useful classification of hypertension has been recently described by the Joint National Committee of the WHO/International Society of Hypertension (Table 20.11). By means of these criteria, the prevalence of hypertension is observed in about 25% of population.

Hypertension is generally classified into 2 types:

1. Primary or essential hypertension in which the cause of increase in blood pressure is unknown. Essential hypertension constitutes about 90-95% patients of hypertension.

2. Secondary hypertension, in which the increase in blood pressure is caused by diseases of the kidneys, endocrines or some other organs. Secondary hypertension comprises 5-10% cases of hypertension.

According to the clinical course, both essential and secondary hypertension may be benign or malignant.

- **Benign hypertension** is moderate elevation of blood pressure and the rise is slow over the years. About 90-95% patients of hypertension have benign hypertension.
- **Malignant hypertension** is marked and rapid increase of blood pressure to 200/140 mm Hg or more and the patients have papilloedema, retinal haemorrhages and hypertensive encephalopathy. Less than 5% of hypertensive patients develop malignant hypertension and life expectancy after diagnosis in these patients is generally less than 2 years if not treated effectively.

Etiology and Pathogenesis

The etiology and pathogenesis of secondary hypertension that comprises less than 10% cases has been better understood, whereas the mechanism of essential hypertension that constitutes about 90% of cases remains largely obscure. In general, normal blood pressure is regulated by 2 haemodynamic forces—*cardiac output* and *total peripheral vascular resistance.* Factors which alter these two factors result in hypertension. The role of kidney in hypertension, particularly in secondary hypertension, by elaboration of renin and subsequent formation of angiotensin II, is well established (renin-angiotensin system).

With this background knowledge, we next turn to the mechanisms involved in the two forms of hypertension (Table 20.12).

ESSENTIAL (PRIMARY) HYPERTENSION. By definition, the cause of essential hypertension is unknown but a number of factors are related to its development. These are as under:

1. Genetic factors. The role of heredity in the etiology of essential hypertension has long been suspected. The evidences in support are the familial aggregation, occurrence of hypertension in twins, epidemiologic data, experimental animal studies and identification of hypertension susceptibility gene (angiotensinogen gene).

2. Racial and environmental factors. Surveys in the US have revealed higher incidence of essential hypertension in blacks than in whites. A number of environ-

TABLE 20.11: Clinical Classification of Hypertension.*

CATEGORY	SYSTOLIC (mm Hg)	DIASTOLIC (mm Hg)
Normal	< 130	< 85
High normal	130-139	85-89
Hypertension		
mild (stage 1)	140-159	90-99
moderate (stage 2)	160-179	100-109
severe (stage 3)	180-209	110-119
very severe (stage 4)	≥ 210	≥ 120
Malignant hypertension	> 200	≥ 140

*WHO/International Society of Hypertension (ISH) Special Report, 1995.

TABLE 20.12: Etiologic Classification of Hypertension.

A. ESSENTIAL HYPERTENSION (90%)

1. Genetic factors
2. Racial and environmental factors
3. Risk factors modifying the course

B. SECONDARY HYPERTENSION (10%)

1. *Renal*
   - i) Renovascular
   - ii) Renal parenchymal diseases
2. *Endocrine*
   - i) Adrenocortical hyperfunction
   - ii) Hyperparathyroidism
   - iii) Oral contraceptives
3. *Coarctation of Aorta*
4. *Neurogenic*

mental factors have been implicated in the development of hypertension including salt intake, obesity, skilled occupation, higher living standards and patients in high stress.

3. Risk factors modifying the course of essential hypertension. There is sufficient evidence to show that the course of essential hypertension that begins in middle life is modified by a number of factors. These are as under:

i) Age. Younger the age at which hypertension is first noted but left untreated, lower the life expectancy.

ii) Sex. Females with hypertension appear to do better than males.

iii) Atherosclerosis. Accelerated atherosclerosis invariably accompanies essential hypertension. This could be due to contributory role of other independent factors like cigarette smoking, elevated serum cholesterol, glucose intolerance and obesity.

iv) Other risk factors. Other factors which alter the prognosis in hypertension include: smoking, excess of alcohol intake, diabetes mellitus, persistently high diastolic pressure above 115 mm Hg and evidence of end-organ damage (i.e. heart, eyes, kidney and nervous system).

The *pathogenetic mechanism* in essential hypertension is explained by many theories. These are:

1. *High plasma level of catecholamines.*
2. *Increase in blood volume* i.e. arterial overfilling (volume hypertension) and arteriolar constriction (vasoconstrictor hypertension).
3. *Increased cardiac output.*
4. *Low-renin essential hypertension* found in approximately 20% patients due to altered responsiveness to renin release.
5. *High renin essential hypertension* seen in about 15% cases due to decreased adrenal responsiveness to angiotensin II.

SECONDARY HYPERTENSION. Mechanisms underlying hypertension with identifiable cause have been studied more extensively. Based on the etiology, these are described under four headings: renal hypertension, endocrine hypertension, hypertension associated with coarctation of aorta and neurogenic causes.

1. RENAL HYPERTENSION. Hypertension produced by renal diseases is called renal hypertension. Renal hypertension is subdivided into 2 groups:

i) Renal vascular hypertension e.g. in occlusion of a major renal artery, pre-eclampsia, eclampsia, polyarteritis nodosa and fibromuscular dysplasia of renal artery.

ii) Renal parenchymal hypertension e.g. in various types of glomerulonephritis, pyelonephritis, interstitial nephritis, diabetic nephropathy, amyloidosis, polycystic kidney disease and renin-producing tumours.

In either case, renal hypertension can be produced by one of the 3 inter-related pathogenetic mechanisms:

- activation of renin-angiotensin system,
- sodium and water retention, and
- decreased release of vasodepressor materials.

a) Activation of renin-angiotensin system. Renin is a proteolytic enzyme produced and stored in the granules of the juxtaglomerular cells surrounding the afferent arterioles of glomerulus (page 673). The release of renin is stimulated by renal ischaemia, sympathetic nervous system stimulation, depressed sodium concentration, fluid depletion and decreased potassium intake. Released renin is transported through blood stream to the liver where it acts upon substrate angiotensinogen, an α_2-globulin synthesised in the liver, to form angiotensin I, a decapeptide. Angiotensin I is converted into angiotensin II, an octapeptide, by the action of convertase in the lungs. Angiotensin II is the most potent naturally-occurring vasoconstrictor substance and its pressor action is mainly attributed to peripheral arteriolar vasoconstriction. The other main effect of angiotensin II is to stimulate the adrenal cortex to secrete aldosterone that promotes reabsorption of sodium and water.

Thus, the renin-angiotensin system is concerned mainly with 3 functions:

i) Control of blood pressure by altering plasma concentration of angiotensin II and aldosterone.
ii) Regulation of sodium and water content.
iii) Regulation of potassium balance.

The renin-angiotensin mechanism is summarised in Fig. 20.22.

b) Sodium and water retention. Blood volume and cardiac output, both of which have a bearing on blood pressure, are regulated by blood levels of sodium which is significant for maintaining extracellular fluid volume. Blood concentration of sodium is regulated by 3 mechanisms:

i) *Release of aldosterone* from activation of renin-angiotensin system, as already explained.

ii) *Reduction in GFR* due to reduced blood flow as occurs in reduced renal mass or renal artery stenosis. This results in proximal tubular reabsorption of sodium.

iii) *Release of atriopeptin hormone* from atria of the heart in response to volume expansion. These peptides cause increased GFR and inhibit sodium reabsorption.

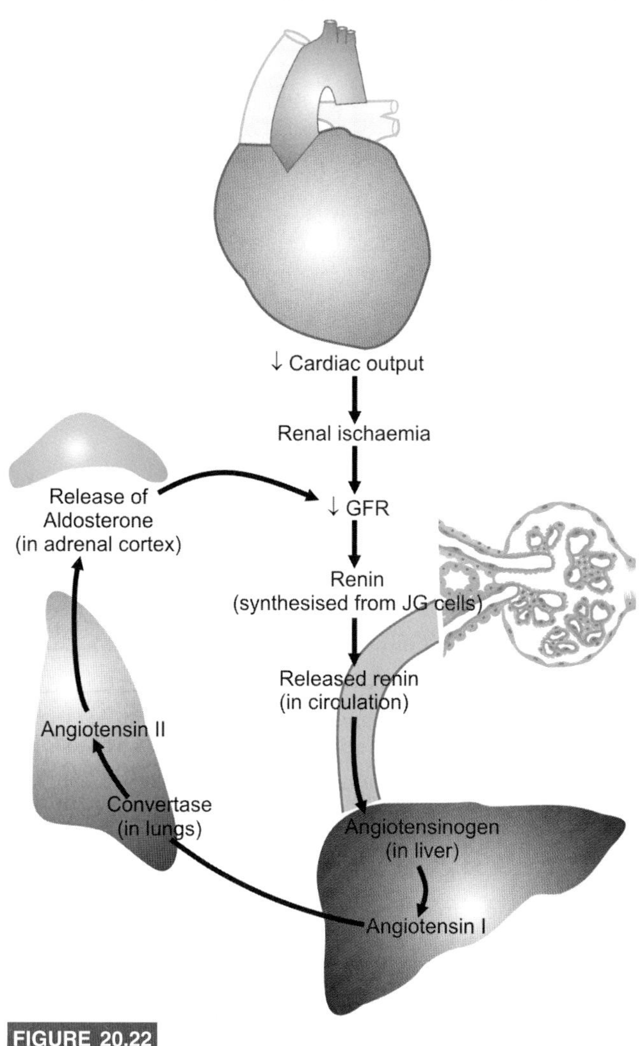

FIGURE 20.22

The renin-angiotensin mechanism.

c) **Release of vasodepressor material.** A number of vasodepressor materials and antihypertensives counterbalance the vasopressor effect of angiotensin II. These substances include: prostaglandins (PGE2, PGF2, PGA or medullin) released from interstitial cells of the medulla, urinary kallikrein-kinin system and platelet-activating factor.

2. *ENDOCRINE HYPERTENSION.* A number of hormonal secretions may produce secondary hypertension. These are:

i) *Adrenal gland*—e.g. in primary aldosteronism, Cushing's syndrome, adrenal virilism and pheochromocytoma.

ii) *Parathyroid gland*—e.g. hypercalcaemia in hyperparathyroidism.

iii) *Oral contraceptives*—Oestrogen component in the oral contraceptives stimulates hepatic synthesis of renin substrate.

3. *COARCTATION OF AORTA.* Coarctation of the aorta causes systolic hypertension in the upper part of the body due to constriction itself (Chapter 12). Diastolic hypertension results from changes in circulation.

4. *NEUROGENIC.* Psychogenic, polyneuritis, increased intracranial pressure and section of spinal cord are all uncommon causes of secondary hypertension.

EFFECTS OF HYPERTENSION

Systemic hypertension causes major effects in three main organs—heart and its blood vessels, nervous system, and kidneys. The renal effects in the form of benign and malignant nephrosclerosis are discussed below, whereas hypertensive effects on other organs are described elsewhere in the respective chapters.

Benign Nephrosclerosis

Benign nephrosclerosis is the term used to describe the kidney of benign phase of hypertension. Mild benign nephrosclerosis is the most common form of renal disease in persons over 60 years of age but its severity increases in the presence of hypertension and diabetes mellitus.

PATHOLOGIC CHANGES. ***Grossly,*** both the kidneys are affected equally and are reduced in size and weight, often weighing about 100 gm or less. The capsule is often adherent to the cortical surface. The surface of the kidney is finely granular and shows V-shaped areas of scarring.* The cut surface shows firm kidney and narrowed cortex (Fig. 20.23,A).

Microscopically, there are primarily diffuse vascular changes which produce parenchymal changes secondarily as a result of ischaemia. The histologic changes are, thus, described as vascular and parenchymal (Fig. 20.23,B):

*The various acquired causes of *'small contracted kidney'* and their characteristic gross macroscopic appearance may be recollected here. These are: 1. Chronic GN (granular appearance); 2. Chronic pyelonephritis (U-shaped scars); and 3. Benign nephrosclerosis (V-shaped scars). Although granular, U- and V-shaped scars correspond to the respective macroscopic patterns, an easy way to remember is: *'granular'* for *g*lomerular scars of chronic GN; *'U-scars'* for *u*neven scars of chronic pyelonephritis; and *'V-scars'* for *v*ascular scars of benign nephrosclerosis. Less common causes are: amyloidosis of the kidney, myeloma kidney and diabetic nephropathy.

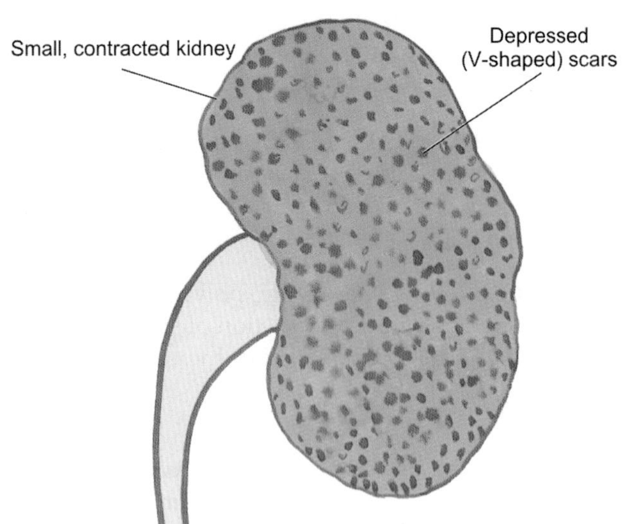

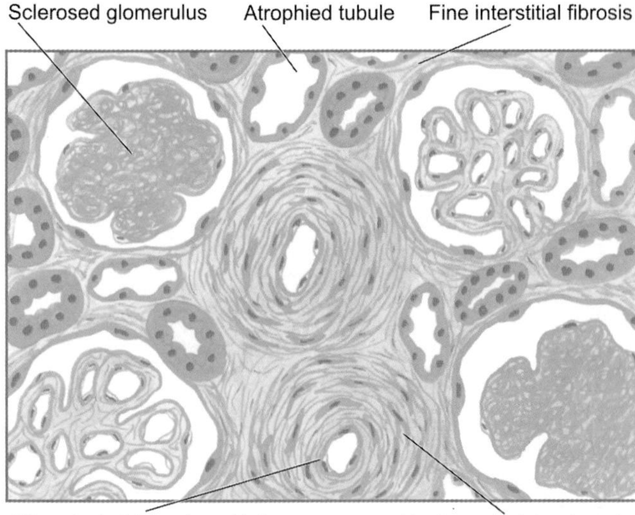

A, SMALL CONTRACTED KIDNEY   B, BENIGN NEPHROSCLEROSIS

FIGURE 20.23

Benign nephrosclerosis. A, Gross appearance, showing characteristic *'small contracted kidney'* with depressed V-shaped scars. B, Microscopic appearance. The vascular changes are hyaline arteriolosclerosis and intimal thickening of small blood vessels in the glomerular tuft. The parenchymal changes include sclerosed glomeruli, tubular atrophy and fine interstitial fibrosis.

i) Vascular changes: Changes in blood vessels involve arterioles and arteries up to the size of arcuate arteries. There are 2 types of changes in these blood vessels:

a) *Hyaline arteriolosclerosis* that results in homogeneous and eosinophilic thickening of the wall of small blood vessels.

b) *Intimal thickening* due to proliferation of smooth muscle cells in the intima.

ii) Parenchymal changes: As a consequence of ischaemia, there is variable degree of atrophy of parenchyma. This includes: glomerular shrinkage, deposition of collagen in Bowman's space, periglomerular fibrosis, tubular atrophy and fine interstitial fibrosis.

CLINICAL FEATURES. There is variable elevation of the blood pressure with headache, dizziness, palpitation and nervousness. Eye ground changes may be found but papilloedema is absent. Renal function tests and urine examination are normal in early stage. But in long-standing cases, there may be mild proteinuria with some hyaline or granular casts. Rarely, renal failure and uraemia may occur.

Malignant Nephrosclerosis

Malignant nephrosclerosis is the form of renal disease that occurs in malignant or accelerated hypertension. Malignant nephrosclerosis is uncommon and usually occurs as a superimposed complication in 5% cases of pre-existing benign essential hypertension or in those having secondary hypertension with identifiable cause such as in chronic renal diseases. However, the pure form of disease also occurs, particularly at younger age with preponderance in males.

PATHOLOGIC CHANGES. Grossly, the appearance of the kidney varies. In a case of malignant hypertension superimposed on pre-existing benign nephrosclerosis, the kidneys are small in size, shrunken and reduced in weight and have finely granular surface. However, the kidneys of a patient who develops malignant hypertension in pure form are enlarged, oedematous and have petechial haemorrhages on the surface producing so called *'flea-bitten kidney'*.* Cut

*Recall the other causes of *flea-bitten kidney:* acute post-streptococcal GN, rapidly progressive GN, haemolytic-uraemic syndrome, thrombotic thrombocytopenic purpura and Henoch-Schonlein purpura.

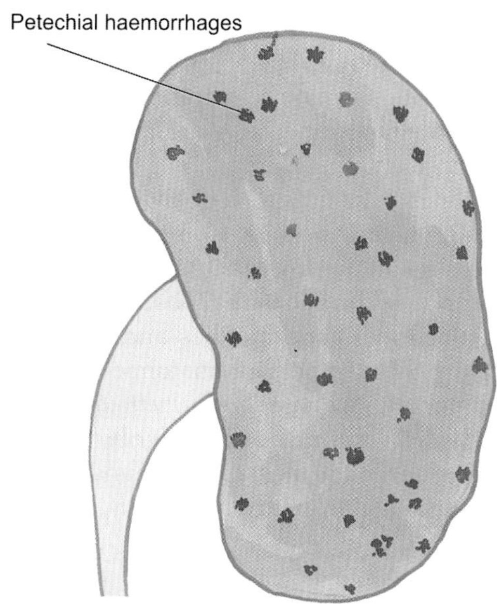

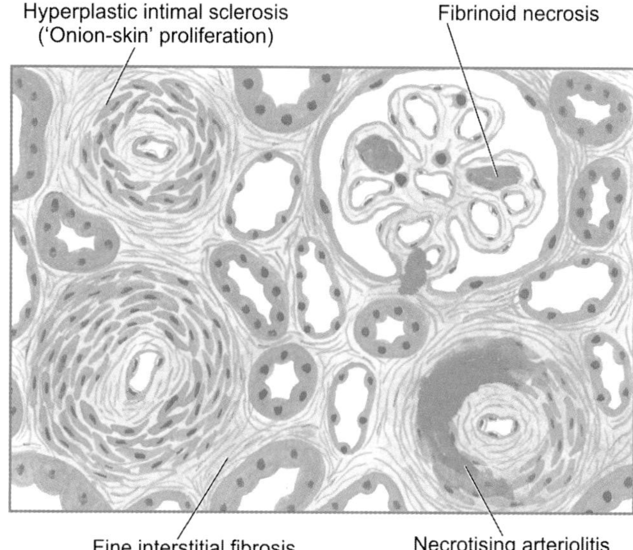

A, FLEA-BITTEN KIDNEY   B, MALIGNANT NEPHROSCLEROSIS

FIGURE 20.24

Malignant nephrosclerosis. A, Gross appearance, showing characteristic *'flea bitten kidney'* due to tiny petechial haemorrhages on the surface. B, Microscopic appearance. The vascular changes are necrotising arteriolitis and hyperplastic intimal sclerosis or onionskin proliferation. The parenchymal changes are tubular loss, fine interstitial fibrosis and foci of infarction necrosis.

surface shows red and yellow mottled appearance (Fig. 20.24,A).

Microscopically, most commonly the changes are superimposed on benign nephrosclerosis. These changes are as under (Fig. 20.24,B):

i) Vascular changes: These are more severe and involve the arterioles. The two characteristic vascular changes seen are as under:

a) *Necrotising arteriolitis* develops on hyaline arteriolosclerosis. The vessel wall shows fibrinoid necrosis, a few acute inflammatory cells and small haemorrhages.

b) *Hyperplastic intimal sclerosis* or *onionskin proliferation* is characterised by concentric laminae of proliferated smooth muscle cells, collagen and basement membranes.

ii) Ischaemic changes: The effects of vascular narrowing on the parenchyma include tubular loss, fine interstitial fibrosis and foci of infarction necrosis.

CLINICAL FEATURES. The patients of malignant nephrosclerosis have malignant or accelerated hypertension with blood pressure of 200/140 mm Hg or higher. Headache, dizziness and impaired vision are commonly found. The presence of papilloedema distinguishes malignant from benign phase of hypertension. The urine frequently shows haematuria and proteinuria. Renal function tests show deterioration during the course of the illness. Azotaemia (high BUN and serum creatinine) and uraemia develop soon if malignant hypertension is not treated aggressively. Approximately 90% of patients die within one year from causes such as uraemia, congestive heart failure and cerebrovascular accidents.

II. THROMBOTIC MICROANGIOPATHY

Thrombotic renal disease encompasses a group of diseases having in common the formation of thrombi composed by platelets and fibrin in arterioles and glomeruli of the kidney and culminating clinically in acute renal failure. Causes of thrombotic microangiopathy of renal microvasculature are listed in Table 20.13.

The common clinical manifestations include microangiopathic haemolytic anaemia, thrombocytopenia, DIC, and eventually renal failure.

PATHOGENESIS In all such cases, endothelial injury appears to be the trigger for vascular changes. The injured endothelial surface causes the following effects:

TABLE 20.13: Causes of Thrombotic Microangiopathy.

1. Infections
   (*E.coli, Shigella, Pseudomonas)*
2. Drugs
   (e.g. mitomycin, cisplatin, cyclosporine)
3. Autoimmune disease
   (scleroderma, SLE)
4. Thrombotic thrombocytopenic purpura
5. Haemolytic-uraemic syndrome
6. Pregnancy and pre-eclampsia
7. Malignant hypertension

- Passage of plasma constituents to the subendothelial zone of microvasculature.
- Promotes thrombosis.

Morphologically, the lesions closely resemble those of malignant nephrosclerosis. The features include:

- Fibrinoid necrosis of arterioles.
- Thrombi in renal microvasculature.
- Oedema of intima of arterioles.
- Consolidation, necrosis and congestion of glomeruli.

If the renal lesions are massive, the prognosis is generally lethal.

III. RENAL CORTICAL NECROSIS

Renal cortical necrosis is infarction of renal cortex varying from microscopic foci to a situation where most of the renal cortex is destroyed. The medulla, the juxtamedullary cortex and a rim of cortex under the capsule are usually spared. The condition develops most commonly as an obstetrical emergency (e.g. in eclampsia, pre-eclampsia, premature separation of the placenta). Other causes include septic shock, poisoning, severe trauma etc.

The lesions may be present focally, patchily or diffusely. The gross and microscopic characteristics of infarcts of cortex are present. Patients present with sudden oliguria or anuria and haematuria. If the process has involved renal cortex extensively, acute renal failure and uraemia develop and prognosis is grave.

OBSTRUCTIVE UROPATHY

Obstruction in the urinary tract is common and important because it increases the susceptibility to infection and stone formation. Obstruction can occur at any age and in either sex. The cause of obstruction may lie at any level of the urinary tract—renal pelvis, ureters, urinary bladder and urethra. The obstruction at any of these anatomic locations may be intraluminal, intramural or extramural. Important causes are listed in Table 20.14 and illustrated in Fig. 20.25.

The obstruction may be unilateral or bilateral, partial or complete, sudden or insidious. Complete bilateral obstruction may result in irreversible renal failure, whereas long-standing chronic partial obstruction may cause various functional abnormalities and anatomic changes. There are three important anatomic sequelae of obstruction, namely: *hydronephrosis, hydroureter and hypertrophy of the bladder.* But before describing these conditions, an account of the most common and important cause of obstructive uropathy, *urolithiasis,* is given below.

UROLITHIASIS

Urolithiasis or formation of urinary calculi at any level of the urinary tract is a common condition. Urinary calculi are worldwide in distribution but are particularly common in some geographic locales such as in parts of the United States, South Africa, India and South-East Asia. It is estimated that approximately 2% of the population experiences renal stone disease at sometime in their life with male-female ratio of 2:1. The peak incidence is observed in 2nd to 3rd decades of life. Renal calculi are characterised clinically by colicky pain *(renal colic)* as they pass down along the ureter and manifest by haematuria.

Types of Urinary Calculi

There are 4 main types of urinary calculi—calcium containing, mixed (struvite), uric acid and cystine stones, and a small number of rare types (Table 20.15).

1. CALCIUM STONES. Calcium stones are the most common comprising about 75% of all urinary calculi. They may be pure stones of calcium oxalate (50%) or calcium phosphate (5%), or mixture of calcium oxalate and calcium phosphate (45%).

Etiology. Etiology of calcium stones is variable.

i) About 50% of patients with calcium stones have *idiopathic hypercalciuria without hypercalcaemia.*

ii) Approximately 10% cases are associated with *hypercalcaemia* and *hypercalciuria,* most commonly due to hyperparathyroidism or a defect in the bowel (i.e. absorptive hypercalciuria) or in the kidney (i.e. renal hypercalciuria).

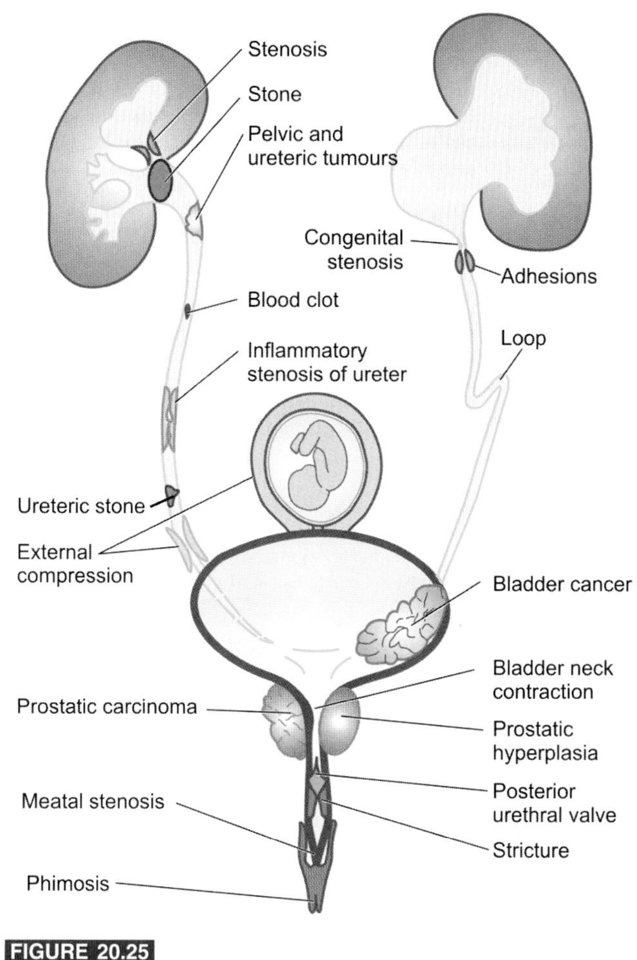

FIGURE 20.25

Causes of obstructive uropathy.

iii) About 15% of patients with calcium stones have *hyperuricosuria with a normal blood uric acid level* and without any abnormality of calcium metabolism.

iv) In about 25% of patients with calcium stones, the cause is unknown as there is no abnormality in urinary excretion of calcium, uric acid or oxalate and is referred to as *'idiopathic calcium stone disease'*.

Pathogenesis. The mechanism of calcium stone formation is explained on the basis of imbalance between the degree of supersaturation of the ions forming the stone and the concentration of inhibitors in the urine. Most likely site where the crystals of calcium oxalate and/or calcium phosphate are precipitated is the tubular lining or around some fragment of debris in the tubule acting as nidus of the stone. The stone grows, as more and more crystals are deposited around the nidus. A number of other predisposing factors contributing to formation of calcium stones are alkaline urinary pH, decreased urinary volume and increased excretion of oxalate and uric acid.

TABLE 20.14: Causes of Obstructive Uropathy.

A. Intraluminal

1. Calculi
2. Tumours (e.g. cancer of kidney and bladder)
3. Sloughed renal papilla
4. Blood clots
5. Foreign body

B. Intramural

1. Pelvi-ureteric junction (PUJ) obstruction
2. Vesicoureteric obstruction
3. Urethral stricture
4. Urethral valves
5. Inflammation (e.g. phimosis, cystitis etc)
6. Neuromuscular dysfunction

C. Extramural

1. Pregnant uterus
2. Retroperitoneal fibrosis
3. Tumours (e.g. carcinoma of cervix, rectum, colon, caecum etc)
4. Prostatic enlargement, prostatic carcinoma and prostatitis
5. Trauma

Morphology. Calcium stones are usually small (less than a centimeter), ovoid, hard, with granular rough surface. They are dark brown due to old blood pigment deposited in them as a result of repeated trauma caused to the urinary tract by these sharp-edged stones.

2. MIXED (STRUVITE) STONES. About 15% of urinary calculi are made of magnesium-ammonium-calcium phosphate, often called *struvite.* That is why mixed stones are also called as *'struvite stones'* or 'triple phosphate stones'.

Etiology. Struvite stones are formed as a result of infection of the urinary tract with urea-splitting organisms that produce urease such as by species of *Proteus,* and occasionally *Klebsiella, Pseudomonas* and *Enterobacter.* These are, therefore, also known as infection-induced stones. However, *E. coli* does not form urease.

Morphology. Struvite stones are yellow-white or grey. They tend to be soft and friable and irregular in shape. 'Staghorn stone' which is a large, solitary stone that takes the shape of the renal pelvis where it is often formed is an example of struvite stone.

3. URIC ACID STONES. Approximately 6% of urinary calculi are made of uric acid. Uric acid calculi are radiolucent unlike radio-opaque calcium stones.

Etiology. Uric acid stones are frequently formed in cases with hyperuricaemia and hyperuricosuria such as due

TABLE 20.15: Salient Features of Urinary Calculi.

TYPE	INCIDENCE	ETIOLOGY	PATHOGENESIS
1. *Calcium stones*	75%	Hypercalciuria with or without hypercalcaemia; idiopathic	Supersaturation of ions in urine, alkaline pH of urine; low urinary volume, oxaluria and hyperuricosuria
2. *Mixed (struvite) stones*	15%	Urinary infection with urea-splitting organisms like *Proteus*	Alkaline urinary pH produced by ammonia from splitting of urea by bacterially produced urease
3. *Uric acid stones*	6%	Hyperuricosuria with or without hyperuricaemia (e.g. in primary and secondary gout)	Acidic urine (pH below 6) decreases the solubility of uric acid in urine and favours its precipitation
4. *Cystine stones*	2%	Genetically-determined defect in cystine transport	Cystinuria containing least soluble cystine precipitates as cystine crystals
5. *Other types*	< 2%	Inherited abnormalities of amino acid metabolism	Xanthinuria

to primary gout or secondary gout due to myeloproliferative disorders (e.g. in leukaemias), especially those on chemotherapy, and administration of uricosuric drugs (e.g. salicylates, probenacid). Other factors contributing to their formation are acidic urinary pH (below 6) and low urinary volume.

Pathogenesis. The solubility of uric acid at pH of 7 is 200 mg/dl while at pH of 5 is 15 mg/dl. Thus, as the urine becomes more acidic, the solubility of uric acid in urine decreases and precipitation of uric acid crystals increases favouring the formation of uric acid stones. Hyperuricosuria is the most important factor in the production of uric acid stones, while hyperuricaemia is found in about half the cases.

Morphology. Uric acid stones are smooth, yellowish-brown, hard and often multiple. On cut section, they show laminated structure.

4. CYSTINE STONES. Cystine stones comprise less than 2% of urinary calculi.

Etiology. Cystine stones are associated with cystinuria due to a genetically-determined defect in the transport of cystine and other amino acids across the cell membrane of the renal tubules and the small intestinal mucosa.

Pathogenesis. The resultant excessive excretion of cystine which is least soluble of the naturally-occurring amino acids leads to formation of crystals and eventually cystine calculi.

Morphology. Cystine stones are small, rounded, smooth and often multiple. They are yellowish and waxy.

5. OTHER CALCULI. Less than 2% of urinary calculi consist of other rare types such as due to inherited abnormality of xanthine metabolism resulting in xanthinuria and consequently xanthine stones.

Table 20.15 summarises the salient features of various types of urinary calculi.

HYDRONEPHROSIS

Hydronephrosis is the term used for dilatation of renal pelvis and calyces due to partial or intermittent obstruction to the outflow of urine (Fig. 20.25). Hydronephrosis develops if one or both the pelviureteric sphincters are incompetent, as otherwise there will be dilatation and hypertrophy of the urinary bladder but no hydronephrosis. Hydroureter nearly always accompanies hydronephrosis. Hydronephrosis may be *unilateral or bilateral.*

Unilateral Hydronephrosis

This occurs due to some form of ureteral obstruction at the level of pelviureteric junction (PUJ). The causes are:

1. **Intraluminal** e.g. a calculus in the ureter or renal pelvis.

2. **Intramural** e.g. congenital PUJ obstruction, atresia of ureter, inflammatory stricture, trauma, neoplasm of ureter or bladder.

3. **Extramural** e.g. obstruction of upper part of ureter by inferior renal artery or vein, pressure on ureter from outside such as carcinoma cervix, prostate, rectum, colon or caecum and retroperitoneal fibrosis.

Bilateral Hydronephrosis

This is generally the result of some form of urethral obstruction but can occur from the various causes listed above if the lesions involve both sides. The causes are:

TABLE 20.15: Urinary Calculi (continued)

MORPHOLOGY

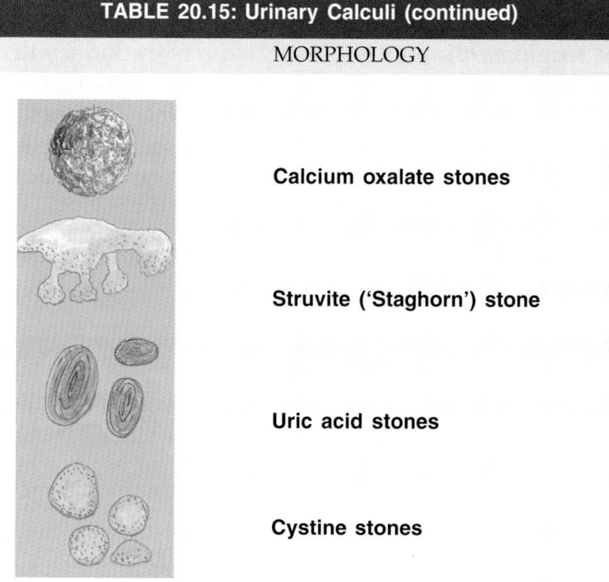

Figure facing Table 20.15

1. **Congenital** e.g. atresia of the urethral meatus, congenital posterior urethral valve.

2. **Acquired** e.g. bladder tumour involving both ureteric orifices, prostatic enlargement, prostatic carcinoma and prostatitis, bladder neck stenosis, inflammatory or traumatic urethral stricture and phimosis.

PATHOLOGIC CHANGES. The pathologic changes vary depending upon whether the obstruction is sudden and complete, or incomplete and intermittent. The latter situation is more common.

Grossly, the kidneys may have moderate to marked enlargement. Initially, there is *extrarenal hydronephrosis* characterised by dilatation of renal pelvis medially in the form of a sac (Fig. 20.26,A). As the obstruction persists, there is progressive dilatation of pelvis and calyces and pressure atrophy of renal parenchyma. Eventually, the dilated pelvi-calyceal system extends deep into the renal cortex so that a thin rim of renal cortex is stretched over the dilated calyces and the external surface assumes lobulated appearance. This advanced stage is called as *intrarenal hydronephrosis* (Fig. 20.26,B). An important point of distinction between the sectioned surface of advanced hydronephrosis and polycystic kidney disease (page 680) is the direct continuity of dilated cystic spaces (i.e. dilated calyces) with the renal pelvis in the former.

Microscopically, the wall of hydronephrotic sac is thickened due to fibrous scarring and chronic inflammatory cell infiltrate. There is progressive atrophy of tubules and glomeruli alongwith interstitial fibrosis. Stasis of urine in hydronephrosis causes infection *(pyelitis)* resulting in filling of the sac with pus, a condition called *pyonephrosis.*

TUMOURS OF KIDNEY

Both benign and malignant tumours occur in the kidney, the latter being more common. These may arise from *renal tubules* (adenoma, adenocarcinoma), *embryonic tissue* (mesoblastic nephroma, Wilms' tumour), *mesenchymal tissue* (angiomyolipoma, medullary interstitial tumour) and from the *epithelium of the renal pelvis* (urothelial carcinoma). Besides these tumours, the kidney may be the site of the secondary tumours.

Table 20.16 provides a list of kidney tumours; the important forms of renal neoplasms are described below.

BENIGN TUMOURS

Benign renal tumours are usually small and are often an incidental finding at autopsy or nephrectomy.

Cortical Adenoma

Cortical tubular adenomas are more common than other benign renal neoplasms. They are frequently multiple and associated with chronic pyelonephritis or benign nephrosclerosis.

Grossly, these tumours may form tiny nodules up to 3 cm in diameter. They are encapsulated and white or yellow.

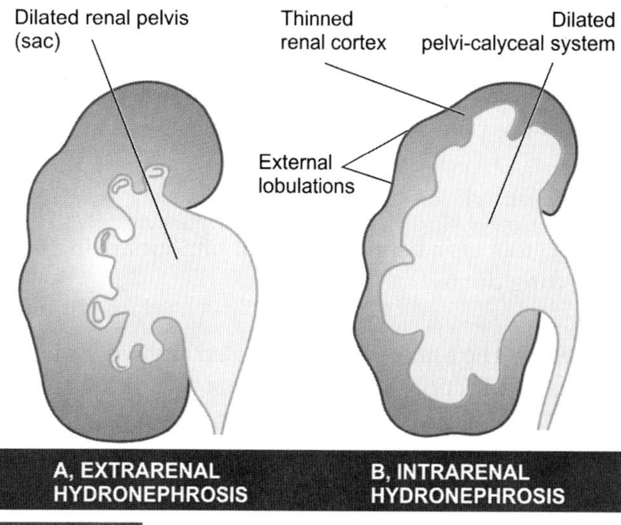

FIGURE 20.26

Hydronephrosis, stages in its evolution.

TABLE 20.16: Classification of Kidney Tumours.

BENIGN	MALIGNANT
A. EPITHELIAL TUMOURS OF RENAL PARENCHYMA	
Adenoma	Adenocarcinoma
Oncocytoma	(hypernephroma, renal cell carcinoma)
B. EPITHELIAL TUMOURS OF RENAL PELVIS	
Transitional cell papilloma	Transitional cell carcinoma
	Others (squamous cell carcinoma, adenocarcinoma of renal pelvis, undifferentiated carcinoma of renal pelvis)
C. EMBRYONAL TUMOURS	
Mesoblastic nephroma	Wilms' tumour (nephroblastoma)
Multicystic nephroma	
D. NON-EPITHELIAL TUMOURS	
Angiomyolipoma	Sarcomas (rare)
Medullary interstitial tumour (fibroma)	
E. MISCELLANEOUS	
Juxtaglomerular cell tumour (Reninoma)	
F. METASTATIC TUMOURS	

Microscopically, they are composed of tubular cords or papillary structures projecting into cystic space. The cells of the adenoma are usually uniform, cuboidal with no atypicality or mitosis. However, size of the tumour rather than histologic criteria is considered more significant parameter to predict the behaviour of the tumour—those larger than 3 cm in diameter are potentially malignant and metastasising.

Oncocytoma

Oncocytoma is a benign epithelial tumour arising from collecting ducts.

Grossly, The tumour is encapsulated and has variable size. Cut section is homogeneous and has characteristic mahogany-brown or tan colour.

Microscopically, the tumour cells are plump with abundant, finely granular, acidophilic cytoplasm and round nuclei. Electron microscopy demonstrates numerous mitochondria in the cytoplasm.

Other Benign Tumours

- **Angiomyolipoma** is a hamartoma of the kidney that contains differentiated tissue element derived from blood vessels, smooth muscle and fat. Patients of tuberous sclerosis, a multisystem disease characterised by skin lesions, CNS and renal involvement, frequently have bilateral angiomyolipomas.

- **Mesoblastic nephroma** is a congenital benign tumour.

Grossly, the tumour resembles a uterine leiomyoma in having whorled appearance.
Microscopically, it shows cellular growth of spindle cells derived from secondary mesenchyme.

- **Multicystic nephroma** is another uncommon tumour of early infancy.

Grossly, it is a solitary, unilateral well demarcated tumour of varying size. Cut surface shows characteristic multilocular appearance.
Microscopically, the cysts are lined by tubular epithelium while the stroma between the cysts contains mesenchymal tissue with some immature blastemal or abortive tubules. Some authors consider this entity as fully-differentiated variant of Wilms' tumour. However, clinically multicystic nephroma is always benign compared to Wilms' tumour.

- **Medullary interstitial cell tumour** is a tiny nodule in the medulla composed of fibroblast-like cells in hyalinised stroma. These tumours used to be called *renal fibromas* but electron microscopy has revealed that the tumour cells are not fibrocytes but are medullary interstitial cells.

- **Juxtaglomerular tumour or reninoma** is a rare tumour of renal cortex consisting of sheets of epithelioid cells with many small blood vessels. The tumour secretes excessive quantities of renin and, thus, the patients are likely to have hypertension.

MALIGNANT TUMOURS

The two most common primary malignant tumours of the kidney are *adenocarcinoma* and *Wilms' tumour.* A third less common tumour is *urothelial carcinoma* of renal pelvis which is described in the next section alongwith similar tumours of the lower urinary tract.

Adenocarcinoma of Kidney *(Synonyms: Renal cell carcinoma, Hypernephroma, Grawitz tumour)*

Hypernephroma is an old misnomer under the mistaken belief that the tumour arises from adrenal rests because of the resemblance of the tumour cells with clear cells of the adrenal cortex. It is now known that the renal cell carcinoma (RCC) is an adenocarcinoma arising from tubular epithelium. This cancer comprises 70 to 80% of all renal cancers and occurs most commonly in 50 to 70 years of age with male preponderance (2:1).

ETIOLOGY AND PATHOGENESIS. Various etiologic factors implicated in the etiology of RCC are as follows:

1. **Tobacco.** Tobacco is the major risk factor for RCC, whether chewed or smoked. Cigarette smokers have 2-times higher risk of developing RCC.

2. **Additional risk factors.** These include:

i) Exposure to asbestos, heavy metals and petrochemical products.

ii) In women, obesity and oestrogen therapy.

iii) Hereditary and acquired cystic diseases of the kidney.

iv) Analgesic nephropathy.

v) Hereditary and family history are associated with 4-5 times higher risk.

vi) Hypertension.

Majority of cases of RCC are sporadic but about 5% cases are inherited in which *carcinogenesis* has been studied in detail. Carcinongenesis in RCC is explained on the basis of following:

1. *von Hippel-Lindau (VHL) disease:* It is an autosomal dominant cancer syndrome that includes: haemangioblastoma of the cerebellum, retinal angiomas, multiple RCC (clear cell type), pheochromocytoma and cysts in different organs. Patients of VHL disease have germline mutations of tumour suppressor *VHL* gene located on chromosome 3, commonly as homozygous loss of *VHL* gene.

2. *Hereditary clear cell RCC:* These are cases of clear cell type RCC confined to the kidney without other manifestations of VHL but having autosomal dominant inheritance.

3. *Papillary RCC:* This form of RCC is characterised by bilateral and multifocal cancer with papillary growth pattern. Genetic abnormality in these cases lies in *MET* gene located on chromosome 7.

4. *Chromophobe RCC*: These cases have genetic defects in the form of multiple losses of whole chromosomes i.e. they have extreme degree of hypodiploidy.

CLASSIFICATION. Based on cytogenetics of sporadic and familial tumours, RCC has been reclassified into clear cell, papillary, granular cell, chromophobe, sarcomatoid and collecting duct type (Table 20.17).

PATHOLOGIC CHANGES. Grossly, the RCC commonly arises from the poles of the kidney as a solitary and unilateral tumour, more often in the upper pole. The tumour is generally large, golden yellow and circumscribed. Papillary tumours may be multifocal and bilateral, besides grossly visible papillae. Cut section of the tumour commonly shows large areas of ischaemic necrosis, cystic change and foci of haemorrhages. Another significant characteristic is the frequent presence of tumour thrombus in the renal vein which may extend into the vena cava (Fig. 20.27,A).

Chapter Twenty

TABLE 20.17: Classification of Renal Cell Carcinoma

TYPE	INCIDENCE	GENETICS	MAIN HISTOLOGY
1. *Clear cell type (non-papillary)*	70%	Sporadic and familial (Homozygous loss of *VHL* gene located on chromosome 3)	Clear cytoplasm (due to glycogen and lipid), well differentiated
2. *Papillary type*	15%	Familial and sporadic (Familial cases: mutation in *MET* gene on chromosome 7; sporadic cases trisomy of chromosome 7, 16, 17 and loss of Y chromosome)	Papillary pattern, psammoma bodies
3. *Granular cell type*	8%	Sporadic and familial	Abundant acidophilic cytoplasm, marked atypia
4. *Chromophobe type*	5%	Multiple chromosome losses, hypodiploidy	Mixture of pale clear cells with perinuclear halo and granular cells
5. *Sarcomatoid type*	1.5%	—	Whorls of atypical anaplastic spindle cells
6. *Collecting duct type*	0.5%	—	Tubular and papillary pattern

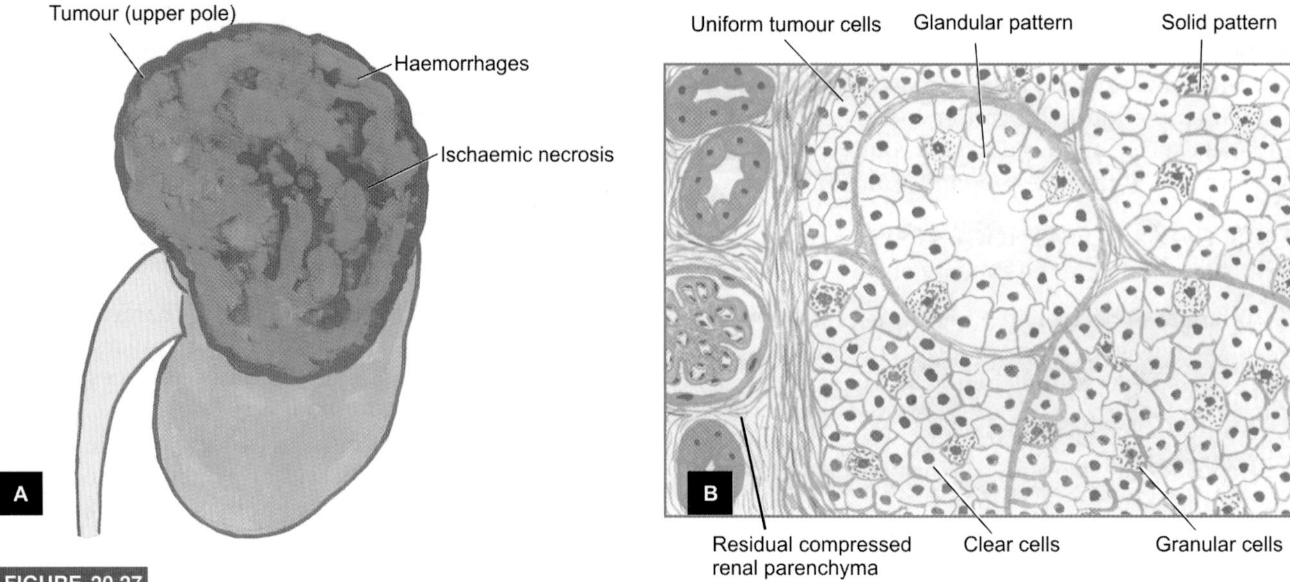

FIGURE 20.27

Renal cell carcinoma A, Grossly shows a large circumscribed tumour in the upper pole. The sectioned surface shows golden-yellow tumour with areas of ischaemic necrosis, cystic changes and haemorrhages. B, Microscopy shows solid masses and acini of uniform-appearing tumour cells. Clear cells predominate in the tumour and there are some granular cells. The stroma is composed of fine and delicate fibrous tissue.

Histologically, the features of various types of RCC are as under:

1. *Clear cell type RCC (70%):* This is the most common pattern. The clear cytoplasm of tumour cells is due to removal of glycogen and lipid from the cytoplasm during processing of tissues. The tumour cells have a variety of patterns: solid, trabecular and tubular, separated by delicate vasculature. Majority of clear cell tumours are well differentiated (Fig. 20.27,B) (COLOUR PLATE XXVIII: CL 110).
2. *Papillary type RCC (15%):* The tumour cells are arranged in papillary pattern over the fibrovascular stalks. The tumour cells are cuboidal with small round nuclei. Psammoma bodies may be seen.
3. *Granular cell type RCC (8%):* The tumour cells have abundant acidophilic cytoplasm. These tumours have more marked nuclear pleomorphism, hyperchromatism and cellular atypia.
4. *Chromophobe type RCC (5%):* This type shows admixture of pale clear cells with perinuclear halo and acidophilic granular cells. The cytoplasm of these tumour cells contains many vesicles.
5. *Sarcomatoid type RCC (1.5%):* This is the most anaplastic and poorly differentiated form. The tumour is characterised by whorls of atypical spindle tumour cells.
6. *Collecting duct type RCC (0.5%):* This is a rare type that occurs in the medulla. It is composed of a single layer of cuboidal tumour cells arranged in tubular and papillary pattern.

CLINICAL FEATURES. Renal cell carcinoma is generally a slow-growing tumour and the tumour may have been present for years before it is detected. The classical evidence for diagnosis of renal cell carcinoma is the triad of *gross haematuria, flank plain* and *palpable abdominal mass.* The most common presenting abnormality is haematuria that occurs in about 60% of cases. By the time the tumour is detected, it has spread to distant sites via haematogenous route to lungs, brain and bone, and locally to liver and perirenal lymph nodes.

Systemic symptoms of fatiguability, weight loss, cachexia and intermittent fever unassociated with evidence of infection are found in many cases at presentation. A number of paraneoplastic syndromes due to ectopic hormone production by the renal cell carcinoma have been described. These include *polycythaemia* (by erythropoietin), *hypercalcaemia* (by parathyroid hormone and prostaglandins), *hypertension* (by renin), effects of *feminisation* or *masculinisation* (by gonadotropins) and *Cushing's syndrome* (by glucocorticoids).

The **prognosis** in renal cell carcinoma depends upon the extent of tumour involvement at the time of diagnosis. The overall 5-year survival rate is about 45%. Presence of metastases lowers the survival rate.

Wilms' Tumour
(Synonym: Nephroblastoma)

Nephroblastoma or Wilms' tumour is an embryonic tumour derived from primitive renal epithelial and mesenchymal components. It is the most common abdominal malignant tumour of young children, seen most commonly between 1 to 6 years of age with equal sex incidence.

PATHOLOGIC CHANGES. ***Grossly,*** the tumour is usually quite large, spheroidal, replacing most of the kidney. It is generally solitary and unilateral but 5-10% cases may have bilateral tumour. On cut section, the tumour shows characteristic variegated appearance—soft, fishflesh-like grey-white to cream-yellow tumour with foci of necrosis and haemorrhages and grossly identifiable myxomatous or cartilaginous elements (Fig. 20.28,A). Invasion into renal vein is grossly evident in half the cases.
Microscopically, nephroblastoma shows mixture of primitive epithelial and mesenchymal elements. Most of the tumour consists of small, round to spindled, anaplastic, sarcomatoid tumour cells. In these areas are present abortive tubules and poorly-formed glomerular structures (Fig. 20.28,B). Sometimes, mesenchymal elements such as smooth and skeletal muscle, cartilage and bone, fat cells and fibrous tissue, may be seen (COLOUR PLATE XXVIII: CL 111).

CLINICAL FEATURES. The most common presenting feature is a palpable abdominal mass in a child. Other common abnormalities are haematuria, pain, fever and hypertension. The tumour rapidly spreads via blood, especially to lungs.

The **prognosis** of the tumour with combination therapy of nephrectomy, post-operative irradiation and chemotherapy, has improved considerably and the 5-year survival now is above 75%.

Secondary Tumours

Leukaemic infiltration of the kidneys is a common finding, particularly in chronic myeloid leukaemia. Kidney is a common site for blood-borne metastases from different primary sites, chiefly from cancers of lungs, breast and stomach.

LOWER URINARY TRACT

NORMAL STRUCTURE

The lower urinary tract consists of *ureters, urinary bladder* and *urethra.*

URETERS are tubular structures, 30 cm in length and half a centimeter in diameter, and extend from the renal

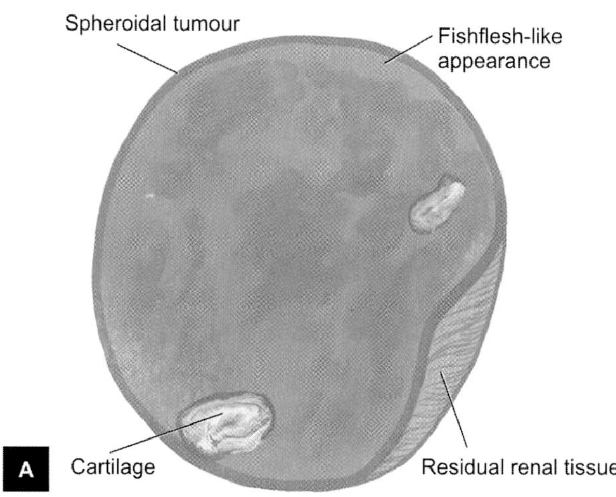

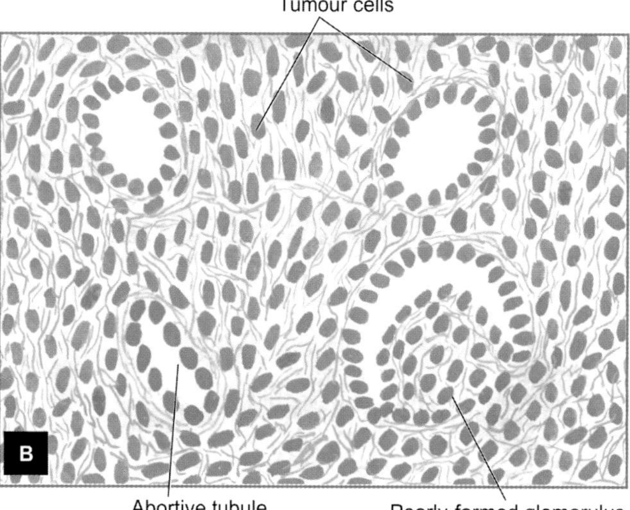

FIGURE 20.28

Nephroblastoma (Wilms' tumour). A, The tumour forms a large spherical mass replacing most of the kidney. The sectioned surface shows variegated appearance—fishflesh-like, grey-white tumour with some areas of necrosis and haemorrhages and some macroscopically evident mesenchymal elements. B, Microscopy shows predominance of small round to spindled sarcomatoid tumour cells. A few abortive tubules and poorly-formed glomerular structures are present in it.

pelvis (pelvi-ureteric junction) to the urinary bladder (vesico-ureteric junction). Normally they enter obliquely into the bladder, so that ureter is compressed during micturition, thus preventing vesico-ureteric reflux. Ureters lie retroperitoneally throughout their course.

Histologically, ureter has an outer fibrous investing layer which overlies a thick muscular layer and is lined internally by transitional epithelium or urothelium similar to the lining of the renal pelvis above and bladder below.

URINARY BLADDER lies extraperitoneally and the peritoneum is reflected on its superior surface. Normally, the capacity of bladder is about 400 to 500 ml without over-distension. Micturition is partly a reflex and partly a voluntary act under the control of sympathetic and parasympathetic innervation.

Histologically, the greater part of the bladder wall is made up of muscular layer (detrusor muscle) having 3 coats—internal, middle and external. The *trigone* muscle is derived from the prolongation of the longitudinal muscle layer of each ureter. The inner layer of bladder consists of urothelium up to 6 layers in thickness.

URETHRA runs from the bladder up to the external meatus. The *male urethra* consists of 3 parts—prostatic, membranous and penile. It is lined in the prostatic part by urothelium but elsewhere by stratified columnar epithelium except near its orifice where the epithelium is stratified squamous. The urethral mucosa rests on highly vascular submucosa and outer layer of striated muscle. There are numerous small mucous glands in the urethral mucosa. The *female urethra* is shorter and runs from the bladder parallel with the anterior wall of the vagina. The mucous membrane in female urethra is lined throughout by columnar epithelium except near the bladder where the epithelium is transitional. The other layers and mucous glands are similar to those in male urethra.

CONGENITAL ANOMALIES

Vesicoureteric reflex is the most common anomaly described already on page 706. A few others are considered below.

DOUBLE URETER. This is a condition in which the entire ureter or only the upper part is duplicated. Double ureter is invariably associated with a double renal pelvis, *one* in the upper part and the *other* in the lower part of the kidney. If double ureter affects the entire length, then there are two separate openings into the bladder on one side but more commonly they are joined in the intravesical portion and open by a single ureteric orifice.

URETEROCELE. Ureterocele is cystic dilatation of the terminal part of the ureter which lies within the bladder wall. The cystic dilatation lies beneath the bladder mucosa and can be visualised by cystoscopy.

ECTOPIA VESICAE (EXSTROPHY). This is a rare condition owing to congenital developmental deficiency of anterior wall of the bladder and is associated with splitting of the overlying anterior abdominal wall. This results in exposed interior of the bladder. There may be prolapse of the posterior wall of the bladder through the defect in the anterior bladder and abdominal wall. The condition in males is often associated with *epispadias* in which the urethra opens on the dorsal aspect of penis. If the defect is not properly repaired, the exposed bladder mucosa gets infected repeatedly and may undergo squamous metaplasia with increasing tendency to develop carcinoma of the bladder.

URACHAL ABNORMALITIES. Rarely, there may be persistence of urachus in which urine passes from the bladder to the umbilicus. More often, part of urachus remains patent which may be the umbilical end, bladder end, or central portion. Persistence of central portion gives rise to *urachal cyst* lined by transitional or squamous epithelium. Adenocarcinoma may develop in urachal cyst.

INFLAMMATIONS

Urinary tract infection (UTI) is common, especially in females and has been described already alongwith its morphologic consequences (page 706). Inflammation of the tissues of urinary tract (ureteritis, cystitis and urethritis) are considered here.

Ureteritis

Infection of the ureter is almost always secondary to pyelitis above, or cystitis below. Ureteritis is usually mild but repeated and longstanding infection may give rise to chronic ureteritis.

Cystitis

Inflammation of the urinary bladder is called cystitis. Primary cystitis is rare since the normal bladder epithelium is quite resistant to infection. Cystitis may occur by spread of infection from upper urinary tract as seen following renal tuberculosis, or may spread from the urethra such as in instrumentation. Cystitis is caused by a variety of bacterial and fungal infections as discussed in the etiology of pyelonephritis (page 706). The most common pathogenic organism in urinary tract infection is *E. coli*, followed in decreasing frequency by *Enterobacter, Klebsiella, Pseudomonas* and *Proteus*. Infection with *Candida albicans* may occur in the bladder in immunosuppressed patients. Besides bacterial and fungal organisms, parasitic infestations such as with *Schistosoma haematobium* is common in the Middle-East countries, particularly in Egypt. *Chlamydia* and *Mycoplasma* may occasionally cause cystitis. In addition, radiation, direct exposure to chemical irritant, foreign bodies and local trauma may all initiate cystitis.

Cystitis, like UTI, is more common in females than in males because of the shortness of urethra which is liable to faecal contamination and due to mechanical trauma during sexual intercourse. In males, prostatic obstruction is a frequent cause of cystitis. All forms of cystitis are clinically characterised by a *triad* of symptoms—*frequency* (repeated urination), *dysuria* (painful or burning micturition) and *low abdominal pain*. There may, however, be systemic manifestations of bacteraemia such as fever, chills and malaise.

PATHOLOGIC CHANGES. Cystitis may be acute or chronic.

ACUTE CYSTITIS. ***Grossly,*** the bladder mucosa is red, swollen and haemorrhagic. There may be suppurative exudate or ulcers on the bladder mucosa.

Microscopically, this form of cystitis is characterised by intense neutrophilic exudate admixed with lymphocytes and macrophages. There is oedema and congestion of mucosa.

CHRONIC CYSTITIS. Repeated attacks of acute cystitis lead to chronic cystitis.

Grossly, the mucosal epithelium is thickened, red and granular with formation of polypoid masses. Long-standing cases result in thickened bladder wall and shrunken cavity.

Microscopically, there is patchy ulceration of the mucosa with formation of granulation tissue in the regions of polypoid masses. Submucosa and muscular coat show fibrosis and infiltration by chronic inflammatory cells. A form of chronic cystitis characterised by formation of lymphoid follicles in the bladder mucosa is termed *cystitis follicularis*.

A few other special forms of cystitis having distinct clinical and morphological appearance are described below.

INTERSTITIAL CYSTITIS (HUNNER'S ULCER). This variant of cystitis occurs in middle-aged women. The patients get repeated attacks of severe and excruciating pain on distension of the bladder, frequency of micturition and great decrease in bladder capacity. Cystoscopy often reveals a localised ulcer. The *etiology* of the condition is unknown but it is thought to be neurogenic in origin.

Microscopically, the submucosa and muscle coat show increased fibrosis and chronic inflammatory infiltrate, chiefly lymphocytes, plasma cells and eosinophils.

CYSTITIS CYSTICA. As a result of long-standing chronic inflammation, there occurs a downward projection of epithelial nests known as *Brunn's nests* from the deeper layer of bladder mucosa. These epithelial cells may appear as small cystic inclusions in the bladder wall, or may actually develop columnar metaplasia with secretions in the lumen of cysts.

MALAKOPLAKIA. This is a rare condition most frequently found in the urinary bladder but can occur in the ureters, kidney, testis and prostate, and occasionally in the gut. The *etiology* of the condition is unknown but probably results from persistence of chronic inflammation with defective phagocytic process by the macrophages. Malakoplakia occurs more frequently in immunosuppressed patients and recipients of transplants.

Grossly, the lesions appear as soft, flat, yellowish, slightly raised plaques on the bladder mucosa. They may vary from 0.5 to 5 cm in diameter.

Microscopically, the plaques are composed of massive accumulation of foamy macrophages with occasional multinucleate giant cells and some lymphocytes. These macrophages have granular PAS-positive cytoplasm and some of them contain cytoplasmic laminated concretions of calcium phosphate called *Michaelis-Gutmann bodies*. These bodies ultrastructurally represent lysosomes filled with partly digested debris of bacteria phagocytosed by macrophages which have not been digested fully by them due to defective phagocytosis.

POLYPOID CYSTITIS. Polypoid cystitis is characterised by papillary projections on the bladder mucosa due to submucosal oedema and can be confused with transitional cell carcinoma. The condition occurs due to indwelling catheters and infection.

Urethritis

Urethritis may be *gonococcal* or *non-gonococcal*.

■ **Gonococcal (gonorrhoeal) urethritis** is an acute suppurative condition caused by gonococci *(Neisseria gonorrhoeae)*. The mucosa and submucosa are eventually converted into granulation tissue which becomes fibrosed and scarred resulting in urethral stricture.

■ **Non-gonococcal urethritis** is more common and is most frequently caused by *E. coli*. The infection of urethra often accompanies cystitis in females and prostatitis in males. Urethritis is one of the components in the triad of Reiter's syndrome which comprises arthritis, conjunctivitis and urethritis (Chapter 4). The pathologic changes are similar to inflammation of the lower urinary tract elsewhere but strictures are less common than following gonococcal infection of the urethra.

TUMOURS

The urinary bladder and renal pelvis are more common sites for urinary tract tumours than the ureters and urethra. Majority of urinary tract tumours are epithelial. Both benign and malignant tumours occur; the latter being more common.

TUMOURS OF THE BLADDER

Epithelial (Urothelial) Bladder Tumours

More than 90% of bladder tumours arise from transitional epithelial (urothelium) lining of the bladder in continuity with the epithelial lining of the renal pelvis, ureters, and the major part of the urethra. Though many workers consider all transitional cell tumours as transitional cell carcinoma, others distinguish true transitional cell papilloma from grade I transitional cell carcinoma.

Bladder cancer comprises about 3% of all cancers. Most of the cases appear beyond 5th decade of life with preponderance in males.

ETIOPATHOGENESIS. Urothelial tumours in the urinary tract are typically multifocal and the pattern of disease becomes apparent over a period of years. A number of environmental and host factors are associated with increased risk of bladder cancer. These are as under:

1. Industrial occupations. Workers in industries that produce aniline dyes, rubber, plastic, textiles, and cable have high incidence of bladder cancer. Bladder cancer may occur in workers in these factories after a prolonged exposure of about 20 years. The carcinogenic substances responsible for bladder cancer in these cases are the metabolites of β-naphthylamine and benzene.

2. Schistosomiasis. There is increased risk of bladder cancer, particularly squamous cell carcinoma, in patients having bilharzial infestation *(Schistosoma haematobium)* of the bladder. Schistosomiasis is common in Egypt and accounts for high incidence of bladder cancer in that country. It is thought to induce local irritant effect and initiate squamous metaplasia followed by squamous cell carcinoma.

3. Dietary factors. Certain carcinogenic metabolites of tryptophan are excreted in urine of patients with bladder cancer. These metabolites have been shown to induce bladder cancer in experimental animals. The role of artificial sweeteners like saccharin, coffee or caffeine and chronic alcoholism in the etiology of bladder cancer in man is controversial.

4. Local lesions. A number of local lesions in the bladder predispose to the development of bladder cancer. These include ectopia vesicae (extrophied bladder), vesical diverticulum, leukoplakia of the bladder mucosa and urinary diversion in defunctionalised bladder. All these conditions are associated with squamous metaplasia and high incidence of bladder cancer.

5. Smoking. Tobacco smoking is associated with 2 to 3 fold increased risk of developing bladder cancer, probably due to increased urinary excretion of carcinogenic substances.

6. Drugs. Immunosuppressive therapy with cyclophosphamide and patients having analgesic-abuse (phenacetin-) nephropathy have high risk of developing bladder cancer.

Multicentric nature of urothelial cancer and high rate of recurrence has led to the hypothesis that a *field effect* in the urothelium is responsible for this form of cancer. Several chromosomal aberrations have been described in bladder cancer in different stages.

PATHOLOGIC CHANGES. Grossly, urothelial tumours may be single or multiple. About 90% of the tumours are papillary (non-invasive or invasive), whereas the remaining 10% are flat indurated (non-invasive or invasive). The papillary tumours have free floating fern-like arrangement with a broad or narrow pedicle. The non-papillary tumours are bulkier with ulcerated surface (Fig. 20.29). More common locations for either of the two types are the

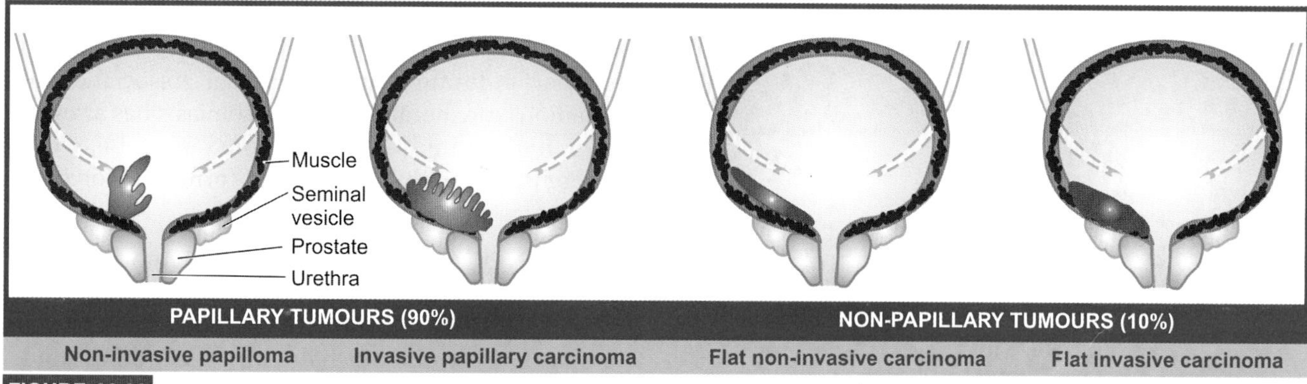

FIGURE 20.29

Macroscopic patterns of epithelial bladder tumours.

trigone, the region of ureteral orifices and on the lateral walls.

Histologically, urothelial tumours are of 3 cell types—transitional cell, squamous cell, and glandular (Table 20.18).

A. TRANSITIONAL CELL TUMOURS. Approximately 90% of all epithelial tumours of the bladder are transitional cell tumours. As stated before, transitional cell papilloma is distinguished by some workers from grade I transitional cell carcinoma (TCC), whereas others do not consider this as a distinct entity. Here, we follow the widely accepted classification of Mostofi (1960) adopted by the American Bladder Tumour Registry that divides TCC into 3 grades.

1. Transitional cell papilloma. Papillomas may occur singly or may be multiple. They are generally small, less than 2 cm in diameter, papillary with branching pattern. Each papilla is composed of fibrovascular stromal core covered by normal-looking transitional cells having normal number of layers (not more than six) in thickness. The individual cells resemble the normal transitional cells and do not vary in size and shape. Mitoses are absent and basal polarity is retained. It must be emphasised that the designation transitional cell papilloma is purely a histological diagnosis but does not imply an innocent biologic behaviour. In fact, it may recur and behave in a malignant manner.

TABLE 20.18: Histologic Classification of Epithelial (Urothelial) Tumours (Mostofi, 1960).

A. **Transitional cell tumours (90%)**
   1. Transitional cell papilloma
   2. Transitional cell carcinoma (grade I, II and III)

B. **Carcinoma *in situ***

C. **Squamous cell carcinoma (5%)**

D. **Adenocarcinoma (Rare)**

E. **Mixed carcinoma (5%)**

2. Transitional cell carcinoma. This is the commonest cancer of the bladder and is divided into 3 grades depending upon 2 features: the *degree of anaplasia* and the *extent of invasion.*

- The *criteria for anaplasia* are: increased cellularity, nuclear crowding, deranged cellular polarity, failure of normal orientation from base to the surface, variation in cell size and shape, variation in nuclear chromatin pattern, mitotic figures and giant cells.
- The *criteria for invasion* in papillary as well as non-papillary tumours are: penetration of the basement membrane of bladder mucosa.

Based on these salient features, the characteristics of three grades of transitional cell carcinoma are as under:

Grade I: The tumour cells are clearly transitional type but show increased number of layers of cells *(c.f.* transitional cell papilloma). The individual cells are generally regular but are slightly larger and show mild hyperchromatism.

Grade II (Fig. 20.30): The tumour cells are still recognisable as of transitional cell origin and the number of layers of cells is increased. The individual tumour cells are less regular, larger in size, and show pronounced nuclear hyperchromatism, mitotic activity and loss of polarity. The tumour may or may not be invasive (COLOUR PLATE XXVIII: CL 112).

Grade III: This is the anaplastic or undifferentiated grade of the tumour which is always invasive

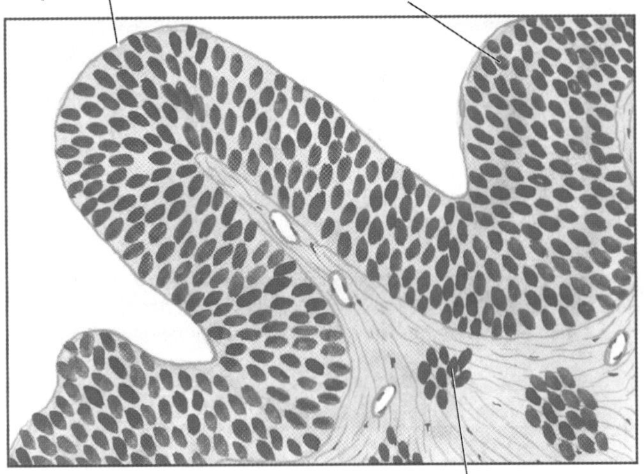

FIGURE 20.30

Microscopic features of grade II transitional cell carcinoma. There is increase in the number of layers of epithelium. The cells are still recognisable as of transitional origin and show features of anaplasia.

extending into the bladder wall to variable depth depending upon the clinical stage (described later). The tumour cells are no longer recognisable as of transitional origin. The individual tumour cells show pronounced features of anaplasia such as marked pleomorphism, hyperchromatism, total loss of polarity with loosened surface cells exfoliated in the bladder lumen.

There may be foci of squamous or glandular metaplasia in any grade of the tumour.

B. CARCINOMA *IN SITU*. Foci of epithelial hyperplasia, dysplasia and carcinoma in situ are seen in other parts of the bladder in non-invasive as well as in invasive carcinomas. Similar foci may be present in the ureters and renal pelvis. The malignant potential of epithelial hyperplasia and dysplasia is uncertain but carcinoma *in situ* is certainly precancerous and is currently included as grade 0 transitional cell carcinoma. Carcinoma *in situ* is characterised by highly anaplastic malignant cells confined to layers superficial to basement membrane of the bladder mucosa. These pathologic changes can be induced in experimental animals by chemical carcinogens. Therefore, it is reasonable to assume that these stages are precursors of invasive bladder cancer.

C. SQUAMOUS CELL CARCINOMA. Squamous cell carcinoma comprises about 5% of the bladder carcinomas. Unlike transitional cell carcinomas which are mostly papillary and non-ulcerating, most squamous carcinomas of the bladder are sessile, nodular, infiltrating and ulcerating. Association of squamous carcinoma and schistosomiasis has already been highlighted. The carcinoma may be well-differentiated with keratin pearl formation, or may be anaplastic.

D. ADENOCARCINOMA. Adenocarcinoma of the bladder is rare. Adenocarcinoma has association with exostrophy of the bladder with glandular metaplasia, or may arise from urachal rests, periurethral and periprostatic glands, or from cystitis cystica. The tumour is characterised by glandular and tubular pattern with or without mucus production.

E. MIXED CARCINOMA. About 50% of epithelial tumours of the bladder show mixed pattern, usually of transitional and squamous cell combination.

STAGING OF BLADDER CANCER. The clinical behaviour and prognosis of bladder cancer can be assessed by the following simple staging system:

Stage 0: Carcinoma confined to the mucosa.

Stage A: Carcinoma invades the lamina propria but not the muscularis.

Stage B1: Carcinoma invades the superficial muscle layer.

Stage B2: Carcinoma invades the deep muscle layer.

Stage C: Carcinoma invades the perivesical tissues.

Stage D1: Carcinoma shows regional metastases.

Stage D2: Carcinoma shows distant metastases.

Non-epithelial Bladder Tumours

These may be benign or malignant.

BENIGN. The most common benign mesenchymal tumour of the bladder is leiomyoma. Other less common examples are neurofibroma, haemangioma and granular cell myoblastoma.

MALIGNANT. Rhabdomyosarcoma is the most frequent malignant mesenchymal tumour. It exists in 2 forms:

Adult form occurring in adults over 40 years of age and resembles the rhabdomyosarcoma of skeletal muscle.

Childhood form occurring in infancy and childhood and appears as large polypoid, soft, fleshy, grapelike mass and is also called *sarcoma botryoides* or *embryonal rhabdomyosarcoma.* It is morphologically characterised by masses of embryonic mesenchyme consisting of masses of highly pleomorphic stellate cells in myxomatous background. Similar tumours occur in the female genital tract (Chapter 22).

TUMOURS OF RENAL PELVIS AND URETERS

Almost all the tumours of the renal pelvis and ureters are of epithelial origin. They are of the same types as are seen in the urinary bladder. However, tumours in the ureters are quite rare.

TUMOURS OF URETHRA

Tumours of the urethra are rare except for the urethral caruncle which is a tumour-like lesion.

URETHRAL CARUNCLE. Urethral caruncle is not uncommon. It is an inflammatory lesion present on external urethral meatus in elderly females.

Grossly, the caruncle appears as a solitary, 1 to 2 cm in diameter, pink or red mass, protruding from urethral meatus. It is quite friable and ulcerated.

Microscopically, the mass may be covered by squamous or transitional epithelium or there may be ulcerated surface. The underlying tissues show proliferating blood vessels, fibroblastic connective tissue and intense acute and chronic inflammatory infiltrate. Thus, the histologic appearance closely resembles a *pyogenic granuloma.*

URETHRAL CARCINOMA. Carcinoma of the urethra is uncommon. In most cases it occurs in the distal urethra near the external meatus and thus is commonly squamous cell carcinoma. Less often, there may be transitional cell carcinoma or adenocarcinoma arising from periurethral glands.

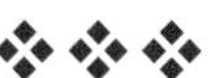

The Male Reproductive System and Prostate

21

TESTIS AND EPIDIDYMIS

NORMAL STRUCTURE

Contents of the scrotal sac include the testicle and epididymis alongwith lower end of the spermatic cord and the tunica vaginalis that forms the outer serous investing layer. The epididymis is attached to body of the testis posteriorly. Thus, the testicle and epididymis may be regarded as one organ.

Structurally, the main components of the testicle are the seminiferous tubules which when uncoiled are of considerable length.

Histologically, the seminiferous tubules are formed of a lamellar connective tissue membrane and contain several layers of cells (Fig. 21.1,A). In the adult, the cells lining the seminiferous tubules are of 2 types:

1. *Spermatogonia* or germ cells which produce spermatocytes, spermatids and mature spermatozoa.
2. *Sertoli cells* which are larger and act as supportive cells to germ cells, produce oestrogen and androgen and also form the basement membrane of the seminiferous tubules.

The seminiferous tubules drain into collecting ducts which form the rete testis from where the secretions pass into the vasa efferentia. Vasa efferentia opens at the upper end of the epididymis. The lower end of the epididymis is prolonged into a thick muscular tube, the vas deferens, that transports the secretions into the urethra.

The fibrovascular stroma present between the seminiferous tubules contains varying number of *interstitial cells of Leydig*. Leydig cells have abundant cytoplasm containing lipid granules and elongated Reinke's crystals. These cells are the main source of testosterone and other androgenic hormones in males. Thus, Sertoli and Leydig cells are hormone-producing cells homologous to their ovarian counterparts, granulosa-theca cells, and are termed *specialised stromal cells of* the gonads.

CONGENITAL ANOMALIES

Cryptorchidism

Cryptorchidism or undescended testis is a condition in which the testicle is arrested at some point in its descent. Its incidence is about 0.2% in adult male population. In 70% of cases, the undescended testis lies in the inguinal ring, in 25% in the abdomen and, in the remaining 5%, it may be present at other sites along its descent from intra-abdominal location to the scrotal sac.

ETIOLOGY. The exact etiology is not known in majority of cases. However, a few apparent causes associated with cryptorchidism are as under:

1. **Mechanical factors** e.g. short spermatic cord, narrow inguinal canal, adhesions to the peritoneum.
2. **Genetic factors** e.g. trisomy 13, maldevelopment of scrotum or cremaster muscles.

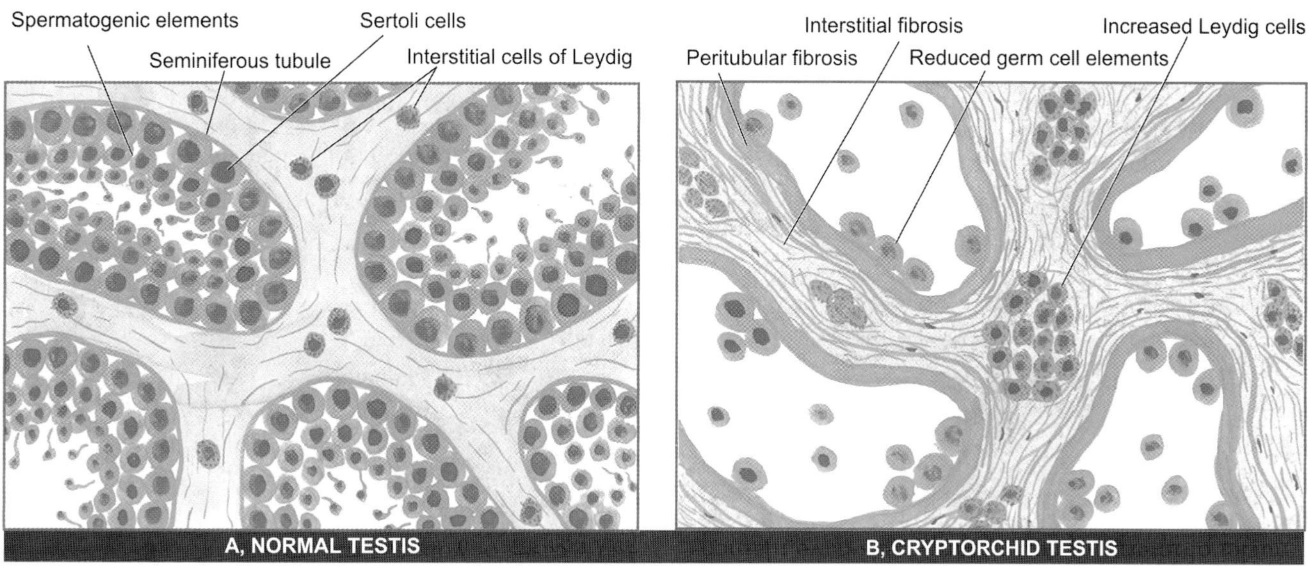

FIGURE 21.1

Microscopic appearance of cryptorchid testis (B) contrasted with that of normal testis (A).

3. **Hormonal** factors e.g. deficient androgenic secretions.

PATHOLOGIC CHANGES. Cryptorchidism is unilateral in majority of cases but in 25% of patients, it is bilateral.

Grossly, the cryptorchid testis is small in size, firm and fibrotic.

Histologically, contrary to previous beliefs, the changes of atrophy begin to appear by about 2 years of age. These changes are as under (Fig. 21.1,B) (COLOUR PLATE III: CL 9):

1. *Seminiferous tubules:* There is progressive loss of germ cell elements so that the tubules may be lined by only spermatogonia and spermatids but foci of spermatogenesis are discernible in 10% of cases. The tubular basement membrane is thickened. Advanced cases show hyalinised tubules with a few Sertoli cells only, surrounded by prominent basement membrane.
2. *Interstitial stroma:* There is usually increase in the interstitial fibrovascular stroma and conspicuous presence of Leydig cells, seen singly or in small clusters.

CLINICAL FEATURES. As such, cryptorchidism is completely asymptomatic and is discovered only on physical examination. However, if surgical correction by orchiopexy is not undertaken by about 2 years of age, or certainly in the prepubertal period, significant adverse clinical outcome may result as under:

1. **Sterility-infertility.** Bilateral cryptorchidism is associated with sterility while unilateral disease may result in infertility.
2. **Inguinal hernia.** A concomitant inguinal hernia is frequently present alongwith cryptorchidism.
3. **Malignancy.** Cryptorchid testis is at 35 times increased risk of developing testicular malignancy, most commonly seminoma and embryonal carcinoma, than a normally descended testis. The risk of malignancy is greater in intra-abdominal testis than in testis in the inguinal canal.

Male Infertility

The morphologic pattern of testicular atrophy described above for cryptorchidism can result from various other causes of male infertility. These causes can be divided into 3 groups: pre-testicular, testicular and post-testicular.

A. PRE-TESTICULAR CAUSES:

1. **Hypopituitarism.** Pre-pubertal or post-pubertal hypopituitarism such as from tumour, trauma, infarction, cyst and genetic deficiency of FSH and LH secretion.
2. **Oestrogen excess.** *Endogenous* excess such as from hepatic cirrhosis, adrenal tumour, Sertoli and Leydig cell tumour; or *exogenous* excess such as in the treatment of carcinoma of the prostate.

3. Glucocorticoid excess. *Endogenous* excess may occur in Cushing's syndrome while *exogenous* excess may occur in the treatment of ulcerative colitis, bronchial asthma, rheumatoid arthritis etc.

4. Other endocrine disorders. Hypothyroidism and diabetes mellitus are associated with hypospermatogenesis.

B. TESTICULAR CAUSES:

1. **Agonadism** i.e. total absence of the testes.

2. **Cryptorchidism** or undescended testis described above.

3. **Maturation arrest** i.e. failure of spermatogenesis beyond one of the immature stages.

4. **Hypospermatogenesis** i.e. presence of all the maturation stages of spermatogenesis but in decreased number.

5. **Sertoli cell-only syndrome.** Congenital or acquired absence of all germ cells so that the seminiferous tubules are lined by Sertoli cells only.

6. **Klinefelter's syndrome.** An XXY intersexuality characterised by primary hypogonadism, azoospermia, gynaecomastia, eunuchoid built and subnormal intelligence.

7. **Mumps orchitis** occurring as a complication of parotitis (Chapter 18).

8. **Irradiation damage** resulting in permanent germ cell destruction.

C. POST-TESTICULAR CAUSES:

1. **Congenital block** e.g. absence or atresia of vas deferens.

2. **Acquired** block e.g. due to gonorrhoea and surgical intervention.

3. **Impaired sperm motility** in the presence of normal sperm counts e.g. immotile cilia syndrome (Chapter 15).

INFLAMMATIONS

Inflammation of the testis is termed as orchitis and of epididymis as epididymitis; the latter being more common. A combination epididymo-orchitis may also occur. A few important types are described below.

Non-specific Epididymitis and Orchitis

Non-specific epididymitis and orchitis, or their combination, may be acute or chronic. The common routes of spread of infection are via the vas deferens, or via lymphatic and haematogenous routes. Most frequently, the infection is caused by urethritis, cystitis, prostatitis and seminal vesiculitis. Other causes are mumps, smallpox, dengue fever, influenza, pneumonia and filariasis. The common infecting organisms in sexually-active men under 35 years of age are *Neisseria gonorrhoeae* and *Chlamydia trachomatis,* whereas in older individuals the common organisms are urinary tract pathogens like *Escherichia coli* and *Pseudomonas.*

PATHOLOGIC CHANGES. ***Grossly,*** in acute stage the testicle is firm, tense, swollen and congested. There may be multiple abscesses, especially in gonorrhoeal infection. In chronic cases, there is usually variable degree of atrophy and fibrosis.
Histologically, acute orchitis and epididymitis are characterised by congestion, oedema and diffuse infiltration by neutrophils, lymphocytes, plasma cells and macrophages or formation of neutrophilic abscesses. Acute inflammation may resolve, or may progress to chronic form. In chronic epididymo-orchitis, there is focal or diffuse chronic inflammation, disappearance of seminiferous tubules, fibrous scarring and destruction of interstitial Leydig cells. Such cases usually result in permanent sterility.

Granulomatous (Autoimmune) Orchitis

Non-tuberculous granulomatous orchitis is a peculiar type of unilateral, painless testicular enlargement in middle-aged men that may resemble a testicular tumour clinically. The exact etiology and pathogenesis of the condition are not known though an autoimmune basis is suspected.

PATHOLOGIC CHANGES. ***Grossly,*** the affected testis is enlarged with thickened tunica. Cut section of the testicle is greyish-white to tan-brown.
Histologically, there are circumscribed non-caseating granulomas lying within the seminiferous tubules. These granulomas are composed of epithelioid cells, lymphocytes, plasma cells, some neutrophils and multinucleate giant cells. The origin of the epithelioid cells is from Sertoli cells lining the tubules. The tubules show peritubular fibrosis which merges into the interstitial tissue that is infiltrated by lymphocytes and plasma cells.

Tuberculous Epididymo-orchitis

Tuberculosis invariably begins in the epididymis and spreads to involve the testis. Tuberculous epididymo-orchitis is generally secondary tuberculosis from elsewhere in the body. It may occur either by direct spread from genitourinary tuberculosis such as tuberculous seminal vesiculitis, prostatitis and renal tuberculosis, or may reach by haematogenous spread of infection such as from tuberculosis of the lungs. Primary genital tuberculosis may occur rarely.

*PATHOLOGIC CHANGES. **Macroscopically,*** discrete, yellowish, caseous necrotic areas are seen.
Microscopically, numerous tubercles which may coalesce to form large caseous mass are seen. Characteristics of typical tubercles such as epithelioid cells, peripheral mantle of lymphocytes, occasional multinucleate giant cells and central areas of caseation necrosis are seen. Numerous acid-fast bacilli can be demonstrated by Ziehl-Neelsen staining. The lesions produce extensive destruction of the epididymis and may form chronic discharging sinuses on the scrotal skin. In late stage, the lesions heal by fibrous scarring and may undergo calcification.

Spermatic Granuloma

Spermatic granuloma is the term used for development of inflammatory lesions due to invasion of spermatozoa into the stroma. Spermatic granuloma may develop due to trauma, inflammation and loss of ligature following vasectomy.

*PATHOLOGIC CHANGES. **Grossly,*** the sperm granuloma is a small nodule, 3 mm to 3 cm in diameter, firm, white to yellowish-brown.
Histologically, it consists of a granuloma composed of histiocytes, epithelioid cells, lymphocytes and some neutrophils. Characteristically, the centre of spermatic granuloma contains spermatozoa and necrotic debris. The late lesions have fibroblastic proliferation at the periphery and hyalinisation.

Elephantiasis

Elephantiasis is enormous thickening of the scrotal skin resembling the elephant's hide and results in enlargement of the scrotum. The condition results from filariasis in which the adult worm lives in the lymphatics, while the larvae travel in the blood. The most important variety of filaria is *Wuchereria bancrofti.* The condition is common in all tropical countries. The vector is generally the Culex mosquito. The patients may remain asymptomatic or may manifest with fever, local pain, swelling, rash, tender lymphadenopathy and blood eosinophilia. An asthma-like respiratory complaint may develop in some cases.

*PATHOLOGIC CHANGES. **Grossly,*** the affected leg and scrotum are enormously thickened with enlargement of regional lymph nodes. The affected area of skin may show dilated dermal lymphatics and varicosities.
Histologically, the changes begin with lymphatic obstruction by the adult worms. The worm in alive, dead or calcified form may be found in the dilated lymphatics or in the lymph nodes. Dead or calcified worm in lymphatics is usually followed by lymphangitis with intense infiltration by eosinophils. Sometimes, granulomatous reaction may be evident. In advanced cases, chronic lymphoedema with tough subcutaneous fibrosis and epidermal hyperkeratosis develops which is termed elephantiasis.

MISCELLANEOUS LESIONS

Torsion of Testis

Torsion of the testicle may occur either in a fully-descended testis or in an undescended testis. The latter is more common and more severe. It results from sudden cessation of venous drainage and arterial supply to the testis, usually following sudden muscular effort or physical trauma. Torsion is common in boys and young men.

PATHOLOGIC CHANGES. The pathologic changes vary depending upon the duration and severity of vascular occlusion. There may be coagulative necrosis of the testis and epididymis, or there may be haemorrhagic infarction. The inflammatory reaction is generally not so pronounced.

Varicocele

Varicocele is the dilatation, elongation and tortuosity of the veins of the pampiniform plexus in the spermatic cord. It is of 2 types: primary (idiopathic) and secondary.

- **Primary or idiopathic form** is more frequent and is common in young unmarried men. It is nearly always on the left side as the loaded rectum presses the left vein. Besides, the left spermatic vein enters the renal vein at right angles while the right spermatic vein enters the vena cava obliquely.
- **Secondary form** occurs due to pressure on the spermatic vein by enlarged liver, spleen or kidney. It is commoner in middle-aged people.

Hydrocele

A hydrocele is abnormal collection of serous fluid in the tunica vaginalis. It may be acute or chronic, congenital or acquired. The usual causes are trauma, systemic oedema such as in cardiac failure and renal disease, and as a complication of gonorrhoea, syphilis and tuberculosis.

The hydrocele fluid is generally clear and straw-coloured but may be slightly turbid or haemorrhagic. The hydrocele sac may have single loculus or may have multiple loculi. The wall of the hydrocele sac is composed of fibrous tissue infiltrated with lymphocytes and plasma cells.

Haematocele

Haematocele is haemorrhage into the sac of the tunica vaginalis. It may result from direct trauma, from injury to a vein by the needle, or from haemorrhagic diseases.

In recent haematocele, the blood coagulates and the wall is coated with ragged deposits of fibrin. In long-standing cases, the tunica vaginalis is thickened with dense fibrous tissue and occasionally may get partly calcified.

TESTICULAR TUMOURS

Testicular tumours are the cause of about 1% of all cancer deaths. They are more frequent in white male population but are less common in Africans and Asians. They have *trimodal* age distribution—a peak during infancy, another during late adolescence and early adulthood, and a third peak after 60 years of age.

CLASSIFICATION

The most widely accepted classification is the histogenetic classification proposed by the World Health Organisation (Table 21.1). Based on this, all testicular tumours are divided into: *germ cell tumours, sex cord-stromal tumours* and *mixed forms.* Vast majority of the testicular tumours (95%) arise from germ cells or their precursors in the seminiferous tubules, while less than 5% originate from sex cord-stromal components of the testis. From clinical point of view, gem cell tumours of testis are distinguished into 2 main groups—seminomatous and non-seminomatous (Table 21.2).

TABLE 21.1: Classification of Testicular Tumours.

I. GERM CELL TUMOURS
1. Seminoma
2. Spermatocytic seminoma
3. Embryonal carcinoma
4. Yolk sac tumour (*Syn.* endodermal sinus tumour, orchio blastoma, infantile type embryonal carcinoma)
5. Polyembryoma
6. Choriocarcinoma
7. Teratomas
   (i) Mature
   (ii) Immature
   (iii) With malignant transformation
8. Mixed germ cell tumours

II. SEX CORD-STROMAL TUMOURS
1. Leydig cell tumour
2. Sertoli cell tumour (Androblastoma)
3. Granulosa cell tumour
4. Mixed forms

III. COMBINED GERM CELL-SEX CORD-STROMAL TUMOURS
Gonadoblastoma

IV. OTHER TUMOURS
1. Malignant lymphoma (5%)
2. Rare tumours

ETIOLOGIC FACTORS

The cause of testicular germ cell tumours is unknown, but the following factors have been implicated:

1. Cryptorchidism. The probability of a germ cell tumour developing in an undescended testis is 35 times greater than in a normally-descended testis. About 10% of testicular germ cell tumours are associated with cryptorchidism. The high incidence is attributed to higher temperature to which the undescended testis in the groin or abdomen is exposed. Intra-abdominal testis is at greater risk than the inguinal testis. There is increased incidence of tumour in the contralateral normally-descended testis. There are no data to confirm or deny whether surgical repositioning or orchiopexy of a cryptorchid testis alters the incidence of testicular tumour. However, surgical correction is still helpful since it is easier to detect the tumour in scrotal testis than in an abdominal or inguinal téstis.

2. Other developmental disorders. Dysgenetic gonads associated with endocrine abnormalities such as androgen insensitivity syndrome have higher incidence of development of germ cell tumours.

3. Genetic factors. Genetic factors play a role in the development of germ cell tumours supported by the observation of high incidence in other family members, twins and in white male populations while blacks in

TABLE 21.2: Distinguishing Features of Seminomatous (SGCT) and Non-seminomatous (NSGCT) Germ Cell Tumours of Testis.

FEATURE	SGCT	NSGCT
1. *Primary tumour*	Larger, confined to testis for sufficient time; testicular contour retained	Smaller, at times indistinct; testicular contour may be distorted
2. *Metastasis*	Generally to regional lymph nodes	Haematogenous spread early
3. *Response to radiation*	Radiosensitive	Radioresistant
4. *Serum markers*	hCG; generally low levels	hCG, AFP, or both; high levels
5. *Prognosis*	Better	Poor

Africa have a very low incidence. However, no definite pattern of inheritance has been recognised.

4. **Other factors.** A few less common factors include the following:

i) Orchitis. A history of mumps or other forms of orchitis may be given by the patient with germ cell tumour.

ii) Trauma. Many patients give a history of trauma prior to the development of the tumour but it is not certain how trauma initiates the neoplastic process.

iii) Carcinogens. A number of carcinogens such as use of certain drugs (e.g. LSD, hormonal therapy for sterility, copper, zinc etc), exposure to radiation and endocrine abnormalities may play a role in the development of testicular tumours.

HISTOGENESIS

Pathogenesis of testicular tumours remains controversial except that vast majority of these tumours originate from germ cells. Based on current concepts on histogenesis of testicular tumours, following agreements and disagreements have emerged (Fig 21.2):

1. **Developmental disorders:** Disorders such as cryptorchidism, gonadal dysgenesis and androgen insensitivity syndrome are high risk factors for development of testicular germ cell tumours. These observations point to developmental defect in gonadogenesis. In more than 90% of testicular germ cell tumours irrespective of histologic type (as also ovarian germ cell tumours), an isochromosome of short arm of chromosome 12, abbreviated as *i(12p)*, is found suggesting a common molecular pathogenesis of all germ cell tumours.

2. **CIS/ITGCN:** A preinvasive stage of carcinoma *in situ* (CIS) termed *intratubular germ cell neoplasia* generally precedes the development of most of the invasive testicular germ cell tumours in adults. CIS originates from spermatogenic elements. Areas of CIS are found in seminiferous tubules adjacent to most seminomas, embryonal carcinomas and other mixed germ cell tumours. However, CIS is not found in seminiferous tubules adjoining yolk sac carcinoma of childhood, benign teratoma in children and adolescents, and spermatocytic seminoma indicating different pathogenetic mechanisms.

3. **'Three hit' process:** Germ cells in seminiferous tubules undergo activation *('first hit')* before undergoing malignant transformation confined to seminiferous tubules (CIS) *('second hit')* and eventually into invasive stage by some epigenetic phenomena *('third hit')*. Though this sequential tumorigenesis explains the development of seminomatous tumours, it is yet not clear whether non-seminomatous germ cell tumours develop directly or through intermediate stage.

CLINICAL FEATURES AND DIAGNOSIS

The usual presenting clinical symptoms of testicular tumours are gradual gonadal enlargement and a dragging sensation in the testis. Metastatic involvement may produce secondary symptoms such as pain, lymphadenopathy, haemoptysis and urinary obstruction.

SPREAD. Since testicular germ cell tumours originate from totipotent germ cells, it is not unusual to find metastases of histologic types different from the primary growth. Testicular tumours may spread by both lymphatic and haematogenous routes:

- *Lymphatic spread* occurs to retroperitoneal para-aortic lymph nodes, mediastinal lymph nodes and supraclavicular lymph nodes.
- *Haematogenous spread* primarily occurs to the lungs, liver, brain and bones.

TUMOUR MARKERS. Germ cell tumours of the testis secrete polypeptide hormones and certain enzymes which can be detected in the blood. Two tumour markers widely used in the diagnosis, staging and monitoring the follow-up of patients with testicular tumours

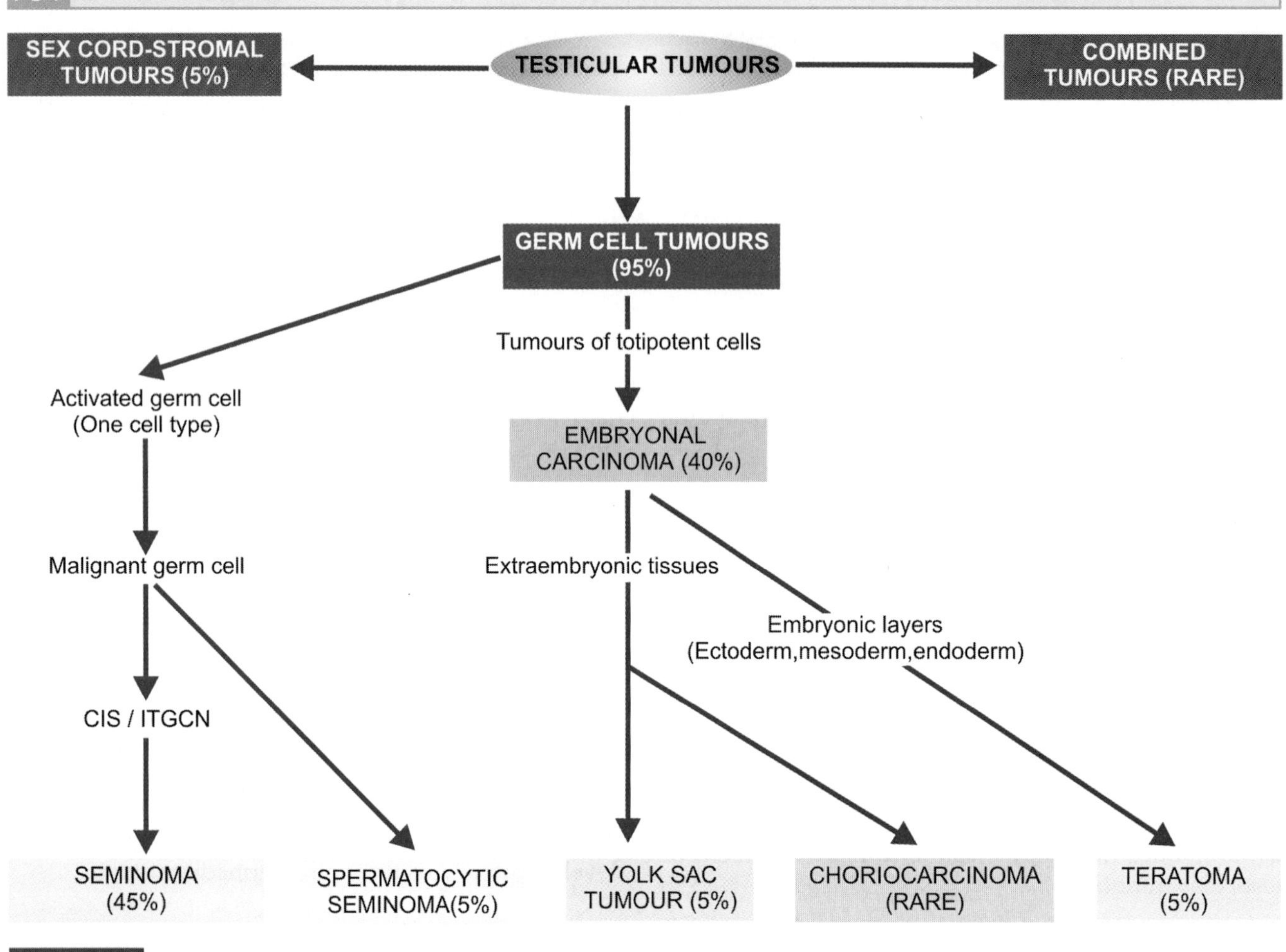

FIGURE 21.2

Histogenesis of testicular tumours.

are: human chorionic gonadotropin (hCG) and alpha-foetoprotein (AFP). In addition, carcinoembryonic antigen (CEA), human placental lactogen (HPL), placental alkaline phosphatase, testosterone, oestrogen and luteinising hormone may also be elevated.

■ **hCG** is synthesised by placental syncytio-trophoblast such as in various non-seminomatous germ cell tumours of the testis (e.g. in choriocarcinoma, yolk sac tumour and embryonal carcinoma). However, ectopic hCG production may occur in a variety of non-testicular non-germ cell tumours as well.

■ **AFP** is normally synthesised by the foetal liver cells, yolk sac and foetal gut. Its levels are elevated in testicular tumours associated with yolk sac components. However, elevated serum AFP levels are also found in liver cell carcinoma.

PROGNOSIS. For selecting post-orchiectomy treatment (radiation, surgery, chemotherapy or all the three) and for monitoring prognosis, 3 clinical stages are defined:

Stage I: tumour confined to the testis.

Stage II: distant spread confined to retroperitoneal lymph nodes below the diaphragm.

Stage III: distant metastases beyond the retroperitoneal lymph nodes.

Seminomas tend to remain localised to the testis (stage I) while non-seminomatous germ cell tumours more often present with advanced clinical disease (stage II and III). Seminomas are extremely radiosensitive while non-seminomatous germ cell tumours are radioresistant. In general, seminomas have a better prognosis with 90% cure rate while the non-seminomatous tumours behave in a more aggressive manner and have poor prognosis.

After these general comments, specific testicular tumours are as described below.

GERM CELL TUMOURS

Germ cell tumours comprise approximately 95% of all testicular tumours and are more frequent before the

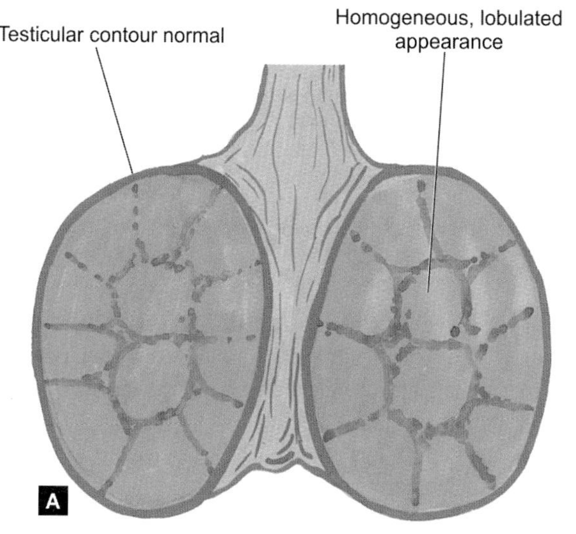

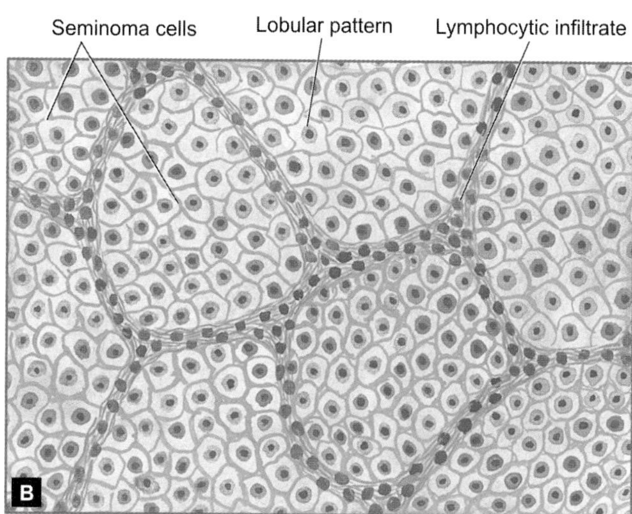

FIGURE 21.3

Seminoma. A, Typical gross appearance of cut surface of the involved testis. B, Microscopy of the tumour shows lobules of monomorphic seminoma cells separated by delicate fibrous stroma containing lymphocytic infiltration.

age of 45 years. *Testicular germ cell tumours are almost always malignant.* Nearly half of them contain more than one histologic type. Germ cell tumours are also found in the ovary (page 771), retroperitoneum and mediastinum.

Intratubular Germ Cell Neoplasia

The term intratubular germ cell neoplasia (ITGCN) is used to describe the preinvasive stage of germ cell tumours, notably intratubular seminoma and intratubular embryonal carcinoma. Others have used carcinoma *in situ* (CIS) stage of germ cell tumours as synonymous term.

Histologically, the malignant atypical tumour cells are restricted to the seminiferous tubules without evident invasion into the interstitium.

Seminoma

Seminoma is the commonest malignant tumour of the testis and corresponds to dysgerminoma in the female (page 773). It constitutes about 45% of all germ cell tumours, and in another 15% comprises the major component of mixed germ cell tumour. The tumour has a peak incidence in the 4th decade of life and is rare before puberty. Undescended testis harbours seminoma more frequently as compared to other germ cell tumours. About 10% pure seminomas are associated with elevated hCG levels in serum.

PATHOLOGIC CHANGES. Grossly, the involved testis is enlarged up to 10 times its normal size but tends to maintain its normal contour since the tumour rarely invades the tunica. The larger tumour replaces the entire testis, whereas the smaller tumour appears as circumscribed mass in the testis. Cut section of the affected testis shows homogeneous, grey-white lobulated appearance (Fig. 21.3,A). Necrosis and haemorrhage in the tumour are rare.

Microscopically, the tumour has the following characteristics (Fig. 21.3,B) (COLOUR PLATE XXIX: CL 113):

1. Tumour cells. The seminoma cells generally lie in cords, sheets or columns forming lobules. Typically, in a classic seminoma, the tumour cells are fairly uniform in size with clear cytoplasm and well-defined cell borders. The cytoplasm contains variable amount of glycogen that stains positively with PAS reaction. The nuclei are centrally located, large, hyperchromatic and usually contain 1-2 prominent nucleoli. Tumour giant cells may be present. Mitotic figures are infrequent. However, about 10% of seminomas have increased mitotic activity and have aggressive behaviour and are referred to as *anaplastic seminomas.*

2. Stroma. The stroma of seminoma is delicate fibrous tissue which divides the tumour into lobules. The stroma shows a characteristic lymphocytic infiltration, indicative of immunologic response of the host to the tumour. About 20% of the tumours show granulomatous reaction in the stroma.

The *prognosis* of seminoma is better than other germ cell tumours. The tumour is highly radiosensitive.

Spermatocytic Seminoma

Spermatocytic seminoma is both clinically and morphologically a distinctive tumour from classic seminoma and is, therefore, classified separately in the WHO classification. It is an uncommon tumour having an incidence of about 5% of all germ cell tumours. Spermatocytic seminoma usually occurs in older patients, generally in 6th decade of life. The tumour is bilateral in 10% of patients.

PATHOLOGIC CHANGES. Grossly, spermatocytic seminoma is homogeneous, larger, softer and more yellowish and gelatinous than the classic seminoma. ***Histologically,*** the distinctive features are as under:

1. Tumour cells. The tumour cells vary considerably in size from lymphocyte-like to huge mononucleate or multinucleate giant cells. Majority of the tumour cells are, however, of intermediate size. The cells have eosinophilic cytoplasm devoid of glycogen. The nuclei of intermediate and large cells have filamentous pattern. Mitoses are often frequent.

2. Stroma. The stroma lacks lymphocytic and granulomatous reaction seen in classic seminoma.

The *prognosis* of spermatocytic seminoma is excellent since the tumour is slow-growing and rarely metastasises. The tumour is believed to be radiosensitive.

Embryonal Carcinoma

Pure embryonal carcinoma constitutes 30% of germ cell tumours but areas of embryonal carcinoma are present in 40% of germ cell tumours. These tumours are more common in 2nd to 3rd decades of life. About 90% cases are associated with elevation of AFP or hCG or both. They are more aggressive than the seminomas.

PATHOLOGIC CHANGES. Grossly, embryonal carcinoma is usually a small tumour in the testis. It distorts the contour of the testis as it frequently invades the tunica and the epididymis. The cut surface of the tumour is grey-white, soft with areas of haemorrhages and necrosis.

Microscopically, the following features are seen:

1. The tumour cells are arranged in a variety of *patterns*—glandular, tubular, papillary and solid.
2. The *tumour cells* are highly anaplastic carcinomatous cells having large size, indistinct cell borders, amphophilic cytoplasm and prominent hyperchromatic nuclei showing considerable variation in nuclear size. Mitotic figures and tumour giant cells are frequently present. Haemorrhage and necrosis are common.
3. The *stroma* is not as distinct as in seminoma and may contain variable amount of primitive mesenchyme.

Embryonal carcinoma is more aggressive and less radiosensitive than seminoma. Chemotherapy is considered more effective in treating this tumour.

Yolk Sac Tumour
(Synonyms: Endodermal Sinus Tumour, Orchioblastoma, Infantile Embryonal Carcinoma)

This characteristic tumour is the most common testicular tumour of infants and young children up to the age of 4 years. In adults, however, yolk sac tumour in pure form is rare but may be present as the major component in 40% of germ cell tumours. AFP levels are elevated in 100% cases of yolk sac tumours.

PATHOLOGIC CHANGES. Grossly, the tumour is generally soft, yellow-white, mucoid with areas of necrosis and haemorrhages.

Microscopically, yolk sac tumour has the following features (COLOUR PLATE XXIX: CL 114):

1. The tumour cells form a variety of *patterns*—loose reticular network, papillary, tubular and solid arrangement.
2. The *tumour cells* are flattened to cuboid epithelial cells with clear vacuolated cytoplasm.
3. The tumour cells may form distinctive perivascular structures resembling the yolk sac or endodermal sinuses of the rat placenta called *Schiller-Duval bodies.*
4. There may be presence of both intracellular and extracellular PAS-positive *hyaline globules,* many of which contain AFP.

Polyembryoma

Polyembryoma is defined as a tumour composed predominantly of embryoid bodies. Embryoid bodies are structures containing a disc and cavities surrounded by loose mesenchyme simulating an embryo of about 2 weeks' gestation. Polyembryoma is extremely rare but embryoid bodies may be present with embryonal carcinoma and teratoma.

Choriocarcinoma

Pure choriocarcinoma is a highly malignant tumour composed of elements consisting of syncytiotrophoblast and cytotrophoblast.

However, pure form is extremely rare and occurs more often in combination with other germ cell tumours. The patients are generally in their 2nd decade of life. The primary tumour is usually small and the patient may manifest initially with symptoms of metastasis. The serum and urinary levels of hCG are greatly elevated in 100% cases.

PATHOLOGIC CHANGES. ***Grossly,*** the tumour is usually small and may appear as a soft, haemorrhagic and necrotic mass.

Microscopically, the characteristic feature is the identification of intimately related syncytiotrophoblast and cytotrophoblast without formation of definite placental-type villi.

- *Syncytiotrophoblastic cells* are large with many irregular and bizarre nuclei and abundant eosinophilic vacuolated cytoplasm which stains positively for hCG. These cells often surround masses of cytotrophoblastic cells.
- *Cytotrophoblastic cells* are polyhedral cells which are more regular and have clear or eosinophilic cytoplasm with hyperchromatic nuclei.

Teratoma

Teratomas are complex tumours composed of tissues derived from more than one of the three germ cell layers—endoderm, mesoderm and ectoderm. Testicular teratomas are more common in infants and children and constitute about 40% of testicular tumours in infants, whereas in adults they comprise 5% of all germ cell tumours. However, teratomas are found in combination with other germ cell tumours (most commonly with embryonal carcinoma) in about 45% of mixed germ cell tumours. About half the teratomas have elevated hCG or AFP levels or both.

PATHOLOGIC CHANGES. Testicular teratomas are classified into 3 types:

1. Mature (differentiated) teratoma
2. Immature teratoma
3. Teratoma with malignant transformation.

Grossly, most teratomas are large, grey-white masses enlarging the involved testis. Cut surface shows characteristic variegated appearance—grey-white solid areas, cystic and honey-combed areas, and foci of cartilage and bone (Fig. 21.4,A). Dermoid tumours commonly seen in the ovaries are rare in testicular teratomas.

Microscopically, the three categories of teratomas show different appearances:

1. Mature (differentiated) teratoma. Mature teratoma is composed of disorderly mixture of a variety of well-differentiated structures such as cartilage, smooth muscle, intestinal and respiratory epithelium, mucous glands, cysts lined by squamous and transitional epithelium, neural tissue, fat and bone. This type of mature or differentiated teratoma is the most common, seen more frequently in infants and children and has favourable prognosis. But similar mature and benign-appearing tumour in adults is invariably associated with small hidden foci of immature elements so that their clinical course in adults is unpredictable. It is believed that *all testicular teratomas in the adults are malignant.*

As mentioned above, dermoid cysts similar to those of the ovary are rare in the testis.

2. Immature teratoma. Immature teratoma is composed of incompletely differentiated and primitive or embryonic tissues alongwith some mature elements (Fig. 21.4,B). Primitive or embryonic tissue commonly present are poorly-formed cartilage, mesenchyme, neural tissues, abortive eye, intestinal and respiratory tissue elements etc. Mitoses are usually frequent.

3. Teratoma with malignant transformation. This is an extremely rare form of teratoma in which one or more of the tissue elements show malignant transformation. Such malignant change resembles morphologically with typical malignancies in other organs and tissues and commonly includes rhabdomyosarcoma, squamous cell carcinoma and adenocarcinoma.

Mixed Germ Cell Tumours

About 60% of germ cell tumours have more than one of the above histologic types (except spermatocytic seminoma) and are called mixed germ cell tumours. The clinical behaviour of these tumours is worsened by inclusion of more aggressive tumour component in a less malignant tumour. Interestingly, metastases of the mixed germ cell tumours may not exactly reproduce the histologic types present in the primary tumour.

The most common combinations of mixed germ cell tumours are:

1. teratoma, embryonal carcinoma, yolk sac tumour and syncytiotrophoblast;

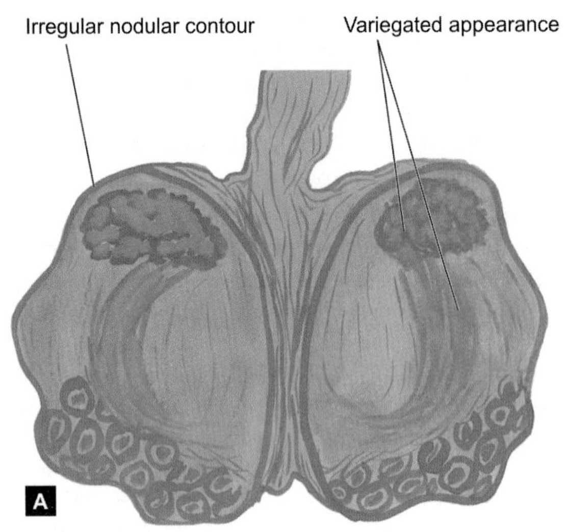

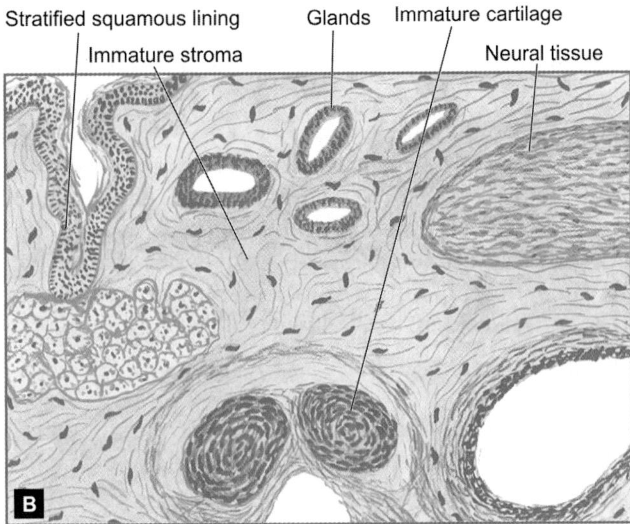

FIGURE 21.4

Immature teratoma. A, Typical gross appearance on cut section. The tumour produces an irregular, nodular enlargement of the testis, while the sectioned surface shows characteristic variegated appearance. B, Microscopy shows incompletely differentiated tissue elements.

2. embryonal carcinoma and teratoma (teratocarcinoma); and
3. seminoma and embryonal carcinoma.

SEX CORD-STROMAL TUMOURS

Tumours arising from specialised gonadal stroma are classified on the basis of histogenesis. The primitive mesenchyme which forms the specialised stroma of gonads in either sex gives rise to theca, granulosa and lutein cells in the female, and Sertoli and interstitial Leydig cells in the male. Since the cell of origin of primitive mesenchyme is identical, Sertoli and interstitial Leydig cell tumours may occur in the ovaries (in addition to theca cell, granulosa cell and lutein cell tumours). Likewise, the latter three tumours may occur in the testis (in addition to Sertoli cell and Leydig cell tumours). All these tumours secrete various hormones. The biologic behaviour of these tumours generally cannot be determined on histological grounds alone.

Leydig (Interstitial) Cell Tumour

Leydig cell tumours are quite uncommon. They may occur at any age but are more frequent in the age group of 20 to 50 years. Characteristically, these cells secrete androgen, or both androgen and oestrogen, and rarely corticosteroids. Bilateral tumours may occur typically in congenital adrenogenital syndrome.

PATHOLOGIC CHANGES. Grossly, the tumour appears as a small, well-demarcated and lobulated nodule. Cut surface is homogeneously yellowish or brown.

Histologically, the tumour is composed of sheets and cords of normal-looking Leydig cells. These cells contain abundant eosinophilic cytoplasm and Reinke's crystals and a small central nucleus.

Most of Leydig cell tumours are benign. Only about 10% may invade and metastasise.

Sertoli Cell Tumours (Androblastoma)

Sertoli cell tumours correspond to arrhenoblastoma of the ovary. They may occur at all ages but are more frequent in infants and children. These tumours may elaborate oestrogen or androgen and may account for gynaecomastia in an adult, or precocious sexual development in a child.

PATHOLOGIC CHANGES. Grossly, the tumour is fairly large, firm, round, and well circumscribed. Cut surface of the tumour is yellowish or yellow-grey.

Microscopically, Sertoli cell tumour is composed of benign Sertoli cells arranged in well-defined tubules.

Majority of Sertoli cell tumours are benign but about 10% may metastasise to regional lymph nodes.

Granulosa Cell Tumour

This is an extremely rare tumour in the testis and resembles morphologically with its ovarian counterpart (Chapter 22).

MIXED GERM CELL-SEX CORD STROMAL TUMOURS

An example of combination of both germ cells and sex cord stromal components is gonadoblastoma.

Gonadoblastoma

Dysgenetic gonads and undescended testis are predisposed to develop such combined proliferations of germ cells and sex cord-stromal elements. The patients are commonly intersexuals, particularly phenotypic females. Most of the gonadoblastomas secrete androgen so as to produce virilisation in female phenotype. A few, however, secrete oestrogen.

PATHOLOGIC CHANGES. Grossly, the tumour is of variable size, yellowish-white and soft.
Microscopically, gonadoblastoma is composed of 2 principal cell types—large germ cells resembling seminoma cells, and small cells resembling immature Sertoli, Leydig and granulosa cells. Call-Exner bodies of a granulosa cell tumour may be present.

Prognosis largely depends upon the malignant potential of the type of germ cell components included.

OTHER TUMOURS

Malignant Lymphoma

Malignant lymphomas comprises 5% of testicular malignancies and is the most common testicular tumour in the elderly. Bilaterality is seen in half the cases. Most common are large cell non-Hodgkin's lymphoma of B cell type.

Rare Tumours

In addition to the testicular tumours described above, some other uncommon tumours in this location include: plasmacytoma, leukaemic infiltration, carcinoid tumour, haemangioma, primary sarcomas and metastatic tumours.

PENIS

NORMAL STRUCTURE

The penis is covered by skin, foreskin (prepuce) and stratified squamous mucosa. The structure of penis consists of 3 masses of erectile tissue—the two corpora cavernosa, one on each side dorsally, and the corpus spongiosum ventrally through which the urethra passes. The expanded free end of the corpus spongiosum forms the glans.

The lumen of the urethra in sectioned surface of the penis appears as an irregular cleft in the middle of the corpus spongiosum. In the prostatic part, it is lined by transitional epithelium, but elsewhere it is lined by columnar epithelium except near its orifice where stratified squamous epithelium lines it.

CONGENITAL ANOMALIES

Some of the clinically significant congenital anomalies of the penis are phimosis, hypospadias and epispadias.

Phimosis

Phimosis is a condition in which the prepuce is too small to permit its normal retraction behind the glans. It may be congenital or acquired. *Congenital phimosis* is a developmental anomaly whereas *acquired phimosis* may result from inflammation, trauma or oedema leading to narrowing of preputial opening. In either case, phimosis interferes with cleanliness and predisposes to the development of secondary infection, preputial calculi and squamous cell carcinoma.

Paraphimosis is a condition in which the phimotic prepuce is forcibly retracted resulting in constriction over the glans penis and subsequent swelling.

Hypospadias and Epispadias

Hypospadias is a developmental defect of the urethra in which the urethral meatus fails to reach the end of the penis, but instead, opens on the ventral surface of the penis. Similar developmental defect with resultant urethral opening on the dorsal surface of the penis is termed *epispadias.* Hypospadias and epispadias may cause urethral constriction with consequent infection and may also interfere with normal ejaculation and insemination. Both these urethral anomalies are more frequently associated with cryptorchidism.

INFLAMMATIONS

Glans and prepuce are frequently involved in inflammation in a number of specific and non-specific conditions. The specific inflammations include various sexually-transmitted diseases such as hard chancre in syphilis, chancroid caused by *Haemophilus ducreyi,* gonorrhoea caused by gonococci, herpes progenitalis, granuloma inguinale (donovanosis), and lymphopathia venereum caused by *Chlamydia trachomatis.* Non-specific inflammations are designated as balanoposthitis.

Balanoposthitis

Balanoposthitis is the term used for non-specific inflammation of the inner surface of the prepuce *(balanitis)* and adjacent surface of the glans *(posthitis)*. It is caused by a variety of microorganisms such as staphylococci, streptococci, coliform bacilli and gonococci. Balanoposthitis usually results from lack of cleanliness resulting in accumulation of secretions and smegma. It is a common accompaniment of phimosis. The type of inflammation may be acute or chronic, sometimes with ulceration on the mucosal surface of the glans.

Balanitis Xerotica Obliterans

Balanitis xerotica obliterans is a white atrophic lesion on the glans penis and the prepuce and is a counterpart of the *lichen sclerosus et atrophicus* in the vulva described on page 748.

TUMOURS

Benign and malignant tumours as well as certain premalignant lesions may occur on the penis. These are discussed below:

BENIGN TUMOURS

Condyloma Acuminatum

Condyloma acuminatum or venereal wart is a benign tumour caused by human papilloma virus (HPV) types 6 and 11. The tumour may occur singly, or there may be conglomerated papillomas. A more extensive, solitary, exophytic and cauliflower-like warty mass is termed *giant condyloma or Buschke-Löwenstein tumour or verrucous carcinoma*.

PATHOLOGIC CHANGES. The condyloma is commonly located on the coronal sulcus on the penis or the perineal area.

Grossly, the tumour consists of solitary or multiple, warty, cauliflower-shaped lesions of variable size with exophytic growth pattern.

Histologically, the lesions are essentially like common warts (verruca vulgaris). The features include formation of papillary villi composed of connective tissue stroma and covered by squamous epithelium which shows hyperkeratosis, parakeratosis, and hyperplasia of prickle cell layer. Many of the prickle cells show clear vacuolisation of the cytoplasm (*koilocytosis*) indicative of HPV infection.

Giant condyloma shows upward as well as downward growth of the tumour but is otherwise histologically identical to condyloma acuminatum. Though histologically benign, clinically the giant condyloma is associated with recurrences and behaves as intermediate between truly benign condyloma acuminatum and squamous cell carcinoma.

PREMALIGNANT LESIONS (CARCINOMA *IN SITU)*

In the region of external male genitalia, three lesions display cytological changes of malignancy confined to epithelial layers only without evidence of invasion. These conditions are: Bowen's disease, erythroplasia of Queyrat and bowenoid papulosis.

Bowen's Disease

Bowen's disease is located on the shaft of the penis and the scrotum besides the sun-exposed areas of the skin (page 805).

Grossly, it appears as a solitary, circumscribed plaque lesion with ulceration.

Histologically, the changes are superficial to the dermo-epidermal border. The epithelial cells of the epidermis show hyperplasia, hyperkeratosis, parakeratosis and scattered bizarre dyskeratotic cells.

A fair proportion of cases of Bowen's disease are associated with internal visceral cancers.

Erythroplasia of Queyrat

The lesions of erythroplasia of Queyrat appear on the penile mucosa.

Grossly, the lesions are pink, shiny and velvety soft.

Histologically, the thickened and acanthotic epidermis shows variable degree of dysplasia.

Unlike Bowen's disease, there is no relationship between erythroplasia of Queyrat and internal malignancy.

Bowenoid Papulosis

The lesions of bowenoid papulosis appear on the penile shaft and adjacent genital skin.

Grossly, they are solitary or multiple, shiny, red-brown papular lesions.

Histologically, there is orderly maturation of epithelial cells in hyperplastic epidermis with scattered hyperchromatic nuclei and dysplastic cells.

MALIGNANT TUMOURS

Squamous Cell Carcinoma

The incidence of penile carcinoma shows wide variation in different populations. In the United States, the overall incidence of penile cancer is less than 2% of all cancers but it is 3-4 times more common in blacks than in whites. In China, its incidence is about 18%. Carcinoma of the

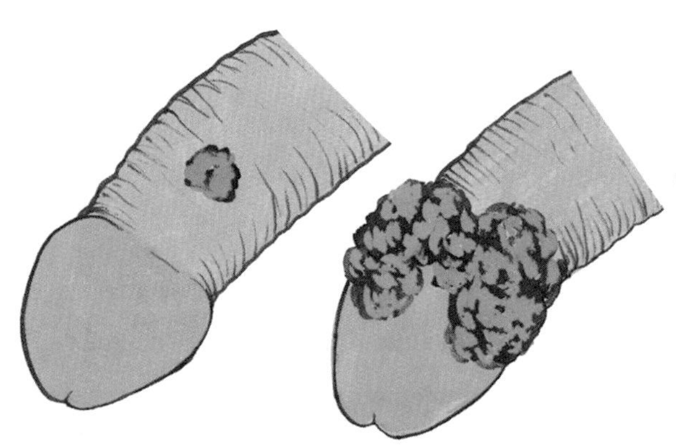

FIGURE 21.5

Squamous cell carcinoma of the penis, showing flat-ulcerating (A) and cauliflower-papillary (B) patterns of growth at common locations.

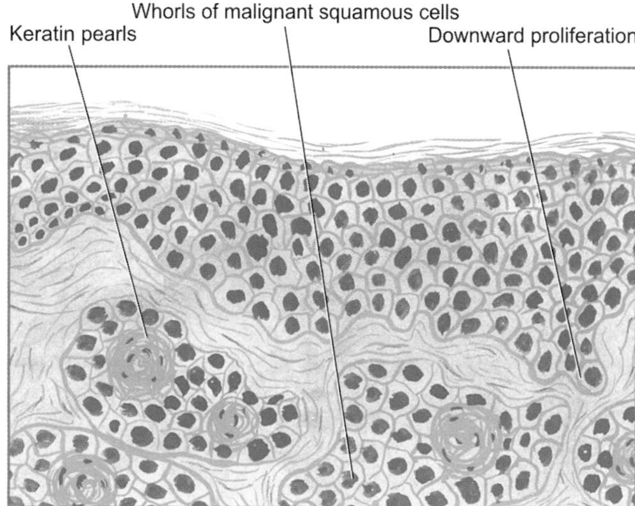

FIGURE 21.6

Squamous cell carcinoma. Microscopic features show whorls of malignant squamous cells with central keratin pearls.

penis is quite rare in Jews and Muslims who have a ritual of circumcision early in life. In India, cancer of the penis is rare in Muslims who practice circumcision as a religious rite in infancy, whereas Hindus who do not normally circumcise have higher incidence. Circumcision provides protection against penile cancer due to prevention of accumulation of smegma which is believed to be carcinogenic. The greatest incidence of penile cancer is between 45 and 60 years.

PATHOLOGIC CHANGES. ***Grossly,*** the tumour is located, in decreasing frequency, on frenum, prepuce, glans and coronal sulcus. The tumour may be cauliflower-like and papillary, or flat and ulcerating (Fig. 21.5).

Histologically, squamous cell carcinoma of both fungating and ulcerating type is generally well differentiated to moderately-differentiated type (Fig. 21.6) which resembles in morphology to similar cancer elsewhere in the body (COLOUR PLATE X: CL 38).

The tumour metastasises via lymphatics to regional lymph nodes. Visceral metastases by haematogenous route are uncommon and occur in advanced cases only.

PROSTATE

NORMAL STRUCTURE

The prostate gland in the normal adult weighs approximately 20 gm. It surrounds the commencement of the urethra in the male and is composed of 5 lobes during embryonic development—anterior, middle, posterior and two lateral lobes. But at birth, the five lobes fuse to form 3 distinct lobes—two major lateral lobes and a small median lobe (Fig. 21.7, A).

Histologically, the prostate is composed of tubular alveoli (acini) embedded in fibromuscular tissue mass. The glandular epithelium forms infoldings and consists of 2 layers—a basal layer of low cuboidal cells and an inner layer of mucus-secreting tall columnar cells. The alveoli are separated by thick fibromuscular septa containing abundant smooth muscle fibres.

The prostate has numerous blood vessels and nerves. In addition to nervous control, the prostate is an endocrine-dependent organ. Based on hormonal responsiveness, the prostate is divided into 2 separate parts:

- *the inner periurethral female part* which is sensitive to oestrogen and androgen; and
- *outer subcapsular true male part* which is sensitive to androgen.

While benign nodular hyperplasia occurs in the periurethral part distorting and compressing the centrally located urethral lumen, the prostatic carcinoma usually arises from the outer subcapsular part in which case it does not compress the urethra (Fig. 21.7, B, C).

Prostate is involved in 3 important pathologic processes: prostatitis, nodular hyperplasia and carcinoma.

PROSTATITIS

Inflammation of the prostate i.e. prostatitis, may be acute, chronic and granulomatous types.

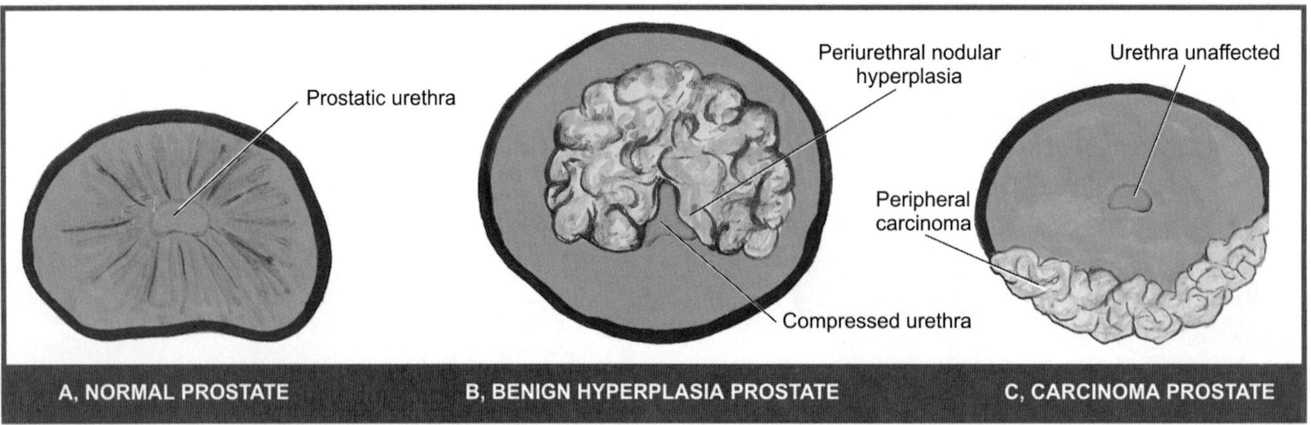

FIGURE 21.7

Normal prostate, benign nodular hyperplasia and prostatic carcinoma. The nodule in case of benign nodular hyperplasia located in the inner periurethral part compresses the prostatic urethra (B) while prostatic carcinoma generally arises in the peripheral glands and, thus, does not compress the urethra (C).

Acute Prostatitis

Acute focal or diffuse suppurative inflammation of the prostate is not uncommon. It occurs most commonly due to ascent of bacteria from the urethra, less often by descent from the upper urinary tract or bladder, and occasionally by lymphogenous or haematogenous spread from a distant focus of infection. The infection may occur spontaneously or may be a complication of urethral manipulation such as by catheterisation, cystoscopy, urethral dilatation and surgical procedures on the prostate. The common pathogens are those which cause UTI, most frequently *E. coli,* and others such as *Klebsiella, Proteus, Pseudomonas, Enterobacter,* gonococci, staphylococci and streptococci. The diagnosis is made by culture of urine specimen.

*PATHOLOGIC CHANGES. **Grossly,*** the prostate is enlarged, swollen and tense. Cut section shows multiple abscesses and foci of necrosis.

Histologically, the prostatic acini are dilated and filled with neutrophilic exudate. There may be diffuse acute inflammatory infiltrate. Oedema, hyperaemia and foci of necrosis frequently accompany acute inflammatory involvement.

Chronic Prostatitis

Chronic prostatitis is more common and foci of chronic inflammation are frequently present in the prostate of men above 40 years of age. Chronic prostatitis is usually asymptomatic but may cause allergic reactions, iritis, neuritis or arthritis.

Chronic prostatitis is of 2 types—bacterial and abacterial.

- **Chronic bacterial prostatitis** is caused in much the same way and by the same organisms as the acute prostatitis. It is generally a consequence of recurrent UTI. Diagnosis is made by detection of more than 10-12 leucocytes per high power field in expressed prostatic secretions, and by positive culture of urine specimen and prostatic secretions. This condition is more difficult to treat since antibiotics penetrate the prostate poorly.
- **Chronic abacterial prostatitis** is more common these days. There is no history of recurrent UTI and culture of urine and prostatic secretions is always negative, though leucocytosis is demonstrable in prostatic secretions. The pathogens implicated are *Chlamydia trachomatis* and *Ureaplasma urealyticum.*

PATHOLOGIC CHANGES. Pathologic changes in both bacterial and abacterial prostatitis are similar. ***Grossly,*** the prostate may be enlarged, fibrosed and shrunken.

Histologically, the diagnosis of chronic prostatitis is made by foci of lymphocytes, plasma cells, macrophages and neutrophils within the prostatic substance. Corpora amylacea, prostatic calculi and foci of squamous metaplasia in the prostatic acini may accompany inflammatory changes. Seminal vesicles are invariably involved.

Granulomatous Prostatitis

Granulomatous prostatitis is a variety of chronic prostatitis, probably caused by leakage of prostatic secretions into the tissue, or could be of autoimmune origin.

PATHOLOGIC CHANGES. Grossly, the gland is firm to hard, giving the clinical impression of prostatic carcinoma on rectal examination.

Histologically, the inflammatory reaction consists of macrophages, lymphocytes, plasma cells and some multinucleate giant cells. The condition may be confused with tuberculous prostatitis.

NODULAR HYPERPLASIA

Non-neoplastic tumour-like enlargement of the prostate, commonly termed benign nodular hyperplasia (BNH) or benign enlargement of prostate (BEP), is a very common condition in men and considered by some as normal ageing process. It becomes increasingly more frequent above the age of 50 years and its incidence approaches 75-80% in men above 80 years. However, symptomatic BEP producing urinary tract obstruction and requiring surgical treatment occurs in 5-10% of cases only.

ETIOLOGY. The cause of BEP has not been fully established. However, a few etiologic factors such as *endocrinologic, racial, inflammation* and *arteriosclerosis* have been implicated but endocrine basis for hyperplasia has been more fully investigated and considered a strong possibility in its genesis. It has been found that both sexes elaborate androgen and oestrogen, though the level of androgen is high in males and that of oestrogen is high in females. With advancing age, there is decline in the level of androgen and a corresponding rise of oestrogen in the males. The periurethral inner prostate which is primarily involved in BEP is responsive to the rising level of oestrogen, whereas the outer prostate which is mainly involved in the carcinoma is responsive to androgen. A plausible hypothesis suggested is that there is synergistic stimulation of the prostate by both hormones—the *oestrogen* acting to sensitise the prostatic tissue to the growth promoting effect of *dihydroxytestosterone* derived from plasma testosterone.

PATHOLOGIC CHANGES. Grossly, the enlarged prostate is nodular, smooth and firm and weighs 2-4 times its normal weight i.e. may weigh up to 40-80 gm. The appearance on cut section varies depending upon whether the hyperplasia is predominantly of the glandular or fibromuscular tissue. In *primarily glandular BEP* the tissue is yellow-pink, soft, honeycombed, and milky fluid exudes, whereas in *mainly fibromuscular BEP* the cut surface is firm, homogeneous and does not exude milky fluid. The hyperplastic nodule forms a mass mainly in the inner periurethral prostatic gland so that the surrounding prostatic tissue forms a false capsule which enables the surgeon to enucleate the nodular masses. The left-over peripheral prostatic tissue may sometimes undergo recurrent nodular enlargement or may develop carcinoma later.

Histologically, in every case, there is hyperplasia of all three tissue elements in varying proportions—glandular, fibrous and muscular (Fig. 21.8) (COLOUR PLATE XXIX: CL 115):

- *Glandular hyperplasia* predominates in most cases and is identified by exaggerated intra-acinar papillary infoldings with delicate fibrovascular cores. The lining epithelium is two-layered: the inner tall columnar mucus-secreting with poorly-defined borders, and the outer cuboidal to flattened epithelium with basal nuclei.
- *Fibromuscular hyperplasia* when present as dominant component appears as aggregates of spindle cells forming an appearance akin to fibromyoma of the uterus.

In addition to glandular and/or fibromuscular hyperplasia, other histologic features frequently found include foci of lymphocytic aggregates, small areas of infarction, corpora amylacea and foci of squamous metaplasia.

CLINICAL FEATURES. Clinically, the symptomatic cases develop symptoms due to complications such as

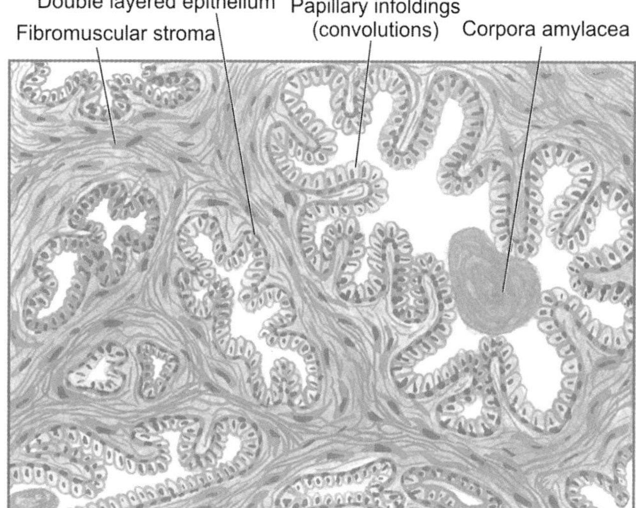

FIGURE 21.8

Nodular hyperplasia of the prostate, microscopic appearance. There are areas of intra-acinar papillary infoldings (convolutions) lined by two layers of epithelium with basal polarity of nuclei.

urethral obstruction and secondary effects on the bladder (e.g. hypertrophy, cystitis), ureter (e.g. hydroureter) and kidneys (e.g. hydronephrosis). The presenting features include frequency, nocturia, difficulty in micturition, pain, haematuria and sometimes, the patients present with acute retention of urine requiring immediate catheterisation.

CARCINOMA OF PROSTATE

Cancer of the prostate is the second most common form of cancer in males, followed in frequency by lung cancer. It is a disease of men above the age of 50 years and its prevalence increases with increasing age so that more than 50% of men 80 years old have asymptomatic (latent) carcinoma of the prostate. Many a times, carcinoma of the prostate is small and detected as microscopic foci in a prostate removed for BEP or found incidentally at autopsy. Thus, it is common to classify carcinoma of the prostate into the following 4 types:

1. **Latent carcinoma.** This is found unexpectedly as a small focus of carcinoma in the prostate during autopsy studies in men dying of other causes. Its incidence in autopsies has been variously reported as 25-35%.

2. **Incidental carcinoma.** About 15-20% of prostatectomies done for BEP reveal incidental carcinoma of the prostate.

3. **Occult carcinoma.** This is the type in which the patient has no symptoms of prostatic carcinoma but shows evidence of metastases on clinical examination and investigations.

4. **Clinical carcinoma.** Clinical prostatic carcinoma is the type detected by rectal examination and other investigations and confirmed by pathologic examination of biopsy of the prostate.

ETIOLOGY. The cause of prostatic cancer remains obscure. However, a few factors have been suspected. These are as under:

1. **Endocrinologic factors.** Androgens are considered essential for development and maintenance of prostatic epithelium. But how androgens are responsible for causing malignant transformation is not yet clear. However, the etiologic role of androgens is supported by the following indirect evidences:

i) Orchiectomy causes arrest of metastatic prostatic cancer disease (testis being the main source of testosterone).

ii) Administration of oestrogen causes regression of prostatic carcinoma.

iii) Cancer of the prostate is extremely rare in eunuchs and in patients with Klinefelter's syndrome.

iv) Cancer of the prostate begins at the stage of life when androgen levels are high. However, the cancer may remain latent with decline in androgen level with advancing age.

2. **Racial and geographic influences.** There are some racial and geographic differences in the incidence of prostatic cancer. It is uncommon in Japanese and Chinese, while the prevalence is high in Americans. American blacks have a markedly higher incidence as compared to whites.

3. **Environmental influences.** It is possible that some common, as yet unidentified, environmental factors and carcinogens may play a role in the evolution of prostatic cancer.

4. **Nodular hyperplasia.** Though nodular prostatic hyperplasia has been suggested by some as precursor for development of prostatic cancer, it is considered unlikely. Most prostatic cancers develop in the periphery of the gland while BEP occurs in the periurethral part of the gland. Any concomitant occurrence of the two diseases may be considered as aging process. Approximately 15-20% of nodular hyperplastic prostates harbour carcinoma.

5. **Genetic factors.** The possibility of genetic basis of prostatic cancer has been suggested by the observations of familial clustering and in first degree relatives. Recently prostatic cancer susceptibility gene has been identified in familial cases.

HISTOGENESIS. Histogenesis of prostatic adenocarcinoma has been documented recently as arising from premalignant stage of *prostatic intraepithelial neoplasia (PIN)*. PIN refers to multiple foci of cytologically atypical luminal cells overlying diminished number of basal cells in prostatic ducts and is a forerunner of invasive prostatic carcinoma. Based on cytologic atypia, PIN may be low grade to high grade. PIN of high grade progresses to prostatic adenocarcinoma.

PATHOLOGIC CHANGES. ***Grossly,*** the prostate may be enlarged, normal in size or smaller than normal. In 95% of cases, prostatic carcinoma is located in the peripheral zone, especially in the posterior lobe. The malignant prostate is firm and fibrous. Cut section is homogeneous and contains irregular yellowish areas. ***Microscopically,*** 4 histologic types are described—adenocarcinoma, transitional cell carcinoma, squamous cell carcinoma and undifferentiated carcinoma.

Chapter Twenty One

However, *adenocarcinoma* is the most common type found in 96% of cases and is the one generally referred to as carcinoma of the prostate. The other three histologic types are rare and resemble in morphology with similar malignant tumours elsewhere in the body.

The histologic characteristics of adenocarcinoma of the prostate are as under (Fig. 21.9) (COLOUR PLATE XXIX: CL 116):

1. Architectural disturbance: In contrast to convoluted appearance of the glands seen in normal and hyperplastic prostate, there is loss of intra-acinar papillary convolutions. The groups of acini are either closely packed in back-to-back arrangement without intervening stroma or are haphazardly distributed.

2. Stroma: Normally, fibromuscular sling surrounds the acini, whereas malignant acini have little or no stroma between them. The tumour cells may penetrate and replace the fibromuscular stroma.

3. Gland pattern: Most frequently, the glands in well-differentiated prostatic adenocarcinoma are small or medium-sized, lined by a single layer of cuboidal or low columnar cells. Moderately-differentiated tumours have cribriform or fenestrated glandular appearance. Poorly-differentiated tumours have little or no glandular arrangement but instead show solid or trabecular pattern.

4. Tumour cells: In many cases, the individual tumour cells in prostatic carcinoma do not show usual morphologic features of malignancy. The tumour cells may be clear, dark and eosinophilic cells. *Clear cells* have foamy cytoplasm, *dark cells* have homogeneous basophilic cytoplasm, and *eosinophilic cells* have granular cytoplasm. The cells may show varying degree of anaplasia and nuclear atypia but is generally slight.

5. Invasion: One of the important diagnostic features of malignancy in prostate is the early and frequent occurrence of invasion of intra-prostatic *perineural spaces.* Lymphatic and vascular invasion may be present but are difficult to detect.

SPREAD. The tumour spreads within the gland by direct extension, and to distant sites by metastases.

Direct spread. Direct extension of the tumour occurs into the prostatic capsule and beyond. In late stage, the tumour may extend into the bladder neck, seminal vesicles, trigone and ureteral openings.

Metastases. Distant spread occurs by both lymphatic and haematogenous routes. The rich lymphatic network

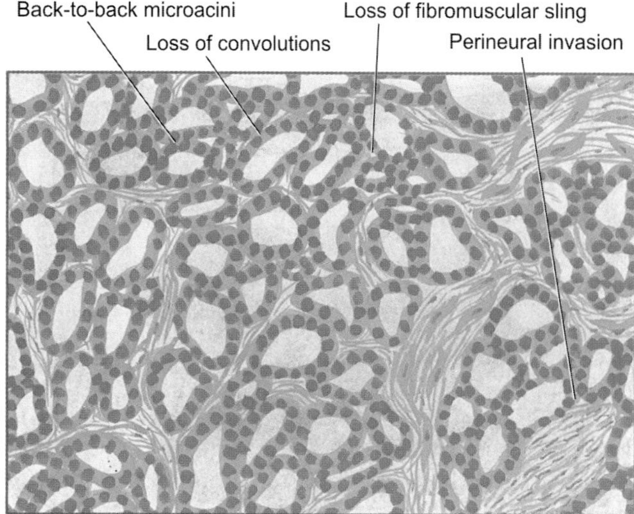

FIGURE 21.9

Carcinoma of the prostate, small acinar type.

surrounding the prostate is the main mode of spread to the sacral, iliac and para-aortic lymph nodes. The earliest metastasis occur to the obturator lymph node. Haematogenous spread leads most often to osteoblastic *osseous metastases,* especially to pelvis, and lumbar spine; other sites are lungs, kidneys, breast and brain. The route of blood-borne metastases may be retrograde spread by prostatic venous plexus or via systemic circulation.

CLINICAL FEATURES. By the time symptoms appear, the carcinoma of prostate is usually palpable on rectal examination. In such symptomatic cases, clinical features are: urinary obstruction with dysuria, frequency, retention of urine, haematuria, and in 10% of cases pain in the back due to skeletal metastases. Per-rectal examination shows a hard and nodular gland fixed to the surrounding tissues.

Clinical staging of carcinoma prostate takes into account the following:

- The tumour found incidentally or a clinically unsuspected cancer in prostate removed for benign disorder *(Stage A).*
- The tumour palpable by rectal digital examination but confined to the prostate *(Stage B).*
- The tumour has extended locally beyond the prostate into the surrounding tissues *(Stage C).*
- The tumour is associated with distant metastases *(Stage D).*

Such clinical staging has good correlation with histologic grading and, thus, has a prognostic significance. *Mostofi's (WHO) histologic grading* categorising prostate cancer into grade I (well-differentiated), grade II (moderately differentiated) and grade III (poorly differentiated) has largely been replaced with *Gleason's microscopic grading system* which is based on two features:

i) the degree of glandular differentiation; and

ii) the growth pattern of the tumour in relation to the stroma.

These features are assessed by low-power examination of the prostatic tissue. For clinical staging of prostate cancer, *TNM system* is considered international standard.

The diagnosis of prostatic carcinoma is made by cytologic, biochemical, radiologic, ultrasonographic and pathologic methods. Two **tumour markers** employed commonly for diagnosis and monitoring the prognosis of prostatic carcinoma are as under:

- **Prostatic acid phosphatase (PAP)** is secreted by prostatic epithelium. Elevation of serum level of PAP is found in cases of prostatic cancer which have extended beyond the capsule or have metastasised. A reading of 3-5 KA units (normal 1-3 KA units) is highly suspicious but above 5 KA units is diagnostic of prostatic carcinoma. PAP can also be demonstrated in the normal prostatic tissues.

- **Prostate-specific antigen (PSA)** can be detected by immunohistochemical method in the malignant prostatic epithelium as well as in the serum. PSA assay is also useful in deciding whether the metastasis originated from the prostate or not. PSA assay is also helpful in distinguishing high-grade prostatic cancer from urothelial carcinoma, colonic carcinoma, lymphoma and prostatitis. PSA level is generally higher in low-grade tumours than in high-grade tumours.

Treatment of prostatic carcinoma consists of surgery, radiotherapy and hormonal therapy. The hormonal dependence of cancer of prostate consists of depriving the tumour cells of growth-promoting influence of testosterone. This can be achieved by orchiectomy and by administration of oestrogen.

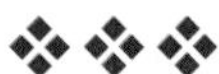

The Female Genital Tract

22

VULVA

NORMAL STRUCTURE

The vulva consists of structures of ectodermal origin—labia majora, labia minora, mons pubis, clitoris, vestibule, hymen, Bartholin's glands and minor vestibular glands. The mons pubis and labia majora are covered externally by skin with hair follicles, sebaceous glands and sweat glands including apocrine glands. The inner surface of labia majora, labia minora and vestibule are covered by stratified squamous epithelium. The clitoris is made up of vascular erectile tissue. Bartholin's or vulvovaginal glands are located one on each side of the mass of tissue forming labia majora. The glands are racemose type and their secretions are released during sexual excitement.

Since vulva is of ectodermal origin, the common inflammatory conditions affecting it are similar to those found on the skin generally. A few specific conditions such as Bartholin's cyst and abscess, vulvar dystrophy and certain tumours are described below.

BARTHOLIN'S CYST AND ABSCESS

Inflammation of Bartholin's vulvovaginal glands (Bartholin's adenitis) may occur due to bacterial infection, notably gonorrhoeal infection. Infection may be *acute* or *chronic*.

■ **Acute Bartholin's adenitis** occurs from obstruction and dilatation of the duct by infection resulting in formation of a Bartholin's abscess. The condition presents with intense pain, swelling and fluctuant mass which can be incised and drained.

Microscopic examination shows the usual appearance of acute suppurative inflammation with neutrophilic infiltration, hyperaemia, oedema and epithelial degeneration.

■ **Chronic Bartholin's adenitis** results from a less virulent infection so that the process is slow and prolonged. Alternatively, the chronic process evolves from repeated attacks of less severe acute inflammation which may be short of abscess formation and resolves incompletely. In either case, the chronic inflammatory process terminates into fluid-filled Bartholin's cyst. The resulting cyst may be quite large, 3-5 cm in diameter and readily palpable in the perineum, but may remain asymptomatic for years.

Histologic examination shows variable lining of the cyst varying from the transitional epithelium of the normal duct to a flattened lining because of increased intracystic pressure. The cyst wall may show chronic inflammatory infiltrate and a few mucus-secreting acini.

NON-NEOPLASTIC EPITHELIAL DISORDERS

The older term vulvar dystrophy has been replaced by non-neoplastic epithelial disorders of skin and mucosa of vulva. The term is applied to chronic lesions of the vulva characterised clinically by white, plaque-like, pruritic mucosal thickenings and pathologically by disorders of epithelial growth. Clinicians often use the term *'leukoplakia'* for such white lesions. But white lesions may represent other depigmented conditions as well, such as vitiligo, inflammatory dermatoses, carcinoma in *situ,* Paget's disease or even invasive carcinoma and thus usage of the term leukoplakia by pathologists is not desirable.

Currently, non-neoplastic epithelial disorders of skin of vulva includes 2 lesions:

1. Lichen sclerosus (older term: atrophic dystrophy).
2. Squamous hyperplasia (older term: hyperplastic dystrophy).

The two types of lesions may coexist in the same patient.

Lichen Sclerosus

Lichen sclerosus may occur anywhere in the skin (Chapter 24) but is more common and more extensive in the vulva in post menopausal women. The lesions appear as multiple, small, coalescent, yellowish-blue macules or papules which produce thin and shiny parchment-like skin. The lesions may extend from vulva onto the perianal and perineal area. Clinically, the patient, usually a post-menopausal woman, complains of intense pruritus which may produce excoriation of the affected skin. Eventually, there is progressive shrinkage and atrophy resulting in narrowing of the introitus, clinically referred to as *kraurosis vulvae.*

PATHOLOGIC CHANGES. Microscopically, the following characteristics are seen (Fig. 22.1,A):

1. Hyperkeratosis of the surface layer.
2. Thinning of the epidermis with disappearance of rete ridges.
3. Amorphous homogeneous degenerative change in the dermal collagen.
4. Chronic inflammatory infiltrate in the mid-dermis.

Lichen sclerosus is *not* a premalignant lesion and responds favourably to topical treatment with androgens.

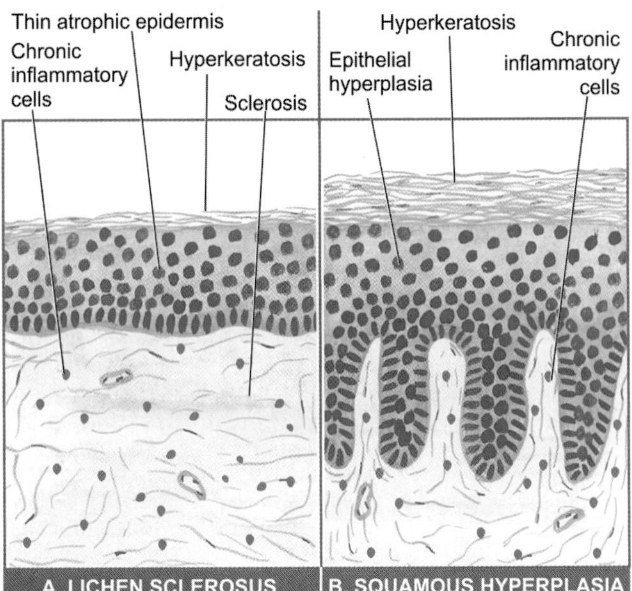

FIGURE 22.1

Non-neoplastic epithelial disorders of vulval skin.

Squamous Hyperplasia

Squamous hyperplasia is characterised by white, thickened vulvar lesions which are usually itchy. The cause is unknown but symptomatic relief results from use of topical treatment with corticosteroids.

PATHOLOGIC CHANGES. The histologic characteristics are as under (Fig. 22.1,B):

1. Hyperkeratosis.
2. Hyperplasia of squamous epithelium with elongation of rete ridges.
3. Increased mitotic activity of squamous layers but cytologically no atypia.
4. Chronic inflammatory infiltrate in the underlying dermis.

A small proportion of cases of hyperplastic dystrophy (1-4%) may show cytologic atypia and produce vulvar dysplasia which may progress to vulvar carcinoma *in situ* and invasive carcinoma.

VULVAL TUMOURS

Vulva is the site of a variety of benign and malignant neoplasms which are in common with skin neoplasms elsewhere in the body. These include papillomas, fibromas, neurofibromas, angiomas, lipomas, sweat gland tumours, squamous cell carcinoma, verrucous carcinoma, malignant melanoma and mesenchymal sarcomas. However, a few tumours peculiar to the vulva such as stromal polyps, papillary hidradenoma, condyloma acuminatum, extra-mammary Paget's disease, vulval carcinoma and intra-epithelial neoplasia are discussed below. Mention has already been made above about dysplasia and carcinoma *in situ* in the vulva.

Stromal Polyps

Stromal (fibroepithelial) polyps or acrochordons may form in the vulva or vagina. There may be single or multiple polypoid masses.

Histologically, they are covered by an orderly stratified squamous epithelium. The stroma consists of loose fibrous and myxomatous connective tissue with some adipose tissue and blood vessels.

Papillary Hidradenoma (Hidradenoma Papilliferum)

This is a benign tumour arising from apocrine sweat glands of the vulva. Most commonly, it is located in the labia or in the perianal region as a small sharply circumscribed nodule.

Histologically, the tumour lies in the dermis under a normal epidermis. The tumour consists of papillary structures composed of fibrovascular stalk and covered by double layer of epithelial cells—a layer of flattened myoepithelial cells and an overlying layer of columnar cells.

Condyloma Acuminatum

Condyloma acuminata or venereal warts are benign papillary lesions of squamous epithelium which can be transmitted venereally to male sex partner. They may be solitary but more frequently are multiple forming soft warty masses. The common locations are the anus, perineum, vaginal wall, vulva and vagina. They are induced by human papilloma virus (HPV), particularly type 6 and 11.

Histologically, they are identical to their counterparts on male external genitalia (Chapter 21). The features consist of a tree-like proliferation of stratified squamous epithelium, showing marked acanthosis, hyperkeratosis, parakeratosis, papillomatosis and perinuclear vacuolisation of epithelium called *koilocytosis,* indicative of HPV infection. The papillary projections consist of fibrovascular stoma.

Condylomas are benign lesions and regress spontaneously except in immunosuppressed individuals.

Extra-Mammary Paget's Disease

Paget's disease of the vulva is a rare condition which has skin manifestations like those of Paget's disease of the nipple (Chapter 23). The affected skin appears as map-like, red, scaly, elevated and indurated area, most frequently on the labia majora.

Histologically, extra-mammary Paget's disease is identified by the presence of large, pale, carcinoma cells lying singly or in small clusters within the epidermis and adnexal structures. These cells characteristically have halo which stains positively with PAS, alcian blue and mucicarmine and are thus believed to be of apocrine epithelial origin.

Unlike Paget's disease of the breast in which case there is always an underlying ductal carcinoma, extra-mammary Paget's disease is confined to epidermis in most cases and only a small proportion of cases have an underlying adenocarcinoma. Prognosis is good if there is no invasion but occasional cases progress into invasive carcinoma.

Carcinoma and Vulval Intraepithelial Neoplasia

Squamous cell carcinoma and vulval intraepithelial neoplasia (VIN) are morphologically similar to those in the cervix and vagina. The etiologic role of certain viruses in carcinogenesis, particularly HPV types 16 and 18, in these sites is well known (high risk types). Mention has already been made about the preceding stage of vulval epithelial disorders, particularly squamous hyperplasia, in the development of these lesions. Vulval carcinoma constitutes 3% of all female genital tract cancers. The usual age for development of cancer or VIN is the 4th to 6th decade.

Grossly, VIN and vulval carcinoma in early stage is a 'white' lesion (leukoplakia) while later the area develops an exophytic or endophytic (ulcerative) growth pattern. A staging system for vulval cancer based on 2 cm in greatest dimension has been described.

Microscopically, these lesions are squamous cell type with varying anaplasia and depth of invasion depending upon the stage. HPV-positive tumours are more often poorly-differentiated squamous cell carcinoma while HPV-negative are well-differentiated keratinising type. *Verrucous carcinoma* is a rare variant which is a fungating tumour but is locally malignant.

Clinical staging for vulval carcinoma (Table 22.1) based on tumour size and extent of spread has been

TABLE 22.1: FIGO Clinical Staging of Carcinoma of the Vulva.

Stage		
Stage	0	Carcinoma *in situ*
Stage	I	Tumour confined to the vulva and/or perineum; 2 cm or less in diameter.
Stage	II	Tumour confined to the vulva and/or perineum; more than 2 cm in diameter.
Stage	III	Tumour of any size with (1) adjacent spread to the lower urethra and/ or vagina, or the anus, and/or (2) unilateral regional lymph node metastasis.
Stage	IVA	Tumour invades any of the following-upper urethra, bladder mucosa, rectal mucosa, pelvic bone, and/or bilateral regional node metastasis.
Stage	IVB	Any distant metastasis including pelvic lymph nodes.

described by International Federation of Gynaecology and Obstetrics termed FIGO staging.

VAGINA

NORMAL STRUCTURE

The vagina consists of a collapsed cylinder extending between vestibule externally and the cervix internally.

Histologically, the vaginal wall consists of 3 layers: an *outer* fibrous, a *middle* muscular and an *inner* epithelial. The muscular coat has a double layer of smooth muscle. The epithelial layer consists of stratified squamous epithelium which undergoes cytologic changes under hormonal stimuli. Oestrogen increases its thickness such as during reproductive years, whereas the epithelium is thin in childhood, and atrophic after menopause when oestrogen stimulation is minimal.

Primary diseases of the vagina are uncommon. The only conditions which require to be described here are vaginitis and certain tumours.

VAGINITIS

The adult vaginal mucosa is relatively resistant to gonococcal infection because of its histology. However, certain other infections are quite common in the vagina. These are:

- Bacterial e.g. streptococci, staphylococci, *Escherichia coli, Haemophilus vaginalis.*
- Fungal e.g. *Candida albicans.*
- Protozoal e.g. *Trichomonas vaginalis.*
- Viral e.g. Herpes simplex.

The most common causes of vaginitis are *Candida* (moniliasis) and *Trichomonas* (trichomoniasis). The hyphae of *Candida* can be seen in the vaginal smears. Similarly, the protozoa, *Trichomonas,* can be identified in smears. These infections are particularly common in pregnant and diabetic women and may involve both vulva and vagina.

TUMOURS

Vaginal cysts such as Gartner's duct (Wolffian) cyst lined by glandular epithelium and vaginal inclusion cyst arising from inclusion of vaginal epithelium are more common benign vaginal neoplasms. Other uncommon benign tumours are papillomas, fibromas, lipomas, angiomas and leiomyomas and resemble their counterparts elsewhere in the body. Primary malignancies of the vagina are rare and include carcinoma (squamous cell carcinoma and adenocarcinoma) and embryonal rhabdomyosarcoma (sarcoma botyroides).

Carcinoma of Vagina

Primary carcinoma of the vagina is an uncommon tumour. Squamous cell dysplasia or vaginal intraepithelial neoplasia occur less frequently as compared to the cervix or vulva and can be detected by Pap smears. Invasive carcinoma of the vagina includes two types:

1. **Squamous cell carcinoma** of vagina constitutes less than 2% of all gynaecologic malignancies and is similar in morphology as elsewhere in the female genital tract. The role of HPV type 16 in its etiology and the possibility of an extension from cervical carcinoma to the vagina have been emphasised.

2. **Adenocarcinoma of the vagina** is much less than squamous cell carcinoma of the vagina. It may be endometrioid or mucinous type. The significance of association of diethylstilbestrol administered during pregancy to the mother with development of adenocarcinoma of the vagina in the daughter has been discussed in Chapter 8.

Clinical staging of carcinoma of vagina proposed by FIGO is given in Table 22.2.

TABLE 22.2: FIGO Clinical Staging of Carcinoma of the Vagina.

Stage		
Stage	0	Carcinoma *in situ.*
Stage	I	Carcinoma is limited to the vaginal wall.
Stage	II	Carcinoma has involved the subvaginal tissue but has not extended to the pelvic wall.
Stage	III	Carcinoma has extended to the pelvic wall
Stage	IV	Carcinoma has extended beyond the true pelvis or has clinically involved the mucosa of the bladder or rectum.
Stage	IVA	Spread of the growth to adjacent organs and/ or direct extension beyond the true pelvis.
Stage	IVB	Spread to distant organs.

Embryonal Rhabdomyosarcoma (Sarcoma Botyroides)

This is an unusual and rare malignant tumour occurring in infants and children under 5 years of age. The common location is anterior vaginal wall. Similar tumours may occur in the urinary bladder (Chapter 20), orbit, external auditory canal and biliary tract.

PATHOLOGIC CHANGES. Grossly, the tumour is characterised by bulky and polypoid grape-like mass (*botyroides* = grape) that fills and projects out of the vagina.

Histologically, the features are as under:

1. Groups of round to fusiform tumour cells are characteristically lying underneath the vaginal epithelium, called *cambium layer* of tumour cells.
2. The central core of polypoid masses is composed of loose and myxoid stroma with many inflammatory cells.

The tumour invades extensively in the pelvis and metastasises to regional lymph nodes and distant sites such as to lungs and liver. Radical surgery combined with chemotherapy offers some benefit.

CERVIX

NORMAL STRUCTURE

The cervix consists of an *internal os* communicating with the endometrial cavity above, and an *external os* opening into the vagina below. *Ectocervix* (exocervix) or *portio vaginalis* is the part of the cervix exposed to the vagina and is lined by stratified squamous epithelium, whereas the endocervix is continuous with the endocervical canal and is lined by a single layer of tall columnar mucus-secreting epithelium. The endocervical mucosa is thrown into folds resulting in formation of clefts and tunnels, commonly referred to as cervical glands. The junction of the ectocervix and endocervix—*junctional mucosa,* consists of gradual transition between squamous and columnar epithelia (squamo-columnar junction) and is clinically and pathologically significant landmark. The cervical mucus varies during the menstrual cycle, being viscus after menses, but under the influence of oestrogen becomes thin which on drying forms fern-like pattern on glass slide. The cervical mucosa undergoes changes under the influence of hormones and during pregnancy.

Lesions of the cervix are rather common. Of great significance are cervicitis, certain benign tumours, dysplasia, carcinoma *in situ* and invasive carcinoma.

CERVICITIS

Some degree of cervical inflammation is present in virtually all multiparous women and some nulliparous women. The normal intact ectocervical stratified epithelium is usually more resistant to infection whereas the endocervical columnar epithelium bears the brunt of the initial inflammation.

Cervicitis may be specific or nonspecific, acute or chronic. *Specific cervicitis* may be caused by tuberculosis, syphilis, granuloma inguinale, lymphogranuloma venereum, chlamydia and chancroid. *Nonspecific cervicitis* is more frequent and is generally divided into acute and chronic forms, the latter being quite common.

ACUTE CERVICITIS. Acute cervicitis is usually associated with puerperium or gonococcal infection. Other causes are primary chancre and infection with herpes simplex.

Grossly, the cervix shows everted endocervical mucosa which is red and oedematous.

Histologically, there is infiltration of the subepithelial and periglandular tissue with neutrophils, and there is oedema and congestion. The mucosa may be ulcerated and haemorrhagic.

CHRONIC CERVICITIS. Chronic nonspecific cervicitis is encountered quite frequently and is the common cause of leukorrhoea. The most common organisms responsible for chronic cervicitis are the normal mixed vaginal flora that includes streptococci, enterococci (e.g. *E. coli*) and staphylococci. Other infecting organisms include gonococci, *Trichomonas vaginalis, Candida albicans* and herpes simplex. Factors predisposing to chronic cervicitis are sexual intercourse, trauma of childbirth, instrumentation and excess or deficiency of oestrogen.

Grossly, there is eversion of ectocervix with hyperaemia, oedema and granular surface. Nabothian (retention) cysts may be grossly visible from the surface as pearly grey vesicles.

Histologically, chronic cervicitis is characterised by extensive subepithelial inflammatory infiltrate of lymphocytes, plasma cells, large mononuclear cells and a few neutrophils. There may be formation of lymphoid follicles termed *follicular cervicitis.* The surface epithelium may be normal, or may show squamous metaplasia. The squamous epithelium of the ectocervix in cases of uterine prolapse may develop surface keratinisation and hyperkeratosis, so called *epidermidisation.* Areas of squamous metaplasia and hyperkeratosis may be mistaken on cursory microscopic look for a well-differentiated squamous carcinoma.

TUMOURS

Both benign and malignant tumours are common in the cervix. In addition, cervix is the site of 'shades of grey' lesions that include cervical dysplasia and carcinoma *in situ* (cervical intraepithelial neoplasia, CIN), currently termed squamous intraepithelial lesions (SIL). Benign tumours of the cervix consist most commonly of cervical polyps. Uncommon benign cervical tumours are leiomyomas, papillomas and condyloma acuminatum which resemble in morphology with similar tumours elsewhere in the genital tract. The most common malignant tumour is epidermoid carcinoma of the cervix.

Cervical Polyps

Cervical polyps are localised benign proliferations of endocervical mucosa though they may protrude through the external os. They are found in 2-5% of adult women and produce irregular vaginal spotting.

PATHOLOGIC CHANGES. Grossly, cervical polyp is a small (upto 5 cm in size), bright red, fragile growth which is frequently pedunculated but may be sessile.
Microscopically, most cervical polyps are endocervical polyps and are covered with endocervical epithelium which may show squamous metaplasia. Less frequently, the covering is by squamous epithelium of the portio vaginalis. The stroma of the polyp is composed of loose and oedematous fibrous tissue with variable degree of inflammatory infiltrate and contains dilated mucus-secreting endocervical glands.

Microglandular Hyperplasia

Microglandular hyperplasia is a benign condition of the cervix in which there is closely packed proliferation of endocervical glands without intervening stroma. The condition is caused by progestrin stimulation such as during pregnancy, postpartum period and in women taking oral contraceptives. Morphologically, condition may be mistaken for well-differentiated adenocarcinoma.

Squamous Intraepithelial Lesion (SIL) (Cervical Intraepithelial Neoplasia, CIN)

TERMINOLOGY. Presently, the terms dysplasia, CIN, carcinoma *in situ*, and SIL are used synonymously (Fig. 22.2):

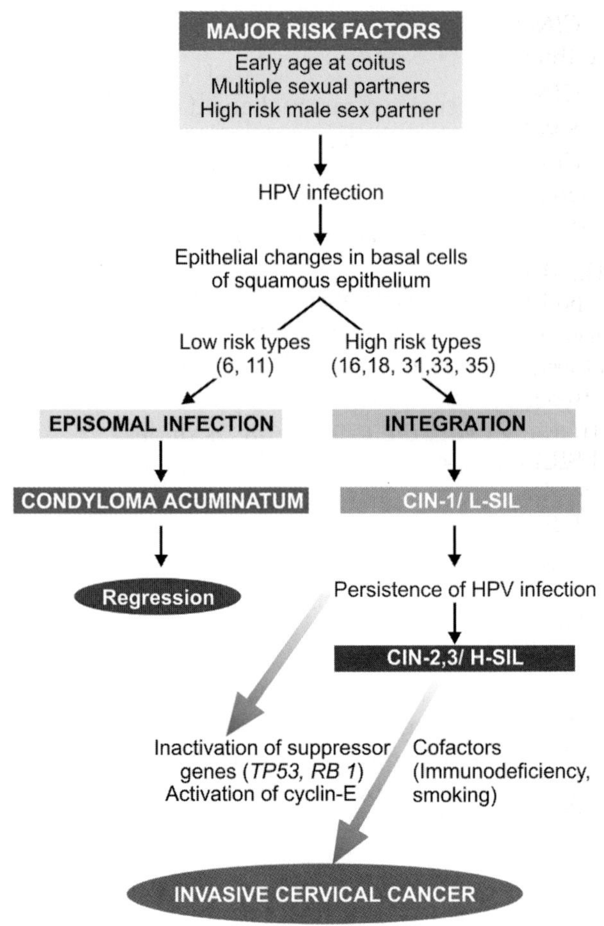

FIGURE 22.2
Role of human papillomavirus (HPV) in the pathogenesis of cervical neoplasia.

DYSPLASIA. The term 'dysplasia' (meaning 'bad moulding') is commonly used for atypical cytologic changes in the layers of squamous epithelium, the changes being progressive (Chapter 3). Depending upon the thickness of squamous epithelium involved by atypical cells, dysplasia is conventionally graded as *mild, moderate* and *severe*. Carcinoma *in situ* is the full-thickness involvement by atypical cells, or in other words carcinoma confined to layers above the basement membrane. At times, severe dysplasia may not be clearly demarcated from carcinoma *in situ*. It is well accepted that invasive cervical cancer evolves through progressive stages of dysplasia and carcinoma *in situ*.

CIN. An alternative classification is to group various grades of dysplasia and carcinoma *in situ* together into cervical intraepithelial neoplasia (CIN) which is similarly graded from grade I to III. According to this concept, the criteria are as under:

- *CIN-1* represents less than one-third involvement of the thickness of epithelium (mild dysplasia);
- *CIN-2* is one-third to two-third involvement (moderate dysplasia); and
- *CIN-3* is full-thickness involvement or equivalent to carcinoma *in situ* (severe dysplasia and carcinoma *in situ*).

SIL. More recently, the National Cancer Institute (NCI) of the US has proposed the *Bethesda System* for reporting cervical and vaginal cytopathology. According to the Bethesda system, the three grades of CIN are readjusted to two grades of squamous intraepithelial lesions (SIL) termed as low-grade SIL (L-SIL) and high-grade SIL (H-SIL) based on cytomorphologic features and HPV types implicated in their etiology as under:

- *L-SIL* corresponds to CIN-1 and is a flat condyloma, having koilocytic atypia, usually related to HPV 6 and 11 infection (i.e. includes mild dysplasia and HPV infection).
- *H-SIL* corresponds to CIN-2 and 3 and has abnormal pleomorphic atypical squamous cells. HPV 16 and 18 are implicated in the etiology of H-SIL (i.e. includes moderate dysplasia, severe dysplasia, and carcinoma *in situ*).

A comparison of these classifications is shown in Table 22.3.

CIN/SIL is a classical example of progression of malignancy through stepwise epithelial changes and that it can be detected early by simple Papanicolaou cytologic test ('Pap smear') (Chapter 29, page 927). The use of Pap smear followed by colposcopy and biopsy confirms the diagnosis which has helped greatly in instituting early effective therapy and thus has reduced the incidence of cervical cancer in the West.

CIN or SIL can develop at any age though it is rare before puberty. Low grade reversible changes arise in young women between 25 and 30 years old, whereas progressive higher grades of epithelial changes develop a decade later. Hence, the desirability of periodic Pap smears on all women after they become sexually active.

ETIOPATHOGENESIS. The biology of CIN/SIL and its relationship to invasive carcinoma of the cervix is well understood by epidemiologic, virologic, cytogenetic, immunologic and ultrastructural studies and is outlined in Fig. 22.2.

1. Epidemiologic studies. Based on epidemiology of large population of women with cervical cancer, several risk factors have been identified which include the following 4 most important factors:

i) Women having *early age of sexual activity.*

ii) Women having *multiple sexual partners.*

iii) Women with *persistent HPV infection* with high risk types of oncogenic virus.

iv) *Potential role of high risk male* sexual partner such as promiscuous male having previous multiple sexual partners, having history of penile condyloma, or male who had previous spouse with cervical cancer.

In addition to the above factors, other epidemiologic observations reveal high incidence of cervical cancer in lower socioeconomic strata, in multiparous women, promiscuous women, cigarette smoking, use of oral contraceptives, HIV infection and immunosuppression, while a low incidence is noted in virgins and nuns.

2. Virologic studies. Human papilloma virus (HPV) infection is strongly implicated in the etiology of cervical cancer. By recombinant DNA hybridisation techniques it has been proved that:

- HPV, most commonly of types 16 and 18, and less often types 31, 33 and 35, together termed *high risk types,* are present in cases of cervical cancer in 75-100% cases.
- HPV types 6 and 11 called *low risk types* are found most frequently in condylomas.
- *Mixed high and low risk types* of HPV may be found in dysplasias.

3. Cytogenetic studies. Cytogenetic studies have shown that low risk HPV types do not integrate in the host cell genome. On the other hand, high risk HPV types are integrated into cervical epithelial cells where they activate cell cycle gene, *cyclin E,* and inactivate tumour suppressor genes, *TP53* and *RB-1 gene,* thus permitting uncontrolled cellular proliferation. However, all women who harbour HPV infection with high risk

TABLE 22.3: Classification of Cervical Intraepithelial Neoplasia/Squamous Intraepithelial Lesion (CIN/SIL).

BETHESDA SYSTEM	HPV TYPES	MORPHOLOGY	CIN	DYSPLASIA
L-SIL	6, 11	Koilocytic atypia, flat condyloma	CIN-1	Mild
H-SIL	16, 18	Progressive cellular atypia, loss of maturation	CIN-2, CIN-3	Moderate, severe, carcinoma *in situ*

L-SIL = low-grade squamous intraepithelial lesions; H-SIL = high-grade squamous intraepithelial lesion; CIN= cervical intraepithelial neoplasia.

type do not develop invasive cancer of the cervix. Women who have persistence of this infection or those who have another cofactor such as cigarette smoking or immunodeficiency, are at greater risk to develop progression of lesions.

4. Immunologic studies. Circulating tumour specific antigens and antibodies are detected in patients of cervical cancer. Antibodies to virus specific antigens are identified on tumour cells and in sera of such patients.

5. Ultrastructural studies. The changes observed on ultrastructural studies of cells in CIN/SIL reveal increased mitochondria and free ribosomes, and depletion of normally accumulated glycogen in the surface cells. The latter change forms the basis of *Schiller's test* in which the suspected cervix is painted with solution of iodine and potassium iodide. The cancerous focus, if present, fails to stain because of lack of glycogen in the surface cells.

PATHOLOGIC CHANGES. Grossly, no specific picture is associated with cellular atypia found in dysplasias or carcinoma *in situ* except that the changes begin at the squamo-columnar junction or transitional zone. The diagnosis can be suspected on the basis of Schiller's test described above.

Histologically, distinction between various grades of CIN is quite subjective, but, in general dysplastic cells are distributed in the layers of squamous epithelium for varying thickness, and accordingly graded as mild, moderate and severe dysplasia, and carcinoma in *situ* (Fig. 22.3,A).

- In *mild dysplasia (CIN-1),* the abnormal cells extend upto one-third thickness from the basal to the surface layer;
- In *moderate dysplasia (CIN-2)* upto two-thirds;
- In *severe dysplasia (CIN-3),* these cells extend from 75-90% thickness of epithelium; and
- In *carcinoma in situ (again CIN-3),* the entire thickness from the basement membrane to the surface shows dysplastic cells.

The atypical cells migrate to the surface layers from where they are shed off (exfoliated) into vaginal secretions in Pap smear. The individual dysplastic or abnormal cells in these grades of atypia show various cytologic changes such as: crowding of cells, pleomorphism, high nucleocytoplasmic ratio, coarse and irregular nuclear chromatin, numerous mitoses and scattered dyskaryotic cells **(COLOUR PLATE IV: CL 13, 14).**

The diagnosis of dysplasia and carcinoma *in situ* or CIN/SIL is best made by *exfoliative cytologic studies* (Chapter 29). The degree of atypicality in the exfoliated surface epithelial cells can be objectively graded on the basis of 3 principal features (Fig. 22.3,B):

1. More severe nuclear dyskaryotic changes such as increased hyperchromasia and nuclear membrane folding.
2. Decreased cytoplasmic maturation i.e. less cytoplasm as the surface cells show less maturation.
3. In lower grades of dysplasia (CIN-1/L-SIL) predominantly superficial and intermediate cells are shed off whereas in severe dysplasia and in carcinoma *in situ* (CIN-3/H-SIL) the desquamated cells are mainly small, dark basal cells.

CERVICAL SCREENING AND BETHESDA SYSTEM OF CYTOLOGIC EXAMINATION. With introduction of effective Pap screening programme in the Western countries, incidence of invasive cervical cancer has declined greatly. However, worldwide cervical cancer remains second most common cancer in women, next to breast cancer. Although accurate statistics are not available from India, but it is perhaps the leading cause of death in women. In the Pap screening programme, patients having abnormal Pap smear are appropriately followed up and, therefore, it requires clinician's understanding of current Bethesda system for evaluation by the cytologist/cytotechnician as regards its value and limitations.

Cervical screening recommendations include annual cervical smear in all sexually active women (above age of 18 years) having any risk factors listed above. However, if three consecutive Pap smears are negative in 'high risk women' or satisfactory in 'low risk women', frequency of Pap screening is reduced. There is no upper age limit for cervical screening.

The broad principles of ***Bethesda system*** of cytologic evaluation are as under:

- Pap smears are evaluated as regards *adequacy of specimen* i.e. satisfactory for evaluation, satisfactory but limited, or unsatisfactory for evaluation giving reason.
- General diagnosis is given in the form of *normal or abnormal smear.*
- *Descriptive diagnosis* is given in abnormal smears that includes: benign cellular changes, reactive cellular changes, and abnormalities of epithelial cells.
- Cellular abnormalities include: *ASCUS* (atypical squamous cells of undetermined significance), *L-SIL* (mentioning HPV infection and CIN-1 present or not), *H-SIL* (stating CIN-2 or CIN-3) and *squamous cell carcinoma.*

Invasive Cervical Cancer

Invasive cervical cancer in about 80% of cases is epidermoid (squamous cell carcinoma). The incidence of

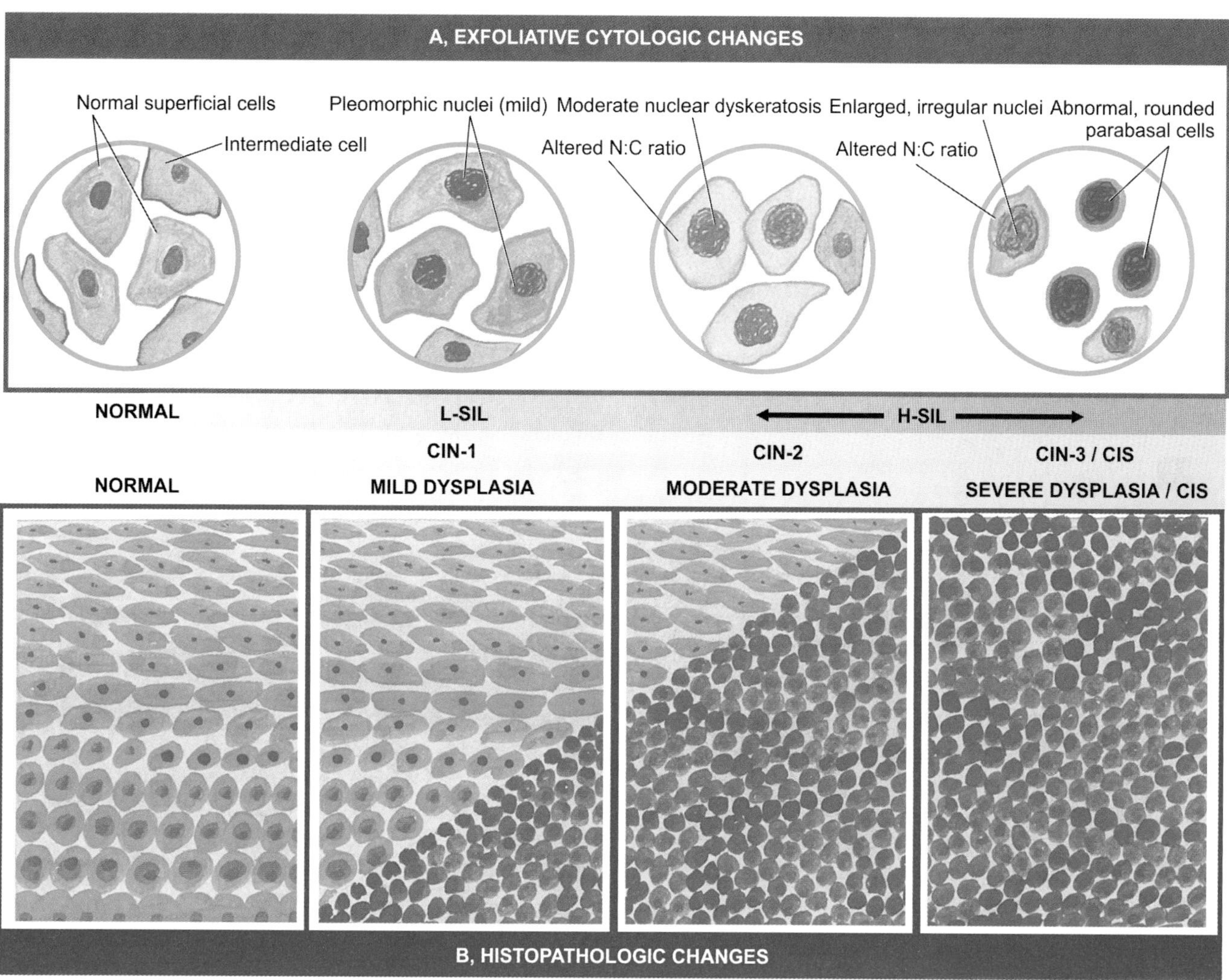

FIGURE 22.3

Cervical intraepithelial neoplasia (CIN) and squamous intraepithelial lesions (SIL). A, schematic representation of histologic changes (below). The grades of CIN-1 or mild dysplasia (L-SIL), CIN-2 (moderate dysplasia) and CIN-3 (severe dysplasia and carcinoma *in situ*) (together grouped as H-SIL) show progressive increase in the number of abnormal cells parallel to the increasing severity of grades. B, exfoliative cytologic studies in various grades of cellular changes (above).

invasive carcinoma of the cervix has shown a declining trend in developed countries due to increased use of Pap smear technique for early detection and diagnosis but the incidence remains high in countries with low living standards. The risk factors and etiologic factors are the same as for CIN discussed above. The peak incidence of invasive cervical cancer is in 4th to 6th decades of life.

PATHOLOGIC CHANGES. Grossly, invasive cervical carcinoma may present 3 types of patterns: fungating, ulcerating and infiltrating. The fungating or exophytic pattern appearing as cauliflower-like growth infiltrating the adjacent vaginal wall is the most common type (Fig. 22.4,A). Characteristically, cervical carcinoma arises from the squamo-columnar junction. The advanced stage of the disease is characterised by widespread destruction and infiltration into adjacent structures including the urinary bladder, rectum, vagina and regional lymph nodes. Distant metastases occur in the lungs, liver, bone marrow and kidneys. ***Histologically,*** the following patterns are seen:

1. Epidermoid (Squamous cell) carcinoma. This type comprises vast majority of invasive cervical carcinomas (about 80%).

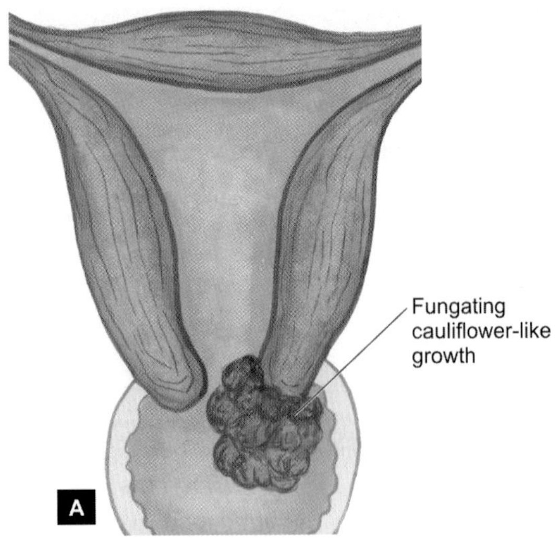

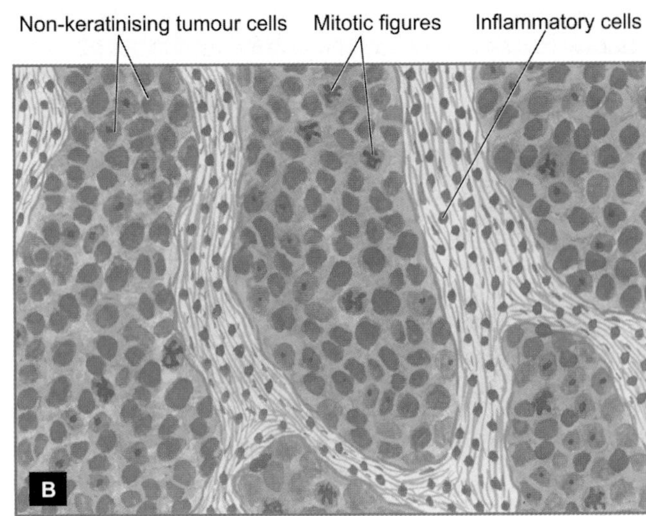

FIGURE 22.4

Invasive carcinoma of the cervix. A, common gross appearance of a fungating or exophytic, cauliflower-like tumour. B, common histologic type is epidermoid (squamous cell) carcinoma showing the pattern of a moderately-differentiated non-keratinising large cell carcinoma.

- The most common pattern (70%) is moderately-differentiated non-keratinising large cell type and has better prognosis.
- Next in frequency (25%) is well-differentiated keratinising epidermoid carcinoma (Fig. 22.4,B).
- Small cell undifferentiated carcinoma (neuro-endocrine or oat cell carcinoma) is less common (5%) and has a poor prognosis.

2. **Adenocarcinoma.** Adenocarcinomas comprise about 10% of cases. These may be well-differentiated mucus-secreting adenocarcinoma, or clear cell type containing glycogen but no mucin.

3. **Others.** The remaining 5% cases are a variety of other patterns such as adenosquamous carcinoma, verrucous carcinoma and undifferentiated carcinoma.

CLINICAL STAGING. Classification of cervical cancer described by the Cancer Committee of the International Federation of Gynaecology and Obstetrics (FIGO classification) is widely adopted by the clinicians and pathologists and is given in Table 22.4.

MYOMETRIUM AND ENDOMETRIUM

NORMAL STRUCTURE

The *myometrium* is the thick muscular wall of the uterus which is covered internally by uterine mucosa called the *endometrium.* The endometrium extends above the level of the internal os where it joins the endocervical

TABLE 22.4: FIGO Clinical Staging of Carcinoma of the Cervix Uteri.

Stage	0	Carcinoma *in situ*
Stage	I	Carcinoma strictly confined to the cervix
	IA	Preclinical carcinomas diagnosed only by microscopy Maximum size 5 mm deep and 7 mm across measured from the base of epithelium.
	IA1	Stromal invasion of less than 3 mm in depth and 7 mm in horizontal axis (minimally invasive).
	IA2	Stromal invasion of 3 to 5 mm depth and horizontal 7 mm or less (microinvasive).
	IB	Clinical lesion confined to the cervix or preclinical lesions greater than stage IA.
	IB1	Clinical lesions no greater than 4 cm in size.
	IB2	Clinical lesions greater than 4 cm in size.
Stage	II	Carcinoma extends beyond the cervix but has not extended to the pelvic wall. Involvement of the vagina limited to upper two-thirds.
	IIA	No obvious parametrial involvement.
	IIB	Obvious parametrial involvement.
Stage	III	The carcinoma has extended to the pelvic wall. The tumour invades the lower third of vagina.
	IIIA	No extension to the pelvic wall.
	IIIB	Extension to the pelvic wall and/or hydro-nephrosis or nonfunctioning kidney.
Stage	IV	The carcinoma has extended beyond the true pelvis or has clinically involved the mucosa of the bladder or rectum.
	IVA	Spread of the growth to adjacent organs.
	IVB	Spread to distant organs.

epithelium. The myometrium is capable of marked alterations in its size, capacity and contractility during pregnancy and labour. The endometrium responds in a cyclic fashion to the ovarian hormones with resultant monthly menstruation and has remarkable regenerative capacity.

The lesions pertaining to the corpus uteri and the endometrium are numerous and constitute vast majority of gynaecologic conditions. However, some of the important pathologic entities are discussed below, but first, the changes in normal menstrual cycle.

NORMAL CYCLIC CHANGES

The normal endometrial cycle begins with proliferative phase lasting for about 14 days under the influence of oestrogen, followed by ovulation on or around 14th day, and consequent secretory phase under the influence of progesterone. The cycle ends with endometrial shedding and the next cycle begins anew.

The histologic changes in different phases of the menstrual cycle vary.

Histologically, the endometrium essentially consists of 3 structures: the endometrial lining epithelium, endometrial glands and stroma.

- **The epithelial lining** undergoes increase in its thickness from cuboidal to tall columnar appearance at ovulation and subsequently regresses.
- **The endometrial glands** with their lining provide most of the information on phase of the menstrual cycle. In the immediate postmenstrual period, the glands are straight and tubular, having columnar lining with basal nuclei. This phase is under the predominant influence of oestrogen and lasts for about 14 days and is called *proliferative phase*. The evidence of ovulation is taken from the appearance of convolutions in the glands and subnuclear vacuolation in the cells indicative of secretions. The secretory changes remain prominent for the next 7 days after ovulation for implantation of the ovum if it has been fertilised. Otherwise, the secretory activity wanes during the following 7 days with increased luminal secretions and a frayed and ragged luminal border of the cells lining the glands. This phase is under the predominant influence of progesterone and is called *secretory phase*. Eventually, the endometrium is sloughed away at *menstruation* followed by beginning of the fresh cycle.
- **The endometrial stroma** in the pre-ovulatory phase or proliferative phase is generally dense and compact, composed of oval to spindled cells. In the post-ovulatory phase or secretory phase, the stroma is loose and oedematous, composed of large, pale and polyhedral cells. The true *decidual reaction* of the stroma occurs if the pregnancy has taken place. However, decidual reaction may be suggested in the absence of pregnancy due to extreme response to progesterone. Thus, it may be impossible to distinguish an advanced progestational endometrium from early pregnancy except for the presence of trophoblastic tissue.

EFFECTS OF HORMONES

In addition to the changes that take place during the normal menstrual cycle, the endometrium undergoes morphologic changes when hormonal preparations are administered, or during pregnancy and menopause.

Oestrogen and Progesterone

Oestrogen produces the characteristic changes of proliferative phase at the time of menopause and in young women with anovulatory cycles as occurs in Stein-Leventhal syndrome. The therapeutic addition of progesterone produces secretory pattern in an oestrogen-primed endometrium. Oestrogen-progesterone combination hormonal therapy is employed for control of conception. The sequential type of oestrogen-progesterone oral contraceptives act by producing prolonged oestrogenic effect past the time of ovulation and implantation so that the secretion is delayed until about 25th day, followed by progestational effect and shedding. Repeated cyclic administration with combination therapy such as after long-term use of oral contraceptives produces inactive-looking, small and atrophic endometrial glands, and compact decidua-like stroma.

Pregnancy

The implantation of a fertilised ovum results in interruption of the endometrial cycle. The endometrial glands are enlarged with abundant glandular secretions and the stromal cells become more plump, polygonal with increased cytoplasm termed *decidual reaction*. About 25% cases of uterine or extrauterine pregnancy show hyperactive secretory state called *Arias-Stella reaction*. It is characterised by hyperchromatic, atypical, tall cells lining the glands and the glandular epithelium may show multilayering and budding which may be mistaken for an adenocarcinoma.

Menopause

The onset of menopause is heralded with hormonal transition and consequent varying morphologic changes in the endometrium. Most commonly, the *senile endometrium,* as it is generally called, is thin and atrophic with inactive glands and fibrous stroma. However, some of the glands may show cystic dilatation. Sometimes, retrogressive hyperplasia is seen which is characterised by Swiss-cheese pattern of glands resembling endometrial hyperplasia but composed of inactive retrogressive lining epithelium. There is intermingling of cystic and dilated glands with small and atrophic glands. Postmenopausal endometrium may show actual active hyperplasia under the stimulatory influence of post-menopausal oestrogen originating from the ovary or adrenal gland.

DYSFUNCTIONAL UTERINE BLEEDING (DUB)

Dysfunctional uterine bleeding (DUB) may be defined as excessive bleeding occurring during or between menstrual periods without a causative uterine lesion such as tumour, polyp, infection, hyperplasia, trauma, blood dyscrasia or pregnancy. DUB occurs most commonly in association with anovulatory cycles which are most frequent at the two extremes of menstrual life i.e. either when the ovarian function is just beginning (menarche) or when it is waning off (menopause). Anovulation is the result of prolonged and excessive oestrogenic stimulation without the development of progestational phase. The causes for *anovulation* at different ages are as follows:

1. In *prepuberty:* precocious puberty of hypothalamic, pituitary or ovarian origin.
2. In *adolescence:* anovulatory cycles at the onset of menstruation.
3. In *reproductive age:* complications of pregnancy, endometrial hyperplasia, carcinoma, polyps, leiomyomas and adenomyosis.
4. At *premenopause:* anovulatory cycles, irregular shedding, endometrial hyperplasia, carcinoma and polyps.
5. At *perimenopause:* endometrial hyperplasia, carcinoma, polyps and senile atrophy.

It has been observed that women who ovulate may also occasionally have anovulatory cycles. In addition to anovulatory cycles, DUB may occur in *inadequate luteal phase* that manifests clinically as infertility *(ovulatory dysfunctional bleeding).* In such cases, the premenstrual endometrial biopsy shows histologic lag of more than 2 days.

ENDOMETRITIS AND MYOMETRITIS

Inflammatory involvement of the endometrium and myometrium are uncommon clinical problems; myometritis is seen less frequently than endometritis and occurs in continuation with endometrial infections. Endometritis and myometritis may be acute or chronic.

- The **acute form** generally results from 3 types of causes—puerperal (following full-term delivery, abortion and retained products of conception), intrauterine contraceptive device (IUCD), and extension of gonorrheal infection from the cervix and vagina.
- The **chronic form** is more common and occurs by the same causes which result in acute phase. In addition, *tuberculous endometritis* is an example of specific chronic inflammation, uncommon in the Western countries but not so uncommon in developing countries. Its incidence in India is reported to be approximately in 5% of women.

PATHOLOGIC CHANGES. In *acute endometritis and myometritis,* there is progressive infiltration of the endometrium, myometrium and parametrium by polymorphs and marked oedema. *Chronic nonspecific endometritis and myometritis* are characterised by infiltration of plasma cells alongwith lymphocytes and macrophages. *Tuberculous endometritis* is almost always associated with tuberculous salpingitis and shows small non-caseating granulomas.

ADENOMYOSIS

Adenomyosis is defined as abnormal distribution of histologically benign endometrial tissue within the myometrium alongwith myometrial hypertrophy. The term *adenomyoma* is used for actually circumscribed mass made up of endometrium and smooth muscle tissue. Adenomyosis is found in 15-20% of all hysterectomies. Pathogenesis of the condition remains unexplained. The possible underlying cause of the invasiveness and increased proliferation of the endometrium into the myometrium appears to be either a metaplasia or oestrogenic stimulation due to endocrine dysfunction of the ovary. Clinically, the patients of adenomyosis generally complain of menorrhagia, colicky dysmenorrhoea and menstrual pain in the sacral or sacrococcygeal regions.

PATHOLOGIC CHANGES. Grossly, the uterus may be slightly or markedly enlarged. On cut section, there is diffuse thickness of the uterine wall with presence of coarsely trabecular, ill-defined areas of haemorrhages.

Microscopically, the diagnosis is based on the finding of normal, benign endometrial islands composed of glands as well as stroma deep within the muscular layer. The minimum distance between the endometrial islands within the myometrium and the basal endometrium should be one low-power microscopic field (2-3 mm) for making the diagnosis. Associated muscle hypertrophy is generally present.

ENDOMETRIOSIS

Endometriosis refers to the presence of endometrial glands and stroma in abnormal locations outside the uterus. Endometriosis and adenomyosis are closely interlinked, so much so that some gynaecologists have termed adenomyosis as *endometriosis interna* and the other category termed as *endometriosis externa* for similar appearance at the extrauterine sites. But the two varieties differ as regards age, fertility and histogenesis and thus endometriosis should be regarded as a distinct clinicopathologic entity.

The chief locations where the abnormal endometrial development may occur are as follows (in descending order of frequency): ovaries, uterine ligaments, rectovaginal septum, pelvic peritoneum, laparotomy scars, and infrequently in the umbilicus, vagina, vulva, appendix and hernial sacs.

The **histogenesis** of endometriosis has been a debatable matter for years. Currently, however, the following 3 theories of its histogenesis are described:

1. *Transplantation or regurgitation theory* is based on the assumption that ectopic endometrial tissue is transplanted from the uterus to an abnormal location by way of fallopian tubes due to regurgitation of menstrual blood.
2. *Metaplastic theory* suggests that ectopic endometrium develops *in situ* from local tissues by metaplasia of the coelomic epithelium.
3. *Vascular or lymphatic dissemination* explains the development of endometrial tissue at extrapelvic sites by these routes.

Endometriosis is characteristically a disease of reproductive years of life. Clinical signs and symptoms include intrapelvic bleeding from implants, severe dysmenorrhoea, pelvic pain, dyspareunia and infertility.

PATHOLOGIC CHANGES. Grossly, the appearance of endometriosis varies widely depending upon the location and extent of the disease. Typically, the foci of endometriosis appear as blue or brownish-black underneath the surface of the sites mentioned. Often, these foci are surrounded by fibrous tissue resulting in adherence to adjacent structures. The ovary is the most common site of endometriosis and shows numerous cysts varying in diameter from 0.1 to 2.5 cm. Ovarian involvement is often bilateral. Larger cysts, 3-5 cm in diameter, filled with old dark brown blood form *'chocolate cysts'* of the ovary.

Histologically, the diagnosis is simple and rests on identification of foci of endometrial glands and stroma, old or new haemorrhages, haemosiderin-laden macrophages and surrounding zone of inflammation and fibrosis.

ENDOMETRIAL HYPERPLASIAS

Endometrial hyperplasia is a condition characterised by proliferative patterns of glandular and stromal tissues and commonly associated with prolonged, profuse and irregular uterine bleeding in a menopausal or postmenopausal woman. It may be emphasised here that the syndrome of DUB with which endometrial hyperplasia is commonly associated is a clinical entity, while hyperplasia is a pathologic term. Hyperplasia results from prolonged oestrogenic stimulation with absence of progestational activity. Such conditions include Stein-Leventhal syndrome, functioning granulosa-theca cell tumours, adrenocortical hyperfunction and prolonged administration of oestrogen. Endometrial hyperplasia is clinically significant due to the presence of cytologic atypia which is closely linked to endometrial carcinoma.

The following classification of endometrial hyperplasias is widely employed by most gynaecologic pathologists:

1. Simple hyperplasia (Cystic hyperplasia)
2. Complex hyperplasia (Adenomatous hyperplasia)
3. Atypical hyperplasia.

SIMPLE HYPERPLASIA (CYSTIC HYPERPLASIA). Commonly termed cystic glandular hyperplasia (CGH), this form of endometrial hyperplasia is characterised by the presence of varying-sized glands, many of which are large and cystically dilated and are lined by atrophic epithelium. Mitoses are scanty. The stroma between the glands is sparsely cellular and oedematous (Fig. 22.5,A) **(COLOUR PLATE XXX: CL 117).**

There is minimal risk (1%) of adenocarcinoma developing in cystic hyperplasia.

COMPLEX HYPERPLASIA (ADENOMATOUS HYPERPLASIA). This type of hyperplasia shows distinct proliferative pattern. The glands are increased

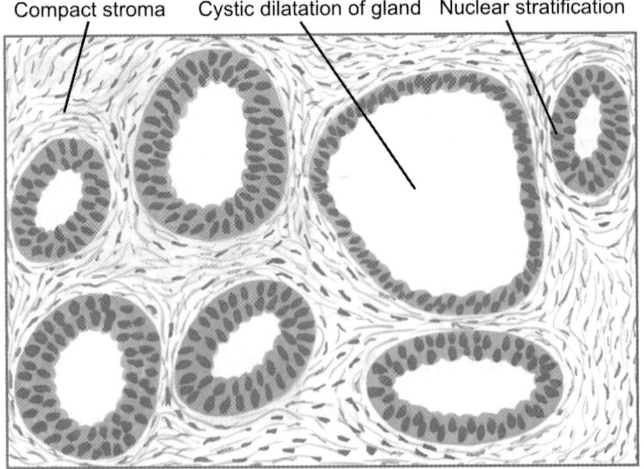

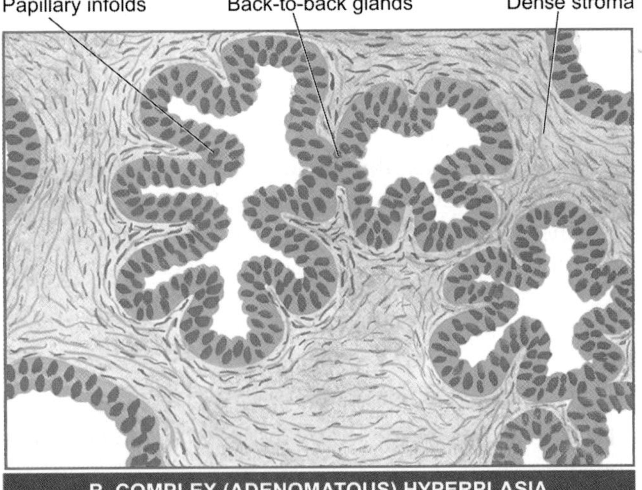

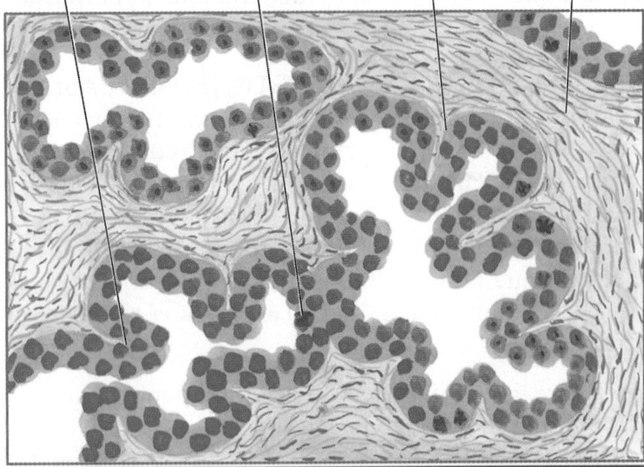

FIGURE 22.5

Three forms of endometrial hyperplasias.

in number, exhibit variation in size and are irregular in shape. The glands are lined by multiple layers of tall columnar epithelial cells with large nuclei which have not lost basal polarity and there is no significant atypia. The glandular epithelium at places is thrown into papillary infolds or out-pouchings into adjacent stroma i.e. there is crowding and complexity of glands without cytologic atypia. The stroma is generally dense, cellular and compact (Fig. 22.5,B).

The malignant potential of adenomatous hyperplasia in the absence of cytologic atypia is 3%.

ATYPICAL HYPERPLASIA. Some authors have suggested the terms such as anaplasia or carcinoma *in situ* for this form of endometrial hyperplasia but these terms are generally not favoured. Atypical hyperplasia is distinguished from adenomatous hyperplasia by the presence of 'atypical cells' in the hyperplastic epithelium. The extent of cytologic atypia may be mild, moderate or severe. The cytologic features present in these cells include loss of polarity, large size, irregular and hyperchromatic nuclei, prominent nucleoli, and altered nucleocytoplasmic ratio (Fig. 22.5,C).

Atypical hyperplasia is a precancerous condition and its malignant transformation is related to the degree of cytologic atypia. About 20-25% cases of untreated atypical hyperplasia progress to carcinoma.

TUMOURS OF ENDOMETRIUM AND MYOMETRIUM

Tumours arising from endometrium and myometrium may be benign or malignant. They may originate from different tissues such as:

- *Endometrial glands*—endometrial polyps, endometrial carcinoma.
- *Endometrial stroma*—stromal nodules, stromal sarcoma.
- *Smooth muscle of the myometrium*—leiomyoma, leiomyosarcoma.
- *Mullerian mesoderm*—mixed mesodermal or mullerian tumours.

Out of these, endometrial polyps, endometrial carcinoma, leiomyomas and leiomyosarcomas are relatively more common and are described below.

Endometrial Polyps

'Uterine polyp' is clinical term used for a polypoid growth projecting into the uterine lumen and may be composed of benign lesions (e.g. endometrial or mucous polyp, leiomyomatous polyp and placental polyp), or malignant polypoid tumours (e.g. endometrial carcinoma, choriocarcinoma and sarcoma). The most common variety, however, is the one having the structure like that of endometrium and is termed *endometrial or mucous polyp.* They are more common in the perimenopausal age group. Small endometrial polyps generally remain asymptomatic and are detected incidentally. The larger ones may ulcerate, degenerate and result in clinical bleeding.

PATHOLOGIC CHANGES. Grossly, endometrial polyps may be single or multiple, usually sessile and small (0.5 to 3 cm in diameter) but occasionally they are large and pedunculated.
Histologically, they are essentially made up of mixture of endometrial glands and stroma. The histologic pattern of the endometrial tissue in the polyp may resemble either functioning endometrium or hyperplastic endometrium of cystic hyperplasia type; the latter being more common. Rarely, a large endometrial polyp may undergo malignant change.

Endometrial Carcinoma

Carcinoma of the endometrium has become more common than the invasive carcinoma of the cervix in women in the United States. Whereas the decline in the incidence of cervical cancer is due to early detection and cure of *in situ* stage, increased frequency of endometrial carcinoma may be due to longevity of women's life to develop this cancer of older females. The peak incidence at onset is 6th to 7th decades of life and is rare below the age of 40 years. The most important presenting complaint is abnormal bleeding in the postmenopausal woman or excessive flow in the premenopausal years.

ETIOPATHOGENESIS. The exact etiology of endometrial cancer remains unknown. However, a few factors associated with increased frequency of its development are oestrogen excess, obesity, diabetes, hypertension and nulliparous state. There is irrefutable evidence of *relationship of endometrial carcinoma with prolonged oestrogenic stimulation.* These evidences are as under:

1. Endometrial carcinoma has association with endometrial hyperplasia in which there is hyperoestrogenism and frequent anovulatory cycles.
2. Endometrial carcinoma is characteristically a disease of postmenopausal women. At this age, there is excessive synthesis of oestrogen in the body from adrenal as well as from ovarian sources.
3. Women having oestrogen-secreting tumours (e.g. granulosa cell tumour) have increased risk of developing endometrial cancer.
4. Patients receiving prolonged oestrogen therapy are at higher risk of developing this cancer.
5. Prolonged administration of oestrogen to laboratory animals can produce endometrial hyperplasia and carcinoma.
6. Women with gonadal agenesis rarely develop endometrial carcinoma.

Papillary serous variant of endometrial carcinoma is associated with mutation in *TP53* tumour suppressor gene while endometrioid carcinoma has mutation in *PTEN* gene located on chromosome 10.

PATHOLOGIC CHANGES. Grossly, endometrial carcinoma may have 2 patterns—localised *polypoid tumour,* or a *diffuse tumour;* the latter being more common (Fig. 22.6). The tumour protrudes into the endometrial cavity as irregular, friable and grey-tan mass. Extension of the growth into myometrium may be identified by the presence of soft, friable and granular tissue in cut section. In advanced disease, the involvement may extend beyond the physiologic limits—into the cervical canal, into the peritoneum, besides lymphatic metastases and haematogenous metastases to distant sites such as lungs, liver, bones and other organs.
Histologically, most endometrial carcinomas are adenocarcinomas. Depending upon the pattern of glands and individual cell changes, these may be well-differentiated, moderately-differentiated or poorly-differentiated.

- *Well-differentiated adenocarcinoma* is characterised by increase in the number of glands which are closely packed sometimes showing 'back-to-back crowding' due to obliterated intervening stroma. The glandular epithelium shows stratification, formation of tufting and papillae and atypical changes. Most growths are well-differentiated (Fig. 22.7).
- *Moderately-differentiated adenocarcinoma* shows all the above features alongwith presence of some solid sheets of malignant cells.
- *Poorly-differentiated adenocarcinoma* is characterised by presence of solid sheets and ribbons of malignant epithelial cells which show marked cytologic atypia and frequent mitoses. Glandular pattern is hard to find.

Cases can also be categorised as regards histologic grade as follows:
G1: Well-differentiated (predominantly glandular).
G2: Moderately-differentiated (glandular and partly solid areas).
G3: Poorly-differentiated (predominantly solid).

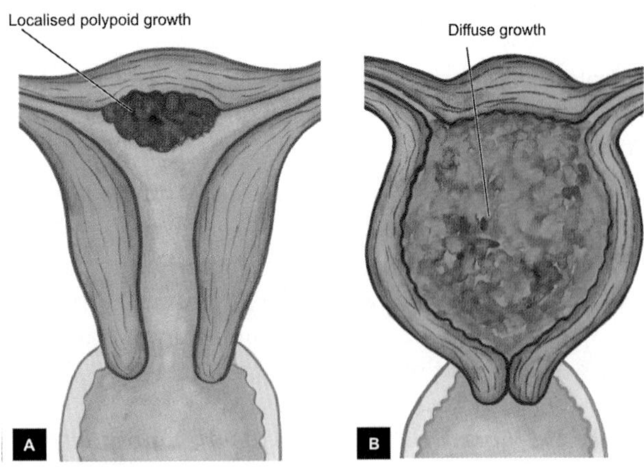

FIGURE 22.6

Endometrial carcinoma, the common macroscopic patterns. A, localised polypoid growth. B, diffuse growth.

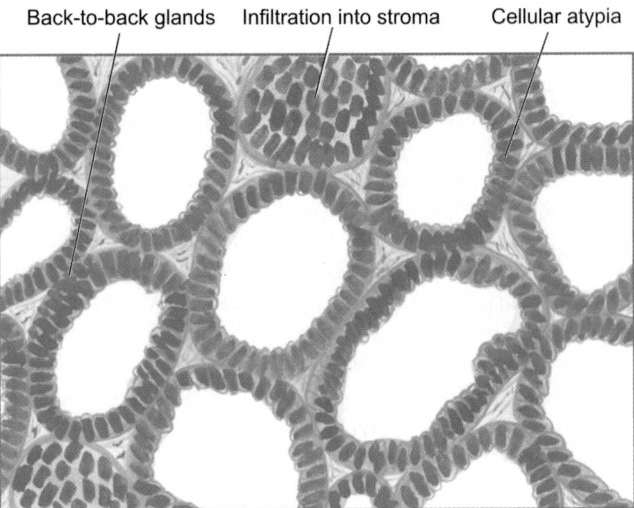

FIGURE 22.7

Endometrial carcinoma. The most common histologic pattern is well-differentiated adenocarcinoma showing closely packed ("back-to-back") glands with cytologic atypia.

Uncommon histologic variants of endometrial carcinoma are: adenocarcinoma with squamous metaplasia (adenoacanthoma), adeno-squamous carcinoma (when both components are frankly malignant), clear cell carcinoma, mucinous adenocarcinoma and papillary serous carcinoma.

Carcinoma of the endometrium is categorised into four stages as per FIGO classification given in Table 22.5.

Leiomyoma

Leiomyomas or fibromyomas, commonly called *fibroids* by the gynaecologists, are the most common uterine tumours of smooth muscle origin, often admixed with variable amount of fibrous tissue component. About 20% of women above the age of 30 years harbour uterine myomas of varying size. Vast majority of them are benign and cause no symptoms. Malignant transformation occurs in less than 0.5% of leiomyomas. Symptomatic cases may produce abnormal uterine bleeding, pain, symptoms due to compression of surrounding structures and infertility.

TABLE 22.5: FIGO Clinical Staging of Carcinoma of the Endometrium.

Stage	IA	Tumour limited to endometrium.
	IB	Invasion to less than one-half the myometrium.
	IC	Invasion to more than one-half the myometrium.
Stage	IIA	Endocervical glandular involvement only.
	IIB	Cervical stromal invasion.
Stage	IIIA	Tumour invades serosa and/or adnexa and/or positive peritoneal cytology.
	IIIB	Metastases to pelvic and/or para-aortic lymph nodes.
Stage	IVA	Tumour invasion of bladder and/or bowel mucosa.
	IVB	Distant metastases including intra-abdominal and/or inguinal lymph nodes.

The cause of leiomyomas is unknown but the possible stimulus to their proliferation is oestrogen. This is evidenced by increase in their size in pregnancy and high dose oestrogen-therapy and their regression following menopause and castration. Other possible factors implicated in its etiology are human growth hormone and sterility.

PATHOLOGIC CHANGES. Leiomyomas are most frequently located in the uterus where they may occur within the myometrium *(intramural or interstitial),* the serosa *(subserosal),* or just underneath the endometrium *(submucosal).* Subserosal and submucosal leiomyomas may develop pedicles and protrude as pedunculated myomas. Leiomyomas may involve the cervix or broad ligament.

Grossly, irrespective of their location, leiomyomas are often multiple, circumscribed, firm, nodular, grey-white masses of variable size. On cut section, they exhibit characteristic whorled pattern (Fig. 22.8,A).

Histologically, they are essentially composed of 2 tissue elements—whorled bundles of smooth muscle cells admixed with variable amount of connective tissue. The smooth muscle cells are uniform in size and shape with abundant cytoplasm and central oval nuclei (Fig. 22.8,B) (COLOUR PLATE I: CL 2).

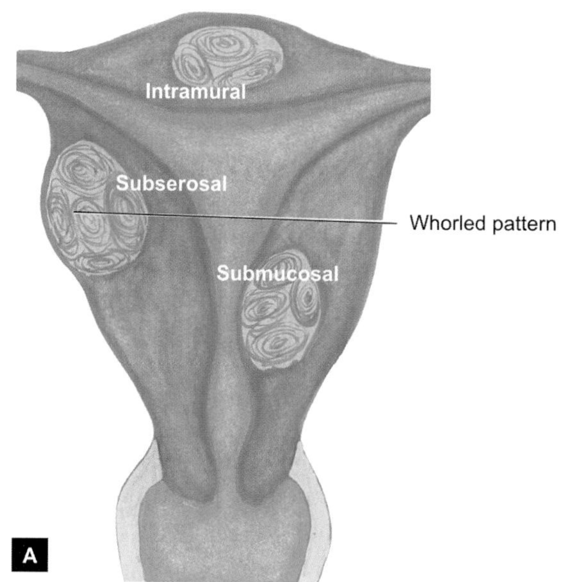

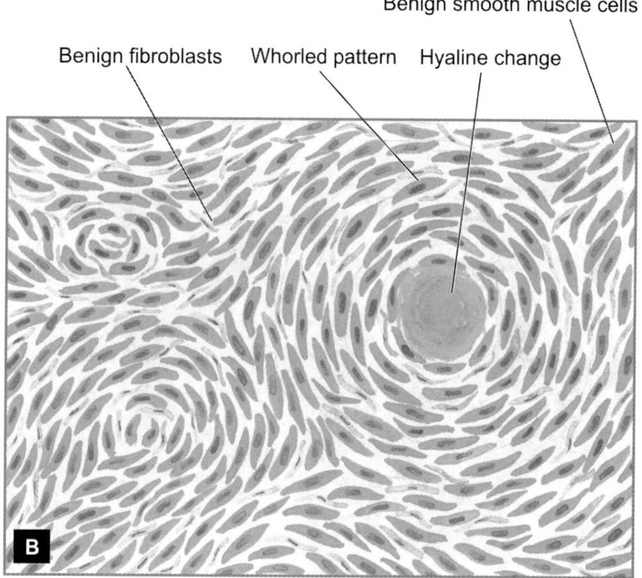

FIGURE 22.8

Leiomyomas. A, common locations. Cut surface shows characteristic whorled appearance. B, microscopy shows whorls of smooth muscle cells which are spindle-shaped, having abundant cytoplasm and oval nuclei.

Cellular leiomyoma has preponderance of smooth muscle elements and may superficially resemble leiomyosarcoma but is distinguished from it by the absence of mitoses (see below).

The pathologic appearance may be altered by secondary changes in the leiomyomas. These include: hyaline degeneration, cystic degeneration, infarction, calcification, infection and suppuration, necrosis, fatty change, and rarely, sarcomatous change.

Leiomyosarcoma

Leiomyosarcoma is an uncommon malignant tumour as compared to its rather common benign counterpart. The incidence of malignancy in pre-existing leiomyoma is less than 0.5% but primary uterine sarcoma is less common than that which arises in the leiomyoma. The peak age incidence is seen in 4th to 6th decades of life. The symptoms produced are nonspecific such as uterine enlargement and abnormal uterine bleeding.

PATHOLOGIC CHANGES. Grossly, the tumour may form a diffuse, bulky, soft and fleshy mass, or a polypoid mass projecting into lumen.

Histologically, though there are usually some areas showing whorled arrangement of spindle-shaped smooth muscle cells having large and hyperchromatic nuclei, the hallmark of diagnosis and prognosis is the number of mitoses per high power field (HPF). The essential diagnostic criteria are: more than 10 mitoses per 10 HPF with or without cellular atypia, or 5-10 mitoses per 10 HPF with cellular atypia. More the number of mitoses per 10 HPF, worse is the prognosis.

Leiomyosarcoma is liable to recur after removal and eventually metastasises to distant sites such as lungs, liver, bone and brain.

FALLOPIAN TUBES

NORMAL STRUCTURE

The fallopian tube or oviducts are paired structures, each extending from superior angle of the uterus laterally to the region of the ovaries and running in the superior border of the broad ligaments forming mesosalpinx. Each tube is 7-14 cm long and is divided into 4 parts—*interstitial portion* in the uterine cornual wall; narrow *isthmic portion;* wider *ampullary region;* and funnel-like distal *infundibulum.* The infundibulum is fringed by fimbriae, the longest of which called fimbria ovarica is attached to the ovary.

Histologically, the wall of tube has 4 coats—*serous* forming the peritoneal covering, *subserous* consisting of fibrovascular tissue, *muscular* composed of longitudinal and circular smooth muscle layers, and *tubal mucosa* having 3 types of cells namely: ciliated, columnar and dark intercalated cells. The tubal serosal covering may contain tiny nodular masses of mesothelial cells forming *Walthard's cell rests.*

The major conditions involving the fallopian tubes are inflammations, ectopic tubal gestation, and endometriosis.

INFLAMMATIONS

Salpingitis and Pelvic Inflammatory Disease

Pelvic inflammatory disease (PID) by definition is a clinical syndrome characterised by signs and symptoms of ascending infection beginning in the vulva or vagina and spreading through the entire genital tract. Although ascending route of infection is the most common mode of spread, PID may occur following abortion and puerperium, with use of intrauterine contraceptive devices, or from local intra-abdominal infections such as appendicitis with peritonitis. In addition, haematogenous spread may occur, though this route is more important in the pathogenesis of tuberculosis.

Most commonly, PID occurs as a venereally-transmitted infection, chiefly caused by *Chlamydia trachomatis* and *Neisseria gonorrhoeae.* Post-abortal and postpartum infections are mainly caused by staphylococci, streptococci, coliform bacteria, clostridia and pneumococci.

Patients generally complain of lower abdominal and pelvic pain which is often bilateral, dysmenorrhoea, menstrual abnormalities and fever with tachycardia. Long-standing chronic PID may lead to infertility and adhesions between small intestine and pelvic organs.

PATHOLOGIC CHANGES. Grossly, the fallopian tubes are invariably involved bilaterally. The distal end is blocked by inflammatory exudate and the lumina are dilated. There may be formation of loculated tubo-ovarian abscess involving the tube, ovary, broad ligament and adjacent part of uterus.

Microscopically, the appearance varies with the duration of inflammatory process.

- The process begins with *acute salpingitis* characterised by oedema and intense acute inflammatory infiltrate of neutrophils involving the tubal mucosa as well as wall. The lumen is filled with purulent exudate consisting of leucocytes and sloughed off epithelial cells.
- The purulent process may extend to involve tube as well as ovary causing salpingo-oophoritis and forming *tubo-ovarian abscess.*
- The escape of purulent exudate into the peritoneal cavity produces *pelvic peritonitis* and *pelvic abscess.*
- *Pyosalpinx* is distension of the fallopian tube with pus due to occluded fimbrial end.
- End-result of pyosalpinx after resorption of the purulent exudate is *hydrosalpinx* in which the tube is thin-walled, dilated and filled with clear watery fluid.
- Acute salpingitis may resolve with treatment but some cases pass into *chronic salpingitis* with infiltrate of polymorphs, lymphocytes and plasma cells and fibrosis.
- *Salpingitis isthmica nodosa* used to be considered another manifestation of chronic salpingitis but currently accepted pathogenesis of this lesion appears to be similar to that of adenomyosis. Nevertheless, the appearance is characterised by multiple nodules containing spaces which are lined by benign tubal epithelium. Inflammatory changes are scanty or absent.

Tuberculous Salpingitis

Tuberculous salpingitis is almost always secondary to focus elsewhere in the body. The tubercle bacilli reach the tube, most commonly by haematogenous route, generally from the lungs, but occasionally from the urinary tract or abdominal cavity. Tubal tuberculosis is always present when there is tuberculosis of other female genital organs such as of endometrium, cervix and lower genital tract. Though infrequent in developed countries of the world, the incidence of tubal tuberculosis in developing countries like India is estimated to be about 5%. It affects more commonly young women in their active reproductive life and the most common complaint is infertility.

PATHOLOGIC CHANGES. Grossly, the tube is dilated and contains purulent exudate though the fimbrial end is generally patent. The tubal peritoneum as well as the peritoneum in general is studded with yellowish tubercles.

Microscopically, typical caseating granulomas and chronic inflammation are identified in the tubal serosa, muscularis and mucosa.

ECTOPIC TUBAL PREGNANCY

The term ectopic tubal pregnancy is used for implantation of a fertilised ovum in the tube. Though ectopic pregnancy may rarely occur in the uterine horn, cornu, ovary and abdominal cavity, tubal pregnancy is by far the most common form of ectopic gestation. Several factors which predispose to ectopic tubal pregnancy are: PID, previous tubal surgery, use of IUCD and congenital anomalies of the female genital tract. The most frequent site of tubal pregnancy is the ampullary portion and the least common is interstitial pregnancy. Ectopic tubal pregnancy is a potentially hazardous problem because of rupture which is followed by intraperitoneal haemorrhage.

TUMOURS AND TUMOUR-LIKE LESIONS

Tumours in the fallopian tubes are rare. Relatively more common are hydatids of Morgagni or parovarian cysts which are unilocular, thin-walled cysts hanging from the tubal fimbriae. Rare tumours include adenomatoid tumours, leiomyomas, teratomas, adenocarcinomas and choriocarcinoma all of which are similar in morphology to such tumours elsewhere in the body.

OVARIES

NORMAL STRUCTURE

The ovaries are paired bean-shaped organs hanging from either tube by a mesentery called the mesovarium, the lateral suspensory ligament and the ovarian ligament. The lateral suspensory ligament of the ovary contains blood vessels, lymphatics and plexuses of nerves. Each ovary measures 2.5-5 cm in length, 1.5-3 cm in breadth and 0.7-1.5 cm in width and weighs 4-8 gm.

Histologically, the ovarian structure consists of covering by coelomic epithelium, outer cortex and inner medulla (Fig. 22.9).

Coelomic epithelium. The surface of the ovary is covered by a single layer of cuboidal epithelial cells.

Cortex. During active reproductive life, the cortex is broad and constitutes the predominant component of the ovary. The cortex contains numerous ovarian follicles and their derivative structures. Each follicle consists of a central *germ cell ovum* surrounded by specialised gonadal stroma. This stroma consists of *granulosa cells* encircling the ovum, and concentrically-arranged plump spindle-shaped *theca cells.* In infancy, the granulosa cells form a single layer of cuboidal cells around the ovum but later form several layers. Granulosa cells may form *Call-Exner bodies* normally as well as in certain neoplastic conditions. Call-Exner bodies have a central small round mass of dense pink material surrounded by a rosette of granulosa cells. The granulosa component is avascular and draws its nutrition from the highly vascular theca component. The theca component has 2 parts—luteinised theca layer called *theca interna,* and outer condensed ovarian stroma called *theca externa.* Granulosa cells and follicle-associated (luteinised) theca cells produce oestrogen. Fully mature ovarian follicle called *graafian follicle* bursts releasing the ovum and becomes transformed into corpus luteum which is the principle source of progesterone that brings about secretory endometrial pattern. The corpus luteum is later replaced by corpus albicans. In addition to specialised gonadal stroma and follicles, the cortex contains unspecialised ovarian stroma consisting of spindle-shaped connective tissue cells and smooth muscle fibres.

Medulla. The ovarian medulla is primarily made up of connective tissue fibres, smooth muscle cells and numerous blood vessels, lymphatics and nerves. In addition, the medulla may also contain clusters of hilus cell (or hilar-Leydig cells) which may have androgenic role in contrast to oestrogenic role of the ovarian cortex.

The major pathologic lesions of the ovary are the non-neoplastic cysts and ovarian tumours.

NON-NEOPLASTIC CYSTS

The most common of the non-neoplastic cysts of the ovary are tubo-ovarian inflammatory mass (discussed above) and follicular and luteal cysts. Polycystic ovarian disease of Stein-Leventhal syndrome is another cause of cystic ovary.

Follicular and Luteal Cysts

Normally follicles and corpus luteum do not exceed a diameter of 2 cm. When their diameter is greater than 3 cm, they are termed as cysts.

■ **Follicular cysts** are frequently multiple, filled with clear serous fluid and may attain a diameter upto 8 cm. When large, they produce clinical symptoms.

> ***Histologically,*** they are lined by granulosa cells. Occasionally, however, there may be difficulty in distinguishing between a large cyst of coelomic epithelial origin *(serous cyst)* lined by flattened epithelial cells and a cyst of follicular origin. Such cases are appropriately designated as *'simple cysts'.*

■ **Luteal cysts** are formed by rupture and sealing of corpus haemorrhagicum. The wall of these cysts is composed of yellowish luteal tissue *(lutein* = yellow pigment).

> ***Histologically,*** luteal cysts are commonly lined by luteinised granulosa cells. Lining by predominantly

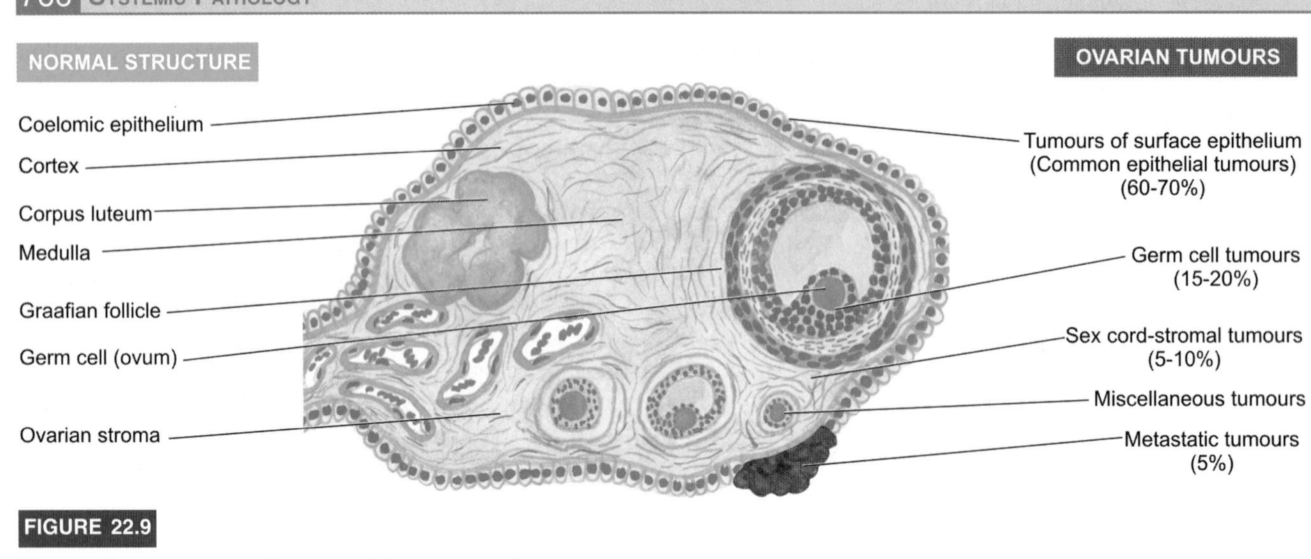

FIGURE 22.9
The structure of ovary to illustrate origin of ovarian tumours.

luteinised theca cells may also be seen in cystic ovaries in association with hydatidiform mole and choriocarcinoma, and rarely, in normal pregnancy. *Corpus albicans cyst* is a variant of corpus luteum cyst in which there is hyalinisation in the wall and distension of the cavity with fluid.

Polycystic Ovary Disease (Stein-Leventhal Syndrome)

This is a syndrome characterised by oligomenorrhoea, anovulation, infertility, hirsutism and obesity in young women having bilaterally enlarged and cystic ovaries. The principal biochemical abnormalities in most patients are excessive production of androgens, and low levels of pituitary follicle stimulating hormone (FSH). These endocrinologic abnormalities were previously attributed to primary ovarian dysfunction as evidenced by excellent results from wedge resection of the ovary. But current concept of pathogenesis is the unbalanced release of FSH and LH by the pituitary. FSH is inhibited to low levels by testosterone but the level of LH is sufficient to cause luteinisation of ovarian theca and granulosa cells which then secrete androgen inappropriately and produce an abnormal state of anovulation. A hereditary basis for the syndrome has been suggested in some cases.

PATHOLOGIC CHANGES. Grossly, the ovaries are usually involved bilaterally and are at least twice the size of the normal ovary. They are grey-white in colour and studded with multiple small (0.5-1.5 cm in diameter) bluish cysts just beneath the cortex. The medullary stroma is abundant, solid and grey.
Histologically, the outer cortex is thick and fibrous. The subcortical cysts are lined by prominent luteinised theca cells and represent follicles in various stages of maturation but there is no evidence of corpus luteum.

OVARIAN TUMOURS

The ovary is third most common site of primary malignancy in the female genital tract, preceded only by endometrial and cervical cancer. Both benign and malignant tumours occur in the ovaries.

ETIOPATHOGENESIS

Unlike the other two female genital cancers (cervix and endometrium), not much is known about the etiology of ovarian tumours. However, a few risk factors have been identified which include the following:

1. **Nulliparity.** There is higher incidence of ovarian cancer in unmarried women and married women with low or no parity.
2. **Heredity.** About 5% cases of ovarian cancer occur in women with family history of ovarian or breast cancer. Women with hereditary breast-ovarian cancer susceptibility have mutation in *BRCA* gene—*BRCA-1* (located on chromosome 17) and *BRCA-2* (located on chromosome 13). The risk in *BRCA-1* carriers is higher compared to that in *BRCA-2* carriers. Interestingly, men in such families have an increased risk of prostate cancer. In addition to *BRCA* mutation, other molecular abnor-

TABLE 22.6: Classification of Ovarian Tumours.

1. **TUMOURS OF SURFACE EPITHELIUM (COMMON EPITHELIAL TUMOURS) (60-70%)**
   - A. Serous tumours
     1. Serous cystadenoma
     2. Borderline serous tumour
     3. Serous cystadenocarcinoma
   - B. Mucinous tumours
     1. Mucinous cystadenoma
     2. Borderline mucinous tumour
     3. Mucinous cystadenocarcinoma
   - C. Endometrioid tumours
   - D. Clear cell (mesonephroid) tumours
   - E. Brenner tumours

II. **GERM CELL TUMOURS (15-20%)**
   - A. Teratomas
     1. Benign (mature, adult) teratoma
        - Benign cystic teratoma (dermoid cyst)
        - Benign solid teratoma
     2. Malignant (immature) teratoma
     3. Monodermal or specialised teratoma
        - Struma ovarii
        - Carcinoid tumour
   - B. Dysgerminoma
   - C. Endodermal sinus (yolk sac) tumour
   - D. Choriocarcinoma
   - E. Others (embryonal carcinoma, polyembryoma, mixed germ cell tumours)

III. **SEX CORD-STROMAL TUMOURS (5-10%)**
   - A. Granulosa-theca cell tumours
     1. Granulosa cell tumour
     2. Thecoma
     3. Fibroma
   - B. Sertoli-Leydig cell tumours (Androblastoma, arrhenoblastoma)
   - C. Gynandroblastoma

IV. **MISCELLANEOUS TUMOURS**
   - A. Lipid cell tumours
   - B. Gonadoblastoma

V. **METASTATIC TUMOURS (5%)**
   - A. Krukenberg tumour
   - B. Others

malities in ovarian cancers include mutation of *TP53* tumour suppressor gene and overexpression of *ERBB-2* and *K-RAS* genes.

3. **Complex genetic syndromes.** Besides the above two main factors, several complex genetic syndromes are associated with ovarian tumours as follows:

i) *Peutz-Jeghers syndrome* with ovarian sex cord-stromal tumours.

ii) *Gonadal dysgenesis* with gonadoblastoma.

iii) *Nevoid basal cell carcinoma* with ovarian fibromas.

CLINICAL FEATURES AND CLASSIFICATION

In general, benign ovarian tumours are more common, particularly in young women between the age of 20 and 40 years, and account for 80% of all ovarian neoplasms. Malignant tumours may be primary or metastatic; ovary being a common site for metastases from various other cancers. Primary malignant ovarian tumours are more common in older women between the age of 40 and 60 years.

Although certain specific tumours have distinctive features such as elaboration of hormones, most benign and malignant ovarian tumours are discovered when they grow sufficiently to cause abdominal discomfort and distension. Urinary tract and gastrointestinal tract symptoms are frequently associated due to compression by the tumour. Ascites is common in both benign and malignant ovarian tumours. Menstrual irregularities may or may not be present. Some ovarian tumours are bilateral. Malignant tumours usually spread beyond the ovary to other sites before the diagnosis is made.

A simplified classification proposed by the WHO with minor modifications has been widely adopted (Table 22.6). According to this classification, ovarian tumours arise from normally-occurring cellular components of the ovary (Fig. 22.9). Five major groups have been described:

I. Tumours of surface epithelium (common epithelial tumours)
II. Germ cell tumours
III. Sex cord-stromal tumours
IV. Miscellaneous tumours
V. Metastatic tumours

I. TUMOURS OF SURFACE EPITHELIUM (COMMON EPITHELIAL TUMOURS)

Tumours derived from the surface (coelomic) epithelium called common epithelial tumours form the largest group of ovarian tumours. This group constitutes about 60-70% of all ovarian neoplasms and 90% of malignant ovarian tumours. The common epithelial tumours are of 3 major types—*serous, mucinous* and *endometrioid,* though mixtures of these epithelia may occur in the same tumour. These tumours frequently have prominent cystic component which may have a single or multiple loculations and hence the descriptive prefix *cystadeno-* in these tumours. In addition, surface epithelial tumours may differentiate along urothelium to form *Brenner tumour,* and along mesonephroid pattern forming *clear cell (mesonephroid) adenocarcinoma.*

Depending upon the aggressiveness, the surface epithelial tumours are divided into 3 groups: *clearly*

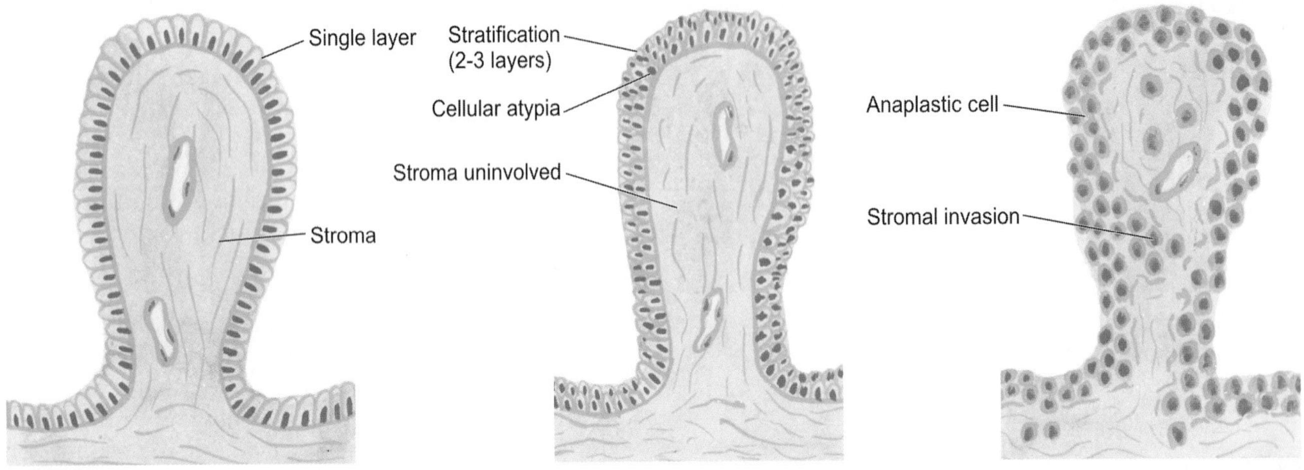

FIGURE 22.10

General histologic criteria to distinguish benign, borderline and malignant surface epithelial tumours of the ovary.

benign, clearly malignant, and *borderline* or *low-grade malignant tumours.* In general, the criteria for diagnosis of these 3 grades of aggressiveness are as follows (Fig. 22.10):

- **Clearly benign tumours** are lined by a single layer of well-oriented columnar epithelium. Papillary projections, if present, are covered by the same type of epithelium without any invasion into fibrovascular stromal stalk.
- **Clearly malignant tumours** have anaplastic epithelial component, multilayering, loss of basal polarity and unquestionable stromal invasion. The prognosis of these tumours is very poor.
- **Borderline tumours** or tumours with low malignant potential have some morphological features of malignancy, apparent detachment of cellular clusters from their site of origin and essential absence of stromal invasion. Morphological features of malignancy which may be present in varying combinations include: stratification (2-3 layers) of the epithelial cells but generally maintained basal polarity of nuclei, moderate nuclear abnormalities, and some mitotic activity. This group has a much better prognosis than frankly malignant tumours of the ovary.

Serous Tumours

Serous tumours comprise the largest group constituting about 20% of all ovarian tumours and 40% of malignant ovarian tumours. They are called serous tumours because of the presence of clear, watery, serous fluid in these predominantly cystic tumours. About 60% of serous tumours are benign, 15% borderline and 25% malignant. Only 20% of benign tumours occur bilaterally, whereas 65% of both borderline and malignant serous tumours have bilateral ovarian involvement. Serous tumours occur most commonly in 2nd to 5th decades of life, the malignant forms being more frequent in later life.

Histogenesis of the serous tumours is from the surface (coelomic) epithelium or mesothelium which differentiates along tubal-type of epithelium.

PATHOLOGIC CHANGES. Grossly, the benign, borderline and malignant serous tumours are large (above 5 cm in diameter) and spherical masses. Small masses are generally unilocular while the larger serous cysts are multiloculated similar to the mucinous variety, but differ from the latter in containing serous fluid rather than the viscid fluid of mucinous tumours. *Malignant serous tumours* may have solid areas in the cystic mass. Exophytic as well as intracystic papillary projections may be present in all grades of serous tumours but are more frequent in malignant tumours and are termed papillary serous cystadenocarcinomas (Fig. 22.11,A).

Histologically, the features are as follows:

1. **Serous cystadenoma** is characteristically lined by properly-oriented low columnar epithelium which is

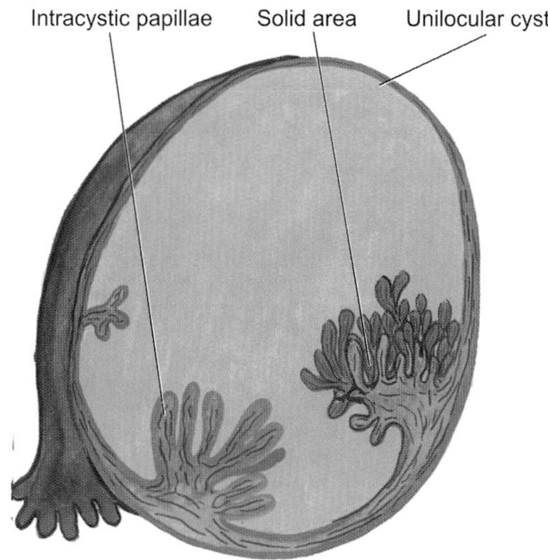

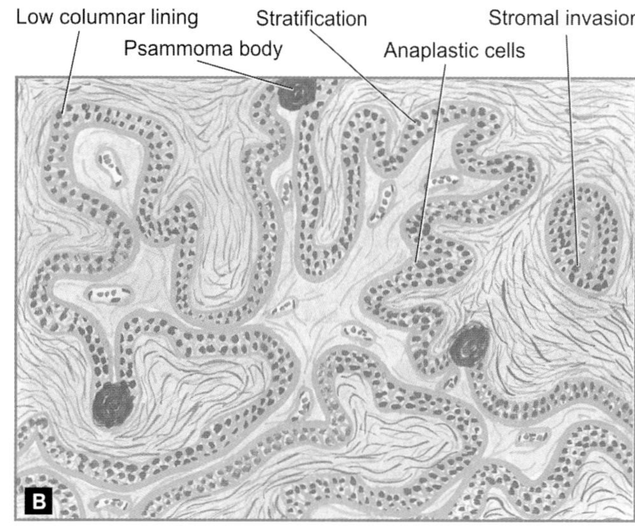

FIGURE 22.11

Papillary serous cystadenocarcinoma of the ovary. A, Gross appearance as seen on cut section showing a unilocular cyst with intracystic papillae. B, Microscopic features include stratification of low columnar epithelium lining the inner surface of the cyst and a few psammoma bodies. The stroma shows invasion by clusters of anaplastic tumour cells.

sometimes ciliated and resembles tubal epithelium. Microscopic papillae may be found.

2. Borderline serous tumour usually has stratification (2-3 layers) of benign serous type of epithelium. There is detachment of cell clusters from their site of origin and moderate features of malignancy but there is absence of stromal invasion.

3. Serous cystadenocarcinoma has multilayered malignant cells which show loss of polarity, presence of solid sheets of anaplastic epithelial cells and definite evidence of stromal invasion. Papillae formations are more frequent in malignant variety and may be associated with psammoma bodies but mere presence of psammoma bodies is not indicative of malignancy (Fig. 22.11,B) (COLOUR PLATE XXX: CL 119).

Mucinous Tumours

Mucinous tumours are somewhat less common than serous tumours and constitute about 20% of all ovarian tumours and 10% of all ovarian cancers. Over 80% are benign, 10-15% are borderline and 5-10% are malignant. These predominantly cystic tumours contain mucin which was previously described as pseudomucin. Well-differentiated borderline mucinous tumours are associated with mucinous ascites termed *pseudomyxoma peritonei* (page 594). Mucinous tumours as compared with serous tumours are more commonly unilateral. Benign mucinous tumours occur bilaterally in 5% of cases while borderline and malignant are bilateral in 20%. Mucinous tumours occur principally between 2nd and 5th decades of life. Mucinous carcinoma usually develops in women above the age of 40 years.

Histogenesis of mucinous tumours, in line with that of serous tumours, is from the coelomic epithelium that differentiates along endocervical type or intestinal type of mucosa.

PATHOLOGIC CHANGES. ***Grossly,*** mucinous tumours are larger than serous tumours. They are smooth-surfaced cysts with characteristic multiloculations containing thick and viscid gelatinous fluid (Fig. 22.12,A). Benign tumours generally have thin wall and septa dividing the loculi are also thin and often translucent, but malignant varieties usually have thickened areas. In younger patients, an element of teratoma may be recognised in the firm areas of the tumour.

Histologically, the most distinctive feature is the characteristic tall columnar nonciliated epithelium lining the loculi (Fig. 22.12,B). Other features are as under:

1. Mucinous cystadenoma is lined by a single layer of these cells having basal nuclei and apical mucinous vacuoles. There is very little tendency to papillary proliferation of the epithelium (COLOUR PLATE XXX: CL 120).

2. Borderline mucinous tumour is identified by the same histologic criteria as for borderline serous tumour i.e. stratification (usually 2-3 cell thick) of typical epithelium without stromal invasion.

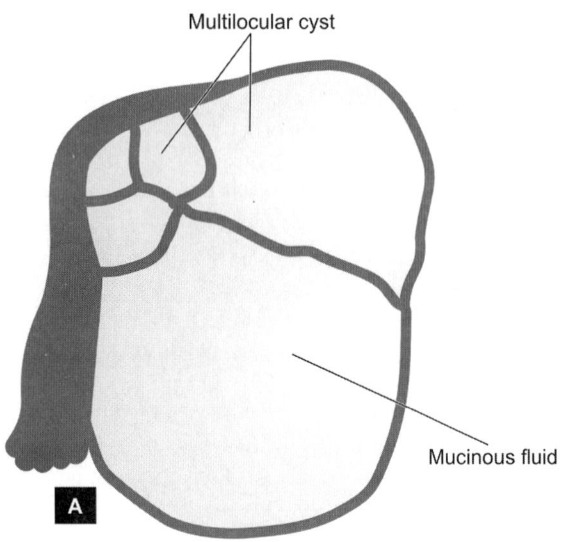

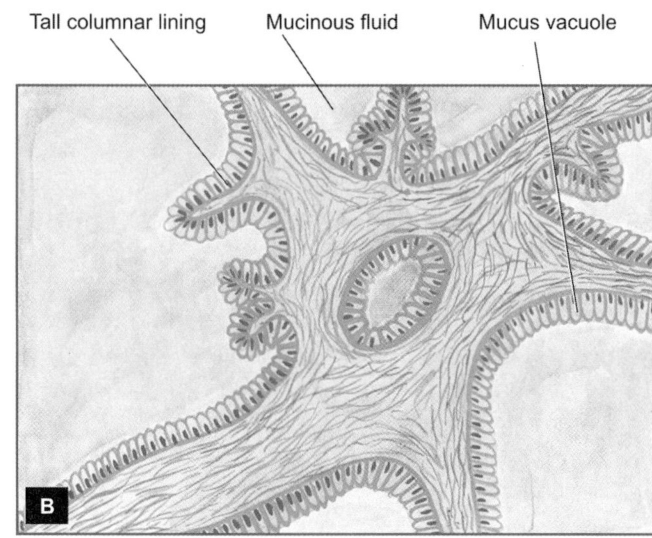

FIGURE 22.12

Mucinous cystadenoma of the ovary. A, gross appearance on cut section revealing a multiloculated cyst without papillae. B, histologically, the cyst wall and the septa are lined by a single layer of tall columnar mucin-secreting epithelium with basally-placed nuclei and large apical mucinous vacuoles.

3. **Mucinous cystadenocarcinoma** likewise is characterised by piling up of malignant epithelium, at places forming solid sheets, papillary formation, adenomatous pattern and infiltration into stroma with or without pools of mucin.

Endometrioid Tumours

Endometrioid tumours comprise about 5% of all ovarian tumours. Most of them are malignant accounting for about 20% of all ovarian cancers. Benign and borderline forms are very rare. They are called endometrioid carcinomas because of the close resemblance of histologic pattern to that of uterine endometrial adenocarcinoma. About 40% of endometrioid carcinomas have bilateral ovarian involvement. About 15-30% of cases of endometrioid carcinoma have coexistent endometrial adenocarcinoma.

Histogenesis of these tumours in majority of cases is believed to be from ovarian coelomic epithelium differentiating towards endometrial type of epithelium. Some authors, however, on the basis of presence of endometriosis in a few cases of endometrioid tumours, have suggested malignant transformation of endometriosis.

PATHOLOGIC CHANGES. ***Grossly,*** these tumours are partly solid and partly cystic and may have foci of haemorrhages, especially in benign variety.

Histologically, the endometrioid adenocarcinoma is distinguished from serous and mucinous carcinomas by typical glandular pattern that closely resembles that of uterine endometrial adenocarcinoma. There may be foci of squamous metaplasia justifying the diagnosis of adenoacanthoma. Papillary pattern and foci of serous and mucinous carcinoma may also be found. Benign variety closely resembles endometriosis with cystic change. There are no clearly defined criteria for borderline endometrioid tumours.

Clear Cell (Mesonephroid) Tumours

Clear cell (mesonephroid) tumours are almost always malignant and comprise about 5% of all ovarian cancers. Rare benign variety is called *clear cell adenofibroma.* They are termed clear cell or mesonephroid carcinomas because of the close histologic resemblance to renal adenocarcinoma. They have also been called as mesonephroma or mesonephric carcinoma because of the questionable relationship to the mesonephric structures.

PATHOLOGIC CHANGES. ***Grossly,*** these tumours are large, usually unilateral, partly solid and partly cystic. Less than 10% are bilateral.

Histologically, clear cell or mesonephroid carcinoma is characterised by tubules, glands, papillae, cysts and solid sheets of tumour cells resembling cells of renal adenocarcinoma i.e. clear cells having abundant eosinophilic cytoplasm rich in glycogen.

Brenner Tumour

Brenner tumours are uncommon and comprise about 2% of all ovarian tumours. They are characteristically solid ovarian tumours. Less than 10% of Brenner tumours are bilateral. Most Brenner tumours are benign. Rarely, borderline form is encountered and is called 'proliferating Brenner tumour' and one with carcinomatous change is termed 'malignant Brenner tumour'.

Histogenesis of the tumour is from coelomic epithelium by metaplastic transformation into transitional epithelium (urothelium).

PATHOLOGIC CHANGES. Grossly, Brenner tumour is typically solid, yellow-grey, firm mass of variable size. Occasionally, a few scattered tiny cysts may be present on cut section.

Histologically, Brenner tumour consists of nests, masses and columns of epithelial cells, scattered in fibrous stroma of the ovary. These epithelial cells resemble urothelial cells which are ovoid in shape, having clear cytoplasm, vesicular nuclei with characteristic nuclear groove called 'coffee-bean' nuclei.

II. GERM CELL TUMOURS

Ovarian germ cell tumours arising from germ cells which produce the female gametes (i.e. ova) account for about 15-20% of all ovarian neoplasms. The neoplastic germ cells may follow one of the several lines of differentiation as shown in Fig. 22.13. Nearly 95% of them are benign and vast majority of them are benign cystic teratomas (dermoid cysts) and occur chiefly in young females. The remainder are malignant germ cell tumours comprising a variety of morphologic forms occurring chiefly in children and young adults and are highly aggressive tumours. Most germ cell tumours of the ovaries have their counterparts in the testis (Chapter 21) and sometimes in the mediastinum but their frequency differs from one site to the other. For instance, benign cystic teratoma or dermoid cyst so common in ovaries is extremely rare in the testis.

Teratomas

Teratomas are tumours composed of different types of tissues derived from the three germ cell layers—ectoderm, mesoderm and endoderm, in different combi-

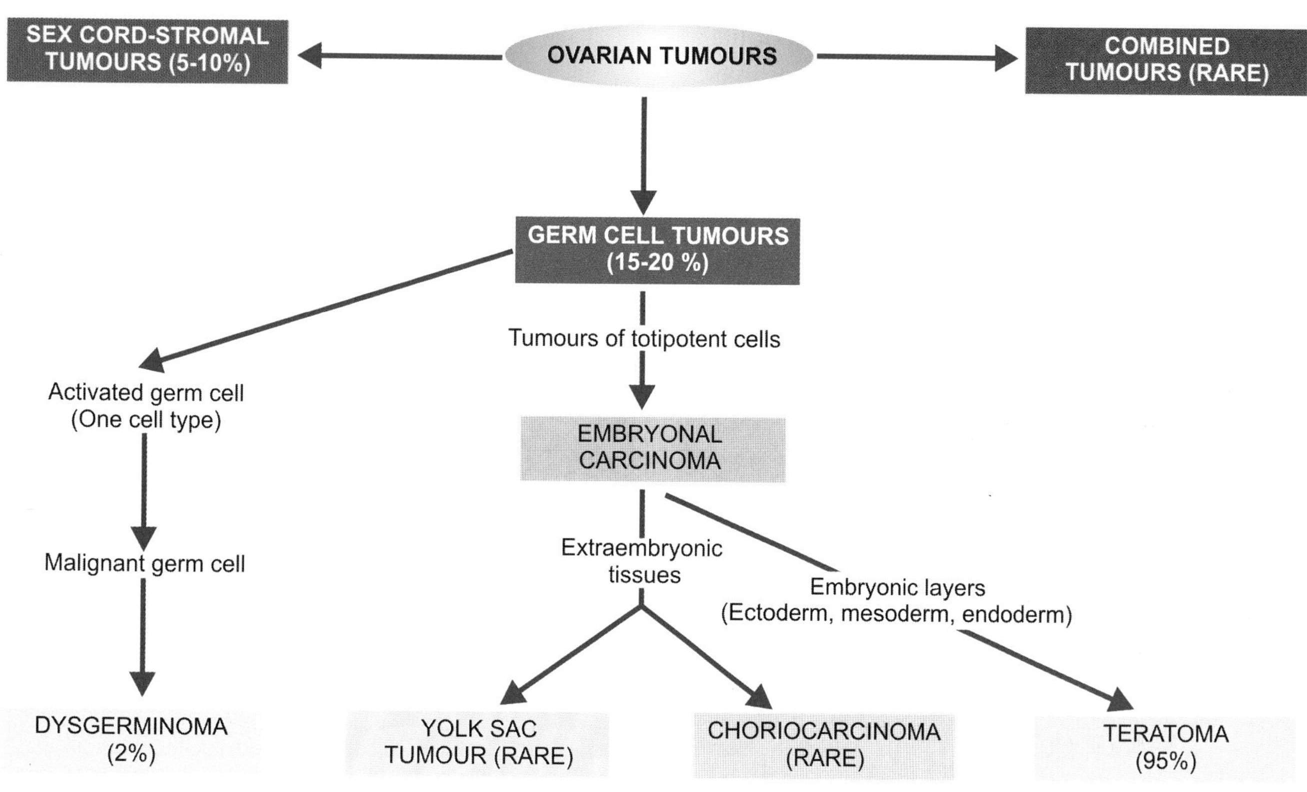

FIGURE 22.13

Histogenetic classification of germ cell tumours of the ovary.

nations. They are divided into 3 types: mature (benign), immature (malignant), and monodermal or highly specialised teratomas.

MATURE (BENIGN) TERATOMA. The vast majority of ovarian teratomas are benign and cystic and have the predominant ectodermal elements, often termed clinically as *dermoid cyst.* Infrequently, mature teratoma may be solid and benign and has to be distinguished from immature or malignant teratoma. Benign cystic teratomas are more frequent in young women during their active reproductive life. The tumour is bilateral in 10% of cases. In view of wide spectrum of tissue elements found in these teratomas, their *histogenesis* has been a matter of speculation for centuries. More recently, cytogenetic studies have revealed that these tumours arise from a single germ cell (ovum) after its first meiotic division.

*PATHOLOGIC CHANGES. **Grossly,*** benign cystic teratoma or dermoid cyst is characteristically a unilocular cyst, 10-15 cm in diameter, usually lined by skin and hence its name. On sectioning, the cyst is filled with paste-like sebaceous secretions and desquamated keratin admixed with masses of hair. The cyst wall is thin and opaque grey-white. Generally, in one area of the cyst wall, a solid prominence is seen (Rokitansky's protuberance) where tissue elements such as tooth, bone, cartilage and various other odd tissues are present (Fig. 22.14,A). Less often, the cyst may contain mucoid material.

Microscopically, the most prominent feature is the lining of the cyst wall by stratified squamous epithelium and its adnexal structures such as sebaceous glands, sweat glands and hair follicles (Fig. 22.14,B). Though ectodermal derivatives are most prominent features, tissues of mesodermal and endodermal origin are commonly present. Various other tissue components frequently found are bronchus, intestinal epithelium, cartilage, bone, tooth, smooth muscle, neural tissue, salivary gland, retina, pancreas and thyroid tissue. Thus, viewing a benign cystic teratoma in different microscopic fields reveals a variety of mature differentiated tissue elements, producing *kaleidoscopic patterns* (COLOUR PLATE XXXI: CL 121). Less than 1% of patients with a dermoid cyst develop malignant transformation of one of the tissue components, most commonly squamous cell carcinoma.

IMMATURE (MALIGNANT) TERATOMA. Immature or malignant teratomas are rare and account for approximately 0.2% of all ovarian tumours. They are predominantly solid tumours that contain immature or embryonal structures in contrast to the mature or adult structures of the benign teratomas. They are more common in prepubertal adolescents and young women under 20 years of age.

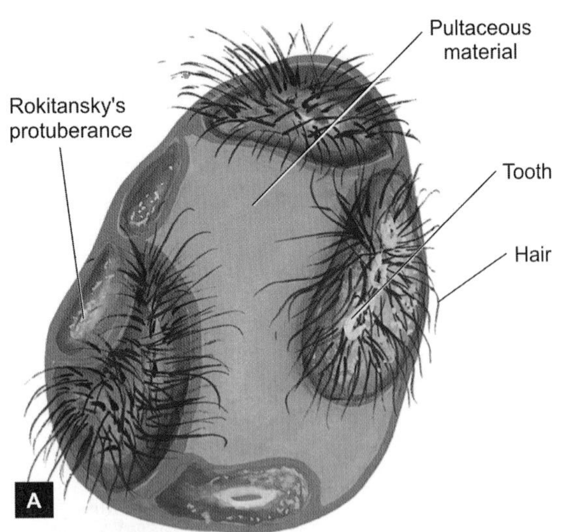

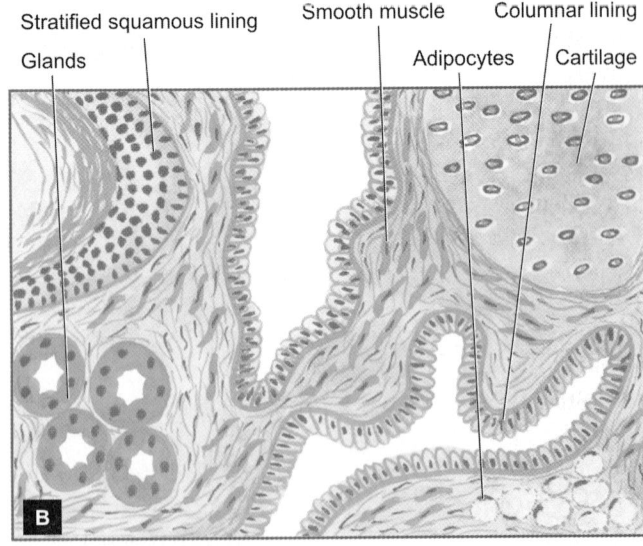

FIGURE 22.14

Benign cystic teratoma (dermoid cyst) of the ovary A, Gross appearance. B, Microscopy shows characteristic lining of the cyst wall by epidermis and its appendages.

*PATHOLOGIC CHANGES. **Grossly,*** malignant teratoma is a unilateral solid mass which on cut section shows characteristic variegated appearance revealing areas of haemorrhages, necrosis, tiny cysts and heterogeneous admixture of various tissue elements.

Microscopically, parts of the tumour may show mature tissues, while most of it is composed of immature tissues having an embryonic appearance. Immature tissue elements may differentiate towards cartilage, bone, glandular structures, neural tissue etc, and are distributed in spindle-shaped myxoid or undifferentiated sarcoma cells. An important factor in grading and determining the prognosis of immature teratoma is the relative amount of immature neural tissue. Immature neural tissue can undergo maturation even at the site of metastases over a period of years. Immature teratoma may contain areas of other germ cell tumours such as endodermal sinus tumour, embryonal carcinoma and choriocarcinoma.

Grade I tumours having relatively mature elements and confined to the ovary have a good prognosis, whereas grade III immature teratomas with metastases have an extremely poor prognosis.

MONODERMAL (SPECIALISED) TERATOMA. Monodermal or highly specialised teratomas are rare and include 2 important examples—struma ovarii and carcinoid tumour.

- **Struma ovarii.** It is a teratoma composed exclusively of thyroid tissue, recognisable grossly as well as microscopically. Most often, the tumour has the appearance of a follicular adenoma of the thyroid. Rarely, struma ovarii may be hyperfunctioning and produce hyperthyroidism.
- **Carcinoid tumour.** This is an ovarian teratoma arising from argentaffin cells of intestinal epithelium in the teratoma. Ovarian carcinoid may also hyperfunction and produce 5-HT and consequent carcinoid syndrome.
- **Struma-carcinoid** is a rare combination of struma ovarii and ovarian carcinoid.

Dysgerminoma

Dysgerminoma is an ovarian counterpart of seminoma of the testes (page 735). Dysgerminomas comprise about 2% of all ovarian cancers. They occur most commonly in 2nd to 3rd decades. About 10% of them are bilateral. About 10% of patients with dysgerminoma have elevated hCG level in the plasma. All dysgerminomas are malignant and are extremely radiosensitive.

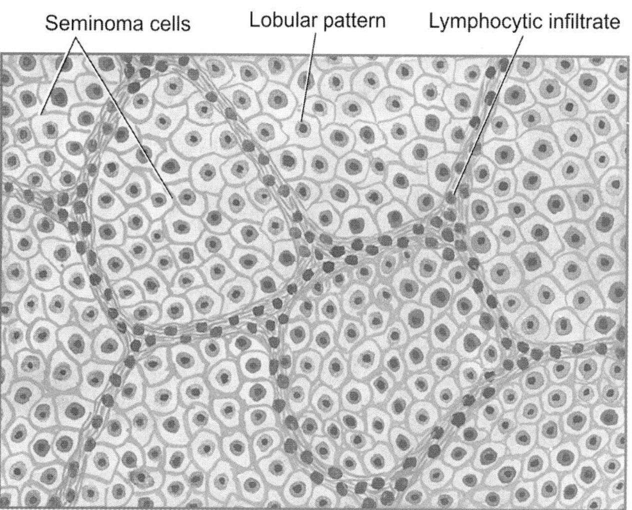

FIGURE 22.15

Dysgerminoma. The histologic appearance is identical to that of seminoma of the testis. Masses of large uniform tumour cells are separated by scanty fibrous stroma that is infiltrated by lymphocytes.

*PATHOLOGIC CHANGES. **Grossly,*** dysgerminoma is a solid mass of variable size. Cut section of the tumour is grey-white to pink, lobulated, soft and fleshy with foci of haemorrhages and necrosis.

Histologically, their structure is similar to that of seminoma of the testis (Fig. 22.15). The tumour cells are arranged in diffuse sheets, islands and cords separated by scanty fibrous stroma. The tumour cells are uniform in appearance and large, with vesicular nuclei and clear cytoplasm rich in glycogen. The fibrous stroma generally contains lymphocytic infiltrate and sometimes may have sarcoid granulomas.

Endodermal Sinus (Yolk Sac) Tumour

Endodermal sinus tumour or yolk sac tumour is the second most common germ cell tumour occurring most commonly in children and young women. More often, endodermal sinus tumour is found in combination with other germ cell tumours rather than in pure form. The tumour is rich in alphafetoprotein (AFP) and alpha-1-antitrypsin. The tumour is usually unilateral but may metastasise to the other ovary. It is a highly aggressive and rapidly growing tumour.

*PATHOLOGIC CHANGES. **Grossly,*** the tumour is generally solid with areas of cystic degeneration.

Histologically, like its testicular counterpart, the endodermal sinus tumour is characterised by the presence of papillary projections having a central blood vessel with perivascular layer of anaplastic embryonal germ cells. Such structures resemble the endodermal sinuses of the rat placenta (Schiller-Duval body) from which the tumour derives its name (COLOUR PLATE XXIX: CL 114). It is common to find intracellular and extracelluar PAS-positive hyaline globules which are composed of AFP.

Choriocarcinoma

Choriocarcinoma in females is of 2 types—*gestational and non-gestational.* Gestational choriocarcinoma of placental origin is more common and considered separately later (page 778), while non-gestational choriocarcinoma of ovarian origin is rare. Primary ovarian choriocarcinoma more often occurs in combination with other germ cell tumours than in pure form. The patients are usually young girls under the age of 20 years. Morphologically, ovarian choriocarcinoma is identical to gestational choriocarcinoma. Ovarian choriocarcinoma is more malignant than that of placental origin and disseminates widely via blood stream to the lungs, liver, bone, brain and kidneys. The marker for both types of choriocarcinoma is hCG.

Other Germ Cell Tumours

Certain other germ cell tumours occasionally encountered in the ovaries are embryonal carcinoma, polyembryoma and mixed germ cell tumours. All these tumours are morphologically identical to similar tumours occurring in the testes (Chapter 21).

III. SEX CORD-STROMAL TUMOURS

Sex cord-stromal tumours of the ovaries comprise 5-10% of all ovarian neoplasms. They arise from specialised ovarian stromal cells of the developing gonads. Thus, these include tumours originating from granulosa cells, theca cells and Sertoli-Leydig cells. Since sex cord-stromal cells have functional activity, most of these tumours elaborate steroid hormones which may have feminising effects or masculinising effects.

Granulosa-Theca Cell Tumours

Granulosa-theca cell tumours comprise about 5% of all ovarian tumours. The group includes: pure granulosa cell tumours, pure thecomas, combination of granulosa-theca cell tumours and fibromas.

GRANULOSA CELL TUMOUR. Pure granulosa cell tumours may occur at all ages. These tumours invade locally but occasionally may have more aggressive and malignant behaviour. Recurrences after surgical removal are common. Most granulosa cell tumours secrete oestrogen which may be responsible for precocious puberty in young girls, or in older patients may produce endometrial hyperplasia, endometrial adenocarcinoma and cystic disease of the breast. Rarely, granulosa cell tumour may elaborate androgen which may have masculinising effect on the patient.

Grossly, granulosa cell tumour is a small, solid, partly cystic and usually unilateral tumour. Cut section of solid areas is yellowish-brown.

Microscopically, the granulosa cells are arranged in a variety of patterns including micro- and macrofollicular, trabecular, bands and diffuse sheets. The microfollicular pattern is characterised by the presence of characteristic rosette-like structures, Call-Exner bodies, having central rounded pink mass surrounded by a circular row of granulosa cells (Fig. 22.16).

Morphologic appearance alone is a poor indicator of clinical malignancy but presence of metastases and invasion outside the ovary are considered better indicators of aggressive behaviour.

THECOMA. Pure thecomas are almost always benign. They occur more frequently in post-menopausal women. Thecomas are typically oestrogenic. Endometrial

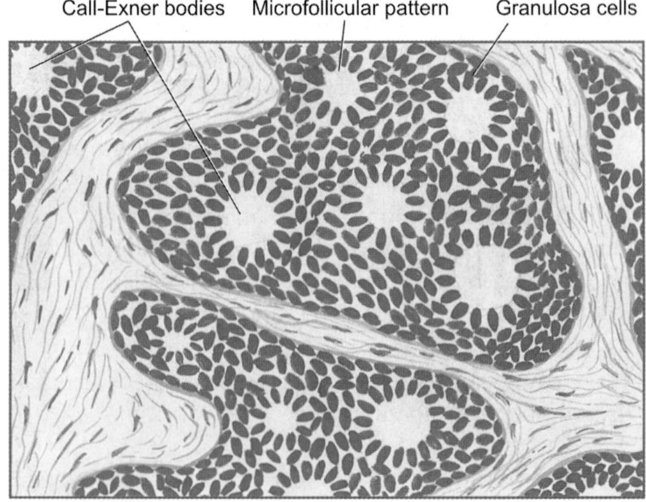

FIGURE 22.16

Granulosa cell tumour, showing uniform granulosa cells and numerous rosette-like Call-Exner bodies containing central amorphous pink material surrounded by granulosa cells.

Chapter Twenty Two

hyperplasia, endometrial carcinoma and cystic disease of the breast are some of its adverse effects. Occasionally a thecoma may secrete androgen and cause virilisation.

Grossly, thecoma is a solid and firm mass, 5-10 cm in diameter. Cut section is yellowish.
Microscopically, thecoma consists of spindle-shaped theca cells of the ovary admixed with variable amount of hyalinised collagen. The cytoplasm of theca cells is lipid-rich and vacuolated which reacts with lipid stains.

GRANULOSA-THECA CELL TUMOUR. Mixture of both granulosa and theca cell elements in the same ovarian tumour is seen in some cases with elaboration of oestrogen.

FIBROMA. Fibromas of the ovary are more common and account for about 5% of all ovarian tumours. These tumours are hormonally inert but some of them are associated with pleural effusion and benign ascites termed Meig's syndrome.

Grossly, these tumours are large, firm and fibrous, usually unilateral masses.
Histologically, they are composed of spindle-shaped well-differentiated fibroblasts and collagen. Sometimes, combination of fibroma and thecoma is present called fibrothecoma.

Sertoli-Leydig Cell Tumours (Androblastoma, Arrhenoblastoma)

Tumours containing Sertoli and Leydig cells in varying degree of maturation comprise Sertoli-Leydig cell tumours, also called androblastomas or arrhenoblastomas. Their histogenesis remains obscure. Characteristically, they produce androgens and musculinise the patient. Less often, they may elaborate oestrogen. Their peak incidence is in 2nd to 3rd decades of life.

Grossly, Sertoli-Leydig cell tumour resembles a granulosa-theca cell tumour.
Histologically, these tumours recapitulate to some extent the structure of the testis. Three histologic types are distinguished:
1. *Well-differentiated* androblastoma composed almost entirely of Sertoli cells or Leydig cells forming well-defined tubules.
2. *Tumours with intermediate differentiation* have a biphasic pattern with formation of solid sheets in which abortive tubules are present.
3. *Poorly-differentiated or sarcomatoid variety* is composed of spindle cells resembling sarcoma with interspersed scanty Leydig cells.

Gynandroblastoma

Gynandroblastoma is an extremely rare tumour in which there is combination of patterns of both granulosa-theca cell tumour and Sertoli-Leydig cell tumour. The term gynandroblastoma stands for combination of female *(gyn)* and male *(andro).*

IV. MISCELLANEOUS TUMOURS

LIPID CELL TUMOURS. There is a small group of ovarian tumours that appears as soft yellow or yellow-brown nodules which on histologic examination are composed of large lipid-laden cells. These cells resemble Leydig, lutein and adrenal cortical cells. The examples of these tumours are: hilus cell tumours, adrenal rest tumours and luteomas. These tumours elaborate steroid hormones and are responsible for various endocrine dysfunctions such as Cushing's syndrome and virilisation.

GONADOBLASTOMA. This is a rare tumour occurring exclusively in dysgenetic gonads, more often in phenotypic females and in hermaphrodites. Dysfunctions include virilism, amenorrhoea and abnormal external genitalia.

Microscopically, gonadoblastoma is composed of mixture of germ cell and sex cord components.

V. METASTATIC TUMOURS

About 10% of ovarian cancers are secondary carcinomas. Metastasis may occur by lymphatic or haematogenous route but direct extension from adjacent organs (e.g. uterus, fallopian tube and sigmoid colon) too occurs frequently. Bilaterality of the tumour is the most helpful clue to diagnosis of metastatic tumour. Most common primary sites from where metastases to the ovaries are encountered are: carcinomas of the breast, genital tract, gastrointestinal tract (e.g. stomach, colon appendix, pancreas, biliary tract) and haematopoietic malignancies.

The **Krukenberg tumour** is a distinctive bilateral tumour metastatic to the ovaries by transcoelomic spread characterised by the presence of mucus-filled signet ring cells accompanied by sarcoma-like proliferation of ovarian stroma (Fig. 22.17). This tumour is generally secondary to a gastric carcinoma (Chapter 18) but other primary sites where mucinous carcinomas

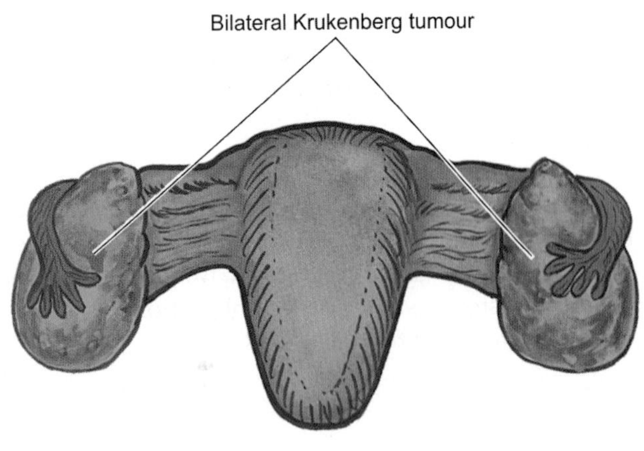

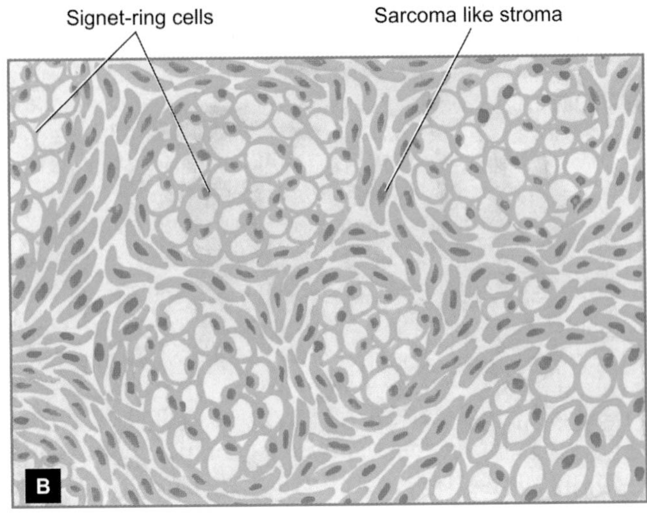

FIGURE 22.17

Krukenberg tumour. A, characteristic bilateral metastatic ovarian cancer. B, histologic features include mucin-filled signet-ring cells and sarcoma-like proliferation of the ovarian stroma.

occur (e.g. colon, appendix and breast) may also produce Krukenberg tumour in the ovary. Rarely, a tumour having the pattern of Krukenberg tumour is primary in the ovary.

FIGO staging of ovarian cancer is given in Table 22.7.

TABLE 22.7: FIGO Clinical Staging of Carcinoma of the Carcinoma of the Ovary.		
Stage	I	Growth limited to ovaries.
	IA	Growth limited to one ovary; no ascites; capsule intact.
	IB	Growth limited to both ovaries; no ascites; capsule intact.
	IC	Tumour classified as either stage IA or IB but with tumour in the surface of one or both ovaries, or with ascites containing malignant cells.
Stage	II	Growth involving one or both ovaries, with pelvic extension
	IIA	Extension and/or metastases to the uterus and/or tubes.
	IIB	Extension to other pelvic tissues.
	IIC	Tumour either stage IIA or IIB but with tumour on the surface of one or both ovaries, or with capsule ruptured, or with ascites containing malignant cells.
Stage	III	Tumour invading one or both ovaries with peritoneal implants outside the pelvis.
	IIIA	Tumour grossly limited to the true pelvis with negative nodes but with microscopic seeding of abdominal peritoneal surfaces.
	IIIB	Tumour of one or both ovaries with histologically confirmed implants of abdominal peritoneal surfaces, not exceeding 2 cm in diameter; nodes are negative.
	IIIC	Abdominal implants greater than 2 cm in diameter and/or positive retroperitoneal or inguinal nodes.
Stage	IV	Growth involving one or both ovaries, with distant metastases.

PLACENTA

NORMAL STRUCTURE

At term, the normal placenta is blue red, rounded, flattened and discoid organ 15-20 cm in diameter and 2-4 cm thick. It weighs 400-600 gm or about one-sixth the weight of the newborn. The umbilical cord is about 50 cm long and contains two umbilical arteries and one umbilical vein attached at the foetal surface. The placenta is derived from both maternal and foetal tissues. The *maternal portion* of the placenta has irregular grooves dividing it into cotyledons which are composed of sheets of decidua basalis and remnants of blood vessels. The *foetal portion* of the placenta is composed of numerous functional units called chorionic villi and comprise the major part of placenta at term. The villi consist of a loose fibrovascular stromal core and a few phagocytic (Hoffbauer's) cells. The villous core is covered by an inner layer of cytotrophoblast and outer layer of syncytiotrophoblast. The basement membrane separating the foetal capillaries in the villous core and the trophoblast forms zones where nutrients and metabolites are transported between the mother and the foetus. Such zones are called vasculosyncitial membranes. The placenta secretes a number of hormones and enzymes into the maternal blood. These include: human chorionic gonadotropin (hCG), human placental lactogen (HPL), chorionic thyrotropin and adrenocorticotropin hormone which partake in oestrogen and progesterone metabolism.

Diseases related to pregnancy and placenta are numerous and form the subject matter of discussion in obstetrics. Certain conditions such as inflammation of the placenta and chorionic membranes (placentitis and chorioamnionitis), placental abnormalities (e.g. placenta accreta, placenta praevia and twin placenta etc), toxaemia of pregnancy (eclampsia and pre-eclampsia) and products of gestation seen in abortions need mere mention only. However, gestational trophoblastic diseases resulting from benign and malignant overgrowth of trophoblast, namely: hydatidiform mole (complete and partial mole) and choriocarcinoma respectively, are significant morphologic lessions and are discussed below and their features contrasted in Table 22.8.

HYDATIDIFORM MOLE

The word 'hydatidiform' means *drop of water* and 'mole' for a *shapeless mass.* Hydatidiform mole is a condition characterised by 2 features—hydropic change of the chorionic villi, and trophoblastic proliferation. Most workers consider hydatidiform mole as a benign tumour of placental tissue with potential for developing into choriocarcinoma, while some authors have described mole as a degenerative lesion though capable of neoplastic change. The incidence of molar pregnancy is high in teenagers and in older women. For unknown reasons, frequency of hydatidiform mole varies in different regions of the world; the incidence in Asia and Central America is about 10 times higher than in the United States. The incidence is higher in poorer classes.

Hydatidiform mole may be non-invasive or invasive. Two types of non-invasive moles are distinguished—complete (classic) and partial. The pathogenesis of these 2 forms is different:

■ **Complete (classic) mole** by cytogenetic studies has been shown to be derived from the father (androgenesis) and shows 46, XX or rarely 46, XY chromosomal

TABLE 22.8: Comparative Features of Major Forms of Gestational Trophoblastic Disease.

FEATURE	COMPLETE MOLE	PARTIAL MOLE	CHORIOCARCINOMA
1. *Karyotype*	46,XX or rarely 46,XY	Triploid i.e. 69,XXY or 69,XXX	46,XY or variable
2. *Clinical findings*			
i) Diagnosis	Mole	Missed abortion	Abortion; molar, ectopic or normal pregnancy
ii) Vaginal bleeding	Marked	Mild	Marked, abnormal
iii) Uterus size	Large	Small	Generally not bulky
3. *hCG levels*			
i) Serum hCG	High	Low	Persistently high
ii) hCG in tissues	Marked	Mild	Localised in syncytiotrophoblast only
4. *Embryo*	Not present	May be present	Not present
5. *Gross appearance*			
i) Vesicles	Large and regular	Smaller and irregular	No vesicles
ii) Villi	Present	Present	Always absent
6. *Microscopy*			
i) Villous size	Uniform	Variable	None present
ii) Hydropic villi	All	Some	None
iii) Trophoblastic proliferation	Diffuse, all three (cytotrophoblast, intermediate trophoblast and syncytiotrophoblast)	Focal, syncytiotrophoblast only	Both cytotrophoblast and syncytiotrophoblast
iv) Atypia	Diffuse	Minimal	Marked
v) Blood vessels	Generally absent	Present	Present and abnormal
7. *Persistence after initial therapy*	20%	7%	May metastasise rapidly if not treated
8. *Behaviour*	2% may develop choriocarcinoma	Choriocarcinoma almost never develops	Survival rate with chemotherapy 70%

pattern. Complete mole bears relationship to choriocarcinoma.

■ **The partial mole** is mostly triploid (i.e. 69,XXY or 69,XXX) and rarely tetraploid. Partial mole rarely develops into choriocarcinoma.

Clinically, the condition appears in 4th-5th month of gestation and is characterised by increase in uterine size, vaginal bleeding and often with symptoms of toxaemia. Frequently, there is history of passage of grape-like masses per vaginum. About 1% of women with molar pregnancy develop it again in a subsequent pregnancy.

The single most significant investigation is the serial determination of hCG which is elevated more in both blood and urine as compared with the levels in normal pregnancy. Removal of the mole is accompanied by fall in hCG levels. A more ominous behaviour is associated with no fall in hCG levels after expulsion of the mole. About 10% of patients with complete mole develop into invasive moles and 2.5% into choriocarcinoma.

PATHOLOGIC CHANGES. The pathologic findings in non-invasive (complete and partial) and invasive mole are different (Table 22.8):

COMPLETE (CLASSIC) MOLE: ***Grossly,*** the uterus is enlarged and characteristically filled with grape-like vesicles upto 3 cm in diameter (Fig. 22.18,A). The vesicles contain clear watery fluid. Rarely, a macerated foetus may be found.

Microscopically, the features are quite typical. These are (Fig. 22.18,B) (COLOUR PLATE XXX: CL 118):

■ Large, round oedematous villi.

■ Hydropic degeneration and decreased vascularity of villous stroma.

■ Trophoblastic proliferation in the form of masses and sheets of both cytotrophoblast and syncytiotrophoblast.

PARTIAL MOLE: ***Grossly,*** the uterus is generally smaller than expected and contains some cystic villi, while part of the placenta appears normal. A foetus with multiple malformations is often present.

Microscopically, some of the villi show oedematous change while others are normal or even fibrotic. Trophoblastic proliferation is usually slight and focal.

INVASIVE (DESTRUCTIVE) MOLE (CHORIOADENOMA DESTRUENS): ***Grossly,*** invasive mole shows invasion of the molar tissue into the uterine wall which may be a source of haemorrhage. Rarely, molar tissue may invade the blood vessels and reach the lungs.

Microscopically, the lesion is benign and identical to classic mole but has potential for haemorrhage. It is always associated with persistent elevation of hCG levels.

CHORIOCARCINOMA

Gestational choriocarcinoma is a highly malignant and widely metastasising tumour of trophoblast (non-

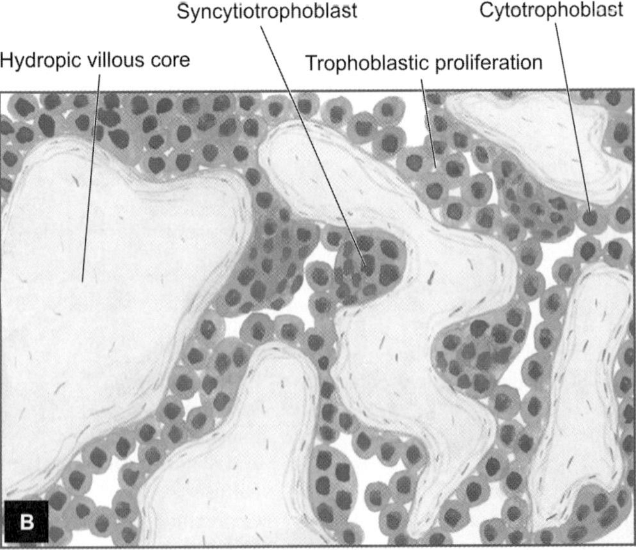

FIGURE 22.18

A, Uterus containing hydatidiform mole. B, Hydatidiform mole characterised by hydropic and avascular enlarged villi with trophoblastic proliferation in the form of masses and sheets.

gestational type is described on page 774). Approximately 50% of cases occur following hydatidiform mole, 25% following spontaneous abortion, 20% after an otherwise normal pregnancy, and 5% develop in an ectopic pregnancy. Choriocarcinoma follows the geographic pattern of hydatidiform mole, being more common in Asia and Africa than in the United States and Europe.

Clinically, the most common complaint is vaginal bleeding following a normal or abnormal pregnancy. Occasionally, the patients present with metastases in the brain or lungs. The diagnosis is confirmed by demonstration of persistently high levels of hCG in the plasma and urine. Widespread haematogenous metastases are early and frequent in choriocarcinoma if not treated and are found chiefly in the lungs, vagina, brain, liver and kidneys.

PATHOLOGIC CHANGES. ***Grossly,*** the tumour appears as haemorrhagic, soft and fleshy mass. Sometimes, the tumour may be small, often like a blood clot, in the uterus.

Microscopically, the characteristic features are as under:

- Absence of identifiable villi.
- Masses and columns of highly anaplastic and bizarre cytotrophoblast and syncytiotrophoblast cells which are intermixed.
- Invariable presence of haemorrhages and necrosis.
- Invasion of the underlying myometrium and other structures, blood vessels and lymphatics.

Gestational choriocarcinoma and its metastases respond very well to chemotherapy while non-gestational choriocarcinoma is quite resistant to therapy and has worse prognosis. With chemotherapy, the cure rate of choriocarcinoma has remarkably improved from dismal 20 to 70% survival rate and almost total cure in localised tumours. The effectiveness of treatment is also monitored by serial hCG determinations.

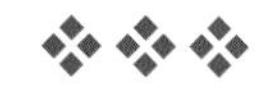

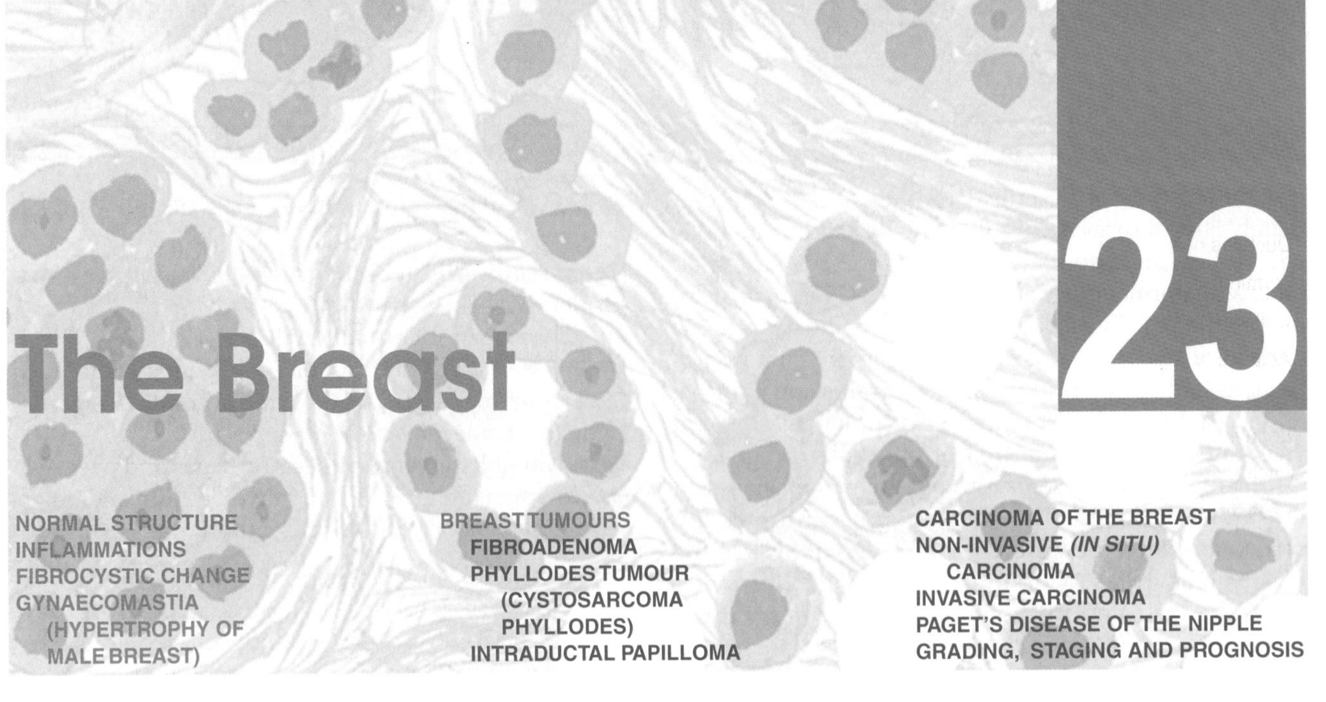

23 The Breast

NORMAL STRUCTURE

The breast is a modified skin appendage which is functional in the females during lactation but is rudimentary in the males. Microanatomy of the breast reveals 2 types of tissue components: *epithelial* and *stromal* (Fig. 23.1). In a fully-developed non-lactating female breast, the epithelial component comprises less than 10% of the total volume but is more significant pathologically since majority of lesions pertain to this portion of the breast.

EPITHELIAL COMPONENT. The epithelial component of the breast consists of the breast lobules and the collecting duct system. The breast is divided into about 20 *lobes.* Each lobe consists of *breast lobules* which drain their secretions through its *collecting duct system* and opens into the nipple through its own main excretory duct, *lactiferous duct.* The segment of lactiferous duct subjacent to the nipple shows a small dilatation called *lactiferous sinus.* Each lactiferous duct has its own collecting duct system which has branches of smaller diameter, ultimately terminating peripherally as *terminal ducts* in the breast lobules which are the main secretory functional units of the mammary tissue during lactation. The breast lobules are composed of *acini* or *ductules* which are lined by cuboidal epithelium during resting mammary gland but develop secretory vacuoles in the last trimester of pregnancy. The terminal ducts too are lined by a single layer of cuboidal epithelium; relatively larger ducts have double-layered epithelial lining which becomes pseudostratified in the major ducts. The main lactiferous ducts are lined by stratified squamous epithelium. In addition to the epithelial cells, the intermediate collecting ducts are supported by myoepithelial cells.

STROMAL COMPONENT. The supportive stroma of the breast consists of variable amount of loose connective tissue and adipose tissue during different stages of reproductive life. The stromal tissue of the breast is present at 2 locations: intralobular and interlobular stroma. *Intralobular stroma* encloses each lobule, and its acini and ducts, and is chiefly made of loose connective tissue, myxomatous stroma and a few scattered lymphocytes. *Interlobular stroma* separates one lobule from the other and is composed mainly of adipose tissue and some loose connective tissue.

The most important disease of the breast is cancer. However, there are a few inflammatory lesions, benign tumours and tumour-like lesions which may be confused clinically with breast cancer. These pathologic lesions are described first, followed by an account of carcinoma of the breast.

INFLAMMATIONS

Inflammation of the breast is called mastitis. Important types of mastitis are acute mastitis and breast abscess, chronic mastitis, mammary duct ectasia (or plasma cell mastitis), traumatic fat necrosis and galactocele.

Acute Mastitis and Breast Abscess

Acute pyogenic infection of the breast occurs chiefly during the first few weeks of lactation and sometimes by eczema of the nipples. Bacteria such as staphylococci and streptococci gain entry into the breast by development of cracks and fissures in the nipple. Initially a localised area of acute inflammation is produced which, if not effectively treated, may cause single or multiple

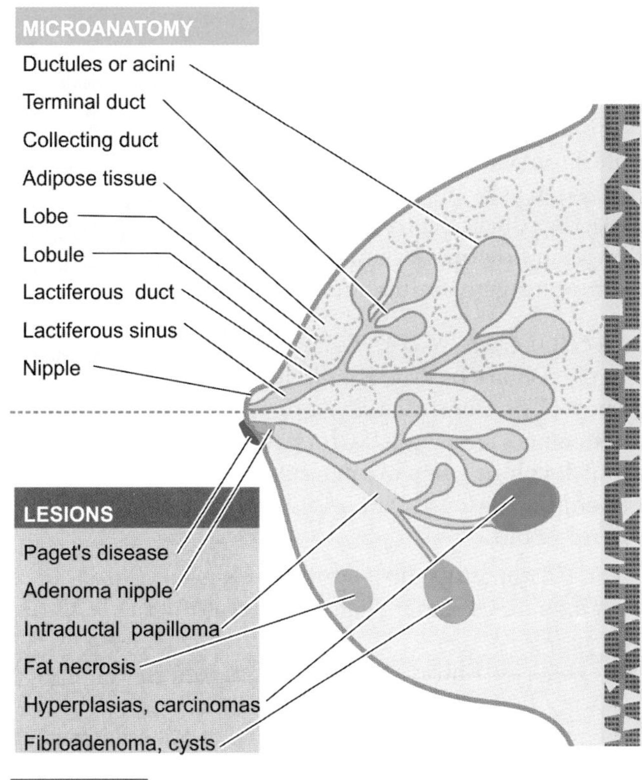

FIGURE 23.1

Microanatomy of the breast and major lesions at various sites.

breast abscesses. Extensive necrosis and replacement by fibrous scarring of the breast with retraction of the nipple may result.

Granulomatous Mastitis

Although chronic non-specific mastitis is uncommon, chronic granulomatous inflammation in the breast may occur as a result of the following:

1. *Systemic granulomatous disease* e.g. as part of systemic sarcoidosis, Wegener's granulomatosis.
2. *Infections* e.g. tuberculosis which is not so uncommon in developing countries like India and may be misdiagnosed clinically as breast cancer owing to axillary nodal involvement. Tubercle bacilli reach the breast by haematogenous, lymphatic or direct spread, usually from the lungs or pleura. Pathologically, typical caseating tubercles with discharging sinuses through the surface of the breast are found. ZN staining may demonstrate acid-fast bacilli. Fungal infection of the breast may occur in immunocompromised patients.
3. *Silicone breast implants* implanted on either breast cancer patients after mastectomy or as breast augmentation cosmetic surgery may rupture or silicone may slowly leak into surrounding breast tissue. This incites chronic inflammatory reaction of lymphocytes, macrophages and foreign body giant cells. Eventually, a surrounding fibrous capsule forms and after long period it may even be calcified.
4. *Idiopathic granulomatous mastitis* is an uncommon form of reaction around lobules and ducts in the absence of any known etiology. Exact pathogenesis is not known but probably it is a form of hypersensitivity reaction to luminal secretion of the breast epithelium during lactation.

Mammary Duct Ectasia (Plasma Cell Mastitis)

Mammary duct ectasia is a condition in which one or more of the larger ducts of the breast are dilated and filled with inspissated secretions. These are associated with periductal and interstitial chronic inflammatory changes. Duct ectasia affects women in their 4th to 7th decades of life. The patients may remain asymptomatic or there may be nipple discharge, retraction of the nipple due to fibrous scarring and clinically palpable dilated ducts in the subareolar area. The lesion may be mistaken for carcinoma of the breast. The etiology of the condition remains unknown but it appears to begin with periductal inflammation followed by destruction of the elastic tissue to cause ectasia and periductal fibrosis.

PATHOLOGIC CHANGES. Grossly, the condition appears as a single, poorly-defined indurated area in the breast with ropiness on the surface. Cut section shows dilated ducts containing cheesy inspissated secretions.

Histologically, the features are as under:

1. Dilated ducts with either necrotic or atrophic lining by flattened epithelium and lumen containing granular, amorphous, pink debris and foam cells.
2. Periductal and interstitial chronic inflammation, chiefly lymphocytes, histiocytes with multinucleate histiocytic giant cells. Sometimes, plasma cells are present in impressive numbers and the condition is then termed *plasma cell mastitis.*
3. Occasionally, there may be obliteration of the ducts by fibrous tissue and varying amount of inflammation and is termed *obliterative mastitis.*

Fat Necrosis

Focal fat necrosis of an obese and pendulous breast followed by an inflammatory reaction is generally initiated by trauma. The condition presents as a well defined mass with indurated appearance.

Grossly, the excised lump has central pale cystic area of necrosis.

Histologically, there is disruption of the regular pattern of lipocytes with formation of lipid-filled spaces surrounded by neutrophils, lymphocytes, plasma cells and histiocytes having foamy cytoplasm and frequent foreign body giant cell formation. In late stage, there is replacement fibrosis and even calcification.

Galactocele

A galactocele is cystic dilatation of one or more ducts occurring during lactation. The mammary duct is obstructed and dilated to form a thin-walled cyst filled with milky fluid. Rarely, the wall of galactocele may get secondarily infected.

FIBROCYSTIC CHANGE

The term fibrocystic change of the female breast is a histologic entity characterised by:

i) cystic dilatation of terminal ducts;

ii) relative increase in inter- and intralobular fibrous tissue; and

iii) variable degree of epithelial proliferation in the terminal ducts.

It was previously termed *fibrocystic disease* but is currently considered as an exaggerated physiologic phenomena and not a disease, or was called as *benign mammary dysplasia* under the mistaken belief that all forms are dysplastic or precancerous condition, and hence has attracted considerable interest.

It is the most common benign breast condition producing vague 'lumpy' breast rather than palpable lump in the breast of adult women. Its incidence has been reported to range from 10-20% in adult women. Most of the patients with fibrocystic change are between 3rd and 5th decades of life, with dramatic decline in its incidence after menopause suggesting the role of oestrogen in its pathogenesis.

It is important to identify the spectrum of histology or cytology findings by FNAC in fibrocystic changes since only some subset of changes have an increased risk of development of breast cancer. Presently, the spectrum of histologic changes are divided into two clinicopathologically relevant groups:

A. Nonproliferative changes (or cyst formation and fibrosis, or simple fibrocystic change);

B. Proliferative changes (includes epithelial hyperplasia and sclerosing adenosis).

A. Nonproliferative Fibrocystic Changes (Cyst Formation and Fibrosis, Simple Fibrocystic Change)

Formation of cysts of varying size and increase in fibrous stroma are the most common features of fibrocystic disease. Cysts are formed by dilatation of obstructed collecting ducts, obstruction being caused by periductal fibrosis following inflammation or fibrous overgrowth from oestrogen stimulation.

PATHOLOGIC CHANGES. Grossly, the cysts are rarely solitary but are usually multifocal and bilateral. They vary from microcysts to 5-6 cm in diameter. The usual large cyst is rounded, translucent with bluish colour prior to opening (blue-dome cyst). On opening, the cyst contains thin serous to haemorrhagic fluid.

Microscopically, the features of simple fibrocystic change are as under (Fig. 23.2) (COLOUR PLATE XXXI: CL 122):

1. The cyst lining shows a variety of appearances. Often, the epithelium is flattened or atrophic. Frequently, there is apocrine change or apocrine metaplasia in the lining of the cyst resembling the cells of apocrine sweat glands. Occasionally, there is simultaneous epithelial hyperplasia (discussed below) forming tiny intracystic papillary projections of piled up epithelium.

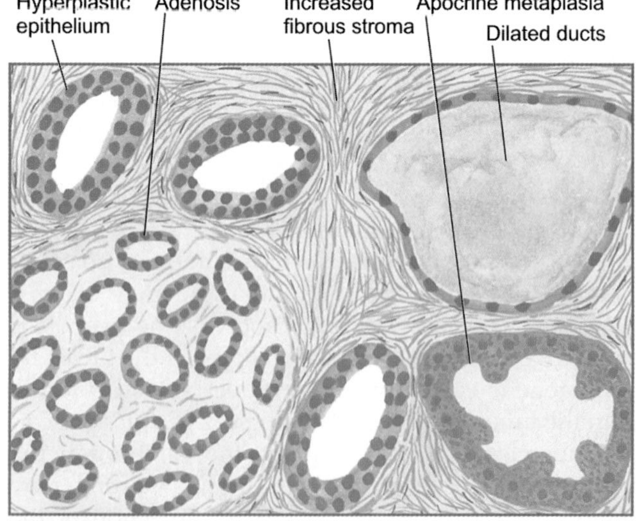

FIGURE 23.2

Simple fibrocystic change showing cystic dilatation of ducts and increase in fibrous stroma. There is mild epithelial hyperplasia in terminal ducts.

2. There is increased fibrous stroma surrounding the cysts and variable degree of stromal lymphocytic infiltrate.

B. Proliferative Fibrocystic Changes (Epithelial Hyperplasia and Sclerosing Adenosis)

EPITHELIAL HYPERPLASIA. Epithelial hyperplasia (or epitheliosis in the British literature) is defined as increase in the layers of epithelial cells over the basement membrane to three or more layers in the ducts *(ductal hyperplasia)* or lobules *(lobular hyperplasia)*. The latter condition, lobular hyperplasia, must be distinguished from adenosis (discussed separately) in which there is increase in the number of ductules or acini without any change in the number or type of cells lining them. Epithelial hyperplasia may be totally benign or may have atypical features. It is the latter type of hyperplasia which is precancerous and is associated with increased risk of developing breast cancer.

Microscopically, epithelial hyperplasia is characterised by epithelial proliferation to more than its normal double layer. In general, ductal hyperplasia is termed as *epithelial hyperplasia of usual type* and may show various grades of epithelial proliferations, while *lobular hyperplasia* involving the ductules or acini is always atypical.

1. **Mild hyperplasia** of ductal epithelium consists of at least three layers of cells above the basement membrane, present focally or evenly throughout the duct (Fig. 23.2).
2. **Moderate and florid hyperplasia** of ductal type is associated with tendency to fill the ductal lumen with proliferated epithelium. Such epithelial proliferations into the lumina of ducts may be focal, forming papillary epithelial projections called *ductal papillomatosis,* or may be more extensive, termed *florid papillomatosis,* or may fill the ductal lumen leaving only small fenestrations in it.
3. Of all the ductal hyperplasias, **atypical ductal hyperplasia** is more ominous and has to be distinguished from intraductal carcinoma (page 787). The proliferated epithelial cells in the atypical ductal hyperplasia partially fill the duct lumen and produce irregular microglandular spaces or *cribriform pattern.* The individual cells are uniform in shape but show loss of polarity with indistinct cytoplasmic margin and slightly elongated nuclei.
4. **Atypical lobular hyperplasia** is closely related to lobular carcinoma *in situ* (page 788) but differs from the latter in having cytologically atypical cells only in half of the ductules or acini.

SCLEROSING ADENOSIS. Sclerosing adenosis is benign proliferation of small ductules or acini and intralobular fibrosis. The lesion may be present as diffusely scattered microscopic foci in the breast parenchyma, or may form an isolated palpable mass which may simulate an infiltrating carcinoma, both clinically and pathologically.

Grossly, the lesion may be coexistent with other components of fibrocystic disease, or may form an isolated mass which has hard cartilage-like consistency, resembling an infiltrating carcinoma.
Microscopically, there is proliferation of ductules or acini and fibrous stromal overgrowth. The histologic appearance may superficially resemble infiltrating carcinoma but differs from the latter in having maintained lobular pattern and lack of infiltration into the surrounding fat.

Prognostic Significance

Since there is a variable degree of involvement of epithelial and mesenchymal elements in fibrocystic change, following prognostic derivations can be made:
1. *Nonproliferative fibrocystic changes* of fibrosis and cyst formation donot carry any increased risk of developing invasive breast cancer.
2. Identification of *general proliferative fibrocystic changes* are associated with 1.5 to 2 times increased risk for development of invasive breast cancer.
3. *Multifocal and bilateral proliferative changes* in the breast pose increased risk to both the breasts equally.
4. Within the group of proliferative fibrocystic changes, *atypical hyperplasia,* in partilcular, carries 4 to 5 times increased risk to develop invasive breast cancer later. This risk is further more if there is a history of breast cancer in the family.

GYNAECOMASTIA (HYPERTROPHY OF MALE BREAST)

Unilateral or bilateral enlargement of the male breast is known as gynaecomastia. Since the male breast does not contain secretory lobules, the enlargement is mainly due to proliferation of ducts and increased periductal stroma. Gynaecomastia occurs in response to hormonal stimulation, mainly oestrogen. Such excessive oestrogenic activity in males is seen in young boys between 13 and 17 years of age *(pubertal gynaecomastia),* in men over 50 years *(senescent gynaecomastia),* in endocrine diseases associated with increased oestrogenic or decreased androgenic activity e.g. in hepatic cirrhosis, testicular tumours, pituitary tumours, carcinoma of the lung, exogenous oestrogen therapy as in carcinoma of the prostate and testicular atrophy in Klinefelter's syndrome *(secondary gynaecomastia)*; and lastly, enlargement without any obvious cause *(idiopathic gynaecomastia)*.

PATHOLOGIC CHANGES. ***Grossly,*** one or both the male breasts are enlarged having smooth glistening white tissue.

Microscopically, there are 2 main features:

1. Proliferation of branching ducts which display epithelial hyperplasia with formation of papillary projections at places.
2. Increased fibrous stroma with, myxoid appearance.

BREAST TUMOURS

Tumours of the female breast are common and clinically significant but are rare in men. Among the important benign breast tumours are fibroadenoma, phyllodes tumour (cystosarcoma phyllodes) and intraductal papilloma. Carcinoma of the breast is an important malignant tumour which occurs as non-invasive (carcinoma *in situ*) and invasive cancer with its various morphologic varieties.

FIBROADENOMA

Fibroadenoma or adenofibroma is a benign tumour of fibrous and epithelial elements. It is the most common benign tumour of the female breast. Though it can occur at any age during reproductive life, most patients are between 15 to 30 years of age. Clinically, fibroadenoma generally appears as a solitary, discrete, freely mobile nodule within the breast. Rarely, fibroadenoma may contain *in situ* or invasive lobular or ductal carcinoma, or the carcinoma may invade the fibroadenoma from the adjacent primary breast cancer.

PATHOLOGIC CHANGES. ***Grossly,*** typical fibroadenoma is a small (2-4 cm diameter), solitary, well-encapsulated, spherical or discoid mass. The cut surface is firm, grey-white, slightly myxoid and may show slit-like spaces formed by compressed ducts. Occasionally, multiple fibroadenomas may form part of fibrocystic disease and is termed *fibroadenomatosis*. Less commonly, a fibroadenoma may be fairly large in size, upto 15 cm in diameter, and is called *giant fibroadenoma* but lacks the histologic features of cystosarcoma phyllodes (see below).

Microscopically, fibrous tissue comprises most of a fibroadenoma. The arrangements between fibrous overgrowth and ducts may produce two types of patterns which may coexist in the same tumour. These are intracanalicular and pericanalicular patterns (Fig. 23.3):

- **Intracanalicular pattern** is one in which the stroma compresses the ducts so that they are reduced to slit-like clefts lined by ductal epithelium or may appear as cords of epithelial elements surrounding masses of fibrous stroma (COLOUR PLATE XXXI: CL 123).
- **Pericanalicular pattern** is characterised by encircling masses of fibrous stroma around the patent or dilated ducts.

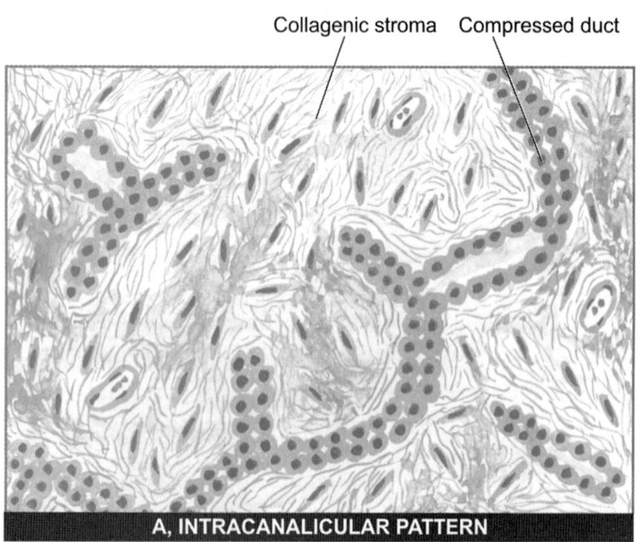

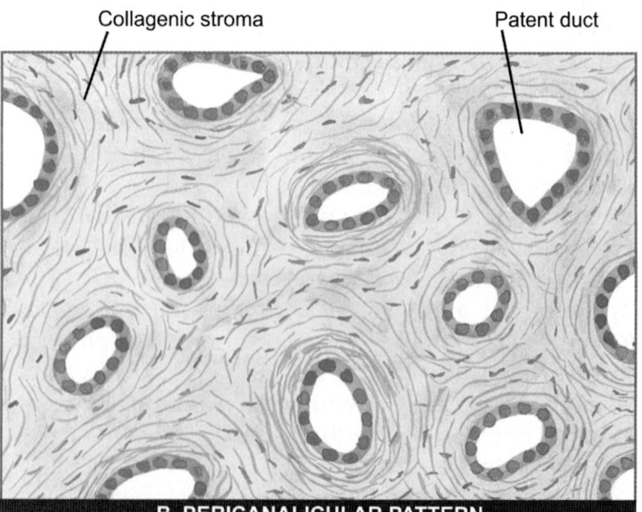

FIGURE 23.3

Fibroadenoma of the breast, microscopic patterns.

The fibrous stroma may be quite cellular, or there may be areas of hyalinised collagen. Sometimes, the stroma is loose and myxomatous. Occasionally, the fibrous tissue element in the tumour is scanty, and the tumour is instead predominantly composed of closely-packed ductular or acinar proliferation and is termed *tubular adenoma.* If such an adenoma is composed of acini with secretory activity, it is called *lactating adenoma* seen during pregnancy or lactation. *Juvenile fibroadenoma* is an uncommon variant of fibroadenoma which is larger and rapidly growing mass seen in adolescent girls but fortunately does not recur after excision.

PHYLLODES TUMOUR (CYSTOSARCOMA PHYLLODES)

Cystosarcoma phyllodes was the nomenclature given by Müller in 1838 to an uncommon bulky breast tumour with leaf-like gross appearance (*phyllodes*=leaf-like) having an aggressive clinical behaviour. Most patients are between 30 to 70 years of age. Grossly, the tumour resembles a giant fibroadenoma but is distinguished histologically from the latter by more cellular connective tissue. The WHO classification of breast tumours has proposed the term 'phyllodes tumour' in place of misleading term of 'cystosarcoma phyllodes'. Phyllodes tumour can be classified into *benign, borderline* and *malignant* on the basis of histologic features. Local recurrences are much more frequent than metastases.

PATHOLOGIC CHANGES. ***Grossly,*** the tumour is generally large, 10-15 cm in diameter, round to oval, bosselated, and less fully encapsulated than a fibroadenoma. The cut surface is grey-white with cystic cavities, areas of haemorrhages, necrosis and degenerative changes.

Histologically, the phyllodes tumour is composed of an extremely hypercellular stroma, accompanied by proliferation of benign ductal structures. Thus, phyllodes tumour resembles fibroadenoma except for enhanced stromal cellularity. The histologic criteria used to distinguish benign, borderline and malignant categories of phyllodes tumour are as under:

- frequency of mitoses;
- cellular atypia;
- cellularity; and
- infiltrative margins.

About 20% of phyllodes tumours are histologically malignant and less than half of them may metastasise.

INTRADUCTAL PAPILLOMA

Intraductal papilloma is a benign papillary tumour occurring most commonly in a lactiferous duct or lactiferous sinus near the nipple. Clinically, it produces serous or serosanguineous nipple discharge. It is most common in 3rd and 4th decades of life.

PATHOLOGIC CHANGES. ***Grossly,*** intraductal papilloma is usually solitary, small, less than 1 cm in diameter, commonly located in the major mammary ducts close to the nipple. Less commonly, there are multiple papillomatosis which are more frequently related to a papillary carcinoma.

Histologically, an intraductal papilloma is characterised by multiple papillae having well-developed fibrovascular stalks attached to the ductal wall and covered by benign cuboidal epithelial cells supported by myoepithelial cells. An intraductal papillary carcinoma is distinguished from intraductal papilloma in having severe cytologic atypia, pleomorphism, absence of myoepithelial cells, multilayering and presence of mitotic figures.

CARCINOMA OF THE BREAST

Cancer of the breast is among the commonest of human cancers throughout the world. Its incidence and mortality are particularly high in developed countries. In the United States, carcinoma of the breast constitutes about 25% of all cancers in females and causes approximately 20% of cancer deaths among females. Cancer of the male breast, on the other hand, is quite rare and comprises 0.2% of malignant tumours (ratio between male-female breast cancer is 1:100). The incidence of breast cancer is highest in the perimenopausal age group and is uncommon before the age of 25 years.

Clinically, the breast cancer usually presents as a solitary, painless, palpable lump which is detected quite often by self-examination. Higher the age, more are the chances of breast lump turning out to be malignant. Thus, all breast lumps, irrespective of the age of the patient must be removed surgically. Currently, emphasis is on early diagnosis by mammography, xero-radiography and thermography. Techniques like fine needle aspiration cytology (FNAC), stereotactic biopsy and frozen section are immensely valuable to the surgeon for immediate pathological diagnosis.

Etiology

Though extensive clinical and experimental research as well as epidemiologic studies have been carried out in the field of breast cancer, its exact etiology remains elusive. However, based on current status of our knowledge, the following risk factors are considered significant in its etiology:

1. Geography. The incidence of breast cancer is about six times higher in developed countries than the developing countries, with the notable exception of Japan. These geographic differences are considered to be related to consumption of large amount of animal fats and high caloric diet by Western populations than the Asians (including Japanese) and Africans.

2. Genetic factors. Recently, much work has been done on the influence of family history and inherited mutations in breast cancer:

i) *Family history:* First-degree relatives (mother, sister, daughter) of women with breast cancer have 2 to 6-fold higher risk of development of breast cancer. The risk is proportionate to a few factors:

- number of blood relatives with breast cancer;
- younger age at the time of development of breast cancer;
- bilateral cancers; and
- high risk cancer families having breast and ovarian carcinomas.

ii) *Genetic mutations:* About 10% breast cancers have been found to have inherited mutations. These mutations include the following, most important of which is *br*east *ca*ncer (*BRCA*) susceptibility gene in inherited breast cancer:

- *BRCA 1 gene* located on chromosome 17, a DNA repair gene, is implicated in both breast and ovarian cancer in inherited cases. *BRCA1* deletion is seen in about two-third of women with inherited breast cancer having family history but *BRCA1* mutation is uncommon in sporadic cases. Men who have mutated *BRCA1* have increased risk of developing prostate cancer but not of male breast.
- *BRCA 2 gene* located on chromosome 13, another DNA repair gene, in its mutated form, has a similarly higher incidence of inherited cancer of the breast (one-third cases) and ovary in females, and prostate in men. In both *BRCA1* and *BRCA2*, both copies of the genes (homozygous state) must be inactivated for development of breast cancer.
- *Mutation in TP53 tumour suppressor gene* on chromosome 17 as an acquired defect accounts for 40% cases of sporadic breast cancer in women but rarely in women with family history of breast cancer. *TP53* mutation is also seen in Li-Fraumeni syndrome having multiple cancers including breast cancer in young women; others are tumours of the brain, sarcomas, and adrenal cortical tumours.
- *Other mutations* seen less commonly in breast cancer include ataxia telangiectasia gene, *PTEN* (*p*hosphate and *ten*sin) tumour suppressor gene.

3. Oestrogen excess. There is sufficient evidence to suggest that excess endogenous oestrogen or exogenously administered oestrogen for prolonged duration is an important factor in the development of breast cancer. Evidences in support of increased risk with oestrogen excess are as follows:

i) Women with prolonged reproductive life, with menarche setting in at an early age and menopause relatively late have greater risk.

ii) Higher risk in unmarried and nulliparous women than in married and multiparous women.

iii) Women with first childbirth at a late age (over 30 years) are at greater risk.

iv) Lactation is said to reduce the risk of breast cancer.

v) Bilateral oophorectomy reduces the risk of development of breast cancer.

vi) Functioning ovarian tumours (e.g. granulosa cell tumour) which elaborate oestrogen are associated with increased incidence of breast cancer.

vii) Oestrogen replacement therapy administered to postmenopausal women may result in increased risk of breast cancer.

viii) However, there is no definite increased risk with balanced oestrogen-progesterone preparations used in oral contraceptives.

ix) Men who have been treated with oestrogen for prostatic cancer have increased risk of developing cancer of the male breast.

Normal breast epithelium possesses oestrogen and progesterone receptors. The breast cancer cells secrete many growth factors which are oestrogen-dependent. In this way, the interplay of high circulating levels of oestrogen, oestrogen receptors and growth factors brings about progression of breast cancer.

4. Environmental and dietary factors. Among the environmental influences associated with increased risk of breast cancer are consumption of large amounts of animal fats, high calorie foods, cigarette smoking and alcohol. The identification of a transmissible retrovirus, mouse mammary tumour virus (MMTV), also called *Bittner milk factor* transmitted from the infected mother-mice to the breast-fed daughter-mice prompted researchers to look for similar agent in human breast cancer (Chapter 8). Though no such agent has yet been identified, there are reports of presence of reverse transcriptase in breast cancer cells.

5. Fibrocystic change. Fibrocystic change, particularly when associated with atypical epithelial hyperplasia, has about 5-fold higher risk of developing breast cancer subsequently.

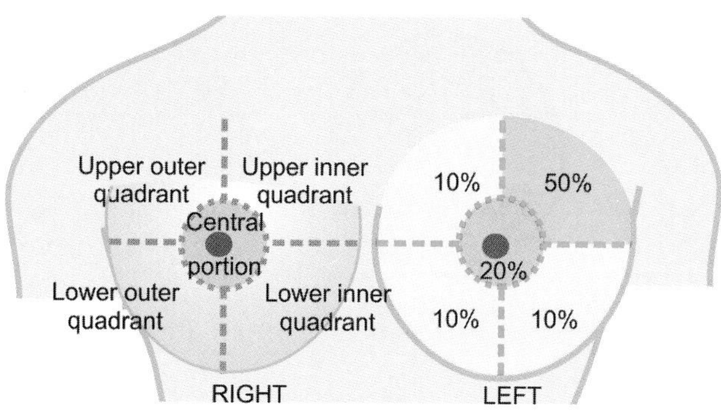

FIGURE 23.4

Anatomic considerations in breast cancer.

TABLE 23.1: Classification of Carcinoma of the Breast.

A. NON-INVASIVE *(IN SITU)* CARCINOMA
1. Intraductal carcinoma
2. Lobular carcinoma *in situ*

B. INVASIVE CARCINOMA
1. Infiltrating (invasive) duct carcinoma-NOS (not otherwise specified)
2. Infiltrating (invasive) lobular carcinoma
3. Medullary carcinoma
4. Colloid (mucinous) carcinoma
5. Papillary carcinoma
6. Tubular carcinoma
7. Adenoid cystic (invasive cribriform) carcinoma
8. Secretory (juvenile) carcinoma
9. Inflammatory carcinoma
10. Carcinoma with metaplasia

C. PAGET'S DISEASE OF THE NIPPLE

General Features and Classification

Cancer of the breast occurs more often in left breast than the right and is bilateral in about 4% cases. Anatomically, upper outer quadrant is the site of tumour in half the breast cancers; followed in frequency by central portion, and equally in the remaining both lower and the upper inner quadrant as shown in Fig. 23.4.

Carcinoma of the breast arises from the ductal epithelium in 90% cases while the remaining 10% originate from the lobular epithelium. For variable period of time, the tumour cells remain confined within the ducts or lobules (non-invasive carcinoma) before they invade the breast stroma (invasive carcinoma). While there are only 2 types of *non-invasive carcinoma*—intraductal carcinoma and lobular carcinoma *in situ*, there is a great variety of histological patterns of *invasive carcinoma breast* which have clinical correlations and prognostic implications. Table 23.1 presents different types of carcinoma of the breast as proposed in the WHO classification with some modifications. The important morphological types are described below.

A. NON-INVASIVE *(IN SITU)* CARCINOMA

In general, non-invasive or *in situ* carcinoma is characterised histologically by presence of tumour cells within the ducts or lobules without evidence of invasion. Two types of carcinoma *in situ* are recognised: intraductal carcinoma and lobular carcinoma *in situ*.

1. Intraductal Carcinoma

Carcinoma *in situ* confined within the larger mammary ducts is called intraductal carcinoma. The tumour initially begins with atypical hyperplasia of ductal epithelium followed by filling of the duct with tumour cells. Clinically, it produces a palpable mass in 30-75% of cases and presence of nipple discharge in about 30% patients. Approximately a quarter of patients of intraductal carcinoma treated with excisional biopsy alone develop ipsilateral invasive carcinoma during a follow-up period of 10 years while the chance of a contralateral breast cancer developing in patients with intraductal carcinoma is far less than that associated with *in situ* lobular carcinoma.

PATHOLOGIC CHANGES. Grossly, the tumour may vary from a small poorly-defined focus to 3-5 cm diameter mass. On cut section, the involved area shows cystically dilated ducts containing cheesy necrotic material *(comedo pattern)*, or the intraductal tumour may be polypoid and friable resembling intraductal papilloma *(papillary pattern)*.

Histologically, the proliferating tumour cells within the ductal lumina may have 4 types of patterns in different combinations: solid, comedo, papillary and cribriform (Fig. 23.5,A):

i) *Solid pattern* is characterised by filling and plugging of the ductal lumina with tumour cells.

ii) *Comedo pattern* is centrally placed necrotic debris surrounded by neoplastic cells in the duct.

iii) *Papillary pattern* has formation of intraductal papillary projections of tumour cells which lack a fibrovascular stalk so as to distinguish it from intraductal papilloma.

iv) *Cribriform pattern* is recognised by neat punched out fenestrations in the intraductal tumour.

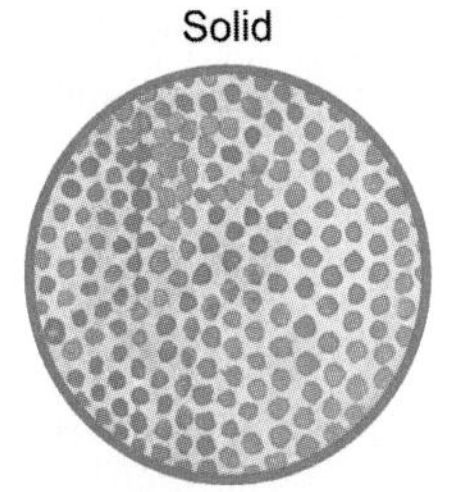

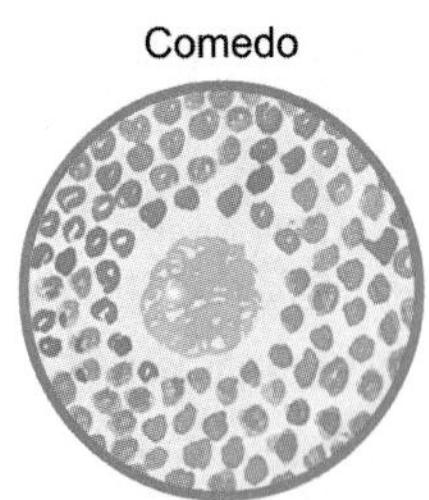

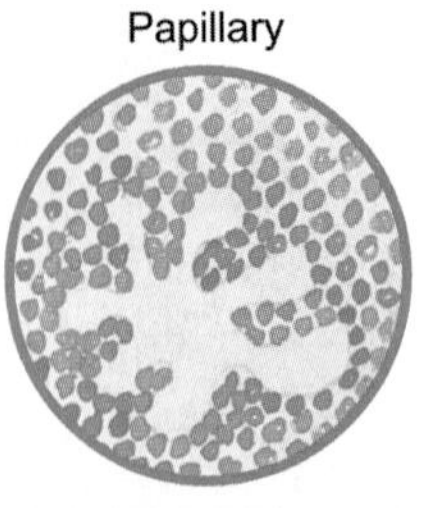

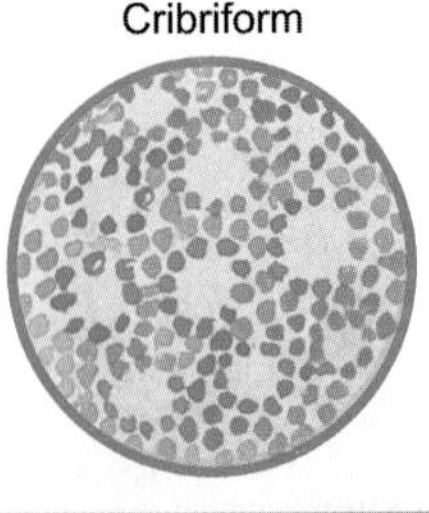

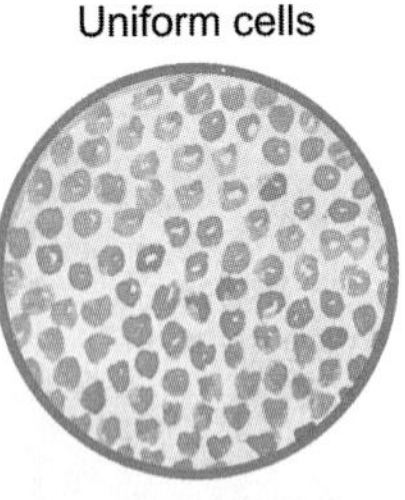

FIGURE 23.5

Non-invasive *(in situ)* carcinoma of breast.

2. Lobular Carcinoma *in Situ*

Lobular carcinoma *in situ* is not a palpable or grossly visible tumour. Patients of *in situ* lobular carcinoma treated with excisional biopsy alone develop invasive cancer of the ipsilateral breast in about 25% cases in 10 years as in intraductal carcinoma but, in addition, have a much higher incidence of developing a contralateral breast cancer (30%).

*PATHOLOGIC CHANGES. **Grossly,*** no visible tumour is identified.

Histologically, *in situ* lobular carcinoma is characterised by filling up of terminal ducts and ductules or acini by rather uniform cells which are loosely cohesive and have small, rounded nuclei with indistinct cytoplasmic margins (Fig. 23.5,B).

B. INVASIVE CARCINOMA

The invasive breast cancer has various morphologic types which have clinical and prognostic correlates. In general, 90% of breast cancers are of larger ductal origin, while the remaining 10% arise from lobular epithelium.

1. Infiltrating (Invasive) Duct Carcinoma-NOS

Infiltrating duct carcinoma-NOS *(not otherwise specified)* is the classic breast cancer and is the most common histologic pattern accounting for 70% cases of breast cancer. In fact, this is the pattern of cancer for which the terms 'cancer' and 'carcinoma' were first coined by Hippocrates. Clinically, majority of infiltrating duct carcinomas have a hard consistency due to dense collagenous stroma (scirrhous carcinoma). They are found more frequently in the left breast, often in the upper outer quadrant (Fig. 23.4). Retraction of the nipple and attachment of the tumour to underlying chest wall may be present.

*PATHOLOGIC CHANGES. **Grossly,*** the tumour is irregular, 1-5 cm in diameter, hard cartilage-like mass that cuts with a grating sound. The sectioned surface of the tumour is grey-white to yellowish with chalky streaks and often extends irregularly into the surrounding fat (Fig. 23.6,A).

Histologically, as the name NOS suggests, the tumour is different from other special types in lacking a regular and uniform pattern throughout the lesion. A variety of histologic features commonly present are as under (Fig. 23.6,B) (COLOUR PLATE XXXI: CL 124):

i) Anaplastic tumour cells forming solid nests, cords, poorly-formed glandular structures and some intraductal foci.

ii) Infiltration by these patterns of tumour cells into diffuse fibrous stroma and fat.

iii) Invasion into perivascular and perineural spaces as well as lymphatic and vascular invasion.

2. Infiltrating (Invasive) Lobular Carcinoma

Invasive lobular carcinoma comprises about 5% of all breast cancers. This peculiar morphologic form differs from other invasive cancers in being more frequently bilateral; and within the same breast, it may have multicentric origin.

*PATHOLOGIC CHANGES. **Grossly,*** the appearance varies from a well-defined scirrhous mass to a poorly-defined area of induration that may remain undetected by inspection as well as palpation.

Histologically, there are 2 distinct features (Fig. 23.7):

i) Pattern—A characteristic single file (Indian file) linear arrangement of stromal infiltration by the tumour cells with very little tendency to gland formation is seen. Infiltrating cells may be arranged concentrically around ducts in a target-like pattern.

ii) Tumour cytology—Individual tumour cells resemble cells of *in situ* lobular carcinoma. They are

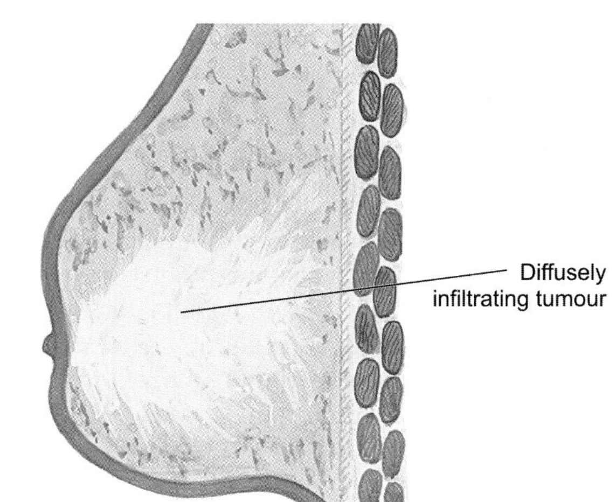

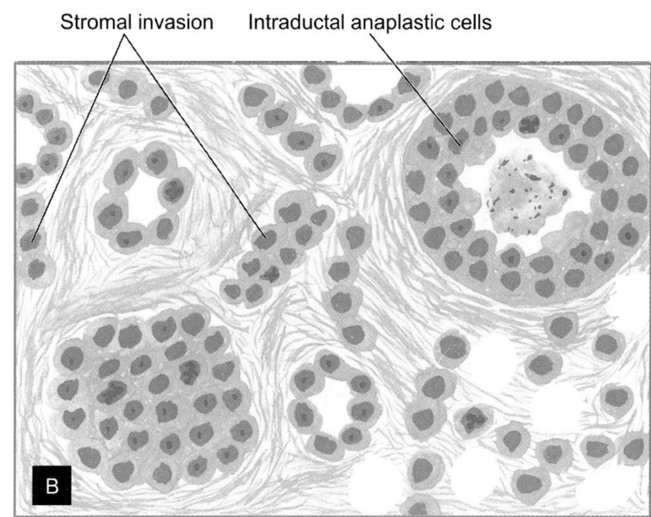

FIGURE 23.6

Infiltrating duct carcinoma-NOS.

A, Sectioned surface of breast showing gross appearance of the tumour. B, Microscopic features include formation of solid nests, cords, gland-like structures and intraductal growth pattern of anaplastic tumour cells. There is infiltration of densely-collagenised stroma by these cells in a haphazard way.

round and regular with very little pleomorphism and infrequent mitoses. Some tumours may show signet-ring cells distended with cytoplasmic mucin.

3. Medullary Carcinoma

Medullary carcinoma is a variant of ductal carcinoma and comprises about 1% of all breast cancers. The tumour has a significantly better prognosis than the usual infiltrating duct carcinoma, probably due to good host immune response in the form of lymphoid infiltrate in the tumour stroma.

*PATHOLOGIC CHANGES. **Grossly,*** the tumour is characterised by a large, well-circumscribed, rounded mass that is typically soft and fleshy or brain-like and hence the alternative name of 'encephaloid carcinoma'. Cut section shows areas of haemorrhages and necrosis.

Histologically, medullary carcinoma is characterised by 2 distinct features:

i) Tumour cells—Sheets of large, pleomorphic tumour cells with abundant cytoplasm, large vesicular nuclei and many bizarre and atypical mitoses are diffusely spread in the scanty stroma.

ii) Stroma—The loose connective tissue stroma is scanty and usually has a prominent lymphoid infiltrate.

4. Colloid (Mucinous) Carcinoma

This is an uncommon pattern of breast cancer occurring more frequently in older women and is slow-growing. Colloid carcinoma has better prognosis than the usual infiltrating duct carcinoma.

*PATHOLOGIC CHANGES. **Grossly,*** the tumour is usually a soft and gelatinous mass with well-demarcated borders.

Histologically, colloid carcinoma contains large amount of extracellular epithelial mucin and acini

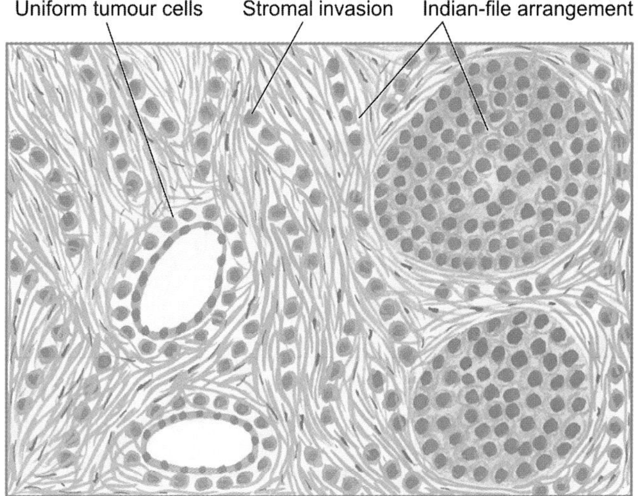

FIGURE 23.7

Invasive lobular carcinoma. Characteristic histologic features are: one cell wide files of round regular tumour cells ('Indian file' arrangement) infiltrating the stroma and arranged circumferentially around ducts in a target-like pattern.

filled with mucin. Cuboidal to tall columnar tumour cells, some showing mucus vacuolation, are seen floating in large lakes of mucin.

5. Papillary Carcinoma

Papillary carcinoma is a rare variety of infiltrating duct carcinoma in which the stromal invasion is in the form of papillary structures.

6. Tubular Carcinoma

Tubular carcinoma is another uncommon variant of invasive ductal carcinoma which has more favourable prognosis.

Histologically, the tumour is highly well-differentiated and has an orderly pattern. The tumour cells are regular and form a single layer in well-defined tubules. The tubules are quite even and distributed in dense fibrous stroma.

7. Adenoid Cystic (Invasive Cribriform) Carcinoma

Adenoid cystic or invasive cribriform carcinoma is a unique histologic pattern of breast cancer with excellent prognosis.

Histologically, there is stromal invasion by islands of cells having characteristic cribriform (fenestrated) appearance.

8. Secretory (Juvenile) Carcinoma

This pattern is found more frequently in children and has a better prognosis. The tumour is generally circumscribed which on histologic examination shows abundant intra- and extracellular PAS-positive clear spaces due to secretory activity of tumour cells.

9. Inflammatory Carcinoma

Inflammatory carcinoma of the breast is a clinical entity and does not constitute a histological type. The term has been used for breast cancers in which there is redness, oedema, tenderness and rapid enlargement. Inflammatory carcinoma is associated with extensive invasion of dermal lymphatics and has a dismal prognosis.

10. Carcinoma with Metaplasia

Rarely, invasive ductal carcinomas may have various types of metaplastic alterations such as squamous metaplasia, cartilagenous and osseous metaplasia, or their combinations. Development of squamous cell carcinoma of the breast parenchyma is exceedingly rare and must be separated from lesions of epidermis or nipple region.

C. PAGET'S DISEASE OF THE NIPPLE

Paget's disease of the nipple is an eczematoid lesion of the nipple, often associated with an invasive or non-invasive ductal carcinoma of the underlying breast. The nipple bears a crusted, scaly and eczematoid lesion with a palpable subareolar mass in about half the cases. Most of the patients with palpable mass are found to have infiltrating duct carcinoma, while those with no palpable breast lump are usually subsequently found to have intraductal carcinoma. Prognosis of patients with ductal carcinoma having Paget's disease is less favourable than of those who have ductal carcinoma without Paget's disease.

The *pathogenesis* of Paget's disease of the breast is explained by the following 2 hypotheses:

1. The tumour cells from the underlying ductal carcinoma have migrated up into the lactiferous ducts and invaded the epidermis producing skin lesions.
2. An alternate theory, though less reliable than the former, is that Paget's disease represents a form of carcinoma *in situ* of the epidermis itself.

PATHOLOGIC CHANGES. Grossly, the skin of the nipple and areola is crusted, fissured and ulcerated with oozing of serosanguineous fluid from the erosions.

Histologically, the skin lesion is characterised by the presence of Paget's cells singly or in small clusters in the epidermis. These cells are larger than the epidermal cells, spherical, having hyperchromatic nuclei with cytoplasmic halo that stains positively with mucicarmine. In these respects, Paget's cells are adenocarcinoma-type cells. In addition, the underlying breast contains invasive or non-invasive duct carcinoma which shows no obvious direct invasion of the skin of nipple.

GRADING, STAGING AND PROGNOSIS

Histologic grading and clinical staging of breast cancer determines the management and clinical course in these patients.

HISTOLOGIC GRADING. The breast cancers are subdivided into various histologic grades depending upon the following parameters:

1. Histologic type of tumour. Based on classification described in Table 23.1, breast cancer can be subdivided into 3 histologic grades:

i) *Non-metastasising*—Intraductal and lobular carcinoma *in situ*.

ii) *Less commonly metastasising*—Medullary, colloid, papillary, tubular, adenoid cystic (invasive cribriform), and secretory (juvenile) carcinomas.

iii) *Commonly metastasising*—Infiltrating duct, invasive lobular, and inflammatory carcinomas.

2. Microscopic grade. Widely used system for microscopic grading of breast carcinoma is that of Nottingham modification of the Bloom-Richardson system. It is based on 3 features:

i) Tubule formation

ii) Nuclear pleomorphism

iii) Mitotic count.

3. Tumour size. There is generally an inverse relationship between diameter of primary breast cancer at the time of mastectomy and long-term survival.

4. Axillary lymph node metastasis. Survival rate is based on the number and level of lymph nodes involved by metastasis. More the number of regional lymph nodes involved, worse is the survival rate. Involvement of the lymph nodes from proximal to distal axilla (i.e. *level I*—superficial axilla, to *level III*—deep axilla) is directly correlated with the survival rate. In this regards, identification and dissection of sentinel lymph node followed by histopathologic examination has attained immense prognostic value (*Sentinel lymph node* is the first node in the vicinity to receive drainage from primary cancer i.e. it stands 'sentinel' over the tumour).

5. Oestrogen and progesterone receptors. Oestrogen is known to promote the breast cancer. Presence or absence of oestrogen receptors on the tumour cells can help in predicting the response of breast cancer to endocrine therapy. Accordingly, patients with high levels of oestrogen receptors on breast tumour cells have a better prognosis. A recurrent tumour that is receptor-positive is more likely to respond to anti-oestrogen therapy than one that is receptor-negative.

6. DNA content. Tumour cell subpopulations with aneuploid DNA content as evaluated by flow cytometry have a worse prognosis than purely diploid tumours.

CLINICAL STAGING. The American Joint Committee (AJC) on cancer staging has modified the TNM (primary Tumour, Nodal, and distant Metastasis) staging proposed by UICC (Union International for Control of Cancer), (Table 23.2).

Spread of breast cancer to axillary lymph nodes occurs early. Later, however, distant spread by lymphatic route to internal mammary lymphatics, mediastinal lymph nodes, supraclavicular lymph nodes, pleural lymph nodes and pleural lymphatics may occur. Common sites for haematogenous metastatic spread from breast cancer are the lungs, liver, bones, adrenals, brain and ovaries. Breast is one of the most suspect source of inapparent primary carcinoma in women presenting with metastatic carcinoma.

TABLE 23.2: AJC Clinical Staging of Breast Cancer.

Stage TIS:	*In situ* carcinoma (*in situ* lobular, intraductal, Paget's disease of the nipple without palpable lump)
Stage I:	Tumour 2 cm or less in diameter No nodal spread
Stage II:	Tumour > 2 cm in diameter Regional lymph nodes involved
Stage III A:	Tumour $\geq$ 5 cm in diameter Regional lymph nodes involved on same side
Stage III B:	Tumour $\geq$ 5 cm in diameter Supraclavicular and infraclavicular lymph nodes involved
Stage IV:	Tumour of any size With or without regional spread but with distant metastasis

PROGNOSTIC FACTORS IN BREAST CANCER. Based on current knowledge gained by breast cancer screening programmes in the West employing mammography and stereotactic biopsy, various breast cancer risk factors and prognostic factors have been described. These prognostic factors are divided into following 3 groups:

1. Potentially pre-malignant lesions. These conditions are as under:

i) *Atypical ductal hyperplasia* is associated with 4-5 times increased risk than women of the same age. Such lesions are commonest in the age group of 45-55 years.

ii) *Clinging carcinoma* is a related lesion in the duct but different from carcinoma *in situ* and has lower risk of progression to invasive cancer than *in situ* carcinoma.

iii) *Fibroadenoma* is a long-term risk factor (after over 20 years) for invasive breast cancer, the risk being about twice compared to controls.

2. Breast carcinoma *in situ*. Following factors act as determinants:

i) *Ductal carcinoma in situ* (comedo and non-comedo subtypes) is diagnosed on the basis of three histologic features—nuclear grade, nuclear morphology and necrosis, while *lobular neoplasia* includes full spectrum of changes of lobular carcinoma *in situ* and atypical lobular

TABLE 23.3: Summary of Prognostic Markers and Predictive Factors for Invasive Breast Cancer.

FACTOR	FAVOURABLE PROGNOSIS	POOR PROGNOSIS
I. *Routine histopathology criteria:*		
i) *Histologic type*	Medullary ca., tubular ca., mucinous (colloid) ca.; lobular ca. of low grade	Inflammatory ca.
ii) *Tumour size (two dimensions)*	Nodal metastasis 10-20% in 1 cm size tumour; 10 years survival 90% in node negative	Size larger than 1 cm
iii) *Histologic (Nottingham) grading (Score range of 3-9; based on degree of tubule formation-1-3 score, regularity of nuclei-1-3 score, and mitoses-1-3 score)*	Low grade (grade I) tumour = score 3-5, moderate grade (grade II) tumour = score 6-7	High grade (grade III) tumour = score 8-9
iv) *Axillary nodal status*	Node negative: recurrence rate after 10 years 10-30%; Number of nodes: less than 4; sentinel node negative	Node positive: recurrence rate after 10 years 70%; number of nodes: more than 4; sentinel node positive
v) *Lymphatic and/ or vascular invasion (both extratumoral)*	Negative for both: good	Positive for one or both: poor
vi) *Others:*		
a) Tumour circumscription	Good	Poor
b) Inflammatory reaction	May have some role	Controversial
c) Stromal elastosis	Absence good	Presence poor
d) Intraductal component	Presence good	Absence poor
e) Skin involvement	Absence good	Presence poor
II. *Hormone receptor status:*		
Oestrogen-progesterone receptors (ER-PR)	ER-PR positive better response to adjuvant therapy	ER-PR negative poor response to adjuvant therapy
III. *Biological indicators:*		
i) *Mitotic index (by Ki67, MIB-1)*	Low mitotic count	High mitotic count
ii) *DNA ploidy analysis (aneuploidy, diploidy)*	Not related	Not related
iii) *C-ERBB2 (HER2-NEU)*	Lack of amplification good	Presence of amplification
iv) *Epidermal growth factor receptor (EGFR)*	Underexpression	Overexpression
v) *Angiogenesis (VEGF, CD31, CD34, microvessel density counts)*	Angiogenic activity low	High angiogenic activity
vi) *Oncogene disregulation*		
a) BRCA1, BRCA2	*BRCA* negative	*BRCA* positive
b) TP53	*TP53* positive respond better to chemotherapy and radiotherapy	*TP53* negative respond spoorly to chemotherapy and radiotherapy
c) BCL2	*BCL2* positive good	*BCL2* negative poor
d) Cathepsin D	Absence indicates good prognosis	Presence renders poor prognosis

hyperplasia. Ductal carcinoma *in situ* is more important and demands most attention. Comedo type of *in situ* carcinoma has higher recurrence rate.

ii) *Breast conservative therapy* is used more frequently nowadays in carcinoma *in situ* which requires consideration of three factors for management: *margins, extent of disease,* and *biological markers.* The biological markers such as *TP53* and *BCL 2* have low positivity in high-grade *in situ* ductal carcinoma and likelihood of recurrences after conservative surgery.

3. **Invasive breast cancer.** Prognostic and predictive factors for invasive breast cancer have been extensively studied by univariate analysis (examining single factor separately) as well as by multivariate analysis (comparing the value of various factors included in a study). These can be broadly divided into 3 groups:
1. routine histopathology criteria;
2. hormone receptor status; and
3. biological indicators.

A summary combining all these factors is given in Table 23.3.

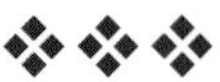

24 The Skin

NORMAL STRUCTURE

The skin or the integument is the external organ that protects against mechanical trauma, UV light and infection. In addition, the skin is concerned with thermoregulation, conservation and excretion of fluid, sensory perception and, of course, has aesthetic role.

The histology of normal skin shows some variation in different parts of the body. In general, it is composed of 2 layers, the epidermis and the dermis, which are separated by an irregular border. Cone-shaped dermal papillae extend upward into the epidermis forming peg-like *rete ridges* of the epidermis. Fig. 24.1 represents a diagram of the main structures identifiable in a section of the normal skin and Fig. 24.2 shows the various layers of the epidermis.

EPIDERMIS

The epidermis is composed of the following 5 layers from base to the surface:

1. Basal cell layer (stratum germinatum). The basal cell layer consists of a single layer of keratinocytes that forms the junction between the epidermis and dermis. The nuclei of these cells are perpendicular to the epidermal basement membrane. These are hyperchromatic and normally contain a few mitoses indicating that the superficial epidermal layers originate from the basal cell layer. These cells are interconnected with each other and with the overlying squamous cells by *desmosomes.* Depending upon the complexion of the individual, melanocytes which are a type of dendritic cells, are seen interspersed in the keratinocytes of the basal layer. *Melanocytes* have small nuclei with clear cytoplasm containing melanin granules and are usually spaced as every tenth cell in the basal layer. They are always positive with dopa reaction (page 46). The other type of dendritic cells in the basal layer are *Langerhans cells* which belong to mononuclear-phagocyte system.

2. Prickle cell layer (Stratum spinosum, Stratum malpighii). This layer is composed of several layers of polygonal prickle cells or squamous cells. The layers become flat as they near the surface so that their long axis appears parallel to the skin surface. These cells possess intercellular bridges or tonofilaments. These intercellular cytoplasmic tonofilaments contain PAS-positive material that is precursor of keratin.

3. Granular cell layer (stratum granulosum). This layer consists of 1 to 3 layers of flat cells containing keratohyaline basophilic granules which are PAS-negative. Granular cell layer is much thicker in palms and soles.

4. Stratum lucidum. This layer is present exclusively in palms and soles as a thin homogeneous, eosinophilic, non-nucleate zone.

5. Horny layer (Stratum corneum). The stratum corneum is also normally devoid of nuclei and consists of eosinophilic layers of keratin.

Intraepidermal nerve endings are present in the form of *Merkel cells* which are touch receptors.

DERMIS

The dermis consists of 2 parts—the superficial *pars papillaris* or *papillary dermis,* and the deeper *pars reticularis* or

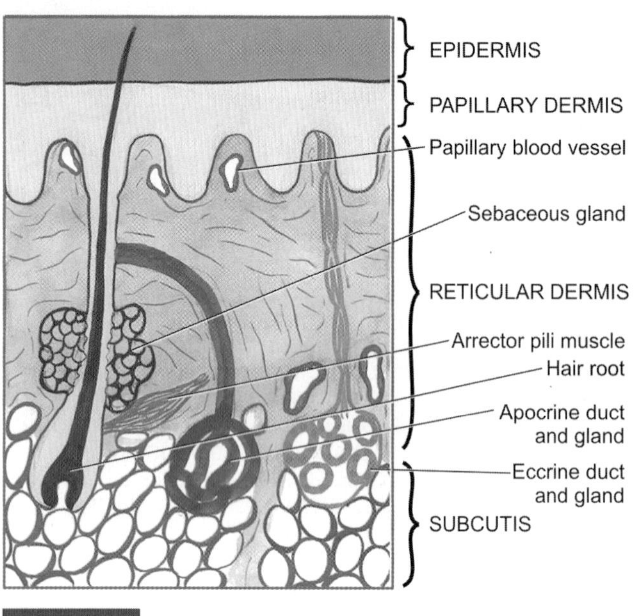

FIGURE 24.1

Main structures identified in a section of the normal skin.

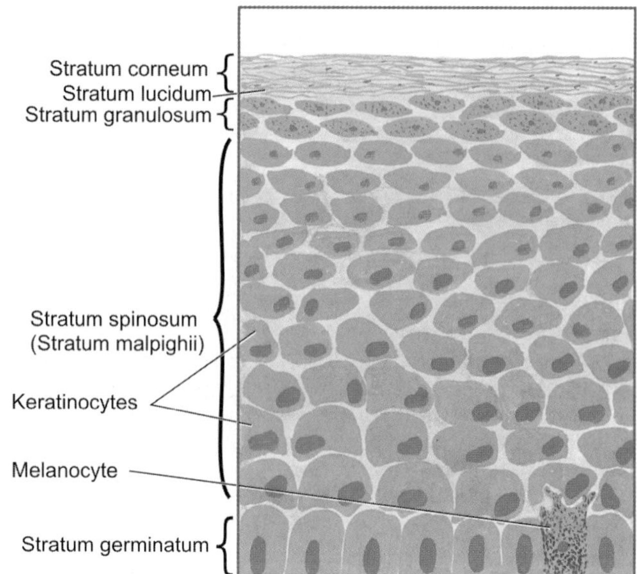

FIGURE 24.2

Different layers comprising the normal epidermis.

reticular dermis. The dermis is composed of fibrocollagenic tissue containing blood vessels, lymphatics and nerves. In the skin of fingers, arteriovenous shunts or *glomera* are normally present. The specialised nerve endings present at some sites perform specific functions. These are as under:

- *Pacinian corpuscles* concerned with pressure are present in the deep layer of skin.
- *Meissner corpuscles* are touch receptors, located in the papillae of skin of palms, soles, tips of fingers and toes.
- *Ruffini corpuscles* are cold receptors found in the external genitalia.
- *End-bulbs of Krause* are cold receptors found in the external genitalia.

Besides these structures, the dermis contains cutaneous appendages or adnexal structures. These are sweat glands, sebaceous glands, hair follicles, arrectores pilorum and nails.

1. SWEAT GLANDS. These are of 2 types—eccrine and apocrine.

i) Eccrine glands. They are present all over the skin but are most numerous on the palms, soles and axillae. They are coiled tubular glands lying deep in the dermis. Their ducts pass through the epidermis on the surface of the skin as pores via which they empty their secretion i.e. sweat. The glands are lined by two main types of secretory cells: basal, acidophilic, *clear or chief cells,* and the superficial, basophilic, *dark granular cells.* The secretory cells are surrounded by myoepithelial cells.

ii) Apocrine glands. Apocrine glands are encountered in some areas only—in the axillae, in the anogenital region, in the external ear as modified glands called ceruminous glands, in the eyelids as Moll's glands, and in the breast as mammary glands. Apocrine glands are also tubular glands but have larger lumina. Apocrine glands have a single layer of secretory cells which contain acidophilic, PAS-positive, prominent granular cytoplasm. The type of secretion in apocrine glands is decapitation secretion as if the cytoplasm of the secretory cells is pinched off (*apo* = off).

2. SEBACEOUS (HOLOCRINE) GLANDS. Sebaceous glands are found everywhere on the skin except on the palms and soles. They are often found in association with hair but can be seen in a few areas devoid of hair as modified sebaceous glands such as in the external auditory meatus, nipple and areola of male and female breast, labia minora, prepuce, and meibomian glands of the eyelids. Sebaceous glands are composed of lobules of sebaceous cells containing small round nuclei and abundant fatty, network-like cytoplasm.

3. HAIR. The hair grows from the bottom of the follicle. It has, therefore, an intracutaneous portion present in the hair follicle and the shaft. The hair follicle consists of epithelial and connective tissue components. The hair shaft is made up of an outer sheath and pigmented cortex and inner medulla.

4. ARRECTORES PILORUM. These are small bundles of smooth muscle attached to each hair follicle. When the muscle contracts, the hair becomes more erect, the follicle is dragged upwards so as to become prominent on the surface of the skin producing what is known as *'goose skin'*.

5. NAILS. The nails are thickenings of the deeper part of the stratum corneum that develop at specially modified portion of the skin called nail bed. The nail is composed of clear horny cells, resembling stratum lucidum but are much more keratinised.

HISTOPATHOLOGIC TERMS

Before describing pathology of common skin diseases, the following pathologic terms in common use need to be defined for proper understanding:

Acanthosis: Thickening of the epidermis due to hyperplasia of stratum malpighii.

Acantholysis: Loss of cohesion between epidermal cells with formation of intraepidermal space containing oedema fluid and detached epithelial cells.

Dyskeratosis: Abnormal development of epidermal cells resulting in rounded cells devoid of their prickles and having pyknotic nuclei. Dyskeratosis is a feature of premalignant and malignant lesions and is rarely seen in benign conditions.

Hyperkeratosis: Thickening of the horny layer.

Parakeratosis: Abnormal keratinisation of the cells so that the horny layer contains nucleated keratinocytes rather than the normal non-nucleate keratin layer.

Spongiosis: Intercellular oedema of the epidermis which may progress to vesicle formation in the epidermis.

Pigment incontinence: Loss of melanin pigment from damaged basal cell layer so that the pigment accumulates in the melanophages in the dermis.

DERMATOSES

Dermatosis is the common term used for any skin disorder. Dermatosis may be of various types such as genetic, inflammatory, infectious, granulomatous, connective tissue, bullous and scaling type. A few common examples of each of these groups are described below.

I. GENETIC DERMATOSES

1. ICTHYOSIS. Two important forms of icthyosis are: *icthyosis vulgaris* which is an autosomal dominant disorder; and *sex-linked icthyosis* which is a sex-(X) linked recessive disorder.

■ **Icthyosis vulgaris** is more common and appears a few months after birth as scaly lesions on the extensor surfaces of the extremities.

Histologically, the characteristic feature is association of hyperkeratosis with thin or absent granular layer.

■ **Sex-linked icthyosis** begins shortly after birth and affects extensor as well as flexor surfaces but palms and hands are spared.

Histologically, there is hyperkeratosis with normal or thickened granular cell layer and acanthosis.

2. KERATOSIS PALMARIS *ET PLANTARIS*. The condition occurs as both autosomal dominant and autosomal recessive forms. It mainly affects the palms and soles as localised or diffuse lesions.

Histologically, there is marked hyperkeratosis, hypergranulosis, acanthosis and mild inflammatory infiltrate in the upper dermis.

3. XERODERMA PIGMENTOSUM. This is an autosomal recessive disorder in which sun-exposed skin is more vulnerable to damage. The condition results from decreased ability to repair the sunlight-induced damage to DNA. Patients of xeroderma pigmentosum are more prone to develop various skin cancers like squamous cell carcinoma, basal cell carcinoma and melanocarcinoma.

Histologically, the changes include hyperkeratosis, thinning and atrophy of stratum malpighii, chronic inflammatory cell infiltrate in the dermis and irregular accumulation of melanin in the basal cell layer. Changes of skin cancers mentioned above may be present in advanced stage.

4. DARIER'S DISEASE (KERATOSIS FOLLICULARIS). The condition is either transmitted as autosomal dominant disorder or as a mutation. In typical cases, there is extensive papular eruption.

Histologically, the characteristic changes are hyperkeratosis, papillomatosis and dyskeratosis. Dyskeratosis result in the formation of *'corps ronds'* (present in the granular layer as a central homogeneous basophilic dyskeratotic mass surrounded by a clear halo) and *'grains'* (having grain-shaped elongated nuclei surrounded by homogeneous dyskeratotic material) and there is appearance of suprabasal clefts containing acantholytic cells. The dermis often shows chronic inflammatory cell infiltrate.

5. URTICARIA PIGMENTOSA. Urticaria pigmentosa may occur as congenital form or may appear without any family history in the adolescents. Clinically, the condition presents as extensive pigmented macules.

Histologically, the epidermis is normal except for an increase in melanin pigmentation in the basal cell layer. The characteristic feature is the presence of numerous mast cells in the dermis.

6. **ATAXIA TELANGIECTASIA.** An autosomal recessive disorder, ataxia appears in infancy, while telangiectasia appears in childhood. The lesions are located on the conjunctivae, cheeks, ears and neck. These children are more prone to develop infections, especially of lungs, and lymphoma-leukaemia.

Histologically, the papillary dermis shows numerous dilated blood vessels.

II. NON-INFECTIOUS INFLAMMATORY DERMATOSES

A very large number of skin diseases have acute or chronic inflammation as a prominent feature. A few selected examples of non-infectious acute and chronic inflammatory dermatoses are presented here which have not been covered in other groups of dermatoses.

1. **DERMATITIS (ECZEMA).** The pathologic term dermatitis is synonymous with the clinical term eczema. Both refer to inflammatory response to a variety of agents acting on the skin from outside or from within the body such as chemicals and drugs, hypersensitivity to various antigens and haptens etc. Accordingly, clinical types such as contact dermatitis, atopic dermatitis, drug-induced dermatitis, photo-eczematous dermatitis and primary irritant dermatitis are described. Many idiopathic varieties of skin disorders such as pompholyx, seborrheic dermatitis, exfoliative dermatitis (erythroderma) and neurodermatitis (lichen simplex chronica) are also included under this heading. In general, these conditions are clinically characterised by itching, erythema with oedema, oozing and scaling. However, irrespective of the clinical type of dermatitis, the histopathologic picture is similar.

Histologically, dermatitis reaction may be acute, subacute or chronic:

- **Acute dermatitis** is characterised by considerable spongiosis (intercellular oedema) that may lead to formation of intraepidermal vesicles or bullae. The vesicles and bullae as well as the oedematous epidermis are permeated by acute inflammatory cells. The upper dermis shows congested blood vessels and mononuclear inflammatory cell infiltrate, especially around the small blood vessels.
- **Subacute dermatitis** may follow acute dermatitis. Spongiosis and vesicles are smaller than in acute dermatitis. The epidermis shows moderate acanthosis and varying degree of parakeratosis in the horny layer with formation of surface crusts containing degenerated leucocytes, bacteria and fibrin. The dermis contains perivascular mononuclear infiltrate. The classical example of subacute dermatitis is *nummular dermatitis.*
- **Chronic dermatitis** shows hyperkeratosis, parakeratosis and acanthosis with elongation of the rete ridges and broadened dermal papillae. Vesicles are absent but slight spongiosis may be present. The upper dermis shows perivascular chronic inflammatory infiltrate and fibrosis. The most characteristic example of chronic dermatitis is *lichen simplex chronicus.*

2. **URTICARIA.** Urticaria or hives is the presence of transient, recurrent, pruritic wheals (i.e. raised erythematous areas of oedema). Hereditary angioneurotic oedema is an uncommon variant of urticaria in which there is recurrent oedema not only on the skin but also on the oral, laryngeal and gastrointestinal mucosa (page 99).

Histologically, there is dermal oedema and a perivascular mononuclear infiltrate. There is localised mast cell degranulation by sensitisation with specific IgE antibodies but no increase in dermal mast cells (*c.f.* mastocytosis in which there is increase in dermal mast cells).

3. **MILIARIA.** Miliaria is a condition in which there is cutaneous retention of sweat due to obstruction of sweat ducts. There are 2 types of miliaria: miliaria crystallina and miliaria rubra.

- **Miliaria crystallina** occurs when there is obstruction of sweat duct within the stratum corneum. It occurs in areas of skin exposed to sun or may occur during a febrile illness.

Histologically, there are intracorneal or subcorneal vesicles which are in continuity with underlying sweat ducts.

- **Miliaria rubra** occurs when there is obstruction of sweat ducts within the deeper layers of the epidermis. It is seen more often in areas of skin covered by clothes following profuse sweating and the lesions are itchy.

Histologically, there are spongiotic vesicles in the stratum malpighii similar to those seen in dermatitis.

These vesicles are in continuity with a sweat duct. Adjacent dermis usually shows chronic inflammatory infiltrate.

4. PANNICULITIS (ERYTHEMA NODOSUM AND ERYTHEMA INDURATUM). Panniculitis is inflammation of the subcutaneous fat. Panniculitis may be acute or chronic. Generally, panniculitis appears as nodular lesions, predominantly on the lower legs. The following types of panniculitis are described:

- **Erythema nodosum,** acute or chronic, is the most common form. The lesions consist of tender red nodules, 1-5 cm in diameter, seen more often on the anterior surface of the lower legs. Erythema nodosum is often found in association with bacterial or fungal infections, drug intake, inflammatory bowel disease and certain malignancies.
- **Erythema induratum** is a less common variety. The lesions are chronic, painless, slightly tender, recurrent and found on the calves of lower legs.

Histologically, the early lesions show necrotising vasculitis involving the blood vessels in the deep dermis and subcutis. In chronic stage, there is inflammatory infiltrate consisting of lymphocytes, histiocytes and multinucleate giant cells. The infiltrate is located in the septa separating the lobules of fat.

5. ACNE VULGARIS. Acne vulgaris is a very common chronic inflammatory dermatosis found predominantly in adolescents in both sexes. The lesions are seen more commonly on the face, upper chest and upper back. The appearance of lesions around puberty is related to physiologic hormonal variations. The condition affects the hair follicle, the opening of which is blocked by keratin material resulting in formation of *comedones.* Comedones may be open having central black appearance due to oxidation of melanin called *black heads,* or they may be in closed follicles referred to as *white heads.* A closed comedone may get infected and result in pustular acne.

Histologically, a comedone consists of keratinised cells, sebum and bacteria. The hair follicle containing a comedone is surrounded by lymphocytic infiltrate in papular acne, and neutrophilic infiltrate in pustular acne. Sometimes, the wall of the distended follicle is disrupted so that the contents escape into the dermis where they may incite granulomatous reaction.

III. INFECTIOUS DERMATOSES

Micro-organisms like bacteria, viruses and fungi are responsible for a large number of dermatoses. Some common examples of each category are described below.

1. IMPETIGO. Impetigo is a common superficial bacterial infection caused by staphylococci and streptococci. The condition may occur in children or in adults and more commonly involves hands and face. The lesions appear as vesico-pustules which may rupture and are followed by characteristic yellowish crusts.

Histologically, the characteristic feature is the subcorneal pustule which is a collection of neutrophils under the stratum corneum. Often, a few acantholytic cells and gram-positive bacteria are found within the pustule. The upper dermis contains severe inflammatory reaction composed of neutrophils and lymphoid cells.

2. VERRUCAE (WARTS). Verrucae or warts are common viral lesions of the skin. They are caused by human papillomaviruses (HPV) that belong to papovavirus group, a type of DNA oncogenic virus (page 228). More than 80 HPV types have been identified. But it must be appreciated that various types of HPVs produce not only different morphologic lesions but also have variable oncogenic potential (Table 24.1). The infection with HPV is acquired by direct contact or by autoinoculation. Verrucae may undergo spontaneous regression in a few months to 2 years, or may spread to other sites. Depending upon the clinical appearance and location, they are classified into different types described below.

i) **Verruca vulgaris** is the most common human wart. The lesions are often multiple, less than 1 cm in size, circumscribed, firm, elevated papules occurring more commonly on the dorsal surfaces of hands and fingers.

TABLE 24.1: Correlation of HPV Types with Disease.

	DISEASE	COMMON TYPE	MALIGNANT POTENTIAL
1.	Common wart (verruca vulgaris)	1, 2	41
2.	Palmoplantar wart	1, 2	—
3.	Flat wart (Verruca plana)	3, 10	41
4.	Anogenital warts (condyloma acuminatum)	6, 11	30, 45
5.	Bowen's disease	16	31
6.	Bowenoid papulosis	16	39, 45
7.	Laryngeal papilloma	6, 11	—
8.	Conjunctival papilloma	6, 11, 16	16
9.	Epidermodysplasia verruciformis	2, 3, 9, 10	5, 8
10.	Cervical carcinoma	16, 18	16, 18, 31, 33

ii) Verruca plana on the other hand, is flat or slightly elevated wart, common on the face and dorsal surface of hands.

iii) Palmoplantar warts occur on the palms and soles. They are covered with a thick callus. They may, therefore, resemble calluses or a verrucous carcinoma.

iv) Epidermodysplasia verruciformis resembles verruca plana but differs by having familial occurrence with autosomal recessive inheritance. The genome of HPV types 5 and 8 have been found in some of these tumours. Epidermodysplasia verruciformis is of special clinical significance as it may undergo malignant change, usually into Bowen's disease, and occasionally into squamous cell carcinoma.

v) Condyloma acuminatum (or venereal wart or anogenital wart) occurs on the penis, on the vulva and around the anus (page 740). The lesions appear as soft, papillary, cauliflower-like mass that may grow fairly large in size (giant condyloma acuminata). In rare cases, transformation into verrucous carcinoma may occur.

Histologically, all types of verrucae have some common features as under (Fig. 24.3):

i) Papillomatosis (papillary folds).

ii) Acanthosis (hyperplasia of stratum malpighii containing foci of vacuolated cells in the upper stratum malpighii.

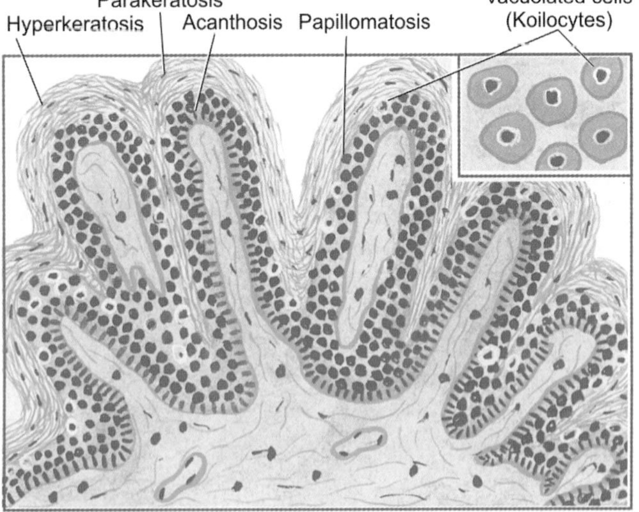

FIGURE 24.3

Typical appearance of a verruca. The histologic features include papillomatosis, acanthosis, hyperkeratosis with parakeratosis and elongated rete ridges appearing to point towards the centre. Foci of vacuolated cells (koilocytes) are found in the upper stratum malpighii. *Inset* shows koilocytes and virus-infected keratinocytes containing prominent keratohyaline granules.

iii) Hyperkaratosis with parakeratosis.

iv) Clumped keratohyaline granules in the granular cells in the valleys between adjacent papillae.

v) Elongation of rete ridges with their lower tips bent inwards.

vi) Virus-infected epidermal cells contain prominent vacuolation (koilocytosis) and keratohyaline granules of intracytoplasmic keratin aggregates due to viral cytopathic effects. These cells on electron microscopy reveal numerous intranuclear viral particles.

3. MOLLUSCUM CONTAGIOSUM. Molluscum contagiosum is a common self-limiting contagious lesion caused by a poxvirus which is a DNA virus. It is more common in children and young adults. Infection is acquired by direct contact. Clinically, the lesions are often multiple, discrete, waxy, papules, about 5 mm in diameter and are seen more frequently on the face and trunk. In a fully-developed lesion, small amount of paste-like material can be expressed on pressing.

Histologically, typical lesion consists of sharply circumscribed cup-like epidermal lesion growing down into the dermis. The proliferating epidermal cells contain the pathognomonic intracytoplasmic eosinophilic inclusion bodies called *molluscum bodies.* These bodies contain numerous viral particles.

4. VIRAL EXANTHEMATA. Viral exanthemata are a group of contagious conditions in which the epidermal cells are destroyed by replicating viruses causing eruption or rash. There are predominantly two groups of viruses which may cause exanthem. These are: the *poxvirus group* (e.g. smallpox or variola, cowpox or vaccinia), and the *herpesvirus group* (e.g. chickenpox or varicella, herpes zoster or shingles, herpes simplex). Clinically, these conditions have different presentations but the eruptive lesions may look alike and are, therefore, considered together.

Variola (smallpox) has been globally eradicated since 1978. The route of infection is via upper respiratory tract or mouth followed by viraemia and characteristic skin lesions. **Vaccinia (cowpox)** is primarily a disease of the teats and udders of cows but humans are infected by milking the infected animals. **Varicella (chickenpox)** and **herpes zoster (shingles)** are both caused by a common virus, varicella-zoster virus. Chickenpox is transmitted by the respiratory route followed by viraemia and successive crops of lesions. Herpes zoster is different manifestation of infection with the same viral agent after years of latency. It is a disease of the nerves and the tissues supplied by the nerves. The condition is characterised by sharp burning pain, often disproportionate to the rash. **Herpes simplex,** caused by HSV-1, and another related herpetic infection, **herpes genitalis,** caused by HSV-2, are characterised by transmission by direct physical contact and prolonged latency. The vesicular lesions are often located on the skin, especially the facial skin around lips and external nares; other sites are mucosal surfaces and eyes.

Histologically, the characteristic feature of viral exanthemata is the formation of intra-epidermal vesicles or bullae due to cytopathic effects of viruses. In the early stage, there is proliferation of epidermal cells and formation of multinucleate giant cells. This is followed by intracellular oedema and ballooning degeneration that progresses on to rupture of the cells with eventual formation of vesicles or bullae.

5. SUPERFICIAL MYCOSES. Superficial fungal infections of the skin are localised to stratum corneum (page 189). These include some of the common dermatophytes such as: *Trichophyton rubrum* and *Pityrosporum.* Clinically, these fungal infections are labelled according to the region involved. These are:

i) Tinea capitis occurring on the scalp, especially in children.

ii) Tinea barbae affecting the region of beard in adult males.

iii) Tinea corporis involving the body surface at all ages.

iv) Tinea cruris occurs most frequently in the region of groin in obese men, especially in hot weather.

v) Tinea pedis or 'athlete foot' is located in the web spaces between the toes.

vi) Onychomycosis shows disintegration of the nail substance.

vii) Tinea versicolor caused by *Malassezia furfur* generally affects the upper trunk.

Histologically, fungal hyphae (or mycelia) and spores of dermatophytes are present in the stratum corneum of skin, nails or hair. Hyphae may be septate or nonseptate. Spores are round to oval bodies which grow by budding. Special stains can be used to demonstrate the fungi. These are: *periodic acid-Schiff (PAS) reaction* which stains the fungi deep pink to red, and *methenamine silver nitrate method* that stains fungi black.

IV. GRANULOMATOUS DISEASES

In many skin diseases, the host may respond by granulomatous inflammation to a variety of microbial agents and nonmicrobial material. Tuberculosis of the skin is the classical example in which typical tubercles are formed; other conditions are leprosy, syphilis, sarcoidosis, deep fungal infection etc. These conditions have already been discussed in Chapter 6. Nonmicrobial agents which can incite granulomatous inflammation are keratin, hair, thorns, talc, minerals like beryllium, asbestos and tattoo pigment etc.

Two representative examples of granulomatous inflammation—*lupus vulgaris* which is a variety of skin tuberculosis, and *granuloma annulare* seen in diabetics, are described here.

1. LUPUS VULGARIS. The lesions of lupus vulgaris, the prototype of skin tuberculosis, are found most commonly on the head and neck, especially skin of the nose. They are yellowish-brown to reddish-brown tiny nodules (apple-jelly nodules).

Histologically, the nodules consist of well-defined tubercles lying in the upper dermis. They consist of accumulation of epithelioid cells surrounded by lymphoid cells. Caseation necrosis may be slight or absent. Langhans' and foreign body type of giant cells are often present. Tubercle bacilli are present in very small numbers that are hard to demonstrate by acid-fast staining.

2. GRANULOMA ANNULARE. The lesions of granuloma annulare are often numerous. Dermal nodules are arranged in a ring-like fashion, commonly on the hands and feet. The condition appears to have correlation with diabetes mellitus.

Histologically, the centre of the lesion shows a well demarcated focus of complete collagen degeneration. These foci are surrounded by an infiltrate composed largely of histiocytes and some mononuclear inflammatory cells forming a palisade arrangement and are therefore also referred to as palisading granulomas.

V. CONNECTIVE TISSUE DISEASES

Group of diseases caused by self-antigens or autoimmune diseases are included under connective tissue diseases. A list of such diseases alongwith their etiology and pathogenesis is given in Chapter 4. Morphology of skin lesions of two important representative examples—*lupus erythematosus* and *systemic sclerosis (scleroderma),* is given below. Another connective tissue disease of unknown etiology, lichen sclerosus et atrophicus, is also considered here.

1. LUPUS ERYTHEMATOSUS. Two types of lupus erythematosus are recognised—a chronic form, *discoid* *lupus erythematosus (DLE)* which is confined to the skin; and a systemic form, *systemic lupus erythematosus (SLE)* that has widespread visceral vascular lesions. The discoid variety is more common which is generally benign, while systemic form may be fatal, usually from renal involvement. The diagnosis is made on the basis of clinical, serologic and pathologic changes. The characteristic cutaneous lesions in DLE consist of well-defined erythematous discoid patches associated with scaling and atrophy and often limited to the face. In contrast, cutaneous lesions in SLE are present only in a small proportion of cases and consist of erythematous, slightly oedematous patches which are without significant scaling and without atrophy.

Histologically, cutaneous lesion in DLE and SLE may not be distinguishable in all cases. The important features are as follows:

i) Hyperkeratosis with keratotic plugging.
ii) Thinning and flattening of rete malpighii.
iii) Hydropic degeneration of basal layer.
iv) Patchy lymphoid infiltrate around cutaneous adnexal structures.
v) Upper dermis showing oedema, vasodilatation and extravasation of red cells.

Direct immunofluorescence reveals granular deposits of immunoglobulins, most commonly IgG and IgM, and components of complement on the basement membrane of the affected skin in both DLE and SLE. High serum titres of antinuclear antibodies and demonstration of LE cells (page 78) are other notable features, especially in SLE.

2. SYSTEMIC SCLEROSIS (SCLERODERMA). Two types of systemic sclerosis or scleroderma are identified: a localised form called *morphea,* and a generalised form called *progressive systemic sclerosis.* A variant of progressive systemic sclerosis is *CREST syndrome.* (C=calcinosis, R=Raynaud's phenomenon, E=esophageal dismotility, S=sclerodactyly and T=telangiectasia). Etiology and pathogenesis of these conditions are already described (page 79). Morphea consists of lesions limited to the skin and subcutaneous tissue, while progressive systemic sclerosis consists of extensive involvement of the skin and the subcutaneous tissue and has visceral lesions too. The lesions generally begin in the fingers and distal extremities and then extend proximally to involve the arms, shoulders, neck and face.

Histologically, there is thickening of the dermal collagen extending into the subcutaneous tissue. There is pronounced chronic inflammatory infiltrate in the affected area. The epidermis is often thin, devoid of rete ridges and adnexal structures, and there is hyalinised thickening of the walls of dermal arterioles and capillaries. Subcutaneous calcification may develop.

3. LICHEN SCLEROSUS *ET ATROPHICUS.* This condition involves genital skin most frequently and is often the only site of involvement. It occurs in both sexes, more commonly in women than in men. It is termed *kraurosis vulvae* in women while the counterpart in men is referred to as *balanitis xerotica obliterans.* Occasionally, the condition may coexist with morphea. Clinically, the condition may simulate malignancy.

Histologically, the characteristic features are as under:

i) Hyperkeratosis with follicular plugging.
ii) Thinning and atrophy of the epidermis.
iii) Hydropic degeneration of the basal layer.
iv) Upper dermis showing oedema and hyaline appearance of collagen.
v) Inflammatory infiltrate in mid-dermis.

VI. NON-INFECTIOUS BULLOUS DERMATOSES

This is a group of skin diseases characterised by bullae and vesicles. A *bulla* is a cavity formed in the layers of the skin and containing blood, plasma, epidermal cells or inflammatory cells, while a *vesicle* is a small bulla less than 5 mm in diameter. *Blister* is the common term used for both bulla and vesicle. The blister can be located at different sites such as subcorneal, intra-epidermal (suprabasal or subcorneal) and subepidermal. These blisters can appear in infectious as well as in noninfectious dermatoses. A few common examples of noninfectious dermatoses are pemphigus, pemphigoid, dermatitis herpetiformis and erythema multiforme and are illustrated in Fig. 24.4.

1. PEMPHIGUS. Pemphigus is an autoimmune bullous disease of skin and mucosa which has 4 clinical and pathologic variants: pemphigus vulgaris, pemphigus vegetans, pemphigus foliaceous and pemphigus erythematosus.

All forms of pemphigus have acantholysis as common histologic feature. Sera from these patients contain IgG antibodies to cement substance of skin and mucosa.

i) Pemphigus vulgaris is the most common type characterised by the development of flaccid bullae on the skin and oral mucosa. These bullae break easily leaving behind denuded surface.

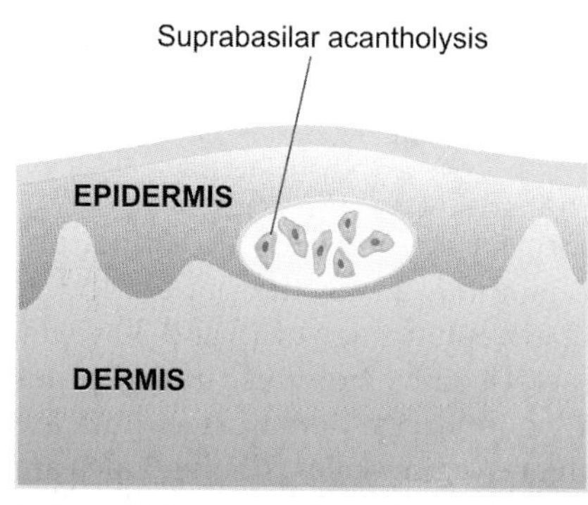

A, PEMPHIGUS VULGARIS

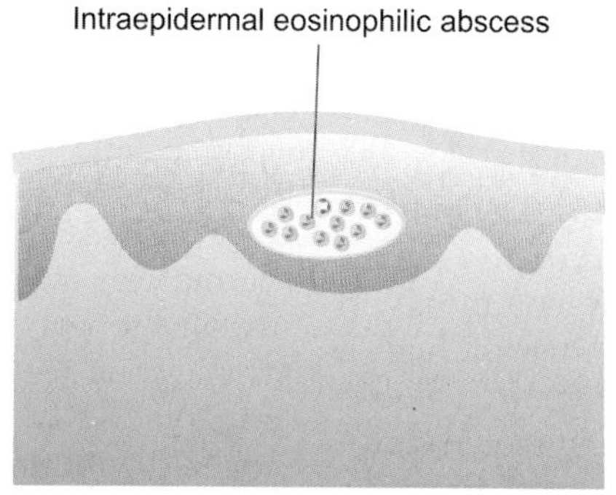

B, PEMPHIGUS VEGETANS

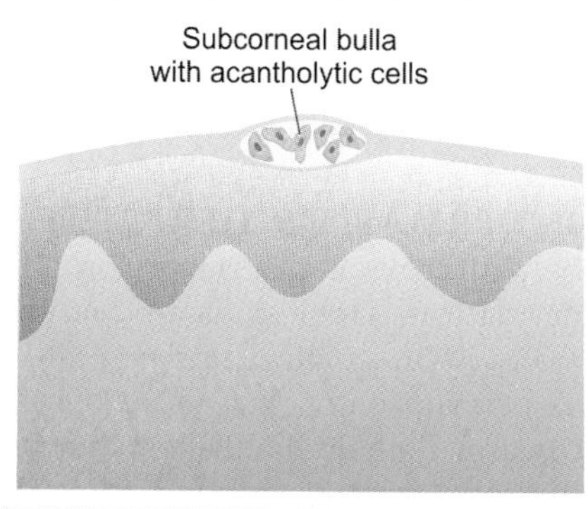

C, PEMPHIGUS FOLIACEOUS

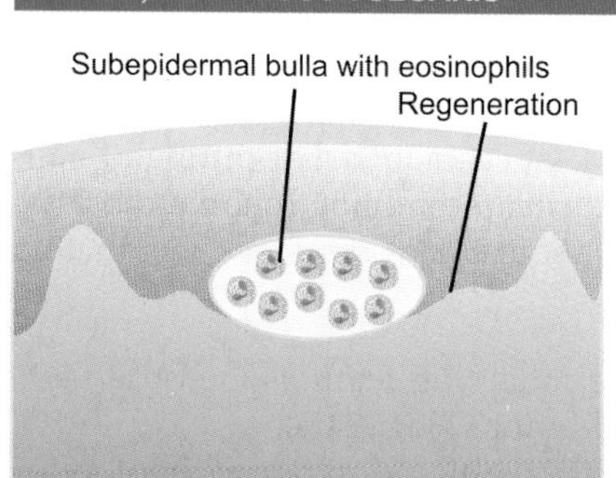

D, PEMPHIGOID

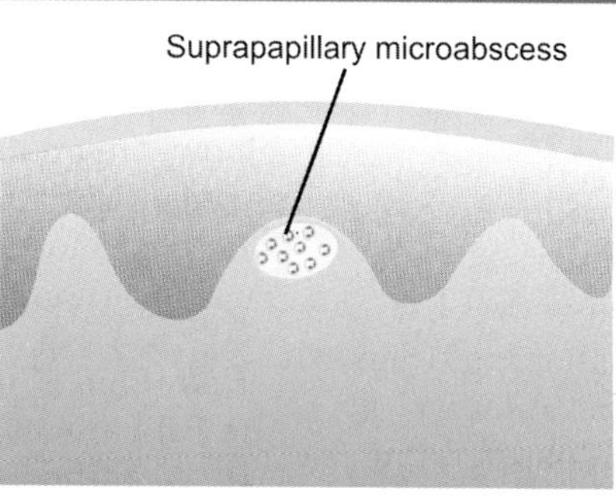

E, DERMATITIS HERPETIFORMIS

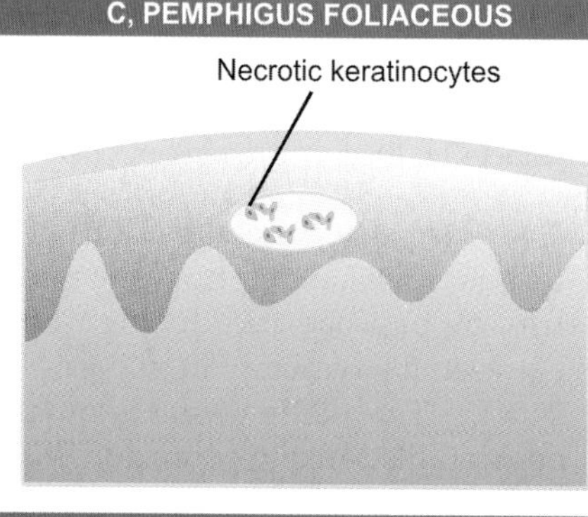

F, ERYTHEMA MULTIFORME

FIGURE 24.4

Location of bullae and vesicles in non-infectious bullous dermatoses. A, *Pemphigus vulgaris:* The bulla is predominantly suprabasilar in position and contains acantholytic cells. B, *Pemphigus vegetans*: An intraepidermal abscess composed of eosinophils is seen. C, *Pemphigus* foliaceous: The bulla is superficial in subcorneal position and contains acantholytic cells. D, *Pemphigoid:* The bulla is subepidermal with regeneration of the epidermis at the periphery. E, *Dermatitis herpetiformis:* There is a papillary microabscess composed of neutrophils. F, *Erythema Multiforme:* The affected area shows necrotic keratinocytes and inflammatory cells.

Histologically, the bullae are suprabasal in location so that the basal layer remains attached to dermis like a row of tombstones. The bullous cavity contains serum and acantholytic epidermal cells (Fig. 24.4,A).

ii) Pemphigus vegetans is an uncommon variant consisting of early lesions resembling pemphigus vulgaris. But later, verrucous vegetations are found on the skin and oral mucosa instead of bullous lesions.

Histologically, there is considerable acanthosis and papillomatosis. Intraepidermal abscesses composed almost entirely of eosinophils are diagnostic of pemphigus vegetans (Fig. 24.4,B).

iii) Pemphigus foliaceous is characterised by quite superficial bullae which leave shallow zones of erythema and crust.

Histologically, superficial subcorneal bullae are found which contain acantholytic epidermal cells (Fig. 24.4,C).

iv) Pemphigus erythematosus is an early form of pemphigus foliaceous. The distribution of clinical lesions is similar to lupus erythematosus involving face.

Histologically, the picture is identical to that of pemphigus foliaceous.

2. PEMPHIGOID. This is a form of bullous disease affecting skin or the mucous membranes. Three variants have been described—*localised form* occurring on the lower extremities; *vesicular form* consisting of small tense blisters; and *vegetating form* having verrucous vegetations found mainly in the axillae and groins.

Histologically, the characteristic distinguishing feature from pemphigus is the subepidermal location of the non-acantholytic bullae. With passage of time, there is some epidermal regeneration from the periphery at the floor of the bulla. The bullous cavity contains fibrin network and many mononuclear inflammatory cells and some eosinophils (Fig. 24.4,D).

Dermal changes seen in inflammatory bullae consist of infiltrate of mononuclear cells, a few eosinophils and neutrophils.

3. DERMATITIS HERPETIFORMIS. Dermatitis herpetiformis is a form of chronic, pruritic, vesicular dermatosis. The lesions are found more commonly in males in 3rd to 4th decades of life. The disease has an association with gluten-sensitive enteropathy (coeliac disease). Both dermatitis herpetiformis and gluten-sensitive enteropathy respond to a gluten-free diet. The pathogenesis of the disease is not quite clear but probably individuals with certain histocompatibility types develop IgA and IgG antibodies to gliadin which is a fraction of gluten present in the flour (page 590).

Histologically, the early lesions of dermatitis herpetiformis consist of neutrophilic micro-abscesses at the tips of papillae, producing separation or blister between the papillary dermis and the epidermis (Fig. 24.4,E). The older blisters contain fair number of eosinophils causing confusion with bullous pemphigoid. Direct immunofluorescence shows granular deposits of IgA at the papillary tips in dermatitis herpetiformis.

4. ERYTHEMA MULTIFORME. This is an acute, self-limiting but recurrent dermatosis. The condition occurs due to hypersensitivity to certain infections and drugs, and in many cases, it is idiopathic. As the name suggests, the lesions are *multiform* such as macular, papular, vesicular and bullous. Quite often, the lesions have symmetric involvement of the extremities. *Stevens-Johnson syndrome* is a severe, at times fatal, form of involvement of skin and mucous membranes of the mouth, conjunctivae, genital and perianal area. Another variant termed *toxic epidermal necrolysis* consists of diffuse necrosis of the epidermis and mucosa, exposing the dermis giving the skin a scalded appearance.

Histologically, the changes vary according to the clinical multiform stage.

i) *Early lesions* show oedema and lymphocytic infiltrate at the dermoepidermal junction. The superfical dermis shows perivascular lymphocytic infiltrate.

ii) *Later stage* is associated with migration of lymphocytes upwards into the epidermis resulting in epidermal necrosis and blister formation (Fig. 24.4,F).

VII. SCALING DERMATOSES

The skin surface in some chronic inflammatory dermatoses is roughened due to excessive and abnormal scale formation and desquamation. Common examples of this group are psoriasis and lichen planus. Hereditary icthyosis having similar scaly lesions has already been described.

1. PSORIASIS. Psoriasis is a chronic inflammatory dermatosis that affects about 2% of the population. It usually appears first between the age of 15 and 30 years. The lesions are characterised by brownish-red papules and plaques which are sharply demarcated and are covered with fine, silvery white scales. As the scales are removed by gentle scrapping, fine bleeding points appear termed *Auspitz sign.* Commonly involved sites are the scalp, upper back, sacral region and extensor surfaces of the extremities, especially the knees and elbows. In about 25% of cases, peculiar pitting of nails is seen. Psoriatic arthritis resembling rheumatoid arthritis is produced in about 5% of cases but rheumatoid factor is absent.

Histologically, the following features are observed in fully-developed lesions (Fig. 24.5):

i) Acanthosis with regular downgrowth of rete ridges to almost the same dermal level with thickening of their lower portion.

ii) Elongation and oedema of the dermal papillae with broadening of their tips.

iii) Suprapapillary thinning of stratum malpighii.

iv) Absence of granular cell layer.

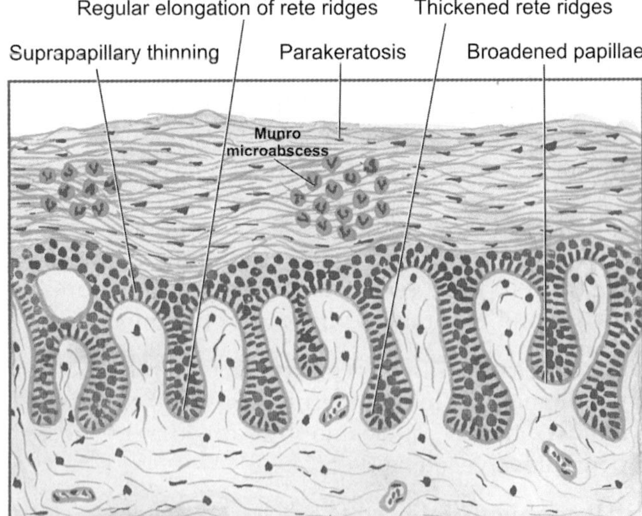

FIGURE 24.5

Psoriasis. There is regular elongation of the rete ridges with thickening of their lower portion. The papillae are elongated and oedematous with suprapapillary thinning of epidermis. There is marked parakeratosis with diagnostic Munro microabscesses in the parakeratotic layer.

v) Prominent parakeratosis.
vi) Presence of Munro microabscesses in the parakeratotic horny layer is diagnostic of psoriasis.

2. LICHEN PLANUS. Lichen planus is a chronic dermatosis characterised clinically by irregular, violaceous, shining, flat-topped, pruritic papules. The lesions are distributed symmetrically with sites of predilection being flexor surfaces of the wrists, forearms, legs and external genitalia. Buccal mucosa is also involved in many cases of lichen planus.

Histologically, the characteristic features are as under (Fig. 24.6):
i) Marked hyperkeratosis.
ii) Focal hypergranulosis.
iii) Irregular acanthosis with elongated saw-toothed rete ridges.
iv) Liquefactive degeneration of the basal layer.
v) A band-like dermal infiltrate of mononuclear cells, sharply demarcated at its lower border and closely hugging the basal layer.

VIII. METABOLIC DISEASES OF SKIN

Skin is involved in a variety of systemic metabolic derangements. The examples include the following:
1. Amyloidosis (primary as well as secondary, page 83).

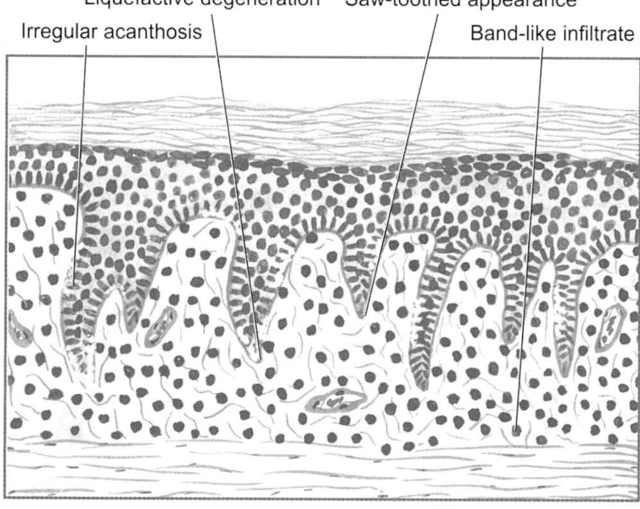

FIGURE 24.6

Lichen planus. There is hyperkeratosis, focal hypergranulosis and irregular acanthosis with elongated saw-toothed rete ridges. The basal layer shows liquefactive degeneration. The upper dermis shows a band-like mononuclear infiltrate with a sharply-demarcated lower border.

2. Lipoid proteinosis is rare.
3. Porphyria of various types (page 48).
4. Calcinosis cutis
5. Gout due to urate deposits or tophi (page 878).
6. Ochronosis due to alkaptonuria (page 47).
7. Mucinosis seen in myxoedema (page 97).
8. Idiopathic haemochromatosis with skin pigmentation (page 47).

Many of these conditions have been discussed elsewhere in the book; calcinosis cutis is briefly considered below.

CALCINOSIS CUTIS. There are four types of calcification in the skin:
i) Metastatic calcinosis cutis
ii) Dystrophic calcinosis cutis
iii) Idiopathic calcinosis cutis
iv) Subepidermal calcified nodule

i) Metastatic calcinosis cutis develops due to hypercalcaemia or hyperphosphataemia as discussed on page 57.

ii) Dystrophic calcinosis cutis results when there is deposition of calcium salts at damaged tissue.

iii) Idiopathic calcinosis cutis resembles dystrophic type but is not associated with any underlying disease. A special manifestation of idiopathic calcinosis cutis is *tumoral calcinosis* in which there are large subcutaneous calcified masses, often accompanied by foreign body giant cell reaction. Calcium may discharge from the surface of the lesion. *Idiopathic calcinosis of the scrotum* consists of multiple asymptomatic nodules of the scrotal skin.

iv) Subepidermal calcified nodule or *cutaneous calculus* is a single raised hard calcified nodule in the upper dermis.

TUMOURS AND TUMOUR-LIKE LESIONS

The skin is the largest organ of the body. Tumours and tumour-like lesions may arise from different components of the skin such as surface epidermis, epidermal appendages and dermal tissues. Each of these tissues may give rise to benign and malignant tumours as well as tumour-like lesions. Besides these, there is a group of conditions and lesions which are precancerous. Another group of tumours have their origin from elsewhere in the body but are cellular migrants to the skin. A comprehensive list of tumours and tumour-like lesions of the skin is presented in Table 24.2. It is beyond the scope of this book to describe all these tumours and lesions, for which the interested reader may consult specialised work on dermatopathology. Some important and common examples of these conditions are considered here.

TABLE 24.2: Tumours and Tumour-like Lesions of the Skin.

I. EPIDERMAL TUMOURS

A. Benign tumours
1. Squamous papilloma
2. Seborrhoeic keratosis
3. Fibroepithelial polyps
4. Keratoacanthoma

B. Epithelial cysts
1. Epidermal cyst
2. Pilar (trichilemmal, sebaceous) cyst
3. Dermoid cyst
4. Steatocystoma multiplex

C. Pre-malignant lesions
1. Solar keratosis (actinic keratosis, senile keratosis)
2. Bowen's disease
3. Xeroderma pigmentosum
4. Erythroplasia of Queyrat

D. Malignant tumours
1. Squamous cell carcinoma
2. Basal cell carcinoma (Rodent ulcer)
3. Metatypical (Basosquamous) carcinoma

II. ADNEXAL (APPENDAGEAL) TUMOURS

A. Tumours of hair follicles
1. Trichoepithelioma (Brooke's tumour)
2. Pilomatricoma (Calcifying epithelioma of Malherbe)
3. Trichofolliculoma
4. Trichilemmoma

B. Tumours of sebaceous glands
1. Naevus sebaceus
2. Sebaceous adenoma
3. Sebaceous carcinoma

C. Tumours of sweat glands
1. Eccrine tumours
i) Eccrine poroma
ii) Eccrine hidradenoma
iii) Eccrine spiradenoma
2. Apocrine tumours
i) Papillary hidradenoma
ii) Cylindroma (Turban tumour)
3. Sweat gland carcinoma

III. MELANOCYTIC TUMOURS
1. Naevocellular naevi
2. Malignant melanoma

IV. DERMAL TUMOURS
1. Dermatofibroma and malignant fibrous histiocytoma
2. Dermatofibrosarcoma protuberans
3. Xanthoma
4. Lipoma and liposarcoma
5. Leiomyoma and leiomyosarcoma
6. Haemangiomas, lymphangiomas and angiosarcoma (page 300)

Contd.

Contd.

7. Glomangioma (page 302)
8. Kaposi's sarcoma (page 303)

V. CELLULAR MIGRANT TUMOURS
1. Mycosis fungoides
2. Langerhans' cell histiocytosis (page 463)
3. Mastocytosis
4. Lymphomas and leukaemias (Chapter 14)
5. Plasmacytoma (page 459)

I. TUMOURS AND CYSTS OF THE EPIDERMIS

A. Benign Tumours

1. SQUAMOUS PAPILLOMA. Squamous papilloma is a benign epithelial tumour of the skin. Though considered by many authors to include common viral warts (verrucae) and condyloma acuminata, true squamous papillomas differ from these viral lesions. If these 'viral tumours' are excluded, squamous papilloma is a rare tumour.

Histologically, squamous papillomas are characterised by hyperkeratosis, acanthosis with elongation of rete ridges and papillomatosis. The *verrucae,* in addition to these features, have foci of vacuolated cells in the acanthotic stratum malpighii, vertical tiers of parakeratosis between the adjacent papillae and irregular clumps of keratohyaline granules in the virus-infected granular cells lying in the valleys between the papillae (page 797) (Fig. 24.7) (COLOUR PLATE X: CL 37).

2. SEBORRHEIC KERATOSIS. Seborrheic keratosis is a very common lesion in middle-aged adults. There may be only one lesion, but more often these are many. The common locations are trunk and face. They are sharply-demarcated, brownish, smooth-surfaced, measuring a few millimeters in diameter.

Histologically, the pathognomonic feature is a sharply-demarcated exophytic tumour overlying a straight line from the normal epidermis at one end of the tumour to the normal epidermis at the other end. The other features are hyperkeratosis, acanthosis and papillomatosis as seen in squamous cell papillomas.

3. FIBROEPITHELIAL POLYPS. Also known by other names such as 'skin tags', 'acrochordons' and 'soft fibromas', these are the most common cutaneous lesions. They are often multiple, soft, small (a few mm in size), bag-like tumours commonly seen on the neck, trunk and axillae.

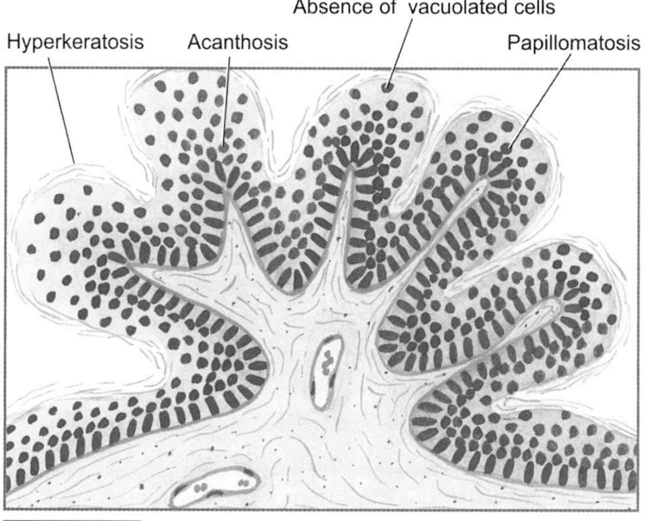

FIGURE 24.7

Squamous cell papilloma. Please note that it differs from verruca by not having vacuolated cells in stratum malpighii.

Histologically, the tumours are composed of loosely-arranged fibrovascular cores with overlying hyperplastic epidermis.

B. Epithelial Cysts

Various cysts in the skin may arise from downgrowth of the epidermis and the appendages. These cysts often contain paste-like pultaceous material containing keratin, sebaceous secretions and lipid-containing debris. Depending upon the structure of the cyst wall, these cysts are of various types as under:

1. **EPIDERMAL CYST.** These intradermal or subcutaneous cysts may occur spontaneously or due to implantation of the epidermis into the dermis or subcutis (implantation cysts).

Histologically, epidermal cysts have a cyst wall composed of true epidermis with laminated layers of keratin. Rupture of the cyst may incite foreign body giant cell inflammatory reaction in the wall.

2. **PILAR (TRICHILEMMAL, SEBACEOUS) CYST.** These cysts clinically resemble epidermal cysts but occur more frequently on the scalp and are more common than the epidermal cysts.

Histologically, the cyst wall is composed of palisading squamous epithelial cells. These cells undergo degeneration towards the cyst cavity. Rupture of the cyst wall is common and leads to foreign body giant cell inflammatory reaction. Calcification in the cyst wall is often present.

3. **DERMOID CYST.** These are subcutaneous cysts often present at birth. Dermoid cysts are more common on the face.

Histologically, the cyst wall contains epidermis as well as appendages such as hair follicles, sebaceous glands and sweat glands.

4. **STEATOCYSTOMA MULTIPLEX.** This is an inherited autosomal dominant disorder having multiple cystic nodules, 1-3 cm in size. They are more common in the axillae, sternum and arms.

Histologically, the cyst walls are composed of several layers of epithelial cells and contain lobules of sebaceous glands in the cyst wall.

C. Pre-malignant Lesions

1. **SOLAR KERATOSIS (ACTINIC KERATOSIS, SENILE KERATOSIS).** Solar (sun-induced) or actinic (induced by a variety of rays) keratoses are the multiple lesions occurring in sun-exposed areas of the skin in fair-skinned elderly people. Similar lesions may be induced by exposure to ionising radiation, hydrocarbons and arsenicals. The condition is considered to be a forerunner of invasive squamous cell and/or basal cell carcinoma. Clinically, the lesions are tan-brown, erythematous, about 1 cm in diameter with rough, sandpaper-like surface and are seen more commonly on the dorsum of the hands and on the balded portion of the skin.

Histologically, solar keratoses are squamous cell carcinoma *in situ* with the following characteristic features:

i) Considerable hyperkeratosis.
ii) Marked acanthosis.
iii) Dyskeratosis and dysplasia of the epidermal cells showing features such as hyperchromatism, loss of polarity, pleomorphism and increased number of mitotic figures.
iv) Non-specific chronic inflammatory cell infiltrate in the upper dermis encroaching upon the basement membrane of the epidermis.

2. **BOWEN'S DISEASE.** Bowen's disease is also a carcinoma *in situ* of the entire epidermis but differs from solar keratosis in having often solitary lesion that

may occur on sun-exposed as well as sun-unexposed skin. The condition may occur anywhere on the skin but is found more often on the trunk, buttocks and extremities. Clinically, the lesions of Bowen's disease are sharply circumscribed, rounded, reddish-brown patches which enlarge slowly.

Histologically, the characteristic features are as under:
i) Marked hyperkeratosis.
ii) Pronounced parakeratosis.
iii) Marked epidermal hyperplasia with disappearance of dermal papillae.
iv) Scattered bizarre dyskeratotic cells distributed throughout the epidermis.

Bowen's disease, unlike solar keratosis which invariably leads to invasive cancer, may remain confined to the surface for many years.

3. XERODERMA PIGMENTOSUM. This condition is a hypersensitivity of the skin to sunlight that is determined by a recessive gene. The disorder may lead to multiple malignancies of the skin such as basal cell carcinoma, squamous cell carcinoma and malignant melanoma. Xeroderma pigmentosum has already been described under *genetic dermatoses.*

D. Malignant Tumours

1. SQUAMOUS CELL CARCINOMA. Squamous cell carcinoma may arise on any part of the skin and mucous membranes lined by squamous epithelium but is more likely to occur on sun-exposed parts in older people. Various predisposing conditions include:
i) xeroderma pigmentosum;
ii) solar keratosis;
iii) chronic inflammatory conditions such as chronic ulcers and draining osteomyelitis;
iv) old burn scars (Marjolin's ulcers);
v) chemical burns;
vi) psoriasis;
vii) HIV infection;
viii) ionising radiation;
ix) industrial carcinogens (coal tars, oils etc); and
x) in the case of cancer of oral cavity, chewing betel nuts and tobacco.

Cancer of scrotal skin in chimney-sweeps was the first cancer in which an occupational carcinogen (soot) was implicated. *'Kangari cancer'* of the skin of inner side of thigh and lower abdomen common in natives of Kashmir is another example of skin cancer due to chronic irritation (*Kangari* is an earthenware pot containing glowing charcoal used by Kashmiris close to their abdomen to keep them warm).

Although squamous carcinomas can occur anywhere on the skin, most common locations are the face, pinna of the ears, back of hands and mucocutaneous junctions such as on the lips, anal canal and glans penis. Cutaneous squamous carcinoma arising in a pre-existing inflammatory and degenerative lesion has a higher incidence of developing metastases.

PATHOLOGIC CHANGES. Macroscopically, squamous carcinoma of the skin and squamous-lined mucosa can have one of the following two patterns:
i) More commonly, an *ulcerated growth* with elevated and indurated margin is seen.
ii) Less often, a raised *fungating or polypoid verrucous* lesion without ulceration is found (Fig. 24.8,A).

Microscopically, squamous cell carcinoma is an invasive carcinoma of the surface epidermis characterised by the following features (Fig. 24.8,B) (COLOUR PLATE X: CL 38):
i) There is irregular downward proliferation of epidermal cells into the dermis.
ii) Depending upon the grade of malignancy, the masses of epidermal cells show atypical features such as variation in cell size and shape, nuclear hyperchromatism, absence of intercellular bridges, individual cell keratinisation and occurrence of atypical mitotic figures.
iii) Better-differentiated squamous carcinomas have whorled arrangement of malignant squamous cells forming horn pearls. The centres of these horn pearls may contain laminated, keratin material.
iv) Higher grades of squamous carcinomas, however, have fewer or no horn pearls and may instead have highly atypical cells.
v) An uncommon variant of squamous carcinoma may have spindle-shaped tumour cells *(spindle cell carcinoma).*
vi) Adenoid changes may be seen in a portion of squamous cell carcinoma *(adenoid squamous cell carcinoma).*
vii) *Verrucous carcinoma* is a low grade squamous cell carcinoma in which the superficial portion of the tumour resembles verruca (hyperkeratosis, parakeratosis, acanthosis and papillomatosis) but differs from it in having downward proliferation into deeper portion of the tumour.
viii) All variants of squamous cell carcinoma show inflammatory reaction between the collections of tumour cells, while in *pseudocarcinomatous hyperplasia* there is permeation of the epithelial proliferations by inflammatory cells.

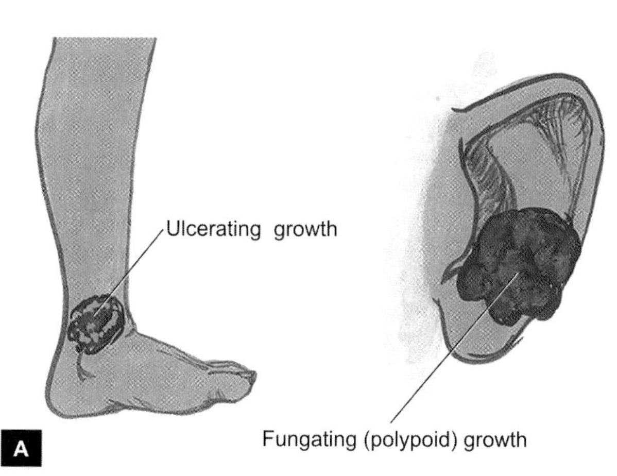

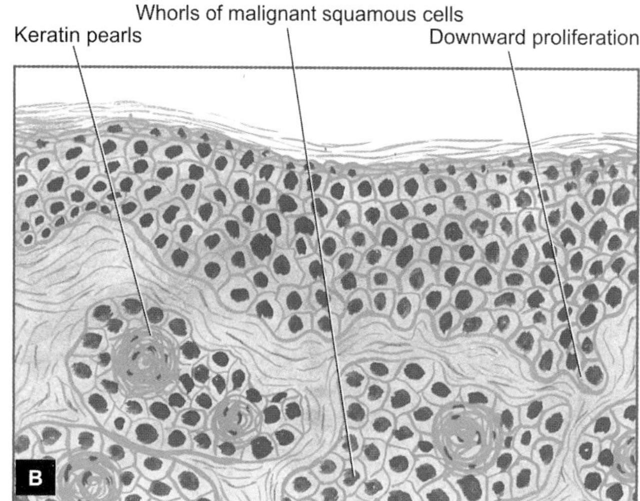

FIGURE 24.8

Squamous cell carcinoma. A, Main macroscopic patterns. B, Microscopic features of well-differentiated squamous cell carcinoma. The dermis is invaded by downward proliferating epidermal masses of cells which show atypical features. A few horn pearls with central laminated keratin are present. There is marked inflammatory reaction in the dermis between the masses of tumour cells.

A system of grading of squamous cell carcinoma called **Broders' grading** has been proposed that depends upon the percentage of anaplastic cells present in a tumour (page 209). Accordingly, following 4 grades are recognised:

Grade I : Less than 25% anaplastic cells

Grade II : 25-50% anaplastic cells

Grade III : 50-75% anaplastic cells

Grade IV : More than 75% anaplastic cells.

However, it is important to take into account other factors for grading the tumour such as: the degree of atypicality of the tumour cells, presence or absence of keratinisation and the depth of penetration of the lesion. Therefore, based on combination of these factors, it is customary with pathologists to label squamous cell carcinomas with descriptive terms such as: well-differentiated, moderately-differentiated, undifferentiated, keratinising, non-keratinising, spindle cell type etc.

2. BASAL CELL CARCINOMA (RODENT ULCER). Typically, the basal cell carcinoma is a locally invasive, slow-growing tumour of middle-aged that rarely metastasises. It occurs exclusively on hairy skin, the most common location (90%) being the face, usually above a line from the lobe of the ear to the corner of the mouth (Fig. 24.9). Basal cell carcinoma is seen more frequently in white-skinned people and in those who have prolonged exposure to strong sunlight like in those living in Australia and New Zealand (page 225).

PATHOLOGIC CHANGES. ***Macroscopically,*** the most common pattern is a nodulo-ulcerative basal cell carcinoma in which a slow-growing small nodule undergoes central ulceration with pearly, rolled margins. The tumour enlarges in size by burrowing and by destroying the tissues locally like a rodent and hence the name 'rodent ulcer' (Fig. 24.9,A). However, less frequently non-ulcerated nodular pattern, pigmented basal cell carcinoma and fibrosing variants are also encountered.

Histologically, the most characteristic feature is the proliferation of basaloid cells (resembling basal layer of epidermis). A variety of patterns of these cells may be seen: solid masses, masses of pigmented cells, strands and nests of tumour cells in morphea pattern, keratotic masses, cystic change with sebaceous differentiation, and adenoid pattern with apocrine or eccrine differentiation. The most common pattern is *solid basal cell carcinoma* in which the dermis contains irregular masses of basaloid cells having characteristic peripheral palisaded appearance of the nuclei (Fig. 24.9,B) (COLOUR PLATE XII: CL 45). A superficial multicentric variant composed of multiple foci of tumour cells present in the dermis, especially in the trunk, has also been described.

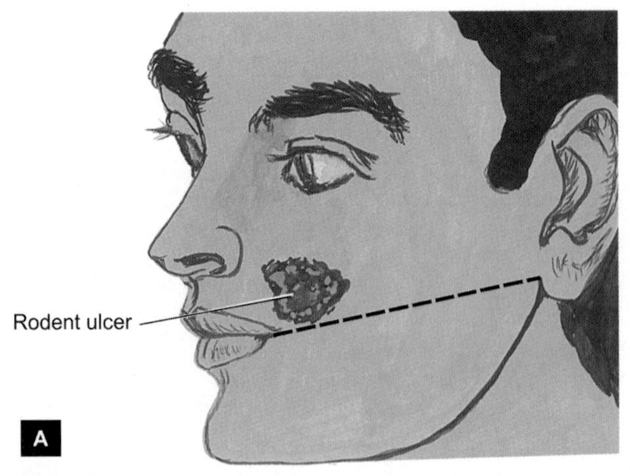

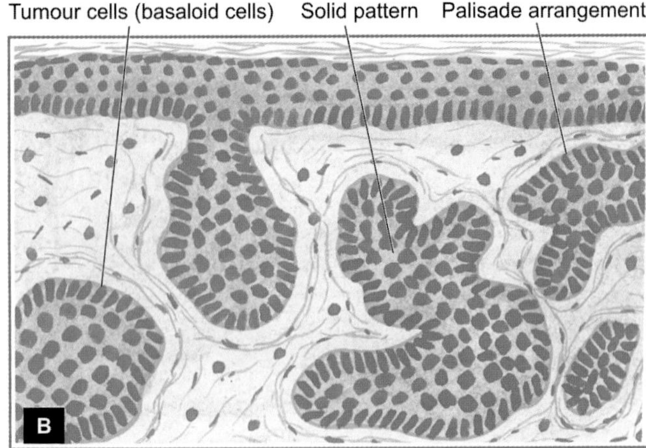

FIGURE 24.9

A, Common location and macroscopic appearance of basal cell carcinoma (rodent ulcer). B, Solid basal cell carcinoma. The dermis is invaded by irregular masses of basaloid cells with characteristic peripheral palisaded appearance.

3. METATYPICAL CARCINOMA (BASOSQUAMOUS CELL CARCINOMA). Metatypical or basosquamous cell carcinoma is the term used for a tumour in which the cell type and arrangement of cells cause difficulty in deciding between basal cell carcinoma and squamous cell carcinoma. The tumour masses are composed of malignant squamous cells with horn pearls and the outer row of dark-staining basal cells. These tumours have a high malignant potential and may occasionally metastasise.

II. ADNEXAL (APPENDAGEAL) TUMOURS

Tumours arising from epidermal adnexa or appendages can differentiate towards hair follicles, sebaceous glands and sweat glands (apocrine and eccrine glands). Most of the adnexal tumours are benign but a few malignant variants also exist.

A. Tumours of Hair Follicle

These are uncommon benign tumours. Two important examples are trichoepithelioma and pilomatricoma.

1. TRICHOEPITHELIOMA (BROOKE'S TUMOUR). This tumour may occur as a solitary lesion or as multiple inherited lesions, predominantly on the face, scalp and neck.

Histologically, the tumour is often circumscribed. The most characteristic histologic feature is the presence of multiple horn cysts having keratinised centre and surrounded by basophilic cells resembling basal cells. These horn cysts simulate abortive pilar structures which are interconnected by epithelial tracts.

2. PILOMATRICOMA (CALCIFYING EPITHELIOMA OF MALHERBE). Pilomatricoma usually occurs as a solitary lesion, more often on the face and upper extremities. It may be seen at any age. The lesions vary in size from 0.5-5 cm and appear as well-demarcated dark red nodules.

Histologically, the circumscribed tumour is located in deeper dermis and subcutis. The masses of tumour cells embedded in cellular stroma characteristically consist of 2 types of cells: the *peripheral basophilic cells* resembling hair matrix cells, and the *inner shadow cells* having central unstained shadow in place of the lost nucleus. Areas of calcification are present within lobules of shadow cells in three-fourth of the tumours.

B. Tumours of Sebaceous Glands

Tumours originating from sebaceous glands are commonly benign (e.g. naevus sebaceus and sebaceous adenoma) but sebaceous carcinoma may occasionally occur.

1. NAEVUS SEBACEUS. Naevus sebaceus of Jadassohn occurs mainly on the scalp or face as a solitary lesion that may be present at birth. Initially, the lesion appears as a hairless plaque, but later it becomes verrucous and nodular.

Histologically, naevus sebaceus is characterised by hyperplasia of immature sebaceous glands and pilar structures. The overlying epidermis shows papillary acanthosis.

2. SEBACEOUS ADENOMA. Sebaceous adenoma occurs in middle-aged persons, most commonly on the face.

Histologically, it is sharply demarcated from the surrounding tissue. The tumour is composed of irregular lobules of incompletely differentiated sebaceous glands.

3. SEBACEOUS CARCINOMA. Sebaceous carcinoma is a rare tumour that may occur anywhere in the body except the palms and soles. Variants of sebaceous carcinoma are carcinoma of the Meibomian glands of the eyelids and carcinoma of the ceruminous glands in the external meatus.

Histologically, the tumour is composed of variable-sized lobules of poorly-differentiated cells containing some sebaceous cells. The tumour cells show marked cytologic atypia such as pleomorphism and hyperchromasia.

C. Tumours of Sweat Glands

A large number of lesions develop from sweat gland structures, either from apocrine or eccrine glands. These are more commonly benign but sweat gland carcinoma may also occur.

1. ECCRINE TUMOURS. Depending upon the portion of eccrine sweat gland from which the tumour takes origin, the eccrine tumours are of 3 types:
i) arising from intraepidermal portion of the duct e.g. eccrine poroma;
ii) arising from intradermal portion of the duct e.g. hidradenoma; and
iii) arising from secretory coils e.g. eccrine spiradenoma.

■ **Eccrine poroma.** This tumour arises from intraepidermal portion of the sweat gland duct. The tumour is found more commonly on the sole and hands.

Histologically, it consists of tumour cells arising from the lower portion of the epidermis and extending downward into dermis as broad anastomosing bands. The tumour cells are, however, different from squamous cells. They are smaller in size, cuboidal in shape and have deeply basophilic nucleus.

■ **Eccrine hidradenoma.** Hidradenoma originates from the intradermal portion of the eccrine sweat duct. The tumour may occur anywhere in the body.

Histologically, hidradenoma consists of solid masses and cords of tumour cells which may have an occasional duct-like structure containing mucin. The tumour cells are round to polygonal and may have clear or eosinophilic cytoplasm.

■ **Eccrine spiradenoma.** This is found as a solitary, painful, circumscribed nodule in the dermis.

Histologically, the tumour consists of lobules which are surrounded by a thin capsule. The tumour lobules contain 2 types of epithelial cells like in the secretory coils of the eccrine sweat gland. Peripheral cells are small with dark nuclei, while the centre of lobules contains large cells with pale nuclei. An occasional area may show glandular structures.

2. APOCRINE TUMOURS. Apocrine sweat glands may give rise to tumours; the two common examples being papillary hidradenoma and cylindroma.

■ **Papillary hidradenoma.** Papillary hidradenoma or hidradenoma papilliferrum is usually located as a small lesion commonly in women in the skin of the anogenital area.

Histologically, it is a circumscribed tumour in the dermis under a normal epidermis. Papillary hidradenoma represents an adenoma with apocrine differentiation and containing papillary, tubular and cystic structures. The tumour cells lining these structures resemble apocrine epithelium with features of decapitation secretions.

■ **Cylindroma.** Also called as 'turban tumour' due to its common location on the scalp, cylindroma may occur as both solitary and multiple lesions.

Histologically, the tumour is composed of irregular islands of tumour cells creating a pattern resembling jigsaw puzzle. The islands are surrounded by a hyaline sheath. The tumour cells comprising the islands consist of 2 types of epithelial cells: *peripheral small cells* with dark nuclei, and *inner large cells* with light staining nuclei. Some of the islands may contain tubular lumina containing amorphous material.

3. SWEAT GLAND CARCINOMA. Rarely, the eccrine and apocrine gland tumours described above may turn malignant. All these carcinomas are adenocarcinomas and must be distinguished from metastatic adenocarcinoma in the skin.

III. MELANOCYTIC TUMOURS

Melanocytic tumours may arise from one of the three cell types: naevus cells, epidermal melanocytes and dermal melanocytes.

- Benign tumours originating from *naevus cells* are called naevocellular naevi.
- The examples of benign tumours *arising from epidermal melanocytes* are lentigo, freckles, pigmentation associated with Albright's syndrome and *cafe-au-lait* spots of neurofibromatosis (page 919).
- Benign tumours *derived from dermal melanocytes* are Mongolian spots, naevi of Ota and of Ito and the blue naevus.
- *Malignant melanoma* is the malignant counterpart of melanocytic tumours.

The important examples amongst these are described below.

1. NAEVOCELLULAR NAEVI. Pigmented naevi or moles are extremely common lesions on the skin of most individuals. They are often flat or slightly elevated lesions; rarely they may be papillomatous or pedunculated. Most naevi appear in adolescence and in early adulthood due to hormonal influence but rarely may be present at birth. They are mostly tan to brown and less than 1 cm in size.

Histologically, irrespective of the histologic types, all naevocellular naevi are composed of 'naevus cells' which are actually identical to melanocytes but differ from melanocytes in being arranged in clusters or nests. Naevus cells are cuboidal or oval in shape with homogeneous cytoplasm and contain large round or oval nucleus. Melanin pigment is abundant in the naevus cells present in the lower epidermis and upper dermis, but the cells in the mid-dermis and lower dermis hardly contain any melanin (COLOUR PLATE X: CL 39).

The important *histological variants* of naevi are as under:

i) Lentigo is the replacement of the basal layer of the epidermis by melanocytes (Fig. 24.10,B).

ii) Junctional naevus is the one in which the naevus cells lie at the epidermal-dermal junction. The naevus cells form well-circumscribed nests.

iii) Compound naevus is the commonest type of pigmented naevus. These lesions, in addition to the junctional activity as in junctional naevi, show nests of naevus cells in the dermis to a variable depth (Fig. 24.10,A)

iv) Intradermal naevus shows slight or no junctional activity. The lesion is mainly located in the upper dermis as nests and cords of naevus cells. Multinucleate naevus cells are common.

v) Spindle cell (epithelioid) naevus or juvenile melanoma is a compound naevus with junctional activity.

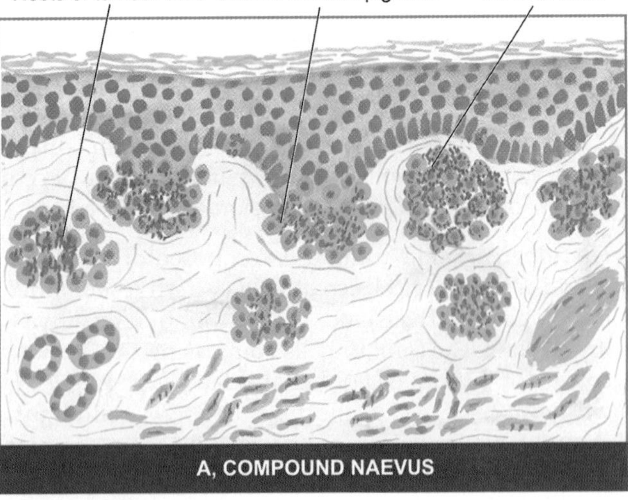

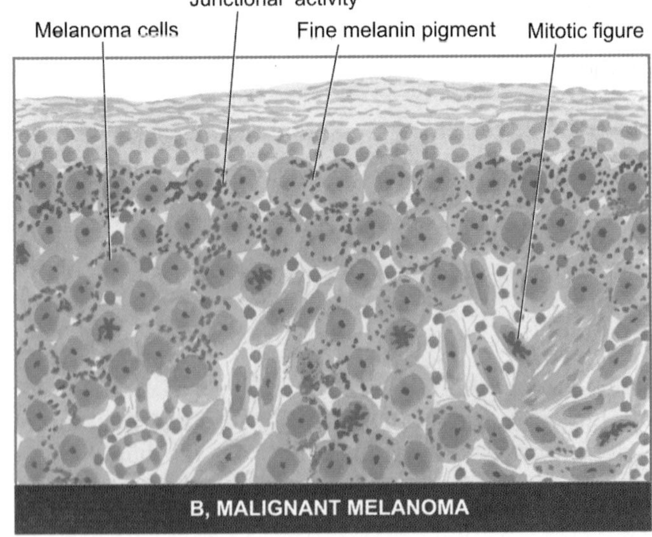

FIGURE 24.10

A, Compound naevus showing nests of naevus cells which are typically uniform and present in dermis as well as epidermis. Melanin pigment in naevus cells is coarse and irregular. B, Malignant melanoma shows junctional activity at the dermal-epidermal junction. Tumour cells resembling epithelioid cells with pleomorphic nuclei and prominent nucleoli are seen as solid masses in the dermis. Many of the tumour cells contain fine granular melanin pigment.

The naevus cells are, however, elongated and epithelioid in appearance which may or may not contain melanin. Juvenile melanoma is important since it is frequently confused with malignant melanoma histologically.

vi) Blue naevus is characterised by dendritic spindle naevus cells rather than the usual rounded or cuboidal naevus cells. These cells are often quite rich in melanin pigment.

vii) Dysplastic naevi are certain atypical naevi which have increased risk of progression to malignant melanoma. These lesions are larger than the usual acquired naevi, are often multiple, and appear as flat macules to slightly elevated plaques with irregular borders and variable pigmentation. Many of the cases are familial and inheritable.

Histologically, dysplastic naevi have melanocytic proliferation at the epidermo-dermal junction with some cytologic atypia.

2. MALIGNANT MELANOMA. Malignant melanoma or melanocarcinoma arising from melanocytes is one of the most rapidly spreading malignant tumour of the skin that can occur at all ages but is rare before puberty. The tumour spreads locally as well as to distant sites by lymphatics and by blood. The etiology is unknown but there is role of excessive exposure of white skin to sunlight e.g. higher incidence in New Zealand and Australia where sun exposure in high. Besides the skin, melanomas may occur at various other sites such as oral and anogenital mucosa, oesophagus, conjunctiva, orbit (page 522) and leptomeninges. The common sites on the skin are the trunk *(in men),* legs *(in women)*; other locations are face, soles, palms and nail-beds.

Some high risk factors associated with increased incidence of malignant melanoma are:
i) persistent change in appearance of a mole;
ii) presence of pre-existing naevus (especially dysplastic naevus),
iii) family history of melanoma in a patient of atypical mole;
iii) higher age of the patient; and
iv) more than 50 moles 2 mm or more in diameter.

Molecular studies in familial and hereditary cases have revealed germline mutation in *CDKN2A* gene which encodes for cyclin-dependent kinase inhibitor, mutational loss of *PTEN* gene and mutation in several other tumour suppressor genes but not *TP53*.

Clinically, melanoma often appears as a flat or slightly elevated naevus which has variegated pigmentation, irregular borders and, of late, has undergone secondary changes of ulceration, bleeding and increase in size. Many of the malignant melanomas, however, arise *de novo* rather than from a pre-existing naevus. Malignant melanoma can be differentiated from benign pigmented lesions by subtle features which dermatologists term as ABCD of melanoma; these are summed up in Table 24.3.

Depending upon the clinical course and prognosis, cutaneous malignant melanomas are of the following 4 types:

i) Lentigo maligna melanoma. This often develops from a pre-existing lentigo (a flat naevus characterised by replacement of basal layer of epidermis by naevus cells). It is essentially a malignant melanoma *in situ.* It is slow-growing and has good prognosis.

ii) Superficial spreading melanoma. This is a slightly elevated lesion with variegated colour and ulcerated

TABLE 24.3: Distinguishing Features of Benign Mole and Malignant Melanoma.

FEATURE	BENIGN MOLE	MALIGNANT MELANOMA
1. *Clinical features*		
i) Symmetry	Symmetrical	A = Asymmetry
ii) Border	well-demarcated	B = Border irregularity
iii) Colour	Uniformly pigmented	C = Colour change
iv) Diameter	Small, less than 6 mm	D = Diameter more than 6 mm
2. *Common locations*	Skin of face, mucosa	Skin; mucosa of nose, bowel, anal region
3. *Histopathology*		
i) Architecture	Nests of cells	Various patterns: solid sheets, alveoli, nests, islands
ii) Cell morphology	Uniform looking naevus cells	Malignant cells, atypia, mitoses, nucleoli
iii) Melanin pigment	Irregular, coarse clumps	Fine granules, uniformly distributed
iv) Inflammation	May or may not be present	Often present
4. *Spread*	Remains confined, poses cosmetic problem only	Haematogenous and/or lymphatic spread early

surface. It often develops from a superficial spreading melanoma *in situ* (pagetoid melanoma) in 5 to 7 years. The prognosis is worse than for lentigo maligna melanoma.

iii) Acral lentigenous melanoma. This occurs more commonly on the soles, palms and mucosal surfaces. The tumour often undergoes ulceration and early metastases. The prognosis is worse than that of superficial spreading melanoma.

iv) Nodular melanoma. This often appears as an elevated and deeply pigmented nodule that grows rapidly and undergoes ulceration. This variant carries the worst prognosis.

Histologically, irrespective of the type of malignant melanoma, the following characteristics are observed (Fig. 24.10,B) (COLOUR PLATE X: CL 40):

i) Origin. The malignant melanoma, whether arising from a pre-existing naevus or starting *de novo,* has marked junctional activity at the epidermo-dermal junction and grows downward into the dermis.

ii) Tumour cells. The malignant melanoma cells are usually larger than the naevus cells. They may be epithelioid or spindle-shaped, the former being more common. The tumour cells have amphophilic cytoplasm and large, pleomorphic nuclei with conspicuous nucleoli. Mitotic figures are often present and multinucleate giant cells may occur. These tumour cells may be arranged in various patterns such as solid masses, sheets, island, alveoli etc.

iii) Melanin. Melanin pigment may be present (melanotic) or absent (amelanotic melanoma) without any prognostic influence. The pigment, if present, tends to be in the form of uniform fine granules (unlike the benign naevi in which coarse irregular clumps of melanin are present). At times, there may be no evidence of melanin in H&E stained sections but the Fontana-Masson stain or *dopa reaction* reveals melanin granules in the cytoplasm of tumour cells.

iv) Inflammatory infiltrate. Some amount of inflammatory infiltrate is present in the invasive melanomas. Infrequently, partial spontaneous regression of the tumour occurs due to destructive effect of dense inflammatory infiltrate.

The prognosis for patients with malignant melanoma is related to the depth of invasion of the tumour in the dermis. Depending upon the depth of invasion below the granular cell layer in millimeters, *Clark* has described 5 levels:

Level I: Malignant melanoma cells confined to the epidermis and its appendages.

Level II: Extension into the papillary dermis.

Level III: Extension of tumour cells upto the interface between papillary and reticular dermis.

Level IV: Invasion of reticular dermis.

Level V: Invasion of the subcutaneous fat.

Metastatic spread of malignant melanoma is very common and takes place via lymphatics to the regional lymph nodes and through blood to distant sites like lungs, liver, brain, spinal cord, and adrenals. Rarely, the primary lesion regresses spontaneously but metastases are present widely distributed.

IV. TUMOURS OF THE DERMIS

All the tissue elements of the dermis such as fibrous tissue, adipose tissue, neural tissue, endothelium and smooth muscle are capable of transforming into benign and malignant tumours. Many of the examples of these tumours are discussed in Chapter 27 but a few representative dermal neoplasms are described below.

1. DERMATOFIBROMA AND MALIGNANT FIBROUS HISTIOCYTOMA. These soft tissue tumours are composed of cells having mixed features of fibroblasts, myofibroblasts, histiocytes and primitive mesenchymal cells. The histogenesis of these tumours is not quite clear but probably they arise from multidirectional differentiation of the primitive mesenchymal cells. The tumours appear at any age but are more common in advanced age. The commonest sites are the lower and upper extremities, followed in decreasing frequency, by abdominal cavity and retroperitoneum. The benign variant is also known by various synonyms like dermatofibroma, histiocytoma, sclerosing haemangioma, fibroxanthoma and xanthogranuloma. Benign histiocytomas are often small but malignant fibrous histiocytomas may be of enormous size. They are circumscribed but unencapsulated.

Histologically, the tumours are composed of spindle-shaped fibrohistiocytoid cells which are characteristically arranged in cartwheel or storiform pattern. The benign variety contains uniform spindle-shaped cells with admixture of numerous foamy histiocytes. The malignant fibrous histiocytoma shows pleomorphic tumour cells and some multinucleate giant cells in a stroma that may show myxoid change and inflammatory infiltrate.

2. DERMATOFIBROSARCOMA PROTUBERANS. This is a low grade fibrosarcoma that rarely metastasises but is locally recurrent. The tumour usually forms a solid nodule, within the dermis and subcutaneous fat, protruding the epidermis outwards. Sometimes multiple nodules may form.

Histologically, the tumour is very cellular and is composed of uniform fibroblasts arranged in a cartwheel or storiform pattern. A few mitoses are often present. The overlying epidermis is generally thinned and may be ulcerated. The subcutaneous fat is frequently invaded by the tumour cells.

3. XANTHOMAS. These are solitary or multiple tumour-like lesions, often associated with high levels of serum cholesterol and phospholipids. Many of the cases result from familial hyperlipidaemia. They may occur at different sites such as buttocks, knees, elbows, tendo-achilles, palmar creases and on the eyelids (referred to as xanthelasma).

Histologically, xanthomas are composed of dermal collections of benign-appearing foamy histiocytes. Multinucleate tumour giant cells surrounded by lipid-laden cytoplasm are often present.

V. CELLULAR MIGRANT TUMOURS

All the tumours described above arise from progenitor cells in the skin only. However, there are some tumours which have their precursor cells elsewhere in the body, but are cellular immigrants to the skin. The examples are Langerhans' cell histiocytosis (page 463), mycosis fungoides, mastocytosis, lymphomas and leukaemias (Chapter 14). Mycosis fungoides is considered here.

MYCOSIS FUNGOIDES (CUTANEOUS T-CELL LYMPHOMA). Mycosis fungoides or cutaneous T-cell lymphoma (CTCL) is the commonest form of lymphoma in the skin but in advanced stage, mycosis fungoides may disseminate to the lymph nodes and other organs. Clinically, mycosis fungoides may manifest in 3 stages:

i) Premycotic stage in which the lesions are erythematous, red-brown, scaly and pruritic, resembling eczema or psoriasis.

ii) Infiltrative stage has slightly elevated, bluish-red, firm plaques.

iii) Fungoid (Tumour) stage is characterised by red-brown nodules of tumour which often undergo ulceration.

The condition is found more frequently beyond 4th decade of life. Lesions may affect different body surfaces but more often involve the trunk, extremities, face and scalp.

Histologically, the condition has the following characteristics:

i) Initially, lower portion of the epidermis contains hyperchromatic enlarged lymphocytes. In about half the cases, there is formation of intraepidermal clusters of atypical lymphoid cells forming *Darier-Pautrier's microabscesses* which is a misnomer as it does not contain pus cells.

ii) Later, there are band-like sharply demarcated aggregates of polymorphous cellular infiltrate in the dermis including atypical lymphoid cells (Sézary-Lutzner cells) and multinucleated cells.

iii) The individual mycosis cells are malignant T lymphocytes which have hyperchromatic and cerebriform nuclei and express CD4 and HLA-DR antigen.

The etiology of mycosis fungoides or cutaneous T cell-lymphoma has been found to be the same as for adult T cell lymphoma-leukaemia syndrome which is human T cell-leukaemia virus-I (HTLV-I) as discussed on page 229.

Sézary syndrome is a variant of CTCL, often due to dissemination of underlying CTCL to the blood and infiltration into the skin causing generalised erythroderma, lymphadenopathy and hepatosplenomegaly.

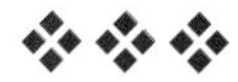

The Endocrine System

25

GENERAL PRINCIPLES

The development, structure and functions of human body are governed and maintained by 2 mutually interlinked systems—*the endocrine system* and *the nervous system* (Chapter 28); a third system combining features of both these systems is appropriately called *neuroendocrine system*.

NEUROENDOCRINE SYSTEM

This system forms a link between the endocrine and nervous systems. The cells of this system elaborates polypeptide hormones; owing to these biochemical properties, it has also been called as *APUD cell system* (for Amine Precursor Uptake and Decarboxylation properties). However, though having common biochemical properties, the cells of this system are widely distributed in the body in different anatomic areas and hence is currently called *dispersed neuroendocrine system*. Cells comprising this system are as under:

1. *Neuroendocrine cells* are present in the gastric and intestinal mucosa and elaborate peptide hormones.
2. *Neuroganglia cells* lie in the ganglia cells in the sympathetic chain and elaborate amines.
3. *Adrenal medulla* elaborates epinephrine and norepinephrine.
4. *Parafollicular C cells* of the thyroid secrete calcitonin.
5. *Islets of Langerhans* in the pancreas (included in both endocrine and neuroendocrine systems) secrete insulin.
6. *Isolated cells in the left atrium* of the heart secrete atrial natriuretic (salt-losing) peptide hormone.

In addition to above, other non-endocrine secretions include neurotransmitter substances such as *acetylcholine* and *dopamine* released from neural synapses, and *erythropoietin* and *vitamin D3* elaborated from the kidney.

THE ENDOCRINE SYSTEM

Anatomically, the endocrine system consists of 6 distinct organs: pituitary, adrenals, thyroid, parathyroids, gonads, and pancreatic islets (also included in neuroendocrine system). Understanding the patholgy of these endocrine organs requires the knowledge of overall framework of hormone secretions, their actions and broad principles of feedback mechanisms.

Broadly speaking, human hormones are divided into 5 major classes which are further grouped under two headings depending upon their site of interactions on the target cell receptors (whether cell membrane or nuclear):

Group I: Those interacting with cell-surface membrane receptors:

1. *Amino acid derivatives:* thyroid hormone, catecholamines.
2. *Small neuropeptides:* gonadotropin-releasing hormone (GnRH), thyrotropin-releasing hormone (TRH), somatostatin, vasopressin.

Group II: Those interacting with intracellular nuclear receptors:

3. *Large proteins:* insulin, luteinising hormone (LH), parathormone hormone.
4. *Steroid hormones:* cortisol, estrogen.
5. *Vitamin derivatives:* retinol (vitamin A) and vitamin D.

The *synthesis* of these hormones and their precursors takes place through a prescribed genetic pathway that involves: transcription → mRNA → protein synthesis → post-translational protein processing → intracellular sorting/membrane integration → secretion.

Major functions of hormones are as under:

i) *Growth and differentiation of cells:* by pituitary hormones, thyroid, parathyroid, steroid hormones.
ii) *Maintenance of homeostasis:* thyroid (by regulating BMR), parathormone, mineralocorticoids, vasopressin, insulin.
iii) *Reproduction:* sexual development and activity, pregnancy, foetal development, menopause etc.

A basic feature of all endocrine glands is the existence of both negative and positive **feedback control system** that stimulates or regulates hormone production in a way that levels remain within the normal range (abbreviated as S or R respectively with the corresponding hormone e.g. TSH-TRH pathway, GnRH-LH/FSH pathway etc). This system is commonly termed *hypothalamic-pituitary hormone axis* for different hormones (Fig. 25.1). The stimulatory or regulatory action by endocrine hormonal secretions may follow paracrine or autocrine pathways. *Paracrine regulation* means that the

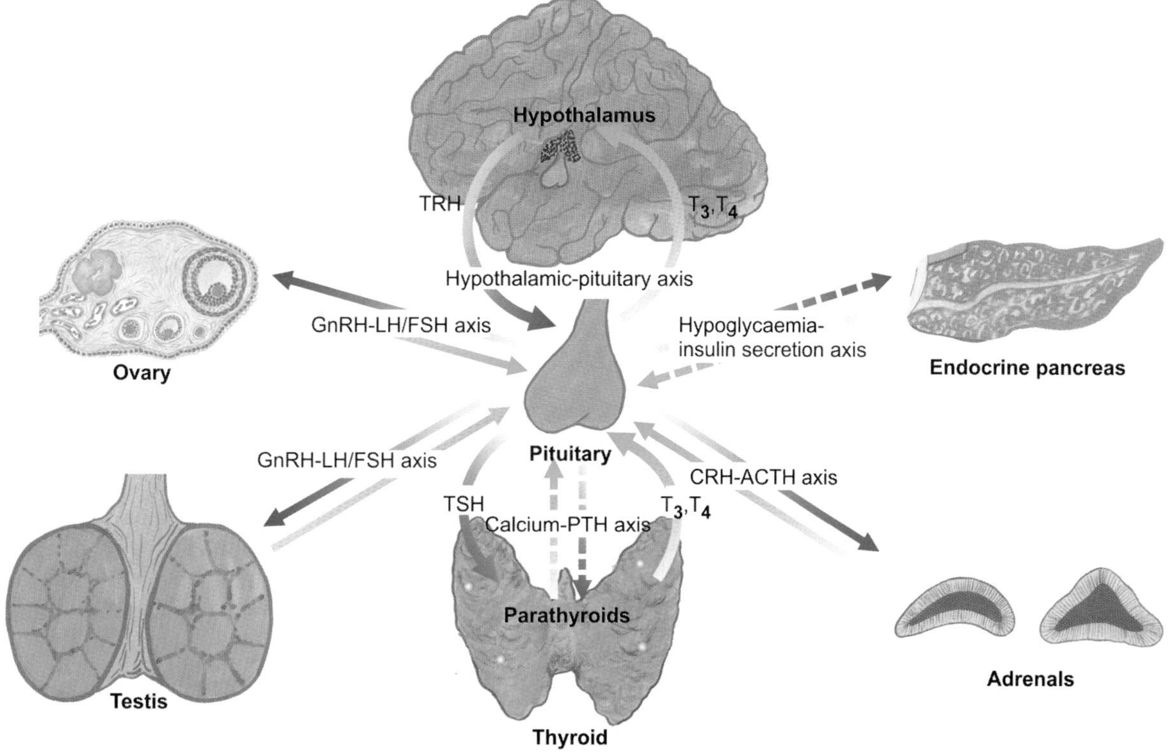

FIGURE 25.1

Endocrine organs and the existence of feedback controls. Both positive and negative feedback controls exist for each endocrine gland having a regulating (R) and stimulating (S) hormone. Those acting through hypothalamic-pituitary axis include: thyroid hormones on TRH-TSH axis, cortisol on CRH-ACTH axis, gonadal steroids on GnRH-LH/FSH axis and insulin-like GH on GHRH-GH axis. Those independent of pituitary control (shown by dotted arrows) have also feedback controls by: calcium on PTH, and hypoglycaemia on insulin release by pancreatic islets.

stimulatory/regulatory factors are released by one type of cells but act on another adjacent cell of the system, while *autocrine regulation* refers to action of the factor on the same cell that produced it.

With this brief overview of principles of physiology of hormones, we now turn to the study of diseases of the endocrine organs. In general, pathologic processes affecting endocrine glands with resultant hormonal abnormalities may occur from following processes:

- **Hyperfunction:** This results from excess of hormone secreting tissues e.g. hyperplasia, tumours (adenoma, carcinoma), ectopic hormone production, excessive stimulation from inflammation (often autoimmune), infections, iatrogenic (drugs-induced, hormonal administration).
- **Hypofunction:** Deficiency of hormones occurs from destruction of hormone-forming tissues from inflammations (often autoimmune), infections, iatrogenic (e.g. surgical removal, radiation damage), developmental defects (e.g. Turner's syndrome, hypoplasia), enzyme deficiency, haemorrhage and infarction (e.g. Sheehan's syndrome), nutritional deficiency (e.g. iodine deficiency).
- **Hormone resistance:** There may be adequate or excessive production of a hormone but there is peripheral resistance, often from inherited mutations in receptors (e.g. defect in membrane receptors, nuclear receptors or receptor for signal transduction).

PITUITARY GLAND

NORMAL STRUCTURE

ANATOMY. The pituitary gland or hypophysis in an adult weighs about 500 mg and is slightly heavier in females. It is situated at the base of the brain in a hollow called *sella turcica* formed out of the sphenoid bone. The gland is composed of 2 major anatomic divisions: anterior lobe (adenohypophysis) and posterior lobe (neurohypophysis).

1. The **anterior lobe or adenohypophysis** is an ectodermal derivative formed from Rathke's pouch which is an upward diverticulum from the primitive buccal cavity. The adenohypophysis has no direct neural connection but has indirect connection through capillary portal circulation by which the anterior pituitary receives the blood which has already passed through the hypothalamus.

2. The **posterior lobe or neurohypophysis** is a downgrowth from the primitive neural tissue. The neurohypophysis, therefore, has direct neural connection superiorly with the hypothalamus.

HISTOLOGY AND FUNCTIONS. The histology and functions of the anterior and posterior lobes of the pituitary gland are quite distinct.

A. ANTERIOR LOBE (ADENOHYPOPHYSIS). It is composed of round to polygonal epithelial cells arranged in cords and islands having fibrovascular stroma. These epithelial cells, depending upon their staining characteristics and functions, are divided into 3 types, each of which performs separate functions:

1. Chromophil cells with acidophilic granules: These cells comprise about 40% of the anterior lobe and are chiefly located in the lateral wings. The acidophils are further of 2 types:

i) *Somatotrophs (GH cells)* which produce growth hormone (GH); and

ii) *Lactotrophs (PRL cells)* which produce prolactin (PRL).

Cells containing both GH and PRL called *mammosomatotrophs* are also present.

2. Chromophil cells with basophilic granules: These cells constitute about 10% of the anterior lobe and are mainly found in the region of median wedge. The basophils include 3 types of cells:

i) *Gonadotrophs (FSH-LH cells)* which are the source of the FSH and LH or interstitial cell stimulating hormone (ICSH).

ii) *Thyrotrophs (TSH cells)* are the cells producing TSH.

iii) *Corticotrophs (ACTH-MSH cells)* produce ACTH, melanocyte stimulating hormone (MSH), β-lipoprotein and β-endorphin.

3. Chromophobe cells without visible granules: These cells comprise the remainder 50% of the adenohypophysis. These cells by light microscopy contain no visible granules, but on electron microscopy reveal sparsely granulated corticotrophs, thyrotrophs and gonadotrophs.

All these functions of the adenohypophysis are under the indirect *control* of the hypothalamus through stimulatory and inhibitory factors synthesised by the hypothalamus which reach the anterior lobe through capillary portal blood.

B. POSTERIOR LOBE (NEUROHYPOPHYSIS). The neurohypophysis is composed mainly of interlacing nerve fibres in which are scattered specialised glial cells called *pituicytes*. These nerve fibres on electron microscopy contain granules of neurosecretory material made up of 2 octapeptides—*vasopressin or antidiuretic hormone* (ADH), and *oxytocin*, both of which are produced by neurosecretory cells of the hypothalamus but are stored in the cells of posterior pituitary.

1. ADH causes reabsorption of water from the renal tubules and is essential for maintenance of osmolality of the plasma. Its deficiency results in diabetes insipidus characterised by uncontrolled diuresis and polydipsia.

2. Oxytocin causes contraction of mammary myoepithelial cells resulting in ejection of milk from the lactating breast and causes contraction of myometrium of the uterus at term.

It is obvious from the description above that pituitary, though a tiny organ, is concerned with a variety of diverse functions in the body. The pituitary gland and hypothalamus are so closely interlinked that diseases of the pituitary gland involve the hypothalamus, and dysfunctions of the hypothalamus cause secondary changes in the pituitary. The pituitary gland is involved in several diseases which include: *non-neoplastic* such as inflammations, haemorrhage, trauma, infarction and many other endocrine diseases; and *neoplastic* diseases. However, functionally and morphologically diseases of the pituitary can be classified as below, each of which includes diseases of anterior and posterior pituitary and hypothalamus, separately:

i) Hyperpituitarism
ii) Hypopituitarism
iii) Pituitary tumours

HYPERPITUITARISM

Hyperpituitarism is characterised by oversecretion of one or more of the pituitary hormones. Such hypersecretion may be due to diseases of the anterior pituitary, posterior pituitary or hypothalamus. For all practical purposes, however, hyperfunction of the anterior pituitary is due to the development of a hormone-secreting pituitary adenoma (discussed later), and rarely, a carcinoma. For each of the hormonal hyperfunction of the anterior pituitary, posterior pituitary and hypothalamus, a clinical syndrome is described. A few important syndromes are as follows:

A. Hyperfunction of Anterior Pituitary

Three common syndromes of adenohypophyseal hyperfunction are: gigantism and acromegaly, hyperprolactinaemia and Cushing's syndrome.

1. GIGANTISM AND ACROMEGALY. Both these clinical syndromes result from sustained excess of growth hormone (GH), most commonly by somatotroph (GH-secreting) adenoma.

Gigantism. When GH excess occurs prior to epiphyseal closure, gigantism is produced. Gigantism, therefore, occurs in prepubertal boys and girls and is much less frequent than acromegaly. The main clinical feature in gigantism is the excessive and proportionate growth of the child. There is enlargement as well as thickening of the bones resulting in considerable increase in height and enlarged thoracic cage.

Acromegaly. Acromegaly results when there is overproduction of GH in adults following cessation of bone growth and is more common than gigantism. The term 'acromegaly' means increased growth of extremities. There is enlargement of hands and feet, coarseness of facial features with increase in soft tissues, prominent supraorbital ridges and a more prominent lower jaw which when clenched results in protrusion of the lower teeth in front of upper teeth *(prognathism)*. Other features include enlargement of the tongue and lips, thickening of the skin and kyphosis. Sometimes, a few associated features such as TSH excess resulting in thyrotoxicosis, and gonadotropin insufficiency causing amenorrhoea in the females and impotence in the male, are found.

2. HYPERPROLACTINAEMIA. Hyperprolactinaemia is the excessive production of prolactin (PRL), most commonly by lactotroph (PRL-secreting) adenoma, also called prolactinoma. Occasionally, hyperprolactinaemia results from hypothalamic inhibition of PRL secretion by certain drugs (e.g. chlorpromazine, reserpine and methyl-dopa). In the female, hyperprolactinaemia causes *amenorrhoea-galactorrhoea syndrome* characterised clinically by infertility and expression of a drop or two of milk from breast, not related to pregnancy or puerperium. In the male, it may cause *impotence* or *reduced libido.* These features result either from associated inhibition of gonadotropin secretion or interference in gonadotropin effects.

3. CUSHING'S SYNDROME. Pituitary-dependent Cushing's syndrome results from ACTH excess. Most frequently, it is caused by corticotroph (ACTH-secreting) adenoma. Cushing's syndrome is discussed under diseases of the adrenal gland on page 821.

B. Hyperfunction of Posterior Pituitary and Hypothalamus

Lesions of posterior pituitary and hypothalamus are uncommon. Two of the syndromes associated with hyperfunction of the posterior pituitary and hypothalamus are: inappropriate release of ADH and preco–cious puberty.

1. INAPPROPRIATE RELEASE OF ADH. Inappropriate release of ADH results in its excessive secretion which manifests clinically by passage of concentrated urine due to increased reabsorption of water and loss of sodium in the urine, consequent hyponatraemia, haemodilution and expansion of intra- and extracellular fluid volume. Inappropriate release of ADH occurs most often in paraneoplastic syndrome e.g. in oat cell carcinoma of the lung, carcinoma of the pancreas, lymphoma and thymoma. Infrequently, lesions of the hypothalamus such as trauma, haemorrhage and meningitis may produce ADH hypersecretion. Rarely, pulmonary diseases such as tuberculosis, lung abscess, pneumoconiosis, empyema and pneumonia may cause overproduction of ADH.

2. PRECOCIOUS PUBERTY. A tumour in the region of hypothalamus or the pineal gland may result in premature release of gonadotropins causing the onset of pubertal changes prior to the age of 9 years. The features include premature development of genitalia both in the male and in the female, growth of pubic hair and axillary hair. In the female, there is breast growth and onset of menstruation.

HYPOPITUITARISM

In hypopituitarism, there is usually deficiency of one or more of the pituitary hormones affecting either anterior pituitary, or posterior pituitary and hypothalamus.

A. Hypofunction of Anterior Pituitary

Adenohypophyseal hypofunction is invariably due to destruction of the anterior lobe of more than 75% because the anterior pituitary possesses a large functional reserve. This may result from anterior pituitary lesions or pressure and destruction from adjacent lesions. Lesions of the anterior pituitary include nonsecretory (chromophobe) adenoma, metastatic carcinoma, craniopharyngioma, trauma, postpartum ischaemic necrosis (Sheehan's syndrome), empty-sella syndrome, and rarely, tuberculosis. Though a number of syndromes associated with deficiency of anterior pituitary hormones have been described, two important syndromes are: panhypopituitarism and dwarfism.

1. PANHYPOPITUITARISM. The classical clinical condition of major anterior pituitary insufficiency is called panhypopituitarism. Three most common causes of panhypopituitarism are: non-secretory (chromophobe) adenoma (discussed later), Sheehan's syndrome and Simmond's disease, and empty-sella syndrome.

Sheehan's syndrome and Simmond's disease. Pituitary insufficiency occurring due to postpartum pituitary (Sheehan's) necrosis is called Sheehan's syndrome, whereas occurrence of similar process without preceding pregnancy as well as its occurrence in males is termed Simmond's disease. The main pathogenetic mechanism underlying Sheehan's necrosis is the enlargement of the pituitary occurring during pregnancy which may be followed by hypotensive shock precipitating ischaemic necrosis of the pituitary. Other mechanisms hypothesised are: DIC following delivery, traumatic injury to vessels, and excessive haemorrhage. Patients with long-standing diabetes mellitus appear to be at greater risk of developing this complication.

The first *clinical manifestation* of Sheehan's syndrome is failure of lactation following delivery which is due to deficiency of prolactin. Subsequently, other symptoms develop which include loss of axillary and pubic hair, amenorrhoea, sterility and loss of libido. Concomitant deficiency of TSH and ACTH may result in hypothyroidism and adrenocortical insufficiency.

The ***pathologic changes*** in the anterior pituitary in Sheehan's syndrome during early stage are ischaemic necrosis and haemorrhage, while later necrotic tissue is replaced by fibrous tissue.

Empty-sella syndrome. Empty-sella syndrome is characterised by the appearance of an empty sella and features of panhypopituitarism. Most commonly, it results from herniation of subarachnoid space into the sella turcica due to an incomplete diaphragma sella creating an empty sella. Other less common causes are Sheehan's syndrome, infarction and scarring in an adenoma, irradiation damage, or surgical removal of the gland.

2. PITUITARY DWARFISM. Severe deficiency of GH in children before growth is completed results in retarded growth and pituitary dwarfism. Most commonly, isolated GH deficiency is the result of an inherited autosomal recessive disorder. Less often it may be due to a pituitary adenoma or craniopharyngioma, infarction and trauma to the pituitary. The clinical features of inherited cases of pituitary dwarfism appear after one year of age. These include proportionate retardation in growth of bones, normal mental state for age, poorly-developed genitalia, delayed puberty and episodes of hypoglycaemia. Pituitary dwarf must be distinguished from hypothyroid dwarf (cretinism) in which there is achondroplasia and mental retardation (page 827).

B. Hypofunction of Posterior Pituitary and Hypothalamus

Insufficiency of the posterior pituitary and hypothalamus is uncommon. The only significant clinical syndrome due to hypofunction of the neurohypophysis and hypothalamus is diabetes insipidus.

DIABETES INSIPIDUS. Deficient secretion of ADH causes diabetes insipidus. The causes of ADH deficiency are: inflammatory and neoplastic lesions of the hypothalamo-hypophyseal axis, destruction of neurohypophysis due to surgery, radiation, head injury, and lastly, are those cases where no definite cause is known and are labelled as idiopathic. The main features of diabetes insipidus are excretion of a very large volume of dilute urine of low specific gravity (below 1.010), polyuria and polydipsia.

PITUITARY TUMOURS

Tumours of the anterior pituitary are more common than those of the posterior pituitary and hypothalamus. The most common of the anterior pituitary tumours are adenomas; primary and metastatic carcinomas being rare. Craniopharyngioma and granular cell tumour (choristoma) are the other benign pituitary tumours found occasionally.

All pituitary tumours, whether benign or malignant, cause symptoms in 2 ways: by pressure effects, and by hormonal effects.

1. Pressure effects. These are caused by expansion of the lesion resulting in destruction of the surrounding glandular tissue by pressure atrophy. This causes erosion and enlargement of sella turcica, upward extension of the tumour damaging the optic chiasma, optic nerves, neurohypophysis and adjacent cranial nerves, and rarely, downward extension into the nasopharynx.

2. Hormonal effects. Depending upon their cell types, pituitary adenomas produce excess of pituitary hormones and the corresponding clinical syndromes of hyperpituitarism. Infarction and destruction of adenoma may cause symptoms of hypopituitarism.

Pituitary Adenomas

Adenomas are the most common pituitary tumours. They are conventionally classified according to their haematoxylin-eosin staining characteristics of granules into acidophil, basophil and chromophobe adenomas. However, this *morphologic classification* is considered quite inadequate because of the significant functional characteristics of each type of adenoma including the chromophobe adenoma, which on H & E staining does not show visible granules. As a result of advances in the ultrastructural and immunocytochemical studies, a functional classification of pituitary adenoma has been made possible. A recent classification of pituitary adenomas based on functional features as correlated with morphologic features of older classification is given in Table 25.1. The syndromes produced by the tumours have been described already.

PATHOLOGIC CHANGES. Grossly, pituitary adenomas range in size from small foci of less than 10 mm in size (termed microadenoma) to large adenomas several centimeters in diameter. They are spherical, soft and encapsulated.

Histologically, by light microscopy of H & E stained sections, an adenoma is composed predominantly of one of the normal cell types of the anterior pituitary i.e. acidophil, basophil or chromophobe cells. These cells may have 3 types of patterns: diffuse, sinusoidal and papillary.

1. *Diffuse pattern* is composed of polygonal cells arranged in sheets with scanty stroma.
2. *Sinusoidal pattern* consists of columnar or fusiform cells with fibrovascular stroma around which the tumour cells are arranged.

TABLE 25.1: Morphologic and Functional Classification of Pituitary Adenomas.

FUNCTIONAL TYPE	FREQUENCY	HORMONES PRODUCED	CLINICAL SYNDROME
1. *Lactotroph adenoma (Prolactinoma)*	20-30%	PRL	Hypogonadism, galactorrhoea
2. *Somatotroph adenoma*	5%	GH	Acromegaly/gigantism
3. *Mixed somatotroph-lactotroph adenoma*	5%	PRL, GH	Acromegaly, hypogonadism, galactorrhoea
4. *Corticotroph adenoma*	10-15%	ACTH	Cushing's syndrome
5. *Gonadotroph adenoma*	10-15%	FSH-LH	Inactive or hypogonadism
6. *Thyrotroph adenoma*	1%	TSH	Thyrotoxicosis
7. *Null cell adenoma/ oncocytoma*	20%	Nil	Pituitary failure
8. *Pleurihormonal adenoma*	15%	Multiple hormones	Mixed

3. *Papillary pattern* is composed of columnar or fusiform cells arranged about fibrovascular papillae.

Functionally, most common pituitary adenomas, in decreasing order of frequency, are: lactotroph (PRL-secreting) adenoma, somatotroph (GH-secreting) adenoma and corticotroph (ACTH-secreting) adenoma. Infrequently, mixed somatotroph-lactotroph (GH-PRL-secreting) adenoma, gonadotroph (FSH-LH-secreting) adenomas and null-cell (endocrinologically inactive) adenomas or oncocytoma are found. Pleurihormonal-pituitary adenoma, on the other hand, may have multiple hormone elaborations. Functional classification of pituitary adenoma can be done by carrying out specific immunostains against the hormone products.

Pituitary adenoma may also occur as a part of multiple endocrine neoplasia type I (MEN-I) in which adenomas of pancreatic islets, parathyroids and the pituitary are found (page 854). Clinically, the patients are characterised by combination of features of Zollinger-Ellison's syndrome, hyperparathyroidism and hyperpituitarism.

Pituitary adenocarcinoma is rare and is demonstrated by metastasis only.

Craniopharyngioma

Craniopharyngioma is a benign tumour arising from remnants of Rathke's pouch. It is more common in children and young adults. The tumour, though benign, compresses as well as invades the adjacent structures extensively.

PATHOLOGIC CHANGES. Grossly, the tumour is encapsulated, adherent to surrounding structures and is typically cystic, reddish-grey mass.
Histologically, craniopharyngioma closely resembles ameloblastoma of the jaw (page 542). There are 2 distinct histologic features:
1. Stratified squamous epithelium frequently lining, a cyst and containing loose stellate cells in the centre; and
2. Solid ameloblastous areas.

Granular Cell Tumour (Choristoma)

Though tumours of the posterior pituitary are rare, granular cell tumour or choristoma is the most common tumour of the neurohypophysis. It is composed of a mass of cells having granular eosinophilic cytoplasm similar to the cells of the posterior pituitary. It is believed to arise as a result of developmental anomaly and hence the name choristoma. Generally, it remains asymptomatic and discovered as an incidental autopsy finding.

ADRENAL GLAND

NORMAL STRUCTURE

ANATOMY. The adrenal glands lie at the upper pole of each kidney. Each gland weighs approximately 4 gm in the adult but in children the adrenals are proportionately larger. On sectioning, the adrenal is composed of 2 distinct parts: an outer yellow-brown *cortex* and an inner grey *medulla.* The anatomic and functional integrity of adrenal cortices are essential for life, while it does not hold true for adrenal medulla.

HISTOLOGY AND PHYSIOLOGY. Microscopically and functionally, cortex and medulla are quite distinct.

ADRENAL CORTEX. It is composed of 3 layers:

1. **Zona glomerulosa** is the outer layer and comprises about 10% of the cortex. It consists of cords or columns of polyhedral cells just under the capsule. This layer is responsible for the synthesis of *mineralocorticoids,* the most important of which is aldosterone, the salt and water regulating hormone.
2. **Zona fasciculata** is the middle layer and constitutes approximately 70% of the cortex. It is composed of columns of lipid-rich cells which are precursors of various *steroid hormones* manufactured in the adrenal cortex such as glucocorticoids (e.g. cortisol) and sex steroids (e.g. testosterone).
3. **Zona reticularis** is the inner layer which makes up the remainder of the adrenal cortex. It consists of cords of more compact cells than those of zona fasciculata but has similar functional characteristics of synthesis and secretion of *glucocorticoids* and *androgens.*

The synthesis of glucocorticoids and adrenal androgens is under the control of ACTH from hypothalamus-anterior pituitary. In turn, ACTH release is under the control of a hypothalamic releasing factor called corticotropin-releasing factor. Release of aldosterone, on the other hand, is independent of ACTH control and is largely regulated by the serum levels of potassium and renin-angiotensin mechanism (page 99).

ADRENAL MEDULLA. The adrenal medulla is a component of the dispersed neuroendocrine system derived from primitive neuroectoderm; the other components of this system being *paraganglia* distributed in the vagi, paravertebral and visceral autonomic ganglia. The cells comprising this system are neuroendocrine cells, the major function of which is synthesis and secretion of catecholamines (epinephrine and norepinephrine). Various other peptides such as calcitonin, somatostatin and vasoactive intestinal polypeptide (VIP) are also secreted by these cells. The major metabolites of catecholamines are metanephrine, normetanephrine, vanillyl mandelic acid (VMA) and homovanillic acid (HVA). In case of damage to the adrenal medulla, its function is taken over by other paraganglia.

Diseases affecting the two parts of adrenal glands are quite distinctive in view of distinct morphology, and function of the adrenal cortex and medulla. While the disorders of the *adrenal cortex* include adrenocortical hyperfunction (hyperadrenalism), adrenocortical insufficiency (hypoadrenalism) and adrenocortical tumours, the main lesions affecting the *adrenal medulla* are the medullary tumours.

ADRENOCORTICAL HYPERFUNCTION (HYPERADRENALISM)

Hypersecretion of each of the three types of corticosteroids elaborated by the adrenal cortex causes distinct corresponding hyperadrenal clinical syndromes:

1. *Cushing's syndrome* caused by excess of glucocorticoids (i.e. cortisol); also called *chronic hypercortisolism.*
2. *Conn's syndrome* caused by oversecretion of mineralocorticoids (i.e. aldosterone); also called *primary hyperaldosteronism.*
3. *Adrenogenital syndrome* characterised by excessive production of adrenal sex steroids (i.e. androgens); and also called *adrenal virilism.*

Mixed forms of these clinical syndromes may also occur.

Cushing's Syndrome (Chronic Hypercortisolism)

Cushing's syndrome is caused by excessive production of cortisol of whatever cause. The full clinical expression of the syndrome, however, includes contribution of the secondary derangements.

ETIOPATHOGENESIS. There are 4 major etiologic types of Cushing's syndrome which should be distinguished for effective treatment.

1. Pituitary Cushing's syndrome. About 60-70% cases of Cushing's syndrome are caused by excessive secretion of ACTH due to a lesion in the pituitary gland, most commonly a corticotroph adenoma or multiple corticotroph microadenomas. This group of cases was first described by Harvey Cushing, an American neurosurgeon, who termed the condition as Cushing's disease. Also included in this group are cases with hypothalamic origin of excessive ACTH levels without apparent pituitary lesion. All cases with pituitary Cushing's syndrome are characterised by bilateral adrenal cortical hyperplasia and elevated ACTH levels. These cases show therapeutic response on administration of high doses of dexamethasone which suppresses ACTH secretion and causes fall in plasma cortisol level.

2. Adrenal Cushing's syndrome. Approximately 20-25% cases of Cushing's syndrome are caused by disease in one or both the adrenal glands. These include adrenal cortical adenoma, carcinoma, and less often, cortical hyperplasia. This group of cases is characterised by low serum ACTH levels and absence of therapeutic response to administration of high doses of glucocorticoid.

3. Ectopic Cushing's syndrome. About 10-15% cases of Cushing's syndrome have an origin in ectopic ACTH elaboration by non-endocrine tumours. Most often, the tumour is an oat cell carcinoma of the lung but other lung cancers, malignant thymoma and pancreatic tumours have also been implicated. The plasma ACTH level is high in these cases and cortisol secretion is not suppressed by dexamethasone administration.

4. Iatrogenic Cushing's syndrome. Prolonged therapeutic administration of high doses of glucocorticoids or ACTH may result in Cushing's syndrome e.g. in organ transplant recipients and in autoimmune diseases. These cases are generally associated with bilateral adrenocortical insufficiency.

CLINICAL FEATURES. Cushing's syndrome occurs more often in patients between the age of 20-40 years with three times higher frequency in women than in men. The severity of the syndrome varies considerably, but in general the following features characterise a case of Cushing's syndrome:

1. Central or truncal *obesity* contrasted with relatively thin arms and legs, buffalo hump due to prominence of fat over the shoulders, and rounded oedematous moonface.
2. Increased *protein breakdown* resulting in wasting and thinning of the skeletal muscles, atrophy of the skin and subcutaneous tissue with formation of purple striae on the abdominal wall, osteoporosis and easy bruisability of the thin skin to minor trauma.
3. *Systemic hypertension* is present in 80% of cases because of associated retention of sodium and water.
4. *Impaired glucose tolerance* and diabetes mellitus are found in about 20% cases.
5. Amenorrhoea, hirsutism and infertility in many women.
6. Insomnia, depression, confusion and psychosis.

Conn's Syndrome (Primary Hyperaldosteronism)

This is an uncommon syndrome occurring due to overproduction of aldosterone, the potent salt-retaining hormone.

ETIOPATHOGENESIS. The condition results primarily due to adrenocortical diseases such as:

1. Adrenocortical adenoma, producing aldosterone.
2. Bilateral adrenal hyperplasia, especially in children (congenital hyperaldosteronism).
3. Rarely, adrenal carcinoma.

Primary hyperaldosteronism from any of the above causes is associated with low plasma renin levels. *Secondary hyperaldosteronism,* on the contrary, occurs in response to high plasma renin level due to overproduction of renin by the kidneys such as in renal ischaemia, reninoma or oedema.

CLINICAL FEATURES. Conn's syndrome is more frequent in adult females. Its principal features are as under:

1. *Hypertension,* usually mild to moderate diastolic hypertension.
2. *Hypokalaemia* and associated muscular weakness, peripheral neuropathy and cardiac arrhythmias.
3. *Retention of sodium and water.*
4. *Polyuria* and *polydipsia* due to reduced concentrating power of the renal tubules.

Adrenogenital Syndrome (Adrenal Virilism)

Adrenal cortex secretes a smaller amount of sex steroids than the gonads. However, adrenocortical hyperfunction may occasionally cause sexual disturbances.

ETIOPATHOGENESIS. Hypersecretion of sex steroids, mainly androgens, may occur in children or in adults:

1. *In children,* it is due to congenital adrenal hyperplasia in which there is congenital deficiency of a specific enzyme.
2. *In adults,* it is caused by an adrenocortical adenoma or a carcinoma. Cushing's syndrome is often present as well.

CLINICAL FEATURES. The clinical features depend upon the age and sex of the patient.

1. *In children,* there is distortion of the external genitalia in girls, and precocious puberty in boys.
2. *In adults,* the features in females show virilisation (e.g. hirsutism, oligomenorrhoea, deepening of voice, hypertrophy of the clitoris); and in males may rarely cause feminisation.
3. There is generally increased excretion of 17-ketosteroids in the urine.

ADRENOCORTICAL INSUFFICIENCY (HYPOADRENALISM)

Adrenocortical insufficiency may result from deficient synthesis of cortical steroids from the adrenal cortex or may be secondary to ACTH deficiency. Three types of adrenocortical hypofunction are distinguished:

1. *Primary adrenocortical insufficiency* caused primarily by the disease of the adrenal glands. Two forms are described: acute or 'adrenal crisis', and chronic or 'Addison's disease'.
2. *Secondary adrenocortical insufficiency* resulting from diminished secretion of ACTH.
3. *Hypoaldosteronism* characterised by deficient secretion of aldosterone.

PRIMARY ADRENOCORTICAL INSUFFICIENCY

Primary adrenal hypofunction occurs due to defect in the adrenal glands and normal pituitary function. It may develop in 2 ways:

A. Acute primary adrenocortical insufficiency or 'adrenal crisis'.
B. Chronic primary adrenocortical insufficiency or 'Addison's disease'.

A. Primary Acute Adrenocortical Insufficiency (Adrenal Crisis)

Sudden loss of adrenocortical function may result in an acute condition called *adrenal crisis.*

ETIOPATHOGENESIS. Causes of acute insufficiency are as under:

1. Bilateral adrenalectomy e.g. in the treatment of cortical hyperfunction, hypertension and in selected cases of breast cancer.
2. Septicaemia e.g. in endotoxic shock and meningococcal infection producing grossly haemorrhagic and necrotic adrenal cortex termed adrenal apoplexy. The acute condition so produced is called *Waterhouse-Friderichsen's syndrome.*
3. Rapid withdrawal of steroids.
4. Any form of acute stress in a case of chronic insufficiency i.e. in Addison's disease.

CLINICAL FEATURES. Clinical features of acute adrenocortical insufficiency are due to deficiency of mineralocorticoids and glucocorticoids. These are as follows:

1. Deficiency of mineralocorticoids (i.e. aldosterone deficiency) result in salt deficiency, hyperkalaemia and dehydration.
2. Deficiency of glucocorticoids (i.e. cortisol deficiency) leads to hypoglycaemia, increased insulin sensitivity and vomitings.

B. Primary Chronic Adrenocortical Insufficiency (Addison's Disease)

Progressive chronic destruction of more than 90% of adrenal cortex on both sides results in an uncommon clinical condition called Addison's disease.

ETIOPATHOGENESIS. Any condition which causes marked chronic adrenal destruction may produce Addison's disease. These include: tuberculosis, autoimmune or idiopathic adrenalitis, histoplasmosis, amyloidosis, metastatic cancer, sarcoidosis and haemochromatosis. However, currently the first two causes—tuberculosis and autoimmune chronic destruction of adrenal glands, are implicated in majority of cases of Addison's disease. Irrespective of the cause, the adrenal glands are bilaterally small and irregularly shrunken. Histologic changes, depending upon the cause, may reveal specific features as in tuberculosis and histoplasmosis, or the changes may be in the form of nonspecific lymphocytic infiltrate as in idiopathic (autoimmune) adrenalitis.

CLINICAL FEATURES. Clinical manifestations develop slowly and insidiously. The usual features are:

1. Asthenia i.e. progressive weakness, weight loss and lethargy as the cardinal symptoms.
2. Hyperpigmentation, initially most marked on exposed areas, but later involves unexposed parts and mucous membranes as well.
3. Arterial hypotension.
4. Vague upper gastrointestinal symptoms such as mild loss of appetite, nausea, vomiting and upper abdominal pain.
5. Lack of androgen causing loss of hair in women.
6. Episodes of hypoglycaemia.
7. Biochemical changes include reduced GFR, acidosis, hyperkalaemia and low levels of serum sodium, chloride and bicarbonate.

SECONDARY ADRENOCORTICAL INSUFFICIENCY

Adrenocortical insufficiency resulting from deficiency of ACTH is called secondary adrenocortical insufficiency.

ETIOPATHOGENESIS. ACTH deficiency may appear in 2 settings :

1. *Selective ACTH deficiency* due to prolonged administration of high doses of glucocorticoids. This leads to suppression of ACTH release from the pituitary gland and selective deficiency.
2. *Panhypopituitarism* due to hypothalamus-pituitary diseases is associated with deficiency of multiple trophic hormones (page 818).

CLINICAL FEATURES. The clinical features of secondary adrenocortical insufficiency are like those of Addison's disease except the following:

1. These cases lack hyperpigmentation because of suppressed production of melanocyte-stimulating hormone (MSH) from the pituitary.
2. Plasma ACTH levels are low-to-absent in secondary insufficiency but are elevated in Addison's disease.
3. Aldosterone levels are normal due to stimulation by renin.

HYPOALDOSTERONISM

Isolated deficiency of aldosterone with normal cortisol level may occur in association with reduced renin secretion.

ETIOPATHOGENESIS. The causes of such hyporeninism are:

1. Congenital defect due to deficiency of an enzyme required for its synthesis.
2. Prolonged administration of heparin.
3. Certain diseases of the brain.
4. Excision of an aldosterone-secreting tumour.

CLINICAL FEATURES. The patients of isolated hypoaldosteronism are adults with mild renal failure and diabetes mellitus. The predominant features are hyperkalaemia and metabolic acidosis.

TUMOURS OF ADRENAL GLANDS

Primary tumours of the adrenal glands are uncommon and include distinct adrenocortical tumours and medullary tumours. However, adrenal gland is a more common site for metastatic carcinoma.

ADRENOCORTICAL TUMOURS

The commonest cortical tumour is adenoma. Cortical carcinoma is uncommon.

Cortical Adenoma

Adenomas of adrenal cortex are indistinguishable from hyperplastic nodules except that lesions smaller than 2 cm diameter are labelled *hyperplastic nodules.* A cortical adenoma is a benign and slow-growing tumour. It is usually small and nonfunctional. A few large adenomas may, however, produce excess of cortisol, aldosterone or androgen. Association of cortical adenomas with systemic hypertension has been suggested by some workers. Occasionally, a cortical adenoma may be a part of multiple endocrine neoplasia type I (MEN-I) in which patients have associated adenomas of parathyroid, islet cells and anterior pituitary (page 854).

*PATHOLOGIC CHANGES. **Grossly,*** an adenoma is usually a small, solitary, spherical and encapsulated tumour which is well-delineated from the surrounding normal adrenal gland. Cut section is typically bright yellow.

Microscopically, the tumour cells are arranged in trabeculae and generally resemble the cells of zona fasciculata. Less frequently, the cells of adenoma are like those of zona glomerulosa or zona reticularis.

Cortical Carcinoma

Carcinoma of the adrenal cortex is an uncommon tumour occurring mostly in adults. It invades locally as well as spreads to distant sites. Most cortical carcinomas secrete one of the adrenocortical hormones excessively.

*PATHOLOGIC CHANGES. **Grossly,*** an adrenal carcinoma is generally large, spherical and well-demarcated tumour. On cut section, it is predominantly yellow with intermixed areas of haemorrhages, necrosis and calcification.

Microscopically, the cortical carcinoma may vary from well-differentiated to anaplastic growth. Well-differentiated carcinoma consists of foci of atypia in an adenoma, while anaplastic carcinoma shows large, pleomorphic and bizarre cells with high mitotic activity.

MEDULLARY TUMOURS

The most significant lesions of the adrenal medulla are neoplasms. These include uncommon benign tumours such as pheochromocytoma and myelolipoma, and more common tumours arising from embryonic nerve cells such as neuroblastoma and ganglioneuroma. These tumours together with extra-adrenal paraganglioma are described below.

Pheochromocytoma (Chromaffin Tumour)

Pheochromocytoma (meaning *dusky brown tumour*) is generally a benign tumour arising from the adrenal medulla. The extra-adrenal pheochromocytomas arising from other paraganglia are preferably called *paragangliomas,* named along with the anatomic site of origin, as described later.

Pheochromocytoma may occur at any age but most patients are 20-60 years old. Most pheochromocytomas are slow-growing and benign but about 5% of the tumours are malignant, invasive and metastasising. These tumours are commonly sporadic but 10-20% are associated with familial syndromes of multiple endocrine neoplasia (MEN) having bilaterality and association with medullary carcinoma of the thyroid, hyperparathyroidism, pituitary adenoma, mucosal neuromas and von Recklinghausen's neurofibromatosis in varying combinations.

The *clinical features* of pheochromocytoma are predominantly due to secretion of catecholamines, both epinephrine and norepinephrine. The most common feature is hypertension. Other manifestations due to sudden release of catecholamines are congestive heart failure, myocardial infarction, pulmonary oedema, cerebral haemorrhage, and even death. The diagnosis is established by measuring 24-hour urinary catecholamines or their metabolites such as metanephrine and VMA.

*PATHOLOGIC CHANGES. **Grossly,*** the tumour is soft, spherical, about 5 cm in diameter, and well-demarcated from the adjacent adrenal gland. On cut section, the tumour is grey to dusky brown with areas of haemorrhages, necrosis, calcification and cystic change. On immersing the tumour in dichromate fixative, it turns brown-black due to oxidation of catecholamines in the tumour and hence the name chromaffin tumour.

Microscopically, the tumour has the following characteristics:

1. The tumour cells are arranged in solid columns, sheets, trabeculae or clumps.
2. The tumour cells are large, polyhedral and pleomorphic with abundant granular amphophilic or basophilic cytoplasm and vesicular nuclei.
3. The tumour cells of pheochromocytoma stain positively with neuroendocrine substances such as neuron-specific enolase (NSE) and chromogranin.
4. The tumour has abundant fibrovascular stroma.

Myelolipoma

Myelolipoma is an uncommon benign adrenal medullary tumour found incidentally at autopsy. Less often, it may produce symptoms due to excessive hormone elaboration.

*PATHOLOGIC CHANGES. **Grossly,*** a myelolipoma is usually a small tumour, measuring 0.2-2 cm in diameter.

Microscopically, it consists of well-differentiated adipose tissue in which are scattered clumps of haematopoietic cells.

Neuroblastoma

Neuroblastoma, also called as sympathicoblastoma, is a common malignant tumour of embryonic nerve cells, occurring most commonly in children under 5 years of age. Vast majority of cases occur within the abdomen (in the adrenal medulla and paravertebral autonomic ganglia) and rarely in the cerebral hemisphere. Most cases are sporadic but familial occurrence with autosomal dominant transmission is also seen.

The *clinical manifestations* of neuroblastoma are related to its rapid local growth, metastatic spread or development of hormonal syndrome. Local symptoms include abdominal distension, fever, weight loss and malaise. Foci of calcification may be observed on radiologic examination of the abdomen. Metastatic spread occurs early and widely through haematogenous as well as lymphatic routes and involves bones (especially skull), liver, lungs and regional lymph nodes. Neuroblastoma produces variable amounts of catecholamines and its metabolites such as vanillyl mandelic acid (VMA) and homovanillic acid (HVA), which can be detected in the 24-hour urine. Less often, the patient develops carcinoid-like syndrome, probably due to production of kinins or prostaglandins by the tumour. The features in such a case include watery diarrhoea, flushing of the skin and hypokalaemia. Rarely, the tumour may produce sufficient catecholamines to cause hypertension.

Prognosis of neuroblastoma depends upon a few variables:

1. *Age* of the child below 2 years is associated with better prognosis.
2. Extra-abdominal *location* of the tumour have better outlook than abdominal masses.
3. *Patients in clinical stage* I (confined to the organ of origin) or stage II (tumour extending in continuity beyond the organ of origin but not crossing the midline) have better prognosis than higher stages with distant metastases.
4. Tumours with amplification of *MYC oncogene* and *TP53* are associated with poor prognosis.

PATHOLOGIC CHANGES. Grossly, the tumour is generally large, soft and lobulated mass with extensive areas of necrosis and haemorrhages. The tumour is usually diffusely infiltrating into the adjacent tissues. Cut surface of the tumour is grey-white and may reveal minute foci of calcification.

Microscopically, neuroblastoma has the following characteristics (Fig. 25.2):

1. The tumour cells are small, round and oval, slightly larger than lymphocytes, and have scanty and poorly-defined cytoplasm and hyperchromatic nuclei.
2. The tumour cells stain positively with immunohistochemical markers such as neuron-specific enolase (NSE), neurofilaments (NF) and chromogranin.

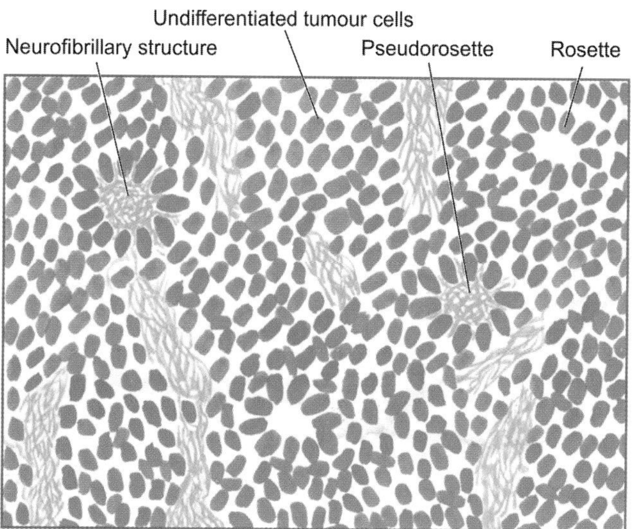

FIGURE 25.2

Neuroblastoma, microscopic appearance. It shows small, round to oval cells forming irregular sheets separated by fibrovascular stroma. A few Homer-Wright's pseudorosettes are also present.

3. They are generally arranged in irregular sheets separated by fibrovascular stroma.
4. Classical neuroblastomas show Homer-Wright's rosettes (pseudorosettes) which have a central fibrillar eosinophilic material surrounded by radially arranged tumour cells. The central fibrillar material stains positively by silver impregnation methods indicating their nature as young nerve fibrils.

Ganglioneuroma

A ganglioneuroma is a mature, benign and uncommon tumour occurring in adults. It is derived from ganglion cells, most often in the posterior mediastinum, and uncommonly in other peripheral ganglia and brain. The tumour produces symptoms because of its size and location. Catecholamines and their metabolites can be detected in large amounts in the 24-hour urine specimen of patients with ganglioneuroma.

PATHOLOGIC CHANGES. Grossly, the tumour is spherical, firm and encapsulated.

Microscopically, it contains large number of well-formed ganglionic nerve cells scattered in fibrillar stroma and myelinated and non-myelinated nerve fibres.

Extra-adrenal Paraganglioma (Chemodectoma)

Parasympathetic paraganglia located in extra-adrenal sites such as the carotid bodies, vagus, jugulotympanic and aorticosympathetic (pre-aortic) paraganglia may produce neoplasms, collectively termed *paragangliomas* with the anatomic site of origin e.g. carotid body paraganglioma, intravagal paraganglioma, jugulo-tympanic paraganglioma etc. These tumours are also called chemodectomas because of their responsiveness to chemoreceptors. They are uncommon tumours found in adults and rarely secrete excess of catecholamines, except aorticosympathetic paraganglioma (also termed extra-adrenal pheochromocytoma). Paragangliomas are generally benign but recurrent tumours. A small proportion of them may metastasise widely.

THYROID GLAND

NORMAL STRUCTURE

ANATOMY. Embryologically, the thyroid gland arises from a midline invagination at the root of the tongue and grows downwards in front of trachea and thyroid cartilage to reach its normal position. Failure to descent may produce *anomalous lingual thyroid.* The thyroglossal duct that connects the gland to the pharyngeal floor normally disappears by 6th week of embryonic life. In adults, its proximal end is represented by foramen caecum at the base of the tongue and distal end by the pyramidal lobe of the thyroid. Persistence of the remnants of thyroglossal duct in the adults may develop into *thyroglossal cyst* (page 531). The C-cells of the thyroid originate from the neuroectoderm.

The thyroid gland in an adult weighs 15-40 gm and is composed of two lateral lobes connected in the midline by a broad isthmus which may have a pyramidal lobe extending upwards. Cut section of normal thyroid is yellowish and translucent.

HISTOLOGY. The thyroid is composed of lobules of colloid-filled spherical follicles or acini. The lobules are enclosed by fibrovascular septa. The follicles are the main functional units of the thyroid. They are lined by cuboidal epithelium with numerous fine microvilli extending into the follicular colloid that contains the glycoprotein, *thyroglobulin.* The follicles are separated from each other by delicate fibrous tissue that contains blood vessels, lymphatics and nerves. Calcitonin-secreting C-cells or parafollicular cells are dispersed within the follicles and can only be identified by silver stains and immunohistochemical methods.

FUNCTIONS. The major function of the thyroid gland is to maintain a high rate of metabolism which is done by means of iodine-containing thyroid hormones, thyroxine (T_4) and tri-iodothyronine (T_3).

The thyroid is one of the most labile organs in the body and responds to numerous stimuli such as puberty, pregnancy, physiologic stress and various pathologic states. This functional lability of the thyroid is respon–sible for transient hyperplasia of the thyroidal epithelium. Under normal conditions, the epithelial lining of the follicles may show changes in various phases of function as under:

1. **Resting phase** characterised by large follicles lined by flattened cells and filled with deeply staining homogeneous colloid e.g. in colloid goitre and iodine-treated hyperthyroidism.
2. **Secretory phase** in which the follicles are lined by cuboidal epithelium and the colloid is moderately dark pink e.g. in normal thyroid.
3. **Resorptive phase** is characterised by follicles lined by columnar epithelium and containing lightly stained vacuolated and scalloped colloid e.g. in hyperthyroidism.

The *synthesis and release* of the two main circulating thyroid hormones, T_3 and T_4 are regulated by hypophyseal thyroid-stimulating hormone (TSH) and involves the following steps:

1. **Iodine trapping** by thyroidal cells involves absorbing of iodine from the blood and concentrating it more than twenty-fold.
2. **Oxidation** of the iodide takes place within the cells by a thyroid peroxidase.
3. **Iodination** occurs next, at the microvilli level between the oxidised iodine and the tyrosine residues of thyroglobulin so as to form mono-iodotyrosine (MIT) and di-iodotyrosine (DIT).
4. **Coupling** of MIT and DIT in the presence of thyroid peroxidase forms tri-iodothyronine (T_3) and thyroxine (T_4).

The thyroid hormones so formed are released by endocytosis of colloid and proteolysis of thyroglobulin within the follicular cells resulting in discharge of T_3 and T_4 into circulation where they are bound to thyroxine-binding globulin.

A number of *thyroid function tests* are currently available. These include:

- determination by radioimmunoassay (RIA) of serum levels of T_3, T_4;
- TSH and TRH;
- assessment of thyroid activity by its ability to uptake radioactive iodine (RAIU); and
- to assess whether thyroid lesion is a nonfunctioning ('cold nodule') or hyperactive mass ('hot nodule').

Diseases of the thyroid include: functional disorders (hyperthyroidism and hypothyroidism), thyroiditis, Graves' disease, goitre and tumours. The relative frequency of some of these diseases varies in different geographic regions according to the iodine content of the diet consumed. One of the important investigation tool available in current times is the widespread use of FNAC for thyroid lesions which has avoided the large number of unwanted diagnostic biopsies.

FUNCTIONAL DISORDERS

Two significant functional disorders characterised by distinct clinical syndromes are described. These are: *hyperthyroidism (thyrotoxicosis)* and *hypothyroidism.*

HYPERTHYROIDISM (THYROTOXICOSIS)

Hyperthyroidism, also called thyrotoxicosis, is a hypermetabolic clinical and biochemical state caused by excess production of thyroid hormones. The condition is more frequent in females and is associated with rise in both T_3 and T_4 levels in blood, though the increase in T_3 is generally greater than that of T_4.

ETIOPATHOGENESIS. Hyperthyroidism may be caused by many diseases but three most common causes are: Graves' disease (diffuse toxic goitre), toxic multinodular goitre and a toxic adenoma. Less frequent causes are hypersecretion of pituitary TSH by a pituitary tumour, hypersecretion of TRH, thyroiditis, metastatic tumours of the thyroid, struma ovarii, congenital hyperthyroidism in the newborn of mother with Graves' disease, HCG-secreting tumours due to mild thyrotropic effects of HCG (e.g. hydatidiform mole, choriocarcinoma and testicular tumours), and lastly, by excessive doses of thyroid hormones or iodine called *jodbasedow disease.*

CLINICAL FEATURES. Patients with hyperthyroidism have a slow and insidious onset, varying in severity from case to case. The usual symptoms are emotional instability, nervousness, palpitation, fatigue, weight loss in spite of good appetite, heat intolerance, perspiration, menstrual disturbances and fine tremors of the outstretched hands. Cardiac manifestations in the form of tachycardia, palpitations and cardiomegaly are invariably present in hyperthyroidism. The skin of these patients is warm, moist and flushed. Weakness of skeletal muscles and osteoporosis are common. Typical eye changes in the form of exophthalmos are a common feature in Graves' disease. The serum T_3 and T_4 levels are elevated but TSH secretion is usually inhibited.

A sudden spurt in the severity of hyperthyroidism termed *'thyroid storm'* or *'thyroid crisis'* may occur in patients who have undergone subtotal thyroidectomy before adequate control of hyperthyroid state, or in a hyperthyroid patient under acute stress, trauma and with severe infection. These patients develop high grade fever, tachycardia, cardiac arrhythmias and coma and may die of congestive heart failure or hyperpyrexia.

HYPOTHYROIDISM

Hypothyroidism is a hypometabolic clinical state resulting from inadequate production of thyroid hormones for prolonged periods, or rarely, from resistance of the peripheral tissues to the effects of thyroid hormones. The clinical manifestations of hypothyroidism, depending upon the age at onset of disorder, are divided into 2 forms:

1. *Cretinism* or *congenital hypothyroidism* is the development of severe hypothyroidism during infancy and childhood.
2. *Myxoedema* is the adulthood hypothyroidism.

Cretinism

A cretin is a child with severe hypothyroidism present at birth or developing within first two years of postnatal life. This is the period when brain development is taking place so that in the absence of treatment the child is both physically and mentally retarded. The word *'Cretin'* is derived from the French, meaning *Christ-like* because these children are so mentally retarded that they are incapable of committing sins.

ETIOPATHOGENESIS. The causes of congenital hypothyroidism are as follows:

1. *Developmental anomalies* e.g. thyroid agenesis and ectopic thyroid.
2. *Genetic defect* in thyroid hormone synthesis e.g. defect in iodine trapping, oxidation, iodination, coupling and thyroglobulin synthesis.
3. *Foetal exposure* to iodides and antithyroid drugs.
4. *Endemic cretinism* in regions with endemic goitre due to dietary lack of iodine (*sporadic cretinism,* on the other hand, is due to developmental anomalies and genetic defects in thyroid hormone synthesis described above).

CLINICAL FEATURES. The clinical manifestations usually become evident within a few weeks to months of birth. The presenting features of a cretin are: slow to thrive, poor feeding, constipation, dry scaly skin, hoarse cry and bradycardia. As the child ages, clinical picture of fully-developed cretinism emerges characterised by impaired skeletal growth and consequent dwarfism, round face, narrow forehead, widely-set eyes, flat and broad nose, big protuberant tongue and protuberant abdomen. Neurological features such as deaf-mutism, spasticity and mental deficiency are more evident in sporadic cretinism due to developmental anomalies and dyshormonogenetic defects.

Characteristic laboratory findings include a rise in TSH level and fall in T_3 and T_4 levels.

Myxoedema

The adult-onset severe hypothyroidism causes myxoedema. The term myxoedema connotes non-pitting oedema due to accumulation of hydrophilic mucopolysaccharides in the ground substance of dermis and other tissues.

ETIOPATHOGENESIS. There are several causes of myxoedema listed below but the first two are the most common causes:

1. Ablation of the thyroid by surgery or radiation.
2. Autoimmune (lymphocytic) thyroiditis (termed primary idiopathic myxoedema).
3. Endemic or sporadic goitre.
4. Hypothalamic-pituitary lesions.
5. Thyroid cancer.
6. Prolonged administration of antithyroid drugs.
7. Mild developmental anomalies and dyshormonogenesis.

CLINICAL FEATURES. The onset of myxoedema is slow and a fully-developed clinical syndrome may appear after several years of hypothyroidism. The striking features are cold intolerance, mental and physical lethargy, constipation, slowing of speech and intellectual function, puffiness of face, loss of hair and altered texture of the skin.

The laboratory diagnosis in myxoedema is made by low serum T_3 and T_4 levels and markedly elevated TSH levels as in the case of cretinism but cases with suprathyroid lesions (hypothalamic-pituitary disease) have low TSH levels.

THYROIDITIS

Inflammation of the thyroid, thyroiditis, is more often due to non-infectious causes and is classified on the basis of onset and duration of disease into acute, subacute and chronic as under:

I. Acute thyroiditis:

1. Bacterial infection e.g. *Staphylococcus, Streptococcus.*
2. Fungal infection e.g. *Aspergillus, Histoplasma, Pneumocystis.*
3. Radiation injury

II. Subacute thyroiditis:

1. Subacute granulomatous thyroiditis (de Quervain's thyroiditis, giant cell thyroiditis, viral thyroiditis)
2. Subacute lymphocytic (postpartum, silent) thyroiditis
3. Tuberculous thyroiditis

III. Chronic thyroiditis:

1. Autoimmune thyroiditis (Hashimoto's thyroiditis or chronic lymphocytic thyroiditis)
2. Riedel's thyroiditis (or invasive fibrous thyroiditis).

However, the first group i.e. acute infectious thyroiditis, is uncommon. The more common types are discussed below.

HASHIMOTO'S (AUTOIMMUNE, CHRONIC LYMPHOCYTIC) THYROIDITIS

Hashimoto's thyroiditis, also called diffuse lymphocytic thyroiditis, struma lymphomatosa or goitrous autoimmune thyroiditis, is characterised by 3 principal features:

- diffuse goitrous enlargement of the thyroid;
- lymphocytic infiltration of the thyroid gland; and
- occurrence of thyroid autoantibodies.

Hashimoto's thyroiditis occurs more frequently between the age of 30 and 50 years and shows an approximately ten-fold preponderance among females. Though rare in children, about half the cases of adolescent goitre are owing to autoimmune thyroiditis. Hashimoto's thyroiditis is the most common cause of *goitrous hypothyroidism* in regions where iodine supplies are *adequate.* Regions where iodine intake is highest have higher incidence of Hashimoto's thyroiditis e.g. in Japan and the United States.

ETIOPATHOGENESIS. Hashimoto's thyroiditis is an autoimmune disease is well established. Hashimoto, a Japanese surgeon, described it in 1912 as the first autoimmune disease of any organ. Autoimmune pathogenesis of Hashimoto's thyroiditis is explained by the following observations:

1. Other autoimmune disease association: Like in other autoimmune diseases, Hashimoto's disease has been found in association with other autoimmune diseases such as Graves' disease, SLE, Sjögren's syndrome, rheumatoid arthritis, pernicious anaemia and Type 1 (juvenile-onset) diabetes mellitus.

2. Immune destruction of thyroid cells: The sequence of immune phenomena is initial activation of CD4+ T helper cells. These cells then induce infiltration of CD8+ T cytotoxic cells in the thyroid parenchyma as well as activate B cells to form autoantibodies, which bring about immune destruction of thyroid parenchyma.

3. Detection of autoantibodies: The following autoantibodies against different thyroid cell antigens are detectable in the sera of most patients with Hashimoto's thyroiditis:

i) Thyroid microsomal autoantibodies (against the microsomes of the follicular cells).

ii) Thyroglobulin autoantibodies.

iii) TSH receptor autoantibodies.

iv) Less constantly found are thyroid autoantibodies against follicular cell membranes, thyroid hormones themselves, and colloid component other than thyroglobulin.

4. Inhibitory TSH-receptor antibodies: TSH-receptor antibody seen on the surface of thyroid cells in Hashimoto's thyroiditis is inhibitory to TSH, producing hypothyroidism. Similar antibody is observed in Graves' disease where it causes hyperthyroidism. It appears that TSH-receptor antibody may act both to depress or stimulate the thyroid cells to produce hypo- or hyperthyroidism respectively. Thus, these patients may have alternate episodes of hypo- or hyperthyroidism.

5. Genetic basis: The disease has higher incidence in first-degree relatives of affected patients. Hashimoto's thyroiditis is seen more often with HLA-DR3 and HLA-DR5 subtypes.

PATHOLOGIC CHANGES. Pathologically, two varieties of Hashimoto's thyroiditis are seen: *classic form*, the usual and more common, and *fibrosing variant* found in only 10% cases of Hashimoto's thyroiditis.

Grossly, the *classic form* is characterised by diffuse, symmetric, firm and rubbery enlargement of the thyroid which may weigh 100-300 gm. Sectioned surface of the thyroid is fleshly with accentuation of normal lobulations but with retained normal shape of the gland. The *fibrosing variant* has a firm, enlarged thyroid with compression of the surrounding tissues.

Histologically, the *classic form* shows the following features (Fig. 25.3):

1. There is extensive infiltration of the gland by lymphocytes, plasma cells, immunoblasts and macrophages, with formation of lymphoid follicles having germinal centres.
2. There is decreased number of thyroid follicles which are generally atrophic and are often devoid of colloid.
3. The follicular epithelial cells are transformed into their degenerated state termed Hurthle cells (also called Askanazy cells, or oxyphil cells, or oncocytes). These cells have abundant oxyphilic or eosinophilic

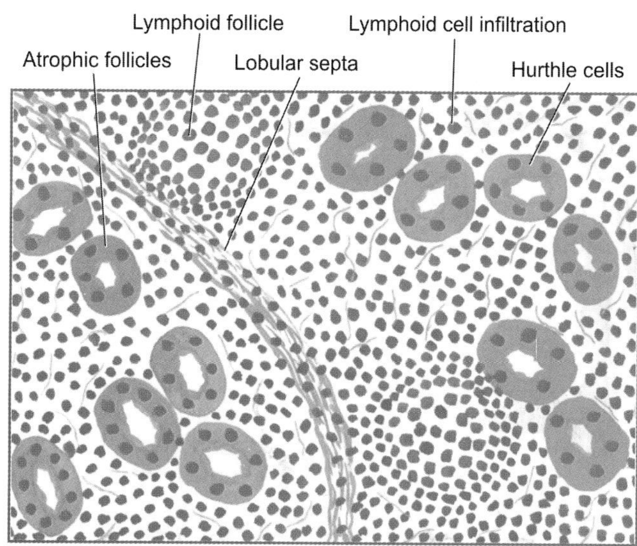

FIGURE 25.3

Hashimoto's thyroiditis. Histologic features include: lymphoid cell infiltration with formation of lymphoid follicles having germinal centres; small, atrophic and colloid-deficient follicles; presence of Hurthle cells which have granular oxyphil cytoplasm and large irregular nuclei; and slight fibrous thickening of lobular septa.

and granular cytoplasm due to large number of mitochondria and contain large bizarre nuclei.

4. There is slight fibrous thickening of the septa separating the thyroid lobules.

The less common *fibrosing variant* of Hashimoto's thyroiditis shows considerable fibrous replacement of thyroid parenchyma and a less prominent lymphoid infiltrate.

CLINICAL FEATURES. The presenting feature of Hashimoto's thyroiditis is a painless, firm and moderate goitrous enlargement of the thyroid gland, usually associated with hypothyroidism, in an elderly woman. At this stage, serum T_3 and T_4 levels are decreased and RAIU is also reduced. A few cases, however, develop hyperthyroidism, termed *hashitoxicosis,* further substantiating the similarities in the autoimmune phenomena between Hashimoto's thyroiditis and Graves' thyrotoxicosis. There is no increased risk of developing thyroid carcinoma in Hashimoto's thyroiditis but there is increased frequency of malignant lymphoma in these cases.

SUBACUTE LYMPHOCYTIC THYROIDITIS

Subacute lymphocytic (or painless or silent or post-partum) thyroiditis is another variety of autoimmune thyrioditis. Clinically, it differs from subacute granulomatous in being non-tender thyroid enlargement. It occurs frequently 3-6 months after delivery.

Microscopically, the features are as under:
1. Dense multifocal infiltrate of lymphocytes and plasma cells in the parenchyma.
2. Collapse of thyroid follicles.
3. Rarely, presence of lymphoid follicles with germinal centres, simulating Hashimoto's thyroiditis.

SUBACUTE GRANULOMATOUS THYROIDITIS

Granulomatous thyroiditis, also called de Quervain's or subacute, or giant cell thyroiditis, is a distinctive form of self-limited inflammation of the thyroid gland. Etiology of the condition is not known but clinical features of a prodromal phase and preceding respiratory infection suggest a possible viral etiology. The disease is more common in young and middle-aged women and may present clinically with painful moderate thyroid enlargement with fever, features of hyperthyroidism in the early phase of the disease, and hypothyroidism if the damage to the thyroid gland is extensive. The condition is self-limiting and shows complete recovery of thyroid function in about 6 months.

PATHOLOGIC CHANGES. Grossly, there is moderate enlargement of the gland which is often asymmetric or focal. The cut surface of the involved area is firm and yellowish-white.
Microscopically, the features vary according to the stage of the disease:
- *Initially,* there is acute inflammatory destruction of the thyroid parenchyma and formation of micro-abscesses.
- *Later,* the more characteristic feature of granulomatous appearance is produced. These granulomas consist of central colloid material surrounded by histiocytes and scattered multinucleate giant cells.
- More *advanced* cases may show fibroblastic proliferation.

Morphologically similar appearance may be produced in cases where vigorous thyroid palpation may initiate mechanical trauma to follicles, so-called *palpation thyroiditis.*

RIEDEL'S THYROIDITIS

Riedel's thyroiditis, also called Riedel's struma or invasive fibrous thyroiditis, is a rare chronic disease characterised by stony-hard thyroid that is densely adherent to the adjacent structures in the neck. The condition is clinically significant due to compressive clinical features (e.g. dysphagia, dyspnoea, recurrent laryngeal nerve paralysis and stridor) and resemblance with thyroid cancer. Riedel's struma is seen more commonly in females in 4th to 7th decades of life. The etiology is unknown but possibly Riedel's thyroiditis is a part of *multifocal idiopathic fibrosclerosis* (page 606). This group of disorders includes: idiopathic retroperitoneal, mediastinal and retro-orbital fibrosis, and sclerosing cholangitis, all of which may occur simultaneously with Riedel's thyroiditis.

PATHOLOGIC CHANGES. Grossly, the thyroid gland is usually contracted, stony-hard, asymmetric and firmly adherent to the adjacent structures. Cut section is hard and devoid of lobulations.
Microscopically, there is extensive fibrocollagenous replacement, marked atrophy of the thyroid parenchyma, focally scattered lymphocytic infiltration and invasion of the adjacent muscle tissue by the process.

GRAVES' DISEASE (DIFFUSE TOXIC GOITRE)

Graves' disease, also known as Basedow's disease, primary hyperplasia, exophthalmic goitre, and diffuse toxic goitre, is characterised by a triad of features:
- hyperthyroidism (thyrotoxicosis);
- diffuse thyroid enlargement; and
- ophthalmopathy.

The disease is more frequent between the age of 30 and 40 years and has five-fold increased prevalence among females.

ETIOPATHOGENESIS. Graves' disease is an autoimmune disease and, as already stated, there are many immunologic similarities between this condition and Hashimoto's thyroiditis. These are as follows:

1. HLA association. Like in Hashimoto's thyroiditis. Graves'disease too has genetic predisposition. A familial occurrence has been observed. Graves' disease has been found strongly associated with HLA-DR3 (Hashimoto's thyroiditis has both HLA-DR3 and HLA-DR5 association, page 828).

2. Autoimmune disease association. Graves' disease may be found in association with other organ-specific autoimmune diseases. Hashimoto's thyroiditis and Graves' disease are frequently present in the same families and the two diseases may coexist in the same patient.

3. Other factors. Besides these two factors, other factors observed in Graves' disease are higher prevalence in women (7 to 10 times), association with emotional stress and smoking.

4. **Autoantibodies.** Autoantibodies against thyroid antigens are detectable in the serum of these patients

too but their sites of action are different from that of Hashimoto's thyroiditis. In Graves' disease, TSH-receptor autoantigen is the main antigen against which *autoantibodies* are mostly directed. These are as under:
i) *Thyroid-stimulating immunoglobulin (TSI):* It binds to TSH receptor and stimulates increased release of thyroid hormone.
ii) *Thyroid growth-stimulating immunoglobulins (TGI)*: It stimulates proliferation of follicular epithelium.
iii) *TSH-binding inhibitor immunoglobulins (TBII)*: It is inhibitory to binding of TSH to its own receptor. Depending upon its action as inhibitory or stimulatory to follicular epithelium, it may result in alternate episodes of hypo- and hyperthyroidism.

However, it is not quite clear what stimulates B cells to form these autoantibodies in Graves' disease. Possibly, intrathyroidal CD4+ helper T cells are responsible for stimulating B cells to secrete autoantibodies.

The pathogenesis of Graves' infiltrative ophthalmopathy is also of autoimmune origin. The evidence in support is the intense lymphocytic infiltrate around the ocular muscles and detection of circulating autoantibodies against muscle antigen that cross-react with thyroid microsomes.

PATHOLOGIC CHANGES. Grossly, the thyroid is moderately, diffusely and symmetrically enlarged and may weigh up to 70-90 gm. On cut section, the thyroid parenchyma is typically homogeneous, red-brown and meaty and lacks the normal translucency. ***Histologically,*** the following features are found (Fig. 25.4):

1. There is considerable epithelial hyperplasia and hypertrophy as seen by increased height of the follicular lining cells and formation of papillary infoldings of piled up epithelium into the lumina of follicles which are small.
2. The colloid is markedly diminished and is lightly staining, watery and finely vacuolated.
3. The stroma shows increased vascularity and accumulation of lymphoid cells.

However, the pathologic changes in gross specimen as well as on histologic examination are considerably altered if preoperative medication has been administered. Iodine administration results in accumulation of colloid in the follicles and decrease in vascularity and height of follicular cells, while antithyroid drugs such as thiouracil cause marked hyperplasia.

CLINICAL FEATURES. Graves' disease generally develops slowly and insidiously. The patients are usually young women who present with symmetric, moderate enlargement of the thyroid gland with features of

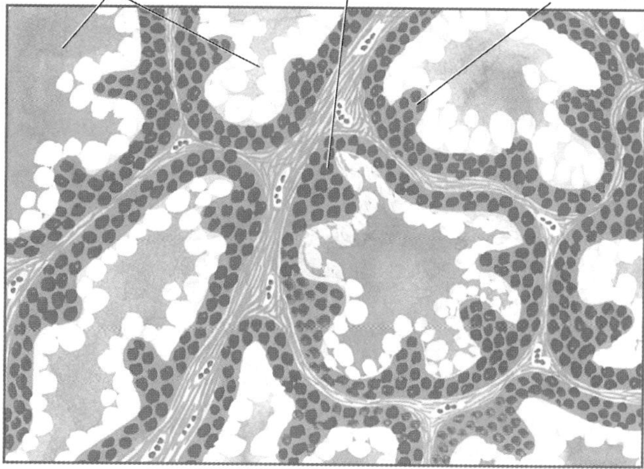

FIGURE 25.4

Graves' disease. The follicles are small and are lined by tall columnar epithelium, which is piled up at places forming papillary infoldings. Colloid is nearly absent and appears lightly staining, watery and finely vacuolated.

thyrotoxicosis (page 827), ophthalmopathy and dermatopathy. The *ocular abnormalities* are lid lag, upper lid retraction, stare, weakness of eye muscles and proptosis. In extreme cases, the lids can no longer close and may produce corneal injuries and ulcerations. *Dermatopathy* in Graves' disease most often consists of pretibial (localised) myxoedema in the form of firm plaques. Like in Hashimoto's thyroiditis, there is no increased risk of development of thyroid cancer in Graves' disease.

GOITRE

The term goitre is defined as thyroid enlargement caused by compensatory hyperplasia and hypertrophy of the follicular epithelium in response to thyroid hormone deficiency. The end-result of this hyperplasia is generally a *euthyroid state* (in contrast to thyrotoxicosis occurring in diffuse toxic goitre or Graves' disease) though at some stages there may be hypo- or hyperthyroidism. Two morphologic forms of goitre are distinguished:
A. Diffuse goitre (simple nontoxic goitre or colloid goitre).
B. Nodular goitre (multinodular goitre or adenomatous goitre).

Pathogenesis of Goitre

The pathogenetic mechanisms of both forms of goitre can be considered together since nodular goitre is generally regarded as the end-stage of long-standing simple

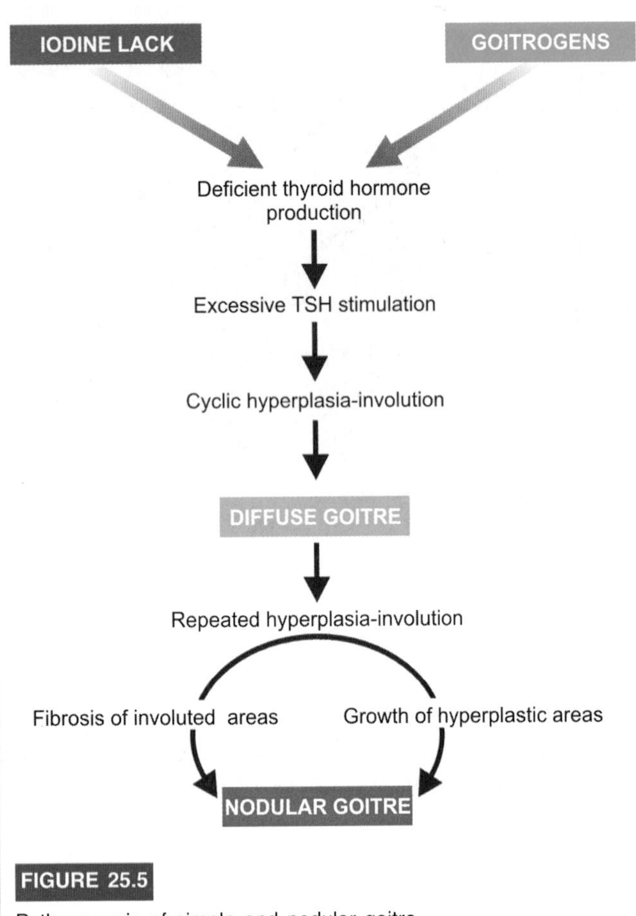

FIGURE 25.5

Pathogenesis of simple and nodular goitre.

goitre (Fig. 25.5). The fundamental defect is deficient production of thyroid hormones due to various etiologic factors described below, but most common is *dietary lack of iodine.* Deficient thyroid hormone production causes excessive TSH stimulation which leads to hyperplasia of follicular epithelium as well as formation of new thyroid follicles. Cyclical hyperplastic stage followed by involution stage completes the picture of *simple goitre.* Repeated and prolonged changes of hyperplasia result in continued growth of thyroid tissue while involuted areas undergo fibrosis, thus completing the picture of *nodular goitre.*

Diffuse Goitre (Simple Non-toxic Goitre, Colloid Goitre)

Diffuse, nontoxic simple or colloid goitre is the name given to diffuse enlargement of the thyroid gland, unaccompanied by hyperthyroidism. Most cases are in a state of euthyroid though they may have passed through preceding stage of hypothyroidism due to inadequate supply of iodine. TSH levels are invariably elevated. In general, goitre is more common in females. Simple goitre often appears at puberty or in adolescence, following which it may either regress or may progress to nodular goitre.

ETIOLOGY. Epidemiologically, goitre occurs in 2 forms: endemic, and non-endemic or sporadic.

Endemic goitre. Prevalence of goitre in a geographic area in more than 10% of the population is termed endemic goitre. Such endemic areas are several high mountainous regions far from the sea where iodine content of drinking water and food is low such as in the regions of the Himalayas, the Alps and the Ande. Of late, however, the prevalence in these areas has declined due to prophylactic use of iodised salt.

Though most endemic goitres are caused by dietary lack of iodine, some cases occur due to goitrogens and genetic factors. *Goitrogens* are substances which interfere with the synthesis of thyroid hormones. These substances are drugs used in the treatment of hyperthyroidism and certain items of food such as cabbage, cauliflower, turnips and cassava roots.

Sporadic goitre. Non-endemic or sporadic simple goitre is less common than the endemic variety. In most cases, the etiology of sporadic goitre is unknown. A number of causal influences have been attributed. These include:

- Suboptimal iodine intake in conditions of increased demand as in puberty and pregnancy.
- Genetic factors.
- Dietary goitrogenes.
- Hereditary defect in thyroid hormone synthesis and transport (dyshormonogenesis).
- Inborn errors of iodine metabolism.

PATHOLOGIC CHANGES. Grossly, the enlargement of the thyroid gland in simple goitre is moderate (weighing upto 100-150 gm), symmetric and diffuse. Cut surface is gelatinous and translucent brown (Fig. 25.6,A).

Histologically, two stages are distinguished:

1. *Hyperplastic stage* is the early stage and is characterised by tall columnar follicular epithelium showing papillary infoldings and formation of small new follicles.
2. *Involution stage* generally follows hyperplastic stage after variable period of time. This stage is characterised by large follicles distended by colloid and lined by flattened follicular epithelium (Fig. 25.6,B).

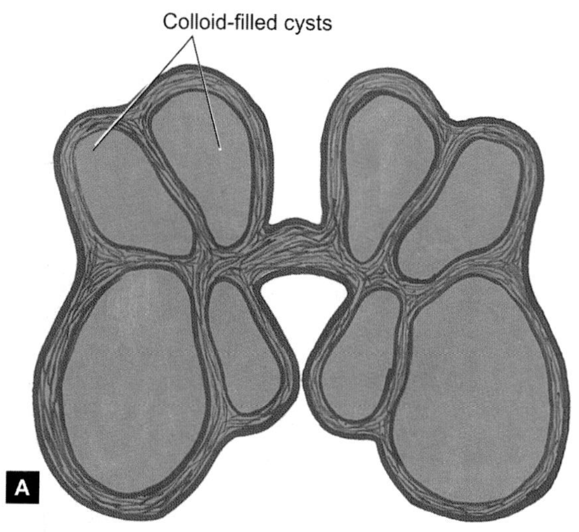

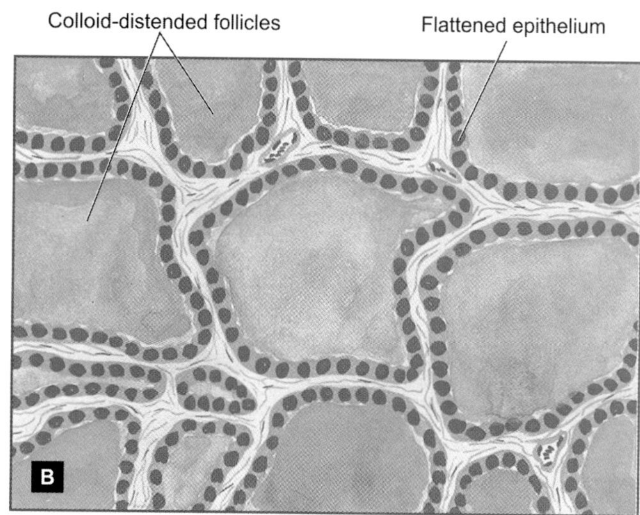

FIGURE 25.6

Simple (diffuse nontoxic or colloid) goitre. A, Sectioned appearance of thyroid gland. B, Microscopy shows large follicles distended by colloid and lined by flattened follicular epithelium.

Nodular Goitre (Multinodular Goitre, Adenomatous Goitre)

As already stated, nodular goitre is regarded as the end-stage of long-standing simple goitre. It is characterised by most extreme degree of tumour-like enlargement of the thyroid gland and characteristic nodularity. The enlargement of the gland may be sufficient to cause not only cosmetic disfigurement, but in many cases may cause dsyphagia and choking due to compression of oesophagus and trachea. Most cases are in a euthyroid state but about 10% cases may develop thyrotoxicosis resulting in toxic nodular goitre or Plummer's disease. However, thyrotoxicosis of *Plummer's disease* (toxic nodular goitre) differs from that of Graves' disease (diffuse toxic goitre) in lacking features of ophthalmopathy and dermatopathy. Such 'hot nodules' may be picked up by scintiscan or by RAIU studies. Since nodular goitre is derived from simple goitre, it has the same female preponderance but affects older individuals because it is a late complication of simple goitre.

ETIOLOGY. Etiologic factors implicated in endemic and non-endemic or sporadic variety of simple goitre are involved in the etiology of nodular goitre too. However, how nodular pattern is produced is not clearly understood. Possibly, epithelial hyperplasia, generation of new follicles, and irregular accumulation of colloid in the follicles—all contribute to produce increased tension and stress in the thyroid gland causing rupture of follicles and vessels. This is followed by haemorrhages, scarring and sometimes calcification, resulting in development of nodular pattern.

PATHOLOGIC CHANGES. Grossly, the thyroid in nodular goitre shows asymmetric and extreme enlargement, weighing 100-500 gm or even more. The *five* cardinal macroscopic features are (Fig. 25.7,A):

1. nodularity with poor encapsulation;
2. fibrous scarring;
3. haemorrhages;
4. focal calcification; and
5. cystic degeneration.

Cut surface generally shows multinodularity but occasionally there may be only one or two nodules which are poorly-circumscribed (unlike complete encapsulation of thyroid adenoma, described below). ***Histologically,*** the same heterogenicity as seen on macroscopic structure is seen. These features are (Fig. 25.7,B) (COLOUR PLATE XXXII: CL 125):

1. Partial or incomplete encapsulation of nodules.
2. The follicles varying from small to large and lined by flat to high epithelium. A few may show macropapillary formation.
3. Areas of haemorrhages, haemosiderin-laden macrophages and cholesterol crystals.
4. Fibrous scarring with foci of calcification.
5. Micro-macrocystic change.

The features of diffuse and nodular goitre are summarised in Table 25.2.

THYROID TUMOURS

Most primary tumours of the thyroid are of follicular epithelial origin; a few arise from parafollicular C-cells. The most common benign thyroid neoplasm is a

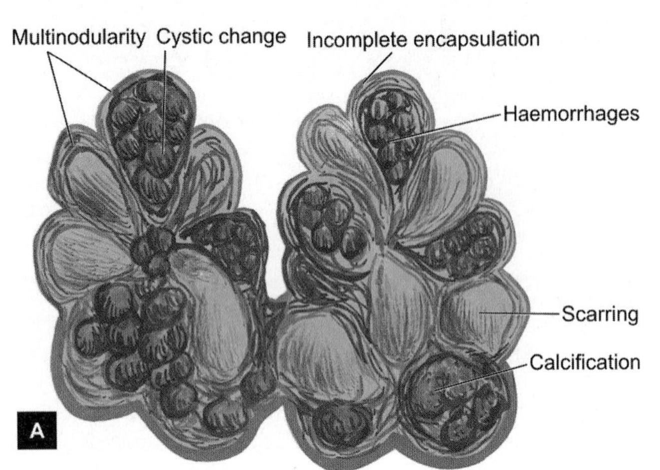

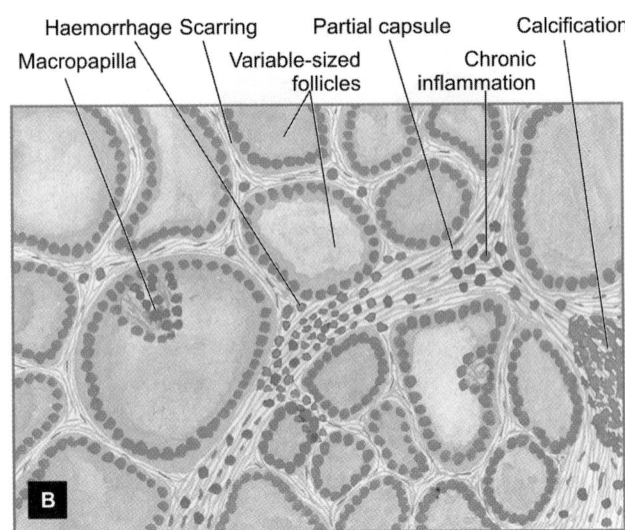

FIGURE 25.7

Nodular goitre. A, Sectioned surface showing characteristic asymmetric enlargement of the gland with multinodularity. B, The predominant histologic features are: nodularity, extensive scarring with foci of calcification, areas of haemorrhages and variable-sized follicles lined by flat to high epithelium and containing abundant colloid.

follicular adenoma. Malignant tumours of the thyroid are less common but thyroid carcinoma is the most common type, though rarely lymphomas and sarcomas also occur.

FOLLICULAR ADENOMA

Follicular adenoma is the most common benign thyroid tumour occurring more frequently in adult women. Clinically, it appears as a solitary nodule which can be found in approximately 1% of the population. Besides the follicular adenoma, other conditions which may produce clinically apparent solitary nodule in the thyroid are a dominant nodule of nodular goitre and thyroid carcinoma. It is thus important to distinguish adenomas from these two conditions. Though most adenomas cause no clinical problem and behave as a 'cold nodule', rarely they may produce mild hyperthyroidism and appear as 'hot nodule' on RAIU studies. Adenoma, however, rarely ever becomes malignant.

PATHOLOGIC CHANGES. Grossly, the follicular adenoma is characterised by *four* features so as to distinguish it from a nodule of nodular goitre:

1. solitary nodule;
2. complete encapsulation;
3. clearly distinct architecture inside and outside the capsule; and

TABLE 25.2: Contrasting Features of Simple and Nodular Goitre.

FEATURE	DIFFUSE GOITRE	NODULAR GOITRE
1. *Nomenclature*	Simple goitre, hyperplastic goitre, nontoxic goitre	Multinodular, adenomatous goitre
2. *Etiology*	Graves' disease, thyroiditis, puberty	Endemic thyroiditis, cancer
3. *Pathogenesis*	Hyperplasia-involution	Repeated cycles of hyperplasia with growth and involution with fibrosis
4. *Composition*	Cellular-rich	Colloid-rich
5. *Gross*	Moderate, symmetric, diffuse enlargement, colloid-filled follicles, gelatinous	Nodular asymmetric, haemorrhages, scarring, cystic change, calcification
6. *Microscopy*	Hyperplastic phase: papillary infoldings, Involution stage: large colloid filled follicles with flat epithelium	Incomplete encapsulation, nodularity, variable-sized follicles, fibrous scarring, haemorrhages, calcification, cyst formation
7. *Functional status*	Hyperthyroidism, euthyroid	Hypothyroidism, euthyroid

4. compression of the thyroid parenchyma outside the capsule

Usually, an adenoma is small (upto 3 cm in diameter) and spherical. On cut section, the adenoma is grey-white to red-brown, less colloidal than the surrounding thyroid parenchyma and may have degenerative changes such as fibrous scarring, focal calcification, haemorrhages and cyst formation.

Histologically, the tumour shows complete fibrous encapsulation. The tumour cells are benign follicular epithelial cells forming follicles of various sizes or may show trabecular, solid and cord patterns with little follicle formation. Accordingly, the following 6 types of growth patterns are distinguished, though more than one pattern may be present in a single tumour:

1. *Microfollicular (foetal) adenoma* consists of small follicles containing little or no colloid and separated by abundant loose stroma (Fig. 25.8) (COLOUR PLATE XXXII: CL 126).
2. *Normofollicular (simple) adenoma* has closely packed follicles like that of normal thyroid gland.
3. *Macrofollicular (colloid) adenoma* contains large follicles of varying size and distended with colloid.
4. *Trabecular (embryonal) adenoma* resembles embryonal thyroid and consists of closely packed solid or trabecular pattern of epithelial cells with an occasional small abortive follicle.

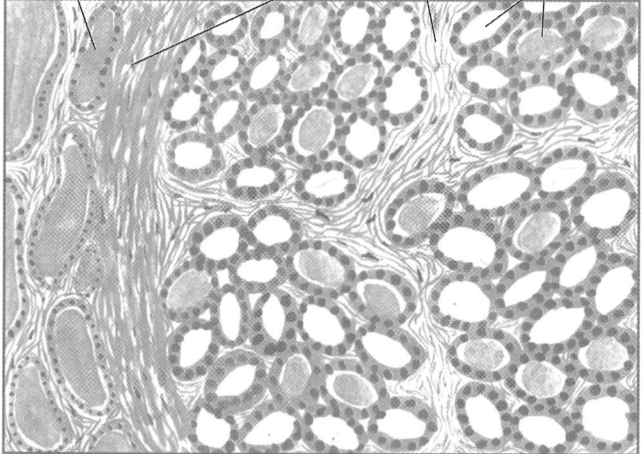

FIGURE 25.8

Follicular adenoma, foetal (microfollicular) type. The tumour is well-encapsulated with compression of surrounding thyroid parenchyma. The tumour consists of small follicles lined by cuboidal epithelium and contain little or no colloid and separated by abundant loose stroma.

5. *Hurthle cell (oxyphilic) adenoma* is an uncommon variant composed of solid trabeculae of large cells having abundant granular oxyphilic cytoplasm and vesicular nuclei. The tumour cells do not form follicles and contain little stroma.
6. *Atypical adenoma* is the term used for a follicular adenoma which has more pronounced cellular proliferation so that features may be considered indicative of malignancy such as pleomorphism, increased mitoses and nuclear atypia. These tumours, however, do not show capsular and vascular invasion—features which distinguish it from follicular carcinoma.

THYROID CANCER

Approximately 95% of all primary thyroid cancers are carcinomas. Primary lymphomas of the thyroid comprise less than 5% of thyroid cancers and majority of them possibly evolve from autoimmune (lymphocytic) thyroiditis (page 828). Sarcomas of the thyroid are extremely rare. About 20% of patients dying of metastasising malignancy have metastatic deposits in the thyroid gland, most commonly from malignant melanoma, renal cell carcinoma and bronchogenic carcinoma.

Carcinoma of the thyroid gland has 4 main morphologic types with distinctly different clinical behaviour and variable prevalence. These are: papillary, follicular, medullary and undifferentiated (anaplastic) carcinoma (Table 25.3).

In line with most other thyroid lesions, most carcinomas of the thyroid too have female preponderance. Irrespective of the histologic types, two types of factors are implicated in the pathogenesis of thyroid cancer: environmental and genetic.

1. Environmental factors: The single most important environmental factor associated with increased risk of developing thyroid carcinoma after many years is exposure to external radiation of high dose. Evidences in support include: high incidence of thyroid cancer in individuals irradiated in early age for enlarged thymus and for skin disorders, in Japanese atomic bomb survivors, and in individuals living in the vicinity of nuclear accident sites.

2. Genetic factors: Familial clustering of thyroid cancer has been observed. Molecular studies reveal a variety of mutations:

i) *Mutation in RET gene* on chromosome 10 seen in papillary thyroid carcinoma (gene overexpression) and medullary carcinoma (point mutation). This mutation renders the tyrosine kinase receptor under the target of

TABLE 25.3: Contrasting Features of Main Histologic Types of Thyroid Carcinoma.

FEATURE	PAPILLARY CARCINOMA	FOLLICULAR CARCINOMA	MEDULLARY CARCINOMA	ANAPLASTIC CARCINOMA
1. *Frequency*	75-80%	10-20%	5%	5%
2. *Age*	All ages	Middle to old age	Middle to old age; familial too	Old age
3. *Female/male ratio*	3:1	2.5:1	1:1	1.5:1
4. *Cell of origin*	Follicular	Follicular	Parafollicular	Follicular
5. *Gross*	Small, multifocal	Moderate size, nodular	Moderate size	Invasive growth
6. *Pathognomonic microscopy*	Nuclear features, papillary pattern	Vascular and capsular invasion	Solid nests, amyloid stroma	Undifferentiated, spindle-shaped, giant cells
7. *Regional metastases*	Common	Rare	Common	Common
8. *Distant metastases*	Rare	Common	Rare	Common
9. *10-year survival*	80-95%	50-70%	60-70%	5-10% (median survival about 2 months)

other tumour-promoting factors such as radiation exposure in papillary carcinoma or C-cell hyperplasia in medullary carcinoma.

ii) *Mutation in RAS gene* is seen in 20-30% cases of all types of thyroid tumours, benign as well as malignant.

Papillary Carcinoma

Papillary carcinoma is the most common type of thyroid carcinoma, comprising 75-85% of cases. It can occur at all ages including children and young adults but the incidence is higher with advancing age. The tumour is found about three times more frequently in females than in males. The following associations have been observed to explain the etiology of papillary carcinoma:

1. **External radiation.** Exposure to radiation to children and adults has been found to be associated with higher incidence of development of papillary carcinoma later. It has been found that children living in the contaminated vicinity of Chernobyl nuclear disaster 1986, have increased prevalence of papillary carcinoma of thyroid.

2. **Iodine excess.** In regions where endemic goitre is widespread, addition of iodine to diet has resulted in increase in incidence of papillary cancer.

3. **Genetic factors.** An association with HLA-DR7 has been found. A mutation in chromosome 10 has been observed in more than half of the cases of thyroid cancer from Chernobyl accident site.

Papillary carcinoma is typically a slow-growing malignant tumour, most often presenting as an asymptomatic solitary nodule. Involvement of the regional lymph nodes is common but distant metastases to organs are rare. Some cases first come to attention by spread to regional lymph nodes and cause cervical lymphadenopathy. *'Lateral aberrant thyroid'* is the term used for occurrence of thyroid tissue in the lateral cervical lymph node, which in most patients represents a well-differentiated metastasis of an occult papillary carcinoma of the thyroid.

PATHOLOGIC CHANGES. ***Grossly,*** papillary carcinoma may range from microscopic foci to nodules upto 10 cm in diameter and is generally poorly delineated. Cut surface of the tumour is greyish-white, hard and scar-like (Fig. 25.9,A). Sometimes the tumour is transformed into a cyst, into which numerous papillae project and is termed *papillary cystadenocarcinoma.*

Histologically, the following features are present (Fig. 25.9,B) **(COLOUR PLATE XXXII: CL 127).**

1. **Papillary pattern.** Papillae composed of fibrovascular stalk and covered by single layer of tumour cells is the predominant feature. Papillae are often accompanied by follicles.

2. **Tumour cells.** The tumour cells have characteristic nuclear features due to dispersed nuclear chromatin imparting it *ground glass or optically clear appearance* and clear or oxyphilic cytoplasm. These tumour cells, besides covering the papillae, may form follicles and solid sheets.

3. **Invasion.** The tumour cells invade the capsule and intrathyroid lymphatics but invasion of blood vessels is rare.

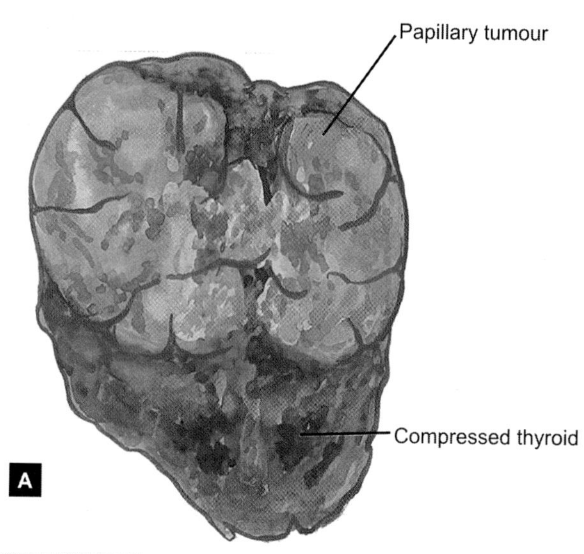

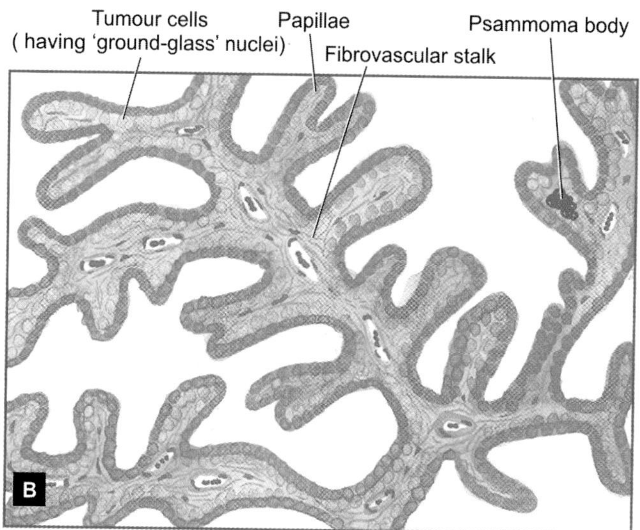

FIGURE 25.9

Papillary carcinoma of the thyroid. A, Gross appearance of papillary tumour replacing upper part of the thyroid gland. B, Microscopy shows branching papillae having flbrovascular stalk covered by a single layer of cuboidal cells having ground-glass nuclei. Colloid-filled follicles and solid sheets of tumour cells are also present.

4. **Psammoma bodies.** Half of papillary carcinomas show typical small, concentric, calcified spherules called psammoma bodies in the stroma.

The prognosis of papillary carcinoma is good: 10-year survival rate is 80-95%, irrespective of whether the tumour is pure papillary or mixed papillary-follicular carcinoma.

Follicular Carcinoma

Follicular carcinoma is the other common type of thyroid cancer, next only to papillary carcinoma and comprises about 10-20% of all thyroid carcinomas. It is more common in middle and old age and has preponderance in females (female-male ratio 2.5:1). In contrast to papillary carcinoma, follicular carcinoma has a positive correlation with endemic goitre but the role of external radiation in its etiology is unclear.

Follicular carcinoma presents clinically either as a solitary nodule or as an irregular, firm and nodular thyroid enlargement. The tumour is slow-growing but more rapid than the papillary carcinoma. In contrast to papillary carcinoma, regional lymph node metastases are rare but distant metastases by haematogenous route are common, especially to lungs and bones.

*PATHOLOGIC CHANGES. **Grossly,*** follicular carcinoma may be either in the form of a solitary adenoma-like circumscribed nodule or as an obvious cancerous irregular thyroid enlargement. The cut surface of the tumour is grey-white with areas of haemorrhages, necrosis and cyst formation and may extend to involve adjacent structures.

Microscopically, the features are as under:

1. *Follicular pattern:* Follicular carcinoma, like follicular adenoma, is composed of follicles of various sizes and may show trabecular or solid pattern. The tumour cells have hyperchromatic nuclei and the cytoplasm resembles that of normal follicular cells (Fig. 25.10). However, variants like *clear cell type* and *Hurthle cell (oxyphilic) type* of follicular carcinoma may occur. The tumour differs from papillary carcinoma in lacking: papillae, ground-glass nuclei of tumour cells and psammoma bodies.
2. *Vascular invasion and direct extension:* Vascular invasion and direct extension to involve the adjacent structures (e.g. into the capsule) are significant features but lymphatic invasion is rare.

The prognosis of follicular carcinoma is between that of papillary and undifferentiated carcinoma: 10-year survival rate is 50-70%.

Medullary Carcinoma

Medullary carcinoma is a less frequent type derived from parafollicular or C-cells present in the thyroid and

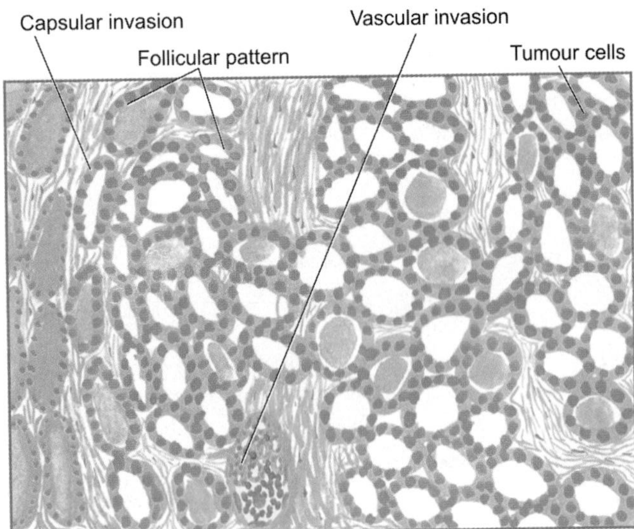

FIGURE 25.10

Follicular carcinoma, showing encapsulated tumour with invasion of a capsular vessel. The follicles lined by tumour cells are of various sizes.

comprises about 5% of thyroid carcinomas. It is equally common in men and women. There are 3 distinctive features which distinguish medullary carcinoma from the other thyroid carcinomas. These are: its familial occurrence, secretion of calcitonin and other peptides, and amyloid stroma.

1. Familial occurrence. Most cases of medullary carcinoma occur sporadically, but about 10% have a genetic background with mutation in chromosome 10. The familial form of medullary carcinoma has association with pheochromocytoma and parathyroid adenoma (multiple endocrine neoplasia, MEN II A), or with pheochromocytoma and multiple mucosal neuromas (MEN II B). The sporadic cases occur in the middle and old age (5th-6th decades) and are generally unilateral, while the familial cases are found at younger age (2nd-3rd decades) and are usually bilateral and multicentric.

2. Secretion of calcitonin and other peptides. Like normal C-cells, tumour cells of medullary carcinoma secrete calcitonin, the hypocalcaemic hormone. In addition, the tumour may also elaborate prostaglandins, histaminase, somatostatin, vasoactive intestinal peptide (VIP) and ACTH. These hormone elaborations are responsible for a number of clinical syndromes such as carcinoid syndrome, Cushing's syndrome and diarrhoea.

3. Amyloid stroma. Most medullary carcinomas have amyloid deposits in the stroma which stains positively with usual amyloid stains such as Congo red. The amyloid deposits are believed to represent stored calcitonin derived from neoplastic C-cells in the form of prohormone.

Most cases of medullary carcinoma present as solitary thyroid nodule but sometimes an enlarged cervical lymph node may be the first manifestation.

PATHOLOGIC CHANGES. Macroscopically, the tumour may either appear as a unilateral solitary nodule *(sporadic form)*, or have bilateral and multicentric involvement *(familial form)*. However, sporadic neoplasms also eventually spread to the contralateral lobe. Cut surface of tumour in both forms shows well-defined tumour areas which are firm to hard, grey-white to yellow-brown with areas of haemorrhages and necrosis.

Histologically, the features are as under (Fig. 25.11) (COLOUR PLATE XXXII: CL128) :

1. *Tumour cells:* Like other neuroendocrine tumours (e.g. carcinoid, islet cell tumour, paraganglioma etc), medullary carcinoma of the thyroid too has a well-defined organoid pattern, forming nests of tumour cells separated by fibrovascular septa . Sometimes, the tumour cells may be arranged in sheets, ribbons pseudopapillae or small follicles. The tumour cells are uniform and have the structural and functional characteristics of C-cells. Less often, the neoplastic cells are spindle-shaped.

2. *Amyloid stroma:* The tumour cells are separated by amyloid stroma derived from altered calcitonin which can be demonstrated by immunostain for calcitonin.

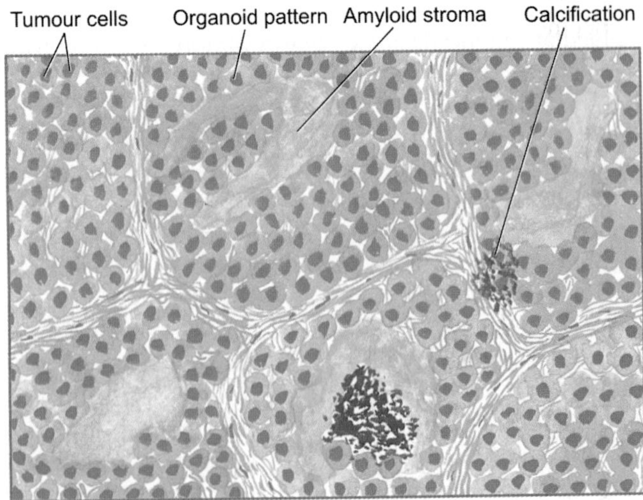

FIGURE 25.11

Medullary carcinoma. Microscopy shows organoid pattern of oval tumour cells and abundant amyloid stroma.

The staining properties of amyloid are similar to that seen in systemic amyloidosis and may have areas of irregular calcification but without regular laminations seen in psammoma bodies.

3. *C-cell hyperplasia:* Familial cases generally have C-cell hyperplasia as a precursor lesion but not in sporadic cases.

Most medullary carcinomas are slow-growing. Regional lymph node metastases may occur but distant organ metastases are infrequent. The prognosis is better in familial form than in the sporadic form: overall 10-year survival rate is 60-70%.

Anaplastic Carcinoma

Undifferentiated or anaplastic carcinoma of the thyroid comprises less than 5% of all thyroid cancers and is one of the most malignant tumour in humans. The tumour is predominantly found in old age (7th-8th decades) and is slightly more common in females than in males (female-male ratio 1.5:1). The tumour is widely aggressive and rapidly growing. The features at presentation are usually those of extensive invasion of adjacent soft tissue, trachea and oesophagus. These features include: dyspnoea, dysphagia and hoarseness, in association with rapidly-growing tumour in the neck. The tumour metastasises both to regional lymph nodes and to distant organs such as the lungs.

PATHOLOGIC CHANGES. ***Grossly,*** the tumour is generally large and irregular, often invading the adjacent strap muscles of the neck and other structures in the vicinity of the thyroid. Cut surface of the tumour is white and firm with areas of necrosis and haemorrhages.

Histologically, the tumour is too poorly-differentiated to be placed in any other histologic type of thyroid cancer, but usually shows a component of either papillary or follicular carcinoma in better differentiated areas. The tumour is generally composed of 3 types of cells occurring in varying proportions: small cells, spindle cells and giant cells. When one of these cell types is predominant, the histologic variant of undifferentiated carcinoma is named accordingly. Thus, there are 3 histologic variants:

1. Small cell carcinoma: This type of tumour is composed of closely packed small cells having hyperchromatic nuclei and numerous mitoses. This variant closely resembles malignant lymphoma.

2. Spindle cell carcinoma: These tumours are composed of spindle cells resembling sarcoma. Some tumours may contain obvious sarcomatous component such as areas of osteosarcoma, chondrosarcoma or rhabdomyosarcoma.

3. Giant cell carcinoma: This type is composed of highly anaplastic giant cells showing numerous atypical mitoses, bizarre and lobed nuclei and some assuming spindle shapes.

The prognosis is poor: 5-year survival rate is less than 10% and median survival after the diagnosis is about 2 months.

PARATHYROID GLANDS

NORMAL STRUCTURE

ANATOMY. The parathyroid glands are usually 4 in number: the *superior pair* derived from the 3rd branchial pouch and *inferior pair* from the 4th branchial pouch of primitive foregut. Both pairs are usually embedded in the posterior aspect of the thyroid substance but separated from it by a connective tissue capsule. In the adults, each gland is an oval, yellowish-brown, flattened body, weighing 35-45 mg. There may, however, be variation in the number, location and size of parathyroid glands.

HISTOLOGY AND FUNCTIONS. ***Microscopically,*** parathyroid glands are composed of solid sheets and cords of parenchymal cells and variable amount of stromal fat. The parenchymal cells are of 3 types: *chief cells, oxyphil cells* and *water-clear cells.* The chief cells are most numerous and are the major source of parathyroid hormone. The latter two types of cells appear to be derived from the chief cells and have sparse secretory granules but are potentially capable of secreting parathyroid hormone.

The major *function* of the parathyroid hormone, in conjunction with calcitonin and vitamin D, is to regulate serum calcium levels and metabolism of bone. Parathyroid hormone tends to elevate serum calcium level and reduce serum phosphate level. Secretion of parathyroid hormone takes place in response to serum levels of calcium by a feedback mechanism—lowered serum calcium stimulates secretion of parathyroid hormone, while elevated serum calcium causes decreased secretion of the hormone. The role of parathyroid hormone in regulating calcium metabolism in the body is at the following 3 levels:

1. Parathyroid hormone *stimulates osteoclastic activity* and results in resorption of bone and release of calcium. Calcitonin released by C-cells, on the other hand, opposes parathyroid hormone by preventing resorption of bone and lowering serum calcium level.

2. Parathyroid hormone acts *directly on renal tubular epithelial cells* and increases renal reabsorption of calcium and inhibits reabsorption of phosphate; calcitonin enhances renal excretion of phosphate.
3. Parathyroid hormone increases renal production of the *most active metabolite of vitamin D,* 1, 25-dihydrocholecalciferol, which in turn increases calcium absorption from the small intestine.

The major parathyroid disorders are its functional disorders (hyper- and hypoparathyroidism) and neoplasms.

HYPERPARATHYROIDISM

Hyperfunction of the parathyroid glands occurs due to excessive production of parathyroid hormone. It is classified into 3 types—primary, secondary and tertiary.

- *Primary hyperparathyroidism* occurs from oversecretion of parathyroid hormone due to disease of the parathyroid glands.
- *Secondary hyperparathyroidism* is caused by diseases in other parts of the body.
- *Tertiary hyperparathyroidism* develops from secondary hyperplasia after removal of the cause of secondary hyperplasia.

Primary Hyperparathyroidism

Primary hyperparathyroidism is not uncommon and occurs more commonly with increasing age. It is especially likely to occur in women near the time of menopause.

ETIOLOGY. Common causes of primary hyperparathyroidism are as follows:
1. Most commonly, parathyroid adenomas in approximately 80% cases.
2. Carcinoma of the parathyroid glands in 2-3% patients.
3. Primary hyperplasia in about 15% cases (usually chief cell hyperplasia).

Also included above are the familial cases of multiple endocrine neoplasia (MEN) syndromes where parathyroid adenoma or primary hyperplasia is one of the components.

CLINICAL FEATURES. The patients with primary hyperparathyroidism have the following characteristic biochemical abnormalities:
1. Elevated levels of parathyroid hormone
2. Hypercalcaemia
3. Hypophosphataemia
4. Hypercalciuria

Clinical presentation of individuals with primary hyperparathyroidism may be in a variety of ways:
1. Most commonly, *nephrolithiasis* and or/*nephrocalcinosis* (page 714). These dysfunctions result from excessive excretion of calcium in the urine due to hypercalcaemia induced by increased parathyroid hormone level.
2. *Metastatic calcification*, especially in the blood vessels, kidneys, lungs, stomach, eyes and other tissues (page 57).
3. *Generalised osteitis fibrosa cystica* due to osteoclastic resorption of bone and its replacement by connective tissue (page 861).
4. *Neuropsychiatric disturbances* such as depression, anxiety, psychosis and coma.
5. *Hypertension* is found in about half the cases.
6. *Other changes* such as pancreatitis, cholelithiasis and peptic ulcers due to hypercalcaemia and high parathyroid hormone level are less constant features.

Secondary Hyperparathyroidism

Secondary hyperparathyroidism occurs due to increased parathyroid hormone elaboration secondary to a disease elsewhere in the body. Hypocalcaemia stimulates compensatory hyperplasia of the parathyroid glands and causes secondary hyperparathyroidism.

ETIOLOGY. Though any condition that causes hypocalcaemia stimulates excessive secretion of parathyroid hormone, the important causes of secondary hyperparathyroidism are as under:
1. *Chronic renal insufficiency* resulting in retention of phosphate and impaired intestinal absorption of calcium.
2. *Vitamin D deficiency* and consequent rickets and osteomalacia may cause parathyroid hyperfunction.
3. *Intestinal malabsorption syndromes* causing deficiency of calcium and vitamin D.

CLINICAL FEATURES. The main biochemical abnor–mality in secondary hyperparathyroidism is mild hypocalcaemia, in striking contrast to hypercalcaemia in primary hyperparathyroidism. The patients with secondary hyperparathyroidism have signs and symptoms of the disease which caused it. Usually, secondary hyperparathyroidism is a beneficial compensatory mechanism, but more severe cases may be associated with renal osteodystrophy (i.e. features of varying degree of osteitis fibrosa, osteomalacia, osteoporosis and osteosclerosis in cases of chronic renal insufficiency) and soft tissue calcification (Fig. 25.12).

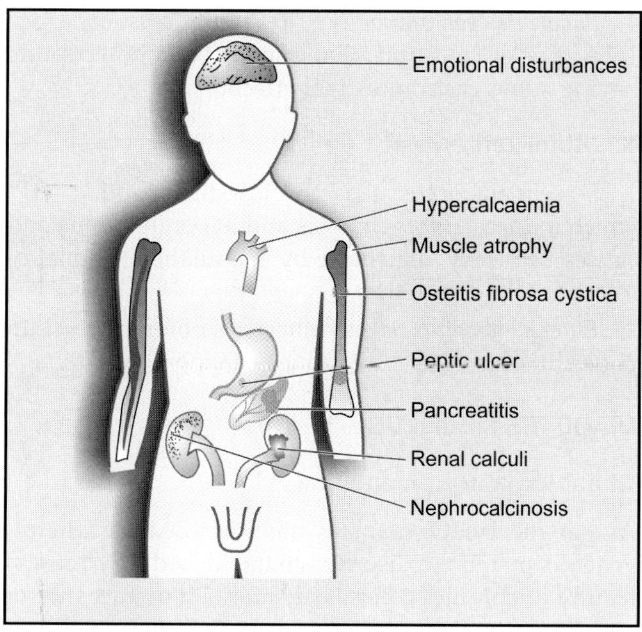

FIGURE 25.12

Major clinical manifestations of hyperparathyroidism.

Tertiary Hyperparathyroidism

Tertiary hyperparathyroidism is a complication of secondary hyperparathyroidism in which the hyperfunction persists in spite of removal of the cause of secondary hyperplasia. Possibly, a hyperplastic nodule in the parathyroid gland develops which becomes partially autonomous and continues to secrete large quantities of parathyroid hormone without regard to the needs of the body.

HYPOPARATHYROIDISM

Deficiency or absence of parathyroid hormone secretion causes hypoparathyroidism. Hypoparathyroidism is of 3 types—*primary, pseudo-* and *pseudopseudo-hypoparathyroidism.*

Primary Hypoparathyroidism

Primary hypoparathyroidism is caused by disease of the parathyroid glands. Most common causes of primary hypoparathyroidism are: surgical procedures involving thyroid, parathyroid, or radical neck dissection for cancer. Other causes are uncommon and include idiopathic hypoparathyroidism of autoimmune origin in children and may occur as sporadic or familial cases. These cases are generally associated with other autoimmune diseases.

CLINICAL FEATURES. The main biochemical dysfunctions in primary hypoparathyroidism are hypocalcaemia, hyperphosphataemia and hypocalciuria. The clinical manifestations of these abnormalities are:

1. increased neuromuscular irritability and tetany;
2. calcification of the lens and cataract formation;
3. abnormalities in cardiac conduction;
4. disorders of the CNS due to intracranial calcification; and
5. abnormalities of the teeth.

Pseudo-hypoparathyroidism

In pseudo-hypoparathyroidism, the tissues fail to respond to parathyroid hormone though parathyroid glands are usually normal. It is a rare inherited condition with an autosomal dominant character. The patients are generally females and are characterised by signs and symptoms of hypoparathyroidism and other clinical features like short stature, short metacarpals and metatarsals, flat nose, round face and multiple exostoses. Since renal tubules cannot adequately respond to parathyroid hormone, there is hypercalciuria, hypocalcaemia and hyperphosphataemia.

Pseudopseudo-hypoparathyroidism

Pseudopseudo-hypoparathyroidism is another rare familial disorder in which all the clinical features of pseudo-hypoparathyroidism are present except that these patients have no hypocalcaemia or hyperphosphataemia and the tissues respond normally to parathyroid hormone. Pseudopseudo-hypoparathyroidism has been considered an incomplete form of pseudo-hypoparathyroidism.

PARATHYROID TUMOURS

Parathyroid adenoma and carcinoma are the neoplasms found in parathyroid glands, the former being much more common than the latter.

Parathyroid Adenoma

The commonest tumour of the parathyroid glands is an adenoma. It may occur at any age and in either sex but is found more frequently in adult life. Most adenomas are first brought to attention because of excessive secretion of parathyroid hormone causing features of hyperparathyroidism as described above.

PATHOLOGIC CHANGES. ***Grossly,*** a parathyroid adenoma is small (less than 5 cm diameter) encapsulated, yellowish-brown, ovoid nodule and weighing up to 5 gm or more.

Microscopically, majority of adenomas are predominantly composed of chief cells arranged in sheets or cords. Oxyphil cells and water-clear cells may be found intermingled in varying proportions. Usually, a rim of normal parathyroid parenchyma and fat are present external to the capsule which help to distinguish an adenoma from diffuse hyperplasia.

Parathyroid Carcinoma

Carcinoma of the parathyroid is rare and produces manifestations of hyperparathyroidism which is often more pronounced. Carcinoma tends to be irregular in shape and is adherent to the adjacent tissues. Most parathyroid carcinomas are well-differentiated. It may be difficult to distinguish carcinoma of parathyroid gland from an adenoma but local invasion of adjacent tissues and distant metastases are helpful criteria of malignancy in such cases.

ENDOCRINE PANCREAS

The human pancreas, though anatomically a single organ, histologically and functionally, has 2 distinct parts—the exocrine and endocrine. The exocrine part of the gland and its disorders have already been discussed in Chapter 19. The discussion here deals with the endocrine pancreas and its two main disorders: *diabetes mellitus* and *islet cell tumours.*

NORMAL STRUCTURE

The endocrine pancreas consists of microscopic collections of cells called islets of Langerhans found scattered within the pancreatic lobules, as well as individual endocrine cells found in duct epithelium and among the acini. The total weight of endocrine pancreas in the adult, however, does not exceed 1-1.5 gm (total weight of pancreas 60-100 gm). The islet cell tissue is greatly concentrated in the tail than in the head or body of the pancreas. Islets possess no ductal system and they drain their secretory products directly into the circulation. Ultrastructurally and immunohistochemically, 4 *major* and 2 *minor* types of islet cells are distinguished, each type having its distinct secretory product and function. These are as follows:

A. Major cell types:

1. *Beta (B) cells* comprise about 70% of islet cells and secrete insulin, the defective response or deficient synthesis of which causes diabetes mellitus.

2. *Alpha (A) cells* comprise 20% of islet cells and secrete glucagon which induces hyperglycaemia.

3. *Delta (D) cells* comprise 5-10% of islet cells and secrete somatostatin which suppresses both insulin and glucagon release.

4. *Pancreatic polypeptide (PP) cells or F cells* comprise 1-2% of islet cells and secrete pancreatic polypeptide having some gastrointestinal effects.

B. Minor cell types:

1. *D1 cells* elaborate vasoactive intestinal peptide (VIP) which induces glycogenolysis and hyperglycaemia and causes secretory diarrhoea by stimulation of gastrointestinal fluid secretion.

2. *Enterochromaffin cells* synthesise serotonin which in pancreatic tumours may induce carcinoid syndrome.

DIABETES MELLITUS

Definition and Epidemiology

As per the WHO, diabetes mellitus (DM) is a hetrogeneous metabolic disorder characterised by common feature of chronic hyperglycaemia with disturbance of carbohydrate, fat and protein metabolism.

DM is a leading cause of morbidity and mortality the world over. It is estimated that approximately 1% of population suffers from DM. The incidence is rising in the developed countries of the world, especially of type 2 DM, due to rising incidence of obesity and reduced activity levels. DM is expected to continue as a major health problem owing to its serious complications, especially end-stage renal disease, IHD, gangrene of the lower extremities and blindness in the adults.

Classification and Etiology

The older classification systems dividing DM into primary (idiopathic) and secondary types, juvenile-onset and maturity onset types, and insulin-dependent (IDDM) and non-insulin independent (NIDDM) types, have become obsolete and undergone major revision due to extensive understanding of etiology and pathogenesis of DM in recent times.

As outlined in Table 25.4 based on etiology, currently DM is classified into two broad categories (type 1 and type 2), a few uncommon specific etiologic types, and gestational DM. Brief comments on these etiologic terminologies as contrasted with former nomenclatures of DM are given below:

TYPE 1 DM. It constitutes about 10% cases of DM. It was previously termed as juvenile-onset diabetes (JOD) due to its occurrence in younger age, and was called insulin-dependent DM (IDDM) because these patients had absolute requirement for insulin replacement as treatment. However, in the new classification, neither

TABLE 25.4: Etiologic Classification of Diabetes Mellitus (as per American Diabetes Association, 2000).

I. **Type 1 diabetes mellitus (10%)** (earlier called Insulin-dependent, or juvenile-onset diabetes)

Type IA DM: Immune-mediated

Type IB DM: Idiopathic

II. **Type 2 diabetes mellitus (80%)** (earlier called non-insulin-dependent, or maturity-onset diabetes)

III. **Other specific types of diabetes (10%)**

A. Genetic defect of β-cell function due to mutations in various enzymes (earlier called maturity-onset diabetes of the young or MODY) (e.g. hepatocyte nuclear transcription factor HNF, glucokinase)

B. Genetic defect in insulin action (e.g. type A insulin resistance)

C. Diseases of exocrine pancreas (e.g. chronic pancreatitis, pancreatic tumours, post-pancreatectomy)

D. Endocrinopathies (e.g. acromegaly, Cushing's syndrome, pheochromocytoma)

E. Drug- or chemical-induced (e.g. steroids, thyroid hormone, thiazides, β-blockers etc)

F. Infections (e.g. congenital rubella, cytomegalovirus)

G. Uncommon forms of immune-mediated DM (stiff man syndrome, anti-insulin receptor antibodies)

H. Other genetic syndromes (e.g. Down's syndrome, Klinefelter's syndrome, Turner's syndrome)

IV. **Gestational diabetes mellitus**

age nor insulin-dependence are considered as absolute criteria. Instead, based on underlying etiology, type 1 DM is further divided into 2 subtypes:

Subtype 1A (immune-mediated) DM characterised by autoimmune destruction of β-cells which usually leads to insulin deficiency.

Subtype 1B (idiopathic) DM is characterised by insulin deficiency with tendency to develop ketosis but these patients are negative for autoimmune markers.

Though type 1 DM occurs commonly in patients under 30 years of age, autoimmune destruction of β-cells can occur at any age. In fact, 5-10% patients who develop DM above 30 years of age are of type 1A DM and hence the term JOD has become obsolete.

TYPE 2 DM. This type comprises about 80% cases of DM. It was previously called maturity-onset diabetes, or non-insulin dependent diabetes mellitus (NIDDM) of obese and non-obese type.

Although type 2 DM predominantly affects older individuals, it is now known that it also occurs in obese adolescent children; hence the term MOD for it is inappropriate. Moreover, many type 2 DM patients also require insulin therapy to control hyperglycaemia or to prevent ketosis and thus are not truly non-insulin dependent contrary to its former nomenclature.

The contrasting features of the two main forms of diabetes mellitus are presented in Table 25.5.

OTHER SPECIFIC ETIOLOGIC TYPES OF DM. Besides the two main types, about 10% cases of DM have a known specific etiologic defect; these are listed in Table 25.4. One important subtype in this group is *maturity-onset diabetes of the young (MODY)* which has autosomal dominant inheritance, early onset of hyperglycaemia and impaired insulin secretion.

GESTATIONAL DM. About 4% pregnant women develop DM due to metabolic changes during pregnancy. Although they revert back to normal glycaemia after delivery, these women are prone to develop DM later in their life.

Pathogenesis

Depending upon etiology of DM, hyperglycaemia may result from:

- reduced insulin secretion;
- decreased glucose use by the body; and
- increased glucose production.

Pathogenesis of two main types of DM and its complications is distinct. In order to understand it properly, it is essential to relearn physiology of normal insulin synthesis and secretion.

NORMAL INSULIN METABOLISM. *The major stimulus for both synthesis and release of insulin is glucose.* The steps involved in biosynthesis, release and actions of insulin are as follows:

Synthesis. Insulin is synthesised in the β-cells of pancreatic islets of Langerhans (Fig. 25.13,A):

i) It is initially formed as *pre-proinsulin* which is single-chain 86-amino acid precursor polypeptide.

ii) Subsequent proteolysis removes the amino terminal signal peptide, forming *proinsulin*.

iii) Further cleavage of proinsulin gives rise to *A (21 amino acids) and B (30 amino acids) chains* of insulin, linked together by connecting segment called *C-peptide*, all of which are stored in the secretory granules in the β-cells. As compared to A and B chains of insulin, C-peptide is less susceptible to degradation in the liver and is therefore used as a marker to distinguish endogenously synthesised and exogenously administered insulin.

iv) For therapeutic use, *human insulin* is now produced by recombinant DNA technology.

Release. Glucose is the key regulator of insulin secretion from β–cells by a series of steps (Fig. 25.13,A):

i) Hypoglycaemia (glucose level below 70 mg/dL or below 3.9 mmol/L) stimulates transport into β-cells of a *glu*cose *t*ransporter, *GLUT2*. Other stimuli influencing

TABLE 25.5: Contrasting Features of Type 1 and Type 2 Diabetes Mellitus.

	FEATURE	TYPE 1 DM	TYPE 2 DM
1.	*Frequency*	10-20%	80-90%
2.	*Age at onset*	Early (below 35 years)	Late (after 40 years)
3.	*Type of onset*	Abrupt and severe	Gradual and insidious
4.	*Weight*	Normal	Obese/non-obese
5.	*HLA*	Linked to HLA DR3, HLA DR4, HLA DQ	No HLA association
6.	*Family history*	< 20%	About 60%
7.	*Genetic locus*	Unknown	Chromosome 6
8.	*Diabetes in identical twins*	50% concordance	80% concordance
9.	*Pathogenesis*	Autoimmune destruction of β-cells	Insulin resistance, impaired insulin secretion
10.	*Islet cell antibodies*	Yes	No
11.	*Blood insulin level*	Decreased insulin	Normal or increased insulin
12.	*Islet cell changes*	Insulitis, β-cell depletion	No insulitis, later fibrosis of islets
13.	*Amyloidosis*	Infrequent	Common in chronic cases
14.	*Clinical management*	Insulin and diet	Diet, exercise, oral drugs, insulin
15.	*Acute complications*	Ketoacidosis	Hyperosmolar coma

insulin release include nutrients in the meal, ketones, amino acids etc.

ii) An islet transcription factor, *glucokinase,* causes glucose phosphorylation, and thus acts as a step for controlled release of glucose-regulated insulin secretion.

iii) Metabolism of glucose to glucose-6-phosphate by glycolysis generates *ATP*.

iv) Generation of ATP *alters the ion channel activity* on the membrane. It causes inhibition of ATP-sensitive K^+ channel on the cell membrane and opening up of calcium channel with resultant influx of calcium, which stimulates insulin release.

Action. Half of insulin secreted from β-cells into portal vein is degraded in the liver while the remaining half enters the systemic circulation for action on the target cells (Fig. 25.13,B):

i) Insulin from circulation binds to its receptor on the target cells. This *insulin receptor* has intrinsic tyrosine kinase activity.

ii) This, in turn, activates post-receptor intracellular signalling pathway molecules, *insulin receptor substrates (IRS) 1 and 2 proteins,* which initiate sequence of phosphorylation and dephosphorylation reactions.

iii) These reactions on the target cells are responsible for the main *mitogenic and anabolic actions of insulin*—glycogen synthesis, glucose transport, protein synthesis, lipogenesis.

iv) Besides the role of glucose in maintaining equilibrium of insulin release, *low insulin level in the fasting state* promotes hepatic gluconeogenesis and glycogenolysis, reduced glucose uptake by insulin-sensitive tissues and promotes mobilisation of stored precursors, so as to prevent hypoglycaemia.

PATHOGENESIS OF TYPE 1 DM. *The basic phenomena in type 1 DM is destruction of β-cell mass, usually leading to absolute insulin deficiency.* While type 1B DM remains idiopathic, pathogenesis of type 1A DM is immune-mediated and has been extensively studied. Currently, pathogenesis of type 1A DM is explained on the basis of 3 mutually-interlinked mechanisms: genetic susceptibility, autoimmune factors, and certain environmental factors (Fig. 25.14,A).

1. Genetic susceptibility. Type 1A DM involves inheritance of multiple genes to confer susceptibility to the disorder:

i) It has been observed in *identical twins* that if one twin has type 1A DM, there is about 50% chance of the second twin developing it, but not all. This means that some additional modifying factors are involved in development of DM in these cases.

ii) About half the cases with genetic predisposition to type 1A DM have the *susceptibility gene* located in the HLA region of chromosome 6 (MHC class II region), particularly HLA DR3, HLA DR4 and HLA DQ locus.

It appears that in a HLA-associated susceptible individual, β–cells act as autoantigens and activate CD4+ T lymphocytes, bringing about immune destruction of pancreatic β–cells.

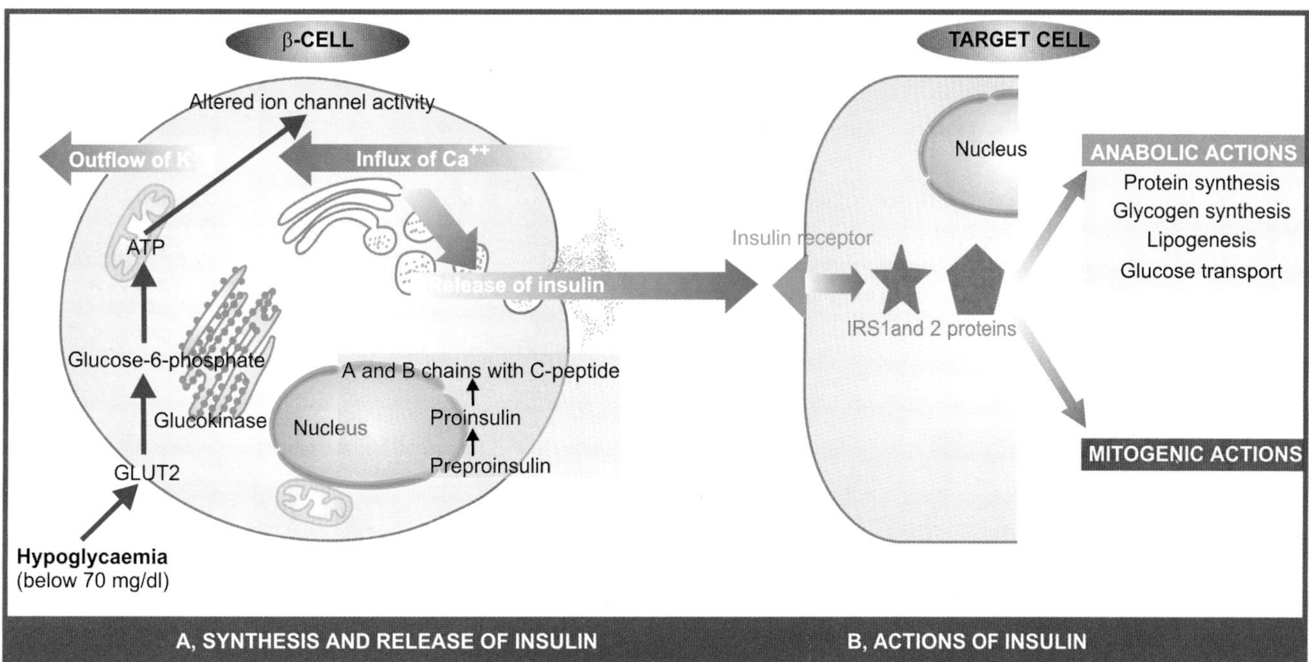

FIGURE 25.13

A, Pathway of normal insulin synthesis and release in β-cells of pancreatic islets. B, Chain of events in action of insulin on target cell.

2. Autoimmune factors. Studies on humans and animal models on type 1A DM have shown several immunologic abnormalities:

i) Presence of *islet cell antibodies* against GAD (glutamic acid decarboxylase), insulin etc, though its assay largely remained as a research tool due to tedious method.

ii) Occurrence of lymphocytic infiltrate in and around the pancreatic islets termed *insulitis*. It chiefly consists of CD8+ T lymphocytes with variable number of CD4+ T lymphocytes and macrophages.

iii) *Selective destruction of β-cells* while other islet cell types (glucagon-producing alpha cells, somatostatin-producing delta cells, or polypeptide-forming PP cells) remain unaffected. This is mediated by T-cell mediated cytotoxicity or by apoptosis.

iv) Role of *T cell-mediated autoimmunity* is further supported by transfer of type 1A DM from diseased animal by infusing T lymphocytes to a healthy animal.

v) Association of type 1A DM with *other autoimmune diseases* in about 10-20% cases such as Graves' disease, Addison's disease, Hashimoto's thyroiditis, pernicious anaemia.

vi) Remission of type 1A DM in response to immunosuppressive therapy such as administration of cyclosporin A.

3. Environmental factors. Epidemiologic studies in type 1A DM suggest the involvement of certain environmental factors in its pathogenesis, though role of none of them has been conclusively proved. In fact, the trigger may precede the occurrence of the disease by several years. It appears that certain viral and dietary proteins share antigenic properties with human cell surface proteins and trigger the immune attack on β-cells by a process of molecular mimicry. These factors include the following:

i) *Certain viral infections* preceding the onset of disease e.g. mumps, measles, coxsackie B virus, cytomegalovirus and infectious mononucleosis.

ii) *Experimental induction* of type 1A DM with certain chemicals has been possible e.g. alloxan, streptozotocin and pentamidine.

iii) *Geographic and seasonal variations* in its incidence suggest some common environmental factors.

iv) Possible relationship of early exposure to *bovine milk proteins* and occurrence of autoimmune process in type 1A DM is being studied.

SUMMARY: Pathogenesis of type 1A DM can be summed up by interlinking the above three factors as under:

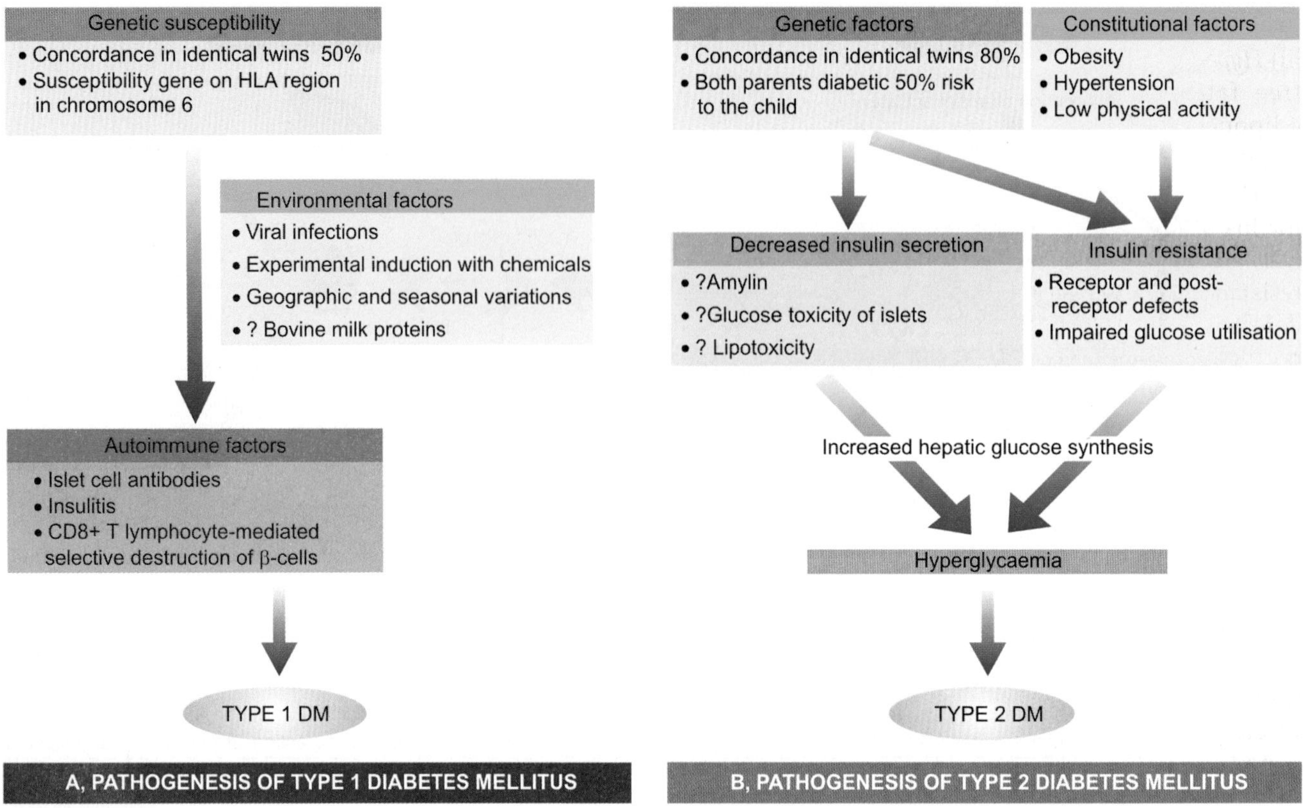

FIGURE 25.14

Schematic mechanisms involved in pathogenesis of two main types of diabetes mellitus.

1. At birth, individuals with *genetic susceptibility* to this disorder have normal β-cell mass.
2. Destruction of β–cell mass occurs by *autoimmune phenomena* and takes months to years. Clinical features of diabetes manifest after more than 80% of β-cell mass has been destroyed.
3. The trigger for autoimmune process appears to be some *infectious or environmental factor* which specifically targets β-cells.

PATHOGENESIS OF TYPE 2 DM. The basic metabolic defect in type 2 DM is either a delayed insulin secretion relative to glucose load *(impaired insulin secretion)*, or the peripheral tissues are unable to respond to insulin *(insulin resistance)*.

Type 2 DM is a heterogeneous disorder with a more complex etiology and is far more common than type 1, but much less is known about its pathogenesis. A number of factors have been implicated though, but HLA association and autoimmune phenomena are not implicated. These factors are as under (Fig. 25.14,B):

1. Genetic factors. Genetic component has a stronger basis for type 2 DM than type 1A DM. Although no definite and consistent genes have been identified, multifactorial inheritance is the most important factor in development of type 2 DM:

i) There is approximately 80% chance of developing diabetes in the other *identical twin* if one twin has the disease.

ii) A person with one parent having type 2 DM is at an increased risk of getting diabetes, but if *both parents* have type 2 DM the risk in the offspring rises to 40%.

2. Constitutional factors. Certain environmental factors such as obesity, hypertension, and level of physical activity play contributory role and modulate the phenotyping of the disease.

3. Insulin resistance. One of the most prominent metabolic features of type 2 DM is the lack of responsiveness of peripheral tissues to insulin, especially of skeletal muscle and liver. Obesity, in particular, is strongly associated with insulin resistance and hence type 2 DM. Mechanism of hyperglycaemia in these cases is explained as under:

i) Resistance to action of insulin *impairs glucose utilisation* and hence hyperglycaemia.

ii) There is *increased hepatic synthesis* of glucose.

iii) *Hyperglycaemia in obesity* is related to high levels of free fatty acids and cytokines (e.g. TNF-α and adiponectin) affect peripheral tissue sensitivity to respond to insulin.

The precise underlying molecular defect responsible for insulin resistance in type 2 DM has yet not been fully identified. Currently, it is proposed that insulin resistance may be possibly due to one of the following defects:

- Polymorphism in various *post-receptor intracellular signal pathway molecules.*
- *Elevated free fatty acids* seen in obesity may contribute e.g. by impaired glucose utilisation in the skeletal muscle, by increased hepatic synthesis of glucose, and by impaired β–cell function.

Insulin resistance syndrome is a complex of clinical features occurring from insulin resistance and its resultant metabolic derangements that includes hyperglycaemia and compensatory hyperinsulinaemia. The clinical features are in the form of accelerated cardiovascular disease and may occur in both obese as well as non-obese type 2 DM patients. The features include: mild hypertension (related to endothelial dysfunction) and dyslipidaemia (characterised by reduced HDL level, increased triglycerides and LDL level).

4. Impaired insulin secretion. In type 2 DM, insulin resistance and insulin secretion are interlinked:

i) Early in the course of disease, in response to insulin resistance there is compensatory increased secretion of insulin (*hyperinsulinaemia*) in an attempt to maintain normal blood glucose level.

ii) Eventually, however, there is *failure of β–cell function* to secrete adequate insulin, although there is some secretion of insulin i.e. cases of type 2 DM have mild to moderate deficiency of insulin (which is much less severe than that in type 1 DM) but not its total absence.

The exact genetic mechanism why there is a fall in insulin secretion in these cases is unclear. However, following possibilities are proposed:

- Islet amyloid polypeptide (*amylin*) which forms fibrillar protein deposits in pancreatic islets in longstanding cases of type 2 DM may be responsible for impaired function of β-cells islet cells.
- Metabolic environment of chronic hyperglycaemia surrounding the islets *(glucose toxicity)* may paradoxically impair islet cell function.
- Elevated free fatty acid levels (*lipotoxicity*) in these cases may worsen islet cell function.

5. Increased hepatic glucose synthesis. One of the normal roles played by insulin is to promote hepatic storage of glucose as glycogen and suppress gluconeogenesis. In type 2 DM, as a part of insulin resistance by peripheral tissues, liver also shows insulin resistance i.e. in spite of hyperinsulinaemia in the early stage of disease, gluconeogenesis in the liver is not suppressed. This results in increased hepatic synthesis of glucose which contributes to hyperglycaemia in these cases.

SUMMARY: In essence, hyperglycaemia in type 2 DM is not due to destruction of β-cells but is instead a failure of β-cells to meet the requirement of insulin in the body. Its pathogenesis can be summed up by interlinking the above factors as under:

1. Type 2 DM is a more *complex multifactorial disease.*
2. There is greater role of *genetic defect and heredity.*
3. The two main mechanisms for hyperglycaemia in type 2 DM—*insulin resistance and impaired insulin secretion*, are interlinked.
4. While *obesity* plays a role in pathogenesis of insulin resistance, impaired insulin secretion may be from many constitutional factors.
5. *Increased hepatic synthesis of glucose* in initial period of disease contributes to hyperglycaemia.

Pathologic Changes in Pancreatic Islets

Pathologic changes in islets have been demonstrated in both types of diabetes, though the changes are more distinctive in type 1 DM.

1. INSULITIS: In type 1 DM, characteristically, in early stage there is lymphocytic infiltrate, mainly by T cells, in the islets which may be accompanied by a few macrophages and polymorphs. Diabetic infants born to diabetic mothers, however, have eosinophilic infiltrate in the islets.

In type 2 DM, there is no significant leucocytic infiltrate in the islets but there is variable degree of fibrous tissue in the islets.

2. ISLET CELL MASS: In type 1 DM, as the disease becomes chronic there is progressive depletion of β–cell mass, eventually resulting in total loss of pancreatic β–cells.

In type 2 DM, β-cell mass is either normal or mildly reduced. Infants of diabetic mothers, however, have hyperplasia and hypertrophy of islets as a compensatory response to maternal hyperglycaemia.

3. β-CELL DEGRANULATION: In type 1 DM, EM shows degranulation of remaining β-cells of islets.

In type 2 DM, no such change is observed.

4. AMYLOIDOSIS: In type 1 DM, deposits of amyloid around islets are absent.

In type 2 DM, characteristically chronic long-standing cases show deposition of amyloid material around the capillaries of the islets causing compression and atrophy of islet tissue.

Clinical Features

It can be appreciated that hyperglycaemia in DM does not cause a single disease but is associated with numerous diseases and symptoms, especially due to complications. Two main types of DM can be distinguished clinically to the extent shown in Table 25.5. However, overlapping of clinical features occurs as regards the age of onset, duration of symptoms and family history. Pathophysiology in evolution of clinical features is schematically shown in Fig. 25.15.

Type 1 DM:

i) Patients of type 1 DM usually manifest at early age, generally below the age of 35.

ii) The onset of symptoms is often abrupt.

iii) At presentation, these patients have polyuria, polydipsia and polyphagia.

iv) The patients are not obese but have generally progressive loss of weight.

v) These patients are prone to develop metabolic complications such as ketoacidosis and hypoglycaemic episodes.

Type 2 DM:

i) This form of diabetes generally manifests in middle life or beyond, usually above the age of 40.

ii) The onset of symptoms in type 2 DM is slow and insidious.

iii) Generally, the patient is asymptomatic when the diagnosis is made on the basis of glucosuria or hyperglycaemia during physical examination, or may present with polyuria and polydipsia.

iv) The patients are frequently obese and have unexplained weakness and loss of weight.

v) Metabolic complications such as ketoacidosis are infrequent.

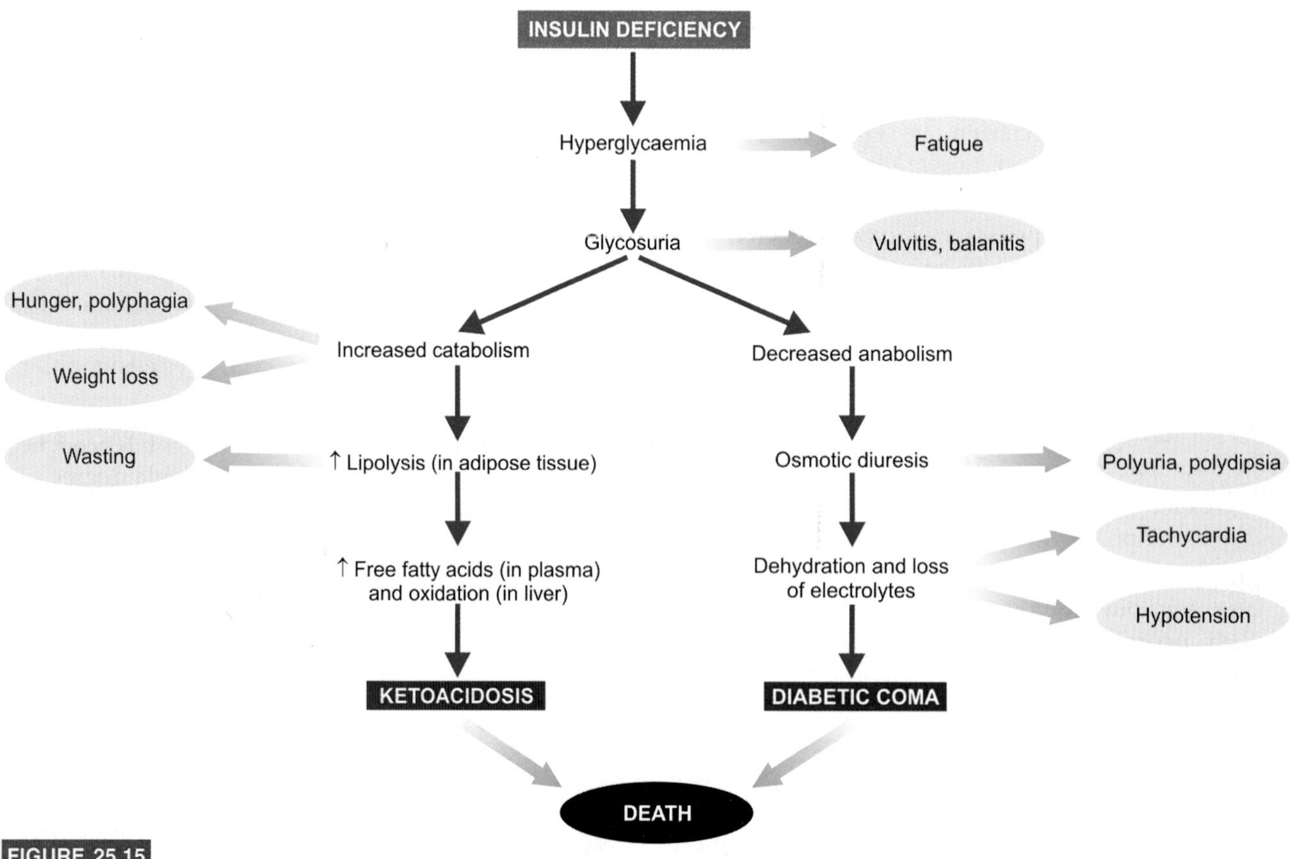

FIGURE 25.15

Pathophysiological basis of common signs and symptoms due to uncontrolled hyperglycaemia in diabetes mellitus.

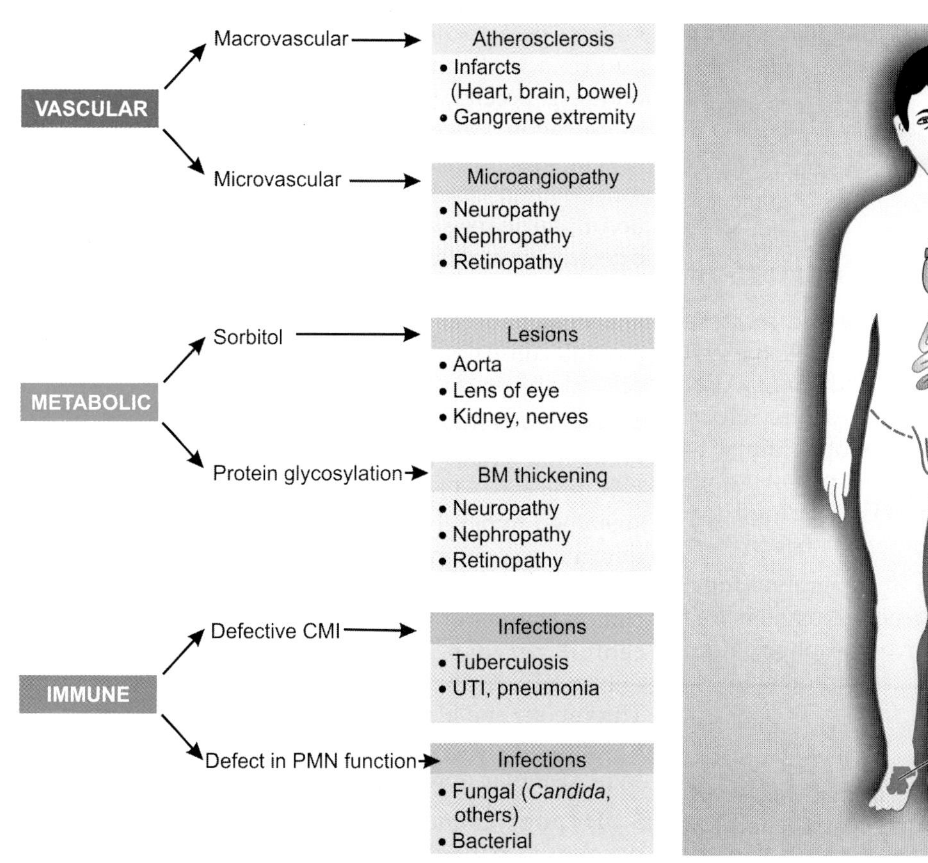

A, PATHOGENESIS OF LONG TERM COMPLICATIONS OF DIABETES

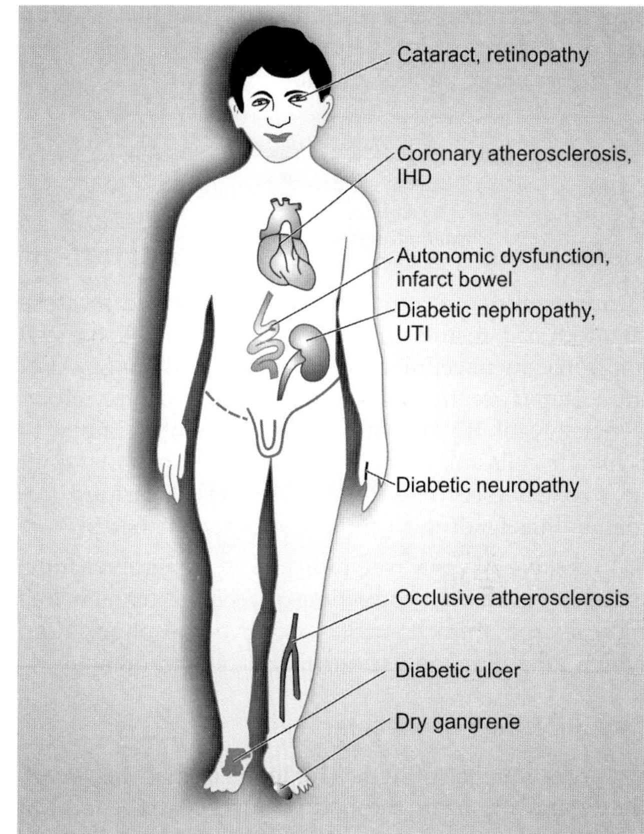

B, SECONDARY SYSTEMIC COMPLICATIONS OF DIABETES

FIGURE 25.16

Long-term complications of diabetes mellitus. A, Pathogenesis. B, Secondary systemic complications.

Pathogenesis of Complications

It is now known that in both type 1 and 2 DM, *severity and chronicity of hyperglycaemia* forms the main pathogenetic mechanism for 'microvascular complications' (e.g. retinopathy, nephropathy, neuropathy); therefore control of blood glucose level constitutes the mainstay of treatment for minimising development of these complications. Longstanding cases of type 2 DM, however, in addition, frequently develop 'macrovascular complications' (e.g. atherosclerosis, coronary artery disease, peripheral vascular disease, cerebrovascular disease) which are more difficult to explain on the basis of hyperglycaemia alone.

The following biochemical mechanisms have been proposed to explain the development of complications of diabetes mellitus (Fig. 25.16,A):

1. Non-enzymatic protein glycosylation: The free amino group of various body proteins binds by non-enzymatic mechanism to glucose; this process is called *glycosylation* and is directly proportionate to the severity of hyperglycaemia. Various body proteins undergoing chemical alterations in this way include haemoglobin, lens crystalline protein, and basement membrane of body cells. An example is the measurement of a fraction of haemoglobin called glycosylated haemoglobin (HbA_{1C}) as a test for monitoring glycaemic control in a diabetic patient during the preceding 100 to 120 days which is lifespan of red cells (page 361) . Similarly, there is accumulation of labile and reversible glycosylation products on collagen and other tissues of the blood vessel wall which subsequently become stable and irreversible by chemical changes and form advanced glycosylation end-products (AGE). The AGEs bind to receptors on different cells and produce a variety of biologic and chemical changes e.g. thickening of vascular basement membrane in diabetes.

2. Polyol pathway mechanism: This mechanism is responsible for producing lesions in the aorta, lens of the eye, kidney and peripheral nerves. These tissues have an enzyme, aldose reductase, that reacts with glucose to form sorbitol and fructose in the cells of the hyperglycaemic patient as under:

$$\text{Glucose} + \text{NADH} + \text{H}^+ \xrightarrow{\text{aldose reductase}} \text{Sorbitol} + \text{NAD}^+$$

$$\text{Sorbitol} + \text{NAD} \xrightarrow[\text{dehydrogenase}]{\text{sorbitol}} \text{Fructose} + \text{NADH} + \text{H}^+$$

Intracellular accumulation of sorbitol and fructose so produced results in entry of water inside the cell and consequent cellular swelling and cell damage. Also, intracellular accumulation of sorbitol causes intracellular deficiency of myoinositol which promotes injury to Schwann cells and retinal pericytes. These polyols result in disturbed processing of normal intermediary metabolites leading to complications of diabetes.

3. Excessive oxygen free radicals. In hyperglycaemia, there is increased production of reactive oxygen free radicals from mitochondrial oxidative phosphorylation which may damage various target cells in diabetes.

Complications of Diabetes

As a consequence of hyperglycaemia of diabetes, every tissue and organ of the body undergoes biochemical and structural alterations which account for the major complications in diabetics which may be *acute metabolic* or *chronic systemic*.

Both types of diabetes mellitus may develop complications which are broadly divided into 2 major groups:

I. *Acute metabolic complications:* These include diabetic ketoacidosis, hyperosmolar nonketotic coma, and hypoglycaemia.

II. *Late systemic complications:* These are atherosclerosis, diabetic microangiopathy, diabetic nephropathy, diabetic neuropathy, diabetic retinopathy and infections.

I. ACUTE METABOLIC COMPLICATIONS. Metabolic complications develop acutely. While ketoacidosis and hypoglycaemic episodes are primarily complications of type 1 DM, hyperosmolar nonketotic coma is chiefly a complication of type 2 DM (also see Fig. 25.15).

1. Diabetic ketoacidosis. Ketoacidosis is almost exclusively a complication of type 1 DM. It can develop in patients with severe insulin deficiency combined with glucagon excess. Failure to take insulin and exposure to stress are the usual precipitating causes. Severe lack of insulin causes lipolysis in the adipose tissues, resulting in release of free fatty acids into the plasma. These free fatty acids are taken up by the liver where they are oxidised through acetyl coenzyme-A to ketone bodies, principally acetoacetic acid and β-hydroxybutyric acid. Such free fatty acid oxidation to ketone bodies is accelerated in the presence of elevated level of glucagon. Once the rate of ketogenesis exceeds the rate at which the ketone bodies can be utilised by the muscles and other tissues, ketonaemia and ketonuria occur. If urinary excretion of ketone bodies is prevented due to dehydration, systemic metabolic ketoacidosis occurs. Clinically, the condition is characterised by anorexia, nausea, vomitings, deep and fast breathing, mental confusion and coma. Most patients of ketoacidosis recover.

2. Hyperosmolar nonketotic coma. Hyperosmolar nonketotic coma is usually a complication of type 2 DM. It is caused by severe dehydration resulting from sustained hyperglycaemic diuresis. The loss of glucose in urine is so intense that the patient is unable to drink sufficient water to maintain urinary fluid loss. The usual clinical features of ketoacidosis are absent but prominent central nervous signs are present. Blood sugar is extremely high and plasma osmolality is high. Thrombotic and bleeding complications are frequent due to high viscosity of blood. The mortality rate in hyperosmolar nonketotic coma is high.

3. Hypoglycaemia. Hypoglycaemic episode may develop in patients of type 1 DM. It may result from excessive administration of insulin, missing a meal, or due to stress. Hypoglycaemic episodes are harmful as they produce permanent brain damage, or may result in worsening of diabetic control and rebound hyperglycaemia, so called *Somogyi's effect*.

II. LATE SYSTEMIC COMPLICATIONS. A number of systemic complications may develop after a period of 15-20 years in either type of diabetes. These late complications are largely responsible for morbidity and premature mortality in diabetes mellitus. These complications are briefly outlined below as they are discussed in detail in relevant chapters (Fig. 25.16,B).

1. Atherosclerosis. Diabetes mellitus of both type 1and type 2 accelerates the development of atherosclerosis so that consequent atherosclerotic lesions appear earlier than in the general population, are more extensive, and are more often associated with complicated plaques such as ulceration, calcification and thrombosis (page 286). The cause for this accelerated atherosclerotic process is not known but possible contributory factors are hyperlipidaemia, reduced HDL levels, nonenzymatic glycosylation, increased platelet adhesiveness, obesity and associated hypertension in diabetes.

The possible ill-effects of accelerated atherosclerosis in diabetes are early onset of coronary artery disease, silent myocardial infarction, cerebral stroke and gangrene of the toes and feet. Gangrene of the lower extremities is 100 times more common in diabetics than in non-diabetics.

2. Diabetic microangiopathy. Microangiopathy of diabetes is characterised by basement membrane thickening of small blood vessels and capillaries of different organs and tissues such as the skin, skeletal muscle, eye and kidney. Similar type of basement membrane-like material is also deposited in nonvascular tissues such as peripheral nerves, renal tubules and Bowman's capsule. The pathogenesis of diabetic microangiopathy as well as of peripheral neuropathy in diabetics is believed to be due to recurrent hyperglycaemia that causes *increased glycosylation* of haemoglobin and other proteins (e.g. collagen and basement membrane material) resulting in thickening of basement membrane.

3. Diabetic nephropathy. Renal involvement is a common complication and a leading cause of death in diabetes. Four types of lesions are described in diabetic nephropathy (page 701):

i) *Diabetic glomerulosclerosis* which includes diffuse and nodular lesions of glomerulosclerosis.

ii) *Vascular lesions* that include hyaline arteriolosclerosis of afferent and efferent arterioles and atheromas of renal arteries.

iii) *Diabetic pyelonephritis* and *necrotising renal papillitis.*

iv) *Tubular lesions or Armanni-Ebstein lesion.*

4. Diabetic neuropathy. Diabetic neuropathy may affect all parts of the nervous system but symmetric peripheral neuropathy is most characteristic. The basic pathologic changes are segmental demyelination, Schwann cell injury and axonal damage (page 918). The pathogenesis of neuropathy is not clear but it may be related to diffuse microangiopathy as already explained, or may be due to accumulation of sorbitol and fructose as a result of hyperglycaemia, leading to deficiency of myoinositol.

5. Diabetic retinopathy. Diabetic retinopathy is a leading cause of blindness. There are 2 types of lesions involving retinal vessels: *background* and *proliferative* (page 519). Besides retinopathy, diabetes also predisposes the patients to early development of cataract and glaucoma.

6. Infections. Diabetics have enhanced susceptibility to various infections such as tuberculosis, pneumonias, pyelonephritis, otitis, carbuncles and diabetic ulcers. This could be due to various factors such as impaired leucocyte functions, reduced cellular immunity, poor blood supply due to vascular involvement and hyperglycaemia *per se.*

Diagnosis of Diabetes

Hyperglycaemia remains the fundamental basis for the diagnosis of diabetes mellitus. In *symptomatic cases,* the diagnosis is not a problem and can be confirmed by finding glucosuria and a random plasma glucose concentration above 200 mg/dl (Fig. 25.17,D).

- The severity of clinical symptoms of polyuria and polydipsia is directly related to the degree of hyperglycaemia.
- In *asymptomatic cases,* when there is persistently elevated fasting plasma glucose level, diagnosis again poses no difficulty.
- The problem arises in asymptomatic patients who have normal fasting glucose level in the plasma but are suspected to have diabetes on other grounds and are thus subjected to oral glucose tolerance test (GTT). If abnormal GTT values are found, these subjects are said to have *'chemical diabetes'*. The WHO-American Diabetes Association (2000) have suggested definite diagnostic criteria for early diagnosis of diabetes mellitus (Table 25.6).

The following investigations are helpful in establishing the diagnosis of diabetes mellitus:

I. URINE TESTING. Urine tests are cheap and convenient but the diagnosis of diabetes cannot be based on urine testing alone since there may be false-positives and false-negatives. They can be used in population screening surveys. Urine is tested for the presence of glucose and ketones.

1. Glucosuria. *Benedict's qualitative test* detects any reducing substance in the urine and is not specific for glucose. More sensitive and glucose specific test is *dipstick* method based on enzyme-coated paper strip which turns purple when dipped in urine containing glucose.

The main disadvantage of relying on urinary glucose test alone is the individual variation in renal threshold. Thus, a diabetic patient may have a negative urinary glucose test and a nondiabetic individual with low renal threshold may have a positive urine test.

Besides diabetes mellitus, *glucosuria* may also occur in certain other conditions such as: renal glycosuria, alimentary (lag storage) glucosuria, many metabolic disorders, starvation and intracranial lesions (e.g. cerebral tumour, haemorrhage and head injury). However, two of these conditions—renal glucosuria and alimentary glucosuria, require further elaboration here.

TABLE 25.6: Revised Criteria for Diagnosis of Diabetes by Oral GTT (as per WHO-American Diabetes Association, 2000).

PATIENT STATUS	PLASMA GLUCOSE VALUE*	DIAGNOSIS
1. Fasting value	below 110 mg/dl (< 6.1 mmol/L)	Normal fasting value
2. Fasting value	110-126 mg/dl (6.1-7.0 mmol/L)	Impaired fasting glucose (IFG)**
3. Fasting value	126 mg/dl (7.0 mmol/L) or more	Diabetes mellitus
4. Two-hour after 75 g oral glucose load	140-200 mg/dl (7.8-11.1 mmol/L)	Impaired glucose tolerance (IGT)**
5. Two-hour after 75 g oral glucose load	200 mg/dl (11.1 mmol/L) or more	Diabetes mellitus
6. Random value	200 mg/dl (11.1 mmol/L) or more in a symptomatic patient	Diabetes mellitus

Note: * Plasma glucose values are 15% higher than whole blood glucose value.
** Individuals with IFG and IGT are at increased risk for development of type 2 DM later.

■ *Renal glucosuria (Fig. 25.17,B):* After diabetes, the next most common cause of glucosuria is the reduced renal threshold for glucose. In such cases although the blood glucose level is below 180 mg/dl (i.e. below normal renal threshold for glucose) but glucose still appears regularly and consistently in the urine due to lowered renal threshold.

Renal glucosuria is a benign condition unrelated to diabetes and runs in families and may occur temporarily in pregnancy without symptoms of diabetes.

■ *Alimentary (lag storage) glucosuria (Fig. 25.17,C):* A rapid and transitory rise in blood glucose level above the normal renal threshold may occur in some individuals after a meal. During this period, glucosuria is present. This type of response to meal is called 'lag storage curve' or more appropriately 'alimentary glucosuria'. A characteristic feature is that unusually high blood glucose level returns to normal 2 hours after meal.

2. **Ketonuria.** Tests for ketone bodies in the urine are required for assessing the severity of diabetes and not for diagnosis of diabetes. However, if both glucosuria and ketonuria are present, diagnosis of diabetes is almost certain. *Rothera's test* (nitroprusside reaction) and *strip test* are conveniently performed for detection of ketonuria.

Besides uncontrolled diabetes, ketonuria may appear in individuals with prolonged vomitings, fasting state or exercising for long periods.

II. SINGLE BLOOD SUGAR ESTIMATION. For diagnosis of diabetes, blood sugar determinations are absolutely necessary. *Folin-Wu method* of measurement of all reducing substances in the blood including glucose is now obsolete. Currently used are *O-toluidine, Somogyi-Nelson* and *glucose oxidase* methods. Whole blood or plasma may be used but *whole blood values are 15% lower than plasma values.*

A grossly elevated single determination of plasma glucose may be sufficient to make the diagnosis of diabetes. A *fasting plasma glucose value above 126 mg/dl (7 mmol/L) is certainly indicative of diabetes.* In other cases, oral GTT is performed (Fig. 25.17).

III. ORAL GLUCOSE TOLERANCE TEST. The patient who is scheduled for oral GTT is instructed to eat a high carbohydrate diet for at least 3 days prior to the test and come after an overnight fast on the day of the test (for at least 8 hours). A fasting blood sugar sample is first drawn. Then 75 gm of glucose dissolved in 300 ml of water is given. Blood and urine specimen are collected at half-hourly intervals for at least 2 hours. Blood or plasma glucose content is measured and urine is tested for glucosuria to determine the approximate renal threshold for glucose. Venous whole blood concentrations are 15% lower than plasma glucose values.

Currently accepted criteria for diagnosis of DM (as per WHO-American Diabetes Association, 2000) are given in Table 25.6.

■ Individuals with fasting value of plasma glucose higher than 126 mg/dl and 2-hour value after 75 gm oral glucose higher than 200 mg/dl are labelled as *diabetics* (Fig. 25.17,D).

■ In a symptomatic case the random blood glucose value above 200 mg/dl is diagnosed as diabetes mellitus.

■ Normal cut off value for fasting blood glucose level is considered as 110 mg/dl. Cases with fasting blood glucose value between 110 and 126 mg/dl are considered as *impaired fasting glucose tolerance (IGT);* these cases are at increased risk of developing diabetes later and therefore kept under observation for repeating the test. During pregnancy, however, a case of IGT is treated as a diabetic.

IV. OTHER TESTS. A few other tests are sometimes performed in specific conditions in diabetics and for research purposes:

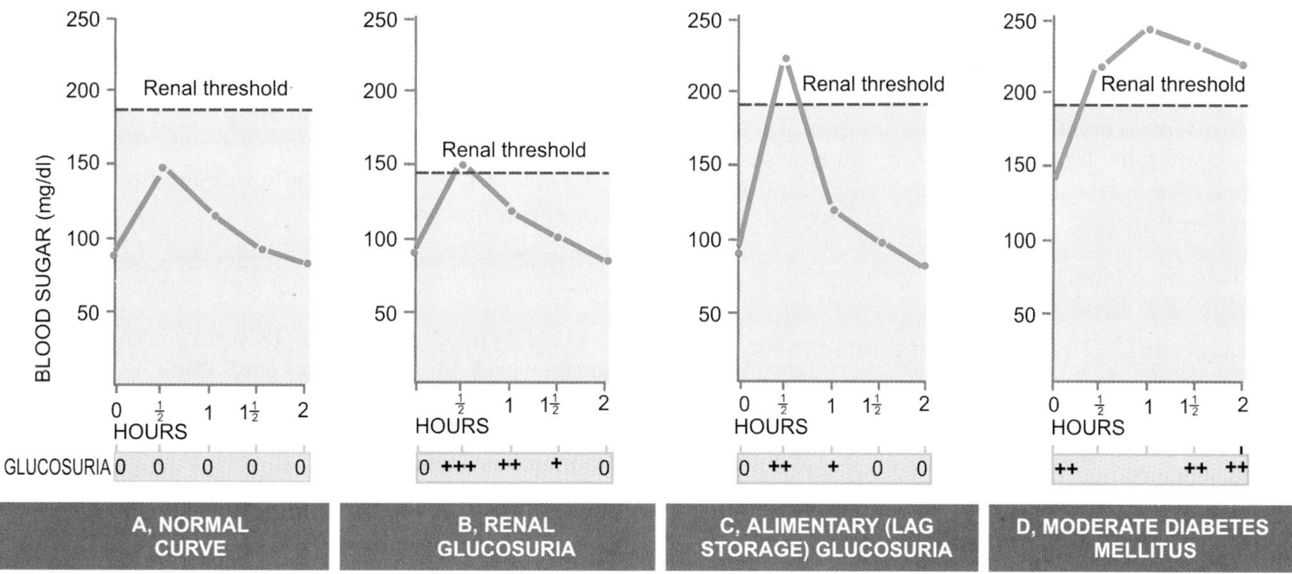

FIGURE 25.17

The glucose tolerance test, showing blood glucose curves (venous blood glucose) and glucosuria after 75 gm of oral glucose.

1. **Glycosylated haemoglobin (HbA_{1C}).** Measurement of blood glucose level in diabetics suffers from variation due to dietary intake of the previous day. Long-term objective assessment of degree of diabetic control is better done by measurement of glycosylated haemoglobin (HbA_{1C}), a minor haemoglobin component present in normal persons. This is because the non-enzymatic glycosylation of haemoglobin takes place over 120 days, life span of red blood cells. HbA_{1C} assay, therefore, gives an estimate of diabetic control for the preceding 6-10 weeks.

2. **Extended GTT.** The oral GTT is extended to 3-4 hours for appearance of symptoms of hyperglycaemia. It is a useful test in cases of reactive hypoglycaemia of early diabetes.

3. **Intravenous GTT.** This test is performed in persons who have intestinal malabsorption or in postgastrectomy cases.

4. **Cortisone-primed GTT.** This provocative test is a useful investigative aid in cases of potential diabetics.

5. **Insulin assay.** Plasma insulin levels can be measured by radioimmunoassay and ELISA techniques.

6. **C-peptide assay.** This test is even more sensitive than insulin assay because its levels are not affected by insulin therapy.

ISLET CELL TUMOURS

Islet cell tumours are rare as compared with tumours of the exocrine pancreas. Islet cell tumours are generally small and may be hormonally inactive or may produce hyperfunction. They may be benign or malignant, single or multiple. They are named according to their histogenesis such as: B-cell tumour (insulinoma), G-cell tumour (gastrinoma), A-cell tumour (glucagonoma) D-cell tumour (somatostatinoma), vipoma (diarrhoeagenic tumour from D_1 cells which elaborate VIP), pancreatic polypeptide (PP)-secreting tumour, and carcinoid tumour. However, except insulinoma and gastrinoma, all others are extremely rare and require no further comments.

Insulinoma (β-Cell Tumour)

Insulinomas or beta (β)-cell tumours are the most common islet cell tumours. The neoplastic β-cells secrete insulin into the blood stream which remains unaffected by normal regulatory mechanisms. This results in characteristic attacks of hypolgycaemia with blood glucose level falling to 50 mg/dl or below, high plasma insulin level (hyperinsulinism) and high insulin-glucose ratio. The central nervous manifestations are conspicuous which are promptly relieved by intake of glucose. Besides insulinoma, however, there are other causes of hypoglycaemia such as: in starvation, partial gastrectomy, diffuse liver disease, hypopituitarism and hypofunction of adrenal cortex.

PATHOLOGIC CHANGES. Grossly, insulinoma is usually solitary and well-encapsulated tumour which may vary in size from 0.5 to 10 cm. Rarely, they are multiple.

Microscopically, the tumour is composed of cords and sheets of well-differentiated β cells which do not differ from normal cells. Electron microscopy reveals typical crystalline rectangular granules in the neoplastic cells. It is extremely difficult to assess the degree of anaplasia to distinguish benign from malignant B-cell tumour.

Gastrinoma (G-Cell Tumour, Zollinger-Ellison Syndrome)

Zollinger and Ellison described diagnostic triad consisting of:

- fulminant peptic ulcer disease;
- gastric acid hypersecretion; and
- presence of non-β pancreatic islet cell tumour.

Such non-β pancreatic islet cell tumour is the source of gastrin, producing hypergastrinaemia and hence named gastrinoma. Definite G cells similar to intestinal and gastric G cells which are normally the source of gastrin in the body, have not been identified in the normal human pancreas but neoplastic cells of certain islet cell tumours have ultrastructural similarities.

PATHOLOGIC CHANGES. Majority of gastrinomas occur in the wall of the duodenum. They may be benign or malignant. Gastrinomas are associated with peptic ulcers at usual sites such as the stomach, first and second part of the duodenum, or sometimes at unusual sites such as in the oesophagus and jejunum. About one-third of patients have multiple endocrine neoplasia—multiple adenomas of the islet cells, pituitary, adrenal and parathyroid glands.

MULTIPLE ENDOCRINE NEOPLASIA (MEN) SYNDROMES

Multiple adenomas and hyperplasias of different endocrine organs are a group of genetic diorders which produce heterogeneous clinical features called multiple endocrine neoplasia (MEN) syndromes. Presently, 4 distinct types of MEN syndromes are distinguished. These are briefly outlined below along with major disease associations:

1. MEN type 1 syndrome (Wermer's syndrome) includes adenomas of the parathyroid glands, pancreatic islets and pituitary. The syndrome is inherited as an autosomal dominant trait. There is 50% chance of transmitting the predisposing gene, *MEN 1* (or *menin*) gene, to the child of an affected person. MEN 1 is characterised by the following features:

1. *Parathyroid:* Hyperplasia or adenoma; hyperparathyroidism is the most common (90%) clinical manifestation.

2. *Pancreatic islet cells:* Hyperplasia or adenoma seen in 80% cases; frequently with Zollinger-Ellison syndrome.

3. *Pituitary:* Hyperplasia or adenoma in 65% cases; manifest as acromegaly or hypopituitarism.

4. *Adrenal cortex:* Uncommonly involved by adenoma or pheochromocytoma.

5. *Thyroid:* Less commonly involved by adenoma or hyperplasia.

2. MEN type 2 syndrome (Sipple's syndrome) is characterised by medullary carcinoma thyroid and pheochromocytoma. Genetic abnormality in these cases is mutation in *RET* gene in almost all cases. MEN 2 has two major syndromes:

- **MEN type 2A** is the combination of medullary carcinoma thyroid, pheochromocytoma and hyperparathyroidism. MEN type 2A has further *three subvariants*:

i) MEN 2A with familial medullary carcinoma thyroid;

ii) MEN 2A with cutaneous lichen amyloidosis; and

iii) MEN 2A with Hirschsprung's disease.

- **MEN type 2B** the combination of medullary carcinoma thyroid, pheochromocytoma, mucosal neuromas, intestinal ganglioneuromatosis, and marfanoid features.

3. Mixed syndromes include a variety of endocrine neoplastic combinations which are distinct from those in MEN type 1 and type 2. A few examples are as under:

- von Hippel-Lindau syndrome from mutation in *VHL* gene is association of CNS tumours, renal cell carcinoma, pheochromocytoma and islet cell tumours.
- Type 1 neurofibromatosis from inactivation of neurofibromin protein and activation of *RAS* gene, is associated with MEN type 1 or type 2 features.

POLYGLANDULAR AUTOIMMUNE (PGA) SYNDROMES

Immunologic syndromes affecting two or more endocrine glands and some non-endocrine immune disturbances produce syndromic presentation termed polyglandular autoimmune (PGA) syndromes. PGA syndromes are of two types:

- PGA type I occurring in children is characterised by mucocutaneous candidiasis, hypoparathyroidism, and adrenal insufficiency.
- PGA type II (Schmidt syndrome) presents in adults and commonly comprises of adrenal insufficiency, autoimmune thyroiditis, and type 1 diabetes mellitus.

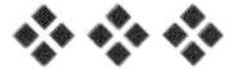

The Musculoskeletal System

26

SKELETAL SYSTEM

The skeleton consists of cartilage and bone. Cartilage has a role in growth and repair of bone, and in the adults forms the articular skeleton responsible for movement of joints. Bone is a specialised form of connective tissue which performs the function of providing mechanical support and is also a mineral reservoir for calcium homeostasis. There are 206 bones in the human body, and depending upon their size and shape may be long, flat, tubular etc.

NORMAL STRUCTURE OF BONE

Bone is divided into 2 components (Fig. 26.1):

■ **Cortical or compact bone** comprises 80% of the skeleton and is the dense outer shell responsible for structural rigidity. It consists of haversian canals with blood vessels surrounded by concentric layers of mineralised collagen forming osteons which are joined together by cement lines (Fig. 26.1,A).

■ **Trabecular or cancellous bone** composes 20% of the skeleton and has trabeculae traversing the marrow space (Fig. 26.1,B). Its main role is in mineral homeostasis.

HISTOLOGY. Bone consists of large quantities of extracellular matrix which is loaded with calcium hydroxyapatite and relatively small number of bone cells which are of 3 main types: osteocytes, osteoblasts and osteoclasts, besides osteoid matrix.

1. Osteoblasts. Osteoblasts are uninucleate cells found abundantly along the new bone-forming surfaces. They synthesise bone matrix. The serum levels of bone-related *alkaline phosphatase* (other being hepatic alkaline phosphatase) is a marker for osteoblastic activity. Its levels are raised in puberty during period of active bone growth and in pathologic conditions associated with high osteoblastic activity such as in fracture repair and Paget's disease of the bone.

2. Osteocytes. Osteocytes are those osteoblasts which get incorporated into bone matrix during its synthesis. Osteocytes are found within small spaces called lacunae lying in the bone matrix. The distribution of the osteocytic lacunae is a reliable parameter for distinguishing between woven and lamellar bone.

■ **Woven bone** is immature and rapidly deposited bone containing large number of closely-packed osteocytes and consists of irregular interlacing pattern of collagen fibre bundles in bone matrix. Woven bone is seen in foetal life and in children under 4 years of age.

■ **Lamellar bone** differs from woven bone in having smaller and less numerous osteocytes and fine and

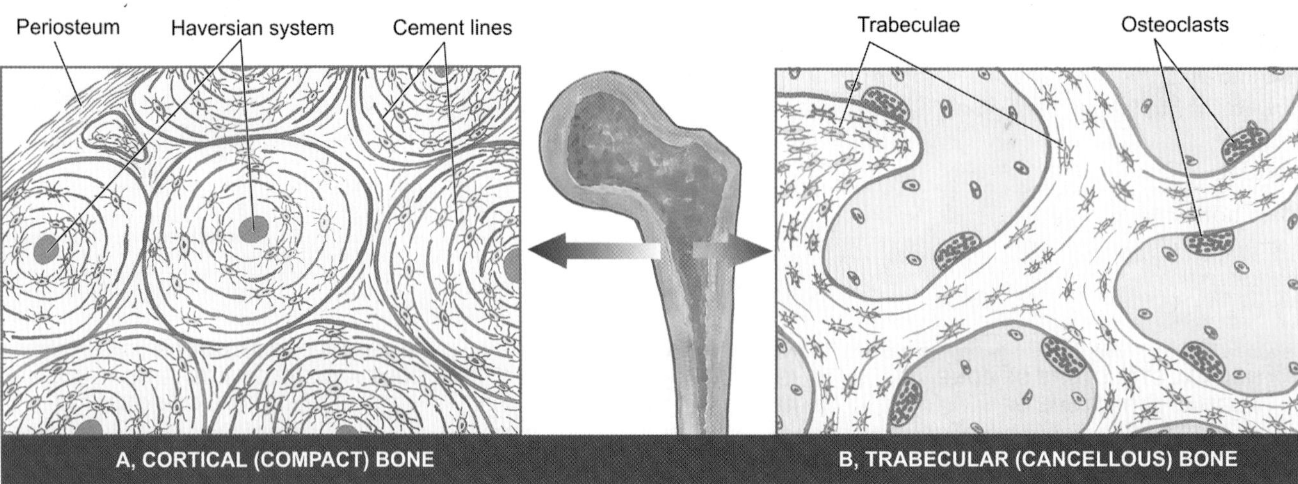

FIGURE 26.1

A, The normal structure of cortical (compact) bone and B, trabecular (cancellous) bone in transverse section. The cortical bone forming the outer shell shows concentric lamellae alongwith osteocytic lacunae surrounding central blood vessels, while the trabecular bone forming the marrow space shows trabeculae with osteoclastic activity at the margins.

parallel or lamellar sheets of collagen fibres. Lamellar bone usually replaces woven bone or pre-existing cartilage.

3. **Osteoclasts.** Osteoclasts are large multinucleate cells of mononuclear-macrophage origin and are responsible for bone resorption. The osteoclastic activity is determined by bone-related serum *acid phosphatase* levels (other being prostatic acid phosphatase). Osteoclasts are found along the endosteal surface of the cortical (compact) bone and the trabeculae of trabecular (cancellous) bone.

4. **Osteoid matrix.** The osteoid matrix of bone consists of 90-95% of collagen type I and comprises nearly half of total body's collagen. Virtually whole of body's hydroxyproline and hydroxylysine reside in the bone. The architecture of bone collagen reflects the rate of its synthesis and may be woven or lamellar, as described above.

BONE FORMATION AND RESORPTION. Bone is not a static tissue but its formation and resorption are taking place during period of growth as well as in adult life. Bone deposition is the result of osteoblasts while bone resorption is the function of osteoclasts. Bone formation may take place directly from collagen called *membranous ossification* seen in certain flat bones, or may occur through an intermediate stage of cartilage termed *endochondral ossification* found in metaphysis of long bones. In either case, firstly an uncalcified osteoid matrix is formed by osteoblasts which is then mineralised in 12-15 days. This delay in mineralisation results in formation of about 15 μm thick osteoid seams at calcification fronts (About > 1 μm of matrix osteoid is formed daily). Uncalcified osteoid appears eosinophilic in H & E stains and does not stain with von Kossa reaction, while mineralised osteoid is basophilic in appearance and stains black with von Kossa reaction (a stain for calcium). Areas of active bone resorption have scalloped edges of bone surface called Howship's lacunae and contain multinucleated osteoclasts. In this way, osteoblastic formation and osteoclastic resorption continue to take place into adult life in a balanced way termed *bone modelling*. The important role of vitamin D_1, parathyroid hormone and calcitonin in calcium metabolism has already been discussed on page 255.

NORMAL STRUCTURE OF CARTILAGE

Unlike bone, the cartilage lacks blood vessels, lymphatics and nerves. It may have focal areas of calcification. Cartilage consists of 2 components: cartilage matrix and chondrocytes.

■ **Cartilage matrix.** Like bone, cartilage too consists of organic and inorganic material. Inorganic material of cartilage is calcium hydroxyapatite similar to that in bone matrix but the organic material of cartilage is distinct from bone. It consists of very high content of water (80%) and remaining 20% consists of type II collagen and proteoglycans. High water content of cartilage matrix is responsible for function of articular cartilage and lubrication. Proteoglycans are macromolecules having proteins complexed with polysaccharides termed glycosaminoglycans. Cartilage glycosaminoglycans consist of chondroitin sulfate and keratan sulfate, the former being most abundant comprising 55-90% of cartilage matrix varying on the age of the cartilage.

■ **Chondrocytes.** Primitive mesenchymal cells which form bone cells form chondroblasts which give rise to chondrocytes. However, calcified cartilage is removed by the osteoclasts.

Depending upon location and structural composition, cartilage is of 3 types:

1. *Hyaline cartilage* is the basic cartilaginous tissue comprising articular cartilage of joints, cartilage in the growth plates of developing bones, costochondral cartilage, cartilage in the trachea, bronchi and larynx and the nasal cartilage. Hyaline cartilage is the type found in most cartilage-forming tumours and in the fracture callus.

2. *Fibrocartilage* is a hyaline cartilage that contains more abundant type II collagen fibres. It is found in annulus fibrosus of intervertebral disc, menisci, insertions of joint capsules, ligament and tendons. Fibrocartilage may also be found in some cartilage-forming tumours and in the fracture callus.

3. *Elastic cartilage* is hyaline cartilage that contains abundant elastin. Elastic cartilage is found in the pinna of ears, epiglottis and arytenoid cartilage of the larynx.

Diseases of skeletal system include infection (osteomyelitis), disordered growth and development (skeletal dysplasias), metabolic and endocrine derangements, and tumours and tumour-like conditions.

OSTEOMYELITIS

An infection of the bone is termed osteomyelitis (myelo = marrow). A number of systemic infectious diseases may spread to the bone such as enteric fever, actinomycosis, mycetoma (madura foot), syphilis, tuberculosis and brucellosis. However, two of the conditions which produce significant pathologic lesions in the bone, namely pyogenic osteomyelitis and tuberculous osteomyelitis, are described below.

Pyogenic Osteomyelitis

Suppurative osteomyelitis is usually caused by bacterial infection and rarely by fungi. Haematogenous pyogenic osteomyelitis occurs most commonly in the long bones of infants and young children (5-15 years of age), particularly in the developing countries of the world. In the developed world, however, where institution of antibiotics is early and prompt, haematogenous spread of infection to the bone is uncommon. In such cases, instead, direct extension of infection from the adjacent area, frequently involving the jaws and skull in adults, is more common mode of spread. Bacterial osteomyelitis may be a complication at all ages in patients with compound fractures, surgical procedures involving prosthesis or implants, gangrene of a limb in diabetics, debilitation and immunosuppression. Though any etiologic agent may cause osteomyelitis, *Staphylococcus aureus* is implicated in a vast majority of cases. Less frequently, other organisms such as streptococci, *Escherichia coli, Pseudomonas, Klebsiella* and anaerobes are involved. Mixed infections are common in post-traumatic cases of osteomyelitis. There may be transient bacteraemia preceding the development of osteomyelitis so that blood cultures may be positive.

Clinically, the child with acute haematogenous osteomyelitis has painful and tender limb. Fever, malaise and leucocytosis generally accompany the bony lesion. Radiologic examination confirms the bony destruction.

Occasionally, osteomyelitis remains undiscovered until it becomes chronic. Draining sinus tracts may form which may occasionally be the site for development of squamous carcinoma. Persistence and chronicity of osteomyelitis over a period of time may lead to development of amyloidosis.

PATHOLOGIC CHANGES. Depending upon the duration, osteomyelitis may be *acute, subacute* or *chronic.* The basic pathologic changes in any stage of osteomyelitis are: suppuration, ischaemic necrosis, healing by fibrosis and bony repair. The ***sequence of pathologic changes*** is as under (Fig. 26.2):

1. The infection begins in the metaphyseal end of the *marrow cavity* which is largely occupied by *pus.* At this stage, microscopy reveals congestion, oedema and an exudate of neutrophils (**COLOUR PLATE XXXIII: CL 129**).
2. The tension in the marrow cavity is increased due to pus and results in spread of infection along the marrow cavity, into the endosteum, and into the haversian and Volkmann's canal, causing *periosteitis.*
3. The infection may reach the subperiosteal space forming *subperiosteal abscesses.* It may penetrate through the cortex creating draining skin sinus tracts.
4. Combination of suppuration and impaired blood supply to the cortical bone results in erosion, thinning and infarction necrosis of the cortex called *sequestrum* (Fig. 26.3).

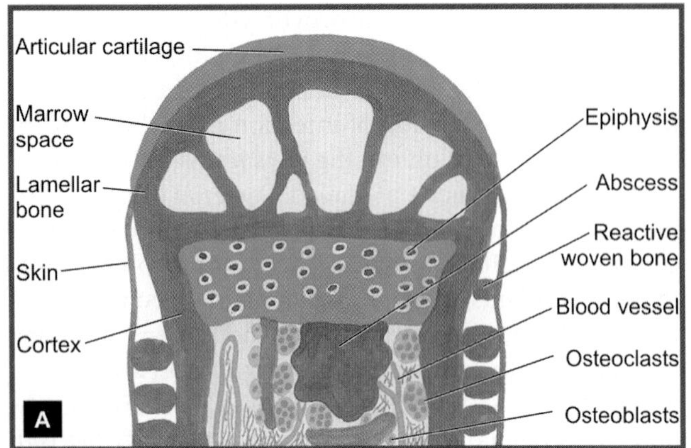

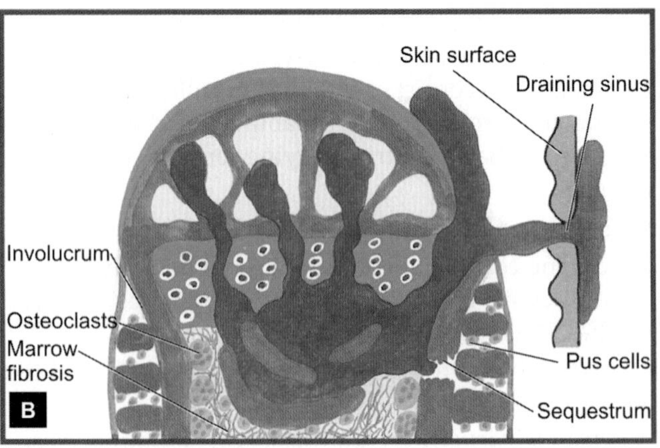

FIGURE 26.2

Pathogenesis of pyogenic osteomyelitis. A, The process begins as a focus of microabscess in a vascular loop in the marrow which expands to stimulate resorption of adjacent bony trabeculae. Simultaneously, there is beginning of reactive woven bone formation by the periosteum. B, The abscess expands further causing necrosis of the cortex called sequestrum. The formation of viable new reactive bone surrounding the sequestrum is called involucrum. The extension of infection into the joint space, epiphysis and the skin produces a draining sinus.

5. With passage of time, there is formation of new bone beneath the periosteum present over the infected bone. This forms an encasing sheath around the necrosed bone and is known as *involucrum*. Involucrum has irregular surface and has perforations through which discharging sinus tracts pass.
6. Long continued neo-osteogenesis gives rise to dense sclerotic pattern of osteomyelitis called *chronic sclerosing nonsuppurative osteomyelitis of Garré.*
7. Occasionally, acute osteomyelitis may be contained to a localised area and walled off by fibrous tissue and granulation tissue. This is termed *Brodie's abscess.*
8. Occasionally, *vertebral osteomyelitis* may occur in which case infection begins from the disc (discitis) and spreads to involve the vertebral bodies (Fig. 26.4,A).

FIGURE 26.3

Chronic suppurative osteomyelitis. Histologic appearance shows necrotic bone and extensive purulent inflammatory exudate.

COMPLICATIONS. Osteomyelitis may result in the following complications:

1. Septicaemia.
2. Acute bacterial arthritis.
3. Pathologic fractures.
4. Development of squamous cell carcinoma in long-standing cases.
5. Secondary amyloidosis in long-standing cases.
6. Vertebral osteomyelitis may cause vertebral collapse with paravertebral abscess, epidural abscess, cord compression and neurologic deficits.

Tuberculous Osteomyelitis

Tuberculous osteomyelitis, though rare in developed countries, continues to be a common condition in under-developed and developing countries of the world. The tubercle bacilli, *M. tuberculosis,* reach the bone marrow and synovium most commonly by haematogenous dissemination from infection elsewhere, usually the lungs, and infrequently by direct extension from the pulmonary or gastrointestinal tuberculosis (page 162). The disease affects adolescents and young adults more often. Most frequently involved are the spine and bones of extremities.

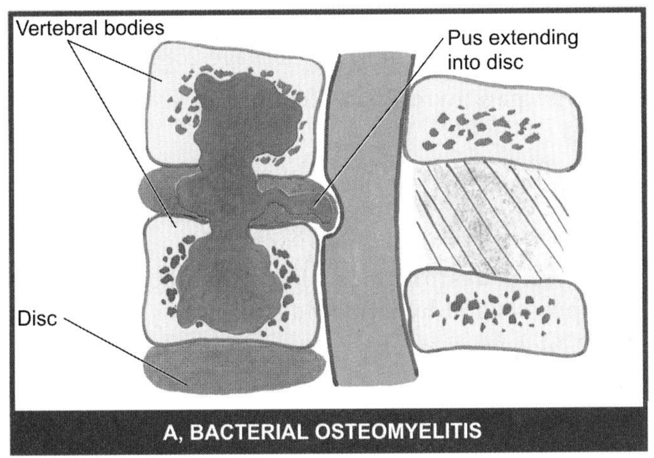

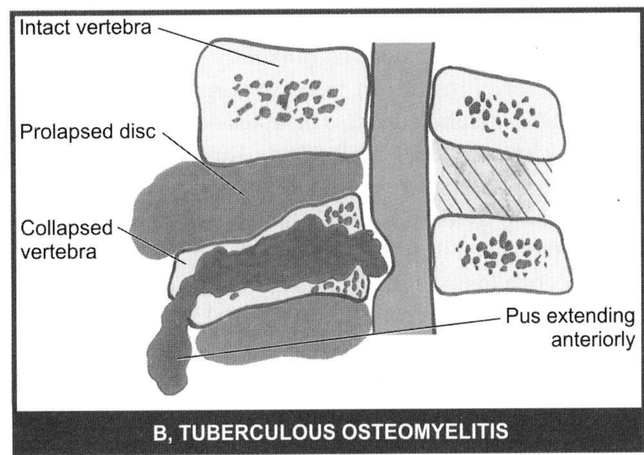

FIGURE 26.4
Osteomyelitis of the vertebral body.

PATHOLOGIC CHANGES. The bone lesions in tuberculosis have the same general histological appearance as in tuberculosis elsewhere and consist of central caseation necrosis surrounded by tuberculous granulation tissue. The tuberculous lesions appear as a focus of bone destruction and replacement of the affected tissue by caseous material and formation of multiple discharging sinuses through the soft tissues and skin. Involvement of joint spaces and intervertebral disc are frequent. Tuberculosis of the spine, *Pott's disease,* often commences in the vertebral body and may be associated with compression fractures and destruction of intervertebral discs, producing permanent damage and paraplegia. Extension of caseous material alongwith pus from the lumbar vertebrae to the sheaths of psoas muscle produces *psoas abscess* or *lumbar cold abscess* (Fig. 26.4,B). The cold abscess may burst through the skin and form sinus. Long-standing cases may develop systemic amyloidosis.

FRACTURE HEALING

Fracture of the bone initiates a series of tissue changes which eventually lead to restoration of normal structure and function of the affected bone. Fracture of a bone is commonly associated with injury to the soft tissues. The various types of fractures and their mechanism of healing are discussed alongwith healing of specialised tissues in Chapter 6 (page 177).

DISORDERS OF BONE GROWTH AND DEVELOPMENT (SKELETAL DYSPLASIAS)

A number of abnormalities of skeleton are due to disordered bone growth and development and are collectively termed *skeletal dysplasias.* These include both local and systemic disorders.

- *Local defects* involve a single bone or a group of bones such as: absence or presence in diminished form, fused with neighbouring bones (e.g. syndactyly), and formation of extra bones (e.g. supernumerary ribs).
- However, more importantly, skeletal dysplasias include *systemic disorders* involving particular epiphyseal growth plate. These include: achondroplasia (disorder of chondroblasts), osteogenesis imperfecta (disorder of osteoblasts), osteopetrosis (disorder of osteoclasts) and foetal rickets (disorder of mineralisation). Though multiple exostoses (osteochondromas) is a hereditary lesion, it is described later alongwith solitary sporadic exostosis on page 869.

Achondroplasia

Achondroplasia is an autosomal dominant genetic abnormality. There is selective interference with normal endochondral ossification at the level of epiphyseal cartilaginous growth plates of long bones. Thus, the long bones are abnormally short but the skull grows normally leading to relatively large skull. Achondroplasia is the commonest cause of dwarfism.

Osteogenesis Imperfecta

Osteogenesis imperfecta is an autosomal dominant or recessive disorder of synthesis of type I collagen that constitutes 90-95% of bone matrix. The disorder, thus, involves not only the skeleton but other extra-skeletal tissues as well containing type I collagen such as sclera, eyes, joints, ligaments, teeth and skin. The skeletal manifestations of osteogenesis imperfecta are due to defective osteoblasts which normally synthesise type I collagen. This results in thin or non-existent cortices and irregular trabeculae *(too little bone)* so that the bones are very fragile and liable to multiple fractures. The growth plate cartilage is, however, normal. The condition may be evident at birth (osteogenesis imperfecta congenita) when it is more severe, or may appear during adolescence (osteogenesis imperfecta tarda) which is a less incapacitating form. Extraskeletal lesions of osteogenesis imperfecta include blue and translucent sclerae, hearing loss due to bony abnormalities of middle and inner ear, and imperfect teeth.

Osteopetrosis

Osteopetrosis, also called *marble bone disease,* is an autosomal dominant or recessive disorder of increased skeletal mass or osteosclerosis caused by a hereditary defect in osteoclast function. The condition may appear in 2 forms: autosomal recessive (malignant infantile form) and autosomal dominant (benign adult form). Failure of normal osteoclast function of bone resorption coupled with continued bone formation and endochondral ossification results in net overgrowth of calcified dense bone *(too much bone)* which occupies most of the available marrow space. Despite increased density of the bone, there is poor structural support so that the skeleton is susceptible to fractures. Besides the skeletal abnormalities, the infantile malignant form is characterised by effects of marrow obliteration such as anaemia, neutropenia, thrombocytopenia, hepatosplenomegaly with extramedullary haematopoiesis, hydrocephalus and neurologic involvement with consequent deafness, optic atrophy and blindness. Metabolically, hypocalcaemia occurs due to defective osteoclast function.

Histologically, the number of osteoclasts is increased which have dysplastic, bizarre and irregular nuclei and are dysfunctional.

METABOLIC AND ENDOCRINE BONE DISEASES

A large number of metabolic and endocrine disorders produce generalised skeletal disorders. These include the following:

1. **Osteoporosis**—resulting from quantitative reduction in otherwise normal bone.

2. **Osteomalacia and rickets**—characterised by qualitative abnormality in the form of impaired bone mineralisation due to deficiency of vitamin D in adults and children respectively (page 256).

3. **Scurvy**—caused by deficiency of vitamin C resulting in subperiosteal haemorrhages (page 258).

4. **Hyperparathyroidism**—leading to osteitis fibrosa cystica (page 840).

5. **Pituitary dysfunctions**—hyperpituitarism causing gigantism and acromegaly and hypopituitarism resulting in dwarfism (page 817).

6. **Thyroid dysfunctions**—hyperthyroidism causing osteoporosis and hypothyroidism leading to cretinism (page 827).

7. **Renal osteodystrophy**—occurring in chronic renal failure and resulting in features of osteitis fibrosa cystica, osteomalacia and areas of osteosclerosis.

8. **Skeletal fluorosis**—occurring due to excess of sodium fluoride content in the soil and water in an area.

Many of the conditions listed above have been discussed in respective chapters already; others are considered below.

Osteoporosis

Osteoporosis or osteopenia is a common clinical syndrome involving multiple bones in which there is quantitative reduction of bone tissue mass but the bone tissue mass is otherwise normal. This reduction in bone mass results in fragile skeleton which is associated with increased risk of fractures and consequent pain and deformity. The condition is particularly common in elderly people and more frequent in postmenopausal women. The condition may remain asymptomatic or may cause only backache. However, more extensive involvement is associated with fractures, particularly of distal radius, femoral neck and vertebral bodies. Osteoporosis may be difficult to distinguish radiologically from other osteopenias such as osteomalacia, osteogenesis imperfecta, osteitis fibrosa of hyperparathyroidism, renal osteodystrophy and multiple myeloma. Radiologic evidence becomes apparent only after more than 30% of bone mass has been lost. Levels of serum calcium, inorganic phosphorus and alkaline phosphatase are usually within normal limits.

PATHOGENESIS. Osteoporosis is conventionally classified into 2 major groups: primary and secondary.

■ **Primary osteoporosis** results primarily from osteopenia without an underlying disease or medication. Primary osteoporosis is further subdivided into 2 types: *idiopathic type* found in the young and juveniles and is less frequent, and *involutional type* seen in postmenopausal women and aging individuals and is more common. The exact mechanism of primary osteoporosis is not known but there is a suggestion that it is the result of an excessive osteoclastic resorption and slow bone formation. A number of risk factors have been attributed to cause this imbalance between bone resorption and bone formation. These include the following:

1. *Genetic factors*—more marked in whites and Asians than blacks.
2. *Sex*—more frequent in females than in males.
3. *Reduced physical activity*—as in old age.
4. *Deficiency of sex hormones*—oestrogen deficiency in women as in postmenopausal osteoporosis and androgen deficiency in men.
5. *Combined deficiency of calcitonin and oestrogen.*
6. *Hyperparathyroidism.*
7. *Deficiency of vitamin D.*
8. *Local factors*—which may stimulate osteoclastic resorption or slow osteoblastic bone formation.

■ **Secondary osteoporosis** is attributed to a number of factors and conditions (e.g. immobilisation, chronic anaemia, acromegaly, hepatic disease, hyperparathyroidism, hypogonadism, thyrotoxicosis and starvation), or as an effect of medication (e.g. hypercortisonism, administration of anticonvulsant drugs and large dose of heparin).

PATHOLOGIC CHANGES. Except disuse or immobilisation osteoporosis which is localised to the affected limb, other forms of osteoporosis have systemic skeletal distribution. Most commonly encountered osteoporotic fractures are: vertebral crush fracture, femoral neck fracture and wrist fracture. There is enlargement of the medullary cavity and thinning of the cortex.

Histologically, osteoporosis may be active or inactive type.

■ **Active osteoporosis** is characterised by increased bone resorption and formation i.e. *accelerated turnover.* There is increase in the number of osteoclasts with increased resorptive surface as well as increased quantity of osteoid with increased osteoblastic surfaces. The width of osteoid seams is normal.

■ **Inactive osteoporosis** has the features of minimal bone formation and reduced resorptive activity i.e. *reduced turnover.* Histological changes of inactive osteoporosis include decreased number of osteoclasts with decreased resorptive surfaces, and normal or reduced amount of osteoid with decreased osteoblastic surface. The width of osteoid seams is usually reduced or may be normal.

Osteitis Fibrosa Cystica

Hyperparathyroidism of primary or secondary type results in oversecretion of parathyroid hormone which causes increased osteoclastic resorption of the bone. General aspects of hyperparathyroidism are discussed on page 840. Here, skeletal manifestations of hyperparathyroidism are considered. Severe and prolonged hyperparathyroidism results in osteitis fibrosa cystica. The lesion is generally induced as a manifestation of primary hyperparathyroidism, and less frequently, as a result of secondary hyperparathyroidism such as in chronic renal failure (renal osteodystrophy).

The clinical manifestations of bone disease in hyperparathyroidism are its susceptibility to fracture, skeletal deformities, joint pains and dysfunctions as a result of deranged weight bearing. The bony changes may disappear after cure of primary hyperparathyroidism such as removal of functioning adenoma. The chief biochemical abnormality of excessive parathyroid hormone is hypercalcaemia, hypophosphataemia and hypercalciuria.

PATHOLOGIC CHANGES. The bone lesions of primary hyperparathyroidism affect the long bones more severely and may range from minor degree of generalised bone rarefaction to prominent areas of bone destruction with cyst formation or brown tumours.

Grossly, there are focal areas of erosion of cortical bone and loss of lamina dura at the roots of teeth.

Histologically, the following sequential changes appear over a period of time:

■ Earliest change is *demineralisation* and *increased bone resorption* beginning at the subperiosteal and endosteal surface of the cortex and then spreading to the trabecular bone.

■ There is replacement of bone and bone-marrow by fibrosis coupled with increased number of bizarre osteoclasts at the surfaces of moth-eaten trabeculae and cortex *(osteitis fibrosa).*

■ As a result of increased resorption, microfractures and microhaemorrhages occur in the marrow cavity leading to development of cysts *(osteitis fibrosa cystica).*

■ Haemosiderin-laden macrophages and multinucleate giant cells appear at the areas of haemorrhages producing an appearance termed as *'brown tumour'* or *'reparative giant cell granuloma of hyperparathyroidism'* requiring differentiation from giant cell tumour or osteoclastoma (page 871). However, the so-called brown tumours, unlike osteoclastoma, are not true tumours but instead regress or disappear on surgical removal of hyperplastic or adenomatous parathyroid tissue.

Renal Osteodystrophy (Metabolic Bone Disease)

Renal osteodystrophy is a loosely used term that encompasses a number of skeletal abnormalities appearing in cases of chronic renal failure and in patients treated by dialysis for several years (page 678). Renal osteodystrophy is more common in children than in adults. Clinical symptoms of bone disease in advanced renal failure appear in less than 10% of patients but radiologic and histologic changes are observed in fairly large proportion of cases.

PATHOGENESIS. Renal osteodystrophy involves two main events: *hyperphosphataemia* and *hypocalcaemia* which, in turn, leads to parathormone elaboration and resultant osteoclastic activity and major lesions of renal osteodystrophy—osteomalacia (rickets in children), secondary hyperparathyroidism, osteitis fibrosa cystica, osteosclerosis and metastatic calcification.

The mechanisms underlying renal osteodystrophy are schematically illustrated in Fig. 26.5 and briefly outlined below:

1. Hyperphosphataemia: In CRF, there is impaired renal excretion of phosphate, causing phosphate retention and hyperphosphataemia. Hyperphosphataemia, in turn, causes hypocalcaemia which is responsible for secondary hyperparathyroidism.

2. Hypocalcaemia: Hypocalcaemia may also result from the following:

- Due to renal dysfunction, there is decreased conversion of vitamin D metabolite 25(OH) cholecalciferol to its active form 1,25 $(OH)_2$ cholecalciferol.
- Reduced intestinal absorption of calcium.

3. Parathormone secretion: Hypocalcaemia stimulates secretion of parathormone, eventually leading to secondary hyperparathyroidism which, in turn, causes increased osteoclastic activity.

4. Metabolic acidosis: As a result of decreased renal function, acidosis sets in which may cause osteoporosis and bone decalcification.

5. Calcium phosphorus product > 70: When the product of biochemical value of calcium and phosphate is higher than 70, metastatic calcification may occur at extraosseous sites.

6. Dialysis-related metabolic bone disease: Long-term dialysis employing use of aluminium-containing dialysate is currently considered to be a major cause of metabolic bone lesions. Aluminium interferes with deposition of calcium hydroxyapatite in bone and results in osteomalacia, secondary hyperparathyroidism and osteitis fibrosa cystica. In addition, accumulation of

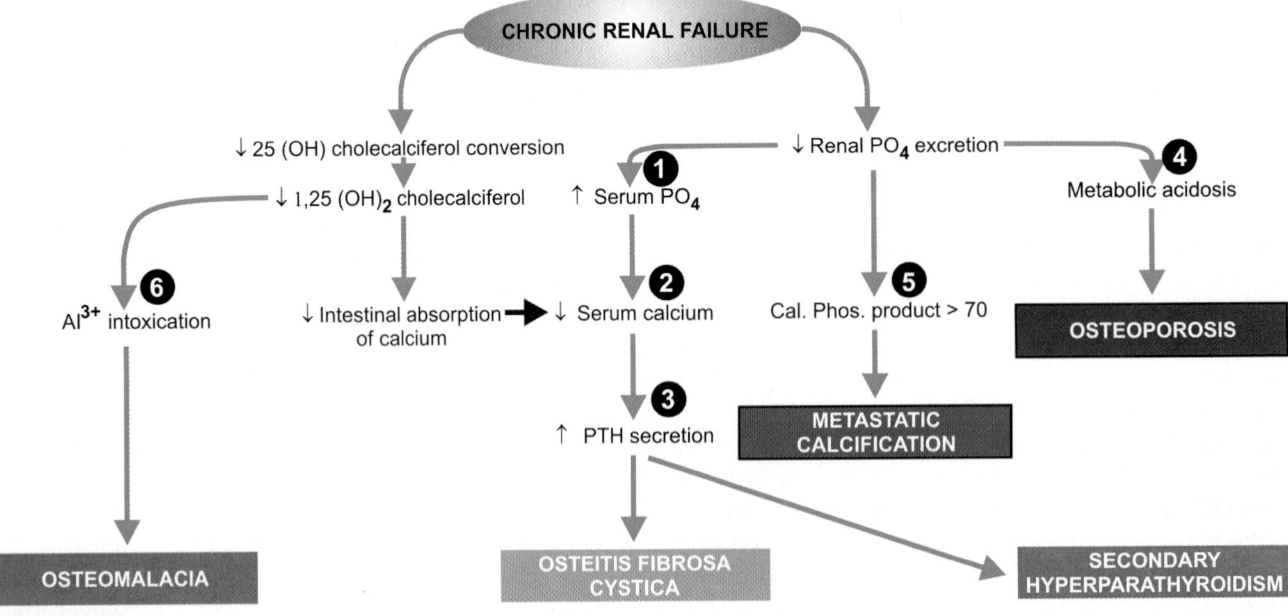

FIGURE 26.5

Pathogenesis of renal osteodystrophy in chronic renal failure. Circled serial numbers in the graphic representation correspond to the sequence described in the text on pathogenesis.

β_2-microglobulin amyloid in such cases causes dialysis-related amyloidosis (page 88).

PATHOLOGIC CHANGES. The following skeletal lesions can be identified in renal osteodystrophy:

1. *Mixed osteomalacia-osteitis fibrosa* is the most common manifestation of renal osteodystrophy resulting from disordered vitamin D metabolism and secondary hyperparathyroidism.
2. *Pure osteitis fibrosa* results from metabolic complications of secondary hyperparathyroidism.
3. *Pure osteomalacia* of renal osteodystrophy is attributed to aluminium toxicity.
4. *Renal rickets* resembling the changes seen in children with nutritional rickets with widened osteoid seams may occur (page 256).
5. *Osteosclerosis* is characterised by enhanced bone density in the upper and lower margins of vertebrae.
6. *Metastatic calcification* is seen at extraosseous sites such as in medium-sized blood vessels, periarticular tissues, myocardium, eyes, lungs and gastric mucosa (page 57).

Skeletal Fluorosis

Fluorosis of bones occurs due to high sodium fluoride content in soil and water consumed by people in some geographic areas and is termed endemic fluorosis. Such endemic regions exist in some tropical and subtropical areas; in India it exists in parts of Punjab and Andhra Pradesh. The condition affects farmers who consume drinking water from wells. Non-endemic fluorosis results from occupational exposure in manufacturing industries of aluminium, magnesium, and superphosphate.

PATHOGENESIS. In fluorosis, fluoride replaces calcium as the mineral in the bone and gets deposited without any regulatory control. This results in heavily mineralised bones which are thicker and denser but are otherwise weak and deformed (just as in osteopetrosis). In addition, there are also deposits of fluoride in soft tissues, particularly as nodules in the interosseous membrane. The patient develops skeletal deformities and mottling of teeth.

*PATHOLOGIC CHANGES. **Grossly,*** the long bones and vertebrae develop nodular swellings present both inside the bones and on the surface.

Microscopically, these nodules are composed of heavily mineralised irregular osteoid admixed with fluoride which requires confirmation chemically.

PAGET'S DISEASE OF BONE (OSTEITIS DEFORMANS)

Paget's disease of bone* or osteitis deformans was first described by Sir James Paget in 1877. Paget's disease of bone is an osteolytic and osteosclerotic bone disease of uncertain etiology involving one (monostotic) or more bones (polyostotic). The condition affects predominantly males over the age of 50 years. Though the etiology remains obscure, recently there has been a suggestion that osteitis deformans is a form of slow-virus infection by paramyxovirus detected in osteoclasts. Autosomal dominant inheritance has also been proposed on the basis of observation of disease in families.

Clinically, the *monostotic form* of the disease may remain asymptomatic and the lesion is discovered incidentally or on radiologic examination. *Polyostotic form,* however, is more widespread and may produce pain, fractures, skeletal deformities, and occasionally, sarcomatous transformation. Typically, there is marked elevation of serum alkaline phosphatase and normal to high serum calcium level.

PATHOLOGIC CHANGES. Monostotic Paget's disease involves most frequently: tibia, pelvis, femur, skull and vertebra, while the order of involvement in polyostotic Paget's disease is: vertebrae, pelvis, femur, skull, sacrum and tibia. Three sequential stages are identified in Paget's disease:

1. **Initial osteolytic stage:** This stage is characterised by areas of osteoclastic resorption produced by increased number of large osteoclasts.
2. **Mixed osteolytic-osteoblastic stage:** In this stage, there is imbalance between osteoblastic laying down of new bone and osteoclastic resorption so that mineralisation of the newly-laid matrix lags behind, resulting in development of characteristic *mosaic pattern* of osteoid seams or cement lines. The narrow space between the trabeculae and cortex is filled with collagen which gradually becomes less vascular.
3. **Quiscent osteosclerotic stage:** After many years, excessive bone formation results so that the bone becomes more compact and dense producing osteosclerosis. However, newly-formed bone is poorly mineralised, soft and susceptible to fractures. Radiologically, this stage produces characteristic *cotton-wool appearance* of the affected bone.

---

*It is pertinent to recall here that James Paget described Paget's disease at three different anatomic sites which are not mutually interlinked in any way: Paget's disease of nipple (page 790), Paget's disease of vulva (page 749) and Paget's disease of bone.

TABLE 26.1: Classification of Tumour-like Lesions of Bone.

1. Fibrous dysplasia
2. Fibrous cortical defect (metaphyseal fibrous defect, non-ossifying fibroma)
3. Solitary bone cyst (simple or unicameral bone cyst)
4. Aneurysmal bone cyst
5. Ganglion cyst of bone (intraosseous ganglion)
6. Brown tumour of hyperparathyroidism (reparative granuloma) (page 840)
7. Histiocytosis-X (Langerhans' cell histiocytosis) (page 463)

TUMOUR-LIKE LESIONS OF BONE

In the context of bones, several non-neoplastic conditions resemble true neoplasms and have to be distinguished from them clinically, radiologically and morphologically. Table 26.1 gives a list of such tumour-like lesions. A few common conditions are described below.

Fibrous Dysplasia

Fibrous dysplasia is not an uncommon tumour-like lesion of the bone. It is a benign condition, possibly of developmental origin, characterised by the presence of localised area of replacement of bone by fibrous connective tissue with a characteristic whorled pattern and containing trabeculae of woven bone. Radiologically, the typical focus of fibrous dysplasia has well-demarcated ground-glass appearance.

Three types of fibrous dysplasia are distinguished—monostotic, polyostotic, and Albright syndrome.

- **Monostotic fibrous dysplasia.** Monostotic fibrous dysplasia affects a solitary bone and is the most common type, comprising about 70% of all cases. The condition affects either sex and most patients are between 20 and 30 years of age. The bones most often affected, in descending order of frequency, are: ribs, craniofacial bones (especially maxilla), femur, tibia and humerus. The condition generally remains asymptomatic and is discovered incidentally, but infrequently may produce tumour-like enlargement of the affected bone.

- **Polyostotic fibrous dysplasia.** Polyostotic form of fibrous dysplasia affecting several bones constitutes about 25% of all cases. Both sexes are affected equally but the lesions appear at a relatively earlier age than the monostotic form. Most frequently affected bones are: craniofacial, ribs, vertebrae and long bones of the limbs. Approximately a quarter of cases with polyostotic form have more than half of the skeleton involved by disease. The lesions may affect one side of the body or may be distributed segmentally in a limb. Spontaneous fractures and skeletal deformities occur in childhood polyostotic form of the disease.

- **Albright syndrome.** Also called McCune-Albright syndrome, this is a form of polyostotic fibrous dysplasia associated with endocrine dysfunctions and accounts for less than 5% of all cases. Unlike monostotic and polyostotic varieties, Albright syndrome is more common in females. The syndrome is characterised by polyostotic bone lesions, skin pigmentation (*cafe-au-lait* macular spots) and sexual precocity, and infrequently other endocrinopathies.

PATHOLOGIC CHANGES. All forms of fibrous dysplasia have an identical pathologic appearance.

Grossly, the lesions appear as sharply-demarcated, localised defects measuring 2-5 cm in diameter, present within the cancellous bone, having thin and smooth overlying cortex. The epiphyseal cartilages are generally spared in the monostotic form but involved in the polyostotic form of disease. Cut section of the lesion shows replacement of normal cancellous bone of the marrow cavity by gritty, grey-pink, rubbery soft tissue which may have areas of haemorrhages, myxoid change and cyst formation.

Histologically, the lesions of fibrous dysplasia have characteristic benign-looking fibroblastic tissue arranged in a loose, whorled pattern in which there are irregular and curved trabeculae of woven (non-lamellar) bone. There may be numerous osteoclasts in relation to bony trabeculae. Rarely, malignant change may occur in fibrous dysplasia, most often an osteogenic sarcoma.

Fibrous Cortical Defect (Metaphyseal Fibrous Defect, Non-ossifying Fibroma)

Fibrous cortical defect or metaphyseal fibrous defect is a rather common benign tumour-like lesion occurring in the metaphyseal cortex of long bones in children. Most commonly involved bones are upper or lower end of tibia or lower end of femur. The lesion is generally solitary but rarely there may be multiple and bilaterally symmetrical defects. Radiologically, the lesion is eccentrically located in the metaphysis and has a sharply-delimited border. The pathogenesis of fibrous cortical defect is unknown. Possibly, it arises as a result of some developmental defect at the epiphyseal plate, or could be a tumour of histiocytic origin because of close resemblance to fibrohistiocytic tumours (page 889).

Clinically, fibrous cortical defect causes no symptoms and is usually discovered accidentally when X-ray of the region is done for some other reason.

PATHOLOGIC CHANGES. Grossly, the lesion is generally small, less than 4 cm in diameter, granular and brown. Larger lesion (5-10 cm) occurring usually in response to trauma is referred to as non-ossifying fibroma.

Microscopically, fibrous cortical defect consists of cellular masses of fibrous tissue showing storiform pattern. There are numerous multinucleate osteoclast-like giant cells, haemosiderin-laden macrophages and foamy cells. That is why the lesion is also termed histiocytic xanthogranuloma or fibrous xanthoma of bone.

Solitary (Simple, Unicameral) Bone Cyst

Solitary, simple or unicameral bone cyst is a benign condition occurring in children and adolescents, most frequently located in the metaphyses at the upper end of humerus and femur. The cyst expands the bone causing thinning of the overlying cortex. The pathogenesis is unknown. Clinically, solitary bone cyst may remain asymptomatic or may cause pain and fracture.

PATHOLOGIC CHANGES. Grossly, the simple cyst of the bone is generally unilocular with smooth inner surface. The cavity is filled with clear fluid. ***Histologically,*** the cyst wall consists of thin collagenous tissue having scattered osteoclast giant cells and newly formed reactive bony trabeculae. Fracture alters the appearance and produces sanguineous fluid in the cavity, and haemorrhages, haemosiderin deposits and macrophages in the cyst wall.

Aneurysmal Bone Cyst

Aneurysmal bone cyst, true to its name, is an expanding osteolytic lesion filled with blood (*aneurysm* = dilatation, distension). The condition is seen more commonly in young patients under 30 years of age. Most frequently involved bones are shafts of metaphyses of long bones or the vertebral column. The radiographic appearance shows characteristic ballooned-out expansile lesion underneath the periosteum. The pathogenesis is not clear but it has been suggested by some authors that the condition probably arises from persistent local alteration in haemodynamics. Clinically, the aneurysmal bone cyst may enlarge over a period of years and produce pain, tenderness and pathologic fracture.

PATHOLOGIC CHANGES. Grossly, the lesion consists of a large haemorrhagic mass covered over by thinned out reactive bone (Fig. 26.6,A). ***Histologically,*** the cyst consists of blood-filled aneurysmal spaces of variable size, some of which are endothelium-lined. The spaces are separated by connective tissue septa containing osteoid tissue, numerous osteoclast-like multinucleate giant cells and trabeculae of bone (Fig. 26.6,B). The condition has to be distinguished histologically from giant cell tumour or osteoclastoma (page 871) and telangiectatic osteosarcoma (page 868).

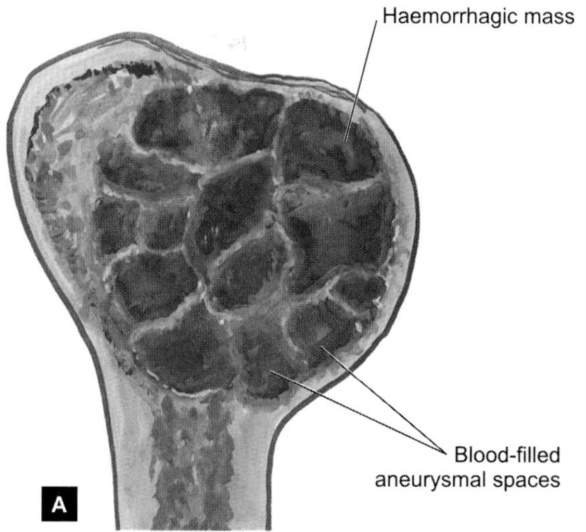

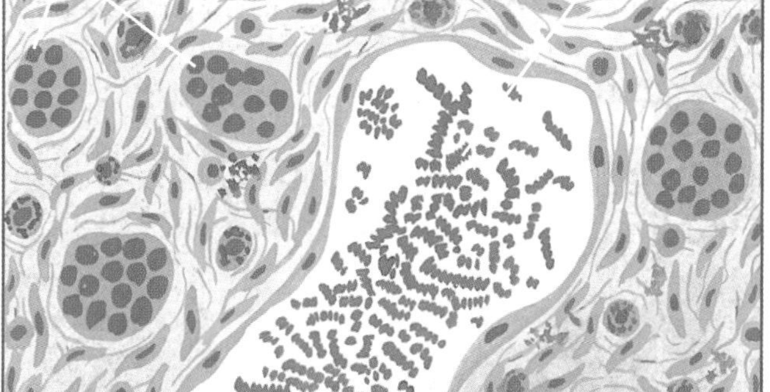

FIGURE 26.6

Aneurysmal bone cyst. A, Characteristic gross appearance of ballooned-out expansile lesion. B, Histologic hallmark of lesion is presence of aneurysmal spaces filled with blood, party lined by endothelium and separated by connective tissue septa containing osteoclast-like giant cells along the wall of vascular spaces.

Ganglion Cyst of Bone

Ganglion cyst of bone or intraosseous ganglion is a benign condition occurring in middle-aged patients. It usually involves lower end of the tibia or humerus. Radiographically, it appears as well-defined osteolytic area within the bone with surrounding zone of sclerosis close to the joint space.

PATHOLOGIC CHANGES. ***Grossly,*** the ganglion cyst of bone is often multiloculated and is mucus-filled. ***Histologically,*** it resembles the usual soft tissue ganglion but lacks a synovial lining (page 881).

BONE TUMOURS

Bone tumours are comparatively infrequent but they are clinically quite significant since some of them are highly malignant. Bone tumours may be primary or metastatic. Since histogenesis of some bone tumours is obscure, the WHO has recommended a widely accepted classification of primary bone tumours based on both histogenesis and histologic criteria. Table 26.2 lists the various types of bone tumours arising from different tissue components—osseous and non-osseous, indigenous to the bone. However, in the discussion below, only osseous bone tumours are considered, while non-osseous bone tumours are described elsewhere in the book. The anatomic origin of common primary bone tumours is illustrated in Fig. 26.7.

It may be mentioned here that the diagnosis of any bone lesion is established by a combination of clinical, radiological and pathological examination, supplemented by biochemical and haematological investigations wherever necessary. These include: serum levels of calcium, phosphorus, alkaline phosphatase and acid phosphatase. Specific investigations like plasma and urinary proteins and bone marrow examination in case of myeloma, urinary catecholamines in metastatic neuroblastoma and haematologic profile in lymphoma and leukaemic involvement of bone, are of considerable help.

BONE-FORMING (OSTEOBLASTIC) TUMOURS

Bone-forming or osteoblastic group of bone tumours is characterised by the common property of synthesis of osteoid or bone, or both, directly by the tumour cells (osteogenesis). Formation of reactive bone and endochondral ossification should not be construed as osteogenesis. Benign bone-forming tumours include: osteoma, osteoid osteoma and osteoblastoma, while the malignant counterpart is osteosarcoma (osteogenic sarcoma).

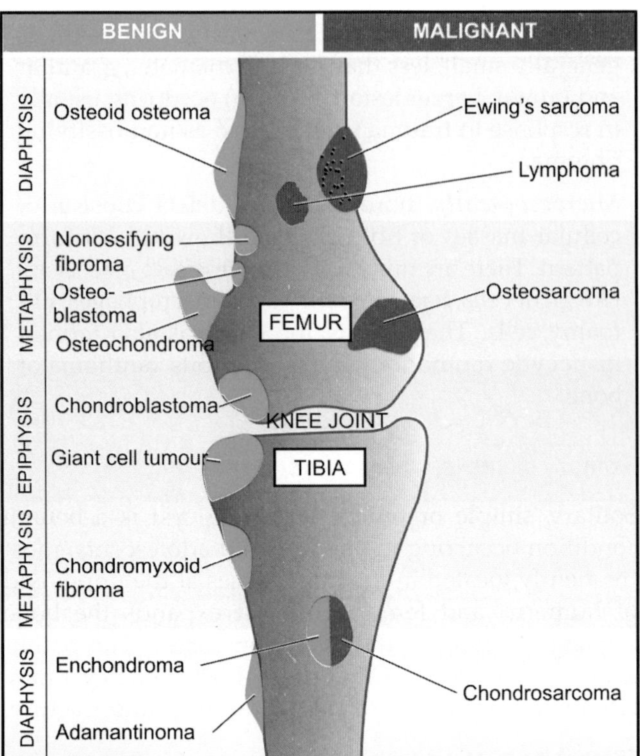

FIGURE 26.7

Anatomic locations of common primary bone tumours.

Osteoma

An osteoma is a rare benign, slow-growing lesion, regarded by some as a hamartoma rather than a true neoplasm. Similar lesions may occur following trauma, subperiosteal haematoma or local inflammation. Osteoma is almost exclusively restricted to the skull and facial bones. It may grow into paranasal sinuses or protrude into the orbit. An osteoma may form a component of Gardner's syndrome (page 601). Radiologic appearance is of a dense ivory-like bony mass.

PATHOLOGIC CHANGES. The lesion is composed of well-differentiated mature lamellar bony trabeculae separated by fibrovascular tissue.

Osteoid Osteoma and Osteoblastoma

Osteoid osteoma and osteoblastoma (or giant osteoid osteoma) are closely related benign tumours occurring in children and young adults. Osteoid osteoma is more common than osteoblastoma. There are no clear-cut histologic criteria to distinguish the two. The distinction between them is based on clinical features, size and radiographic appearance.

TABLE 26.2: Classification of Primary Bone Tumours.

HISTOLOGIC DERIVATION	BENIGN	MALIGNANT
A. OSSEOUS TUMOURS		
I. *Bone-forming (osteogenic, osteoblastic) tumours*	Osteoma (40-50 yrs) Osteoid osteoma (20-30 yrs) Osteoblastoma (20-30 yrs)	Osteosarcoma (10-20 yrs) Parosteal (juxtacortical) osteosarcoma (50-60 yrs)
II. *Cartilage-forming (chondrogenic) tumours*	Enchondroma (20-50 yrs) Osteochondroma (20-50 yrs) (Osteocartilaginous exostosis) Chondroblastoma (10-20 yrs) Chondromyxoid fibroma (20-30 yrs)	Chondrosarcoma (40-60 yrs)
III. *Haematopoietic (marrow) tumours*	—	Myeloma (50-60 yrs) Lymphoplasmacytic lymphoma (50-60 yrs)
IV. *Unknown*	Giant cell tumour (20-40 yrs) (osteoclastoma)	Malignant giant cell tumour (30-50 yrs) Ewing's sarcoma (5-20 yrs) Adamantinoma of long bones (page 542)
V. *Notochordal tumour*	—	Chordoma (40-50 yrs)
B. NON-OSSEOUS TUMOURS		
I. *Vascular tumours*	Haemangioma	Haemangioendothelioma Haemangiopericytoma Angiosarcoma
II. *Fibrogenic tumours*	Non-ossifying fibroma (metaphyseal fibrous defect)	Fibrosarcoma
III. *Neurogenic tumours*	Neurilemmoma and neurofibroma	Neurofibrosarcoma
IV. *Lipogenic tumours*	Lipoma	Liposarcoma
V. *Histiocytic tumours*	Fibrous histiocytoma	Malignant fibrous histiocytoma

Figures in brackets indicate common age of occurrence.

- **Osteoid osteoma** is generally small (usually less than 1 cm) and painful tumour, located in the cortex of a long bone. The tumour is clearly demarcated having surrounding zone of reactive bone formation so that radiographically it appears as a small radiolucent central focus or nidus surrounded by dense sclerotic bone.
- **Osteoblastoma,** on the other hand, is larger in size (usually more than 1 cm), painless, located in the medulla, commonly in the vertebrae, ribs, ilium and long bones, and there is absence of reactive bone formation.

Histologically, the distinction between osteoid osteoma and osteoblastoma is not obvious. In either case, the lesion consists of trabeculae of osteoid, rimmed by osteoblasts and separated by highly vascularised connective tissue stroma. Later, some of the trabeculae are mineralised and calcified.

Osteosarcoma

Osteosarcoma or osteogenic sarcoma is the most common primary malignant tumour of the bone. The tumour is characterised by formation of *osteoid or bone, or both, directly by sarcoma cells.* The tumour is thought to arise from primitive osteoblast-forming mesenchyme. Depending upon their locations within the bone, osteosarcomas are classified into 2 main categories: *medullary* (central) and *parosteal* (juxtacortical). The latter is an uncommon variety with a better prognosis and is described separately.

Medullary or central osteosarcoma is the more common type and is generally referred to as 'osteosarcoma' if not specified. The tumour occurs in young patients between the age of 10 and 20 years. Males are affected more frequently than females. The tumour arises in the metaphysis of long bones. Most common sites, in descending order of frequency, are: the lower end of femur and upper end of tibia (i.e. around knee joint about 60%); the upper end of humerus (10%); pelvis and the upper end of femur (i.e. around hip joint about 15%); and less often in jaw bones, vertebrae and skull. Rarely an osteosarcoma may occur in extraskeletal soft tissues.

Based upon the pathogenesis, osteosarcoma is divided into 2 types: primary and secondary.

■ *Primary osteosarcoma* is more common and occurs in the absence of any known underlying disease. Its etiology is unknown but there is evidence linking this form of osteosarcoma with genetic factors (e.g. hereditary mutation of chromosome 13 in common with retinoblastoma locus), period of active bone growth (occurrence of the tumour in younger age), and certain environmental influences (e.g. radiation and an oncogenic virus). Cases of hereditary retinoblastoma have a very high prevalence risk of development of osteosarcoma.

Many sporadic osteosarcomas show mutation in *TP53* tumour suppressor gene; some have over-expression of *MDM2* gene. Patients of hereditary retinoblastoma are predisposed to develop osteosarcoma implicating *RB* gene in their pathogenesis.

■ *Secondary osteosarcoma,* on the other hand, develops following pre-existing bone disease e.g. Paget's disease of bone, fibrous dysplasia, multiple osteochondromas, chronic osteomyelitis, infarcts and fractures of bone. The tumour has a more aggressive behaviour than the primary osteosarcoma.

Medullary osteosarcoma is a highly malignant tumour. The tumour arises centrally in the metaphysis, extends longitudinally for variable distance into the medullary cavity, expands laterally on either side breaking through the cortex and lifting the periosteum. If the periosteum is breached the tumour grows relentlessly into the surrounding soft tissues. The only tissue which is able to stop its spread, *albeit* temporarily, is the cartilage of epiphyseal plate. The radiographic appearance is quite distinctive: characteristic *'sunburst pattern'* due to osteogenesis within the tumour and presence of *Codman's triangle* formed at the angle between the elevated periosteum and underlying surface of the cortex (Fig. 26.8,A).

Clinically, the usual osteosarcoma presents with pain, tenderness and an obvious swelling of affected extremity. Serum alkaline phosphatase level is generally raised but calcium and phosphorus levels are normal. The tumour metastasises rapidly and widely to distant sites by haematogenous route and disseminates commonly to the lungs, other bones, brain and various other sites.

*PATHOLOGIC CHANGES. **Grossly,*** the tumour appears as a grey-white, bulky mass at the metaphyseal end of a long bone of the extremity. The articular end of the bone is generally uninvolved in initial stage. Codman's triangle, though identified radiologically, may be obvious on macroscopic examination (Fig. 26.8,A). Cut surface of the tumour is grey-white with areas of haemorrhages and necrotic bone. Tumours which form abundance of osteoid, bone and cartilage may have hard, gritty and mucoid areas.

Histologically, osteosarcoma shows considerable variation in pattern from case to case and even within a tumour from one area to the other. However, the following two features characterise all osteosarcomas (Fig. 26.8,B) (COLOUR PLATE XXXIII: CL 132):

1. **Sarcoma cells:** The tumour cells of osteosarcomas are undifferentiated mesenchymal stromal cells which show marked pleomorphism and polymorphism i.e. variation in size as well as shape. The tumour cells may have various shapes such as spindled, round, oval and polygonal and bizarre tumour giant cells. The tumour cells have variable size and show hyperchromatism and atypical mitoses.

2. **Osteogenesis:** The anaplastic sarcoma cells form osteoid matrix and bone directly which are found interspersed in the areas of tumour cells. In addition to osteoid and bone, the tumour cells may produce cartilage, fibrous tissue or myxoid tissue.

A variant of the usual osteosarcoma is *telangiectatic osteosarcoma* in which the tumour has large, cavernous, dilated vascular channels.

Parosteal (Juxtacortical) Osteosarcoma

Parosteal or juxtacortical osteosarcoma is an uncommon form of osteosarcoma having its origin from the external surface of the bone (*parosteal* or *juxtacortical* means outer to cortex). The tumour should be distinguished from the more common medullary osteosarcoma because of its better prognosis and different presentation. The tumour occurs in older age group, has no sex predilection and is slow growing. Its common locations are metaphysis of long bones, most frequently lower end of the femur and upper end of the humerus. X-ray examination usually reveals a dense bony mass attached to the outer cortex of the affected long bone.

*PATHOLOGIC CHANGES. **Grossly,*** the tumour is lobulated and circumscribed, calcified mass in the subperiosteal location.

Microscopically, though the features which characterise the usual osteosarcoma (sarcomatous stroma and production of neoplastic osteoid and bone) are present, the tumour shows a high degree

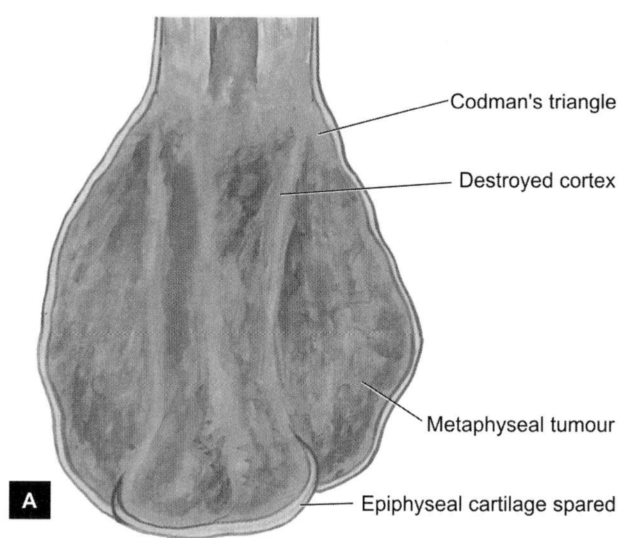

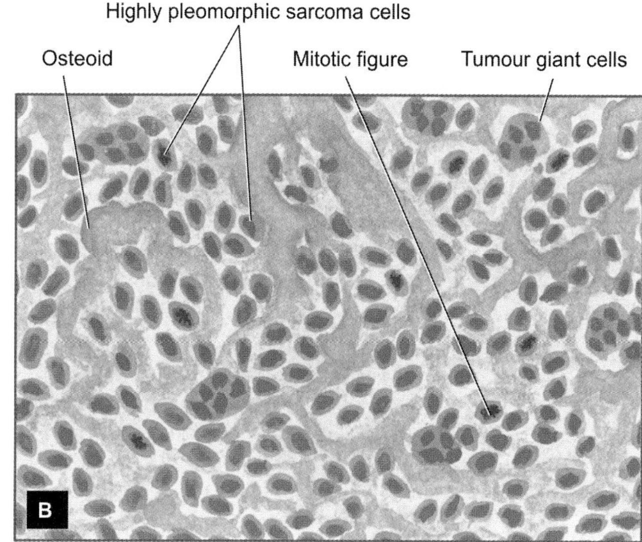

FIGURE 26.8

Osteosarcoma. A, Typical macroscopic appearance of tumour in the lower metaphysis of femur. B, Hallmarks of microscopic picture of the usual osteosarcoma are the sarcoma cells characterised by variation in size and shape of tumour cells, bizarre mitosis and multinucleate tumour giant cells, and osteogenesis i.e. production of osteoid matrix and bone directly by the tumour cells.

of structural differentiation, accounting for distinctly better prognosis in these cases.

CARTILAGE-FORMING (CHONDROBLASTIC) TUMOURS

The tumours which are composed of frank cartilage or derived from cartilage-forming cells are included in this group. It comprises benign lesions like osteocartilaginous exostoses (osteochondromas), enchondroma, chondroblastoma and chondromyxoid fibroma, and a malignant counterpart chondrosarcoma.

Osteocartilaginous Exostoses (Osteochondromas)

Osteocartilaginous exostoses or osteochondromas are the commonest of benign cartilage-forming lesions. Though designated and discussed with neoplasms, exostosis or osteochondroma is not a true tumour but is regarded as a disorder of growth and development (page 869). It may occur as a *'solitary sporadic exostosis'* or there may be *'multiple hereditary exostoses'*.

Exostoses arise from metaphyses of long bones as exophytic lesions, most commonly lower femur and upper tibia (i.e. around knee) and upper humerus but may also be found in other bones such as the scapula or ilium. They are discovered most commonly in late childhood or adolescence and are more frequent in males. They may remain asymptomatic and discovered as an incidental radiographic finding or may produce obvious deformity. Both solitary and multiple exostoses may undergo transformation into chondrosarcoma but the risk is much greater with multiple hereditary exostoses.

PATHOLOGIC CHANGES. Grossly, osteochondromas have a broad or narrow base (i.e. may be either sessile or pedunculated) which is continuous with the cortical bone. They protrude exophytically as mushroom-shaped, cartilage-capped lesions enclosing well-formed cortical bone and marrow (Fig. 26.9). ***Microscopically,*** they are composed of outer mature cartilage resembling epiphyseal cartilage and the inner mature lamellar bone and bone marrow.

Enchondroma

Enchondroma is the term used for the benign cartilage-forming tumour that develops centrally within the interior of the affected bone, while chondroma refers to the peripheral development of lesion similar to osteochondromas. Enchondromas may occur singly or they may be multiple, forming a non-hereditary disorder called *enchondromatosis* or *Ollier's disease.* The coexistence of multiple enchondromas with multiple soft tissue haemangiomas constitutes a familial syndrome called *Maffucci's syndrome.* Most common locations for enchondromas are short tubular bones of the hands and

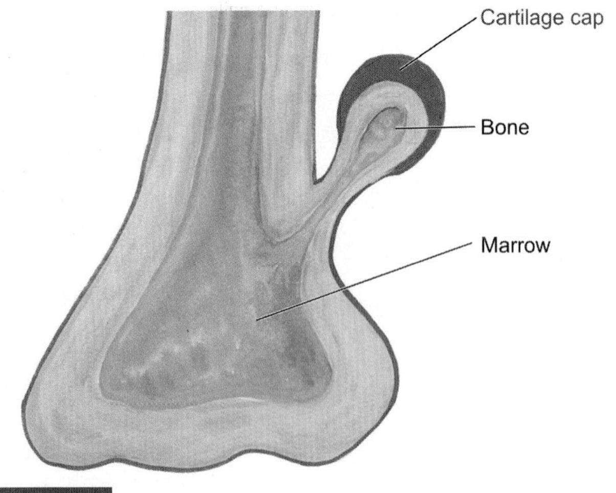

FIGURE 26.9

Characteristic appearance of a solitary osteocartilaginous exostosis (osteochondroma).

feet, and less commonly, they involve the ribs or the long bones. They may appear at any age and in either sex. Enchondromas, like osteochondromas, may remain asymptomatic or may cause pain and pathologic fractures. X-ray reveals a radiolucent, lobulated tumour mass with spotty calcification. Malignant transformation of solitary enchondroma is rare but multiple enchondromas may develop into chondrosarcoma.

PATHOLOGIC CHANGES. ***Grossly,*** the enchondroma is lobulated, bluish-grey, translucent, cartilaginous mass lying within the medullary cavity.

Histologically, the tumour has characteristic lobulated appearance. The lobules are composed of normal adult hyaline cartilage separated by vascularised fibrous stroma. Foci of calcification may be evident within the tumour. Enchondroma is distinguished from chondrosarcoma by the absence of invasion into surrounding tissues and lack of cytologic features of malignancy (COLOUR PLATE XXXIV: CL 133).

Chondroblastoma

Chondroblastoma is a relatively rare benign tumour arising from the epiphysis of long bones adjacent to the epiphyseal cartilage plate. Most commonly affected bones are upper tibia and lower femur (i.e. about knee) and upper humerus. The tumour usually occurs in patients under 20 years of age with male preponderance (male-female ratio 2:1). The radiographic appearance is of a sharply-circumscribed, lytic lesion with multiple small foci of calcification. Chondroblastoma may be asymptomatic, or may produce local pain, tenderness and discomfort. The behaviour of the tumour is benign though it may recur locally after curettage.

PATHOLOGIC CHANGES. ***Grossly,*** chondroblastoma is a well-defined mass, up to 5 cm in diameter, lying in the epiphysis. The tumour is surrounded by thin capsule of dense sclerotic bone. Cut surface reveals a soft chondroid tumour with foci of haemorrhages, necrosis and calcification.

Histologically, the tumour is highly cellular and is composed of small, round to polygonal mononuclear cells resembling chondroblasts and also contains multinucleate osteoclast-like giant cells. There are small areas of cartilaginous intercellular matrix and focal calcification.

Chondromyxoid Fibroma

Chondromyxoid fibroma is an uncommon benign tumour of cartilaginous origin arising in the metaphysis of long bones. Most common locations are upper end of tibia and lower end of femur i.e. around the knee joint. Majority of tumours appear in 2nd to 3rd decades of life with male preponderance. Radiologically, the tumour appears as a sharply-outlined radiolucent area with foci of calcification and expansion of affected end of the bone. The lesion may be asymptomatic, or may cause pain, swelling and discomfort in the affected joint. The lesions may recur after curettage. Thus, there are many similarities with chondroblastoma.

PATHOLOGIC CHANGES. ***Grossly,*** chondromyxoid fibroma is sharply-demarcated, grey-white lobulated mass, not exceeding 5 cm in diameter, lying in the metaphysis. The tumour is often surrounded by a layer of dense sclerotic bone. Cut surface of the tumour is soft to firm and lobulated but calcification within the tumour is not as common as with other cartilage-forming tumours.

Histologically, the tumour has essentially lobulated pattern. The lobules are separated by fibrous tissue and variable number of osteoclast-like giant cells. The lobules themselves are composed of immature cartilage consisting of spindle-shaped or stellate cells with abundant myxoid or chondroid intercellular matrix.

In view of close histogenetic relationship between chondromyxoid fibroma and chondroblastoma, occasional tumours show a combination of histological features of both.

Chondrosarcoma

Chondrosarcoma is a malignant tumour of chondroblasts. In frequency, it is next in frequency to osteosarcoma but is relatively slow-growing and thus has a much better prognosis than that of osteosarcoma. Two types of chondrosarcoma are distinguished: *central* and *peripheral.*

- **Central chondrosarcoma** is more common and arises within the medullary cavity of diaphysis or metaphysis. This type of chondrosarcoma is generally primary i.e. occurs *de novo.*
- **Peripheral chondrosarcoma** arises in the cortex or periosteum of metaphysis. It may be primary or secondary occurring on a pre-existing benign cartilaginous tumour such as osteocartilaginous exostoses (osteochondromas), multiple enchondromatosis, and rarely, chondroblastoma.

Both forms of chondrosarcoma usually occur in patients between 3rd and 6th decades of life with slight male preponderance. In contrast to benign cartilaginous tumours, majority of chondrosarcomas are found in the central skeleton (i.e. in the pelvis, ribs and shoulders) and around the knee joint. Radiologic appearance is of hugely expansile and osteolytic growth with foci of calcification. Clinically, the tumour is slow-growing and comes to attention because of pain and gradual enlargement over the years. Lower grades of the tumour recur following surgical removal but higher grades cause metastatic dissemination, commonly to the lungs, liver, kidney and brain.

PATHOLOGIC CHANGES. ***Grossly,*** chondrosarcoma may vary in size from a few centimeters to extremely large and lobulated masses of firm consistency. Cut section of the tumour shows translucent, bluish-white, gelatinous or myxoid appearance with foci of ossification (Fig. 26.10,A).

Histologically, the hallmarks of chondrosarcoma are invasive character and formation of lobules of anaplastic cartilage cells showing cytologic features of malignancy such as hyperchromatism, pleomorphism, two or more cells in the lacunae and tumour giant cells (Fig. 26.10,B). However, sometimes distinction between a well-differentiated chondrosarcoma and a benign chondroma may be difficult and in such cases location, clinical features and radiological appearance are often helpful (COLOUR PLATE XXXIV: CL 134).

Rare variants of chondrosarcoma are mesenchymal chondrosarcoma, dedifferentiated chondrosarcoma and clear cell chondrosarcoma.

GIANT CELL TUMOUR (OSTEOCLASTOMA)

Giant cell tumour or osteoclastoma is a distinctive neoplasm with uncertain histogenesis and hence classified separately. The tumour arises in the epiphysis of long bones close to the articular cartilage. Most

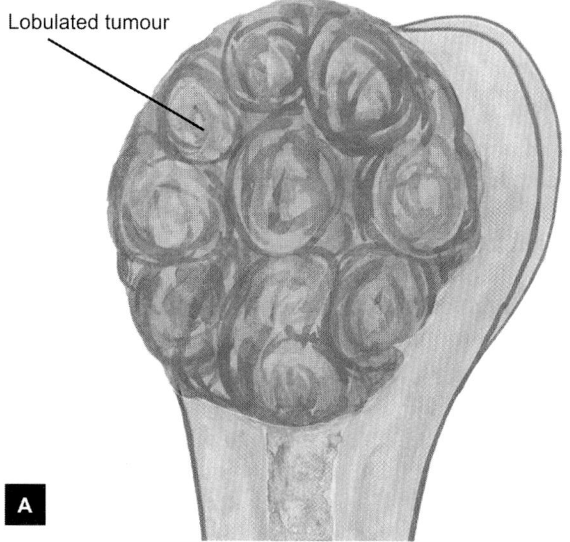

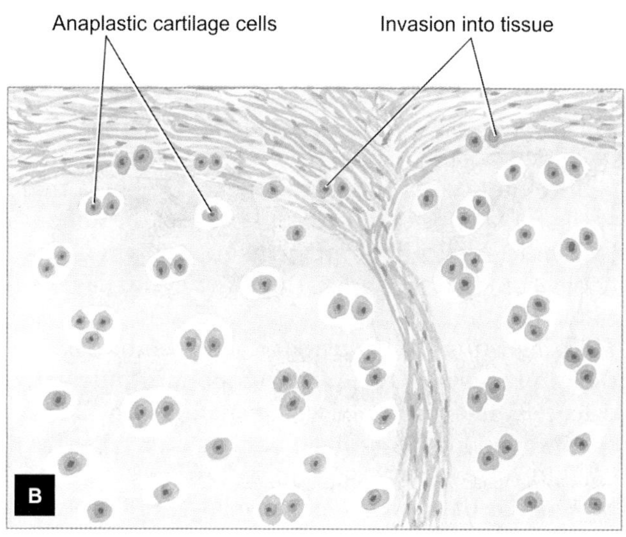

FIGURE 26.10

Chondrosarcoma. A, Gross appearance showing a large lobulated and translucent tumour on cut section (upper end of humerus). B, Histologic features include invasion of the tumour into adjacent soft tissues and cytologic characteristics of malignancy in the tumour cells.

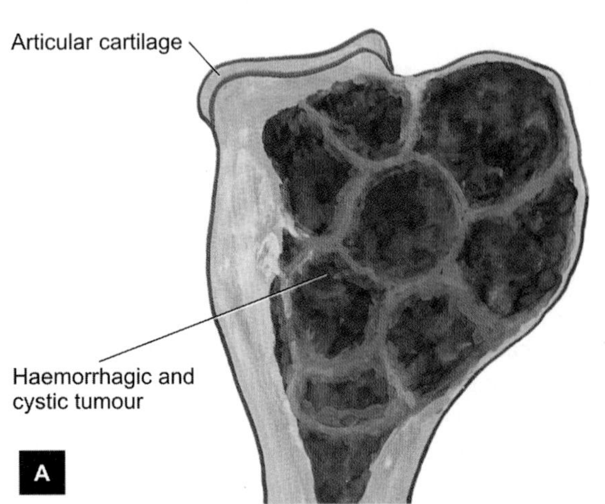

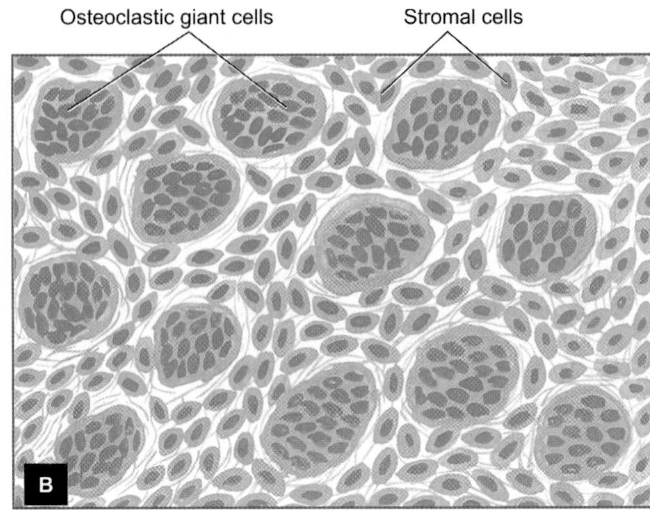

FIGURE 26.11

Giant cell tumour (osteoclastoma). A, sectioned appearance of tumour in the upper end of tibia showing expansion of epiphysis and haemorrhagic and honey-combed tumour. B, Microscopy reveals osteoclast-like multinucleate giant cells which are regularly distributed among the mononuclear stromal cells.

common sites of involvement are lower end of femur and upper end of tibia (i.e. about the knee), lower end of radius and upper end of fibula. Giant cell tumour occurs in patients between 20 and 40 years of age with no sex predilection. Clinical features at presentation include pain, especially on weight-bearing and movement, noticeable swelling and pathological fracture. Radiologically, giant cell tumour appears as a large, lobulated and osteolytic lesion at the end of an expanded long bone with characteristic *'soap bubble'* appearance.

PATHOLOGIC CHANGES. Grossly, giant cell tumour is eccentrically located in the epiphyseal end of a long bone which is expanded. The tumour is well-circumscribed, dark-tan and covered by a thin shell of subperiosteal bone. Cut surface of the tumour is characteristically haemorrhagic, necrotic, and honey-combed due to focal areas of cystic degeneration (Fig. 26.11,A).

Histologically, the hallmark of giant cell tumour is the presence of large number of multinucleate osteoclast-like giant cells which are regularly scattered throughout the stromal mononuclear cells (Fig. 26.11,B) (COLOUR PLATE XXXIII: CL 131):

- **Giant cells** often contain as many as 100 benign nuclei and have many similarities to normal osteoclasts. These cells have very high acid phosphatase activity.
- **Stromal cells** are mononuclear cells and are the real tumour cells and their histologic appearance determines the biologic behaviour of the tumour. Typically, they are uniform, plump, spindle-shaped or round to oval cells with numerous mitotic figures.
- **Other features** of the stroma include its scanty collagen content, rich vascularity, areas of haemorrhages and presence of macrophages.

Giant cell tumour of bone has certain peculiarities which deserve further elaboration. These are: its *cell of origin, its differentiation from other giant cell lesions* and its *biologic behaviour.*

- **Cell of orign.** Though designated as giant cell tumour or osteoclastoma, the true tumour cells are round to spindled mononuclear cells and not osteoclast-like giant cells. Histogenesis of tumour cells is uncertain but possibly they are of mesenchymal origin. The available evidence suggests that osteoclasts are perhaps derived from fusion of monocytes and are reactive in nature.
- **Other giant cell lesions.** This peculiar tumour with above description is named 'giant cell tumour' but giant cells are present in several other benign tumours and tumour-like lesions from which the giant cell tumour is to be distinguished. These *benign giant cell lesions* are: chondroblastoma, brown tumour of hyperparathyroidism, reparative giant cell granuloma, aneurysmal bone cyst, simple bone cyst and metaphyseal fibrous defect (non-ossifying fibroma).

■ **Biologic behaviour.** Giant cell tumours are best described as aggressive lesions. About 40 to 60% of them recur after curettage, sometimes after a few decades of initial resection. Approximately 4% cases result in distant metastases, mainly to lungs. Metastases are histologically benign and there is usually history of repeated curettages and recurrences. Thus attempts at histologic grading of giant cell tumour do not yield satisfactory results. One of the factors considered significant in malignant transformation of this tumour is the role of radiotherapy resulting in development of post-radiation bone sarcoma though primary *(de novo)* malignant or dedifferentiated giant cell tumour may also occur.

EWING'S SARCOMA AND PRIMITIVE NEUROECTODERMAL TUMOUR (PNET)

Ewing's sarcoma is a highly malignant small round cell tumour occurring in patients between the age of 5 and 20 years with predilection for occurrence in females. Since its first description by Ewing in 1921, the histogenesis of this tumour has been a debatable issue. At different times, the possibilities suggested for the cell of origin are endothelial, pericytic, bone marrow, osteoblastic, mesenchymal, and more recently is settled for primitive neuroectodermal cells. Thus, currently Ewing's sarcoma includes:

i) classic (skeletal) Ewing's sarcoma;

ii) soft tissue Ewing's sarcoma; and

iii) primitive neuroectodermal tumour (PNET).

The three are linked together by a common neural origin and by a common cytogenetic translocation abnormality t(11; 22) (q24; q12). This suggests a phenotypic spectrum in these conditions varying from undifferentiated Ewing's sarcoma to PNET positive for rosettes and neural markers (neuron-specific enolase NSE, S-100). However, PNET ultimately has a worse prognosis.

The skeletal Ewing's sarcoma arises in the medullary canal of diaphysis or metaphysis. The common sites are shafts and metaphysis of long bones, particularly femur, tibia, humerus and fibula, although some flat bones such as pelvis and scapula may also be involved.

Clinical features include pain, tenderness and swelling of the affected area accompanied by fever, leucocytosis and elevated ESR. These signs and symptoms may lead to an erroneous clinical diagnosis of osteomyelitis. However, X-ray examination reveals a predominantly osteolytic lesion with patchy subperiosteal reactive bone formation producing characteristic *'onion-skin'* radiographic appearance.

*PATHOLOGIC CHANGES. **Grossly,*** Ewing's sarcoma is typically located in the medullary cavity and produces expansion of the affected diaphysis (shaft) or metaphysis, often extending into the adjacent soft tissues. The tumour tissue is characteristically grey-white, soft and friable (Fig. 26.12,A).

Histologically, Ewing's tumour is a member of *small round cell tumours* which includes other tumours such as: PNET, neuroblastoma, embryonal rhabdomyosarcoma, lymphoma-leukaemias, and metastatic small cell carcinoma. Ewing's tumour shows the following microscopic characteristics (Fig. 26.12,B) (COLOUR PLATE XXXIII: CL 130):

1. **Pattern.** The tumour is divided by fibrous septa into irregular lobules of closely-packed tumour cells. These tumour cells are characteristically arranged around capillaries.

2. **Tumour cells.** The individual tumour cells comprising the lobules are small and uniform resembling lymphocytes and have ill-defined cytoplasmic outlines, scanty cytoplasm and round nuclei having 'salt and pepper' chromatin and frequent mitoses. Based on these cytological features the tumour is also called *round cell tumour* or *small blue cell tumour.* The cytoplasm contains glycogen that stains with periodic acid-Schiff (PAS) reaction. The tumour cells may be arranged around blood vessels forming *pseudorosettes.*

3. **Other features.** The tumour is richly vascularised and lacks the intercellular network of reticulin fibres. There may be areas of necrosis and acute inflammatory cell infiltration. Focal areas of reactive bone formation may be present.

Ewing's sarcoma metastasises early by haematogenous route to the lungs, liver, other bones and brain. Involvement of other bones has prompted a suggestion of *multicentric origin* of Ewing's sarcoma. The tumour has to be distinguished microscopically from *other small round cell tumours of bone* such as malignant lymphoma, metastatic neuroblastoma, myeloma, leukaemic deposits and metastatic carcinoma. The prognosis of Ewing's sarcoma used to be dismal (5-year survival rate less than 10%). But currently, use of combined regimen consisting of radiotherapy and systemic chemotherapy has improved the outcome greatly (5-year survival rate 40-75%).

CHORDOMA

Chordoma is a slow-growing malignant tumour arising from remnants of notochord. Notochord is the primitive axial skeleton which subsequently develops into the

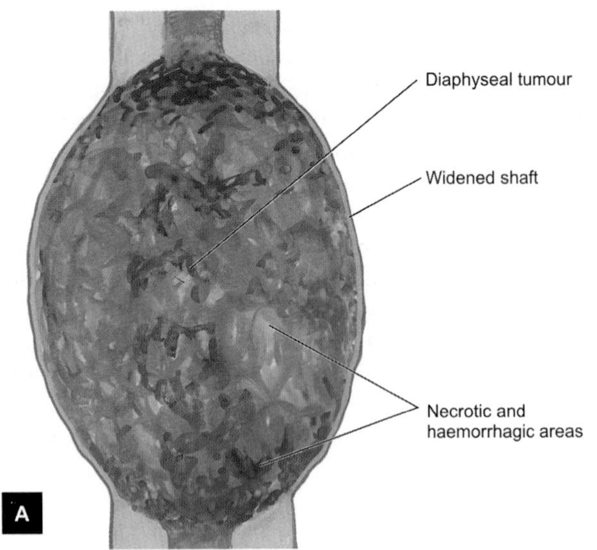

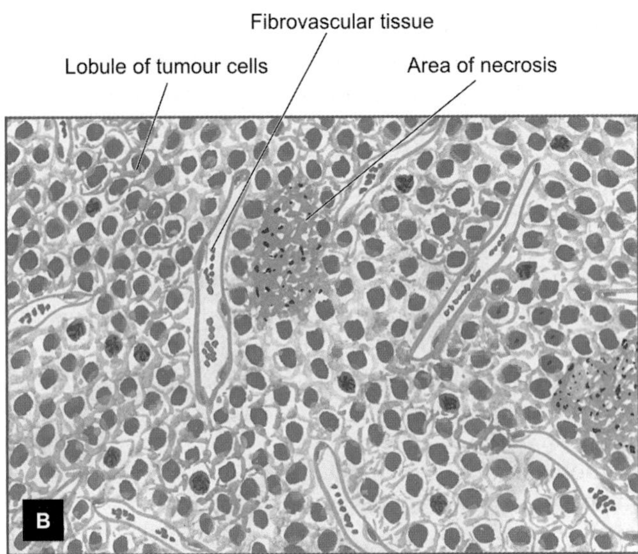

FIGURE 26.12

Ewing's sarcoma. A, Sectioned appearance of a diaphyseal (shaft) tumour in the femur showing characteristic grey-white and soft tumour in expanded medullary cavity. B, Characteristic microscopic features are irregular lobules of uniform small tumour cells with indistinct cytoplasmic outlines which are separated by fibrous tissue septa having rich vascularity. Areas of necrosis and inflammatory infiltrate are also included.

spine. Normally, remnants of notochord are represented by notochordal or physaliphorous (*physalis* = bubble, *phorous* = bearing) cells present in the nucleus pulposus and a few clumps within the vertebral bodies. Chordomas thus occur in the axial skeleton, particularly sacral and spheno-occipital region, and infrequently in the vertebrae. Chordoma is usually found in patients over the age of 40 years with no sex predilection. Radiographically, the tumour usually appears as an osteolytic lesion. Symptoms of spinal cord compression may be present. The tumour grows slowly and infiltrates adjacent structures but metastases develop rarely. Recurrences after local excision are frequent and the tumour almost invariably proves fatal.

PATHOLOGIC CHANGES. Grossly, the tumour is soft, lobulated, translucent and gelatinous with areas of haemorrhages.

Microscopically, chordoma is composed of highly vacuolated physaliphorous cells surrounded by a sea of intercellular mucoid material. Histologic differentiation between chordoma and chondrosarcoma or mucin-secreting carcinoma may sometimes be difficult.

METASTATIC BONE TUMOURS

Metastases to the skeleton are more frequent than the primary bone tumours. Metastatic bone tumours are exceeded in frequency by only 2 other organs—lungs and liver. Most skeletal metastases are derived from haematogenous spread.

Bony metastases of carcinomas predominate over the sarcomas. Some of the common *carcinomas* metastasising to the bones are of: breast, prostate, lung, kidney, stomach, thyroid, cervix, body of uterus, urinary bladder, testis, melanoma and neuroblastoma of adrenal gland. Examples of *sarcomas* which may metastasise to bone are: embryonal and alveolar rhabdomyosarcoma, Ewing's sarcoma and osteosarcoma.

Skeletal metastases may be single or multiple. Most commonly involved bones are: the spine, pelvis, femur, skull, ribs and humerus. Usual radiographic appearance is of an *osteolytic* lesion. *Osteoblastic* bone metastases occur in cancer of the prostate, carcinoid tumour and small cell carcinoma of lung.

Metastatic bone tumours generally reproduce the microscopic picture of primary tumour. Many a times, evidence of skeletal metastases is the first clinical manifestation of an occult primary cancer in the body.

JOINTS

NORMAL STRUCTURE

The joints are of 2 types—*diarthrodial or synovial joints* with a joint cavity, and *synarthrodial or nonsynovial joints* without a joint cavity. Most of the diseases of joints affect diarthrodial or synovial joints. In diarthrodial joints, the ends of two bones are held together by joint capsule with ligaments and tendons inserted at the outer surface of the capsule. The articular surfaces of bones are covered by hyaline cartilage which is thicker in weight-bearing areas than in nonweight-bearing areas. The joint space is lined by synovial membrane or synovium which forms synovial fluid that lubricates the joint during movements. The synovium may be smooth or thrown into numerous folds and villi. The synovial membrane is composed of inner layer of 1-4 cell thick synoviocytes and outer layer of loose vascular connective tissue. On electron microscopy, two types of synoviocytes are distinguished: type A and type B. *Type A* synoviocytes are more numerous and are related to macrophages and produce degradative enzymes, while *type B* synthesise hyaluronic acid.

Diseases of joints are numerous and joints are involved in several systemic disorders as well. In the following discussion, only those joint diseases which are morphologically significant are described. Synovial tumours are discussed in the next chapter together with other soft tissue tumours.

OSTEOARTHRITIS

Osteoarthritis (OA), also called osteoarthrosis or degenerative joint disease, is the most common form of chronic disorder of synovial joints. It is characterised by progressive degenerative changes in the articular cartilages over the years, particularly in weight-bearing joints.

TYPES AND PATHOGENESIS. OA occurs in 2 clinical forms—primary and secondary.

- **Primary OA** occurs in the elderly, more commonly in women than in men. The process begins by the end of 4th decade and then progressively and steadily increases producing clinical symptoms. Little is known about the etiology and pathogenesis of primary OA. The condition may be regarded as a reward of longevity. Probably, wear and tear with repeated minor trauma, heredity, obesity, aging *per se,* all contribute to focal degenerative changes in the articular cartilage of the joints. Genetic factors favouring susceptibility to develop OA have been observed though there are no consistent chromosomal alterations.
- **Secondary OA** may appear at any age and is the result of any previous wear and tear phenomena involving the joint such as previous injury, fracture, inflammation, loose bodies and congenital dislocation of the hip.

The manifestations of OA are most conspicuous in large joints such as hips, knee and back. However, the pattern of joint involvement may be related to the type of physical activity such as ballet-dancers' toes, karate fingers etc. Minor degree of OA may remain asymptomatic. In symptomatic cases, clinical manifestations are joint stiffness, diminished mobility, discomfort and pain. The symptoms are more prominent on waking up from bed in the morning. Degenerative changes in the interphalangeal joints lead to hard bony and painless enlargements in the form of nodules at the base of terminal phalanx called *Heberden's nodes.* These nodes are more common in females and heredity seems to play a role. In the spine, osteophytes of OA may cause compression of cervical and lumbar nerve root with pain, muscle spasms and neurologic abnormalities.

PATHOLOGIC CHANGES. As mentioned above, the weight-bearing joints such as hips, knee and vertebrae are most commonly involved but interphalangeal joints of fingers may also be affected. The pathologic changes occur in the articular cartilages, adjacent bones and synovium (Fig. 26.13,B):

1. Articular cartilages. The regressive changes are most marked in the weight-bearing regions of articular cartilages. Initially, there is loss of cartilaginous matrix (proteoglycans) resulting in progressive loss of normal metachromasia. This is followed by focal loss of chondrocytes, and at other places, proliferation of chondrocytes forming clusters. Further progression of the process causes loosening, flaking and fissuring of the articular cartilage resulting in breaking off of pieces of cartilage exposing subchondral bone. Radiologically, this progressive loss of cartilage is apparent as narrowed joint space.

The molecular mechanism of damage to cartilage in OA appears to be the breakdown of collagen type II, probably by IL-1, TNF and nitric oxide.

2. Bone. The denuded subchondral bone appears like polished ivory. There is death of superficial osteocytes and increased osteoclastic activity causing rarefaction, microcyst formation and occasionally microfractures of the subjacent bone. These changes result in remodelling of bone and changes in the shape of joint surface leading to flattening and mushroom-like appearance of the articular end of the bone. The margins of the joints respond to cartilage damage by *osteophyte* or *spur formation.* These are cartilaginous outgrowths at the joint margins which later get ossified. Osteophytes give the appearance of lipping of the affected joint. Loosened and fragmented osteophytes may form free 'joint mice' or loose bodies.

3. Synovium. Initially, there are no pathologic changes in the synovium but in advanced cases there

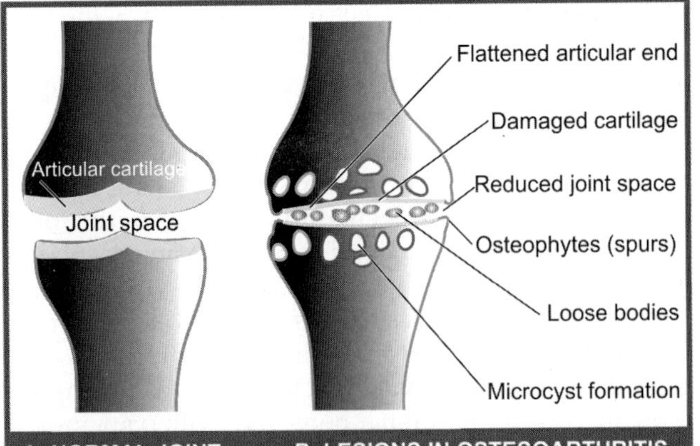

FIGURE 26.13

Fully-developed lesions in osteoarthritis (B), contrasted with appearance of a normal joint (A).

is low-grade chronic synovitis and villous hypertrophy. There may be some amount of synovial effusion associated with chronic synovitis.

RHEUMATOID ARTHRITIS

Rheumatoid arthritis (RA) is a chronic multisystem disease of unknown cause. Though the most prominent manifestation of RA is inflammatory arthritis of the peripheral joints, usually with a symmetrical distribution, its systemic manifestations include haematologic, pulmonary, neurological and cardiovascular abnormalities.

RA is a common disease having peak incidence in 3rd to 4th decades of life, with 3-5 times higher preponderance in females. The condition has high association with HLA-DR4 and HLA-DR1 and familial aggregation. The onset of disease is insidious, beginning with prodrome of fatigue, weakness, joint stiffness, vague arthralgias and myalgias. This is followed by pain and swelling of joints usually in symmetrical fashion, especially involving joints of hands, wrists and feet. Unlike migratory polyarthritis of rheumatic fever, RA usually persists in the involved joint. Approximately 20% of patients develop rheumatoid nodules located over the extensor surfaces of the elbows and fingers.

About 80% of cases are seropositive for *rheumatoid factor (RF)*. However, RF titres are elevated in certain unrelated diseases too such as in: viral hepatitis, cirrhosis, sarcoidosis and leprosy. Advanced cases show characteristic radiologic abnormalities such as narrowing of joint space and ulnar deviation of the fingers and radial deviation of the wrist. Other laboratory findings include mild normocytic and normochromic anaemia, elevated ESR, mild leucocytosis and hypergammaglobulinaemia. Extra-articular manifestations infrequently produce symptoms, but when present complicate the diagnosis.

ETIOPATHOGENESIS. Present concept on etiology and pathogenesis proposes that RA occurs in an *immunogenetically predisposed individual to the effect of microbial agents acting as trigger antigen.* More recently, the role of *superantigens* which are produced by several microorganisms with capacity to bind to HLA-DR molecules (MHC-II region) has been proposed (Fig. 26.14).

I. Immunologic derangements. A number of observations in patients and experimental animals indicate the role of immune processes, particularly autoimmune phenomenon, in the development of RA. These include the following:

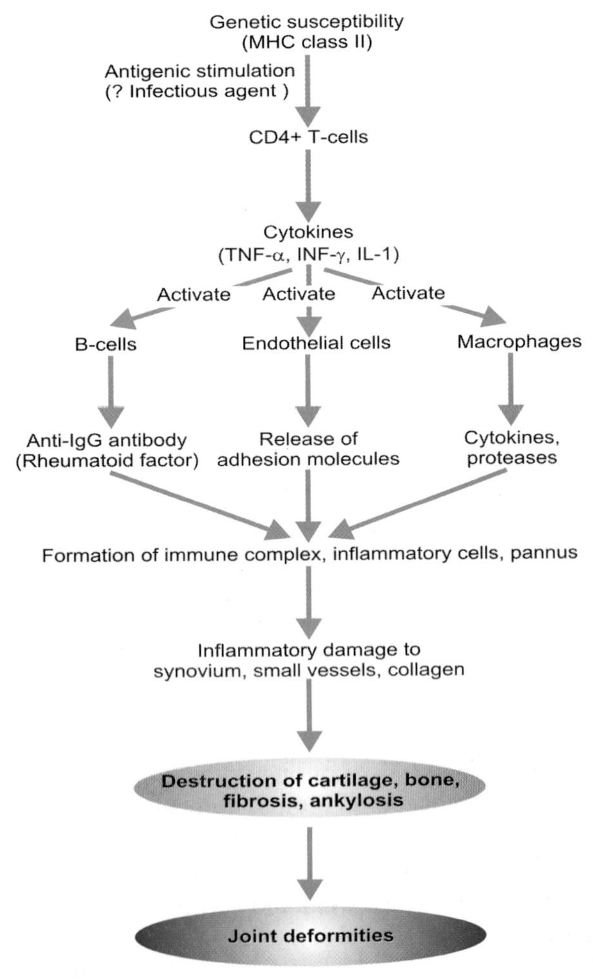

FIGURE 26.14

Pathogenesis of rheumatoid arthritis.

1. Detection of circulating autoantibody called rheumatoid factor (RF) against Fc portion of autologous IgG in about 80% cases of RA. RF antibodies are heterogeneous and consist of IgM and IgG class.

2. The presence of antigen-antibody complexes (IgG-RF complexes) in the circulation as well as in the synovial fluid.

3. The presence of other autoantibodies such as antinuclear factor (ANF), antibodies to collagen type II, and antibodies to cytoskeleton.

4. Antigenicity of proteoglycans of human articular cartilage.

5. The presence of γ-globulin, particularly IgG and IgM, in the synovial fluid.

6. Association of RA with amyloidosis.

7. Activation of cell-mediated immunity as evidenced by presence of numerous inflammatory cells in the synovium, chiefly CD4+ T lymphocytes and some macrophages.

II. Trigger events. Though the above hypothesis of a possible role of autoimmunity in the etiology and pathogenesis of RA is generally widely accepted, controversy continues as regards the trigger events which initiate the destruction of articular cartilage. Various possibilities which have been suggested are as follows:

1. The existence of an infectious agent such as mycoplasma, Epstein-Barr virus (EBV), cytomegalovirus (CMV) or rubella virus, either locally in the synovial fluid or systemic infection some time prior to the attack of RA.

2. The possible role of HLA-DR4 and HLA-DR1 in initiation of immunologic damage.

The proposed events in **immunopathogenesis** of RA is schematically shown in Fig. 26.14. Briefly, it consists of the following sequence:

- In response to antigenic exposure (? infectious agent) in a genetically predisposed individual (HLA-DR), *CD4+ T-cells* are activated.
- These cells elaborate *cytokines;* the important ones being tumour necrosis factor (TNF)-α, interferon (IF)-γ and interleukin (IL)-1.
- These cytokines *activate* endothelial cells, B lymphocytes and macrophages.
- Activation of B-cells releases IgM antibody against IgG (i.e. anti-IgG); this molecule is termed *rheumatoid factor (RF).*
- IgG and IgM immune complexes trigger *inflammatory damage* to the synovium, small blood vessels and collagen.
- Activated endothelial cells express *adhesion molecules* which stimulate collection of inflammatory cells.
- Activation of macrophages releases more cytokines which cause damage to joint tissues and vascularisation of cartilage termed *pannus formation.*
- Eventually damage and destruction of bone and cartilage are followed by *fibrosis* and *ankylosis* producing joint deformities.

PATHOLOGIC CHANGES. The predominant pathologic lesions are found in the joints and tendons, and less often, extra-articular lesions are encountered.

ARTICULAR LESIONS. RA involves first the small joints of hands and feet and then symmetrically affects the joints of wrists, elbows, ankles and knees. The proximal interphalangeal and metacarpophalangeal joints are affected most severely. Frequently cervical spine is involved but lumbar spine is spared.

Histologically, the characteristic feature is diffuse proliferative synovitis with formation of pannus. The microscopic changes are as under (Fig. 26.15):

1. Numerous folds of large villi of synovium.

2. Marked thickening of the synovial membrane due to oedema, congestion and multilayering of synoviocytes.

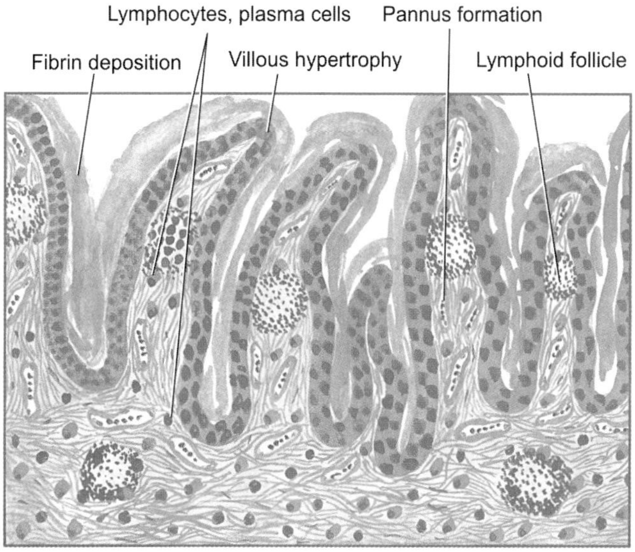

FIGURE 26.15

Rheumatoid arthritis. The characteristic histologic features are villous hypertrophy of the synovium and marked mononuclear inflammatory cell infiltrate in synovial membrane with formation of lymphoid follicles at places.

3. Intense inflammatory cell infiltrate in the synovial membrane with predominence of lymphocytes, plasma cells and some macrophages, at places forming lymphoid follicles.
4. Foci of fibrinoid necrosis and fibrin deposition.

The pannus progressively destroys the underlying cartilage and subchondral bone. This invasion of pannus results in demineralisation and cystic resorption of underlying bone. Later, fibrous adhesions or even bony ankylosis may unite the two opposing joint surfaces. In addition, persistent inflammation causes weakening and even rupture of the tendons.

EXTRA-ARTICULAR LESIONS. Nonspecific inflammatory changes are seen in the blood vessels (acute vasculitis), lungs, pleura, pericardium, myocardium, lymph nodes, peripheral nerves and eyes. But one of the characteristic extra-articular manifestation of RA is occurrence of rheumatoid nodules in the skin. *Rheumatoid nodules* are particularly found in the subcutaneous tissue over pressure points such as the elbows, occiput and sacrum. The centre of these nodules consists of an area of fibrinoid necrosis and cellular debris, surrounded by several layers of palisading large epithelioid cells, and peripherally there are numerous lymphocytes, plasma cells and macrophages. Similar nodules may be found in the lung parenchyma, pleura, heart valves, myocardium and other internal organs.

There are some *variants* of RA:

1. **Juvenile RA** found in adolescent patients under 16 years of age is characterised by acute onset of fever and predominant involvement of knees and ankles. Pathologic changes are similar but RF is rarely present.

2. **Felty's syndrome** consists of polyarticular RA associated with splenomegaly and hypersplenism and consequent haematologic derangements.

3. **Ankylosing spondylitis or rheumatoid spondylitis** is rheumatoid involvement of the spine, particularly sacro-iliac joints, in young male patients. The condition has a strong HLA-B27 association and may have associated inflammatory diseases such as inflammatory bowel disease, anterior uveitis and Reiter's syndrome.

SUPPURATIVE ARTHRITIS

Infectious or suppurative arthritis is invariably an acute inflammatory involvement of the joint. Bacteria usually reach the joint space from the blood stream but other routes of infection by direct contamination of an open wound or lymphatic spread may also occur. Immunocompromised and debilitated patients are increasingly susceptible to suppurative arthritis. The common causative organisms are gonococci, meningococci pneumococci, staphylococci, streptococci, *H. influenzae* and gram-negative bacilli. Clinically, the patients present with manifestations of any local infection such as redness, swelling, pain and joint effusion. Constitutional symptoms such as fever, neutrophilic leucocytosis and raised ESR are generally associated.

PATHOLOGIC CHANGES. The haematogenous infectious joint involvement is more often monoarticular rather than polyarticular. The large joints of lower extremities such as the knee, hip and ankle, shoulder and sternoclavicular joints are particularly favoured sites. The process begins with hyperaemia, synovial swelling and infiltration by polymorphonuclear and mononuclear leucocytes alongwith development of effusion in the joint space. There may be formation of inflammatory granulation tissue and onset of fibrous adhesions between the opposing articular surfaces resulting in permanent ankylosis.

TUBERCULOUS ARTHRITIS

Tuberculous infection of the joints results most commonly from haematogenous dissemination of the organisms from pulmonary or other focus of infection. Another route of infection is direct spread from tuberculous osteomyelitis close to the joint. The disease may occur in adults but is found more commonly in children.

PATHOLOGIC CHANGES. Tuberculous involvement of the joints is usually monoarticular type but tends to be more destructive than the suppurative arthritis. Most commonly involved sites are the spine, hip joint and knees, and less often other joints are affected. Tuberculosis of the spine is termed *Pott's disease* or *tuberculous spondylitis*.

Grossly, the affected articular surface shows deposition of grey-yellow exudate and occasionally tubercles are present. The joint space may contain tiny grey-white loose bodies and excessive amount of fluid.

Histologically, the synovium is studded with solitary or confluent caseating tubercles. The underlying articular cartilage and bone may be involved by extension of tuberculous granulation tissue and cause necrosis *(caries)*.

GOUT AND GOUTY ARTHRITIS

Gout is a disorder of purine metabolism manifested by the following features, occurring singly or in combination:

1. Increased serum uric acid concentration *(hyperuricaemia).*
2. Recurrent attacks of characteristic type of acute arthritis in which crystals of *monosodium urate monohydrate* may be demonstrable in the leucocytes present in the synovial fluid.
3. Aggregated deposits of monosodium urate monohydrate *(tophi)* in and around the joints of the extremities.
4. *Renal disease* involving interstitial tissue and blood vessels.
5. Uric acid *nephrolithiasis.*

The disease usually begins in 3rd decade of life and affects men more often than women. A family history of gout is present in a fairly large proportion of cases indicating role of inheritance in hyperuricaemia. Clinically, the natural history of gout comprises 4 stages: asymptomatic hyperuricaemia, acute gouty arthritis, asymptomatic intervals of intercritical periods, and chronic tophaceous stage. In addition, gout nephropathy and urate nephrolithiasis may occur (page 704).

TYPES AND PATHOGENESIS. The fundamental biochemical hallmark of gout is *hyperuricaemia.* A serum uric acid level in excess of 7 mg/dl, which represents the upper limit of solubility of monosodium urate in serum at 37°C at blood pH, is associated with increased risk of development of gout. Thus, *pathogenesis of gout is pathogenesis of hyperuricaemia.*

Hyperuricaemia and gout may be classified into 2 types: *metabolic* and *renal,* each of which may be *primary* or *secondary.* Primary refers to cases in which the underlying biochemical defect causing hyperuricaemia is not known, while secondary denotes cases with known causes of hyperuricaemia.

1. Hyperuricaemia of metabolic origin. This group comprises about 10% cases of gout which are characterised by overproduction of uric acid. There is either an accelerated rate of purine biosynthesis *de novo,* or an increased turnover of nucleic acids. The causes of *primary metabolic gout* include a number of specific enzyme defects in purine metabolism which may be either of unknown cause or are inborn errors of metabolism. The *secondary metabolic gout* is due to either increased purine biosynthesis or a deficiency of glucose-6-phosphatase.

2. Hyperuricaemia of renal origin. About 90% cases of gout are the result of reduced renal excretion of uric acid. Altered renal excretion could be due to reduced glomerular filtration of uric acid, enhanced tubular reabsorption or decreased secretion. The causes of gout of renal origin include diuretic therapy, drug-induced (e.g. aspirin, pyrazinamide, nicotinic acid, ethambutol and ethanol), adrenal insufficiency, starvation, diabetic ketosis, and disorders of parathyroid and thyroid. Renal disease *per se* rarely causes secondary hyperuricaemia such as in polycystic kidney disease and leads to urate nephropathy.

PATHOLOGIC CHANGES. The pathologic manifestations of gout include: acute gouty arthritis, chronic tophaceous arthritis, tophi in soft tissues, and renal lesions as under:

1. Acute gouty arthritis. This stage is characterised by acute synovitis triggered by precipitation of sufficient amount of needle-shaped crystals of monosodium urate from serum or synovial fluid. There is joint effusion containing numerous polymorphs, macrophages and microcrystals of urates. The mechanism of acute inflammation appears to include phagocytosis of crystals by leucocytes, activation of the kallikrein system, activation of the complement system and urate-mediated disruption of lysosomes within the leucocytes leading to release of lysosomal products in the joint effusion. Initially, there is monoarticular involvement accompanied with intense pain, but later it becomes polyarticular alongwith constitutional symptoms like fever. Acute gouty arthritis is predominantly a disease of lower extremities, affecting most commonly *great toe.* Other joints affected, in order of decreasing frequency, are: the instep, ankles, heels, knees, wrists, fingers and elbows.

2. Chronic tophaceous arthritis. Recurrent attacks of acute gouty arthritis lead to progressive evolution into chronic arthritis. The deposits of urate encrust the articular cartilage. There is synovial proliferation, pannus formation and progressive destruction of articular cartilage and subchondral bone. Deposits of urates in the form of tophi may be found in the periarticular tissues.

3. Tophi in soft tissue. A *tophus* (meaning 'a porous stone') is a mass of urates measuring a few millimeters to a few centimeters in diameter. Tophi may be located in the periarticular tissues as well as subcutaneously such as on the hands and feet. Tophi are surrounded by inflammatory reaction consisting of macrophages, lymphocytes, fibroblasts and foreign body giant cells (Fig. 26.16).

4. Renal lesions. Chronic gouty arthritis frequently involves the kidneys. Three types of renal lesions are described in the kidneys: acute urate nephropathy, chronic urate nephropathy and uric acid nephrolithiasis.

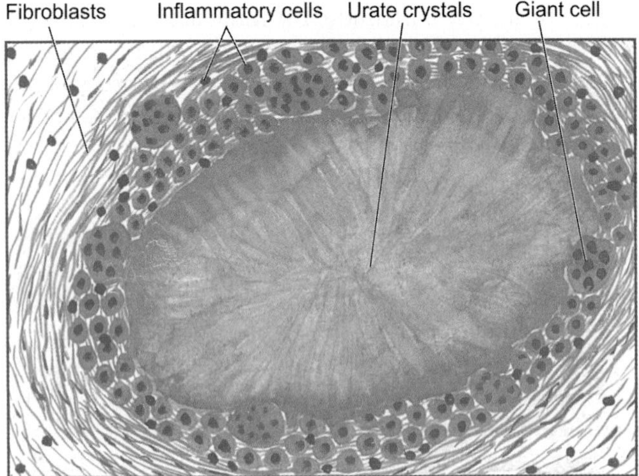

FIGURE 26.16

A gouty tophus, showing central aggregates of urate crystals surrounded by macrophages, lymphocytes, fibroblasts and occasional giant cells.

i) *Acute urate nephropathy* is attributed to the intra-tubular deposition of monosodium urate crystals resulting in acute obstructive uropathy.
ii) *Chronic urate nephropathy* refers to the deposition of urate crystals in the renal interstitial tissue.
iii) *Uric acid nephrolithiasis* is related to hyper-uricaemia resulting in hyperuricaciduria (page 715).

PSEUDOGOUT (PYROPHOSPHATE ARTHROPATHY)

Pseudogout refers to an inflammatory joint involvement due to deposition of calcium pyrophosphate in the joint space. The condition is seen in middle-aged and elderly individuals of either sex. The pain is usually less severe and involvement of big toe is rare. The pathogenesis is unclear but several factors have been implicated. These include: associated metabolic disease (e.g. hyper-parathyroidism, hypothyroidism, gout, ochronosis, Wilson's disease and haemochromatosis), heredity, familial occurrence, rheumatoid arthritis and osteoarthritis.

PATHOLOGIC CHANGES. The involvement may be monoarticular or polyarticular but large joints such as knees, hips and shoulders are more often affected. The joint effusion contains crystals of calcium pyrophosphate. There is acute inflammatory response and deposits of rhomboid crystals on the articular cartilage, ligaments, tendons and joint capsule, termed *chondrocalcinosis*.

PIGMENTED VILLONODULAR SYNOVITIS AND GIANT CELL TUMOUR OF TENDON SHEATH (NODULAR TENOSYNOVITIS)

The terms 'pigmented villonodular synovitis' and 'nodular tenosynovitis' represent diffuse and localised form respectively of the same underlying process. The localised form of lesion is also termed *xanthofibroma* or *benign synovioma*. When the giant cells are numerous in localised tenosynovitis, the condition is called *giant cell tumour of tendon sheath*.

The origin and histogenesis of these conditions are unknown. They were initially regarded as inflammatory in origin and hence the name synovitis. But currently cytogenetic studies have shown clonal proliferation of cells indicating that these lesions are neoplastic. Clinically, they present with pain, swelling and limitation of movement of the affected joint and may be easily mistaken for rheumatoid or infective arthritis. The lesions are adequately treated by excision but recurrences are common.

PATHOLOGIC CHANGES. Though the two conditions have many morphologic similarities, they are best described separately.

■ **Giant cell tumour of tendon sheath (Nodular tenosynovitis).** The localised nodular tenosynovitis is seen most commonly in the tendons of fingers.

Grossly, it takes the form of a solitary, circumscribed, pedunculated, small and lobulated nodule, measuring less than 2 cm in diameter. It is closely attached to and sometimes grooved by the underlying tendon. On section, the lesion is yellowish-brown.

Histologically, it is well encapsulated and is composed of sheets of small oval to spindle-shaped cells, foamy xanthoma cells, scattered multinucleate giant cells and irregular bundles of collagen. Many of the spindle-shaped cells are haemosiderin-laden.

■ **Pigmented villonodular tenosynovitis.** This is a diffuse form of synovial overgrowth seen most commonly in the knee and hip.

Grossly, the synovium has characteristic sponge-like reddish-brown or tan appearance with intermingled elongated villous projections and solid nodules.

Histologically, the changes are modified by recurrent injury. The enlarged villi are covered by hyperplastic synovium and abundant subsynovial infiltrate of lymphocytes, plasma cells and macrophages, many of which are lipid-laden and haemosiderin-laden. Multinucleate giant cells are scattered in these areas.

CYST OF GANGLION

A ganglion is a small, round or ovoid, movable, subcutaneous cystic swelling. The most common location is dorsum of wrist but may be found on the dorsal surface of foot near the ankle. Histogenesis of the ganglion is disputed. It may be the result of herniated synovium, embryologically displaced synovial tissue, or post-traumatic degeneration of connective tissue.

PATHOLOGIC CHANGES. ***Grossly,*** a ganglion is a small cyst filled with clear mucinous fluid. It may or may not communicate with the joint cavity or tendon where it is located.
Microscopically, the cyst has a wall composed of dense or oedematous connective tissue which is sometimes lined by synovial cells but more often is lined by necrotic cells.

BURSITIS

Inflammation of bursa is termed bursitis. Bursae are synovial-lined sacs found over bony prominences. Bursitis occurs following mechanical trauma or inflammation. It may result following single injury such as *olecranon bursitis* and *prepatellar bursitis,* but is more often due to repeated injuries from excessive pressure such as in *housemaid's knee* or *tennis elbow.*

PATHOLOGIC CHANGES. ***Grossly,*** the bursal sac is thick-walled and may contain watery, mucoid or granular brown material.
Histologically, the bursal wall is composed of dense fibrous tissue lined by inflammatory granulation tissue. The wall is infiltrated by lymphocytes, plasma cells and macrophages and may show focal calcium deposits.

SKELETAL MUSCLES

NORMAL STRUCTURE

Striated skeletal muscles consist of bundles of fibres called *fascicles,* each of which is surrounded by connective tissue sheath termed *perimysium.* Perimysium contains blood vessels and nerve supply of the muscle fascicles. Each muscle fibre is enveloped by delicate fibrous stroma called *endomysium.*

Individual muscle fibre is an elongated multinucleated syncytium-like cell about 100 μm in diameter and several centimeters in length. The muscle nuclei are spindle-shaped and lie at the periphery of fibre under the sarcolemma, the plasma membrane of muscle fibre. The cytoplasm of the muscle fibre contains myofilaments which are contractile elements. Myofilaments are of 2 types—*myosin* comprising thick filaments and *actin* constituting thin filaments. These together produce cross-striations in muscle fibres seen in longitudinal sections on light microscopy. *Sarcomeres* are the partitions of myofilaments into equal zones. Each sarcomere represents the distance between consecutive *Z bands* and contains the *central A* (anisotropic) band, and the *lateral I* (isotropic) bands.

The major *functions* of striated skeletal muscle are to convert chemical energy into mechanical energy, to act as a store of energy and proteins, and to play a role in the metabolism of the body. The muscle, however, cannot function as a contractile organ without a nerve supply. For this purpose, there are **motor units,** each of which consists of the following:

1. *motor neuron cell body* located in the spinal cord anterior horn, or a cranial nerve nucleus;
2. the *axon* of the motor neuron in the peripheral or cranial nerve;
3. the *neuromuscular junction;* and
4. the *muscle fibres* innervated by the motor neuron.

The muscle fibre contraction occurs by action potential generated by chemical transmission of the impulse across the synaptic gap by acetylcholine.

Skeletal muscles are affected in a number of systemic diseases and pathologic processes such as ischaemia and toxic (Zenker's) necrosis; atrophy and hypertrophy; degeneration and regeneration; and polymyositis, dermatomyositis, and various forms of infective myositis (e.g. viral myositis, pyogenic myositis, gas gangrene and parasitic involvements such as cysticercosis). Most of the conditions are considered already in different chapters. Here, two important groups of specific diseases—neurogenic and myopathic diseases, are considered. A classification of neuromuscular disorders based on the part of the motor unit involved is presented in Table 26.3.

TABLE 26.3: Classification of Neuromuscular Diseases.

SITE OF MOTOR UNIT	DISEASE
I. *Anterior horn cell*	
1. Without upper motor neuron involvement	Spinal muscular atrophy
2. With upper motor neuron involvement	Amyotrophic lateral sclerosis
II. *Peripheral nerve*	
1. Unifocal	Carpal-tunnel syndrome
2. Multifocal	Mononeuritis multiplex
3. Diffuse	Diabetic neuropathy
III. *Neuromuscular junction*	Myasthenia gravis
IV. *Muscle*	Duchenne's muscular dystrophy

NEUROGENIC DISEASES

The group of neurogenic diseases affecting skeletal muscles is characterised by a combination of muscular weakness and fatiguability. The most common of these is myasthenia gravis; others are congenital myasthenia, an acquired Eaton-Lambert syndrome associated with carcinoma of the lung, and denervation atrophy.

MYASTHENIA GRAVIS

Myasthenia gravis (MG) is a neuromuscular disorder of autoimmune origin in which the acetylcholine receptors (AChR) in the motor end-plates of the muscles are damaged. The term *'myasthenia'* means muscular weakness and *'gravis'* implies serious; thus both together denote the clinical characteristics of the disease. MG may be found at any age but adult women are affected more often than adult men in the ratio of 3:2. The condition presents clinically with muscular weakness and fatiguability, initially in the ocular musculature but later spreads to involve the trunk and limbs. There is about 10% mortality in MG which is due to severe generalised disease and involvement of respiratory muscles. Several other autoimmune diseases have been found associated with MG such as autoimmune thyroiditis, rheumatoid arthritis, SLE, pernicious anaemia and collagen-vascular diseases.

PATHOGENESIS. The pathogenesis of MG is best understood in the context of normal muscle metabolism.

- **Normally,** acetylcholine is synthesised in the motor nerve terminal and stored in vesicles that are released spontaneously when an action potential reaches the nerve terminal. Acetylcholine from released vesicles combines with AChRs, initiating an action potential which is propagated along the muscle fibre triggering muscle contraction (Fig. 26.17,A).

- **In MG,** the basic defect is reduction in the number of available AChRs at the postsynaptic muscle membrane. In addition, the postsynaptic folds are flattened (Fig. 26.17,B). These changes result in decreased neuromuscular transmission leading to failure to trigger muscle action potentials and consequent weakened muscle contraction. The neuromuscular abnormalities in MG are mediated by autoimmune response. About 85-90% patients of MG have anti-AChR-antibodies in their sera. These antibodies reduce the number of available AChRs either by blocking the active sites of the receptors or by damaging the post-synaptic muscle membrane in collaboration with complement. The exact mechanism how autoimmune response is initiated is not completely understood but the thymus appears to play a role in this process (page 467). Majority of patients of MG may have either thymoma or thymic hyperplasia; thymectomy is helpful in ameliorating the condition. The thymus possibly sensitises B cells to produce anti-AChR antibodies.

*PATHOLOGIC CHANGES. **Grossly,*** the muscles appear normal until late in the course of disease when they become wasted.

By ***light microscopy,*** a few clumps of lymphocytes may be found around small blood vessels. Degenerating muscle fibres are present in half the cases.

Electron microscopy reveals reduction in synaptic area of the motor axons due to flattening or simpli-

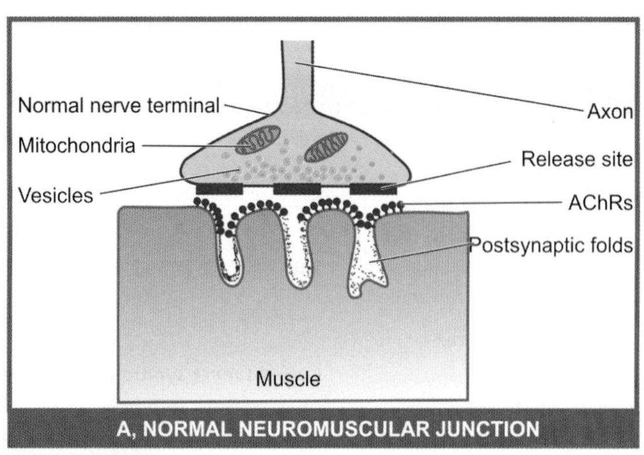

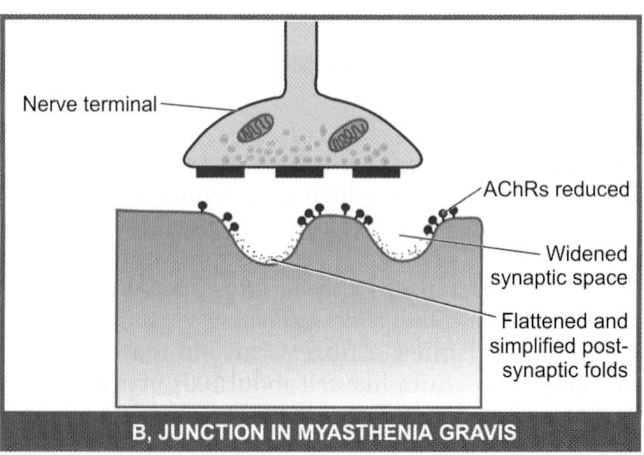

FIGURE 26.17

Neuromuscular junction in normal transmission (A) and in myasthenia gravis (B). The junction in MG shows reduced number of AChRs, flattened and simplified postsynaptic folds, a widened synaptic space but a normal nerve terminal.

fication of postsynaptic folds. The number of AChRs is greatly reduced (Fig. 26.17,B). By immunocytochemistry combined with electron microscopy, it is possible to demonstrate the complex of IgG and complement at the neuromuscular junctions.

DENERVATION ATROPHY

If the muscle or a part of muscle is deprived of its motor nerve supply, the affected muscle undergoes atrophy. In demyelination, on the other hand, there is conduction block in the nerve impulse but no denervation and hence muscle atrophy does not occur.

Denervating diseases are characterised by axonal degeneration and consequent muscle atrophy. These include *amyotrophic lateral sclerosis* as an example of anterior horn cell disease, and *peripheral neuropathy* causing injury to myelinated axon. The clinical manifestations of denervation atrophy are combination of muscular weakness and reduced muscle bulk. In amyotrophic lateral sclerosis, there are characteristic fasciculations of muscles of the shoulder and tongue.

PATHOLOGIC CHANGES. Denervation atrophy is pathologically characterised by groups of small angulated muscle fibres alternating with groups of plump, normal or even hypertrophic fibres with intact innervation. Further progression of the process may produce superimposed changes of muscular dystrophy.

MYOPATHIC DISEASES (MYOPATHIES)

Myopathies are primary skeletal muscle diseases resulting in chronic muscle weakness. These are divided into 5 broad groups: hereditary (muscular dystrophies), inflammatory, endocrine, metabolic and toxic myopathies. Only the hereditary myopathies, also termed muscular dystrophies, are briefly considered below.

MUSCULAR DYSTROPHIES

Muscular dystrophies are a group of genetically-inherited primary muscle diseases, having in common, progressive and unremitting muscular weakness. Six major forms of muscular dystrophies are described: *Duchenne's, Becker's, myotonic, facio-scapulohumeral, limb-girdle and oculo-pharyngeal type.* Each type of muscular dystrophy is a distinct entity having differences in inheritance pattern, age at onset, clinical features, other organ system involvements and clinical course. These differences are summarised in Table 26.4. However, in general, muscular

TABLE 26.4: Contrasting Features of Muscular Dystrophies.

	TYPE	INHERITANCE	AGE AT ONSET	CLINICAL FEATURES	OTHER SYSTEMS INVOLVED	COURSE
1.	*Duchenne's type*	X-linked recessive	By age 5	Symmetric weakness; initially pelvifemoral; later weakness of girdle muscles; pseudo-hypertrophy of calf muscles	Cardiomegaly; reduced intelligence	Progressive; death by age 20 due to respiratory failure
2.	*Becker's type*	X-linked recessive	By 2nd decade	Slow progressive weakness of girdle muscle (minor variant of Duchenne's type)	Cardiomegaly	Benign
3.	*Myotonic type*	Autosomal dominant	Any decade	Slow progressive weakness and myotonia of eyelids, face, neck, distal limb muscles	Cardiac conduction defects; mental impairment; cataracts; frontal baldness; gonadal atrophy	Benign
4.	*Facioscapulo-humeral type*	Autosomal dominant	2nd-4th decade	Slowly progressive weakness of facial, scapular and humeral muscles	Hypertension	Benign
5.	*Limb-girdle type*	Autosomal recessive	Early child-hood to adult	Slowly progressive weakness of shoulder and hip girdle muscles	Cardiomyopathy	Variable progression
6.	*Oculo-pharyngeal type*	Autosomal dominant	5th-6th decade	Slowly progressive weakness of extraocular eyelid, face and pharyngeal muscles	—	Rarely progressive

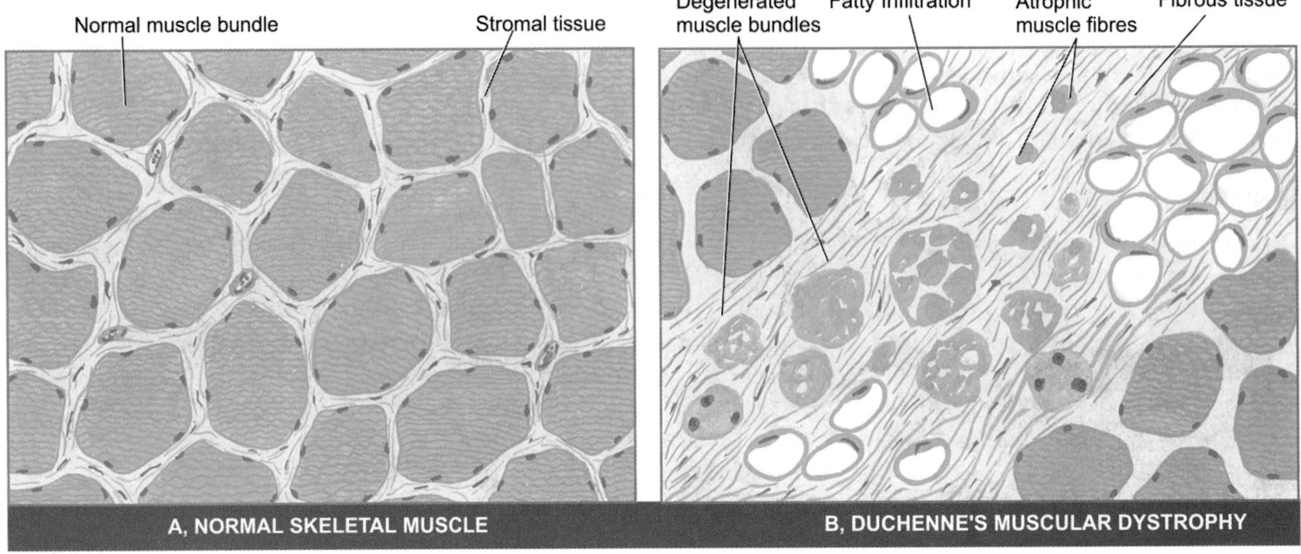

FIGURE 26.18

A, Normal skeletal muscle. B, Duchenne's muscular dystrophy showing hyaline fibres, fibre degeneration, loss of fibres and replacement by interstitial fibrosis and adipose tissue.

dystrophies manifest in childhood or in early adulthood. Family history of neuromuscular disease is elicited in many cases.

PATHOLOGIC CHANGES. Common to all forms of muscular dystrophies are muscle fibre necrosis, regenerative activity, replacement by interstitial fibrosis and adipose tissue (Fig. 26.18).

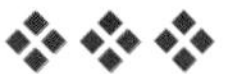

Soft Tissue Tumours

27

GENERAL FEATURES

INTRODUCTION. For the purpose of classification of this group of tumours, the WHO has defined soft tissues as including all non-epithelial extra-skeletal tissues of the body except the reticuloendothelial system, the glia and the supporting tissues of specific organs and viscera. Thus, tissues included in soft tissues are: fibrous tissue, adipose tissue, muscle tissue, synovial tissue, blood vessels and neuroectodermal tissues of the peripheral and autonomic nervous system. The lesions of these tissues are embryologically derived from mesoderm, except those of peripheral nerve which are derived from ectoderm. Tumours of smooth muscle tissue, blood vessels and nerves are described elsewhere in the book, while tumours and tumour-like lesions composed of other soft tissues are discussed here.

In general, the benign tumours of soft tissues are designated by a prefix indicating the tissue of origin followed by suffix *-oma* and malignant counterparts by adding the suffix *-sarcoma.* Benign soft tissue tumours are about 100 times more common than sarcomas. Sarcomas rarely arise from malignant transformation of a pre-existing benign tumour. Instead, sarcomas originate from the primitive mesenchymal cells having the capacity to differentiate along different cell pathways. It may be recalled here that soft tissue sarcomas metastasise most frequently by the haematogenous route and disseminate commonly to the lungs, liver, bone and brain. Lymph node metastases are often late and are associated with widespread dissemination of the tumour. Histologic differentiation and grading of soft tissue sarcomas are important because of varying clinical behaviour, prognosis and response to therapy.

A few important principles apply to majority of soft tissue tumours:

- Superficially-located tumours tend to be benign while *deep-seated lesions* are more likely to be malignant.
- *Large-sized tumours* are generally more malignant than small ones.
- A *rapidly-growing tumour* often behaves as a malignant tumour than the one that develops slowly.
- Malignant tumours have frequently *increased vascularity* while benign tumours are selectively avascular.
- Although soft tissue tumours may arise anywhere in the body but in general *more common locations* are: lower extremity (40%), upper extremity (20%), trunk and retroperitoneum (30%) and head and neck (10%).
- In general *males* are affected more commonly than females.
- Approximately 15% of soft tissue tumours occur in *children* and includes some specific examples of soft tissue sarcomas e.g. rhabdomyosarcoma, synovial sarcoma.

ETIOLOGY AND PATHOGENESIS. Etiology of soft tissue tumours remains largely unknown; however a few common features characterise many soft tissue tumours:

1. Frequently there is history of antecedent *trauma* which may bring the tumour to attention of the patient.
2. Molecular and cytogenetic studies in many soft tissue tumours reveal *chromosomal abnormalities and mutations* in genes which can be used as a marker for diagnosis

and histogenesis e.g. translocations, various fusion genes etc.

3. Most of the soft tissue tumours occur *sporadically;* however there are a few examples which are components of *genetic syndromes* e.g. neurofibromatosis type 1, Li-Fraumeni syndrome, Osler-Weber-Rendu syndrome etc.

CLASSIFICATION AND DIAGNOSTIC CRITERIA. Soft tissue tumours are generally classified clinically on the basis of tissue produced by the tumour e.g. fibrous, lipogenic etc. However, accurate pathological diagnosis of soft tissue tumours is based on histogenesis which is important for determining the prognosis and can be made by the following plan:

1. Cell patterns: Several morphological patterns in which tumour cells are arranged are peculiar in different tumours e.g.

i) Smooth muscle tumours: interlacing fascicles of pink staining tumour cells.

ii) Fibrohistiocytic tumours: characteristically have storiform pattern in which spindle tumour cells radiate from the centre in a spokewheel manner.

iii) Herringbone pattern: is seen in fibrosarcoma in which the tumour cells are arranged like the vertebral column of seafish.

iv) Pallisaded arrangement: characteristically is seen in schwannomas in which the nuclei of tumour cells are piled upon each other.

v) Biphasic pattern: is the term used for a combination arrangement of two types—fascicles and epithelial-like; e.g. in synovial sarcoma.

2. Cell types: After looking at the pattern of cells described above, preliminary categorisation of soft tissue tumours is done on the basis of cell types comprising the soft tissue tumour:

i) Spindle cells: These are the most common cell types in most sarcomas. However, there are subtle differences in different types of spindle cells e.g.

a) *fibrogenic tumours* have spindle cells with light pink cytoplasm and tapering-ended nuclei;

b) *neurogenic (schwann cell) tumours* have tumour cells similar to fibrogenic cells but have curved nuclei;

c) *leiomyomatous tumours* have spindle cells with blunt-ended (cigar-shaped) nuclei and more intense eosinophilic cytoplasm; and

d) *skeletal muscle tumours* have spindle cells similar to leiomyomatous cells but in addition have cytoplasmic striations.

ii) Small round cells: Some soft tissue sarcomas are characterised by dominant presence of small round cells or blue cells and are accordingly termed as malignant small round cell tumours, round cell sarcomas, or blue cell tumours (due to presence of lymphocyte-like nuclear size and dense blue chromatin). For example:

a) rhabdomyosarcoma (embryonal and alveolar types);
b) primitive neuroectodermal tumour (PNET),
c) Ewing's sarcoma;
d) neuroblastoma; and
e) malignant lymphomas.

A few examples of epithelial tumours such as small cell carcinoma and malignant carcinoid tumours are also included in the differential diagnosis of small round cell tumours.

iii) Epithelioid cells: Some soft tissue tumours have either epithelioid cells as the main cells (e.g. epithelioid sarcoma) or have epithelial-like cells as a part of biphasic pattern of the tumour (e.g. synovial sarcoma).

3. Immunohistochemistry: Soft tissue tumours are distinguished by application of immunohistochemical stains. Antibody stains are available against almost each cell constituent. Based on differential diagnosis made on routine morphology, the panel of antibody stains is chosen for applying on paraffin sections for staining. Some common examples are:

i) smooth muscle actin (SMA) for smooth muscle tumours;
ii) vimentin as common marker to distinguish mesenchymal cells from epithelium;
iii) desmin for skeletal muscle cells;
iv) S-100 for nerve fibres;
v) factor VIII antigen for vascular endothelium; and
vi) LCA (leucocyte common antigen) common marker for lymphocytes.

4. Electron microscopy: EM as such is mainly a research tool and does not have much diagnostic value in soft tissue tumours but can be applied sometimes to look for tonofilaments or cell organelles.

5. Cytogenetics: As mentioned above, many soft tissue tumours have specific genetic and chromosomal changes which can be done for determining histogenesis, or for diagnosis and prognosis.

STAGING AND GRADING. Pathological grading of soft tissue tumours based on degree of cytologic atypia is similar to grading for other tumours (grade 0 to 4). However, a different staging system for soft tissue sarcomas *(Enneking's staging)* based on grade and location of tumour given below is accepted by oncologists:

- *Low grade or stage I* (combines histologic grades 1 and 2). Stage I is further divided into stage IA and IB depending upon whether one tissue compartment or more than one compartment is involved.
- *High grade or stage II* (combines histologic grades 3 and 4), and is similarly further divided into stage IIA

and IIB depending upon involvement of one or more than one tissue compartment.

- *Satge III* is given to any histologic grade of soft tissue tumour having distant metastases.

After these brief general comments, a few important examples of tumours of different types of mesenchymal tissue origin are described below.

TUMOURS AND TUMOUR-LIKE LESIONS OF FIBROUS TISSUE

Fibromas, fibromatosis and fibrosarcoma are benign, tumour-like, and malignant neoplasms respectively, of fibrous connective tissue.

FIBROMAS

True fibromas are uncommon tumours in soft tissues. Many fibromas are actually examples of hyperplastic fibrous tissue rather than true neoplasms. On the other hand, combinations of fibrous growth with other mesenchymal tissue elements are more frequent e.g. neurofibroma, fibromyoma etc.

Three types of fibromas are distinguished:

1. **Fibroma durum** is a benign, often pedunculated and well-circumscribed tumour occurring on the body surfaces and mucous membranes. It is composed of fully matured and richly collagenous fibrous connective tissue (COLOUR PLATE XI: CL 43).

2. **Fibroma molle or fibrolipoma,** also termed **soft fibroma,** is similar type of benign growth composed of mixture of mature fibrous connective tissue and adult-type fat.

3. **Elastofibroma** is a rare benign fibrous tumour located in the subscapular region. It is characterised by association of collagen bundles and branching elastic fibres.

FIBROMATOSIS

'Fibromatosis' is the term used for tumour-like lesions of fibrous tissue which continue to proliferate actively and may be difficult to differentiate from sarcomas. These lesions may, therefore, be regarded as non-metastasising fibroblastic tumours which tend to invade locally and recur after surgical excision. In addition, electron microscopy has shown that the cells comprising these lesions have features not only of fibroblasts, but of both fibroblasts and smooth muscle cells, so called *myofibroblasts.* Depending upon the anatomic locations and the age group affected, fibromatoses are broadly grouped as under:

A. Infantile or juvenile fibromatoses include: fibrous hamartoma of infancy, fibromatosis colli, diffuse infantile fibromatosis, juvenile aponeurotic fibroma, juvenile nasopharyngeal angiofibroma and congenital (generalised and solitary) fibromatosis.

B. Adult type of fibromatoses are: palmar and plantar fibromatosis, nodular fascitis, cicatricial fibromatosis, keloid, irradiation fibromatosis, penile fibromatosis (Peyronie's disease), abdominal and extra-abdominal desmoid fibromatosis, and retroperitoneal fibromatosis.

Obviously, it is beyond the scope of the present discussion to cover all these lesions. Some of the important forms of fibromatoses are briefly discussed here.

KELOID. A keloid is a progressive fibrous overgrowth in response to cutaneous injury such as burns, incisions, insect bites, vaccinations and others. Keloids are found more often in Negroes. Their excision is frequently followed by recurrences.

Grossly, the keloid is a firm, smooth, pink, raised patch from which extend claw-like processes (keloid-claw).

Histologically, it is composed of thick, homogeneous, eosinophilic hyalinised bands of collagen admixed with thin collagenous fibres and large active fibroblasts. The adnexal structures are atrophic or destroyed.

There are some differences between a *keloid* and a *hypertrophic scar.* A hypertrophic scar of the skin is more cellular and has numerous fibroblasts than a keloid and is composed of thinner collagenous fibres. A keloid is a progressive lesion and liable to recurrences after surgical excision.

NODULAR FASCITIS. Nodular fascitis, also called pseudosarcomatous fibromatosis, is a form of benign and reactive fibroblastic growth extending from superficial fascia into the subcutaneous fat, and sometimes into the subjacent muscle. The most common locations are the upper extremity, trunk and neck region of young adults. Local excision is generally curative. Less than 5% cases may have local recurrence.

Grossly, the lesion appears as a solitary well-cirumscribed nodule (true to its name) in the superficial fascia. The size may vary from a centimeter to several centimeters in diameter.

Microscopically, various morphologic patterns may be seen but most common is a whorled or S-shaped pattern of fibroblasts present in oedematous background. The individual cells are spindle-shaped, plump fibroblasts showing mild nuclear atypia. Typical mitoses are frequent but atypical mitoses are not present.

PALMAR AND PLANTAR FIBROMATOSES. These fibromatoses, also called Dupuytren-like contractures are the most common form of fibromatoses occurring superficially.

■ **Palmar fibromatosis** is more common in the elderly males occurring in the palmar fascia and leading to flexion contractures of the fingers (Dupuytren's contracture). It appears as a painless, nodular or irregular, infiltrating, benign fibrous subcutaneous lesion. In almost half the cases, the lesions are bilateral.

■ **Plantar fibromatosis** is a similar lesion occurring on the medial aspect of plantar arch. However, plantar lesions are less common than palmar type and do not cause contractures as frequently as palmar lesions. They are seen more often in adults and are infrequently multiple and bilateral. Essentially similar lesions occur in the shaft of the penis *(penile fibromatosis* or *Peyronie's disease)* and in the soft tissues of the knuckles *(knuckle pads).*

Histologically, all these forms of fibromatoses have similar appearance. The nodules are composed of fibrovascular tissue having plump, tightly-packed fibroblasts which have high mitotic rate. Ultrastructurally, some of the fibroblasts have features of myofibroblasts having contractile nature. The palmar lesions frequently extend into soft tissues causing contractures. Both palmar and plantar lesions may remain stationary at nodular stage, progress, or regress spontaneously. Recurrence rate after surgical excision in both forms is as high as 50-60%.

DESMOID FIBROMATOSES. Desmoid fibromatoses or musculo-aponeurotic fibromatoses, commonly referred to as desmoid tumours, are of 2 types: abdominal and extra-abdominal. Both types are, however, histologically similar. Clinically, both types behave in an aggressive way and have to be distinguished from sarcomas. Recurrences are frequent and multiple. The pathogenesis of these lesions is not known but among the factors implicated are the role of antecedent trauma, genetic influences and relationship to oestrogen as evidenced by occurrence of these lesions in pregnancy.

■ **Abdominal desmoids** are locally aggressive infiltrating tumour-like fibroblastic growths, often found in the musculo-aponeurotic structures of the rectus muscle in the anterior abdominal wall in women during or after pregnancy.

■ **Extra-abdominal desmoids,** on the other hand, are more common in men and are widely distributed such as in the upper and lower extremities, chest wall, back, buttocks and head and neck region.

■ **Intra-abdominal desmoids** present at the root of the small bowel mesentery are associated with Gardner's syndrome (consisting of fibromatosis, familial intestinal polyposis, osteomas and epidermal cysts).

Grossly, desmoids are solitary, large, grey-white, firm and unencapsulated tumours infiltrating the muscle locally. Cut surface is whorled and trabeculated.
Microscopically, their appearance is rather misleadingly bland in contrast with aggressive local behaviour. They are composed of uniform-looking fibroblasts arranged in bands and fascicles. Pleomorphism and mitoses are infrequent. The older regions of the tumour have hypocellular hyalinised collagen.

FIBROSARCOMA

The number of soft tissue tumours diagnosed as fibrosarcoma has now dropped, partly because of reclassification of fibromatoses which have aggressive and recurrent behaviour, and partly due to inclusion of many of such tumours in the group of fibrous histiocytomas (described below).

Fibrosarcoma is a slow-growing tumour, affecting adults between 4th and 7th decades of life. Most common locations are the lower extremity (especially thigh and around the knee), upper extremity, trunk, head and neck, and retroperitoneum (Fig. 27.1,A). The tumour is capable of metastasis, chiefly via the blood stream.

Grossly, fibrosarcoma is a grey-white, firm, lobulated and characteristically circumscribed mass. Cut surface of the tumour is soft, fishflesh-like, with foci of necrosis and haemorrhages.
Histologically, the tumour is composed of uniform, spindle-shaped fibroblasts arranged in intersecting fascicles. In well-differentiated tumours, such areas produce *'herring-bone pattern'* (herring-bone is a sea fish) (Fig. 27.1) (COLOUR PLATE XI: CL 44). Poorly-differentiated fibrosarcoma, however, has highly pleomorphic appearance with frequent mitoses and bizarre cells.

Chapter Twenty Seven

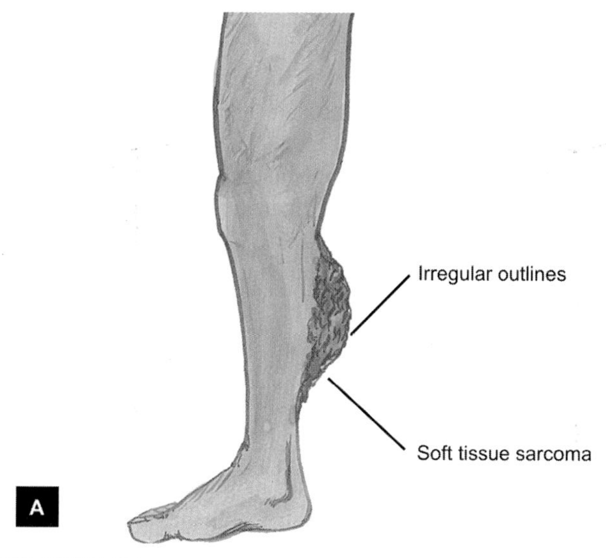

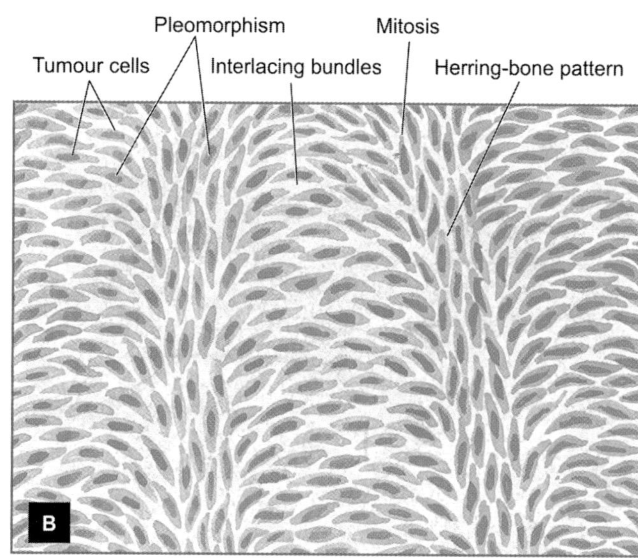

FIGURE 27.1

Fibrosarcoma. A, Common clinical location. B, Microscopy shows a well-differentiated tumour composed of spindle-shaped cells forming interlacing fascicles producing a typical herring-bone pattern.

FIBROHISTIOCYTIC TUMOURS

The group of fibrohistiocytic tumours is characterised by distinctive light microscopic features that include presence of cells with fibroblastic and histiocytic features in varying proportion and identification of characteristic *cart-wheel or storiform pattern* in which the spindle cells radiate outward from the central focus. The histogenesis of these cells is uncertain but possibly they arise from primitive mesenchymal cells which are capable of differentiating along different cell lines. The group includes full spectrum of lesions varying from *benign* (benign fibrous histiocytoma) to *malignant* (malignant fibrous histiocytoma), with dermatofibrosarcoma protuberans occupying the *intermediate* (low-grade malignancy) position.

BENIGN FIBROUS HISTIOCYTOMA

Depending upon the location and predominant pattern, benign fibrous histiocytomas include a number of diverse entities such as dermatofibroma, sclerosing haemangioma, fibroxanthoma, xanthogranuloma, giant cell tumour of tendon sheath and pigmented villonodular synovitis. All these tumours have mixed composition of benign fibroblastic and histiocytic pattern of cells and have been described in relevant sections already.

DERMATOFIBROSARCOMA PROTUBERANS

Dermatofibrosarcoma protuberans is a low-grade malignant cutaneous tumour of fibrohistiocytic origin. The tumour recurs locally, and in rare instances gives rise to distant metastases. Most frequent location is the trunk.

Grossly, the tumour forms a firm, solitary or multiple, satellite nodules extending into the subcutaneous fat and having thin and ulcerated skin surface.

Histologically, the tumour is highly cellular and is composed of fibroblasts arranged in a cart-wheel or storiform pattern.

MALIGNANT FIBROUS HISTIOCYTOMA

Malignant fibrous histiocytomas represent approximately 20-30% of all soft tissue sarcomas. It is the most common soft tissue sarcoma and is the most frequent sarcoma associated with radiotherapy. The tumour occurs more commonly in males and more frequently in the age group of 5th to 7th decades. Most common locations are lower and upper extremities and retroperitoneum. It begins as a painless, enlarging mass, generally in relation to skeletal muscle, deep fascia or subcutaneous tissue. The tumour is believed to arise from primitive mesenchymal cells which are capable of differentiating towards both fibroblastic and histiocytic cell lines.

Grossly, malignant fibrous histiocytoma is a multilobulated, well-circumscribed, firm or fleshy mass, 5-10 cm in diameter. Cut surface is grey-white, soft and myxoid.

Histologically, there is marked variation in appearance from area to area within the same tumour. In general, there is admixture of spindle-shaped *fibroblast-like cells* and mononuclear round to oval *histiocyte-like cells* which may show phagocytic function. There is tendency for the spindle shaped cells to be arranged in characteristic cart-wheel or storiform pattern. The tumour cells show varying degree of pleomorphism, hyperchromatism, mitotic activity and presence of multinucleate bizarre tumour giant cells. Usually there are numerous blood vessels and some scattered lymphocytes and plasma cells (Fig. 27.2). The myxoid variant shows areas of loose myxoid stroma in the cellular areas.

Prognosis is determined by the location of the tumour. Deep-seated malignant fibrous histiocytomas such as of the retroperitoneum have poorer prognosis than those of the subcutaneous soft tissue which come to attention earlier. Metastases are frequent, most often to the lungs and regional lymph nodes. Five-year survival rate is approximately 30-50%.

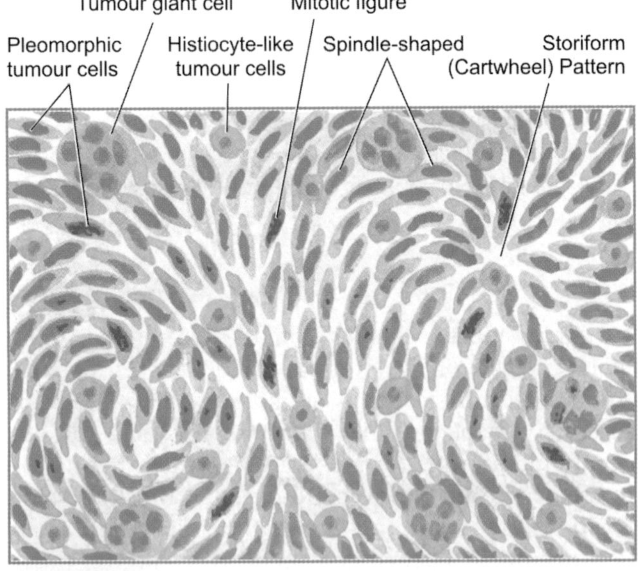

FIGURE 27.2

Malignant fibrous histiocytoma. The tumour shows admixture of spindle-shaped pleomorphic cells forming storiform (cart-wheel) pattern and histiocyte-like round to oval cells. Bizarre pleomorphic multinucleate tumour giant cells and some mononuclear inflammatory cells are also present.

TUMOURS OF ADIPOSE TISSUE

Lipomas and liposarcomas are the common examples of benign and malignant tumours respectively of adipose tissue. Uncommon varieties of adipose tissue tumours include hibernoma, a benign tumour arising from brown fat, and lipoblastoma (foetal lipoma) resembling foetal fat and found predominantly in children under 3 years of age.

LIPOMA

Lipoma is the commonest soft tissue tumour. It appears as a solitary, soft, movable and painless mass which may remain stationary or grow slowly. Lipomas occur most often in 4th to 5th decades of life and are frequent in females. They may be found at different locations in the body but most common sites are the subcutaneous tissues in the neck, back and shoulder. A lipoma rarely ever transforms into liposarcoma.

Grossly, a subcutaneous lipoma is usually small, round to oval and encapsulated mass. The cut surface is soft, lobulated, yellowish-orange and greasy.

Histologically, the tumour is composed of lobules of mature adipose cells separated by delicate fibrous septa. A thin fibrous capsule surrounds the tumour (Fig. 27.3) **(COLOUR PLATE XI: CL 41).**

A variety of admixture of lipoma with other tissue components may be seen. These include: fibrolipoma (admixture with fibrous tissue), angiolipoma (combination with proliferating blood vessels) and myelolipoma (admixture with bone marrow elements as seen in adrenals). Infrequently, benign lipoma may infiltrate the striated muscle (infiltrating or intramuscular lipoma). Spindle cell lipoma and pleomorphic (atypical) lipoma are the other unusual variants of lipoma. The latter type may be particularly difficult to distinguish from well-differentiated liposarcoma.

LIPOSARCOMA

Liposarcoma is one of the common soft tissue sarcomas, perhaps next in frequency only to malignant fibrous histiocytoma. Unlike lipoma which originates from mature adipose cells, liposarcoma arises from primitive mesenchymal cells, the *lipoblasts.* The peak incidence is in 5th to 7th decades of life. In contrast to lipomas which are more frequently subcutaneous in location, liposarcomas often occur in the deep tissues. Most frequent sites are intermuscular regions in the thigh, buttocks and retroperitoneum.

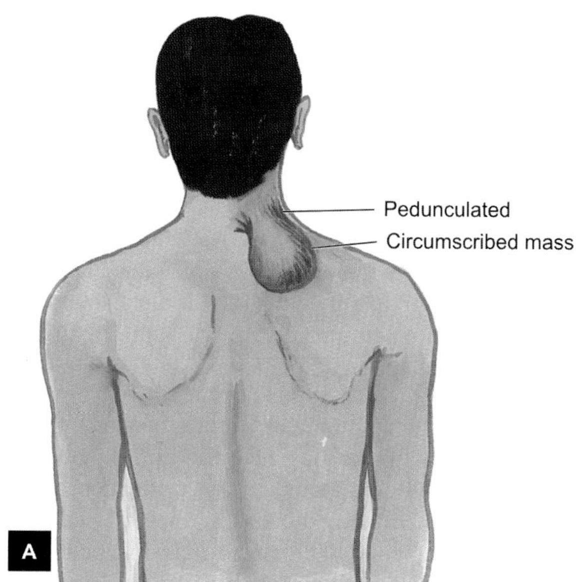

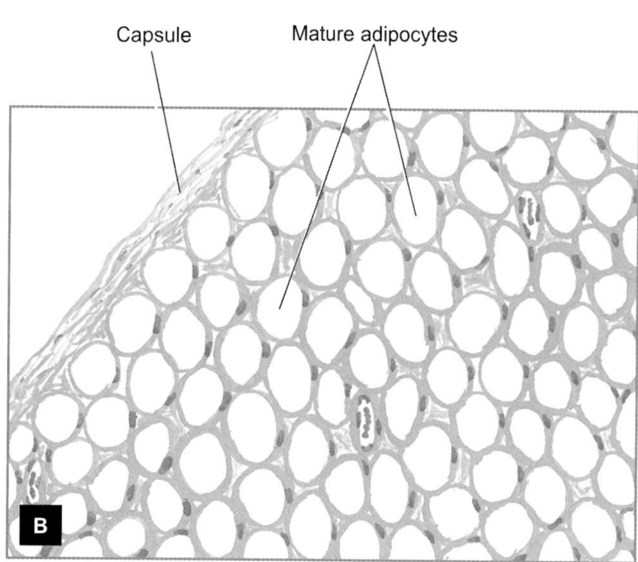

FIGURE 27.3

Lipoma. A, Common clinical location. B, Microscopy of the tumour shows a thin capsule and underlying lobules of mature adipose cells separated by delicate fibrous septa.

Grossly, liposarcoma appears as a nodular mass, 5 cm or more in diameter. The tumour is generally circumscribed but infiltrative. Cut surface is grey-white to yellow, myxoid and gelatinous. Retroperitoneal masses are generally much larger.

Histologically, the hallmark of diagnosis of liposarcoma is the identification of variable number of *lipoblasts* which may be univacuolated or multivacuolated (Fig. 27.4). The vacuoles represent fat in the cytoplasm. Four major histologic varieties of liposarcomas are distinguished: well-differentiated, myxoid, round cell, and pleomorphic (COLOUR PLATE XI: CL 42):

1. *Well-differentiated liposarcoma* resembles lipoma but contains uni- or multi-vacuolated lipoblasts.
2. *Myxoid liposarcoma* is the most common histologic type. It is composed of monomorphic, fusiform or stellate cells representing primitive mesenchymal cells, lying dispersed in mucopolysaccharide-rich ground substance. Occasional tumour giant cells may be present. Prominent meshwork of capillaries forming chicken-wire pattern is a conspicuous feature.
3. *Round cell liposarcoma* is composed of uniform, round to oval cells having fine multivacuolated cytoplasm with central hyperchromatic nuclei. Round cell liposarcoma may resemble a signet-ring carcinoma but mucin stains help in distinguishing the two.
4. *Pleomorphic liposarcoma* is highly undifferentiated and the most anaplastic type. There are numerous large tumour giant cells and bizarre lipoblasts.

The *prognosis* of liposarcoma depends upon the location and histologic type. In general, well differentiated and myxoid varieties have excellent prognosis, while pleomorphic liposarcoma has significantly poorer prognosis. Round cell and pleomorphic variants metastasise frequently to the lungs, other visceral organs and serosal surfaces.

SKELETAL MUSCLE TUMOURS

Rhabdomyoma and rhabdomyosarcoma are the benign and malignant tumours respectively of striated muscle.

RHABDOMYOMA

Rhabdomyoma is a rare benign soft tissue tumour. It should not be confused with glycogen-containing lesion of the heart designated as cardiac rhabdomyoma which is probably a hamartomatous lesion and not a true tumour. Soft tissue rhabdomyomas are predominantly located in the head and neck, most often in the upper neck, tongue, larynx and pharynx.

Histologically, the tumour is composed of large, round to oval cells, having abundant, granular, eosinophilic

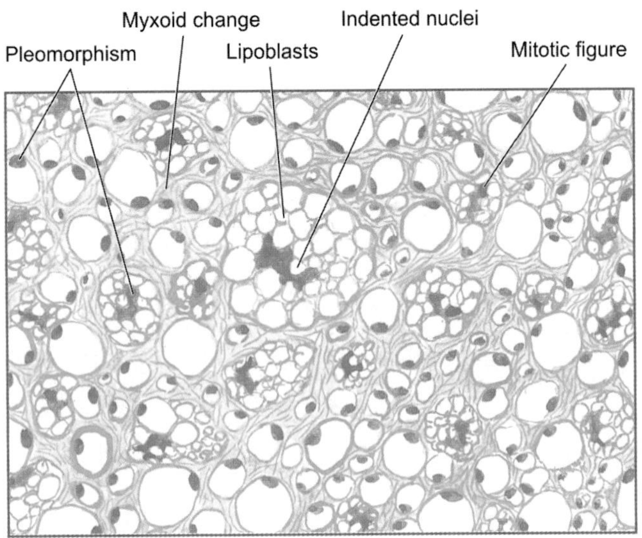

FIGURE 27.4

Liposarcoma, showing characteristic, univacuolated and multivacuolated lipoblasts with bizarre nuclei.

cytoplasm which is frequently vacuolated and contains glycogen. Cross-striations are generally demonstrable in some cells with phosphotungstic acid-haematoxylin (PTAH) stain. The tumour is divided into adult and foetal types, depending upon the degree of resemblance of tumour cells to normal muscle cells.

RHABDOMYOSARCOMA

Rhabdomyosarcoma is a much more common soft tissue tumour than rhabdomyoma, and is the commonest soft tissue sarcoma in children and young adults. It is a highly malignant tumour arising from rhabdomyoblasts in varying stages of differentiation with or without demonstrable cross-striations. Depending upon the growth pattern and histology, 4 types are distinguished: embryonal, botryoid, alveolar and pleomorphic.

1. EMBRYONAL RHABDOMYOSARCOMA. The embryonal form is the most common of the rhabdomyosarcomas. It occurs predominantly in children under 12 years of age. The common locations are in the head and neck region, most frequently in the orbit, urogenital tract and the retroperitoneum.

Grossly, the tumour forms a gelatinous mass growing between muscles or in the deep subcutaneous tissues but generally has no direct relationship to the skeletal muscle.
Histologically, the tumour cells have resemblance to embryonal stage of development of muscle fibres. There is considerable variation in cell types. Generally, the tumour consists of a mixture of small, round to oval cells and spindle-shaped strap cells having tapering bipolar cytoplasmic processes in which cross-striations may be evident. The tumour cells form broad fascicles or bands. Mitoses are frequent.

2. BOTRYOID RHABDOMYOSARCOMA. Botryoid variety is regarded as a variant of embryonal rhabdomyosarcoma occurring in children under 10 years of age. It is seen most frequently in the vagina, urinary bladder and nose (page 751).

Grossly, the tumour forms a distinctive grape-like gelatinous mass protruding into the hollow cavity.
Histologically, the tumour grows underneath the mucosal layer, forming the characteristic *cambium layer* of tumour cells. The tumour is hypocellular and myxoid with predominance of small, round to oval tumour cells.

3. ALVEOLAR RHABDOMYOSARCOMA. Alveolar type of rhabdomyosarcoma is more common in older children and young adults under the age of 20 years. The most common locations, unlike the embryonal variety, are the extremities.

Grossly, the tumour differs from embryonal type in arising directly from skeletal muscle and grows rapidly as soft and gelatinous mass.
Histologically, the tumour shows characteristic alveolar pattern resembling pulmonary alveolar spaces. These spaces are formed by fine fibrocollagenous septa. The tumour cells lying in these spaces and lining the fibrous trabeculae are generally small, lymphocyte-like with frequent mitoses and some multinucleate tumour giant cells (Fig. 27.5). Cross-striation can be demonstrated in about a quarter of cases.

4. PLEOMORPHIC RHABDOMYOSARCOMA. This less frequent variety of rhabdomyosarcoma occurs predominantly in older adults above the age of 40 years. They are most common in the extremities, most frequently in the lower limbs.

Grossly, the tumour forms a well-circumscribed, soft, whitish mass with areas of haemorrhages and necrosis.
Histologically, the tumour cells show considerable variation in size and shape. The tumour is generally composed of highly anaplastic cells having bizarre appearance and numerous multinucleate giant cells. Various shapes include racquet shape, tadpole appear-

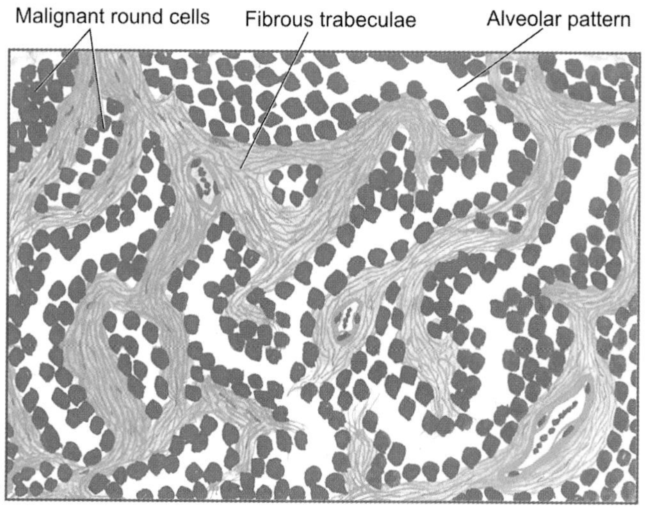

FIGURE 27.5

Alveolar rhabdomyosarcoma. The tumour is divided into alveolar spaces composed of fibrocollagenous tissue. The fibrous trabeculae are lined by small, dark, undifferentiated tumour cells, with some cells floating in the alveolar spaces. A few multinucleate tumour giant cells are also present.

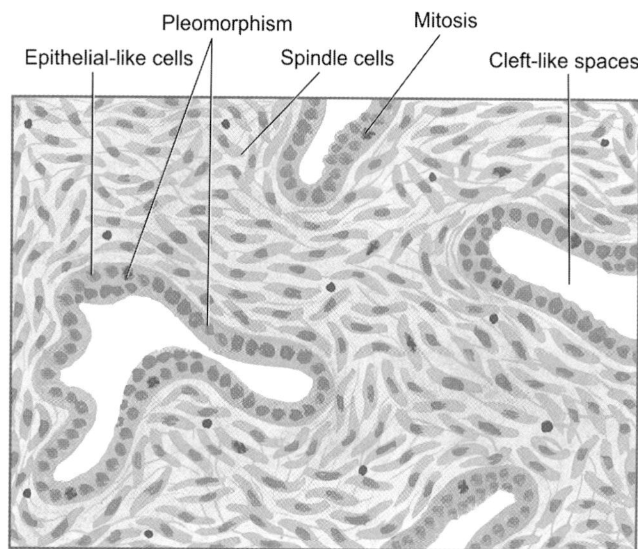

FIGURE 27.6

Classic synovial sarcoma, showing characteristic biphasic cellular pattern. The tumour is composed of epithelial-like cells lining cleft-like spaces and gland-like structures, and spindle cell areas forming fibrosarcoma-like growth pattern.

ance, large strap cells, and ribbon shapes containing several nuclei in a row. Cross-striations can be demonstrated with PTAH stain in a few tumours.

TUMOURS OF UNCERTAIN HISTOGENESIS

Some soft tissue tumours have a distinctive morphology but their exact histogenesis is unclear. A few examples are described below.

SYNOVIAL SARCOMA (MALIGNANT SYNOVIOMA)

Whether true benign tumours of synovial tissue exist is controversial. Pigmented villonodular synovitis and giant cell tumours of tendon sheaths, both of which are tumour-like lesions of synovial tissues are discussed already on page 880. Synovial sarcoma or malignant synovioma, on the other hand, is a distinctive soft tissue sarcoma arising from synovial tissues close to the large joints, tendon sheaths, bursae and joint capsule but almost never arising within joint cavities. Most common locations are the extremities, most frequently the lower extremity. However, synovial sarcoma is also found in regions where synovial tissue is not present such as in the anterior abdominal wall, parapharyngeal region and the pelvis. The *histogenesis* of tumour is, therefore, believed to be from multipotent mesenchymal cells which may differentiate along different cell lines. The tumour principally occurs in young adults, usually under 40 years of age. The tumour grows slowly as a painful mass but may metastasise via blood stream, chiefly to the lungs.

Grossly, the tumour is of variable size and is grey-white, round to multilobulated and encapsulated. Cut surface shows fishflesh-like sarcomatous appearance with foci of calcification, cystic spaces and areas of haemorrhages and necrosis.

Microscopically, *classic synovial sarcoma* shows a characteristic *biphasic cellular pattern* composed of clefts or gland-like structures lined by cuboidal to columnar epithelial-like cells and plump to oval spindle cells (Fig. 27.6). Reticulin fibres are present about the spindle cells but absent within the epithelial foci. The spindle cell areas form interlacing bands similar to those seen in fibrosarcoma. Myxoid matrix, calcification and hyalinization are frequently present in the stroma. Mitoses and multinucleate giant cells are infrequent.

An uncommon variant of synovial sarcoma is *monophasic pattern* in which the epithelial component is exceedingly rare and thus the tumour may be difficult to distinguish from fibrosarcoma.

ALVEOLAR SOFT PART SARCOMA

Alveolar soft part sarcoma is a histologically distinct, slow-growing malignant tumour of uncertain histogenesis. The tumour may occur at any age but affects children and young adults more often. Most alveolar soft part sarcomas occur in the deep tissues of the extremities, along the musculofascial planes, or within the skeletal muscles.

Grossly, the tumour is well-demarcated, yellowish and firm.

Microscopically, the tumour shows characteristic alveolar pattern. Organoid masses of tumour cells are separated by fibrovascular septa. The tumour cells are large and regular and contain abundant, eosinophilic, granular cytoplasm which contains diastase-resistant PAS-positive material. This feature distinguishes the tumour from paraganglioma, with which it closely resembles.

GRANULAR CELL MYOBLASTOMA

Granular cell tumour is a benign tumour of unknown histogenesis. It may occur at any age but most often affected are young to middle-aged adults. The most frequent locations are the tongue and subcutaneous tissue of the trunk and extremities.

Grossly, the tumour is generally small, firm, grey-white to yellow-tan nodular mass.

Histologically, tumour consists of nests or ribbons of large, round or polygonal, uniform cells having finely granular, acidophilic cytoplasm and small dense nuclei. The tumours located in the skin are frequently associated with pseudoepitheliomatous hyperplasia of the overlying skin.

EPITHELIOID SARCOMA

This soft tissue sarcoma occurring in young adults is peculiar in that it presents as an ulcer with sinuses, often located on the skin and subcutaneous tissues as a small swelling. The tumour is slow growing but metastasising.

Grossly, the tumour is somewhat circumscribed and has nodular appearance with central necrosis.

Microscopically, the tumour cells comprising the nodules have epithelioid appearance by having abundant pink cytoplasm and the centres of nodules show necrosis and thus can be mistaken for a granuloma.

CLEAR CELL SARCOMA

Clear cell sarcoma, first described by Enginzer, is seen in skin and subcutaneous tissues, especially of hands and feet.

Morphologically, it closely resembles malignant melanoma, and is therefore also called melanoma of soft tissues.

TUMOUR-LIKE LESIONS

Besides the soft tissue tumours, there are some proliferative conditions of the soft tissues which resemble clinically and morphologically with soft tissue tumours. Important examples are nodular fascitis (pseudosarcomatous fascitis) and myositis ossificans. The former condition has already been described under fibromatous lesions while the latter is discussed below.

MYOSITIS OSSIFICANS

Myositis ossificans is a benign, tumour-like lesion characterised by osteoid and heterotopic bone formation in the soft tissues. It is a misnomer since the lesion neither occurs exclusively in the skeletal muscle as the name leads one to believe, nor are the inflammation or ossification always essential.

Myositis ossificans is generally preceded by history of antecedent trauma to a skeletal muscle or its tendon. The trauma may be minor and repetitive e.g. to the adductor muscles of the thigh of a horseman, or may be single injury followed by haemorrhage into the muscle. The patient generally complains of pain, tenderness and swelling. Richly vascularised granulation tissue replaces the affected muscle or tendon. Then follows development of osteoid and bone at the periphery, giving characteristic X-ray appearance.

Grossly, the lesion appears as unencapsulated, gritty mass replacing the muscle.

Histologically, the central region of the mass shows loosely-arranged fibroblasts having high mitotic activity. Towards the periphery, there is presence of osteoid matrix and formation of woven mineralised bone with trapped skeletal muscle fibres and regenerating muscle (myogenic) giant cells. The appearance is sufficiently atypical to suggest osteosarcoma but osteosarcoma lacks maturation phenomena seen in myositis ossificans. This is why the condition is also called *pseudomalignant osseous tumour* of the soft tissues.

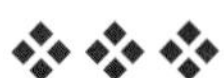

Chapter Twenty Seven

The Nervous System 28

CENTRAL NERVOUS SYSTEM

NORMAL STRUCTURE

The skull and the vertebrae form a rigid compartment encasing the delicate brain and spinal cord. The average weight of the brain is about 1400 gm in men and 1250 gm in women. The two main divisions of the brain, the cerebrum and the cerebellum, are quite distinct in structure. There is absence of lymphatic drainage in the brain. There are 2 types of tissues in the nervous system:

1. *Neuroectodermal tissues* which include neurons (nerve cells) and neuroglia, and together form the predominant constituent of the CNS.
2. *Mesodermal tissues* are microglia, dura mater, the leptomeninges (pia-arachnoid), blood vessels and their accompanying mesenchymal cells.

The predominant tissues comprising the nervous system and their general response to injury are considered below:

1. NEURONS. The neurons are highly specialised cells of the body which are incapable of dividing after the first few weeks of birth. Thus, brain damage involving the neurons is irreversible. Neurons vary considerably in size and shape. Their size may range from the small granular cells of the cerebellum to large Betz cells of the motor cortex. Some neurons are round, others oval or fusiform but the prototype of cortical neuron is pyramidal in shape. A neuron consists of 3 main parts: the cell body, an axon and numerous dendrites (Fig. 28.1,A). The *cell body* (or perikaryon) is the main constituent of the neuron from which an axon and numerous dendritic processes extend. The cell bodies may be arranged in layers as in the cerebral cortex, or may be aggregated as in the basal ganglia. The cell body possesses a large, round, centrally-placed nucleus having finely granular nuclear chromatin and a prominent nucleolus. The cytoplasm contains polygonal, basophilic structures called Nissl substance. It consists of aggregates of RNA, sheaves of rough endoplasmic reticulum and intervening groups of free ribosomes. Besides Nissl substance, other special features of the cytoplasm of neuronal cell body are the presence of microtubules, synaptic vesicles and neurofilaments which are a form of intermediate filaments specific to neurons. Lipofuscin may be present due to ageing. Neuromelanin is found in neurons in the substantia nigra and pigmented nucleus of the pons.

Neurons respond to injury in a variety of ways depending upon the etiologic agent and the pathologic processes. These include central chromatolysis, atrophy and degeneration of neurons and axons, and intraneuronal storage of substances.

2. NEUROGLIA. The neuroglia provides supportive matrix and maintenance to the neurons. It includes 3 types of cells: astrocytes, oligodendrocytes and ependymal cells (Fig. 28.1,B). Neuroglia is generally referred to as *glia;* the tumours originating from it are termed *gliomas,* and reactive proliferation of the astrocytes being called *gliosis.*

i) Astrocytes. The astrocytes are stellate cells with numerous fine branching processes. In routine haemato-

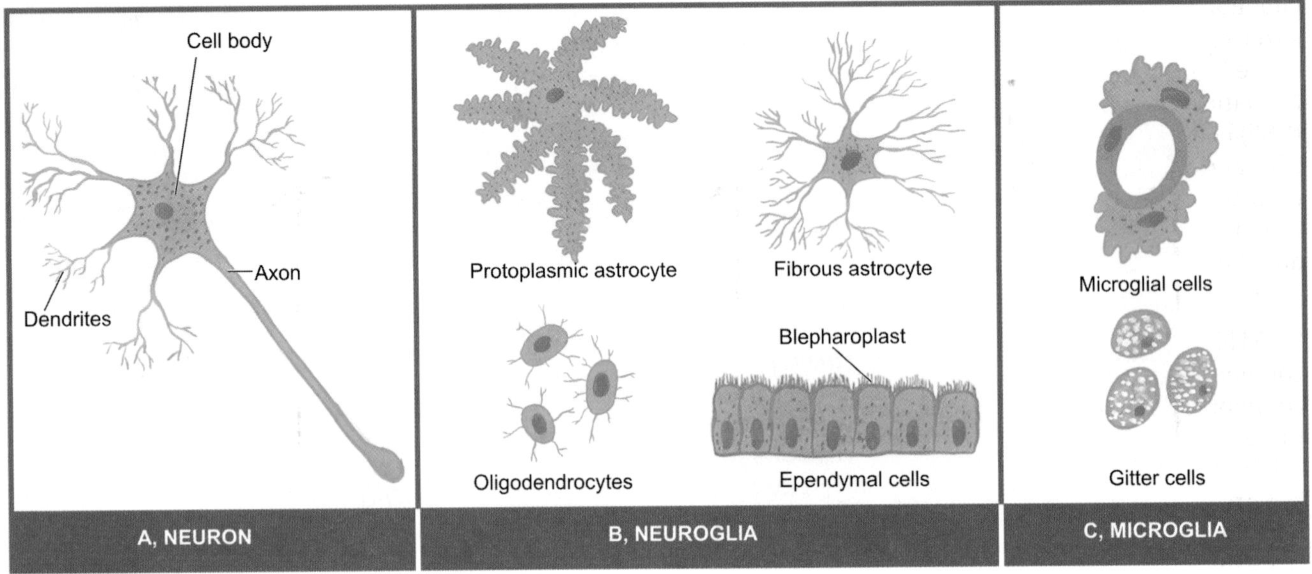

FIGURE 28.1

Cells comprising the nervous system.

xylin and eosin stains, an astrocyte has round or oval vesicular nucleus, but unlike neuron, lacks a prominent nucleolus. The cytoplasm is generally scanty. The processes radiate from the cell body. Depending upon the type of processes, two types of astrocytes are distinguished:

- *Protoplasmic astrocytes* have branched processes and are found mostly in the grey matter.
- *Fibrous astrocytes* have long, thin processes and are present mainly in the white matter.

Some astrocytic processes are directed towards neurons and their processes, which others surround capillaries by terminal expansions called *foot processes.* The astrocytic processes may not be visible by routine stains but can be demonstrated by phosphotungstic acid haematoxylin (PTAH) stain. Ultrastructurally, these processes are composed of abundant intermediate filaments, mostly vimentin.

The main functions of astrocytes in health are physiological and biochemical support to the neurons and interactions with capillary endothelial cells to establish blood brain barrier. In case of damage to the brain, astrocytes act like fibroblasts of other tissues. The astrocytes in respond to injury undergo hyperplasia and hypertrophy termed 'gliosis' which is an equivalent of scar elsewhere in the body. *Gemistocytic astrocytes* are early reactive astrocytes having prominent pink cytoplasm. Long-standing progressive gliosis results in the development of *Rosenthal fibres* which are eosinophilic, elongated or globular bodies present on the astrocytic processes. *Corpora amylacea* are basophilic, rounded, sometimes laminated bodies, present in elderly people in the white matter and result from accumulation of starch-like material in the degenerating astrocytes.

ii) Oligodendrocytes. Oligodendrocytes are so named because of their short and fewer processes when examined by light microscopy with special stains. In haematoxylin-eosin stained sections, these cells appear as small cells with a darkly-staining nucleus resembling that of small lymphocyte. The cytoplasm appears as a clear halo around the nucleus. Oligodendrocytes are present throughout the brain in grey as well as white matter and are most numerous of all other cells in the CNS. In grey matter, they are clustered around the neurons and are called *satellite cells.* In white matter, they are present along the myelinated nerve fibres and are termed *interfascicular oligodendroglia.*

The major function of oligodendrocytes is formation and maintenance of myelin. Thus, in this respect they are counterparts of Schwann cells of the peripheral nervous system. Diseases of oligodendrocytes are, therefore, disorders of myelin and myelinisation such as inherited leucodystrophies and acquired demyelinating diseases.

iii) Ependymal cells. The ependymal cells are epithelium-like and form a single layer of cells lining the ventricular system, the aqueduct, the central canal of the spinal cord and cover the choroid plexus. They are cuboidal to columnar cells and have ciliated luminal surface, just beneath which are present small bodies termed *blepharoplasts.* The ependymal cells influence the formation and composition of the cerebrospinal fluid (CSF) by processes of active secretion, diffusion, absorption and exchange. The function of cilia is not very clear but probably they play a role in the circulation of CSF. The ependymal cells respond to injury by cell loss and the space left is filled by proliferation of underlying glial fibres.

3. **MICROGLIA.** The microglia is the nervous system counterpart of the monocyte-macrophage system. The commonly used term 'microglia' is inappropriate since these cells, unlike neuroglia, are not of neuroectodermal origin. Microglial cells (or Hortega cells) are not fixed but are mobile cells. These cells are found throughout the brain and are often present close to the blood vessels. Normally, microglial cells appear as small inconspicuous cells with bean-shaped vesicular nuclei, scanty cytoplasm and long cytoplasmic processes (Fig. 28.1,C). In response to injury or damage, however, these cells have capability to enlarge in size, proliferate and develop elongated nuclei, so called *rod cells.* Microglial cells may actually assume the shape and phagocytic function of macrophages and form *gitter cells.* The foci of necrosis and areas of selective hypoxic damage to the neurons are surrounded by microglial cells which perform phagocytosis of damaged and necrosed cells; this is known as *neuronophagia.*

Neuropil is the term used for the fibrillar network formed by processess of all the neuronal cells.

4. **THE DURA MATER.** The dura mater is a tough fibrous covering of the brain which is closely attached to the skull on its inner layer of endocranial periosteum. In the region of spinal canal, it encloses a potential space, the *epidural space,* between the bone and the dura. The dura is composed of dense collagen, fused with periosteum of the skull.

5. **THE PIA-ARACHNOID (LEPTOMENINGES).** The leptomeninges (*lepto*=thin, slender) consisting of the pia and arachnoid mater form the delicate vascular membranous covering of the central nervous system. The pia mater is closely applied to the brain and its convolutions, while the arachnoid mater lies between the pia mater and the dura mater without dipping into sulci. Thus, a space is left between the two layers of leptomeninges, known as *subarachnoid space,* which contains the CSF. The major arteries and veins run in the subarachnoid space and small nutrient arteries pass into the cortex. Extension of the subarachnoid space between the wall of blood vessels entering the brain and their pial sheaths form a circumvascular space called *Virchow-Robin space.* Another important potential space is enclosed between the dura and the arachnoid membrane known as *subdural space.*

DEVELOPMENTAL ANOMALIES

These malformations are the result of various inherited and acquired factors. The acquired conditions include viral infections of the mother and foetus (e.g. rubella), intake of drugs (e.g. thalidomide), exposure to ionising radiation and foetal anoxia. There are a large number of developmental malformations of the CNS but only a few important and common ones are mentioned here. Congenital hydrocephalus is considered separately alongwith other types of hydrocephalus.

Spinal Cord Defects

Spina bifida is the term applied to the malformations of the vertebral column involving incomplete embryologic closure of one or more of the vertebral arches (rachischisis), most frequently in the lumbosacral region. The vertebral defect is frequently associated with defect in the neural tube structures and their coverings. The bony defect may be of varying degree. The least serious form is **spina bifida occulta** in which there is only vertebral defect but no abnormality of the spinal cord and its meninges. The site of bony defect is marked by a small dimple, or a hairy pigment mole in the overlying skin. The larger bony defect, however, appears as a distinct cystic swelling over the affected site called **spina bifida cystica.** The latter is associated with herniation of the meninges or the spinal cord, or both.

Herniation of the meninges alone through the bony defect, **meningocele,** is a less common variety. The herniated sac in meningocele consists of dura and arachnoid. The commonest and more serious form is, however, **meningomyelocele** in which spinal cord or its roots also herniate through the defect and are attached to the posterior wall of the sac. In this defect, the dura and the skin in the sac are deficient. A more serious variant of meningomyelocele is associated with hydrocephalus and Arnold-Chiari malformation. A rare form of the defect is **myelocele** or **syringomyelocele** in which there is defective closure of the spinal canal so that the sac consists of an open flat neural tissue plate without skin covering and the CSF leaking through it. Meningomyelocele and myelocele are frequently associated with neurologic defects of varying degree which include bladder and bowel dysfunction, motor and sensory defects, and paraplegia.

The existence of defect in bony closure in the region of occipital bone or fronto-ethmoid junction may result in **cranial meningocele** and **encephalocele.**

Syringomyelia and Syringobulbia

These are probably congenital malformations since they manifest clinically later in life and often develop in association with certain acquired lesions involving the CNS. Syringomyelia and syringobulbia are characterised by development of a *syrinx* or a tubular cavity in the spinal cord and medulla respectively. The cavity may be fusiform or irregular. It usually begins in the grey matter of the spinal cord dorsal to the central canal. The syrinx is usually surrounded by glial tissue. If the cavity communicates with the spinal canal, it is lined by ependymal cells. Since the fibres of lateral spino-thalamic tract are frequently involved in the cavity, the clinical effects include loss of pain and temperature sensation in the affected region.

Arnold-Chiari Malformations

Arnold-Chiari malformation is the term used for a group of malformations of the brain involving the brainstem and cerebellum. The primary defect is elongation of the medulla and part of the vermis of the cerebellum resulting from failure of the pontine flexure to form. Approximately 50% of children with hydrocephalus have the Arnold-Chiari malformation. Four types are described, of which type II malformation is the most common and is most frequently associated with congenital hydrocephalus. Most patients of Arnold-Chiari malformation have, in addition, meningomyelocele. The major components of type II Arnold-Chiari malformation are:

1. elongation of the medulla with part of fourth ventricle in the cervical canal;
2. distortion of the medulla forming a characteristic S-shaped bend at the junction with the cervical spinal cord; and
3. lengthening and herniation of the cerebellar vermis and cerebellar tonsils through the foramen magnum resulting in formation of a mass over the upper cervical cord.

Combination of these abnormalities results in stenosis of the aqueduct or obstruction of the foramina of Luschka and Magendie causing internal hydrocephalus discussed below.

HYDROCEPHALUS

Hydrocephalus is the term used for increased volume of CSF within the skull, accompanied by dilatation of the ventricles. In majority of cases of hydrocephalus, there is increased intracranial pressure. This type of hydrocephalus involving ventricular dilatation is termed *internal hydrocephalus.* A localised collection of CSF in the subarachnoid space is called *external hydrocephalus.* Before considering the types, causes and mechanisms involved in the hydrocephalus, it is essential to briefly review the source and circulation of CSF.

Source and Circulation of CSF

CSF is mainly produced by choroid plexus in the lateral, third and fourth ventricle, and a small part is formed on the surface of the brain and spinal cord. The total volume of CSF is about 120-150 ml. CSF formed in the lateral ventricles flows through the foramina of Munro to the third ventricle and from there by the aqueduct of Sylvius to the fourth ventricle. The fluid then passes through the foramina of Magendie and Luschka of the fourth ventricle to reach the subarachnoid space of the brain. It then spreads through the subarachnoid space over the surface of the spinal cord. It is absorbed into the blood by the arachnoid villi present along the dural venous sinuses (Fig. 28.2).

Types and Etiopathogenesis

Hydrocephalus is classified into primary and secondary types, the former being much more common, both types have distinct etiology and pathogenesis.

PRIMARY HYDROCEPHALUS. Primary hydrocephalus is defined as actual increase in the volume of CSF within the skull alongwith elevated intracranial pressure. There are 3 possible mechanisms of primary hydrocephalus:

1. Obstruction to the flow of CSF.
2. Overproduction of CSF.
3. Deficient reabsorption of CSF.

However, obstruction to the flow of CSF is by far the commonest cause and is termed *obstructive hydrocephalus.* The terms *non-communicating* and *communicating hydrocephalus* are used to denote the site of obstruction.

Non-communicating hydrocephalus. When the site of obstruction of CSF pathway is in the third ventricle or at the exit foramina in the fourth ventricle, the ventricular system enlarges and CSF cannot pass into the subarachnoid space. This is termed as non-communi-

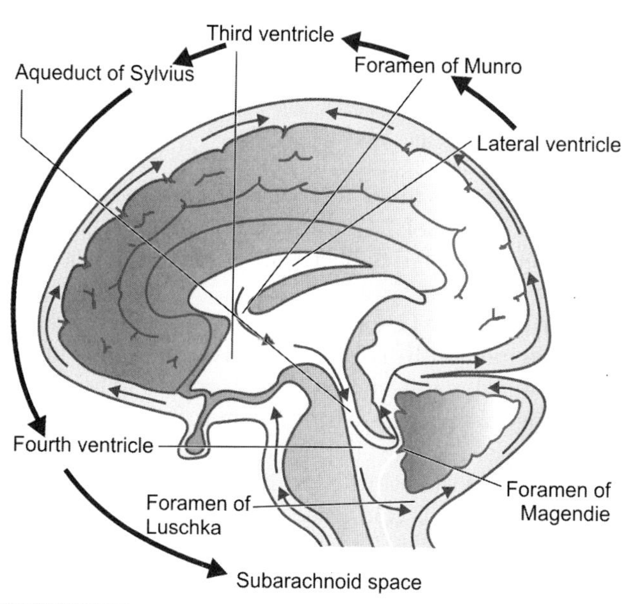

FIGURE 28.2
Normal circulation of CSF.

cating hydrocephalus. Among the common causes are the following:

i) *Congenital non-communicating hydrocephalus* e.g. stenosis of the aqueduct, Arnold-Chiari malformation, progressive gliosis of the aqueduct and intra-uterine meningitis.

ii) *Acquired non-communicating hydrocephalus* may occur from expanding lesion within the skull. These conditions are as under:

- Tumours adjacent to the ventricular system e.g. ependymoma, choroid plexus papilloma, medulloblastoma and others.
- Inflammatory lesions e.g. cerebral abscess, meningitis.
- Haemorrhage e.g. parenchymal haemorrhage, intraventricular haemorrhage, and epidural and subdural haematoma.

Communicating hydrocephalus. When obstruction to the flow of CSF is in the subarachnoid space at the base of the brain, it results in enlargement of the ventricular system but CSF flows freely between dilated ventricles and the spinal canal. This is called communicating hydrocephalus. The causes of communicating hydrocephalus are non-obstructive which are as follows:

i) *Overproduction of CSF* e.g. choroid plexus papilloma.

ii) *Deficient reabsorption of CSF* e.g. following meningitis, subarachnoid haemorrhage and dural sinus thrombosis.

SECONDARY HYDROCEPHALUS. Secondary hydrocephalus is much less common and is defined as compensatory increase of CSF due to loss of neural tissue without associated rise in intracranial pressure (normal pressure hydrocephalus) e.g. from cerebral atrophy and infarction.

*PATHOLOGIC CHANGES. **Grossly,*** there is dilatation of the ventricles depending upon the site of obstruction. There is thinning and stretching of the brain. The scalp veins overlying the enlarged head are engorged and the fontanelle remain open. ***Histologically,*** severe hydrocephalus may be associated with damage to ependymal lining of the ventricles and periventricular interstitial oedema.

INFECTIONS

A large number of pathogens comprising various kinds of bacteria, fungi, viruses, rickettsiae and parasites can cause infections of the nervous system. The micro-organisms may gain entry into the nervous system by one of the following routes:

1. **Via blood stream.** Spread of infection by the arterial route from another focus is the most common mode of spread of infection in the nervous system. Less often, the spread may occur by retrograde venous route and by lodgement of septic emboli in the brain.

2. **Direct implantation.** Spread of infection by direct implantation occurs following skull fractures or through defects in the bony and meningeal coverings of the nervous system.

3. **Local extension.** Extension of infection from contiguous focus such as otitis media and frontal or mastoid sinusitis may occur.

4. **Along nerve.** Certain viruses such as herpes simplex, herpes zoster and rabies spread along cranial and peripheral nerves and ascend to the CNS.

In general, resultant lesions are in the form of either diffuse inflammation of the meninges (meningitis) and of brain parenchyma (encephalitis), or combination of both (meningoencephalitis). In addition, other inflammatory lesions of CNS include: brain abscess, epidural abscess, subdural empyema, septic thromboembolism of dural sinuses and encephalomyelitis. Some of the morphologically significant lesions are described below.

MENINGITIS

Meningitis is inflammatory involvement of the meninges. Meningitis may involve the dura called *pachymeningitis,* or the leptomeninges (pia-arachnoid) termed *leptomeningitis.* The latter is far more common, and unless otherwise specified, meningitis would mean leptomeningitis.

Pachymeningitis is invariably an extension of the inflammation from chronic suppurative otitis media or from fracture of the skull. An *extradural abscess* may form by suppuration between the bone and dura. Further spread of infection may penetrate the dura and form a *subdural abscess.* Other effects of pachymeningitis are localised or generalised leptomeningitis and *cerebral abscess.*

Leptomeningitis, commonly called meningitis, is usually the result of infection but infrequently chemical meningitis and carcinomatous meningitis by infiltration of the subarachnoid space by cancer cells may occur. Infectious meningitis is broadly classified into 3 types: acute pyogenic, acute lymphocytic (viral, aseptic) and chronic (bacterial or fungal).

Acute Pyogenic Meningitis

Acute pyogenic or acute purulent meningitis is acute infection of the pia-arachnoid and of the CSF enclosed in the subarachnoid space. Since the subarachnoid space is continuous around the brain, spinal cord and the optic nerves, infection spreads immediately to whole of the cerebrospinal meninges as well as to the ventricles.

ETIOPATHOGENESIS. The causative organisms vary with age of the patient.

1. *Escherichia coli* infection is common in neonates with neural tube defects.
2. *Haemophilus influenzae* is commonly responsible for infection in infants and children.
3. *Neisseria meningitidis* causes meningitis in adolescent and young adults and is causative for epidemic meningitis.
4. *Streptococcus pneumoniae* is causative for infection at extremes of age and following trauma.

The **routes** of infection are as follows:

1. Most commonly by the blood stream.
2. From an adjacent focus of infection.
3. By iatrogenic infection such as introduction of micro-organisms at operation or during lumbar puncture.

PATHOLOGIC CHANGES. ***Grossly,*** pus accumulates in the subarachnoid space so that normally clear CSF becomes turbid or frankly purulent. The turbid fluid is particularly seen in the sulci and at the base of the brain where the space is wide. In fulminant cases, some degree of ventriculitis is also present having a fibrinous coating on their walls and containing turbid CSF. In addition, purulent material may interfere with CSF flow and result in obstructive hydrocephalus.
Microscopically, there is presence of numerous polymorphonuclear neutrophils in the subarachnoid space as well as in the meninges, particularly around the blood vessels. Gram-staining reveals varying number of causative bacteria.

CLINICAL FEATURES AND DIAGNOSIS. Acute bacterial meningitis is a medical emergency. The immediate clinical manifestations are fever, severe headache, vomiting, drowsiness, stupor, coma, and occasionally, convulsions. The most important clinical sign is stiffness of the neck on forward bending.

The *diagnosis* is confirmed by examining CSF as soon as possible. The diagnostic alterations in the CSF in acute pyogenic meningitis are as under:

1. Naked eye appearance of cloudy or frankly purulent CSF.
2. Elevated CSF pressure (above 180 mm water).
3. Polymorphonuclear neutrophilic leucocytosis in CSF (between 10-10,000/μl).
4. Raised CSF protein level (higher than 50 mg/dl).
5. Decreased CSF sugar concentration (lower than 40 mg/dl).
6. Bacteriologic examination by Gram's stain or by CSF culture reveals causative organism.

Acute Lymphocytic (Viral, Aseptic) Meningitis

Acute lymphocytic meningitis is a viral or aseptic meningitis, especially common in children and young adults. Among the etiologic agents are numerous viruses such as enteroviruses, mumps, ECHO viruses, coxsackie virus, Epstein-Barr virus and herpes simplex II. However, evidence of viral infection may not be demonstrable in about a third of cases.

PATHOLOGIC CHANGES. ***Grossly,*** some cases show swelling of the brain while others show no distinctive change.
Microscopically, there is mild lymphocytic infiltrate in the leptomeninges.

CLINICAL FEATURES AND DIAGNOSIS. The clinical manifestations of viral meningitis are much the same as in bacterial meningitis with features of acute onset meningeal symptoms and fever. But viral meningitis has a benign and self-limiting clinical course of short duration and is invariably followed by complete recovery without the life-threatening complications of bacterial meningitis.

The *CSF findings* in viral meningitis are as under:

1. Naked eye appearance of clear or slightly turbid CSF.
2. CSF pressure increased (above 250 mm water).
3. Lymphocytosis in CSF (10-100 cells/μl).
4. CSF protein usually normal or mildly raised.
5. CSF sugar concentration usually normal.
6. CSF bacteriologically sterile.

Chronic (Tuberculous and Cryptococcal) Meningitis

There are two principal types of chronic meningitis—one bacterial (tuberculous meningitis) and the other fungal (cryptococcal meningitis). Both types cause chronic granulomatous reaction and may produce parenchymal lesions.

- *Tuberculous meningitis* occurs in children and adults through haematogenous spread of infection from tuberculosis elsewhere in the body, or it may simply be a manifestation of miliary tuberculosis. Less commonly, the spread may occur directly from tuberculosis of a vertebral body.
- *Cryptococcal meningitis* develops particularly in debilitated or immunocompromised persons, usually as a result of haematogenous dissemination from a pulmonary lesion. Cryptococcal meningitis is especially an important cause of meningitis in patients with AIDS.

PATHOLOGIC CHANGES. Grossly, in tuberculous meningitis, the subarachnoid space contains thick exudate, particularly abundant in the sulci and the base of the brain. Tubercles, 1-2 mm in diameter, may be visible, especially adjacent to the blood vessels. The exudate in cryptococcal meningitis is scanty, translucent and gelatinous.

Microscopically, tuberculous meningitis shows exudate of acute and chronic inflammatory cells, and granulomas with or without caseation necrosis and giant cells. Acid-fast bacilli may be demonstrated. Late cases show dense fibrous adhesions in the subarachnoid space and consequent hydrocephalus. Cryptococcal meningitis is characterised by infiltration by lymphocytes, plasma cells, an occasional granuloma and abundant characteristic capsulated cryptococci.

CLINICAL FEATURES AND DIAGNOSIS. Tuberculous meningitis manifests clinically as headache, confusion, malaise and vomiting. The clinical course in cryptococcal meningitis may, however, be fulminant and fatal in a few weeks, or be indolent for months to years.

The *CSF findings* in chronic meningitis are as under:

1. Naked eye appearance of a clear or slightly turbid CSF which may form fibrin web on standing.
2. Raised CSF pressure (above 300 mm water).
3. Mononuclear leucocytosis consisting mostly of lymphocytes and some macrophages (100-1000 cells/μl).
4. Raised protein content.
5. Lowered glucose concentration.
6. Tubercle bacilli may be found on microscopy of centrifuged deposits by ZN staining in tuberculous meningitis, and pathognomonic capsulated cryptococci in India ink preparation of CSF in cases of cryptococcal meningitis.

Table 28.1 summarises the CSF findings in the three important types of meningitis in comparison with those in health.

ENCEPHALITIS

Parenchymal infection of brain is termed encephalitis. Encephalitis may be the result of bacterial, viral, fungal and protozoal infections.

Bacterial Encephalitis

Bacterial infection of the brain substance is usually secondary to involvement of the meninges rather than a primary bacterial parenchymal infection. This results in bacterial cerebritis that progresses to form *brain abscess.* However, *tuberculosis* and *neurosyphilis* are the two primary bacterial involvements of the brain parenchyma.

BRAIN ABSCESS. Brain abscesses may arise by one of the following routes:

1. By direct implantation of organisms e.g. following compound fractures of the skull.
2. By local extension of infection e.g. chronic suppurative otitis media, mastoiditis and sinusitis.
3. By haematogenous spread e.g. from primary infection in the heart such as acute bacterial endocarditis, and from lungs such as in bronchiectasis.

Clinically, there is usually evidence of reactivation of infection at the primary site preceding the onset of cerebral symptoms. The features of abscess are fever, headache, vomiting, seizures and focal neurological deficits depending upon the location of the abscess. Brain abscess is most common in cerebral hemispheres and less frequent in the cerebellum and basal ganglia.

TABLE 28.1: CSF Findings in Health and Various Types of Meningitis.

FEATURE	NORMAL	ACUTE PYOGENIC (BACTERIAL) MENINGITIS	ACUTE LYMPHO-CYTIC (VIRAL) MENINGITIS	CHRONIC (TUBERCULOUS) MENINGITIS
1. *Naked eye appearance*	Clear and colourless	Cloudy or frankly purulent	Clear or slightly turbid	Clear or slightly turbid, forms fibrin coagulum on standing
2. *CSF pressure*	60-150 mm water	Elevated (above 180 mm water)	Elevated (above 250 mm water)	Elevated (above 300 mm water)
3. *Cells*	0-4 lymphocytes/µl	10-10,000 neutrophils/µl	10-100 lymphocytes/µl	100-1000 lymphocytes/µl
4. *Proteins*	15-45 mg/dl	Markedly raised	Raised	Raised
5. *Glucose*	50-80 mg/dl	Markedly reduced	Normal	Reduced
6. *Bacteriology*	Sterile	Causative organisms present	Sterile	Tubercle bacilli present

Grossly, it appears as a localised area of inflammatory necrosis and oedema surrounded by fibrous capsule.
Microscopically, the changes consist of liquefactive necrosis in the centre of the abscess containing pus. It is surrounded by acute and chronic inflammatory cells, neovascularisation, oedema, septic thrombosis of vessels, fibrous encapsulation and zone of gliosis, The CSF and overlying meninges also show evidence of acute and chronic inflammation.

TUBERCULOMA. Tuberculoma is an intracranial mass occurring secondary to dissemination of tuberculosis elsewhere in the body. Tuberculomas may be solitary or multiple.

Grossly, it has a central area of caseation necrosis surrounded by fibrous capsule.
Microscopically, there is typical tuberculous granulomatous reaction around the central caseation necrosis. A zone of gliosis generally surrounds the tuberculoma. Advanced cases may show areas of calcification.

NEUROSYPHILIS. Syphilitic lesions of the CNS used to be common and serious, but more recently there is evidence of atypical neurosyphilis in cases of AIDS. The lesions in syphilis may be in the form of *syphilitic meningitis* found in secondary syphilis, and *neurosyphilis* consisting of tabes dorsalis and generalised paralysis of the insane occurring in tertiary stage (page 167).

■ **Syphilitic meningitis.** This is a form of chronic meningitis characterised by distinctive perivascular inflammatory reaction of plasma cells and endarteritis obliterans.

■ **Tabes dorsalis (Locomotor ataxia).** There is slowly progressive degeneration of the posterior roots of the spinal nerves and the posterior columns of the spinal cord by the spirochaetes. These changes produce loss of coordination of muscles and joints resulting in locomotor ataxia. These changes produce loss of coordination of muscles and joints resulting in locomotor ataxia. There is also loss of pain sensation and presence of Argyll-Robertson pupils which react to accommodation but not to light.

■ **General paralysis of the insane.** This is the result of diffuse parenchymal involvement by the spirochaetes with widespread lesions in the nervous system. The symptoms consist of motor, sensory and psychiatric abnormalities.

Viral Encephalitis

A number of viruses can infect the CNS and produce either aseptic meningitis (described already) or viral encephalitis, but sometimes combination of both termed meningoencephalitis, is present. Most viral infections of the CNS are the end-result of preceding infection in other tissues and organs. There is usually a preceding phase of extraneural viral replication before involvement of the nervous system occurs.

Most of the viruses reach the nervous system via blood stream before which they enter the body by various routes e.g. infection of the skin and mucous membrane (in herpes simplex and herpes zoster-varicella), by the alimentary tract (in enteroviruses including polio virus), by arthropod bite (in arbovirus), by transplacental infection (in cytomegalovirus), and through body fluids in AIDS (in HIV infection). Rabies virus travels along the peripheral nerves to reach the

CNS. Herpes zoster-varicella is a distinct primary disease (chickenpox) but the virus remains latent for a long time before it gets reactivated to cause severe hyperalgesia and pain along the distribution of nerve related to acutely inflamed posterior root ganglia (herpes zoster). All these viral infections enumerated so far cause *acute viral encephalitis. Slow virus diseases* are another group of CNS infections in which the agents have not only a long latent period but the disease also develops slowly and may produce subacute sclerosing panencephalitis, progressive multifocal leucoencephalopathy, progressive rubella panencephalopathy and subacute spongiform encephalopathy.

PATHOLOGIC CHANGES. Although histologic changes vary from one viral infection of the CNS to the other but, in general, the characteristic features of viral diseases of the CNS are as under:

1. Parenchymal infiltrate, chiefly in perivascular location, of mononuclear cells consisting of lymphocytes, plasma cells and macrophages.
2. Microscopic clusters of microglial cells and presence of neuronophagia.
3. Intranuclear inclusion bodies in most viral diseases and specific cytoplasmic inclusions of Negri bodies in rabies.

HIV Encephalopathy (AIDS-Dementia Complex)

Late in the course of AIDS, a group of signs and symptoms of CNS disease appear termed HIV encephalopathy or AIDS-dementia complex. One major clinical feature of this entity is the occurrence of *dementia* i.e. fall in the cognitive ability of the individual compared to previous level. The condition is believed to be the result of direct effect of HIV on the CNS. Clinically, the disease develops in about 25% cases of AIDS while autopsy studies reveal presence of HIV-encephalopathy in 80-90% cases of AIDS.

Histologically, the changes are more in subcortical area of the brain and consist of gliosis, multinucleate giant cell encephalitis, and vacuolar myelopathy.

Table 28.2 lists important forms of CNS diseases in patients with AIDS.

Progressive Multifocal Leucoencephalopathy

Progressive multifocal leucoencephalopathy (PML) is a slow viral infection of the CNS caused by a papovavirus called *JC virus* (not to be confused with CJ disease or mad-cow disease; JC virus here stands for the initials of the patient first infected). PML develops in immunocompromised individual like CMV and Toxoplasma encephalitis does, and is, therefore, an important form of encephalitis due to increasing number of cases of AIDS.

TABLE 28.2: Major Forms of CNS Diseases in AIDS.

DISEASE	INCIDENCE
1. HIV-encephalopathy (AIDS-dementia complex)	25%
2. Toxoplasmosis	15%
3. Cryptococcal meningitis	9%
4. Progressive multifocal leucoencephalopathy	4%
5. Neurosyphilis	1%
6. CNS lymphoma	1%
7. Tuberculous meningitis	1%

PML infects oligodendrocytes and causes progressive demyelination at multifocal areas scattered throughout the CNS.

Grossly, the lesions consist of focal, irregular gelatinous areas most prominent at the junction of grey and white matter. Main areas affected are cerebrum, brainstem, cerebellum, and sometimes spinal cord.

Microscopically, the features consist of the following:

- focal areas of demyelination;
- many lipid-laden macrophages in the centre of foci; and
- enlarged oligodendroglial nuclei containing purple viral inclusions at the periphery of the lesion.

Spongiform Encephalopathy (Creutzfeldt-Jakob Disease)

Spongiform encephalopathy, also called Creutzfeldt-Jakob disease (CJD) or mad-cow disease, though included under the group of viral encephalitis but is caused by accumulation of prion proteins. *Prion proteins* are a modified form of normal structural proteins present in the mammalian CNS and are peculiar in two respects: they lack nucleic acid (DNA or RNA), and they can be transmitted as an infectious proteinaceous particles (Dr Prusiner was awarded the Nobel Prize in medicine in 1997 for his discovery on prion proteins).

Majority of cases occur sporadically though familial predisposition with autosomal dominant inheritance has also been reported in 5-15% cases. Other methods of transmission are by iatrogenic route (e.g. by tissue transplantation from an infected individual) and by human consumption of BSE (bovine spongiform encephalopathy)-infected beef; the last-named route came to be called as mad-cow disease and hit the headlines when BSE was reported in the UK sometime back.

Clinically, CJD is characterised by rapidly progressive dementia with prominent association of myoclonus. CJD is invariably fatal with mean survival of about 7 months after diagnosis.

Grossly, the changes are too rapid to become noticeable but brain atrophy may be seen in long-standing cases.

Microscopically, the hallmark is spongiform change i.e. there are small round vacuoles in the neuronal cells. These changes are predominantly seen in the cortex and other grey matter areas. Spongiform changes result in neuronal loss and glial cell proliferation but significantly without any inflammation or white matter involvement.

Fungal and Protozoal Encephalitis

Mycotic diseases of the CNS usually develop by blood stream from systemic deep mycoses elsewhere in the body. They are particularly more common in immunosuppressed individuals such as in AIDS, patients of lymphomas and other cancers. Some of the fungi which may disseminate to the CNS are *Candida albicans, Mucor, Aspergillus fumigatus, Cryptococcus neoformans, Histoplasma capsulatum and Blastomyces dermatitidis.* These fungal infections may produce one of the three patterns: fungal chronic meningitis, vasculitis and encephalitis.

Besides fungal infections, CNS may be involved in protozoal diseases such as in malaria, toxoplasmosis, amoebiasis and trypanosomiasis.

CEREBROVASCULAR DISEASES

Cerebrovascular diseases are all those diseases in which one or more of the blood vessels of the brain are involved in the pathologic processes. Various pathologic processes commonly implicated in cerebrovascular diseases are: thrombosis, embolism, rupture of a vessel, hypoxia, hypertensive arteriolosclerosis, atherosclerosis, arteritis, trauma, aneurysm and developmental malformations. These processes can result in 2 main types of parenchymal diseases of the brain:

A. Ischaemic brain damage:

a) Generalised reduction in blood flow resulting in *global hypoxic-ischaemic encephalopathy*

b) Local vascular obstruction causing *infarcts.*

B. Intracranial haemorrhage:

a) Haemorrhage in the brain parenchyma *(intracerebral haemorrhage)*

b) Haemorrhage in the subarachnoid space *(subarachnoid haemorrhage).*

The *stroke syndrome* is the cardinal feature of cerebrovascular disease. The term stroke is used for sudden and dramatic development of focal neurologic deficit, varying from trivial neurologic disorder to hemiplegia and coma. Other less common effects of vascular disease include: transient ischaemic attacks (TIA), vascular headache (e.g. in migraine, hypertension and arteritis), local pressure of an aneurysm and increased intracranial pressure (e.g. in hypertensive encephalopathy and venous thrombosis).

A. ISCHAEMIC BRAIN DAMAGE

Ischaemic necrosis in the brain results from ischaemia caused by considerable reduction or complete interruption of blood supply to neural tissue which is insufficient to meet its metabolic needs. The brain requires sufficient quantities of oxygen and glucose so as to sustain its aerobic metabolism, mainly by citric acid (Krebs') cycle which requires oxygen. Moreover, neural tissue has limited stores of energy reserves so that cessation of continuous supply of oxygen and glucose for more than 3-4 minutes results in permanent damage to neurons and neuroglial cells.

Deprivation of oxygen (anoxia) to the brain may occur in 4 different ways:

1. *Anoxic anoxia,* in which there is low inspired pO_2.
2. *Anaemic anoxia,* in which the oxygen-carrying haemoglobin is reduced.
3. *Histotoxic anoxia,* in which there is direct toxic injury as occurs in cyanide poisoning.
4. *Stagnant (ischaemia) anoxia,* in which the damage is caused by cessation of blood with resultant local accumulation of metabolites and changes in pH.

In all these different forms of anoxia, the end-result is ischaemic brain damage which may have one of the following two patterns:

1. *Global hypoxic-ischaemic encephalopathy,* resulting from generalised cerebral hypoperfusion.
2. *Cerebral infarction,* resulting from severe localised reduction or cessation of blood supply.

Global Hypoxic-Ischaemic Encephalopathy

The brain receives 20% of cardiac output for maintaining its vital aerobic metabolism. A number of factors determine the maximum length of time the CNS can *survive irreversible ischaemic damage.* These include:

i) severity of the hypoxic episode;

ii) presence of pre-existing cerebrovascular disease;

iii) age of the patient; and
iv) body temperature.

In normal individuals, the brain continues to be perfused adequately upto systolic arterial pressure of 50 mmHg by an auto-regulatory vascular control mechanism. However, fall of systemic arterial systolic pressure below this critical value results in rapid fall in cerebral perfusion pressure and eventual ischaemic encephalopathy. Such types of medical emergencies occur at the time of cardiac arrest followed by relatively delayed resuscitation, severe episode of hypotension, carbon monoxide intoxication and status epilepticus. Hypoxic encephalopathy may be followed by a post-ischaemic confusional state and complete recovery or a state of coma and even a persistent vegetative life and brain death.

Depending upon the proneness of different cells of the brain to the effects of ischaemia-hypoxia, three types of lesion may occur:

1. Selective neuronal damage: Neurons are most vulnerable to damaging effect of ischaemia-hypoxia and irreversible injury. In particular, oligodendroglial cells are most susceptible, followed by astrocytes while microglial cells and vascular endothelium survive the longest. The reason for undue vulnerability of neurons to hypoxia can be explained by various factors:
i) different cerebral circulatory blood flow;
ii) presence of acidic excitatory neurotransmitters called *excitotoxins;*
iii) excessive metabolic requirement of these neurons; or
iv) increased sensitivity of neurons to lactic acid.

2. Laminar necrosis: Global ischaemia of cerebral cortex results in uneven damage because of different cerebral vasculature which is termed laminar or pseudolaminar necrosis. In this, superficial areas of cortical layers escape damage while deeper layers are necrosed.

3. Watershed infarcts: Circulatory flow in the brain by anterior, middle and posterior cerebral arteries has overlapping circulations. In ischaemia-hypoxia, perfusion of overlapping zones, being farthest from the blood supply, suffers maximum damage. This results in wedge-shaped areas of coagulative necrosis called watershed or borderzone infarcts. Particularly vulnerable is the border zone of the cerebral cortex between the anterior and middle cerebral arteries, producing para-sagittal infarction.

PATHOLOGIC CHANGES. The pathologic appearance of the brain in hypoxic encephalopathy varies depending upon the duration and severity of hypoxic episode and the length of survival.

■ **Survival for a few hours:** No pathologic changes are visible.

■ **Survival 12-24 hours:** No macroscopic change is discernible but microscopic examination reveals early neuronal damage in the form of eosinophilic cytoplasm and pyknotic nuclei, so called red neurons.

■ **After 2-7 days:** ***Grossly,*** there is focal softening. The area supplied by distal branches of the cerebral arteries suffers from the most severe ischaemic damage and may develop *border zone* or *watershed infarcts* in the junctional zones between the territories supplied by major arteries.

Microscopically, the nerve cells die and disappear and are replaced by reactive fibrillary gliosis. There are minor variations in the distribution of neuronal damage to the cortex; the loss of pyramidal cell layer is more severe than that of granular cell layer producing laminar necrosis.

■ **Longer duration:** Use of modern ventilators has led to maintenance of cardiorespiratory function in the presence of total brain necrosis unassociated with vital reaction.

Cerebral Infarction

Cerebral infarction is a localised area of tissue necrosis caused by local vascular occlusion—arterial or venous. Occasionally, it may be the result of non-occlusive causes such as compression on the cerebral arteries from outside and from hypoxic encephalopathy. Clinically, the signs and symptoms associated with cerebral infarction depend upon the region infarcted. In general, the focal neurologic deficit termed stroke, is present. However, significant atherosclerotic cerebrovascular disease may produce transient ischaemic attacks (TIA).

1. Arterial occlusion. Occlusion of the cerebral arteries by either thrombi or emboli is the most common cause of cerebral infarction. Thrombotic occlusion of the cerebral arteries is most frequently the result of atherosclerosis, and rarely, from arteritis of the cranial arteries. Embolic arterial occlusion is commonly derived from the heart, most often from mural thrombosis complicating myocardial infarction, from atrial fibrillation and endocarditis. The size and shape of an infarct are determined by the extent of anastomotic connections with adjacent arterial branches. For instance,

■ The circle of Willis provides a complete collateral flow for internal carotid and vertebral arteries.

■ The middle and anterior cerebral arteries have partial anastomosis of their distal branches. Their complete occlusion may cause infarcts.

■ The small terminal cerebral arteries, on the contrary, are end-arteries and have no anastomosis. Hence, occlusion of these branches will invariably lead to an infarct.

2. **Venous occlusion.** Venous infarction in the brain is an infrequent phenomenon due to good communications of the cerebral venous drainage. However in cancer, due to increased predisposition to thrombosis, superior sagittal thrombosis may occur leading to bilateral, parasagittal, multiple haemorrhagic infarcts.

3. **Non-occlusive causes.** Compression of the cerebral arteries from outside such as occurs during herniation may cause cerebral infarction. Mechanism of watershed (border zone) cerebral infarction in hypoxic encephalopathy has already been explained above.

In any case, the extent of damage produced by any of the above causes depends upon:
i) rate of reduction of blood flow;
ii) type of blood vessel involved; and
iii) extent of collateral circulation.

PATHOLOGIC CHANGES. Cerebral infarcts may be anaemic or haemorrhagic.
Grossly, an *anaemic infarct* becomes evident 6-12 hours after its occurrence. The affected area is soft and swollen and there is blurring of junction between grey and white matter. Within 2-3 days, the infarct undergoes softening and disintegration. Eventually, there is central liquefaction with peripheral firm glial reaction and thickened leptomeninges, forming a cystic infarct (Fig. 28.3). A *haemorrhagic infarct* is red and superficially resembles a haematoma. It is usually the result of fragmentation of occlusive arterial emboli or venous thrombosis.
Histologically, the sequential changes are as under:
1. Initially, there is eosinophilic neuronal necrosis and lipid vacuolisation produced by breakdown of myelin. Simultaneously, the infarcted area is infiltrated by neutrophils.
2. After the first 2-3 days, there is progressive invasion by macrophages and there is astrocytic and vascular proliferation.
3. In the following weeks to months, the macrophages clear away the necrotic debris by phagocytosis followed by reactive astrocytosis, often with little fine fibrosis (Fig. 28.4). A haemorrhagic infarct has some phagocytes containing haemosiderin.
4. Ultimately, after 3-4 months an old cystic infarct is formed which shows a cyst traversed by small blood vessels and has peripheral fibrillary gliosis. Small cavitary infarcts are called *lacunar infarcts* and are commonly found as a complication of systemic hypertension.

B. INTRACRANIAL HAEMORRHAGE

Haemorrhage into the brain may be traumatic, non-traumatic, or spontaneous. There are two main types of spontaneous intracranial haemorrhage:
1. Intracerebral haemorrhage, which is usually of hypertensive origin.
2. Subarachnoid haemorrhage, which is commonly aneurysmal in origin.

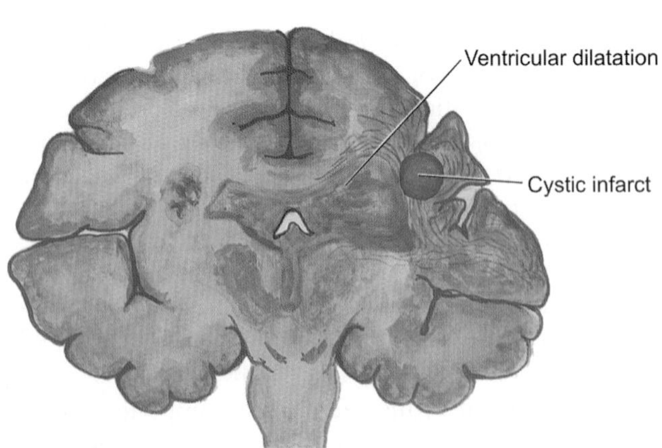

FIGURE 28.3
An old cystic infarct in the brain (coronal section). There is shrinkage of scarred area with ipsilateral ventricular dilatation.

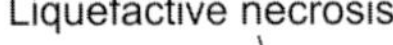

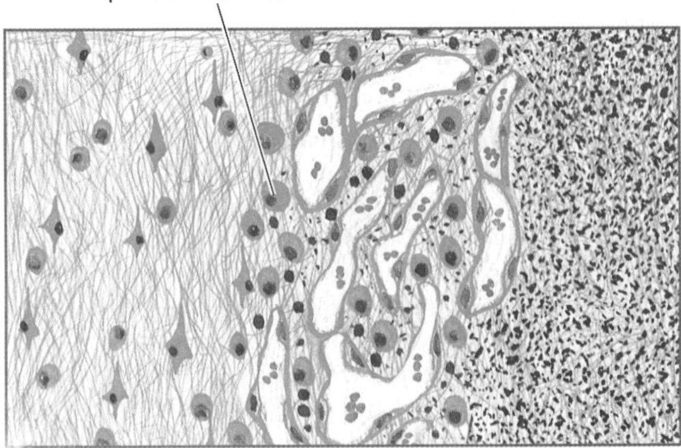

FIGURE 28.4
An anaemic infarct of a few days duration. The histologic changes are reactive astrocytosis, a few reactive macrophages and neovascularisation in the wall of the cystic lesion. The outer cortical layer is, however, intact.

In addition to hypertension and rupture of an aneurysm, other causes of spontaneous intracranial haemorrhage include vascular malformations which produce mixed intracerebral and subarachnoid haemorrhage, haemorrhagic diathesis and haemorrhage into tumours.

Intracerebral Haemorrhage

Spontaneous intracerebral haemorrhage occurs mostly in patients of hypertension. Most hypertensives over middle age have microaneurysms in very small cerebral arteries in the brain tissue. Rupture of one of the numerous microaneurysms is believed to be the cause of intracerebral haemorrhage. Unlike subarachnoid haemorrhage, it is not common to have recurrent intracerebral haemorrhages.

The common sites of hypertensive intracerebral haemorrhage are the region of the basal ganglia (particularly the putamen and the internal capsule), pons and the cerebellar cortex. Clinically the onset is usually sudden with headache and loss of consciousness. Depending upon the location of the lesion, hemispheric, brainstem or cerebellar signs will be present. About 40% of patients die during the first 3-4 days of haemorrhage, mostly from haemorrhage into the ventricles. The survivors tend to have haematoma that separates the tissue planes which is followed by resolution and development of an *apoplectic cyst* accompanied by loss of function.

PATHOLOGIC CHANGES. Grossly and ***microscopically***, the haemorrhage consists of dark mass of clotted blood replacing brain parenchyma. The borders of the lesion are sharply-defined and have a narrow rim of partially necrotic parenchyma. Small ring haemorrhages in the Virchow-Robin space in the border zone are commonly present. Ipsilateral ventricles are distorted and compressed and may contain blood in their lumina. Rarely, blood may rupture through the surface of the brain into the subarachnoid space. After a few weeks to months, the haematoma undergoes resolution with formation of a slit-like space called *apoplectic cyst* and containing yellowish fluid. Its margins are yellow-brown and contain haemosiderin-laden macrophages and a reactive zone of fibrillary astrocytosis.

Subarachnoid Haemorrhage

Haemorrhage into the subarachnoid space is most commonly caused by rupture of an aneurysm, and rarely, rupture of a vascular malformation.

A general discussion of aneurysms is given on page 294. Of the three types of aneurysms affecting the larger intracranial arteries, namely berry, mycotic and fusiform, ***berry aneurysms*** are most important and most common. Berry aneurysms are saccular in appearance with rounded or lobulated bulge arising at the bifurcation of intracranial arteries and varying in size from 2 mm to 2 cm or more. They account for 95% of aneurysms which are liable to rupture. Berry aneurysms are rare in childhood but increase in frequency in young adults and middle life. They are, therefore, not congenital anomalies but develop over the years from developmental defect of the media of the arterial wall at the bifurcation of arteries forming thin-walled saccular bulges. Although most berry aneurysms are sporadic in occurrence, there is an increased incidence of their presence in association with congenital polycystic kidney disease and coarctation of the aorta. About a quarter of berry aneurysms are multiple.

In more than 85% cases of subarachnoid haemorrhage, the cause is massive and sudden bleeding from a berry aneurysm on or near the circle of Willis. The four most common sites are (Fig. 28.5):

1. in relation to anterior communicating artery;
2. at the origin of the posterior communicating artery from the stem of the internal carotid artery;
3. at the first major bifurcation of the middle cerebral artery; and
4. at the bifurcation of the internal carotid into the middle and anterior cerebral arteries.

The remaining 15% cases of subarachnoid haemorrhage are the result of rupture in the posterior circulation,

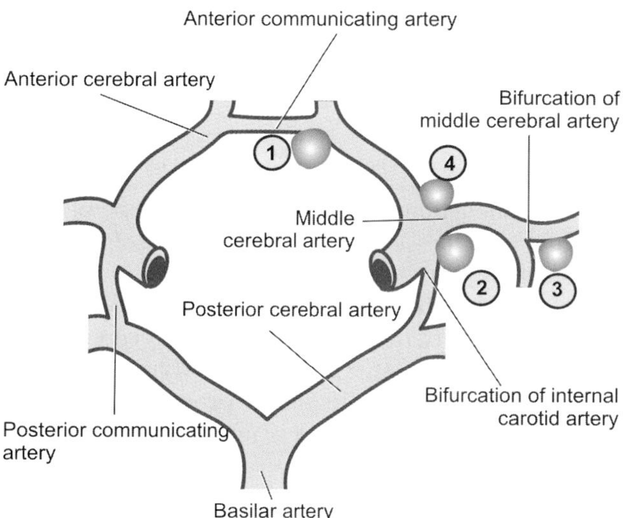

FIGURE 28.5

The circle of Willis showing principal sites of berry (saccular) aneurysms. The serial numbers indicate the frequency of involvement.

vascular malformations and rupture of mycotic aneurysms that occurs in the setting of bacterial endocarditis. In all types of aneurysms, the rupture of thin-walled dilatation occurs in association with sudden rise in intravascular pressure but chronic hypertension does not appear to be a risk factor in their development or rupture.

Clinically, berry aneurysms remain asymptomatic prior to rupture. On rupture, they produce severe generalised headache of sudden onset which is frequently followed by unconsciousness and neurologic defects. Initial mortality from first rupture is about 20-25%. Survivors recover completely but frequently suffer from recurrent episodes of fresh bleeding.

PATHOLOGIC CHANGES. Rupture of a berry aneurysm frequently spreads haemorrhage throughout the subarachnoid space with rise in intracranial pressure and characteristic blood-stained CSF. An intracerebral haematoma may develop if the blood tracks into the brain parenchyma. The region of the brain supplied by the affected artery frequently shows infarction, partly attributed to vasospasm.

TRAUMA TO THE CNS

Trauma to the CNS constitutes an important cause of death and permanent disability in the modern world. Important causes of head injuries are: motor vehicle accidents, accidental falls and violence. Traumatic injuries to the CNS may result in three consequences which may occur in isolation or in combination:

- epidural haematoma;
- subdural haematoma; and
- parenchymal brain damage.

A. Epidural Haematoma

Epidural haematoma is accumulation of blood between the dura and the skull following fracture of the skull, most commonly from rupture of middle meningeal artery. The haematoma expands rapidly since accumulating blood is arterial in origin and causes compression of the dura and flattening of underlying gyri (Fig. 28.6,A). The patient develops progressive loss of consciousness if haematoma is not drained early.

B. Subdural Haematoma

Subdural haematoma is accumulation of blood between the dura and subarachnoid and develops most often from rupture of veins which cross the surface convexities of the cerebral hemispheres. Subdural haematoma may be acute or chronic.

- **Acute subdural haematoma.** Acute subdural haematoma develops following trauma and consists of clotted blood, often in the frontoparietal region. There is no significant compression of gyri (Fig. 28.6,B). Since the accumulated blood is of venous origin, symptoms appear slowly and may become chronic with passage of time if not fatal.

- **Chronic subdural haematoma.** Chronic subdural haematoma occurs often with brain atrophy and less commonly following trauma. Chronic subdural haematoma is composed of liquid blood. Separating the haematoma from underlying brain is a membrane composed of granulation tissue.

C. Parenchymal Brain Damage

Trauma to the CNS may result in damage to brain parenchyma and includes the following forms:

1. Concussion. Concussion is caused by closed head injury and is characterised by transient neurologic dysfunction and loss of consciousness. Invariably, there is complete neurologic recovery after some hours to days.

No significant morphologic change is noticed but more severe concussion may cause diffuse axonal injury (discussed below).

2. Diffuse axonal injury. Diffuse axonal injury is the most common cause of persistent coma or vegetative state following head injury. The underlying cause is sudden angular acceleration or deceleration resulting in widespread axonal shearing in the deep white matter of both the hemispheres.

Grossly, the changes are minimal to small multiple haemorrhages.

3. Contusions and lacerations. Contusions and lacerations are the result of direct damage to the brain parenchyma, particularly cerebral hemispheres, as occurs in the soft tissues. Most often, they are the result of blunt trauma. The overlying skull may or may not be fractured. Traumatic subarachnoid haemorrhage invariably accompanies cerebral contusions.

Microscopically, brain parenchyma at the affected site is haemorrhagic, necrotic and fragmented. On healing, these lesions appear as shrunken areas with golden brown haemosiderin pigment on the surface.

4. Traumatic intracerebral haemorrhage. On trauma to the CNS, the parenchymal vessels of the hemispheres may get torn and cause multiple intracerebral haemorrhages.

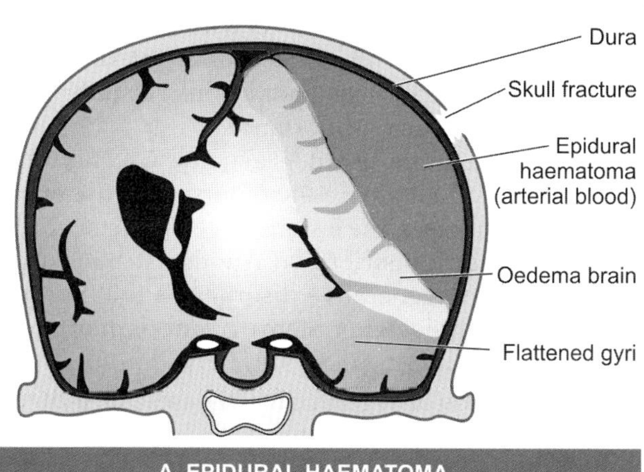

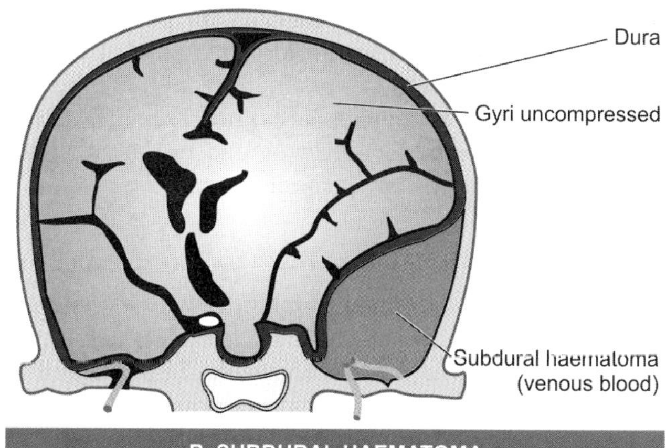

FIGURE 28.6

Epidural and subdural haematoma. A, Epidural haematoma often results from rupture of artery following skull fracture resulting in accumulation of arterial blood between the skull and the dura. B, Subdural haematoma often results from rupture of veins crossing the cerebral convexities and is characterised by accumulation of venous blood between the dura and the arachnoid.

5. **Brain swelling.** Head injury may be accompanied by localised or diffuse brain swelling.

DEMYELINATING DISEASES

Demyelinating diseases are an important group of neurological disorders which have, in common, the pathologic features of focal or patchy destruction of myelin sheaths in the CNS accompanied by an inflammatory response. Demyelination may affect peripheral nervous system as well. Some degree of axonal damage may also occur but demyelination is the predominant feature. The exact cause for demyelination is not known but currently viral infection and autoimmunity are implicated in its pathogenesis.

Loss of myelin may occur in certain other conditions as well, but without an inflammatory response. These conditions have known etiologies such as: genetically-determined defects in the myelin metabolism (leucodystrophies), slow virus diseases of oligodendrocytes (progressive multifocal leucoencephalopathy), and exposure to toxins (central pontine myelinolysis). All these entities are currently not classified as demyelinating diseases. Only those conditions in which the myelin sheath or the myelin-forming cells (i.e. oligodendrocytes and Schwann cells) are primarily injured and are associated with considerable inflammatory exudate are included under the term 'demyelinating diseases'. Pathologically and clinically, two demyelinating diseases are distinguished:

1. Multiple or disseminated sclerosis
2. Perivenous encephalomyelitis.

Multiple (Disseminated) Sclerosis

Multiple or disseminated sclerosis is the most common of the CNS demyelinating diseases. The usual age at onset is 20 to 40 years. The disease presents as recurrent attacks of focal neurologic disorder with predilection for involvement of the spinal cord, optic nerve and brain. The first attack usually begins with a single sign or symptom, most commonly optic neuritis, followed by recovery. As the disease becomes more progressive, remissions become infrequent and incomplete. The etiology of multiple sclerosis remains unknown but a role for genetic susceptibility, infectious agent and immunologic mechanism has been proposed.

PATHOLOGIC CHANGES. The pathologic hallmark is the presence of many scattered discrete areas of demyelination termed *plaques.*

Grossly, plaques appear as grey-pink, swollen, sharply defined, usually bilaterally symmetric areas in the white matter.

Microscopically, the features vary according to the age of the plaque:

1. In *active enlarging plaques*, the histologic features are accumulation of lymphocytes and macrophages around venules and at the plaque margin where demyelination is occurring. In addition, there is loss of oligodendrocytes and presence of reactive astrocytosis with numerous lipid-laden macrophages (microglia) in the plaque. The axons in the plaque are generally intact.

2. In *old inactive plaques,* there is no perivascular inflammatory cell infiltrate and nearly total absence of oligodendrocytes. Demyelination in the plaque area is complete as there is only limited regeneration of myelin. Gliosis is well-developed but astrocytes are less prominent. Some axonal loss may be present.

Perivenous Encephalomyelitis

Perivenous encephalomyelitis includes two uncommon diseases: *acute disseminated encephalomyelitis* and *acute necrotising haemorrhagic leucoencephalitis.* Both are monophasic diseases characterised by perivenous mononuclear inflammatory cell infiltration. Both diseases occur following a viral infection, vaccination or a respiratory illness. Both conditions are looked upon as human counterpart of experimental allergic encephalomyelitis (EAE) and are considered to be allergic reaction against myelin antigen.

■ **Acute disseminated encephalomyelitis** occurs usually following viral infection (measles, mumps, rubella, chickenpox), whooping cough or vaccination. The disease begins abruptly with headache and delirium followed by lethargy and coma. Signs of meningeal irritation and fever may be present. Prognosis for recovery is generally good.

■ **Acute necrotising haemorrhagic leucoencephalitis** is a rare disease occurring more often after a respiratory infection. The clinical course is similar to that of acute disseminated encephalomyelitis except for its suddeness of onset and rapidity of progression, sometimes leading to death within 48 hours.

MISCELLANEOUS DISEASES

Included under the heading of miscellaneous diseases of the CNS are degenerative, metabolic and nutritional diseases. These groups alongwith the list of diseases included in each group are briefly outlined below without going into the details of individual diseases. Interested reader should consult pertinent text on neuropathology and neurology.

Degenerative Diseases

Degenerative diseases are disorders of unknown etiology and pathogenesis, characterised pathologically by progressive loss of CNS neurons and their processes accompanied by fibrillary astrocytosis. The identification of these diseases depends upon exclusion of diseases with known etiologies such as metabolic disturbances, vascular diseases, nutritional deficiencies or infection. A considerable proportion of degenerative disorders are genetic in origin, with either dominant or recessive inheritance; others occur sporadically. Family history is, of course, of great importance.

The degenerative disorders usually begin insidiously and have a gradual progressive course over many years. In virtually all cases, the lesions have characteristic bilaterally symmetric distribution. Another striking characteristic of the degenerative disorders is that particular anatomic or physiologic system of neurons may be selectively affected, leaving others entirely intact.

Classification of degenerative diseases into individual syndromes is based on clinical aspects and anatomic distribution of the lesions. Some of the more common degenerative diseases are listed in Table 28.3. Two of the important examples—Alzheimer's disease and parkinsonism are discussed below.

ALZHEIMER'S DISEASE. Alzheimer's disease is the most common cause of dementia in the elderly. The condition occurs after 5th decade of life and incidence progressively increases with advancing age. The exact cause is not known but a few factors are implicated in its etiology which include positive family history and deposition of Aβ amyloid derived from amyloid precursor protein (APP) forming *neuritic 'senile' plaques* and *neurofibrillary tangles.*

Grossly, the brain is often reduced in weight and bilaterally atrophic.

Microscopically, the main features are as under:

i) *Senile neuritic plaque* is the most conspicuous lesion and consists of focal area which has a central core containing Aβ amyloid.

ii) *Neurofibrillary tangle* is a filamentous collection of neurofilaments and neurotubules within the cytoplasm of neurons.

iii) *Amyloid angiopathy* is deposition of the same amyloid in the vessel wall which is deposited in the amyloid core of the plaque.

iv) *Granulovacuolar degeneration* is presence of multiple, small intraneuronal cytoplasmic vacuoles, some of which contain one or more dark granules called *Hirano bodies.*

PARKINSONISM. Parkinsonism is a syndrome of chronic progressive disorder of motor function and is clinically characterised by tremors which are most conspicuous at rest and worsen with emotional stress; other features are rigidity and disordered gait and posture. Parkinsonism is caused by several degenerative diseases, the most important being Parkinson's disease; other causes of parkinsonism are trauma, toxic agents, and drugs (dopamine antagonists).

TABLE 28.3: Common Degenerative Diseases.

REGION AFFECTED	DISEASE	MAIN FEATURES	PREDOMINANT PATHOLOGY
I. *Cerebral cortex*	Alzheimer's disease	Progressive senile dementia	Cortical atrophy, senile plaques (neurites), neurofibrillary tangles, amyloid angiopathy
	Pick's disease	Pre-senile dementia	Lobar cortical atrophy, ballooning degeneration of neurons (Pick's cells)
II. *Basal ganglia and brainstem*	Huntington's disease	Progressive dementia with choreiform movements	Atrophy of frontal lobes, fibrillary astrocytosis
	Parkinson's disease	Abnormalities of posture and movement	Aggregates of melanin-containing nerve cells in brainstem, intracytoplasmic neuronal inclusions (Lewy bodies)
III. *Spinal cord and cerebellum*	Cerebellar cortical degeneration	Progressive cerebellar ataxia	Loss of Purkinje cells in cerebellar cortex
	Olivopontocerebellar atrophy	Cerebellar ataxia	Combination of atrophy of cerebellar cortex, inferior olivary nuclei and pontine nuclei
	Spinocerebellar atrophy (Friedreich's ataxia)	Gait ataxia, dysarthria	Degeneration of spinocerebellar tracts, peripheral axons and myelin sheaths
IV. *Motor neurons (UMN and LMN)*	Motor neuron disease (Amyotrophic lateral sclerosis)	Syndromes of muscular weakness and wasting without sensory loss	Progressive loss of motor neurons, both in the cerebellar cortex (UMN) and in the anterior horn of spinal cord (LMN)
	Werdnig-Hoffmann's disease	Spinal muscular atrophy in infants	Loss of lower motor neurons, denervation atrophy of muscles

Grossly, the brain is atrophic or may be normal externally.

Microscopically, the hallmark is depigmentation of substantia nigra and locus ceruleus due to loss of neuromelanin pigment from neurons and accumulation of neuromelanin pigment in the glial cells. Some of the residual neurons in these areas contain intracytoplasmic, eosinophilic, elongated inclusions called *Lewy bodies.*

Metabolic Diseases

Metabolic diseases of the CNS result from neurochemical disturbances which are either inherited or acquired. *Hereditary metabolic disorders* predominantly manifest in infancy or childhood and include genetically-determined disorders of carbohydrate, lipid, amino acid and mineral metabolism. *Acquired or secondary metabolic diseases* are the disturbances of cerebral function due to disease in some other organ system such as the heart and circulation, lungs and respiratory function, kidneys, liver, endocrine glands and pancreas. In addition, endogenous metabolic diseases may be caused by toxic injuries induced by metals, gases, chemicals, and drugs. The pathologic changes in each of these conditions are quite diverse and include oedema, neuronal storage, degenerative changes, and sometimes parenchymal necrosis.

The predominant types of hereditary and acquired metabolic disorders are as under:

A. HEREDITARY METABOLIC DISEASES:

1. Neuronal storage diseases—characterised by storage of a metabolic product in the neurons due to specific enzyme deficiency. Common examples are: gangliosidoses (e.g. Tay-Sachs disease or GM2 gangliosidosis), mucopolysaccharidoses, Gaucher's disease and Niemann-Pick disease). These conditions are described on page 270.

2. Leucodystrophies—are diseases of white matter characterised by diffuse demyelination and gliosis. They are caused by deficiency of one of the enzymes required for formation and maintenance of myelin. That is why these conditions are also called *dysmyelinating diseases.* Common types of leucodystrophies are: sudanophilic leucodystrophy, adrenoleucodystrophy, metachromatic leucodystrophy and globoid cell leucodystrophy (Krabbe's disease).

3. Other inborn errors of metabolism—e.g. Wilson's disease (hepatolenticular degeneration), glycogen-storage diseases, phenylketonuria and galactosaemia.

B. ACQUIRED METABOLIC DISEASES:

These include the following:

1. Anoxic-ischaemic encephalopathy

2. Hypoglycaemic encephalopathy
3. Hyperglycaemic coma
4. Acute hepatic encephalopathy (Reye's syndrome)
5. Chronic hepatic encephalopathy
6. Kernicterus
7. Uraemic encephalopathy
8. Encephalopathy due to electrolyte and endocrine disturbances.

All these conditions have already been discussed in the relevant chapters.

Nutritional Diseases

Neurologic disorders may be caused by malnutrition from lack of adequate diet in many underdeveloped countries and many poor socio-economic groups. In the United States and Europe, however, nutritionally-induced disease is chiefly found in association with chronic alcoholism or due to defect in absorption, transport or metabolism of dietary nutrients.

The general aspects of deficiency diseases have been covered in Chapter 9. Some of the common neurologic diseases included in the category of deficiency diseases are:

1. Wernicke's encephalopathy and Korsakoff's psychosis (vitamin B_1 or thiamine deficiency).
2. Subacute combined degeneration of the spinal cord (vitamin B_{12} deficiency).
3. Folic acid deficiency (page 378).
4. Spinocerebellar syndrome (vitamin E deficiency).
5. Pellagra (niacin deficiency).
6. Alcoholic cerebellar degeneration.

TUMOURS OF THE CNS

Tumours of the CNS may originate in the brain or spinal cord (primary tumours), or may spread from another primary site of cancer (metastatic tumours). More than one-quarter of the CNS tumours are secondary metastases arising in patients undergoing treatment for systemic cancer. Primary CNS tumours are the second commonest form of cancer in infants and children under the age of 15 years, exceeded in frequency only by leukaemia. Both benign and malignant CNS tumours are capable of producing neurologic impairment depending upon their site.

Primary CNS tumours or intracranial tumours include: tumours arising from *constituent cells of the brain* (with the sole exception of microglial cells) and from *the supporting tissues.* In childhood, tumours arise from more primitive cells (e.g. neuroblastoma, medulloblastoma).

TABLE 28.4: Classification of Intracranial Tumours.

I.	**TUMOURS OF NEUROGLIA (GLIOMAS)**
1.	Astrocytoma
2.	Oligodendroglioma
3.	Ependymoma
4.	Choroid plexus papilloma
II.	**TUMOURS OF NEURONS**
1.	Neuroblastoma (page 824)
2.	Ganglioneuroblastoma
3.	Ganglioneuroma
III.	**TUMOURS OF NEURONS AND NEUROGLIA**
	Ganglioglioma
IV.	**POORLY-DIFFERENTIATED AND EMBRYONAL TUMOURS**
1.	Medulloblastoma
2.	Neuroblastoma (page 824)
3.	PNET (page 873)
V.	**TUMOURS OF MENINGES**
1.	Meningioma
2.	Meningeal sarcoma
VI.	**NERVE SHEATH TUMOURS**
1.	Schwannoma (neurilemmoma)
2.	Neurofibroma
3.	Malignant nerve sheath tumour
VII.	**OTHER PRIMARY INTRAPARENCHYMAL TUMOURS**
1.	Haemangioblastoma
2.	Primary CNS lymphoma
3.	Germ cell tumours
VIII.	**MISCELLANEOUS TUMOURS**
1.	Malignant melanoma (page 811)
2.	Craniopharyngioma (page 820)
3.	Pineal cell tumours
4.	Pituitary tumours
IX.	**TUMOUR-LIKE LESIONS**
	(epidermal cyst, dermoid cyst, colloid cyst)
X.	**METASTATIC TUMOURS**

A classification of intracranial tumours abbreviated from the WHO classification is given in Table 28.4. The anatomic distribution of common intracranial tumours is illustrated in Fig. 28.7. A few important morphologic types are described below.

GLIOMAS

The term glioma is used for all tumours arising from neuroglia, or more precisely, from neuroectodermal epithelial tissue. Gliomas are the most common of the primary CNS tumours and collectively account for 40% of all intracranial tumours. They include: tumours arising *from astrocytes* (astrocytomas and glioblastoma multiforme); *from oligodendrocytes* (oligodendroglioma); *from ependyma* (ependymoma); and *from choroid plexus* (choroid plexus papilloma). Gliomas may be well-differentiated or poorly-differentiated. However, glio-

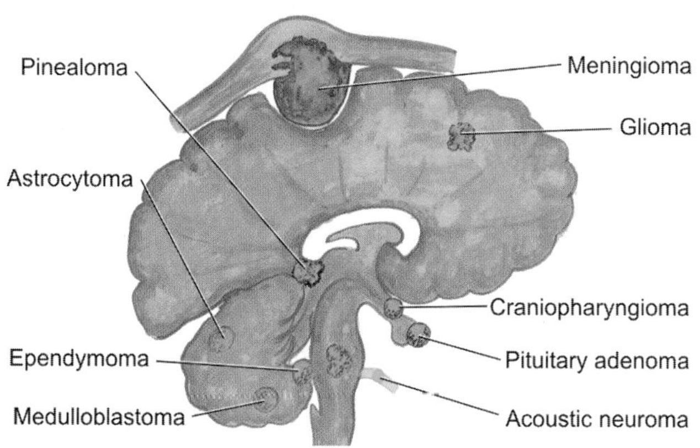

FIGURE 28.7

The anatomic distribution of common intracranial tumours.

mas are never truly well-demarcated or encapsulated and thus all grades of gliomas infiltrate the adjacent brain tissue. Gliomas are disseminated to other parts of the CNS by CSF but they rarely ever metastasise beyond the CNS.

Astrocytoma and Glioblastoma Multiforme

Astrocytomas are the most common type of gliomas. In general, they are found in the late middle life with a peak in 6th decade of life. They occur predominantly in the cerebral hemispheres, and occasionally in the spinal cord. In children and young adults, pilocytic astrocytomas arise in the optic nerves, cerebellum and brainstem. Astrocytomas have tendency to progress from low grade to higher grades of anaplasia. Low-grade astrocytomas evolve slowly over several years whereas higher grades (anaplastic astrocytoma and glioblastoma multiforme) bring about rapid clinical deterioration of the patient.

PATHOLOGIC CHANGES. Pathologically, astrocytomas are divided into 3 progressive histologic grades: low-grade astrocytoma, anaplastic astrocytoma, and glioblastoma multiforme.

1. LOW-GRADE ASTROCYTOMA. ***Grossly,*** it is a poorly defined, grey-white tumour of variable size. The tumour distorts the underlying brain tissue and merges with the surrounding tissue.

Histologically, it is composed of well-differentiated astrocytes separated by variable amount of fibrillary background of astrocytic processes. Based on the type of astrocytes, three subtypes are distinguished: *fibrillary, protoplastic* and *gemistocytic astrocytoma.*

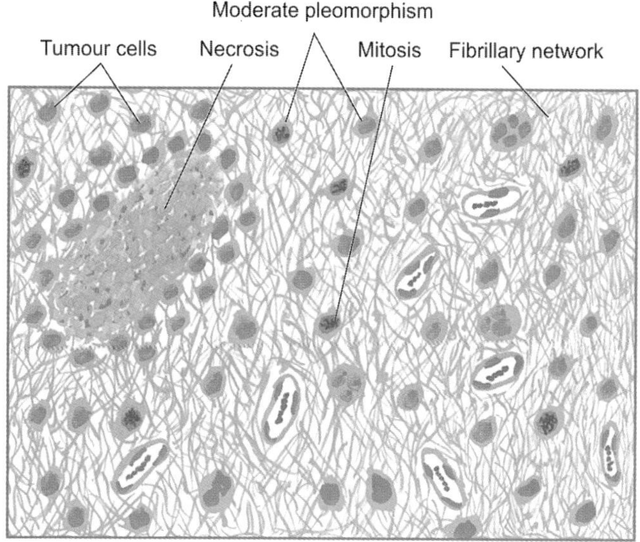

FIGURE 28.8

Anaplastic astrocytoma, revealing hypercellularity of pleomorphic astrocytic cells, mitoses and vascular proliferation in fibrillary background. Areas of necrosis are also present.

PILOCYTIC ASTROCYTOMA. It is a distinctly benign astrocytoma occurring in children and young adults.

Grossly, it is usually cystic or solid and circumscribed.

Microscopically, it is predominantly composed of fusiform pilocytic astrocytes having unusually long, wavy fibrillary processes.

2. ANAPLASTIC ASTROCYTOMA. ***Grossly,*** it may not be distinguishable from the low-grade astrocytoma.

Histologically, it contains features of anaplasia such as hypercellularity, pleomorphism, nuclear hyperchromatism and mitoses. Another characteristic feature of anaplastic variety of astrocytoma is the proliferation of vascular endothelium (Fig. 28.8).

3. GLIOBLASTOMA MULTIFORME. ***Grossly,*** it shows variegated appearance, with some areas showing grey-white appearance while others are yellow and soft with foci of haemorrhages and necrosis. The surrounding normal brain tissue is distorted and infiltrated by yellow tumour tissue.

Histologically, the features are as under:

i) Highly anaplastic and cellular appearance. The cell types show marked variation consisting of fusiform cells, small poorly-differentiated round cells, pleomorphic cells and giant cells. Mitoses are quite frequent and glial fibrils are scanty.

ii) Areas of tumour necrosis around which tumour cells may form pseudopalisading.
iii) Microvascular endothelial proliferation is marked.

The diagnosis of various types of astrocytomas can be generally made by routine H & E morphology but in difficult situations and poorly differentiated cases, immunohistochemical staining with glial fibrillary protein (GFAP) or by electron microscopic demonstration of glial filaments can be established.

Oligodendroglioma

Oligodendroglioma is an uncommon glioma of oligodendroglial origin and may develop in isolation or may be mixed with other glial cells. The tumour commonly presents in 3rd to 4th decades of life. It occurs in the cerebral hemispheres, most commonly in the frontal lobes or within the ventricles. X-ray examination and CT scan reveal a well-defined mass with numerous small foci of calcification. The tumour is generally slow-growing.

PATHOLOGIC CHANGES. ***Grossly,*** oligodendroglioma is well-circumscribed, grey-white and gelatinous mass having cystic areas, foci of haemorrhages and calcification.
Microscopically, the tumour is characterised by uniform cells with round to oval nuclei surrounded by a clear halo of cytoplasm and well-defined cell membranes. Tumour cells tend to cluster around the native neurons forming *satellitosis.* Typically, there are varying degree of endothelial cell hyperplasia and foci of calcification. Anaplastic change may occur as in other gliomas.

Ependymoma

Ependymoma is not an uncommon tumour, derived from the layer of epithelium that lines the ventricles and the central canal of the spinal cord. It occurs chiefly in childhood and young adulthood (below 20 years of age). Typically, it is encountered in the fourth ventricle (posterior fossa tumour). Other locations are the lateral ventricles, the third ventricle, and in the case of adults, the spinal cord in the region of lumbar spine. Clinically, by virtue of their frequent location in the floor of the fourth ventricle, ependymomas are associated with obstructive hydrocephalus. The usual biologic behaviour is of a slow-growing tumour over a period of years.

PATHOLOGIC CHANGES. ***Grossly,*** ependymoma is a well-demarcated tumour but complete surgical removal may not be possible due to close proximity to vital structures in the medulla and pons.

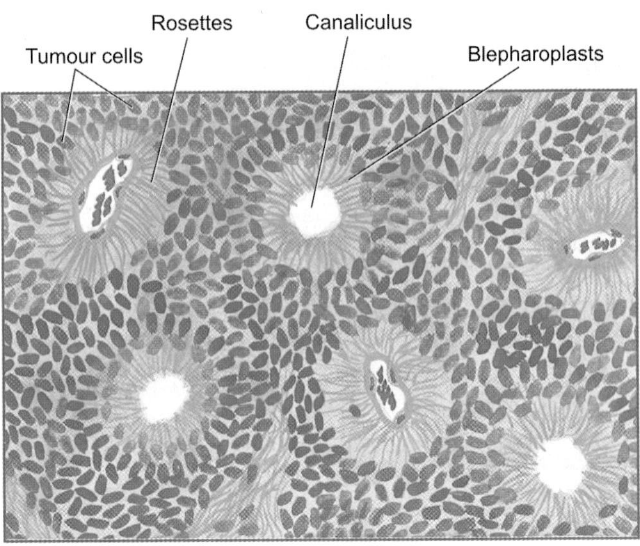

FIGURE 28.9

Ependymoma showing uniform ependymal tumour cells forming rosettes and a canaliculus.

Microscopically, the tumour is composed of uniform epithelial (ependymal) cells forming rosettes, canals and perivascular pseudorosettes. By light microscopy under high magnification, PTAH-positive structures, blepharoplasts, representing basal bodies of cilia may be demonstrated in the cytoplasm of tumour cells (Fig. 28.9). Most tumours are well-differentiated but anaplastic variants are also recognised.

Two variants of ependymoma deserve special mention: myxopapillary type and subependymoma.

1. Myxopapillary ependymoma. Characteristically, it occurs in the region of cauda equina and originates from the filum terminale in adults. True to its name, it contains myxoid and papillary structures interspersed in the typical ependymal cells. It is a slow-growing tumour.

2. Subependymoma. It occurs as a small, asymptomatic, incidental solid nodule in the fourth and lateral ventricle of middle-aged or elderly patients. Areas of microcysts and calcification may be encountered. ***Histologically,*** it is composed of nests of uniform ependymal cells in a stroma of very dense, acellular, finely fibrillar background. Subependymoma is typically a very slow-growing tumour.

Choroid Plexus Papilloma

Tumours derived from choroid plexus epithelium are uncommon intracranial tumours. They are found in the distribution of the choroid plexus. In children, they occur most frequently in the lateral ventricles, whereas in adults fourth ventricle is the most common site. They are invariably benign tumours and rarely ever undergo malignant transformation.

PATHOLOGIC CHANGES. ***Grossly,*** the tumour projects as rounded, papillary mass into one of the ventricles.

Histologically, choroid plexus papilloma is a papillary tumour resembling normal choroid plexus with a vascular connective tissue core covered by a single layer of cuboidal epithelium which lies upon a basement membrane.

POORLY-DIFFERENTIATED AND EMBRYONAL TUMOURS

CNS tumours composed of primitive undifferentiated cells include medulloblastoma and glioblastoma, and rarely, neuroblastoma (page 824) and retinoblastoma (page 523). Except for medulloblastoma, other examples of these tumours have been described elsewhere in the text.

Medulloblastoma

Medulloblastoma is the most common variety of primitive neuroectodermal tumour. It comprises 25% of all childhood brain tumours but a quarter of cases occur in patients over the age of 20 years. The most common location is the cerebellum in the region of roof of fourth ventricle, in the midline of cerebellum, in the vermis, and in the cerebellar hemispheres. Medulloblastoma is a highly malignant tumour and spreads to local as well as to distant sites. It invades locally and by the CSF to meninges, ventricles and subarachnoid space and has a tendency for widespread metastases to extraneural sites such as to lungs, liver, vertebrae and pelvis.

PATHOLOGIC CHANGES. ***Grossly,*** the tumour typically protrudes into the fourth ventricle as a soft, grey-white mass or invades the surface of the cerebellum.

Microscopically, medulloblastoma is composed of small, poorly-differentiated cells with ill-defined cytoplasmic processes and a tendency to be arranged around blood vessels and occasionally forms pseudorosettes (Homer-Wright rosettes). Another characteristic of the tumour is differentiation into glial or neuronal elements.

OTHER PRIMARY INTRAPARENCHYMAL TUMOURS

Important examples of some other primary intraparenchymal are haemangioblastoma, CNS lymphoma and germ cell tumours.

Haemangioblastoma

Haemangioblastoma is a tumour of uncertain origin and constitutes about 2% of all intracranial tumours. It is seen more commonly in young adults and is commoner in males. It may occur sporadically or be a part of von Hippel-Lindau syndrome (along with cysts in the liver, kidney, and benign/malignant renal tumour). About a quarter of haemangioblastomas secrete erythropoietin and cause polycythaemia.

Grossly, the tumour is usually a circumscribed cystic mass with a mural nodule. The cyst contains haemorrhagic fluid.

Microscopically, the features are as under:

i) Large number of thin-walled blood vessels lined by plump endothelium.

ii) Vascular spaces are separated by groups of polygonal lipid-laden foamy stromal cells.

Primary CNS Lymphoma

Lymphomas in the brain may occur as a part of disseminated non-Hodgkin's lymphoma (Chapter 14) or may be a primary CNS lymphoma. The incidence of the primary CNS lymphoma has shown a rising trend in patients of AIDS and other immunosuppressed conditions. They occur in men above 5th decade of life. Primary CNS lymphoma has a poor prognosis.

Grossly, the tumour is frequently periventricular in location and may appear nodular or diffuse.

Microscopically, the features are as under:

i) Characteristically, the tumour grows around blood vessels i.e. has an angiocentric growth pattern. Reticulin stain highlights this feature well.

ii) Typically, CNS lymphomas are diffuse, large cell type with high mitotic activity.

iii) They are generally B-cell type.

Germ Cell Tumours

Rarely, germ cell tumours may occur in the brain, especially in children. Common locations are suprasellar region and pineal area. Some common examples of such tumours are germinoma (seminoma/dysgerminoma), teratoma and embryonal carcinoma. Morphologically, they are similar to their counterparts elsewhere.

TUMOURS OF MENINGES

The most common tumour arising from the pia-arachnoid is meningioma accounting for 20% of intracranial tumours.

Meningioma

Meningiomas arise from the cap cell layer of the arachnoid. Their most common sites are in the front half of the head and include: lateral cerebral convexities, midline along the falx cerebri adjacent to the major venous sinuses parasagittally, and olfactory groove. Less frequent sites are: within the cerebral ventricles, foramen magnum, cerebellopontine angle and the spinal cord. Meningiomas are generally solitary. They have an increased frequency in patients with neurofibromatosis 2 and are often multiple in them. They are usually found in 2nd to 6th decades of life, with slight female preponderance. Most are benign and can be removed successfully. Rarely, a malignant meningioma may metastasise, mainly to the lungs.

PATHOLOGIC CHANGES. Grossly, meningioma is well-circumscribed, solid, spherical or hemispherical mass of varying size (1-10 cm in diameter). The tumour is generally firmly attached to the dura and indents the surface of the brain but rarely ever invades it (Fig. 28.10). The overlying bone usually shows hyperostosis. Cut surface of the tumour is firm and fibrous, sometimes with foci of calcification.

Microscopically, meningiomas are divided into 5 subtypes: meningotheliomatous (syncytial), fibrous (fibroblastic), transitional (mixed), angioblastic and anaplastic (malignant).

1. **Meningotheliomatous (syncytial) meningioma.** This pattern of meningioma resembles the normal arachnoid cap cells. The tumour consists of solid masses of polygonal cells with poorly-defined cell membranes (i.e. syncytial appearance). The cells have round to oval, central nuclei with abundant, finely granular cytoplasm. Some amount of collagenous stroma is present that divides the tumour into irregular lobules.

2. **Fibrous (fibroblastic) meningioma.** A less frequent pattern is of a spindle-shaped fibroblastic tumour in which the tumour cells form parallel or interlacing bundles. Whorled pattern and psammoma bodies are less common features of this type.

3. **Transitional (mixed) meningioma.** This pattern is characterised by a combination of cells with syncytial and fibroblastic features with conspicuous whorled pattern of tumour cells, often around central capillary-sized blood vessels. Some of the whorls contain psammoma bodies due to calcification of the central core of whorls (Fig. 28.11). Other forms of degenerative changes like xanthomatous and myxomatous degeneration may also be encountered, in transitional variety (COLOUR PLATE XXXIV: CL 135).

The first three histologic patterns constitute a spectrum of lesions rather than three distinct entities.

4. **Angioblastic meningioma.** An angioblastic meningioma includes 2 patterns: *haemangioblastic pattern* resembling haemangioblastoma of the cerebellum, and *haemangiopericytic pattern* which is indistinguishable from haemangiopericytoma elsewhere in the body.

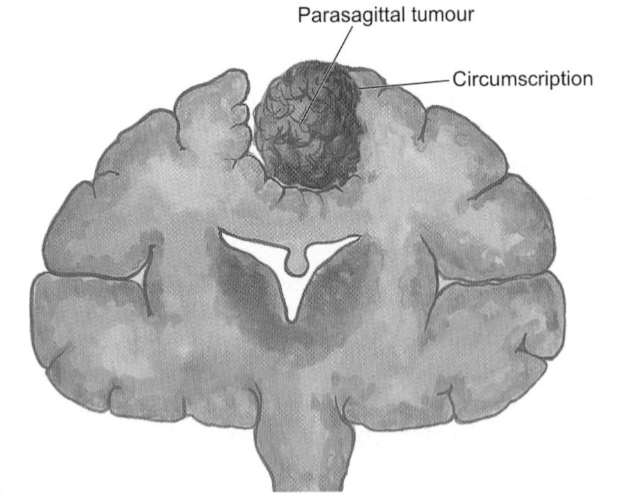

FIGURE 28.10

Meningioma, seen as firm, lobulated mass located parasagittally and indenting the surface of the brain.

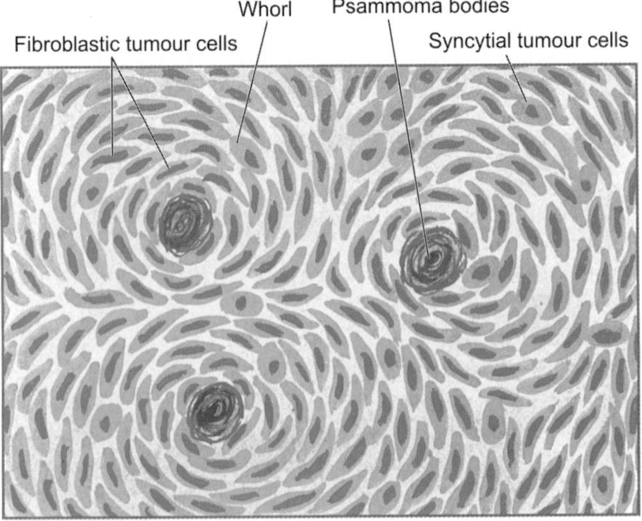

FIGURE 28.11

The cells have features of both syncytial and fibroblastic type and form whorled appearance. Some of the whorls contain psammoma bodies.

Both types of angioblastic meningiomas have high rate of recurrences.

5. Anaplastic (malignant) meningioma. Rarely, a meningioma may display features of anaplasia and invade the underlying brain or spinal cord. This pattern of meningioma is associated with extraneural metastases, mainly to the lungs.

METASTATIC TUMOURS

Approximately a quarter of intracranial tumours are metastatic tumours. The clinical features are like those of a primary brain tumour. Most common primary tumours metastasising to the brain are: carcinomas of the lung, breast, skin (malignant melanoma), kidney and the gastrointestinal tract and choriocarcinoma. Infiltration from lymphoma and leukaemias may also occur.

PATHOLOGIC CHANGES. Grossly, the metastatic deposits in the brain are usually multiple, sharply-defined masses at the junction of grey and white matter (Fig. 28.12). A less frequent pattern is carcinomatous meningitis or meningeal carcinomatosis in which there is presence of carcinomatous nodules on the surface of the brain and spinal cord, particularly encountered in carcinomas of the lung and breast.

Histologically, metastatic tumours in the brain recapitulate the appearance of the primary tumour of origin with sharp line of demarcation from adjoining brain tissue. It is usually surrounded by a zone of oedema.

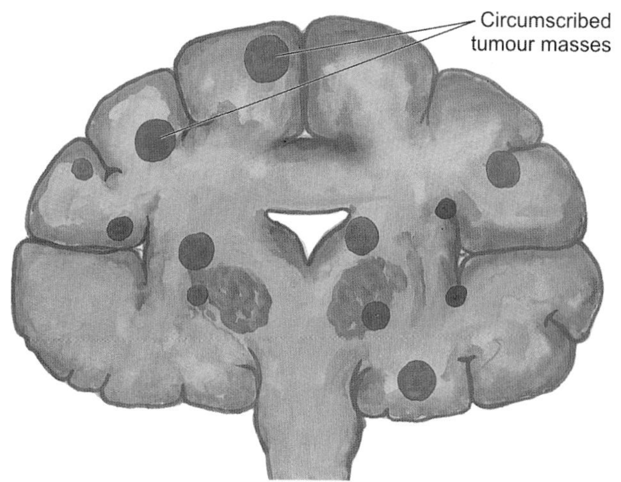

FIGURE 28.12

Metastatic tumour deposits in the brain. They are commonly multiple, well-defined and usually located at the grey and white matter junction.

PERIPHERAL NERVOUS SYSTEM

NORMAL STRUCTURE

The peripheral nervous system (PNS) consists of cranial and spinal nerves, sympathetic and parasympathetic autonomic nervous system and the peripheral ganglia. The PNS is involved in electric transmission of sensory and motor impulses to and from the CNS. A peripheral nerve is surrounded by an outer layer of fibrous tissue, the *epineurium.* Each nerve is made of several fascicles enclosed in multilayered membrane of flattened cells, the *perineurium.* Each fascicle is composed of bundles of connective tissue, the *endoneurium.* There are 2 main types of nerve fibres or axons comprising a peripheral nerve—myelinated and non-myelinated. *Myelinated axons* are thicker (diameter greater than 2 μm) and are surrounded by a chain of Schwann cells which produce myelin sheath. *Non-myelinated axons* have diameter of 0.2-3 μm and about ten non-myelinated fibres may be enclosed by a Schwann cell. *Nodes of Ranvier* on myelinated fibres are the boundaries between each Schwann cell surrounding the fibre (Fig. 28.13,A). Myelinated axons have their origin from neurons in the posterior root ganglia and the anterior horn cell of the spinal cord, whereas non-myelinated axons arise from neurons in the posterior root ganglia and in the autonomic ganglia.

PATHOLOGIC REACTIONS TO INJURY

The peripheral nerves, unlike brain, have regenerative capacity as has been discussed on page 179. The pathologic reactions of the PNS in response to injury may be in the form of one of the types of degenerations causing *peripheral neuropathy* or formation of a *traumatic neuroma.* There are 3 main types of degenerative processes in the PNS—Wallerian degeneration, axonal degeneration and segmental demyelination.

WALLERIAN DEGENERATION. Wallerian degeneration occurs after transection of the axon which may be as a result of knife wounds, compression, traction and ischaemia. Following transection, initially there is accumulation of organelles in the proximal and distal ends of the transection sites. Subsequently, the axon and myelin sheath distal to the transection site undergo disintegration upto the next node of Ranvier, followed by phagocytosis (Fig. 28.13,B). The process of regeneration occurs by sprouting of axons and proliferation of Schwann cells from the proximal end.

AXONAL DEGENERATION. In axonal degeneration, degeneration of the axon begins at the peripheral terminal and proceeds backward towards the nerve cell

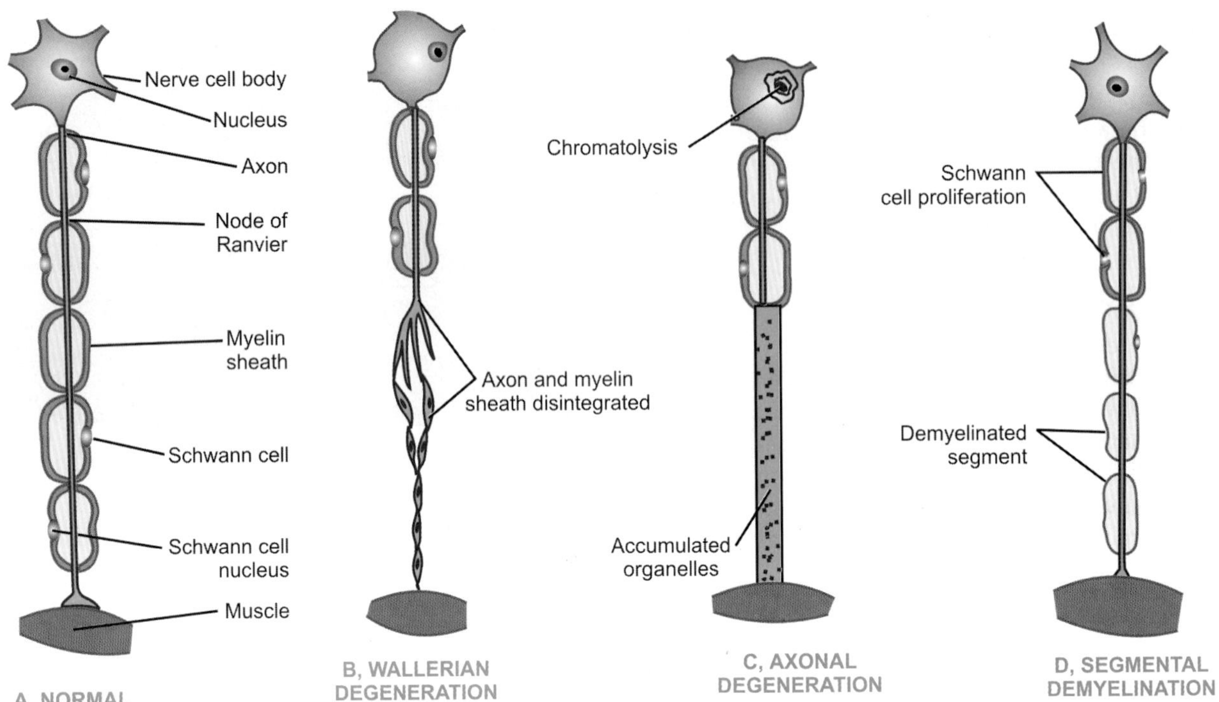

FIGURE 28.13

Pathologic reaction of peripheral nerve to injury.

body (Fig. 28.13,C). The cell body often undergoes chromatolysis. There is Schwann cell proliferation in the region of axonal degeneration. The loss of axonal integrity occurs, probably as a result of some primary metabolic disturbance within the axon itself. Changes similar to those seen in Wallerian degeneration are present but regenerative reaction is limited or absent.

SEGMENTAL DEMYELINATION. Segmental demyelination is similar to demyelination within the brain (page 909). Segmental demyelination is demyelination of the segment between two consecutive nodes of Ranvier, leaving a denuded axon segment. The axon, however, remains intact. Schwann cell proliferation generally accompanies demyelination (Fig. 28.13,D). This results in remyelination of the affected axon. Repeated episodes of demyelination and remyelination are associated with concentric proliferation of Schwann cells around axons producing *'onion bulbs'* found in hypertrophic neuropathy.

TRAUMATIC NEUROMA. Normally, the injured axon of a peripheral nerve regenerates at the rate of approximately 1 mm per day. However, if the process of regeneration is hampered due to an interposed haematoma or fibrous scar, the axonal sprouts together with Schwann cells and fibroblasts form a peripheral mass called as traumatic or stump neuroma.

PERIPHERAL NEUROPATHY

Peripheral neuropathy is the term used for disorders of the peripheral nerves of any cause. It may be polyneuropathy, mononeuropathy multiplex, and mononeuropathy.

■ **Polyneuropathy** is characteristically symmetrical with noticeable sensory features such as tingling, pricking, burning sensation or dysaesthesia in feet and toes. Motor features in the form of muscle weakness and loss of tendon reflexes may be present. Involvement of the autonomic nervous system may be associated. Most cases have origin in acquired metabolic and toxic causes such as thiamine deficiency, diabetes, amyloidosis, autoimmune demyelinating disease (Guillain-Barré syndrome), and administration of toxins and certain therapeutic agents (e.g. vincristine, isoniazid). Besides these, a number of hereditary polyneuropathies are described.

Pathologically, polyneuropathy may be the result of axonal degeneration (axonopathy) or segmental demyelination (demyelinating polyneuropathy). In each type, acute, subacute and chronic forms are distinguished. *Guillain-Barré syndrome* is the classical example of acute demyelinating polyneuropathy which has probably an autoimmune etiology.

■ **Mononeuropathy multiplex or multifocal neuropathy** is defined as simultaneous or sequential multifocal involvement of nerve trunks which are not in continuity. The involvement may be partial or complete and may evolve over days or years. Multifocal neuropathy represents part of spectrum of chronic acquired demyelinating neuropathy.

■ **Mononeuropathy,** on the other hand, is focal involvement of a single nerve. It is generally the result of local causes such as direct trauma, compression and entrapment.

NERVE SHEATH TUMOURS

Tumours of the peripheral nerves are commonly benign and include schwannoma (neurilemmoma) and neurofibroma. Both of them arise from Schwann cells but neurofibroma contains large amount of collagen. Rarely, their malignant counterpart, malignant peripheral nerve sheath tumour, develops particularly in patients with von Recklinghausen's neurofibromatosis.

Schwannoma (Neurilemmoma)

Schwannomas or neurilemmomas arise from cranial and spinal nerve roots. An *acoustic schwannoma* or *acoustic neuroma* is an intracranial schwannoma located within the internal auditory canal originating from vestibular portion of the acoustic nerve (page 487). *Intraspinal schwannomas* are found as intradural tumours in the thoracic region. In the peripheral nerves, they occur as solitary nodule on any sheathed sensory, motor, or autonomic nerve. Multiple schwannomas are uncommon and occur in von Recklinghausen's disease (see below). Schwannomas are tumours of adults except in von Recklinghausen's disease.

PATHOLOGIC CHANGES. ***Grossly,*** a schwannoma is an encapsulated, solid, sometimes cystic, tumour that produces eccentric enlargement of the nerve root from where it arises.

Microscopically, the tumour is composed of fibrocellular bundles forming whorled pattern. There are areas of dense and compact cellularity *(Antoni A pattern)* alternating with loose acellular areas *(Antoni B pattern)*. Areas of Antoni A pattern show palisaded nuclei called *Verocay bodies* (Fig. 28.14). Nerve fibres are usually found stretched over the capsule but not within the tumour. Areas of degeneration contain haemosiderin and lipid-laden macrophages (COLOUR PLATE XXXIV: CL 136). Schwann cells characteristically express S-100 protein. A schwannoma rarely ever becomes malignant.

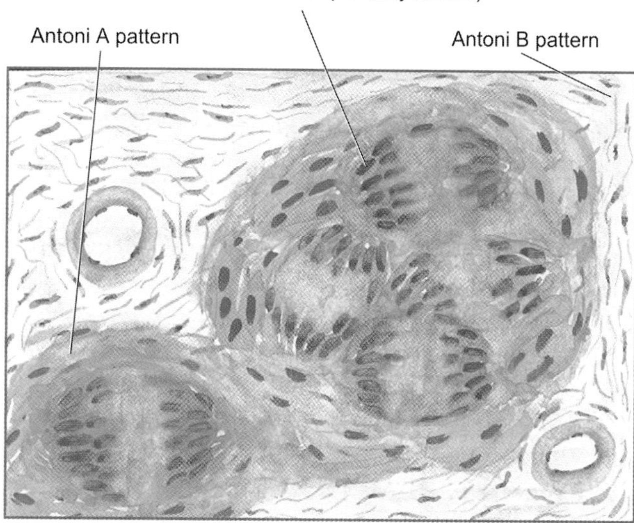

FIGURE 28.14

Schwannoma (neurilemmoma), showing whorls of densely cellular (Antoni A) and loosely cellular (Antoni B) areas with characteristic nuclear palisading (Verocay bodies).

Neurofibroma and von Recklinghausen's Disease

Neurofibromas may occur as solitary, fusiform cutaneous tumour of a single nerve, but more often are multiple associated with von Recklinghausen's disease. Solitary neurofibroma is a tumour of adults but multiple neurofibromas or neurofibromatosis is a hereditary disorder with autosomal dominant inheritance. Solitary neurofibroma is generally asymptomatic but patients with von Recklinghausen's disease have a triad of features:

■ multiple cutaneous neurofibromas

■ numerous pigmented skin lesions (*'cafe au lait'* spots); and

■ pigmented iris hamartomas.

Neurofibromatosis type 1 is a genetic disorder having mutation in chromosome 17 while type 2 has mutation in chromosome 22.

PATHOLOGIC CHANGES. ***Grossly,*** neurofibroma is an unencapsulated tumour producing fusiform enlargement of the affected nerve. Neurofibromatosis in von Recklinghausen's disease is characterised by numerous nodules of varying size, seen along the small cutaneous nerves but may also be found in visceral branches of sympathetic nerves. Neurofibromatosis may involve a group of nerves or may occur as multiple, oval and irregular swellings along the length of a nerve (plexiform neurofibroma).

Microscopically, a neurofibroma is composed of bundles and interlacing fascicles of delicate and elongated spindle-shaped cells having wavy nuclei. The cellular area is separated by loose collagen and mucoid material. Residual nerve fibres (neurites) may be demonstrable (Fig. 28.15). Histologic appearance of Antoni B pattern of schwannoma may be seen in neurofibroma and cause diagnostic difficulty. Immunohistochemically, neurofibroma is positive for epithelial membrane antigen (EMA) and some tumours express S-100 protein as schwannomas do.

Neurofibromas have tendency for local recurrences after excision. Neurilemmoma virtually never turns malignant, while sarcomatous transformation in neurofibroma, particularly in neurofibromatosis, is not unusual. It is estimated that about 3% of patients with von Recklinghausen's neurofibromatosis develop malignant transformation of one of the nodules. Rarely, neurogenic sarcoma may develop spontaneously in the absence of pre-existing von Recklinghausen's disease.

The contrasting features to distinguish neurofibroma from schwannoma are listed in Table 28.5.

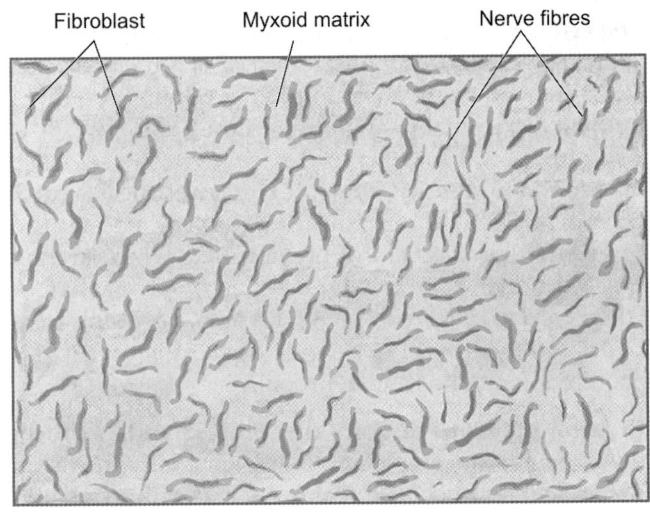

FIGURE 28.15

Neurofibroma, showing interlacing bundles of spindle-shaped cells separated by mucoid matrix. The cells have wavy nuclei and a residual nerve fibre (neurite) is also identified.

Malignant Peripheral Nerve Sheath Tumour

Malignant peripheral nerve sheath tumour (MPNST) is a poorly differentiated spindle cell sarcoma of the peripheral nerves occurring most often in adults. The tumour may arise *de novo* or from malignant transformation of a pre-existing neurofibroma than a schwannoma, generally at an early age (20-40 years). About 50% of the tumours are seen in patients with neurofibromatosis type 1, while some develop at sites of previous irradiation.

TABLE 28.5: Contrasting Features of Neurilemmoma (Schwannoma) and Neurofibroma.

FEATURE	NEURILEMMOMA	NEUROFIBROMA
1. *Location*	Cerebellopontine angle (vestibular branch of 8th nerve); extradural sites	Dermis; along the nerve trunk
2. *Number*	Generally solitary	Solitary or multiple neurofibromatosis
3. *Genetics*	Bilateral in association with type 2 neurofibromatosis having autosomal dominant inheritance (chromosome 22 disorder)	Multiple associated with type 1 neurofibromatosis having autosomal dominant inheritance (chromosome 17 disorder)
4. *Gross appearance*	Firm, encapsulated, c/s tan, translucent	Soft, well demarcated but unencapsulated, c/s mucoid, translucent
5. *Microscopy*	Compact areas (Antoni A) and myxomatous areas (Antoni B), palisading tumour cells (Verocay bodies)	Dense collagen fibres and abundant extracellular mucoid material
6. *Infiltration*	Encapsulated along the edge of nerve without invading it	May infiltrate the peripheral nerve
7. *Immunohistochemistry*	S-100 protein	EMA; sometimes S-100 protein
8. *Behaviour*	Invariably benign	May turn malignant

PATHOLOGIC CHANGES. Grossly, the tumour appears as an unencapsulated fusiform enlargement of a nerve.

Microscopically, the tumour has the appearance of a fibrosarcoma. The tumour has frequent mitosis and areas of necrosis. *Triton tumour* is the name use for MPNST which has areas of poorly-differentiated rhabdomyosarcoma, cartilage and bone.

Local recurrence and haematogenous metastasis are common with this tumour.

Diagnostic Cytopathology

29

Rohit Sharma, MD*, *Amanjit*, MD,DNB**

INTRODUCTION

As mentioned in the beginning of this book, diagnostic surgical pathology developed as a branch around the turn of 19th Century. Its basis was application of knowledge of morphological details of cells for diagnosis of disease in biopsy material. This generated interest by workers towards obtaining cellular material by non-biopsy techniques to arrive at the diagnosis. As a result, cytopathologic diagnosis was initially introduced purely as *Exfoliative Cytology* in the 1920s by Dr. George N. Papanicolaou. Subsequently, *Aspiration Biopsy* was introduced in the 1930s, and evolved over the next three decades (mainly in Europe) to become the mainstay branch of diagnostic cytology known as *Interventional Cytology.*

In general, diagnostic cytology pertains to the interpretation of cells from the human body that either exfoliate (desquamate) spontaneously from epithelial surfaces, or are obtained from various organs/tissues by different clinical procedures. While histopathologic diagnosis is based on interpretation of changes in tissue architecture, the cytopathologic diagnosis rests upon alterations in morphology observed in single cells or groups of cells.

Role of Diagnostic Cytology

Among the numerous applications of cytodiagnostic techniques, the following are more important:

1. Diagnosis and management of cancer. In the field of oncology, establishing a 'tissue diagnosis' (i.e. pathologic diagnosis based on microscopic evidence of malignancy) is an essential pre-requisite for proper management of a cancer patient.

i) Cytodiagnosis in its traditional role is a *valuable adjunct* to histopathology for establishing the vital tissue diagnosis e.g. diagnosis of lymphomas where imprint smears prove valuable, and in some respects superior to histopathology in typing the lymphoma.

ii) Cytologic techniques also provide a *preliminary diagnosis* of cancer for later confirmation by histopathology e.g. detection of ovarian cancer cells in ascitic fluid.

iii) In some fields, cytodiagnosis has replaced histopathology as the *primary source/method* of establishing a tissue diagnosis e.g. in breast cancer, where positive cytologic report is considered sufficient for planning the management, obviating the need for diagnostic surgical biopsy.

iv) Cytodiagnosis has a major role in the detection and diagnosis of clinically silent *early cancer* e.g. carcinoma *in situ* of the uterine cervix.

v) In the management of cancer, cytodiagnosis may help in assessing *response to therapy* e.g. cervical smears for response to radiotherapy in carcinoma cervix, and urinary cytology for response to chemotherapy in carcinoma of the urinary bladder.

vi) In the *follow-up* of previously diagnosed/known cases of cancer, it is of particular value in detecting dissemination (metastatic spread) or recurrence of tumour.

2. Identification of benign neoplasms. This application is derived from its ability to distinguish between

*Senior Consultant Cytopathology, Apollo Hospital, Colombo (Sri Lanka)

**Senior Lecturer, Department of Pathology, Government Medical College, Chandigarh-160030 India benign and malignant neoplasms e.g. fibroadenoma of the breast *versus* carcinoma.

3. Intraoperative pathologic diagnosis. In this role, cytodiagnosis complements histopathologic diagnosis e.g. imprint smears alongwith frozen section for breast lumps.

4. Diagnosis of non-neoplastic/inflammatory conditions. Cytodiagnosis allows recognition of specific conditions which do not routinely require surgical intervention e.g. Hashimoto's thyroiditis.

5. Diagnosis of specific infections. A variety of bacterial, viral, protozoal and fungal infections can be identified by cytologic methods e.g. tubercle bacilli in lymph node aspirates, herpetic inclusions and *Trichomonas* in cervico-vaginal smears, fungal hyphae in touch preparations from draining sinuses.

6. Cytogenetics. Cytodiagnostic techniques can be employed for chromosomal studies including leucocyte and tissue cultures and for demonstrating sex-chromatin e.g. buccal smear for Barr body.

7. Assessment of hormonal status in women. Vaginal smears accurately reflect changes in female sex hormonal levels e.g. to confirm the onset of menopause.

8. Identification of tissues/cells. For example, identification of spermatogenic elements in aspirates from the testes in cases of male infertility.

For cytomorphological *recognition of cancer, nuclear characteristics* are used to determine the presence or absence of malignancy (Table 29.1). *Cytoplasmic characteristics* help in *typing the malignancy* e.g.keratinisation in squamous cell carcinoma, mucin droplets in adenocarcinoma, melanin pigment in melanomas.

TABLE 29.1: Nuclear Criteria of Malignancy.

1. *Nuclear size*	:	Usually larger than benign nuclei; variation in size (anisonucleosis) more significant.
2. *Nucleus-cytoplasmic (N:C) ratio*	:	Increased.
3. *Nuclear shape*	:	Moderate to marked variation.
4. *Nuclear membrane*	:	Irregular thickening, angulation and indentations.
5. *Nuclear chromatin*	:	Hyperchromatic (less significant), uneven distribution, coarse irregular angulated chromatin clumping, parachromatin clearing (more significant).
6. *Nucleoli*	:	Increased size and number less significant; irregular angular outlines more significant.
7. *Number of nuclei*	:	Multinucleation unreliable; nuclear character more important.
8. *Mitoses*		Increased mitoses unreliable; abnormal mitoses significant.

Branches of Diagnostic Cytology

Two branches of diagnostic cytology are currently recognised: exfoliative and interventional.

EXFOLIATIVE CYTOLOGY. This is the older branch that essentially involves the study of cells spontaneously shed off (as a result of continuous growth of epithelial linings) from epithelial surfaces into body cavities or body fluids. Exfoliative cytology is facilitated by the fact that the rate of exfoliation is enhanced in disease-states thereby yielding a larger number of cells for study. In addition, cells for study may also be obtained by scraping, brushing, or washing various mucosal surfaces (abrasive cytology).

INTERVENTIONAL CYTOLOGY. This is the branch in which samples are obtained by clinical procedures or surgical intervention. It is dominated by, and is virtually synonymous with, Fine Needle Aspiration Cytology (FNAC) which is also known as Aspiration Biopsy Cytology (ABC). In interventional cytology, the cytopathologist often performs the clinical procedure himself and interacts with the patient in contrast to exfoliative cytology where the samples are prepared/ forwarded by the clinician and the cytopathologist interprets them in isolation.

Contrasting features and differences between exfoliative and interventional cytology are presented in Table 29.2.

EXFOLIATIVE CYTOLOGY

Type of samples that can be obtained from different organ systems for exfoliative cytodiagnosis are listed in Table 29.3. Apparently, a comprehensive review of each type of sample is beyond the scope of this text. Cytology of female genital tract is discussed in detail below while brief mention is made about other samples.

I. FEMALE GENITAL TRACT

Samples (smears) from the female genital tract have traditionally been known as 'Pap smears'. These smears may be prepared by different methods depending upon the purpose for which they are intended:

i) *Lateral vaginal smears (LVS)* obtained by scraping the upper third of the lateral walls of the vagina are ideal for cytohormonal assessment.

TABLE 29.2: Differences between Exfoliative and Interventional Cytology.

FEATURE	EXFOLIATIVE CYTOLOGY	INTERVENTIONAL CYTOLOGY
1. *Cell samples*	Exfoliated from epithelial surfaces	Obtained by intervention/aspiration
2. *Smears*	Require screening to locate suitable cells for study	Abundance of cells for study in most smears
3. *Diagnostic basis*	Individual cell morphology	Cell patterns and morphology of groups of cells
4. *Morphologic criteria of diagnostic significance*	Nuclear characteristics most important	Nuclear characteristics important; cytoplasmic character and background equally significant

ii) *Vaginal 'pool' or 'vault' smears* are obtained by scraping or aspirating material from the posterior fornix of the vagina and are recommended for detection of endometrial and ovarian cancer.

iii) *Cervical smears* obtained by cotton swabs or Ayre's spatula from the portio of the cervix are ideal for detection of cervical carcinoma.

iv) *Combined (Fast) smears* are a combination of vaginal pool and cervical scrapings. They offer the advantages of both and are recommended for routine population screening as they allow detection of up to 97% of cervical cancers and about 90% of endometrial cancers when properly prepared.

v) *Triple smears (cervical-vaginal-endocervical or CVE)* contain three distinct samples representing the ectocervix, vagina and endocervix on three separate areas of the same slide. These smears are also recommended for routine screening as they allow localisation of lesions but are difficult to prepare.

vi) *Endocervical and endometrial smears* may also be prepared by aspirating the contents of the endocervical canal and endometrial cavity respectively.

TABLE 29.3: Types of Samples for Exfoliative Cytology: Obtainable from Different Organ Systems/Body Sites.

1. *Female genital tract*	— Lateral vaginal smears (LVS) — Vaginal 'pool' smears — Cervical smears — Combined (fast) smears — Triple smears (CVE) — Endocervical/Endometrial aspiration
2. *Respiratory tract*	— Sputum — Bronchial washings/brushing/ bronchio-alveolar lavage (BAL)
3. *Gastrointestinal tract*	— Endoscopic lavage/brushing
4. *Urinary tract*	— Urinary sediment — Bladder washings — Retrograde catheterisation — Prostatic massage (secretions)
5. *Body fluids*	— Effusions — Fluids of small volume i. Cerebrospinal fluid (CSF) ii. Synovial fluid iii. Amniotic fluid iv. Hydrocele fluid v. Seminal fluid (semen) vi. Nipple discharge
6. *Other samples*	— Buccal smears (for sex chromatin)

CELLS IN NORMAL COMBINED SMEARS. Normally, combined smear contains two types of cells: epithelial and others (Fig. 29.1):

Epithelial cells: There are 4 types of squamous epithelial cells in the cervical smear: *superficial, intermediate, parabasal and basal cells.* Morphological features of these cells are summed up in Table 29.4. A few variants of morphological forms and other epithelial cells are as under:

- *Navicular cells* are boat-shaped intermediate cells with folded cell borders. These cells appear in latter half of the menstrual cycle, during pregnancy and menopause.
- *Lactation cells* are parabasal cells with strongly acidophilic cytoplasm. These cells are seen so long as lactation persists.
- *Endocervical cells* appear either as single dispersed nuclei due to degeneration, or as clusters of columnar cells giving it honey-combed appearance. Nuclei of endocervical cells are vesicular, with fine granular chromatin and contain 1-2 nucleoli, while the cytoplasm is slightly basophilic or vacuolated.
- *Endometrial cells* are seen upto 12th day of menstrual cycle. They are slightly smaller than endocervical cells, appear as tight rounded clusters of overlapping cells with moderately dark oval nuclei and scanty basophilic, vacuolated cytoplasm.
- *Trophoblastic cells* are seen following abortion or after delivery.

Other cells: Besides epithelial cells, other cells in cervical smears are leucocytes and Döderlein bacilli.

- *Leucocytes* in cervical smear include polymorphonuclear neutrophils (in large numbers normally),

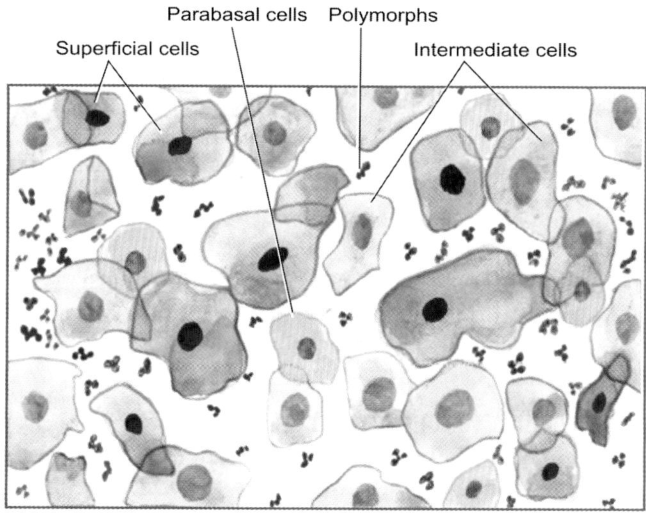

FIGURE 29.1

Various types of cells seen in Pap smear.

lymphocytes (isolated and entrapped in mucus normally), plasma cells (in chronic cervicitis), macrophages (normally in first 10 days of the menstrual cycle) and multinucleate cells (in specific inflammation).

- *Döderlein bacilli (Bacillus vaginalis/Lactobacillus acidophilis)*, which belong to the group of lactobacilli, are the predominant organisms of the normal vaginal flora. It is a slender, gram-positive, rod-like, organism staining pale blue with the Papanicolaou technique. These organisms utilise the glycogen contained in the cytoplasm of intermediate and parabasal cells resulting in their disintegration (cytolysis). They are most numerous in the luteal phase and during pregnancy.

APPLICATIONS OF PAP SMEAR

Cytohormonal Evaluation

Assessment of hormonal status is best carried out from lateral vaginal smears although vaginal 'pool' or fast smears may also be used. Ideally, at least 3 smears obtained on alternate days should be scrutinised and cytologic indices determined for each smear for accurate assessment.

Several indices are available for description of cytohormonal patterns. The most commonly used are as under:

i) *Acidophilic index (AI):* The relative proportion of cells containing acidophilic (pink) and basophilic (blue) cytoplasm are determined by AI.

ii) *Pyknotic index (PI):* The percentage of cells having small, dark, shrunken nuclei (less than 6 μm in size) is determined by PI. The PI is more reliable than AI as it is not influenced by many of the cytoplasmic artefacts e.g. acidophilia caused by drying of smears prior to fixation that affects the latter.

iii) *Maturation index (MI):* MI is the most widely used method. One hundred squamous cells are counted and grouped according to their type—parabasal, intermediate, or superficial (basal cells are virtually absent from normal vaginal smears). Their proportions are expressed as a percentage; for example 10/80/10 represents parabasal, intermediate and superficial cells respectively. Some representative MIs at different stages of life are listed in Table 29.5.

Abnormal Combined Smears

In order to evolve a system acceptable to clinicians and cytopathologists, National Cancer Institute Workshop

TABLE 29.4: Squamous Epithelial Cells Found in Normal Combined (Fast) Smears.

CELL TYPE	SIZE	NUCLEI	CYTOPLASM	MORPHOLOGY
Superficial	30-60 μm	< 6 μm dark, pyknotic	Polyhedral, thin, broad, acidophilic or cyanophilic with keratohyaline granules.	
Intermediate	20-40 μm	6-9 μm vesicular	Polyhedral or elongated, thin, cyanophilic with folded edges.	
Parabasal	15-25 μm	6-11 μm vesicular	Round to oval, thick, well-defined, basophilic with occasional small vacuoles.	
Basal	13-20 μm	Large, (> one-half of cell volume), hyperchromatic, may have small nucleoli	Round to oval, deeply basophilic.	

in 1988 developed *The Bethesda System* for uniformity in evaluation as well as limitations of reporting in cervicovaginal cytopathology; this was subsequently modified in 1991 and further updated in 2001. Mention has already been made about criteria adopted in the Bethesda system in Chapter 22 (page 754). Briefly, it has three basic components:

1. **Specimen adequacy:** It is an important component of quality assurance and provides feedback regarding sampling technique. It implies properly labelled, adequately fixed smears having sufficient number of evenly spread, well preserved cells on microscopic evaluation.

2. **General categorisation:** It includes categorising the smear in one of the three broad categories: within normal limits, benign cellular changes, and epithelial cell abnormalities.

3. **Descriptive diagnosis:** Final aspect of the Bethesda system includes detailed description of the benign cellular changes or epithelial cell abnormalities in the smear.

Based on it, the cellular changes in cervical smears are discussed below under 2 headings: benign (non-neoplastic) cellular changes and epithelial cell abnormalities.

BENIGN CELLULAR CHANGES (NON-NEOPLASTIC):

i) NON-SPECIFIC INFLAMMATORY CHANGES. Inflammatory changes not associated with any specific infection/identifiable infectious agent (i.e. non-specific inflammation) are commonly seen in smears of the female genital tract (COLOUR PLATE XXXV: CL 137).

TABLE 29.5: Representative Maturation Indices at Different Stage of Life.

STAGE	MATURATION INDEX* (%)	COMMENT
Neonatal	0/90/10	As in pregnancy
Infancy	90/10/0	With infections shows midzone shift
Preovulatory	0/40/60	Shift-to-right
Post-ovulatory	0/70/30	Midzone shift
Pregnancy	0/95/5	Midzone shift
Postpartum	90/10/0	Shift-to-left
Menopausal (early)	0/80/10	Estatrophy
Menopausal (late)	95/5/0	Teleatrophy

MI = Parabasal/intermediate/superficial

- *Acute inflammatory changes* are characterised by an increase in the number of parabasal cells (due to disruption of superficial layers of the epithelium resulting in exposure of deeper layers), cytoplasmic acidophilia and vacuolisation, leucocytic migration into cytoplasm, and perinuclear halos with nuclear pyknosis or enlargement.
- *Chronic inflammatory changes (Reactive changes)* manifest in squamous cells as nuclear enlargement, hyperchromatism, and nucleolar prominence, with multinucleation in some instances. Endocervical cells may show reparative hyperplasia and/or squamous metaplasia.

ii) SPECIFIC INFLAMMATORY CHANGES. Specific inflammatory changes may be associated with a variety of infectious agents, the common among which are listed in Table 29.6.

a) *Bacterial agents:*

- *N. gonorrhoeae* (the gonococcus) is a gram-negative diplococcus which is an intracellular micro-organism. It may be observed under oil-immersion within intermediate or parabasal squamous cells and polymorphonuclear leucocytes as tiny paired coffee-bean organisms. However, a definitive diagnosis requires bacterial culture.
- *Gardnerella vaginalis,* a gram-negative rod, is a frequent cause of bacterial vaginitis. It manifests in smears as blue stained cocco-bacillary organism covering and imparting a grainy appearance to affected squamous cells (so called 'clue cells') against a clean background devoid of *Döderlein bacilli.*
- Tuberculosis of the female genital tract usually manifests as tuberculous salpingitis or endometritis, but may involve the uterine cervix. While *Mycobacterium tuberculosis* cannot be identified in Papanicolaou stained smears, tuberculous granulomas composed of epithelioid macrophages with accompanying Langhans' giant cells may occasionally be identified.

b) *Viral agents:*

- Genital infection by *herpes simplex virus (HSV)* commonly affects the squamous epithelium of the vulva, vagina and cervix, but may ascend to involve endocervical and endometrial epithelium. Infected cells show enlarged nuclei with watery, 'ground-glass' chromatin, multinucleation with internuclear moulding, and intranuclear acidophilic inclusions.
- *Human papilloma virus (HPV)* is one of the commonest sexually-transmitted infections. HPV causes wart-like condyloma acuminatum and is also associated with precancerous lesions of ectocervical epithelium. Smears from infected subjects show aggregates of rounded to

TABLE 29.6: Common Infections Detectable on Pap Smears.

Bacterial agents:
Neisseria gonorrhoeae
Gardnerella vaginalis
Mycobacterium tuberculosis

Viral agents:
Herpes simplex virus (HSV)
Human papilloma virus (HPV)

Fungal agents:
Candida albicans
Torulopsis glabrata

Parasitic agents:
Trichomonas vaginalis
Entamoeba histolytica

oval squamous cells with blunted cell margins, peripheral cytoplasmic condensation and crisply outlined perinuclear halos, with dysplastic or degenerative changes of nuclei; these changes are collectively termed 'koilocytotic changes.'

c) *Fungal agents:*

■ Moniliasis (infection by *Candida albicans)* is the commonest fungal infection of the female genital tract and is particularly associated with diabetes, pregnancy and use of antibacterial agents (which alter the vaginal flora). Candida appears in smears in two forms—the *yeast form* (unicellular) appears as round to oval budding organisms with inconspicuous capsules, and the *fungal form* (pseudohyphae) as thin, elongated, pseudoseptate, bamboo-like filaments.

■ *Torulopsis glabrata* causes less than 10% of mycotic vaginal infections. It is related to Candida, appears in smears as round budding organisms with thick capsule-like halos, and does not form pseudohyphae *in vivo.*

d) *Parasitic agents:*

■ Up to 25% of adult women are estimated to harbour *Trichomonas vaginalis* in their lower genital tract. Smears from infected women may not show any cytomorphological changes or may show non-specific acute inflammatory changes. The protozoan appears in the background as a fuzzy, grey-green, round or elliptical structure 8 to 20 µm in size, containing a small vesicular nucleus (COLOUR PLATE XXXV: CL 137 *inbox*).

■ *Entamoeba histolytica* (in trophozoite form) appears in Pap smears as basophilic, round to oval structures, 15 to 20 µm in size, with ingested erythrocytes and a round eccentric nucleus with a central karyosome.

Epithelial Cell Abnormalities—Neoplastic

Carcinoma of the uterine cervix still ranks high in the list as the most frequent cancer in third world countries and is the leading cause of morbidity and mortality. The vast majority of cervical cancers are of the squamous or epidermoid type, and the diagnosis of squamous cell carcinoma of the cervix may be considered the single most important role of exfoliative cytology.

Neoplastic epithelial changes are described below under 2 headings: squamous cell abnormalities and glandular cell abnormalities.

1. SQUAMOUS CELL ABNORMALITIES: The fully-developed invasive squamous cell carcinoma of the uterine cervix is preceded by a pre-invasive intraepithelial neoplastic process that is recognisable on histologic and cytologic examination.

Morphogenesis and nomenclature. The earliest recognisable change is *hyperplasia* of basal or reserve cells which normally constitute a single layer at the deepest part of the epithelium. The proliferating reserve cells next develop certain atypical features i.e. hyperchromasia and increased nuclear size. The continuing proliferation of these atypical cells with loss of polarity, a concomitant increase in mitotic activity, and progressive involvement of more and more layers of the epithelium is known as *dysplasia* (disordered growth). When dysplasia involves the full thickness of the epithelium and the lesion morphologically resembles squamous cell carcinoma without invasion of underlying stroma, it is termed *carcinoma in situ (CIS).* CIS further evolves through the stage of *microinvasive carcinoma* (with depth of stromal invasion not exceeding 3 mm) into full-blown *invasive squamous cell carcinoma* (see Fig. 22.3, page 755).

Previously depending on the degree of epithelial involvement, three grades of dysplasia were recognised: mild, moderate and severe. As the stages of dysplasia and CIS represented a continuous spectrum of lesions seen in the precancerous state, they were collectively termed 'cervical intraepithelial neoplasia' (CIN) and categorised as under:

CIN I	Mild dysplasia	Primitive (atypical) cells proliferating in lower third of epithelium.
CIN II	Moderate dysplasia	Involvement up to middle-third of epithelium.
CIN III	Severe dysplasia	Involvement of upper-third of epithelium.
	Carcinoma *in situ* (CIS)	Involvement of full thickness of epithelium.

Presently, the Bethesda system divides squamous cell abnormalities into four categories:

■ *Atypical squamous cells of undetermined significance (ASCUS)* which represents cellular changes falling short of intraepithelial lesion.

■ *Low-grade squamous intraepithelial lesion (L-SIL)* that includes CIN-I and cellular changes associated with HPV infection.

■ *High-grade squamous intraepithelial lesion (H-SIL)* includes CIN grade II and III as well as CIS.

■ Squamous cell carcinoma.

Cytomorphology. Precancerous states can be distinguished from invasive carcinoma on the basis of cytomorphological features observed in smears (COLOUR PLATE IV: CL 13,14).

In dysplastic epithelium, stratification and maturation of cytoplasm occurs above the layers of proliferating primitive cells. While, nuclear abnormalities persist. Cells exfoliating from the surface, thus, display cytoplasmic maturation and differentiation with nuclear atypia and are known as *dyskaryotic cells.*

The character and type of dyskaryotic cells observed in smears reflect the severity of dysplasia. In mild dysplasia, maturation occurs in the upper two thirds of the epithelium and exfoliated dyskaryotic cells are of the superficial type. With increasing dysplasia, the proliferating primitive cells reach closer to the epithelial surface, less cytoplasmic maturation/differentiation occurs, and dyskaryotic intermediate and parabasal cells are observed in smears. Progression to CIS manifests as subtle alterations in cell arrangement and morphology (with predominantly basal and parabasal cells in smears), while the onset of invasive carcinoma is heralded by the appearance of macronucleoli, cytoplasmic orangeophilia and presence of tumour diathesis (dirty, necrotic background).

2. GLANDULAR CELL ABNORMALITIES. The Bethesda system categorises glandular abnormalities as under:

■ *Atypical glandular cells of undetermined significance(AGUS)* which represent nuclear atypia of endocervical and endometrial cells exceeding repartive changes.

■ *Endocervical* and *endometrial adenocarcinoma*, both of which can be detected from Pap smears. Cytomorphological features allowing distinction between these two types of malignancies are summed up in Table 29.7.

■ Cells from *extrauterine cancers* may also be present in Pap smears, the majority originating from the ovaries. Clues to the extrauterine origin of cancer cells include: the absence of a tumour diathesis, arrangement of cancer cells in glandular and papillary configuration (accompanied by psammoma bodies in some instances), and absence of dysplastic changes in coexistent cervico-endometrial cells.

Automation in Cervical Cytology

Introduction of automated devices like PapNet for primary screening is a major technologic achievement in recent times. Automation offers routine pre-screening of hundreds of Pap smears, decreasing the workload of cytopathologists and at the same time providing quality assurance. It can be applied to conventional Pap smears or *thin-preps* (discussed later).

II. RESPIRATORY TRACT

Cellular material from the respiratory tract may be obtained as a result of spontaneous expectoration (sputum) or by aspiration/brushing during bronchoscopic procedures.

1. SPUTUM EXAMINATION. 'Sputum' is produced by a spontaneous deep cough bringing up material from

TABLE 29.7: Cytomorphological Features of Endocervical and Endometrial Adenocarcinoma.

FEATURE	ENDOCERVICAL CARCINOMA	ENDOMETRIAL CARCINOMA
1. ***Background***	Clean	Dirty, bloody
2. ***Cell yield***	High (found mainly on cervical smears)	Low (found mainly on vaginal smears)
3. ***Cell arrangement***	Clusters or sheets with 'side-by-side' grouping	Three-dimensional 'cell ball' or grape-like clusters
4. ***Cytoplasm***		
i) Amount	Moderate (often in columnar configuration)	Small
ii) Character	Granular, well-stained, often producing mucin	Finely vacuolated, transluscent, with ingested leucocytes
5. ***Nuclei***		
i) Size	Large	Fairly small
ii) Character	Finely granular chromatin (mild hyperchromasia)	Coarse chromatin (marked hyperchromasia)
iii) Nucleoli	Macronucleoli	Micronucleoli

small airways and alveoli. The cough reflex may also be triggered artificially by aerosol-inhalation of cough-stimulating substances (e.g. propylene glycol with hypertonic saline). Sputum examination is advantageous as samples are easily obtained and the cellular content is representative of the entire respiratory tract (satisfactory specimens allow diagnosis of over 80% of lung cancers). However, a large number of cells have to be scrutinised and the specimen does not allow localisation of the lesion within the respiratory tract.

2. BRONCHIAL ASPIRATION (WASHINGS) AND BRONCHIAL BRUSHING. Cellular material obtained by aspiration brushing or bronchio-alveolar lavage (BAL) during bronchoscopy allows localisation of lesions to specific areas of the respiratory tract. Moreover, specimens are easier to study as the cellularity is less than that of sputum. However, bronchoscopic procedures are unpleasant for patients, time-consuming, require considerable expertise, and are unsuitable for routine screening purposes.

III. GASTROINTESTINAL TRACT

Lesions in the oral cavity may be sampled by scraping the surface with wooden and metal tongue-depressors. For the oesophagus and stomach, samples are obtained under direct vision by brushing or lavage through fibreoptic endoscopes. Samples from the stomach may also be obtained by blind lavage through a Ryle's tube using isotonic saline or Ringer's solution. Samples from the colon are obtained by brushing during colonoscopy or lavage following enema to clean the colon.

IV. URINARY TRACT

1. URINARY SEDIMENT CYTOLOGY. Cytological evaluation of the urinary tract is most often carried out by examining the sediment of voided or catheterised specimens of urine. It is convenient for the patient and a useful method for study of both the upper and lower urinary tracts, provided the samples are collected and processed in the correct manner (page 932). While voided specimens are satisfactory in men, catheterisation is often preferred in women to avoid contamination by vaginal cells and menstrual blood.

2. BLADDER IRRIGATION (WASHINGS). Washings of the urinary bladder obtained at cystoscopy are preferred in symptomatic patients when bladder tumours are suspected. The procedure provides excellent cytological preparations but is not suitable for routine screening.

3. RETROGRADE CATHETERISATION. For suspected lesions of the upper urinary tract, voided urine is usually satisfactory. While renal parenchymal cells are infrequent in urine, material obtained from the renal pelvis and ureter contains adequate quantity of these cells. In some instances, retrograde catheterisation and brushing of the ureter and renal pelvis are utilised for localisation of lesions.

4. PROSTATIC MASSAGE. Prostatic secretions are obtained by prostatic massage and the sample is collected directly onto a glass slide and smeared. The procedure is rarely used nowadays with the advent of direct sampling of the prostate by FNAC.

Diagnostic Utility of Urinary Cytology

While evaluating the utility of urinary cytology in the diagnosis of urothelial tumours, some points have to be kept in mind:

1. *Papillary tumours of low-grade* are lined by urothelium showing no morphological abnormalities or only slight cellular and nuclear abnormalities. Such tumours cannot be identified on cytologic material with any degree of certainty.

2. *High-grade papillary tumours,* sessile tumours and carcinoma *in situ* where urothelial cells exhibit cytomorphological abnormalities are readily diagnosed by urinary cytology.

3. Urothelial tumours are often synchronous or metachronous and may involve *different regions of the urinary tract.* Urinary cytology is, thus, of immense value in the follow-up of patients with previously diagnosed urothelial tumours.

V. BODY FLUIDS

The cytology of body fluids can conveniently be discussed under two headings:

A. Effusions in body cavities; and

B. Fluids of small volume.

A. EFFUSIONS

Effusion refers to the accumulation of fluid in any of the three body cavities (pleural, pericardial and peritoneal). An effusion in the peritoneal cavity is also known as ascites. Effusions have traditionally been classed as transudates or exudates. This distinction is important in diagnostic cytology as malignant effusions are invariably exudates with a protein content greater than 3g/dl (page 98).

Diagnostic cytology of effusions (on samples obtained by paracentesis) is mainly related to the identification of malignancy, and wherever possible, its classification (COLOUR PLATE XXXV: CL 138). In benign effusions, cytological findings are mostly non-specific.

B. FLUIDS OF SMALL VOLUME

Of the miscellaneous fluids included in this category, the most common samples submitted for cytological evaluation are cerebrospinal fluid (CSF) and seminal fluid (semen).

Cerebrospinal Fluid (CSF)

CSF examination is an important part of complete neurologic evaluation, both in non-neoplastic and neoplastic diseases of the central nervous system. Samples are usually obtained by lumbar puncture. Factors that are critical to the successful cytological evaluation of CSF are as under:

i) Speed in delivery to the laboratory and immediate processing, as diagnostic material may disintegrate within an hour resulting in false-negative diagnosis.

ii) Correct cytological processing and technique, as the cell yield of CSF is generally low and faulty technique may result in loss of cellular material or poor morphology.

Normal CSF. CSF is an ultrafiltrate of plasma with a total volume of about 150 ml (in the adult). Cell content is low (0-4/μl) comprising mainly lymphocytes or monocytes.

CSF in non-neoplastic diseases. Changes in CSF in various non-neoplastic diseases are presented in Table 29.1 (page 902).

CSF in neoplastic disease. Neoplasms that are in direct contact with the CSF are most likely to shed cells which are recoverable for scrutiny. Metastatic cancers (leukaemia, lymphoma and adenocarcinoma), medulloblastomas, and ependymomas shed the greatest amount of material. Though meningioma occurs in the subarachnoid space, it rarely exfoliates sufficient material for diagnosis. Low-grade gliomas do not generally shed sufficient cells although high-grade gliomas may yield adequate cellular material for diagnosis.

2. Seminal Fluid (Semen)

Examination of seminal fluid (semen analysis) is one of the tests for investigating infertile couples, and is also used to check the adequacy of vasectomy. Samples are obtained by masturbation or coitus interruptus after at least 4 days of sexual abstinence and assessed on the following lines:

1. **Volume.** Normal volume is between 2.5 and 5 ml.

2. **Viscosity and pH.** When ejaculated, semen is fairly viscid but liquefies in about 10 to 30 minutes. It is usually alkaline (pH about 8).

3. **Motility.** Normally, within 2 hours of ejaculation at least 60% of the spermatozoa are vigorously motile; in 6 to 8 hours 25 to 40% are still motile.

4. **Count.** Counting is done in a Neubauer chamber after suitable dilution. Normally, 60 million or more spermatozoa are present per ml.

5. **Morphology.** Stained smears are used to assess morphology. Normally, not more than 20% of spermatozoa are morphologically abnormal (e.g. double-head, pointed-head, or swollen).

6. **Fructose.** Seminal fructose estimation (normal levels 150-600 mg/dl) complements cytological analysis. Low levels of seminal fructose indicate obstruction at the level of ejaculatory ducts.

Results of semen analysis need to be interpreted with caution as infertility is caused by several factors in the couple. Other causes of infertility need to be evaluated before it is ascribed to abnormalities in semen. Even specimens with several abnormal features need not necessarily be the cause of infertility.

VI. BUCCAL SMEARS FOR SEX CHROMATIN BODIES

Sex-specific chromatin bodies are observed in interphase nuclei and comprise the Barr body (X chromatin) and the fluorescent or F body (Y chromatin). The number of Barr bodies observed in interphase nuclei is one less than the number of X chromosome (n–1), whereas the number of F bodies observed is equal to the number of Y chromosomes present (n). In effect, the Barr body is specific for females and the F body for males (page 264).

1. DEMONSTRATION OF THE BARR BODY (X CHROMATIN). In buccal smears, the Barr body appears as a plano-convex mass about 1 μm in diameter applied to the inner surface of the nuclear membrane. The interphase nuclei of one hundred intermediate squamous epithelial cells are scrutinised. In normal females, Barr bodies are present in at least 20% of nuclei. Males have a Barr body count of less than 2%. Vaginal smears may also be used for Barr body counts (page 264).

2. DEMONSTRATION OF THE F BODY (Y CHROMATIN). Demonstration of the F body requires fluorescent staining in contrast to the Barr body which may be observed on routine Papanicolaou-stained smears. On staining buccal smears with quinacrine mustard, the intensely fluorescent F body is observed in about 60% of interphase nuclei in males and in less than 8% of nuclei in females. The F body is also demonstrable in the nuclei of lymphocytes in a peripheral blood film stained with quinacrine mustard.

3. **COUNTING OF DRUM-STICK APPENDAGE.** The presence and frequency of drum-stick appendages attached to nuclei of polymorphonuclear leucocytes on a peripheral blood film may also be used for determining sex. At least 500 neutrophilic leucocytes are scrutinised in a Romanowsky-stained blood film. Genetic females show drumsticks in 3-6% of neutrophils. In males, the frequency of drumsticks is less than 0.3%.

TECHNIQUES IN EXFOLIATIVE CYTOLOGY

A brief resume of methods for collection of specimens and processing of samples for exfoliative cytodiagnosis is outlined below under 4 headings: collection, fixation and fixatives, processing in the laboratory, and staining.

A. Collection of Samples

1. **PREPARATION OF COMBINED (FAST) SMEARS.** Smears should not be taken during menstrual bleeding. The patient should not douche for at least 24 hours before the smear is obtained.

i) Smears are obtained under *direct vision* after introducing a Cusco's speculum with the patient in lithotomy position.

ii) Ideally, *lubricants* and medical jellies should not be used for introducing the speculum. If required, the speculum may be moistened with a few drops of normal saline (use of lubricants results in contamination of the smear).

iii) The posterior fornix of the vagina is aspirated with a *blunt-ended glass pipette* fitted with a rubber bulb. A drop of the aspirate is placed at the unlabelled end of a glass slide.

iv) The ectocervix is sampled with the *Ayre's spatula* (Fig. 29.2). The longer limb of the spatula is fitted into the external os and the spatula rotated through 360° to sample the entire cervix. The scraped material on the spatula is then placed on the drop aspirated from the vaginal pool and the smear prepared with the spatula itself or with the tip of the gloved finger (cotton swabs may be used instead of the Ayre's spatula, although the quality of smears is not as good).

v) Thin uniform smears should be prepared and the slide immediately *immersed in fixative* to avoid artefacts in cells caused by drying.

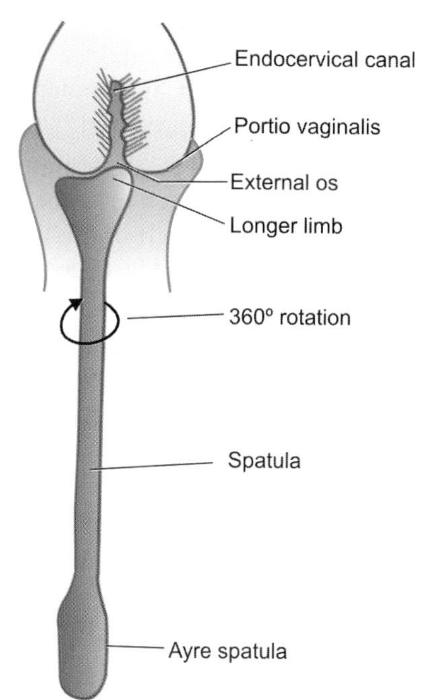

FIGURE 29.2
Method of obtaining cervical material for fast smears.

vi) Smears should be *transported* to the laboratory in the fixative in a Coplin's jar.

Slides should ideally be labelled by using a diamond pencil. If labels of sticking plaster are used, the labels must not come into contact with the fixative.

2. **LIQUID-BASED CYTOLOGY PREPARATIONS (THIN PREPS).** This is a special technique for preparation of gynaecologic and non-gynaecologic samples which provides uniform monolayered dispersion of cells on smears, without overlapping or clump formation. It is a pre-requisite for quantitative analysis and automated devices.

3. **PREPARATION OF LATERAL VAGINAL SMEARS (LVS).** The LVS is obtained by scraping the lateral walls of the upper third of the vagina (at the level of the cervical external os) with the flat surface of a wooden tongue depressor and smearing the material directly onto labelled slides. The patient is prepared and positioned as described for the Fast smear.

4. **COLLECTION OF SPUTUM.** Fresh, unfixed, early morning specimens resulting from overnight accumulation of secretions are best for diagnostic purposes. A minimum of three specimens collected on three successive days should be examined (ideally, five specimens).

The patient is instructed to cough deeply on waking up and to expectorate all sputum into a clean, dry, wide-mouthed glass container or a petridish. Care should be taken to avoid spitting into the container. The container is capped or covered, labelled and transported to the laboratory where smears are prepared.

5. **BRONCHIAL MATERIALS.** All aspirated bronchial secretions, lavage and brushings must be despatched to the laboratory without delay. If immediate despatch is not possible, the sample should be collected in fixative (50% ethanol in volumes equal to that of the sample).

6. **BUCCAL SMEARS.** The mouth is rinsed with water or normal saline and the buccal mucosa scraped vigorously with a wooden or metal tongue depressor. The material is smeared directly onto labelled glass slides which are placed in fixative.

7. **GASTRIC LAVAGE.** The patient is prepared by overnight fasting. Water is allowed up to one hour before the procedure. In patients with pyloric obstruction, the stomach is emptied the evening before and washed repeatedly with normal saline or Ringer's solution till returns are clear.

i) For lavage, the Ryle's tube is passed using glycerin as a lubricant.

ii) Stomach contents are aspirated and discarded.

iii) 500 ml of normal saline or Ringer's solution are instilled and re-aspirated in small portions while the patient is rotated from side-to-side (the stomach may also be massaged).

iv) The lavage fluid is collected in an equal volume of chilled 95% ethanol for despatch to the laboratory (alcohol is chilled to 4°C in a refrigerator).

Chymotrypsin in acetate buffer (pH 5.6) or papain in phosphate buffer (pH 7.3) may be used as lavage fluids. These enzymes dissolve mucus and enhance cell recovery/yields in aspirates.

8. **URINE.** Fresh catheterised specimens are preferred in female patients while voided urine is satisfactory in males.

After initial morning voiding (which is discarded), samples of about 50 to 100 ml are collected on three consecutive days. Hydration by forced intake of fluids (1 glass of water every 30 minutes over 3 hour period) is recommended by some workers for production of high volume specimens. If delay is anticipated in despatch to the laboratory, the sample should be collected in an equal volume of 50% ethanol.

The initial morning specimen is discarded as cells deteriorate extremely quickly in acidic urine, and the morphology of cells accumulating overnight in bladder urine is distorted to an extreme degree. For the same reason, 24-hour collections of urine are useless for cytodiagnostic purposes.

9. **EFFUSIONS.** Pericardial, pleural and peritoneal fluids are obtained by paracentesis. As these fluids are often exudative in character, they may clot after removal from respective cavities. Anticoagulants may be used to prevent coagulation—heparin (3-5 units per ml), 3.8% sodium citrate (1 ml per 10 ml), or EDTA (1 mg per ml) may be used for this purpose.

If the fluids cannot be processed within 12 hours of collection, an equal volume of 50% ethanol or 10% formalin should be added.

10. **CEREBROSPINAL FLUID (CSF).** CSF samples should be despatched without delay to the laboratory for immediate processing as the cells contained are extremely fragile. A gap of even 1 hour between removal and processing may result in loss of diagnostic cellular material.

11. **SEMEN.** Samples of seminal fluid obtained by masturbation are best collected at the laboratory. Samples obtained by coitus interruptus are collected in clean, dry test tubes (or vials) and transported to the laboratory within 30 minutes. The patient is instructed to note the time of ejaculation.

B. Fixation and Fixatives

All material for cytological examination must be properly fixed to ensure preservation of cytomorphological details. Methods of fixation vary depending upon the type of staining employed (e.g. Papanicolaou or Romanowsky staining). Material for exfoliative cytodiagnosis is usually *wet-fixed* (i.e. smears are immersed in fixative without allowing them to dry) for use with the Papanicolaou or haematoxylin and eosin stains. Sometimes, smears are *air-dried* for use with the Romanowsky stains (as used in haematologic studies). In Romanowsky staining, fixation is effected during the staining procedure.

1. **ROUTINE FIXATIVES.** The ideal fixative for routine use is Papanicolaou's fixative comprising a solution of equal parts of ether and 95% ethanol. However, the flammability of ether makes it hazardous. Most laboratories use 95% ethanol alone with excellent results. Where ethanol is not available, 100% methanol, 95% denatured alcohol, or 85% isopropyl alcohol (isopropanolol) may be used.

Smears prepared at the bedside as well as those prepared in the laboratory from fluid samples are immediately placed in 95% ethanol *without allowing them to dry prior to fixation.* Drying causes distortion of cells and induces cytoplasmic staining artefacts. Fixation time of 10 to 15 minutes at room temperature is adequate. (Smears may also be left in the fixative for 24 hours or more without detriment to cytomorphological detail). Smears should be transported to the laboratory in the fixative (screw-capped Coplin jars are best for this purpose).

2. COATING FIXATIVES. Coating fixatives are applied as aerosol-sprays or with a dropper to the surface of freshly prepared smears. While commercial preparations (e.g. cytospray) are available, a standard hairspray with a high alcohol content is also a suitable alternative. Smears while still wet, are placed face-up on a table and sprayed with the nozzle held at a distance of 10 to 12 inches. A period of 10 minutes is sufficient for drying of coated smears, which may then be wrapped or put in a box for transport to the laboratory. Coating fixatives are ideal when unstained smears are to be transported over long distances.

3. SPECIAL PURPOSE FIXATIVES. Buffered neutral formalin, Bouin's fluid and picric acid are used for specific purposes when required. Formalin vapour fixation is also employed for some staining procedures.

4. PRESERVATION OF FLUID SAMPLES. Samples of fluids are best submitted to the laboratory in a fresh state for immediate processing. Where a delay is anticipated in despatch to the laboratory or in processing, the sample is collected in a suitable preservative for 'prefixation' so that cellular morphology is preserved. When the samples have been processed and smears prepared, 'fixation' is effected as described earlier.

Fluid samples with a high protein content (e.g. pericardial, pleural and peritoneal fluids) may be preserved under refrigeration for up to 12 hours without prefixation. However, fluids with a low protein content (e.g. urine and cerebrospinal fluid) deteriorate in 1 to 2 hours even if refrigerated. Fluids with low pH (e.g. gastric lavage samples) must be collected in pre-cooled preservative since cells deteriorate extremely rapidly in such specimens.

The best *preservative for general use* is 50% ethanol in volumes equal to that of the sample. Ninety-five per cent ethanol precipitates proteins and hardens the sediment making smear preparation difficult; it is used only for gastric aspirates. Pericardial, pleural and peritoneal fluids may be pre-fixed with an equal volume of 10% formalin if ethanol is not available. Solutions containing ether and acetone are not used as preservatives as they cause extreme hardening of the sediment making smear preparation virtually impossible.

C. Processing of Samples in the Laboratory

1. PREPARED SMEARS. Smears prepared at the bedside and wet-fixed in ethanol need no further processing in the laboratory prior to staining.

2. SPUTUM. The sample is prepared as under:

i) The sample is placed in a petridish and inspected against a dark background.

ii) Bloody, discoloured or solid particles are removed with wooden applicator sticks and placed on glass slides. Strands of ropy mucus are also selected (exfoliated cells adhere to mucus strands).

iii) Clean glass slides are used to crush the particles/ mucus and spread the material evenly.

iv) Four such smears are prepared and immediately placed in 95% ethanol for fixation.

3. FLUID SPECIMENS. Large volumes of fluid received are allowed to stand in the refrigerator for half to one hour. After that, all except the bottom 200 ml is discarded. The retained fluid is then processed. In specimens containing excessive amounts of blood, erythrocytes may be lysed by the addition of 1 ml of glacial acetic acid for every 50 ml of specimen.

Commonly employed techniques for processing of fluids are as under:

i) Preparation of sediment smears from centrifuged samples.

ii) Cytocentrifuge preparations (cytospin).

iii) Membrane filter preparations.

Sediment smears. The sample is poured into 50 ml centrifuge tubes and centrifuged at 600 g for 10 minutes. (To achieve a relative centrifugal force of 600 g, the speed of the centrifuge in revolutions per minute varies with the rotating radius of the centrifuge. With a rotating radius of 25 cm the required speed is 1500 rpm).

Following centrifugation, the supernatant is decanted and smears prepared from the sediment or cell button by recovering the material with a glass pipette or a platinum wire loop. Smear preparation from samples collected in a preservative require albuminised slides as cell adhesiveness is reduced by prefixation. Smears are wet-fixed in 95% ethanol (or air-dried in some instances).

Cytocentrifuge and membrane filter preparations. These methods are most useful for small volume fluids of low cell content. The interested reader is referred to specialised texts for descriptions of these methods.

D. Staining of Smears

Three staining procedures are commonly employed: Papanicolaou and haematoxylin and eosin (H&E) stains are used for *wet-fixed smears* while Romanowsky stains are used for *air-dried smears.*

1. PAPANICOLAOU STAIN. Papanicolaou staining is the best method for routine cytodiagnostic studies. Three solutions are used comprising a nuclear stain and two cytoplasmic counter-stains. Harris' haematoxylin is the nuclear stain. Orange G (OG-6) and eosin-alcohol (EA-65 or EA-50) are the two cytoplasmic counterstains which impart the orange and cyanophilic tints to cytoplasm respectively.

2. H&E STAIN. The stain is essentially the same as that used for histological sections. Harris' haematoxylin is the nuclear stain, and eosin is the cytoplasmic counter-stain.

3. ROMANOWSKY STAINS. Romanowsky stains used in haematological preparations may also be used for cytological smear preparations. Leishman's, May-Grünwald-Giemsa (MGG) and Wright's stains are most commonly used.

INTERVENTIONAL CYTOLOGY

In interventional cytology, samples are obtained by aspiration or surgical biopsy. This branch includes FNAC, imprint cytology, crush smear cytology and biopsy sediment cytology.

I. FINE NEEDLE ASPIRATION CYTOLOGY

Interventional cytology is virtually synonymous with Fine Needle Aspiration Cytology or FNAC. The technique has gained wide acceptance only over the past three decades and is increasingly being used to sample a wide variety of body tissues. Almost all organ systems are accessible to the fine needle and the versatility of the technique has enormously increased the scope of diagnostic cytology.

Morphological descriptions of various lesions sampled by FNAC are beyond the scope of this work. Interested readers are referred to the specialised texts listed at the end of the book. The applications and advantages of FNAC, its procedure, complications and limitations are detailed below.

A. Applications of FNAC

In routine practice, FNAC is most often used for diagnosis of palpable mass lesions. Palpable lesions commonly sampled are: breast masses (COLOUR PLATE XXXV: CL 139, 140), enlarged lymph nodes (Fig. 29.3,A) (COLOUR PLATE XXXVI: CL 141), enlarged thyroid (Fig. 29.3, B) (COLOUR PLATE XXXVI: CL 142), and superficial soft tissue masses. The salivary glands, palpable abdominal lesions and the testicles are also frequently sampled for FNAC. Other sites/lesions accessible to FNAC are: the prostate, pelvic organs, bone and joint spaces, lungs, retroperitoneum and orbit.

Lymphocytes
Langhans' giant cell
Epithelioid cell granuloma
Caseation necrosis
Polymorphs

A, TUBERCULOUS LYMPHADENITIS (H & E STAIN)

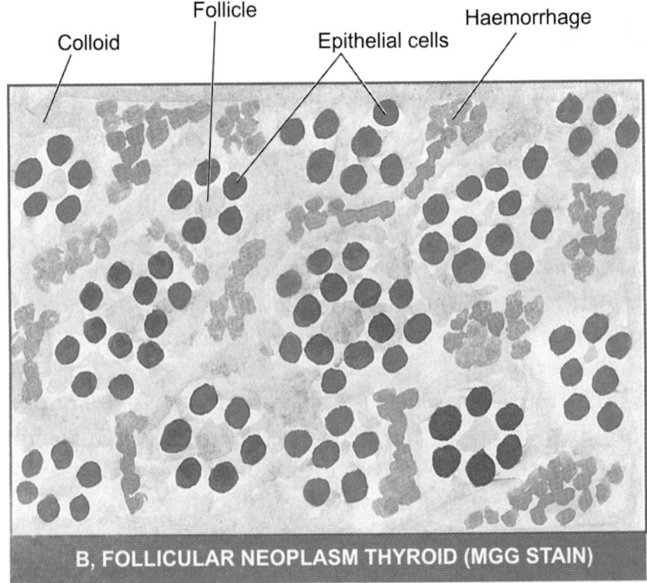

B, FOLLICULAR NEOPLASM THYROID (MGG STAIN)

FIGURE 29.3

Microscopic appearance of FNA in tuberculosis of lymph node (A) and in follicular neoplasm of thyroid (B).

B. Advantages of FNAC

i) FNAC is an office/OPD procedure and *no hospitalisation* is required, while surgical biopsies are obtained in the operation theatre and hospitalisation is often required.

ii) *No anaesthesia* is required (except in specific circumstances), while surgical biopsy is performed under local or general anaesthesia.

iii) The procedure is *quick, safe and painless.*

iv) *Multiple attempts* (or repeating the procedure) are possible without inconvenience, whereas repeating a surgical biospy is uncomfortable and inconvenient for the patient.

v) Results are obtained *rapidly* with reports being available in a matter of hours (2 to 24 hours depending on the urgency), while histopathological reports are available after a longer duration (2 to 4 days on account of time required for processing and sectioning of tissues).

vi) It is a low-cost procedure which is *cost-effective.*

vii) As the cytopathologist performs the procedure himself, he gains *first-hand knowledge* of the clinical findings which facilitates interpretation of slides and enhances diagnostic accuracy.

C. General Procedure for FNAC

1. Materials

For performing FNAC, a syringe with a well-fitting needle, some microscopic glass slides and a suitable fixative are the only material required in most instances (Fig. 29.4).

NEEDLES. Fine needles range from 25 to 20 gauge (0.6 mm to 0.9 mm outer diameter). The standard 21 gauge disposable needle of 38 mm length is suitable for routine transcutaneous FNAC of palpable masses; 25 or 24 gauge disposable needles of 25 mm length are used for lymph nodes and in children. Larger needles, 80 to 160 mm in length, are required for sampling the lung and abdominal viscera; 22 to 20 gauge Chiba spinal puncture needles may be profitably employed for this purpose. Needles of up to 200 mm length are used for transrectal and transvaginal FNAC of the prostate and ovary respectively. Aspiration of bony lesions may require 18 gauge (1 mm outer diameter) needles although superficial lytic lesions are adequately sampled with a 21 gauge needle.

SYRINGES. Syringes of 10 to 20 ml capacity are suitable. Syringe holders (such as the Franzen handle, Fig. 29.4,B) permit a single-hand grip during aspiration, employing disposable syringes. For needles with metal hubs (e.g. spinal puncture needles), disposable syringes should be used to ensure a proper fit between the needle hub and syringe nozzle.

GLASS SLIDES AND FIXATIVE. Four or six standard microscopic glass slides and a Coplin jar containing 95% ethyl alcohol (as a fixative) are the only other equipment required for routine FNAC.

2. Method of Aspiration

Transcutaneous FNAC of palpable masses is routinely performed without anaesthesia as per the following procedure (aspiration of sites/lesions requiring anaesthesia or special technique are discussed separately).

A, FRANZEN HANDLE

B, SYRINGE AND 22G NEEDLE

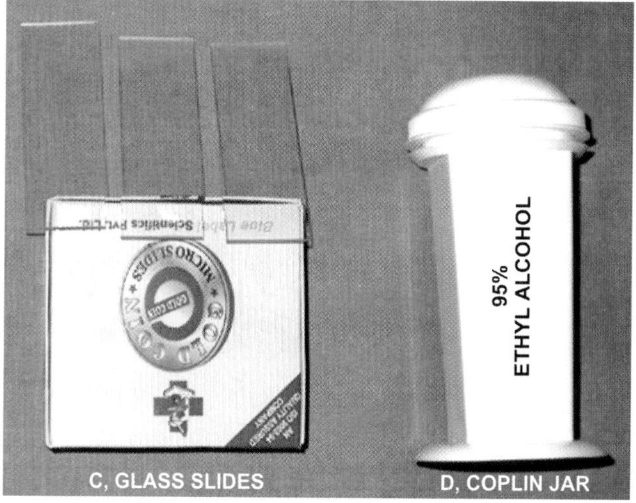

FIGURE 29.4

Equipments required for transcutaneous FNAC.

i) The patient is asked to *lie down* in a position that best exposes the target area.

ii) The target area is thoroughly *palpated* and the firmest portion of the lesion/mass delineated.

iii) The skin is *cleaned* with an alcohol pad.

iv) The mass is *fixed* by the palpating hand of the operator or by an assistant (gloves may be used for the protection of the operator and the assistant).

v) The needle is *inserted* into the target area. On reaching the lesion the plunger of the syringe is retracted and at least 10 ml of suction applied while moving the needle back and forth within the lesion; the direction (angle) of the needle may be changed to access different areas of the lesion (Fig. 29.5).

vi) Aspiration is *terminated* when aspirated material or blood becomes visible at the base/hub of the needle. For diagnostic purposes, cellular material contained within the needle is more than adequate; material drawn into the barrel of the syringe is not recovered since it is of no use for cytologic diagnosis.

vii) On completion of aspiration, suction is *released* and pressure within the syringe allowed to equalise before withdrawing the needle. Withdrawing the needle with negative pressure/suction results in blood being aspirated and cellular material being sucked into the barrel of the syringe, thus lost to interpretation.

viii) Following withdrawal of the needle from the lesion, *pressure* is applied to the site of puncture by the assistant/patient for 2 to 3 minutes in order to arrest bleeding and prevent haematoma formation.

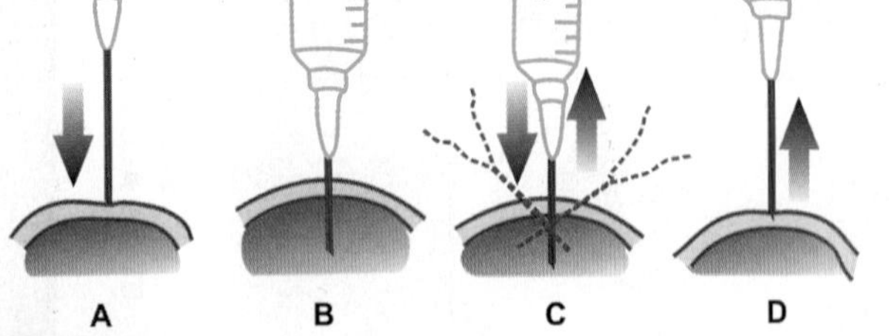

ix) Aspirated material is *recovered* by detaching the needle from the syringe and filling the syringe with air; the syringe and needle are then reconnected and the aspirate expressed onto one end of a glass slide.

FIGURE 29.5

Procedure for FNAC of palpable masses. Needle is introduced into the mass (A). Plunger is retracted after needle enters the mass (B). Suction is maintained while needle is moved back and forth within the mass (C). Suction is released and plunger returned to original position before needle is withdrawn (D).

3. Preparation of Smears

Preparation of smears is crucial to the success of FNAC. Poorly-prepared smears with distorted cellular morphology will frustrate the best efforts of the most competent cytopathologist, and often result in errors of interpretation or in failure to arrive at any specific diagnosis. The procedure consists of the following steps:

i) Aspirates deposited on the slide are *inspected* with the naked eye.

ii) Semisolid particulate aspirates are *crush-smeared* by flat pressure with a glass slide or a thick coverslip (Fig. 29.6,A). Even and gentle pressure is required to avoid traumatising cells. Droplets of fluid or bloody material are gathered under the edge of the angled smearing slide/coverslip (Fig. 29.6,B) and pulled like a blood smear (Fig. 29.6,C). Particulate material, which collects along the edges and at the end of the smear, is then crush-smeared by flattening the smearing slide (Fig. 29.6,D).

iii) Prepared smears are either *wet-fixed* or *air-dried*. Half the number of smears are immediately immersed in 95% ethanol, transported to the laboratory in the fixative, and used for Papanicolaou or haematoxylin and eosin (H&E) staining. The remaining smears are air-dried, wrapped in tissue paper for transport to the laboratory, and stained by Romanowsky stains (Leishman's, May-Grünwald-Giemsa). Most cytopathologists use both wet-fixed and air-dried smears as the former provides excellent nuclear detail while the latter yields information about the cytoplasm and the background. The general properties of wet-fixed and air-dried smears are enumerated in Table 29.8.

4. Special Studies

Aspirates may also be studied by special stains/techniques for specific purposes as under:

i) **SPECIAL STAINS.** Wet-fixed smears are used for a variety of special stains such as Alcian blue, mucicarmine and PAS (for mucin and carbohydrates); methyl violet or congo red (for amyloid); and bacterial/fungal stains (for infectious agents).

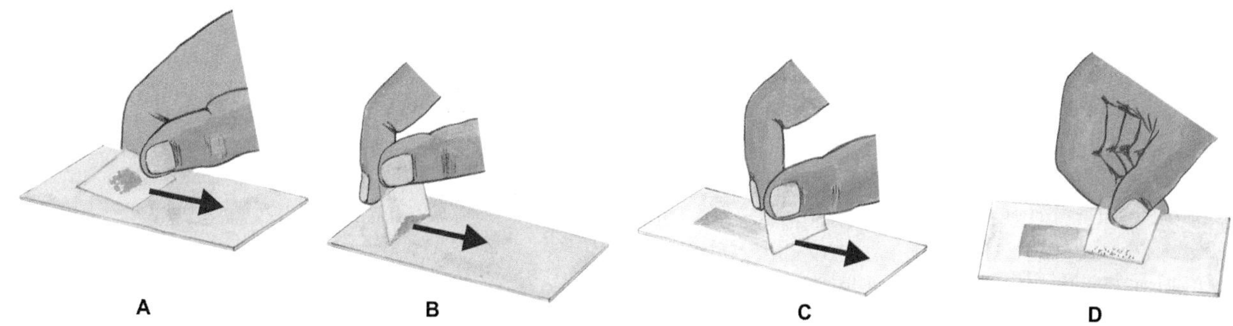

FIGURE 29.6

Preparation of smears. Semisolid aspirates are crush-smeared by flat pressure with cover slip or glass slide (A). Fluid or blood droplet is collected along edge of spreader (B), and pulled as for peripheral blood films (C). Particles at the end of the smear are crush-smeared (D).

ii) MICROBIOLOGICAL STUDIES. Aspirates may also be submitted for viral, fungal, mycobacterial and bacterial culture. When infection is suspected, an additional aspirate is obtained and expressed into a sterile culture tube. If additional aspiration is not feasible, the needle is flushed with sterile isotonic saline or foetal calf serum and the rinsed fluid submitted for microbial culture.

iii) CELL BLOCK. Aspirated material may be processed as surgical pathology material by preparing paraffin blocks from cell button of the centrifuged deposit. Sections provide recognition of histologic patterns and can also be used for ancillary techniques (COLOUR PLATE XXIV: CL 144).

iv) IMMUNOCYTOCHEMICAL STUDIES. The smears or cell block sections can be studied for immunocytochemical stains by employing panel of antibodies selected on the basis of differential diagnosis made after routine morphologic examination of smears (COLOUR PLATE XXIV: CL 144 *inbox*).

v) IMAGE ANALYSIS AND MORPHOMETRY. These techniques when applied to cytological smears bring quantitation and objectivity to cytodiagnosis. They determine the cellular parameters like N/C ratio, nuclear area, shape and size of nuclei and nucleoli etc.

vi) FLOW CYTOMETRY. Determination of ploidy status and S phase fraction of tumour cells using flow cytometry enhances the diagnostic and prognostic information available on routine cytology.

vii) ULTRASTRUCTURAL STUDIES. Aspirates obtained by FNAC are also suitable for electron microscopy (both TEM and SEM).

viii) MOLECULAR BIOLOGIC TECHNIQUES. These techniques are now being widely applied to cytopathology also. Detection of oncogenes like *ERBB-2* in breast cancer and *BCL-2* in lymphomas has been reported in aspiration samples.

5. Aspiration of Specific Lesions/Body Sites

In addition to the general procedure for FNAC described above, aspiration from certain specific sites/lesions require greater expertise and additional material as outlined below.

i) CYSTS. Cysts of the neck, thyroid, breast and other sites are often encountered during FNAC. During

TABLE 29.8: General Properties of Wet-Fixed and Air-Dried Smears.

FEATURE	WET-FIXED	AIR-DRIED
1. *Staining*	Papanicolaou, H&E	Leishman, May-Grünwald-Giemsa
2. *Cell size*	Comparable to tissue sections	Exaggerated
3. *Nuclear detail*	Excellent	Fair
4. *Nucleoli*	Well demonstrated	Not always discernible
5. *Cytoplasmic details*	Poorly demonstrated	Well demonstrated
6. *Stromal components*	Poorly demonstrated	Well demonstrated
7. *Partially necrotic material*	Single intact cells, well defined	Cell details poorly defined

aspiration, the entire fluid content is evacuated by drawing into the syringe and collected in test tube for centrifugation and smear preparation. If a residual mass is palpable after removal of fluid, a fresh syringe is used for additional aspiration of the mass in the usual manner.

ii) THYROID. Lesions of the thyroid are aspirated with the patient either sitting up or lying supine with the neck extended. Solitary nodules are fixed between two palpating fingers, while a diffusely enlarged lobe is fixed by asking the patient to swallow and applying two fingers to the base of the lobe to hold it against the trachea. The patient is asked to avoid swallowing during aspiration. Subsequently, firm pressure is applied to the puncture site for about 3 minutes to prevent haematoma formation (COLOUR PLATE XXXVI: CL 142).

iii) LUNG AND RETROPERITONEUM. FNAC of these two sites is usually carried out under the guidance of radiological imaging techniques. Local anaesthesia (1% xylocaine) is advisable with infiltration of skin and deeper tissues. Spinal puncture needles (22 or 20 gauge) are used. Since these long needles are flexible they are rotated during insertion to enable an accurate approach to the target lesion.

iv) PROSTATE. The prostate is sampled transrectally during per-rectal examination with the patient in lithotomy position. A custom-made or commercially available needle guide (such as the Franzen needle guide) may be used. Alternatively, a 16 gauge blunt-tipped venous cannula may serve as a needle guide. The cannula is taped to the index finger of the gloved hand with its tip just proximal to the pulp of the index-finger, and a fingercot drawn over it. The prostatic lesion is palpated with the pulp of the finger and sampled by puncturing through the finger cot with a long 22 gauge needle introduced through the cannula.

v) TESTIS. Local anaesthesia is advisable when FNAC of the testis is carried out for infertility as pain may be considerable when suction is applied. Spermatic cord block is employed for the purpose. Infiltration of scrotal skin is not required. For suspected testicular tumours, local anaesthesia is not required; however, thinner needles (25 or 24 gauge) are advocated by some workers to avoid seeding of tumour along the needle track.

vi) ABDOMINAL FAT ASPIRATION. FNA of the para-umbilical abdominal adipose tissue is currently accepted method for diagnosis of secondary systemic amyloidosis. Amyloid is demonstrated as rings around fat cells by the conventional Congo red staining (congophilia) and apple-green birefringence when viewed under polarising microscopy (COLOUR PLATE XXIV: CL 143).

6. Radiological Imaging Aids for FNAC

Non-palpable lesions require some form of localisation by radiological aids for FNAC to be carried out. *Plain X-ray films* are usually adequate for lesions within bones and for some lesions within the chest. FNAC of the chest may also be attempted under *image amplified fluoroscopy* which allows visualisation of needle placement on the television monitor. *Computerised tomography (CT scans)* can also be used for lesions within the chest and abdomen. The most versatile radiological aid is *ultrasonography (USG)* which allows direct visualisation of needle placement in real time and is free from radiation hazards. It is an extremely valuable aid for FNAC of thyroid nodules, soft tissue masses, intra-abdominal lesions and for intrathoracic lesions which abut the chest wall, but is of no help in deep intrathoracic lesions or in bony lesions.

D. Complications and Hazards of FNAC

FNAC is associated with relatively few complications. Possible hazards and more commonly encountered complications are as follows:

1. **Haematomas.** Bleeding from the puncture site and haematoma formation are the commonest complications of the procedure, particularly in the breast and the thyroid. Firm finger pressure for 2 to 3 minutes immediately after the procedure greatly reduces the frequency of these complications.

2. **Infection.** Introduction of infection is not a significant hazard; even trans-abdominal aspiration does not result in peritoneal contamination despite puncture of bowel walls. Transrectal aspiration in cases of acute prostatitis may, however, result in bacteraemia and septicaemia.

3. **Pneumothorax.** Transcutaneous aspiration of the lung causes pneumothorax in about 20% of cases; most resolve spontaneously although intercostal intubation may be required in some instances. Transient haemoptysis may also be associated with lung aspiration.

4. **Dissemination of tumour.** Generalised dissemination of malignant cells via lymphatics and blood vessels following FNAC is a theoretical possibility but no instances have been recorded. Local dissemination by seeding of malignant cells along the needle tract is a rare complication and has been reported in cancers of the lung, prostate and pancreas. Aspiration of malignant ovarian

cysts may result in release of cyst contents into the peritoneal cavity with peritoneal implants.

E. Precautions and Contraindications of FNAC

While FNAC is generally a safe procedure, precautions have to be taken when aspiration is contemplated of some sites under certain circumstances:

1. **Bleeding disorders.** Thrombocytopenia *per se* is not a contraindication to FNAC. In patients with coagulopathies such as haemophilia, aspiration of joint spaces, chest and abdominal viscera is contraindicated; superficial lesions may be aspirated and pressure applied to the puncture site for at least 5 minutes following the procedure.
2. **Liver.** Estimation of prothrombin time is an essential pre-requisite for aspiration of the liver. FNAC is not advisable if prothrombin index (PTI) is less than 80%. Obstructive jaundice is a relative contraindication for FNAC on account of the risk of bile peritonitis.
3. **Lung.** FNAC of the lung should not be undertaken in elderly patients with emphysema or pulmonary hypertension because of the enhanced risk of pneumothorax and haemoptysis respectively.
4. **Pancreas.** FNAC is contraindicated in acute pancreatitis as it aggravates the inflammatory process.
5. **Prostate.** Transrectal aspiration in acute prostatitis may cause bacteraemia/septicaemia and is contraindicated.
6. **Testis.** Aspiration is extremely painful in acute epididymo-orchitis and should be deferred till such time the acute inflammatory process subsides. The patient is treated with anti-inflammatory agents and antibiotics and FNAC undertaken at a later date.
7. **Adrenal.** FNAC of a suspected pheochromo-cytoma is inadvisable as it may sometimes provoke extreme fluctuations in blood pressure.

F. Limitations of FNAC

The main limitation of FNAC lies in the fact that only a small population of cells is sampled by the procedure. The reliability of the test, thus, depends upon the adequacy of the sample and its representative character. An inadequate sample which is not representative of the true lesion results in a 'false-negative' diagnosis. If the FNAC report is 'negative' despite a strong clinical suspicion of malignancy, the patient should be investigated further. FNAC may be repeated or a surgical biopsy performed to obtain a tissue diagnosis in such instances.

Lack of requisite clinical information (e.g. size, site and character of mass) or relevant investigative results (e.g. X-ray findings) further limit the utility of FNAC. Knowledge of the exact site from where the aspirate has been obtained is crucial to the accurate interpretation of FNAC smears and lack of this information severely compromises the ability of the cytopathologist to provide a diagnosis

II. IMPRINT CYTOLOGY

In imprint cytology, touch preparations from cut surfaces of fresh unfixed surgically excised mass lesions are examined. Imprints may also be obtained from draining sinuses or ulcerated areas.

For surgically resected specimens (e.g. lymph nodes) smears are prepared by bisecting or slicing the specimen and lightly touching/pressing a glass slide onto the freshly exposed surface without smearing it. Smears cannot be prepared from fixed specimens. Smears are wet-fixed or air-dried and stained as per routine.

The main advantage of the imprint smear is that the cell distribution reflects, and to some extent, recapitulates tissue architecture thus aiding in interpretation. The technique is used in the intraoperative diagnosis of malignancy as a complement to frozen-section, and is also valuable as an adjunct to histopathology in the typing of lymphomas.

III. CRUSH SMEAR CYTOLOGY

Crush smear preparations of tissue particles obtained by craniotomy have been used in the diagnosis of brain tumours. These smears are preferred by some workers as they allow recognition of tissue architecture to some degree, in addition to better cytological details.

IV. BIOPSY SEDIMENT CYTOLOGY

Biopsy sediment cytology entails the examination of sediment obtained by centrifugation of fixatives/fluids in which surgical biopsy specimens are despatched to the laboratory. The method may be useful in the rapid diagnosis of bone tumours as histological sections are usually obtained after many days on account of the delay necessitated by decalcification. For soft tissue specimens, the technique offers no particular advantage.

In conclusion, both exfoliative cytology and FNA cytology have now become a part of diagnostic pathology. It is imperative for the student in pathology as well as the clinician to be familiar with the advantages and limitations of cytologic diagnosis. It is acknowledged that a marked decline in incidence of cervical cancer in many western countries is attributable to highly successful preventive Pap smear screening programme. Similarly, large number of surgical diagnostic procedures are now avoided by rational use of FNAC. However, in view of unique responsibility of pathologist in patient management, reporting cytopathologist should be adequately trained in the skill and should not hesitate to ask for ancillary diagnostic techniques, or advise the use of core biopsy or open biopsy, wherever appropriate.

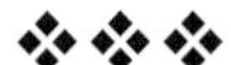

Normal Values

Appendix

WEIGHTS AND MEASUREMENTS OF NORMAL ORGANS
LABORATORY VALUES OF CLINICAL SIGNIFICANCE
CLINICAL CHEMISTRY OF BLOOD
OTHER BODY FLUIDS
HAEMATOLOGICAL VALUES

WEIGHTS AND MEASUREMENTS OF NORMAL ORGANS

In order to understand the significance of alterations in weight and measurement of an organ in disease, it is important to be familiar with the normal values. In the foregoing chapters normal figures are given alongside the normal structure of each organ/system that precedes the discussion of pathologic states affecting it. Here, a comprehensive list of generally accepted normal weights and measurements of most of the normal organs in fully-developed, medium-sized individual and a normal healthy newborn are compiled in Table A-1.

Single value and value within brackets are indicative of the average figure for that organ. Measurements have been given as width × breadth (thickness) × length. An alphabetic order has been followed.

TABLE A-1: Weights and Measurement of Normal Organs.

ORGAN	IN ADULTS	AT BIRTH (wherever applicable)
Adrenal gland:		
Weight	4–5 gm	8-11 gm
Brain:		
Weight (in males)	1400 gm	320-420 gm
Weight (in females)	1250 gm	—
Measurements (sagittal × vertical)	16.5 × 12.5 cm	—
Volume of cerebrospinal fluid	120–150 ml	—
Heart:		
Weight (in males)	300–350 gm	17-30 gm
Weight (in females)	250–300 gm	—
Thickness of right ventricular wall	0.3–0.5 cm	—
Thickness of left ventricular wall	1.3–1.5 cm	—
Circumference of mitral valve	10 cm	—
Circumference of aortic valve	7.5 cm	—
Circumference of pulmonary valve	8.5 cm	—
Circumference of tricuspid valve	12 cm	—
Volume of pericardial fluid	10–30 ml	—
Intestines:		
Length of duodenum	30 cm	—
Total length of small intestine	550–650 cm	—
Length of large intestine	150–170 cm	—
Kidneys:		
Weight each (in males)	150 gm	20-30 gm
Weight each (in females)	135 gm	—
Measurements	3.5 × 5.5 × 11.5 cm	—

Contd...

TABLE A-1: Weights and Measurement of Normal Organs. *(Contd...)*

ORGAN	IN ADULTS	AT BIRTH (wherever applicable)
Liver:		
Weight (in males)	1400–1600 (1500) gm	100-160 gm
Weight (in females)	1200–1400 (1300) gm	—
Measurements	27 × 8 × 20 cm	—
Lungs:		
Weight (right lung)	375–500 (450) gm	35-55 gm
Weight (left lung)	325–450 (400) gm	—
Volume of pleural fluid	< 15 ml	—
Oesophagus:		
Length (cricoid cartilage to cardia)	25 cm	—
Distance from incisors to gastro-oesophageal junction	40 cm	—
Ovaries:		
Weight (each)	4–8 (6) gm	—
Measurements	1 × 2.5 × 4.5 cm	—
Pancreas:		
Total weight	60–100 (80) gm	3-6 gm
Weight of endocrine pancreas	1–1.5 gm	—
Measurements	3.8 × 4.5 × 18 cm	—
Parotid glands:		
Weight (each)	30 gm	—
Pituitary gland (hypophysis):		
Weight	500 mg	—
Placenta:		
Weight at term	400–600 gm	—
Prostate:		
Weight	20 gm	—
Stomach:		
Length	25–30 cm	—
Spleen:		
Weight	125–175 (150) gm	6-14 gm
Measurements	3.5 × 8.5 × 13 cm	
Testis and epididymis:		
Weight each (in adults)	20–27 gm	—
Thymus:		
Weight	5–10 gm	10-35 gm
Thyroid:		
Weight	15–40 gm	—
Uterus:		
Weight (in nonpregnant woman)	35–40 gm	—
Weight (in parous woman)	75–125 gm	—

LABORATORY VALUES OF CLINICAL SIGNIFICANCE

Currently, the concept of 'normal values' and 'normal ranges' is replaced by 'reference values' and 'reference limits' in which the variables for establishing the values for the reference population in a particular test are well defined. Reference ranges are valuable guidelines for the clinician. However, the following cautions need to be exercised in their interpretation:

- *Firstly,* they should not be regarded as absolute indicators of health and ill-health since values for healthy individuals often overlap with values for persons afflicted with disease.
- *Secondly,* laboratory values may vary with the method and mode of standardisation used; reference ranges given below are based on the generally accepted values by the standard methods in laboratory medicine.
- *Thirdly,* although in most laboratories in the West and in all medical and scientific journals, international units (IU) conforming to the SI system are followed, but conventional units continue to be used in many laboratories in the developing countries.

The WHO as well as International Committee for Standardisation in Haematology (ICSH) have recommended adoption of SI system by the scientific community throughout world. In this section, laboratory values are given in both conventional and international units. Conversion from one system to the other can be done as follows:

$$\text{mg/dl} = \frac{\text{mmol/L} \times \text{atomic weight}}{10}$$

$$\text{mmol/L} = \frac{\text{mg/dl} \times 10}{\text{atomic weight}}$$

According to the SI system, the prefixes and conversion factors for metric units of length, weight and volume are as given in Table A-2.

Appendix

TABLE A-2: Prefixes and Conversion Factors in SI System.

PREFIX	PREFIX SYMBOL	FACTOR	UNITS OF LENGTH	UNITS OF WEIGHT	UNITS OF VOLUME
kilo-	k	10^3	kilometre (km)	kilogram (kg)	kilolitre (kl)
		1	metre (m)	gram (g)	litre (l)
deci-	d	10^{-1}	decimetre (dm)	decigram (dg)	decilitre (dl)
centi-	c	10^{-2}	centimetre (cm)	centigram (cg)	centilitre (cl)
milli-	m	10^{-3}	millimetre (mm)	milligram (mg)	millilitre (ml)
micro-	μ	10^{-6}	micrometre (μm)	microgram (μg)	microlitre (μl)
nano-	n	10^{-9}	nanometre (nm)	nanogram (ng)	nanolitre (nl)
pico-	p	10^{-12}	picometre (pm)	picogram (pg)	picolitre (pl)
femto-	f	10^{-15}	femtometre (fm)	femtogram (fg)	femtolitre (fl)
alto-	a	10^{-18}	altometre (am)	altogram (ag)	altolitre (al)

The laboratory values given here are divided into three sections: clinical chemistry of blood (Table A-3), other body fluids (Table A-4), and haematologic values (Table A-5). In general, an alphabetic order has been followed.

TABLE A-3: Clinical Chemistry of Blood.

COMPONENT	FLUID	REFERENCE VALUE CONVENTIONAL	SI UNITS
Alcohol, ethyl	Serum/whole blood	Negative	Negative
mild to moderate intoxication		80-200 mg/dl	
marked intoxication		250-400 mg/dl	
severe intoxication		>400 mg/dl	
Aminotransferases (transaminases)			
aspartate (AST, SGOT)	Serum	0-35 U/L	0-0.58 μkat*/L
alanine (ALT, SGPT)	Serum	0-35 U/L	0-0.58 μkat/L
Ammonia	Plasma	10-80 μg/dl	6-47 μmol/L
Amylase	Serum	60-180 U/L	0.8-3.2 μkat/L
Bicarbonate (HCO_3^-)	Whole blood	21-30 mEq/L	21-28 mmol/L
Bilirubin			
total	Serum	0.3-1.0 mg/dl	5.1-17 μmol/L
direct (conjugated)	Serum	0.1-0.3 mg/dl	1.7-5.1 μmol/L
indirect (unconjugated)	Serum	0.2-0.7 mg/dl	3.4-12 μmol/L
Blood volume			
total		60-80 ml/kg body weight	
red cell volume, males		30 ml/kg body weight	
females		25 ml/kg body weight	
Plasma volume, males		39 ml/kg body weight	
females		40 ml/kg body weight	
Bromsulphalein (BSP) test			
5 mg/kg body weight	Serum	<5% retention in serum after 45 min	
Calcium, ionised	Serum	4.5-5.6 mg/dl	1.1-1.4 mmol/L
Calcium, total	Plasma	9.0-10.5 mg/dl	2.2-2.6 mmol/L
CO_2 content	Whole blood	21-30 mEq/L (arterial)	21-30 mmol/L (arterial)

*μkat (kat stands for katal meaning catalytic activity) is a modern unit of enzymatic activity.

Contd...

Appendix

TABLE A-3: Clinical Chemistry of Blood *(Contd...)*

COMPONENT	FLUID	REFERENCE VALUE	
		CONVENTIONAL	SI UNITS
Chloride (Cl^-)	Serum	98-106 mEq/L	98-106 mmol/L
Cholesterol	Serum		
total desirable for adults		<200 mg/dl	<5.2 mmol/L
borderline high		200-239 mg/dl	5.20-6.18 mmol/L
high undesirable		>240 mg/dl	>6.21 mmol/L
LDL-cholesterol, desirable range		<130 mg/dl	<3.36 mmol/L
HDL-cholesterol, protective range		>60 mg/dl	>1.15 mmol/L
triglycerides		<160 mg/dl	<1.8 mmol/L
Copper	Serum	70-140 μg/dl	13-24 μmol/L
Creatine kinase (CK)	Serum		
males		25-90 U/L	0.42-1.50 μkat/L
females		10-70 IU/L	0.17-1.17 μkat/L
Creatine kinase-MB (CK-MB)	Serum	0-7 μg/L	
Creatinine	Serum	0.5-1.5 mg/dl	53-133 μmol/L
Electrophoresis, protein	Serum	*See under proteins*	
Fatty acids, free non-esterified	Plasma	<180 mg/dl	<18mg/L
Gamma-glutamyl trans-peptidase (transferase) (γ-GT)	Serum	4-60 IU/L	0.07-1.00 μmol/L
Gases, arterial			
HCO_3^-	Whole blood	21-30 mEq/L	21-28 mmol/L
pH	Whole blood	7.38-7.44	7.38-7.44
pCO_2	Whole blood	35-45 mmHg	4.7-5.9 kPa
pO_2	Whole blood	80-100 mmHg	11.0-13.0 kPa
Glucose (fasting)	Plasma		
normal		70-110 mg/dl	< 6.1 mmol/L
impaired fasting glucose (IFG)		110-126 mg/dl	6.1-7.0 mmol/L
diabetes mellitus		>126 mg/dl	>7.0 mmol/L
Glucose (2-hr post-prandial)	Plasma		
normal		<140 mg/dl	<7.8 mmol/L
impaired glucose tolerance (IGT)		140-200 mg/dl	7.8-11.1 mmol/L
diabetes mellitus		>200 mg/dl	>11.1 mmol/L
Immunoglobulins	Serum		
IgA		90-325 mg/dl	
IgD		0-8 mg/dl	
IgE		<0.025 mg/dl	
IgG		800-1500 mg/dl	
IgM		45-150 mg/dl	
Lactate dehydrogenase (LDH)	Serum	100-190 U/L	1.7-3.2 μkat/L
Lactate/pyruvate ratio		10/1	
Lipids	Serum	*See under cholesterol*	
Non-protein nitrogen (NPN)	Serum	<35 mg/dl	
Oxygen (% saturation)			
arterial blood	Whole blood	94-100%	
venous blood	Whole blood	60-85%	
pH		Blood	7.38-7.44

Contd...

TABLE A-3: Clinical Chemistry of Blood *(Contd...)*

COMPONENT	FLUID	REFERENCE VALUE CONVENTIONAL	SI UNITS
Phosphatases			
acid phosphatase	Serum	0-5.5 U/L	0.90 nkat/L
alkaline phosphatase	Serum	30-120 U/L	0.5-2.0 nkat/L
Phosphorus, inorganic	Serum	3-4.5 mg/dl	1.0-1.4 mmol/L
Potassium	Serum	3.5-5.0 mEq/L	3.5-5.0 mmol/L
Proteins	Serum		
total		5.5-8 g/dl	
albumin		3.5-5.5 g/dl (50-60%)	
globulin		2.0-3.5 g/dl (40-50%)	
α1 globulin		0.2-0.4 g/dl	
α2 globulin		0.5-0.9 g/dl	
β globulin		0.6-1.1 g/dl	
γ globulin		0.7-1.7 g/dl	
A/G ratio		1.5-3 : 1	
Renal blood flow		1200 ml/min	
Sodium	Serum	136-145 mEq/L	136-145 mmol/L
Thyroid function tests			
radioactive iodine uptake (RAIU) 24-hr		5-30%	
thyroxine (T4)	Serum	5-12 μg/dl	64-154 nmol/L
triiodothyronine (T3)	Serum	70-190 ng/dl	1.1-2.9 nmol/L
thyroid stimulating hormone (TSH)	Serum	0.4-5.0 μU/ml	0.4-5.0 mU/L
Troponins, cardiac (cTn)			
troponin I (cTnI)	Serum	0-0.4 ng/ml	0-0.4 μg/L
troponin T (cTnT)	Serum	0-0.1 ng/ml	0-0.1 μg/L
Urea	Blood	20-40 mg/dl	3.3-6.6 mmol/L
Urea nitrogen (BUN)	Blood	10-20 mg/dl	
Uric acid	Serum		
males		2.5-8.0 mg/dl	150-480 μmol/L
females		1.5-6.0 mg/dl	90-360 μmol/L

TABLE A-4: Other Body Fluids.

COMPONENT	FLUID	REFERENCE VALUE CONVENTIONAL	SI UNITS
Body volume, water			
total		50-70% (60%)	
intracellular		33%	
extracellular		27%	
interstitial fluid including lymph fluid		12%	
intravascular fluid or blood plasma		5%	
fluid in mesenchymal tissues		9%	
transcellular fluid		1%	

Contd...

TABLE A-4: Other Body Fluids *(Contd...)*

COMPONENT	FLUID	REFERENCE VALUE CONVENTIONAL	SI UNITS
Catecholamines	24-hr urinary excretion		
epinephrine		< 10 ng/day	
free catecholamines		<100 μg/day	
metanephrine		<1.3 mg/day	
vanillyl mandelic acid (VMA)		<8 mg/day	
Cerebrospinal fluid (CSF)	CSF		
CSF volume		120-150 ml	
CSF pressure		60-150 mm water	
leucocytes		0-5 lymphocytes/μl	
pH		7.31-7.34	
glucose		40-70 mg/dl	
proteins		20-50 mg/dl	
FIGLU	24-hr urine	<3 mg/day	<17.2 μmol/day
Gastric analysis	Gastric juice		
24-hr volume		2-3 L	
pH		1.6-1.8	1.6-1.8
basal acid output (BAO)		1-5 mEq/hr	1-5 mmol/hr
maximal acid output (MAO) after injection of stimulant		5-40 mEq/hr	5-40 mmol/hr
BAO/MAO ratio		<0.6	
Glomerular filtration rate (GFR)	Urine	180 L/day (about 125 ml/min)	
5-HIAA	24-hr urinary excretion	2-8 mg/day	
17-Ketosteroids	24-hr urinary excretion		
males		7-25 mg/day	
females		4-15 mg/day	
Seminal fluid	Semen		
liquefaction		Within 20 min	
sperm morphology		>70% normal, mature spermatozoa	
sperm motility		>60%	
pH		>7.0 (average 7.7)	
sperm count		60-150 million/ml	$60\text{-}150 \times 10^6$/ml
volume		1.5-5.0 ml	
Stool examination	Stool		
coproporphyrin		400-1000 mg/day	
faecal fat excretion		<6.0 g/day	
occult blood		Negative (<2 ml blood /day)	
urobilinogen		40-280 mg/day	
Schilling's test (intrinsic factor test)	24-hr urinary excretion	>10% of ingested dose of 'hot' vitamin B_{12} *(Details on page 383)*	
Urine examination	24-hr volume	600-1800 ml (variable)	
specific gravity	urine (random)	1.002-1.028 (average 1.018)	
protein excretion	24-hr urine	<150 mg/day	
protein, qualitative	urine (random)	Negative	
glucose excretion	24-hr urine	50-300 mg/day	
glucose, qualitative	urine (random)	Negative	
porphobilinogen	urine (random)	Negative	
urobilinogen	24-hr urine	1.0-3.5 mg/day	
Urobilinogen	Urine (random)	Present in 1: 20 dilution	
D-Xylose excretion	Stool	5-8 g within 5 hrs after oral dose of 25 g	

Appendix

TABLE A-5: Normal Haematologic Values.

COMPONENT	FLUID	REFERENCE VALUE CONVENTIONAL	SI UNITS
Myelogram		*See Table 13.2 on page 359*	
Erythrocytes and Haemoglobin			
Erythrocyte count	Blood		
males		4.5-6.5 × 10^{12}/L (mean 5.5 × 10^{12}/L)	
females		3.8-5.8 × 10^{12}/L (mean 4.8 × 10^{12}/L)	
Erythrocyte diameter		6.7-7.7 μm (mean 7.2 μm)	
Erythrocyte thickness			
peripheral		2.4 μm	
central		1.0 μm	
Erythrocyte indices (Absolute values)	Blood	*(also see page 361)*	
mean corpuscular haemoglobin (MCH)		27-32 pg	
mean corpuscular volume (MCV)		77-93 fl	
mean corpuscular haemoglobin concentration (MCHC)		30-35 g/dl	
Erythrocyte life-span	Blood	120 days	
Erythrocyte sedimentation rate (ESR)	Blood		
Westergren 1st hr, males		0-15 mm	
females		0-20 mm	
Wintrobe, 1st hr, males		0-9 mm	
females		0-20 mm	
Ferritin	Serum		
males		15-200 ng/ml	15-200 μg/L
females		12-150 ng/ml	15-150 μg/L
Folate			
body stores		2-3 mg	
daily requirement		100-200 μg	
red cell level	Red cells	150-450 ng/ml	
Serum level	Serum	6-12 ng/ml	11-57 nmol/L
Free erythrocyte protoporphyrin (FEP)	Red cells	20 μg/dl	
Haematocrit (PCV)		Blood	
males		40-54%	0.47 ± 0.07 L/L
females		37-47%	0.42 ± 0.05 L/L
Haptoglobin	Serum	60-270 mg/dl	0.6-2.7 g/L
Haemoglobin (Hb)			
adult haemoglobin (HbA)	Whole blood		
males		13.0-18.0 g/dl	130-180 g/L
females		11.5-16.5 g/dl	115-165 g/L
plasma Hb (quantitative)		0.5-5 mg/dl	5-50 mg/L
haemoglobin A_2 (HbA_2)		1.5-3.5%	
haemoglobin, foetal (HbF) in adults		<1%	
HbF, children under 6 months		<5%	
Iron, total	Serum	80-180 μg/dl	10.7-26.9 μmol/L
total iron binding capacity (TIBC)	Serum	250-460 μg/dl	44.8-71.6 μmol/L
iron saturation	Serum	20-45% (mean 33%)	
Iron intake		10-15 mg/day	
Iron loss			
males		0.5-1.0 mg/day	
females		1-2 mg/day	

Contd...

Appendix

TABLE A-5: Normal Haematologic Values *(Contd...)*			
		REFERENCE VALUE	
COMPONENT	FLUID	CONVENTIONAL	SI UNITS
Iron, total body content			
males		50 mg/kg body weight	
females		35 mg/kg body weight	
Iron, storage form (ferritin and haemosiderin)		30% of body iron	
Osmotic fragility	Blood		
slight haemolysis		at 0.45 to 0.39 g/dl NaCl	
complete haemolysis		at 0.33 to 0.36 g/dl NaCl	
mean corpuscular fragility		0.4-0.45 g/dl NaCl	
Reticulocytes	Blood		
adults		0.5-2.5%	
infants		2-6%	
Transferrin	Serum	1.5-2.0 mg/dl	
Vitamin B_{12}			
body stores		10-12 mg	
daily requirement		2-4 μg	
serum level	Serum	200-900 pg/ml	200-900 pmol/L
Leucocytes in Health			
Total leucocyte count (TLC)	Blood		
adults		4,000-11,000/μl	
infants (full term, at birth)		10,000-25,000/μl	
infants (1 year)		6,000-16,000/μl	
Differential leucocyte count (DLC)	Blood film		
P (polymorphs or neutrophils)		40-75% (2,000-7,500/μl)	
L (lymphocytes)		20-50% (1,500-4,000/μl)	
M (monocytes)		2-10% (200-800/μl)	
E (eosinophils)		1-6% (40-400/μl)	
B (basophils)		< 1% (10-100/μl)	
Muramidase	Serum	5-20 μg/ml	
Platelets and Coagulation			
Bleeding time (BT)			
Ivy's method	Prick blood	2-7 min	
template method		2.5-9.5 min	
Clot retraction time	Clotted blood		
qualitative		Visible in 60 min (complete in <24-hr)	
quantitative		48-64% (55%)	
Clotting time (CT) Whole blood			
Lee and White method		4-9 min at 37°C	
Euglobin lysis time			72 hr
Fibrinogen	Plasma	200-400 mg/dl	2-4 g/L
Fibrin split (or degradation) products (FSP or FDP)	Plasma	<10 μg/ml	<10 mg/L
Partial thromboplastin time with kaolin (PTTK) or activated partial thromboplastin time (APTT)	Plasma	30-40 sec	
Prothrombin time (PT) (Quick's one-stage method)	Plasma	10-14 sec	
Thrombin time (TT)	Plasma	<20 sec (control ± 2 sec)	
Platelet count	Blood	150,000-400,000/μl	

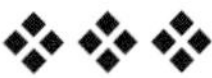

Appendix

Further Reading

In compilation of the material in this textbook, books and original works of several authors listed below have been consulted which are gratefully acknowledged. In order to stimulate an inquisitive and indulgent reader, additional references are given chapterwise below, which are preceded by some general references used as the resource material for the book. An *author index* in alphabetic order has been followed.

GENERAL (COMMON TO ALL CHAPTERS)

Boyd, William: *Pathology—Structure and Function in Disease,* 8th ed. Philadelphia, Lea & Febiger, 1970.

Braunwald E *et al: Harrison's Principles of Internal Medicine* (2 vols), 15th ed. New York, McGraw-Hill Health Profession Division, 2001.

Cormack DH: *Ham's Histology,* 9th ed. Philadelphia, JB Lippincott Company, 1987.

Cotran RS, Kumar V, Robbins SL: *Robbins Pathologic Basis of Disease,* 6th ed. Philadelphia, WB Saunders Company, 1999.

Damjanov I, Linder J: *Andersen's Pathology* (2 vols), 10th ed. St Louis, Mosby, 1996.

Datta BN: *Textbook of Pathology,* 2nd ed. New Delhi, Jaypee Brothers, 2004.

Edwards CRR *et al: Davidson's Practice of Medicine,* 17th ed. ELBS-Churchill Livingstone, 1995.

Fauci AS *et al: Harrison's Principles of Internal Medicine* (2 vols), 14th ed. New York, McGraw Hill Health Profession Division, 1998.

Ganong WF: *Review of Medical Physiology,* 15th ed. Appleton and Lange, 1991.

Kumar V, Cotran RS, Robbins SL: *Basic Pathology,* 7th ed. Philadelphila, WB Saunders Company, 2003.

Lowe DG, Underwood JCE: *Recent Advances in Histopathology,* number 20. Philadelphia, Churchill Livingstone, 2004.

MacSween RNM, Whaley K: *Muir's Textbook of Pathology,* 13th ed. Kent, ELBS with Edward Arnold, 1992.

Mann CV, Russel RCG: *Bailey and Love's Short Practice of Surgery,* 21st ed. ELBS-Chapman & Hall, 1991.

McGee *et al: Oxford Textbook of Pathology* (3 vols), 1st ed. Oxford, Oxford University Press, 1992.

Mills SE *et al: Sternberg's Diagnostic Surgical Pathology,* 4th ed. Philadelphia, Lippincott Williams & Wilkins, 2004.

Nayak NC *et al: Pathology of Diseases.* New Delhi, Jaypee Brothers, 2000.

Ritchie AC: *Boyd's Textbook of Pathology* (2 vols), 9th ed. Philadelphia, Lea & Febiger, 1990.

Rosai J: *Ackerman's Surgical Pathology* (2 vols), 8th ed. St Louis, Mosby, 1996.

Rubin *et al: Rubin's Pathology,* 4th ed. Philadelphia, Lippincott Williams & Wilkins, 2004.

Stevens A, Lowe J: *Pathology,* 1st ed. London, Mosby, 1995.

Thibobeau GA, Patton KT: *Anthony's Textbook of Anatomy and Physiology,* 17th ed. Delhi, Elsevier, 2004.

Underwood, JCE: *General and Systemic Pathology,* 2nd ed. Edinburgh, Churchill Livingstone, 1992.

Walter JB, Israel MS: *General Pathology,* 7th ed. Edinburgh, Churchill Livingstone, 1997.

SECTION I: GENERAL PATHOLOGY

CHAPTER 1: INTRODUCTION TO PATHOLOGY

Deodhare SG: *YM Bhende's General Pathology* and *Pathology of Systems* (2 vols), 6th ed. Mumbai, Popular Prakashan, 2002.

Firkin BG, Whiteworth, JA: *Dictionary of Medical Eponyms,* 2nd ed. New York, The Patheron Publishing Group, 1988.

Lyons AS: *Medicine—An Illustrated History.* New York, Abradele Publishers, 1987.

Rosen G: Beginning of surgical biopsy. *Am J Surg Pathol* 1: 361, 1977.

Rutkow IM: *Surgery—An Illustrated History.* St. Louis, Mosby, 1993.

CHAPTER 2: TECHNIQUES FOR STUDY OF PATHOLOGY

Bancroft JD, Gamble M: *Theory and Practice of Histopathological Techniques,* 5th ed. London, Churchill Livingstone, 2002.

Codling BW: Audit, quality assurance and quality control. In *Recent Advances in Histopathology,* number 16, Anthony PP *et al* (Eds). London, Churchill Livingstone, pp 293, 1994.

Friedman BA: Informatics as a separate section within a department of pathology. *Am J Clin Pathol* 94 (suppl 1): 52, 1990.

Gershon D: DNA diagnostic tools for the 21st Century. *Nature Med* 1: 102, 1995.

Herey JB: *Clinical Diagnosis and Management by Laboratory Methods,* 19th ed. Philadelphia, WB Saunders Company, 1996.

Kerr MA, Thorpe R: *Immunochemistry Lab Fascicle.* Oxford, Blackwell Scientific Publications, 1994.

Kirkpatrick P, Marshall RJ: Technical advances in histopathology. In *Recent Advances in Histopathology,* number 15, Anthony PP *et al* (Eds). Philadelphia, Churchill Livingstone, pp 241, 1992.

Knight BH: The histopathologist and the law. In *Recent Advances in Histopathology,* number 17, Anthony PP *et al* (Eds). London, Churchill Livingstone, pp 233, 1997.

Leong ASY: *Applied Immunohistochemistry for the Surgical Pathologist.* London, Edward Arnold, 1993.

Macey MG: *Flow Cytometry: Clinical Applications.* London, Blackwell Scientific Publications, 1994.

Mason DY, Gatter KC: Immunohistochemistry in histological diagnosis. In *Recent Advances in Histopathology,* number 16, Anthony PP *et al* (Eds). London, Churchill Livingstone, pp 263, 1994.

Sehgal S *et al: Methodology Book on Molecular Pathology and HLA* (International Academy of Pathology, Indian Division), Department of Immunopathology, Postgraduate Institute of Medical Education & Research, Chandigarh, 1997.

Wright TR: The development of the frozen section technique, the evolution of surgical biopsy and the origin of surgical pathology. *Bull Med Histol* 59: 295, 1985.

CHAPTER 3: CELL INJURY AND CELLULAR ADAPTATIONS

Blackburn EH: Switching and signaling at telomere. *Cell* 106: 661, 2001.

Cummings MC *et al:* Apoptosis. *Am J Surg Pathol* 21: 88, 1997.

Grace PA: Ischaemic-reperfusion injury. *Br J Surg* 81: 637, 1994.

Jazwinski SM: Longevity, genes and aging. *Science* 273: 54, 1996.

Knight JA: Diseases related to oxygen-derived free radicals. *Ann Clin Lab Sci* 25: 111, 1995.

Majno G, Joris I: Apoptosis, oncosis and necrosis: an overview of cell death. *Am J Pathol* 146: 3, 1995.

Martin GM: The genetics of aging. *Hosp Pract* 32: 47, 1997.

Toyokuni S: Reactive oxygen species-induced molecular damage and its application in pathology. *Pathol Int* 49: 91, 1999.

Wyllie AH: Apoptosis: In *Recent Advances in Histopathology,* number 17, Anthony PP *et al* (Eds). London, Churchill Livingstone, pp 1, 1997.

CHAPTER 4: IMMUNOPATHOLOGY INCLUDING AMYLOIDOSIS

Benson MD, Uemichi T: Transthyretin amyloidosis. *Amyloid* 3: 44, 1996.

Blumenfeld W, Hildebrandt RH: Fine needle aspiration of abdominal fat for the diagnosis of amyloidosis. *Acta Cytol* 37: 170, 1993.

Chapel H, Haeney M: *Essentials of Clinical Immunology,* 3rd ed. London, Blackwell Scientific Publications, 1993.

Cohen AS, Sipe JD: Amyloidosis: In *Clinical Immunology,* RR Rich *et al* (Eds). St Louis, Mosby, pp 1264, 1995.

Cohen OJ *et al:* Host factors in the pathogenesis of HIV disease. *Immunol Res* 159: 31, 1997.

Davidson A, Diamond B: Autoimmune diseases. *New Engl J Med* 345: 240, 2001.

Ferrara JL, Deeg HJ: Graft-versus-host disease: review of mechanisms of disease. *N Engl J Med* 324: 667, 1991.

Glenner GG: Amyloid deposits and amyloidosis—the beta fibrillosis. *N Eng J Med* 302: 1283, 1333, 1980.

Guy CD, Jones CK: Abdominal fat pad aspiration biopsy for tissue confirmation of systemic amyloidosis. Specificity, positive predictive value and diagnostic pitfalls. *Diagn Cytopathol* 24: 181, 2001.

McCune J: The dynamics of CD4+ T-cell depletion in HIV disease. *Nature* 410: 974, 2001.

Millard PR, Esiri MM: The pathology of AIDS, an update: In *Recent Advances in Histopathology,* number 15. Philadelphia, Churchill Livingstone, pp 67, 1992.

Moore RD, Chaisson RE: Natural history of opportunistic diseases in an HIV-infected urban clinical cohort. *Ann Intern Med* 124: 633, 1996.

Pickens MM: The changing concept of amyloid. *Arch Pathol Lab Med* 125: 38-43, 2001.

Price RW: Neurologic complications of HIV infection. *Lancet* 348: 445, 1996.

Sipe JD: Amyloidosis. *Crit Rev Clin Lab Sci* 31: 325, 1995.

Verghese *et al:* Transfusion-associated AIDS and other infections, Govt. of India, Delhi. NICD Publications, Shamnath Marg, 1990.

CHAPTER 5: HAEMODYNAMIC DISORDERS

Brady AJ: Nitric acid, myocardial infarction and septic shock. *Int J Cardiol* 50: 269, 1995.

Dahlbeck B: Blood coagulation. *Lancet* 355: 1627, 2000.

Evans JJ, Kransz T: Pathogenesis and pathology of shock. In *Recent Advances in Histopathology,* number 16, Anthony PP *et al* (Eds). Philadelphia, Churchill Livingstone, pp 21, 1994.

Ganong WF: *Review of Medical Physiology,* 15th ed. London, Prentice-Hall International lnc, 1991.

McManus ML *et al:* Regulation of cell volume in health and disease—review article. *New Engl J Med* 333: 1260, 1995.

Mecik BG, Ortel TL: Clinical and laboratory evolution of the hypercoagulable states. *Clin Chest Med* 16: 375, 1995.

Miller MJ: *Pathophysiology—Principles of Disease.* Philadelphia, WB Saunders Company, 1983.

Rosendaal FR: Risk factors for venous thrombosis: prevalence, risk and interactions. *Semin Hematol* 34: 171, 1997.

CHAPTER 6: INFLAMMATION AND HEALING

Baggiolini M: Chemokines in medicine and pathology. *J Intern Med* 250: 90, 2001.

Dvorak HF *et al:* Vascular permeability factor/vascular endothelial growth factor, microvascular hyperpermeability and angiogenesis. *Am J Pathol* 146: 1029, 1995.

Evans SW, Whicher JT: The cytokines: physiological and pathophysiological aspects. *Adv Clin Chem* 30: 1, 1993.

Martin P: Wound healing—aiming for perfect skin regeneration. *Science* 276: 75, 1997.

Prockop DJ, Kivirikko KI: Collagens: molecular biology, diseases and potentials for therapy. *Annu Rev Biochem* 64: 403, 1995.

Risau W: Mechanism of angiogenesis. *Nature* 380: 671, 1997.

Vernon RB, Sage EH: Between molecules and morphology: extracellular matrix and creation of vascular form. *Am J Pathol* 147: 873, 1995.

CHAPTER 7: INFECTIOUS AND PARASITIC DISEASES

Human plague-United States 1993-94. *JAMA* 271: 1312, 1994.

Meslin FX: Surveillance and control of emerging zoonoses. *World Health Statistics Quarterly* 45: 200, 1992.

Pasloske BL, Howard RJ: Malaria, the red cell and the endothelium. *Annu Rev Med* 45: 283, 1994.

Swartz MN: Recognition and management of anthrax- an update. *N Engl J Med* 345: 1621, 2001.

Talib VH *et al:* Dengue: the killer. *Indian J Pathol Microbiol* 40(1): 3, 1997.

Talib VH *et al:* Plague in India (1994): Was it really plague in India? *Indian J Pathol Microbiol* 38(2): 131, 1995.

Von Lichtenberg F: *Pathology of Infectious Diseases.* New York, Raven Press, 1991.

CHAPTER 8: NEOPLASIA

Ahr A *et al:* Identification of high risk breast cancer patients by gene expression profiling. *Lancet* 359: 131, 2002.

Agarwala SS: Paraneoplastic syndromes. *Med Clin North Am* 80: 173, 1996.

Bertram JS: Molecular biology of cancer. *Mol Aspects Med* 21: 167, 2001.

Butel JS: Viral carcinogenesis: revelation of molecular mechanisms and etiology of human disease. *Carcinogenesis* 21: 405, 2000.

Cawkwell L, Quirke P: Molecular genetics of cancer. In *Recent Advances in Histopathology,* number 16, Anthony PP *et al* (Eds). Philadelphia, Churchill Livingstone, pp 1, 1994.

Clemons M, Goss P: Estrogen and the risk of breast cancer. *N Engl J Med* 344: 276, 2001.

Cohen JI: Epstein-Barr virus infections. *N Engl J Med* 343: 481, 2000.

Deodhare SG: *YM Bhende's General Pathology and Pathology of Systems* (2 vols), 6th ed. Mumbai, Popular Prakashan, 2002.

Eichhorst ST, Krammer PH: Derangement of apoptosis in cancer. *Lancet* 358: 345, 2001.

Folkman J: Clinical application of research on angiogenesis. *N Engl J Med* 333: 1757, 1995.

Greider CW, Blackburn EH: Telomeres, telomerase and cancer. *Sci Am* 274: 92, 1996.

Hanahan D, Weinberg RA: The hallmarks of cancer. *Cell* 100: 57, 2000.

Heim S, Mitelman F: Cytogenetics of solid tumours, In *Recent Advances in Histopathology,* number 15, Anthony PP *et al* (Eds). Philadelphia, Churchill Livingstone, pp 37, 1992.

Herrington CS: Human papilloma viruses and cervical neoplasia I. Classification, virology, pathology and epidemiology. *J Clin Pathol* 47: 1066, 1994.

Jiang WG: E-cadherin and its associated protein catenins, cancer invasion and metastasis. *Br J Surg* 83: 437, 1996.

Kerbel RS: Tumour angiogenesis: past, present and the near future. *Carcinogenesis* 21: 505, 2000.

Lichtenstein P *et al:* Environmental and heritable factors in causation of cancers. *N Engl J Med* 343: 78, 2000.

Pamies RJ. Crawford DR: Tumour markers, an update. *Med Clin North Am* 80: 185, 1996.

Renkvist N *et al:* A listing of human tumour antigens recognised by T cells. *Cancer Immunol Immunother* 50: 3, 2001.

Smith NM, Keeling JW: Paediatric solid tumours. In *Recent Advances in Histopathology,* number 17, Anthony PP *et al* (Eds). London, Churchill Livingstone, pp 191, 1997.

Tarin D: Prognostic markers and mechanisms of metastasis. In *Recent Advances in Histopathology,* number 17, Anthony PP *et al* (Eds). London, Churchill Livingstone, pp 15, 1997.

Webb CP, Van de Woude GF: Genes that regulate metastases and angiogenesis. *J Neurooncol* 50: 71, 2000.

Williams GM: Mechanisms of chemical carcinogenesis and application to human cancer risk assesssment. *Toxicology* 166: 3, 2001.

Zur Hausen H: Papilloma virus infections. A major cause of human cancers. *Biochem Biophys Acta* 1288 F 55, 1996.

CHAPTER 9: ENVIRONMENTAL AND NUTRITIONAL DISEASES

Buehlmann AA, Froesch ER: *Pathophysiology.* New York, Springer-Verlag, 1979.

Ganong WF: *Review of Medical Physiology,* 15th ed. London, Prentice-Hall Inc, 1991.

Glanz SA, Parmley WW: Passive smoking and heart disease. *JAMA* 273: 1047, 1995.

Greenberg ER, Sporn MB: Antioxidant vitamins, cancer and cardiovascular disease. *N Engl J Med* 334: 1189, 1996.

Keele CA, Neil E, Joel N: *Samson Wright's Applied Physiology,* 13th ed. Delhi, Oxford University Press, 1983.

Kopelman PG: Obesity as a medical problem. *Nature* 404: 635, 2000.

McBride PE: The health consequences of smoking: cardiovascular diseases. *Med Clin N Am* 76: 333, 1992.

Miller MJ: *Pathophysiology—Principles of Disease.* Philadelphia, WB Saunders Company, 1983.

Nishiyama H *et al:* The incidence of malignant lymphoma and multiple myeloma in Hiroshima and Nagasaki atomic bomb survivors. *Cancer* 32: 1301, 1973.

Pi-Sunyer FX: Medical hazards of obesity. *Ann Inter Med* 119: 655, 1993.

Sodeman WA, Sodeman TM: *Sodeman's Pathologic Physiology. Mechanisms of Diseases,* 6th ed. Philadelphia, WB Saunders Company, 1979.

CHAPTER 10: GENETIC AND PAEDIATRIC DISEASES

Gilbert-Barness (Ed). *Potters' Pathology of the Foetus and Infant.* New York, Mosby, 1996.

Glew RH *et al:* Lysosomal storage diseases. *Lab Invest* 53: 250, 1985.

Green DM *et al:* Wilms' tumour. *CA Cancer J Clin* 46: 46, 1996.

Matthay KK: Neuroblastoma: a clinical challenge and biologic puzzle. *CA Cancer J Clin* 45: 1795, 1995.

Smith NM, Keeling JW: Paediatric solid tumours. In *Recent Advances in Histopathology,* number 17, Anthony PP *et al* (Eds). London, Churchill Livingstone, pp 191, 1997.

Zwarthoff EC: Neurofibromatosis and associated tumour-suppressor genes. *Pathol Res Pract* 192: 647, 1996.

SECTION II: SYSTEMIC PATHOLOGY

CHAPTER 11: BLOOD VESSELS AND LYMPHATICS

Atherosclerosis (special issue): *Arch Pathol Lab Med* 1112, 1988.

Berlinder JA *et al:* Atherosclerosis: Basic mechanisms, oxidation, inflammation and genetics. *Circulation* 91: 2488, 1995.

Erust CB: Abdominal aortic aneurysms. *N Engl J Med* 328: 1167, 1993.

Gimbrone MA Jr *et al:* Endothelial dysfunction, haemodynamic forces and atherogenesis. *Ann N Y Acad Sci* 902: 230, 2000.

Jennette JC, Falk RJ: Antineutrophil cytoplasmic autoantibodies: discovery, specificity, disease associations and pathogenic potential. *Adv Pathol Lab Med* 8: 313, 1995.

Parmus DV: The arteritides. *Histopathology* 25: 1, 1995.

Rose R: The pathogenesis of atherosclerosis: a perspective for 1990s. *Nature* 362: 801, 1993.

Rose R: The pathogenesis of atherosclerosis—an inflammatory disease. *N Engl J Med* 340: 115, 1999.

Silver MD: *Cardiovascular Pathology,* 2nd ed. London, Churchill Livingstone, 1991.

Stary HC *et al:* A definition of advanced types of atherosclerotic lesions and a histological classification of atherosclerosis: A report from the committee on vascular lesions of the council on arteriosclerosis. *Circulation* 92: 1355, 1995.

CHAPTER 12: THE HEART

Chopra P: *Illustrated Textbook of Cardiovascular Pathology.* New Delhi, Jaypee Brothers Medical Publisher(P) Ltd., 2003.

Frazer WJ *et al:* Rheumatic Aschoff nodule revisited. *Histopathology* 27: 457, 1995.

Fuster V *et al:* Acute coronary syndromes: biology. *Lancet* 353 (suppl II): 59, 1999.

Fuster V *et al:* The pathogenesis of coronary artery disease and the acute coronary syndromes. *N Engl J Med* 326; 242, 1992.

Gallaghar PJ: The investigation of cardiac death. In *Recent Advances in Histopathology,* number 16, Anthony PP *et at* (Eds). Philadelphia, Churchill Livingstone, pp 123, 1994.

Kushwaha SS *et al:* Restrictive cardiomyopathy. *N Engl J Med* 336: 267, 1997.

Mylonkis E, Calderwood SB: Infecive endocarditis in adults. *N Engl J Med* 345: 1318, 2001.

Sethi KK, Verma P: Chlamydial pneumonia and coronary heart disease (Editorial). *Cardiol Today* 2: 9, 1999.

Schrier RW *et al:* Haemodynamics in congestive heart failure. *N Engl J Med* 341: 577, 1999.

Schwartz SM *et al:* The intima: Soil for atherosclerosis and restenosis. *Circ Res* 77: 445, 1995.

Silver MD: *Cardiovascular Pathology,* 2nd ed. London, Churchill Livingstone, 1991.

Tegos TJ *et al:* The genesis of atherosclerosis and risk factors: a review. *Angiology* 52: 89, 2001.

Van de Werf: Cardiac troponins in acute coronary syndromes. *N Engl J Med* 335: 1338, 1996.

CHAPTER 13: THE HAEMATOPOIETIC SYSTEM

Bennet JM *et al:* Proposed revised criteria for classification of acute myeloid leukaemia—A report of French-American-British cooperative Group. *Ann Int Med* 103: 629, 1985.

Beutler *et al: William's Haematology,* 6th ed. New York, McGraw-Hill Publishing Company, 2001.

Beutler E, Luzzatto L: Hemolytic anaemia. *Semin Hematol* 36: 38, 1999.

Brenner MK, Hoffbrand AV: *Recent Advances in Haematology,* number 7. London, Churchill Livingstone, 1993.

Brenner MK, Hoffbrand AV: *Recent Advances in Haematology,* number 8. London, Churchill Livingstone, 1996.

Dacie JV, Lewis SM: *Practical Haematology,* 7th ed. London, Churchill Livingstone, 1991.

Firkin *et al: de Gruchy's Clinical Haematology in Medical Practice,* 5th ed. Bombay, Oxford University Press (Indian ed), 1994.

Greer JP *et al: Wintrobe's Clinical Haematology* (2 vols), 11th ed. Philadelphia, Lippincott Williams & Wilkins, 2004.

Harris NL *et al:* A revised European-American classification of lymphoid neoplasms: a proposal from the International Lymphoma Study Group. *Blood* 84: 1361, 1994.

Harris NL *et al:* World Health Organisation classification of neoplastic diseases of the haematopoietic and lymphoid tissues: report of the Clinical Advisory Committee, Airlie House, Virginia, Nov 1997. *J Clin Oncol* 17: 3835, 1999.

Hoffbrand AV, Brenner MK: *Recent Advances in Haematology,* number 6. London, Churchill Livingstone, 1992.

CHAPTER 14: THE LYMPHOID SYSTEM

Freedman AS, Nadler LM: Immunologic markers in non-Hodgkin's lymphoma. *Haematol Oncol Clin North Am* 5: 871, 1991.

Harris NL *et al:* A revised European-American classification of lymphoid neoplasms: a proposal from the International Lymphoma Study Group. *Blood* 84: 1361, 1994.

Harris NL *et al:* World Health Organisation classification of neoplastic diseases of the haematopoietic and lymphoid tissues: report of the Clinical Advisory Committee, Airlie House, Virginia, Nov 1997. *J Clin Oncol* 17: 3835, 1999.

Issacson PG, Norton AJ: *Extranodal Lymphomas.* Edinburgh, Churchill Livingstone, 1994.

Kuppers R *et al:* Cellular origin of human B-cell lymphomas. *N Engl J Med* 341: 1520, 1999.

Lauder 1: T-cell malignant lymphomas. In *Recent Advances in Histopathology,* number 15, Anthony PP *et al* (Eds). Philadelphia, Churchill Livingstone, pp 93, 1992.

Lieberman PH *et al:* Evaluation of malignant lymphomas using three classifications and the Working Formulations. *Am J Med* 81: 365, 1986.

Miller T, Grogan T: Lymphoma. *Hematology/Oncology Clin N Am,* Vol 11. Philadelphia: WB Saunders, 1997.

Shipp MA: Prognostic factors in aggressive non-Hodgkin's lymphoma: Who has high risk disease? *Blood* 83: 1165, 1994.

William CL *et al:* Langerhans' cell histiocytosis (histiocytosis X)—a clonal proliferative disease. *N Engl J Med* 331: 154, 1994.

CHAPTER 15: THE RESPIRATORY SYSTEM

Barnes PJ: Chronic obstructive pulmonary disease. *N Engl J Med* 343: 269, 2000.

Drobienwski FA *et al:* Tuberculosis and AIDS. *J Med Microbiol* 43: 85, 1995.

Evans MD, Pryor WA: Cigarette smoking, emphysema and damage to alpha-1-anti protease inhibitor. *Am J Physiol* 246: 493, 1994.

ICMR Bulletin: Silicosis–an uncommonly diagnosed common occupational disease, 29: 9, 1999.

Leslie KO, Colby TV: Pathology of lung cancer. *Curr Opin Pul Med* 3: 252, 1997.

Morsman B, Gee J: Asbestos-related diseases. *N Engl J Med* 320: 1721, 1989.

Murin S, Hilbert J, Reilly SJ: Cigarette smoke and the lung. *Clin Res Allergy Immunol* 15: 307, 1997.

Patel A *et al:* Paraneoplastic syndromes associated with lung cancer. *Mayo Clin Proc* 68: 278, 1993.

Sethi JM: Smoking and chronic pulmonary diseases. *Clin Chest Med* 21: 67, 2000.

Spencer H, Hasleton PS: *Spencer's Pathology of the Lung.* New York, Mc-Graw Hill, 1996.

WHO-Histological Typing of Lung Cancer. Geneva, WHO, 1999.

CHAPTER 16: THE EYE, ENT AND NECK

Neel HB III. Nasopharyngeal carcinoma. *Oncol* 6: 87, 1992.

Miller SJH: *Parson's Diseases of the Eye,* 18th ed. London, Churchill Livingstone, 1990.

Vokes EE *et al:* Head and neck cancer. *N Engl J Med* 328: 184, 1993.

WHO-Histological Typing of Upper Respiratory Tract Tumours, number 19. Geneva, WHO, 1978.

Yanoff M, Fine BS: *Ocular Pathology,* 4th ed. London, Mosby-Wolfe, 1996.

Zimmerman LE, Sobin LH: *WHO-Histological Typing of Tumours of the Eye and its Adnexa,* number 24. Geneva, WHO, 1980.

CHAPTER 17: THE ORAL CAVITY AND SALIVARY GLANDS

Crissmann JD, Zarbo RJ: Dysplasia, in situ carcinoma and progression to invasive carcinoma of the upper aerodigestive tract. *Am J Surg Pathol* 13: 5, 1989.

Forastiere A *et al:* Head and neck cancer. *N Engl J Med* 345: 1890, 2001.

Kapadia SB: Salivary gland tumours. In *Proceedings of III International CME & Update in Surgical Pathology,* Gupta RK (Ed). Lucknow, SGPGI, 1998.

Mac Donald DG, Browne RM: Tumours of odontogenic epithelium. In *Recent Advances in Histopathology,* number 17, Anthony PP *et al* (Eds). London, Churchill Livingstone, pp 139, 1997.

Seifert G: *WHO Histological Typing of Salivary Gland Tumours,* 2nd ed. Berlin, Springer-Verlag, 1991.

Shah JP, Ihde JK: Salivary Gland Tumours. *Curr Probl Surg* 27: 779, 1990.

Simpson RHW: Salivary gland tumours. In *Recent Advances in Histopathology,* number 17, Anthony PP *et al* (Eds). London, Churchill Livingstone, pp 167, 1997.

CHAPTER 18: THE GASTROINTESTINAL TRACT

Blaser MJ, Parsonnet J: The bacteria behind ulcers. *Sci Am* 274: 104, 1996.

Brandtzaeg P *et al:* Immunopathology of human inflammatory bowel disease. *Semin Immunopathol* 18: 555, 1997.

Fernhead NS *et al:* The ABC of APC. *Hum Mol Genet* 10: 721, 2001.

Fuchs CS, Mayor RJ: Gastric carcinoma. *N Engl J Med* 333: 32, 1995.

Haggitt RC: Barrett's oesophagus, dysplasia and adenocarcinoma. *Hum Pathol* 25: 982, 1994.

Jass JR, Sobin LH: *WHO Histological Typing of Intestinal Tumours,* 2nd ed. Berlin, Springer-Verlag, 1989.

MacGowan *et al: Helicobacter pylori* and gastric acid, biological and therapeutic implications. *Gastroenterology* 110: 926, 1996.

Morson DC *et al: Gastrointestinal Pathology,* 3rd ed. Oxford, Blackwell Scientific Publications, 1992.

Oota K, Sobin LH: *WHO-Histological Typing of Gastric and Oesophageal Tumours,* number 18. Geneva, WHO, 1977.

Papadakis KA, Targan SR: Current theories on the causation of inflammatory bowel disease. *Gastroenterol Clin* 28: 283, 1999.

Podolsky DK: Inflammatory bowel disease. *N Engl J Med* 325: 929, 1991.

Thomas RM, Sobin LH: Gastrointestinal cancer. *Cancer* 75: 154, 1995.

Whitehead R: *Gastrointestinal and Oesophageal Pathology,* 2nd ed. London, Churchill Livingstone, 1995.

CHAPTER 19: THE LIVER, BILIARY TRACT AND EXOCRINE PANCREAS

Bhandari BN, Wright TL: Hepatitis C: an overview. *Annu Rev Med* 46: 309, 1995.

Carey MC: Pathogenesis of gallstones. *Am J Surg* 165: 410, 1993.

Feitelson MA, Zern MA: Hepatitis and chronic liver disease. *Clin Lab Med* 16, 1996.

Ferrell L: Liver pathology: cirrhosis, hepatitis and primary liver tumours: an update and diagnostic problems. *Mod Pathol* 13: 679, 2000.

Ishak KG: Pathologic features of chronic hepatitis: a review and update. *Am J Clin Pathol* 113: 40, 2000.

Joshi VV: Indian childhood cirrhosis. *Perspec Pediatric Pathol* 11: 175, 1987.

Lauer GM, Walker BD: Hepatitis C virus infection. *N Engl J Med* 345: 41, 2001.

Ludwig J: *Practical Liver Biopsy Interpretation—Diagnostic Algorithms.* ASCP, Chicago, 1992.

Nayak NC *et al:* Obliterative portal venopathy. *Arch Pathol* 87: 359, 1969.

Scheuer PJ: *Liver Biopsy Interpretation,* 4th ed. London, Bailliere Tindall, 1988.

Sheila Sherlock: *Diseases of the Liver and Biliary System,* 10th ed. Oxford, Blackwell Scientific Publications, 1997.

Van Doorn LJ: Molecular biopsy of the hepatitis C virus. *J Med Virol* 43: 345, 1994.

Yu MW, Chen CJ: Hepatitis B and C viruses in the development of hepatocellular carcinoma. *Crit Rev Oncol Haematol* 17: 71, 1994.

CHAPTER 20: THE KIDNEY AND LOWER URINARY TRACT

Bostwick DG, Eble JN: *Urologic Surgical Pathology.* St Louis, Mosby, 1997.

Epstein JI *et al:* The WHO/ International Society of Urologic Pathologic consensus classification of urothelial (transitional cell) neoplasms of the urinary bladder. *Am J Surg Pathol* 22: 1435, 1998.

Freedman BI *et al:* The link between hypertension and nephrosclerosis. *Am J Kidney Dis* 25: 207, 1995.

Heptinstall RH: *Pathology of the Kidney* (3 vols). London, Little, Brown and Company, 1992.

Hrick DE *et al:* Glomerulonephritis. *N Engl J Med* 339: 888, 1998.

Joshi VV: Cystic lesions of the kidney. In *Proceedings of III International CME & Update in Surgical Pathology,* Gupta RK (Ed). Lucknow, SGPGI, 1998.

Lamm DL, Torti FM: Bladder cancer 1996. *CA* 46: 93, 1996.

Mostofi FK *et al. WHO-Histological Typing of Urinary Bladder Tumours,* number 10. Geneva, WHO, 1977.

Mostofi FK *et al: WHO-Histological Typing of Kidney Tumours,* number 25. Geneva, WHO, 1981.

Phillips JL *et al:* The genetic basis of renal epithelial tumours: advances in research and its impact on prognosis and therapy. *Curr Opin Urol* 11: 463, 2001.

Webb JN: Aspects of tumours of the urinary bladder and prostate gland. In *Recent Advances in Histopathology,* number 15, Anthony PP *et al* (Eds). Philadelphia, Churchill Livingstone, pp 157, 1992.

CHAPTER 21: THE MALE REPRODUCTIVE SYSTEM AND PROSTATE

Chevelle JC: Classification and pathology of testicular germ cell and sex cord stromal tumours. *Urol Clin Am* 26: 585, 1999.

Chitale A, Vadera V: *Pathology of Urinary and Male Genital System.* New Delhi, BI Churchill Livingstone, 1992.

Garnik MB, Fair WR: Prostate cancer: emerging concepts. Part I. *Ann Intern Med* 125: 118, 1996.

Gleason DF: Atypical hyperplasia, benign hyperplasia and well-differentiated adenocarcinoma of the prostate. *Am J Surg Pathol* 9: 53, 1985.

Grigor KM: Germ cell tumours of testis. In *Recent Advances in Histopathology,* number 15, Anthony PP *et al* (Eds). Philadelphia, Churchill Livingstone, pp 1277, 1992.

Mostofi FK *et al:* Pathology of carcinoma of the prostate. *Cancer* 70 (suppl 1): 235, 1992.

Mostofi FK *et al: WHO-Histological Typing of Prostate Tumours,* number 22. Geneva, WHO, 1980.

Mostofi FK, Sobin LH: *WHO-Histological Typing of Testis Tumours,* number 16. Geneva, WHO, 1977.

Stenman UH *et al:* Prostate specific antigen. *Semin Cancer Biol* 9: 83, 1999.

Ulbright TM: Germ cell neoplasms of the testis. *Am J Surg Pathol* 17: 1075, 1993.

CHAPTER 22: THE FEMALE GENITAL TRACT

Bethesda system for reporting cervical/vaginal cytological diagnosis. *Am J Surg Pathol* 16: 914, 1992.

Coppleson *et al: Gynaecologic Oncology* (2 vols), 2nd ed. London, Churchill Livingstone, 1992.

Hennandoz E, Atkinson BF: *Clinical Gynaecologic Pathology.* Philadelphia, WB Saunders, 1996.

Kosary C: FIGO stage, histology, histologic grade, age and race as prognostic factors in determining survival for cancers of the female gynaecological system. An analysis of 1973-87 SEER cases of cancers of the endometrium, cervix, ovary, vulva and vagina. *Semin Surg Oncol* 10: 31, 1994.

Kurman RJ: *Blaustein's Pathology of the Female Genital Tract,* 4th ed. New York, Springer-Verlag, 1994.

Lowe DG, Buckley CH, Fox H: Advances in gynaecologic pathology. In *Recent Advances in Histopathology,* number 17, Anthony PP *et al* (Eds). London, Churchill Livingstone, pp 113, 1997.

Mazur MT, Kurman RJ: *Diagnosis of Endometrial Biopsies and Curettings.* New York, Springer-Verlag, 1995.

Ostor AG: Natural history of cervical intraepithelial neoplasia, a critical review. *Int J Gynaecol Pathol* 12: 186, 1993.

Pernoll ML: *Current Obstetric and Gynaecologic Diagnosis and Treatment,* 7th ed. London, Prentice-Hall International, 1991.

Rollason TP: Aspects of ovarian pathology. In *Recent Advances in Histopathology,* number 15, Anthony PP *et al* (Eds). Philadelphia, Churchill Livingstone, pp 195, 1992.

Rose PG: Medical progress: endometrial carcinoma. *N Engl J Med* 335: 640, 1996.

Scully RE *et al: WHO-Histological Classification by Female Genital Tract Tumours,* 2nd ed. Berlin, Springer-Verlag, 1994.

Scully RE *et al:* Tumours of the ovary, maldeveloped gonads, fallopian tube and broad ligament. *Atlas of Tumour Pathology,* 3rd ed. AFIP fscicle 23, Washington, 1998.

CHAPTER 23: THE BREAST

Anderson TJ, Page DL: Risk assessment in breast cancer. In *Recent Advances in Histopathology,* number 17, Anthony PP *et al* (Eds). London, Churchill Livingstone, pp 69, 1997.

Arver B *et al:* Hereditary breast cancer: a review. *Semin Cancer Biol* 10: 271, 2000.

Azzopardi *et al: Problems in Breast Pathology.* Philadelphia, WB Saunders Company, 1979.

Haagensen CD: *Diseases of the Breast,* 3rd ed. Philadelphia, WB Saunders Company, 1996.

Harris JR *et al:* Breast cancer. *N Engl J Med* 327: 319 (also 390 and 473), 1992.

Skolinick AA: New data suggest needle biopsies could replace surgical biopsies for diagnosing breast cancer. *JAMA* 271: 1724, 1994.

Tavassoli FA: *Pathology of the Breast.* Edinburgh, Churchill Livingstone, 1992.

Trojani M: *A Colour Atlas of Breast Histopathology.* London, Chapman and Hall Medical, 1991.

WHO-Histological Typing of Breast Tumours, 2nd ed, number 2. Geneva, WHO, 1981.

CHAPTER 24: THE SKIN

Elder D *et al: Lever's Histopathology of the Skin,* 8th ed. Philadelphia, Lippincott-Raven, 1997.

McKee PH: *Pathology of the Skin with Clinical Correlations,* 2nd ed. London, Mosby-Wolfe, 1996.

Mihm MC: The clinical diagnosis, classification and histogenetic concepts of the early stages of cutaneous malignant melanomas. *N Engl J Med* 284: 1078, 1971.

Rabinowitz LO, Zaim M: A clinicopathologic approach to granulomatous dermatoses. *J Am Acad Dermatol* 35: 588, 1996.

Seldan REJ *et al: WHO-Histological Typing of Skin Tumours,* number 12. Geneva, WHO, 1974.

Shelton RM: Skin cancer: a review and atlas for medical providers. *Mt Sinai J Med* 68: 243, 2001.

CHAPTER 25: THE ENDOCRINE SYSTEM

Atkintson MA, Maclaren NK: The pathogenesis of insulin-dependent diabetes mellitus. *N Engl J Med* 331: 1428, 1994.

Atkinson MA, Eisenbarth GS: Type I diabetes: new perspectives on disease pathogenesis and treatment. *Lancet* 358: 221, 2001.

Dayan CM, Daniel GH: Chronic autoimmune thyroiditis. *N Engl J Med* 335: 99, 1996.

Kovacs K, Horvath E: Pathology of pituitary tumours. *Endocrinol Metab Clin North Am* 16: 529, 1987.

Livolsi VA: Papillary neoplasms of the thyroid: pathologic and prognostic features. *Am J Clin Pathol* 97: 426, 1992.

Ostenson CG: The pathophysiology of type 2 diabetes mellitus: an overview. *Acta Physiol Scand* 171: 241, 2001.

Phay JE *et al:* Multiple endocrine neoplasia. *Semin Surg Oncol* 18: 324, 2000.

Porte D Jr, Kahn SE: Beta cell dysfunction and failure in type 2 diabetes: potential mechanisms. *Diabetes* 50 (suppl 1): S-160, 2001.

WHO-Histological Typing of Thyroid Tumours, number 11. Geneva, WHO, 1979.

Williams ED *et al: WHO-Histological Typing of Endocrine Tumours,* number 23. Geneva, WHO, 1980.

CHAPTER 26: THE MUSCULOSKELETAL SYSTEM

Gallacher SJ: Paget's disease of bone. *Curr Opin Rheumatol* 5: 351, 1993.

Kretschmar CS: Ewing's sarcoma and the peanut tumours. *N Engl J Med* 331: 294, 1994.

Lipsky PE, Davis LS: The central involvement of T cells in rheumatoid arthritis. *Immunologist* 6: 121, 1998.

Marcove RC, Arlen M: *Atlas of Bone Pathology with Clinical and Radiographic Correlations.* Philadelphia, JB Lippincott Company, 1992

Schajowicz F *et al: WHO Histological Typing of Bone Tumours,* 2nd ed. Berlin, Springer-Verlag, 1993.

Smith NM, Keeling JW: Paediatric solid tumours. In *Recent Advances in Histopathology,* number 17, Anthony PP *et al* (Eds). London, Churchill Livingstone, pp 191, 1997.

Snaith ML: ABC of rheumatology: gout, hyperuricaemia, and crystal arthritis. *BMJ* 310: 521, 1995.

Unni KK: *Dahlin's Bone Tumours,* 5th ed. Philadelphia, Lippincott-Raven, 1996.

CHAPTER 27: SOFT TISSUE TUMOURS

Ashley DJB: *Evan's Histological Appearance of Tumours,* 4th ed. London, Churchill Livingstone, 1996.

Fletcher CDM: Soft tissue tumours—an update. In *Recent advances in Histopathology,* number 15, Anthony PP *et al* (Eds). London, Churchill Livingstone, pp 113, 1992.

Leyvraz S *et al:* Histological diagnosis and grading of soft tissue sarcomas. *Semin Surg Oncol* 4: 3, 1988.

Weiss SW, Goldblum JR: *Enzinger and Weiss's Soft Tissue Tumours,* 4th ed. St Louis, Mosby, 2001.

CHAPTER 28: THE NERVOUS SYSTEM

Burger PC, Scheithauer BW: *Atlas of Tumors of the Central Nervous System.* Washington DC, AFIP. 1994.

Forn LS: Neuropathology of Parkinson's disease. *J Neuropathol Exp Neurol,* 55: 259, 1996.

Graham DI, Lantos PL (Eds): *Grrenfield's Neuropathology,* 6th ed. London, Arnold, 1997.

Kleinues P *et al: WHO Classification of Tumours: Pathology and Genetics of Tumours of the Nervous System.* Lyon IARC Press, 2000.

LevyLahad E, Bird TD: Genetic factors in Alzheimer's disease: a review of recent advances. *Ann Neurol* 40: 829, 1996.

Mastrianni JA, Roos RP: The prion diseases. *Semin Neurol* 20: 337, 2000.

Price RW: Neurological complications of HIV infection. *Lancet* 348: 445, 1996.

Prusiner SB: Human prion disease and neurodegeneration. *Current Topics Microbiol Immunol* 207: 1, 1996.

Prusiner SB: The prion diseases. *Sci Am* 272: 48, 1995.

Will R *et al:* A new variant of Creutzfeldt-Jakob disease in the UK. *Lancet* 347: 921, 1996.

Wilterdink JL, Easton JD: Vascular event rates in patients with atherosclerotic cerebrovascular disease. *Arch Neurol* 49: 857, 1992.

CHAPTER 29: DIAGNOSTIC CYTOPATHOLOGY

Astarita RW: *Practical Cytopathology.* New York, Churchill Livingstone, 1990.

Atkinson BF: *Atlas of Diagnostic Cytopathology.* Philadelphia, WB Saunders Company, 1992.

Bibbo M: *Comprehensive Cytopathology,* 2nd ed. Philadelphia, WB Saunders, 1997.

Erozan YS, Bonfiglio TA: *Fine Needle Aspiration of Subcutaneous Organs and Masses.* Philadelphia, Lippincott-Raven, 1996.

Gray W: *Diagnostic Cytopathology,* Edinburgh, Churchill Livingstone, 1995.

Grubb C: *Diagnostic Cytopathology—A Text and Colour Atlas.* London, Churchill Livingstone, 1988.

Koss LG: *Diagnostic Cytology and the Histopathological Basis* (2 vols), 4th ed. Philadelphia, Lippincott Company, 1994.

Naib ZM: *Cytopathology,* 4th ed. Boston, Little, Brown and Company, 1996.

Orell SR *et al: Manual and Atlas of Fine Needle Aspiration Cytology,* 3rd ed. Edinburgh, Churchill Livingstone, 1999.

APPENDIX : NORMAL VALUES

Anderson WAD, Kissane JM: *Pathology,* 9th ed. St Louis, The CV Mosby Company, 1977.

Boyd, William: *Pathology—Structure and Function in Diseases,* 8th ed. Philadelphia, Lea & Febiger, 1970.

Braunwald E *et al: Harrison's Principles of Internal Medicine* (2 vols), 15th ed. New York, McGraw-Hill Health Profession Division, 2001.

Dacie JV, Lewis SM: *Practical Haematology,* 7th ed. London, Churchill Livingstone, 1991.

Gilbert-Barness E: *Potter's Pathology of the Fetus and Infant* (2 vols). St Louis, Mosby, 1997.

Gowenlock AH: McLauchian DM: *Varley's Practical Clinical Biochemistry,* 6th ed. Oxford, Heinmann Professional Publishing Company, 1988.

Greer JP *et al: Wintrobe's Clinical Haematology* (2 vols), 11th ed. Philadelphia, Lippincott Williams & Wilkins, 2004.

Henry JB: *Clinical Diagnosis and Management by Laboratory Methods,* 20th ed. New Delhi, Harcourt (India) Private Limited, 2001.

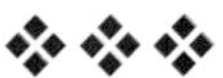

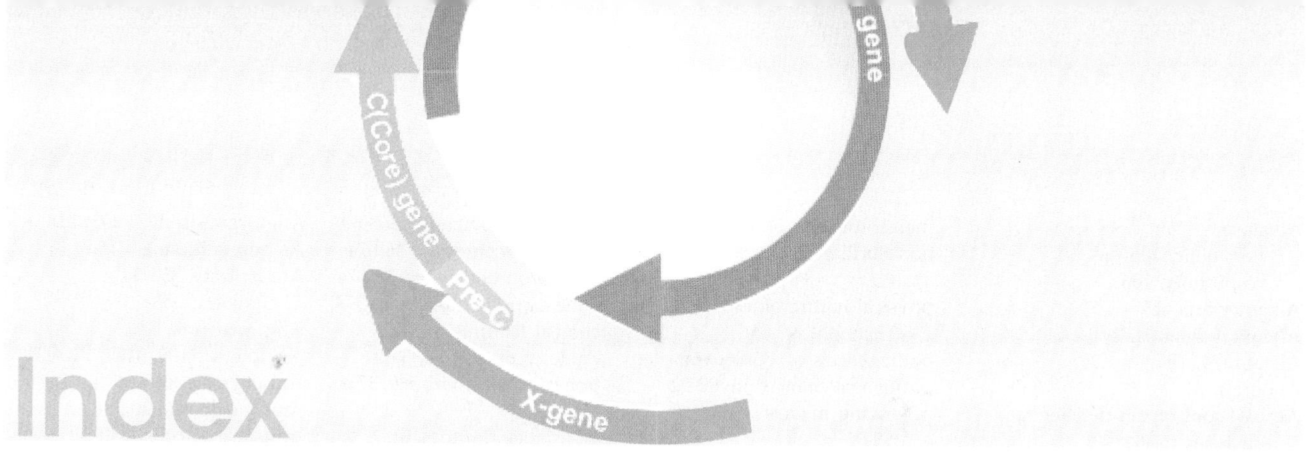

Index

*The letter **t** after page number in the index below denotes Table and the letter **f** stands for Figure on that page.*

A

Index

Index

D

Index

E

F

G

H

Index

Index

N

Index

Index

Q

R

S

READER SUGGESTIONS SHEET

Please help us to improve the quality of our publications by completing and returning this sheet to us.

Title/Author: **Textbook of Pathology** *by* **Dr Harsh Mohan**

Your name and address:

Phone and Fax:

e-mail address:

How did you hear about this book? [please tick appropriate box (es)]

- ☐ Direct mail from publisher
- ☐ Conference
- ☐ Bookshop
- ☐ Book review
- ☐ Lecturer recommendation
- ☐ Friends
- ☐ Other (please specify)
- ☐ Website

Type of purchase: ☐ Direct purchase ☐ Bookshop ☐ Friends

Do you have any brief comments on the book?

Please return this sheet to the name and address given below.

JAYPEE BROTHERS

MEDICAL PUBLISHERS (P) LTD

EMCA House, 23/23B Ansari Road, Daryaganj

New Delhi 110 002, India